DISEASES AND ICD-9CM CODES *(Continued)*

Gynecomastia 611.1
Head Trauma 854
Headache 784.0
Hearing Loss 389.9
Heart Failure 428.9
Hemangioma 228.00
Hemolytic Uremic Syndrome 283.11
Hemophilia 286.0
Hemoptysis 786.3
Hemorrhagic Disease 287.9
Hepatitis 573.3
Hepatosplenomegaly 571.8
Hereditary Elliptocytosis 282.1
Hereditary Spherocytosis 282.0
Herpes Simplex Virus Infections 054.9
Hip Dysplasia 755.63
Hirschsprung Disease 751.3
Hirsutism 704.1
Hodgkin Disease 201.9
Human Immunodeficiency Virus Infection 042
Hydrocephalus 331.4
Hypercalciuria 275.4
Hyernatremic Dehydration 276.0
Hyperparathyroidism 252.0
Hypertension 401
Hyperthyroidism 242.9
Hypocalcemia 275.4
Hypoglycemia 251.2
Hypogonadotropic Hypogonadism 253.4
Hypoparathyroidism 252.1
Hypopituitarism 253.2
Hypoplastic Anemias 284.9
Hypoplastic Left Heart Syndrome 746.7
Hypospadias 752.61
Hypothyroidism, Acquired 244.9
Hypothyroidism, Congenital 243
Immunodeficiency Disorders 279.3
Increased Intracranial Pressure 348.2
Inflammatory Bowel Disease 558.9
Insulin-Dependent Diabetes Mellitus 250.00
Iron Deficiency Anemia 280.9
Jaundice 782.4
Juvenile Arthritis 714.30
Juvenile Dermatomyositis 710.3
Kawasaki Syndrome 446.1
Kyphosis 737.10
Learning Disabilities 315.2
Legg-Calvé-Perthes Disease 732.1
Lethargy 780.7
Lipid Metabolism Disorders 272.9
Liver Failure 572.8
Liver Tumors 155.2
Low Birth Weight 765.0
Lower Respiratory Infections 519.8
Lymphadenopathy 785.6

Marfan Syndrome 759.82
Mastocytosis 757.33
Mastoiditis 383.9
McCune-Albright Syndrome 756.59
Meconium Aspiration 770.1
Megaloblastic Anemia 281.9
Melanoma 172.9
Meningitis 322.9
Menstrual Disorders 626.9
Mental Retardation 319
Microangiopathic Hemolytic Anemia 283.19
Microcephaly 742.1
Microcytic Anemias 280.9
Micropenis (Hypogenitalism) 752.64
Migraine Syndromes 346.0
Mitral Valve Prolapse 424.0
Movement Disorders 333.90
Multisystem Trauma 359.1
Mumps 072.9
Muscular Dystrophies 359.1
Mycobacteria, Atypical 031.9
Myelogenous Leukemia, Chronic 205.1
Myocarditis 429.0
Nasolacrimal Duct Obstruction 375.56
Neck Mass 784.2
Neglect 995.52
Nephrotic Syndrome 581.9
Neuroblastoma 194.0 (M9500/3)
Neurofibromatosis 237.70
Neutropenia 288.0
Neutrophilic Leukocytosis (Neutrophilia) 288.8
Non-Hodgkin Lymphoma 202.8
Nystagmus 379.50
Obesity 278.00
Orbital Cellulitis 376.01
Osgoode-Schlatter Disease 732.4
Osteomyelitis 730.2
Osteosarcoma 170.9
Otitis Externa (Swimmer's Ear) 380.10
Otitis Media 382.9
Painful Knee 719.46
Pallor 782.61
Parasitic Infections 136.9
Patent Ductus Arteriosus 747.0
Pectus Excavatum 754.81
Peptic Ulcer Disease 533.9
Pericarditis 423.9
Pharyngitis 462
Physical Abuse 995.54
Pigmented Skin Lesions 709.00
Pityriasis Rosea 696.3
Platelet Disorders (Thrombocytopenia) 287.1
Plethora 782.62
Pleural Effusions 511.9
Pneumonia 486

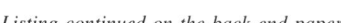

D0911488

Listing continued on the back end paper

Saunders
Manual
of Pediatric
Practice

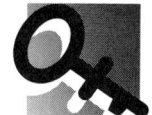

Saunders Manual of Pediatric Practice

LAURENCE FINBERG, M.D.

Professor and Chairman Emeritus of Pediatrics
State University of New York at Brooklyn
Brooklyn, New York
Clinical Professor of Pediatrics
University of California, San Francisco
San Francisco, California
Clinical Professor of Pediatrics
Stanford University School of Medicine
Stanford, California

Joann Quane-Finberg, Managing Editor

W.B. SAUNDERS COMPANY
A Division of Harcourt Brace & Company
Philadelphia   London   Toronto   Montreal   Sydney   Tokyo

W.B. SAUNDERS COMPANY
A Division of Harcourt Brace & Company

The Curtis Center
Independence Square West
Philadelphia, Pennsylvania 19106

Library of Congress Cataloging-in-Publication Data

Saunders manual of pediatric practice / [edited by] Laurence Finberg.

p.   cm.

ISBN 0–7216–6537–3

1. Pediatrics—Handbooks, manuals, etc.   I. Finberg, Laurence.
   [DNLM: 1. Pediatrics.   WS 100 S257 1998]

RJ48.S34   1998   618.92—dc21

DNLM/DLC   97-5188

SAUNDERS MANUAL OF PEDIATRIC PRACTICE   ISBN 0–7216–6537–3

Last digit is the print number: 9   8   7   6   5   4   3   2   1

To all the residents with whom I have worked over many years, as we learned together.

With a special acknowledgment to an outstanding, achieving group of young men and women who served as Chief Residents.

Section Editors

Preventive Pediatrics
Laurence Finberg, M.D.
*Clinical Professor of Pediatrics
Departments of Pediatrics*
University of California, San Francisco;
Stanford University,
Stanford, California

Ethical Issues in Pediatrics
Alan R. Fleischman, M.D.
*Senior Vice President, The New York Academy of Medicine;
Clinical Professor of Pediatrics and Clinical Professor of
Epidemiology and Social Medicine*
Albert Einstein College of Medicine
The Bronx, New York

Nutrition
Laurence Finberg, M.D.
Clinical Professor of Pediatrics
University of California, San Francisco,
School of Medicine
San Francisco, California

Neonatology
Leonard Glass, M.D.
*Professor and Interim Chairman; Director, Division of
Neonatology, State University of New York*
Health Science Center at Brooklyn
Brooklyn, New York

Adolescent Medicine
S. Kenneth Schonberg, M.D.
*Professor of Pediatrics, Albert Einstein College of
Medicine; Director, Division of Adolescent Medicine*
Montefiore Medical Center
The Bronx, New York

Behavior/Psychology
Michael S. Jellinek, M.D.
*Professor of Psychiatry and of Pediatrics, Harvard Medical
School; Chief, Child Psychiatry Service*
Massachusetts General Hospital
Boston, Massachusetts

Genetics/Metabolism
Marc Yudkoff, M.D.
*Professor of Pediatrics, University of Pennsylvania School
of Medicine; Associate Chief, Division of Child
Development*
Children's Hospital of Philadelphia and Children's Seashore
House
Philadelphia, Pennsylvania

Immunology/Allergy and Rheumatic Disease
Mark Ballow, M.D.
*Professor, Department of Pediatrics, State University of
New York at Buffalo, School of Medicine and Biomedical
Sciences, Buffalo, New York; Chief, Division of Allergy/
Immunology and Pediatric Rheumatology*
The Children's Hospital of Buffalo
Buffalo, New York

Infectious Disease
Robert Finberg, M.D.
*Professor of Medicine, Harvard School of Medicine;
Head of Infectious Disease Services*
Dana-Farber Cancer Hospital
Boston, Massachusetts

Hematology/Oncology
Sreedhar P. Rao, M.D.
*Professor of Clinical Pediatrics; Director, Pediatric
Hematology/Oncology, State University of New York*
Health Science Center at Brooklyn,
Brooklyn, New York

Paul A. Meyers, M.D.
*Associate Professor of Clinical Pediatrics, Cornell
University Medical College; Associate Attending
Pediatrician*
Memorial Sloan-Kettering Cancer Center
New York, New York

Gastroenterology
Ronald Kleinman, M.D.
Associate Professor of Pediatrics, Harvard Medical School;
Chief, Pediatric Gastroenterology and Nutrition;
Associate Chief of Pediatrics
Massachusetts General Hospital
Boston, Massachusetts

Cardiology
Ronald M. Lauer, M.D.
Professor of Pediatrics and Preventive Medicine,
Division of Pediatric Cardiology
University of Iowa School of Medicine
Iowa City, Iowa

Respiratory Disorders
Howard Eigen, M.D.
Professor of Pediatrics; Associate Chairman for Clinical
Affairs; Director, Section of Pulmonology and Critical Care
Indiana University School of Medicine
Indianapolis, Indiana

Nephrology/Urology
Stanley Hellerstein, M.D.
Professor of Pediatrics, University of Missouri School of
Medicine; Pediatric Nephrologist
The Children's Mercy Hospital
Kansas City, Missouri

Endocrinology
Paul H. Saenger, M.D.
Professor of Pediatrics; Head, Division of Pediatric
Endocrinology
Albert Einstein College of Medicine and
Montefiore Medical Center
The Bronx, New York

Neurology
Gerald S. Golden, M.D.
Adjunct Professor of Neurology
University of Pennsylvania School of Medicine
Philadelphia, Pennsylvania

Dermatology
Lawrence A. Schachner, M.D.
Professor, Department of Dermatology; Professor,
Department of Pediatrics
University of Miami School of Medicine
Miami, Florida

Medical Ophthalmology
Constance E. West, M.D.
Pediatric Ophthalmologist, Children's Hospital Medical
Center and Cincinnati Eye Institute
Cincinnati, Ohio

Medical Ear/Nose/Throat
Robert J. Ruben
Professor of Pediatrics
Albert Einstein College of Medicine; Professor and
Chairman, Department of Otolaryngology
Montefiore Medical Center, The Bronx, New York

Medical Orthopedics
Paul G. Dyment, M.D.
Professor of Pediatrics, Vice Chancellor for
Academic Affairs
Tulane University School of Medicine
New Orleans, Louisiana

Emergency Pediatrics
Binita R. Shah, M.D.
Professor of Clinical Pediatrics, Children's Medical Center
of Brooklyn, State University of New York Health Science
Center at Brooklyn; Director, Pediatric Emergency
Medicine
Kings County Hospital Center
Brooklyn, New York

Poisonings and Environmental Hazards
Laurence Finberg, M.D.
Clinical Professor of Pediatrics
University of California, San Francisco,
School of Medicine
San Francisco, California

Contributors

David Abramson, M.D., F.A.C.S.
Clinical Professor of Opthalmology, Cornell University Medical College, New York Hospital, New York, New York
Retinoblastoma

Stephen Ajl, M.D.
Clinical Associate Professor of Pediatrics, State University of New York Health Science Center at Brooklyn, College of Medicine, Brooklyn, New York
The Normal Newborn Infant

Assunta Albanese, M.Phil., M.D., M.R.C.P.
Honorary Research Fellow, The Institute of Child Health and Great Ormond Street Hospital for Children; Specialist Registrar in Paediatrics, Hammersmith Hospital, London, England
Constitional Delay of Growth and Puberty

Elizabeth M. Alderman, M.D.
Assistant Professor of Pediatrics, Albert Einstein College of Medicine; Assistant Attending, Director of Adolescent Ambulatory Services, Montefiore Hospital, The Bronx, New York
Contraception

Uri S. Alon, M.D.
Professor of Pediatrics, University of Missouri at Kansas City School of Medicine; Pediatric Nephrologist, The Children's Mercy Hospital, Kansas City, Missouri
Renal Tubular Acidosis; Fanconi Syndrome; Bartter Syndrome; Hypercalciuria and Urinary Tract Stone Disease; Acute Renal Failure; Hypertensive Crisis; Urinalysis

Jack Andrish, M.D.
Staff Surgeon, Department of Orthopaedic Surgery; Member, Section of Pediatric Orthopaedics; Section of Sports Medicine, Cleveland Clinic Foundation, Cleveland, Ohio
Limp; Painful Knee

Richard Antaya, M.D.
Chief Resident of Dermatology, Duke University Medical Center, Durham, North Carolina
Alopecias; Acne; Damaging Effects of Solar Radiation

Roberta T. Arceci, M.D., Ph.D.
Jacob G. Schmidlapp Professor of Pediatrics, University of Cincinnati College of Medicine; Director, Hematology/Oncology, Children's Hospital Medical Center, Cincinnati, Ohio
Acute Myeloid Leukemia

Dianne L. Atkins, M.D.
Associate Professor, Department of Pediatrics, University of Iowa College of Medicine, Iowa City, Iowa
Tachyarrhythmia; Bradyarrhythmia; Defibrillation

Mark Ballow, M.D.
Professor, Department of Pediatrics, State University of New York at Buffalo, School of Medicine and Biomedical Sciences; Chief, Division of Allergy/Immunology and Pediatric Rheumatology, The Children's Hospital of Buffalo, Buffalo, New York
Host Defense Systems; Disorders of the Complement System; Disorders of the Phagocytic System; Disorders of the B-Cell Immune System; Disorders of the T-Cell Immune System

Phillipe Bareille, M.D.
Research Fellow in Endocrinology, Institute of Child Health, Research Fellow in Endocrinology, The Middlesex Hospital, London, England
Constitutional Short Stature; Familial Short Stature

Tamar Barlam, M.D.
Instructor in Medicine, Harvard Medical School; Senior Associate in Medicine, Department of Infectious Diseases; Beth Israel Deaconess Medical Center, Boston, Massachusetts
Sexually Transmitted Diseases

Lewis A. Barness, M.D.
Professor of Pediatrics, University of South Florida College of Medicine, Tampa, Florida
Sudden Infant Death

Sharon R. Beier, M.D.
Postdoctoral Fellow in Adolescent Medicine, Albert Einstein School of Medicine; Montefiore Medical Center, The Bronx, New York
Eating Disorders

Jennifer Bell, M.D.
Associate Professor of Clinical Pediatrics, Columbia University College of Physicians and Surgeons; Associate Attending Pediatrician, Presbyterian Hospital, New York, New York
Tall Stature

Jacques Benaim, M.D.
Division of Adolescent Medicine, Montefiore Medical Center, The Bronx, New York
Suicide

Aurora J. Bennett, M.D.
Assistant Professor of Psychiatry, University of Cincinnati College of Medicine; Director of Child Psychiatry, Consultation Liaison Service, Children's Hospital Medical Center, Cincinnati, Ohio
A Developmental Understanding of Chronic Illness

James T. Bennett, M.D.
Professor and Chief of Pediatric Orthopaedics, Tulane University School of Medicine, New Orleans, Louisiana
Dysplasia of the Hip; Scoliosis and Kyphosis

D. Woodrow Benson, Jr., M.D., Ph.D.
Professor of Pediatrics, Northwestern University Medical School, Chicago, Illinois
The Electrocardiogram: Preliminary Interpretation

Eugene V. Beresin, M.A., M.D.
Assistant Professor of Psychiatry, Harvard Medical School; Director of Child and Adolescent Psychiatry Residency Training, Massachusetts General Hospital, Boston; McLean Hospital, Belmont, Massachusetts
Difficult Families

Jeffrey Bergelson, M.D.
Assistant Professor of Pediatrics, University of Pennsylvania School of Medicine; Division of Infectious Diseases, The Children's Hospital of Philadelphia, Philadelphia, Pennsylvania
Meningitis; Encephalitis; Brain Abscess; Endocarditis; Myocarditis; Pericarditis; Upper Respiratory Infections; Lower Respiratory Infections

Joseph Biederman, M.D.
Professor, Harvard Medical School; Chief of the Joint Program in Pediatric Psychopharmacology, Massachusetts General Hospital, Boston, Massachusetts Upper Respiratory Infections; Lower Respiratory Infections
Attention-Deficit/Hyperactivity Disorder

Harvey P. Bieler, M.D.
Lecturer in Pediatrics, Section of Pulmonology and Critical Care Medicine, Indiana University School of Medicine; Attending Pediatric Pulmonologist and ICU Staff Physician, James Whitcomb Riley Hospital for Children, Indianapolis, Indiana
Hemoptysis; Pleural Effusions; Congenital Malformations

Douglas L. Blowey, M.D.
Assistant Professor of Pediatrics and Pharmacology, University of Missouri—Kansas City; The Children's Mercy Hospital, Kansas City, Missouri
Isolated Hematuria; Acute Glomerulonephritis; Polycystic Kidney Disease; End-Stage Renal Disease

Farid Boulad, M.D.
Assistant Professor, Cornell University Medical College; Clinical Assistant Attending, Bone Marrow Transplant Service, Department of Pediatrics, Memorial Sloan-Kettering Cancer Center, New York, New York
Chronic Myelaginous Leukemia

Rosalind Brown, M.D., C.M.
Associate Professor of Pediatrics, University of Massachusetts Medical School; Director, Division of Pediatric Endocrinology/Diabetes, University of Massachusetts Medical Center, Worcester, Massachusetts
Maternal Antibody–Induced Neonatal Thyroid Dysfunction

John C. Bucuvalas, M.D.
Associate Professor, Pediatric Gastroenterology and Nutrition, University of Cincinnati College of Medicine; Attending Physician, Associate Medical Director of Liver Transplantation, Children's Hospital Medical Center, Cincinnati, Ohio
Biliary Atresia; Viral Hepatitis; End-Stage Liver Disease and Cirrhosis

Sandra K. Burchett, M.D.
Assistant Professor of Pediatrics, Harvard Medical School; Division of Infectious Diseases, Children's Hospital, Boston, Massachusetts
Congenital Infections

Miles J. Burke, M.D.
Associate Professor of Ophthalmology, University of Cincinnati College of Medicine; Director, Department of Pediatric Ophthalmology, Children's Hospital Medical Center, Cincinnati, Ohio
Strabismus

Penina Burnstein, M.D.
Clinical Assistant Professor of Dermatology, State University of New York Health Science Center at Brooklyn College of Medicine; Attending, Pediatric Dermatology Clinic, Kings County Hospital Center, Brooklyn, New York
Genodermatoses

James Bussel, M.D.
Associate Professor of Pediatrics and Pediatric Hematology/Oncology, New York Hospital–Cornell University Medical Center, New York, New York
The Child with a Bleeding Tendency; Hemophilia; Platelet Disorders (Thrombocytopenia); Thrombophilia

Cecilia C. Capriles, M.D.
Fellow in Pediatric Endocrinology, Harvard Medical School; Massachusetts General Hospital, Boston, Massachusetts
Insulin-Dependent Diabetes Mellitus

Marc S. C. Cheah, M.D.*
Associate Professor, Children's Medical Center of Brooklyn, State University of New York Health Science Center at Brooklyn, Brooklyn, New York
Neutrophilic Leukocytosis (Neutrophilia); Polycythemia; Childhood Neutropenia

Nai-Kong V. Cheung, M.D., Ph.D.
Associate Professor, Cornell Medical College; Associate Member and Attending, Memorial Sloan-Kettering Cancer Center; New York, New York
Neuroblastoma

---

*Deceased.

George P. Chrousos, M.D.
Clinical Professor of Pediatrics and Physiology, Georgetown University Medical Center, Washington, D.C.; Chief, Section on Pediatric Endocrinology; Director, Pediatric Endocrinology Training Program, National Institute of Child Health and Human Development, National Institutes of Health, Bethesda, Maryland
Cushing Syndrome and Cushing Disease

Andrew Clark, M.D.
Instructor in Psychiatry, Harvard Medical School; Clinical Associate in Psychiatry, Massachusetts General Hospital, Boston, Massachusetts
Posttraumatic Stress Disorder

Michael E. Cohen, M.D.
Professor of Neurology and Pediatrics; Chairman, Department of Neurology, State University of New York at Buffalo, Buffalo, New York
Brain Tumors

Meryl S. Cohen, M.D.
Clinical Assistant in Pediatrics, The Children's Hospital of Philadelphia; University of Pennsylvania School of Medicine; Assistant Cardiologist, The Children's Hospital of Philadelphia, Philadelphia, Pennsylvania
Hypoplastic Left Heart Syndrome

David L. Coulter, M.D.
Associate Professor of Pediatrics and Neurology, Director of Pediatric Neurology, Boston University School of Medicine; Director of Pediatric Neurology, Boston Medical Center, Boston, Massachusetts
Cerebrovascular Disorders; Head Trauma; Coma; Increased Intracranial Pressure

Susan M. Coupey, M.D.
Professor of Pediatrics, Albert Einstein College of Medicine; Associate Director, Division of Adolescent Medicine, Department of Pediatrics, Montefiore Medical Center, The Bronx, New York
Eating Disorders

Finella Craig, M.B., M.R.C.P.
Research Fellow in Endocrinology/Oncology, Great Ormond Street Hospital for Children, London, England
Familial Short Stature

Susan Davis, M.D., Ph.D.
Senior Lecturer, Monash University; Director of Research, The Jean Hailes Foundation, Melbourne, Victoria, Australia
Menstrual Disorders; Premature Ovarian Failure

Joan DiMartino-Nardi, M.D.
Associate Professor, Albert Einstein College of Medicine; Associate Director, Division of Pediatric Endocrinology, Montefiore Medical Center, The Bronx, New York
Onset of Puberty

Theresa L. Dise, M.D.
Assistant Professor of Pediatrics, Tulane University School of Medicine, New Orleans, Louisiana
Flatfeet and Tibial Torsion

Sean P. Donahue, M.D., Ph.D.
Assistant Professor of Ophthalmology, Neurology, and Pediatrics, Vanderbilt University Medical Center, Nashville, Tennessee
Conjunctivitis; Orbital and Preseptal Cellulitis

David J. Driscoll, M.D.
Professor of Pediatrics; Head, Section of Pediatric Cardiology, Mayo Medical School and Mayo Clinic, Rochester, Minnesota
Tetralogy of Fallot

Patricia K. Duffner, M.D.
Professor of Neurology and Pediatrics, State University of New York at Buffalo School of Medicine; Attending, Children's Hospital of Buffalo; Associate Director, Child Neurology, Children's Hospital of Buffalo, Buffalo, New York
Brain Tumors

Ira J. Dunkel, M.D.
Instructor, Department of Pediatrics, Cornell University Medical College; Assistant Attending, New York Hospital, Memorial Sloan-Kettering Cancer Center, New York, New York
Brain Tumors

Paul G. Dyment, M.D.
Professor of Pediatrics and Vice Chancellor for Academic Affairs, Tulane University School of Medicine, New Orleans, Louisiana
Osgood-Schlatter Disease and Other Apophysitides

Robert M. Ehrlich, M.D., F.R.C.P.(C.)
Professor Emeritus, Department of Pediatrics, University of Toronto, Faculty of Medicine; Senior Staff Physician, Division of Endocrinology, Hospital for Sick Children, Toronto, Canada
Congenital Hypothyroidism; Acquired Hypothyroidism; Hyperthyroidism

Howard Eigen, M.D.
Professor of Pediatrics; Associate Chairman for Clinical Affairs; Director, Section of Pulmonology and Critical Care, Indiana University School of Medicine; Indianapolis, Indiana
Stridor; Bronchiolitis; Pulmonary Hemosiderosis; Respiratory Failure; Blood Gas Analysis; Thoracentesis

Leon Eisenberg, M.D.
Maude and Lillian Presley Professor of Social Medicine and Professor of Psychiatry Emeritus, Harvard Medical School; Honorary Psychiatrist, Massachusetts General Hospital, Boston, Massachusetts
Cognitive Development

Gerald Erenberg, M.D.
Director, Learning Assessment Clinic, Cleveland Clinic Foundation, Cleveland, Ohio
Movement Disorders; Migraine Syndromes; Sleep Disorders

Robert H. Feldt, M.D., M.S.
Professor of Pediatrics, Mayo Medical School, Rochester, Minnesota
Atrioventricular Canal Defects

Laurence Finberg, M.D.
Clinical Professor of Pediatrics, University of California, San Francisco, School of Medicine, San Francisco, California
Feeding Guidelines; Growth and Development; Anticipatory Guidance; Concepts and Diet Analysis; Deficiencies and Excesses of Food Components; Nutritional Rickets; Fluid and Electrolytes; Treatment and Prevention of Dehydration; Acute Severe Dehydration; Hypernatremic Dehydration; Measurement of Body Fat–Triceps Skinfold; Total Parenteral Nutrition (TPN); Clinically Important Trisomies; Metabolic Bone Disorders; Congenital Syphilis; Poliomyelitis; Poisonings and Environmental Hazards

Robert Finberg, M.D.
Professor of Medicine, Harvard Medical School; Chief of Infectious Diseases, Dana-Farber Cancer Institute, Boston, Massachusetts
Earache; Sore Throat, Cervical Adenitis, and Mumps; Approach to the Child with Fever and Rash; Upper Respiratory Infections; Lower Respiratory Infections; Herpes Virus Infections; Cellulitis; Enteritis; Osteomyelitis and Septic Arthritis; Hepatitis; Fungal Infections; Infection in the Immunocompromised Host; Animal Exposures

Jonathan L. Finlay, M.B., Ch.B.
Associate Professor of Pediatrics, Cornell University Medical College; Vice-Chairman, Department of Pediatrics; Associate Attending, Department of Pediatrics, Memorial Sloan-Kettering Cancer Center; New York, New York
Hodgkin Disease; Non-Hodgkin Lymphoma; Brain Tumors

Irma Fiordalisi, M.D.
Associate Professor of Pediatrics, Pediatric Critical Care, East Carolina University School of Medicine; Director, Pediatric Intensive Care Unit, Children's Hospital of Eastern North Carolina, Pitt County Memorial Hospital, Greenville, North Carolina
Diabetic Ketoacidemia

Alan R. Fleischman, M.D.
Senior Vice President, The New York Academy of Medicine; Clinical Professor of Pediatrics and Clinical Professor of Epidemiology and Social Medicine, Albert Einstein College of Medicine, The Bronx, New York
Ethical Issues in Pediatrics

Linda Forsythe, M.D.
Instructor in Psychiatry, Harvard Medical School; Clinical Assistant in Psychiatry, Massachusetts General Hospital, Boston, Massachusetts
The Adopted Child; The Depressed Child

Jean A. Frazier, M.D.
Instructor in Psychiatry, Harvard Medical School and Massachusetts General Hospital; Director of Psychiatric Disorders Program through the Joint Program of Pediatric Psychopharmacology at Massachusetts General Hospital and McLean Hospital, Belmont, Massachusetts
Mental Retardation; Autism, Asperger Syndrome, and Schizophrenia

Donna Futterman, M.D.
Associate Professor of Pediatrics, Albert Einstein College of Medicine; Director, Adolescent AIDS Program, Montefiore Medical Center, The Bronx, New York
Human Immunodeficiency Virus Infection

John Gaebler, M.D.
Associate Professor of Pediatrics, Indiana University School of Medicine; Member, Infectious Disease Section, James Whitcomb Riley Hospital, Indianapolis, Indiana
Pharyngitis and Tonsillitis

Sharon Gardner, M.D.
Instructor in Pediatrics, Cornell University Medical Center and Memorial Sloan-Kettering Cancer Center, New York, New York
Hodgkin Disease

Joseph M. Gertner, M.B., M.R.C.P.
Professor of Pediatrics, Cornell University Medical College, New York, New York
Hypopituitarism

Tal Geva, M.D.
Assistant Professor, Pediatrics and Pathology, Harvard Medical School; Associate in Cardiology, Children's Hospital, Boston, Massachusetts
Single Ventricle

Anita Gewurz, M.D.
Division of Pediatrics and Immunology, Rush Presbyterian–St. Luke's Medical Center, Chicago, Illinois
Anaphylaxis and Serum Sickness Reactions; Adverse Drug Reactions; Insect Allergies

Fereshteh Ghavimi, M.D.
Associate Professor, Clinical Pediatrics, Cornell University Medical Center; Assistant Member and Associate Attending Pediatrician, Memorial Sloan-Kettering Cancer Center, New York, New York
Rhabdomyosarcoma

James B. Gibson, M.D., Ph.D.
Assistant Professor of Pediatrics, University of Arkansas College of Medicine; Arkansas Children's Hospital, Little Rock, Arkansas
Disorders of Carbohydrate Metabolism

Enid Gilbert-Barness, M.B.B.S., M.D.
Professor of Pathology and Laboratory Medicine, Pediatrics and Obstetrics and Gynecology, University of South Florida College of Medicine; Director, Pediatric Pathology, Tampa General Hospital, Tampa, Florida
Sudden Infant Death

Leonard Glass, M.D.
Professor and Interim Chairman; Director, Division of Neonatology, State University of New York Health Science Center at Brooklyn, Brooklyn, New York
Symptoms of the Newborn; Infants of Diabetic Mothers; Neonatal Pneumonia

Elizabeth Gloster, M.D.
Associate Professor of Clinical Pathology, State University of New York Health Science Center at Brooklyn; Blood Bank Director and Attending Pathologist, University and Kings County Hospitals, Brooklyn, New York
Blood Transfusion

David Gold, M.D.
Assistant Professor of Pediatrics, Albert Einstein College of Medicine, The Bronx, New York; Pediatric Gastroenterologist, Schneider Children's Hospital, New Hyde Park, New York
Gastroesophageal Reflux

Gerald S. Golden, M.D.
Adjunct Professor of Neurology, University of Pennsylvania School of Medicine, Philadelphia, Pennsylvania
Neurologic Symptoms; The Floppy Infant; Neonatal Seizures; Learning Disabilities; Attention-Deficit/Hyperactivity Disorder; Microcephaly; Hydrocephalus; Craniosynostosis; Neural Tube Defects; Agenesis of the Corpus Callosum; Spinal Cord Disorders with Late Onset; Neurofibromatosis; Tuberous Sclerosis; Sturge-Weber Syndrome; von Hippel–Lindau Disease; Neurologic Examination; Neurologic Examination of the Neonate; Lumbar Puncture

Karl C. Golnik, M.D.
Department of Ophthalmology, University of Cincinnati College of Medicine; Cincinnati Eye Institute, Cincinnati, Ohio
Nystagmus

Carol Greene, M.D.
Associate Professor of Pediatrics, University of Colorado Health Sciences Center; Director, Inherited Metabolic Diseases Clinic, The Childrens Hospital, Denver, Colorado
Lysosomal Storage Disorders

Fenella Greig, M.D., D.PHIL.
Clinical Associate Professor of Pediatrics and Director of Pediatric Diabetes and Endocrinology, Mount Sinai School of Medicine; New York, New York
Dietary Management of Childhood Diabetes Mellitus

Moses Grossman, M.D.
Emeritus Professor of Pediatrics, University of California, San Francisco School of Medicine, San Francisco, California
Immunizations

Andrea Hagani, M.D.
Fellow, Pediatric Hematology/Oncology, Memorial Sloan-Kettering Cancer Center and The New York Hospital; New York, New York
The Child with a Bleeding Tendency; Hemophilia; Platelet Disorders (Thrombocytopenia); Thrombophilia

Paul Harmatz, M.D.
Associate in Gastroenterology and Nutrition, Children's Hospital Oakland, Oakland, California
Constipation, Encopresis, and Hirschsprung Disease; Allergic Gastroenteropathy Including Celiac Disease; Acute Appendicitis

Glenn D. Harris, M.D.
Associate Professor of Pediatrics, Pediatric Critical Care and Diabetes, East Carolina University School of Medicine; Children's Hospital of Eastern North Carolina, Pitt County Memorial Hospital, Greenville, North Carolina
Diabetic Ketoacidemia

Stanley Hellerstein, M.D.
Professor of Pediatrics, University of Missouri School of Medicine at Kansas City; Pediatric Nephrologist, The Children's Mercy Hospital, Kansas City, Missouri
Symptoms of Renal Disorders; The Urinary Tract; Urinary Tract Infection and Vesicoureteric Reflux; Voiding Disorders; Tests of Kidney Function

David B. Herzog, M.D.
Professor of Psychiatry, Harvard Medical School; Director, Eating Disorders Unit, Massachusetts General Hospital, Boston, Massachusetts
Eating Disorders

Peter W. Hiatt, M.D.
Assistant Professor and Director, Cystic Fibrosis Center, Department of Pediatrics, Baylor College of Medicine; Texas Children's Hospital, Houston, Texas
Wheezing; Adult Respiratory Distress Syndrome

Raymond L. Hintz, M.D.
Professor of Pediatrics, Stanford University School of Medicine; Head, Division of Pediatric Endocrinology, Stanford University Medical Center, Stanford, California
Idiopathic Short Stature

Jay A. Hochman, M.D.
Fellow, Pediatric Gastroenterology and Nutrition, University of Cincinnati College of Medicine; Children's Hospital Medical Center, Cincinnati, Ohio
Biliary Atresia

Neal Hoffman, M.D.
Assistant Professor of Pediatrics, Albert Einstein College of Medicine; Attending Physician, Division of Adolescent Medicine, Montefiore Medical Center, The Bronx, New York
Sexually Transmitted Diseases

Paul L. Hofman, M.B.Ch.B., F.R.A.C.P.
Fellow, Pediatric Endocrinology, James Whitcomb Riley Hospital for Children, Indianapolis, Indiana
Premature Thelarche

Arno R. Hohn, M.D.
Professor of Pediatrics, University of Southern California School of Medicine; Head, Division of Pediatric Cardiology, Children's Hospital of Los Angeles and Los Angeles County/USC Hospital, Los Angeles, California
Hypertension

Michelle S. Howenstine, M.D.
Associate Clinical Professor, Department of Pediatrics, University of South Florida College of Medicine, Tampa; Medical Director, Section of Pediatric Pulmonology, All Children's Hospital, St. Petersburg, Florida
Croup; Pneumonia; Foreign Body Aspiration; Epiglottitis

Robert N. Husson, M.D.
Assistant Professor of Pediatrics, Harvard Medical School; Associate in Medicine, Children's Hospital, Boston, Massachusetts
Tuberculosis and Atypical Mycobacteria

Laura S. Inselman, M.D.
Associate Professor of Pediatrics, Jefferson Medical College of Thomas Jefferson University, Philadelphia, Pennsylvania; Active Attending Pulmonologist and Medical Director, Respiratory Care Department and Pulmonary Function Laboratory, Du Pont Hospital for Children, Alfred I. Du Pont Institute of the Nemours Foundation, Wilmington, Delaware
Tuberculosis; Sarcoidosis

Michael S. Jellinek, M.D.
Professor of Psychiatry and of Pediatrics, Harvard Medical School; Chief, Child Psychiatry Service, Massachusetts General Hospital, Boston, Massachusetts
The Adopted Child; The Depressed Child; Anxiety Disorders; Divorce; Posttraumatic Stress Disorder; Questionnaire Approaches to the Recognition and Assessment of Psychosocial Problems

Rima Jibaly, M.D.
Instructor in Pediatrics, Pediatric Gastroenterology and Nutrition Fellow, Children's Medical Center of Brooklyn, Brooklyn, New York
Toxic Megacolon

Robert H. Johr, M.D.
Associate Clinical Professor of Dermatology and Pediatrics; Director, Pigmented Lesion Clinic, University of Miami School of Medicine, Miami, Florida
Normal Neonatal Skin; Neonatal Skin Abnormalities; Seborrheic Dermatitis; Vesiculopustular Rashes; Sarcoidosis; Mastocytosis; Granuloma Annulare; Melanoma; Nevocellular (Melanocytic) Nevi; Miscellaneous Pigmented Lesions; Potassium Hydroxide (KOH) Preparation; Patch Testing; Scabies Preparation; Tzanck Preparation; Wood Lamp Examination

Edward L. Kaplan, M.D.
Professor of Pediatrics, University of Minnesota, Minneapolis, Minnesota
Rheumatic Fever

Richard A. Kaplan, M.D., Ph.D.
Director, Pediatric Nephrology and Hypertension, Lutheran General Children's Hospital, Park Ridge, Illinois
Hemolytic Uremic Syndrome; Chronic Renal Failure

Mary Kaufman, M.D.
Clinical Professor of Pediatrics, State University of New York Health Science Center at Brooklyn College of Medicine; Retired Chairman of Pediatrics; Director, Pediatric Hematology/Oncology, Long Island College Hospital, Brooklyn, New York
Hemorrhagic Disease of the Newborn; Hemophilia; von Willebrand Disease; Disseminated Intravascular Coagulation

Richard I. Kelley, M.D., Ph.D.
Associate Professor of Pediatrics, Johns Hopkins University School of Medicine; Director of Metabolism, The Kennedy Krieger Institute, Baltimore, Maryland
Disorders of Lipid Metabolism

Bradley Kessler, M.D.
Assistant Professor of Pediatrics, Albert Einstein College of Medicine, New York; Attending, Pediatric Gastroenterology, Schneider Children's Hospital; Long Island Jewish Medical Center, New Hyde Park, New York
Pyloric Stenosis

Michael H. Kohrman, M.D., M.S.
Associate Professor of Neurology and Pediatrics, State University of New York School of Medicine and Biomedical Sciences, Buffalo, New York
Seizures; Status Epilepticus

Stanley J. Kogan, M.D.
Clinical Professor of Urology, Cornell University School of Medicine, New York; New York Medical College, Valhalla; Attending Pediatric Urologist, New York Hospital; Westchester Medical Center, Valhalla; Montefiore/Einstein Medical Center, The Bronx, New York
Hypospadias

Bernice R. Krafchik, M.B., Ch.B., F.R.C.P.C.
Professor, Department of Paediatrics, University of Toronto Faculty of Medicine; Head, Division of Dermatology, Hospital for Sick Children, Toronto, Canada
Diaper Dermatitis; Atopic Dermatitis (Eczema); Urticaria; Erythema Multiforme and Stevens-Johnson Syndrome; Hemangioma and Vascular Malformation; Psoriasis; Pityriasis Rosea

Brian H. Kushner, M.D.
Attending Physician, Memorial Sloan-Kettering Cancer Center, New York, New York
Neuroblastoma

Stephan Ladisch, M.D.
Professor of Pediatrics and Biochemistry/Molecular Biology, George Washington University School of Medicine; Director, Center for Cancer and Transplantation Biology, Children's Research Institute, Children's National Medical Center, Washington, D.C.
Langerhans Cell Histiocytosis

Fred S. Lamb, M.D., Ph.D.
Assistant Professor of Pediatric Cardiology and Pediatric Critical Care, University of Iowa Hospitals and Clinics, Iowa City, Iowa
Heart Failure

Michael P. LaQuaglia, M.D., F.A.C.S., F.A.A.P.
Chief, Pediatric Surgery, Memorial Sloan-Kettering Cancer Center, New York, New York
Soft Tissue Sarcomas; Liver Tumors

Teresita A. Laude, M.D.
Associate Professor of Pediatrics and Associate Professor of Dermatology; Director, Division of Pediatric Dermatology, State University of New York Health Science Center at Brooklyn, Brooklyn, New York
Skin Infections; Genodermatoses

Ronald M. Lauer, M.D.
Professor of Pediatrics and Preventive Medicine, Division of Pediatric Cardiology, University of Iowa College of Medicine and University of Iowa Hospitals and Clinics, Iowa City, Iowa
Symptoms of Cardiovascular Disorders; Ventricular Septal Defects

Gobind Laungani, M.D.
Clinical Associate Professor, State University of New York Health Science Center at Brooklyn, Brooklyn, New York
Genitourinary Disorders

Sheela G. Laungani, M.D.
Clinical Associate Professor, State University of New York Health Science Center at Brooklyn, Brooklyn, New York
Genitourinary Disorders; Resuscitation of the Newborn

Peter Lee, M.D., Ph.D.
Professor of Pediatrics, University of Pittsburgh School of Medicine; Program Director, General Clinical Research Center, Children's Hospital of Pittsburgh, Pittsburgh, Pennsylvania
Hypogonadotropic Hypogonadism; Micropenis (Hypogenitalism)

Fred Leickly, M.D.
Clinical Associate Professor of Pediatrics, Indiana University School of Medicine; James Whitcomb Riley Hospital for Children, Indianapolis, Indiana
Bronchitis; Status Asthmaticus

Jeremiah Levine, M.D.
Associate Professor, Albert Einstein College of Medicine, The Bronx; Co-Chief, Department of Gastroenterology and Nutrition, Schneider Children's Hospital, Long Island Jewish Medical Center, New Hyde Park, New York
Achalasia; Pyloric Stenosis; Helicobacter pylori–*Associated Peptic Ulcer Disease*

Lynne L. Lentsky, M.D.
Associate Professor of Pediatrics, Harvard Medical School; Chief, Pediatric Endocrine Unit, Massachusetts General Hospital, Boston, Massachusetts
Insulin-Dependent Diabetes Mellitus

L. Glen Lewis, M.D.
Assistant Professor of Pediatrics, University of Cincinnati School of Medicine; Division of Pediatric Gastroenterology and Nutrition, Children's Hospital Medical Center, Cincinnati, Ohio
End-Stage Liver Disease and Cirrhosis

Barbara Linder, M.D., Ph.D.
Assistant Professor of Pediatrics, Albert Einstein College of Medicine; Montefiore Medical Center, The Bronx, New York
Hypoglycemia; Steroid Withdrawal

Barbara Lippe, M.D.
Professor Emeritus of Pediatrics, University of California, Los Angeles, School of Medicine, Los Angeles, California; Senior Medical Director, Peptide Hormones/Metabolic Diseases, Pharmacia & Upjohn, Kalamazoo, Michigan
Turner Syndrome

Thomas R. Lloyd, M.D.
Associate Professor, Division of Pediatric Cardiology, University of Michigan Medical School; Director, Cardiac Catheterization Laboratories, C.S. Mott Children's Hospital, Ann Arbor, Michigan
Pulmonary Stenosis

Janet Loch-Donahue, M.D.
Emergency Physician, St. Thomas Hospital, Nashville, Tennessee
Orbital and Preseptal Cellulitis

Larry T. Mahoney, M.D.
Professor of Pediatrics, University of Iowa College of Medicine; Director, Pediatric Cardiology, University of Iowa Hospitals and Clinics, Iowa City, Iowa
Coarctation of the Aorta

Joseph A. Majzoub, M.D.
Associate Professor in Pediatrics, Harvard Medical School; Chief, Division of Endocrinology, Children's Hospital, Boston, Massachusetts
Diabetes Insipidus

Michael J. Maloney, M.D.
Associate Professor of Psychiatry and Pediatrics, University of Cincinnati School of Medicine; Director, Division of Child and Adolescent Psychiatry, Children's Hospital Medical Center, Cincinnati, Ohio
A Developmental Understanding of Chronic Illness

Michael Marble, M.D.
Assistant Professor of Pediatrics, Human Genetics Program, Hayward Genetics Center, Tulane University School of Medicine, New Orleans, Louisiana
Skeletal Dysplasias

Morri E. Markowitz, M.D.
Professor of Pediatrics, Albert Einstein College of Medicine; Attending Physician, Montefiore Medical Center, The Bronx, New York
Parathyroid Disorders; Pseudohypoparathyroidism; Hyperparathyroidism; Neonatal Hypocalcemia

William L. Marshall, M.D.
Instructor in Medicine, Harvard Medical School; Attending Physician in Infectious Disease, Brigham and Women's Hospital/Dana-Farber Cancer Institute, Boston, Massachusetts
Human Immunodeficiency Virus

Bruce J. Masek, Ph.D.
Assistant Professor of Psychology (Psychiatry), Harvard Medical School; Director, Behavioral Medicine Program, Department of Child Psychiatry, Children's Hospital; Massachusetts General Hospital, Boston, Massachusetts
Behavioral Symptoms and Management Strategies for Common Problems

Paul A. Meyers, M.D.
Associate Professor of Clinical Pediatrics, Cornell University Medical College; Associate Attending Pediatrician, Memorial Sloan-Kettering Cancer Center, New York, New York
Osteosarcoma; Ewing Sarcoma

Scott T. Miller, M.D.
Associate Professor of Clinical Pediatrics, State University of New York Health Science Center at Brooklyn; Attending Physician, University Hospital of Brooklyn, Kings County Hospital, Brooklyn, New York
Sickle Cell Disease; Thalassemias

Walter L. Miller, M.D.
Professor of Pediatrics and Director, Child Health Research Center, University of California, San Francisco, School of Medicine, San Francisco, California
21-Hydroxylase Deficiency; Other Congenital Adrenal Hyperplasias; Addison Disease

Jill H. Morriss, M.D.
Associate Professor, University of Iowa College of Medicine, Iowa City, Iowa
Patent Ductus Arteriosus; Aortic Stenosis

James N. Moy, M.D.
Assistant Professor, Department of Immunology/Microbiology, Rush Medical College; Director, Division of Allergy and Immunology, Cook County Children's Hospital, Chicago, Illinois
Asthma; Angioedema/Urticaria; Allergic Rhinitis; Food Allergies

Gary A. Mueller, M.D.
Assistant Professor of Pediatrics; Associate Director, Division of Pediatric Pulmonary Medicine, Wright State University School of Medicine; Medical Director, Department of Respiratory Therapy; Medical Director, Pulmonary Function Laboratory, Children's Medical Center, Dayton, Ohio
Pulmonary Function Testing

Kevin Mulhern, M.D.
Assistant Professor of Medicine, University of Iowa College of Medicine, Iowa City, Iowa
Mitral Valve Prolapse; Marfan Syndrome

J. Michael Murphy, Ed.D.
Assistant Professor of Psychology, Harvard Medical School; Staff Psychologist, Massachusetts General Hospital, Boston, Massachusetts
Questionnaire Approaches to the Recognition and Assessment of Psychosocial Problems

J. Patrick Murphy, M.D.
Associate Professor of Surgery, University of Missouri—Kansas City School of Medicine, Kansas City, Missouri; Associate Clinical Professor of Surgery, University of Kansas School of Medicine, Kansas City, Kansas; Chief of Pediatric Urology, Children's Mercy Hospital, Kansas City, Missouri
Neonatal Urinary Tract Dilation; Cryptorchidism; Trauma to the Urinary Tract

Sakkubai Naidu, M.D.
Associate Professor, Departments of Pediatrics and Neurology, Johns Hopkins University School of Medicine; Pediatric Neurologist, The Kennedy Krieger Institute, Baltimore, Maryland
Neurodegenerative Disorders; Subacute Sclerosing Panencephalitis; Rett Syndrome

Wendy Neal, M.D.
Post-doctorate Fellow in Adolescent Medicine, Albert Einstein College of Medicine/Montefiore Medical Center, The Bronx, New York
Substance Abuse

Robert P. Nelson, M.D.
Associate Professor of Medicine and Pediatrics, Division of Allergy and Clinical Immunology, University of South Florida College of Medicine, Tampa; All Children's Hospital, St. Petersburg, Florida
Pneumonia

Karin M. Nussbaum, B.A.
Research Coordinator, Eating Disorders Unit, Massachusetts General Hospital, Boston, Massachusetts
Eating Disorders

K. M. O'Neil, M.D.
Assistant Clinical Professor of Pediatrics, State University of New York at Buffalo School of Medicine and Biomedical Sciences; Director, Pediatric Rheumatology Service, The Children's Hospital of Buffalo, Buffalo, New York
Juvenile Arthritis; Systemic Lupus Erythematosus; Juvenile Dermatomyositis and Polymyositis; Scleroderma; Vasculitis Syndromes of Childhood; Infection-Associated Rheumatic Syndromes

Robert H. Pantell, M.D.
Professor of Pediatrics, University of California, San Francisco, School of Medicine, San Francisco, California
Fever in Infants Less than 3 Months of Age

Ora Hirsch Pescovitz, M.D.
Professor of Pediatrics, Physiology/Biophysics, Indiana University School of Medicine; Director, Pediatric Endocrinology/Diabetology, James Whitcomb Riley Hospital for Children, Indianapolis, Indiana
Premature Thelarche

Michael Pettei, M.D.
Associate Professor of Pediatrics, Albert Einstein School of Medicine, The Bronx; Co-Chief, Division of Gastroenterology and Nutrition, Schneider Children's Hospital, Long Island Jewish Medical Center, New Hyde Park, New York
Gastroesophageal Reflux

Steve Piecuch, M.D.
Clinical Assistant Professor of Pediatrics, State University of New York Health Science Center at Brooklyn, Brooklyn, New York
Birth Injuries; Neonatal Infections; Gastrointestinal Disorders

Neil S. Prose, M.D.
Associate Professor of Medicine (Dermatology) and Pediatrics, Duke University Medical Center, Durham, North Carolina
Alopecias; Acne; Damaging Effects of Solar Radiation

Marlene Rabinovitch, M.D.
Professor of Pediatrics, Pathology, and Medicine, University of Toronto Faculty of Medicine; Director, Division of Cardiovascular Research, The Hospital for Sick Children, Toronto, Canada
Eisenmenger Syndrome

Simon Rabinowitz, Ph.D., M.D.
Clinical Associate Professor of Pediatrics; Chief, Pediatric Gastroenterology and Nutrition, Children's Medical Center of Brooklyn, Brooklyn, New York
Gastrointestinal Hemorrhage; Liver Failure; Toxic Megacolon; Gastrointestinal Endoscopy

Sreedhar P. Rao, M.D.
Professor of Clinical Pediatrics; Director, Pediatric Hematology/Oncology; State University of New York Health Science Center at Brooklyn, Brooklyn, New York
Pallor; Jaundice; Anemia; Lymphadenopathy; Neck Mass; Abdominal Mass; Hepatosplenomegaly; Iron Deficiency Anemia and Other Microcytic Anemias; Aplastic Anemia; Hypoplastic Anemia; Glucose 6-Phosphate Dehydrogenase Deficiency; Pyruvate Kinase Deficiency; Microangiopathic Hemolytic Anemia; Autoimmune Hemolytic Anemia; Examination of Peripheral Blood; Examination of Bone Marrow

Paula K. Rauch, M.D.
Assistant Professor, Harvard Medical School; Co-Director, Child Psychiatry Consultation Service, Massachusetts General Hospital, Boston, Massachusetts
Death in the Family

Edward O. Reiter, M.D.
Professor of Pediatrics, Tufts University School of Medicine, Boston; Chairman, Department of Pediatrics, Baystate Medical Center Children's Hospital, Springfield, Massachusetts
Undescended Testes

Frederick J. Rescorla, M.D.
Associate Professor of Surgery, Indiana University School of Medicine; Staff Surgeon, James Whitcomb Riley Hospital for Children, Indianapolis, Indiana
Pectus Excavatum; Pneumothorax

Michael Rosenbaum, M.D.
Associate Professor of Pediatrics, Columbia University College of Physicians and Surgeons, New York, New York
Obesity

Ron G. Rosenfeld, M.D.
Professor and Chairman, Department of Pediatrics; Professor, Department of Cell and Developmental Biology, Oregon Health Sciences University; Physician-in-Chief, Doernbecher Children's Hospital, Portland, Oregon
Growth Hormone Resistance Syndromes

Warren Rosenfeld, M.D.
Professor of Pediatrics, State University of New York at Stony Brook Health Sciences Center; Chairman of Pediatrics, Winthrop-University Hospital, Mineola, New York
Respiratory Distress Syndrome; Bronchopulmonary Dysplasia; Transient Tachypnea of the Newborn; Meconium Aspiration; Air Leaks

Robert L. Rosenfield, M.D.
Professor of Pediatrics and Medicine, The University of Chicago Pritzker School of Medicine; Head, Section of Pediatric Endocrinology, The University of Chicago Children's Hospital, Chicago, Illinois
Hirsutism and Hyperandrogenism in Adolescent Girls

Sheldon P. Rothenberg, M.D.
Professor of Medicine; Chief, Division of Hematology/Oncology, State University of New York Health Science Center at Brooklyn, Brooklyn, New York
Megaloblastic Anemia

James A. Royall, M.D.
C.R. Anthony Professor of Pediatrics, University of Oklahoma College of Medicine; Chief, Section of Pediatric Pulmonology; Faculty, Section of Pediatric Critical Care, Children's Hospital at Oklahoma, Oklahoma City, Oklahoma
Cardiogenic Shock/Hypertensive Crisis

Robert J. Ruben, M.D.
Professor and Chairman, Department of Otolaryngology; Professor of Pediatrics, Albert Einstein College of Medicine and Montefiore Medical Center, The Bronx, New York
Symptoms of ENT Disorders; Otitis Media; Serous Otitis Media; Chronic Otitis Media and Mastoiditis; Otitis Externa (Swimmer's Ear); Hearing Tests; Tympanocentesis; Removing Cerumen

Nathan Rudolph, M.B.B.Ch.
Professor of Pediatrics, State University of New York Health Science Center at Brooklyn; Associate Director of Neonatology, Children's Medical Center of Brooklyn, Brooklyn, New York
Low Birth Weight; Parenteral Nutrition of the Neonate; Screening

Barry Russman, M.D.
Professor of Pediatrics and Neurology, University of Connecticut School of Medicine, Farmington; Director, Rehabilitation Medicine; Staff Neurologist, Connecticut Children's Medical Center, Hartford, Connecticut
Cerebral Palsy; Muscular Dystrophies; Spinal Muscular Atrophy

Paul H. Saenger, M.D.
Professor of Pediatrics; Head, Division of Pediatric Endocrinology, Montefiore Medical Center/Albert Einstein College of Medicine; The Bronx, New York
Gynecomastia; Premature Adrenarche; Brief Guide to Work-up of the Child with Short Stature; Ambiguous Genitalia; Undescended Testes

Stephen P. Sanders, M.D.
Professor of Pediatrics; Chief, Division of Pediatric Cardiology, Duke University Medical Center, Durham, North Carolina
Transposition of the Great Vessels

Lawrence A. Schachner, M.D.
Professor, Department of Dermatology, Department of Pediatrics; Director, Division of Pediatric Dermatology, University of Miami School of Medicine, Miami, Florida
Normal Neonatal Skin; Neonatal Skin Abnormalities; Seborrheic Dermatitis; Vesicopustular Rashes; Sarcoidosis; Mastocytosis; Granuloma Annulare; Melanoma; Nevocellular (Melanocytic) Nevi; Miscellaneous Pigmented Lesions; Potassium Hydroxide (KOH) Preparation; Patch Testing; Scabies Preparation; Tzanck Preparation; Wood Lamp Examination

David Schleifer, B.A.
Pediatric Pharmacology Clinic, Massachusetts General Hospital, Boston, Massachusetts
Attention Deficit/Hyperactivity Disorder

Thomas D. Scholz, M.D.
Assistant Professor of Pediatrics, University of Iowa College of Medicine, Iowa City, Iowa
Atrial Septal Defects

Joel M. Schwartz, M.D.
Professor of Clinical Medicine, State University of New York Health Science Center at Brooklyn; Director of Hematology and Oncology, Coney Island Hospital, Brooklyn, New York
Hereditary Spherocytosis and Hereditary Elliptocytosis

Binita R. Shah, M.D.
Professor of Clinical Pediatrics, State University of New York at Brooklyn Health Science Center; Children's Medical Center of Brooklyn; Director, Pediatric Emergency Medicine, Kings County Hospital Center, Brooklyn, New York
Comatose Child; Child with Multisystem Trauma; Child Poisoned by Unknown Substance

Joseph Shrand, M.D.
Instructor of Psychiatry, Harvard Medical School, Boston; Director, Child and Adolescent Ambulatory Services, McLean Hospital, Belmont, Massachusetts
Triage of Psychiatrically Ill Children

Ari M. Simckes, M.D.
Assistant Professor of Pediatrics, University of Missouri—Kansas City School of Medicine; Section of Pediatric Nephrology, The Children's Mercy Hospital, Kansas City, Missouri
Isolated Asymptomatic Proteinuria; Nephrotic Syndrome; Bladder Catheterization; Suprapubic Aspiration (Bladder Tap)

John D. Snyder, M.D.
Professor of Clinical Pediatrics, Division of Hepatology, University of California, San Francisco, School of Medicine, San Francisco, California
Acute Diarrhea; Persistent Diarrhea; Inflammatory Bowel Disease: Ulcerative Colitis and Crohn Disease

Thomas J. Spencer, M.D.
Assistant Professor, Harvard Medical School; Staff Psychiatrist, Massachusetts General Hospital, Boston, Massachusetts
Attention Deficit/Hyperactivity Disorder

Paul Stanger, M.D.
Professor of Pediatrics (Cardiology), University of California, San Francisco, School of Medicine, San Francisco, California
Truncus Arteriosus

Richard Stanhope, M.D., D.C.H., F.R.C.P.
Senior Lecturer in Paediatric Endocrinology, Institute of Child Health; Consultant Paediatric Endocrinologist, Great Ormond Street Hospital for Children, London, England
Constitutional Short Stature; Familial Short Stature; Constitutional Delay of Growth and Puberty

Peter G. Steinherz, M.D.
Professor of Pediatrics, Cornell University Medical College; Member and Attending Pediatrician, Memorial Sloan-Kettering Cancer Center, New York, New York
Acute Lymphoblastic Leukemia; Wilms Tumor

John C. Stevens, M.D.
Clinical Associate Professor of Pediatrics, Section of Pulmonology, Indiana University School of Medicine; Attending Pediatric Pulmonologist, James Whitcomb Riley Hospital for Children, Indianapolis, Indiana
Chronic Cough; Cystic Fibrosis

Julia L. Stevens, M.D.
Assistant Professor, Department of Ophthalmology, University of Kentucky College of Medicine; A.B. Chandler Medical Center, Lexington, Kentucky
Amblyopia; Retinopathy of Prematurity

Constantine A. Stratakis, M.D., D.Sc.
Assistant Professor of Pediatrics, Pediatric Endocrinology, and Genetics, Georgetown University, Washington, D.C.; Senior Staff Scientist, National Institute of Child Health and Human Development, National Institutes of Health, Bethesda, Maryland
Cushing Syndrome and Cushing Disease

Muriel Sugarman, M.D.
Clinical Instructor in Psychiatry, Harvard Medical School; Assistant in Psychiatry, Massachusetts General Hospital, Boston, Massachusetts
Physical Abuse and Neglect; Sexual Abuse

Masato Takahashi, M.D.
Professor of Pediatrics, University of Southern California School of Medicine; Attending Cardiologist, Children's Hospital, Los Angeles, California
Kawasaki Syndrome

Shanti Thirumalai, M.D., M.R.C.P.(U.K.)
Assistant Professor, Division of Pediatric Neurology, University of South Carolina School of Medicine; Attending Physician, Richland Memorial Hospital, Columbia, South Carolina
Neurodegenerative Disorders; Subacute Sclerosing Panencephalitis; Rett Syndrome

Jeffrey A. Towbin, M.D.
Associate Professor of Pediatrics (Cardiology) and Molecular and Human Genetics, Baylor College of Medicine, Texas Children's Hospital, Houston, Texas
Myocarditis; Pericarditis

Guochuan E. Tsai, M.D., Ph.D.
Assistant Professor, Harvard Medical School; Assistant in Psychiatry, Massachusetts General Hospital, Boston, Massachusetts
Anxiety Disorders

Gloria B. Valencia, M.D.
Clinical Associate Professor, State University of New York Health Science Center at Brooklyn; Attending Neonatologist; Kings County Hospital Center, Brooklyn, New York
Neonatal Jaundice; Infant Transport

Cornelis Van Dop, M.D., Ph.D.
Associate Professor of Pediatrics, University of California, Los Angeles, School of Medicine, Los Angeles, California
McCune-Albright Syndrome

Stella Van Praagh, M.D.
Associate in Cardiology, Emeritus, Department of Cardiology, Children's Hospital, Boston, Massachusetts
Single Ventricle

L. George Veasy, M.D.
Professor of Pediatrics, University of Utah School of Medicine; Physician-in-Chief (Retired), Primary Children's Medical Center, Salt Lake City, Utah
Cardiac Auscultation

Fredric H. Warren, M.D.
Associate Professor of Orthopaedics, Tulane University, New Orleans, Louisiana
Slipped Capital Femoral Epiphysis; Genu Varum and Genu Valgum; Legg-Calvé-Perthes Disease

Paul M. Weinberg, M.D.
Associate Professor of Pediatrics and Radiology, University of Pennsylvania School of Medicine; Senior Cardiologist; Consultant in Radiology (MRI) and Pathology; Director, Cardiac Registry, The Children's Hospital of Philadelphia, Philadelphia, Pennsylvania
Hypoplastic Left Heart Syndrome

Toba Weinstein, M.D.
Assistant Professor, Albert Einstein College of Medicine, The Bronx; Pediatric Gastroenterologist, Schneider Children's Hospital, Long Island Jewish Medical Center, New Hyde Park, New York
Achalasia; Helicobactor Pylori–Associated Peptic Ulcer Disease

Peter F. Weller, M.D., F.A.C.P.
Professor of Medicine, Harvard Medical School; Co-Chief, Infectious Diseases, Beth Israel Deaconess Medical Center, Boston, Massachusetts
Selected Parasitic Infections

Robert J. Wells, M.D.
Professor of Clinical Pediatrics, University of Cincinnati College of Medicine; Children's Hospital Medical Center, Cincinnati, Ohio
Acute Myeloid Leukemia

Constance E. West, M.D.
Pediatric Ophthalmologist, Children's Hospital Medical Center and Cincinnati Eye Institute, Cincinnati, Ohio
Nasolacrimal Duct Obstruction; Retinoblastoma; Ocular Trauma

Timothy E. Wilens, M.D.
Associate Professor, Harvard Medical School; Staff Psychiatrist, Massachusetts General Hospital, Boston, Massachusetts
Attention Deficit/Hyperactivity Disorder

Steven M. Willi, M.D.
Assistant Professor of Pediatrics, Medical University of South Carolina College of Medicine, Charleston, South Carolina
Hypoglycemia

Robert R. Wolfe, B.S.Ch.E., M.D.
Professor of Pediatric Cardiology, University of Colorado School of Medicine, Director of Pediatric Exercise Laboratory; Director of Pediatric Cardiology Outreach, Denver Children's Hospital, Denver, Colorado
Pulmonary Atresia

Norma Wollner, M.D.
Professor of Pediatrics, Cornell University Medical College; Attending Pediatrician; Director, Pediatric Day Hospital, Memorial Sloan-Kettering Cancer Center, New York, New York
Non-Hodgkin Lymphoma

Alice C. Yao, M.D.
Professor of Pediatrics, Pediatric Cardiology, and Neonatology, State University of New York at Brooklyn Health Science Center; Attending Pediatrician, Attending Neonatologist and Cardiologist, Children's Medical Center of Brooklyn at University Hospital of Brooklyn, Brooklyn, New York
Cardiovascular Disorders

Nada Yazigi, M.D.
Mt. Sinai Hospital Medical Center, Chicago, Illinois
Viral Hepatitis

Marc Yudkoff, M.D.
Professor of Pediatrics, University of Pennsylvania School of Medicine; Associate Chief, Division of Child Development, Children's Hospital of Philadelphia and Children's Seashore House, Philadelphia, Pennsylvania
Disorders of Amino Acid Metabolism

Jean Homrighausen Zander, R.N., M.S.N.
Formerly Clinical Instructor and Lecturer (Adjunct), Indiana University School of Nursing; Staff Nurse, Pediatric ICU, James Whitcomb Riley Hospital for Children, Indianapolis, Indiana
Pulmonary Home Care

Donald Zimmerman, M.D.
Associate Professor of Pediatrics, Mayo Medical School; Section Head, Pediatric Endocrinology; Consultant in Pediatric Endocrinology and Metabolism, Mayo Clinic, Rochester, Minnesota
Thyroid Cancer

Foreword

At some point the reader of SAUNDERS MANUAL OF PEDIATRIC PRACTICE may reasonably ask: In this age of electronic data processing, is the textbook needed to support the clinician's knowledge base? I believe that the answer is a clear YES! The complexity of modern medical practice demands that the good physician rely extensively on external sources of information. The time is long past (if it ever existed) when the information necessary for competent office or bedside care could be contained in the physician's head. Despite incredible progress in electronic data handling systems, the book remains the most portable, readily available, economical, and convenient source of information for the busy student or clinician.

This is an unusual book. Writing a guide to serve as an office or bedside companion to the child's physician is a challenge. Few authors or editors have been able to discipline themselves to restrict their product, tending instead to be so comprehensive that they go far beyond the bedside or office needs of the student or clinician, or, worse, presenting their material as an exhaustively complete list of facts. By contrast, SAUNDERS MANUAL OF PEDIATRIC PRACTICE represents a clear, concise, and authoritative resource for the child's physician, assembled so as to provide in-depth information quickly to the reader. The style chosen for this text makes it easy to locate information about a clinical problem or situation. It is also written in a readable, almost conversational style.

The tasks of the physician who would provide health care to children are multiple. That person must acquire general knowledge of medicine and of the special needs of immature subjects; develop skill in gathering data from the child and other sources to define the patient's current status, and, by observation and conversation, gather and integrate specific information with medical knowledge of normal and disease states. From this process, conclusions must be reached, decisions made, and actions taken.

SAUNDERS MANUAL OF PEDIATRIC PRACTICE gives high priority to exact and concisely stated information. The author and contributors make the evaluative process both simple and stimulating by grouping information in the way the physician will want to use it. As often as possible, a topic is addressed by a presentation of background, related facts, and practical applications in a single unit. Illustrative information is included intermittently to stimulate a deeper understanding of the basis of diagnosis and treatment.

The target audience is the medical professional (pediatrician, family and generalist physician, pediatric nurse, nurse practitioner) who accepts the responsibility of providing medical care to children. This book recognizes that the adult learner is inquiring and goal oriented as he or she builds new knowledge and skills on previous experience. Most of us learn by doing, but knowledge and understanding must precede action. The practice of a profession requires the acquisition of knowledge, skills, and attitudes through multiple learning modes. The medical caregiver must go beyond the application of factual knowledge to make innovative applications of information to the solution of individual clinical problems. Great teachers (Socrates, Hippocrates, Maimonides, Jesus, Osler) taught through analysis of experience, using dialogue, parables, and problem examples. This technique, which teases the student's mind and makes the learner an enthusiastic participant in the learning process, is used to advantage in SAUNDERS MANUAL OF PEDIATRIC PRACTICE.

The sections on water and salt metabolism (Chapters 10 to 13) are particularly good examples of the book's didactic style. The author, writing in an area where he is an acknowledged expert, builds understanding of the physiology of the body's internal milieu and relates this basic knowledge to the management of disturbances due to acute illness, deprivation, or genetic anomalies. The reader is thus encouraged to approach a clinical problem via physiologic reasoning rather than predetermined formula or habit.

In summary, the modest title—SAUNDERS MANUAL OF PEDIATRIC PRACTICE—belies the breadth and depth of information to be found in this scholarly text. In most sections, there are four divisions for convenience: symptoms, disorders, critical states, and relevant procedures. Each of the disorders is described in the same format, making it easy to find the information that the clinician seeks. All should find this style useful for quick reference as well as for thoughtful analysis.

C.W. DAESCHNER, JR., M.D.
Professor and Chairman of Pediatrics, Emeritus
University of Texas Medical Branch
Galveston, Texas

Preface

SAUNDERS MANUAL OF PEDIATRIC PRACTICE is designed to assist clinicians caring for children so that they can make accurate assessments of their patients and provide appropriate therapy. Chapters are presented in outline format, and key information is boxed and highlighted in a second color so that the user of this book can obtain information quickly in the office or at the bedside. Because I firmly believe that understanding a disease process is important to designing the best management of a disorder, a brief summary of pathophysiology or pathogenesis accompanies each entity, when appropriate.

There are 351 topics presented in SAUNDERS MANUAL OF PEDIATRIC PRACTICE. Most chapters discuss specific diseases, but there are also chapters on symptoms and on procedures commonly performed in the office setting. Diseases are usually presented in the following format: definition; etiology and epidemiology; pathophysiology; clinical, laboratory, and radiographic findings; treatment; and prevention. Each chapter includes about five recent or classic references for those who may need additional information. Also, SAUNDERS MANUAL OF PEDIATRIC PRACTICE has many tables throughout, each presenting a maximum of information in an easily retrievable format.

Pediatrics has always had a major component of prevention in its practice. Thus, SAUNDERS MANUAL OF PEDIATRIC PRACTICE has chapters on infant and childhood feeding, accidents and poisoning avoidance, and counseling.

These matters are part of virtually every patient encounter and thus are covered herein.

Children differ from adults anatomically, physiologically, biochemically, immunologically, and psychologically. Each body system—as well as many subsystems—matures at its unique rate. We have tried to reflect this influence of growth and maturation, the essence of pediatric knowledge, in a practical and usable way.

Even as new discoveries in genetics and molecular biology lead to new insights and improved therapies, the knowledge that we possess now needs to be available to those who care for children. We have tried to provide that, mindful that by the time of publication one can anticipate further advances.

I am deeply grateful to the Section Editors and the many contributors who have conformed to the stylistic strictures placed on them. Many of them have been my colleagues as students, house staff, and faculty—some of them serving in all these roles. All have performed nobly, as expected, and mostly on schedule.

Much credit goes to Joann Quane-Finberg for managing the flow of manuscripts in and out of our office and for deciphering my handwriting. Many thanks also to Judith Fletcher and Leslie Hoeltzel for the excellent service and good cheer at W.B. Saunders Company.

LAURENCE FINBERG, M.D.

Contents

Part V   Adolescent Medicine
Kenneth S. Schonberg, Editor

Part VI   Behavior/Psychology
Michael S. Jellinek, Editor

Part VII   Genetics/Metabolism
Marc Yudkoff, Editor

Part XIII   Respiratory Disorders
Howard Eigen, Editor

Part XVII   Dermatology
Lawrence A. Schachner, Editor

1 **Feeding Guidelines**

Laurence Finberg

Infant Feeding

The origins of pediatrics as a specialty date to concerns about infant feeding during the Industrial Revolution, when poor women were able to earn money in ways other than by serving as wet nurses and women were able to find remunerative employment, which limited their availability for breast feeding. The values of breast feeding include the nutritional, the immunologic, and the psychological. The composition of milks and other diets will be discussed along with age-specific recommendations and techniques of feeding. The underlying science, insofar as it is known, is reviewed in the section on nutrition.

1. Breast feeding

   a. The composition of human milk evolved, as for other mammals, as a compromise between the survival value of the infant and the continued survival of the mother, who must nurture the young through a long period of immaturity. The main components of human milk are listed in Table 1–1. The water content is high and, in comparison with cow milk, the solute load very low—a significant protection against diseases that cause dehydration manifested by anorexia, vomiting, and diarrhea. As an example, the protein proportion of calories is low (6 to 8 per cent), but the nutritional quality is very high and obviously sufficient for infants born at or near term (although too low for the <1500 g premature infant).

   The fat content of breast milk is high: 51 per cent of calories, with adequate amounts of linolenic and linoleic acids. About 14.2 per cent of the fat is polyunsaturated, 41.6 percent monosaturated, and 44.2 per cent saturated.

   The carbohydrate (CHO) is lactose, 41 per cent of calories. This nutrient transports some minerals and plays an important role as the substrate for the bacterial flora that emerges in the intestine of the breast-fed infant, namely *Lactobacillus bifidus*. The bacteria, in turn, benefit the infant host by repressing growth of gram-negative organisms that are potential pathogens.

   The vitamin content is complete except for vitamin D, the natural source of which is sunlight, stimulating cells in the dermis to produce the prohormone cholecalciferol. Breast-fed infants should routinely be given vitamin D supplementation (400 U/day) unless smog-free sunlight is assured for those with light-colored skin (see Chapter 1).

   The mineral content is appropriate for the term or near-term infant except for iron. The small amount of iron in human milk is exceptionally well absorbed, and the term infant has iron stored in the blood sufficient for an average of 3 months. By 5 months at most, breast-fed infants require another source of iron from solid foods. The phosphorus content is adequate for the term infant but is low for the low birth weight (<1500 g) infant.

   b. Immunologic

   Breast milk contains secretory IgA antibodies that prevent microorganisms from adhering to the intestinal cell wall. Live macrophages, lysozyme, and lactoferrin present in the milk may also play a protective role against intestinal infection. There are data that show fewer episodes of otitis media and other respiratory illness occur in breast-fed infants. This may be the result of *breast feeding* (single provider and positioning) rather than a property of *breast milk*. The anti-infection benefits are maximal for the first 3 months.

   c. Psychological

   The process of successful breast feeding provides a very satisfying experience for mother and infant. Nontheless, a woman who cannot or does not wish to breast feed may achieve a similar sense of accomplishment while providing affectionate care for her baby.

   d. Contraindications

   Among the very few contraindications to breast feeding are HIV infection and active tuberculosis in the mother. Antineoplastic and antithyroid drug therapy for the mother are others. A very high store of PCBs or organic mercury in the mother's fat tissue is a contraindication seen in unusual circumstance. The lower levels of pesticides similarly stored are below the danger level.

   e. Technique

   The stimulus to a good milk supply is suckling to empty the breasts. Feeding should be commenced, when possible, a few hours after birth. Initially only 5 minutes or so at each breast is required until the milk supply is established at 2 to 3 days. The milk

TABLE 1–1.   CONTENT OF HUMAN MILK VS. COW MILK

COMPONENT	UNITS	HUMAN MILK	COW MILK
Energy	calories/L	740	671
Protein	%/cal	8	22
Fat	%/cal	51	49
CHO	%/cal	41	29
Casein	g/L	3.7	25
Lactalbumin	g/L	3.6	2.4
Lactoglobulin	g/L	3.4	1.7
Na	mEq/L	6	22
Cl	mEq/L	10	30
K	mEq/L	12	37
Ca	mEq/L	340	1200
P	mEq/L	150	930

TABLE 1–2. CONTENT OF INFANT FEEDINGS

NAME	% OF CALORIES P	Fat	CHO	cal/ml	Na mEq/L	mEq/100 cal	Cl mEq/L	mEq/100 cal	K mEq/L	mEq/100 cal	Ca mg/L	mg/100 cal	P mg/L	mg/100 cal	RENAL SOLUTE mOsm/100 cal
Human milk	8	51	41	0.67	6	0.9	10	1.4	12	1.8	340	51	150	22.4	12
Whole cow milk	22	49	29	0.67	22	3.3	30	4.5	37	5.5	1200	180	930	139	33
Skim cow milk	40	5	55	0.34	22	6.6	30	9.0	37	11	1200	360	930	278	66
Evaporated cow milk: H_2O 1:1 + 5 g CHO/dl	17	37	46	0.9	22	2.4	30	3.3	37	4.1	1200	133	930	103	24
EM:H_2O 1:1 + 10 g CHO/dl	11	33	56	1.1	22	2	30	2.7	37	3.4	1200	109	930	85	20
Infant formula*	10	50	40	0.67	8	1.2	12	1.8	15	2.4	520	78	400	60	16
Infant formula† 5 g CHO/dl	8	42	50	0.87	8	0.9	12	1.4	15	1.7	520	60	400	46	12
Protein hydrolysate; no lactose	13	36	51	0.67	13	1.9	16	2.4	18	2.7	600	90	400	60	19

*Representative of the major commercial infant formulas.

†The infant feedings above illustrate the problem in trying to reduce sodium and other renal solute while maintaining an adequate protein intake. The practical minimum of protein is about 8% of total daily calories when from a high quality animal source (12–15% from vegetable sources). When cow milk or other protein is used (as contrasted to human), it is wiser to use a higher minimum because digestion and absorption may be inefficient, though theoretically an even lower protein percentage intake may be successful. The usual modifier for feedings is carbohydrate which produces no renal solute. Renal solute comes from protein, primarily as urea; and from minerals, primarily sodium salts. Note that when the sodium load is reduced by carbohydrate dilution so is the phosphorus load which may also be important in other conditions. Note also that skim milk, when a major portion of the diet, is a particularly poor feeding, providing a maximum stress to water balance. (From Finberg L, Kravath RE, Hellerstein S (eds): Water and Electrolytes in Pediatrics: Physiology, Pathophysiology, and Treatment, 2nd ed. Philadelphia, WB Saunders, 1993.)

ejection reflex and let-down (milk engorgement in the presence of the infant) are signs of successful initiation of feeding. The infant should feed approximately every 3 hours and should be offered both breasts, emptying at least one. For the first 6 weeks it is best not to offer a supplementary or alternative feeding. After that time a relief bottle may be used to provide greater maternal freedom without loss of milk supply. Pumping of the breast milk with temporary storage and later feeding may also be used to increase the mother's mobility and her ability to work, if desired.

2. Formula Feeding

a. Proprietary infant formula

This product is regulated in the United States by the standards set by the Infant Formula Act of 1980 (revised 1986). Several manufacturers produce a nutritious milk derived from cow milk, with vegetable fat substituted for butter and with the mineral and vitamin content adjusted for a complete feeding. Iron and vitamin D are included. An inadvisable low-iron formulation is also available; some practitioners continue to prescribe it in the mistaken belief, from misinterpretation of data, that iron in recommended levels causes gastointestinal symptoms. Careful studies thoroughly contradict this belief.

b. Evaporated milk mixtures

Once the standard feeding for formula-fed infants, these feedings are now used for about 5 per cent of infants in the United States. Their advantage is that they have the lowest cost of any milk feeding. When the evaporated milk is reconstituted by the addition of water it is cow milk with the protein altered (by heat) to provide a soft curd and with vitamin D added (400 U/reconstituted liter [quart]). Because of the high renal solute (Table 1–2) and high phosphate content it is desirable to dilute the milk with an additional 5 per cent carbohydrate by weight to reduce the solute and phosphate per calorie. The added carbohydrate may be sucrose, corn syrup (e.g., Karo), or dextromaltose. It is customary to also add water to dilute the energy concentration to that of natural human or cow milk, approximately 0.68 cal/ml. Iron supplementation is achieved by introducing solid foods with iron by 5 months. The intake volume should not exceed 1 L (quart) per day lest iron deficiency be promoted. There is no vitamin C in evaporated milk and therefore must be supplemented.

c. Whole cow milk

Although the pasteurized, homogenized, vitamin D–supplemented milk commercially available today is better, and better tolerated, than the raw or even pasteurized milk of many years ago, it still has the disadvantages of a high renal solute load and no iron; when taken in amounts of a liter or more per day, it can cause intestinal bleeding. Most experts believe that it should not be introduced as the milk of the diet until 1 year of age, although small amounts after 6 months of age are clearly not harmful.

3. Supplements

a. Vitamin D for breast-fed infants—400 U/day.

b. Vitamin C for evaporated milk formula–fed infants—30 mg/day. Orange juice may be substituted—120 ml (4 oz) daily after a few weeks of age.

c. Iron should be added by introduction of solid foods at 5 months. This may be delayed a little longer for those fed the fortified infant formula.

d. Fluoride supplementation is advisable after 6 months for prevention of dental caries. Some advocate earlier usage of 0.25 mg daily for breast-fed infants and for those in locales where the water supply has <0.3 ppm of fluoride. Information about the latter is available from the local health department.

4. Solid foods

   a. The infant's swallowing ability matures at about 5 months for handling solid foods. This coincides with the time that many mothers can no longer provide full energy needs from their supply of breast milk.

   b. It is best to introduce new foods one at a time. The slightly sweet pureed fruits and vegetables are good beginning foods, although iron-fortified cereal has often been given as the earliest solid. In any event, iron-containing food should be introduced early. The best such food—meats—are often not well liked by infants, but mixtures of meat and vegetables are better accepted. Egg yolk may be given after 5 to 6 months, but egg white should be withheld until at least 1 year of age, as it is a potential allergen that may cause fatal anaphylaxis. By 9 months of age it is appropriate to have at least 35 to 40 per cent of calories derived from sources other than breast milk or formula.

Feeding in the Second Year of Life and for Toddlers

1. The diet after the first year should be similar in composition to that of the older child or adult, except that it must be prepared in such a way that the child can chew and swallow easily and without danger. The rate of growth will have slowed markedly so that the weight gain for the second year will be only 2 to 3 kg at most. Accordingly, the appetite is reduced, and there may be occasional periods when the intake becomes low for a few days or only a few favorite foods seem to be wanted. This behavior is normal and calls for no corrective measures. Parents should avoid making eating the focus of conflict with the child. Food should be offered and, if not eaten in a reasonable period, should be withdrawn without comment.

2. Foods likely to be aspirated or to cause choking are to be consistently avoided. Peanuts in particular (although not peanut butter in small quantity) and nuts in general can be delayed until age 5 or 6 years. Pieces of sausage (hot dogs) present a choking danger. These precautions continue through the toddler years, with changes in the form of food offered following the child's ability to handle them.

Middle Childhood and Adolescence

1. Growth needs

   The diet at this stage becomes similar to that proper for an adult. Energy intake should be sufficient to support growth, generally along the percentile growth curve established during the first few years. Variety in foods is the key to optimal nutrition. Energy, protein, and accessory substances should receive primary attention. If a vegetarian regimen is chosen, it should be one that permits milk and eggs as a source of animal protein. If only vegetable sources are to be offered, the percentage of protein calories must be higher (15 per cent vs. 10 per cent). Also, supplemental vitamin B_{12} must be given in some form, as this vitamin does not occur in vegetables. The principal vegetables must be combined—a grain and a bean—to avoid amino acid deficiency. Grains are generally deficient for human nutrition in lysine, and beans are deficient in methionine. Depending on preparation, corn may be deficient in tryptophane. Adolescents have an increased energy requirement starting in prepuberty and extending through the period of rapid growth. Adequate calcium should be ensured, especially for girls.

2. Prevention of adult degenerative disease

   Current advice to adults stresses avoidance of hypercholesterolemia. The advice consists of limiting calories of fat to 30 per cent of intake, with one third of this (10 per cent) as polyunsaturated fat, one third as monosaturated, and no more than 10 per cent of calories as saturated fat. Whether these recommendations are important in childhood is unknown. Certainly, for the first 2 years or so they would be unwise, because the high energy–containing fat is needed to support growth for the volume of food that an infant can consume. After that, if there is evidence of susceptibility to atherosclerotic disease based on a history of early (<50 years) heart disease in a first-degree relative or of known high cholesterol levels in a parent, it may be appropriate to advise the adult on a prudent diet regimen for the child. Controversy exists about this and related issues for children. The advice, if given, will be harmless provided that the family does not reduce fat calories so far that growth is impeded. Regular visits, at least annually with height and weight measurements, are mandatory if such a regimen is undertaken.

Bibliography

Kleinman RE (ed): Pediatric Nutrition Handbook, 4th ed. Elk Grove Village, IL, American Academy of Pediatrics, 1997.

Lawrence RA: Breast Feeding: A Guide for the Medical Profession, 4th ed. St. Louis, CV Mosby, 1994.

2 Immunizations

Moses Grossman

Routine immunization of all children is universally accepted as a fundamental step in the prevention of many childhood diseases. Smallpox has been eradicated from the world. Poliomyelitis has been eliminated from the Western Hemisphere. Measles has become a rare disease in the developed world. Recent advances in molecular biology and genetics hold a bright promise of major advances to come. Varicella vaccine has recently been released. Many vaccines are being improved, and many new vaccines are in the development pipeline. The advances in vaccine development need to be matched by our improved ability to administer these immunizations in a timely manner to all children and by our continued ability to pay for them.

Authoritative statements about immunization can be found in the recommendations of the Committee on Infectious Diseases of the American Academy of Pediatrics (Red Book) and of the Advisory Committee on Immunization Practices published in the *Morbidity and Mortality Weekly Report* of the Centers for Disease Control and Prevention (CDC).

Active Immunization

Active immunization involves the administration of an antigen resulting in the production of protective antibodies. Many antigens are used: viruses, both killed and attenuated; portions of viruses; bacteria, both modified and killed; and bacterial products. Thus, successful active immunization requires that the antigen be in optimal condition and be appropriately delivered to the host, who in turn is able to produce protective antibodies.

1. The vaccine
   a. The conditions of vaccine storage supplied on the label must be strictly observed. Live attenuated viruses need to remain live and to replicate when administered, in order to induce antibody formation. Correct administration of vaccines is equally crucial. Vaccines are designed, made, and licensed with a particular mode of administration in mind (oral, intramuscular [IM], or subcutaneous [SC]). Protective antibody production depends on correct administration.
   b. Almost all vaccines may have some undesirable effects in addition to their protective ones. These adverse effects can be very minor, such as low-grade fever or soreness at the site of administration. The adverse effects can also be major, such as paralysis. The protection afforded by a vaccine is usually not complete. Many vaccines are 90 to 95 per cent effective. The balance between protection and adverse reactions is often called the risk-benefit ratio.
   c. The clonal nature of the immune system permits the simultaneous administration of multiple antigens, with protective antibodies developing to each of these antigens. Our current childhood immunization schedule is based on this principle.
   d. The maintenance of protective levels of antibodies often depends on continuing or episodic exposure to the antigen. This is achieved by periodic boosters.

2. The host
   Active immunization requires the host to produce antibodies in response to an antigenic stimulus. This ability could be impaired by a number of factors, such as:
   a. Congenital immunodeficiency. Although the condition is relatively rare, some children are born with defects of the immune system, often genetically mediated, such as the severe combined immunodeficiency syndrome. Affected infants are unable to produce antibodies. Furthermore, they may have very severe side effects after the administration of live virus vaccines because of their inability to handle even an attenuated virus infection.
   b. Acquired immunodeficiency. The principal cause of acquired immunodeficiency is HIV infection. The infected host's ability to reach a protective level of antibodies is dependent on the stage of the disease and is very compromised in the advanced stages. Other viral infections, such as measles, often produce a mild, temporary immune defect.
   c. Age. The normal infant can respond to protein antigens at any age. However, adequate response to a polysaccharide antigen does not occur until the child is 18 to 24 months old. Thus capsular antigens have to be conjugated with protein to allow early administration.
   d. The nutritional state of the infant has a significant impact on response to immunization.
   e. Allergy to vaccine components may produce mild to very severe side effects.

3. Legal obligations
   a. Record keeping. The health provider is required to maintain a permanent record of the vaccines administered to each child, including dates and the exact type of vaccine used. These records are very important in order to keep each child's immunization up to date, to administer appropriate boosters, to support school entry, and to enable the family to be compensated in case of a severe reaction. It is also important to provide the family with an ongoing duplicate immunization record.
   b. Informed consent. Parental permission for immunizations is required both ethically and legally. Benefits as well as risks need to be explained. The CDC has camera-ready forms in various languages available for the practitioner.

c. Reporting adverse reactions to the standard immunizing agents for children is required by federal law. The Vaccine Adverse Effects Reporting System can be reached at 1-800-822-7967.

d. Vaccine injury compensation for serious adverse reactions is available through a special program within the Health Resources and Services Administration in Rockville, MD.

4. Vaccines in routine use in childhood

a. The vaccines discussed in this chapter are recommended for the universal immunization of all children in the United States as of the beginning of 1996. Most of these immunizations are also required for school entry. The immunizing agents are listed in Table 2–1. The currently recommended schedule for immunization is given in Figure 2–1.

b. It is important to accomplish immunizations in a timely manner. Frequent review of immunization status and catching up on missed immunizations are important for the child's health as well as for public health.

5. Vaccines for selective use

Several vaccines are not used universally but are recommended only for certain peculiarly susceptible children.

a. Influenza vaccine. This should be used annually to protect children with significant cardiopulmonary disease. The split virus (viral components) is more suitable for children.

b. Pneumococcal polysaccharide vaccine should be used to protect children with sickle cell disease as well as asplenic children. Currently the vaccine can be used only for children over 2 years of age. A protein-conjugated vaccine, expected in the near future, will be usable in infancy.

c. BCG (bacille Calmette-Guérin) is an attenuated strain of *Mycobacterium bovis*. It is used extensively throughout the world for protection against tuberculosis. In the United States it is used infrequently and only in special family settings.

d. Rabies vaccine, a tissue culture–grown attenuated virus, is used for the protection of children exposed to rabies through animal bites.

Passive Immunization

Passive immunization entails the administration of antibody to the susceptible host with a view of preventing an infection to which the recipient has already been exposed or expects to be exposed in the near future. The principal *advantage* of passive immunization is that the antibodies are preformed and can be protective as soon as they are administered. This is particularly helpful when exposure has already occurred and protective antibodies cannot be expected in response to active immunization to afford timely protection. The principal *disadvantage* of passive immunization is that the administered antibodies usually last only 6 to 8 weeks. Additionally, the protection is limited to humoral antibodies and almost exclusively to the IgG class of antibodies. Passive antibodies can be administered as human immune globulin or as sera of animal origin.

1. Human immune globulin

Human immune globulin is manufactured from pooled (at least 1000 donors per lot of final product) adult human plasma. The level of specific protective antibodies of each lot is variable. The human plasma is prescreened to ensure the absence of infectious agents. Peak antibody levels are achieved 3 to 5 days after intramuscular (IM) administration. The half-life of the material is 3 to 4 weeks. Regular immune globulin should always be administered intramuscularly. Several types of immune globulin are available.

a. Regular immune globulin is used for the prevention of hepatitis A as well as measles.

TABLE 2–1. ROUTINE CHILDHOOD IMMUNIZATIONS

VACCINE	SYMBOL	ACTIVE COMPONENT	NOTES
Hepatitis B	Hep B	Recombinant surface antigen of hepatitis B virus	Minor reactions only.
Diphtheria	D	Diphtheria toxoid	Usually administered as DTP combination.
	d	Adult type diphtheria toxoid	Further combinations with Hib and Hep B also available.
Tetanus	T	Tetanus toxoid	
Pertussis	P	Whole cell killed *B. pertussis* bacteria	Acellular pertussis (aP) has fewer side
	aP	Acellular—several immunogens derived from *B. pertussis*	effects.
Haemophilus influenzae type b	Hib	Polysaccharide capsule conjugated to protein	Three conjugated vaccines are licensed. Schedules are slightly different.
Poliomyelitis	OPV	Attenuated live virus (3 types)	Schedules combining OPV and IPV may
	IPV	Inactivated (killed) virus (3 types)	be recommended in near future. Immunocompromised individuals (including HIV-infected children) should not receive OPV.
Measles	MMR	Inactivated live viruses	Immunocompromised individuals should
Mumps		Usually given in combination, but single components are	not receive live vaccines. However,
Rubella		available	measles vaccine is recommended for HIV-positive children because the hazard of the disease is greater.
Varicella-zoster	VZV	Inactivated live virus	Immunocompromised individuals should not receive live vaccines.

OPV, Oral polio vaccine; IPV, inactivated polio vaccine.

Vaccines are listed under the routinely recommended ages. ⬜Bars⬜ *indicate range of acceptable ages for vaccination.* ⬛Shaded bars⬛ *indicate catch-up vaccination: at 11-12 years of age, hepatitis B vaccine should be administered to children not previously vaccinated, and Varicella Zoster Virus vaccine should be administered to children not previously vaccinated who lack a reliable history of chickenpox.*

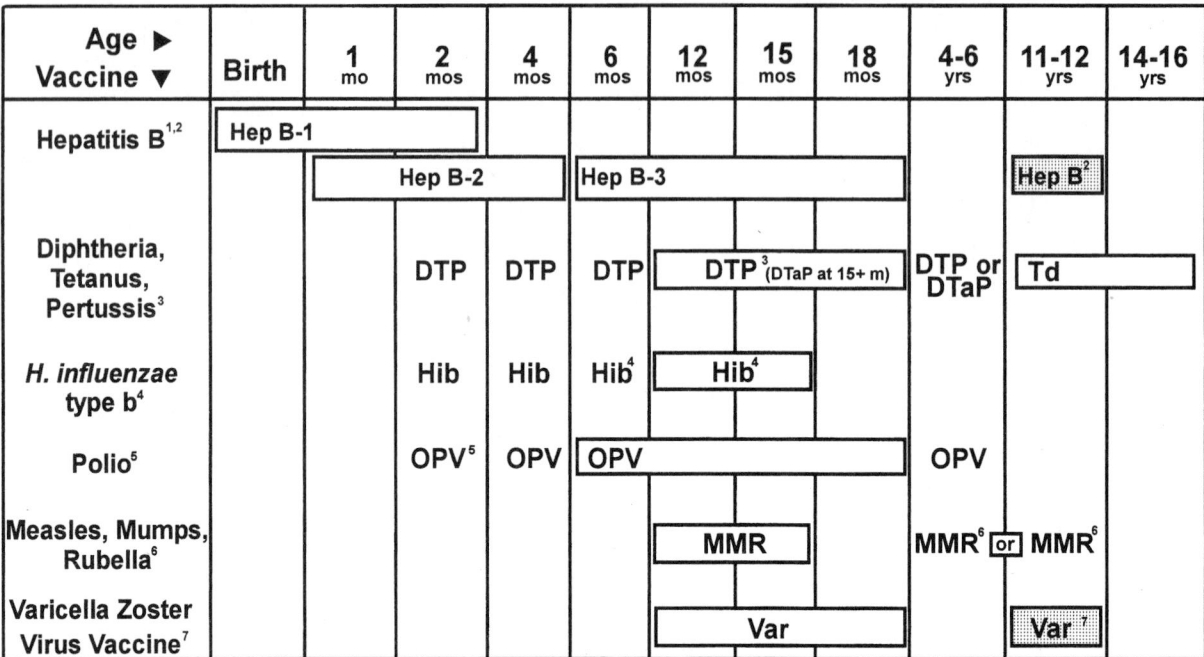

Approved by the Advisory Committee on Immunization Practices (ACIP), the American Academy of Pediatrics (AAP), and the American Academy of Family Physicians (AAFP).

[1] Infants born to HBsAg-negative mothers should receive 2.5 µg of Merck vaccine (Recombivax HB) or 10 µg of SmithKline Beecham (SB) vaccine (Engerix-B). The 2nd dose should be administered ≥1 mo after the 1st dose.
Infants born to HBsAg-positive mothers should receive 0.5 mL hepatitis B immune globulin (HBIG) within 12 hrs of birth, and either 5 µg of Merck vaccine (Recombivax HB) or 10 µg of SB vaccine (Engerix-B) at a separate site. The 2nd dose is recommended at 1-2 mos of age and the 3rd dose at 6 mos of age.
Infants born to mothers whose HBsAg status is unknown should receive either 5 µg of Merck vaccine (Recombivax HB) or 10 µg of SB vaccine (Engerix-B) within 12 hrs of birth. The 2nd dose of vaccine is recommended at 1 mo of age and the 3rd dose at 6 mos of age.

[2] Adolescents who have not previously received 3 doses of hepatitis B vaccine should initiate or complete the series at the 11-12 year-old visit. The 2nd dose should be administered at least 1 mo after the 1st dose, and the 3rd dose should be administered at least 4 mos after the 1st dose and at least 2 mos after the 2nd dose.

[3] DTP4 may be administered at 12 mos of age, if at least 6 mos have elapsed since DTP3. DTaP (diphtheria and tetanus toxoids and acellular pertussis vaccine) is licensed for the 4th and/or 5th vaccine dose(s) for children aged ≥15 mos and may be preferred for these doses in this age group. Td (tetanus and diphtheria toxoids, adsorbed, for adult use) is recommended at 11-12 years of age if at least 5 years have elapsed since the last dose of DTP, DTaP, or DT.

[4] Three *H. influenzae* type b (Hib) conjugate vaccines are licensed for infant use. If PRP-OMP (PedvaxHIB [Merck]) is administered at 2 and 4 mos of age, a dose at 6 mos is not required. After completing the primary series, any Hib conjugate vaccine may be used as a booster.

[5] Oral poliovirus vaccine (OPV) is recommended for routine infant vaccination. Inactivated poliovirus vaccine (IPV) is recommended for persons with a congenital or acquired immune deficiency disease or an altered immune status as a result of disease or immunosuppressive therapy, as well as their household contacts, and is an acceptable alternative for other persons. The primary 3-dose series for IPV should be given with a minimum interval of 4 wks between the 1st and 2nd doses and 6 mos between the 2nd and 3rd doses.

[6] The 2nd dose of MMR is routinely recommended at 4-6 yrs of age or at 11-12 yrs of age, but may be administered at any visit, provided at least 1 mo has elapsed since receipt of the 1st dose.

[7] Varicella zoster virus vaccine (Var) can be administered to susceptible children any time after 12 months of age. Unvaccinated children who lack a reliable history of chickenpox should be vaccinated at the 11-12 year-old visit.

Figure 2–1 Recommended Childhood Immunization Schedule, United States, July–December 1996.

b. Intravenous immune globulin (IGIV) is further purified gamma globulin suitable for intravenous use. It is considerably more expensive and is intended to be used in large quantities. It is not suitable for intramuscular administration. The current indications for this product are limited—for the protection of very small premature babies, HIV-infected babies, and bone marrow transplantation recipients. It is also used as replacement therapy in antibody deficiency disorders and for the management of Kawasaki disease.

c. Specific immune globulins are prepared from the pooled plasma of donors who have a very high level of the particular antibody. This is achieved either by selection of donors (varicella-zoster) or by actively immunizing donors (tetanus). The following specific immune globulins are available:

(1) Hepatitis B immune globulin (HBIG)

(2) Rabies immune globulin (RIG)

(3) Tetanus immune globulin (TIG)

(4) Varicella-zoster immune globulin (VZIG)

(5) Botulinum immune globulin is available but has not yet been licensed.

These specific agents are for intramuscular use. Additionally, intravenous cytomegalovirus immune globulin (CMV IVG) is available.

d. Adverse reactions. The adverse reactions to IM globulin are usually minor, such as pain at the site of administration. Rarely, more severe reactions may occur, such as chills, fever, and, very rarely, anaphylaxis and shocklike symptoms. Intravenous globulin results in somewhat more frequent reactions (5 per cent). These for the most part are also minor and self limited: fever, chills, myalgia, nausea. Vasomotor reactions and anaphylaxis may also occur on very rare occasions.

2. Animal antisera

These products are generally prepared from the serum of hyperimmunized horses. They are always inferior to products prepared from human plasma, and the latter should be used in preference, if available. The recipient should *always be tested for sensitivity* to animal serum, and suitable anaphylaxis precautions must be taken. The following products are available:

a. Botulinum antitoxin types A, B, E.

b. Diphtheria antitoxin

c. Tetanus antitoxin

d. Antirabies serum

Foreign Travel

Travel abroad, particularly to tropical and developing countries, often entails increased exposure to infections. Thus, a review and update of immunizations prior to departure is in order.

1. Routine immunizations. Many of the common childhood diseases such as measles are much more common abroad than in the United States. A review of the current immunization status and the need for boosters should therefore be undertaken.

2. Special immunizations. These should be considered, depending on the itinerary, the current requirements of the countries to be visited, and the presence of outbreaks. The CDC publication *Health Information for International Travel* as well as a CDC hotline provide current information about these issues. Immunizations to be considered include the following:

a. Yellow fever immunization is advisable and often required by some countries as a condition for entry. This live attenuated virus vaccine presents an increased hazard for infants younger than 6 months of age.

b. Japanese encephalitis is spread by mosquitos and occurs in certain parts of Asia. An inactivated virus vaccine is available.

c. Gastrointestinal infections are particularly common among travelers and best prevented by careful handling of food. Typhoid vaccine is available for certain travelers. Cholera vaccine provides very low protection and is not recommended.

d. Meningococcal vaccine should be considered for children traveling to areas of high prevalence.

e. Immune globulin might be considered for protection against acquiring hepatitis A infection. Hepatitis A vaccine is now licensed also.

f. In considering immunization requirements for travelers, the possible need for malaria prophylaxis should be reviewed.

Developing Vaccines

1. Vaccine development is proceeding at a rapid pace. Many new vaccines are in various stages of development. Among them are vaccines against Lyme disease, malaria, herpes simplex, respiratory syncytial virus, and rotavirus.

2. The conjugation of pneumococcal and meningococcal polysaccharide vaccines to proteins will enable these protective vaccines to be used in infants.

3. One of the many challenges of vaccine development is to ensure that such new vaccines will be usable and affordable in developing countries, where they are most needed.

B Bibliography

Ad Hoc Working Group for the Development of Standards for Pediatric Immunization Practices: Standards for pediatric immunization practices. JAMA 1993;269:1817–1822.

American Academy of Pediatrics: Report of Committee on Infectious Diseases. Elk Grove Village, IL, American Academy of Pediatrics, 1994.

Centers for Disease Control: General recommendations on immunization. MMWR 1994;43:RR1.

Centers for Disease Control: Recommended childhood immunization schedule—United States, 1995. MMWR 1995;44:RR-5.

Gilsdorf JR: Vaccines: Moving into the molecular era. J Pediatr 1994;125:339.

3 Growth and Development

Laurence Finberg

Following the growth and development of the infant and child is the essence of pediatric practice, involving the child's interaction with the environment and, particularly, the ways that diseases impact and are impacted on. Accordingly, knowledge of the normal range of variation for physical measures and developmental milestones is essential.

1. Anthropomorphic measures
   a. Height (length) and weight

   Probably the best way to follow linear growth and mass accretion is the use of growth curves showing percentile tracks (Figs. 3–1 through 3–6). Each patient's measurements should be plotted sequentially over the entire growth period. For the first 2 years the linear measure is length; after 2 years, height is measured. Head circumference measurement is also valuable, particularly during the first year. The growth curve charts are perhaps the single most important tool for pediatric use.

   Movement across two percentile tracks, particularly on the linear curve, should prompt the clinician to search diligently for a cause. Failure to thrive means either primary nutritional deprivation or illness, usually chronic. The underlying disorder may be renal, gastrointestinal, neurologic, cardiac, or metabolic or may be systemic infection; the box at left below gives examples for the early years.

   b. Dentition

   The deciduous teeth erupt sequentially and are shed in approximately the order shown in Table 3–1, followed by eruption of the secondary dentition. Calcification of the deciduous teeth begins in the fifth fetal month. Calcification of the permanent teeth begins in the third to fourth month of life for the incisors and continues sequentially for up to 10 years for initiation and up to 20 ± 2 years for completion of the third molars.

2. Developmental milestones

   As the child grows, he or she also matures. There are progressive changes in motor function, language development, other cognitive functions, and social adaptation. These changes, with moderate variation, occur as shown in Tables 3–2 and 3–3.

System	Disease Examples
Renal	Renal tubular acidosis
	Congenital cystic disease
Gastrointestinal	Celiac disease
	Inflammatory bowel disease
Neurologic	Diencephalic syndrome
	Tay-Sachs disease
Cardiac	Acyanotic congenital heart disorder
Metabolic	Hypothyroidism
	Hyperthyroidism
	Fructose intolerance
Infections	Tuberculosis
	HIV

TABLE 3–1. USUAL DENTITION MILESTONES

DECIDUOUS TEETH	AGE AT ERUPTION		AGE AT SHEDDING	
	Maxillary	Mandible	Maxillary	Mandible
Central incisors	6–8 mo	5–7 mo	7–8 yr	6–7 yr
Lateral incisors	6–11 mo	7–10 mo	8–9 yr	7–8 yr
Cuspids	16–20 mo	16–20 mo	11–12 yr	9–11 yr
First molars	10–16 mo	10–16 mo	10–11 yr	10–12 yr
Second molars	20–30 mo	10–16 mo	10–11 yr	10–12 yr

PERMANENT TEETH				
Central incisors	7–8 yr		6–7 yr	
Lateral incisors	8–9 yr		7–8 yr	
Cuspids	11–12 yr		9–11 yr	
First bicuspids	10–11 yr		10–12 yr	
Second bicuspids	10–12 yr		11–13 yr	
First molars	6–7 yr		6–7 yr	
Second molars	12–13 yr		12–13 yr	
Third molars	17–22 yr		17–22 yr	

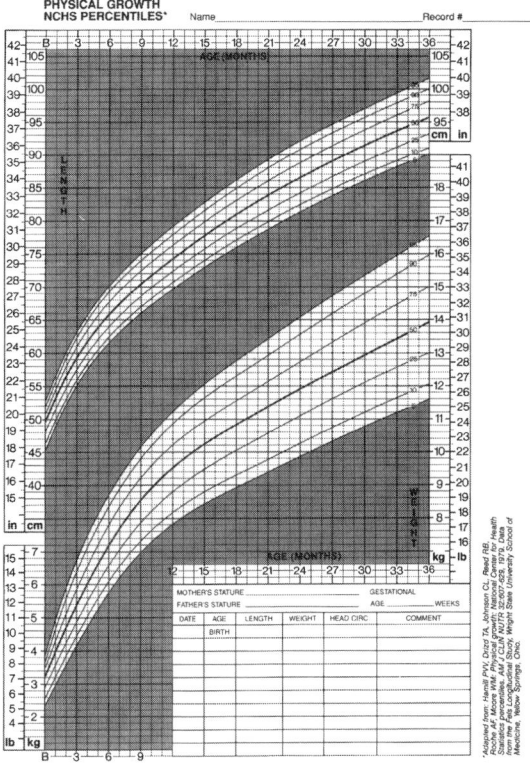

Figure 3–1

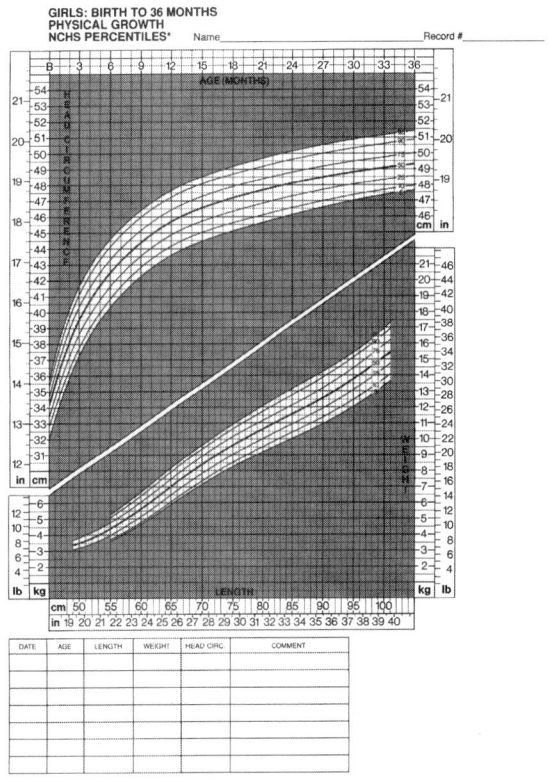

Figure 3–2

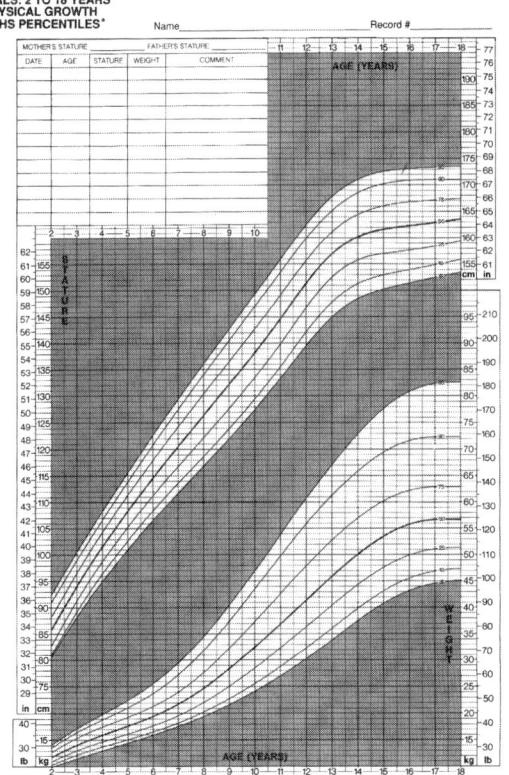

Figure 3–3

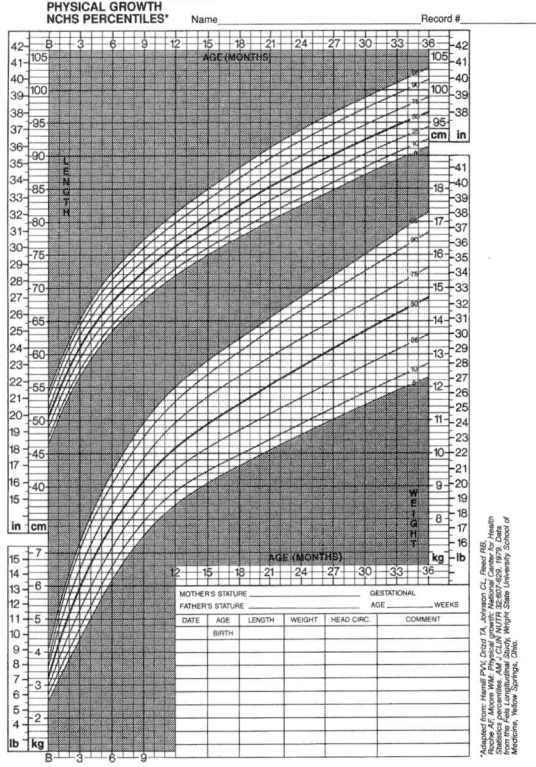

Figure 3–4

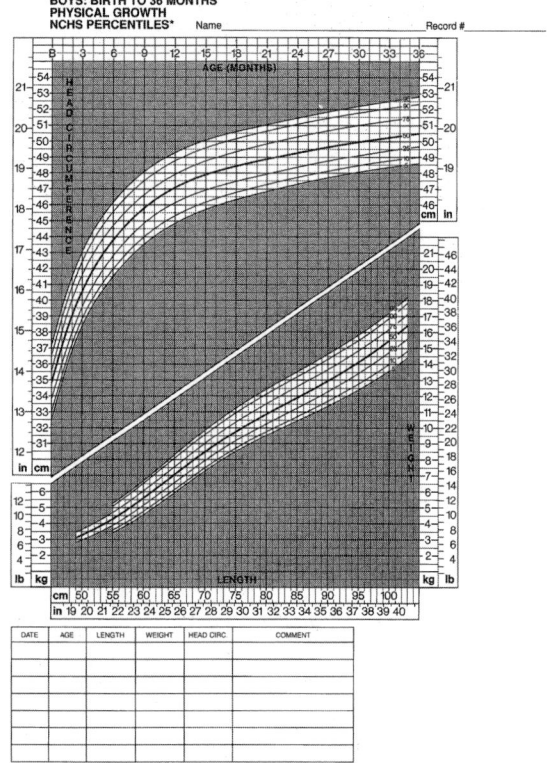

Figure 3–5

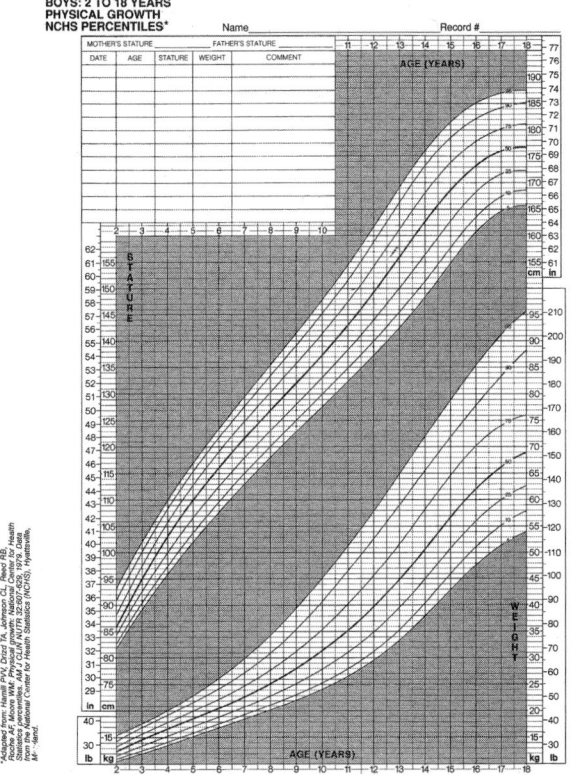

Figure 3–6

TABLE 3–2. EMERGING PATTERNS OF BEHAVIOR DURING THE FIRST YEAR OF LIFE*

NEONATAL PERIOD (1ST 4 WK)

Prone:	Lies in flexed attitude; turns head from side to side; head sags on ventral suspension
Supine:	Generally flexed and a little stiff
Visual:	May fixate face or light in line of vision; "doll's-eye" movement of eyes on turning of the body
Reflex:	Moro response active; stepping and placing reflexes; grasp reflex active
Social:	Visual preference for human face

AT 4 WK

Prone:	Legs more extended; holds chin up; turns head; head lifted momentarily to plane of body on ventral suspension
Supine:	Tonic neck posture predominates; supple and relaxed; head lags on pull to sitting position
Visual:	Watches person; follows moving object
Social:	Body movements in cadence with voice of other in social contact; beginning to smile

AT 8 WK

Prone:	Raises head slightly farther; head sustained in plane of body on ventral suspension
Supine:	Tonic neck posture predominates; head lags on pull to sitting position
Visual:	Follows moving object 180 degrees
Social:	Smiles on social contact; listens to voice and coos

AT 12 WK

Prone:	Lifts head and chest, arms extended; head above plane of body on ventral suspension
Supine:	Tonic neck posture predominates; reaches toward and misses objects; waves at toy
Sitting:	Head lag partially compensated on pull to sitting position; early head control with bobbing motion; back rounded
Reflex:	Typical Moro response has not persisted; makes defensive movements or selective withdrawal reactions
Social:	Sustained social contact; listens to music; says "aah," "ngah"

AT 16 WK

Prone:	Lift head and chest, head in approximately vertical axis; legs extended
Supine:	Symmetric posture predominates, hands in midline; reaches and grasps objects and brings them to mouth
Sitting:	No head lag on pull to sitting position; head steady, tipped forward; enjoys sitting with full truncal support
Standing:	When held erect, pushes with feet
Adaptive:	Sees pellet, but makes no move to it
Social:	Laughs out loud; may show displeasure if social contact is broken; excited at sight of food

AT 28 WK

Prone:	Rolls over; pivots; crawls or creep-crawls (Knobloch)
Supine:	Lifts head; rolls over; squirming movements
Sitting:	Sits briefly, with support of pelvis; leans forward on hands; back rounded
Standing:	May support most of weight; bounces actively
Adaptive:	Reaches out for and grasps large object; transfers objects from hand to hand; grasp uses radial palm; rakes at pellet
Language:	Polysyllabic vowel sounds formed
Social:	Prefers mother; babbles; enjoys mirror; responds to changes in emotional content of social contact

AT 40 WK

Sitting:	Sits up alone and indefinitely without support, back straight
Standing:	Pulls to standing position; "cruises" or walks holding onto furniture
Motor:	Creeps or crawls
Adaptive:	Grasps objects with thumb and forefinger; pokes at things with forefinger; picks up pellet with assisted pincer movement; uncovers hidden toy; attempts to retrieve dropped object; releases object grasped by other person
Language:	Repetitive consonant sounds (mama, dada)
Social:	Responds to sound of name; plays peek-a-boo or pat-a-cake; waves bye-bye

AT 52 WK (1 YR)

Motor:	Walks with one hand held (48 wk); rises independently, takes several steps (Knobloch)
Adaptive:	Picks up pellet with unassisted pincer movement of forefinger and thumb; releases object to other person on request or gesture
Language:	A few words besides "mama," "dada"
Social:	Plays simple ball game; makes postural adjustment to dressing

*Data are derived from those of Gesell (as revised by Knobloch), Shirley, Provence, Wolf, Bailey, and others.

TABLE 3–3. EMERGING PATTERNS OF BEHAVIOR FROM 1 TO 5 YEARS OF AGE*

15 MO

Motor:	Walks alone; crawls up stairs
Adaptive:	Makes tower of 3 cubes; makes a line with crayon; inserts pellet in bottle
Language:	Jargon; follows simple commands; may name a familiar object (ball)
Social:	Indicates some desires or needs by pointing; hugs parents

18 MO

Motor:	Runs stiffly; sits on small chair; walks up stairs with one hand held; explores drawers and waste baskets
Adaptive:	Makes a tower of 4 cubes; imitates scribbling; imitates vertical stroke; dumps pellet from bottle
Language:	10 words (average); names pictures; identifies one or more parts of body
Social:	Feeds self; seeks help when in trouble; may complain when wet or soiled; kisses parent with pucker

24 MO

Motor:	Runs well; walks up and down stairs, one step at a time; opens doors; climbs on furniture; jumps
Adaptive:	Tower of 7 cubes (6 at 21 mo); circular scribbling; imitates horizontal stroke; folds paper once imitatively
Language:	Puts 3 words together (subject, verb, object)
Social:	Handles spoon well; often tells immediate experiences; helps to undress; listens to stories with pictures

30 MO

Motor:	Goes up stairs alternating feet
Adaptive:	Tower of 9 cubes; makes vertical and horizontal strokes, but generally will not join them to make a cross; imitates circular stroke, forming closed figure
Language:	Refers to self by pronoun "I"; knows full name
Social:	Helps put things away; pretends in play

36 MO

Motor:	Rides tricycle; stands momentarily on one foot
Adaptive:	Tower of 10 cubes; imitates construction of "bridge" of 3 cubes; copies a circle; imitates a cross
Language:	Knows age and sex; counts 3 objects correctly; repeats 3 numbers or a sentence of 6 syllables
Social:	Plays simple games (in "parallel" with other children); helps in dressing (unbuttons clothing and puts on shoes); washes hands

48 MO

Motor:	Hops on one foot; throws ball overhand; uses scissors to cut out pictures; climbs well
Adaptive:	Copies bridge from model; imitates construction of "gate" of 5 cubes; copies cross and square; draws a man with 2 to 4 parts besides head; names longer of 2 lines
Language:	Counts 4 pennies accurately; tells a story
Social:	Plays with several children with beginning of social interaction and role-playing; goes to toilet alone

60 MO

Motor:	Skips
Adaptive:	Draws triangle from copy; names heavier of 2 weights
Language:	Names 4 colors; repeats sentence of 10 syllables; counts 10 pennies correctly
Social:	Dresses and undresses; asks questions about meaning of words; domestic role-playing

*Data are derived from those of Gesell (as revised by Knobloch), Shirley, Provence, Wolf, Bailey, and others. After 5 years of age the Stanford-Binet, Wechsler-Bellevue, and other scales offer the most precise estimates of developmental level. In order to have their greatest values, they should be administered only by an experienced and qualified person.

4 Anticipatory Guidance

Laurence Finberg

Part of the pediatrician's responsibility in following growth and development, administering immunizing injections, and examining for and treating disorders is to anticipate the problems likely to be faced by the growing child and the family. Figure 4–1 gives a guideline schedule of visits as currently advised by the American Academy of Pediatrics.

1. Accident prevention
   a. Car seats for infants and toddlers
   b. Seat belts for older children
   c. Stairway gates for toddlers
   d. Protective covers for electrical outlets
   e. Safe toys only
      (1) No small parts that may be swallowed or aspirated
      (2) Eyes and other parts of stuffed toy animals must be secured against removal
   f. Poison prevention
      (1) Storage of cleaners, disinfectants, paints, and the like out of reach or in locked cabinets
      (2) Medicines in safe or locked cabinets. Childproof containers for frequently used medicines
      (3) Give information re accidental ingestions: e.g., use of syrup of ipecac, purchased after the 6-month visit (see Part XXII for treatment of poisons)
2. Socialization and education
   a. Advise re daycare facilities
   b. Advise re school entry and possible school phobia
   c. Advise on sequence of cognition and normal rate variation
3. Hygiene (first child)
   a. Advise on bathing and handwashing (parent and child)
   b. Care of teeth in the toddler
      (1) Fluoride
      (2) No bottle holders for milk or juice feedings
4. Nutrition appropriate to age with varied diet after first year (see Chapter 1 on feeding)
5. Inform on immunizations (see Chapter 2)
   a. What protection already given
   b. What additional injections are scheduled, and for what purpose
6. Check vision appropriate to age at each visit until reading ability is established and untroubled. Referral when problem detected.
7. Check hearing by history and age-appropriate measures. Referral when problem detected.

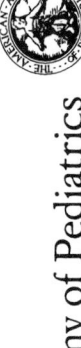

American Academy of Pediatrics

RECOMMENDATIONS FOR PREVENTIVE PEDIATRIC HEALTH CARE

Committee on Practice and Ambulatory Medicine (RE 9535)

Each child and family is unique; therefore, these **Recommendations for Preventive Pediatric Health Care** are designed for the care of children who are receiving competent parenting, have no manifestations of any important health problems, and are growing and developing in satisfactory fashion. **Additional visits may become necessary** if circumstances suggest variations from normal.

These guidelines represent a consensus by the Committee on Practice and Ambulatory Medicine in consultation with national committees and sections of the American Academy of Pediatrics. The Committee emphasizes the great importance of **continuity of care** in comprehensive health supervision and the need to avoid **fragmentation of care.**

A prenatal visit is recommended for parents who are at high risk, for first-time parents, and for those who request a conference. The prenatal visit should include anticipatory guidance and pertinent medical history. Every infant should have a newborn evaluation after birth.

AGE[4]	NEWBORN[1]	2-4d[2]	By 1mo	2mo	4mo	6mo	9mo	12mo	15mo	18mo	24mo	3y	4y	5y	6y	8y	10y	11y	12y	13y	14y	15y	16y	17y	18y	19y	20y	21y
		INFANCY[3]								EARLY CHILDHOOD[3]						MIDDLE CHILDHOOD[3]				ADOLESCENCE[3]								
HISTORY Initial/Interval	●	●	●	●	●	●	●	●	●	●	●	●	●	●	●	●	●	●	●	●	●	●	●	●	●	●	●	●
MEASUREMENTS Height and Weight	●	●	●	●	●	●	●	●	●	●	●	●	●	●	●	●	●	●	●	●	●	●	●	●	●	●	●	●
Head Circumference	●	●	●	●	●	●	●	●	●	●	●																	
Blood Pressure												●	●	●	●	●	●	●	●	●	●	●	●	●	●	●	●	●
SENSORY SCREENING Vision	S	S	S	S	S	S	S	S	S	S	S	O[5]	O	O	O	O	O	S	O	S	S	O	S	S	O	S	O	S
Hearing[6]	S/O	S	S	S	S	S	S	S	S	S	S	O	O	O	O	O	O	S	O	S	S	O	S	S	O	S	O	S
DEVELOPMENTAL/ BEHAVIORAL ASSESSMENT[7]	●	●	●	●	●	●	●	●	●	●	●	●	●	●	●	●	●	●	●	●	●	●	●	●	●	●	●	●
PHYSICAL EXAMINATION[8]	●	●	●	●	●	●	●	●	●	●	●	●	●	●	●	●	●	●	●	●	●	●	●	●	●	●	●	●
PROCEDURES – GENERAL[9] Hereditary/Metabolic Screening[10]	↕																											
Immunization[11]	●			●	●	●		●	●	●			●	●				●	●									●
Lead Screening[12]							●				*																	
Hematocrit or Hemoglobin					*														*									
Urinalysis									*					*														
PROCEDURES – PATIENTS AT RISK Tuberculin Test[15]								*			*			*	*	*	*	*	*	*	*	*	*	*	*	*	*	*
Cholesterol Screening[16]											*	*	*	*	*	*	*	*	*	*	*	*	*	*	*	*	*	*
STD Screening[17]																		*	*	*	*	*	*	*	*	*	*	*
Pelvic Exam[18]																		*	*	*	*	*	*	*	*	*	*	*
ANTICIPATORY GUIDANCE[19]	●	●	●	●	●	●	●	●	●	●	●	●	●	●	●	●	●	●	●	●	●	●	●	●	●	●	●	●
Injury Prevention[20]	●	●	●	●	●	●	●	●	●	●	●	●	●	●	●	●	●	●	●	●	●	●	●	●	●	●	●	●
INITIAL DENTAL REFERRAL[21]												●																

1. Breastfeeding encouraged and instruction and support offered.
2. For newborns discharged in less than 48 hours after delivery.
3. Developmental, psychosocial, and chronic disease issues for children and adolescents may require frequent counseling and treatment visits separate from preventive care visits.
4. If a child comes under care for the first time at any point on the schedule, or if any items are not accomplished at the suggested age, the schedule should be brought up to date at the earliest possible time.
5. If the patient is uncooperative, rescreen within six months.
6. Some experts recommend objective appraisal of hearing in the newborn period. The Joint Committee on Infant Hearing has identified patients at significant risk for hearing loss. All children meeting these criteria should be objectively screened. See the Joint Committee on Infant Hearing 1994 Position Statement.
7. By history and appropriate physical examination; if suspicious, by specific objective developmental testing.
8. At each visit, a complete physical examination is essential, with infant totally unclothed, older child undressed and suitably draped.
9. These may be modified, depending upon entry point into schedule and individual need.
10. Metabolic screening (eg, thyroid, hemoglobinopathies, PKU, galactosemia) should be done according to state law.
11. Schedule(s) per the Committee on Infectious Diseases, published periodically in Pediatrics. Every visit should be an opportunity to update and complete a child's immunizations.
12. Blood lead screen per AAP statement "Lead Poisoning: From Screening to Primary Prevention" (1993).
13. All menstruating adolescents should be screened.
14. Conduct dipstick urinalysis for leukocytes for male and female adolescents.
15. TB testing per AAP statement "Screening for Tuberculosis in Infants and Children" (1994). Testing should be done upon recognition of high risk factors. If results are negative but high risk situation continues, testing should be repeated on an annual basis.
16. Cholesterol screening for high risk patients per AAP "Statement on Cholesterol" (1992). If family history cannot be ascertained and other risk factors are present, screening should be at the discretion of the physician.
17. All sexually active patients should be screened for sexually transmitted diseases (STDs).
18. All sexually active females should have a pelvic examination. A routine pap smear should be offered as part of preventive health maintenance between the ages of 18 and 21 years.
19. Appropriate discussion and counseling should be an integral part of each visit for care.
20. From birth to age 12, refer to AAP's injury prevention program (TIPP®) as described in "A Guide to Safety Counseling in Office Practice" (1994).
21. Earlier initial dental evaluations may be appropriate for some children. Subsequent examinations as prescribed by dentist.

Key: ● = to be performed. * = to be performed for patients at risk. S = subjective, by history. O = objective, by a standard testing method. ↕ = the range during which a service may be provided, with the dot indicating the preferred age.

NB: Special chemical, immunologic, and endocrine testing is usually carried out upon specific indications. Testing other than newborn (eg, inborn errors of metabolism, sickle disease, etc.) is discretionary with the physician.

The recommendations in this publication do not indicate an exclusive course of treatment or serve as a standard of medical care. Variations, taking into account individual circumstances, may be appropriate.

(From Pediatrics Vol. 96, No. 2, August 1995. Copyright 1995 by The American Academy of Pediatrics.)

Figure 4–1

5 Ethical Issues in Pediatrics

Alan R. Fleischman

Ethics is the study of the process of determining the best course of action in the case of conflicting choices. An ethical dilemma places two sets of values in conflict and asks us to come up with an answer or a choice. In medical practice, rarely is the choice between good and evil, but rather between one good and another good. Through the use of ethical principles and analytic inquiry we can ground ethical arguments and attempt to develop generalizable answers to complex problems.

Definitions

1. Respect for persons. The principle of respect for persons supports the right of any person capable of participating in decision making to autonomous determination of what treatments are provided. In addition, this principle incorporates the conviction that persons incapable of deciding for themselves, like most children, are entitled to protection.

2. Surrogate decision making. The process of surrogate decision making is invoked when individuals lack the capacity to make decisions for themselves. This use of a proxy requires that the decision be based not on the individual's choice but rather on another person's view of the right choice. There are two principles that should be used when decisions are made by surrogates:

   a. Substituted judgment. The principle of substituted judgment requires the surrogate to make a decision consistent with the prior wishes and values of the person for whom the decision is being made. This principle respects the former autonomy of a previously capacitated person.

   b. Best interests. The best interests principle is used in making surrogate decisions for those individuals who have never had decision-making capacity or have become incapacitated and have never made their wishes or values known. This patient-centered standard requires the surrogate to make the choice that best promotes the patient's interests.

3. Informed consent. The doctrine of informed consent operationalizes the respect for a person's right to self-determination, if capable, and the use of surrogates to make choices for those who are not capable. Informed consent includes:

   a. The provision of information in understandable language concerning the nature of the problem, the alternative approaches to diagnosis and treatment, and the benefits and risks of the various options.

   b. The assessment of the patient or surrogate's capacity to understand the information and make the decision.

   c. The involvement of the patient, even if incapacitated, to as great an extent as appropriate, in participating in the decision-making process.

   d. The assurance that the decision is made without coercion.

4. Beneficence. The principle of beneficence obligates health care professionals and parents to behave in a selfless manner that maximizes benefits for the patient and minimizes harm. Thus, professionals have the duty to contribute to the health and welfare of patients.

5. Emancipated minor. An emancipated minor is an adolescent who, by law, is considered capable of making independent legal and binding decisions concerning health care. Such adolescents are generally employed and living independently, married, in the military, or the parent of a child.

6. Mature minor. A mature minor, even though unemancipated, is given decision-making authority, without the need for parental involvement and by law in many states, for treatment for certain medical conditions such as sexually transmitted diseases, pregnancy, and drug or alcohol abuse.

7. Nonmaleficence. The principle of nonmaleficence obligates the clinician or scientist to "do no harm." This principle is often invoked as a fundamental tenet of medicine and reminds the health care professional that patients ought not be intentionally harmed or injured. In addition, it establishes the basis for the conduct of physicians to act with due care and in a knowledgeable, skillful, and diligent manner.

8. Distributive justice. The principle of distributive justice demands that fairness be invoked in the distribution of social benefits and burdens under conditions of scarcity. Thus, scientists who seek subjects for research protocols are obligated to include members of all affected communities and not merely choose subjects by convenience.

9. Minimal risk. The concept of minimal risk, as it is applied to research involving children, is defined by federal regulations as "The risks of harm in the proposed research are not greater, considering probability and magnitude, than those ordinarily encountered in daily life and during the performance of routine physical or psychological examinations or tests."

Decision Making for Children

1. Good medical decisions require a balancing of anticipated benefits against immediate and long-term burdens. Competent adults generally perform this task for themselves although often with substantial guidance and support from health care professionals and family members. The vast majority of children are incapable of deciding for themselves and require a parent or guardian to act as surrogate decision maker.

2. The physician has independent obligations to the child to make recommendations that are based on beneficence and to place the child's interests as primary.

3. Decision making should be collaborative, involving the child to an appropriate extent consistent with age and developmental maturity, utilizing the process of informed consent to discuss openly the broad range of options available and the specific recommendations of the physician, recognizing society's deference to parental choice in most circumstances.

4. In the case of adolescents:

    a. Emancipated minors should be treated as autonomous decision makers.

    b. Mature minors should be given deference to make health care decisions, without parental involvement, consistent with local law and custom.

    c. Health care professionals should support the involvement of adolescents in their own health care and foster collaborative decision making among professionals, parents, and the adolescent.

Potential Conflicts

1. Conflicts between physicians and parents

    a. Refusal of beneficial treatment. Medical care that is likely to achieve cure or return the child to health or normal function, such as antibiotics for meningitis, insulin for diabetes, or surgery for appendicitis, rarely poses an ethical conflict. However, there are instances in which parents refuse a recommended treatment that has a strong likelihood of benefit for the child. These situations pose the dilemma of choosing between respecting parental assessment of best interests and promoting the interests of the child as defined by others. The deference that society gives to parental choice in decision making for children is not absolute. When treatment is clearly beneficial and efficacious and refusal will result in immediate or long-term harm to the child, parental objections to treatment should be questioned. These conflicts generally occur as a result of parents' religious beliefs, distrust of the physician, distrust of the standard of medical practice, or as a basic conflict in values. The physician should advocate for those therapies believed to be clearly in the child's interests. If, after sufficient explanation, consultation, and exploration of their concerns, parents continue to refuse treatment, the health care professionals should seek appropriate assistance to determine what course to pursue. This may take the form of consulting an institutional ethics committee or seeking court involvement to decide what is in the best interests of the child or who will make that judgment.

    b. Insistence on treatment. Physicians and parents may disagree about the likelihood of, or the meaning of, benefit of a treatment with an extremely low margin of therapeutic efficacy for a child who is severely compromised. Since the primary justification for medical intervention on children is the ability to benefit the patient, not others, health care professionals may feel constrained by the ethics of their profession to resist parental requests for a treatment that may provide only marginal benefit while prolonging suffering. If a treatment cannot benefit the patient in the narrow, strictly physiologic sense, the physician has no obligation to offer or provide such treatment. If a treatment has a marginal, although questionable, benefit and is being insisted upon by a parent, the physician may not wish to provide such treatment based on the perception of what is in the best interests of the patient. He or she may wish to opt out of the care of this patient by transferring the care to another professional.

2. Conflicts between parents and children

    a. Child abuse and neglect. Parents are responsible for an extremely broad array of children's needs and have the authority to make virtually all decisions for their children regarding nutrition, clothing, housing, education, religion, and medical care. Society's deference to parental choice promotes the value of family integrity, ensures the availability of an identifiable decision maker, and acknowledges the legitimate role that parents play in shaping their children's development. However, society demands that parents exercise this authority responsibly. Children are no longer considered the property of their parents, and society recognizes that children have interests independent of their families. Thus, it is not acceptable for parents to neglect the needs of their children or to harm them physically or emotionally. In every state, if a child is thought to be neglected or abused, it is the legal obligation of physicians and other health care professionals to report these allegations to the appropriate authorities for investigation.

    b. Truth telling. Parents, because of strongly held personal beliefs or the desire to protect, may object to informing their child about his or her disease, the treatment plan, or the prognosis. Physicians have an obligation to ensure that each child receives an appropriate level of information, while helping parents to understand that a conspiracy of silence rarely succeeds, often leaves the child with unanswered questions and fears, and is likely to be harmful to the child's development of trust. In rare circumstances, such as in the case of the diagnosis of AIDS, it may be appropriate to withhold the name of the disease, at parental request, while the child is still too young to understand the potential problems associated with revealing the diagnosis to others. However, even in these cases, the family should be encouraged to share important information about diagnosis and treatment with the child.

    c. Technology dependence. Among chronically ill children there is a small group of patients, perhaps increasing in number, who are dependent on technology such as respirators, intravenous feeding, or dialysis machines. Because they will require technological assistance for many years, or perhaps for the duration of their lives, programs have been created to care for these children at home. Many praiseworthy families have enabled their technology-dependent children to be cared for in the nurturing environment of the home. The family provides the majority of the care for the child, thus decreasing the costs of treatment. This economic saving has resulted in the expectation that all families will be willing and able to care for technology-dependent children at home. We must address and define the limits of parental obligation and sacrifice demanded by society if families are reluctant to take on this burden at home. Social supports, adequate respite care, and financial incentives should be made available to assist families to more readily accept this responsibility. We ought not to force families to reject their chronically ill children by insisting that home care is the only alternative. We need to develop creative options for the chronic care of technology-dependent children, including congregate settings in addition to well-supported home environments.

d. Adolescent issues

(1) Confidentiality. An adolescent may request that the physician maintain confidentiality and not inform a parent concerning an illness. The adolescent may wish to prevent the parent from learning that he or she has a serious illness, may want to hide the behaviors that resulted in acquisition of the disease, or may just wish anonymity. The physician and the patient may be faced with the problem of maintaining confidentiality if the disease progresses. The adolescent should be counseled about the importance of early and continuous support from a caring adult, preferably a parent, and the physician should volunteer to assist the adolescent in informing the parent. If the adolescent insists on maintaining confidentiality, the physician should comply unless such behavior will result in direct harm to the patient. The physician should not violate the adolescent's trust by informing the parents and asking them not to tell the child of their knowledge of the matter.

(2) Refusal of treatment. An adolescent may wish to refuse potentially lifesaving treatment for a serious and ultimately terminal condition over the objection of the parents. If the individual is assessed to be cognitively and psychosocially mature and is able to determine what is in his or her own best interests, the physician should respect the adolescent's position while working with the family to develop a reasonable plan of management. Both the adolescent and the parents should be helped to understand the other's perspective, and the physician generally should advocate for the course of treatment consistent with the adolescent's wishes.

The End of Life

1. Withholding and withdrawal of treatment. At some point in the trajectory of a serious illness in the terminal stages, it may be appropriate to accept that the benefits of continued treatment are far outweighed by the pain and suffering. Graceful acceptance of inevitable death by the health care professionals, parents, and child may become preferable to exerting all efforts to postpone it. At this point, the decision may be made to not initiate new treatments or to withdraw those interventions currently in place. Many physicians believe that withdrawing a treatment is legally and morally less justified and acceptable than withholding one. In the physician-patient relationship with its fiduciary responsibility to provide the most appropriate care and treatment, including the obligation to alleviate suffering, there is little moral distinction between withholding and withdrawing a treatment if the intent and the expected result of either action is the death of the patient. If there is good reason to withhold a particular treatment from a patient, then it is equally defensible to withdraw that treatment if it is no longer providing the intended benefit. There is no question that it is psychologically more difficult for physicians to withdraw a treatment than to withhold one, but this psychologic difference does not create an ethical distinction. In addition, most legal scholars agree that nothing in the law makes stopping treatment a more serious legal issue than not starting it in the first place.

2. Humane care. At the end of life, the primary goal of medical management becomes the promotion of comfort.

a. Pain relief. The severity of pain in children is often underestimated, in part because children have difficulty effectively communicating the extent of their pain. Also, the child may decline to report pain owing to fear that an injection will be used to administer analgesia. Adequate pain medication should be utilized to maintain symptom-free comfort for the child. Since tolerance to pain medication often develops after repeated use, increased dosage or differing modalities for alleviation of pain must be utilized in those children who have a chronic need. Fear of narcotic addiction should not result in depriving a child of adequate pain management. Full and effective doses of pain medication should be given, even if a possible secondary effect is sedation, depression of respiration, and the possible hastening of inevitable death.

b. Hospice care. Many children will experience a less traumatic death at home than in the hospital setting. A home hospice program for the child and family that provides adequate support, pain management, and preparation for the ultimate death may increase the family's sense of comfort, control, and independence.

c. Bereavement counseling. Given the profound impact of the death of any child, the health care professional team should remain available to the family to provide long-term assessment and counseling concerning the loss.

Research Involving Children

1. Research is a careful and diligent search into, or the collection of information about, a particular subject for the purpose of developing important knowledge. It can be distinguished from clinical practice in several ways:

a. Clinical practice is the use of generally accepted treatments that have been shown to be effective and about which the risks and complications are known, even if uncertain. Research is generally the evaluation of unaccepted treatments that have promise but have not been shown to be effective and about which the risks and complications may be unknown.

   b. The ethical basis of clinical practice is the principle of beneficence. The operative principle in research is respect for persons, which enables subjects to voluntarily support the enhancement of knowledge. It is, therefore, critical for the clinician-scientist and the subject of research to not confuse this important difference. Patients and their families, when considering a clinical research protocol, may believe that the scientist is motivated by the best interests of the patient, not realizing that the goal of the research is to enhance knowledge and perhaps is more focused on the interests of future patients than on the present subjects.

2. Ethical standards in the conduct of research

   a. Respect for persons. This principle obligates the scientist to treat each subject as an autonomous agent who has the right to voluntary involvement in the research. Children, who are thought to have diminished autonomy, must be afforded special protections to assure that involvement in research is not unduly burdensome or harmful, since children are unable to consent for themselves.

   b. Nonmaleficence. This principle obligates the scientist to minimize risks to the subjects as much as possible. In addition, it argues that if the subjects are being unduly harmed, the research should be stopped.

   c. Distributive justice. This principle obligates the scientist to design research investigations to include representatives from all affected communities. Both the potential benefits and the potential risks of the research should be distributed fairly among all possible subjects. Research projects should not include subjects who are approached merely out of convenience or because of ease of obtaining consent.

   d. Informed consent. The principle of informed consent requires a scientist to obtain the uncoerced consent from the subject of research or the surrogate and to explain the nature of the research, the benefits, the risks, and the possible alternatives. In addition, the subject must be informed that participation is voluntary, that refusal to participate will not influence other care rendered to the subject, and that withdrawal from the research is possible at any time.

3. Specific issues concerning children

   a. Minimal risk. The concept of minimal risk was developed to anchor the amount of risk acceptable to impose on children enrolled in research projects that offered no therapeutic benefit. Acceptable research involving children includes

     (1) Research not involving greater than minimal risk.

     (2) Research involving greater than minimal risk but with direct therapeutic benefit.

     (3) Research involving a minor increment over minimal risk but having a high likelihood of developing generalizable knowledge.

     (4) Research that presents a unique opportunity to understand, prevent, or alleviate a serious problem affecting children.

   b. Child assent. In addition to the consent or permission of the parent or legal guardian, respect for the role of the child in the decision to participate in the research project is accomplished by obtaining his or her assent. Assent is generally used for children greater than 7 years of age and must include a developmentally appropriate method of informing the child about the research procedures and purposes. For nontherapeutic research, lack of assent from the child should be considered a binding refusal to participate.

   c. Adolescent consent. Although, in many circumstances, mature adolescents may be permitted to consent to medical treatment without parental involvement, it should not be assumed that these same adolescents are permitted to consent to be subjects of research without parental permission. At the present time there is disagreement among experts as to whether adolescents may consent to be subjects of research in protocols related to areas for which they may consent for medical treatment. Individual states and institutions vary in how the federal regulations protecting research subjects are interpreted. At a minimum, for an adolescent to be permitted to consent to be a subject of research, the scientist must assess the capacity of the adolescent and ensure that he or she is fully able to understand the nature of the study and the consequences of participation.

Bibliography

American Academy of Pediatrics Committee on Bioethics: Informed consent, parental permission, and assent in pediatric practice. Pediatrics 1995;95:314–317.

American Academy of Pediatrics Committee on Bioethics: Guidelines on forgoing life-sustaining medical treatment. Pediatrics 1994;93:532–536.

Cassidy R, Fleischman AR (eds): Pediatric Ethics: From Principles to Practice. Reading, UK, Harwood Academic Publishers, 1995.

Fleischman AR, Nolan K, Dubler NN, et al: Caring for gravely ill children. Pediatrics 1994;94:433–439.

Grodin MA, Glantz LH (eds): Children as Research Subjects. New York, Oxford University Press, 1994.

Holder AR: Legal Issues in Pediatrics and Adolescent Medicine, 2nd ed. New Haven, Yale University Press, 1985.

6 Concepts and Diet Analysis

Laurence Finberg

The need to feed infants something other than breast milk arose when the Industrial Revolution sent poor women into the workplace, limiting their availability as wet nurses. The specialty of pediatrics originated during that time to address this nutritional problem but has long since changed its focus. Modern pediatrics is based in the biologic differences between the growing child and the mature adult in health and disease. Nonetheless, nutrition remains a very important part of pediatric knowledge and practice, increasingly so as the possible influence of childhood diet on adult-onset disease comes under consideration. A comprehensive diet must contain adequate water, energy (calories/joules*), protein, and a variety of accessory substances including vitamins, minerals, and some fatty acids. Water is discussed in Chapter 10; the other substances are dealt with here and in Chapter 1 and cross referenced to other sections.

1. Sources of energy
   a. Protein along with water and energy is an absolute requirement for life and growth. Protein consists of large organic nitrogen containing molecules built from amino acids. The 20 amino acids used in building protein molecules are either essential (arginine, cystine, histidine, isoleucine, leucine, lysine, methionine, phenylalanine, threonine, tryptophan, and valine) or nonessential, meaning that they can be synthesized for use (alanine, aspartic acid, cysteine, glutamic acid/glutamine, glycine, proline, serine, taurine,† and tyrosine). Most animal proteins are complete in that they contain all the essential amino acids in sufficient quantity for growth, with no one of them exceeding a threshold for toxicity. No one vegetable taken as a sole source of protein will suffice, because if the deficient amino acid (e.g., lysine in grains, methionine in beans) is made adequate in extraordinary ingestion, the other amino acids will be present in toxic amounts, that is, exceeding the deamination threshold of the liver. However, combinations of vegetables in the diet, such as corn or rice with a bean, will provide adequate nutrition though the minimal percentage of protein calories will be higher. On a human or cow milk feeding an infant can grow on as little as 6 to 8 per cent of calories as protein. To allow for inefficiency of digestion and for increased demands of illness, it is best to have at least 10 per cent of calories as protein. The figure should be 12 to 15 per cent if only vegetables sources are consumed. Protein supplies approximately 4.0 calories/g.
   b. Fat provides a source of high energy to the diet: approximately 9 calories/g (short- and medium-chain fatty acids provide less). Only a small amount of fat, 2 per cent of calories in the form of the unsaturated linolenic or linoleic acid, is essential to growth and maintenance. Because fat is so energy dense it is particularly important in the diet of infants, who have limited capacity for a large volume of food. Animal milks, including breast milk, used for infant feeding typically have 50 per cent of calories from fat.
   c. Carbohydrate, although not an essential nutrient per se, serves a valuable role by providing readily metabolizable energy. Unlike some of the potentially toxic intermediaries of protein or fat, carbohydrate has only water and CO_2 as end products. The energy content is approximately 4 calories/g.
   d. Ethyl alcohol, the only other significant potential source of energy for humans, has no dietary role for children. Other than the small amount produced by bacterial fermentation in the intestine it is best avoided because of its toxic potential.

2. Analysis of diet
   a. Energy is required for heat production, work, metabolism, and, in children, growth. Energy intake above these requirements leads to deposition of excess adipose tissue. Although what constitutes excess cannot be precisely defined for all circumstances, there can be no question that more than 20 per cent of body mass as fat is an excess; the percentage is less for prepubertal children.

Table 6–1 shows average energy expenditures (hence, requirements) at basal conditions for different age groups. For the first year of life, infants require 90 to 110 cal/kg, including requirements for activity and growth.

The only accurate way to analyze a diet for nutritional purposes is to use the energy content as the denominator.

TABLE 6–1.   BASAL CALORIC EXPENDITURE FOR INFANTS AND CHILDREN*

AGE	WEIGHT (kg)	SURFACE AREA (m²)	CALORIC EXPENDITURE (cal/kg)
Newborn	2.5–4	0.2–0.23	50
1 week–6 months	3–8	0.2–0.35	65–70
6–12 months	8–12	0.35–0.45	50–60
1–2 years	10–15	0.45–0.55	45–50
2–5 years	15–20	0.6–0.7	45
5–10 years	20–35	0.7–1.1	40–45
10–16 years	35–60	1.5–1.7	25–40
Adult	70	1.75	15–20

*Water expenditure equals 1 ml/cal.

From Finberg L, Kravath RE, Hellerstein S (eds): Water and Electrolytes in Pediatrics: Physiology, Pathophysiology, and Treatment, 2nd ed. Philadelphia, WB Saunders, 1993.

---

*The calorie is that of the nutritionist, or kilocalorie. One kilocalorie = 4.187 kilojoules.

†Probably essential in premature infants.

The first step is to allocate the appropriate number of calories for a given individual. The next step is to assign the percentage of calories derived from each of the energy sources, and the final step is to assess the water, mineral, and accessory substances per unit of energy/day. In the case of young infants, diet analysis is easier because the diet usually consists of a single food.

    b. Protein minima and maxima at any age generally fall within the range of 10 to 16 per cent of calories.

    c. Fat and carbohydrate calories are interchangeable so long as the linolenic/linoleic acid requirement is met and toxicity from ketosis caused by too much fat is avoided.

    d. The macrominerals, sodium, chloride, and potassium, are safely given as 2 to 3 mEq/100 cal. The actual range for sodium and chloride is from 0.1 to 10.0 mEq/100 cal. The 2–3 value is midrange. Potassium cannot be conserved as readily, so that the figure given should be closely observed.

    e. Trace minerals obviously are needed in very small amounts and can be allocated in mg/day.

    f. Vitamins similarly are needed in small amounts, but the need is proportionate to the energy expended.

The values supplied in the United States by the Food and Nutrition Board of the National Academy of Sciences/National Research Council as recommended dietary allowances are recommendations for intake, not minima or maxima.

B Bibliography

Fomon SJ: Nutrition of Normal Infants. St. Louis, CV Mosby, 1993.

Recommended Dietary Allowances, 10th ed. Washington, DC, National Academy Press, 1989.

Shils ME, Olson JA, Shike M (eds): Modern Nutrition in Health and Disease, 8th ed. Philadelphia, Lea & Febiger, 1994.

7 Deficiencies and Excesses of Food Components

Laurence Finberg

Whereas the previous chapter set forth principles for analyzing nutritional needs, this chapter deals with disease states arising from either lack of a nutritional element or toxicity from an excess.

Energy and Protein

These two factors are discussed as one because the undernutrition syndromes overlap in clinical practice and together are referred to as protein-calorie malnutrition.

Marasmus

Marasmus is the condition of general wasting that occurs when calorie intake is insufficient for any reason but the protein percentage of calories is at least marginally adequate. Infection or other increase in catabolism may convert marasmus to kwashiorkor. Measles and diarrheal disease are frequent culprits.

Clinical Findings and Pathogenesis

The patient will show obvious loss of subcutaneous fat. In addition, lethargy and lack of interest in his or her surroundings is common, especially in infants. The abdominal skin in infants loses elasticity or stands in folds for a minute or so when pinched. When the starvation occurs gradually, simple wasting occurs in infancy and early childhood; stunting of growth will be manifest later. Skin lesions consisting of dry, slightly yellow scaling are often, but not always, seen on the extremities. These are similar to the lesions of pellagra.

Key Clinical Findings: Marasmus

- Apathy

- Loss of subcutaneous fat

- Stunting of growth

Laboratory Findings

Laboratory analyses of usual clinical studies are frequently not remarkable. The urea nitrogen and creatinine levels in serum are low. Hypoglycemia is not usually seen except in extremis. When the condition is severe or of long standing, a hyponatremic state is common. More elaborate laboratory studies reveal a number of hormonal adaptations, but these studies are not required for diagnosis.

Key Laboratory Finding: Marasmus

- Normal serum albumin

Treatment

The child should be fed an adequate caloric intake with appropriate (as in a normal diet) percentages of protein, fat, and carbohydrate plus minerals and vitamins. The caloric intake should be based on the patient's ideal weight. During treatment for severe marasmus, there may be fatty deposition in the liver characterized by clinical hepatomegaly, often seen with a distended abdomen.

Key Treatment: Marasmus

- Feed balanced diet with caloric intake based on ideal weight for age

Kwashiorkor

The word kwashiorkor is derived from the Ga tribal language (Ghana) meaning, in loose translation, disease of the second child. This is because of the occurrence of kwashiorkor in the weanling when another infant supplants the first one at the breast. In this disorder there is protein deficiency with or without energy deficiency.

Clinical Findings and Pathogenesis

There is generalized edema because the serum albumin level falls below the critical concentration needed to sustain Starling (oncotic) forces, a level of 2.4 g/dl or 24 g/L. As in any hypoalbuminemic state, the edema progresses gradually as the elastic skin and subcutaneous tissue yield, lessening tissue back-pressure. Skin lesions of the scalp and extremities are common. The hair loses its pigment so that dark-haired children seem to have red hair (the word kwashiorkor may also mean "red boy"). If there is recovery followed by relapses and again recovery, the hair shows a flag sign of alternating black and reddish yellow. The edema masks the wasting, producing full facial features and swollen extremities.

Key Clinical Findings: Kwashiorkor

- Generalized edema
- Reddish yellow hair
- Skin rash

Laboratory Findings

The diagnostic finding is a low level of albumin. Hypoglycemia is occasionally seen in these patients, and hyponatremia/hypochloremia is common. Potassium and magnesium losses are important but are not measured by their serum levels.

Key Laboratory Finding: Kwashiorkor

- Low serum albumin

Treatment

Refeeding these patients should be done cautiously. If there is concurrent infection, intravenous albumin administration will hasten recovery but is usually not necessary. Frequent feedings are desirable to prevent hypoglycemia. Adequate potassium and magnesium content in foods is important.

Key Treatment: Kwashiorkor

- Refeeding with multiple small feedings per day at caloric intake for age and length (ht).
- Adequate mineral intake, including potassium and magnesium

Obesity

Excess calorie intake leads to obesity, a complex biologic condition with genetic, metabolic, and psychosocial factors. Treatment, simple in concept, proves very difficult in practice. Further discussion is found in Chapter 9.

Vitamins

Fat-Soluble, A, D, E, and K

1. Vitamin A or retinol is contained in fats, particularly fish oil, and in yellow vegetables. Retinol is important to the maintenance of epithelial membranes and plays a specific role in eye tissue.

   a. Deficiency of vitamin A leads to xerophthalmia, a drying of eye tissue that is common in the developing world. Night blindness is another manifestation of deficiency. There is evidence that vitamin A protects against the respiratory damage of measles and perhaps other pulmonary disease, making adequate intake important for both prevention and treatment. The protective dosage is 1500 μg or 5000 IU/day. A therapeutic dose is 1500 μg/kg/day for 5 days.

   b. Excess of vitamin A (20,000 IU/day or 100,000 μg over a few months) causes increased intracranial pressure (pseudotumor cerebri). This can also occur acutely with a single ingested dose of 4500 μg. Chronic hypervitaminosis A produces hyperostosis of the long bones, alopecia, seborrheic skin lesions, anorexia, and pruritus. The only treatment is withdrawal of the vitamin; recovery is usually complete.

2. Vitamin D or cholecalciferol is formed in the skin under stimulus from ultraviolet (UV) rays of sunlight. It may also be taken orally, which is important when long winters or industrial pollution reduce sun exposure. Dark pigment of the skin reduces penetration of UV rays to the layer in the dermis where conversion from 7-dehydrocholesterol, the vitamin D precursor, occurs. The recommended and rickets-preventive dose is 400 u/day or 10 μg. If sun exposure is inadequate, as is common in inner cities, or if the skin is even moderately dark, it is advisable to give a supplement to breast-fed infants. Animal milks, including human milk, contain very little vitamin D. Either fortification, as in infant formula, or supplementation for breast-fed infants is advisable during the first year.

   a. Vitamin D deficiency in children is called rickets, which is discussed further in Chapter 8.

   b. Excess of vitamin D leads to hypercalcemia, which in turn causes hypertension and calcification of tissues, particularly in the kidney. Treatment is that for hypercalcemia (see Chapter 264).

3. Vitamin E or α-tocopherol is an antioxidant present in many foods. Deficiency occurs with fat malabsorption. Hemolytic anemia in premature infants and a neurologic syndrome of cerebellar ataxia and peripheral neuropathy develop with prolonged severe deficiency in disorders producing steatorrhea.

4. Vitamin K is a naphthoquinone appearing in foods as K_1 and as K_2, found also as an active substance pro-

duced by bacterial action in the intestine. Vitamin K is important in the synthesis of several factors, including prothrombin, which is necessary for coagulation (see Chapter 124).

a. Deficiency occurs when there is fat malabsorption or suppression (or especially, both) of intestinal bacterial growth. Diarrheal disease and antibiotic administration are potential causes. Treatment consists of 1 to 2 mg/day for infants with mild deficiency and 5 mg/day of K_1 parenterally for severe prothrombin deficiency.

b. Toxicity of excess vitamin K in most situations has not been described. In newborns, the vitamin K analogs, but not K_1, may aggravate hyperbilirubinemia.

Key Treatment: Vitamin A Deficiency

- Retinol—1500 µg/kg/day × 5 days

Key Treatment: Vitamin K Deficiency

- Vitamin K—1 to 2 mg/day (infants)
- Vitamin K—5 mg/day for severe prothrombin deficiency

Water-Soluble Vitamins; The B Complex

1. Thiamin or B_1 is a cofactor in carbohydrate decarboxylation. It is found in meats, milk, eggs, whole grains, and legumes. The recommended daily intake is 0.3 mg for infants, increasing gradually to 1.5 mg for adolescents.

   a. Deficiency leads to a cardiac and nervous system disorder known as beriberi. Heart failure is characterized by edema and a low-voltage ECG reading. The nervous system damage is first to peripheral nerves, with paresthesias and decreased deep tendon reflexes (DTRs). Later, central nervous system symptoms and signs occur. Hoarseness and aphonia are early symptoms.

Key Clinical Findings: Beriberi

- Hoarseness
- Aphonia
- Heart failure
- Loss of DTRs

Treatment with 10 mg of thiamin daily orally with an initial parenteral dose is quickly effective in relieving symptoms and the heart failure, although several weeks are required for complete resolution.

Key Treatment: Beriberi

- Thiamin—10 mg/day for 2 to 3 weeks

b. Excess thiamin is excreted readily in urine, and no toxicity has been reported.

2. Riboflavin plays an important oxidation-reduction role for enzymes and for synthesis of flavin adenine dinucleotide (FAD) and the mononucleotide FMN. It is present in liver, meats, milk, eggs, green vegetables, and whole grains. The recommended daily intake range is from 0.4 mg for infants to 1.8 mg for adolescents.

   a. Deficiency causes cheilosis, glossitis, and corneal vascularization along with photophobia. Treatment is 5 to 10 mg daily orally, which may be initiated with a parenteral dosage of 2 mg three times a day for 1 or 2 days.

   b. As with thiamin, no excess problem is known.

3. Niacin includes both nicotinic acid and nicotinamide. Tryptophan is a niacin precursor that can partially replace the niacin requirement of 5 to 20 mg daily (which increases gradually from infancy to adolescence). Meats, fish, whole grains, and green vegetables contain niacin.

   a. Deficiency results in pellagra, a disorder symptomatically characterized by the three D's—dermatitis, diarrhea, and dementia. The skin lesions appear in areas exposed to sunlight. In infants, anorexia and apathy are common symptoms. Treatment consists of 50 to 300 mg/day of niacin. A parenteral dose of 100 mg intravenously may be used to initiate therapy. Exposure to sun should be avoided during the active phase.

Key Clinical Findings: Pellagra

- Dermatitis
- Diarrhea
- Dementia

Key Treatment: Pellagra

- Niacin—100 mg IV first dose
- Niacin—50–300 mg/day for 10 days–2 weeks

   b. Excess intake of nicotinic acid causes flushing, and continued high dosage may lead to cholestasis, jaundice, and liver injury.

4. Folic acid or folacin is a group of pteridine ring compounds found in liver, green vegetables, and grains as well as other foods. The daily requirement for infants is 50 µg and for adolescents 400 µg. Folates aid in the synthesis of purines and pyrimidines and also in methylation reactions.

   a. Deficiency results in megaloblastic anemia (see Chapter 114).

   b. Excess is known to be harmful only in individuals with pernicious anemia who are not receiving vitamin B_{12}.

5. Cobalamin (B_{12}), a cobalt-containing compound, is important in red cell maturation (see Chapter 114), in

central nervous system metabolism and in methylmalonic acid mutase disorders (see Chapter 63). Only animal protein foods (meat, eggs, and milk) contain B_{12}. Intestinal bacteria do not provide for host use; the daily requirement is 1 to 2 µg/day.

6. Pyridoxine (B_6), a cofactor for transaminases and decarboxylases, is found in liver, meat, whole grains, and soybeans. The requirement is from 0.2 to 0.3 mg/day for infants and 2 mg/day for adolescents.

   a. Deficiency in infants causes convulsions. Several dependency syndromes have been described, including the convulsive disorder, from high-dosage exposure in fetal life. Peripheral neuritis and anemia are uncommon as manifestations of pyridoxine deficiency. Treatment of the seizure disorder is 100 mg by injection; response is prompt.

Key Treatment: Convulsions Due to Pyridoxine Deficiency

- Pyridoxine—100 mg by injection

   b. Excess causes neuropathy.

7. Biotin a coenzyme for acetyl CoA carboxylase is found in liver, egg yolk, and peanuts and is synthesized by intestinal bacteria. Daily requirement is tiny, but not known.

   a. Deficiency is rare but may be caused by very high intake of egg albumin leading to anorexia, muscle aches, and alopecia. Treatment: avoidance of egg white and a normal food intake.

   b. No known excess toxicity.

8. Pantothenic acid, a component of enzyme CoA, found in most foods. Estimated requirement 5–10 mg/d.

   a. Deficiency only developes when antagonists are taken. Hypertension and weakness may then be seen.

   b. No toxicity reported from excess.

Vitamin C (Ascorbic Acid)

Vitamin C or ascorbic acid is a water-soluble compound found in citrus fruits, in many vegetables, and in human (but not cow) milk. Unlike most animals, humans cannot synthesize ascorbic acid and so must ingest it. The vitamin, a strong reducing agent, is essential for collagen formation and vascular integrity. The requirement is 35 to 50 mg daily.

1. Deficiency, as the name implies, is the disease scurvy. Although vitamin C stores are less than those of fat-soluble vitamins, they are sufficient so that even with total deprivation it takes 5 months for symptomatic scurvy to manifest. Congenital scurvy is unknown because a seriously deficient pregnant woman would spontaneously abort early. Infantile scurvy is now rare in the industrialized world except possibly among people living near the polar region, where fruits and vegetables are scarce. The symptoms of infantile scurvy are caused primarily by bleeding and by failure of formation of bone matrix. Hemorrhage into the subperiosteal space is very painful, and since it commonly occurs in the lower extremity bones, pseudoparalysis results. Bone mineralization is normal, but resorption outpaces formation. The result is a ground-glass appearance on x-rays, with increased density at sites of calcification producing a ring of dense bone around the epiphyses (Wimberger rings) and a brittle dense zone at the metaphyses that often fractures at the corners. Hemorrhage may also occur into the orbit and skin. Mild deficiency may cause a megaloblastic anemia.

Key Clinical Findings: Scurvy

- Bone pain
- Pseudoparalysis
- Megaloblastic anemia

Key Radiologic Findings: Scurvy

- Ground-glass osteopenia
- Wimberger rings

Treatment consists of 100 to 200 mg of ascorbic acid. Response to parenteral administration relieves pain in hours. Oral ascorbic acid or orange juice is also quickly effective.

Key Treatment: Scurvy

- Ascorbic acid—100 to 200 mg single dose to control symptoms
- Ascorbic acid—100 mg daily for 2 weeks

2. Any excess is excreted in urine. Rarely, precipitation with oxalate may occur in the renal collecting system. Tolerance to high dosage, resulting in dependency, has also been reported.

Minerals

Macrominerals

The macrominerals, sodium, potassium, calcium, and the associated anions, are covered in the chapters on electrolytes (see Chapters 10 to 13) and those dealing with the parathyroid gland (see Chapter 264) and rickets (see Chapter 8). For sodium, potassium, and chloride the optimum intake is 2 to 3 mEq/100 cal/day. For calcium the recommended daily intake ranges from 400 mg/day for infants to 600 mg for toddlers, 800 mg for older children and 1200 mg for adolescents. For phosphorus the respective figures are 300, 500, 800, and 1200 mg/day.

Trace Minerals

Trace minerals include a number of metals necessary for growth, maintenance, and biochemical function.

1. Iron is required for hemoglobin formation and is incorporated in cytochromes necessary for cell respiration. It is found in liver, meat, and some vegetables. Other vegetables, such as spinach, have unavailable iron because of fiber or phytates that inhibit absorption. Recommended intake for infants is 6 mg/day; for children, 10 mg;

and for adolescents, 12 mg. (See Chapter 113 for iron deficiency anemia.)

2. Zinc, necessary as an enzyme component, occurs in the same foods as iron. Requirements range from 5 to 15 mg per day. Deficiency results in acrodermatitis enteropathica with diarrhea and skin lesions that also appear as a genetic defect in zinc absorption. Treatment with 1 to 2 mg/kg/day is effective.

3. Copper is another metal active as an enzyme component. Dietary sources are human milk as well as meats and vegetables. Requirements range from 0.4 to 2.5 mg/day through infancy and childhood. Deficiency results in anemia and an osteopenia resembling the changes found in scurvy.

4. Magnesium is an important component of cells and forms metalloenzymes. Like potassium, it is found in all animal and plant cells; unlike potassium, it is well conserved by the body. Deficiency may lead to hypocalcemia and tetany.

5. Other elements needed in small amounts include iodine for thyroxin formation, selenium (an antioxidant), manganese, molybdenum, chromium, and cobalt (B_{12}) as well as minute amounts of arsenic, nickel, silicon, and boron and possibly yet others play a role in biochemical processes.

6. Fluoride, although not necessary for life or growth, is useful for the prevention of dental caries. For this purpose the recommended daily intake from water supply or supplements is 0.25 mg from 4 months to 2 years of age, and 0.5 to 1 mg from 2 years to 16 years. Excess intake results in pitting of the dental enamel or fluorosis.

Bibliography

Kleinman RE (ed): Pediatric Nutrition Handbook, 4th ed. American Academy of Pediatrics, Elk Grove, IL, 1997.

National Research Council: Recommended Dietary Allowances, 10th ed. Washington, DC National Academy Press, 1989.

Shils ME, Olson JA, Shike M (eds): Modern Nutrition in Health and Disease, 8th ed. Philadelphia, Lea & Febiger, 1994.

8 Nutritional Rickets

Laurence Finberg

Definition

Rickets is the failure of calcification of osteoid in the growing child. Failure to calcify osteoid in the adult is called osteomalacia.

Etiology

1. Rickets occurs when the metabolites of vitamin D are deficient. Vitamin D_3 (cholecalciferol) is formed in the skin under stimulus of ultraviolet (UV) light. Sunlight exposure was the only known significant source of vitamin D until early in the twentieth century, when it was discovered that the vitamin is contained in fish liver oil and can be taken orally with good effect. Human milk provides very little Vitamin D.

2. Nutritional rickets may also be caused, although rarely, by deficient intake of calcium or phosphate or some combination of deficiencies of vitamin D, calcium, and phosphate.

3. Rickets appeared in epidemic form in temperate zones when the Industrial Revolution's factories produced smoke that blocked UV rays, probably the first childhood disease produced by environmental pollution.

Epidemiology

1. Infants and children at risk:
   a. Those with dark pigmented skin, which blocks penetration of light
   b. Those who are breast fed and those who receive no oral supplement
   c. Those who live in the inner city
   d. Those in tropical regions who are kept inside or heavily covered and are breast fed.

2. In the United States and Europe, severe nutritional rickets has become rare, although the mild disorder continues in the high-risk population (dark skin, inner city locale, and breast fed with no supplement). All infant formula, evaporated milks, and almost all whole milk sold in the United States contain 400 U (10 μg) of vitamin D per quart.

Pathophysiology

1. Cholecalciferol (D_3) is formed in the skin from 5-dehydrotachysterol. This steroid undergoes hydroxylation in two steps (a plant sterol, ergosterol, may be substituted, since it has an identical potency and metabolic pathway).

   a. At position 25 by the liver, producing calcidiol (25-hydroxycholecalciferol), which is the circulating reserve compound.

   b. At position 1 by the kidney, producing calcitriol (1,25-dihydroxycholecalciferol), the active metabolite. Calcitriol acts at three known sites.

      (1) It promotes absorption of calcium and phosphorus from the intestine.

      (2) It increases reabsorption of phosphate in the kidney.

(3) It acts on bone to release calcium and phosphate.

Calcitriol may facilitate calcification directly as well. The above-named actions increase the concentrations of calcium and phosphate in extracellular fluid (ECF), which in turn leads to the calcification of osteoid, primarily at the metaphyseal growing ends of bones but also throughout the skeleton.

2. Parathyroid hormone facilitates the 1-hydroxylation step in vitamin D metabolism and, along with calcitriol and calcitonin, plays a role in calcium regulation.

3. When calcitriol levels are low, hypocalcemia develops, stimulating parathyroid hormone excess. This in turn produces renal phosphate loss, further reducing calcification potential and producing bone changes of hyperparathyroidism.

4. Early in the course of rickets, the calcium concentration in the serum drops. After the parathyroid response, calcium concentration returns to the normal range with a very low phosphate.

5. Alkaline phosphatase produced by very active osteoblast cells leaks to the ECF, so that its concentration rises to anywhere from moderate elevation to very high levels.

6. Severe malabsorption or disease of liver or kidney may produce the clinical and secondary biochemical picture of nutritional rickets.

7. Anticonvulsant drugs (phenobarbital and phenytoin) accelerate metabolism of calcidiol, which may lead to insufficiency and rickets, particularly in children kept indoors in institutions.

Clinical Findings

1. Generalized muscular hypotonia of unknown mechanism characterizes most patients with clinical (as opposed to biochemical and radiologic) signs of rickets.

2. Craniotabes manifests early in infants. Although this feature may be found normally in premature infants, particularly along suture lines, when rickets is present the sign is pronounced.

3. If rickets progresses, thickening of the skull develops at a later stage, producing frontal bossing, and the closing of the anterior fontanel is delayed. The laying-down of uncalcified osteoid at the metaphysis leads to spreading of those areas, producing knobby deformity. In the chest this results in the rachitic rosary, and the weakened ribs pulled by muscles also produce flaring over the diaphragm known as Harrison's groove.

4. The sternum may be pulled into a pigeon-breast deformity. In more severe instances beyond 2 years of age, vertebral softening leads to kyphoscoliosis. The ends of the long bones show that same knobby thickening.

5. At the ankle, palpation of the tibial malleolus gives the impression of a double epiphysis (Marfan sign). Because the softened long bones may bend, they may fracture one side of the cortex (a "greenstick" fracture). Weight-bearing produces deformities such as bowlegs and knock knees. Some deformity occurs before weight-bearing from strong dorsal muscle pull.

6. Acute infection or fever producing catabolic release of phosphate from cells occasionally precipitates hypocalcemia and tetany as presenting manifestations. In the United States infants with rickets are usually otherwise well nourished. Rickets may occur as part of general malnutrition, although some features are less obvious because of slower skeletal growth.

Key Clinical Findings

- Generalized muscular hypotonia
- Craniotabes
- Thick wrists and ankles
- Rachitic rosary
- Bowlegs (genu varum)

Laboratory Findings

1. Early, the calcium (ionized fraction) will be low, but more often at the time of diagnosis it is in the normal range.

2. The phosphorus level is invariably low for age unless there has been recent partial treatment or recent exposure to sunlight.

3. Alkaline phosphatase values are elevated.

4. Calcidiol levels are low.

5. Parathyroid hormone values are elevated. There is also a generalized aminoaciduria from the parathyroid activity unlike, for example, familial hypophosphatemia.

The last three determinations are not needed for typical instances. In some circumstances, calcitriol levels are normal or high because of parathyroid activity.

Key Laboratory Findings

- Low calcium level early on but normal level at diagnosis
- Phosphorus level invariably low
- Alkaline phosphatase value elevated
- Calcidiol low; parathyroid hormone elevated
- Generalized aminoaciduria

Radiographic Changes

1. The best single x-ray for infants and children under 3 years of age is an anterior view of the knee showing the metaphyseal ends and epiphyses of the femurs and tibias. This site is best because growth is most rapid there, which accentuates the changes.

2. These metaphyses are widened and show cupping because of their normal concavity and "fraying" caused by irregular calcification.

3. Because calcified osteoid is abundant, the provisional calcification zone of the metaphysis is much more distant from the calcification center of the epiphysis than is normal for age.

4. Along the diaphyses the uncalcified osteoid causes the periosteum to appear separated from the diaphysis.

5. There is generalized osteomalacia (seen as osteopenia) with visible coarsening of trabeculae in contrast to the ground-glass osteopenia of scurvy.

Differential Diagnosis

- Familial hypophosphatemia
- Vitamin D–dependent rickets, type 1
- Vitamin D–dependent rickets, type 2 (receptor deficit)
- Metaphyseal dysplasia (Schmidt)

See also Chapters 66 and 347.

Treatment

Treatment with vitamin D may be carried out either gradually over several months or in a single day.

1. If the gradual method is chosen, the dosage should be 125 to 250 μg (5000–10,000 U) daily for 2 to 3 months until healing, documented by x-ray, is well along and the alkaline phosphatase concentration is approaching normal. The success of this method depends on compliance.

2. An alternative and recommended therapy is to give the vitamin D in a single day—15,000 μg (600,000 U) of vitamin D usually divided into four or six oral doses. An intramuscular injection is also available. Vitamin D is well stored in the body and released gradually over many weeks. Neither calcitriol nor calcidiol, each with a short half-life, is suitable.

   a. Single-day therapy avoids problems with compliance and on occasion is helpful in differentiating nutritional rickets from familial hypophosphatemia (FHR). In nutritional rickets, the phosphate level will rise in 96 hours and radiographic healing will be visible in 6 to 7 days. Neither happens with FHR.

   b. One must be careful in the single-day regimen not to use a preparation of vitamin D suspended in propylene glycol. At this dosage the vehicle will be toxic. One may use 50,000 U capsules of ergosterol, softened in water and fed with a blended food such as applesauce.

3. If severe deformities have occurred, orthopedic correction may be required after healing. Most of the deformities will correct with growth. Severe rickets as was once seen in China may so deform the pelvis as to prevent vaginal childbirth.

Key Treatment

- Single-day therapy (preferred)
- Vitamin D (cholecalciferol) 600,000 U (15,000 μg) as either one parenteral dose or divided into four oral doses in 1 day.

Prevention

1. Adequate UV light (as little as 20 minutes a day to the face of a white baby but significantly longer for a baby with melanotic skin) or the oral intake of 10 μg (400 U) daily of a vitamin D preparation plus an adequate dietary supply of calcium and phosphorus will prevent rickets.

2. Human milk contains little vitamin D and, for babies weighing less than 1500 g, too little phosphate. These babies need special supplementation if breast milk is used in their feeding. It is safe and therefore wise to recommend a vitamin D supplement for all breast-fed infants from the first week of life. It is especially important for those in the inner city and those with deeper skin pigmentation.

Key Prevention

- Adequate UV light
- Oral intake of 10 μg (400 U) daily of a vitamin D preparation
- Adequate dietary supply of calcium and phosphorus
- Possibly orthopedic correction if severe deformities have occurred

Bibliography

Harrison HE, Harrison HC: Disorders of Calcium and Phosphate Metabolism in Childhood and Adolescence. Philadelphia, WB Saunders, 1979.

Shah BR, Finberg L: Single-day therapy of nutritional vitamin D–deficiency rickets: A preferred method. J Pediatr 1994; 125:487–490.

Glorieux FH (ed): Rickets. Nestle Nutrition Workshop Series, vol 21. New York, Raven Press, 1991.

9 Obesity

Michael Rosenbaum

Definition

1. Obesity may be defined as a maladaptive increase in the amount of energy stored as fat. Ideally, any definition of obesity in childhood would reflect both the likelihood that the obese child will become an obese adult and the risk of present and potential adiposity-related morbidity.

2. As discussed further on, the risk of persistence of pediatric obesity into adulthood increases with age, independent of the length of time that the child has been obese. The distribution of body fat in a preponderance of central (apple or android pattern) vs. peripheral (pear or gynoid pattern) is more closely correlated with the risk of current and future adiposity-related morbidity (cardiovascular disease, stroke, type II diabetes mellitus) than is total body fatness. Plots of weight, height, and weight-for-height measures vs. normative "standards" are the indices of body fatness that are typically used. Such measures are generally adequate, although they provide no assessment of fat distribution and incorrectly label muscular children as obese. It should also be emphasized that these standards are arbitrary and neither sufficiently sensitive to identify *all* children at risk for adiposity-related morbidity nor sufficiently specific to identify *only* children at such risk. Direct assessment of body fatness by hydrodensitometry (underwater weighing) or various radiologic methods is not feasible in the pediatrician's office. Subscapular skinfold thicknesses are highly correlated with the relative centrality of body fat distribution as well as absolute body fatness; normative standards for this measure are readily available. Subscapular skinfold measurement should be performed in all children, especially those whose weight-for-height is above the 75th percentile. An operational definition of obesity is having a subscapular skinfold thickness above the 75th percentile or experiencing adiposity-related morbidity at any degree of body fatness. Like the normative indices of body fatness based on various permutations of weight-for-height, this standard is somewhat arbitrary and will, of necessity, label 25 per cent of children as obese. Measurement of subscapular skinfold thicknesses is suggested only as a screen to detect the majority of children who are at risk for adiposity-related morbidity.

Etiology

Genetic and environmental factors: The increase in the prevalence of obesity in the United States must reflect the interaction between a genetic predisposition to store excess fat and an environment that permits the phenotypic expression of such a disposition.

1. Genetics: Studies comparing identical vs. fraternal twins and adopted children with their adoptive and their biologic parents indicate that the heritability of body fatness and body fat distribution is 65 to 80 per cent (approximately equal to the heritability of height).

2. Pre- and postnatal influences on obesity: In the United States, obesity is more prevalent among children in urban communities and in smaller families.

Epidemiology

1. The prevalence of obesity among children, defined as triceps skinfold thickness >85th percentile for age and sex based on a survey of United States children from 1961 to 1963, increased from 15 per cent to approximately 25 per cent in a similar survey performed from 1976 to 1980. In a study of adolescents conducted between 1988 and 1991, the prevalence of obesity, defined as body mass index [BMI, weight (kg)/(height)(M)]^2 >85th percentile, based on data obtained in the 1976 to 1980 survey, rose from 15 to 21 per cent.

2. The resistance of obesity to current therapies (including a variety of environmental and behavioral manipulations) is reflected in an overall 80 to 90 per cent recidivism rate among formerly obese adults and children.

3. The prevalence of obesity also varies among different ethnic groups (more prevalent among African Americans), geographic regions (northeast >midwest >south >west; urban >rural), and socioeconomic classes (more prevalent in poorer, less educated families or single parent/older parent families; less prevalent in large families).

   a. Studies of pre- and postnatal under- and overnutrition on subsequent obesity have revealed relatively small effects of the intrauterine environment. Prenatal undernutrition has been studied by examining the prevalence of obesity in children conceived during periods of natural or man-made famine, such as the Nazi-imposed Dutch famine of 1944–1945. There was a small but significant increase in the prevalence of obesity among adults whose mothers were malnourished early in pregnancy.

   b. Though formula-fed babies tend to be longer and heavier than their breast-fed peers, these differences do not persist, and early infant feeding practices do not significantly affect the risk of later obesity. Neither the age at which specific foods are introduced into the diet nor the proportions of fat, carbohydrate, and protein in the diet significantly influence subsequent adult adiposity.

   c. The institution of a well-balanced diet in childhood may form the basis for long-term healthy dietary habits, which will significantly lower cardiovascular disease risk even if they do not substantially affect body composition. Significant negative correlations have been reported between physical activity and body fatness in preschool children, whereas positive correlations have been noted between adiposity and the amount of time spent watching television in adolescence.

Pathophysiology

1. Energy intake and expenditure: The high rate of recidivism to previous levels of fatness, as well as the tendency to maintain a relatively stable body weight over long periods despite wide variations in caloric intake, offers empirical evidence that body weight is regulated. The number of calories needed to maintain body weight is highly variable, so that no a priori judgment of caloric requirements can be made for any child. However, studies of adults have demonstrated that weight maintenance caloric requirements, corrected for differences in body composition, are not significantly different between the obese and never-obese.

   a. The first law of thermodynamics dictates that the accumulation of stored energy (fat) must be due to increased caloric intake relative to energy expenditure. Weight gain to an obese state therefore reflects an unusually low rate of energy expenditure and/or an unusually high rate of caloric consumption; the maintenance of an obese or nonobese weight will occur only when energy intake and expenditure are equal. Feeding behavior consists of "decisions" regarding initiation, composition, and termination of meals; these decisions are influenced by many internal and external factors. Energy expenditure can be viewed as the sum of the energy expended at rest in cardiorespiratory work and maintenance of transmembrane ion gradients (resting energy expenditure), the work of digestion and absorption of nutrients (thermic effect of feeding), and energy expended as physical activity (nonresting energy expenditure).

   b. Decreases in body weight of both obese and nonobese individuals are "resisted" by declines in both resting and nonresting energy expenditure. A formerly obese individual requires 10 to 15 per cent less calories to maintain a "normal" body weight than a never-obese individual of the same body composition. Recent studies of adults during maintenance of a 10 per cent reduced body weight have shown that the activity of the parasympathetic nervous system and the mechanical efficiency of skeletal muscle (calories expended per unit of work) are increased in the weight-reduced state while serum concentrations of thyroid hormones and the activity of the sympathetic nervous system are decreased. These metabolic changes during the maintenance of a reduced body weight are consistent with the observed declines in resting and nonresting energy expenditure and would tend to oppose the maintenance of a reduced body weight.

2. There is suggestive evidence that some individuals destined to become obese may demonstrate increased metabolic efficiency *before* actually becoming obese.

   a. Adults and infants who subsequently become obese have been shown to have a lower rate of energy expenditure than adults and infants of similar weight who do not subsequently become obese. In this sense, weight reduction in some obese individuals may unmask the metabolic state that predisposed them to obesity, and the extra body fat of the obese may mediate a metabolic correction for low energy expenditure.

   b. Classically, investigators of central nervous system regulation of energy intake and expenditure have viewed the brain as having discrete hunger and satiety centers, located respectively in the ventromedial and lateral regions of the hypothalamus. Energy expenditure is often regarded as being independently determined by thyroid hormones and autonomic nervous system activities. In fact, the ventromedial and lateral hypothalamic regions have important effects on feeding behavior *(energy intake)* and autonomic regulation of *energy expenditure*. The central role of the hypothalamus in mediating the regulation of body weight is exemplified by rodents with lesions of the so-called satiety center in the ventromedial hypothalamus. The lesioned rodents become hyperphagic and hypometabolic until they have eaten their way to a higher body weight set point. The human hypothalamus also subserves systems regulating both energy intake and expenditure. Traumatic or infectious injury to the human hypothalamus results in a syndrome characterized by hyperphagia, hyperinsulinism, and hyperactivity of the parasympathetic nervous system.

Clinical and Laboratory Correlates of Obesity in Children

Adiposity-related medical morbidities are summarized in Table 9–1.

1. Some morbidities, such as slipped capital femoral epiphyses, are largely the consequences of excess body weight.
2. Cardiovascular disease, in particular, is more closely correlated with the centrality of body fat distribution than absolute body fatness. Long-term (40 to 50 years) follow-up studies of adolescents show that adiposity-related morbidities, such as hyperlipidemia, that are evident in childhood track well into adulthood and that obesity in childhood constitutes an independent risk factor for adult morbidity and mortality, even if the childhood obesity does not persist.
3. Certain endocrinopathies, such as hypothyroidism, may precipitate weight gain. The vast majority of endocrine disorders associated with obesity are secondary to excess body fat and will diminish with weight loss.
4. There are syndromes in which obesity is part of a distinct symptom complex, often including a primary endocrinopathy and usually including poor statural growth (e.g., hypothyroidism, growth hormone deficiency) and/or very distinct heritable phenotypes (e.g., Prader-Labhart-Willi, Laurence-Moon-Bardet-Biedl) (Table 9–2).
5. Assessment of skeletal maturation by bone age and physical examination for the presence or absence of age-appropriate secondary sexual characteristics as well as syndrome-specific morphology or symptomatology (e.g., hypotension, constipation in hypothyroidism, centripetal distribution of fat in hypercortisolism) will quickly identify these syndromes as causes of obesity.
6. The severe psychologic stress from social stigmatization of obese children by a society that regards obesity as

TABLE 9–1. ADIPOSITY-RELATED MORBIDITIES IN CHILDHOOD

NONENDOCRINE

Cardiovascular	Most common identifiable cause of pediatric hypertension, ↑ total cholesterol, ↑ low-density lipoproteins, ↓ high density lipoproteins
Respiratory	Abnormal respiratory muscle function and central respiratory regulation, poor ventilation/perfusion ratios and difficulty with ventilation during surgery, lower arterial oxygenation, pickwickian syndrome, more frequent and severe upper respiratory infections
Orthopedic	Coxa vara, slipped capital femoral epiphyses, Blount's disease, and Legg-Calvé-Perthes disease
Dermatologic	Intertrigo, furunculosis, acanthosis nigricans
Immunologic	Impaired cell-mediated immunity, polymorphonuclear leukocyte killing capacity, lymphocyte generation of migration inhibiting factor, and maturation rates of monocytes into macrophages

ENDOCRINE

Somatotroph	↓ Basal and stimulated growth hormone release, normal concentration of somatomedins, accelerated linear growth and bone age
Lactotroph	↑ Basal serum prolactin but ↓ prolactin release in response to provocative stimuli
Gonadotroph	Early entrance into puberty with normal circulating gonadotropin concentrations
Thyroid	Normal serum T_4 and reverse T_3, normal or ↑ serum T_3, ↓ TSH-stimulated T_4 release
Adrenal	Normal serum cortisol but ↑ cortisol production and excretion, early adrenarche, ↑ adrenal androgens and DHEA, normal serum catecholamines and 24-hour urinary catecholamine excretion
Gonad	↓ Circulating gonadal androgens due to ↓ sex hormone–binding globulin, dysmenorrhea, dysfunctional uterine bleeding, polycystic ovarian syndrome
Pancreas	↑ Fasting plasma insulin, ↑ insulin and glucagon release, ↑ resistance to insulin-mediated glucose transport

TABLE 9–2. SECONDARY CAUSES OF OBESITY

SYNDROME	STRUCTURAL/BIOCHEMICAL LESION	CLINICAL FEATURES
Prader-Labhart-Willi	Chromosome deletion 15q11–15	Short stature, small hands and feet, mental retardation, neonatal hypotonia and failure to thrive, cryptorchidism, almond-shaped eyes, and fish-mouth
Alström	Unknown	Childhood blindness due to retinal degeneration, nerve deafness, acanthosis nigricans, chronic nephropathy, primary hypogonadism in males only, type II diabetes mellitus, infantile obesity that may diminish in adulthood
Laurence-Moon-Bardet-Biedl	Unknown	Retinitis pigmentosa, mental retardation, polydactyly, hypothalamic hypogonadism; rarely, glucose intolerance, deafness, or renal disease
Carpenter	Unknown	Mental retardation, acrocephaly, poly- or syndactyly, hypogonadism (males only)
Cohen	Unknown	Mental retardation, microcephaly, short stature, dysmorphic facies
Acquired hypothalamic lesions	Infectious (sarcoid, tuberculosis, arachnoiditis, encephalitis), vascular malformations, neoplasms, trauma	Adipocyte hypotrophy with little hyperplasia, headache and visual disturbance, hyperphagia, hypodipsia, hypersomnolence, convulsions, central hypogonadism-hypothyroidism-hypoadrenalism, diabetes insipidus, hyperprolactinemia, hyperinsulinism, type IV hyperlipidemia
Blount	Avascular necrosis or tibial plateau	Bowed legs, tibial torsion
Cushing	Hypercortisolism	Moon facies, central obesity, ↓ lean body mass, glucose intolerance, short stature
Hypothyroidism	Hypothalamic, pituitary, or thyroidal	Hypometabolic state (constipation, hypotension, bradycardia, cold intolerance, cretinism (if congenital)
Pseudohypo-parathyroidism (type II)	Familial (? X-linked) resistance to parathyroid hormone	Mental retardation, short stature, short metacarpals and metatarsals, short thick neck, round facies, subcutaneous calcifications, increased frequency of other endocrinopathies (hypothyroidism, hypogonadism)

the result of self-indulgence and overgratification while considering the ideal to be an almost anorectic thinness may be just as damaging to some children as the medical adiposity-related morbidities. These negative images are so strong that growth failure and pubertal delay due to self-imposed caloric restriction have been reported in some children.

Key Clinical Complications of Obesity

- Slipped femoral epiphysis
- Hypertension

Key Laboratory Findings

- Hyperlipidemia
- Elevated fasting serum glucose

Management

1. Selection
   a. Identification of the child who should be treated: The rate of recidivism to the previous state of adiposity among reduced obese adults and children remains at 80 to 90 per cent. However, the short-term increase in the prevalence of obesity in American children demonstrates the potent effects of environment on this phenotype. The pediatrician should seek to identify the child at risk for adiposity-related morbidity as well as the already obese child, with the goal of encouraging a lifestyle (environment) that will minimize obesity and its comorbidities.
   b. A detailed history and physical examination should be performed to assess each child for current adiposity-related morbidities as well as risk factors for future morbidities (e.g., family history). Anthropometric data should be plotted on height and weight velocity charts, subscapular skinfold thickness charts (Fig. 9–1), and standard curves of absolute height and weight (or BMI), with the aim of detecting increased weight velocity before obesity occurs.
   c. Any child, regardless of body weight, with a strong family history (first-degree relative) of obesity, type II diabetes mellitus, hypertension, hyperlipidemia, or premature myocardial infarction and any child with subscapular skinfold thickness or body weight-for-height indices above the 75th percentile (see Fig. 9–1) should be considered to be at risk for adiposity-related morbidity.
   d. Not all obese children require or will benefit from treatment. The likelihood of persistence of pediatric obesity into adulthood increases with age. The obese 2-year-old is about twice as likely as a non-obese 2-year-old to become an obese adult. In contrast, that risk increases by six or seven fold by adolescence, independent of the duration of the obesity.

   e. Because of the lower risk that obesity will persist, and the higher risk that statural or brain growth will be impaired by caloric restriction, weight reduction should rarely, if ever, be undertaken in infants. Hypothyroidism is an unusual cause of obesity in infants, but the profound neurologic sequelae of untreated hypothyroidism in infancy justify heightened attention to this possibility.
   f. For the older child with obesity-related morbidity (e.g., hypertension), the child with central adiposity (as reflected in the subscapular skinfold thickness), and the child with a strong family history of adiposity-related morbidity (e.g., hyperlipidemia, hypertension, diabetes mellitus), medical evaluation might also include screening for hyperlipidemia and an oral glucose tolerance test to identify the child at risk for diabetes mellitus. Before beginning any type of therapy it is essential to have the cooperation of the child and the family. Clinicians should not assume that the obese child is necessarily depressed or that every obese child is strongly motivated to lose weight.

2. Treatment of the obese child
   a. The major goal of obesity therapy should be to diminish morbidity and morbidity risk rather than to achieve a cosmetically endorsed body habitus. In the otherwise healthy overweight child with no evidence of adiposity-related morbidity, clinicians and parents are generally concerned that the child will become an obese adult. Initial therapy should be directed toward decreasing or eliminating weight growth while allowing height growth to continue so that height eventually becomes appropriate for weight. If this is not possible because weight is at the obese level by adult standards, actual weight loss, as outlined below, should be considered.
   b. Therapeutic weight reduction is clearly indicated for the child with evidence of adiposity-related morbidity. The hypertensive or diabetic child should endeavor to reduce weight or alter body composition within 1 year (sufficient time to permit a safe and gradual weight loss) to the point that the morbidity is no longer evident. The obese child who is experiencing poor self-image, feelings of isolation from peers, and depression should also attempt weight reduction, perhaps with adjunctive psychotherapy.
   c. The initial therapeutic approach should combine exercise and a closely supervised dietary plan, preferably with the involvement of a dietitian. Studies of compliance with weight-reduction plans have emphasized the importance of a family-oriented approach. Any therapeutic regimen should involve the entire family and perhaps the child's school. Frequent physical examination of the child and monitoring of school performance should be included. If appropriate, the significance of any evident reduction in morbidity (e.g., lowering of blood pressure or cholesterol) can be reinforced.
   d. Reasonable goals in the form of a target body weight at the next scheduled appointment should be set at each office visit so that the patient is aware

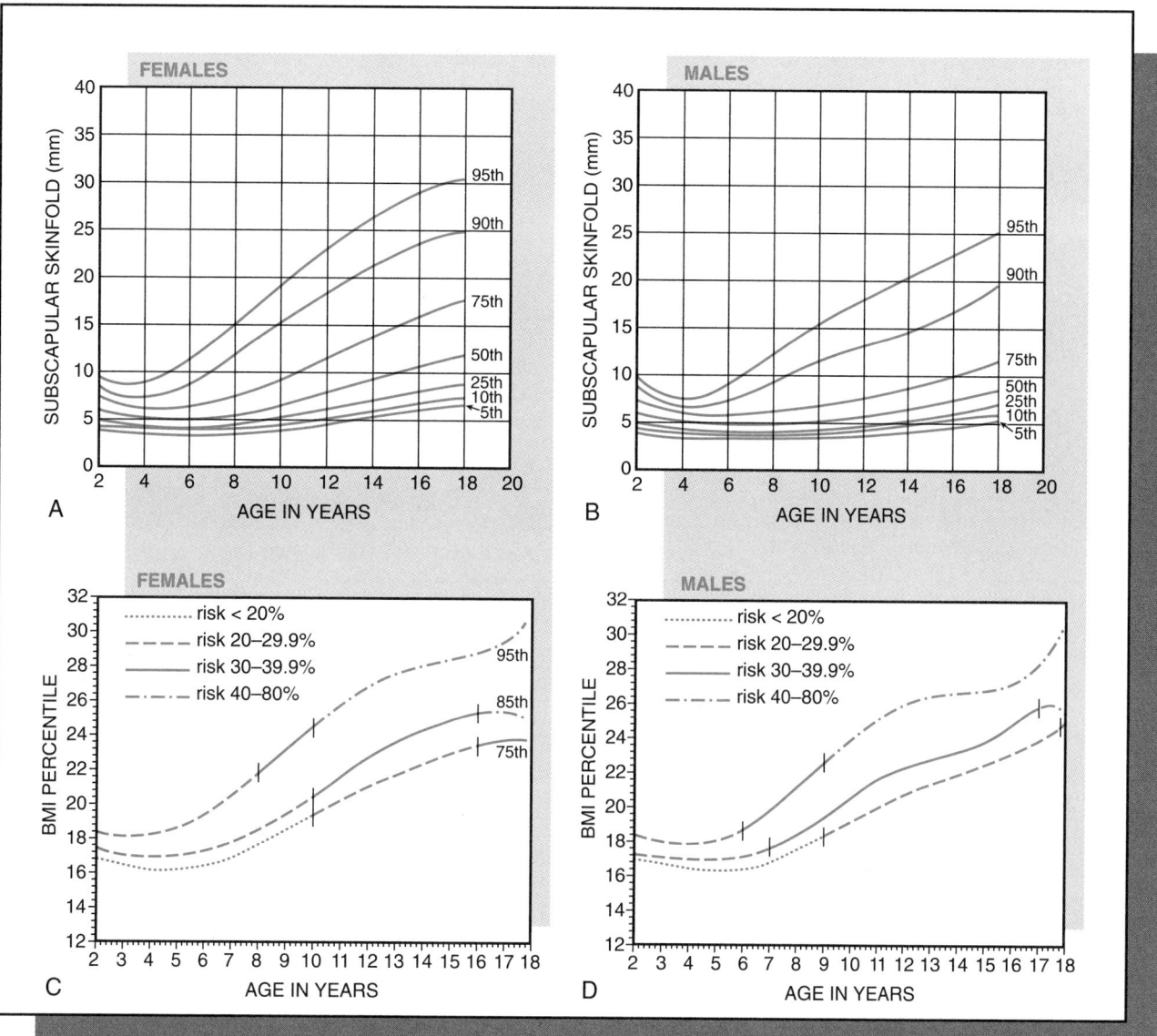

Figure 9–1 *A–B,* Normative values for subscapular skinfolds in children. (From Johnston FE: Sex differences in fat patterning in children and young. *In* Bouchard C, Johnston FE (eds): Fat Distribution During Growth and Later Health Outcomes. New York, Alan R. Liss, 1988, pp 85–102.) *C–D,* Body mass index (BMI) in children based upon the Second National Health and Nutrition Survey. Normative values are shown only for the 75th, 85th, and 95th percentiles of BMI. (Based on Guo SS, Roche AF, Chumlea WC, et al: The predictive value of childhood body mass index values for overweight at age 35y. Am J Clin Nutr 1994, 59:810–819.)

of what is expected. These goals should be modest and attainable even if compliance with diet and exercise regimens is only moderate, since achievement of an interval target weight encourages the patient.

e. Diet

    (1) The wide variation in individual rates of daily energy expenditure makes it inadvisable to prescribe the caloric content of a weight loss diet based solely on anthropometric data. Self-reported caloric intake is generally very inaccurate and the child's ad libitum diet should be directly observed and recorded by the parents for a minimum of 5 consecutive days.

    (2) The prescribed diet should initially provide 300 to 400 kcal/day below weight-maintenance requirements as assessed by dietary history and should result in weight loss of approximately 1 pound/week.

f. Exercise: Regular aerobic exercise will allow the patient to ingest more calories and encourage the long-term continuation of such a regimen. However, the energy cost of even vigorous exercise is low when compared with the caloric density of many fast foods and other snacks, and exercise should not be viewed as a license to eat. Obviously, treats, such as ice cream and potato chips, should not be used as incentives to exercise.

   g. More aggressive therapies

      (1) If the patient is unable to lose weight and/or morbidity persists, consideration should be given to a weight-reduction summer camp, with the obvious caveat that the child must be closely monitored and continue a therapeutic regimen after returning home. A weight-reduction camp will demonstrate to the child with a history of poor compliance with dietary and exercise regimens that weight loss is possible, and such a demonstration may promote future compliance.

      (2) There is no documented role at present for the more radical surgical (e.g., gastric stapling or jejunoileal bypass) or pharmacologic therapies in pediatric obesity. However, in some extremely obese children with life-threatening morbidity (e.g., pickwickian syndrome) in whom all other interventions have failed, it may be appropriate to consider such treatments.

   h. Treatment successes and morbidities: Before prescribing any type of weight reduction, health personnel should ascertain that the risks and difficulties of weight reduction do not exceed the benefits. In the older and otherwise healthy overweight child without a family history of adiposity-related morbidity, the fact that adolescent obesity may constitute an independent risk factor for adult mortality and morbidity must be weighed against the possible morbidities (poor statural growth, precipitation of eating disorders) associated with therapeutic weight reduction. Long-term studies of weight-reduced children and adults have shown that 80 to 90 per cent return to their previous weight percentiles. Obese children and their families must recognize that maintenance of a reduced degree of body fat-

ness will probably require a lifetime of attention to energy intake and expenditure.

Preventive Measures

1. Obesity is only one of many possible risk factors for cardiovascular disease. Since the adverse cardiovascular effects (such as hyperlipidemia, diabetes, and hypertension) are often cumulative, a combination of a cholesterol-lowering diet and program of regular exercise may be sufficient to reduce cardiovascular morbidity even if body weight is not significantly altered.

2. Children with a strong family history of any morbidity that can be exacerbated by obesity should be firmly and repeatedly counseled regarding good dietary and exercise habits, regardless of whether there is a family history of obesity.

Key Treatment

- Balanced diet—300 to 400 cal below daily maintenance weight requirement
- Exercise

Bibliography

American Academy of Pediatrics Nutrition Handbook: Obesity. In press.

Chua SC, Leibel RL: Molecular genetic approaches to obesity. In Bouchard C (ed): Genetics of Obesity. Boca Raton, FL, CRC Press, 1994, pp 213–222.

Fried SK, Edens NK, Rosenbaum M: The regulation of adipose tissue metabolism and growth: implications for the development of human obesity. In Subbiah MIR (ed): Atherosclerosis: A Pediatric Perspective. Boca Raton, FL, CRC Press, 1989, pp 191–217.

Leibel RL, Rosenbaum M, Hirsch J: Changes in energy expenditure resulting from altered body weight. N Engl J Med 1995;332:621–628.

Rosenbaum M, Leibel RL: Pathophysiology of childhood obesity. Adv Pediatr 1988;35:73–137.

10 Fluid and Electrolytes

Laurence Finberg

Although disturbance in hydration was recognized as a medical problem only in 1831, this aspect of physiology has application in every systemic disease, because of the continuous obligatory losses of water and the need to maintain composition of the principal body compartments. Because the activities of water and mineral solutes are governed by thermodynamic physiochemical laws, when the information is sufficient and accurate, mathematical calculations are both rigorous and dependable. This is in contrast to virtually all other biologic processes, which vary not only species to species but also person to person.

For clinical purposes one should always separate calculation of fluid and electrolyte needs into those related to body composition, those related to obligatory normal requirements, and, when disease is present, those losses or gains incurred by the disease process. A single formula combining composition and turnover may be applied only to a particular age and size. Because composition changes relate to mass and requirements relate to energy expended, it is necessary to consider these factors separately.

Composition

The human body is largely composed of water. At all ages from a week after term birth, water constitutes about 70 per cent of the lean body mass. As adipose tissue is added, the well-nourished (nonobese) child or adolescent will have water content of about 60 per cent of weight. The water is divided into two main compartments—the extracellular and the intracellular (Fig. 10–1).

1. The extracellular fluid (ECF), or the sea within us, composes about 25 per cent of the lean body mass (LBM) of an infant; it gradually shrinks to about 20 per cent of the LBM by midchildhood and then remains constant for the remainder of life in the healthy individual.

   a. A subcompartment of the ECF is the intravascular fluid or plasma, which carries nutrients and red cells with oxygen to the tissues and waste products back to excretory organs. The plasma volume, 6 per cent of the LBM, is maintained by the presence of poorly permeable protein molecules that exert an osmotic (oncotic) force opposing the hydrostatic pressure generated by the cardiac pump. Albumin molecules, being smaller than globulin, exert more influence per unit of weight. Although the normal albumin level is only about 2 mOsm/kg of H_2O from 4 to 4.5 g/dl of plasma, it creates enough gradient at the venous end of the capillary to pull back the water (and solute) forced out of the arterial end. The critical level of albumin to prevent edema is about 2.4 g/dl. Below this level, fluid (edema) will expand the ECF at the expense of plasma volume balanced by tissue back-pressure. The slight elasticity of tissue will slowly permit an increasing amount of edema unless the albumin concentration is corrected.

   b. The other subcompartment of the ECF is the interstitial fluid, a transport medium from the plasma to the cells. This fluid contracts with maturation from about 19 to 14 per cent of the LBM by roughly 5 years of age. Both the plasma and the interstitial fluid have sodium, chloride, and bicarbonate ions as their main solutes.

2. The intracellular fluid (ICF) has a strikingly different composition from the ECF (Fig. 10–2). The mechanism responsible for maintaining the difference despite the permeability of the cell membrane to water and the small ions is an energy-dependent transport system, or pump, Na^+/K^+ ATPase, which extrudes most of the sodium from cells. Muscle cells constitute 60 per cent of the cell mass and are representative of 80 to 85 per cent of all cells. Specialized cells (e.g., gastric mucosa,

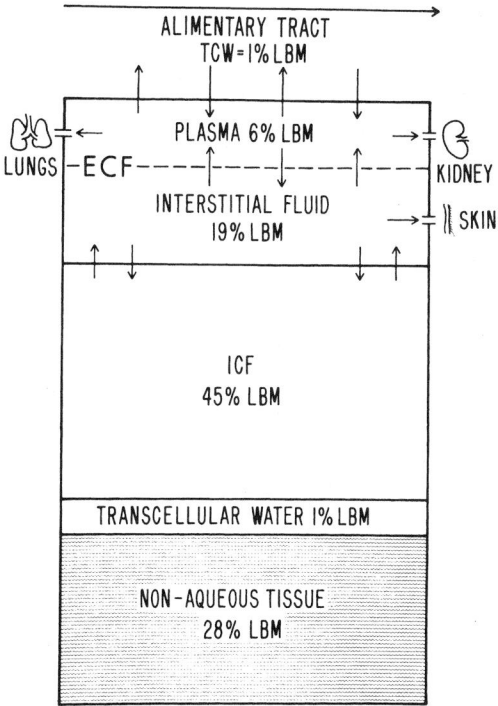

Figure 10–1 Diagram of body fluids in the infant as a proportion of the lean body mass (LBM), showing the rapid movement of water molecules (arrows) among compartments. Part of the transcellular water (TCW) is in the alimentary tract, part is in the urinary tract, and part comprises inaccessible cartilage and bone water. The cerebrospinal fluid (about 4 ml/kg in infants, 140 ml in adults) is included here in the interstitial fluid. ECF = extracellular fluid; ICF = intracellular fluid. (From Finberg L, Kravath RE, Hellerstein S (eds): Water and Electrolytes in Pediatrics: Physiology, Pathophysiology, and Treatment, 2nd ed. Philadelphia, WB Saunders, 1993.)

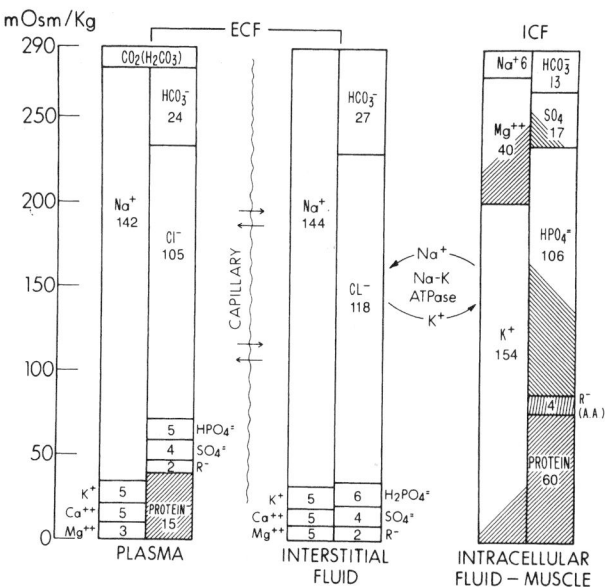

Figure 10–2 Ionic profiles of body fluids: approximate representation of cations and anions of the three principal body fluid compartments. All are electrically neutral and all have the same osmolality despite differences in total charges. The shaded areas represent large molecules or bound ions whose osmolal contribution (mOsm/kg) is quantitatively much less than their electric charge (mEq/kg) but which are of great importance to the distribution of ions because of their impermeability. (From Finberg L, Kravath RE, Hellerstein S (eds): Water and Electrolytes in Pediatrics: Physiology, Pathophysiology, and Treatment, 2nd ed. Philadelphia, WB Saunders, 1993.)

red blood cells, and others) have a somewhat different composition. Although calcium present in mitochondria plays a vital role, the concentration is in microequivalents and therefore does not appear in Figure 10–2. Similarly, there is no milliequivalent concentration of chloride in most cells.

Turnover of Water and Mineral

1. Water
   a. Humans are homothermic; we must maintain a body temperature within narrow limits (36 to 41°C) in order to have optimal function of various systems. As with other warm-blooded species, to do this we expend at rest most of our energy to produce heat (measured as calories or joules) and then lose it to the environment, balancing production and loss to keep a nearly constant body temperature. This expenditure of energy causes accompanying water loss, insensible from the skin and lungs and through the urine. The urinary loss is obligatory because energy production involves some cell breakdown, adding urea and mineral to the ECF. The kidney rectifies this disturbance in plasma concentration by excretion in a watery solution. A small amount of additional water is lost in the stool because of continued intestinal secretion.
   b. With a much larger surface area in relation to mass, the infant loses five times as much water per unit of mass as the adult. If there were no concentration of urine, the loss would be 10 per cent of the body weight per day for the infant under 1 year of age. Even with normal urine concentration, in the first months the loss will be 7.5 per cent of weight if there is no intake, compared with a 1.5 per cent loss in the adult in the same period.
   c. Table 10–1 shows the approximate obligatory water losses as a function of calories expended. Table 10–2 shows the basal calories expended at various ages as the surface area:weight becomes smaller. Neither caloric expenditure nor surface area is readily measured; therefore, Table 10–2 provides the information needed for calculation in either system of measurement. The Calorie is that of the nutritionist (or 1000 cal of the physicist). The urine value assumes a concentration equal to that of body fluids (290 mOsm/kg of H_2O). That is an appropriate value to use in calculation because if the

TABLE 10–1. APPROXIMATE OBLIGATORY WATER LOSSES AS A FUNCTION OF CALORIES EXPENDED

SOURCE OF LOSS	ML/100 CALORIES EXPENDED
Skin	30
Lungs	15
Subtotal insensible loss	45
Urine	50
Stool	5
	100 ml/100 cal expended

TABLE 10–2. BASAL CALORIC EXPENDITURE FOR INFANTS AND CHILDREN*

AGE	WEIGHT (kg)	SURFACE AREA (m²)	CALORIC EXPENDITURE (cal/kg)
Newborn	2.5–4	0.2–0.23	50
1 week–6 months	3–8	0.2–0.35	65–70
6–12 months	8–12	0.35–0.45	50–60
1–2 years	10–15	0.45–0.55	45–50
2–5 years	15–20	0.6–0.7	45
5–10 years	20–35	0.7–1.1	40–45
10–16 years	35–60	1.5–1.7	25–40
Adult	70	1.75	15–20

*Water expenditure equals 1 ml/cal.

infant can concentrate the urine the excess will be easily excreted.
   d. Table 10–2 gives basal calories expended (not ingested) at various ages. The basal state is adjusted to actual conditions for therapeutic purposes by factors learned empirically. The afebrile patient in a hospital bed expends approximately 1.5 times the basal. An increase in temperature of 1°C adds about 13 per cent. In practice, continued moderate to high fever will raise expenditure to about twice basal. Similarly, marked tachypnea or continuous muscle activity will raise the requirement to roughly twice basal. An unlucky patient with high fever all day, rapid breathing, and a continuous convulsion would require three times basal. In neonatal intensive care units, radiant warmers may induce losses in tiny babies of up to 7 to 10 times basal.

2. Mineral solutes
   a. Sodium (Na) and chloride (Cl). These ions are the main skeleton of the ECF. Their content determines the principal partition of body water. If concentrated NaCl is added, the body water will shift from ICF to ECF. Conversely, loss of salt without water (or physiologically more salt than water) will result in a proportionately decreased ECF and increased ICF. There is good homeostatic control for Na and Cl, so that recommended daily maintenance requirements are no more than 2 mEq/100 cal expended, and the tolerance is from 0.1 to 10 mEq/100 cal. The serum concentration of sodium ranges from 135 to 145 mEq/L and the chloride from 96 to 104 mEq/L. These values are not the physiologically active ones inasmuch as there is about 7 per cent solids in serum. For interstitial fluid there is also a Donnan equilibrium with plasma because of negatively charged, relatively impermeable protein. Sodium in interstitial fluid has a concentration range of 146 to 150 mEq/L and chloride from 112 to 120mEq/L.

Because Na and Cl are (for the most part) excluded from cells, their content plays the primary role in determining the division of body fluid between ECF and ICF. Although they are primarily distributed in the ECF or 25 per cent of the LBM, their osmotic distribution is in total body water (indeed, true of any solute) inasmuch as water diffuses across all membranes rapidly to offset establishment of a concentration gradient between compartments. Therefore, if one wishes to raise the concentration of sodium chloride, the calculation must be made on a distribution into 70 per cent of the LBM; in a similar manner the same applies to removal by dialysis.

    b. Potassium (K) is the dominant ICF ion and has a low concentration in the ECF (3.5 to 5.0 mEq/L). High or low concentrations affect myocardial conduction. The ion is plentiful in gastrointestinal secretions and, therefore, losses in diarrheal disease are considerable.

    c. Bicarbonate (HCO_3 and carbonic acid (H_2CO_3 or CO_2) are present in body fluids in a normal ratio of 20:1, maintained by respiration blowing off CO_2 and to a lesser extent by the renal excretion of hydrogen ion. This system constitutes the principal buffer of the blood, maintaining pH at 7.4 ± 0.05. The mathematical relationship is given in the Henderson-Hasselbalch equation.

$$pH = pK + \log \frac{HCO_3}{H_2CO_3}, \text{ where } pK = 6.1$$

When bicarbonate concentration is reduced, compensation occurs by increased rate and/or depth of breathing to reduce the CO_2, maintaining the pH. This condition is called acidosis. When compensation fails to correct, the pH goes down. This is called acidemia. Parallel terminology applies on the alkaline side. Some authors do not make this distinction and use acidosis and alkalosis generically for both states, losing some precision in the process.

    d. Calcium, magnesium, and phosphorus. Calcium is present in plasma in a tightly controlled concentration. With normal values for albumin, the concentration of total calcium is 2.3 to 2.9 mM/L (9 to 10.4 mg/dl), with the active (ionized) fraction about half. Magnesium concentration in the serum is 0.65 to 1.05 mM/L. The metabolism of these ions is discussed elsewhere in connection with disorders of their concentration and deposition. Phosphorus is present as the ions HPO_4^- and $H_2PO_4^-$. This is a buffering system, particularly so for excreted phosphates in the urine. Calcium and phosphate ions are in a steady-state relationship with the skeleton. Their concentration plus hormonal controls determines the building and dissolution of bone mineral.

    e. Other solutes.

The plasma protein carries a negative charge of 12 to 15 mEq/L (see Fig. 10–2). Other organic ions, chiefly sulfate, lactate, and amino acids, make up a small portion of the anions. Un-ionized organic substances, e.g., glucose, are also present, adding to the osmolality.

Bibliography

Finberg L, Kravath RE, Hellerstein S (eds): Water and Electrolytes in Pediatrics: Physiology, Pathophysiology, and Treatment, 2nd ed. Philadelphia, WB Saunders, 1993.

---

11 Treatment and Prevention of Dehydration

Laurence Finberg

Dehydration was first recognized as a significant, possibly life-threatening physiologic disturbance as recently as 1831 when W. B. O'Shaughnessy analyzed the plasma and stools of cholera patients. In pediatrics, dehydration is often seen in infants suffering from intestinal infections. While that group will be emphasized here, the principles enunciated apply to all ages and etiologies. Severe dehydration with medical shock or hypernatremia is further discussed in Chapters 12 and 13.

Etiology

As stated, losses from the gastrointestinal tract in excess of intake are the most common source of dehydration in pediatric patients. Simple thirst, hard work, diabetes (mellitus or insipidus), athletic exertion in the heat, and serious burns and other injury are also possible causes (see the relevant chapters).

Pathogenesis

1. Volume

    Fluid losses in diarrheal stools contain water, sodium, chloride, bicarbonate, and potassium in amounts sufficient to cause deficit of all these substances. The losses may be offset by oral intake for a time, but disease frequently causes anorexia and vomiting, which cuts off replacement of fluid.

2. Body compartments

    In most cases of dehydration, in North America and Western Europe the early losses of bowel secretion lead to loss of extracellular fluid (ECF), with renal compensation maintaining the sodium concentration in the normal range. About 5 per cent of the time, particularly when vomiting and total lack of intake occur early in the illness, water losses physiologically exceed sodium losses, and hypernatremic dehydration results. About 10 to 12 per cent of the time, while the patient is losing water and salt from the disease the caretaker replaces only water, resulting in a hyponatremic state. In hypernatremia the ECF is relatively expanded, the intracellular fluid (ICF) shrunken; in hyponatremia the

ECF is sharply depleted, including the plasma, and the cells relatively hydrated. Usually the relatively increased compartment nevertheless is a deficit.

3. Hydrogen ion metabolism/acid-base

In diarrheal disease a metabolic acidosis/acidemia ensues because of a cascade of factors.

a. Stool water is more alkaline than body fluids, i.e, more bicarbonate. In acute disease this factor is trivial and early compensated for by the kidney while circulation and filtration rate are sustained.

b. Bacterial fermentation producing hydrogen ion may lead to back-diffusion from the intestinal lumen (again, a very small contribution).

c. Early starvation (infants) leads to ketone formation from lipolysis.

d. Decreased perfusion of body tissues from hypovolemia leads to anaerobic glycolysis and lactic acid production.

e. Most importantly, the circulatory impairment from hypovolemia reduces the glomerular filtration rate (GFR) so that the kidney cannot compensate by the excretion of nonvolatile acid. When dehydration reaches this stage, acidosis quickly becomes acidemia; if unchecked in infants, the acidemia may become severe. Note that if plasma volume is maintained, this will not happen.

If dehydration results from upper gastrointestinal obstruction, e.g., pyloric stenosis or duodenal atresia, the chloride loss (not the hydrogen ion) leads to alkalosis.

4. Intracellular losses

Inasmuch as intestinal secretions are rich in potassium, losses of this ion may be considerable, up to 10 to 12 mEq/kg. A normal or even high serum concentration may be present because of low urine output.

5. ECF-skeleton steady state

The release of calcium from bone may be altered during dehydration, resulting in hypocalcemia. This is common in hypernatremic states and may also be seen in the under 3 months age group, in whom calcium homeostasis is immature.

Clinical Symptoms and Signs

An early symptom of dehydration is thirst with dry mouth. Thirst may be nullified by anorexia, and infants cannot communicate the sensation. No objective sign of dehydration appears during acute illness until about 50 ml/kg of body weight has been lost. This, of course, is 5 per cent of the body weight but closer to 7 per cent of body water. In iso- or hyponatremic states the signs are circulatory. The first sign is tachycardia, and next will be mottling and coolness of the extremities. In infants the fontanel sinks, as do the eyeballs at any age. Again, in infants the abdominal skin loses its elasticity and will stand in folds when pinched for several seconds or longer. The most quantitatively useful sign is the capillary refill time (turgor) (Table 11–1). Normal is <2 seconds; 50 to 100 ml/kg loss is 2.5 to 2.9 seconds; 3.0 seconds corresponds to 100 ml/kg (10 per cent of body weight, 14 per cent of body water) loss; medical shock with low-normal blood pressure, >4 seconds implies 120 to 160

TABLE 11–1. DEFICIT ESTIMATE FOR ACUTE DEHYDRATION

CAPILLARY REFILL TIME (SECONDS)	VOLUME LOSS (ml/kg)
<2	0
2–2.9	50–90
3.0–3.5	90–110
3.5–4.0	110–120
>4	150+

From Finberg L, Kravath RE, Hellerstein S (eds): Water and Electrolytes in Pediatrics: Physiology, Pathophysiology, and Treatment, 2nd ed. Philadelphia, WB Saunders, 1993.

ml/kg loss, and at that point blood pressure drops to subnormal levels.

It should be remembered that patients with hypernatremic dehydration show nervous system signs, with circulatory deficit occurring much later after additional losses.

There may be hyperpnea as a sign of acidemia or hypoventilation in the rare alkalemic condition. Potassium losses do not result in symptoms until recovery begins, when ileus and muscle hypotonia may be manifest.

Clinical Dehydration (5% Body Weight Loss)

- Tachycardia
- Prolonged capillary refill
- Loss of skin elasticity (infants)
- Sunken fontanel

Assessment

Use five points of assessment:

1. Volume

a. Estimate the deficits from the capillary refill time, using other signs as confirmative.

b. Estimate the 24-hour obligatory requirements or maintenance by multiplying the basal requirement by 1.5 (see Chapter 10).

c. Observe ongoing abnormal losses from continued disease, if any.

2. Body compartments (osmolality)

Judge from history and physical examination whether dehydration is isonatremic, hyponatremic, or hypernatremic (see Chapter 13). Confirm with laboratory analysis.

If one implements therapy from these two assessments alone, and there is normal renal function, one only has to add potassium to the regimen to achieve clinical success.

3. Hydrogen ion/acid-base

Use base, e.g., bicarbonate, lactate, or acetate ions, as a portion of the anions given, usually one fourth to one third of the total. Use chloride for 67 to 75 per cent.

4. Intracellular ion

As soon as the patient is known to be able to produce urine, add potassium, 3mEq/kg/day to the therapy.

5. ECF/skeleton

Measure calcium level under 3 months and when hypernatremia is suspected. Add to therapy if indicated.

Suggested laboratory determinations include sodium chloride, bicarbonate, potassium, and urea nitrogen. Of all the measures the body weight is the most important; be sure it is accurate.

Assessment

Clinical Analysis Points	Clinical or Laboratory Measure
1. Volume	Body weight, urea nitrogen
2. Body compartment (osmolality)	Serum Na
3. Hydrogen ion/acid-base	Serum HCO_3 (optional: pH, P_{CO_2} and base excess)
4. Intracellular ion	No good measure
5. Skeleton/ECF	Calcium—total or ionized

Implementation

It is important to "front-load" the therapy when there is a circulatory deficit. We divide the therapy into three phases; the emergency phase is skipped if capillary refill <2.5 seconds.

1. Emergency (1 hour): aimed at restoring plasma volume rapidly. The total volume given in this phase is 40 to 50 ml/kg over 1 hour or less. Table 11–2 shows a highly successful approach. Some workers use Ringer's lactate or isotonic saline in this phase. We prefer 10 per cent glucose with added electrolyte to speed urine formation. Five per cent albumin should be used when available (20 ml/kg) for premature infants, very dehydrated infants (loss of >120 ml/kg), and hypernatremic patients with circulatory failure.
2. Repletion

Six to eight hours, including emergency phase, is directed at the ECF or a whole. Plan to give half of 24-hour estimated quantity (plus ongoing abnormal losses) by the end of this time. The vehicle should be 5 per cent glucose, with Na of 65 to 80 mEq/L with K added when urine output is assured. This therapy can be given orally if tolerated.

3. Early recovery

For the next 16 to 18 hours, use the same solutions as above, given slower, to complete 24 hours. Again, if there is a suitable available caregiver, phases b and c can be given orally.

Treatment of Mild to Mild/Moderate Dehydration

1. When no medical shock is present (capillary refill <2.9 seconds), the therapy may be given orally using ORS (World Health Organization) or a suitable commercial solution. During the early or repletion phase the solution should be given rapidly. Vomiting is not a contraindication unless it is intractable (about 5 per cent of the time). There will be enough retained when feeding is persistent. The vomiting will ease when hydration improves. It is best to use a spoon to feed infants rather than a nipple or cup. The initial solution should have 60 to 90 mEq/L of sodium. A maintenance solution should have 40 to 50 mEq/L of sodium. The higher concentrations should be given under supervision and stopped when the deficit is replaced with a shift to a maintenance solution.
2. Oral rehydration and maintenance therapy are to be preferred when practicable, which is when a caretaker, mother, or surrogate is available to feed. The task is so labor-intensive that it is not usually feasible by nursing personnel in industrialized countries unless a family member is free to serve the role.
3. Table 11–3 shows some commercially available oral rehydration and maintenance solutions.
4. When to begin refeeding infants recovering from diarrheal disease has long been debated. Certainly, previously well-nourished infants over 1 year of age may begin taking regular feeds after rehydration is accomplished. In

TABLE 11–2. SCHEME FOR FIRST 24 HOURS OF REHYDRATION FOR ISOTONIC DEHYDRATION OF AN INFANT*

	PHASE I	PHASE II	PHASE III	TOTAL
Phase	Emergency	Repletion	Early recovery	
Duration	1/2 to 1 hour	6 to 7 hours	16 to 18 hours	24 hours
Emphasis for restoration	Plasma volume	ECF volume	ICF volume	All compartments
Fluid composition	a. Plasma or 5% albumin plus 10% glucose b. 10% glucose with Na^+ 75 mEq/L, Cl^- 55 mEq/L, HCO^-_3 20 mEq/L	5% glucose with Na^+ 40 mEq/L, K^+ 20 mEq/L, Cl^- 40 mEq/L, base 20 mEq/L	5% glucose with Na^+ 40 mEq/L, K^+ 20 mEq/L, Cl^- 40 to 45 mEq/L, base$^-$ 15 to 20 mEq/L	Na^+ 9 mEq/kg, K^+ 3 mEq/kg, Cl^- 8.5 mEq/kg
Amount in ml/kg of body weight	a. 20 ml/kg of each solution, totaling 40 ml/kg b. 40 ml/kg	60 ml/kg	100 ml/kg, plus any additional abnormal losses	200 ml/kg "plus"

*Estimated deficit: 10 per cent of weight (100 ml/kg). Estimated ongoing losses: 100 ml/kg.

TABLE 11–3. COMPOSITION OF SOME ORAL ELECTROLYTE SOLUTIONS

	Na⁺ (mEq/L)	K⁺ (mEq/L)	Cl⁻ (mEq/L)	BASE (mEq/L)	GLUCOSE (mmol/L)
Rehydration					
WHO	90	20	80	30	111
Commercial	75	20	60	35	139
Prevention/Maintenance					
Commercial-1	45	20	35	30	139
Commercial-2	50	25	45	30	111

younger infants, especially those under 3 months, a gradual resumption over 2 to 4 days is usually desirable. In this group, if full-formula feedings are given very early, increased stool losses are likely, and recovery becomes compromised. On the other hand, breast feeding may be resumed as soon as the infant will suck. Apple and pear juice should not be offered because they contain sorbitol, a nonabsorbable carbohydrate that enhances water loss.

Key Treatment

- Emergency phase for hypovolemia—1 hour
- Repletion phase for ECF replacement—6–8 hours
- Recovery phase for restoration of all body fluid compartments—16–18 hours

Prevention

Early in the course of diarrheal disease, one of the maintenance solutions may be substituted for milk feedings for a day or two (no more), and dehydration may often be averted. Breast feeding should not be stopped during infant diarrhea unless on rare occasion losses necessitate hospitalization. It should be resumed promptly on rehydration.

B Bibliography

Finberg L, Kravath RE, Hellerstein S (eds): Water and Electrolytes in Pediatrics: Physiology, Pathophysiology, and Treatment, 2nd ed. Philadelphia, WB Saunders, 1993.

12 Acute Severe Dehydration

Laurence Finberg

Critical State

Classic or Isonatremic and Hyponatremic States

Definition

Acute severe dehydration is the loss of body fluids over a short interval, several hours up to 48 hours, totaling approximately 10 per cent of the body weight.

Etiology

1. Losses from the gastrointestinal tract from vomiting and diarrhea are the most common cause of dehydration in pediatric cases. Most patients with this form of dehydration are infants with infectious diarrhea, which may be malabsorptive or secretory. Rarely, a secreting tumor (ganglioneuroma) or a chemical irritant is the cause.
2. Other causes of dehydration include polyuria, burns, weeping skin disease, and simple deprivation of intake (see diabetes mellitus, diabetes insipidus, burns, and Stevens-Johnson syndrome).

Pathogenesis

1. Water lost from the intestinal tract is at first primarily from the extracellular space (ECF) enriched by potassium from intestinal secretion. The plasma, a component of the ECF, loses volume, gradually impairing circulation. This becomes clinically manifest with losses of about 5 per cent of body weight when the process is continuous. Absent intake, this occurs in only a few hours in an infant with moderate diarrheal disease.
2. If some intake is maintained during the early stages, homeostatic mechanisms will retain proportionality of the body's fluid compartments. If water without electrolytes is the only intake, hyponatremia will result. If water intake stops abruptly near the onset, a hypernatremic state is probable (see Chapter 13).
3. Loss of HCO_3 in stool water, lipolysis producing keto acids because of diminished food intake, lactic acid production secondary to anaerobic glycolysis resulting from reduced perfusion, and finally and most importantly, reduced renal perfusion blocking nonvolatile acid excretion lead to acidosis and eventually acidemia.
4. Protracted stool losses lead to loss of intracellular ions. Potassium losses are clinically important. Phosphate and magnesium are important only when the dehydration is superimposed on a severely malnourished state.
5. In infants there may be disturbance of calcium homeostasis.

Critical State *Continued*

Clinical Findings

1. Diarrhea and vomiting are present for as little as a few hours or as much as several days if some intake of liquid is maintained. As in milder dehydration, tears are absent, skin and membranes are dry, and oliguria is present. Because of their high insensible losses per kg, infants are particularly vulnerable to rapid dehydration. Loss of water intake by itself will cause 5 to 7 per cent body weight loss in 24 hours.

2. The earliest clinical sign of progressing disease is tachycardia. Next come other signs of circulatory impairment. The skin of the extremities is cool and mottled; the eyeballs sink into the cranium; and, when still open, the fontanel sinks. The abdominal skin loses its elasticity and stands up in folds when pinched. The most useful sign for quantitating deficit is the capillary refill time (turgor), which usually varies linearly with the degree of deficit. When 10 per cent of weight loss has occurred the refill time will be ≥2 to 2.5 seconds, measured by pressing blood out of tissue under the thumbnail or a fold of abdominal skin and quickly releasing, timing the return of color. When the time exceeds 3 seconds, 12 to 15 per cent of body weight loss is probable.

> ### WARNING
>
> **A hypernatremic state (see Chapter 13) or cardiac failure nullifies this sign. Fever has little effect, but the sign should be elicited in a moderate thermal environment.**

Brachial blood pressure will be low-normal. Should hypotension occur, greater than 15 per cent weight loss has occurred and death is imminent.

3. Acidosis may be inferred from the history. Occasionally hyperpnea or eyeball softness may be detected.
4. Intracellular losses may be inferred from the history.
5. The rare hypocalcemia will be masked by acidemia. Except in hypernatremic states, clinical evidence is not seen unless there is an additional underlying cause.

 Key Clinical Findings

- Tachycardia
- Cool and mottled skin extremities
- Prolonged capillary refill >3 seconds
- Abdominal skin stands in folds (infants)
- Sunken eyeballs and fontanel (infants)

Laboratory Assessment

Routine measurements should be Hbg or Hct, the electrolytes Na, K, Cl, HCO$_3$ (CO$_2$ content), and the serum urea nitrogen (most laboratories for historical reasons mistakenly call this BUN [blood urea nitrogen]). Optional tests include glucose, albumin, calcium, pH, and Pco$_2$.

Laboratory Assessment

Laboratory Value	**Required** *Usefulness*
Hct or Hgb	Check for anemia or hemoconcentration
Na	Assess body space proportionality
Cl	Same and for the type of acidemia
HCO$_3$	Degree of acidosis (-emia)
K	Baseline for later comparison
SUN (BUN)	Rough measure of circulatory disturbance and/or duration of starvation
Optional on Indication	
Glucose	If hypernatremia a possibility
Ca	Same as above
Albumin or total protein	Verify nutritional status and its effect on plasma volume
PO$_4$	Paired with Ca
pH	If there is a concomitant respiratory problem
Pco$_2$	Same as above

Treatment

The goal is rehydration within 24 hours.

1. First summarize the assessment for
   a. Volume: Add estimated deficit and 1.5 × the daily water requirement. If indicated, add for fever, tachypnea, and muscular activity. This is the projected 24-hour volume of water to be given, supplemented by replacement of additional abnormal losses.
   b. Fluid compartmental space (osmolality): If the sodium concentration is judged (or measured) to be in the normal range, allow 150 ml/L concentration of sodium for the deficit fraction of volume and zero for the maintenance portion.
   c. Hydrogen ion: Administer chloride and a base (HCO$_3$, lactate, or acetate) in a ratio of 3 or 4 to 1. It is unnecessary to correct the acidemia specifically, since correction of volume and compartment distribution will permit the kidney and lung to do this. If either organ is independently impaired, specific correction becomes necessary.
   d. Replace potassium *after* urine production is assured, usually after 3 to 5 hours. Give 3 mEq/kg over 18 hours or at an IV fluid concentration of 20 mEq/L.
   e. Calcium homeostasis is not usually a problem.

Critical State *Continued*

2. Phases of treatment—initially intravenously because of the presence of medical shock, defined as ≥10 per cent estimated weight loss with a normal or low-normal blood pressure.

  a. Emergency: The goal is to restore plasma volume and initiate brisk urine flow.

  (1) Alternative plan I—40 to 60 minutes: Plasmanate or 5 per cent albumin 20 ml/kg IV; 15 to 30 minutes: 10 per cent glucose in water 20 ml/kg, IV in 30 minutes.

  (2) Alternative plan II—60 minutes: 40 to 50 ml/kg of 10 per cent glucose with Na, 75 mEq/L; Cl, 50 to 55 mEq/L; and base (HCO$_3$, lactate), 20–25 mEq/L IV.

  (3) Alternative plan III—60 minutes: 40 to 50 ml/kg Ringer's lactate or 0.9 per cent NaCl, IV. This plan restores plasma volume adequately but results in slower production of a brisk urine output, slightly slowing the recovery process. We therefore prefer plan I or II, though others do not.

  b. Repletion of ECF (either IV or oral) 5 to 7 hours. The goal is to give half the estimated first day fluid to complete ECF restoration: 5 per cent glucose with Na, 75 mEq/L; K (only if urine production assured), 20 mEq/L; Cl, 75 mEq/L; base, 20 mEq/L. Replenish milliliter for milliliter any ongoing abnormal losses.

  c. Early recovery: 16 to 18 hours. The goal is ICF replacement. Give the remaining half of the day's allotment, IV or oral, plus replace ongoing abnormal

losses ml/ml. This is the same solution as (b) at a slower rate.

3. Modifications

  If hyponatremia is suspected from history or documented by measurement, the sodium and chloride concentrations in the second and third phases of therapy should be increased by 15 to 25 mEq/L. If the intravenous delivery is switched to oral intake, the glucose concentration in the oral solution should have a molecular ratio to sodium of no more than 2:1 or less than 1:2.

Key Treatment

- Emergency phase hypovolemia

1. 5% albumin—20 ml/kg IV—20 minutes
2. 10% glucose—20 ml/kg IV—30 to 40 minutes
   or
   0.9% NaCl or Ringer's solution
   40–60 ml/kg—60 to 90 minutes

- Repletion and recovery—see text

Bibliography

Finberg L, Kravath RE, Hellerstein S (eds): Water and Electrolytes in Pediatrics: Physiology, Pathophysiology, and Treatment, 2nd ed. Philadelphia, WB Saunders, 1993, Chapters 16 and 17.

Saavedra JM, Harris GD, Li S, Finberg L: Capillary refill (skin turgor) in the assessment of dehydration. Am J Dis Child 1991;145:296.

13 Hypernatremic Dehydration

Laurence Finberg

Critical State

Definition

The physiologic disturbance of hypernatremic dehydration results from lack of water intake, loss of water from disease in physiologic excess of sodium chloride, excess intake of sodium chloride (salt poisoning), or any combination of these. Arbitrarily the condition is defined by a dehydrated state with a concentration of sodium in serum of 150 mEq/L or higher. Since the rate of development is a major determinant of the disturbance, any rapid increase (a few hours) of 10 mEq/L may cause similar physiologic and pathologic

changes regardless of measured concentration. Gradual development of even severe hypernatremia (up to 180 to 190 mEq/L) may be asymptomatic. Hypernatremia without dehydration, other than in experimental conditions, will be transient because the sodium load will lead to water loss in physiologic excess of sodium loss.

Etiology

1. Hypernatremic dehydration most commonly stems from increased body fluid loss from the gastrointestinal

tract secondary to diarrhea and vomiting; it occurs when the disease or the care of an infant results in sharp curtailment of water intake (or, rarely, too high a salt intake).

2. The condition may occur from simple water deprivation or forced salt intake, both known as forms of child abuse.

3. Diabetes insipidus quickly leads to hypernatremia if untreated or if water intake is impaired. This may occur very rapidly in infants or gradually in older children.

4. The inability to communicate or recognize thirst is seen in several types of patients, resulting in deficient water intake.

   a. Infancy

   b. Unconscious state at any age

   c. Severe mental retardation

   d. Absence of thirst center(s) in the brain seen in congenital neurologic midline abnormalities and progressive neurologic encephalopathies leading to conditions such as Ondine's curse.

Pathophysiology

1. When there is a rapid increase in an osmolal gradient between the extracellular fluid (ECF) and the intracellular fluid (ICF) by a solute confined to the ECF, such as sodium chloride ions, water moves instantly from cells to equalize the solute concentrations of ECF and ICF; cell volume shrinks, and the interstitial space and plasma volume increase. Dehydration occurs either from primary losses (e.g., diarrhea) or from urinary losses induced by the hypernatremia.

2. In the central nervous system (CNS) the vascular endothelial cells are joined by tight junctions. Unlike the case in almost all other tissues, sodium and chloride diffusion into the CNS extracellular component is slowed by about 6 hours, so that the extraction of water will be from the entire cranial content, causing the whole brain to shrink away from the rigid skull and reduce the intracranial pressure. Capillaries and venules dilate and may rupture.

When the reverse gradient occurs rapidly, i.e., brain water osmolality greater than plasma, water will flow into the brain, increasing cerebrospinal fluid (CSF) pressure. If the magnitude of the swelling is sufficent, either circulatory impairment with infarction or herniation of the brain may occur. These catastrophic changes seem to occur suddenly because the curve of rising pressure vs. increasing volume, which initially is linear, becomes exponential at a critical point. These considerations are germane to the management of diabetic ketoacidosis and other hyperglycemic states (see Chapter 269).

3. In cells of all tissues, including the CNS, there is a response to diminished cell volume by the accumulation of osmoprotective molecules (often called osmo-

lytes) that defend the cell against further desiccation. In mammals these molcules are amino acids, especially taurine, and myo-inositol. Clinical neurologic symptoms and signs are temporally associated with this phenomenon. Present knowledge suggests that these osmolytes enter the cells from the ECF because of one-way transporters that open in the cell membrane when stimulated by increasing ECF osmolality. If and when whole-body hydration is restored, the osmolytes move out or are metabolized slowly; thus, during rehydration they may for a time continue to draw water into cells beyond the optimal cell volume, representing a hazard to rapid therapy (water intoxication).

4. Other metabolic disturbances involving calcium and glucose metabolism also are seen.

   a. Ionized (hence also total) calcium levels in serum are depressed, although seldom to a clinically significant degree. Rarely, tetany may be seen initally or during therapy as the plasma pH rises. There is a failure to release calcium from bone; beyond this the mechanism is not currently understood.

   b. Hyperglycemia sometimes occurs, occasionally to very high (1000 to 1500 mg/dl or 5.5 to 8.25 mm/L) levels. The mechanism is believed to be suppression of insulin release from the pancreas. The manifestation is not related to latent diabetes mellitus, although it is a transient insulinopenic state.

Pathology

1. When hypernatremia develops rapidly with accompanying brain shrinkage, there is frequently petechial hemorrhage and sometimes more extensive hemorrhage in the brain, followed by clotting and thrombosis. Predictional sites are over the cerebellum and along the superior sagittal sinus. Hemorrhage may occur at any site, including the subarachnoid space, the subdural space, and intracerebrally. Only about a third of patients who come to autopsy show serious hemorrhage. In survivors, 8 per cent show CNS impairment compared with less than 2 per cent in isonatremic dehydration.

2. Hemorrhage is not seen outside the CNS. Cell shrinkage in the renal medulla does sometimes lead to renal tubular necrosis with resultant oliguria or anuria.

Clinical Findings

1. History

The history is of particular importance in arriving at a tentative diagnosis.

   a. In diarrheal disease of infancy the history of early vomiting or other reason for cessation of fluid intake is almost always present. High fever, rapid respiration, and sometimes a dry environment may be contributing factors, increasing pure water loss.

   b. Patients with diabetes insipidus, whether of nephrogenic or central origin, have a history of high colorless urine output.

c. Application of $NaHCO_3$ or salt to the skin has rarely led to hypernatremia.

d. Child abuse by either withholding water or forcing salt intake.

e. Nervous system manifestations as discussed under physical examination.

2. Physical examination

a. The circulation often appears normal other than tachycardia because of the relative preservation of the plasma volume. Capillary refill is usually <2.5 seconds. Shock may (rarely) occur when the volume loss exceeds 100 ml/kg of lean body mass. Capillary refill then will be >3 seconds.

b. Urine output will be close to normal for the same reasons as above.

c. The abdominal skin in infants will not show the signs of classic dehydration: loss of elasticity elicited by pinching, causing to tissue to stand up in folds—rather, there will be a velvety smooth feel. The subcutaneous tissue of the abdomen sometimes has the feel of kneaded dough.

d. The nervous system bears the brunt of the important findings in this physiologic disturbance. A peculiar state of consciousness is usually present—a state of profound lethargy and even somnolence when undisturbed, accompanied by pronounced overreaction to almost any stimulus, tactile, acoustic, or even bright light. The deep tendon reflexes are hyperactive, and there may be slight nuchal rigidity. There may be fasciculations, coma, and convulsions as part of the presentation in the most severe instances. Any evidence of CNS signs has not been associated with losses of 100 ml/kg of lean body mass or approximately 10 per cent of body weight, providing the initial clinical estimate of deficit.

Key Clinical Findings

- History of poor water intake
- Disturbance of consciousness
- Hyperactive reflexes
- Velvety and/or "doughy" abdominal skin (infants)

Laboratory Assessment

The laboratory assessment is similar to that of other acute severe dehydration (see Chapter 12) with the placing of glucose, albumin or total protein, calcium, and phosphorus (PO_4) into the required rather than the optional section. The protein and PO_4 are needed to assess the significance of the total calcium concentration.

Key Laboratory Findings

- Increased Na and Cl concentration in serum (> 150 mEq/L for Na)
- Hyperglycemia (30–50%)
- Slightly low Ca concentration (20%)

Treatment

The goal is gradual restoration of hydration so as not to cause quick shifts of water into the CNS. Table 13–1 applies particularly to infant diarrheal disease and may be modified for unusual conditions in older children or adolescents.

TABLE 13–1. REGIMEN FOR THERAPY OF HYPERNATREMIC DEHYDRATION

CONSIDERATIONS (IN ORDER)	ACTION
1. Volume	a. Estimate the patient's deficit by clinical means, first in milliliters per kilogram, and then multiply by kilograms of weight for total sum. b. Estimate 48 hours' worth of maintenance water following usual clinical rules. c. Add volumes determined in steps a and b for tentative volume of solution for 2 days.
2. Glucose content	Use 2½ (2–3%) to prevent possible problems with hyperglycemia from arising later.
3. Sodium content	Allow 80 to 100 mEq/L for *deficit* fraction of fluid and none for the *maintenance* portion. The resultant concentration is usually 20 to 35 mEq/L. Use this concentration of sodium or simply estimate it at 25 mEq/L.
4. Potassium content	Generally, the maximal safe amount for an IV infusion, or about 40 mEq/L.
5. Anion content	Advised amount of sodium plus potassium equals 60 to 75 mEq/L of cation. Distribute the anions between chloride and base in accordance with clinical judgment. If desired, start with more base and change to more chloride after 6 to 12 hours. Do not use HCO_3 as base, since calcium is to be added. Use acetate or lactate along with chloride.
6. Calcium content	One ampule of 10% calcium gluconate for every 500 ml of infusate.
7. Rate of administration	Administer $\frac{1}{18}$ of volume per hour for 48 hours. In an infant the usual volume will be 275 to 350 ml/kg/48 hours, or about 6 to 7 ml/kg/hour.

From Finberg L, Kravath RE, Hellerstein S: Water and Electrolytes in Pediatrics: Physiology, Pathophysiology, and Treatment, 2nd ed. Philadelphia, WB Saunders, 1993.

Critical State *Continued*

Bibliography

Finberg L, Kravath RE, Hellerstein S (eds): Water and Electrolytes in Pediatrics: Physiology, Pathophysiology, and Treatment, 2nd ed. Philadelphia, WB Saunders, 1993.

McManus ML, Churchwell KB, Strange K: Regulation of cell volume in health and disease. N Engl J Med 1995;333:1260–1266.

Trachtman H, Delpizzo R, Steerman JA, Finberg L: Taurine and osmoprotective molecules in chronic hypernatremic dehydration. Pediatr Res 1988;23:35–39.

14 Measurement of Body Fat–Triceps Skinfold

Laurence Finberg

Procedure

1. In assessing undernourished and overnourished (obese) patients it is frequently useful to have a measure of body fat. A semiquantitative measure is the skinfold thickness as determined by a calibrated caliper. A convenient site is the region over the triceps.
2. The value obtained may be compared with compiled reference values (Table 14–1) and used as a rough guide for an initial assessment. Rough, because a single measurement at a single site does not take into account individual variability in fat deposition or the inherent limitations of the procedure itself. For following the course of reponse to management, however, the procedure has considerable value.

TABLE 14–1. PERCENTILES BASED ON U.S. CHILDREN

AGE IN YEARS	SKINFOLD (mm)				
	5	25	50	75	95
1	6	8	10	12	15
2	7	9	10	12	15
3	6	9	11	12.5	15
5	6	8	10	12	17.5
8	6.5	9	11	15	22.5
12	7.5	10.5	14	18.5	27
16	10	13.5	17	21	32.5*

*The percentile given is for girls; for boys the value is 22.
Abbreviated from the National Center for Health Statistics of the Department of Health and Human Services.

Equipment

The caliper should be sturdy but light, with a jaw pressure maintained at 10 g/mm² over the usual range. The contact surface may vary from 30 to 100 mm. The use of a calibration block is advised.

Sites

Although a number of sites are suitable, including the biceps, subscapular, suprailiac, thigh, and calf areas, we discuss a single site, the area over the triceps muscle. Multiple site measurements will increase accuracy if more precise information is needed.

Technique

The technique is to grasp the skin and subcutaneous tissue 1 cm above the midpoint between the scapula's acromion process and the olecranon process of the ulna along the long axis of the arm. While the arm hangs vertically and is relaxed the caliper is applied posteriorly. One first lifts the skin and fat with the thumb and forefinger and applies the caliper 1 cm distal to the fingers midway between the base and the apex of the fold. While the fold is supported with the fingers, after 3 seconds of application the reading is taken to the nearest 0.5 mm. This is done twice more, and the results are averaged.

Bibliography

Shils ME, Olson JA, Shike M (eds): Modern Nutrition in Health and Disease, 8th ed. Philadelphia, Lea & Febiger, 1994.

15 Total Parenteral Nutrition (TPN)

Laurence Finberg

Procedure

The ability to supply total daily nutrition parenterally requires administration of a very hypertonic solution, which, if given through a peripheral vein, would soon sclerose it. Using newly available Silastic catheters, Dudrick introduced solutions into a large central vein, in which the caliber and flow rapidly dilute the hypertonicity. Alternatively, one may use a peripheral vein with a lower glucose concentration and supplement with separate injections of lipid. The technique described here is for central administration.

Indications

The following are some indications for infants and children.

1. Support for very low birth weight infants
2. Massive bowel resection (short gut)
3. Severe inflammatory bowel disease
4. Persistent vomiting
5. Pseudointestinal obstruction
6. Intestinal villous atrophy, e.g., immune disease
7. Other conditions not amenable to enteral feeding

Technique

1. A suitably sized Silastic, silicone, elastomer, or polyethylene catheter inserted through the external or internal jugular vein into the superior vena with meticulous aseptic precautions.
2. An x-ray should be obtained to verify placement near, but not in, the right auricle. Millipore filters should be used for lipids often administered through a Y connector.

Composition of Solution

The composition of the solution requires all the components of nutrition.

1. The protein is given as an amino acid mixture from a hydrolysate or a crystalline preparation. Percentages vary from 3.5 to 10 per cent. Special preparation may be obtained for premature infants with ratios approximating the composition of human milk. The optimal intake is 1.5 to 3g protein equivalent/kg/day.
2. The carbohydrate used is glucose in high concentration to provide most of the energy requirement. To avoid early hyperglycemia it is advisable to increase the concentration from 10 to 25 per cent in 5 per cent increments over 48 hours.
3. Lipids are given as a fat emulsion. The requirement of α-linoleic acid is achieved by 0.5–1 g/kg of body weight of lipid emulsion; 0.1 g/kg is advisable for linoleic acid.
4. The daily requirement for vitamins should be included (see Table 15–1), or a supplement given at appropriate intervals as indicated below.
5. The necessary macrominerals and trace elements are given in Table 15–1.

Complications

1. Infection from contamination of the delivery system or solution—the most serious

TABLE 15–1. CENTRAL TOTAL PARENTERAL SOLUTION (1 L)*

CONSTITUENT	AMOUNT		FORMULATION
Amino acids	35	gm	500 ml Aminosyn 7%
Dextrose	250	gm	500 ml dextrose U.S.P. 50%
Electrolytes			
Sodium	25	mEq	Sodium chloride concentrate
Chloride	25	mEq	
Potassium	25	mEq	Potassium phosphate
Phosphate	17	mmol	
Calcium	2.5	mEq	Calcium gluconate
Magnesium	2	mEq	Magnesium sulfate
Vitamins			
Vitamin C	50	mg	
Vitamin A	1000	units	
Vitamin D	100	units	
Thiamine HCl	5	mg	
Riboflavin	1	mg	Multiple-vitamin concentrate
Pyridoxine	1.5	mg	
Niacinamide	10.0	mg	
Panthenol	2.5	mg	
Vitamin E	0.5	unit	
Folic acid	0.5	mg	Folic acid
Trace Elements			
Zinc sulfate	0.8	mg	Zinc sulfate
Copper sulfate	0.4	mg	Cupric sulfate
Manganese sulfate	0.4	mg	Manganese sulfate

From Finberg L, Kravath RE, Hellerstein S (eds): Water and Electrolytes in Pediatrics: Physiology, Pathophysiology, and Treatment, 2nd ed. Philadelphia, WB Saunders, 1993.

*This is a solution for patients up to 30 months of age or 15 kg of body weight. Lipid emulsion should be supplemented daily according to energy needs 1 to 4 g/kg. The folic acid and trace minerals are added only to the first liter in a day when more volume is required. Vitamin B_{12} should be given parenterally every 4 weeks. Parenteral vitamin D 5000–15,000 µg every 6 months for long-term TPN users is a useful style of administration.

Procedure *Continued*

2. Hepatic dysfunction with cholestasis
3. Cholelithiasis
4. Metabolic bone disease (rickets) because of low phosphorus intake
5. Lipid overload impairing pulmonary and or hepatic function
6. Thrombus formation.

Bibliography

Dudrick SJ: Total intravenous feeding and growth in puppies. Fed Proc 1966; 25:481.

Finberg L, Kravath RE, Hellerstein S (eds): Water and Electrolytes in Pediatrics: Physiology, Pathophysiology, and Treatment, 2nd ed. Philadelphia, WB Saunders, 1993.

Kleinman RE (ed): Pediatric Nutrition Handbook, 4th ed. American Academy of Pediatrics, Elk Grove, IL, 1997.

Shils ME, Olson JA, Shike M (eds): Modern Nutrition in Health and Disease, 8th ed. Philadelphia, Lea & Febiger, 1994.

16 Symptoms of the Newborn

Leonard Glass

Signs of Illness in the Newborn Infant

- Respiratory distress
- Lethargy
- Cyanosis
- Pallor
- Plethora
- Vomiting
- Constipation
- Diarrhea
- Bloody stool
- Jaundice

| Symptom | **Respiratory Distress** |

Definition

Labored, rapid, or irregular respirations or apnea associated with biochemical evidence of impaired ventilation and/or oxygenation.

Etiology

1. Pulmonary
   - a. Congenital anomalies
     - (1) Choanal atresia
     - (2) Laryngeal and tracheal atresia and stenosis
     - (3) Tracheoesophageal fistula with esophageal atresia
     - (4) Congenital lobar emphysema
     - (5) Pulmonary lymphangiectasia
   - b. Developmental
     - (1) Pulmonary hypoplasia
     - (2) Respiratory distress syndrome (RDS)
     - (3) Transient tachypnea of the newborn (TTN)
   - c. Acquired
     - (1) Congenital pneumonia
     - (2) Meconium aspiration
     - (3) Air leaks (pneumothorax or pneumomediastinum)
     - (4) Bronchopulmonary dysplasia
     - (5) Persistent pulmonary hypertension
     - (6) Narcotic withdrawal
2. Nonpulmonary
   - a. Cardiac
     - (1) Congenital cardiac disease
     - (2) Patent ductus arteriosus
     - (3) Cardiomyopathy
   - b. Other
     - (1) Acute blood loss
     - (2) Hyperviscosity
     - (3) Systemic infection
     - (4) Perforated viscus
     - (5) Intracranial bleeding

Clinical Findings

1. History: A complete knowledge of the prenatal and intrapartum history is vital in identification of the cause of the infant's respiratory distress. The probability of a diagnosis of RDS becomes increasingly likely with decreasing gestational age and is unlikely after 34 weeks of gestation. A history of oligohydramnios may point to pulmonary hypoplasia. Maternal diabetes mellitus may predispose to RDS or be associated with a cardiomyopathy. Prolonged rupture of amniotic membranes with or without fever may be associated with congenital pneumonia. Maternal use of narcotics (heroin or methadone) may cause respiratory depression following delivery. It may also lead to hyperventilation as part of the withdrawal process.

   The presence of meconium in the amniotic fluid may be associated with meconium aspiration syndrome, possibly with an accompanying air leak. Persistent pulmonary hypertension may develop in these infants. Fetal distress during labor may be a sign of perinatal asphyxia, with subsequent respiratory depression occurring because of CNS damage. Significant fetal blood loss, frequently associated with maternal bleeding, may lead to respiratory distress.

2. Initial evaluation: The initial assessment of respiratory status is made in the delivery room. If the infant is obviously preterm and in distress, a presumptive diagnosis of RDS may be made, although congenital pneumonia must also be considered. If the infant appears to be full-term, the diagnosis of RDS is unlikely. The presence of a scaphoid abdomen suggests a diagnosis of diaphragmatic hernia, whereas frothing at the mouth suggests esophageal

atresia. Inspiratory stridor may point to an upper airway obstruction.

If the infant is significantly depressed, artificial ventilation must be instituted. If the 1-minute Apgar score is less than 4, endotracheal intubaton should be performed. If meconium is present in the upper airway, it must be suctioned under direct visualization before ventilation is begun. If a diagnosis of RDS is made, the administration of surfactant in the delivery room must be considered.

3. Subsequent evaluation: The sudden onset of respiratory distress or apneic episodes in an infant who has previously been asymptomatic may be due to systemic infection, aspiration or acquired pneumonia, pneumothorax, pneumomediastinum, gastrointestinal insult, or cardiac decompensation. Dyspnea may be a sign of anemia. Irregular respirations seen in preterm infants may be a manifestation of periodic breathing, which is commonly observed in this group of patients. The tachypnea observed with narcotic (primarily methadone) withdrawal may not be observed until the second to fourth day of life.

Respiratory distress in the neonate must be considered a potentially life-threatening event, and prompt attention must be paid to both establishing a diagnosis and initiating treatment.

Bibliography

Evans HE, Glass L: Signs of neonatal illness. *In* Evans HE, Glass L (eds): Perinatal Medicine. New York, Harper & Row, 1976, pp 418–440.

Symptom | **Lethargy**

Definition

Lethargy or decreased responsiveness may be apparent from the moment of birth or may develop in an infant who had been previously normal. It may be due to either pre- or postnatal factors and may not be immediately apparent to the untrained observer. It may be a transient phenomenon or secondary to a life-threatening illness.

Etiology

1. Antenatal factors
   a. Intrauterine asphyxia
   b. Maternal anesthesia and analgesia
   c. Maternal drugs, e.g., magnesium sulfate, propranolol
   d. Intrauterine infection
2. Postnatal factors
   a. Infection (sepsis and meningitis)
   b. Hypoglycemia
   c. Polycythemia
   d. CNS bleeding
   e. Hypothermia
   f. Hypocalcemia
   g. Metabolic disorders, e.g., organic acidemias and disorders of ammonia metabolism
   h. Bilirubin encephalopathy

Clinical Findings

In the infant who appears depressed at birth, knowledge of intrapartum events is crucial to reaching a correct diagnosis. This includes a history of administration of drugs to the mother, maternal infection, and abnormalities of intrapartum fetal monitoring. When lethargy is observed in an infant who has previously been active, investigation of its cause and appropriate treatment must be undertaken. A careful physical examination, including evaluation of thermal stability, is essential. Evaluation for systemic infection should include a complete blood count, radiograph of the chest, blood and cerebrospinal fluid cultures, and urinalysis. Appropriate antimicrobial therapy should be initiated if infection is suspected, pending results of cultures.

In addition, the diagnostic work-up in the presence of lethargy should include measurements of blood glucose, bilirubin, and calcium concentrations. In preterm infants, cranial sonography is indicated in order to evaluate the possibility of intraventricular or periventricular bleeding. Blood gas determinations are of value, since a significant base deficit may be indicative of either an infection or an organic acidemia.

Symptom | **Cyanosis**

Definition

Central cyanosis occurs when at least 5 g/dl of reduced or abnormal hemoglobin is present in capillary blood. Peripheral cyanosis in the immediate neonatal period may be due to either vasomotor instability or exposure to low environmental temperature without arterial desaturation.

The two mechanisms that account for central cyanosis are (1) the replacement of normal hemoglobin with significant amounts of reduced hemoglobin that cannot combine with oxygen, and (2) the entrance of unsaturated blood from the systemic venous return into the systemic arterial circulation secondary to either intracardiac or intrapulmonary right-to-left shunting.

Etiology

1. Pulmonary
   a. Upper airway obstruction
   b. Parenchymal disease

(1) RDS

(2) Pneumonia

(3) Atelectasis

(4) Meconium aspiration

(5) Pneumothorax/pneumomediastinum

(6) Persistent pulmonary hypertension

(7) Bronchopulmonary dysplasia

2. Hypoventilation secondary to central nervous system dysfunction

a. Hypoxic-ischemic encephalopathy

b. Intraventricular-periventricular hemorrhage

c. Infection

d. Metabolic disorders (e.g., hypoglycemia, hypocalcemia)

3. Cardiac

a. Decreased pulmonary blood flow

(1) Tricuspid atresia

(2) Pulmonary atresia with intact ventricular septum

(3) Critical pulmonic stenosis

(4) Tetralogy of Fallot

(5) Ebstein's anomaly

b. Increased pulmonary blood flow

(1) Transposition of the great arteries

(2) Total anomalous pulmonary venous return

(3) Truncus arteriosus

(4) Hypoplastic left heart syndrome

4. Other

a. Hyperviscosity syndrome

b. Methemoglobinemia

Clinical Picture

Although it is sometimes difficult to determine the cause of cyanosis when this condition is initially encountered, it is important to proceed rapidly with a diagnostic work-up to determine its etiology.

1. If cyanosis is due to a primary pulmonary problem, administration of supplementary oxygen together with the use of assisted ventilation will usually lead to an improvement in oxygenation. Occasionally, as in the case of severe RDS or persistent pulmonary hypertension, cyanosis will persist in spite of these measures. If it is uncertain whether the cyanosis is due to a pulmonary or a cardiac problem, echocardiography should be performed in order to determine the presence of structural cardiac abnormalities and right-to-left blood flow across a patent ductus arteriosus or foramen ovale.

2. If the cyanosis is secondary to a structural cardiac defect with decreased pulmonary blood flow, evaluation for surgical intervention to increase pulmonary blood flow must be done.

3. In all cyanotic infants, frequent measurements of arterial blood pH, P_{CO_2} and Pa_{O_2}, O_2 saturation, hemoglobin, and hematocrit are vital in management of the patient. Since the decreased offloading of oxygen associated with increased levels of reduced hemoglobin may lead to significant tissue damage, it is vital that prompt evaluation and treatment be instituted in all neonates demonstrating cyanosis.

Symptom	**Pallor and Plethora**

Definition

Pallor in the neonate is manifested by an absence of the normal pink appearance of the skin, mucous membranes, and nail beds. Plethora, a state characterized by an excessive amount of blood in the body, is manifested by the deep red or purplish appearance of the skin and mucous membranes.

Etiology

1. Pallor

a. Caused by a decreased number of circulating erythrocytes

(1) Acute blood loss (e.g., rupture or cutting of umbilical cord, abruptio placentae or placenta previa, accidental cutting of placenta during cesarean section, acute bleeding into internal organ or maternal circulation)

(2) Chronic anemia (e.g., isoimmune hemolytic disease, fetomaternal or twin-to-twin transfusion)

b. Caused by impaired circulation with hypotension

(1) Hypoxemia, with decreased perfusion and offloading of oxygen into cells

(2) Congenital cardiac disease (e.g., hypoplastic left heart syndrome, pulmonary atresia)

(3) Infection (group B streptococcal infection)

2. Plethora

a. Increased number of circulating erythrocytes

(1) Twin-to-twin transfusion

(2) Intrauterine hypoxia, with compensatory erythropoiesis

(3) "Milking" of umbilical cord

Clinical Findings

1. Pallor

a. Initial evaluation: In evaluating pallor that is observed shortly after delivery, the cause must be determined promptly and treatment, which may be lifesaving, instituted. Initial evaluation in the delivery room will dictate immediate therapy. If the infant is severely depressed with poor respiratory and cardiac function (usually secondary to antenatal hypoxia and acidosis), immediate resuscitative efforts, including endotracheal intubation, must be undertaken. With restoration of cardiac function and improved circulation, a normal ruddy appearance will usually return. Both the hemoglobin concentration and the hematocrit should be determined. Since a decreased hemoglobin concentration or hematocrit will not occur immediately in the presence of an acute blood loss, normal values do not preclude a diminished number of circulating erythrocytes. In the presence of acute bleeding with diminished blood volume (usually accompanied by systemic hypotension), immediate transfusion with either colloid or whole blood is necessary to restore circulatory integrity. Measurement of systemic blood pressure is required, and hypotension must be treated immediately.

b. Subsequent evaluation: In the infant whose color has been normal and in whom there is a sudden appearance of pallor, the two most likely causes are an acute blood loss or cardiovascular collapse (most often secondary to the onset of sytemic infection). In the infant with isoimmunization secondary to Rh or ABO incompatibility, the appearance of pallor

denotes continued hemolysis. The more insidious appearance of pallor in preterm infants is usually due to the anemia of prematurity.

2. Plethora evaluation

a. In the infant who appears plethoric, a careful physical examination and complete blood count must be performed immediately. Hyperviscosity, with possible adverse effects on the central nervous system, may be associated with hemoglobin concentrations above 22 g/dl and hematocrits above 65 per cent. Physical signs, such as respiratory distress, tremulousness, and irritability, may be due to the increase in blood viscosity. Measurement of blood viscosity is often helpful in making a decision about treatment.

b. Since polycythemia (even in the absence of symptoms) may be associated with adverse neurologic sequelae, treatment with partial exchange transfusion, using a 5 per cent albumin solution, is advised. The aim of this procedure is to reduce the hematocrit to approximately 55 per cent.

Symptom   Vomiting

Definition

Regurgitation of gastric contents; may occur normally or may be associated with a pathologic condition.

Etiology

1. Nonpathologic
   a. Swallowed maternal blood or amniotic fluid
   b. Overfeeding
2. Surgically related
   a. Esophageal atresia
   b. Small bowel atresia
   c. Necrotizing enterocolitis
   d. Perforated viscus
   e. Volvulus
   f. Congenital megacolon
   g. Meconium ileus
3. Nonsurgical
   a. Systemic or localized infection
   b. Intracranial bleeding
   c. Hypoglycemia
   d. Hypocalcemia
   e. Congenital adrenal hyperplasia

Clinical Findings

1. Since vomiting may be a presenting sign of a life-threatening disorder or, on the other hand, may be benign and self-limited, prompt evaluation must be undertaken. If vomiting of mucus is noted shortly after birth, the diagnosis of esophageal atresia must be considered. If a feeding tube cannot be passed into the stomach, a chest radiograph, using either air or a very small quantity of barium

as a contrast medium, should be ordered. If vomiting of blood or amniotic fluid occurs following delivery, aspiration of the stomach using a feeding tube may be curative. If the blood is fresh, performing an alkali denaturization test to determine if it is of maternal or infant origin is indicated.

2. Vomiting may occur after overfeeding, especially in a preterm infant with a limited gastric capacity. If the abdomen is soft and nondistended, feeding volumes can usually be decreased and the infant observed, without any further diagnostic work-up. In the presence of another potentially pathologic clinical sign, such as bilious vomiting, lethargy, abdominal distention, constipation, or jaundice, a further diagnostic evaluation must be undertaken. A condition warranting surgical intervention, such as a perforated viscus, volvulus, small bowel atresia, congenital megacolon, or necrotizing enterocolitis, may be present. Prompt surgical consultation is required, since conditions such as volvulus, perforated viscus, and necrotizing enterocolitis may be immediately life-threatening.

3. If infection is suspected, blood and cerebrospinal fluid cultures are taken together with a complete blood count, and radiographs of the chest and abdomen are done. In preterm infants, cranial sonography should be performed to determine the presence of intracranial bleeding. Serum concentrations of glucose, calcium, sodium, potassium, and chloride should be determined, since aberrations, if noted, must be corrected. Blood gas determinations (pH and P_{CO_2}) should be performed, since disturbances may accompany vomiting.

4. Although female infants with congenital adrenal hyperplasia are usually masculinized, male infants with this condition have normal genitalia. A manifestation of the severe salt-losing variety of congenital adrenal hyperpla-

sia in the neonate is vomiting associated with hyponatremia and hyperkalemia. Serum electrolyte and 17-hydroxyprogesterone concentrations should be determined if this diagnosis is suspected.

5. Oral feedings should be discontinued in infants who are vomiting and parenteral fluids administered until the cause of the vomiting has been found and the vomiting has ceased.

| Symptom | Inappropriate Passage of Meconium or Stool |

Definition

Failure to pass meconium by 48 hours after birth; cessation of passage of stool thereafter; passage of bloody or diarrheal stool.

Etiology

1. Failure to pass meconium or stool
    a. Small or large bowel atresia, imperforate anus
    b. Congenital megacolon
    c. Meconium ileus
    d. Meconium plug syndrome
    e. Malrotation with volvulus
    f. Intestinal perforation
    g. Systemic infection
    h. Necrotizing enterocolitis
    i. Congenital hypothyroidism
    j. Low oral intake of nutrients
2. Diarrhea
    a. Infection
    b. Narcotic withdrawal
    c. Phototherapy
    d. Hyperthyroidism
3. Bloody stool
    a. Swallowed maternal blood
    b. Necrotizing enterocolitis
    c. Anal fissure
    d. Volvulus
    e. Polyps
    f. Meckel diverticulum
    g. Coagulation defect
    h. Infection (shigellosis)

Clinical Findings

1. Failure to pass meconium or stool
    a. It must be determined if the infant has ever been fed (delay in passage of stool may occur in preterm infants who have not received oral feedings), has passed meconium or stool, has ever vomited, or has had abdominal distention. (The presence of bilious vomiting accompanied by abdominal distention suggests a high intestinal obstruction; bilious vomiting without distention suggests a low obstruction.) It should be determined if there is a family history of cystic fibrosis or hypothyroidism. A history of decreased activity or lethargy is suggestive of infection.
    b. On physical examination, the infant's state of activity and presence or absence of jaundice must be determined. Abdominal distention, the presence of masses, tenderness, skin discoloration, and hepatosplenomegaly must be looked for. Anal and rectal examinations should be performed and the presence of a meconium plug and stool in the ampulla determined.
    c. The diagnostic work-up should consist of a complete blood count, appropriate cultures, presence of blood in the stool, radiographs of the chest and abdomen, urinalysis, and serum bilirubin and blood gas determinations (when appropriate). A plain abdominal radiograph will usually demonstrate the level of obstruction and the presence of masses and free air. Occasionally, contrast studies may be required to make a definitive diagnosis.
    d. Because some of the above-named conditions, such as systemic infection and intestinal perforation or volvulus, may be immediately life-threatening, prompt intervention, such as administration of antimicrobial therapy and obtaining a surgical consultation, is indicated.
2. Diarrhea
    Because diarrhea, whatever its cause, may lead to dehydration and acidosis, it is important that appropriate measures be taken to maintain adequate hydration and normal acid-base status while concurrently treating the cause of the diarrhea. Frequent weighing of the infant and determinations of serum electrolyte and acid-base status are necessary in managing the infant with diarrhea.
3. Bloody stool
    Blood in the stool may represent a life-threatening surgical emergency, such as volvulus or necrotizing enterocolitis; a serious coagulation disorder, such as hemophilia or hemorrhagic disease of the newborn; or an infection, such as *Shigella* enteritis. On the other hand, bloody stool may be secondary to swallowed maternal blood or an anal fissure. Careful physical examination, appropriate radiographs and cultures, determination of coagulation factors, and surgical consultation are measures that can be undertaken in the presence of rectal bleeding.

1. Although jaundice is clinically evident in over 50 per cent of all newborn infants and is of little or no clinical importance in the majority, there are instances in which it may be the presenting sign of significant clinical illness.
2. The early onset of jaundice, with a serum bilirubin concentration of ≥5 mg/dl within 24 hours of birth, is usually indicative of a hemolytic process, most often an isoimmune blood group incompatibility. It may also be indicative of intrauterine infection. The onset of jaundice after the first day of life is usually related to the inability of the neonate to conjugate and excrete bilirubin in an efficient manner (physiologic jaundice) but may also be secondary to hemolysis, infection, or some other pathophysiologic entity. This is discussed in Chapter 18.
3. The clinician must be aware that although in most instances the presence of neonatal jaundice requires a minimal diagnostic work-up and no specific treatment, it may be the presenting sign of significant life-threatening illness requiring immediate treatment.

17 The Normal Newborn Infant

Stephen Ajl

History

Prior to examining the newborn infant, the clinician should be aquainted with the maternal history, with special attention to the following points:

1. General
   a. Age
   b. Race and ethnic background
   c. Parity
   d. Past medical history
2. Obstetric history
   a. Abnormal weight gain
   b. Infection (including serologic screening for hepatitis, syphilis, rubella, and, when appropriate, HIV)
   c. Drug use, including drugs of abuse
   d. Diabetes mellitus or other metabolic disorders
   e. Sickle cell anemia or blood dyscrasias
   f. Hypertensive disease
   g. Previous abnormal pregnancies
   h. Fetal monitoring (sonography, amniocentesis)
   i. Drugs administered during labor and delivery
   j. Mode of delivery

Physical Examination

1. The initial physical examination is performed in the delivery room and should include the following:
   a. Presence of meconium in amniotic fluid
   b. Apgar scores at 1 and 5 minutes (see Chapter 33)
   c. Presence of congenital anomalies
   d. Presence of birth injuries
   e. Abnormalities of the placenta and umbilical cord
2. A full physical examination in the nursery must be performed as soon as possible, but no later than 24 hours after birth. Another physical examination is done prior to discharge, at which time a discussion is held with the parents that should include feeding (breast feeding should be encouraged, and the mother should be instructed in its techniques); sleeping position (the supine position is preferable in order to decrease the possibility of sudden infant death syndrome); crying and fussiness; safety issues; bathing; clothing; stooling; umbilical cord care; sneezing and hiccuping; timing of the first follow-up visit; and when to call the pediatrician. The examinations should be performed in the presence of the parents, whenever possible.

   In performing the examination, the heart, lungs, and abdomen are examined first, while the infant is still quiet.
3. Outline of examination
   a. Careful observation of infant
      (1) Presence of congenital anomalies
      (2) Spontaneous movement
      (3) State of consciousness
      (4) Posture
      (5) Respiratory pattern
      (6) Skin color
      (7) Irritability or tremulousness
      (8) Abdominal distention or scaphoid abdomen
      (9) Excessive salivation
   b. Body measurements and vital signs
      (1) Weight
      (2) Length
      (3) Head and chest circumference
      (4) Respiratory and heart rates
      (5) Axillary temperature
      (6) Blood pressure (when indicated)

c. Skin
   (1) Presence of cyanosis, pallor, plethora, erythema, or jaundice
   (2) Purpura or petechiae
   (3) Hemangiomas, nevi, or telangiectasia
   (4) Erythema toxicum or pustular melanosis
   (5) Milia
   (6) Lanugo
   (7) Mottling
   (8) Unusual pigmentation
   (9) Mongolian spots
   (10) Edema or unusual swelling
d. Head
   (1) Size and shape (micro- or macrocephaly, hydrocephaly)
   (2) Cephalhematoma
   (3) Caput succedaneum
   (4) Fontanels (size, shape, and fullness)
e. Eyes
   (1) Spontaneous opening and closing of lids
   (2) Size and anomalies of globe; hypertelorism
   (3) Periorbital edema
   (4) Conjunctival hemorrhage
   (5) Cataracts
   (6) Increased intraocular pressure (congenital glaucoma)
   (7) Presence of red reflex
   (8) Retinal hemorrhage
f. Ears (in addition to physical examination, testing of hearing is recommended)
   (1) Position and shape (abnormalities may be associated with renal anomalies)
   (2) Presence of cartilage
   (3) Preauricular sinuses and skin tags
   (4) Tympanic membranes
g. Nose
   Newborn infants are obligate nose breathers, and failure to recognize choanal atresia, as manifested by unexplained respiratory distress, may have fatal consequences. Diagnosis is made by failure to pass a catheter through the nares into the nasopharynx and is confirmed by CT scan.
   (1) Patency
   (2) Midline defects
   (3) Flaring of alae nasi
h. Mouth and pharynx
   (1) Presence of cleft lip or palate (a bifid uvula may indicate a submucous cleft)
   (2) Macroglossia
   (3) Micrognathia
   (4) Ranula (sublingual dilatation of a salivary gland)
   (5) Natal teeth (these should be extracted)
   (6) Epithelial "pearls" (mucous retention cysts, at junction of soft and hard palates)

   (7) Presence of candidiasis (usually not observed before 1 week of age)
i. Neck
   (1) Webbing
   (2) Fistulas
   (3) Cysts
   (4) Palpable thyroid
   (5) Torticollis
   (6) Clavicular fracture (of no clinical importance when brachial plexus injury is not observed). Since callus formation will begin shortly after discharge, this must be called to the parents' attention.
j. Chest wall
   (1) Symmetry; absence of pectoral muscle
   (2) Retractions
   (3) Pectus excavatum
   (4) Breast tissue and accessory nipples
k. Lungs
   In the neonate, radiographic examination of the lungs is required whenever a pathologic condition is suspected.
   (1) Quality and symmetry of breath sounds
   (2) Presence of crackles
   (3) Presence of bowel sounds (indicative of diaphragmatic hernia)
l. Heart
   If a pathologic condition is suspected, electrocardiogram, echocardiogram, and chest radiograph are required.
   (1) Rate and rhythm
   (2) Location of apical impulse
   (3) Quality of heart sounds
   (4) Murmurs and thrills
m. Blood vessels
   Presence and quality of peripheral pulses (weakness or absence of femoral pulses may be indicative of coarctation of aorta)
n. Abdomen and gastrointestinal tract
   (1) Shape (scaphoid abdomen, distention)
   (2) Gross defects (prune belly, omphalocele)
   (3) Presence of bowel sounds
   (4) Palpable liver, spleen, kidneys, abnormal masses (the liver edge and lower poles of the kidneys may be normally palpated in the neonate)
   (5) Presence of anal orifice
o. Genitalia
   (1) Size of penis
   (2) Location of meatus
   (3) Descent and size of testes
   (4) Presence of hernias and hydrocele
   (5) Size of labia majora, labia minora, and clitoris

(6) Vaginal bleeding and discharge (may be normal in newborn)

(7) Presence of ambiguous genitalia

p. Extremities and spine

(1) Absence of portion of limb, constriction ring, extra digits, or syndactyly

(2) Range of motion and strength of extremities (abnormality may indicate brachial plexus injury or fracture)

(3) Examination of hips for congenital dislocation (performance of Ortolani and Barlow maneuvers)

(4) Deformities of foot (metatarsus adductus, equinovarus, tibial torsion)

(5) Spinal defects (neural tube defects, kyphoscoliosis, fistulas, abnormal tufts of hair)

q. Neurologic examination

The neurologic examination of the newborn infant is based largely on muscle tone and reflex activity and is best performed after the first day of life. It is adversely affected by drugs administered to the mother (e.g., meperidine, magnesium sulfate), perinatal infection, hypoxia, CNS birth injury, intracranial bleeding, anomalies of the CNS, and metabolic disorders (e.g., hypoglycemia). It is used, in conjunction with assessment of physical characteristics, in estimating the gestational age of the infant (Fig. 17–1). The neurologic examination should include

(1) State of consciousness and degree of alertness

(2) Reflexes (Moro, grasp, suck, rooting, Babinski, stepping or placing)

(3) Spontaneous movement

(4) Posture

(5) Muscle tone and activity

r. Estimation of gestational age

Although gestational age is best determined by an accurate maternal history, it can be estimated by assessing several physical and neuromuscular characteristics (see Table 17–1), assigning a score to each of these, and using the total score to estimate gestational age. When body weight, length, and head circumference are plotted against gestational age on standardized graphs, the appropriateness of these three measurements for the infant's gestational age may be determined. Any measurement below the 10th percentile is considered small for gestational age (SGA), and above the 90th percentile, large for gestational age (LGA). Decreased intrauterine growth may be due to maternal hypertension, maternal drug abuse (cocaine, alcohol, tobacco), nonbacterial intrauterine infection, or chromosomal abnormalities. Increased rates of intrauterine growth are observed in infants of diabetic mothers whose disease is inadequately controlled, and these may be associated with hypoglycemia.

Physical Examination of the Newborn Infant

- Observation
- Body measurements and vital signs
- Skin
- Head
- Eyes, ears, nose
- Mouth and pharynx
- Neck
- Chest wall
- Lungs
- Heart
- Blood vessels
- Abdomen and GI tract
- Genitalia
- Extremities and spine
- Neurologic
- Estimation of gestational age

Diagnostic Procedures

1. Maternal testing

Early in the pregnancy, the blood type (Rh and ABO groups) of the mother should be determined, and this information must be available at the time of delivery. Serologic tests for syphilis and hepatitis B and determination of rubella immune status should also be performed. The results of syphilis and hepatitis testing must be on the maternal chart at the time of delivery. If the infant is hepatitis B surface antigen (HB_sAg) positive, hepatitis B immune globulin must be administered within 24 hours of birth. It is now customary in many hospitals to administer the first dose of hepatitis B vaccine during the stay in the newborn nursery. A positive maternal serologic test for syphilis may indicate active infection in the infant if the mother was inadequately treated or untreated, or it may represent passive transplacental passage of antibody. It is recommended that pregnant women be tested for human immunodeficiency virus (HIV) antibody early in pregnancy, since administration of zidovudine during pregnancy, labor, and the early neonatal period significantly reduces transmission of the virus to the fetus in HIV-positive women.

2. Infant testing

a. Metabolic screening

Testing the neonate for phenylketonuria, sickle cell disease, hypothyroidism, galactosemia, and branch-chained amino acidemia should be performed after the first day of life.

b. Blood type, Rh factor, and direct Coombs' test

c. Hematocrit or hemoglobin concentration

NEUROMUSCULAR MATURITY

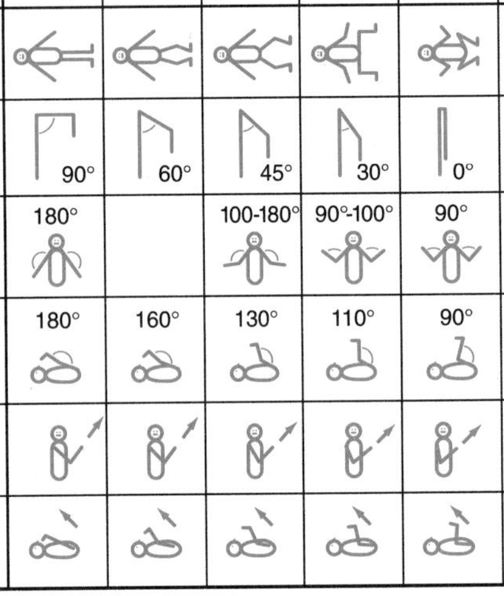

NEUROMUSCULAR MATURITY SIGN	SCORE						RECORD SCORE HERE
	0	1	2	3	4	5	
Posture							
Square window	90°	60°	45°	30°	0°		
Arm recoil	180°		100-180°	90°-100°	90°		
Popliteal angle	180°	160°	130°	110°	90°	<90°	
Scarf sign							
Heel to ear							
					TOTAL NEUROMUSCULAR MATURITY SCORE		

PHYSICAL MATURITY

PHYSICAL MATURITY SIGN	SCORE						RECORD SCORE HERE
	0	1	2	3	4	5	
Skin	gelatinous red. transparent	smooth, pink, visible veins	superficial peeling &/or rash, few veins	cracking, pale area, rare veins	parchment, deep cracking, no vessels	leathery, cracked, wrinkled	
Lanugo	none	abundant	thinning	bald areas	mostly bald		
Plantar creases	no crease	faint red marks	anterior transverse crease only	creases anterior 2/3	creases cover entire sole		
Breast	barely perceptible	flat areola, no bud	stippled areola, 1–2 mm bud	raised areola, 3–4 mm bud	full areola, 5–10 mm bud		
Ear	pinna flat, stays folded	sl. curved pinna: soft with slow recoil	well-curved pinna: soft but ready recoil	formed and firm with instant recoil	thick cartilage, ear stiff		
Genitals (male)	scrotum empty, no rugae		testes descending, few rugae	testes down, good rugae	testes pendulous, deep rugae		
Genitals (female)	prominent clitoris and labia minora		majora and minora equally prominent	majora large, minora small	clitoris and minora completely covered		
					TOTAL PHYSICAL MATURITY SCORE		

SCORE

Neuromuscular _____

Physical _____

Total _____

MATURITY RATING

TOTAL MATURITY SCORE	GESTATIONAL AGE (WEEKS)
5	26
10	28
15	30
20	32
25	34
30	36
35	38
40	40
45	42
50	44

GESTATIONAL AGE (weeks)

By dates _____

By ultrasound _____

By score _____

Figure 17–1 Scoring system for clinical assessment of fetal maturation in newborn infants. (From Ballard JL, Novak KK, Driver M: A simplified score for assessment of fetal maturation of newly born infants. J Pediatr 1979;95:769–774.)

d. Blood glucose concentration, using a glucose oxidase test tape (biochemical determination must be performed if value is less than 40 mg/dl)

e. If maternal drug abuse is suspected, test urine for opiates and cocaine metabolites.

Infant Feeding

Human milk is the ideal nutrient for normal newborn infants, and breast feeding should be actively encouraged. There are instances, however, when breast feeding is discouraged, such as when the mother has an infectious disease that may be transmitted in breast milk (e.g., HIV, active CMV infection), and when the mother is receiving medication that may have an adverse effect on the infant (e.g., antimetabolites).

1. Delivery room

   The normal newborn infant may be put to the breast in the delivery room. This enhances both the flow of colostrum and uterine contraction in the mother.

2. Nursery

   a. Breast feeding

      Although milk production and flow may take several days to become fully established, the nursing infant does not require supplementary formula feedings. Infants should be allowed to nurse ad lib, for up to 15 to 20 minutes on one breast, and then be allowed to nurse on the other breast if still hungry. Intervals between feedings should be 2 to 4 hours, and breasts should be alternated. The infant should be flat against the mother's body while nursing, with at least part of the areola in the mouth. The nursing mother should be guided in this "attaching/latching on" process during the first feeding. Vitamin D supplementation must be given to all breast-fed infants.

   b. Formula feeding

      If the infant is to be formula fed, an iron-containing formula should be used. During the first weeks of life, an infant consumes between 30 and 90 ml at 2- to 3-hour intervals. The commercial formula–fed infant does not require vitamin supplementation.

Circumcision

Circumcision is an elective procedure. There is some evidence that circumcision may be associated with a decreased incidence of urinary tract infection.

Discharge Planning and Follow-Up

1. It is recommended that most healthy term first-born infants born by vaginal delivery remain in the hospital for 48 hours after birth and that those born by cesarean section remain for 96 hours. In many facilities, early discharge of infants at 24 hours of age has been instituted. If early discharge is considered, the following conditions should be met:

   a. Full-term, appropriately grown infant born by normal vaginal delivery

   b. Normal vital signs for at least 12 hours

   c. Passage of urine and at least one meconium stool

   d. At least two normal feedings

   e. No abnormal findings on physical examination

   f. Absence of significant jaundice

   g. No bleeding from circumcision site

2. Discharge planning

   a. Continuity of care must be ensured, so that these early discharged infants are evaluated within 48 hours of discharge.

   b. The mother must receive training with regard to feeding, bathing, cord and skin care, sleeping position, and automobile seats.

   c. All infants should be given follow-up appointments within 2 weeks of discharge, and special attention must be given to families in which there are social and environmental risk factors.

18 Neonatal Jaundice

Gloria B. Valencia

Definition

1. Jaundice is a yellow appearance of the skin secondary to increased concentrations of serum bilirubin.
2. Jaundice becomes clinically apparent when serum concentrations of bilirubin exceed 3 mg/dl. Hyperbilirubinemia may represent increased destruction of erythrocytes, metabolic defects, a decreased capability to excrete bilirubin, or a combination of factors. Immaturity of processes necessary for conjugation and excretion of bilirubin is common among neonates, especially in prematurely born infants. In this group of infants, in whom no pathologic etiology can be found, the condition is commonly called physiologic jaundice.

Etiology

1. Increased destruction of RBCs

   a. Isoimmune (Rh, ABO, or minor blood group incompatibility)

   b. Infection

   c. Inherited disorders (congenital spherocytosis, glucose-6-phosphate dehydrogenase [G6PD] deficiency)

   d. Resorption of blood from cephalhematomas, bleeding into skin, internal organs

   e. Polycythemia

   f. Absorption of swallowed maternal blood

2. Metabolic disorders

   a. Glucuronyltransferase inactivity (Crigler-Najjar syndrome)

   b. Enterohepatic shunting

   c. Breast feeding

   d. Maternal diabetes mellitus

   e. Galactosemia

   f. Hypothyroidism

   g. Intestinal obstruction

   h. Cystic fibrosis

3. Decreased excretion (primarily conjugated bilirubinemia)

   a. Biliary atresia (intra- and extrahepatic)

   b. Hepatitis

   c. Cholestatic jaundice (secondary to total parenteral nutrition)

   d. Choledochal cyst

   e. Tumors

   f. Other rare causes (α_1-antitrypsin deficiency, Dubin-Johnson and Rotor syndromes, galactosemia, tyrosinosis, hypermethioninemia)

Pathophysiology

1. In the fetus, unconjugated bilirubin, which is formed following destruction of red blood cells, is excreted by the placenta. In the presence of Rh isoimmune hemolytic disease, a life-threatening anemia may develop, but the bilirubin itself does not threaten the well-being of the fetus since it is excreted via the placenta. In severely Rh-sensitized fetuses, significant anemia is usually present at birth, but the concentration of unconjugated bilirubin is rarely greater than 5 mg/dl. However, once the placenta is no longer the organ for excretion of bilirubin, blood concentrations rise rapidly, leading to a threat of bilirubin encephalopathy (kernicterus), signs of which in the neonate include lethargy, poor suck, impaired Moro reflex, opisthotonos, rigidity, convulsions, and frequently death. Long-term neurologic damage is a usual sequela to kernicterus. The exact mechanism of damage to brain cells by bilirubin is poorly understood, but several factors, including prematurity, perinatal asphyxia, acidemia, and low serum albumin concentrations, are contributory. Impairment of the blood-brain barrier enhances passage of bilirubin into the brain, thus increasing the likelihood of development of kernicterus.

2. In full-term infants whose jaundice is secondary to a hemolytic process and who are otherwise healthy, the risk of kernicterus may become significant when the serum bilirubin concentration approaches 20 mg/dl. In healthy full-term infants in whom there is no evidence of hemolysis, serum bilirubin concentrations of up to 25 mg/dl may not require exchange transfusion.

3. In infants with less severe manifestations of Rh hemolytic disease (now rarely encountered because of the widespread use of RhoGAM prophylaxis and ABO isoimmunization), the infant is at risk during the first days of life from both anemia and bilirubin encephalopathy. Therapy in potentially affected neonates must be aimed toward preventing these disorders.

Clinical Findings

1. Maternal history

   a. Maternal ABO blood type and Rh status

   b. History of sensitization during pregnancy

   c. Family history of hyperbilirubinemia (e.g., affected siblings)

   d. Maternal diabetes mellitus

   e. Polyhydramnios (indicating possible intestinal obstruction)

   f. Maternal infection (hepatitis, rubella)

2. Intrapartum history

   a. Maternal anesthesia and drug exposure

   b. Apgar score and need for resuscitation

   c. Birth trauma

3. Physical examination

   a. Presence of jaundice

   b. Pallor

   c. Lethargy, poor feeding

   d. Hepatosplenomegaly

   e. Evidence of bleeding (cephalhematoma, petechiae)

   f. Microcephaly

   g. Neurologic status

4. Diagnostic tests

   a. Serum bilirubin concentration (total and conjugated)

   b. Blood types of mother and infant

   c. Direct Coombs' test

   d. Complete blood count, including reticulocyte count and examination of peripheral blood smear

Key Clinical Findings

- Yellow skin and sclerae

- Lethargy in pathologic jaundice

Key Laboratory Tests

- Bilirubin—total and conjugated

- Infant and maternal blood types

- Direct Coombs' test

- Hemogram and peripheral blood smear

- Reticulocyte count

- Serum albumin concentration

Management

1. General principles
   a. The essentials of management of the jaundiced neonate involve prevention of bilirubin encephalopathy and treatment of the anemia accompanying hemolysis. A positive direct Coombs' test or serum bilirubin concentration of ≥5 mg/dl during the first 24 hours of life indicates the presence of a hemolytic process and the possible need for intervention to prevent bilirubin encephalopathy and significant anemia.
   b. If hemolysis secondary to Rh hemolytic disease has occurred in utero and the cord blood bilirubin concentration exceeds 5 mg/dl or the hemoglobin concentration is less than 12 mg/dl, an immediate partial exchange transfusion is required in order to restore red blood cell mass to a normal level. At this point, the infant is in no immediate danger of developing bilirubin encephalopathy. Further exchange transfusions are performed as necessary to remove sensitized red blood cells and bilirubin from the circulation.
   c. Guidelines for the management of hyperbilirubinemia are outlined in Table 18–1.
2. Phototherapy
   a. Naturally occurring bilirubin, a product of the breakdown of heme, is highly insoluble in aqueous solution and is converted to a soluble form (conjugated bilirubin) by a process of glucuronidation in the liver that facilitates excretion in the bile.
   b. Bilirubin maximally absorbs blue light in the range of 420 to 470 nm. When photons of blue light are absorbed by bilirubin in the skin of a neonate, a photochemical reaction occurs, rearranging internal bonding within the bilirubin molecule and converting the bilirubin to a water-soluble form. This water-soluble photobilirubin does not require hepatic conjugation in order to be excreted in the bile and urine.

   c. Phototherapy, using blue or daylight fluorescent bulbs, has become the most common modality of treating neonatal jaundice. The guidelines for using phototherapy are outlined in Table 18–1.
   d. When using phototherapy, care must be taken to shield the infant's eyes, monitor body temperature closely, maintain fluid balance, and determine the serum bilirubin concentration at 4- to 12-hour intervals (depending on the severity of the jaundice).
   e. Phototherapy is usually discontinued when the serum bilirubin concentration drops below 10 mg/dl.
3. Exchange transfusion
   a. Exchange transfusion has been the primary means of treatment for the prevention of bilirubin encephalopathy for the past half century. While the development of immunoprophylaxis for the prevention of Rh hemolytic disease has significantly decreased the need for exchange transfusion in recent years, this form of treatment is required in severe cases of ABO blood group incompatibility and the occasional cases of Rh incompatibility that are still encountered.
   b. Exchange transfusion is performed using either the umbilical vein alone for both removal and infusion of blood or the umbilical artery for removal and the umbilical vein for infusion. The blood used should be fresh and compatible with the blood of both infant and mother. Usually, an amount of blood twice that of the infant's calculated blood volume is exchanged. This results in replacement of approximately 85 per cent of the infant's blood volume. The procedure is usually performed using 10 or 20 ml aliquots of blood, with 1 ml of a 10 per cent calcium gluconate solution given after each 100 ml of exchanged blood. Cardiac rate and rhythm, respiratory rate, and blood pressure must be carefully observed during the procedure.
   c. Serum bilirubin and blood hemoglobin concentrations must be measured both before and after the procedure.
   d. Although exchange transfusion is generally considered to be safe, complications such as bradycardia, arrhythmias, infection, thrombosis, hypocalcemia, fluid overload, and intestinal perforation have been associated with this procedure.
4. Simple transfusion

   In instances in which anemia rather than hyperbilirubinemia is the major sequela of the hemolytic process, replacement of blood using a packed red blood cell transfusion is indicated. Since a prolonged hemolytic process caused by continued presence of the offending antibody may occur following discharge from the nursery in infants with ABO hemolytic disease, careful follow-up of these infants is mandatory.

TABLE 18–1. SUGGESTED THERAPY FOR NEONATAL HYPERBILIRUBINEMIA IN FULL-TERM INFANTS

UNCONJUGATED BILIRUBIN (mg/dl)	<24 HOURS	24–48 HOURS	>48 HOURS
5–10	Begin photoRx; exchange in presence of hemolysis with anemia	PhotoRx	
10–15	Exchange	Exchange PhotoRx may be sufficient	PhotoRx
15–20	Exchange	Exchange	PhotoRx
20–25	Exchange	Exchange	Exchange/<72 hrs PhotoRx in absence of hemolysis
>25	Exchange	Exchange	Exchange

*In preterm infants and full-term infants with a damaged blood-brain barrier, exchange transfusion may be indicated with serum bilirubin concentrations as low as 10 mg/dl.

Key Treatment

- Phototherapy
- Exchange transfusion

Bibliography

American Academy of Pediatrics, Committee on Fetus and Newborn, and American College of Obstetricians and Gynecologists, Committee on Obstetrics, Maternal and Fetal Medicine: Guidelines for Perinatal Care: Evanston, IL: American Academy of Pediatrics and American College of Obstetricians and Gynecologists, 1992, pp 205–210.

Maisels MJ: Jaundice. *In* Avery GB, Fletcher MA, MacDonald MG (eds): Neonatology: Pathophysiology and Management of the Newborn, 4th ed. Philadelphia, JB Lippincott, 1994, pp 630–725.

Tan KL: Efficacy of fluorescent daylight, blue and green lamps in the management of non-hemolytic hyperbilirubinemia. J Pediatr 1989;114:132–137.

19 Infants of Diabetic Mothers

Leonard Glass

Definition

A complex of abnormalities observed in infants born to mothers with inadequately controlled or uncontrolled diabetes mellitus that either was present prior to the onset of pregnancy or developed during pregnancy (gestational diabetes mellitus).

Etiology

During pregnancy, glucose tolerance is normally decreased, leading to increased maternal blood glucose concentrations and enhanced tranplacental transfer of this energy source to the fetus. Up to 5 per cent of all pregnancies are complicated by diabetes mellitus that is first observed during pregnancy (gestational diabetes), while preexisting diabetes mellitus is present in about 0.1 to 0.3 per cent of pregnancies. At least some of the problems observed in infants of diabetic mothers are causally related to the abnormally high maternal blood glucose concentrations.

Pathophysiology

1. Elevated blood glucose concentrations in the pregnant woman lead to fetal hyperglycemia, which stimulates insulin production by fetal pancreatic islet cells. Since insulin is the major fetal growth hormone, increased fetal concentrations lead to increased fetal growth and fat deposition (macrosomia). Increased fetal insulin levels also interfere with synthesis of pulmonary surfactant, predisposing prematurely born infants of diabetic mothers to the respiratory distress syndrome (RDS). Maternal diabetes mellitus, especially the insulin-dependent variety, is associated with an increased incidence of congenital malformations.
2. Poorly controlled maternal diabetes mellitus is associated with increased concentrations of glycosylated hemoglobin (A1C), and an increased risk of perinatal asphyxia. Impairment of fetal oxygenation may be related to these increased concentrations of glycosylated hemoglobin.
3. The neonatal hypoglycemia that is observed in infants of mothers with poorly controlled diabetes mellitus is caused by hyperinsulinism in the face of decreased availability of glucose to the infant following delivery. Severity of hypoglycemia in the neonate is directly proportional to the severity of maternal hyperglycemia. The origin of the hypocalcemia and hypomagnesemia frequently observed in infants of mothers with poorly controlled diabetes is unclear but is probably related to impaired parathyroid function.
4. Impaired intrauterine growth may be observed in infants of insulin-dependent diabetic mothers who have vascular disease and hypertension.
5. A cardiomyopathy may be observed in infants of mothers with inadequately controlled diabetes. This is manifested by thickening of the interventricular septum and left ventricular outlet obstruction. This is probably caused by increased glycogen storage in myocardial muscle fibers and is manifested clinically by the presence of a systolic murmur, cardiac enlargement, and respiratory distress.

Clinical Findings

1. Infants of mothers with inadequately controlled diabetes may be above the 90th percentile for length and weight and may have a typically ruddy facial appearance. There is an increased incidence of congenital anomalies, such as caudal dysplasia and congenital cardiac disease.
2. Hypoglycemia (serum or plasma glucose concentrations ≤35 mg/dl in full-term and 25 mg/dl in preterm infants on the first day of life and less than 40 mg/dl in both term and preterm infants after the first day) secondary to hyperinsulinemia is a frequent finding; manifestations of hypoglycemia include jitteriness, irritability, convulsions, and apnea.
3. Respiratory distress may be present. This may be due to pulmonary immaturity in infants of less than 37 weeks' gestation, meconium aspiration, transient tachypnea of the newborn, or diabetic cardiomyopathy.
4. Hypocalcemia may be asymptomatic or present with symptoms similar to those observed with hypoglycemia.

Key Clinical Findings

- Macrosomia
- Ruddy facial appearance
- Increased incidence of congenital heart disease

Key Laboratory Tests

- Serum glucose
- Arterial blood gases if respiratory distress

Management

1. Infants of diabetic mothers should be admitted to an observation nursery, even if they appear asymptomatic.
2. The initial laboratory evaluation should include a serum glucose determination and complete blood count. Arterial blood gas determinations and chest radiographs should be done when indicated. A screening test for hypoglycemia, using a glucose oxidase test tape, should be performed on admission to the nursery, followed by a biochemical determination.
3. A glucose value of ≤40 mg/dl on the screening test should lead to prompt intervention, pending the results of the biochemical determination.
4. In the presence of hypoglycemia, even if it is asymptomatic, an intravenous infusion of a 10 per cent glucose solution should be started in order to maintain blood glucose concentrations above 40 mg/dl.
5. Oral feedings, if tolerated, should be begun simultaneously. In asymptomatic normoglycemic infants, oral feedings should be started at 3 to 4 hours of age.
6. If oral feedings are not tolerated, an intravenous infusion of 5 per cent glucose solution should be started, at a rate of 6 to 8 mg/kg of body weight/minute.

Key Treatment

- Maintain normoglycemia

Prevention

Maintaining normoglycemia in pregnant diabetics by dietary control and administration of insulin, when indicated, is the best means of preventing the abnormalities observed in these infants. Even with apparent good control in the mother, one or more of these problems may be observed.

Bibliography

Cordero L, Landon MB: Infant of the diabetic mother. Clin Perinatol 1993;20:635–648.

Cowett RM: Hypoglycemia and hyperglycemia in the newborn. *In* Polin RA, Fox WW (eds): Fetal and Neonatal Physiology. Philadelphia, WB Saunders, 1992, pp 406–418.

20 Birth Injuries

Steve Piecuch

External Injury to the Head

Caput Succedaneum

Etiology

A caput succedaneum is a collection of edema fluid and blood in the soft tissue of the skull that accumulates over the presenting part, secondary to the forces of labor. The incidence is increased in prolonged labor and delivery and following vacuum extraction.

Clinical Findings

The edema is nonpitting, and since the caput is external to the periosteum, it may cross suture lines and commonly crosses the midline of the skull. Significant bleeding into a caput is rare, but neonatal jaundice may be aggravated as the blood is resorbed. Skull x-rays are not indicated, and the caput succedaneum usually resolves over a period of several days.

Cephalhematoma

Etiology

A cephalhematoma is a collection of blood under the periosteum of the outer surface of the skull; it is due to rupture of blood vessels running between the skull and the periosteum.

Clinical Findings

1. The incidence of cephalhematoma is approximately 2.5 per cent of live births; 15 per cent are bilateral. The most common location is over the parietal bones. Since the bleeding is subperiosteal, the hematoma does not cross suture lines. A characteristic crater edge may be palpable on the margins of the lesion. Linear skull fractures are found in a minority of infants with cephalhematomas.
2. Occipital cephalhematomas are uncommon but may be confused with encephaloceles because they have a midline location. A cephalhematoma can be differentiated from an encephalocele on physical examination because a cephalhematoma does not transilluminate, is not pulsatile, does not increase in size when the infant strains or cries, and is not associated with an underlying bony defect of the skull. In questionable cases, the diagnosis may be made on the basis of ultrasound examination or CT scan.
3. Cephalhematomas may initially enlarge during the first few days of life but then slowly resolve over a period of several weeks to several months. Significant bleeding may occur into a cephalhematoma, and, uncommonly, a

blood transfusion may be required. Resorption of the accumulated blood may lead to significant jaundice. Infection of a cephalhematoma is rare, and routine aspiration is not indicated.

Key Clinical Findings: Cerebellum

- Soft mass over skull with crater edge

Radiographic Findings

Routine x-rays are not indicated, since most associated fractures are linear and require no specific therapy. If a skull fracture is found, a follow-up x-ray should be done at 2 to 3 months of age to exclude the possibility of a developing leptomeningeal cyst. Skull x-rays may demonstrate hyperostosis of the outer table of the underlying skull that may persist for several months as well as calcification within the clot itself.

Subgaleal Hemorrhage

Etiology

Subgaleal hemorrhage results from bleeding under the scalp aponeurosis.

Clinical Findings

The infant may present with a swelling over the scalp that extends into the posterior neck or in front of the ears. Significant bleeding occurs occasionally, which may necessitate transfusion, and jaundice may develop as the blood is resorbed.

Skull Fractures: Linear

Etiology

Skull fractures are relatively uncommon in the newborn, because the skull is not well mineralized and is very distensible. Although skull fractures are associated with the use of forceps, they may also occur following an uncomplicated spontaneous delivery. In some cases, pressure of the fetal skull against the maternal sacrum may cause in utero skull fracture.

Clinical Findings

1. The infant may be asymptomatic, may have heavy bruising of the head or a cephalhematoma, or may have other evidence of birth trauma. Skull x-rays should not be done routinely after a difficult delivery unless there is evidence suggestive of significant head injury. In such cases, a CT scan may be the preferred study, since it gives information about injury to the underlying brain that skull films do not.
2. Linear skull fractures are in themselves benign and have an excellent prognosis, but an infant found to have a linear skull fracture should be carefully examined to exclude any other evidence of birth injury. Follow-up x-rays should be taken at 2 to 3 months of age to demonstrate healing and exclude a developing leptomeningeal cyst.

Skull Fractures: Depressed

Etiology

Depressed fractures may be associated with the use of forceps but may also be seen following uncomplicated spontaneous delivery; they may occur in utero as well. Most are of the "Ping-Pong ball" variety and are not associated with the loss of bony continuity.

Clinical Findings

The infant may be neurologically normal and present simply with a clinically evident depression in the skull. Bone fragments, hemorrhage, or pressure from the depressed bone may cause injury to the underlying brain. Although some depressed skull fractures require surgical elevation, selected cases may respond to nonoperative manipulation, and in some cases the depression may spontaneously resolve. The prognosis for depressed skull fractures is very good if there are no abnormal neurologic findings or other signs of significant birth injury.

Skull Fractures: Basal

Etiology

Basal skull fractures result from occipital bone separation, leading to direct brain injury and disruption of venous structures with posterior fossa hemorrhage.

Clinical Findings

The resulting posterior fossa hemorrhage can cause brainstem compression with catastrophic neurologic deterioration. This lesion has been managed both surgically and by nonoperative observation in selected cases, but the overall prognosis is guarded, with a significant risk of permanent sequelae or death.

Intracranial Bleeding

Subarachnoid Hemorrhage

Etiology

Subarachnoid hemorrhage may result from hypoxic-ischemic injury as well as from birth trauma.

Clinical Findings

1. Minor degrees of subarachnoid hemorrhage commonly occur in the absence of any neurologic abnormalities and may be discovered when a lumbar puncture is done for an unrelated reason. More extensive hemorrhage may present with seizures, typically in an otherwise well infant on the second day of life. Uncommonly, subarachnoid hemorrhage may be very severe and be associated with significant neurologic deterioration.
2. Subarachnoid hemorrhage can be diagnosed by lumbar puncture or CT scan; ultrasound examination is relatively insensitive. The prognosis for most infants with subarachnoid hemorrhage is good, even for those with seizures. Severe subarachnoid hemorrhage associated with asphyxial injury or significant neurologic abnormalities has a very guarded prognosis, with a high incidence of death or permanent neurologic sequelae.

Epidural Hemorrhage

Etiology

Epidural hemorrhage is due to bleeding between the bone and periosteum of the inner surface of the skull. The source of bleeding may be venous or arterial.

Clinical Findings

This lesion is rare in the newborn and is often associated with a traumatic delivery. An accompanying cephalhematoma or linear skull fracture may be present. The infant may develop signs of increased intracranial pressure. Diagnosis may be made by CT scan. Surgical evacuation may be required, although nonoperative observation may be appropriate in selected cases. The prognosis is guarded.

Subdural Hemorrhage

Etiology

Subdural hemorrhage is usually due to excessive forces of compression on the fetal skull, leading to injury to underlying veins and venous sinuses.

Clinical Findings

1. Bleeding from superficial cerebral veins is relatively common and may be unassociated with abnormal findings in the nursery. Such infants may present later with macrocephaly, anemia, seizures, and developmental delay. Injury to major cerebral veins and sinuses is associated with a more acute onset and is a particular problem in the posterior fossa, where brainstem compression may lead to rapid neurologic deterioration.
2. The diagnosis is made by CT scan or MRI. While selected infants may be managed expectantly, others may require subdural taps or surgical evacuation and repair of the injured vascular structures. Hydrocephalus may develop, the result of either the subdural collections themselves or obstruction to cerebrospinal fluid (CSF) flow. A shunt procedure may be needed in some infants. A subdural effusion presenting later in infancy may be due to birth trauma not detected in the nursery, but child abuse should also be considered.

Injury to the Spinal Cord and Peripheral Nerves

Spinal Cord Injury

Etiology

The neonatal spinal column is more elastic than the cord, and traction may cause the vertebral column to stretch, possibly resulting in injury to the spinal cord. Spinal cord injury is most commonly associated with difficult deliveries, especially deliveries from the breech position, in which there is hyperextension of the fetal head. It may also occur, however, following an uncomplicated spontaneous delivery, presumably as a result of abnormal fetal positioning in utero.

Clinical Findings

1. The typical lesion seen is hemorrhage and edema of the cord; fracture or dislocation of the vertebral column is uncommon. The symptoms and severity are determined by the level of the injury as well as by any accompanying hypoxic-ischemic injury. A high cervical or brainstem injury may be associated with early neonatal death, whereas a lower cervical or thoracic lesion may be compatible with prolonged survival provided that optimal supportive care, including ventilatory assistance, is given.
2. Initially there is a flaccid paralysis and areflexia; spasticity and hyperreflexia develop over a period of weeks or months. Accompanying asphyxial injury may lead to other neurologic abnormalities and may initially cloud the diagnosis. While Werdnig-Hoffmann disease may have a similar presentation, the presence of urinary retention and the loss of sensation in spinal cord injury should assist in distinguishing the two entities. Some newborns have relatively mild injury that is not detected in the nursery, but they present later in infancy with spasticity and hyperreflexia of the lower extremities.
3. Although some improvement may be seen over time, the prognosis for severely affected infants is not good, especially those who require prolonged ventilatory support. Because infants with spinal cord injuries may have problems with urinary retention, repeated respiratory tract infections, and development of contractures and pressure ulcers, a team approach to their care is very important.

Brachial Plexus Palsy

Etiology

Brachial plexus palsy is usually due to stretching forces that cause hemorrhage and edema; less commonly it is caused by avulsion of the nerve roots of the brachial plexus. Although the incidence is increased following difficult deliveries, especially if there is shoulder dystocia, it may also be seen following an uneventful spontaneous delivery.

Clinical Findings

1. Erb palsy, involving C5 and C6, accounts for approximately 80 per cent of brachial plexus palsies. Clinically, the affected limb is adducted and internally rotated at the shoulder, pronated at the elbow, and flexed at the wrist and fingers, with preservation of the grasp reflex. Klumpke palsy involves the roots of C8 and T1, resulting in a limp wrist and hand with an absent grasp reflex. An isolated Klumpke palsy is less common than a combined Erb-Klumpke palsy, which leads to a completely flaccid extremity.
2. A Horner syndrome, with ptosis, miosis, enophthalmos, and delayed pigmentation of the iris, may be seen in lower brachial plexus injury; it is caused by injury to the sympathetic fibers associated with C8. Injury to C3, C4, and C5, leading to phrenic nerve palsy, is seen in approximately 5 per cent of brachial plexus palsies. Brachial plexus palsy is associated with an absent Moro reflex on the affected side, and a fracture of the clavicle or humerus should be ruled out radiologically. It is important to remember that while a fracture may cause findings resembling those of a brachial plexus palsy, the presence of a fracture does not eliminate the possibility of a coexisting brachial plexus injury.

Management

Brachial plexus palsies commonly resolve or significantly improve in the first few days of life. In those that persist, physical therapy may be begun at the end of the second week, by which time any painful neuritis should have resolved. Careful follow-up is necessary, and infants who fail to improve by 2 to 3 months of age should be evaluated for possible nerve root avulsion, which will not heal spontaneously but may be surgically repairable. The prognosis for complete resolution of Erb palsy is excellent, whereas it is more guarded in cases of lower brachial plexus injury. In those infants with continued weakness, ongoing physical therapy is required to prevent contractures, and in some cases orthopedic procedures may be indicated to minimize disability.

Phrenic Nerve Palsy

Etiology

Phrenic nerve palsy is due to stretch injury to the roots of C3, C4, and C5 following injury to C3, C4, and C5.

Clinical Findings

1. The majority of phrenic palsies are right-sided and less than 10 per cent are bilateral. Approximately 80 per cent occur in association with a brachial plexus palsy. The infant may experience significant respiratory difficulties soon after birth, with cyanosis and respiratory acidosis. In some cases the infant's condition stabilizes, while in others there is a progressive respiratory deterioration.
2. The affected diaphragm is elevated, and there is a shift of the heart and the diaphragm to the contralateral side, with a resulting impairment of function of both lungs. The clinical picture may resemble eventration of the diaphragm or even congenital diaphragmatic hernia. The abnormal motion of the diaphragm can be demonstrated on ultrasound or fluoroscopy. In some infants, the elevation of the affected diaphragm is not evident early in the neonatal period, making the diagnosis more difficult.

Management

Affected infants may respond to positioning with the affected side down or to continuous positive airway pressure (CPAP); however, some infants require assisted ventilation. Feeding difficulties are often present, and these infants may develop repeated episodes of aspiration and pneumonia. Recovery may occur over a period of 6 to 12 months, but the need for continued mechanical ventilation is associated with a significant risk of mortality; plication should be considered in such infants.

Facial Palsy

Etiology

Facial palsy may be due to pressure on the facial nerve during birth or from a forceps blade; alternatively, it may result from intrauterine pressure on the nerve from the maternal sacrum or fetal shoulder. Most injuries occur at or near the point of exit of the nerve from the sternomastoid foramen and are due to hemorrhage and edema rather than avulsion.

Clinical Findings

1. The palsy is usually peripheral and involves the upper and lower face. Less commonly, a central facial palsy may be seen, the result of intracranial injury or hemorrhage. The prognosis is excellent; recovery is usual by the end of the first month of life, and the need for surgical intervention is rare. The eye on the affected side may require protection with artificial tears and taping of the lid.
2. Facial palsy should be distinguished from congenital absence of the depressor anguli oris muscle, which is not due to birth trauma. This condition may be associated with other anomalies, particularly cardiac malformations. It should also be distinguished from Möbius syndrome, which is due to bilateral agenesis of the facial nerve and presents with bilateral flaccid facial paralysis.

Intraabdominal Injuries

Hepatic Injury

Etiology

The liver is the most commonly injured intraabdominal organ. The incidence is increased in fetal macrosomia or hepatomegaly and following difficult deliveries, but liver injury may occur in the absence of any obvious precipitating factor. The mechanism of injury may involve direct pressure on the liver itself or thoracic compression displacing the liver downward, leading to stretching and tearing of the ligamentous attachments.

Clinical Findings

The most common injury is a subcapsular hematoma, which typically does not rupture until after the second day. There may be signs of anemia or a palpable right upper quadrant mass prior to rupture, but the infant may be relatively asymptomatic until rupture occurs. Rupture is associated with the development of shock, tense abdominal distention, bluish discoloration of the abdomen, and possibly the presence of a scrotal hematoma.

Diagnosis and Management

An unruptured subcapsular hematoma may be diagnosed by CT scan or ultrasound. Once rupture has occurred, the diagnosis is suggested by the clinical findings and may be confirmed by an abdominal x-ray showing diffuse haziness and by an abdominal paracentesis that is positive for blood. Management involves blood transfusion, correction of any coagulopathy, and surgical repair of the hepatic injury.

Splenic Injury

Etiology

The injury usually results from a tear at the site of ligamentous attachment, most commonly at the lienorenal ligament. The incidence of injury is increased in fetal macrosomia and conditions associated with splenomegaly.

Clinical Findings

Splenic hemorrhage presents earlier than hepatic bleeding and is often massive. The clinical and radiographic findings resemble those of hepatic rupture. If the infant is stable, the diagnosis can be made with ultrasound or CT scan. In the unstable infant, the presence of intraperitoneal blood and the need for emergency laparotomy can be established by paracentesis.

Management

If possible, the spleen should be repaired rather than resected, because of the increased risk of overwhelming infection associated with splenectomy. If splenic salvage is not possible, the infant will require long-term antibiotic prophylaxis, and the parents must be advised to bring the child for medical evaluation should the infant develop fever or other signs of infection.

Adrenal Injury

Etiology

The adrenal gland of the newborn is relatively large, making it prone to traumatic injury. The right adrenal gland is involved in the majority of cases, perhaps owing to its relatively vulnerable location between the liver and vertebral column. The incidence of adrenal injury is increased in fetal macrosomia and in difficult deliveries.

Clinical Findings

1. The bleeding may be minor and confined to the gland or retroperitoneal space; these infants may require only observation and blood transfusion. Uncommonly, there may be rupture into the peritoneal cavity with extensive hemorrhage, and laparotomy may be required to control the bleeding. Bilateral involvement occurs in less than 10 per cent of cases.
2. Adrenal insufficiency may occur if there is extensive hemorrhage, especially if it is bilateral, or if adrenalectomy has been performed. These infants are at risk for adrenal crisis, with vomiting, hypoglycemia, seizures, and shock, and may require maintenance hydrocortisone therapy. Adrenal hemorrhage may be associated with a palpable flank mass, and calcification of the gland may be seen as early as the end of the second week of life. This may be confused with neuroblastoma, but the calcification in neuroblastoma is usually diffusely present throughout the gland.
3. The diagnosis of adrenal hemorrhage may be suggested

by the clinical picture along with the development of calcification. It can be confirmed by ultrasound and CT scan.

Renal Injury

Etiology

Renal injury is very uncommon but may occur with a normal or hydronephrotic kidney.

Clinical Findings

The typical presentation is with anemia, flank mass, hematuria, and signs of intraabdominal hemorrhage. The differential diagnosis includes renal vein thrombosis and renal tumor, but the final diagnosis can be made by ultrasound or CT scan. Management includes blood transfusion and possible laparotomy and surgical repair.

Skeletal Injuries

Fracture of the Clavicle

Etiology

Fracture of the clavicle is not uncommon, and its incidence is increased in fetal macrosomia and shoulder dystocia.

Clinical Findings

The lesion is usually a greenstick fracture involving the middle third of the clavicle. There may be swelling, crepitus, decreased movement of the arm, and absence of the Moro reflex. The lesion may be missed in the nursery and be detected later, when palpable callus is present. There may be an associated Erb palsy.

Key Clinical Findings: Fractured Clavicle

- Swelling and crepitus over clavicle
- Decreased arm movement
- Palpable callus later

Management

Fracture of the clavicle is treated with immobilization, mainly to reduce pain, since excellent healing is the rule, even in the absence of intervention.

Fracture of the Femur

Etiology

Femoral fracture is uncommon. It may occur in a breech delivery when the leg is pulled down but may also occur in the absence of any obvious difficulties with delivery.

Clinical Findings

Most commonly, the fracture is transverse and involves the middle third or upper half of the femur. Obvious swelling or deformity of the thigh may be present. Excellent healing is to be expected.

Fracture of the Humerus

Etiology

Fracture of the humerus is often associated with shoulder dystocia or breech delivery, but it may occur in uncomplicated deliveries as well.

Clinical Findings

The fracture may be transverse or spiral and usually involves the middle third of the shaft. There may be an associated Erb palsy. Complete healing is expected within several weeks.

Bibliography

Kottmeier PK: Birth trauma. *In* Welch KJ, Randolph JG, Ravitch MM, et al (eds): Pediatric Surgery, 4th ed. Chicago, Yearbook Medical, 1986, pp 230–237.

Schullinger JN: Birth trauma. Pediatr Clin North Am 1993;40:1351–1358.

21 Low Birth Weight

Nathan Rudolph

The great advances that have been made in recent years in the management of low birth weight infants have led to a markedly increased survival rate and an improved quality of life for survivors. The following outlines some of the more commonly observed problems in this group of infants and the approach to their management.

Definitions

1. Premature (preterm) infant: an infant born at less than 37 completed weeks of gestation.
2. Low birth weight (LBW) infant: birth weight less than 2500 g, irrespective of gestational age.
3. Very low birth weight (VLBW) infant: birth weight less than 1500 g.
4. Extremely low birth weight (ELBW) infant: birth weight less than 1000 g.
5. Intrauterine growth retardation (IUGR): failure to maintain overall growth and weight gain appropriate for the duration of gestation at any gestational age, as determined by intrauterine evaluation of the fetus, e.g., by sonography, or by clinical evaluation after birth.
6. Symmetric IUGR: growth retardation in which weight gain, linear growth, and head growth (as measured by head circumference) are all affected to a similar extent.
7. Asymmetric IUGR: growth retardation in which head growth is relatively unaffected as compared with weight and length.
8. Small for gestational age (SGA) infant: commonly regarded as an infant who is born with a birth weight below the 10th percentile for a specific period of gestation, using a growth chart that is appropriate for the infant's geographic area or ethnic group. The 5th percentile is often used to delineate a more severe degree of growth retardation. Both term and post-term as well as premature infants can be small for their corresponding gestational ages.
9. Fetal nutritional deprivation syndrome (fetal malnutrition): a condition in which a newborn infant exhibits clinical manifestations of loss of energy stores, such as subcutaneous fat, and in which the infant may or may not be classified as SGA by definition, i.e., the weight may be below or above the 10th percentile for gestational age.

The Premature Infant

Etiology and Epidemiology

1. Of births in the United States, 10.5 to 11 per cent are preterm by gestational age.
2. Approximately 7 per cent of infants born in the United States have birth weights less than 2500 g (LBW). This includes some term neonates.
3. Spontaneous preterm labor and delivery often occur without any obvious cause, although amniotic infection is considered to be a major contributing cause.
4. Conditions that are associated with an increased incidence of prematurity, in addition to chorioamniotic infection, include:
   a. Socioeconomic and racial status: Prematurity and LBW deliveries are more common in lower socioeconomic groups. In the black population in the United States, LBW deliveries are approximately 2.3 times higher than in the white population.
   b. Maternal lifestyle: Teenage pregnancy, drug abuse, and heavy smoking increase the risk of preterm labor.
   c. Multiple gestation: The greater the number of fetuses, the greater the shortening of the period of gestation. This has become a significant problem with the increased use of fertility drugs and in vitro fertilization.
   d. Uteroplacental factors, e.g., incompetent cervix, uterine anomalies, myomas, placenta previa, abruptio placentae, polyhydramnios.
   e. Urinary tract infection.
   f. Medically indicated preterm delivery, e.g., severe

pregnancy-induced hypertension or other maternal illness or a severely compromised fetus.

g. There is an increased risk of premature labor in subsequent pregnancies following a premature delivery.

Factors Associated With Premature Birth

- Chorioamniotic infection
- Low socioeconomic status
- Teenage pregnancy
- Drug abuse
- Smoking
- Multiple pregnancy
- Uterine anomalies and incompetent cervix
- Placenta previa
- Abruptio placentae
- Maternal urinary tract infection
- Maternal hypertension
- Severely compromised fetus

Clinical Findings

1. Clinical signs are very variable and depend on the gestational age and the clinical manifestations of specific problems encountered in each infant.
2. Several methods have been proposed for the clinical estimation of gestational age after birth (see Chapter 16). Most include an evaluation of physical characteristics, neuromuscular maturation, and the stage of development of specified reflexes. The physical features include determination of skin texture and thickness, the presence of lanugo, the extent of cartilage formation in the pinnae, nipple and nipple bud development, genital development, and plantar creases. It has been suggested that neuromuscular maturation may be accelerated in utero by fetal stress.

Clinical Problems Associated With Prematurity

1. Thermoregulation

   The premature infant loses heat rapidly because of a relatively greater surface area to weight ratio, thin skin, and poor subcutaneous fat development. The resting metabolic rate of preterm infants is relatively low compared with that of term infants, and there is a limited ability to respond to a cold stress by increasing heat production.

2. Nutrition and feeding

   a. VLBW and ELBW infants have limited ability to suck and coordinate swallowing and have a relatively small gastric volume at birth.

   b. Immature gastrointestinal digestive and absorptive capacities, as well as lack of complete development of some metabolic pathways, complicate feeding, by both the enteral and the parenteral routes. These complications include delayed development of lactase and variable fat absorption, including absorption of fat-soluble vitamins, such as vitamin E.

c. Large fluid losses may occur from the skin by insensible water loss. These losses are highest in VLBW infants cared for under radiant warmers; they may be as high as 7 to 8 ml/kg/h, or seven to eight times the basal loss rate.

3. Metabolic

   a. Fluid and electrolyte imbalance—hyponatremia, hypernatremia, hyperkalemia. Increased renal tubular losses of sodium lead to hyponatremia, and excessive dehydration secondary to high insensible water losses leads to hypernatremia.

   b. Hypoglycemia—partly as a result of inadequate hepatic glycogen stores. The routine use of intravenous glucose solution infusions has led to a decreased incidence of hypoglycemia in LBW infants.

   c. Hyperglycemia—low insulin secretion in preterm infants receiving parenteral alimentation may produce glycosuria and osmotic diuresis, which accentuate fluid losses.

   d. Hypocalcemia—probably related to parathyroid gland immaturity.

4. Respiratory

   a. Respiratory distress syndrome (RDS): This results from a lack of adequate surfactant production in the developing lung and, in the very immature infant, may be compounded by the fact that the anatomic development of the lung is not sufficiently advanced to permit adequate air exchange.

   b. Apnea of prematurity: Premature infants normally have irregular respiration due to immature central control mechanisms, so that their breathing patterns often exhibit periods of apnea of several seconds' duration. Recurrent apneic episodes lasting longer than 20 seconds, especially when associated with bradycardia and cyanosis, generally require intervention.

   c. Aspiration, secondary to poor coordination of sucking and swallowing or from gastroesophageal reflux, may also manifest as apneic and cyanotic episodes.

   d. Bronchopulmonary dysplasia (BPD): In this condition, there is a continued need for oxygen supplementation for more than 28 days after birth, associated with compatible radiologic and clinical findings. It occurs in premature infants who have required prolonged ventilatory assistance, and it is often associated with chronic airway problems (see Chapter 23).

5. Cardiovascular

   Persistent patency of the ductus arteriosus (PDA) is common and may result in congestive heart failure and ventilator dependence. The incidence of PDA increases with decreasing gestational age.

6. Gastrointestinal and hepatic

   a. Motility disorders: These include delayed emptying time, abdominal distention, infrequent passage of stools, and gastroesophageal reflux.

   b. Necrotizing enterocolitis: A life-threatening complication, often requiring surgical intervention (see Chapter 29).

   c. Jaundice of prematurity—early occurrence of unconjugated hyperbilirubinemia caused by an increased rate of erythrocyte destruction as well as decreased hepatic uptake, conjugation, and excretion of bilirubin.

   d. Cholestatic jaundice—Conjugated hyperbilirubinemia may be associated with the prolonged use of total parenteral nutrition (TPN).

7. Infection

   The underdeveloped immune responses of premature infants render them particularly susceptible to infection. Risks are increased by the prolonged need for parenteral feeding and vascular access. *Staphylococcus epidermidis,* gram-negative bacilli, and *Candida* are among the more common organisms encountered.

8. Central nervous system

   a. Cerebral bleed of prematurity—subependymal bleeding in the highly vascular germinal matrix of one or both cerebral hemispheres. It may remain as a small periventricular hemorrhage (PVH) in this area adjacent to the floor of the anterior horn of the lateral ventricle; it may result in more extensive hemorrhage or infarction of the adjacent parenchyma; or it may rupture through the ependyma into the lateral ventricle, producing intraventricular hemorrhage (IVH). The latter may lead to posthemorrhagic hydrocephalus. In most instances, the bleeding occurs between the second and fifth postnatal days. It is more common in ELBW infants and is not generally encountered after 35 to 36 weeks of gestation, at which time the involutionary process of the germinal matrix has been completed.

   b. Periventricular leukomalacia (PVL)—periventricular areas of white matter necrosis occurring in sick premature infants and probably associated with hypoxia, ischemia, or hypotension. The lesions are generally not identifiable until the third or fourth postnatal week.

   c. A small localized germinal matrix hemorrhage has no clinical manifestations and does not produce clinically significant sequelae. More extensive hemorrhage and brain damage from PVH/IVH or from PVL may result in motor deficits (cerebral palsy) of varying degrees of severity, with or without cognitive impairment.

9. Hematologic

   a. Early anemia of prematurity—An accelerated decline in the hemoglobin concentration and hematocrit during the initial 6 to 10 postnatal weeks occurs because of a short erythrocyte survival time and an attenuated response in erythropoietin production. It may be worsened by repeated blood drawing for laboratory tests.

   b. Late anemia of prematurity is due to iron deficiency in the rapidly growing premature infant and generally presents after the third postnatal month.

10. Ophthalmologic

   a. Retinopathy of prematurity (ROP) may occur in small premature infants following an arrest in the vascularization process of the developing retina that is normally complete by about 34 weeks of gestation.

   b. Excessive oxygen use that produces an elevated blood oxygen tension in a VLBW infant is a major, but not the only, etiologic factor.

   c. In most infants the condition gradually retrogresses spontaneously, but in some babies scarring and areas of retinal detachment with varying degrees of visual loss may occur.

11. Bone mineralization

   Osteopenia and occasionally pathologic fractures and frank rickets may occur in the growing VLBW infant, though they are usually preventable. Among the potential causes are the following:

   a. Hypophosphatemia from inadequate phosphorus intake, absorption, and retention.

   b. Calcium deficiency (e.g., due to increased excretion from prolonged diuretic use).

   c. Deficient hydroxylation of cholecalciferol in severe cholestatic jaundice with hepatic dysfunction.

12. Inguinal hernias

   Indirect inguinal hernias, in both males and females, are common in growing VLBW infants.

13. Psychosocial and ethical problems

   a. In sick VLBW and ELBW infants, the prolonged period of hospitalization and illness, of maternal-infant separation, of disruption of schooling in teenage mothers, and of uncertainty about acute and long-term outcome may combine to produce profound changes in family interaction.

   b. Ethical dilemmas occur fairly frequently in ELBW infants, especially those with gestational ages below 25 weeks, who are of marginal viability. Decisions frequently must be made regarding continuation of intensive care and life support in infants who have extensive brain damage from cerebral parenchymal bleeds or extensive encephalomalacia.

Management of Premature Infants

Antenatal maternal administration of a synthetic glucocorticoid significantly improves the prognosis and long-term outcome for a premature infant between 24 and 34 weeks of gestation. Glucocorticoid treatment is given for 24 to 48 hours 2 to 3 days before delivery. The effects will be manifested by accelerated pulmonary maturation and decreased incidence and severity of RDS; other organ systems (e.g., cardiovascular and renal) will also demonstrate improved function. Antenatal corticosteroid therapy has been shown to decrease the incidence of symptomatic PDA and also to lower the incidence of IVH and PVL.

The systemic approach to the management of problems of the preterm infant after birth includes the following:

1. Maintaining preterm infants in a thermoneutral environment (one with a minimal rate of oxygen consumption) by the use of an enclosed convection incubator or a radiant warmer is associated with increased survival and enhanced growth.

2. Nutrition and feeding

   Larger preterm infants may be able to obtain adequate caloric and fluid requirements by nipple-feeding only. VLBW infants may initially require enteral feeding by intermittent gavage or continuous nasogastric feeding via a nasogastric tube, with or without supplemental parenteral nutrition. Sick babies, especially ELBW infants, frequently require TPN with gradual introduction of continuous nasogastric feeding. Transpyloric tube feeding is not recommended.

   a. Infant-feeding formulas designed specifically for premature babies have been developed. These generally have a higher caloric density (80 cals/dl) and a higher content of protein, calcium, phosphorus, sodium, trace minerals, and vitamins (especially fat-soluble). Some of the fat is present as medium-chain triglycerides.

   b. Human milk fed to premature infants should be fortified with a commercial supplement, particularly to provide additional phosphorus and calcium.

   c. Additional vitamin E supplementation (oral *dl*/α-tocopherol acetate) is suggested for VLBW infants.

3. Fluid and electrolyte control

   a. The initial daily fluid requirement for preterm infants is 75 to 130 ml/kg, increasing progressively to 180 to 200 ml/kg or more in the growing infant or the sick ELBW baby.

   b. Infants managed under a radiant warmer require larger volumes of fluid, and insensible water loss can be minimized by caring for them in a convection incubator.

   c. In sick preterm infants receiving parenteral feeding, serum electrolyte levels, especially of Na^+ and K^+, require close monitoring and appropriate adjustment of daily requirements.

   d. Preterm infants on TPN require a minimum glucose infusion rate of 4 to 6 mg/kg/minute to maintain energy metabolism. When this rate cannot be achieved without producing significant glycosuria, the administration of small amounts of intravenous insulin is recommended (start with 0.02 U/kg/hour).

   e. When enteral feeding has been withheld, IV fluids should contain appropriate amounts of calcium (a daily maintenance of 45 to 90 mg/kg).

4. Respiratory assistance

   a. The endotracheal administration of synthetic or natural surfactant preparations after birth, together with appropriate ventilatory assistance, has revolutionized the management of RDS of prematurity. This is discussed in Chapter 22.

   b. Apneic episodes and bradycardia are generally detected by the use of continuous electronic monitoring of cardiac and respiratory rates and oxygen saturation and by direct observation.

      (1) Infrequent episodes can be managed by physically stimulating the infant when apnea occurs.

      (2) More frequent episodes, especially when accompanied by significant bradycardia and a decline in oxygen saturation, may be treated by the application of nasal CPAP (continuous positive airway pressure), the administration of methylxanthines, maintaining the infant in the prone position, or a judicious increase in the inhaled oxygen concentration (FIO_2). Various combinations of these measures may be appropriate.

      (3) Apneic episodes need to be distinguished from tonic seizures that present with apnea and cyanosis.

      (4) Neonatal sepsis may present with apnea.

   c. Aspiration can be minimized by maintaining the incubator mattress platform at a 15 to 25 degree inclination and by increasing the volume of feedings slowly and in accordance with the infant's tolerance of each increase.

   d. Bronchopulmonary dysplasia (chronic lung disease) is discussed in Chapter 23.

5. Management of a patent ductus arteriosus is discussed in Chapters 30 and 175.

6. Gastrointestinal management

   a. The immature gastrointestinal function and small gastric volume of the premature infant require a gradual and progressive increase in the volume of feeds given. In sick ELBW infants an initial volume of 0.2 to 0.5 ml/hr by continuous nasogastric feeding is appropriate.

   b. Placing the infant in the right lateral position significantly accelerates stomach emptying.

   c. The management of necrotizing enterocolitis is discussed in Chapter 29.

   d. The management of jaundice is discussed in Chapter 18.

7. Infection control

   Rigid infection control measures must be maintained at all times in the neonatal intensive care unit (NICU), since infections, especially nosocomial infections, are the cause of significant morbidity and mortality in the NICU. Management is discussed in Chapter 28.

8. Intracranial hemorrhage

   a. All VLBW infants as well as larger sick premature infants should be monitored routinely by cerebral sonography to detect the occurrence and progression of intraventricular bleeding or PVL.

   b. In infants who develop posthemorrhagic hydrocephalus, serial lumbar punctures or CSF reservoir taps may improve the clinical course but do not decrease the need for eventual ventriculoperitoneal shunting.

9. Hematologic management

a. Routine administration of recombinant erythropoietin to VLBW infants from the first postnatal week has been suggested as a method of attenuating early anemia and decreasing the overall blood transfusion requirement in these patients. This approach remains controversial, although selective use of erythropoietin, supplemented with administration of iron and of vitamin E as an antioxidant, may be warranted.

b. Routine iron supplementation or the use of iron-fortified infant formulas is not recommended in VLBW infants during the first few postnatal weeks, since Fe^{++} acts as a catalyst in free radical formation and can facilitate oxidant injury.

c. It is recommended that iron supplementation be started at 6 to 8 weeks after birth and continue at least during the first year of life.

10. Retinopathy of prematurity (retrolental fibroplasia)

a. In order to prevent retinal damage (retinopathy of prematurity, or ROP), all premature infants receiving oxygen supplementation must be monitored with a pulse oximeter or similar device to ensure that the concentration of inspired oxygen is kept to the minimum level needed to provide adequate oxygenation.

b. Arterial blood gases should be measured periodically on infants being maintained on supplementary oxygen. In ELBW infants, a PaO_2 between 45 and 70 mmHg (usually coinciding with oxygen saturation measurements of 90 to 95 per cent) usually indicates satisfactory oxygenation.

c. All VLBW infants as well as larger sick premature infants who received supplementary oxygen require routine retinoscopic evaluation at 6 to 8 postnatal weeks, with appropriate follow-up as needed.

11. Calcium metabolism

a. Severe osteopenia can generally be prevented by attention to calcium, phosphorus, and vitamin D intake and by monitoring serum levels.

b. Soy-based formulas should not be given to premature infants because of the infant's relatively poor absorption of phosphorus from these formulas.

c. Breast milk fed to premature infants requires supplementation with a commercial fortifier to provide additional phosphorus and calcium.

12. Hernias require surgical correction, which is usually performed just prior to nursery discharge.

13. A social worker is an essential member of the team caring for VLBW infants.

14. Ethical decisions regarding resuscitation and continuation of life support in severely compromised infants are generally made after full agreement has been reached between the parents and caregivers. Occasionally, however, the advice and assistance of a hospital ethics committee is advisable.

Key Treatment

- Maintain thermoneutral environment
- Gradually increase feedings and maintain growth; supply vitamins, including D
- Rigorous infection control
- Erythropoietin for VLBW infants (controversial)
- Selective iron supplementation

Prognosis

The survival of ELBW infants has improved significantly over the past decade, and survival of infants of gestational age 23 to 24 weeks is not unusual. The overall survival rate of infants with birth weights between 500 and 749 g is approximately 45 to 60 per cent, although the incidence of neurodevelopmental sequelae is high. In infants with birth weights of 750 to 999 g, the survival rate is about 75 to 80 per cent; it is 90 to 95 per cent in infants with birth weights between 1000 and 1500 g.

Intrauterine Growth Retardation (Small for Gestational Age)

Etiology

Any condition that influences the well-being of the fetus or interferes with fetal nutrition may impede fetal weight gain and overall growth. The causes can be classified broadly into two categories:

1. Intrinsic or fetal
   a. Chromosomal disorders, e.g., trisomy 18
   b. Multiple congenital anomalies
   c. Intrauterine infections (cytomegalovirus, rubella, toxoplasmosis)
   d. Fetofetal transfusion (donor twin)
   e. Constitutional/familial
2. Extrinsic—maternal, uteroplacental
   a. Inadequate intrauterine space (multiple pregnancies, uterine abnormalities)
   b. Abnormal placentation (abdominal pregnancy, velamentous placenta)
   c. Maternal illness affecting the uteroplacental circulation and delivery of oxygen and nutrients to the fetus (maternal hypertension, toxemia, sickle cell anemia, collagen disorders, diabetes mellitus with vascular disease)
   d. Maternal use of drugs: alcohol, cocaine, tobacco, heroin
   e. Severe maternal undernutrition/starvation, high altitude.

Pathophysiology

1. The effect of adverse conditions on fetal growth depends both on the severity and on the timing and duration of the disturbance.
2. Placental insufficiency initially produces a progressive depletion of liver glycogen and of fat stores in the fetus,

including brown adipose tissue, necessary for thermogenesis following a cold stress. Relatively mild nutritional deprivation will therefore attenuate weight gain only. More prolonged or severe deprivation will retard linear growth as well.

3. Adverse conditions early in gestation (e.g., fetal infections, maternal alcohol use) are more likely to produce symmetric IUGR, in which brain growth is affected as well as somatic growth.

4. Chronic or intermittent hypoxemia associated with placental insufficiency may result in a compensatory polycythemia.

Factors Associated With Intrauterine Growth Retardation

- Chromosomal disorders
- Multiple congenital anomalies
- Intrauterine infections
- Fetofetal transfusion
- Multiple pregnancy
- Abnormal placentation
- Maternal vascular disease; hypertension; toxemia
- Maternal drug use
- Severe maternal malnutrition
- Very high altitude
- Constitutional and familial

Clinical Findings

1. Evaluation of gestational age indicates if the infant is preterm, term, or post term.
2. The skin tends to be dry and wrinkled if placental dysfunction has been present; it may have some areas of peeling and is sometimes meconium-stained.
3. There is a loss of subcutaneous fat.
4. The liver size is frequently decreased.
5. Signs associated with the underlying etiologic condition may be present, e.g., petechiae in intrauterine infections.

Potential Clinical Problems

1. Hypothermia, due to poor subcutaneous fat coverage and loss of brown adipose tissue
2. Hypoglycemia, resulting from depleted liver glycogen stores

3. Polycythemia, which may be accompanied by hyperviscosity
4. Meconium aspiration, especially when placental insufficiency has been compounded by acute fetal distress/hypoxia during labor
5. Neutropenia associated with maternal hypertension and placental insufficiency
6. Hypermagnesemia, secondary to magnesium sulfate therapy of maternal pregnancy-induced hypertension.

Management

1. Maintain infant in a neutral thermal environment.
2. Monitor the blood glucose level and introduce early enteral feeding when feasible, with or without an intravenous glucose infusion, as required.
3. If persistent polycythemia is present, consider a partial exchange transfusion with 5 per cent albumen solution.
4. When no apparent cause for the IUGR has been identified, either clinically or by maternal history, routine screening for an intrauterine infection is appropriate. This should include determination of serum IgM levels and urine examination for cytomegalovirus.

Prognosis

1. The long-term outlook depends on the underlying etiology and the severity of the growth disturbance. When the underlying cause for fetal growth retardation is a chromosomal abnormality, infection, or fetal alcohol syndrome, the long-term prognosis is generally poor.
2. Fetal nutritional deprivation commencing during the third trimester, as is commonly observed in pregnancy-induced hypertension, generally has an excellent long-term prognosis.

 ## Bibliography

Clinical considerations in the use of oxygen. *In* Guidelines for Perinatal Care, 3rd ed. Elk Grove Village, IL, American Academy of Pediatrics and American College of Obstetricians and Gynecologists, 1992, pp 197–203.

Hack M, Taylor HG, Klein N, et al: Schoolage outcomes in children with birth-weights under 750 g. N Engl J Med 1994;331:753–759.

Padbury JF, Gore EM, Polk DH: Extrapulmonary effects of antenatally administered steroids. J Pediatr 1996;128:167–172.

Ryan CA, Finer NN: Antenatal corticosteroid therapy to prevent respiratory distress syndrome. J Pediatr 1995;126:317–319.

Volpe JJ: Intraventricular hemorrhage in the premature infant: current concepts. Part I. Ann Neurol 1989;25:3–11.

22 Respiratory Distress Syndrome

Warren Rosenfeld

The transition from placental intrauterine respiration to extrauterine respiration via the lung requires anatomic and biochemical maturation. Babies born before biochemical maturation of the fetal lung is complete may develop respiratory distress syndrome (RDS). Although abnormal respiratory signs occur with several disorders, RDS specifically refers to the symptom complex caused by either a quantitative or a qualitative lack of surfactant, usually associated with immature anatomic development of the lung.

Epidemiology

1. Approximately 30,000 cases are seen annually in the United States
2. Primarily a disorder of prematurity (usually less than 34 weeks' gestation). Incidence increases with decreasing maturity.
3. Occurs in 75 per cent of patients of less than 1000 g birth weight, in 50 per cent of patients with birth weights of 1000 to 1250 g, and in 25 per cent of patients weighing 1251 to 1500 g.
4. Major cause of neonatal mortality (4000 deaths/year) and morbidity, with a national health care cost of over $1 billion per year.

Pathophysiology

1. The lack of surfactant increases surface tension in the air spaces of the lung, leading to the following changes:
   a. Atelectasis—large portions of the lung are airless
   b. Some areas of overdistention
   c. Pulmonary vascular congestion
   d. Pulmonary hemorrhage
   e. Epithelial injury
   f. Hyaline membranes (eosinophilic proteinaceous material) are nonspecific and require several hours to be formed.
2. Surfactant, produced in the type II pneumocyte, is the surface tension–lowering substance that prevents lung collapse at the end of expiration.
   a. Composition
      (1) Lipids, 90 per cent (87% is phospholipids)
         (a) Dipalmitoyl phosphatidylcholine (36%)
         (b) Unsaturated phosphatidylcholine (32%)
         (c) Phosphatidylglycerol (10%)
         (d) Phosphatidylethanolamine (3%)
         (e) Phosphatidylinositol (2%)
         (f) Other phospholipids (4%)
         (g) Other lipids (3%): cholesterol, diacylglycerol
      (2) Proteins (10%): Surfactant-associated proteins A, B, C, and D. Proteins promote absorption and spreading of phospholipids at the air-water interface in the alveoli and reabsorption of phospholipids to type II alveolar cells.
   b. Surfactant deficiency: quantitative and qualitative deficiency of surfactant leads to:
      (1) Atelectasis
      (2) Decreased functional residual capacity
      (3) Ventilation/perfusion (V/Q) abnormalities
      (4) Decreased lung compliance
      (5) Increased pulmonary vasculature resistance
      (6) Hypoxemia, hypercarbia, metabolic and respiratory acidosis

Clinical Findings

1. Signs are present at birth or soon afterward.
2. Respiratory distress (tachypnea, retractions, grunting, nasal flaring, cyanosis), which, if untreated, can lead to ventilatory failure. Crackles and poor air exchange are observed in unventilated patients.
3. Typical radiograph shows reticular granular infiltrates (airless lung) with air bronchogram that may progress to total "white-out." The radiographic picture may be altered by mechanical ventilation and/or surfactant therapy.
4. In the preventilatory assistance and presurfactant eras, the clinical course worsened over first 3 to 5 days of life; if the patient survived, improvement gradually occurred and patients were asymptomatic by age 7 to 10 days.
5. With the widespread use of ventilatory assistance in the 1970s and the ensuing introduction of surfactant replacement therapy in the 1980s and 1990s, the clinical course of RDS has been shortened; patients usually show continuous improvement following surfactant therapy, with a 3- to 5-day total course of illness.

Key Clinical Findings

- Tachypnea
- Grunting respirations
- Cyanosis

Prevention and Treatment

1. Prenatal: prevention of prematurity
   a. Fetal lung maturity may be assessed by sampling amniotic fluid for the lecithin to sphingomyelin (L/S) ratio or the presence of phosphatidylglycerol (PG).
   b. Systemic corticosteroids administered to the mother in the presence of impending premature labor leads to increased phosphatidylcholine production and enhanced lung maturation.

2. Exogenous surfactant administration

  a. Several surfactant preparations are available for clinical use. Administration is via endotracheal tube.

    (1) Beractant (Survanta)—natural bovine extract, DPPC added; contains surfactant-associated proteins B and C. Dose is 4 ml/kg.

    (2) Synthetic surfactant (Exosurf): synthetic DPPC, ethyl alcohol, tyloxapol; no surface active proteins are present. Dose is 5 ml/kg.

  b. Criteria for administration are not clear-cut; may be administerd as prophylactic or rescue therapy.

    (1) Prophylaxis (prevention): treatment of patients less than 1250 g or those with documented surfactant deficiency, within the first 15 to 30 minutes of life, usually administered in the delivery room.

    (2) Rescue: treatment of patients with confirmed RDS (clinically and radiologically). Usually administered within the first 8 hours of life.

3. Continuous positive airway pressure (CPAP)—delivery of an end-expiratory pressure (usually 3 to 6 cm H_2O) to the neonate's airway during spontaneous respirations, preventing alveolar collapse. Devices used to deliver pressure are nasal prongs or tubes, endotracheal tubes, or face mask.

4. Intermittent mandatory ventilation (IMV): Mechanical ventilation remains the mainstay of supportive care. Maintenance of blood gases in the physiologic range in order to maintain appropriate oxygenation and ventilation is the primary goal of this form of therapy. A wide variety of ventilators are available.

  a. Pressure limited—time cycled

  b. Volume cycled

  c. High frequency (jet or oscillator)

5. Positive end-expiratory pressure (PEEP): delivery of an end-expiratory pressure during mechanical ventilation

6. Supportive therapy

  a. Maintain thermoneutral environment.

  b. Provide appropriate fluids, calories, and electrolytes.

  c. Close patent ductus arteriosus with indomethacin or surgery.

  d. Antibiotics: Since the clinical and radiographic findings of RDS cannot be distinguished from those of bacterial pneumonia (most commonly group B *Streptococcus*), treatment with antibiotics is often appropriate.

Key Treatment

- Exogenous surfactant
- Continuous partial airway pressure
- Intermittent mechanical ventilation with PEEP
- Antibiotics

Complications

1. Airleaks: Rupture of alveoli with dissection of air into the interstitial space and dissecting along perivascular sheaths may lead to

  a. Pulmonary interstitial emphysema

  b. Pneumomediastinum

  c. Pneumothorax

  d. Pneumopericardium

  e. Pneumoperitoneum

2. Bronchopulmonary dysplasia: chronic lung disease that develops after oxygen therapy and/or mechanical ventilation

3. Closure of the ductus arteriosus following delivery ordinarily occurs in 24 to 48 hours. In premature infants, and especially in those with RDS, delayed or no closure may occur.

4. Bleeding into the germinal matrix, a plexus of fragile blood vessels in the periventricular region of the brain, with extension into the ventricular system (intraventricular hemhorrage), frequently occurs in premature infants who have RDS.

Outcome

1. Continued improvement in mortality and morbidity with mortality reduced from 25 per cent to 10 per cent since the clinical introduction of surfactant, with significant increased survival of very low birth weight babies.

2. Decreased morbidity includes decreased airleaks and pulmonary interstitial emphysema.

3. It is currently unclear whether there is a decrease in the incidence of intracranial hemorrhage, PDA, or bronchopulmonary dysplasia.

Bibliography

Avery M, Mead J: Surface properties in relation to atelectasis and hyaline membrane disease. Am J Dis Child 1959;97:517–523.

Corbet A: Clinical trials of synthetic surfactant in respiratory distress syndrome of premature infants. Clin Perinatol 1993;20:761–790.

Mercier CE, Soll RF: Clinical trials of natural surfactant extract in respiratory distress syndrome. Clin Perinatol 1993;20:711–735.

Poulain FR, Clements JA: Pulmonary surfactant therapy. West J Med 1995;162:43–50.

Soll RF, McQueen M: Surfactant treatment of respiratory distress syndrome. *In* Sinclair JC, Bracken MB (eds): Effective Care of the Newborn Infant. Oxford, Oxford University Press, 1992, pp 325–355.

23 Bronchopulmonary Dysplasia

Warren Rosenfeld

Definition

Bronchopulmonary dysplasia is the chronic lung disease that develops in neonates (usually preterm) who are treated with oxygen and mechanical ventilation for a primary lung disorder, most often respiratory distress syndrome (RDS). Approximately 7000 new cases occur yearly, with 10 to 15 percent of these infants dying in the first year of life. BPD has become the most common form of chronic lung disease in infants.

Alternative definitions of bronchopulmonary dysplasia (BPD) have arisen, since the nature of BPD has changed with the advent of exogenous surfactant and other therapeutic interventions.

1. Northway: radiologic, pathologic, and clinical stages
   a. Stages I and II (acute stages): Indistinguishable from RDS in the first 10 days of life.
   b. Stages III and IV (chronic stages): Respiratory symptoms and oxygen needs beyond 28 days. Chest radiographs demonstrate cyst formation, hyperinflation, and atelectasis.
2. Bancalari: Mechanical ventilation for at least the first 3 days of life; respiratory symptoms (tachypnea, rales, and retractions); supplemental oxygen to maintain a PaO$_2$ >50 mmHg; abnormal chest radiograph at 28 days of life.

Epidemiology

Dependent on the definition used and the population studied. Although surfactant treatment has improved overall survival for premature infants, the incidence of BPD in these neonates remains approximately 30 to 40 percent.

Pathogenesis

1. Barotrauma: Initial injury is the result of the primary disease (RDS, pulmonary immaturity). Superimposed mechanical ventilation adds to the lung injury. An inflammatory cascade is then activated, leading to injury and chronic lung disease.
2. Oxygen/Antioxidants: A balance exists between the production of free oxygen radicals (molecules with extra electrons in their outer ring that are toxic to living tissues) and antioxidant defenses (Table 23–1). Balance may be disturbed by increased free radicals (hyperoxia, ischemia/reperfusion, or inflammation) or inadequate antioxidant enzymes.
3. Inflammation: Plays an important role in the pathogenesis of BPD and permits a unified hypothesis for BPD.
4. Infection (*Ureaplasma urealyticum*): Found in 44 percent of cervical cultures of pregnant women and implicated as cause of chorioamnionitis, prematurity, and BPD.
5. Nutrition: Inadequate calories, essential nutrients (vital components for immunologic and antioxidant defenses), vitamin deficiencies (vitamin A), decreased polyunsaturated fatty acids (PUFA).
6. Fluids/Patent ductus arteriosus (PDA): Increased incidence of PDA and BPD have been associated with increased fluid administration. Early closure of the ductus arteriosus (indomethacin or surgical ligation has not substantially affected the incidence of BPD.
7. Genetics: Strong family history of atopy and asthma and HLA$_2$.

Clinical Findings

Infants are evaluated on a clinical and radiographic basis, with the latter reflecting cardiovascular and pulmonary pathology.

1. Cardiovascular changes: Abnormal pulmonary circulation (endothelial cell degeneration and proliferation, medial muscle hypertrophy, peripheral extension of smooth muscle, and vascular obliteration); increased pulmonary vascular pressures and resistance with the development of cor pulmonale.
2. Altered pulmonary mechanics
   a. Initially an increase in pulmonary resistance and airway reactivity.
   b. Later expiratory flow limitation may become more significant.
   c. Increased resistance causes increased work of breathing and V/Q mismatching.
   d. Functional residual capacity may be reduced initially because of atelectasis but may be increased in later stages because of air trapping and hyperinflation.
   e. Reduction of lung compliance.

 Key Clinical Findings

- Cor pulmonale
- Increased pulmonary resistance
- Reduced lung compliance

Pathology

1. Airways: Large upper airways (trachea, main bronchi)
   a. Earliest histologic changes: patchy loss of cilia from columnar epithelial cells.
   b. Mucosal edema and/or necrosis (focal or diffuse) that may lead to frank ulcerations.
   c. Infiltration of inflammatory cells and granulation tissue (area of the endotracheal tube tip).
   d. Mucosal cells regenerate or are replaced by stratified squamous or metaplastic epithelium.
2. Terminal bronchioles and alveolar ducts. Necrotizing bronchiolitis and fibroblast proliferation and activation may lead to peribronchial fibrosis and obliterative fibroproliferative bronchiolitis.

3. Alveoli
   a. Earliest findings involve interstitial and/or alveolar edema.
   b. Later, areas of atelectasis, inflammation, exudate, and fibroblast proliferation.
   c. Finally, areas of atelectasis alternating with areas of marked hyperinflation.

Management

Multidisciplinary approach to improve the complex pathophysiologic changes.

1. Mechanical ventilation: The benefits from continued ventilation should outweigh the risks of continued progression of chronic lung damage.
2. Oxygen: In BPD, chronic hypoxia results in pulmonary vasoconstriction, pulmonary hypertension, and cor pulmonale. PaO_2 should be maintained between 55 and 70 mmHg and SaO_2 from 90 to 95 percent. Oxygen should be withdrawn gradually, but its use may be required for months or years, often following discharge from the nursery.
3. Nutrition
   a. Maximize caloric intake for tissue repair and growth (120 to 140 kcal/kg/day).
   b. Adequate calcium, potassium, and phosphorus intake (especially if receiving furosemide).
   c. Vitamins and trace elements.
4. Medications
   a. Diuretics (furosemide, chlorthiazide, hydrochlorothiazide, spironolactone).
   b. Inhaled agents (albuterol, metaproterenol, isoetharine, atropine, cromolyn, beclomethasone).
   c. Systemic agents (aminophylline, caffeine, terbutaline, dexamethasone, albuterol, nifedipine).
   d. In infants with RDS at high risk for developing BPD, early dexamethasone administration improves pulmonary mechanics, promotes weaning from oxygen and mechanical ventilation, minimizes lung injury, and may improve neurodevelopmental outcome. In infants with documented BPD, dexamethasone acutely reduces tracheal inflammation, improves pulmonary mechanics and clinical pulmonary status, and facilitates weaning from ventilators. Dexamethasone does not appear to result in significant improvements in survival, duration of oxygen treatment, or total length of hospital stay. At the present time, systemic corticosteroid use should be reserved for ventilator-dependent infants with moderate to severe BPD that is resistant to more conventional therapy.
   e. Antibiotics: With respiratory decompensation due to possible infection, appropriate broad-spectrum antibiotics should be used initially. More specific coverage is determined once specific organisms are isolated.
   f. Physical therapy: Appropriate removal of secretions is useful in management of patients with BPD.

Key Treatment

- Oxygen
- Furosemide—cautiously
- Physical therapy

Outcome

1. Most neonates with BPD ultimately achieve normal lung function and thrive. They are, however, at higher risk for death in the first year and for long-term pulmonary and developmental complications.
2. In childhood, respiratory problems (i.e., reactive airway disease) and abnormal neurologic development may occur.
3. Cardiac function: cor pulmonale may develop.
4. Infection: Increased susceptibility to respiratory syncytial virus and influenza.
5. Growth failure and neurodevelopmental abnormalities are increased. In contrast, severity of BPD is not a major predictor of neurologic outcome.

Prevention

1. Corticosteroids for mothers delivering prematurely may reduce the severity and incidence of BPD.
2. Early use of nasal continuous positive airway pressure (CPAP) in RDS may eliminate the need for mechanical ventilation or facilitate extubation.
3. Exogenous surfactant reduces mortality and the severity and incidence of BPD (although the total number of survivors with BPD will increase).
4. Treatment of symptomatic PDA (fluid restriction, diuretics, indomethacin, or surgery).
5. Ventilator pressures and FIO_2 should be reduced as low and as soon as possible.
6. Nutritional support (vitamin A).
7. Prophylactic use of human recombinant antioxidant enzymes.

TABLE 23–1. FREE RADICALS AND ANTIOXIDANT QUENCHERS

RADICAL	SYMBOL	ANTIOXIDANT
Superoxide anion	O_2	Superoxide dismutase, uric acid, vitamin E
Singlet oxygen	$^1O_2$	β-Carotene, uric acid, vitamin E
Hydrogen peroxide	H_2O_2	Catalase, glutathione peroxidase, glutathione
Hydroxyl radical	OH*	Vitamins C, E
Peroxide radical	LOO° (L = lipid)	Vitamins C, E
Hydroperoxyl radical	LOOH (L = lipid)	Glutathione transferase, glutathione peroxidase
Peroxynitrite	ONOO⁻	Superoxide dismutase

Bibliography

Bancalari E, Sosenko I: Pathogenesis and prevention of neonatal chronic lung disease: Recent developments. Pediatr Pulmonol 1990; 8:109.

Davis JM, Rosenfeld W: Chronic lung disease in the newborn: *In*

Avery GB, Fletcher MA, MacDonald MG (eds): Textbook of Neonatology, 4th ed. Philadelphia, JB Lippincott, 1994, pp 453–477.

Davis JM, Rosenfeld WN, Sanders RJ, Gonenne A: The prophylactic effects of human recombinant superoxide dismutase in neonatal lung injury. J Appl Physiol 1993; (74)5:2234.

Frank L, Groseclose EE: Preparation of birth into an O_2 rich environment: The antioxidant enzymes in the developing rabbit lung. Pediatr Res 1984; 18:240.

Northway WH Jr, Rosan C, Porter DY: Pulmonary disease following respiratory therapy of hyaline-membrane disease. N Engl J Med 1967; 76:357.

24 Transient Tachypnea of the Newborn

Warren Rosenfeld

Definition

First reported in 1966, transient tachypnea of the newborn, in which rapid respirations are observed in infants who do not appear very ill, has a characteristic radiograph, is usually of short duration, and has no adverse sequelae. This diagnosis is often (and incorrectly) applied to any transient respiratory problem of no definable etiology and is a diagnosis of exclusion.

Pathophysiology

1. Transient retention of lung fluid secondary to delayed resorption
2. Delay in the normal movement of fetal lung fluid into the interstitial space
3. Delayed clearing of fluid in perivascular sheaths and interlobar sheaths by the lymphatics
4. Retained interstitial fluid compresses airways and decreases compliance.

Clinical Findings

1. Respiratory distress (usually mild)
   a. Tachypnea; 60 to 120 breaths/minute
   b. Grunting
   c. Retractions
   d. Nasal flaring
2. Respiratory distress may be initially severe, with gradual improvement.
3. A decreased PaO_2 and increased $PaCO_2$ may be present initially.
4. Originally described in term or near-term infants; now also described in preterm infants.
5. Contributory maternal history
   a. Heavy sedation
   b. Cesarean section, with absence of labor
   c. Maternal fluid overload

Key Clinical Findings

- Respiratory distress
- Cesarean birth (often)
- Heavily sedated mother at delivery

Radiographic Findings

1. Hyperaeration
2. Prominent vascular markings
3. Mild cardiomegaly
4. Fluid often found in interlobar fissures

Treatment

1. Disease is self-limited and benign (2 to 5 days), and treatment is usually not required. However, other causes of respiratory distress must be looked for.
2. When required, therapy is nonspecific oxygen and assisted ventilation (usually CPAP), as determined by blood gas analysis.

Key Treatment

- Self-limited disorder. No therapy indicated unless hypoxia occurs—then assisted ventilation

Bibliography

Avery ME, Gatewood OB, Brumley G: Transient tachypnea of the newborn: possible delayed resorption of fluid at birth. Am J Dis Child 1986;111:380–385.

Kulm MP, Fletcher BC, de Remo RA: Roentgen findings in transient tachypnea of the newborn. Radiology 1969;92:751–757.

Rawlings JS, Smith FR: Transient tachypnea of the newborn. Am J Dis Child 1984; 138:869–871.

Wiswell TE, Rawlings JS, Smith FR, Good ED: Effect of furosemide on the clinical course of transient tachypnea of the newborn. Pediatrics 1985;75:908–910.

25 Meconium Aspiration

Warren Rosenfeld

Definition

Aspiration of meconium (fetal stool) is a common cause of morbidity and illness in neonates, accounting for 2 per cent of neonatal intensive care unit (NICU) admissions. Meconium initially appears in the fetal ileum during the tenth to sixteenth week of gestation. It consists of a mixture of intestinal secretions, blood, cellular debris, bile, pancreatic secretions, vernix, mucus, lanugo, mucopolysaccharide proteins, mucoprotein, and lipids (8%), and water (72%).

Epidemiology

1. Meconium staining of the skin occurs in 11 to 22 per cent of all deliveries.
2. Meconium aspiration syndrome (MAS) occurs in only 2 to 5 per cent of these deliveries (approximately 6 in 1000 births).

Pathophysiology

1. Meconium that has been passed in utero and mixes with amniotic fluid may be aspirated into the tracheobronchial tree.
2. Intestinal hypoxia and/or ischemia (diversion of blood from the gastrointestinal tract, or diving reflex) increases peristalsis anal sphincter relaxation.
3. It may also represent a normal physiologic event in the maturation of fetal gut. Passage of meconium is rare before 34 weeks of gestation, increases with increasing gestation, and is common in post-term deliveries.
4. Hypoxia and acidemia may be required for aspiration of meconium into the tracheobronchial tree prior to delivery.
5. Aspiration of meconium may occur prior to delivery (often several days prior to delivery in the presence of hypoxia) or during the initial extrauterine breaths following delivery.
6. The hypoxic insult causing the passage of meconium may also cause brain damage.
7. Aspiration of meconium leads to obstruction of large and small airways.
   a. As little as 1 to 5 ml of meconium can cause mechanical obstruction.
   b. Decreased dynamic lung compliance, increased expiratory resistance, and increased functional residual capacity (FRC) all occur within 15 minutes of aspiration.
   c. A ventilation-perfusion (V/Q) mismatch occurs.
   d. Increased pulmonary vascular resistance may lead to the syndrome of persistent pulmonary hypertension of the newborn (PPHN).
   e. Changes occurring after 6 hours include
      (1) Increased lung H_2O (microvascular and endothelial damage)
      (2) Atelectasis and hyperexpansion
      (3) Infiltrates of polymorphonuclear cells in alveolar and interstitial spaces
   (4) Peripheral airway occlusion
      (a) If obstruction is complete, complete atelectasis and significant V/Q abnormalities occur.
      (b) If obstruction is partial, a ball-valve effect occurs, which may lead to air leaks (pneumomediastinum, pneumothorax, pulmonary interstitial emphysema, or PIE).
   (5) Proximal airway occlusion may lead to acute asphyxia and cor pulmonale.
   (6) Pneumonitis, which is initially chemical, may become secondarily infected with bacteria. This can lead to hypoxia, acidosis, and ventilatory failure.

Key Clinical Findings

- Respiratory distress
- Peripheral airway occlusion
- Pneumonitis

Management

1. Postnatal treatment
   Supportive
   a. Oxygen
   b. IV fluids
   c. Mechanical ventilation (required in about 30 per cent of patients with MAS)
   d. Surfactant treatment every 6 hours may be of value in improving oxygenation and decreasing the likelihood of air leaks.
   e. Administration of antibiotics, if infection is suspected
   f. In the presence of severe pulmonary vascular obstruction (PPHN), use of pulmonary vasodilators, such as tolazoline and nitric oxide, is indicated.
   g. Extracorporeal membrane oxygenation (ECMO) is occasionally required to oxygenate patients who are resistant to standard methods of treatment.

Key Treatment

- Oxygen
- Mechanical ventilation
- Consider antibiotics

2. Prevention
   a. Prenatal: In pregnancies complicated by passage of

thick meconium, a rapid intrauterine infusion of isotonic saline followed by a continuous infusion has often been shown to decrease the likelihood of MAS.

b. Delivery room management is discussed in Chapter 33.

Outcome

The overwhelming majority of infants with MAS recover without sequelae. The major long-term sequelae are the result of asphyxial damage to the central nervous system that accompanies the passage of meconium. There is usually no long-term damage to the lungs.

Bibliography

Cunningham K, Bosco BA, Seprington A: Pulmonary interstitial emphysema: A review. Neonatal Network 1992:11;7–16.

Findlay RD, Taeusch HW, Walther FJ: Surfactant replacement therapy for meconium aspiration syndrome. Pediatrics 1996;97:48–52.

Hagerman JR: Meconium staining of amniotic fluid: The need for reassessment of management by obstetricians and pediatricians. Curr Probl Pediatr 1993;23:396–401.

Wiswell TE, Bent RC: Meconium staining and the meconium aspiration syndrome. Unresolved issues. Pediatr Clin North Am 1993:40:955–981.

Wiswell TE, Henley MA: Intratracheal suctioning, systemic infection and meconium aspiration syndrome. Pediatrics 1992; 89:203–206.

26 Air Leaks

Warren Rosenfeld

Air rupturing through the alveolar wall dissects along the perivascular interstitial space. Several factors, including the lung's anatomy and compliance, place stresses on the lung, and the volume and pressure of the dissecting gas determine its ultimate location(s). These include

1. Pulmonary interstitial emphysema (PIE)
2. Pneumomediastinum
3. Pneumothorax
4. Pneumopericardium
5. Pneumoperitoneum

Epidemiology

1. Air leaks that can be detected radiographically occur spontaneously in 1 to 2 per cent of all newborns but cause symptoms in less than 0.05 per cent.
2. The incidence of air leaks increases under the following conditions:
   a. Prematurity and lung immaturity
   b. Respiratory distress syndrome (RDS)
   c. Aspiration syndromes (especially meconium)
   d. Assisted ventilation
   e. Neonatal resuscitation
   f. Congenital anomalies (renal agenesis, hypoplastic lung, diaphragmatic hernia)
3. The incidence of air leaks in infants with RDS decreased significantly in the early 1980s with the routine use of moderately low peak inspiratory pressures in infants requiring ventilatory assistance. With the introduction of surfactant therapy in the late 1980s, there was a further reduction in the incidence of air leaks.

Pathophysiology

Although air leaks may occur spontaneously in the neonate, the majority of clinically significant cases involve barotrauma secondary to resuscitation or overdistention secondary to the ball-valve effect of meconium present in small airways.

1. Overdistention of the lung due to excess lung volume, especially when the lung is noncompliant, may rupture alveolar sac(s). This is thought to occur at the base of the alveolus, contiguous with a pulmonary arterial blood vessel.

2. Air may dissect into the interstitial space and travel along the perivascular sheath. If air remains trapped in the interstitial space, PIE results.

3. Perivascular interstitial air may move along the blood vessel sheath, emerging at the roots of the pulmonary vessels in the mediastinum, resulting in pneumomediastinum.

4. Mediastinal air can rupture into a pleural cavity, causing a pneumothorax. Another rare mechanism causing pneumothorax is direct rupture of subpleural alveoli, allowing air to collect in the pleural space. If air moves in and out of the pleural space with each breath, a nontension pneumothorax is present. When air moves into the pleural space during inspiration but cannot escape during expiration, there is an increased volume of air under increased pressure in the pleural space, forming a tension pneumothorax.

5. Air may rarely track into other extraalveolar sites, including the pericardium (pneumopericardium) and peritoneum (pneumoperitoneum).

6. Trapped interstitial or pleural air
   a. Decreases compliance
   b. Decreases tidal volume
   c. Decreases cardiac return

d. Causes lymphatic congestion
e. Causes airway compression.

Clinical Findings and Management

1. Pneumomediastinum
   a. Respiratory distress, which is usually mild to moderate, is observed. Heart sounds may be distant.
   b. Radiographically, air present in the anterior mediastinum may lift the thymus (sail sign) or outline the lateral borders of the heart.
   c. Treatment is symptomatic; oxygen supplementation may be necessary. The appearance of a pneumomediastinum serves as a warning to adjust ventilator settings to prevent overdistention and further the progression of the air leak.
   d. Spontaneous resolution is usually the outcome unless underlying disease, i.e., RDS, requires continued mechanical support.

2. Pulmonary interstitial emphysema
   a. PIE usually is observed in very low birth weight infants receiving assisted ventilation. It is marked by worsening respiratory status.
   b. Radiographically, there are radiolucencies in interstitial spaces; these may be segmental or lobar or may be present throughout the entire lung(s). The lungs may have a "salt-and-pepper" appearance; flattening of diaphragm may be present.
   c. Treatment consists of adjustment of ventilator settings to decrease overdistention (i.e., decrease PIP, PEEP, inspiratory time). Use of high-frequency ventilation (jet or oscillator) is often effective. If PIE involves a single lobe or segment, selective bronchial intubation may be helpful.
   d. Mortality may be as high as 50 per cent; bronchopulmonary dysplasia is often a complication.

3. Pneumothorax
   a. Nontension pneumothorax may present with mild symptoms, whereas tension pneumothorax causes a sudden and rapid deterioration of respiratory status.
   b. Spontaneous pneumothoraces in healthy term infants may be due to rupture of a congenital bleb and may occur soon after birth. In sick or ventilated patients, they may occur at any time during the course of the illness.
   c. Shift of breath and/or heart sounds to the side opposite the pneumothorax may be observed; shift of the trachea to the side opposite the pneumothorax may be observed; sudden deterioration of respiratory status may occur. Transillumination of the chest may be helpful, but an emergency radiograph is essential.
   d. The radiograph shows a collection of air in the pleural space. If under tension it will cause a shift of the heart and mediastinium to the contralateral side. Since most radiographs are taken with the neonate in the supine position, pleural air may collect anteriorly. This may be confused with pneumomediastinum and can better be detected by a cross-table lateral or lateral decubitus film.
   e. Treatment of nontension pneumothoraces is symptomatic. Tension pneumothorax, however, is a medical emergency. Rapid recognition and treatment are essential.
      (1) Needle aspiration may provide temporary emergency relief.
      (2) Surgical chest tube insertion and drainage is definitive treatment.
   f. If unrecognized, cardiac arrest may ensue, with resultant serious cental nervous system ischemia and hypoxia.

Key Clinical Findings

- Pneumomediastinum
- Pulmonary interstitial emphysema
- Pneumothorax

Key Treatment

- Adjust ventilator to avoid overdistention (emphysema)
- Needle aspiration of tension pneumothorax

Bibliography

Allen RW, Jung AL, Lester PD: Effectiveness of chest tube evaluation of pneumothorax in neonates. J Pediatr 1981;99:629.

Davis CH, Stevens GW: Value of routine radiographic examinations of the newborn based on a study of 702 consecutive babies. Am J Obstet Gynecol 1930;20–73.

Gonzalez F, Harris TR, Black P, Richardson P: Decreased gas flow through pneumothoraces of neonates receiving high frequency jet vs. conventional ventilators. J Pediatr 1987;110:464–466.

Kuhns LR, Bednarek FJ, Wyman ML, et al: Diagnosis of pneumothorax or pneumomediastinum in the neonate by transillumination. Pediatrics 1975;56:355–360.

MacEwan DW, Dunbar JS, Smith RD, Brown B: Pneumothorax in young infants; recognition and evaluation. Can Assoc Radiol J 1971;22:264–269.

27 Neonatal Pneumonia

Leonard Glass

Pneumonia in the neonate may be caused by an infectious agent or may occur secondary to aspiration of meconium or gastric contents. Infectious pneumonia is caused by viruses, bacteria, and fungi; it may be acquired transplacentally, in utero, during the intrapartum period, or postnatally. Aspiration of meconium, leading to chemical pneumonitis, may occur in utero or during delivery.

Transplacental Infection

1. *Treponema pallidum*: Pneumonia secondary to congenital syphilis (pneumonia alba) is rarely observed but, when present, is usually associated with far-advanced disease and death.
2. *Mycobacterium tuberculosis*: Perinatal tuberculosis is extremely rare and is associated with placental involvement. It may be encountered with increased frequency in infants of mothers with AIDS.
3. *Listeria monocytogenes*: Pneumonia secondary to listerial infection is probably underdiagnosed and is associated with systemic symptoms in the neonate.
4. Viral infection: Several viruses listed below are transmitted transplacentally and may cause pneumonia.
   a. Rubella
   b. Cytomegalovirus
   c. Influenza
   d. Adenovirus
   e. Enteroviruses

In Utero Infection

In the presence of maternal chorioamnionitis, the fetus may swallow infected amniotic fluid and aspirate it into the lungs, leading to congenital pneumonia. The most commonly involved bacteria are group B streptococci and gram-negative enteric bacilli.

Intrapartum Transmission

Transmission of agents causing pneumonia during the intrapartum period (labor and delivery) is relatively common. In these infants, symptoms are observed hours or days after transmission. Organisms associated with this mode of transmission include:

1. Group B streptococci
2. Gram-negative enteric bacilli
3. *Chlamydia trachomatis*
4. *Ureaplasma urealyticum*
5. Herpesvirus hominis.

Postnatal Infection

Pneumonia acquired after delivery is usually associated with systemic infection. It is commonly observed in very low birth weight infants who have intravascular catheters and are receiving ventilatory assistance. Respiratory viruses brought into the nursery by visitors and professional staff may lead to a nursery outbreak of pneumonia. Agents associated with postnatally acquired pneumonia include:

1. *Staphylococcus aureus*
2. Coagulase-negative staphylococci (usually catheter related)
3. Group B streptococci
4. *Candida albicans*
5. Respiratory syncytial virus
6. Influenza virus.

Clinical and Radiologic Findings

The clinical presentation of pneumonia includes dyspnea, tachypnea, cyanosis, and, frequently, respiratory failure. It is usually difficult to distinguish pneumonia from other causes of respiratory distress, such as respiratory distress syndrome, bronchopulmonary dysplasia, air leak, and congestive heart failure. Pneumonia secondary to group B streptococci and gram-negative bacilli may coexist with respiratory distress syndrome. Chest radiographs are usually helpful in establishing the diagnosis but are often nonspecific.

Key Clinical Findings

- Tachypnea
- Dyspnea
- Cyanosis

Treatment

When pneumonia is suspected or proven, appropriate antimicrobial therapy should be instituted after obtaining cultures, along with ventilatory assistance and administration of parenteral fluids. Choice of antibiotics is based on clinical judgment prior to obtaining results of cultures and on antibiotic sensitivity studies. When aspiration pneumonia is suspected, administration of antimicrobial therapy is indicated.

Key Treatment

- Antimicrobial therapy appropriate to place and time

Bibliography

Hansen T, Corbet A: Neonatal pneumonias. *In* Taeusch HW, Ballard RA, Avery ME (eds): Diseases of the Newborn. Philadelphia, WB Saunders, 1991, pp 527–535.

Klein JO: Bacterial infections of the respiratory tract. *In* Remington JS, Klein JO: Infectious Diseases of the Fetus and Newborn Infant. Philadelphia, WB Saunders, 1990, pp 657–675.

28 Neonatal Infections

Steve Piecuch

Bacterial and Fungal Infections

Definition

Neonatal sepsis is usually defined as an infection occurring in the first 28 days after birth, associated with systemic signs of infection. Early-onset infections occur in the first week of life and are usually acquired in utero or during labor and delivery. Late-onset infections occur after the first week and may be due to organisms acquired during the birth process, a nursery-acquired nosocomial infection, or an infection acquired after discharge from the nursery. Neonatal sepsis is usually distinguished from congenital infections, which are acquired in utero and are usually due to viruses, protozoa, or spirochetes. Congenital infections may be evident while the infant is still in the nursery, or they may be detected after discharge.

Etiology

1. Group B streptococci and *Escherichia coli* are together responsible for the majority of non-nosocomial neonatal bacterial infections. *Listeria monocytogenes* as well as a variety of other organisms, such as *Streptococcus pneumoniae* and *Haemophilus influenzae*, type b may also cause non-nosocomial infection.
2. Coagulase-negative staphylococci, predominantly *Staphylococcus epidermidis*, and a variety of gram-negative organisms such as *Serratia*, *Acinetobacter*, *Enterobacter* and *Pseudomonas* are commonly responsible for nursery-acquired nosocomial infections.
3. Fungal infection, primarily due to *Candida* species, is a problem of increasing importance in the nursery. Although usually of nosocomial origin, fungal infection may occur in utero. Fungal chorioamnionitis has been described in association with an intrauterine foreign body, such as a retained intrauterine device.

Epidemiology

1. The overall incidence of neonatal bacterial infection is approximately 1 to 4/1000 live births.
2. Fetal infection may be a significant factor in the initiation of premature labor.
3. Although risk factors such as premature birth, prolonged rupture of the membranes, maternal fever, and fetal tachycardia are associated with an increased incidence of neonatal sepsis, infections may also occur in infants without any known risk factors who may appear relatively well immediately after birth.
4. The incidence of nosocomial infections may be increased by overcrowding, lack of proper handwashing, and the use of broad-spectrum antibiotics, which may promote the emergence of resistant microorganisms.
5. Small premature infants, especially those with indwelling vascular catheters and those who require repeated courses of broad-spectrum antibiotics, are particularly prone to fungal infection.

Pathophysiology

1. The newborn infant is at increased risk of infection as a result of a relative impairment of host defenses. Neonatal neutrophil, macrophage, and monocyte function is deficient compared with that of the older child or adult. The neonate's bone marrow neutrophil storage pool is relatively small and subject to depletion, putting the neonate at risk of developing neutropenia in the face of severe infection. There is a similar impairment of cell-mediated immunity and complement function.
2. Since the intrauterine environment is sterile, antibody is not normally produced by the fetus prior to birth. Although the fetus is capable of synthesizing IgM after the twentieth week of gestation in response to intrauterine infection, under normal circumstances the neonate is deficient in both IgM and IgA at birth. Since IgG is actively transported from the mother to the fetus, primarily during the third trimester of pregnancy, the premature infant is born with a relative deficiency of IgG. In addition, the newborn receives only IgG antibody against organisms to which the mother already has immunity. As a result of all these factors, the neonate has a relative impairment of humeral immunity; this is particularly marked in the premature infant.
3. Neonatal infection may occur transplacentally, as with *Listeria monocytogenes*, or may result from maternal chorioamnionitis. Infection may also be acquired during passage through the birth canal or, later, in the nursery or after discharge.

Clinical Findings

1. In some infants the signs of sepsis may be subtle, with mild tachypnea, irritability, lethargy, feeding intolerance, and temperature instability as the only findings. Fever is an unusual presenting sign of neonatal sepsis but may occasionally be observed in full-term infants. Hypothermia is a more frequent sign of systemic infection.
2. Early-onset infection in the newborn, especially when caused by the group B *Streptococcus*, may be fulminant, with respiratory distress, apnea, pallor, and shock. The infant may suffer repeated cardiopulmonary arrests and fail to respond to appropriate antibiotics, despite aggressive support of ventilation and blood pressure. Other infants may have a milder course. Meningitis occurs in a significant minority of infants with early-onset infection.
3. Late-onset infection is typically associated with meningitis and tends to present insidiously with fever, irritability, and a bulging fontanel. The infant with late-onset infection may appear surprisingly well despite the presence of septicemia and meningitis.
4. The presentation of nosocomial infection in the nursery is diverse. A previously stable infant may develop acidosis, leukocytosis, leukopenia, thrombocytopenia, poor feeding, mild tachypnea, or an increasing number of apneic

episodes. In some cases the presentation may be fulminant, resembling that of early-onset infection.

5. Respiratory distress due to sepsis must be distinguished from transient tachypnea of the newborn and respiratory distress syndrome (RDS) of prematurity. These latter conditions may coexist with sepsis. Irritability and poor feeding may be due to birth asphyxia, narcotic withdrawal, or hypoglycemia. Temperature instability may be the result of environmental stress or a malfunctioning incubator or radiant warmer. Cardiac disease may cause respiratory distress; ductus arteriosus–dependent cardiac lesions, such as hypoplastic left heart syndrome, coarctation of the aorta, or interrupted aortic arch, may present with a shocklike state resembling early-onset infection.

Key Clinical Findings: Bacterial and Fungal Infections

- Hypothermia
- Apnea
- Pallor

Laboratory Findings

1. Hematologic
   a. Leukocytosis or leukopenia, thrombocytopenia, an elevated C-reactive protein, and an elevated erythrocyte sedimentation rate all support the diagnosis of infection in the newborn. An elevated immature neutrophil count and an immature to total neutrophil ratio >0.20 are also suggestive of infection. Some infants may have evidence of disseminated intravascular coagulation (DIC), with abnormalities of the prothrombin time, partial thromboplastin time, fibrinogen, fibrin degradation products, and platelets.

2. Bacteriologic
   a. The diagnosis of infection can be made by the presence of a positive culture from a normally sterile site, such as blood, urine, or cerebrospinal fluid (CSF). If the infant was previously treated with antibiotics, or if the mother was treated during labor, cultures may be negative despite the presence of infection. Tests that are based upon antigen detection techniques may be particularly useful in such cases. These tests may also be used in conjunction with other laboratory tests in untreated infants, to identify rapidly those who should receive antibiotic therapy while awaiting culture results.
   b. Surface cultures are used by many clinicians to identify those infants at increased risk of infection as well as to identify those organisms most likely to be responsible. Whether routine surface cultures are cost-effective or add useful clinical information is arguable. If surface cultures are done, it is important to recognize that a positive surface culture represents colonization and not true infection. However, if it is decided to treat an infant for infection and surface cultures have been done, it is important to consider the results of those cultures when selecting the antibiotic regimen.

Key Laboratory Findings: Bacterial and Fungal Infection

- Leukopenia or leukocytosis
- Thrombocytopenia

Radiographic Findings

1. The x-ray findings in neonatal infection may be nonspecific. Affected infants may have radiographic findings suggestive of transient tachypnea with bilateral streakiness and fluid in the minor fissure, or of RDS with a reticulogranular pattern and air bronchograms. It may be difficult to distinguish atelectasis from pneumonia.

2. Cranial ultrasound and CT scans are useful in following infants with meningitis. Abnormal findings are common and may include cerebral edema or infarction, ventricular dilatation, the development of cystic changes or brain atrophy, or the development of subdural collections.

Treatment

1. Supportive care is essential. It is important to prevent hypoxia or hypoglycemia. If oxygen is used in the premature infant, blood gases should be closely monitored to prevent hyperoxia so as to minimize the risk of retinopathy of prematurity. Nasogastric or orogastric decompression may be necessary if there is abdominal distention or vomiting.

2. The critically ill septic infant may require ventilatory support. If there is hypotension or frank shock, the infant may require volume support with isotonic saline, 5 percent albumin solution, or blood. In some cases pressor agents such as dopamine or dobutamine may be required. Careful attention must be paid to the serum electrolytes and urine output.

3. Metabolic acidosis reflects the severity of the underlying infection and should improve as the infant responds to therapy.

4. If there is DIC, replacement therapy with blood, fresh frozen plasma, and platelets may be required, especially if there is active bleeding. As a rule, DIC is best controlled by successful management of the precipitating event.

5. It is important to obtain appropriate cultures prior to beginning antibiotic therapy. As a rule, blood cultures should always be done before starting antibiotics. A urine culture should be done in an infant with suspected late-onset or nosocomial infection; it is often omitted in early-onset infection because blood cultures are expected to be positive in such cases.

6. Because of its relatively low yield in suspected cases of early-onset or nosocomial infection, many clinicians do not include a lumbar puncture in the routine evaluation of such infants. However, late-onset infection is commonly associated with meningitis, and a lumbar puncture should always be done in an infant in whom late-onset sepsis is suspected. In addition, lumbar puncture should be done in any neonate in whom infection appears likely on the basis of clinical or laboratory findings. If an infant is started on antibiotics without a lumbar puncture, and blood cultures are subsequently reported as positive, a lumbar puncture should be done

while the infant is undergoing treatment. While CSF cultures are likely to be negative in such a case, the white blood cell count, and glucose and protein levels, may be abnormal if there is meningitis. Making a diagnosis of meningitis is important, since it will influence both the duration of treatment and the prognosis.

7. The choice of antibiotics is determined by the clinical situation. Early- and late-onset neonatal sepsis are usually treated with ampicillin plus an aminoglycoside such as gentamicin or tobramycin. This combination covers group B *Streptococcus*, *E. coli*, and *Listeria* as well as many other organisms that may cause neonatal infection, such as enterococci, pneumococci, and *H. influenzae*. Some clinicians use a cephalosporin such as cefotaxime along with ampicillin, and others use a cephalosporin alone. If cefotaxime is used alone, infection with *Listeria* will not be covered. It is essential to monitor serum levels if an aminoglycoside is used.

8. Nosocomial infections are usually treated initially with vancomycin plus cefotaxime, in order to cover coagulase-negative staphylococci as well as gram-negative bacteria. Because of increasing concerns about the emergence of vancomycin-resistant organisms, careful clinical judgment must be used in deciding which infants to treat with this agent and for how long, especially if cultures remain negative.

9. Fungal infection may be insidious or fulminant and is commonly associated with splenomegaly or thrombocytopenia, especially in an infant with an indwelling catheter or one who has received multiple courses of antibiotics. Treatment is with amphotericin; some clinicians add flucytosine to the regimen. As a general rule, the empirical use of amphotericin in the absence of a positive fungal culture should be avoided unless the infant is seriously ill and fungal infection is considered likely based on the overall clinical picture.

10. Septic infants may develop neutrophil storage pool depletion, leading to prolonged neutropenia and a resulting impaired ability to fight infection. A number of investigators have demonstrated improved survival in such infants who were given neutrophil transfusions. However, this therapy is not in widespread clinical use, partly because of technical difficulties in obtaining neutrophils for transfusion on short notice.

11. The use of intravenous immunoglobulin in septic infants is appealing, as the newborn, especially the premature one, may lack protective levels of specific IgG. In addition, intravenous immunoglobulin is relatively safe in infants and is readily available. However, a number of carefully conducted clinical trials have failed to produce convincing evidence that this therapy is beneficial. Despite this lack of proven benefit, many clinicians routinely use intravenous immunoglobulin in septic infants, especially in those who are critically ill or who fail to respond to conventional therapy.

Key Treatment: Bacterial and Fungal Infections

- Antimicrobial therapy
- Oxygen for hypoxia

Prevention

1. Since the risk of infection is increased 3 to 10 fold in the premature infant, prevention of prematurity should significantly decrease the incidence of neonatal sepsis.

2. Avoidance of overcrowding, meticulous care of indwelling catheters, and careful attention to handwashing will reduce but will not eliminate nosocomial infections. Nosocomial infections with resistant organisms and with fungi can be reduced by avoiding the inappropriate use of broad-spectrum antibiotics.

3. It is possible to significantly reduce the incidence of early-onset group B streptococcal infection by treating women who are group B streptococcal carriers with prophylactic antibiotics during labor and delivery.

   a. One approach is to culture all women for group B *Streptococcus* at 35 to 37 weeks of pregnancy and to treat all who are positive with penicillin or ampicillin during labor and delivery. If cultures have not been done or if the results are unavailable, prophylactic antibiotics should be given if there is fever (38°C or greater), rupture of membranes for more than 18 hours, or prematurity (less than 37 weeks' gestation).

   b. An alternative approach is to not perform routine cultures but to simply treat all women in the presence of fever, prolonged rupture of membranes, or prematurity.

   c. Women who have had group B streptococcal bacteriuria during pregnancy or who have previously delivered an infant with group B streptococcal infection are at relatively high risk of delivering an infected infant, do not need to have screening cultures done, and should all receive prophylactic antibiotics.

   d. The approach to the infant must be individualized. Infants who are premature or who have clinical evidence of sepsis at delivery should be evaluated for infection and started on antibiotics while culture results are pending. Full-term infants who are well may not need any evaluation or treatment. The clinician must remember that antibiotic prophylaxis does not completely eliminate the risk of neonatal infection and that intrapartum treatment may result in the infant having negative cultures at birth despite the presence of infection. Infants born to mothers colonized with group B streptococcal infection are not candidates for early discharge from the nursery.

Viral and Protozoal Infections

Herpes Simplex Virus
Definition
1. Neonatal herpes is an infection acquired perinatally or, less commonly, postnatally.
2. Congenital herpes is an infection that occurs in utero at a time remote from delivery.
Etiology
1. Most fetal and neonatal infections are due to herpes simplex virus (HSV) type 1, but up to 20 percent of cases are due to HSV 2.

2. Neonatal herpes is usually due to exposure of the infant to maternal virus, either as a result of ascending infection after the membranes have ruptured or during passage through the birth canal. Uncommonly, infection may occur in infants delivered by cesarean section with intact membranes.

3. Approximately 10 percent of neonatal herpes infections occur postnatally, as a result of contact with the mother or another infected individual.

Epidemiology

The incidence of neonatal herpes infections is estimated as 0.1 to 0.5/1000 live births. Premature infants are at increased risk. The estimated risk of infection to an infant born vaginally is approximately 35 to 50 percent if the mother has a primary infection and 4 to 5 percent if the maternal infection is recurrent.

Clinical Findings

1. Congenital herpes infection may present with fetal growth retardation, microcephaly, hepatitis, chorioretinitis, and other abnormalities. A vesicular or bullous rash is usually present.

2. Neonatal herpes infection typically presents in one of three ways.
   a. Disseminated infection presents relatively early, in the first or second week, with respiratory distress, cyanosis, hepatitis, DIC, and shock. Central nervous system (CNS) involvement is common in disseminated disease.
   b. Isolated CNS involvement also occurs, typically presenting between 2 and 4 weeks of age with lethargy, irritability, and seizures. Skin lesions are common in both disseminated and isolated CNS disease, usually in the form of a single vesicle, but lesions may not be present in all patients.
   c. A milder form of infection, localized to the skin, eye, and mouth, also occurs, typically in the third week of life.

Key Clinical Findings: Herpesvirus

- Vesicular rash
- Hepatitis
- Variable CNS disturbances

Laboratory Findings

1. Herpes simplex infection is best diagnosed by culture. Although a positive culture at birth may represent contamination of the infant with virus, a positive culture after 24 to 48 hours is indicative of true infection, as HSV does not cause asymptomatic colonization.

2. Infants may have an abnormal complete blood count, abnormal liver tests, or evidence of DIC.

3. The CSF in infants with CNS involvement may be normal, or there may be a mononuclear pleocytosis with an elevated protein and a normal or low glucose concentration.

Key Laboratory Findings: Herpesvirus

- Culture of virus

Radiographic Findings

Congenitally infected infants may have evidence of microcephaly or intracranial calcifications on brain imaging. The chest x-ray may show pneumonia in infants with disseminated disease.

Treatment

Untreated neonatal herpes infection has a very poor prognosis, with a high mortality rate in both disseminated and CNS disease, and a high rate of serious handicap in survivors. Although the prognosis is better with localized skin, eye, and mouth involvement, some of these infants will have progression of the infection and the development of adverse neurodevelopmental sequelae. Treatment reduces the mortality rate and improves the outcome in survivors. Acyclovir, which is activated by viral thymidine kinase and selectively inhibits viral DNA polymerase, is the drug of choice. Some infants will have recurrent episodes of cutaneous lesions following treatment. The management of these patients must be individualized.

Key Treatment: Herpesvirus

- Acyclovir

Prevention

1. Routinely culturing of virus in pregnant women with a history of genital herpes infections is neither cost-effective nor reliable. The current approach is to deliver women with active genital lesions by cesarean section within 4 to 6 hours of rupture of membranes, preferably before rupture has occurred.

2. Infants born vaginally to mothers with primary lesions are at very high risk of infection. The risk is lower with recurrent lesions and in infants born by cesarean section after the membranes have ruptured. Infants delivered by cesarean section with intact membranes are at low risk of infection. Decisions as to which infants to treat prophylactically must be individualized based on an assessment of the particular infant's risk. If a potentially exposed infant is not treated, the mother should be instructed to carefully observe the infant for skin rash or other signs of infection, and the infant should be closely followed after discharge.

Cytomegalovirus

Definition

Congenital cytomegalovirus (CMV) infection is an infection that occurs in utero. It should be distinguished from perinatal infection acquired during the birth process as well as from postnatal infection.

Etiology

1. Causative organism: cytomegalovirus

2. Congenital infection results from maternal viremia leading to placental and fetal infection in utero. Perinatal infection is acquired from contact with infected maternal genital secretions during delivery. Cytomegalovirus can be acquired postnatally from infected breast milk or blood products. Nosocomial spread within the nursery has also been described but appears to be uncommon.

Epidemiology

Congenital CMV infection occurs in approximately 1 percent of infants. While 90 percent are asymptomatic at birth, approximately 20 percent develop sequelae of the infection. Although congenital infection may result from either a primary maternal infection or the reactivation of a latent infection, the fetus is at greatest risk from a primary infection during the first half of pregnancy. Approximately 50 percent of women of childbearing age in the United States lack protective antibody to CMV and are at risk of primary infection during pregnancy.

Clinical Findings

1. Primary maternal infection may be asymptomatic or may be associated with sore throat, fever, and lymphadenopathy.
2. Most infants with congenital CMV infection are without symptoms during the neonatal period, but these infants may develop long-term sequelae, particularly hearing loss. It is rare for an infant infected as a result of a reactivated maternal infection to have severe neonatal disease.
3. The most common findings in symptomatic infected newborns are hepatosplenomegaly and intrauterine growth retardation.
4. Other findings include pneumonia, petechiae and purpura, chorioretinitis, seizures, microcephaly with periventricular calcifications, and neurodevelopmental delay.
5. The most common sequela of congenital CMV infection is hearing loss.
6. Infants with perinatal or postnatal infections may be asymptomatic or may develop hepatosplenomegaly or pneumonia. Such infants appear to be at very little risk for adverse neurodevelopmental sequelae or hearing loss.
7. Premature infants may develop hepatosplenomegaly, jaundice, and pneumonia as a result of CMV infection acquired by blood transfusion in the nursery.

Key Clinical Findings: Cytomegalovirus

- Hepatosplenomegaly
- Petechiae
- Chorioretinitis
- Periventricular calcifications

Laboratory Findings

1. The symptomatic infant may have abnormal liver tests, conjugated hyperbilirubinemia, or thrombocytopenia.
2. Urine culture is the most reliable diagnostic test. Isolation of virus in the first 3 weeks of life is considered to be proof of a congenital infection. A positive culture later in infancy may reflect congenital infection or infection acquired perinatally or postnatally.
3. Serologic diagnosis is not as reliable as culture. IgM antibody in cord blood or from early in life is suggestive of congenital infection. It may difficult to distinguish between congenital and perinatal or postnatal infection on the basis of IgG antibody titers.

Key Laboratory Findings: Cytomegalovirus

- Thrombocytopenia
- Positive urine culture

Radiographic Findings

1. Brain imaging may demonstrate microcephaly or periventricular calcification.
2. Calcification may also be evident on skull x-ray.

Treatment

There is no antiviral agent of demonstrated clinical use in congenital CMV infection. Ganciclovir has been used in some patients, especially in HIV-infected infants.

Prevention

Women of childbearing age, especially those employed in healthcare and those who work with children, should know their serologic status and avoid contact with infected individuals if seronegative. Patients with CMV infection should be appropriately isolated.

Rubella

Definition

Congenital rubella infection is an intrauterine infection of the fetus that may occur throughout pregnancy. Congenital rubella syndrome refers to a constellation of fetal abnormalities that result from infection early in pregnancy.

Etiology

Maternal viremia from rubella virus results in placental infection, which is followed by a fetal viremia, chronic fetal infection, and fetal injury.

Epidemiology

While immunization has resulted in a dramatic decline in the incidence of rubella, as many as 10 percent of young women may be susceptible.

Clinical Findings

1. Infection during pregnancy is commonly subclinical, but symptoms may include fever, postoccipital and postauricular adenopathy, rash, and arthralgia or arthritis.
2. Congenital rubella infection may lead to stillbirth or fetal growth retardation.
3. Malformations include congenital heart disease; eye abnormalities, including cataract, glaucoma, and retinopathy; microcephaly; mental retardation; and deafness.
4. Other findings include pneumonia, bone lesions, hemolytic anemia, thrombocytopenic purpura, and hepatitis. Fetal injury is common with first-trimester infection; less commonly, retinopathy and hearing loss occur following early second-trimester infection.
5. Long-term sequelae of congenital rubella infection include the late development of chronic lymphocytic thyroiditis and insulin-dependent diabetes mellitus.

Key Clinical Findings: Rubella

- Cataract
- Congenital heart disease
- Blueberry muffin purpura
- Microcephaly

Laboratory Findings

1. The infant may have abnormal liver tests, conjugated hyperbilirubinemia, anemia, and thrombocytopenia.
2. Virus may be isolated from urine, nasopharyngeal secretions, CSF, and other body sites. Viral shedding persists for months in the congenitally infected infant.
3. The presence of specific IgM antibody in early infancy and the persistence of IgG antibody in the second half of the first year of life are both indicative of congenital rubella infection.

Key Laboratory Findings: Rubella

- Abnormal liver tests
- Thrombocytopenia

Radiographic Findings

Bone lesions, described as longitudinal linear areas of rarefaction in the metaphyses of the long bones, are relatively common in congenitally infected infants.

Prevention and Treatment

1. A pregnant woman exposed to rubella who was known to be seropositive prior to pregnancy can be reassured that her fetus is at very low risk. A seronegative woman who develops evidence of rubella infection during the first trimester of pregnancy should be informed of the risks to her fetus and made aware of her options with regard to continuing or terminating the pregnancy.
2. Universal immunization of children against rubella will significantly reduce, but not completely eliminate, potential sources of infection for susceptible pregnant women. Seronegative women of childbearing age should be immunized.
3. Although the vaccine virus does not appear to be teratogenic, women should be advised not to become pregnant for 3 months following immunization, and pregnant women should not be immunized until after delivery.
4. There are concerns that natural or vaccine-induced immunity may wane, and rare cases of congenital rubella have occurred as a result of infection during pregnancy in women who were thought to be immune.
5. There is no treatment that will reduce the risk to the fetus.

Toxoplasmosis

Definition

Congenital toxoplasmosis is caused by fetal infection with the parasite *Toxoplasma gondii*.

Etiology

1. *Toxoplasma gondii* causing primary maternal infection during pregnancy.
2. Infants born to women with underlying immunodeficiency, such as AIDS, may acquire congenital infection as a result of reactivation of a preexisting maternal infection.

Epidemiology

1. The incidence of congenital infection in the United States is approximately 1 to 2 per 1000.
2. Cats are the primary hosts for *Toxoplasma* and shed oocysts in the stool. Animals ingesting the oocysts become infected and form tissue cysts. Humans may acquire infection by contact with soil or with cat feces or by ingesting inadequately cooked meat that contains tissue cysts.
3. The majority of women of childbearing age in the United States are seronegative for *Toxoplasma* and susceptible to primary infection.
4. Primary toxoplasmosis during pregnancy is associated with a 30 to 50 percent risk of fetal infection, with the most severe disease seen in those woman exposed early in pregnancy.

Clinical Findings

1. Maternal infection may be asymptomatic or may be associated with malaise, fever, sore throat, and lymphadenopathy.
2. The majority of congenitally infected infants are asymptomatic at birth but may develop sequelae later in life.
3. Common findings in symptomatic infants include fetal growth retardation, hepatosplenomegaly, and jaundice. Neurologic abnormalities are common, including seizures, psychomotor retardation, and hydrocephalus or microcephaly. Chorioretinitis is common and may lead to severe visual impairment; it may be present at birth or develop later in childhood or in adult life.

Key Clinical Findings: Toxoplasmosis

- Hepatosplenomegaly
- Seizures

Laboratory Findings

1. The presence of IgM or IgA antibody to *Toxoplasma* in an infant, or a rising IgG antibody titer on serial assays, is diagnostic of congenital toxoplasmosis. The absence of specific IgM or IgA antibody does not exclude the diagnosis of congenital infection. The serologic diagnosis of toxoplasmosis is difficult because of problems with the accuracy and reliability of the assays used. The clinician should utilize an appropriate reference laboratory and should be familiar with the capabilities as well as the limitations of that laboratory. Knowing the mother's serologic status is very helpful in evaluating the infant. If the mother was known to be seropositive and immunocompetent prior to pregnancy, the diagnosis of congenital toxoplasmosis can be essentially excluded in her infant. Conversely, if the mother had serologic evidence of acute infection during pregnancy, infection in the infant is very possible.
2. Infected infants may have abnormal liver tests, conjugated hyperbilirubinemia, and anemia.
3. Thrombocytopenia may occur but is less commonly seen than in congenital cytomegalovirus or rubella infection.
4. Cerebrospinal fluid abnormalities, such as pleocytosis or protein elevation, may be seen.

Key Laboratory Findings: Toxoplasmosis

- Presence of IgM or IgA antibody
- Rising titer of IgG

Radiographic Findings

Brain imaging may reveal hydrocephalus, microcephaly, or the presence of intracranial calcifications.

Treatment

Treatment is indicated in all infants with congenital toxoplasmosis. Congenital toxoplasmosis is currently treated with a 1-year course of pyrimethamine and sulfadiazine. The benefits of treatment are limited in severely affected infants. Primary *Toxoplasma* infection during pregnancy can be treated with spiramycin, to reduce the risk of fetal infection. If fetal blood sampling demonstrates active fetal infection, spiramycin will be ineffective, and pyrimethamine and sulfadiazine may be useful.

Key Treatment: Toxoplasmosis

- Pyrimethamine and sulfadiazine for 1 year

Prevention

1. It is possible to routinely screen for toxoplasmosis during pregnancy and at delivery in order to begin treatment in utero or soon after birth and, it is hoped, improve outcome. Whether such screening is cost-effective is unclear. Some women with primary infection during pregnancy may choose abortion.
2. Seronegative women can reduce their risk of infection with *Toxoplasma* by not handling cat feces, by washing their hands carefully after coming in contact with soil, and by not eating undercooked meat. Cats are less likely to acquire *Toxoplasma* if kept indoors and fed only prepared pet food.

Bibliography

Gerdes JS: Clinicopathologic approach to the diagnosis of neonatal sepsis. Clin Perinatol 1991;18:361–381.

Gotoff SP: Sepsis in the newborn. *In* Krugman S, Katz SL, Gershon AA, Wilfert CM (eds): Infectious Diseases of Children. St. Louis, Mosby–Year Book, 1992.

29 Gastrointestinal Disorders

Steve Piecuch

Frequently Encountered Gastrointestinal Disorders in the Neonate

- Hemorrhage
- Intestinal stenosis and atresia
- Malrotation and volvulus
- Congenital megacolon
- Meconium ileus
- Meconium plug syndrome
- Small left colon syndrome
- Necrotizing enterocolitis

Neonatal gastrointestinal (GI) problems range from simple feeding intolerance due to developmental immaturity or the stress of acute illness, to major intraabdominal catastrophes, such as malrotation with midgut volvulus and necrotizing enterocolitis. The major pathologic processes that the pediatrician is likely to encounter are discussed below.

Gastrointestinal Hemorrhage

Definition

Upper GI bleeding is defined as bleeding proximal to the ligament of Treitz and is usually diagnosed on the basis of vomitus or gastric aspirate that contains blood. Lower GI bleeding originates distal to the ligament of Treitz and presents with gross or occult blood in the stool.

Etiology

1. Gastrointestinal bleeding may be seen in neonatal GI disease or accompanying a coagulopathy or thrombocytopenia; alternatively, it may be due to mucosal irritation from suctioning or from indwelling feeding tubes.
2. Stress-related upper GI hemorrhage may be seen in infants with systemic illness such as congenital heart disease or birth asphyxia. Idiopathic upper GI bleeding in apparently well infants may also occur and may be massive, necessitating repeated blood transfusion.

Pathophysiology

Bleeding in disorders such as necrotizing enterocolitis or midgut volvulus is due to injury to the bowel mucosa. Hemorrhagic disease of the newborn may occur if the infant is not given vitamin K at birth, leading to a failure of clotting factor activation. Upper GI bleeding in the stressed infant is presumably due to increased gastric acidity; bowel ischemia and hypoxia may be contributing factors. Idiopathic upper GI bleeding may be due to inapparent stress or may be the result of the increase in gastric acidity that normally occurs on the first day of life.

Clinical Findings

Hemorrhage presents with pallor and tachycardia; hypotension may be a relatively late finding. The vomitus, gastric aspirate, or stool may be grossly bloody or positive for occult blood.

Key Clinical Findings: Gastrointestinal Hemorrhage

- Tachycardia
- Pallor

Laboratory Findings

The infant's hematocrit is expected to be low, but it may be relatively normal if the bleeding is acute and equilibration has not yet occurred. Abnormalities of the prothrombin time (PT), partial thromboplastin time (PTT), fibrinogen, fibrin split products, and platelet count may be present. If bleeding is thought to be due to swallowed maternal blood, an Apt-Downey test should be done to determine if the blood is of neonatal or maternal origin.

Key Laboratory Findings: Gastrointestinal Hemorrhage

- Bloody stool or vomitus
- Low hematocrit
- Prolonged PT and PTT

Radiographic Findings

Radiographic studies may be diagnostic if the bleeding is due to a specific GI disorder, such as necrotizing enterocolitis. In upper GI bleeding that is stress related or idiopathic, plain films and upper GI contrast studies are usually normal.

Treatment

1. Careful monitoring of the infant's hemodynamic status and hematocrit is necessary, and packed red blood cell (RBC) transfusion may be required to correct anemia. Fresh whole blood is preferable to packed RBCs if the infant is actively bleeding and unstable. Volume support with isotonic saline or 5 per cent albumin solution may be necessary while waiting for blood to become available.
2. Fresh frozen plasma may be required if there are abnormalities of the PT and PTT. Hemorrhagic disease of the newborn is expected to respond to 1 to 2 mg of intravenous vitamin K. Immune thrombocytopenia may require treatment with corticosteroids or immune globulin; random donor platelet transfusions are usually not effective. If disseminated intravascular coagulation (DIC) is present, the underlying cause must be identified and treated.
3. Upper endoscopy should be considered in the infant with unexplained upper GI bleeding; it may reveal mucosal ulcerations or erosions. Upper GI bleeding is usually managed with antacids and histamine blockers such as cimetidine or ranitidine. Gastric lavage with saline may be useful but can lead to hypothermia.

Key Treatment: Gastrointestinal Hemorrhage

- Supportive
- Fresh frozen plasma if coagulation studies are abnormal; RBC transfusion if needed

Intestinal Obstruction

Definition

Intestinal obstruction from either stenosis or atresia refers to a narrowing or complete blockage of the intestinal lumen, resulting in bowel obstruction. The duodenum, jejunum and ileum are most commonly affected, with colonic atresia being relatively uncommon. Some patients have multiple areas of atresia.

Etiology

Duodenal obstruction may result from external compression due to an annular pancreas, Ladd band, or preduodenal portal vein or from a failure of duodenal revacuolization. Most cases of jejunoileal and colonic atresias result from intrauterine vascular accidents, volvulus, or intussusception. Infants with jejunoileal atresia may pass meconium, suggesting that this lesion develops relatively late in fetal life. Duodenal atresia is commonly associated with other anomalies, whereas jejunoileal and colonic atresias are not. Cystic fibrosis may be associated with intestinal atresia, either as an isolated finding or as a complication of meconium ileus.

Clinical Findings

The diagnosis may be made in utero by an antenatal ultrasound examination that demonstrates an abnormal bowel pattern or polyhydramnios. The typical postnatal clinical presentations are abdominal distention and vomiting, which is commonly bilious. The passage of meconium does not exclude this diagnosis. The presentation of intestinal stenosis may be delayed into the second postnatal week or later.

Key Clinical Findings: Intestinal Obstruction

- Abdominal distention
- Bilious vomiting

Laboratory Findings

There are no characteristic laboratory findings, although the clinician should be prepared to correct any fluid and electrolyte imbalances that resulted from prolonged vomiting.

Radiographic Findings

The plain abdominal film in a high intestinal atresia may show an abrupt cut-off of the intestinal gas pattern, whereas in a low intestinal atresia there may be only generalized bowel distention. If there has been in utero perforation, the intraperitoneal calcifications of meconium peritonitis may be seen. In intestinal stenosis, the x-ray may demonstrate proximal intestinal distention with decreased or absent distal bowel gas. An upper GI study or barium enema may be required if the diagnosis is not evident from the plain films. A microcolon may be present if there is a low intestinal atresia.

Treatment

The management of intestinal stenosis and atresia is surgical. The pediatrician must pay careful attention to preoperative and postoperative fluid and electrolyte management. The prognosis is dependent on the length of bowel remaining after surgery as well as on the presence of other anomalies. Extensive bowel resection may be complicated by malabsorption and the need for prolonged intravenous nutritional support.

Key Treatment: Intestinal Obstruction

- Surgery

Malrotation

Definition

Malrotation is a developmental anomaly of bowel rotation and fixation, which may result in volvulus and intestinal obstruction.

Etiology

Malrotation is due to a failure of the normal process of midgut rotation and fixation. As a result, the small bowel mesentery is narrow and prone to volvulus, and the abnormally placed cecum is connected to the posterior peritoneum by fibrous Ladd bands.

Pathophysiology

Volvulus leads to intestinal obstruction and to superior mesenteric artery occlusion, which may result in midgut ischemia or infarction. Ladd bands may externally compress and obstruct the duodenum.

Clinical Findings

The neonate with malrotation may present with bilious vomiting. If volvulus has occurred, the abdomen may be tense and tender, and GI bleeding may be seen. Volvulus is a neonatal emergency, and delay in management may lead to ischemic infarction of the entire midgut.

Key Clinical Findings: Malrotation

- Bilious vomiting
- Tense, tender abdomen

Laboratory Findings

There may be electrolyte imbalances as a result of vomiting. Anemia, metabolic acidosis, or evidence of DIC may be seen if there is volvulus with compromise of bowel.

Radiographic Findings

The abdominal plain film may show distention of the proximal bowel, with or without distal bowel gas. In an advanced case, there may be signs of perforation or peritonitis. The findings on upper GI series include an abnormal location of the duodenojejunal junction to the right of the midline and obstruction of the second or third portion of the duodenum. If the upper GI series is not diagnostic, a contrast enema may be useful and may show the cecum and proximal colon abnormally located on the left side of the abdomen.

Treatment

Any derangements of fluid and electrolyte status must be corrected in preparation for surgery. Anemia, acidosis, or DIC may also be present and require specific therapy. In the operating room, if a volvulus is present, it is untwisted and any gangrenous bowel resected. The Ladd bands are lysed, the duodenum placed in the right flank, the small bowel positioned on the right side, and the cecum placed in the left flank. A catheter is passed through the duodenum to rule out a partial obstruction. Prolonged parenteral nutritional support may be required if there has been a significant loss of small bowel.

Key Treatment: Malrotation

- Emergency surgery

Hirschsprung Disease (Congenital Megacolon)

Definition

Hirschsprung disease is an dysmotility syndrome resulting from abnormal innervation of bowel, usually the distal colon.

Etiology

Hirschsprung disease results from a failure of the normal process of craniocaudal migration of the neural crest cells, which give rise to the intestinal ganglion cells. Approximately 75 per cent of cases are confined to the rectum or rectosigmoid; 5 to 10 per cent involve the entire colon, and rare cases of total aganglionosis of the entire large and small bowel have been reported.

Epidemiology

The incidence of Hirschsprung disease is approximately 1 in 5000 births; approximately 80 per cent of patients are male, and the incidence is increased in the presence of Down syndrome. The risk of Hirschsprung disease is increased if a sibling or other family member is affected, but in most cases the family history is negative.

Pathophysiology

The lack of ganglion cells leads to a failure of parasympathetic-mediated relaxation in the involved segment, causing a functional intestinal obstruction. The normal bowel proximal to the point of obstruction may dilate, resulting in a funnel-shaped transition zone. The degree of obstruction varies, and presentation after the neonatal period is not uncommon, even in cases of total colonic aganglionosis.

Clinical Findings

Hirschsprung disease may present in the neonatal period as delayed passage of meconium, as abdominal distention, or as complete intestinal obstruction with bilious vomiting. Physical examination usually reveals absence of stool in the rectum. Hirschsprung disease may be complicated by the development of enterocolitis, with fever, abdominal distention, vomiting, and diarrhea. Although enterocolitis is a greater risk in patients in whom the diagnosis is delayed, it may also occur after an apparently successful initial diverting procedure or definitive pull-through operation.

Key Clinical Findings: Hirschsprung Disease

- Delayed passage of meconium
- Absence of stool in rectum
- Abdominal distention

Laboratory Studies

Suction or full-thickness rectal biopsy findings include absence of ganglion cells and an elevated acetylcholinesterase activity on staining. Anorectal manometry may demonstrate a lack of internal anal sphincter relaxation in response to transient rectal distention, but the reliability of this procedure in the neonate has been questioned. Anemia, leukocytosis, DIC, electrolyte disturbances, and acidosis are seen in enterocolitis.

Key Laboratory Findings: Hirschsprung Disease

- Absence of ganglion cells in rectal biopsy tissue

Radiographic Findings

The plain films may demonstrate distention of the proximal colon. A funnel-shaped transition zone may be seen on barium enema but may be absent in the neonate. In total colonic aganglionosis, ileal distention proximal to the aganglionic bowel may be seen. The colon may be small and may resemble a microcolon in some infants with total colonic aganglionosis, but it may appear normal in others. In some infants with Hirschsprung disease, it is not possible to make the diagnosis by barium enema.

Treatment

Once Hirschsprung disease has been diagnosed, a diverting colostomy or enterostomy proximal to the aganglionic segment is created, and a definitive pull-through procedure is performed at 9 to 12 months of age. Some surgeons may elect to do the pull-through procedure at the time of diagnosis, even in the neonatal period. Enterocolitis is managed with fluid resuscitation, blood transfusion as indicated, rectocolonic saline enemas, and parenteral antibiotics, including coverage for anaerobic bacteria. Oral administration of metronidazole or vancomycin may also be useful.

Meconium Ileus

Definition

Meconium ileus is a lower intestinal obstruction resulting from inspissation of abnormal meconium. Approximately 50 per cent of cases are simple, characterized by intestinal obstruction alone. The remainder are complicated by volvulus, intestinal atresia, or perforation. Almost all cases occur in infants with cystic fibrosis.

Etiology

Abnormal intestinal gland secretions in cystic fibrosis result in meconium with an elevated albumin content that is thick and viscid and causes intestinal obstruction, usually at the level of the terminal ileum.

Epidemiology

Cystic fibrosis is the most common life-threatening genetic disease of Caucasians, with an incidence of 1 in 2500 live births. Cystic fibrosis is relatively uncommon among African Americans and rare among Asians. The incidence of meconium ileus in cystic fibrosis is 5 to 15 per cent, but a family in which one child has meconium ileus has an increased risk of having subsequent children affected.

Pathophysiology

The distal ileal obstruction causes distention of the proximal bowel and the development of a microcolon. Volvulus, ischemia of the bowel, and perforation may also occur. Meconium peritonitis or pseudocyst may result from in utero perforation.

Clinical Findings

The diagnosis may be suspected on the basis of an antenatal ultrasound examination showing dilated proximal loops of bowel, polyhydramnios, or intraabdominal calcifications. "Simple" meconium ileus presents with abdominal distention, bilious vomiting, and failure to pass meconium; onset of symptoms may be delayed for 12 to 24 hours. The abdomen is often described as "doughy," because the distended loops of bowel are filled with meconium rather than air. "Complicated" meconium ileus tends to present earlier, and such infants may have signs of obstruction at the time of birth.

Key Clinical Findings: Meconium Ileus

- Abdominal distention
- Bilious vomiting

Laboratory Studies

Cystic fibrosis is diagnosed on the basis of an elevated sweat chloride concentration. The sweat test is of limited use in neonatal diagnosis because of difficulties in collecting an adequate sample of sweat. The gene responsible for cystic fibrosis is located on chromosome 7, and the delta F508 mutation, which is seen in approximately 70 per cent of cases, has been identified. However, other mutations also occur, and great care must be taken when attempting to diagnose cystic fibrosis on the basis of genetic studies.

Key Laboratory Findings: Meconium Ileus

- Increased Na and Cl concentration in sweat
- Genetic studies

Radiographic Findings

The abdominal plain film may show distention of the proximal bowel, and the right lower abdomen may have a "soap bubble" appearance, which is due to air mixing with the abnormal meconium. An upper GI series demonstrates intestinal obstruction, and a contrast enema demonstrates a microcolon. Intraabdominal calcifications of meconium peritonitis may be seen on the plain film or on ultrasound examination.

Treatment

1. Simple meconium ileus can be managed nonoperatively, using a water-soluble contrast enema. Dilute meglumine diatrizoate (Gastrografin) is instilled into the colon under fluoroscopic guidance and refluxed into the terminal ileum, drawing fluid into the bowel and promoting passage of the meconium. After the enema has been performed, 5 to 10 per cent N-acetylcysteine solution may be administered by nasogastric tube, to further promote the passage of the inspissated meconium. Since Gastrografin is hyperosmolar, the infant's fluid and electrolyte status must be carefully monitored if it is used. Nonoperative therapy is contraindicated in meconium ileus complicated by atresia, volvulus, or perforation, and these infants require laparotomy.

2. Since infants with congenital stenosis of the pancreatic ducts, hypothyroidism, and other conditions may occasionally present in a manner similar to meconium ileus, the clinician must be careful about making a conclusive diagnosis of meconium ileus in an atypical case. The diagnosis of cystic fibrosis should be confirmed by sweat test or genetic studies in all infants with meconium ileus.

Key Treatment: Meconium Ileus

- Water-soluble contrast enema under fluoroscopic guidance

Meconium Plug Syndrome

Definition

Meconium plug syndrome is a colonic obstruction caused by impacted meconium.

Etiology

Meconium plug syndrome is usually idiopathic but may occur in the premature infant and may be associated with hypothyroidism and hypermagnesemia. Some infants initially thought to have meconium plug syndrome are subsequently found to have cystic fibrosis or Hirschsprung disease.

Pathophysiology

Meconium plug syndrome is due to stasis of meconium leading to impaction and obstruction. Underlying intestinal dysmotility may contribute to the development of this problem.

Clinical Findings

Meconium plug syndrome presents as delayed passage of meconium with abdominal distention. It may progress to a picture of complete intestinal obstruction, with bilious vomiting and dilated loops of bowel visible on x-ray.

Key Clinical Finding: Meconium Plug Syndrome

- Delayed passage of meconium

Laboratory Studies

The clinician should rule out the diagnoses of hypermagnesemia and hypothyroidism in patients who appear to have meconium plug syndrome.

Radiographic Findings

The abdominal x-ray may demonstrate bowel distention. A contrast enema shows filling defects in the colon, representing the impacted meconium.

Treatment

Some infants will pass meconium in response to rectal stimulation, but vigorous stimulation or the use of saline enemas should be avoided if there is a question of an underlying organic disorder. In a persistent case, a contrast enema will establish the diagnosis and promote the clearance of the meconium. Either barium or water-soluble contrast material is effective. Infants with meconium plug syndrome should be closely followed after discharge from the nursery, and those with persistent constipation or abdominal distention may require studies to rule out cystic fibrosis and Hirschsprung disease.

Key Treatment: Meconium Plug Syndrome

- Saline enema

Neonatal Small Left Colon Syndrome

Definition

Neonatal small left colon is a developmental anomaly in which the colon is uniformly small from the splenic flexure to the rectum, leading to neonatal obstructive symptoms.

Etiology

The etiology of this disorder is unknown.

Epidemiology

Neonatal small left colon may occur in normal infants, but its incidence is significantly increased in the infant of the diabetic mother.

Pathophysiology

Obstruction in neonatal small left colon is presumably due to colonic stenosis rather than inspissated meconium.

Clinical Findings

Infants with this syndrome present with signs of lower GI obstruction, such as abdominal distention, feeding intolerance, and vomiting.

Laboratory Studies

There are no characteristic laboratory findings.

Radiographic Findings

The plain film of the abdomen shows generalized distention of large and small bowel. The contrast enema shows a left colon that is anatomically small and not simply filled with meconium, as in the meconium plug syndrome. There is usually an abrupt transition zone between the normal and abnormal portions of the colon at the level of the splenic flexure.

Treatment

The contrast enema is usually followed by relief of the obstruction. The mechanism of this effect is not understood, but it is not due to evacuation of impacted meconium. Long-term intestinal function is completely normal.

Necrotizing Enterocolitis

Definition

Necrotizing enterocolitis is an inflammatory lesion of bowel, characterized by abdominal distention, feeding intolerance, and GI bleeding, which may progress to intestinal gangrene with perforation and the development of peritonitis.

Etiology

Necrotizing enterocolitis has been linked to bowel ischemia, improper feeding techniques, and infection. The clearest link is with prematurity, suggesting that an underlying developmental immaturity of bowel is causally important. Necrotizing enterocolitis also occurs in term infants, often in association with conditions that impair intestinal flow, such as asphyxia, polycythemia, or cardiac disease.

Pathophysiology

Direct bowel injury may result from ischemia or the effects of excessive or hyperosmolar feedings. Malabsorbed carbohydrate may promote microbial overgrowth, leading to infection. Ischemia followed by reperfusion may lead to the production of oxygen free radicals that may cause cellular injury. However, necrotizing enterocolitis may also occur in the stable, growing premature infant, in the absence of an obvious precipitating cause.

Clinical Findings

Necrotizing enterocolitis presents with feeding intolerance, abdominal distention, and GI hemorrhage. The abdomen is usually distended, tense, and tender, but in the early stages of the disease the examination may be unremarkable. The infant may develop a palpable abdominal mass or cellulitis of the abdominal wall. A shocklike state may be seen in advanced disease, especially if perforation is present.

Key Clinical Findings: Necrotizing Enterocolitis

- Feeding intolerance
- Distended abdomen
- GI hemorrhage

Laboratory Findings

Leukopenia, thrombocytopenia, and acidosis support the diagnosis but may be seen in septic infants who do not have necrotizing enterocolitis. A progressive metabolic acidosis suggests impending or actual intestinal perforation. Early in the disease the laboratory findings may be unimpressive.

Radiographic Findings

The characteristic radiographic findings in necrotizing enterocolitis include air in the wall of the bowel (pneumatosis intestinalis), air in the hepatic portal venous system, and free intraperitoneal air. A loop of bowel that does not move on serial x-rays is suggestive of intestinal gangrene. The x-ray may show ascites, with centralization of the bowel gas. In early disease, the x-ray may show only bowel distention.

Treatment

1. Therapy is centered on early recognition, withholding of feedings, gastric decompression, and antibiotic therapy. The electrolytes, complete blood count, blood gas, and abdominal x-rays are initially followed every 6 to 8 hours, to detect evidence of deterioriation or intestinal perforation. If the infant is hemodynamically unstable or in DIC, volume support and replacement therapy with blood products may be required. Necrotizing enterocolitis is usually treated for at least 10 to 14 days, and feedings are withheld for the entire period of treatment. Feedings must be resumed very cautiously, as necrotizing enterocolitis may recur.

2. Indications for surgery include intestinal perforation with free intraperitoneal air, cellulitis of the abdominal wall, or a peritoneal tap revealing feculent material or pus. An infant with worsening acidosis or other evidence of deterioration may have gangrenous bowel and may require laparotomy even in the absence of demonstrable free air. At laparotomy, gangrenous bowel is resected and any abscesses are drained. An infant who is too unstable to tolerate a laparotomy may be managed by a peritoneal drainage procedure performed in the neonatal intensive care unit, but in some cases the drainage is inadequate and a formal laparotomy is required. Long-term management may be complicated by problems with malabsorption and the short gut syndrome and by the development of strictures.

Key Treatment: Necrotizing Enterocolitis

- Withholding feedings
- IV fluid and nutrition
- Antibiotics
- Surgery for perforation

Bibliography

GASTROINTESTINAL HEMORRHAGE

Hyams JS, Leichtner AM, Schwartz AN: Recent advances in diagnosis and treatment of gastrointestinal hemorrhage in infants and children. J Pediatr 1985;106:1–9.

Liebman WM, Thaler MM, Bujanover Y: Endoscopic evaluation of upper gastrointestinal bleeding in the newborn. Am J Gastroenterol 1978;69:607–608.

INTESTINAL OBSTRUCTION

Louw JH, Barnard CN: Congenital intestinal atresia: Observations on its origin. Lancet 1955;2:1065–1066.

Paterson-Brown S, Stalewski H, Brereton RJ: Neonatal small bowel atresia, stenosis and segmental dilatation. Br J Surg 1991;78:83–86.

MALROTATION

Torres AM, Ziegler MM: Malrotation of the intestine. World J Surg 1993;17:326–331.

HIRSCHSPRUNG DISEASE (CONGENITAL MEGACO-LON)

Kleinhaus S, Boley SJ, Sheran M, Sieber WK: Hirschsprung's disease: A survey of the members of the Surgical Section of the American Academy of Pediatrics. J Pediatr Surg 1979;14:588–597.

Rescorla FJ, Morrison AM, Engles D, et al: Hirschsprung's disease: Evaluation of mortality and long-term function in 260 cases. Arch Surg 1992; 27:934–942.

Rosenfeld NS, Ablow RC, Markowitz RI, et al: Hirschsprung disease: Accuracy of the barium examination. Radiology 1984;150:393–400.

MECONIUM ILEUS

Rescorla FJ, Grosfeld JL: Contemporary management of meconium ileus. World J Surg 1993;17:318–325.

Ziegler MM: Meconium ileus. Curr Probl Surg 1994;31:737–777.

MECONIUM PLUG SYNDROME

Clatworthy HW Jr, Howard WH, Lloyd J: The meconium plug syndrome. Surgery 1956;39:131–142.

NEONATAL SMALL LEFT COLON SYNDROME

Davis WS, Campbell JB: Neonatal small left colon syndrome. Am J Dis Child 1975;129:1024–1027.

NECROTIZING ENTEROCOLITIS

Ballance W, Dahms B, Shenker N, Kliegman R: Pathology of neonatal necrotizing enterocolitis: a ten year experience. J Pediatr 1990;117:S6–S13.

Kanto W, Hunter J, Stoll B: Recognition and medical management of necrotizing enterocolitis. Clin Perinatol 1994;21:335–346.

Ricketts R: Surgical treatment of necrotizing enterocolitis and the short bowel syndrome. Clin Perinatol 1994;21:365–387.

30 Cardiovascular Disorders

Alice C. Yao

Etiology

1. Structural defects of the heart and blood vessels
2. Failure of adjustment of fetal to postnatal circulation
3. Response to maternal illness (e.g., diabetes mellitus, lupus erythematosus)
4. Exposure to maternal medications (e.g., β-adrenergic blockers, lithium)

Clinical Findings

1. Cyanosis
2. Congestive heart failure
3. Circulatory collapse
4. Arrhythmias
5. Heart murmur

Cyanosis

Pathogenesis

Cardiac cyanosis results from a fixed right-to-left shunt of blood (systemic venous to systemic arterial) through a defect or communication in the heart or blood vessels. The following cardiovascular conditions are usually associated with cyanosis in the neonate.

1. Transposition of the great vessels (TGV)
2. Tetralogy of Fallot (TOF), with pulmonary atresia or severe stenosis
3. Tricuspid atresia or pulmonary atresia with hypoplastic right ventricle
4. Total anomalous pulmonary venous return (TAPVR) with obstruction
5. Truncus arteriosus
6. Transitional circulation disturbance—persistent pulmonary hypertension of the newborn (PPHN).

Clinical and Laboratory Findings

1. Bluish discoloration of the skin, mucous membranes (tongue, oral mucosa), nail beds and extremities, which is aggravated by crying. Central cyanosis must be differentiated from peripheral cyanosis (acrocyanosis), which is caused by vasoconstriction secondary to a cool environmental temperature (see Chapter 16 on signs of illness in the newborn).
2. A low partial pressure of oxygen (Pa_{O_2}), with more than 5 g of unsaturated hemoglobin per 100 ml of blood. Since fetal hemoglobin has a greater affinity for oxygen than does adult hemoglobin (left shift), infants may have an abnormally low Pa_{O_2} in the absence of obvious cyanosis. In order to ensure proper evaluation of the patient, both Pa_{O_2} and oxygen saturation must be determined.

Diagnosis

1. Cardiac cyanosis may be differentiated from the other major causes of cyanosis (pulmonary, metabolic, or neurologic) by administration of 100 per cent oxygen for 10 minutes (hyperoxia test). The failure of the infant to increase arterial P_{O_2} to 100 to 150 mmHg is usually indicative of cardiac origin of the cyanosis. Most cyanotic congenital heart defects are associated with modest increases in arterial P_{O_2} of 10 to 15 mmHg, although no increase may be observed. Rarely, increases to ≥ 150 mmHg have been reported. However, infants with persistent transitional circulation secondary to pulmonary hypertension have right-to-left shunting through a patent ductus arteriosus and foramen ovale and cannot be differentiated from infants with cardiac defects by a hyperoxia test.
2. Cardiac evaluation includes a complete perinatal history, physical examination, chest x-rays, and electrocardiogram

(ECG). However, immediate echocardiography is essential once central cyanosis is recognized. Doppler and color flow mapping studies may provide essential hemodynamic information.

Treatment

1. Immediate

    In order to overcome hypoxemia in the cyanotic infant with congenital cardiac disease, administration of prostaglandin E_1, following echocardiographic diagnosis, is necessary to maintain patency of the ductus arteriosus, prior to creation of a surgical shunt or repair. In infants with PPHN, ventilatory assistance together with administration of a pulmonary artery dilator (e.g., tolazoline or nitric oxide) is required to overcome the hypoxemia. Extracorporeal membrane oxygenation (ECMO) may be required in resistant cases.

2. Definitive

    a. TGV: Arterial switch procedure (total correction) or Rashkind atrial septostomy followed months later by a functional switch in atrial flows (Mustard or Senning procedure).

    b. TOF: Primary repair in full-term infants; in those with severely hypoplastic pulmonary arteries or outflow tract, an aortopulmonary shunt (Blalock-Taussig procedure or its modification) may precede corrective repair.

    c. Tricuspid atresia with hypoplastic right ventricle: shunt procedure to increase pulmonary blood flow; sometimes with atrial septostomy, followed by a Fontan procedure (right atrial to pulmonary artery anastomosis) at a later time. In pulmonary atresia with an intact ventricular septum, a shunt procedure (Blalock-Taussig) to increase pulmonary flow is indicated. A procedure to enlarge the right ventricle may be needed.

    d. TAPVR: Surgical correction can usually be carried out in the newborn term infant but should be delayed for some weeks in the preterm infant.

    e. Truncus arteriosus: Surgical repair may usually be performed depending on the type, with closure of the ventricular septal defect (VSD) and homograft to join the pulmonary arteries.

Key Treatment: Cyanosis

- Supportive
  Oxygen
  Prostaglandin E_1 infusion

- Definitive
  See Part XII, Cardiology

Congestive Heart Failure

Causes

1. When present in utero (usually secondary to fetal nonimmune hydrops) or at birth, it may be related to

    a. Severe tricuspid or other valvular insufficiency, including Ebstein's anomaly of the tricuspid valve or absence of the pulmonary valve in TOF.

    b. Arteriovenous fistula, e.g., cerebral or hepatic.

    c. Complex heart defects such as atrioventricular (AV) canal, unbalanced type, with hypoplastic left ventricle and tricuspid insufficiency.

    d. Arrhythmias: prolonged or recurrent atrial tachycardias or flutter; rarely, complete heart block.

    e. Myocarditis or cardiomyopathy.

2. When heart failure develops after birth, it may result from the foregoing causes as well as from the following:

    a. In premature infants, failure of the ductus arteriosus to close (patent ductus arteriosus, or PDA) leads to increased left-to-right shunting of blood and congestive heart failure. This is rarely a cause of congestive heart failure in full-term infants.

    b. Large VSD; congestive heart failure does not usually appear until the late neonatal period or early infancy.

    c. TAPVR; this condition may not be immediately apparent and must be suspected when there is no obvious cause for the congestive heart failure.

    d. AV canal (commonly observed in infants with Down syndrome).

    e. Postnatal arrhythmias.

Clinical Findings

Common signs of congestive heart failure are tachypnea, tachycardia (except in complete heart block), cardiomegaly, hepatomegaly, and edema.

Key Clinical Findings: Congestive Heart Failure

- Tachycardia

- Tachypnea

- Cardiomegaly

- Hepatomegaly

- Edema

Diagnosis

1. Physical examination
2. Chest x-rays (may show cardiomegaly, hazy lung fields, increased vascularity)
3. Electrocardiogram
4. Echocardiographic examination is required to confirm the clinical diagnosis.
5. Cardiac catheterization and angiocardiography may be needed to confirm the diagnosis in some cases, e.g., complex heart defects.

Treatment

1. Stabilize patient medically:

    a. Fluid restriction; in preterm infants with PDA, limit fluid intake to <150 ml/kg/day. Fluid intake and output and serum electrolytes must be monitored.

    b. Administration of diuretics, e.g., furosemide

c. Ventilatory support for severe pulmonary edema

2. Administration of indomethacin, a prostaglandin synthetase inhibitor, in an intravenous dose of 0.1 to 0.2 mg/kg per dose, administered at 12- to 24-hour intervals, for up to three doses. Slow infusion of indomethacin is advised to prevent acute decreases in cerebral and gastrointestinal blood flow. This infusion usually results in ductal closure in preterm infants, but occasionally, surgical closure may be required.

3. Digitalization: Administration of digoxin (10 to 25 μg/kg, total digitalizing dose for preterm infants, and 20 to 30 μg/kg for term infants), with one half given initially, and one quarter in 8 to 24 hours, for two doses. Maintenance therapy is with one quarter of the total dose given twice daily.

4. Low-solute formula or breast milk.

5. Maintain neutral thermal environment.

6. Correction of anemia by packed red blood cell transfusion (5 ml/kg over 2 to 4 hours) to maintain hematocrit at greater than 40 per cent in order to provide adequate myocardial oxygenation.

7. For defects other than PDA, primary open surgical repair is the treatment of choice once the infant is medically stabilized. Pulmonary artery banding is still occasionally done for large muscular septal defects and for complex AV canals in low birth weight infants.

Key Treatment: Congestive Heart Failure

- Diuretics (e.g., furosemide)
- Indomethacin for PDA
- Digitalis

Cardiovascular Collapse (Shock)

Definition

The systemic blood pressure is more than two standard deviations below the mean for gestational and postnatal age; manifestations include poor peripheral perfusion, mottling of skin, pallor, and metabolic acidosis. Infants may appear normal at birth. In addition to cardiovascular conditions, shock may occur secondary to acute blood loss, systemic infection, or an inherited metabolic disorder.

Etiology

Cardiac causes of shock may not become apparent until the blood flow across a patent ductus arteriosus ceases (ductal dependent lesion) as a result of ductal closure after birth. The following congenital defects may be the cause of shock:

1. Hypoplastic left heart syndrome, with mitral and/or aortic atresia and hypoplastic left ventricle.
2. Critical aortic valve stenosis.
3. Coarctation of the aorta.
4. Interrupted aortic arch, usually with a VSD.
5. Subaortic hypertrophic cardiomyopathy (asymmetric) in infants of diabetic mothers.

Diagnosis

In addition to the hypotension, findings include

1. Tachypnea
2. Dyspnea
3. Prominent right precordial heave
4. Pulse and blood pressure discrepancy between arms and legs
5. Oliguria
6. Weak pulse
7. Systolic murmur that disappears
8. Cardiomegaly and pulmonary venous congestion on chest x-ray.
9. Echocardiography and Doppler examination usually determine the diagnosis.

Key Clinical Findings: Cardiovascular Collapse

- Hypotension
- Dyspnea
- Tachypnea

Treatment

1. Prostaglandin E_1 infusion to maintain patency of ductus arteriosus (in ductal dependent lesions in order to provide systemic blood flow (Table 30–1).
2. Correction of acidosis.
3. Catheter balloon valvuloplasty or surgical valve dilatation for aortic valve stenosis.
4. Surgical repair for coarctation of the aorta or interrupted aortic arch repair surgery.
5. Management of subaortic hypertrophic stenosis in infants of diabetic mothers is usually expectant. However, in the presence of cardiovascular collapse, β-adrenergic blockers such as propranolol are indicated to relieve left ventricular outflow obstruction
6. In hypoplastic left heart syndrome, normal perfusion with prostaglandin E_1 infusion should be maintained while reviewing with the family the treatment options for this usually lethal condition. Available choices are the Norwood procedure, involving a two- or three-staged set of operations during the first 3 years of life, cardiac transplantation, or compassionate care, allowing the patient to die without surgical intervention (the choice of many families).

Key Treatment: Cardiovascular Collapse

- Prostaglandin E_1 infusion
- Correction of acidosis
- Surgical repair when possible

Arrhythmias

Cardiac arrhythmias may be detected antenatally or postnatally, by auscultation or electronically, and may be benign or life-threatening.

TABLE 30–1. CONGENITAL HEART DEFECTS HELPED BY MAINTAINING DUCTAL PATENCY WITH PROSTAGLANDIN E₁

CLASSIFICATION OF LESIONS BY MECHANISM OF DUCTAL DEPENDENCY FOR:

Pulmonary Blood Flow	Systemic Blood Flow	Better Mixing
Pulmonary atresia and severe stenosis with intact VS	Coarctation of the aorta	Transposition of the great vessels with small/absent VSD
Tetralogy of Fallot with severe pulmonary stenosis/atresia	Interrupted aortic arch	Transposition with other cardiac defects such as tricuspid atresia with transposition of great vessels and VSD
Tricuspid atresia with obstruction at the VS or pulmonary valve	Critical aortic stenosis	
Ebstein's anomaly	Hypoplastic left heart syndrome	
Single ventricle with pulmonic stenosis	Total anomalous pulmonary venous drainage with small foramen ovale	

VS, ventricular septum; VSD, ventricular septal defect.

Classification

1. Extrasystoles: Premature atrial contractions (PAC) or premature ventricular contractions (PVC), isolated or occasional, are relatively common, are usually benign, and do not require treatment.
2. Tachyarrhythmias
   a. Supraventricular tachycardia (SVT): Heart rate usually over 230 beats/minute; heart failure occurs within a few hours of onset. It may occur in utero and requires treatment by administration of digoxin to the mother.
   b. Atrial flutter or fibrillation.
   c. Ventricular tachycardia, usually with a wide QRS complex that lacks 1:1 relationship with the P wave; the rate is usually 180 to 200 beats/minute.
3. Bradyarrhythmias
   a. Sinus bradycardia of about 80 to 90 beats/minute during sleep in an otherwise healthy neonate is usually benign. It may also be associated with maternal use of medication, e.g., β-adrenergic blockers.
   b. Apnea-bradycardia is observed in premature infants and is associated with apnea of prematurity.
4. Heart block
   a. Second-degree AV block is associated with dropped beats, e.g., Mobitz I (Wenckebach) and Mobitz II, a more distal block with a wide QRS complex.
   b. Third-degree, or complete, heart block may have rates of less than 50 beats/minute and may produce symptoms in the neonate. It may be associated with structural cardiac defects or may be seen in structurally normal hearts of infants of mothers with systemic lupus erythematosus.

Diagnosis

1. A 12-lead ECG is necessary to make a specific diagnosis of an arrhythmia.
2. An echocardiogram is required to define specific structural anomalies. Fetal echocardiograms should be performed if an arrhythmia is detected antenatally.
3. Holter monitoring for 24 hours may be necessary when the arrhythmia is episodic.
4. Infants with a structurally normal heart and complete heart block should be investigated for lupus erythematosus, together with the mother.

Treatment

1. Supraventricular tachycardia
   a. In utero onset: Digitalization of the mother is often effective; occasionally, direct injection of digoxin into the umbilical vein may be lifesaving.
   b. Onset after birth: SVT may respond to vagal stimulation by applying a cold wet towel to the baby's face while he or she is under continuous ECG monitoring. Digitalization is required if vagal stimulation is unsuccessful. Adenosine has become a widely used drug because of its rapid effectiveness in most instances in converting SVT and atrial flutter to normal sinus rhythm. Cardioversion/electroconversion may be necessary if medical therapy is unsuccessful. SVT from an ectopic atrial focus may require digitalization to slow the ventricular rate (AV conduction), followed by administration of propranolol or other antiarrhythmic drug.
2. Heart block

   Complete heart block may require the insertion of a pacemaker if the ventricular rate is ≤50 beats/minute and the infant is symptomatic. Infants with heart defects may not tolerate rates of ≤80 beats/minute and require pacing.

Key Treatment: Arrhythmias

- Vagal stimulation
- Digitalis
- Adenosine

Heart Murmurs

1. Transient murmurs: During the first days after birth, a systolic murmur of tricuspid regurgitation or patent ductus arteriosus may be heard in the normal neonate. It usually disappears after the first few days of life. Ductal closure may take longer in the preterm infant; persistence of ductal patency is common in premature infants.
2. Persistent systolic murmurs
   a. Tetralogy of Fallot
   b. Pulmonic stenosis, valvular or peripheral branches

c. VSD (The murmur associated with a small muscular defect may not be apparent for several days, will usually cause no symptoms, and most often closes spontaneously during the first year of life.)

d. Atrioventricular canal

e. Aortic stenosis

Diagnosis

1. Physical examination
   a. Localize cardiac apex (to detect cardiomegaly).
   b. Detect parasternal heave (indicative of right ventricular pressure load).
   c. Hyperdynamic precordium (indicates ventricular volume overloading, as in VSD)
   d. A loud, single, and palpable second heart sound (present in TOF and in pulmonary hypertension)
2. Chest x-rays to assess cardiac size and pulmonary vascularity and venous congestion
3. Echocardiography with Doppler color flow mapping to provide structural and hemodynamic diagnosis.

Management

Infants should be followed regularly by primary care physicians in consultation with cardiologists. Syndromes associated with a high incidence of cardiac defects that may require cardiac evaluation include

1. Down syndrome: atrioventricular canal
2. VACTERL syndrome: VSD
3. DiGeorge syndrome: truncus arteriosus, interrupted aortic arch, TOF
4. Noonan syndrome: pulmonic stenosis
5. Turner syndrome: coarctation of the aorta, aortic stenosis, hypoplastic left heart
6. Holt-Oram syndrome: atrial or ventricular septal defect.

Bibliography

Castañeda AR, Jones RA, Mayer JE Jr, Hanley FL (eds): Cardiac Surgery of the Neonate and Infant. Philadelphia, WB Saunders, 1994, pp 167–185, 222–247, 363–383, 418–438.

Driscoll DJ: Evaluation of the cyanotic newborn. Pediatr Clin North Am 1990;37:1–23.

Kinsella JP, Abman SH: Recent developments in the pathophysiology and treatment of persistent pulmonary hypertension of the newborn. J Pediatr 1995;126:853–864.

Rosenfeld LE: The diagnosis and management of cardiac arrhythmias in the neonatal period. Semin Perinatol 1993;17:135–148.

Yabek SM: Neonatal cyanosis: Reappraisal of response to 100 per cent oxygen breathing. Am J Dis Child 1984;138:880–884.

31 Genitourinary Disorders

Gobind Laungani and *Sheela G. Laungani*

Most genitourinary problems of infancy and childhood are easily diagnosed.

Symptoms referred to the genitourinary system, abnormal urinalysis, and abnormal blood chemistry values help in diagnosing those conditions that are not obvious on routine clinical evaluation. Early diagnosis and treatment are critical for minimizing renal parenchymal injury and thereby preventing loss of renal function.

Hypospadias

The normal urethra is formed between the eighth and fifteenth weeks of gestation by fusion of urethral folds joining the ectodermal ingrowth in the glans penis. Failure of this fusion results in incomplete tubularization, with opening of the urethra on the ventral side, or undersurface, of penis. This abnormal location of the urethral opening is called hypospadias.

Etiology

1. Genetic
   a. Single gene defect
   b. In association with chromosomal anomalies such as Down syndrome or as sex chromosomal defects

2. Endocrine
   a. Maternal ingestion of progesterone in the first trimester of pregnancy
   b. Diminished testosterone response to human chorionic gonadotropin in male fetuses
   c. Abnormal effects of testosterone and dihydrotestosterone on the developing urethra.

Classification

Classification of hypospadias is dependent upon the anatomic location of the external meatus.

1. Glandular—meatus opening at midglans level
2. Coronal—meatus opening at the corona of glans penis
3. Subcoronal—meatus present just proximal to corona of glans penis
4. Meatus at midshaft level
5. Meatus at penoscrotal level
6. Meatus at the perineum.

Eighty per cent of hypospadias cases are at the glandular, coronal, and subcoronal levels.

Clinical Findings

1. Clinical signs and symptoms are unusual. Associated meatal stenosis may cause dysuria and difficulty in void-

ing. A small meatal opening does not always indicate meatal stenosis.
2. Presence of a dorsal hood and absence of preputial skin on the ventral surface of glans penis.
3. Penile chordee, bending with ventral and downward curvature of penis described as "SST look" of glans penis.
4. Associated undescended testes are common.

Key Clinical Findings: Hypospadias

• Dorsal hood
• Chordee

Treatment

1. The ambiguous genitalia associated with penoscrotal, scrotal, and perineal hypospadias require further investigation (see Chapter 250). Renal and pelvic sonography should be performed to identify other associated genitourinary abnormalities.
2. Children with distal hypospadias rarely have associated urinary anomalies and require no further radiologic or endoscopic evaluations.
3. The goal of surgical treatment is to correct penile chordee and bring the external meatus to its normal anatomic location. The degree of penile chordee is determined at the time of surgery prior to the definitive repair of hypospadias. Single-stage repairs are now possible using pedicle skin flaps and bladder and buccal mucosal grafts (Fig. 31–1).

Posterior Urethral Valves

Posterior urethral valves are the most common cause of lower urinary tract obstruction in infants. The degree of ureteric reflux with dilatation of the upper urinary tract and the resulting renal dysplasia determine the long-term outcome. Early diagnosis and treatment may preserve renal function and prevent renal failure.

Embryology

Posterior urethral valves are of congenital origin and may result

1. From abnormal development of normal urethral folds.
2. As a remnant of a congenital membrane at the site of anterior and posterior urethral junction.
3. From abnormal wolffian duct insertion or fusion.

Classification

Posterior urethral valves are classified on the basis of their shape and anatomic location.

1. Type I: Valve in the form of folds extending distally and lateroanteriorly from the verumontanum.
2. Type II: Valve arising from verumontanum and extending proximally toward the bladder neck.
3. Type III: Valve located either in front of or behind the verumontanum, like a diaphragm with a perforation.

Clinical Findings

Clinical presentation depends upon the severity of obstruction caused by the posterior urethral valve. Type II valves are nonobstructive and do not cause any clinical symptoms.
1. In the fetus
   a. Obstructive posterior urethral valve leads to oligohydramnios, which in turn contributes to pulmonary hypoplasia, limb anomalies, Potter's facies, and fetal death.
   b. The diagnosis of posterior urethral valve should

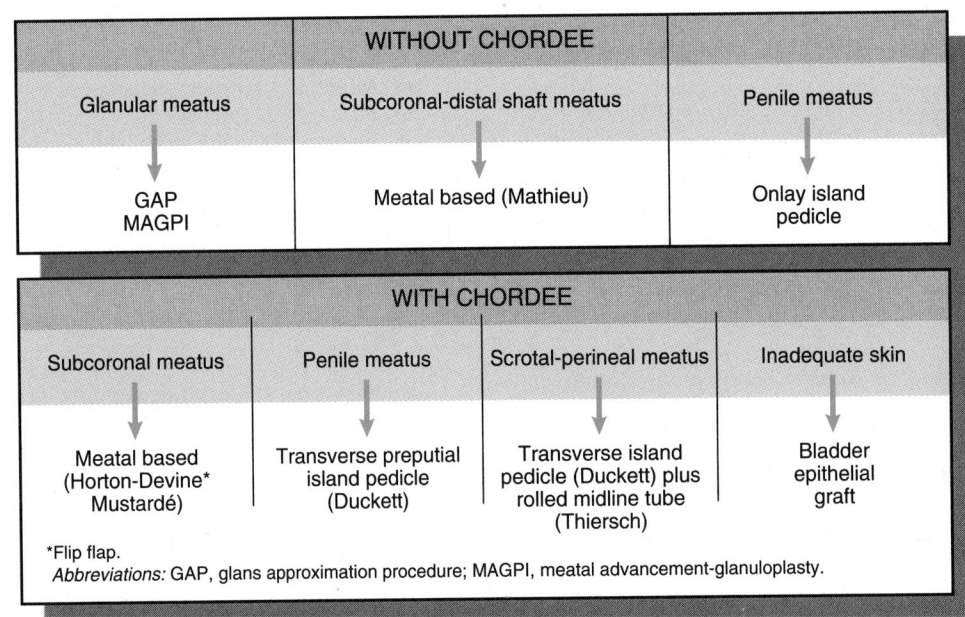

Figure 31–1 Procedures of choice for hypospadias repair. From Belman AB: Hypospadias and other urethral abnormalities. *In* Kelalis PP, King LR, Belman AB (eds): Clinical Pediatric Urology, 3rd ed. Philadelphia, WB Saunders, 1992.
*Flip flap.
GAP = Glans approximation procedure; MAGPI = meatal advancement–glanuloplasty.

be suspected when an antenatal sonogram shows a dilated upper urinary tract and a large bladder.

2. In the newborn infant

a. Slow urinary stream, voiding difficulties, and urinary retention are common symptoms of obstruction. This may lead to a large palpable bladder and hydronephrosis. Signs of azotemia, electrolyte imbalance, dehydration, sepsis, and respiratory distress may develop in severe cases.

b. The diagnostic test for this condition is a voiding cystourethrogram (VCUG). For best results, a VCUG should be done with the infant in an oblique position. A dilated trabeculated bladder with sacculations and diverticula (Christmas tree bladder) is seen together with a hypertrophied bladder neck, dilated posterior urethra, and poor filling of the anterior urethra.

c. Ureteric reflux with ureteral dilatation and hydronephrosis may be unilateral or bilateral. Unilateral reflux is seen more often on the left side. Dilatation of the upper urinary tract seen on renal sonogram may be due to reflux or obstruction of the ureter at the ureterovesical junction (UVJ). Ureteral obstruction is caused by the fibrotic lower end of the ureter or the thick-walled hypertrophied bladder pinching the lower end of the ureter.

d. A DTPA scan with furosemide washout is done to assess differential renal function and supravesicle obstruction.

3. In early childhood this type of obstructive uropathy with azotemia may lead to failure to thrive and end-stage renal disease.

Key Clinical Findings: Posterior Urethral Valves

- Slow urinary stream
- Urinary retention

Key Laboratory Findings: Posterior Urethral Valves

- Hypotemia
- Metabolic acidosis

Treatment

1. Medical

a. Correction of electrolyte imbalance and dehydration

b. Prophylactic use of antibiotics and treatment of diagnosed infection

c. Ventilatory support for respiratory distress, if needed.

2. Surgical

a. Resection of posterior urethral valve

b. Vesicostomy

c. Supravesicle diversion

(1) Cutaneous ureterostomy

(2) Cutaneous pylostomy

(3) Percutaneous nephrostomy

d. Ureteric reimplantation

e. Reduction cystoplasty

f. Augmentation cystoplasty.

The indication for each of these procedures varies depending upon the investigative findings and the condition of the urinary tract.

Prune-Belly Syndrome

The prune-belly syndrome is a triad consisting of deficient or absent abdominal wall, cryptorchidism, and malformation of the urogenital tract. It was described first by Osler in 1901. Associated gastrointestinal, musculoskeletal, cardiac, and pulmonary abnormalities are also observed. This syndrome is usually seen in male newborn infants.

Etiology

1. Possibly hereditary, because the condition is seen among siblings and twins.

2. Obstruction at the junction of anterior and posterior urethra secondary to failure of canalization produces bladder distention with compression of the ventral mesenchymal tissue leading to abdominal wall deficiency and an ill-defined inguinal canal. Bladder distention also causes urachal patency, dilatation of ureters, and dysplastic changes in the kidneys.

Clinical Findings

1. Wrinkled abdominal skin with thin and lax abdominal wall

2. Ease of palpation of intraabdominal and retroperitoneal structures

3. Voiding reflex induced by bladder massage

4. Associated nonurologic problems in other organ systems.

Key Clinical Findings: Prune-Belly Syndrome

- Lax abdominal wall with wrinkled skin
- Cryptorchidism

Radiologic Findings

1. Voiding cystourethrogram (VCUG) showing typical large bladder with patent urachus on the top and wide open bladder neck along with dilated prostatic urethra joining normal anterior urethra. Bilateral free reflux with dilated ureters and collecting systems is also seen.

2. DTPA scan to assess renal function and degree of physiologic obstruction in the upper urinary tract.

3. Chest radiograph to evaluate pulmonary development.

Treatment

1. More than 20 per cent of infants with this syndrome are stillborn or die during the neonatal period. Another 30 to 35 per cent develop renal failure requiring dialysis or renal transplantation, and 45 to 50 per cent will benefit

from treatment aimed at preservation of renal function and management of pulmonary problems.

2. Use of appropriate antibiotics for treatment of sepsis and urinary tract infections
3. Ventilatory support for compromised pulmonary function
4. Vesicostomy to decompress the dilated collecting system and preserve renal function
5. Plication or double breasting procedure done to repair lax abdominal wall
6. Orchidopexy to bring both testicles into the scrotum (primarily for cosmetic reasons). This procedure does not preserve testicular function.

Key Treatment: Prune-Belly Syndrome

- Supportive
- Surgery

Ambiguous Genitalia

The term ambiguous genitalia is used when sex cannot be determined by the anatomic appearance of the external genitalia in a newborn infant. This condition is a social emergency and should be resolved with urgency. A team approach involving the neonatologist, urologist, endocrinologist, and radiologist is necessary to make an appropriate diagnosis, determine the sex for rearing, and provide adequate counseling to the infant's family (see Chapter 243).

Bibliography

HYPOSPADIAS

Belman BA, Kass EJ: Hypospadias repair in children less than 1 year old. J Urol 1982;128:1273.

Gonzales ET Jr, Veeraraghavan KA, Delaune J: The management of distal hypospadias with meatal based vascularized flaps. J Urol 1983;129:119.

Kelalis PP, King LR, Belman AB (eds): Clinical Pediatric Urology, 3rd ed. Philadelphia, WB Saunders, 1992.

Mollard P, Mouriquand P, Bringeon G, Bugmann P: Repair of hypospadias using a bladder mucosal graft in 76 cases. J Urol 1989;142:1548.

POSTERIOR URETHRAL VALVE

Churchill BM, McLorie GA, Khoury AE, et al: Emergency treatment and long term follow-up of posterior urethral valves. Urol Clin North Am 1990;17:343.

Glassberg KI: Current issues regarding posterior urethral valves. Urol Clin North Am 1985;12:175.

Hendren WH: Posterior urethral valves in boys: A broad clinical spectrum. J Urol 1971;106:298.

Waterhouse K: Urethral valves. In Glenn J: Urologic Surgery, 2nd ed. New York, Harper & Row, 1977.

PRUNE-BELLY SYNDROME

Garlinger P, Ott J: Prune-belly syndrome: Possible genetic implications. Birth Defects 1974;10:173.

Nunn IN, Stephens FD: Triad syndrome: A composite anomaly of the abdominal wall, urinary system and testes. J Urol 1961;86:782.

Woodard JR, Parrott TS: Reconstruction of urinary tract in prune-belly uropathy. J Urol 1978;119:824.

---

32 Sudden Infant Death

Enid Gilbert-Barness and *Lewis A. Barness*

Infants may die suddenly and unexpectedly. The cause of death may be determined, but if it cannot be determined, the term SIDS (sudden infant death syndrome) is applied. The cause of death should be ascertained whenever possible for adequate parental counseling, including genetic counseling when applicable.

Definition

SIDS is the sudden death of an infant under 1 year of age that remains unexplained after a thorough case investigation, including a complete autopsy, examination of the death scene, and review of the clinical history.

Etiology and Epidemiology

1. Definable causes of death after a complete autopsy are summarized in Table 32–1.
2. Characteristics of SIDS
   a. Occurrence between 2 and 4 months—85%
   b. Occurrence under 6 months—95%
   c. Occurrence between midnight and 9 A.M.—90%
   d. Increases with birth order
   e. Males >females
   f. Race: In the United States, the incidence is higher in Native Americans and African Americans.
   g. Known risk factors for SIDS are listed in Table 32–2.
3. Incidence of SIDS: 1.6/1000 live births in the United States. In the United Kingdom, incidence was 2.5/1000 live births. After adoption of supine sleeping position for infants, the incidence was 0.7/1000 live births. It is the most common cause of death from 1 month to 6 months of age.

Differential Diagnosis

1. Metabolic disorders associated with sudden infant death (not SIDS) (Table 32–3)

TABLE 32–1. CAUSES OF SIDS

Cardiovascular
 Myocarditis (usually viral)
 Congenital heart disease
 Congenital aortic valvular stenosis
 Endocardial fibroelastosis
 Anomalous origin of the left coronary artery
 Cardiomyopathy
 Rhabdomyoma (in tuberous sclerosis)
Respiratory
 Bronchopneumonia
 Bronchiolitis
Gastrointestinal
 Dehydration with fluid and electrolyte imbalance (usually due
  to diarrhea)
Metabolic disorders
Dehydration with overheating in cystic fibrosis
Adrenal insufficiency
Injury
Abuse
Suffocation

When more than one infant in a family has died suddenly and unexpectedly, a metabolic disorder or child abuse should be suspected.

2. SIDS vs. child abuse: An autopsy examination cannot distinguish between suffocation and SIDS. Physical abuse that produces subdural hematomas or massive hemorrhage into the abdominal organs is evident. Suffocation with a soft object (a pillow or the cupped hand of an adult, for example) is virtually impossible to prove during an autopsy. Shaken baby syndrome can usually be identified by the presence of subdural and retinal hemorrhages.
3. Munchausen syndrome by proxy: A mother or caretaker repeatedly almost suffocates a baby and then comes to an emergency room claiming that the baby suffered an apneic episode. Finally, death from suffocation occurs.

TABLE 32–2. RISK FACTORS FOR SIDS

INFANT

Prematurity <37 weeks and <2500 g
Apgar scores <6 at 5 minutes
Intensive neonatal care requirement
Neonatal respiratory abnormalities
Bronchopulmonary dysplasia
Anemia
Twins
Previous acute life-threatening event (ALTE)
Sibling with SIDS

MATERNAL

Anemia
Smoking*
Alcohol and drug abuse
Maternal age <20 years

OTHER

Prone sleeping position*
Soft bedding
Race
Ethnicity
Socioeconomic status
Cultural influences
Lack of breast feeding*

*The most important preventable risk factors.

TABLE 32–3. METABOLIC DISORDERS ASSOCIATED WITH SUDDEN DEATH

Lactic acidemias
Aminoacidopathies, organic acidurias
Glycogen storage diseases
Carnitine deficiencies
Mitochondrial matrix enzyme defects
 Acyl-CoA dehydrogenase defects
Multiple acyl-CoA-dehydrogenase defects
 Electron transfer flavoprotein (ETF) subunit α deficiency

4. Accidental infant deaths have several recognizable patterns (not SIDS) (Table 32–4).

Pathogenesis

Many pathogenetic mechanisms have been suggested; however, chronic *hypoxemia* may be the initiating cause in many cases. Pathologic changes in the brainstem in the centers for cardiorespiratory control have been identified. Hypoxemia is also reflected in subtle changes in the organs and increased levels of fetal hemoglobin in victims of SIDS. In infants who are so compromised, the *supine sleeping position* may aggravate and augment the risk for SIDS.

Mechanisms for hypoxemia in susceptible infants implicated in the *prone sleeping position* include

1. Rebreathing with resultant CO_2 narcosis.
2. Positional asphyxia
 a. Respiratory obstruction due to backward displacement of the mandible.
 b. High cephalic position of cervical structures in a young infant, with apposition of the soft palate and back of the tongue.
 c. Nasal obstruction due to compression of the nose. (Most infants up to 4 months of age are obligate nasal breathers.)

Prematurely born infants may aerate better in the prone position.

Prevention

1. The baby should sleep in a supine position until at least 6 months of age. The room in which the baby sleeps

TABLE 32–4. ACCIDENTAL INFANT DEATH: FINDINGS IN 36 AUTOPSY CASES

TYPE OF ACCIDENT	NUMBER OF DEATHS
Unsafe sleeping environment	8
Overlying	6
Drowning	4
Scald burn	3
Plastic bag suffocation	3
House fire	3
Motor vehicle collision	3
Foreign body asphyxia	2
Hypothermia	2
Fall from height	1
Alcohol toxicity	1

From: Corey TS, McCloud LC, Nichols GR II, Buchino JJ: Infant death due to unintentional injury—11 year autopsy review. Am J Dis Child 1992;146:968.

should be warm but not hot. If space heaters are used, ventilation must be adequate. Heavy blankets restrict movements and should be avoided.

2. Cribs must meet federal safety standards. New cribs have a label. Hand-me-down cribs should have bars too close together for the infant's head to get caught (2 3/8 inches). The mattress should fit snugly against the crib sides; more than a two-finger space should be filled (e.g., with a rolled-up blanket). Crib bumpers should be avoided, as an infant's head can become wedged between the bumper and the mattress. The crib should not be filled with stuffed animals. Bedding should be firm, with no comforters, pillows, beanbag cushions, sheepskins, or adult water bed.

3. Breast feeding should be maintained as long as possible. Preferably the baby should not sleep in the same bed as an adult. If it is necessary for others to be in the same bed, protective devices to shield the baby should be recommended. The mother should avoid alcohol, tobacco, and other drugs during pregnancy and breast feeding. Smoking should be proscribed in the house.

Bibliography

Committee on Child Abuse and Neglect, 1993–1994: Distinguishing sudden infant death syndrome from child abuse fatalities. Pediatrics 1994;94:124.

Gilbert-Barness E, Barness LA: Sudden infant death: A reappraisal. Contemp Pediatr, 1995;12(4):88–91.

Gilbert-Barness E, Kenison K, Carver J: Fetal hemoglobin and sudden infant death syndrome. Arch Pathol Lab Med 1993;117:177.

Gilbert-Barness E, Hegstrand L, Chandra S, et al: Hazards of mattresses, beds and bedding in deaths of infants. Am J Forensic Med Pathol 1991;12(1):27.

Valdés-Dapena M, Gilbert-Barness E: Sudden death in infants. *In* Gilbert-Barness E (ed): Potter's Pathology of the Fetus and Infant. St. Louis, CV Mosby, 1996.

33 Resuscitation of the Newborn

Sheela G. Laungani

Procedure

Pathophysiology of Perinatal Asphyxia

1. At birth, there is a transition from placental to pulmonary gaseous exchange. Changes occurring in this period include lung expansion, resorption of lung fluid, establishment of air breathing, and conversion of the circulatory pattern from fetal to neonatal, characterized by establishment of pulmonary artery blood flow and elimination of right-to-left shunting of blood across the ductus arteriosus and foramen ovale.

2. Maintenance of adequate tissue oxygenation and elimination of carbon dioxide are essential for this transition. When this process is interfered with either prior to or following birth, damage to all organ systems (including the brain) or death may occur. When significant interference with gaseous exchange occurs either prior to or during the birth process, a defined set of clinical signs may be observed.

3. Following an initial brief period of rapid breathing, respiratory effort ceases. The heart rate begins to fall, muscular tone decreases, and there is a slight rise in blood pressure. This is the period of primary apnea.

4. If the insult continues, respiratory efforts become weak and irregular, with gasps followed by complete apnea. The heart rate and blood pressure continue to drop, and the infant becomes flaccid. This period is called secondary apnea.

5. Inadequate ventilation and oxygenation lead to progressive metabolic and respiratory acidosis, with pulmonary vasoconstriction and right-to-left shunting of blood. Clinically, it is difficult or impossible to distinguish primary from secondary apnea, and it should be assumed that secondary apnea, with the need for immediate resuscitation, is present. Any delay in implementing resuscitation may result in a delay in establishing spontaneous and sustained respirations and increase the likelihood of organ damage (Table 33–1).

Principles and Goals

Principles of resuscitation are based on the knowledge of normal physiologic events. Efforts must be directed toward establishing adequate ventilation and tissue oxygenation and minimizing damage to the brain and other vital organs.

Preparation

1. Identification of high risk deliveries
   a. Timely communication between the obstetrician and pediatrician
   b. Anticipation of the need for resuscitation based on maternal history and antenatal fetal evaluations
2. Preparation of equipment
   a. A radiant warmer, heated and ready for immediate use. Prevention of hypothermia is critical for successful resuscitation, especially in compromised term and all preterm infants.

Procedure *Continued*

TABLE 33–1. DEFINITION OF TERMS

Acidosis:	Metabolic: Accumulation of H⁺ ions with fall in pH and increase in base deficit. Respiratory: Increase in blood P_{CO_2} secondary to hypoventilation.
Apgar score:	Evaluation of the newborn infant using five objective signs (heart rate, respiratory effort, muscle tone, reflex response, and color) each giving a score of 0, 1, 2, performed at 60 seconds and at 5 minutes after birth.
Asphyxia:	A process leading to progressive hypoxia, accumulation of carbon dioxide and lactic acid in the blood, and subsequent acidosis.
Hypoxemia:	Abnormally low blood oxygen tension.
Hypoxia:	Inadequate supply of oxygen at the cellular level, secondary to decreased arterial P_{O_2}, decreased hemoglobin concentration, inadequate blood flow, interference with oxygen unloading, or tissue's ability to use oxygen.

b. All necessary equipment in good working order and medications with appropriate concentrations and volumes for newborn use, e.g, epinephrine 1:10,000 solution.

3. Personnel skilled in resuscitation

One person skilled in complete resuscitation must be present at each delivery. When anticipating an asphyxiated newborn infant or multiple births, a team of at least two persons must be present and must work together.

4. Precautions

   a. Aseptic conditions must be observed when dealing with newborn infants.

   b. All health care professionals must observe universal precautions.

ABCs of Resuscitation

* Establish an open airway
* Initiate breathing
* Support circulation

Continuous evaluation of the infant is necessary for successful resuscitation.

Technique

1. Initial steps:

   a. Place the infant under the radiant warmer.

   b. Dry amniotic fluid from the infant.

   c. Remove wet linen to prevent further evaporative heat loss.

   d. Position the infant and suction the mouth and nose with suction bulb.

   e. Evaluate the infant for respiratory effort, heart rate, and color.

   f. Provide tactile stimulation.

   g. Assign an Apgar score (Table 33–2) indicating the condition of the infant.

   h. Make an appropriate decision concerning further intervention.

2. Next steps:

   a. For an infant with 1-minute Apgar score >8:
   A period of observation and reevaluation at 5 minutes. If the infant continues to do well, no further intervention is necessary. Be cautious about vigorous suctioning and gastric aspiration, which may pose the risk of laryngospasm and cardiac arrhythmias.

   b. For an infant with 1-minute Apgar score of 5 to 7:

      (1) Initiate spontaneous respirations by gentle stimulation.

      (2) Provide oxygen-enriched environment by giving heated and humidified free flow oxygen via mask or anesthesia bag and mask.

      (3) Reevaluate to determine respiratory effort, heart rate, and color.

      (4) No further interventions are necessary if spontaneous respiration has begun, heart rate remains above 100 beats/minute, and there is no cyanosis.

   c. For an infant with Apgar score of 3 or 4:

      (1) Attempt to initiate spontaneous respirations by providing positive pressure ventilation for 15 to 30 seconds with 100 per cent oxygen via bag and mask. It is important to recognize that the success of bag-and-mask ventilation depends upon proper positioning of the infant's head, using an appropriate-size mask applied correctly to the infant's face, and using adequate inspira-

TABLE 33–2. APGAR SCORE

SIGN	0	1	2
Heart rate	Absent	Slow (<100 beats/min)	>100 beats/min
Respirations	Absent	Weak cry, hypoventilation	Good, strong cry
Muscle tone	Limp	Some flexion	Active motion
Reflex irritability	No response	Grimace	Cough or sneeze
Color	Blue or pale	Body pink Extremities blue	Completely pink

tory pressures. A ventilatory rate of 40 to 60 breaths/minute, with inspiratory pressures of 30 to 40 cm of water, is appropriate.

(2) Reevaluate for respiratory effort and heart rate.

(3) If the heart rate is above 100 beats/minute and the infant has spontaneous respirations, discontinue positive pressure ventilation but continue to provide freely flowing oxygen until the infant becomes pink.

(4) If the heart rate remains between 60 and 100 beats/minute and is not increasing, continue positive pressure ventilation with 100 per cent oxygen via bag and mask, continually reassessing the infant.

(5) If the heart rate remains ≤80 beats/minute in spite of positive pressure ventilation with 100 per cent oxygen, chest compressions must be considered. It is important to provide a firm surface or support for the infant's back while administering chest compressions. These must be provided over the lower third of the sternum at a rate of 2 per second, with a one-half second pause after every third compression for ventilation. For effectiveness, the sternum should be compressed 1 to 2 cm without lifting the fingers.

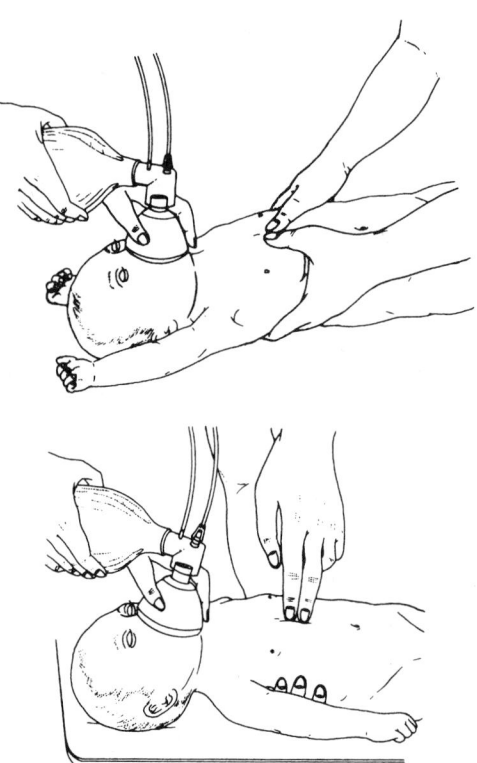

Reproduced with permission. Textbook of Neonatal Resuscitation, 1987, 1990, 1994. Copyright American Heart Association.

The thumb compression technique is the preferred method; an alternative is the two-fingered method.

(6) If, after 30 seconds of chest compression and positive pressure ventilation with 100 per cent oxygen, the heart rate is ≥80 beats/minute, discontinue chest compression but continue positive pressure ventilation with 100 per cent oxygen until the heart rate is ≥100 beats/minute and the infant is breathing spontaneously.

(7) If positive pressure ventilation with 100 per cent oxygen and chest compressions fails to improve the infant's condition, consider endotracheal intubation and drug therapy.

d. For an infant with Apgar score of 0 to 2:

(1) Initiate full resuscitative measures immediately. Do not wait for 1 minute to elapse.

(2) Following a brief period of oropharyngeal suctioning and bag-and-mask ventilation with 100 per cent oxygen, perform endotracheal intubation.

3. Prior to intubation:

a. Select and prepare correct-size endotracheal tube.

b. Use the right size laryngoscope blade and check light bulb.

c. Keep suction equipment (suction pressure not exceeding 100 mmHg), oxygen tubing, and bag and mask ready at all times during intubation.

d. Know the anatomic landmarks in the area of the larynx, and position the infant so that the vocal cords are visualized without difficulty.

4. During intubation:

a. Wait for the vocal cords to open. Do not touch with the tip of the endotracheal tube.

b. To minimize hypoxia, provide freely flowing oxygen, limit intubation attempts to 20 seconds, and ventilate the infant with bag and mask between attempts.

5. Following intubation:

a. Confirm the position of the endotracheal tube, and continue to ventilate the infant with 100 per cent oxygen for about 30 seconds.

b. Reevaluate the heart rate and respiratory effort.

c. If the heart rate remains ≤80 beats/minute in spite of ventilation for 30 seconds, provide chest compressions simultaneously for about 30 seconds.

d. Correction of acidosis with isotonic sodium bicarbonate up to 2 mEq/kg and 10 per cent glucose solution (0.5 to 1 g/kg) may be necessary in order to support myocardial function. Sodium bicarbonate should be used only when resuscitative efforts are prolonged and a significant metabolic acidosis is

Procedure *Continued*

present. Adequate ventilation must be established before sodium bicarbonate is administered.

e. If bradycardia continues with heart rates ≤80 beats/minute or between 60 and 80 and not increasing despite positive pressure ventilation and chest compression, administer 1:10,000 epinephrine (0.1 to 0.3 ml/kg) intravenously via the umbilical vein. If there is no response, epinephrine administration may be repeated every 3 to 5 minutes. If intravenous access is not available, intratracheal administration of epinephrine may be used in a higher dose of 0.1 to 0.2 mg/kg (1 to 2 ml/kg) diluted with isotonic saline solution in a 1:1 ratio.

f. If the infant exhibits signs of hypovolemia (pallor, weak pulses, low blood pressure, and poor response to resuscitation), administration of volume expanders such as 5 per cent albumin solution, isotonic saline, whole blood, or Ringer's lactate solution (10 ml/kg) should be considered. Infant should be reevaluated for additional administrations of volume expanders. In infants with asphyxial myocardial damage, volume expanders should be used cautiously. Measurement of central venous pressure at this time, via a catheter placed in the umbilical vein, may give a better indication of the infant's circulatory status.

6. Umbilical vein catheter placement

A 3.5F or 5F umbilical catheter with a single endhole and a radiopaque marker should be used. The catheter should be inserted into the opening of the umbilical vein on the umbilical stump so as to have the tip of the catheter just below the skin level and a free flow of blood present. If the catheter is inserted any farther, there is a risk of infusing medications into the liver. The catheter should be removed after resuscitation is completed. If vascular access is necessary for continued use, an umbilical artery or peripheral vein should be used.

7. Special situations

a. Meconium in amniotic fluid:

(1) The infant's mouth and hypopharynx should be suctioned by the obstetrician as soon as the head is delivered (before delivery of the shoulders).

(2) Residual meconium in the hypopharynx should be suctioned under direct vision after delivery.

(3) The trachea should then be intubated and meconium suctioned from the lower airway before using positive pressure ventilation.

Note: If the infant is active and crying vigorously at birth, and there is no particulate meconium in the amniotic fluid, tracheal intubation for suctioning may not be necessary. If an infant is severely asphyxiated at birth, it may not be possible to clear the trachea of all meconium before initiating positive pressure ventilation.

b. Diaphragmatic hernia:

In an infant with a confirmed or suspected diagnosis of diaphragmatic hernia, positive pressure ventilation should be given via an endotracheal tube, and an orogastric tube should be inserted for decompression of the stomach.

c. Narcotic depression:

If an infant is depressed because of narcotic administration to the mother during labor, naloxone hydrochloride should be administered to the infant (0.01 mg/kg) as a narcotic antagonist.

d. Prematurity:

(1) Preterm infants lose heat at a much more rapid rate than full-term infants because of a higher body surface to weight ratio and a lack of insulating subcutaneous tissue. Special precautions should be taken in caring for the preterm infant in the delivery room.

(2) In very small preterm infants (≤1000 g), assisted ventilation via an endotracheal tube must be strongly considered. Administration of surfactant to these infants in the delivery room is accomplished in a timely manner when an endotracheal tube is placed.

Postresuscitation Intubation Complications

If the newborn infant suddenly deteriorates, airway compromise should be assumed as a cause and appropriate steps taken to correct the situation.

1. Displaced endotracheal tube
2. Obstructed endotracheal tube
3. Pneumothorax
4. Equipment failure
5. Inadequate ventilatory support
6. Excessive gastric distention from bag-and-mask ventilation.

It is critical for corrective measures to be instituted promptly in order to avoid any further delay in establishing adequate ventilatory support.

 ## Bibliography

American Academy of Pediatrics, Committee on Fetus and Newborn, and the American Academy of Obstetricians and Gynecologists Committee on Obstetrics: Guidelines for Perinatal Care, 3rd ed. American Academy of Pediatrics and College of Obstetricians and Gynecologists, Elk Grove, IL, 1992, pp 84–90.

Bloom RS, Cropley C, and the AHA/AAP Neonatal Resuscitation Program Steering Committee: Textbook of Neonatal Resuscitation, Washington, DC, 1994.

34 Parenteral Nutrition of the Neonate

Nathan Rudolph

Definitions

1. Parenteral nutrition (parenteral alimentation) is the provision of nutrition, which includes carbohydrates, amino acids, lipids, minerals, and vitamins, by the intravenous route.
2. Parenteral nutrition may be *total* (TPN), in which the vascular route is the only method of delivery, or *partial*, when it complements an enteral route.
3. The method of delivery may be
   a. Central, by insertion of a catheter into a large central vein, e.g., a surgically placed Broviac catheter with its tip in the innominate vein or superior vena cava, or, in a neonate, an umbilical vein catheter with its tip in the inferior vena cava.
   b. Peripheral, by insertion of a short catheter into a peripheral vein.
   c. Percutaneously inserted central line (PICC), by peripheral venous insertion of a thin silicone catheter with its tip situated in a large central vein.

Indications

General guidelines for parenteral alimentation in pediatrics are outlined in Table 34–1.

The composition of the parenteral infusion mixture is as follows:

1. Carbohydrate: Dextrose monohydrate is used in a final concentration of 4 to 20 g/dl. For peripheral alimentation, the final concentration must not exceed 12.5 g/dl. The minimum glucose infusion rate in a preterm infant should be no less than 0.25 to 0.35 g/kg/hr (4–6 mg/kg/min), and the initial concentration of dextrose could be 4 to 5 g/dl, depending on fluid requirements. With increasing postnatal age and growth, or in older infants and children, a glucose delivery rate of up to 0.8 to 1.2 g/kg/hr will be appropriate.

2. Protein: Several commercial amino acid solutions are available.
   a. TrophAmine (McGaw, Inc.) is one of the preferred solutions for use in premature and other infants; its amino acid balance is satisfactory, and it also contains taurine, which is considered to be an essential amino acid for sick low birth weight (LBW) infants.
   b. The addition of cysteine hydrochloride to the infusion mixture has been claimed to be advantageous for premature infants, whose ability to metabolize methionine to cysteine may be inadequate.
   c. The growing preterm infant requires 2.5 to 3.5 g/kg/day of amino acid (protein) to maintain growth. Extremely low birth weight (ELBW) infants or sick LBW infants are generally unable to metabolize this quantity of amino acid and may develop metabolic acidosis. During the early postnatal period they should receive 0.5 to 1.0 g/kg/day, which is increased progressively as they stabilize.

3. Minerals
   a. Sodium (Na) is generally added as sodium chloride and sometimes as sodium acetate. The daily quantity of Na infused initially should be 2 to 3 mEq/kg/day, but this will require adjustment depending on serum electrolyte levels, especially in very low birth weight (VLBW) infants, in whom additional quantities might be necessary during the first 1 to 2 postnatal weeks.
   b. Potassium may be added as KCl or as K-phosphate to provide 2 to 3 mEq/kg/day. It might need to be withheld or reduced, however, in an ELBW infant during the first postnatal week.
   c. Calcium and phosphorus
      (1) Because of the limited solubility of the calcium-phosphate complex, it is not usually possible to provide preterm infants with these minerals in TPN at an optimal level that would be equivalent to intrauterine accretion rates.
      (2) Calcium is added as calcium gluconate and phosphorus as potassium phosphate.
      (3) Adequate concentrations in the final solution for an infant are 40 to 60 mg/dl (20–30 mEq/L) calcium, and 30 to 45 mg/dl (10–15 mmol/L) phosphorus, with a preference for the higher level in preterm infants, depending on the solu-

TABLE 34–1. GENERAL CRITERIA FOR USE OF PARENTERAL NUTRITION IN PEDIATRICS

Developmental immaturity of gastrointestinal tract
    Prematurity (VLBW infant)
Inadequate absorptive capacity
    Short bowel syndrome; multiple strictures
Malabsorption syndromes with failure to thrive
    Chronic nonspecific diarrhea of infancy; bovine milk intolerance;
        gluten enteropathy; inflammatory bowel disease
Temporary contraindication to enteral feeding in order to rest the bowel
    Necrotizing enterocolitis; gastrointestinal surgery; inflammatory
        bowel disease
High caloric requirement that cannot be met by increasing enteral intake
    Extensive burns; trauma
Supplement to oral feeding
    Neoplastic disease; AIDS; inflammatory bowel disease

Procedure *Continued*

bility. Approximately one half of these concentrations will generally provide an appropriate daily intake in an older child.

 (4) Calcium-phosphate solubility is affected by a number of factors, including temperature, pH (lower pH increases solubility), type and concentration of amino acid preparation (higher concentrations improve solubility), and addition of cysteine hydrochloride (lowers pH slightly and improves solubility).

 d. Magnesium, as magnesium sulfate, is added to provide 0.25 to 0.5 mEq/kg/day in both infants and children.

 e. Trace minerals

  (1) Copper, zinc, manganese, and chromium are supplied by the addition of an appropriate pediatric trace mineral solution.

  (2) Preterm infants require a higher intake of zinc (approximately 400 mg/kg/day)

  (3) For prolonged TPN, selenium and molybdenum should be added to the solution.

4. A pediatric multivitamin solution is added in an appropriate volume.

5. Lipids

 a. An intravenous lipid emulsion (e.g., Intralipid 10 per cent or 20 per cent [Cutter Medical]) provides calories and essential fatty acids.

 b. The postnatal age for commencing intravenous (IV) lipid infusion in premature infants is controversial. It may be advantageous to delay its use until 5 to 7 days or more after birth, especially in VLBW infants.

 c. The lipid is given concurrently with the TPN mixture by continuous infusion via a Y-adaptor.

 d. In preterm infants IV lipid infusion should commence with 0.5g/kg/day and gradually increase to 2 to 2.5 g/kg. In older infants and children, up to 3 to 3.5 g/kg can be administered.

 e. Since the tocopherols present in Intralipid are primarily isomers with poor biologic vitamin E activity, it is recommended that supplemental vitamin E be given orally to premature infants.

6. Heparin is added to the alimentation solution in a concentration of 1 U/ml of fluid being infused. Heparin decreases the incidence of clotting at the catheter tip. It also stimulates plasma phospholipase activity, which improves clearance of lipids when IV fat is being infused.

Monitoring and Care

1. As far as possible, the TPN line should be maintained only for infusion of alimentation solution.

2. Do not mix medications with the alimentation fluids.

TABLE 34–2. COMPLICATIONS ASSOCIATED WITH PARENTERAL NUTRITION

CATHETER RELATED

Mechanical: Poor position; dislodgement; vessel perforation; tissue injury; bleeding

Thrombosis and embolism: Gangrene of limb or digits; necrotizing enterocolitis; portal hypertension; renal artery/vein thrombosis producing infarction and systemic hypertension; superior vena cava syndrome

Infection: Sepsis; bacterial/fungal endocarditis; osteomyelitis

Air embolism

ASSOCIATED WITH USE OF HYPEROSMOLAR SOLUTIONS

Tissue injury from leakage or malposition: Sloughing of skin and subcutaneous tissues; gangrene of buttock; gangrene of limb; liver abscess

METABOLIC

Hypoglycemia; hyperglycemia, osmotic diuresis

Hypo/hypernatremia; hypo/hyperkalemia

Hypocalcemia; hypophosphatemia; osteopenia; rickets

Metabolic acidosis

Hyperammonemia

IMBALANCE OR INCOMPATIBILITY OF COMPONENTS

Precipitation of calcium phosphate

INADEQUATE NUTRITION

Poor caloric intake; unknown requirements, especially in ELBW infants

CHOLESTATIC JAUNDICE

TPN-associated jaundice, of uncertain etiology—possibly due to delayed introduction of enteral feeding and inspissation of bile, or lack of an unknown nutritional factor, or toxic effect of one or more components of TPN fluid on liver

3. Maintain strict antiseptic techniques to decrease the incidence of sepsis.

4. Biochemical monitoring includes serum electrolyte, urea nitrogen, and glucose levels (initially daily and then two or three times per week); blood gases as necessary; and Ca, P, and Mg (every 2 or 3 days initially, and then about once a week). Plasma proteins and albumin should be measured every 1 to 2 weeks, and if TPN is maintained for a prolonged period, bilirubin and serum amino transferase activity as well.

Complications

These are outlined in Table 34–2.

Bibliography

American Academy of Pediatrics, Committee on Nutrition: Nutritional needs of low-birth-weight infants. Pediatrics 1985; 75:976–986.

Briones ER, Iber FL: Liver and biliary tract changes associated with parenteral nutrition: pathogenesis and prevention. J Am Coll Nutr 1995;14:219–228.

Koo WWK, Tsang RC: Mineral requirements of low-birth-weight infants. J Am Coll Nutr 1991;10:476–486.

35 Infant Transport

Gloria B. Valencia

Procedure

Definition

Perinatal outcome is optimized when a sick newborn infant is cared for at a facility capable of providing, on a continuous basis, all medical services required for intact survival. When the delivery of a sick or potentially compromised neonate is anticipated, a planned delivery should take place at such a facility. If an unanticipated problem arises during labor, the mother should be transferred to a facility with appropriate capabilities. If a low birth weight (LBW) or otherwise compromised infant is born at a facility not capable of providing continuous intensive care, transfer to a fully equipped center should be expedited, following stabilization of the infant at the hospital of birth.

Structure and Administration of Infant and Maternal Transport

1. All hospitals with obstetric services must have written agreements with regional perinatal centers delineating criteria for both consultation and transfer of high-risk mothers and sick neonates, when appropriate. These agreements must also clearly spell out the mechanism for carrying out such transfers.

2. A regional transport program must have full-time medical directors who specialize in fetal-maternal medicine and neonatology, establish policy, and direct operations of the transport service.

3. An appropriately equipped ambulance, together with a staff consisting of a neonatologist, nurse practitioner, and respiratory therapist, should be on call at all times.

Guidelines for Neonatal Transfer

1. The following are the usual indications for transfer of a neonate to a regional center:

   a. Birth weight $\leq$1500 g

   b. Gestational age $\leq$32 weeks

   c. Persistent respiratory distress

TABLE 35–1. NEONATAL RESPIRATORY THERAPY PACK

EQUIPMENT	AMOUNT	EQUIPMENT	AMOUNT
Exterior Pockets		**Interior of Bag (Continued)**	
Oxygen tubing	3	Silicone adapter	2
Infant nasal cannula	1	O$_2$ flow meter nipple	2
Aerosol tubing	1	One-way valve	1
Complete ventilator setup with exhalation valve	1	Gould transducer dome	1
(plus one in incubator)		Set of ECG lead wires	2
Incubator bag	1	25 g ½-inch butterfly	2
Space blanket	1	Tape measure	1
Pulse oximeter sensors (N-25 and I-20)	2 each	Infant MVB bag with O$_2$ tubing (plus one in isolette)	1
Interior of Bag		Suction catheters: 5 French, 6 French, and 8 French	1 each
Airway Supplies		C-size batteries for laryngoscope	2
Laerdal masks	2	Normal saline vials	4
#0	2	Silk tape	1 roll
#1	1	Dermaclear tape	1 roll
#2	1	Oxygen connectors	2
Infant McGill forceps	1 each	Hemostat	2
Laryngoscope handle with #0 and #1 Miller blades		Infant BP cuff (small, medium, and large)	1 each
Set of endotracheal tubes with stylets		Oxygen analyzer membrane kit	2
Other Equipment		Briggs T-adapters	2
		15 mm adapter	2
Benzoin applicators	6	O$_2$ connectors NCG, OES, P-B	1 each
Alcohol swabs	4	O$_2$ connectors (NCG, P-B)	1 each
Adjustable wrench	1	ECG lead pads	3
E-tank wrench	1	Three-way stopcock	2
Cable ties	10	E-Z Heat hot packs	4
Scissors	1	Stethoscope	1
Nine-volt battery	2	1-ml syringe	2
Assorted laryngoscope bulbs	4		
Adjustable Venturi	2		

P, blood pressure; ECG, electrocardiogram; MVB, manual ventilation bag.

Procedure *Continued*

d. Refractory seizures

e. Congenital malformations or inborn errors of metabolism requiring surgery or other special care

f. Congenital cardiac disease, requiring special procedures or surgery

g. Sequelae of hypoxia persisting beyond 2 hours, involving multiple organ systems

h. Unresponsive shock.

2. Other conditions requiring consultation and possible transfer include:

a. Infants of diabetic mothers

b. Infants with hyperbilirubinemia requiring exchange transfusion

c. Infants with birth weights between 1500 and 2000 g and gestational ages between 32 and 36 weeks

d. Intrauterine growth retardation

e. Blood dyscrasias

f. Need for special procedures unavailable at hospital of birth.

3. Responsibility of referring center

   A complete medical summary must accompany the patient, and appropriate consent forms must be signed by the parents.

Equipment

1. Transport ambulance
2. Portable transport incubator with mechanical ventilator
3. Cardiorespiratory monitor with blood pressure transducers
4. Pulse oximeter
5. Intravenous infusion pumps
6. Air-oxygen blender
7. Suction apparatus
8. Neonatal respiratory therapy and medicine packs (Tables 35–1 and 35–2)

Medical Aspects

A neonatologist from the referral center must be on call at all times to receive requests for consultations and transfers. At the time of request, the transport team must be mobilized to enact the transfer. While awaiting the transport team, the transferring hospital should stabilize the patient in the following manner:

1. Maintain thermoneutral state and normalize blood pressure.
2. Maintain appropriate oxygenation, using assisted ventilation if necessary.
3. Administer vitamin K (0.5 mg IM).
4. Take chest radiograph.
5. Begin intravenous infusion and stabilize blood glucose concentration.
6. Insert umbilical arterial catheter, if indicated.
7. Insert nasogastric tube and aspirate stomach.

TABLE 35–2. NEONATAL MEDICINE PACK

DRUG	AMOUNT
Isotonic saline vials	4
Heparin	1
Naloxone	2
Epinephrine 1:10,000 Bristojet	1
Ampicillin, 250 mg	1
Gentamicin	1
Calcium gluconate	1
Dobutamine	1
Norcuron	1
$D_{10}W$	1
Tubex	1
Surfactant	2
Sterile water vials, 20 ml	4
Heparin lock flush	2
KCl	1
Furosemide	1
Lidocaine 1%	1
Dopamine	1
Pavulon	1
Sodium bicarbonate	1
Albumin 5%	2
Vitamin K	1
Neonatal narcotic pack	1
Morphine	2
Chloral hydrate suppository	1
Versed	1
Phenobarbital	3
Diazepam	1
Fentanyl	1

Management During Transport

1. Continuously monitor vital signs and oxygenation status.
2. Maintain thermoneutral state.
3. Intubate infant and begin assisted ventilation, if necessary.
4. Maintain IV infusion and normal blood glucose concentrations.

Responsibilities of Referral Center

1. Continuous communication with referring hospitals
2. Outreach education to all referring hospitals
3. Regular site visits to referring hospitals
4. Conducting transport review conferences
5. Maintaining regional statistics
6. Maintaining quality assurance and continuous quality improvement
7. Sending summary of infant's hospitalization to referring hospital
8. Assuring appropriate follow-up care of infant.

Bibliography

American Academy of Pediatrics, Committee on Fetus and Newborn, and American College of Obstetricians and Gynecologists,

Procedure *Continued*

Committee on Obstetrics, Maternal and Fetal Medicine: Guidelines for Perinatal Care. Evanston, IL, American Academy of Pediatrics and American College of Obstetricians and Gynecologists, 1992, pp 35–47; 246–247.

Bose CL: Neonatal transport. *In* Avery GB, Fletcher MA, MacDonald MG (eds): Neonatology, Pathophysiology and Management of the Newborn, 4th ed. Philadelphia, JB Lippincott, 1994, pp 41–53.

36 Screening

Nathan Rudolph

Procedure

Definition

Screening is a process whereby all newborn infants in a population are tested to identify the presence of selected metabolic or genetic disorders.

Objectives

1. The primary objective of neonatal screening is to prevent or minimize the development of neurologic insults and mental retardation, or of other serious sequelae of specific metabolic defects, by prompt dietary or other therapeutic intervention.
2. A secondary objective is to determine the frequency of specific disorders within population groups.
3. The benefits of the screening program should outweigh the cost.
4. The frequency of false positive results should be minimal, and false negative results should not occur.

Current Status

1. All states in the United States have established mandatory screening of all newborns for specific inherited disorders.
2. States have set up central, automated laboratories for processing and testing biologic samples submitted for screening.
3. The metabolic errors for which neonatal screening is currently being performed in various combinations by different states, and the approximate frequency of their occurrence, are shown in Table 36–1.

TABLE 36–1. METABOLIC DISORDERS FOR WHICH NEWBORN SCREENING IS PERFORMED

DISORDER	SCREENING TEST	APPROXIMATE OVERALL INCIDENCE
Phenylketonuria (PKU)	Phenylalanine	1:15,000*
Maple syrup urine disease	Leucine	1:100,000–200,000*
Homocystinuria	Methionine	1:100,000–200,000*
Galactosemia	GALT,† Galactose	1:60,000
Hypothyroidism	T4; TSH	1:4,000
Biotinidase deficiency	Biotinidase	1:70,000*
Hemoglobinopathy (SS; SC; S- β thalassemia)	Hemoglobin electrophoresis	1:500 African Americans*
Congenital adrenal hyperplasia	17-OH progesterone	1:12,000*

*Considerable variability in frequency occurs among different racial or ethnic groups.
†Galactose-1-phosphate uridyltransferase.

Technique

1. Screening is accomplished by obtaining a sample of blood from each neonate, usually by heel prick, prior to discharge from the hospital.
2. The blood is collected onto circular areas marked on standardized filter paper forms, where it is allowed to saturate both sides of the paper completely in a uniform fashion.
3. After air-drying for at least 4 hours, the blood collection forms are submitted to the central laboratory for testing.
4. Timing of blood collection is important. The optimal time of sampling is between the third and fifth postnatal days, but sampling on the second day is considered acceptable.
5. Babies discharged from hospitals or birthing centers on the first postnatal day require initial sampling on discharge and a second test between the third and fifth days.
6. Infants requiring blood transfusion or exchange transfusion should have blood collected for screening prior to transfusion. Depending on postnatal age at the time of the initial sampling, additional testing may be necessary later.

Procedure *Continued*

7. In premature babies and in sick infants with prolonged hospital stays, an initial specimen is collected between the third and fifth postnatal days, and again on discharge or at 1 month of age, whichever comes first.

8. Some states have extended the newborn metabolic screening process by utilizing the same dried blood samples submitted to the laboratory for other purposes, such as testing for the presence of HIV antibodies (AIDS screening).

Bibliography

Guthrie R, Whitney S: Phenylketonuria detection in the newborn infant as a routine hospital procedure; a trial of a phenylalanine screening method in 400,000 infants. Children's Bureau publication 419, Washington, DC, US Department of Health, Education and Welfare, 1964.

New York State Department of Health: Newborn Screening in New York State; A Guide for Health Professionals, Albany, 1991.

37 Eating Disorders

Sharon R. Beier and *Susan M. Coupey*

Definition

The two common eating disorders, anorexia nervosa and bulimia nervosa, are chronic biopsychosocial syndromes. The primary care physician plays a major role in making the diagnosis, forming a bond of trust with the patient, involving the family, establishing a therapeutic team, and managing the patient's physical health over the often prolonged course of the eating disorder.

Diagnostic Criteria

Anorexia Nervosa: DSM IV Diagnostic Criteria—Anorexia Nervosa (307.1)

(1) Refusal to maintain body weight at or above minimally normal weight for age and height (e.g., weight loss leading to maintenance of body weight less than 85% of that expected; or failure to make expected weight gain during period of growth, leading to body weight less than 85% of that expected).

(2) Intense fear of gaining weight, or becoming fat, even though underweight.

(3) Disturbance in the way in which one's body weight or shape is experienced, undue influence of body weight or shape on self evaluation, or denial of the seriousness of the current low body weight.

(4) In postmenarcheal females, amenorrhea, i.e., the absence of at least three consecutive menstrual cycles. (A woman is considered to have amenorrhea if her periods occur only following hormone, e.g., estrogen, administration.)

(5) Type:
   (a) Restricting type
   (b) Binge-eating/purging type

Bulimia Nervosa: DSM-IV Diagnostic Criteria—Bulimia Nervosa (307.51)

(1) Recurrent episodes of binge eating. An episode of binge eating is characterized by both of the following:
   (a) Eating in a discrete period of time (e.g., within any 2 hour period), an amount of food that definitely is larger than most people would eat during a similar period of time and under similar circumstances.
   (b) A sense of lack of control over eating during the episode (e.g., a feeling that one cannot stop eating or control what or how much one is eating).

(2) Recurrent inappropriate compensatory behavior in order to prevent weight gain, such as self-induced vomiting; misuse of laxatives, diuretics, enemas, and other medications; fasting; or excessive exercise.

(3) The binge eating and inappropriate compensatory behaviors both occur, on average, at least twice a week for 3 months.

(4) Self evaluation is unduly influenced by body shape and weight.

(5) The disturbance does not occur exclusively during episodes of anorexia nervosa.

(6) Type:
   (a) Purging type
   (b) Non-purging type

Epidemiology

Anorexia Nervosa

1. Ninety per cent of patients are female.
2. Ninety per cent of patients are diagnosed before age 25 years.
3. Symptom onset most often begins in early adolescence (age 13 to 14 years) with a secondary peak at age 17 to 18 years. Diagnosis may not occur until 1 to 2 years after onset of symptoms.
4. Most cases occur in the middle and upper socioeconomic classes, in the upwardly mobile, and from industrialized countries where there is an abundance of food. In the United States, the prevalence is estimated at 1 in 300 of 15- to 19-year-old girls and is as high as 1 in 100 girls in elite private schools.

Bulimia Nervosa

1. One to 5 per cent of college women and less than 1 per cent of college men are estimated to have bulimia nervosa.
2. There appears to be an increased genetic risk for affective disorders and alcoholism.

Etiology and Pathogenesis

Anorexia Nervosa

1. Biologic/genetic contributions to the etiology of anorexia nervosa are inferred from findings that there is increased concordance in monozygotic twins, increased incidence in sisters, increased prevalence of affective disorders in families, and increased incidence in females with gonadal dysgenesis.
2. Psychological etiologic factors are evidenced by findings that patients are likely to have personality traits that include shyness, social anxiety, passivity, obsessionality, rigid perfectionism, and self doubts; family characteristics that include enmeshment, overprotectiveness, rigidity, and

lack of conflict resolution; and history of early separation stress and of sexual abuse.

3. Sociocultural stressors of the developing adolescent include affluence in industrial countries where there is an abundance of food, extreme thinness as a standard of feminine beauty, media bombardment with the message that thinness equals success, and media promotion of women as sex objects. There are also the requirements of some sports for the athletes to be thin, including gymnastics, distance running, and ballet.

Bulimia Nervosa

1. Biologic factors possibly important in the etiology include decreased central nervous system levels of a serotonin metabolite, suggesting that there may be a dysregulation of serotonin metabolism resulting in binge eating of high-carbohydrate foods, and a family history of affective disorders, most often depression, and of alcoholism.

2. Psychological factors important in the etiology of bulimia nervosa include history of incest, rape, or sexual abuse and of dysfunctional family interactions, ranging from parental enmeshment to absence. If present, these factors contribute to feelings of being out of control, poor self-esteem, and needing comfort.

3. Sociocultural factors include the strong social pressures to be thin and consequent dissatisfaction with the normal to overweight female body. Bulimia nervosa may begin after unsuccessful attempts at dieting. There may also be a "contagion" factor because there are reports of college women getting together in dormitories and having binging and purging "parties."

Clinical Findings

Anorexia Nervosa
Presenting symptoms include:

1. Excessive weight loss
2. Primary or secondary amenorrhea
3. Gastrointestinal symptoms such as abdominal pain, vomiting, or bloating
4. Growth failure or pubertal delay

Bulimia Nervosa
Presenting symptoms include:

1. Fatigue, weakness, dizziness, headache, or malaise
2. Menstrual disorders, including oligomenorrhea and secondary amenorrhea
3. Sore throat, hoarseness, and dental caries

Key Clinical Findings

- Excessive weight loss
- Amenorrhea
- Fatigue

Differential Diagnosis
1. Thyroid disease
2. Diabetes mellitus
3. Addison disease
4. Inflammatory bowel disease
5. Brain tumors

6. Malignancy
7. Human immunodeficiency virus infection
8. Drug/alcohol abuse
9. Depression
10. Schizophrenia
11. Personality disorders
12. Obsessive/compulsive disorders

Diagnosis

History
The diagnosis of an eating disorder is made by history, which should be taken from both adolescent and parents separately and privately. Areas to be explored in the history include:

1. Weight history
2. Detailed diet history
3. Detailed exercise history
4. Body image history
5. History of self-induced binging; purging; self-medication with laxatives, diuretics, or diet pills
6. Detailed menstrual and/or pubertal history
7. Sexual and/or physical abuse history
8. Family history with particular attention to psychiatric illness, alcoholism, and eating disorders
9. History of substance abuse, voluntary sexual behaviors, compulsive/impulsive behaviors (e.g., rituals, shoplifting)

Physical Examination
A thorough physical examination is important and it is crucial that the physician carefully document height and weight and corresponding percentiles as well as stage of pubertal development.

1. Physical signs in anorexia nervosa

   a. Weight: significant weight loss or failure to make expected gain in height or weight (in pubertal patients)

   b. Vital signs: bradycardia, hypotension, orthostatic hypotension, hypothermia

   c. Extremities: acrocyanosis; edema; cool, mottled discoloration

   d. Skin: lanugo, loss of scalp hair, jaundice and/or dry skin

   e. Musculoskeletal: weakness, loss of muscle mass

   f. Cardiac: arrhythmias

2. Physical signs in bulimia nervosa

   a. Head and neck: bilateral parotid gland swelling, loss of tooth enamel (from acidic stomach contents), dental caries, subconjunctival hemorrhage (from forced vomiting)

   b. Skin: scarring or hyperpigmented calluses on knuckles (Russell's sign) in those who use fingers to induce vomiting; petechiae on face (from forced vomiting)

   c. Gastrointestinal: abdominal distention, ileus, constipation, rectal bleeding, gastritis, esophagitis, esophageal tears

   d. Pulmonary: aspiration pneumonia, pneumomediastinum

   e. Cardiac: arrhythmias

Laboratory/Imaging Findings

1. Results of the following tests are most often normal:
   a. Complete blood cell count with differential (Anemia is very rare; if it is present, one must suspect another diagnosis.)
   b. Erythrocyte sedimentation rate (If it is elevated, suspect another diagnosis.)
   c. Electrolytes (unless very frequent vomiting)
   d. Renal function tests (Blood urea nitrogen [BUN] is usually in the low/normal range even with dehydration.)
   e. Liver function tests (with severe starvation may show mild elevations due to fatty liver)
2. Results of the following tests are sometimes abnormal:
   a. Urinalysis may be alkaline with some ketones and/or protein.
   b. Cholesterol value may be elevated.
   c. Amylase level may be elevated.
   d. Electrocardiogram may indicate bradycardia and low voltage and nonspecific ST and T wave changes.
   e. Computed tomography of the head may show cerebral atrophy.
   f. Bone densitometry may indicate osteopenia.
3. Results of the following tests are usually abnormal:
   a. Luteinizing hormone and follicle-stimulating hormone levels are low.
   b. Thyroid function test results are low.
   c. Cortisol level is high.

Key Laboratory Findings

- Usually no abnormalities of hemogram or usual chemical analyses
- Luteinizing hormone and follicle-stimulating hormone levels low
- Thyroxine (T_4) and triiodothyronine (T_3) levels low
- Cortisol level high

Treatment

The primary care physician has the role of diagnosing the eating disorder, setting weight goals, planning with the patient how to meet them, and negotiating consequences if goals are not met. In addition, he or she makes referrals and coordinates the patient's care among other specialists (e.g., psychotherapist, nutritionist) and cares for intercurrent illnesses as well as managing any physical complications of the eating disorder. Some important aspects of the primary care physician's role in treatment include:

1. Referral to a psychotherapist knowledgeable in diagnosing and treating eating disorders. It is important for the psychotherapist and the primary physician to work closely together. Individual therapy, family therapy, or group therapy alone or in combination may be indicated.

Antidepressants may be helpful adjuncts to treatment, especially for bulimia nervosa.
2. Nutritional management may be done in consultation with a nutritionist or by the primary care physician if he or she is knowledgeable. The patient and family need to be educated about the nutritional requirements necessary to achieve and maintain a healthy weight. For underweight patients with anorexia nervosa, a weight gain goal of 1 pound per week is reasonable for outpatient and up to 3 pounds per week for inpatient treatment. A normally active adolescent girl requires about 1500 kcal/day to maintain her weight, and many patients with anorexia nervosa consume only 600 to 1000 kcal/day.
3. If treatment is begun in an outpatient setting, the primary care physician in collaboration with the psychotherapist needs to set clear criteria with the patient and family regarding when hospitalization may be necessary. This should be part of the process of goal-setting and planning for changing unhealthy behaviors such as binging, vomiting, dieting, excessive exercising, and so on.
4. The primary physician should monitor and manage the physiologic complications of the eating disorder, including starvation; vomiting; excessive laxative, diuretic, or diet pill abuse; amenorrhea; pubertal delay osteopenia; and others.

Key Treatment

- Nutritional management
- Psychiatric consultation and management

Indications for Hospitalization

1. Physiologic
   a. Weight of 30 per cent or more below ideal body weight
   b. Severe metabolic or cardiovascular disturbance
   c. Significant infection in a malnourished patient
   d. An unusual presentation requiring diagnostic confirmation
   e. Failure of outpatient treatment
2. Psychiatric
   a. Severe depression or suicide risk
   b. Acute psychosis
   c. Uncontrollable binging and purging
   d. Acute food refusal
   e. Severe family dysfunction or family crisis

Outcome

Anorexia Nervosa

1. Approximately 50 per cent of patients are cured.
2. Another one third of patients get better but continue to have dysfunctional eating, body image distortion, and impaired social relationships but function well academically and occupationally.
3. About 15 per cent remain chronically ill.

Bulimia Nervosa

1. Bulimia nervosa has only recently been recognized as a disease, so there are no long-term studies of prognosis.
2. Esophageal tears from severe repetitive vomiting, cardiac arrhythmias from hypokalemia due to vomiting and diuretic abuse, cardiomyopathy, and death from ipecac use are some of the lethal complications.
3. Antidepressant medications have been shown to be effective. Twelve-month follow-up studies show recovery rates up to 70 per cent, but frequent relapses are seen.
4. Lower recovery rates are noted in those who need inpatient care or those with concurrent alcohol abuse.

B Bibliography

Boeck MA: Bulimia nervosa. *In* Friedman SB, Fisher M, Schonberg SK (eds): Comprehensive Adolescent Health Care. St. Louis, Quality Medical Publishing, 1992, pp 232–237.

Comerci GD: Eating disorders in adolescents. Pediatr Rev 1988;10:37–47.

Coupey SM: Anorexia nervosa. *In* Friedman SB, Fisher M, Schonberg SK (eds): Comprehensive Adolescent Health Care. St. Louis, Quality Medical Publishing, 1992, pp 217–231.

Kreipe RE: Eating disorders among children and adolescents. Pediatr Rev 1995;16(10).

Shenker IR, Bunnell DW: Bulimia nervosa. *In* McAnarney ER, Kreipe RE, Orr DP, Comerci GD (eds): Textbook of Adolescent Medicine. Philadelphia, WB Saunders, 1992, pp 542–546.

38 Substance Abuse

Wendy Neal

Definition

1. Illicit drug and alcohol use among adolescents in the United States remains at high levels. Most adults who are substance abusers or are substance dependent began using drugs during their teens.
2. Teenagers and preteens usually begin experimentation with inhalants, alcohol, and tobacco. Progression to marijuana use is not infrequent. The use of these "gateway" drugs may be discontinued after a brief period of experimentation or on entrance into adult life. Alternatively, adolescents who regularly use "gateway" substances may develop a physiologic as well as psychological tolerance, with the potential for escalation of the drug use pattern to include the use of barbiturates, opiates, cocaine, and other more dangerous psychoactive substances.

Alcohol

Epidemiology

Annual national surveys and research reveal:

1. Alcohol use has always been and remains very high among American youth.
2. Intoxication secondary to such use is a major cause of morbidity and mortality among adolescents.
3. The 1993 Youth Risk Behavior Surveillance Survey found that nationwide more than 80 per cent of high school students had had a drink of alcohol.
4. The Monitoring the Future survey of 1994 showed that one in seven 8th-graders (14.5 per cent), one in four 10th-graders (23.6 per cent), and more than one in four 12th-graders (28.2 per cent) had had five or more drinks in a row within the previous 2 weeks.
5. Male adolescents report a higher rate of episodic heavy drinking than female adolescents; however, this difference has been narrowing over the past few years.
6. Children of alcoholic parents are four to five times more likely to abuse alcohol than other adolescents.

Pharmacology

1. Ethyl alcohol is produced by fermentation or distillation (higher potency) of the starch or sugar in several fruits and grains (e.g., beer—5 per cent from barley and hops; wine—10 to 15 per cent from grapes; and scotch, rum, gin, and so on—45 per cent from distilled barley, corn, sugar cane, and other grains, tubers, and fruits.
2. After ingestion, alcohol is rapidly absorbed from the gastrointestinal tract into the bloodstream; fatty and high protein foods delay absorption.
3. Alcohol is metabolized in the liver by the enzyme alcohol dehydrogenase.
4. Pharmacologic effects occur approximately 10 minutes after ingestion and peak at 40 to 60 minutes.

Consequences of Use

1. Medical consequences: Alcohol is a central nervous system (CNS) depressant that can cause a spectrum of problems, including:
   a. Euphoria and disinhibition
   b. Impaired judgment
   c. Impaired muscle coordination and slowed reaction time
   d. Impaired sensory function
   e. Loss of motor and emotional control
   f. With overdose—hypoglycemia, respiratory depression, loss of consciousness, and rarely death
2. Social consequences secondary to diminished judgment can lead to:
   a. Engaging in other risk-taking behaviors (e.g., unpro-

tected intercourse, use of other illicit drugs, antisocial behaviors)

b. Automobile accidents. In 1994, 44 per cent of fatal automobile collisions involving adolescents, accounting for nearly 1600 deaths, were secondary to intoxication with alcohol.

c. Higher rates of drownings, fatal falls, homicides, and suicides, which have been shown to be secondary to alcohol intoxication

Treatment

Treatment should be adjusted to the level of alcohol involvement of the particular teenager:

1. Counseling regarding the dangers of alcohol use and, in particular, the consequences of driving while intoxicated should be a part of routine anticipatory guidance for all adolescents.
2. Community support groups (Alcohol Anonymous [AA], Alateen) may be considered for the adolescent whose drinking has become problematic, as manifested by poor school performance, frequent intoxication, and repetitive automobile accidents.
3. Residential treatment centers specializing in the care of alcoholism or drug abuse problems would be appropriate for the adolescent whose drinking is out of control with indications of alcohol dependence.
4. Antabuse, a drug that causes unpleasant side effects (e.g., headaches, nausea, dizziness) when consumed with alcohol, may be used as an adjunct to other therapies in selected, motivated teenagers.

Key Treatment: Alcohol

- Counseling
- Residential treatment
- Antabuse

Cocaine

Epidemiology

1. Use among adolescents peaked approximately a decade ago and then experienced a sharp decline coincident with well-publicized cocaine-related fatalities among prominent sports and entertainment personalities.
2. In recent years there has been a gradual increase in use among adolescents. The 1994 Monitoring the Future data revealed 3.6 per cent of 8th graders, 4.3 per cent of 10th graders, and 5.9 per cent of 12th graders reported having used cocaine.
3. The recent increase in use is attributed to the easy availability of cocaine, the decreased perceived danger of the drug, and the affordability of "crack" cocaine.

Pharmacology

1. Cocaine is a substance extracted from the *Erythroxylum coca* plant that has three main pharmacologic actions:
   a. A local anesthetic
   b. A CNS stimulant
   c. A peripheral sympathomimetic
2. Cocaine is available in various forms:
   a. Cocaine hydrochloride powder—snorted
   b. Liquefied powder—used intravenously; when combined with heroin called a speedball
   c. "Crack" or freebase—smoked

Consequences of Use

1. Medical consequences of use include:
   a. High addictive potential
   b. Seizures
   c. Cardiac arrhythmias
   d. Hypertension
   e. Hyperthermia
   f. Respiratory illnesses and, rarely, respiratory arrest
   g. Nasal sores and bleeding—chronic snorting
   h. Complications of intravenous drug use—i.e., hepatitis, human immunodeficiency virus infection (more often related to sexual activities associated with obtaining cocaine)
   i. Death
2. Social/behavioral consequences of use include:
   a. Marked alteration in mood, which may result in aggressive, antisocial, and risk-taking behaviors, such as violence, criminality, and prostitution (associated with the need to support an expensive drug habit)
   b. Social withdrawal and poor school performance
   c. Depression—suicidal ideation

Treatment

1. There is no specific drug antagonist to cocaine.
2. Acute overdose is managed supportively with particular attention to cardiac and respiratory status.
3. Multiple therapeutic approaches, including family, group, and individual therapy on an outpatient basis would be appropriate for adolescents who are free of heavy drug involvement.
4. Residential treatment centers and therapeutic communities would be most appropriate for adolescents with heavier drug involvement.

Key Treatment: Cocaine

- Acute toxicity–cardiorespiratory support
- Group therapy (for moderate usage)
- Residential treatment

Inhalants

Epidemiology

1. Highest use is reported among preteens and younger teens.
2. In 1994, approximately one in every eight students in the eighth grade reported current inhalant use.
3. Easy availability contributes to extent of use among very young adolescents.

4. Some common household products that may be abused include cleaning fluid, glue, lighter fluid, paints, shoe polish, aerosols, and gasoline.
5. An early pattern of getting high is set, and these products may act as "gateway" substances.

Pharmacology

1. Various patterns of use include:
   a. Sniffing vapors from an open container
   b. "Huffing"—inhaling fumes from a cloth soaked with a volatile substance
   c. "Bagging"—placing or spraying inhalant into a bag then inhaling the concentrated fumes
2. Inhalants are highly lipophilic agents that rapidly enter the circulation and are transported to the brain.

Consequences of Use

A wide range of effects occur depending on material employed and duration of use, including:

1. Euphoria and exhilaration
2. Nausea and vomiting
3. Confusion, ataxia, areflexia
4. Seizures
5. Cardiac arrest secondary to arrhythmias
6. Toxic hepatitis
7. Accidental deaths due to intoxication
8. Tolerance and withdrawal not encountered

Treatment

1. Supportive care is given for acute toxicity.
2. Medical management is geared to the toxic agent.
3. Counseling regarding potential for harm from intoxication and toxicity is provided.
4. When behavior is encountered in an older adolescent or young adult, it is most often a marker of serious psychopathology requiring aggressive intervention.

Key Treatment: Inhalants

• Counseling

Marijuana

Epidemiology

1. Rarely used by adolescents before the 1960s, marijuana has become a popular intoxicant among teenagers worldwide.
2. In 1994, annual use among 8th graders rose to 13 per cent vs. 6.2 per cent in 1991; in 10th graders, it was 25.2 per cent vs. 16.5 per cent; and in 12th graders, it was 30.7 per cent vs. 23.9 per cent.
3. Reported daily use also increased across all grade levels during this time period.

Pharmacology

1. Marijuana is derived from the hemp plant *(Cannabis sativa)*.
2. The active ingredient is δ-9-tetrahydrocannabinol (THC).
3. Hashish, the resinous exudate from top of the female plant, contains a very high concentration of THC.

4. It is rapidly distributed to tissues throughout the body from the bloodstream.
5. It can be smoked or ingested.

Consequences of Use

1. Most medical consequences relate to chronic and heavy use.
2. Acute increase in heart rate and blood pressure is rarely of clinical significance.
3. Panic attacks are similar to those experienced with other intoxicants, including alcohol.
4. A decrease in sperm count and motility with heavy chronic use is reversible with discontinuation of the drug and has not been associated with male infertility; however, reports of concomitant changes in testosterone levels are a concern in the developing adolescent.
5. Initially bronchodilation occurs with subsequent bronchoconstriction (a concern in teenagers with reactive airway disease); precancerous bronchial changes are reported with chronic use.
6. Behavioral consequences are of far greater concern than somatic consequences.
   a. A state of euphoria is induced and motor ability is impaired.
   b. Euphoria and disinhibition occur.
   c. Coordination is decreased, reaction time is delayed, and ability to track moving objects is impaired—all impact on ability to operate a motor vehicle or mechanical equipment.
   d. Deficits in ability to learn and short-term memory occur, which are major concerns in a scholastic setting.
   e. "Amotivational syndrome" with loss of goal-directed activity is associated with chronic use.
   f. Panic attacks and delirium may occur but are uncommon.

Treatment

1. No antidote
2. Supportive care for acute reactions and panic attacks
3. Anticipatory as per alcohol use
4. Therapeutic treatment programs for chronic users

Key Treatment: Marijuana

• Counseling

Opiates and Congeners

Epidemiology

1. Rarely used by adolescents before the 1960s, use of opiates became epidemic in the late 1960s and early 1970s, with a major impact on the society secondary to serious morbidity, mortality, addiction, and criminality associated with the sale and procurement of opiates, particularly heroin. After a sharp decline in adolescent opiate involvement, in recent years a small increase in use has been reported.

2. Current data from high school surveys indicate that less than 1 per cent of students report any long-term use of opiates.

3. Because of the high dropout rate among opiate users, school surveys almost certainly underrepresent the prevalence of use.

Pharmacology

1. Sedative analgesics are naturally derived from opium, yielding morphine and codeine.

2. Semisynthetic preparations include heroin, oxycodone (Percocet), and hydromorphone (Dilaudid).

3. Synthetic compounds include methadone (Dolophine), meperidine (Demerol), propoxyphene (Darvocet), and pentazocine (Talwin).

4. They can be smoked, snorted, injected subcutaneously ("skin popping") or intravenously, and taken orally.

5. Orally administered opiates are rapidly absorbed and undergo first-pass liver extraction and metabolism.

6. Heroin is quickly metabolized to morphine, which is conjugated in the liver and rapidly excreted in the urine.

Consequences of Use

1. Pharmacologic
   a. Intense euphoria
   b. CNS and respiratory depression
   c. Miosis
   d. Constipation
   e. Amenorrhea and anovulatory cycles
   f. Pulmonary edema, hypotension, circulatory collapse—with overdose

2. Related to the route of administration—most major somatic consequences of opiate abuse are infectious and relate to lack of sterile technique in the intravenous administration of the drug.
   a. Hepatitis
   b. Skin abscesses, cellulitis, and thrombophlebitis
   c. Subacute bacterial endocarditis
   d. Human immunodeficiency virus infection leading to the acquired immunodeficiency syndrome
   e. Nasal ulcerations (from "snorting")

3. Social/behavioral
   a. High addiction potential
   b. Involvement in drug subculture with prostitution (the exchange of sex for drugs), criminality, and incarceration commonplace
   c. Violence as a concomitant of the drug subculture

Treatment

1. Acute overdose
   a. Respiratory support
   b. Intravenous naloxone (antagonist)
   c. Chest radiograph for pneumonia or pulmonary edema

2. Physiologic addiction/abstinence syndrome—rarely pronounced in adolescents
   a. Abstinence syndrome is characterized by lacrimation, gooseflesh, dilated pupils, mild hypertension,

tachycardia, elevated temperature, muscle cramps, abdominal pain, diarrhea, insomnia, and, rarely, seizures.

   b. Treatment of abstinence syndrome takes 1 to 2 weeks; options include methadone (initial dose: 20–30 mg PO daily as a single dose reduced by 5 mg every 1 to 2 days until abstinent); alternatively, diazepam (10 mg q6h for 3 to 5 days).

   c. Detoxification alone seldom results in long-term abstinence and therefore should be combined with referral to a drug treatment program.

   d. Most successful long-term treatment programs use therapeutic community model.

   e. Methadone maintenance programs should not be used as a first resort for most adolescents because experience has demonstrated that only a minority of adolescents will be able to use this modality as a stepping stone to complete abstinence; therefore, entrance into such a program may result in a long-term or even lifelong commitment.

Key Treatment: Opiates and Congeners

- Overdosage
  Intravenous naloxone
  Ventilatory support

- Abstinence syndrome
  Methadone

- Long term
  Methadone

Barbiturates

Epidemiology

Barbiturates are not currently (1996) a major drug of abuse among adolescents.

1. Prevalence of abuse has markedly decreased since the 11 per cent rate reported by high school seniors in the 1970s.

2. Among 12th graders in 1994, 7.0 per cent had tried barbiturates.

Pharmacology

1. Parent compound is barbituric acid.

2. Degree of lipid solubility determines onset and duration of action, as well as degree of hypnotic activity.

3. Short-acting drugs have the highest degree of lipid solubility.
   a. Phenobarbital—long acting, 12–24 hours
   b. Secobarbital ("reds")—long acting
   c. Amobarbital ("blues")—intermediate, 8–10 hours
   d. Pentobarbital ("yellow jackets")—short, 4–8 hours

4. Drugs can be taken orally or by subcutaneous injection.

5. Drugs are metabolized in the liver and excreted in the urine.

Consequences of Use

1. Medical—range from mild sedation to coma

a. Ataxia
b. Nystagmus
c. Impaired speech
d. Miosis
e. Decreased gastric motility
f. Severe, at times life-threatening, "abstinence syndrome"
g. Respiratory depression and arrest with overdose
2. Social—highly addictive
a. Effects potentiated by ingestion with alcohol
b. Impaired judgment—increased risk of trauma, accidents, and risk-taking behaviors.

Treatment
1. Overdose
a. Prevent further absorption of drug.
b. Conscious patient: give ipecac; perform gastric lavage; give activated charcoal.
c. Unconscious patient: protect airway before gastric lavage.
d. Supportive therapy: administer fluids; monitor electrolytes, urine output, and serum drug levels.
e. Intubation and respiratory support may be required for severe overdose.
2. Abstinence syndrome
a. Fatal consequence is possible in chronic abusers (>500 mg daily for at least 1 month).
b. Chronic abusers should undergo detoxification in an inpatient setting to prevent serious consequences.
c. Hypotension progresses to shock.
d. Prevention of abstinence syndrome requires administration of a barbiturate in sufficient dosage as to cause mild toxicity and then slow reduction in dose over days.
e. If too little barbiturate is administered, abstinence syndrome may occur; if too much is given, respiratory depression may evolve; close observation and careful monitoring are required.

Key Treatment: Barbiturates

• Toxic dose
  Protect airway
  Provide intravenous fluid infusion
• Abstinence syndrome
  Administer and taper barbiturate dose

Tobacco

Epidemiology
Nicotine dependence should be viewed as a pediatric disease because a large majority of chronically addicted adult smokers began smoking before the age of 18.

1. One fourth of high school students surveyed nationwide (equal number of males and females) report daily cigarette use.

2. More than 10 per cent of high school student (male predominance) report use of smokeless tobacco.

Pharmacology
Nicotine, a natural alkaloid, is the active ingredient in tobacco.

1. Nicotine receptors in the CNS are acted on, producing stimulation and relaxation.
2. Cholinergic synapses in the peripheral nervous system are blocked, yielding sympathomimetic effects.
3. Nicotine is deactivated in the liver and excreted in the kidneys.
4. Higher levels of carbon monoxide in smokers lead to decreased oxygen-carrying capacity.
5. Tars and other carcinogens in tobacco are associated with malignancies.

Consequences of Use
1. Nicotine is both toxic and addictive.
2. Common complaints in adolescents include cough, sputum production, bronchitis, and dyspnea on exertion.
3. Use by pregnant adolescents is associated with prematurity and low birth weight infants.
4. Tolerance and dependence develop quickly.
5. Chronic use is associated with lung cancer and cardiovascular disease, leading causes of premature death in adults.
6. An additional environmental concern is morbidity in nonsmokers from passive inhalation (second-hand smoking).

Treatment
1. Prevention of onset of behavior; discussion of smoking as a routine part of anticipatory guidance for adolescents
2. Urging adolescents who smoke to stop with potential referral to a smoking cessation program
3. Use of nicotine gum or patches alone or in combination with a smoking cessation program

Key Treatment: Tobacco

• Counseling
• Nicotine gum or patches

Laboratory Testing

General Considerations
1. The vast majority of abused substances can be detected in blood or urine for days to weeks after use.
2. Although mandatory drug screening is a routine part of many substance abuse treatment programs, there is major concern regarding the involuntary (nonconsensual) testing of adolescents within routine practice settings; published policy of the American Academy of Pediatrics states that drug testing of the older, competent adolescent should be voluntary.
3. To ensure that test results are accurate and of therapeutic value the laboratory method employed must be reliable and care must be taken to prevent adulteration of the sample by a knowledgeable adolescent.
4. It is most often best to begin with a less expensive and

less sensitive screening test and later confirm positive results with a more expensive and sensitive laboratory procedure.
5. Information obtained from drug screening should be used for therapeutic rather than punitive purposes.

Screening Tests

Screening tests are less sensitive, less expensive, and subject to false-negative and false-positive results.

1. Radioimmunoassay (RIA)
2. Fluorescent polarization immunoassay (FPIA)
3. Enzyme-multiplied immunoassay test (EMIT)
4. Latex agglutination test (ONTRAK)
5. Thin-layer chromatography (TLC)—rarely used

Confirmatory Tests

Confirmatory tests are more sensitive, more expensive, and far less subject to false-positive or false-negative results.

1. Gas chromatography
2. High-performance liquid chromatography
3. Gas chromatography/mass spectrometry—currently most commonly used

Prevention Through Education

1. Coincident with the emergence of substance abuse as a major adolescent problem has been the evolution of a series of prevention initiatives.
2. Evaluation of these prevention initiatives indicates that some are of little or no value whereas others appear to be efficacious.
3. Prevention initiatives may be categorized into four general approaches.
    a. Factual knowledge
        (1) Based on the assumption that increased knowledge of the harmful effects of drugs would be an effective deterrent
        (2) Often uses fear as well as facts
        (3) No data to support efficacy
    b. Affective education
        (1) Designed to enhance self-esteem
        (2) Encourages responsible decision making
        (3) Often does not address issues of peer pressure
        (4) Insufficient emphasis on skills training
        (5) No data to support efficacy
    c. Social influences approach
        (1) Makes students aware of social influences promoting drug use
        (2) Teaches specific skills, including refusal skills
        (3) Corrects misconceptions of societal norms
        (4) Has demonstrated efficacy in reducing the onset of smoking; if not reinforced, effects decay over time
    d. Personal and social skills approach
        (1) Includes the features of the social influences approach
        (2) Emphasizes acquiring generic personal and social skills
        (3) Appears to be generalizable to other areas of behavioral dysfunction
        (4) Data that support short and long-term efficacy

B Bibliography

American Academy of Pediatrics and the Center for Advanced Health Studies: Specific drugs. *In* Schonberg SK (ed): Substance Abuse: A Guide for Health Professionals. Elk Grove Village, IL, American Academy of Pediatrics, 1988, pp 115–176.
Botvin G, Botvin EM: Adolescent tobacco, alcohol, and drug abuse: Prevention strategies, empirical findings, and assessment issues. J Dev Behav Pediatr 1992;13:290–301.
Brown R, Coupey SM: Illicit drugs of abuse. Adolescent Medicine: State of the Art Reviews 1993;4:321–340.
Johnston L, O'Malley PM: National survey results on drug use from the Monitoring the Future study, 1975–1994. U.S. Dept. of Health and Human Services, NIH National Institute on Drug Abuse, NIH publication No. 96-4026, 1995.

39 Contraception

Elizabeth M. Alderman

The United States has the highest adolescent pregnancy rate of all developed nations. Most reports link adolescent pregnancy to the lack of access and use of contraception. Adolescents usually do not seek contraception until at least 1 year after becoming sexually active. The majority of pregnancies in adolescents are unintended. Slightly more adolescents elect to continue a pregnancy to term than to terminate it.

Contraceptive services for adolescents should include confidential and comprehensive healthcare, including gynecologic care, with screening for, and prevention and treatment of, sexually transmitted diseases (STDs).

Factors to Consider When Prescribing Contraception to Adolescents

1. Effectiveness
    a. Inherent
    b. Characteristics of user

2. Safety
   a. Contraindications
   b. Side effects
3. Noncontraceptive benefits
4. Personal considerations
   a. Cost
   b. Stage of reproductive life
   c. Pattern of sexual activity
   d. Access to medical care

Methods of Contraception

Contraceptive methods may be divided into four categories:

- Hormonal
- Barrier
- Fertility awareness
- Emergency contraception (postcoital contraception)

Hormonal Methods

1. Combination oral contraceptive pills (OCPs)
   a. OCPs consist of estrogen and progestin and prevent pregnancy by inhibiting ovulation, preventing implantation, and creating a thick cervical mucus.
   b. If taken daily, they are an extremely effective method of contraception.
   c. However, OCPs do not protect against STDs; thus, condoms should be used concomitantly.
   d. Contraindications to prescribing OCPs include:
      (1) History of thromboembolic disease
      (2) History of cerebrovascular accident
      (3) History of coronary artery disease
      (4) History of breast cancer or any estrogen-dependent neoplasm
      (5) Liver disease and benign hepatic adenoma
      (6) Pregnancy
   e. OCPs must be taken daily, preferably at the same time each day.
   f. The adolescent may experience nausea, breakthrough bleeding or amenorrhea, weight gain, acne, mastalgia, and depression.
   g. Potentially dangerous side effects include loss of vision, deep vein thrombosis, pulmonary embolus, and stroke.
   h. Noncontraceptive benefits of OCPs include alleviating dysmenorrhea, treating simple ovarian cysts, and control of menorrhagia.
2. Depo-medroxyprogesterone acetate (DMPA, Depo-Provera)
   a. DMPA contains only progestin and prevents pregnancy by much the same mechanisms as OCPs.
   b. DMPA is administered as an intramuscular injection of 150 mg every 3 months.
   c. It is an extremely effective method of contraception, but condoms must be used for prevention of STDs.
   d. Common side effects of DMPA include:
      (1) Menstrual irregularity, first as spotting and progressing to amenorrhea

      (2) Weight gain
      (3) Headaches
   e. The product label lists the same contraindications as for OCPs; however, because DMPA does not contain estrogen, it may be a good choice for adolescents who have experienced estrogen-related side effects of OCPs.
   f. After discontinuation of DMPA, the average time of conception is 6 months.
3. Levonorgestrel (Norplant)
   a. This progestin-only contraceptive consists of six thin rods implanted in the upper arm.
   b. Contraception is provided for 5 years, but there is no STD protection.
   c. Side effects and contraindications are similar to those of DMPA except irregular menstrual periods are more common and persistent.
   d. Once the implant is removed, pregnancy may occur.
4. Mini-pill (progestin-only pill)
   a. The mini-pill, as opposed to OCPs, contains only progestin.
   b. Daily compliance, with the pill taken consistently, at the same time each day, is important.
   c. Major side effect is irregular bleeding.
   d. This is a good method for an adolescent who does not wish to experience the estrogenic side effects of OCPs but wants an immediately reversible method of contraception, as opposed to DMPA or levonorgestrel, which rely on time and medical personnel, respectively.

Barrier Methods

1. Barrier methods include:
   a. Condom, both male and female controlled
   b. Diaphragm
   c. Cervical cap
2. Spermicides are included in this section because they augment the contraceptive efficacy of barrier methods.
3. These methods are not only effective in preventing pregnancy in the consistent user but also provide protection against STDs, including infection with the human immunodeficiency virus (HIV).
4. Because these methods must be used with each act of intercourse, their success in preventing pregnancy is extremely user dependent.
5. Male-controlled condoms
   a. Condoms are the oldest and, when used with spermicide, the most effective barrier.
   b. They are the most popular method of contraception in adolescents.
   c. Most condoms are made of latex and are lubricated with nonoxynol-9, a spermicide.
   d. For adolescents with a latex allergy, natural membrane condoms may be used, but these do not protect against STDs. A new type of condom, made of polyurethane, may also be used by those allergic to latex.
   e. Condoms may be bought without a prescription and

are, thus, highly accessible and relatively inexpensive.

f. They are the only method of contraception that requires male participation.

g. The only contraindication to condom use is latex allergy.

6. Female condoms

a. Female condoms are the newest method of contraception.

b. They are made of polyurethane and designed to cover the perineum, fit in the vagina, and thus cover the cervix and vaginal lining.

c. They are cumbersome, but adolescent girls who use them believe that they give them control of an effective barrier contraceptive and method of STD prevention.

d. They may be inserted up to 8 hours before intercourse.

7. Diaphragm

a. A diaphragm is a domelike cover of the cervix.

b. It must be inserted with spermicidal cream or jelly up to 6 hours before intercourse and must be left in place for at least 6 hours afterward with a reapplication of spermicide if intercourse occurs more than once during that time.

c. The diaphragm must be fitted by a medical professional and should be replaced every 1 to 2 years or if the adolescent has lost or gained more than 5 pounds.

d. The diaphragm provides protection against pathogens that cause cervicitis. However, it is not completely protective against HIV infection because the vaginal mucosa is exposed.

e. Diaphragm use is contraindicated in girls with abnormal vaginal anatomy and multiple urinary tract infections.

f. Toxic shock syndrome (TSS) may occur if a diaphragm is left in the vagina for more than 12 hours.

8. Cervical cap

a. The cervical cap fits directly onto the cervix and provides contraception for 48 hours with no additional application of spermicide.

b. It must be fitted by a skilled practitioner and must be replaced every 3 years.

c. Spermicide should be used concurrently.

d. The cervical cap provides some degree of STD protection.

e. Papanicolaou (Pap) smears must be monitored closely in girls using the cap, and its use is contraindicated in girls with abnormal Pap smears.

f. As with the diaphragm, there is a risk of TSS if the device is not removed within 48 hours.

9. Spermicide

a. Spermicides may be used alone or with barrier methods as contraception.

b. They provide a degree of STD protection.

c. Spermicides may be bought over-the-counter as either foams, jellies, creams, or intravaginal suppositories.

d. They must be used at the time of intercourse and reapplied each time.

e. Spermicides may cause genital irritation, and some are allergenic.

Fertility Awareness

1. These methods are the least effective means of preventing pregnancy. They are only useful in girls with regular menstrual cycles.

2. However, fertility awareness methods are very inexpensive and may augment the use of other contraception, especially barrier methods.

3. Calendar charting or rhythm method

a. A female is most fertile around the time of ovulation. Ovulation occurs between days 12 and 16 before the onset of the next menses.

b. A sperm is viable for 2 to 3 days and an ovum is viable for 1 day; hence a girl is most fertile 9 to 16 days before menses.

c. Avoidance of intercourse during this period of fertility is a method of contraception.

4. Basal body temperature (BBT)

a. The adolescent must take her temperature with a special BBT thermometer on awakening in the morning.

b. A decreased BBT usually precedes ovulation.

c. A girl must chart her BBT for a few months to document her own pattern and then avoid intercourse on days of increased fertility.

Emergency Contraception (Postcoital Contraception)

a. A regimen of OCPs may be used within 72 hours, but preferably within 24 hours, of intercourse to prevent an undesired pregnancy.

b. The regimen consists of two doses of either 2 Ovral pills or 4 Lo/Ovral, Nordette, or yellow Triphasil or Tri-Levelen pills, taken 12 hours apart.

c. Before administration of the pills, a pregnancy test must be performed to assess for prior pregnancy.

d. The patient must agree to terminate the pregnancy if the emergency contraception is not effective.

Contraceptive Methods Not Generally Suitable for Adolescents

1. Intrauterine device (IUD)

a. The IUD is a copper, T-shaped device that is placed in the uterus and prevents implantation and development of a viable pregnancy.

b. It is an effective method of contraception, but, because the string that is attached for its removal serves as a nidus for ascending infection, it creates a risk for serious consequences of STD, such as salpingitis, endometritis, and future infertility.

c. The IUD may be considered for the older, monogamous adolescent who has already had children and who does not wish to use one of the hormonal contraceptive methods.

2. Male or female sterilization
   a. These methods are not contraceptive alternatives for adolescents.
   b. This is particularly true for female sterilization, which is generally irreversible.
   c. The adolescent is not at a maturity stage to make such a permanent decision regarding future reproductive potential.

Bibliography

American Academy of Pediatrics: Contraception and adolescents. Pediatrics 1990;86:134–138.

Coupey SM, Klerman LV: Adolescent sexuality. *In* Adolescent State of the Art Reviews, vol 3 (2). Philadelphia, Hanley & Belfus, 1992.

Davis AJ: Contraceptive choices: the adolescent years. Dialogues Contraception 1995;4(6):1–4.

Hatcher RA, Trussell J, Stewart F, et al: Contraceptive Technology, 16th ed. New York, Irvington Publishers, 1994.

40 Sexually Transmitted Diseases

Neal Hoffman

1. Sexually transmitted disease (STD) rates are highest among sexually experienced adolescents compared with any other age group.
2. STD interrelationships
   a. STDs share a common mode of transmission; therefore, a diagnosis of one STD serves as a marker of risk for other STDs.
   b. Many STDs facilitate human immunodeficiency virus (HIV) acquisition and may accelerate the progression of HIV infection; HIV infection alters many clinical aspects of other STDs.
3. Consistent use of latex condoms and other barriers prevents STD transmission.

Viral Infections

Hepatitis B Virus (HBV)
Epidemiology
1. Injection drug use and receptive anal intercourse for both men and women contributes increased risk for hepatitis B infection.
2. The per cent of cases attributable to male-to-male contact has markedly declined, whereas heterosexual transmission has increased.

Clinical Findings
1. HBV has an incubation period of 50 to 180 days.
2. Ten per cent of patients never resolve the 6-week acute illness, thereby becoming chronic carriers.

Key Clinical Findings: Viral Infections

- Hepatomegaly
- Jaundice

Prevention
1. The American Academy of Pediatrics recommends vaccination for all adolescents; screening for past infection is necessary only for those living in endemic areas and those at high risk for HBV infection (e.g., homosexual youth, intravenous drug users, HIV-positive youth, and street youth).
2. The schedule is three injections of the recombinant yeast-derived vaccine at 0, 1, and 6 months; serologic confirmation 1 month after the last dose is only indicated in HIV-infected adolescents.

Human Papillomavirus (HPV)
Epidemiology
1. Genital HPV is most prevalent in women younger than 25 years of age.
2. Two thirds of adolescent women with genital warts also have cervical disease.

Pathophysiology
1. HPV types 6 and 11 are associated with condylomata acuminata and low-grade cervical dysplasia.
2. Types 16, 18, 31, 33, and 35 are most often associated with high-grade dysplasia and invasive carcinoma.

Clinical Findings
1. The majority of infections are subclinical; screening for subclinical infection is not recommended.
2. Most infections do not progress to significant dysplasia, but women younger than 25 years of age with atypia on Papanicolaou (Pap) smear have a threefold greater relative risk of developing severe dysplasia/invasive disease than older women.

Key Clinical Finding: HPV

- Condylomata acuminata in genital region

Management
1. Treatment of subclinical HPV infection is not presently recommended because the virus itself is not eliminated even when clinically evident disease has been removed.
2. The purpose of treating patients with clinically evident

disease is to alleviate symptoms and to limit transmission to sexual partners.

3. Podophyllin (contraindicated in pregnancy), trichloracetic acid applied locally, and cryotherapy remain the primary methods for treatment of penile, vulvar, and perirectal lesions.

4. Trichloracetic acid and cryotherapy can be used for vaginal and rectal warts; podophyllin may be too irritating; cryotherapy and podophyllin can be used at the urethral meatus.

5. More extensive disease can be managed with CO_2 laser or surgery.

6. High-grade cervical dysplasia should be treated with cryotherapy, local excisional biopsy, or conization, depending on the degree of dysplasia, with close follow-up.

7. Yearly external and internal examinations with cervical Pap smear are recommended after age 19, and earlier for those with sexual experience, especially those with genital warts.

8. Colposcopic examination should be done, if cervical cytologic findings are abnormal, to guide biopsies.

9. Women with HIV infection and other forms of immunosuppression may have more accelerated disease, requiring biannual monitoring.

Key Treatment: HPV

- Podophyllin
- Trichloracetic acid
- Cryotherapy

Herpes Simplex Virus (HSV)

Clinical Findings

1. Painful vesicles or ulcers, single or grouped, appear 2 to 21 days after exposure; primary episodes last 1 to 3 weeks, often with fever, malaise, and lymphadenopathy.

2. Recurrences are often preceded by 24 hours of tingling or burning, lasting 7 to 10 days; systemic manifestations are uncommon.

3. Up to half of patients will have asymptomatic shedding of virus.

Key Clinical Findings: HSV

- Vesicles and/or ulcer in genital region
- Lymphadenopathy

Treatment

1. Systemic treatment with acyclovir, rather than topical treatment, can shorten symptom duration if started early in the course of the infection.

2. For primary and recurrent episodes, one can use acyclovir 200 mg orally five times daily for 7 days or until healing is complete; immunocompromised patients may require 400 to 800 mg orally five times daily.

3. Suppressive therapy for more than six episodes per year is recommended, using 200 mg three times daily for as long as 6 to 12 months.

4. Treatment does not eliminate asymptomatic viral shedding.

Key Treatment: HSV

- Acyclovir

BACTERIAL INFECTIONS

Syphilis

Epidemiology

1. The incidence among homosexual men has declined, in contrast to an increase in the incidence among women and heterosexual men.

2. Among adolescents aged 15 to 19 years, the incidence of primary and secondary syphilis in females is nearly four times that in males.

3. The incidence among African American adolescents is twice that of white adolescents.

4. Treponema pallidum is spread by contact with primary chancres and condylomata lata of secondary syphilis.

Clinical Findings

1. The incubation period ranges from 10 to 90 days; nontreponemal tests (e.g., rapid plasma reagin [RPR] or Venereal Disease Research Laboratory [VDRL]) may be negative in up to 50 per cent of patients when the chancre initially appears.

2. The chancre of primary infection, which is often painless, appears as a single papule or as an indurated ulcer with raised borders and a smooth base. It resolves untreated in 3 to 6 weeks and is often unnoticed.

3. When the diagnosis of a genital or anal lesion is uncertain because of a negative serologic test, the patient should be treated for syphilis.

4. Secondary syphilis appears 3 to 6 weeks after the chancre, with a diffuse maculopapular, nonpruritic rash, with variable appearance.

5. Latent syphilis, a clinically silent stage, requires serologic confirmation, whereas the tertiary stage, occurring in half of untreated patients, has many variants.

Key Clinical Findings: Syphilis

- Chancre (rarely seen)
- Rash
- General adenopathy, including epitrochlear

Treatment

1. Treatment of primary, secondary, and early-latent (i.e., less than 1 year) syphilis consists of one intramuscular dose of benzathine penicillin G, 2.4 million units; cephalosporins are not recommended.

2. Doxycycline is an alternative in nonpregnant women, at a dose of 100 mg twice daily for 2 weeks, for penicillin-allergic patients. Erythromycin is an alternative treatment, although its failure to prevent congenital infection has been documented.

3. Treatment of late-latent syphilis requires three consecu-

tive weekly injections of benzathine penicillin G. Neuro-syphilis beyond the acute phase (and late-latent infection in HIV-infected patients with abnormal cerebrospinal fluid findings) must be treated with high-dose intravenous penicillin or a combination of intramuscular penicillin with oral probenecid for 10 to 14 days.

4. Clinical monitoring after therapy should be confirmed with serology; a fourfold increase in a nontreponemal test titer after therapy or a persistence or recurrence of signs or symptoms warrants reevaluation with lumbar puncture. HIV testing is also advised.

5. Re-treatment is recommended, using the regimen for late-latent infection, unless the cerebrospinal fluid examination indicates otherwise.

Key Treatment: Syphilis

- Penicillin
- High-dose penicillin (including during pregnancy)

Gonorrhea and Chlamydial Infection
Epidemiology
1. The age-specific rates for gonorrhea (from infection with *Neisseria gonorrhoeae*) for 15- to 19-year olds remain the highest of any age group; in contrast to the declines seen in the rest of the population, the incidence for gonorrhea has remained the same among African American adolescent women and has increased among African American adolescent men.

2. Estimates of prevalence of chlamydial infections *(Chlamydia trachomatis)* in sexually experienced adolescents range from 8 to 35 per cent for women and 8 to 22 per cent in men.

3. When adjusting for numbers of sexually experienced persons in an age group, the incidence of pelvic inflammatory disease is 1:8 for 15-year olds, compared with 1:80 for 24-year olds.

Pathogenesis
1. Young adolescent females at early stages of puberty may be at higher risk for infection as a result of exposure of endocervical columnar cells extending onto the vaginal cervix that may be more susceptible to infection by *N. gonorrhoeae* and *C. trachomatis*.

2. Thinner, and therefore, more permeable, cervical mucus, as a result of the lack of progesterone production during anovulatory cycles for up to 2 years after the onset of menarche, may explain the increased susceptibility to ascending infection.

Clinical Findings
1. Asymptomatic infection is common among adolescents, such that yearly routine screening for cervical chlamydial infection and gonorrhea is recommended for all sexually experienced adolescents.

2. Yearly screening for asymptomatic infection in males consists of testing the first 10-ml aliquot of urine for leukocyte esterase (a polymerase chain reaction to amplify chlamydial DNA is being studied for this purpose); routine screening for *C. trachomatis* directly from the male urethra is recommended in areas of high prevalence and in high-risk populations.

3. For male and female adolescents who engage in oral-genital, oral-anal, or genital-anal intercourse, cultures of the pharynx, rectum, and male urethra for *N. gonorrhoeae* are indicated for both asymptomatic screening and for purposes of making a diagnosis of clinical disease.

4. Dysuria is common in urethritis from both disorders, but a discharge is more common in gonococcal urethritis; if present, the discharge due to *C. trachomatis* is often clear.

5. Mucopurulent cervicitis is defined as yellowish discharge from the cervical os, accompanied by cervical erosion and friability; more than 10 polymorphonuclear cells can be found using Gram staining.

6. The diagnosis of pelvic inflammatory disease is often difficult but usually includes bilateral lower abdominal and adnexal tenderness and cervical motion tenderness; corroborative findings of low-grade fever, leukocytosis, or elevated sedimentation rate, with or without the identification of an organism from the cervix, are often helpful.

Key Clinical Findings: Gonorrhea and Chlamydial Infection

- Usually asymptomatic (chlamydial infection and sometimes gonorrhea)
- Urethral and/or vaginal discharge
- Pelvic inflammatory disease

Treatment
1. One should treat for both gonorrhea and chlamydial infection in instances of urethritis, pharyngitis, epididymitis, or uncomplicated cervicitis; if diagnostic techniques are unavailable; or if a diagnosis for only gonorrhea has been made, because concurrent infection with *C. trachomatis* is common and diagnostic techniques for *C. trachomatis* may not be adequate at certain institutions.

2. Within an area with a low prevalence of gonorrhea, only specific therapy should be given for chlamydial infection if a definite diagnosis has been made and Gram stain for gram-negative intracellular diplococci and cultures for gonorrhea are negative.

3. Treatment of both infections should be given in all instances of proctitis or salpingitis, even if only one agent can be identified.

4. Hospitalization for at least 7 days is recommended for all adolescent women with salpingitis to ensure completion of therapy, in an attempt to limit future complications, such as infertility and ectopic pregnancy.

5. Treatment of sexual partners is essential to effectively eradicate these infections; routine tests of cure for all are part of standard practice for adolescent patients, unless adherence to treatment can be assured for both the patient and sexual partner.

Key Treatment: Gonorrhea and Chlamydial Infection

- Cephalosporins or quinolones (gonorrhea)
- Doxycycline or azithromycin (chlamydia)

Bibliography

Bell TA, Hein K: Adolescents and sexually transmitted diseases. *In* Holmes KK, Mardh PA, Sparling PF, Wiesner PJ (eds): Sexually Transmitted Diseases. New York, McGraw-Hill, 1984, pp 73–84.

Cates W Jr: Teenagers and sexual risk taking: The best of times and the worst of times. J Adolesc Health 1991;12:84–94.

Centers for Disease Control and Prevention: STD treatment guidelines. MMWR 1993;42:1–102.

Hoffman ND, Hein K: Sexually transmitted diseases. *In* Tonkin R (ed): Current Issues of the Adolescent Patient, vol 2. London, Bailliere Tindall, 1994, pp 301–330.

Remafedi G: Fundamental issues in the care of homosexual youth. Med Clin North Am 1990;74:1169–1179.

Rosenfeld WD: Sexually transmitted diseases in adolescents. Pediatr Ann 1991;20:303–312.

41 Human Immunodeficiency Virus Infection

Donna Futterman

Epidemiology

1. Over 500,000 persons in the United States were diagnosed with the acquired immunodeficiency syndrome (AIDS) by the end of 1995, of whom 1 per cent were adolescents aged 13 to 21.
2. AIDS is the leading cause of death among Americans aged 25 to 44 years.
3. It is estimated that 1 in 4 persons with HIV infection in United States were infected by age 21 years.
4. One third of adolescents with AIDS are females, of whom at least 50 per cent acquired infection by heterosexual sexual contact.
5. Among male adolescents with AIDS, 50 per cent acquired infection by homosexual sexual contact and 25 per cent by infected blood products.
6. Ethnic and racial minority youth are disproportionately represented.

Etiology and Natural History

1. Transmission routes: HIV can be acquired by:
   a. Sexual contact (with same sex or opposite sex partners)
   b. Blood exposure (by shared or unsterilized needles or by blood transfusions before HIV screening in 1985; males with hemophilia account for 25 per cent of adolescent cases of HIV)
   c. Perinatally (in utero or during delivery); many children who were perinatally infected are now surviving into their teen years.
2. HIV multiplies rapidly in the host after infection and causes a gradual decline in immune function; there is an average of 10 years from time of infection to the development of advanced immunosuppression (AIDS) in untreated persons.
3. Measurements of viral load in blood are currently (1997) the most accurate predictor of prognosis. Newer medications have lowered viral load and improved prognoses.
4. CD4-positive T lymphocytes are both a target cell for HIV and the most accurate marker of immunosuppression. A CD4 blood cell count of less than 200/mm³ is an indicator of severe immunodeficiency (AIDS) and risk for opportunistic infection such as *Pneumocystis carinii* pneumonia, cytomegalovirus infection, and toxoplasmosis.
5. The Centers for Disease Control and Prevention (CDC) has established case definitions for AIDS that lists opportunistic infections and CD4 cell counts.
6. The HIV disease course in adolescents generally parallels that seen in adults, because most were infected after their immune system had developed; but the impact of puberty has not yet been systematically studied.

Risk Assessment/HIV Counseling and Testing

1. Recognize that all adolescents who have sexual intercourse without consistent use of latex condoms may be at risk for HIV infection.
2. Youth at increased risk for HIV infection (because of their increased chance of coming into contact with HIV) include:
   a. Illicit substance users (particularly intravenous drug users and crack cocaine users)
   b. Male adolescents who have unprotected sex with other males
   c. Youth having unprotected intercourse and living in areas with high infection rates (endemic areas)
   d. Youth who have had sexually transmitted infections
   e. Homeless and runaway youth
   f. Youth who engage in survival sex (prostitution)
   g. Youth who have been abused
3. All pregnant women should be offered and urged to have HIV testing. HIV counseling and testing (with informed consent) should also be routinely incorporated into adolescent healthcare. Important issues include:
   a. HIV counseling should be developmentally appropriate.
   b. Confidentiality should be maintained according to local laws.

c. The physiologic and mental health benefits of early diagnosis and treatment should be stressed and the risks and fears of an HIV positive diagnosis should be addressed.

d. The youth should be encouraged to identify an adult who can be supportive during the testing process.

e. Written informed consent should be obtained in accordance with local laws with the youth deciding if and when he or she is ready to consent to an HIV test.

f. Risk reduction strategies and skills should be reviewed.

g. All HIV test results should be presented in person.

h. Appropriate health, mental health, and social service referrals should be provided.

HIV Primary Care

Medical and Psychosocial History

1. Assess prior illnesses (especially sexually transmitted diseases [STDs], tuberculosis, HIV seroconversion illness, chronic illnesses), hospitalizations, prior medical care, medications, allergies, and family history.

2. Assess psychosocial history including illnesses, medications, hospitalizations, suicidal thoughts/attempts, substance use, and social history, including family relationships, living status, financial support and health insurance, school and work status, and social supports (especially who knows about their HIV status). Sexual history should also be ascertained, including age of initiation and partner age and gender, types of sexual experiences (oral, genital, and anal intercourse), sexual orientation, condom and birth control use, pregnancy, and parenting history.

3. Review of systems: assess for fatigue, appetite status, weight loss or gain, fevers, night sweats, visual changes, sinusitis, tooth or gum disease, oral infections, cough or shortness of breath, abdominal pain, diarrhea, genital pain, sores or discharge, weakness or abnormal sensations, headaches, or personality, mood, or memory changes.

Primary Care

- History of prior illnesses
- Sexual contact history
- HIV testing
- Sexually transmitted disease testing
- Tuberculin test

Physical Examination

1. Vital signs; height and weight to assess growth curves
2. General: skin, nutritional status, lymph nodes
3. Head, eyes, ears, nose, and throat: careful attention to oral examination for gum, dentition, and fungal/viral infections
4. Lungs, chest, abdomen, extremities, neurologic and mental status examination
5. Genitalia/anus: Tanner staging and thorough inspection including speculum examination for females

Laboratory Assessment

1. HIV status: repeat test for confirmation if written documentation is not obtained.
2. Virologic and immunologic assessment: obtain viral load and CD4 cell count and percentage quarterly and as necessary to monitor effects of medication.
3. Order complete blood cell count, renal and liver function tests, and urinalysis at baseline and at least annually
4. Sexually transmitted disease screening: perform syphilis serology, Chlamydia test, Neisseria gonorrhoeae culture (genital, oral, and anal), Papanicolaou smear (cervical cytology), wet prep for bacterial vaginosis or Trichomonas, and microscopy or culture of lesions for Candida, herpes, syphilis, or chancroid.
5. Perform tuberculin skin test (purified protein derivative [PPD]) with anergy panel.
6. Assess immunity to hepatitis B, toxoplasmosis, and varicella.

Immunizations

1. HIV specific: Pneumovax, influenza (yearly)
2. Adolescent specific: measles, mumps, rubella (MMR); tetanus (Td); and hepatitis B series (if not exposed or immune). Varicella vaccine is not approved for immunocompromised patients.

Medications

1. Antiretroviral medications: six medications are licensed by the Food and Drug Administration, often used in combination; doses vary by weight and are modified for side effects and toxicity, which varies by medication. Medications have demonstrated the ability to prolong life and to improve the quality of life. Eleven medications have been licensed by the FDA as of June 1997.

   a. Nucleoside analogs/reverse transcriptase inhibitors
      (1) Zidovudine (ZDV): 200 mg every 8 hours or 300 mg every 12 hours
      (2) Didanosine (ddI): 125 or 200 mg by weight every 12 hours
      (3) Zalcitabine (ddC): 0.375 or 0.75 mg by weight every 8 hours
      (4) Stavudine (d4T): 20 or 40 mg by weight every 12 hours
      (5) Lamivudine (3TC): 150 mg every 12 hours

   b. Protease inhibitors
      (1) Saquinavir (SQV): 600 mg every 8 hours
      (2) Indinavir (IDV): 800 mg every 8 hours
      (3) Ritonavir (RTV): 600 mg every 12 hours
      (4) Nelfinavir (NLV): 750 mg every 8 hours

   c. Non-nucleoside reverse transcriptase inhibitors
      (1) Nevirapine (NVP): 200 mg every 12 hours
      (2) Delavirdine (DLV): 400 mg every 8 hours.

2. Primary and secondary opportunistic infection prophylaxis

   a. Pneumocystis carinii pneumonia: leading cause of death among patients with AIDS; primary infection highly preventable with prophylaxis initiated when CD4 count is less than 200/mm³: treat with trimethoprim-sulfamethoxazole (TMP/SMX), dapsone, atovaquone, or pentamidine.

b. *Toxoplasmosis gondii* infection: provide prophylaxis for patients with *Toxoplasma* antibodies when CD4 count is less than 100/mm³ with TMP/SMX or dapsone plus pyrimethamine.

c. *Mycobacterium avium complex* infection: prophylaxis is with rifabutin or clarithromycin when CD4 count is less than 75/mm³.

d. *Mycobacterium tuberculosis* infection: provide prophylaxis if PPD test is positive or anergic with isoniazid or rifampin.

e. *Cytomegalovirus* infection: consider prophylaxis if CMV antibody is positive and CD4 count is less than 50/mm³ with ganciclovir.

f. Fungal infections (*Candida, Cryptococcus, Histoplasma,* and *Coccidioides*): consider prophylaxis when CD4 count is less than 50/mm³ with fluconazole.

3. Pregnancy: antiretroviral medications taken during pregnancy, delivery, and postnatally by the newborn can substantially reduce the rate of HIV transmission from mother to her offspring.

Psychosocial Issues

1. Coping: assess how the adolescent is coping with HIV, sources of support and to whom he or she has disclosed the infection (focus on parents/family and sexual partners). Help patient establish positive coping mechanisms.

2. Case management: establish source of coverage for health visits and medications; assess and stabilize living situation, educational and vocational status, and financial support.

3. Living will and health care proxy: develop plans as patient's immune status declines but before terminal phase of illness.

4. Risk reduction: assess for ongoing substance use and unsafe sexual behaviors and promote skills building and motivation to reduce risk for self and others.

B Bibliography

Centers for Disease Control and Prevention: US Public Health Service Guidelines for the prevention of opportunistic infections in persons infected with HIV. MMWR 1995;44:1–34.

El Sadr W, Oleske J, Agins B, et al: Evaluation and management of early HIV infection: Clinical practice guidelines. US Department of Health and Human Services, Agency for Health Care Policy and Research publication No. 94–0572, 1994.

Futterman D, Hein K: Medical management of adolescents with HIV infection. *In* Pizzo P, Wilfert C (eds): Pediatric AIDS, 2nd ed. Baltimore, Williams & Wilkins, 1994, pp 757–772.

Kunins H, Hein K, Futterman D, et al: Guide to HIV/AIDS program development. J Adolesc Health 1993;14(s):1–140.

Sande M, Volberding P (eds): The Medical Management of AIDS. Philadelphia, WB Saunders, 1992.

42 Suicide

Jacques Benhaim

Epidemiology

1. Completed suicide:

   a. Suicide is the third leading cause of death among adolescents, after accidents and homicide.

   b. Since 1950, reported mortality has increased five times for male adolescents and doubled for females.

   c. Yearly mortality approximates 5000.

   d. Sex ratio among completed adolescent suicides: male:female = 4:1

   e. Means: Males: 60 per cent firearms; 20 per cent poisoning; 15 per cent suffocation. Females: 40 per cent firearms; 30 per cent poisoning; 10 per cent suffocation.

2. Attempted suicide:

   a. Estimated ratio of attempts to completions is 50:1 to 200:1.

   b. Incidence is 100,000 to 400,000/year.

   c. Sex ratio among attempters: male:female = 1:4

   d. Twenty-five per cent attempt suicide with intention to die; 50 per cent do not expect to die; 25 per cent not sure

Risk Factors

1. Adolescent issues:

   a. Substance abuse

   b. Chronic illness (in males)

   c. Biologic depression

   d. Psychosis

   e. Gender identity issues: homosexuality

   f. Previous attempts

2. Family issues:

   a. Family disruption: divorce, separation, death of a parent

   b. Family history of attempted or completed suicide

   c. Alcoholism, substance abuse

Symptoms

Issues identified with frequency in adolescents who attempt suicide may be used to alert the practitioner to the potential for suicidal behavior. When such issues emerge the physician is obligated to inquire of the adolescent regarding suicidal ideation. Direct questions regarding thoughts of hurting oneself do not precipitate suicide and may uncover acute suicidal ideation.

1. Vegetative symptoms of depression (i.e., anorexia, insomnia, deep sadness)—relatively uncommon in adolescents
2. Somatic complaints such as headaches, chest pain, abdominal pain
3. Acting out, delinquency, truancy, early onset of sexual activity and promiscuity
4. Substance abuse
5. Running away from home
6. Difficulty concentrating, with consequent decline in performance at school or work
7. Boredom, with loss of interest in age-appropriate activities

Precipitating Event

Circumstances that are most frequently cited by adolescents as the immediate cause of a suicide attempt are often trivial, at least by adult standards and common to the lives of all adolescents, the vast majority of whom do not attempt suicide. They are not to be confused with the long-standing personal or family issues that make a particular adolescent vulnerable to suicidal behavior.

1. A conflict with parents
2. Romantic conflict with boyfriend/girlfriend
3. Loss of a loved one through either death or more commonly physical separation
4. Legal entanglements and incarceration
5. Fight with friends
6. A sexual assault—may act as a precipitant in a previously healthy adolescent

Management of a Suicide Attempt

1. Address all potentially life-threatening consequences of the attempt.
2. Strongly consider hospitalization of all adolescents who have attempted suicide. It is potentially dangerous to immediately discharge an adolescent back into the environment in which he or she just attempted suicide without absolute assurances of adequate follow-up or evaluation.
3. Immediately assess the patient for continued suicidal ideation. The minority of adolescents who continue to express suicidal ideation require close monitoring.
4. Immediately rule out psychosis. Hallucinatory adolescents are at high risk for continued self-destructive behavior.
5. Assess for degree of seriousness of the attempt as an indication of risk of future attempts and a fatal outcome. The following findings are associated with increased seriousness and greater subsequent risk:

   a. Attempt was likely to result in death (i.e., used a gun; took large number of pills; jumped in front of a moving vehicle)
   b. Adolescent did not tell anyone about the attempt (e.g., took pills in a circumstance where discovery was unlikely).
   c. Attempts are repeated.
   d. Patient remains actively suicidal.
6. Use psychiatric and social service consultation to evaluate adolescent and family to determine cause of suicidal behavior and arrive at a disposition tailored to the needs of the individual adolescent.

Key Treatment: Suicide Attempt

- Manage consequences of attempt; toxic, trauma, and so forth
- Hospitalize (usually)
- Assess ideation
- Psychiatric and social service consultation

Potential Dispositions Subsequent to an Attempt

1. Psychiatric hospitalization. This should be reserved for adolescents who are psychotic, who are suffering from a biologic depression and who may be candidates for antidepressant medications, or who for any reason are expressing continued suicidal ideation.
2. Discharge to home with behavioral support/crisis intervention for adolescent and/or family. This is appropriate for the majority of adolescents who are neither psychotic nor continually suicidal and who come from caring and concerned, albeit imperfect, homes.
3. Alternative living situation. This is appropriate for the adolescent coming from an abusive or nonsupportive home. Alternative placement with a family member is a first resort, with foster care and group homes being less desirable alternatives.

 Bibliography

Amanat E, Beck J: Teen-age suicide. *In* The Troubled Adolescent, A Practical Guide. St. Louis, Ishiyaku European, 1994, pp 213–225.

Neinstein LS: Suicide. *In* Neinstein LS (ed): Adolescent Health Care, A Practical Guide, 2nd ed. Baltimore, Williams & Wilkins, 1991, pp 935–940.

Setterberg SR: Suicidal behavior and suicide. *In* Friedman SB, Fisher M, Schonberg SK (eds): Comprehensive Adolescent Health Care. St. Louis, Quality Medical Publishing, 1992, pp 862–867.

Shaffer D, Hicks R: Suicide and suicidal behaviors. *In* McAnarney ER, Kreipe RE, Orr DP, Comerci GD (eds): Textbook of Adolescent Medicine. Philadelphia, WB Saunders, 1992, pp 979–986.

43 Menstrual Disorders

Susan R. Davis

The so-called menstrual disorders include the extremes of the normal menstrual cycle through to clear pathology, but frequently the boundaries between normal and abnormal are blurred. Common menstrual disorders are

- Dysmenorrhea
- Abnormal uterine bleeding
- Premenstrual syndrome
- Menstrual migraine.

Dysmenorrhea

Definition

Dysmenorrhea is painful menstruation (the direct Greek translation is "difficult menstrual flow").

Etiology

1. Primary dysmenorrhea (see discussion)
2. Secondary dysmenorrhea is not normally related to prostaglandin production, with the common underlying causes being pelvic inflammatory disease, endometriosis, (usually more than 3 years post menarche), fibroids (rare in adolescence), uterine outflow obstruction, or pelvic venous congestion syndrome.

Epidemiology

1. Overall, approximately 60 per cent of adolescent girls experience dysmenorrhea; however, the prevalence increases with age such that 39 per cent of 12-year-olds and 72 per cent of 17-year-olds suffer this problem.
2. Reportedly, 14 per cent of adolescents regularly miss school because of this condition. For the first 3 years after menarche, anovulatory cycles are common; hence, dysmenorrhea is less common. Dysmenorrhea is thus more frequent in late adolescence (late teens and early 20s) when ovulation is established.
3. Interestingly, beyond late adolescence the incidence of dysmenorrhea decreases with age. The decline has also been associated with young women becoming sexually active.

Pathophysiology

1. Increased levels of prostaglandins in the endometrium and menstrual fluid result in increased myometrial resting time and induction of uterine contractions causing ischemic pain. Women with primary dysmenorrhea have higher levels of endometrial prostaglandin $F_{2\alpha}$ than asymptomatic women.
2. Menstrual cramps are enhanced by alcohol and nicotine, which increase myometrial activity, and by stress, anxiety, and fear.
3. Cultural attitudes are important modulators of this condition, which is less common among females who have good health and high self esteem and are physically active.

Clinical Findings

1. The classic discomfort of dysmenorrhea is of severe spasmodic crampy lower back and suprapubic pain. Pain is maximal before heavy flow and usually only during the first 12 to 24 hours of heavy menstrual blood loss. Five to 10 per cent of those with primary dysmenorrhea have debilitating pain. Associated symptoms include nausea, vomiting, and diarrhea, possibly secondary to systemic effects of elevated levels of prostaglandins.
2. In contrast, the pain of secondary dysmenorrhea builds up over several days preceding menstruation and continues throughout menstruation.
3. The extent of clinical examination depends on severity of the dysmenorrhea and whether the patient is sexually active. A Papanicoloau smear and cultures are indicated for sexually active individuals. A bimanual rectoabdominal or vaginal examination should be performed.
4. Pelvic ultrasonography should be performed when a bimanual examination is not able to be adequately performed or for further assessment of any abnormal findings.

Treatment

1. The nonsteroidal anti-inflammatory agents (NSAIDs) inhibit prostaglandin endoperoxide synthase, hence their effectiveness in the treatment of primary dysmenorrhea. Unlike the other NSAIDs, mefenamic acid not only inhibits prostaglandin synthase but also antagonizes the action of prostaglandin at the receptor sites. This dual antiprostaglandin action makes mefenamic acid the drug of first choice for the treatment of menstrual pain. Treatment should begin at first sign of menstruation; commencing therapy any earlier does not appear to be of any advantage. Therapy results in an average of 50 per cent reduction of menstrual flow.
2. The combined oral contraceptive pill (OCP) gives complete relief in up to 50 per cent of women and marked relief in a further 30 to 40 per cent. The OCP results in an atrophic decidualized endometrium with reduced prostaglandin production.
3. Girls should also be informed about adjunctive management, such as local heat, relaxation, and massage.
4. Treatment of secondary dysmenorrhea involves diagnosis and treatment of the underlying pathologic condition.

Abnormal Uterine Bleeding

Definitions

1. Dysfunctional uterine bleeding (DUB) is abnormal uterine bleeding not due to pregnancy or pelvic pathologic process.
2. DUB classification:
   Hypermenorrhea (polymenorrhea)—cycles less than 21 days

Oligomenorrhea—cycles more than 35 days
Menorrhagia—menstrual blood loss more than 50 ml
Metromenorrhagia—heavy irregular menses

Etiology and Pathophysiology

1. Complications of pregnancy must be excluded.
2. Pelvic conditions: malignant lesions, fibroids, and pelvic inflammatory disease are rare causes of abnormal bleeding in adolescence.
3. The most common cause of DUB in adolescence is anovulation (Table 43–1). This results in chronic proliferative phase endometrium and irregular breakthrough bleeding. Causes include immaturity of the hypothalamic-pituitary axis and polycystic ovary syndrome. If untreated, the latter may result in endometrial hyperplasia.
4. DUB may occur in ovulating women with either follicular phase or luteal phase defects.
5. Severe platelet dysfunction or coagulopathy frequently results in heavy and sometimes life-threatening vaginal bleeding.

Clinical Findings

1. DUB is frequently painless, irregular, and prolonged.
2. Menstrual blood loss is clinically assessed by the duration of bleeding (>5 days), the number of tampons or pads used (soaking more than five full-sized pads daily), or the passing of menstrual clots (normal menstrual blood contains fibrinolyic compounds and does not clot).
3. The physical examination must include determination of supine and erect blood pressure, attention to signs of anemia, presence of petechiae and purpura, and a thorough abdominal examination. All sexually active girls require a pelvic examination, Papanicolaou smear, and cultures.

Laboratory Findings

1. All patients require a complete blood cell count.
2. Because iron deficiency precedes anemia, ferritin levels (reflecting iron stores) should be measured as well as those of serum iron.
3. The severity of DUB is classified on the basis of impact of blood loss: mild, hemoglobin level greater than or equal to 11 g/dl; moderate, hemoglobin level 9 to 11 g/dl; severe, hemoglobin level less than or equal to 8 g/dl.

Key Laboratory Investigations

- Complete blood cell count
- Iron studies
- Clotting profile
- Serum beta-human chorionic gonadotropin (β-hCG) (if sexually active)
- Thyroid function
- Pelvic ultrasonography (as clinically indicated)

Treatment

1. Reassurance and explanation of the condition
2. Mild to moderate DUB:

TABLE 43–1. ETIOLOGY OF DYSFUNCTIONAL UTERINE BLEEDING

OVARIAN CAUSES

Dysfunctional anovulatory bleeding
Polycystic ovarian syndrome
Follicular phase defects
Luteal phase defects
Low estrogen "threshold" bleeding
Estrogen-secreting follicular cysts

SYSTEMIC DISORDERS

Platelet dysfunction: idiopathic thrombocytopenic purpura; von Willebrand disease
Coagulopathy: primary; secondary to severe hepatic dysfunction
Thyroid disease
Leukemia, lymphoma

---

a. NSAIDs as recommended for dysmenorrhea will reduce menstrual flow up to 50 per cent.
b. Iron supplements to replete iron stores
c. Combined oral contraceptive therapy (OCT) to regulate cycles and decrease menstrual loss. A fixed, low-dose OCP is suitable for girls not actively bleeding. Alternatively, progestogen therapy in the form of medroxyprogesterone acetate, 10 to 30 mg, or norethindrone, 5 to 10 mg, can be prescribed either cyclically or continuously to stop menstruation entirely.

3. Severe DUB requires aggressive management with hospitalization and correction of hemodynamic instability with intravenous fluid replacement and transfusion as indicated.

a. Conjugated equine estrogen, 25 mg, should be administered intravenously every 4 to 6 hours until bleeding stops or four doses are given. Simultaneously, a fixed, high-dose OCP should be given every 6 hours with an antiemetic prophylactically. The frequency of the OCT should be gradually tapered to a once-daily dose after the bleeding ceases.
b. Acute bleeding unresponsive to this management within 24 hours requires dilatation and curettage, followed by high-dose OCT. Once the patient's condition has stabilized, iron supplements should be given and continued at least 3 months beyond normalization of the hemoglobin value.

Premenstrual Syndrome

Definition

Premenstrual syndrome (PMS) is a luteal phase (premenstrual phase) dysphoric disorder with associated distressing physical symptoms not caused by organic disease.

Etiology

1. This is multifactorial. Teenagers are less likely to experience PMS than older women. Those with problems are more likely to have complex psychosocial circumstances or mothers with PMS.
2. Women suffering PMS frequently have underlying personality disorders or emotional tension. However, PMS also affects many women who are otherwise healthy,

well-adjusted individuals, and it is wrong to label all PMS sufferers as environmentally stressed!

3. PMS only occurs in women who ovulate.

Epidemiology

Most regularly ovulating women experience some unpleasant luteal phase symptoms but 3 to 8 per cent of North American women experience significant PMS at some stage in their reproductive years.

Clinical Findings

1. Signs and symptoms of PMS occur premenstrually every month with at least 1 week free of these features after each menses.
   a. Physical signs and symptoms include swollen tender breasts, abdominal bloating and constipation putatively due to progestogen-induced smooth muscle relaxation and bowel dilatation with increased bowel wall edema and gaseous distention, fatigue, acne, and headache. There is no consistent evidence to support weight gain.
   b. Psychological symptoms commonly include irritability, tension, uncontrollable anger, depression, reduced self-esteem, and low libido.
2. The individual's symptoms interfere with work, domestic responsibilities, and normal relationships.

Diagnosis

1. An identifiable psychiatric disorder must be excluded.
2. A symptom rating chart filled in over a minimum of three cycles enables identification and documentation of the cyclicity of the symptoms.

Treatment

1. Symptom documentation, pattern recognition, and patient reassurance are vital for successful management.
2. Review of lifestyle, exercise, and diet is important. Patients need to be encouraged to be positively assertive and in control of their life. Stress reduction and counseling may be beneficial.
3. The combined oral contraceptive therapy is effective in many women.
4. Fluoxetine (Prozac) has been shown to be acutely beneficial at a dose of 20 mg daily. It can be given continuously, but it also appears to be effective when given only in the luteal phase (i.e., commencing on day 14 and taken until menstruation).
5. Medical ovariectomy with gonadotropin releasing hormone agonists ± estrogen replacement may be effective in some women.
6. Some studies suggest calcium supplements combined with 25-hydroxyvitamin D may benefit many patients.
7. Therapies shown to be no better than placebo include vitamin B_6, evening primrose oil, and progestogen therapy. Diuretics should be avoided.

Menstrual Migraine

Definition

Cyclical severe headaches may occur at the onset of or during menstruation.

Etiology

Menstrual migraine is believed to result from the precipitous decline in ovarian hormone levels at the onset of menstruation.

Epidemiology

Sixty per cent of female migraine sufferers report an association with menstruation, and 14 per cent of women with migraine only experience headaches during menstruation.

Clinical Findings

1. Sufferers of menstrual migraine experience recurrent debilitating migrainous headache at the onset of or during menstruation.
2. Women should chart their headaches for at least 3 months to document the relationship with menses.
3. Usually the headaches are classic migraines with frequent auras, photophobia, nausea, and debilitating pain.

Treatment

Continuous low-dose combined OCT therapy is usually effective but chronically results in an atrophic endometrium and breakthrough bleeding. Alternatively, the combined OCT is given for 21 days with estrogen only supplementation for days 22 to 28 (e.g., conjugated equine estrogen 0.625 to 1.25 mg) or an estrogen patch is used during the menstrual phase.

Key Treatment

- Oral contraceptives (combined type)

Bibliography

Coupey S: Menstrual disorders in adolescents. Emerg Med 1994;26(4):21–36.

Speroff L, Glass RH, Kase N: Menstrual cycle disorders. Obstet Gynecol Clin North Am 1990;17(2).

Speroff L, Glass RH, Kase N: Clinical Gynaecological Endocrinology and Infertility, 3rd ed. Baltimore, Williams & Wilkins, 1983.

Steiner M, Steinberg S, Stewart D, et al: Fluoxetine in the treatment of premenstrual syndrome. N Engl J Med 1995;32:1529–1533.

44 Common Behavioral Symptoms and Management Strategies for Common Problems

Bruce J. Masek

Encopresis

Definition

Encopresis is a maladaptive pattern of repeated involuntary or intentional passage of stool into clothing or other inappropriate places. Historically classified as a mental disorder, encopresis is presumed when a physical cause cannot be determined for fecal incontinence. The term currently is delineated into two subtypes: with or without constipation and overflow incontinence.

Epidemiology

Most children with encopresis do not have major psychiatric co-morbidity. However, it is typical to find behavior problems, low self-esteem, and parent-child conflict in association with the disorder. The severity of these issues usually determines whether a referral to a clinical psychologist or psychiatrist is warranted in conjunction with medical therapy or in the case when medical therapy has failed because of noncompliance. For example, the child who appears to be using encopresis to manipulate the environment in a passive-aggressive or passive-dependent way should be referred for psychological evaluation.

Treatment

1. Education: The physiology of defecation and the natural history of constipation need to be explained to parents and child.
   a. A simplified diagram of anorectal anatomy and possibly other tools such as an oblong balloon, play-dough, examination glove, and so on can be used effectively to describe normal and abnormal defecation dynamics.
   b. It is important to stress that no one is to blame for the symptom and critical to counsel parents to try to hold their emotional responses in check and respond neutrally to soiling accidents and intentional non-compliance with various elements of therapy. The importance of this recommendation cannot be overstated because this is the single most effective means of defusing the "power struggle" that often exists between parents and child surrounding the encopresis. Parents typically need practice and support to modify their behavior accordingly.
2. Behavioral plan:
   a. The child needs to be sitting on the toilet, preferably two times per day, for intervals of 5 to 10 minutes. A kitchen timer should be used to motivate the child to stay on a finite task. Some children are resistant to sitting either because of fear of having a bowel movement that will be painful or because of oppositional behavior. In both instances a reward system should be implemented that provides incentives (e.g., stickers that when accumulated can be exchanged for small prizes or privileges) for cooperation with the sitting schedule.
      (1) For the fearful child, the reward system can be used to "shape" sitting on the toilet. At first, stickers are awarded just for standing in the bathroom in underwear for the prescribed time. After 1 or 2 days of success, the criterion is advanced, for example, to sitting on the closed lid of the toilet in underwear and then advanced to sitting on the toilet seat in underwear. The process is repeated with underwear lowered, and steps can be eliminated depending on the responsiveness of the child.
      (2) For the oppositional child, refusal to sit on the toilet should be met neutrally by the parent and a privilege restriction for that day only, for example, bedtime is moved up by the number of minutes in the sitting schedule or television viewing is restricted by the same amount of time. Conversely, the amount of time sitting can be added to bedtime or television viewing for the day as the reward.
   b. Soiling accidents are the responsibility of the child, with parent or caregiver rendering a minimal level of assistance depending on the age and developmental level of the child. It should be explained to the child that it is unhealthy to sit in soiled clothing and it is his or her parents' responsibility to see to it that they are restored to a clean, healthy state. Furthermore, whenever evidence of soiling is detected by a parent, the child needs to clean up and change clothing on the first request. In exchange for this level of cooperation, it is understood that there will be no punishment or admonitions from the parent. However, the world stops, so to speak, for the child until the accident procedure is properly followed. If a parent has to become more than the agreed on "minimally involved" because of oppositional behavior, then the additional time spent handling the situation is deducted from a privilege for that day up to a cumulative limit of 20 to 30 minutes. The key to success in managing accidents is for parents to remain calm and matter-of-fact in their interactions with their child.

Key Treatment: Encopresis

- Regular toileting
- Reward system

131

Assessment

Parents and child should keep a diary of accidents, bowel movements in the toilet, medication intake, and dietary fiber. It is sometimes helpful to record the antecedents and consequences of accidents to look for patterns that could be avoided with a little practical engineering. Telephone contact within a few days of starting the behavioral plan facilitates compliance, and diaries can be returned by mail in a week if a follow-up appointment cannot be scheduled before then. The behavioral plan should be modified based on the data that are coming back, not on impressions or misrepresentation because of noncompliance.

Follow-Up

The physician needs to be a reinforcing agent at every turn in the management of encopresis. For example, approval should be given for a returned diary (even if only partially completed) or any evidence of problem solving by parents or child of a situation not covered in the behavioral plan. Most importantly, parents need to be reinforced for their efforts to provide praise and approval for cooperative behavior and positive attitudes expressed by their child. It is not unusual to make several adjustments to the behavioral plan to maintain its effectiveness over the course of the 6 to 18 months that it often takes before the encopresis is under good control. In the beginning it may require office visits weekly or biweekly to establish a workable behavioral plan. As a final note, most children with encopresis value even brief time spent one-on-one with their pediatrician to receive support for solving the problem.

Enuresis

Definition

Enuresis is the persistence of involuntary or intentional voiding of urine into bed or clothes beyond the age of expected control. In most cases urinary continence is expected by 5 years, or, for children with developmental delays, a mental age of at least 5 years. Enuresis is the most common voiding abnormality in children. There are three subtypes: nocturnal only (nighttime), diurnal only (daytime), or both. To be classified as a mental disorder, the urinary incontinence must not be due to a general medical condition or physical cause and the frequency of wetting causes clinically significant impairment to the child's quality of life.

Etiology

Enuresis is best viewed as a symptom rather than a disorder that can be affected by many etiologic factors. If left untreated, most enuretic children eventually develop complete control. This observation has fueled arguments that enuresis represents delayed neurophysiologic maturation (e.g., small-capacity bladder or unstable bladder) or that it represents a developmental delay in the learning of appropriate bladder control habits. In the latter argument, family history, early sleep pattern, and successful response to behavioral conditioning techniques are offered as evidence that enuresis is not necessarily a function of delayed central nervous system development. It should be noted that the role of sleep patterns in the etiology of enuresis is unclear based on empiric investigation. Urinary infection is an uncommon, but clinically important, cause of enuresis. A very small number of children have diagnosable psychopathology underlying their enuresis; more often this is seen with late-onset enuresis when medical causes have been excluded.

Treatment

1. Behavioral techniques: Behavioral techniques are used extensively in the treatment of enuresis alone and in combination with pharmacologic therapy. Treatment is individualized to the child's wetting pattern, social environment, and family resources and attitudes. As in the case of encopresis, parents must learn how to respond to their child's wetting accidents and noncompliance with treatment responsibilities with emotional neutrality. For the child who wets intermittently during the day, a 1- to 3-hour voiding schedule is useful. Inexpensive digital watches are available that can be set to chime at scheduled voiding times. Most children can assume responsibility for resetting the watch to chime for the next scheduled voiding time. Remaining dry between voiding intervals can be rewarded using a sticker chart and backup reinforcers. It is important that parents monitor the voiding schedule and check for dry clothing closely in the beginning for this technique to work. Unless the child leaks urine continuously throughout the day, there is no reason for him or her to wear anything but regular underwear.

2. Overcorrection: Some children develop the habit of not emptying their bladders completely during voiding and then leak urine for a period of time thereafter that results in damp, but not soaked, underwear. Parents often describe their children in this situation as always in a rush to get in and out of the bathroom and usually waiting to the last possible moment to make the trip in the first place. A technique known as *overcorrection* can be employed that often eliminates this maladaptive pattern. Parents are instructed to have their child return to the bathroom 5 minutes after voiding to "try again" and then return in another 5 minutes. Usually the child voids a small amount of residual urine during one of the return trips. Overcorrection is used at every opportunity until the child learns to take more time and concentrate on emptying the first time, as evidenced by reduced dampness.

3. Nocturnal enuresis: Behavioral treatment of nocturnal enuresis involves the use of a urine alarm to teach the child to respond to a full bladder by awakening and inhibiting further voiding until the child reaches the toilet. In one such system, metal contacts are sewn into the underwear at a place where the first few drops of urine create a "circuit" that activates a loud buzzer (Palco Labs, Santa Cruz, CA). In the beginning, a parent usually has to help the child turn off the alarm, get to the bathroom to finish voiding and change into a dry pair of underwear. Gradually the child is "conditioned" to respond to nociceptive stimuli from the bladder during sleep and inhibit micturition until awake. This method is appropriate for children 6 to 7 years of age or older. The process typically takes 2 to 4 weeks, and initial success is achieved in about 80 per cent of cases. A 25 per cent relapse rate can be expected, but reimplementation of the alarm restores dry nights about 75 per cent of the time. It is not clear whether fluid restriction is critical to success, but a reasonable guideline would be to restrict fluids 90 to 120

minutes before bedtime depending on the child. Most systems come with "star charts" that can be backed up with privileges or rewards by parents. The systems are completely safe because electric current for the alarm is supplied by low-voltage watch batteries.

4. Bladder stretching: If a small-capacity bladder is suspected or documented to be a factor in the enuresis, it may be helpful to teach the child to hold larger volumes of urine using the so-called bladder stretching drill. In this procedure the child is encouraged to drink a large volume of fluid and delay voiding as long as possible. Usually this can be done twice depending on the volume drunk initially and is best reserved for weekend mornings or other convenient times. It is possible to achieve small but significant increases in bladder capacity after six to eight sessions. Of course, this would not be an appropriate strategy for complicated cases of enuresis (e.g., urinary infection or vesicoureteral reflux).

Key Treatment: Enuresis

- Voiding schedule
- Reward system
- Alarm system

Pica

Definition

Pica is the persistent eating of nonnutritive substances that is developmentally inappropriate and not a culturally sanctioned practice. Pica is clinically significant when the behavior leads to medical complications, such as lead poisoning, intestinal obstruction, or nutritional deficiencies. It usually starts at 12 to 18 months and is frequently associated with mental retardation.

Behavior Management

Behavior management of pica follows the principle of using the least restrictive intervention to achieve response suppression.

1. In cases in which pica poses no immediate danger, children can be taught to put food items in their mouth only if they are found on a plate or place mat. Nonfood items are placed nearby but off the place mat. Praise is delivered whenever food from the plate or place mat is put into the mouth, whereas pica is met with a reprimand such as, "no, don't eat that." When pica is encountered naturally, a reprimand such as, "spit that out, it is bad to eat," should be delivered. The child is then directed to place the item in the trash or, if appropriate, a storage container. This procedure should be repeated immediately three or four times as a means of overcorrection.

2. In the case of potentially dangerous pica, it is sometimes necessary to add a mild punishment component. After the reprimand, wiping the child's mouth with a cool damp washcloth, a 10-second physical restraint (holding the child's hands down to the sides), or a 3-minute time-out are effective and minimally restrictive forms of punishment.

3. In almost all cases, parents should be alerted to use a differential reinforcement procedure in which they praise their child at random intervals whenever pica has not occurred during the interval although there was opportunity.

Key Treatment: Pica

- Teach placing only food items in mouth
- Reprimand mouthing of nonfood items
- Forcefully remove dangerous items

Temper Tantrums

Etiology and Epidemiology

A temper tantrum almost needs no definition. At one time or another, most every parent has had to deal with a child who is loudly whining, complaining, or crying, often in combination with flailing arms and stomping feet. The stage is set for a tantrum when a limit is placed on the child's behavior or a performance demand contrary to the child's expectation is made. Persistent temper tantrums are cause for concern, particularly if they begin to occur in public places or if the child's behavior escalates to hitting, biting, or breath holding.

Behavior Management

The very best defense for temper tantrums is a good offense. That is, parents need to work on building a repertoire of appropriate behavior in their children through praise, attention, and physical affection. The applicable axiom is "catch them being good." There are any number of books written for parents on effective discipline and positive parenting that should be recommended as a matter of course. The child's temperament also needs to be factored into the equation. Some children do not respond well to overly enthusiastic praise or harsh reprimands, whereas other children exhibit stubbornness or persistence beyond the physical and emotional capacity of their parents.

1. *Active ignoring:* Active ignoring is the best strategy to deal with mild temper tantrums. All attention, including eye contact (except for the occasional glance to see what the child is doing), verbalizations, and physical contact are completely removed during the temper tantrum. As soon as the child has calmed down, parents need to say something to the effect that they are pleased to see their child is quiet and behaving. It takes practice to perform correctly, and it is a skill that does not come easily for some parents.

2. *Time-out:* Time-out is effective for intolerable or dangerous temper tantrums. Children must be taught how to take a time-out. It is not instinctive for them as parents would want to believe. Time-outs should be brief (3 to 5 minutes for all ages); the time-out environment should be dull and within eyesight of the parent; and the child needs to be quiet and physically in control by the end of the time-out or it is extended until these criteria are met. A kitchen timer (or its equivalent) is essential to make the child aware that the clock is running and the time-out

will be finite. Warning a child that a time-out is coming if he or she does not stop is simply prolonging the temper tantrum. Restitution can be a good thing after the time-out if an apology for aggressive behavior is in order or objects thrown during the temper tantrum need to be picked up. However, after restitution has been made, to maximize the effectiveness of time-out, the rest of the day should be spent trying to reinforce good behavior. Finally, parents should not be fooled by the child who announces that he or she does not mind or even likes time-out. Time-out is not supposed to be a miserable experience for the child—it is supposed to reduce inappropriate behavior over time.

3. *Forced choice:* Forced choice is a useful technique for temper tantrums in public places. This method points out to the child that he or she has a choice in the situation: either he or she can stop the temper tantrum immediately and a rewarding experience will follow in a short time or he or she will be removed from the situation and will go to time-out in the car or the first convenient place away from the excitement. For example, a parent might say: "You have two choices. You can stop crying and we will have a snack together before we go to the next store, or I will carry you to the car for a time-out."

4. *Response cost:* Response cost is another useful technique, particularly for older children in the 8 years and up age range, to control temper tantrums in public places. The child is forewarned about the consequence for engaging in a temper tantrum. That is, the time spent in the temper tantrum will be deducted from television or pre-bedtime. Conversely, behaving appropriately will result in extra time for some privilege.

Key Treatment: Temper Tantrums

- Time-out
- Forced choice

Bibliography

American Psychiatric Association: Diagnostic and Statistical Manual of Mental Disorders, 4th ed. Washington, DC, American Psychiatric Association, 1994.

Clark L: SOS! Help For Parents. Bowling Green, KY, Parents Press, 1985.

Fisher WW, Piazza CC, Bowman LG, et al: A preliminary evaluation of empirically derived consequences for the treatment of pica. J Appl Behav Anal 1994;27:447.

Rushton GH: Wetting and functional voiding. Urol Clin North Am 1995;22:75.

Seth R, Heyman MB: Management of constipation and encopresis in infants and children. Gastroenterol Clin North Am 1994;23:621.

45 Cognitive Development

Leon Eisenberg

Understanding development is the key to understanding human behavior and its biologic underpinnings.

Concepts

1. Although the gestation period is of the same order in higher apes and humans, postnatal maturation in humans is greatly prolonged. The human brain quadruples in size postnatally (from about 350 g in the newborn to about 1450 g in the adult). Histologic studies of the cerebral cortex in infants and young children demonstrate enormous growth in the number and branching of dendrites and the multiplication of synaptic junctions of greater and greater complexity, all occurring while the organism is subject to influence by its biologic and social environment.

2. Extraordinary developmental changes in the brain occur in an organism far more dependent on its caretakers than are other primate young. The very architecture of the cerebral cortex is sculpted by input from a social environment, one that determines the essential attributes of our humanity.

3. Although the genes that control embryonic development shape the initial structure of the infant brain, the infant's experience in the world fine-tunes the final pattern. Such fine-tuning continues through adulthood.

4. Recent progress in the molecular biology of gene-linked neuropsychiatric disorders has been extraordinary. The gene for Canavan disease, a spongy degeneration of the brain, has been cloned; a missense mutation (a glutamine to alanine substitution) results in defective aspartoacyclase hydrolytic activity and leads to a 200-fold increase in *N*-acetylaspartic acid levels in patients.

5. Fragile-X mental retardation syndrome is an X-linked dominant disorder with reduced penetrance (80% in males and 30% in females) and is associated with an expansion of the trinucleotide sequence CGG. In normal persons, the number of repeats is polymorphic, varying from 6 to 52 copies. Nonpenetrant carriers exhibit "premutation" alleles of 52 to 230 repeats; affected individuals display from 230 to more than 1000. Female carriers generally have less severe clinical presentations than affected males and exhibit wide variation in phenotypic expression, which can include

psychiatric manifestations. Mutation category determines the extent of the cognitive deficits in female carriers; whereas only one in three full mutation carriers are of normal intelligence, all of the premutation carriers have intelligence in the normal range. This new knowledge suggests the possibility of preventive measures to intercept what is, after Down syndrome, the most common inherited cause of mental retardation in males.

6. The concepts of brain structure and function revealed by contemporary neuroscience are in accordance with what is known about the development of behavior. We have learned about the luxuriant overgrowth of neurons and their processes in the course of development; activity selects survivors. If it is still the case that the basic ground plan is laid out in the genome, the precise neuroanatomic details are specified by activity-dependent competition between presynaptic axons for common postsynaptic target neurons.

7. The new technology in neuroscience makes possible a degree of precision in measuring localized brain activity in normal humans altogether unimaginable just a few years ago.

   a. Positron emission tomography has demonstrated that different brain loci are in action during different types of working memory tasks. Language functions have a different anatomic distribution in males and females.

   b. Echoplanar functional magnetic resonance imaging has shown that brain activation during phonologic tasks (but not orthographic or semantic tasks) is lateralized to the left inferior frontal gyrus in males, whereas activation occurs more diffusely in both comparable gyri in females. The planum temporale is larger on the left than the right in musicians, with the asymmetry particularly marked in those with perfect pitch. Whether the size differential represents "hypertrophy" from use (as the finding in professional musicians might suggest) or inborn gift (as suggested by the data on perfect pitch) or both remains to be discovered.

Experience and Structure

1. Because the species-typical environment, including the environment of the uterus, reliably supplies the input needed for the development of the central nervous system, these central nervous system structures are as uniform as if they had been predestined in the genome. The visual system is a prime example. Genetically controlled mechanisms generate a coarsely grained topographic map; the fine-tuning of this map requires neural activity.

   a. Two specific instances are found in the formation of the ocular alternation layers in the geniculate nuclei and of the ocular dominance columns in the occipital cortex, the one process prenatal and the other postnatal. Initially, dendritic arborizations from both eyes intermingle. The formation of separate layers in the geniculate for each eye depends on spontaneously generated, asynchronous waves of electrical activity in retinal ganglion cells. If spontaneous reti-

nal electrical activity is abolished by tetrodotoxin, geniculate layers will not form.

   b. In contrast, the formation of the ocular dominance columns in occipital cortex requires that both eyes of the newborn receive precisely focused stimulation from the visual environment during the early months of postnatal life (the sensitive period). If one eye is occluded by an opaque cover, or if its acuity is blurred by a translucent cover, or if it is made strabismic by severing extraocular muscles, the unimpaired eye "captures" most columns in the absence of competition from the deprived eye. The change in occipital cortex is irreversible if occlusion is maintained during the sensitive period; permanent change does not occur in the adult. If the kitten is reared in complete darkness, column formation is delayed and the sensitive period for monocular capture prolonged, but at the expense of diminished visual function.

   c. Deprivation need not be total; human astigmatism, if it is unrecognized and untreated, leads to permanent deficits in visual acuity in the abnormal meridional orientations. It has long been known that amblyopia, in which there are incongruent visual images from the two eyes, results in permanent loss of effective vision from the unused eye in humans if the amblyopia is not corrected within the first 5 years of life.

2. Just as stimulus deprivation leads to anatomic as well as functional loss, enriched stimulation results in increased density of neurons and processes in rat cerebral cortex. Synaptogenesis is keyed to learning. Rats reared in a complex visual environment in contrast to those reared in bare individual cages show an increase in the depth and area of the superficial gray layer of the superior colliculus. Animals forced to learn motor skills have a greater number of synapses per Purkinje cell in cerebellar cortex than comparison animals engaging in the same total amount of rote motor activity without learning. Early manipulation can attenuate the central nervous system deficits associated with aging in the rodent. Handling infant rats increases adrenal output, and the concentration of glucocorticoid receptors in the hippocampus. This results in greater negative feedback in the adrenocortical axis and diminished glucocorticoid secretion in response to stress. In consequence, rats handled in infancy show less neuronal loss in the hippocampus and fewer defects in memory as they age.

The Ontogenetic Niche

1. Nature and nurture stand in reciprocity, not opposition. All children inherit, along with their parents' genes, their parents, their peers, and the places they inhabit. Meredith West and Andrew King have coined the term *ontogenetic* niche to emphasize that development unfolds in an ecologic and social setting that, like its genes, is species-typical for the organism. The ontogenetic niche is a legacy that structures development, a crucial link between parents and offspring, an envelope of life chances.

2. The early steps in the development of language are

akin to the experience-dependent development of the visual system. All healthy human infants are born with the ability to learn language, an ability that is uniquely human; therefore, the potential, by definition, is specified in the genome. Children are able to infer grammatical rules from exemplars without ever being taught grammar per se. That, too, must reflect unique features of the human brain. However, the capacity to use grammar does not spring, like Athena, full-formed from the head of Zeus. Its acquisition and elaboration are dependent on social interaction. Whether a child acquires any language at all, let alone which specific language it acquires, is determined by its linguistic community. The degree of linguistic competence attained is a function of nature, nurture, *and* niche.

3. Auditory learning begins before birth. The human infant in utero hears its mother's voice repeatedly; on testing after birth, it is able to discriminate that voice from other female voices; 4-day-old French infants will suck harder to hear French instead of Russian because of in utero auditory experience. Young infants can detect differences between phonemes in all languages, including those that are not used in their native language.

   a. Within the first 6 to 12 months of life, however, inborn ability for universal phoneme discrimination is altered by experience that "warps" the perceptual space underlying speech. Between 6 and 9 months of age, infants display listening preferences for sound patterns of their native language in lists of words they do not understand. These language traits are most likely based on implicit (nondeclarative) memory. It is as if perceptual maps are "tuned" to native language.

   b. The older child, like the adult, is only able to discriminate the phonemes present in the language(s) it masters. Japanese adults, unlike Japanese infants, cannot hear a difference between the English "l" and "r," two sounds without an independent existence in the Japanese language. This is not the result of neural atrophy; rather, language-specific phonemic categories have suppressed nonspecific auditory sensitivity. The persistence of capacity for discrimination between the sounds of the phonemes can be shown in carefully constructed nonlinguistic experiments.

4. Infants who are reared in institutions staffed by few and inconsistent caretakers display marked retardation on all indices of physical and psychologic maturation. Even if nutrition and cleanliness are maintained at a high level, but without specific enrichment of adult-infant social interactions, the lag in adaptive behavior continues and results in developmental quotients in the defective range. If these conditions are allowed to persist throughout childhood, the youngsters exhibit the psychologic stigmata of mental deficiency and become adults who function as poorly as those with intrinsic brain pathology. It is not known with certainty for how long severe psychosocial deprivation can be tolerated by the organism before the functional retardation becomes irreversible. Rapid and apparently complete recovery can occur after adoption into family life by the end of the first year. The earlier the rescue and the more complete the restitutive measures, the better is the outcome.

5. Extremity of neglect with its inexorable consequences is, of course, the limiting case. It obtains for only a minority of children (e.g., those in Rumanian or Chinese orphanages recently in the news), although it should not be tolerated for a single child, given the means and the knowledge we have at hand. Epidemiologically, the major problem is the far larger numbers of children who experience psychosocial deprivation, lesser in degree than the orphanage prototype, to an extent sufficient to impair sequential acquisition of the full range of cognitive abilities. These are the children of the poor, particularly those of low-status ethnic groups. In the United States, those at greatest hazard are the African American, the Amerindian, the Mexican, and the Puerto Rican, but serious risk is present for Appalachian and other whites in isolated pockets of poverty.

6. Comparative studies of academic achievement find the children of the poor scoring far less well than their middle class age mates, with poor African American children doubly disadvantaged. The gap in school performance becomes progressively greater with ascending age and reaches a crescendo in high percentages of dropping out of school, subsequent unemployability, and social deviance. The most parsimonious explanation of these differences lies in differences in social experience.

7. Programs of early enrichment (e.g., Head Start) minimize but do not completely eliminate the disadvantages associated with poverty and family malfunction; stimulation and social support must continue throughout adolescence if children are to realize the potential in them at birth.

Implications for Guidance

1. Interactionist theory (the ontogenetic niche) has direct relevance to pediatric practice, exotic as it may sound. In anticipatory guidance visits, parents can be helped to understand that talking to their infant is essential to its language development, well before the child can be expected to utter its first words, and that exposure to books by reading stories to the toddler enhances readiness for learning, long before the child will begin to read. When development is slow, the first diagnostic consideration should be an assessment of the adequacy of home circumstances before invoking an intrinsic deficit in the child as the primary cause.

2. Pediatricians should take the lead in insisting on high quality standards for child care services when state regulations are written and in being advocates for the expansion of Head Start "horizontally and vertically" (i.e., to all eligible children at a given age and to children both younger and older than present federal limits).

3. The need for sensory stimulation and social support does not end at school age but continues through adolescence. The need for psychosocial input is like the need for nutrition. Just as feeding a child in infancy does not "prevent" malnutrition in childhood, good preschool pro-

grams, important as they are in getting children off to a healthy start, are no substitutes for good elementary and high school education.

Bibliography

Eisenberg L: Child mental health in the Americas: A public health approach. Bull Pan Am Health Organ 1992;26:230–241.

Frank DA, Klass PE, Earls F, et al: Infants and young children in orphanages. Pediatrics 1996;97:569–578.

Kaback M, Lim-Steele J, Dabholkar D, et al: Tay-Sachs disease carrier screening, prenatal diagnosis and the molecular era: An international perspective. JAMA 1993;270:2307–2315.

Werker JF: Becoming a native listener. Am Scientist 1989;79:54–59.

West MJ, King AP: Settling nature and nurture into an ontogenetic niche. Dev Psychobiol 1987;20:549–562.

---

46 A Developmental Understanding of Chronic Illness

Aurora J. Bennett
Michael J. Maloney

Epidemiology

Ten per cent of children and adolescents live with chronic medical illness (Newacheck and Taylor, 1992). Most of these children successfully cope with the pain, inconvenience, and stress of their chronic disease (Noll, 1997).

Clinical Findings

There are four major factors (Mrazek, 1991) that impact on children's ability to cope with their chronic illness.

Risk Factors

- Illness-specific factors
- Familial coping patterns
- Social/environmental factors
- Developmental factors

---

1. Illness-specific factors

   Prolonged delays in determining a diagnosis, the severity and duration of symptoms, the extent of physical deformity or disability, the prognosis, and the complexity and morbidity associated with the treatment protocols can all heighten the anxiety of the child and family. Each of these factors may overwhelm family routines.

2. Familial coping patterns

   At baseline, families are often dealing with such significant problems as divorce, abuse, and poverty. To these are added the stresses specific to a child's illness.

   a. Parents may blame themselves for an illness secondary to trauma, infection, or genetic predisposition.

   b. Some parents experience peak anxiety in the acute phase of the disease, whereas others feel maximal stress later during prolonged relapses. Chronic relapses interfere with parental job performance and cause social isolation for parents owing to the demands of rigorous treatment protocols.

   c. During a child's hospitalization, the parents become aware of the need to relinquish control of their child to the medical staff. This may be especially difficult for assertive parents who have surveyed the medical literature and center their lives on the care of their child (Gold et al., 1986).

   d. Parents are forced into making medical decisions on behalf of their child with relatively limited understanding of the illness, diagnostic procedures, and treatment protocols.

   e. Parents are apt to compare their child's illness course with that of other children with the same diagnosis. This may lead to their closely scrutinizing all aspects of the medical treatment. Finding fault with the staff may be their only avenue for releasing anger about having to deal with an overwhelming illness.

   f. Some parents feel the need to emotionally pull away from their child because of depression, fear, or guilt, which may result in frequent absence from the hospital in order to escape temporarily their hopeless "medical" role with the child.

   g. During times of illness remission, parents may experience relief from acute worries but may find themselves focusing on longer term issues. These may include medical bills, medical insurance coverage for their child as he or she reaches adulthood, and the child's chances of ever living independently as an adult.

3. Social/environmental factors

   Social/environmental factors involve responses to the child's illness from family, friends, the community, and the medical staff. Any reluctance by these important people to provide acceptance and support for the child and family may further alienate the family from those potentially best equipped to minimize the traumatizing aspects of a chronic illness.

4. Developmental factors

   Consideration of the developmental stage of the child is critical to understanding how a child perceives the illness. Piaget described the cognitive development of children in terms of a sequence of stages from birth

TABLE 46–1. COGNITIVE STAGES OF DEVELOPMENT

Preoperational period (age 2 y to 7 y)
Concrete operations (age 7 y to 11 y)
Formal operations (age 12 y to 18 y)

into adulthood, during which the child progresses from an egocentric and concrete mode of thinking to a logical and abstract form of thought. The child is gradually able to differentiate internal wishes and thoughts from external reality. The cognitive stages of interest to pediatricians are listed in Table 46–1.

a. Preoperational (age 2 years to 7 years)

(1) This period encompasses two patterns of egocentric thought:

(a) Immanent justice—refers to the child's perceiving the illness and its painful treatment as punishment for misdeeds. Shame and fear of retribution may inhibit the child's communication with the medical team.

(b) Magical thinking—refers to the belief that by merely wishing to not be ill, the child will actually become well. The preoperational child believes that by not vocalizing concerns, they will disappear. This may lead to underreporting of important symptoms.

(2) The normal beginning attempts of the preoperational child to assert autonomy are thwarted by the dependency fostered by serious illness and hospitalization.

(3) Fear and anxiety are heightened in the very young ill child because of egocentric thinking along with a limited cognitive ability to comprehend symptoms or their treatment. This may result in regressed behaviors such as soiling, social withdrawal, and opposition to treatment regimens.

b. Concrete operations (age 7 years to 11 years)

(1) Children in this developmental phase have a beginning understanding of the concept of germs and contagion (Schonfeld, 1991) and therefore are less likely to link illness with misbehavior.

(2) Limited contact with chronic illness along with a lack of knowledge about physiology and anatomy continues to fuel heightened anxiety regarding their medical problems.

(3) Interference with school, peer interaction, and growing gaps in motor abilities may exacerbate the sense of isolation and dependency inherent in the long and sometimes arduous course of a chronic illness.

c. Formal operations (age 12 years to 18 years)

(1) Owing to their greater cognitive understanding of physiology and anatomy, adolescents are able to participate in a dialogue with the pediatrician regarding the cause of their illness and the basic

mechanism by which the physician's treatment will lessen their symptoms.

(2) Peer acceptance, body image, sexuality, and identity formation are threatened by an illness that may lead to isolation, disfigurement, and weakened defense mechanisms. The daily struggles to cope with a chronic illness can consume an adolescent's thoughts and energy, leaving minimal reserve to deal with the normal pressures of school, friends, and home.

Laboratory Findings

1. There are no specific laboratory findings that identify the child or adolescent who is not coping well with a medical illness. In fact, it is appropriate to consult a child psychiatrist when there are inconsistencies in the laboratory results, current symptoms, or atypical course, perhaps indicating noncompliance or Munchausen syndrome by proxy.

2. There are a few instances in which laboratory findings can provide direct evidence that a child or adolescent is not complying with treatment, for example, an abnormally high hemoglobin A_1c. Urine or blood toxic screens provide evidence of substance abuse. Otherwise, the pediatrician can best identify impairments in coping based on a detailed history obtained from the child and the family. A detailed mental status examination, to check for depression, psychosis, delirium, or even thoughts of suicide, is an essential tool.

Treatment

The pediatrician, parents, and child form a team that works together to formulate and implement an optimal treatment plan for the child's illness. Maintaining an open dialogue among all team members is integral to a successful implementation of a treatment regimen. The pediatrician assumes a critical role in the team's functioning owing to his or her knowledge of medicine and child development. This medical knowledge can be utilized by the family only if the physician remains sensitive to the presence of the emotional and developmental factors that govern a child and family's adjustment to the illness.

1. It is helpful to utilizing Piaget's developmental framework to understand how children cope with medical problems.

a. Tips for treating the preoperational child (age 2 years to 7 years)

(1) Minimizing separation from parent(s) is the single most important intervention for the very young patient.

(2) Young children are more interested in the explanation of concrete aspects of an upcoming medical procedure, e.g., the physical appearance of the surgery suite, the masks worn by the surgical staff, and so forth, rather than what is actually involved in the procedure.

(3) Utilization of the child life department of a hospital allows play with medical equipment to promote active mastery and a sense of control for the child.

(4) Allowing the child choices in the medical rou-

tine promotes a sense of control and autonomy; for example, "Do you want to do your exercises before or after your lunch?"

(5) Pain is underdiagnosed and undertreated in hospitalized children. Untreated pain reinforces the child's belief that medical procedures are a punishment for misdeeds.

Key Treatment: Chronic Illness (Preoperational Child: 2–7 years)

- Minimize separation from parent
- Explain concrete aspects of procedure (appearances, masks, and so forth)
- Utilize child life staff
- Treat pain adequately

b. Tips for treating the concrete operational child (age 7 years to 11 years)

(1) Promote continuity with school and peers (cards, visits, homework) to maintain a sense of normalcy in the context of a challenging medical illness.

(2) Respond to the child's questions regarding the illness with brief and basic information tailored to his or her cognitive abilities.

(3) Discuss the illness with the child during periods of medical stability when he or she is better able to enter into a dialogue about major concerns.

Key Treatment: Chronic Illness (Operational Child: 7–11 years)

- Promote continuity
- Answer questions appropriate to age
- Discuss illness during stable periods

c. Tips for treating the formal operational child (age 12 years to 18 years)

(1) Encourage active participation in the communication and management of medical symptoms.

(2) Support the adolescent's attempts to integrate a chronic illness into his or her developing identity, yet not be consumed by it.

(3) Encourage discussion of the impact of the illness and its medical treatment on physical appearance, stamina, sexuality, and future functioning.

(4) Contact with peers with a similar illness can promote healthy coping abilities and support.

Key Treatment: Chronic Illness (Formal Operational Child: 11–18 years)

- Encourage active participation
- Integrate illness into developing persona
- Contact with peers similarly affected

2. Delirium is frequently underdiagnosed, yet children with serious illness are prone to this organic syndrome, which may be secondary to sepsis, electrolyte imbalance, medications, or sensory deprivation. Parents and nursing staff are the closest observers of subtle changes in the child's mental status. These findings are critical, since the child may not be able to verbalize what he or she is feeling or perceiving.

3. The possibility of depression should be considered in children who manifest changes in appetite, in sleep, or in the quality of their interactions. These changes may be secondary to organic factors related to their illness, but the possibility of a depressive disorder should be considered. Changes in behavior or mental status that interfere with treatment or pose a risk to the child or others require consultation from a child psychiatrist. This specialist has expertise in the use of psychotropic medications, environmental manipulation, and psychotherapy with children and families to decrease potentially life-threatening behaviors.

4. As time passes, the quality of the dialogue with the pediatrician will evolve parallel with the child's development. When an adolescent becomes more sophisticated cognitively, he or she will look to the pediatrician and family for help in continuing to process the illness as part of his or her identity. The morbidity of a chronic illness can be cumbersome, but the potential for emotional growth can be a lifelong asset for the maturing child.

Bibliography

Bibace R, Walsh ME: Development of children's concepts of illness. Pediatrics 1980;66:912–917.

Gold LM, Kirkpatrick BS, Fricker FJ, et al: Psychosocial issues in pediatric organ transplantation: The parent's perspective. Pediatrics 1986;77:738–744.

Mrazek DA: Chronic pediatric illness and multiple hospitalizations. In Lewis M (ed): Child and Adolescent Psychiatry: A Comprehensive Textbook. Baltimore, Williams & Wilkins, 1991, pp 1041–1050.

Newacheck PW, Taylor WR: Childhood chronic illness: Prevalence, severity, and impact. Am J Public Health 1992;82:364–371.

Noll RB, et al: Peer relationships and emotional well-being of youngsters with sickle cell disease. J Child Dev, 1997.

Schonfeld DJ: The child's cognitive understanding of illness. In Lewis M (ed): Child and Adolescent Psychiatry: A Comprehensive Textbook. Baltimore, Williams & Wilkins, 1991, pp 949–953.

47 Difficult Families

Eugene V. Beresin

The Role of Families in Pediatric Care

1. To a large extent, the pediatrician must rely on family involvement in the delivery of care. Families provide necessary comfort and support for the child both in illness and in health. In outpatient practice, families must understand and implement the prescribed treatment for the child.

2. Having an ill child is one of the most stressful situations a parent can face. Many parents become anxious, tense, and, at times, irritable. Often parents will feel a strong sense of responsibility for their child's illness. These reactions are quite normal and should be considered as such by the pediatrician. Parents who reveal these behaviors are to be distinguished from a variety of "difficult" parents, who are irritating, uncooperative, panic stricken, and, at times, hateful even for the most seasoned pediatrician.

3. The pediatrician, too, is often under stress, wanting the best outcome for the child and family, regardless of the severity of the illness. A range of factors contribute to emotional burdens on the pediatrician both from within and outside his or her practice. Current practice demands typically include a high volume of active clinical cases, long hours, coverage of multiple facilities, and increasing administrative duties. Moreover, the pediatrician, as all physicians, is not immune from an array of family stressors.

4. In certain situations, particularly in acute, serious illness, normal families may behave in ways that are viewed as pathologic. This may be the case in critical times when a child is in intensive care after the diagnosis of a serious or life-threatening illness or in times of extreme uncertainty during the progression of a chronic, potentially fatal disease. Additionally, in routine outpatient practice, there may be a number of iatrogenic factors that tax even the most well-adjusted parents and result in behaviors that may seem disturbed and disturbing to the pediatrician and that tend to transform normal parents into "difficult" parents; thus there is a need for strategies that may be useful in the development of a strong collaborative relationship between parents and pediatrician.

5. Factors that may make normal parents "difficult":

   a. Many normal parents may be perceived as problematic in certain circumstances. There are many possible reasons for this. The problem may be due to the type of illness and the attendant uncertainty surrounding it, external pressures in the parents' lives either in the family or in their environment, stresses due to emotional difficulties in the normal parent, frustrations with the current healthcare delivery system, or problems that are due to the pediatrician's perception and behavior.

   b. Factors deriving from the parent, child, and the family:

      (1) The context in which illness occurs. Certain life events can complicate a parent's reaction to even the most trivial illness. Any major stress may cloud a parent's thinking and obstruct typical compliant behavior. For example, family stress, such as financial pressures, recent moves, personal disputes, or other illnesses in the family may sap a parent's reserve.

      (2) Medical problems tending to cause excessive guilt, such as accidents, injuries, ingestions, or genetic/hereditary illnesses.

      (3) Socioeconomic factors. A wide range of social problems may negatively influence a parent's adaptive response to a child's illness. Common examples include poverty, unemployment, divorce, domestic violence, and lack of close social supports. The single parent, without a partner at home, is particularly at risk of losing an adaptive reserve. The environment in which the child and family live may contribute additional stress. For example, neighborhood problems including gang violence, drug dealing, and political unrest add to a parent's sense of vulnerability.

      (4) Psychiatric conditions in otherwise "functional" parents. A number of parents have neuropsychiatric disorders that are not severe enough to compromise routine living. For example, many parents have mild mental retardation, have learning disabilities, or suffer from periods of depression and anxiety. In most situations, at times with treatment, these parents can adequately care for their children and maintain gainful employment. However, the stress of an ill child may alter their stability and cause them to react in ways that are experienced as "difficult" to the pediatrician. Not all psychiatric disorders produce difficult parents.

   c. Conditions in pediatric practice:

      (1) Long waits in the waiting or examining room; difficulty reaching the pediatrician by phone for consultation.

      (2) Brief visits and/or giving the impression that the pediatrician is too busy or rushed.

      (3) The use of complicated, technical terms when talking to parents. Even the most well-educated parent, when hearing complex language may lose perspective and react with excessive fear.

      (4) Inattention to a parent's real concern, whether it is realistic or not. Too often, parents are worried about a specific problem and need to have their concerns and questions addressed.

Failure to ask what they are worried about leaves them with persistent anxiety.

    (5) Failure to appreciate the normal range of a parent's emotional responses to a child's illness (fear, anger, self-blame).

    (6) Inattention to one's own feelings or uncertainty with a particular clinical situation obstructs effective communication. A certain degree of clinical detachment is critical for effective care. There are many situations when this needed distance is difficult to achieve, resulting in either overinvolvement or detachment, exacerbating fear in the parents.

6. Positive measures to bring out the best in normal parents:

   a. Identify the psychosocial status of the family, including current stressors, support structures, and resources. Communicate this understanding to the parent(s).

   b. Explain, in ways the parent can understand, the nature, course, treatment, and prognosis of a child's illness. Allow time to hear the parent's understanding of the illness, including feelings of blame, guilt, and anxiety. Take the necessary time to clarify origins, educate, and comfort the parents without extending false reassurance. Most parents, despite their emotions, want a clear, candid explanation about the problem.

   c. Allow sufficient time for questions about the illness and its treatment, even if this requires an additional office visit.

   d. Attempt to form a therapeutic alliance around the prescribed treatment, including emotional support and comfort for that child. Articulate concretely what the parent can do to collaborate in the pediatric care.

   e. Avoid abrupt labeling of "difficult" parents, such as viewing all irritating behaviors as pathologic. Snap judgments are quite common and may be somewhat self-serving and/or defensive on the part of the pediatrician. When parents appear "difficult," the pediatrician should welcome the feeling that someone is acting in a problematic fashion and begin to formulate a differential diagnosis as to what the difficulty might mean. This task would entail reviewing some of the causes of difficult behavior as described in this chapter. Once this is done and a strategy is adopted, it is always best to begin identifying the parents' strengths, including their attachment or devotion to their child, their intelligence and/or their natural intuition, and their ability to communicate, such that they can be comforting to their child and effective members of the healthcare team.

   f. Help the parents identify and cope with their emotional reactions to the child's illness. This may require psychiatric or social services consultation.

   g. Identify your own emotional response to the parents and child and avoid letting any excessive positive or negative reactions affect your treatment.

Identifying and Working With Difficult Parents: General Principles

1. Some parents have personality styles that evoke strong negative reactions among clinicians in almost any situation.
2. Groves (1978) reviewed ways physicians can effectively care for "hateful" patients. He noted how certain adult personality types create strong negative reactions among physicians and indicated that it is essential not to deny uncomfortable or hateful feelings, because doing so often results in diagnostic and treatment errors. These evoked responses are often vital clues as to how such persons function interpersonally and the reactions they engender in others. From the pediatrician's standpoint, understanding such personalities can vastly improve developing a working alliance and providing the optimal care for the child and family.
3. Personality-specific strategies are useful for developing a therapeutic alliance with difficult parents.
4. Whenever a pediatrician believes a parent is being difficult, he or she should ask if the parent has ever faced this difficulty before in terms of a child's illness or other crisis. This perspective will help view the patterns of behavior in more objective terms and prevent the feeling that such behavior is specific to the parent. Personalizing difficult parental behavior is a common response and needs to be taken out of the personal realm and treated as part of the challenging clinical situation.
5. The following delineates typical features of the most common difficult parents and interventions suggested to facilitate a good working alliance. The categories described do not always exist in fully expressed forms, and a parent may fit into more than one category. Moreover, the following represent the most extreme cases, and many parents may display the personality traits to varying degrees of severity.

The Demanding Parent

1. Characteristics:

   a. Makes excessive, unreasonable demands, often for preferential treatment.

   b. Prone to be angry and never truly satisfied; hence many are "entitled demanders," who use intimidation, devaluation, and hostility to have their needs met; may be litigious.

   c. Egocentric and grandiose—not uncommonly VIPs, such as executives, physicians, attorneys, high-powered professionals.

   d. Beneath the tough exterior often lies unconscious low self-esteem, dependency, and sensitivity to perceived criticism or rejection.

2. Suggested management:

   a. Avoid, if at all possible, directly attacking or confronting the feelings of entitlement or excessive demands. The reason for this is that the confrontation only heightens the sense of entitlement, which to the demanding parents feels as though they have once again been thwarted in getting what they believe they deserve. If parents can understand their own behavior as a problem, then such behavior on the parents' part may not be viewed as requiring a solution. These parents usually see satisfying entitlement as the problem. If such parents can see that the real problem is receiving care for their child, and this is the true role for the pediatrician, an alliance is much more possible to attain.

b. Understand that the personality style is a defense against insecurity.

c. Acknowledge the right to the best possible medical care, but explain the limits of the pediatric care available.

d. Use senior consultants, but be sure they support your explanations of the limitations of care.

e. Do not bring in psychiatric consultants too late, or the parent will perceive this as a criticism and a breech of your alliance.

The Help-Rejecting Parent

1. Characteristics:

a. Noncompliant and pessimistic.

b. Vigilant and distrusting of the motives, intentions, and actions of the pediatrician. Often these parents have a history of relationships characterized by rejection, abuse, or abandonment.

c. Questions the pediatrician's competency and frequently "tests" the doctor's reliability and trustworthiness.

2. Suggested management:

a. Beware of responding with self-doubt, guilt, resentment, or aversion, which are typical reactions in clinicians.

b. Empathize with the parent around his or her understandable distrust, given the parent's life experience.

c. Provide frequent contact, but set clear limits of your intentions and professional actions.

d. Demonstrate "passing the tests," such as remembering the laboratory tests and results, specifics of the child's history, and so on.

e. Avoid verbalizing or revealing aversion or disdain. Do not fall prey to angry responses, even if provoked. Use colleagues as "sounding boards" to vent your feelings and gain perspective on the parent's irritating style.

f. Never make promises that cannot be kept.

The Denying Parent

1. Characteristics:

a. Uses denial to cope with stress, to manage unbearable fears, to sustain hope.

b. Fails to listen to explanations and instructions.

c. Occasionally refuses use of medications and procedures and resists examination and/or treatment.

2. Suggested management:

a. Be aware of feeling frustrated and helpless and reacting with disdain, viewing the parents as neglectful.

b. Remember that severe denial is a coping strategy to manage a perceived desperate situation and may not be under conscious control.

c. Denying parents should not be managed sternly. No degree of force or threat can break the denial.

d. Approach the parent with gentle understanding, acknowledging how frightening it is to have a sick child.

e. Use calm, direct discourse and avoid excessive emotionality, which is likely to increase denial.

f. Distribute educational material on the child's illness.

g. Encourage parents to speak with other parents of children with similar illnesses.

h. Use of senior consultants may be reassuring.

The Dependent Parent

1. Characteristics:

a. Parents who are insecure and vulnerable may draw strength, emotional support, and stability from an attachment.

b. This dependency may be directed at adults, such as a spouse or pediatrician. It also may be drawn from the child, who becomes "parentified," providing a caretaking role for the parent.

c. Often such parents come from emotionally barren families and had children to fill inner emptiness or increase self-esteem.

d. These parents may view the child's illness as terribly threatening, a potential loss of their lifeline.

e. They may form an intense childlike attachment to the pediatrician, who is perceived as an inexhaustible provider.

f. Contact is sought in any way possible (e.g., frequent phone calls, unexpected office visits).

2. Suggested management:

a. Beware of common reactions of aversion, disparagement, or avoidance.

b. Demonstrate an emphatic understanding of the parent's deep insecurity and need for caretaking.

c. Calmly reassure the parent of your deep involvement, but set firm, clear limits as to your availability. Define the scope and bounds of your role in the child's treatment.

d. Set up regularly scheduled brief meetings.

e. Relate to the parent as an adult, stressing the value and importance of being a parent.

f. Prescribe clear, concrete tasks, defining the role of the parent.

g. Utilize other family members or adult friends to support the dependent parent.

h. Call for social service consultation early in the treatment.

The Obsessive Parent

1. Characteristics:

a. Emotionally constricted, rigid, dogmatic.

b. Excessive focus on the narrow details results in losing the big picture.

c. Compulsion to make the "right" decision based on "facts," yet never have enough data to make any decisions at all.

d. Seemingly endless questions and observations about the child's illness and never satisfied with explanations; chronically worried.

e. Preoccupation with details and logic, resulting in failure to connect emotionally with the child or pediatric team.

f. A personality style that defends against uncertainty and anxiety that feel intolerable.

2. Suggested management:

a. Be aware of feeling irritated or infuriated by flood of questions, as if the parent does not listen or is suspicious of the pediatrician's competence.

b. Approach parent with patience and tolerance, understanding the defense against intense anxiety despite apparent low emotionality.

c. Answer questions directly and logically.

d. Redirect attention to the big picture and emphasize the necessity of being supportive to the child.

The Hysterical Parent

1. Characteristics:

a. Highly dramatic, overly sensitive, and emotional; tends to overreact to many situations.

b. Impressionistic, making broad generalizations based on anxieties and hunches; seems unable to think and act logically.

c. Suggestible and easily distractible.

d. Sexualizes responses—may be seductive.

2. Suggested management:

a. Avoid angry, frustrated reactions to the apparent inability to listen, escalation of emotion, and potential increase in anxiety in the child.

b. Reinforce how vital it is for the child for a diminution of emotions and focused thinking and action.

c. Bring in less overactive relatives to help contain emotionality and high drama.

Understanding Common Themes in Working with Difficult Parents

1. Most difficult parents came from troubled families and were the product of extraordinarily difficult childhoods.

2. There are often family histories of significant trauma on the part of their parents, including abuse, neglect, substance abuse, and/or hostile divorces.

3. There is typically an inability to observe the "difficult" nature of their behavior and its impact on others, including the child, the family, and the pediatric team.

Bibliography

Beresin EV: The difficult parent: *In* Jellinek MS, Herzog DB (eds): Massachusetts General Hospital Handbook: Psychiatric Aspects of General Hospital Pediatrics. Chicago, Year Book Medical, 1990, pp 67–75.

Beresin EV, Jellinek MS, Herzog DB: The difficult parent: Office assessment and management. Curr Probl Pediatr 1990;20:620–633.

Berlin IN: Working with parents of children with chronic disease. *In* Call JD, Cohen RL, Harrison SI, et al (eds): Basic Handbook of Child Psychiatry: V. Advances and New Directions. New York, Basic Books, 1987, pp 565–574.

Groves JE: Taking care of the hateful patient. N Engl J Med 1978;298:883–887.

Jellinek MS: The hospitalized child: General considerations: *In* Hackett TP, Cassem NH (eds): Massachusetts General Hospital Handbook of General Hospital Psychiatry, 2nd ed. Littleton, MA, PSG Publishing Co, 1987, pp 462–476.

48 The Adopted Child

Linda M. Forsythe and *Michael S. Jellinek*

Overview

A pediatrician who appreciates the many facets of adoption is invaluable to adoptive parents and their children. These families may need support, guidance, and intervention around adoption-related issues while medical and developmental needs are being addressed and at periodic well-child visits. In addition, a pediatrician may be asked to consult with a given child or prospective adoptive parents before an adoption or to refer members of the adoptive family for psychologic evaluation or legal assistance.

History

The circumstances of individuals being reared by parents other than their biologic predecessors has been familiar to us since the beginning of civilization. Moses and Oedipus are particularly well-known heroes of such a life story. Other cultural heroes raised by surrogate parents include Superman and Batman. The Roman tradition of adoption was created to ensure an heir. The orphan trains of nineteenth century America carried parentless children west to be adopted by farmers to help work the land. Through much of the past century, the traditional model of adoption was that of an infertile couple providing a solution to another woman's unwanted pregnancy or to another nation's population of war-orphaned children.

Over the past 40 years, with the onset of the children's rights movement and child protection laws, abusive and neglectful parents began to lose parental rights, thereby freeing children for adoption. The number of healthy American infants available for adoption began to dwindle as single parenthood became more acceptable and contraception and abortion became more accessible. Increasingly, adopted children are likely to need special physical, developmental, or emotional assistance. Recruitment efforts and federal adoption subsidies have helped to expand the pool of adoptive parents for these children.

Epidemiology

The prevalence of adoption in the general population of children younger than 18 is about 2 per cent. Every year about 60,000 children join unrelated adoptive families in the United States, which makes up just over half the total number of adoptions yearly. In 1986, fewer than half of the unrelated domestic adoptions involved infants (representing 0.7 per cent of all live births) and about one fourth of the unrelated domestic adoptions involved older children with special needs. Agency adoptions (as opposed to those arranged by private individuals) comprised nearly 70 per cent of domestic adoptions. In 1987, 10,000 children were adopted from 79 foreign countries, with nearly 90 per cent arriving from Asian and Latin American countries. Two thirds were adopted at younger than 1 year of age. Since the mid 1980s, independent, foreign, and special needs adoptions (see Definition of Terms) have increased, making current adoptions more complex than traditional ones. Today, estimates suggest that nearly half of the 100,000 children awaiting placement in adoptive homes are considered as having special needs.

Definition of Terms

Adoption subsidies: federal and state financial support in the form of monthly cash payments, Medicaid coverage, and vouchers for special schools.

Agency adoptions (private and public): a licensed private adoption agency or an authorized public adoption agency completes a home study and places a child who is legally free for adoption. Agency resources should remain available to both the biofamily and the adoptive family even after the adoption is legally finalized.

Closed adoption: a commitment to secrecy on the part of both the biofamily and the adoptive family.

Disruption: when a child is returned to the state after a commitment is made to adopt the child but before the adoption is legally finalized.

Dissolution: when an adopted child is returned to the state after the adoption is legally finalized.

Foster parent: an adult chosen by the child welfare system in whose home other children are placed for care and protection. Some foster children are eventually reunited with their rehabilitated families.

Independent adoptions: physicians, lawyers, the clergy, or others handle the adoption. (In some states an agency must still do the home study.)

Legal risk adoption: when a child, placed with foster parents interested in adopting, is not yet freed from the continuing parental rights of the bioparents.

Open adoption: one in which the biologic and adoptive parents agree in advance to a certain degree of communication–be it an exchange of information without meeting, a meeting without names, a commitment to using a third party intermediary, intermittent or ongoing visitation, or, rarely and in the extreme, a decision to co-parent.

Out-of-home placement: the placement of a child into a respite care, foster care, residential treatment, or psychiatric hospital setting without severing the adoptive family tie or terminating the adoptive parental rights.

Special needs adoptions: related to minority, sibling grouped, mentally or physically handicapped (including major emotional problems), a background of child neglect or abuse, or life in a foster home.

The Adoption Process

Children must be freed for adoption by means of a legal process in which parental rights are either surrendered (usually an uncontested procedure) or terminated (more likely a contested court proceeding). Before the severing of parental rights, a given child might remain in a foster-care setting. Because adoption has become part of the child welfare system, prospective adoptive parents must be screened by an agency before being offered a child. After completion of a home study, prospective adoptive parents may make a commitment to a child, thereby becoming a preadoptive family. At the time of legal finalization, adoption establishes a legal and social relationship between the adult and child by which the child becomes a full member of the family. Adoption offers children who need families the opportunity to be reared by persons who have made a conscious decision to act on their desire to parent. Today, a wide variety of adoptive families are being developed, including some with single or gay or lesbian parents.

Core Psychologic Issues

Adoptive families constitute a diverse population. Although individual characteristics often outweigh any similarities, and issues clearly overlap, it can be conceptually helpful to separate common adoption-related psychological themes:

1. *Loss.* Although adoption is often a win-win situation, it is created in a context of various kinds of loss. Observable losses are known as "overt" losses and relate to specific traumas of abuse, separation, neglect, or multiple changes in caretaker. "Covert" losses, which are more subjective, include feeling deprived of a biologic history, feeling rejected by bioparents or adoptive parents, and having low self-esteem. "Status" losses are associated with the social stigma of differentness or illegitimacy, as when a school-age child is asked to share his or her family tree or when a child's appearance suggests alternative lineage and implies he or she does not belong. As with all types of losses, these must be grieved.

2. *Other core issues, including intimacy, trust, guilt, identity, and control.* All members of the adoption triangle (the adoptee, biologic parents, and adoptive parents) may have unresolved issues relating to each of these emotions. Each person is affected in a different way. For instance, the adoptee may feel guilty that he or she wants to search for a biologic parent, an adoptive parent may feel guilty that he or she was unable to provide biologically related grandchildren, and biologic parents may feel guilty that they were not able to keep the surrendered child. Adoptive parents may misread a toddler's natural pull for independence as a rejection of them as parents. Parents may also underestimate an adopted adolescent's struggle

with identity issues—especially as they relate to interracial, cross-cultural, and older adopted children.

3. *Developmentally linked issues of adoption.* A toddler or preschooler may take great pride in having been "chosen" and relate the stories of their adoption with enthusiasm associated with feeling special. By school age, however, a child's understanding of how families are developed becomes more sophisticated. To be "chosen" implies having been available, which implies having been given up. An adolescent has an even deeper understanding of sexuality, responsibility, and inherited characteristics. They are likely to have curiosity about and identity with known or imagined biologic parents. As adults, adoptees often wish for more medical information.

4. *Telling a child about his or her adoption.* Although professionals continue to debate the issues surrounding what and when to tell, most would agree that any disclosure about a child's past should be done in an empathic tone with an appreciation of the child's cognitive and emotional developmental level. Helpful dialogue about adoption does not occur at a single sitting. It develops over time as relationships themselves continue to deepen.

5. *Acknowledgment vs. denial of difference.* Families that deny obvious differences (e.g., appearance, race, or past experiences) and ones that seem to constantly focus on difference can have psychological difficulties. Minority adolescents in affluent, white families may have difficulty deciding whether to apply to college on minority status.

6. *Parent/child issues around their "goodness of fit."* Great difficulties can result from a disparity of expectations when either the parents expect something the child cannot deliver or the child delivers something the parents did not expect. Sometimes a more emotional child is seen as pathologic when placed with a family of opposite temperament. At other times the agencies are reluctant to give known traumatic or psychiatric history for fear that a potential adoptive parent will be turned away.

Clinical Findings

Adolescence is a critical age for issues of adoption to surface. All adolescents go through a stage of struggling with their identity and negotiating for privacy, independence, and control. The adopted adolescent, however, may be more likely to have an increased interest in how he or she fits in with family, friends, and the rest of the world and how life may have been different. A teenager may start to explore peer groups that he or she believes may represent the type of teenager he or she believes a biologic parent to have been, or may want to begin a search (literal or psychological) for the lost biologic parent, or may see adoptive parent efforts to get him or her to behave as a parental preference for a "wished for" biologic child.

As one 19-year old explained "I, the *real* me, died at age five when my parents adopted me. Ever since then I have been distracted by the fact that my grandparents are not *my* grandparents, my town is not *my* town and my life is not *my* life. I'm a blue-collar guy who has spent his whole life disappointing his white-collar family. Now I've gotten my girlfriend pregnant and feel like running away from everything. . . . But that's just what that guy did with his girlfriend when I was conceived."

Key Clinical Findings (Adolescent Age)

- Search for lost parent
- Search for peer groups of "lost identity"

Adoption and Psychiatric Illness

Adoption itself is not pathologic, nor does it protect a child from psychiatric illness. Although only a fraction of adopted children have disabling psychiatric symptoms, adopted children, adolescents, and their families appear to be overrepresented in mental health clinics, on psychiatric inpatient units, and in residential treatment centers. There is no single reason for these findings. Some research suggests that adoptive parents are known to be more perceptive and more familiar with services in general and therefore are more comfortable seeking treatment for their children. Even so, an appropriate multifactorial model may include some of the previously discussed core psychologic issues and some or all of the following:

1. *Perinatal factors.* The quality of prenatal care and nutrition is included as well as risks associated with prenatal substance abuse and cigarette smoking.

2. *Inherited vulnerabilities.* These may especially relate to the major mental illnessess. For instance, research suggests attention deficit hyperactivity disorder is overrepresented in adoptees.

3. *Attachment-related issues.* A child who has had significant deprivation in the past and exhibits the characteristic sequelae of emotional withdrawal, indiscriminate friendliness, or provocative behavior may have a more serious attachment disorder. Key adoption populations at risk for attachment disorders include children adopted from overseas orphanages and those with multiple traumas and broken attachments.

4. *Effects of early trauma.* These include posttraumatic stress associated with neglect and physical and sexual abuse. One of the greatest challenges to an adoptive family is when the adults become the target of a child's displaced anger for having been abused by a biologic parent.

Prevention and Treatment

1. An astute clinician familiar with several possible implications of the adoption will be invaluable to an adoptive individual or couple as they try to sort things out in a therapeutic way. Early detection of potentially adoption-related issues should be followed by prompt attention using familiar anticipatory guidance techniques, psychoeducation about core adoption-related issues, and information about local postadoptive services, including adoptive-parent support groups and mental health clinic resources.

2. Pediatricians can promote the process of empathic disclosure and helpful dialogue about adoption by educating the parents about their child's evolving cognitive and emotional development. A pediatrician's routine requests for family medical history can either surface as an uncomfortable, provocative time for an adopted child or adoptive parent or as a helpful introduction to other informa-

tion about adoption-related themes. Adopted adolescents wishing to gain more information about biological parents may be stifled by feelings of guilt or worries that they will be viewed by their adoptive parents as ungrateful or disloyal. A pediatrician may be called on to help adoptive parents understand their teenager's natural curiosity.

3. When psychiatric symptoms are more impairing, the pediatrician's role may change to that of gatekeeper for mental health services. In general, the comprehensive biopsychosocial approach to evaluation and treatment of more serious child and family issues is beyond the expertise of the primary care clinician and should be referred to a child psychiatrist who can work with the family to separate out issues that are related to the adoption and those that appear to be independent. After encouraging and preparing an appropriate referral, the pediatrician may monitor the treatment through his or her ongoing relationship with the family.

Key Treatment (Adolescent Age)

- Anticipatory guidance
- Empathic disclosure
- Reassurance of adoptive parents

Outcome

Is adoption itself a risk factor for child and adolescent psychopathology? And adoption compared with what? Compared with those children living in abusive or neglectful settings or in alternative out-of-home placements such as continued institutionalization or foster care, adopted children fare much better. Most adopted individuals remain mentally and physically healthy (with "success rates" of 73 to 86 per cent in some studies). Adoption continues to be a vital resource for children and families as well as for society on the whole. As one 8-year-old said: "Adoption is fun. Adoption is fun . . . 'cause you get to be part of a family."

Bibliography

Adoption Factbook. Washington, DC, National Committee for Adoption, 1989.

Brodzynski DM, Schechter MD (eds): The Psychology of Adoption. New York, Oxford University Press, 1990.

Nickman SL: Losses in adoption: The need for dialogue. Psychoanal Study Child 1985;40:365–398.

Nickman SL, Lewis RG: Adoptive families and professionals: When the experts make things worse. J Am Acad Child Adolesc Psychiatry 1994;33:753–755.

Sherry SN: Adoption and foster family care. In Levine MD, Carey WB, Crocker AC (eds): Developmental-Behavioral Pediatrics. Philadelphia, WB Saunders, 1992, pp 122–127.

49 The Depressed Child

Linda M. Forsythe and *Michael S. Jellinek*

Definition and Overview

1. The fourth edition of the *Diagnostic and Statistic Manual (DSM-IV)*, published by the American Psychiatric Association, acknowledges that in children and adolescents major mood disorders are often in evolution, making for distinctions and presentations that are less clear than their adult counterparts. With this in mind, childhood major depressive disorder (MDD) is characterized by at least 2 weeks of intense and prolonged emotional and behavioral change from baseline to a dysphoric or irritable mood that interferes with interesting or pleasurable activities in the home, at school, or with peers.

2. Although *depression* is a common term used in daily conversation to connote sadness, disappointment, or frustration, the thought of a "depressed child" evokes many different images: a downcast, sad, or gloomy preschooler; a listless, dejected, or disengaged student; or a sullen, irritable adolescent. All pediatricians remember, with frustration, a passive or discouraged child with recurrent abdominal pain or complaints of chronic fatigue. The core symptom, a depressed, sad, irritable, or "bored" mood, is not in itself pathologic but can become so when it interferes with age-specific functioning.

3. Coincident with a depressed mood, a child or adolescent with MDD will show age-specific changes in several of the following:

   a. Appetite—a school-age child may stop gaining weight or an adolescent might become obese or anorexic.

   b. Sleep—with disturbances of insomnia, hypersomnia, or frequent wakings

   c. Energy—including either agitation or lethargy

   d. Social withdrawal—which may look like problems of attachment and separation, loss of spontaneous play, school reluctance, or a sudden drop in academic or after-school performance

   e. Self-esteem—a school-age child might feel inadequate in social situations and settle for the easier role of class clown over the more challenging option of genuine relationships; an adolescent is more likely to describe feelings of guilt, self-reproach, hopelessness, or helplessness.

   f. Concentration—a young child might present with

developmental regression, whereas a school-age child or adolescent is more likely to have difficulty being attentive in class, completing assignments, and making decisions.

    g. Dangerousness—which may include head-banging in infants and an increase in accidents, lying, stealing, or truancy in older children and adolescents

    h. Somatic symptoms—including failure to thrive, enuresis, encopresis, abdominal or head pain

    i. Substance abuse—often associated with peer group changes

    j. Suicidal ideation—which may be obvious or disguised as recurrent thoughts or morbid preoccupation with illness or death.

4. The impulsiveness of childhood can be exceptionally dangerous in the context of a mood disorder. Impulsive ingestions are no less lethal than ingestions that are planned. Inattentiveness without regard for safety (crossing the street without looking) may be a sign of an attentional disability but statistically also increases the risk that an affective disorder will lead to suicide attempts or completions. In adolescence, when peer attachments assume a major role, any break-up or social humiliation might increase suicide risk. Hopelessness and helplessness expressed through actions of a self-harming nature can be dangerously misread as "unintentional" or "accidents."

5. Suicide is one of the leading causes of death among adolescents. Risk factors for adolescent suicide include depression, attention deficit hyperactivity disorder (with characteristic impulsivity), substance abuse, family turmoil, negative life events, sexual orientation (with an associated secret anxiety or fear concerning homosexuality), and a friend or family member with a suicide history. In general, girls are more likely to manifest suicidal ideation and have suicide attempts than are boys. Boys are more likely to use violence and weapons in their suicide attempts and outnumber girls for suicide completion. Research suggests that youths with suicidal ideation at age 15 are 16 times more likely to report lifetime suicide attempts. All references to suicide and death by children and adolescents should be taken seriously, and prompt referral should be made for psychiatric evaluation.

Epidemiology

1. Using relatively strict MDD criteria, the prevalence of MDD in the infant and preschool population is about 1 per cent. In this age bracket, MDD is most confused with failure to thrive, as well as attachment, separation, and behavior problems. The 2 per cent of school-age children who meet criteria for MDD are likely to have a more protracted, recurrent, or severe course. MDD affects nearly 5 per cent of the adolescent population, in whom it presents most like the more familiar adult syndrome and in whom it is most likely to involve suicidality.

2. In selected populations, such as pediatric inpatients, as many as 7 per cent of children and 27 per cent of adolescents meet criteria for MDD. Eight per cent of children with MDD have additional or "co-morbid" disorders such as anxiety, attention deficit, substance abuse, and conduct problems such as lying, stealing, vandalism, and truancy. When these patients seek professional attention for the delinquency or substance use, the associated mood is often overlooked.

Etiology

Research suggests that MDD includes several yet-to-be-defined subgroups with multifactorial interacting causes. Environmental contributions are variable at different developmental stages and are further influenced by what appears to be polygenetic inheritance patterns and organic factors. Children identify with, learn from, and share the mood of their parents. They are greatly affected by losses, especially parental death and divorce. The boundary between extended bereavement and MDD is particularly unclear.

Clinical Findings

The assessment of depressed mood and decreased functional status in developing children requires the use of parent and teacher information and an appreciation for the variety of age-related clinical presentations:

1. *Infant/toddler.* Clinical concern for persistently passive, unresponsive infants as well as for irritable, unsoothable, crying infants has led to speculation about the degree to which temperament can explain the difficulties. For some, the clinical picture is better understood in terms of the early mood dysregulation associated with MDD. As these children develop further, some of them may present as quiet, inhibited toddlers with arrested social development, whereas others may become overactive, impulsive, and irritable preschoolers.

2. *School-aged child.* In school-aged children with MDD, the expected pride associated with industry and enthusiasm may be overwhelmed by humiliation, defeat, irritability, and self-doubt. The child may become isolated, rejected, and accident prone. Familiar temper tantrums of earlier years may reappear, as might morbid preoccupations with bodily injury, illness, abandonment, or death. There may be pediatric office visits for multiple somatic complaints.

3. *Adolescents.* Teenagers with MDD experience hopelessness and have difficulty containing intense negative feelings. In the heat of a crushing rejection, they have both the passion and the means to act on self-destructive urges. They may direct negative actions inward against themselves by disregarding food, sleep, and hygiene; turn to alcohol and drugs for numbing symptomatic relief; or display destructive behaviors. Instead of appearing sad and eliciting sympathy (as adults with MDD might), adolescents with MDD often look angry and are frequently resented. When taking a history, it is especially important to obtain information directly from the adolescent and to try to gain insight into his or her internal state. One might ask, for example, "How big is that anger inside?" or "Do you ever get so mad or so sad that you feel like hurting yourself?"

Key Clinical Findings

- Infant/toddler
  Passive or irritable

- School-aged child
  Self-doubt
  Temper tantrums
  Accident prone

- Adolescent
  Hopelessness
  Drug use

Diagnosis

1. Information about a child's mood—is he or she *mostly* sad and blue? mad and irritable? or fine?—is crucial to the diagnosis of MDD, which, by definition, requires at least a 2-week period of prominent mood-related symptoms. A detailed history of the child's baseline level of functioning, including his or her behaviors at home, performance level at school, and relationships with peers, should be obtained along with any subsequent deviation from this baseline. A cross-situational decrease in function, or significant change in behaviors, can be a key indicator of mood-related stress and disability.

2. Studies suggest that information about a past depressive episode is invaluable because past experiences often herald recurrences. Identifying and clarifying co-morbid symptoms—is the child often intensely worried? profoundly anxious? impulsively inattentive? prone to lie and steal?—improves the quality of subsequent referrals and increases the opportunity for effective treatment selection. Extended family histories can be important predictors of childhood risk. Information should be obtained about personal and family histories of depression, anxiety, attentional deficits, or alcohol or substance use. Significant parental affective disorder is associated with an important constellation of related indicators of impairment and can be used as a powerful predictor of episodes of MDD in adolescents.

3. In addition, routine physical examination is useful to assess medical illnesses as a cause of the symptoms. Screening laboratory tests should be performed when suggested by the history and physical examination and might include complete blood cell count with differential, electrolytes, liver function tests, thyroid function tests, blood urea nitrogen, creatinine, urinalysis, and electrocardiogram.

4. Psychologic testing of children, including projective tests and semi-structured diagnostic interviews, can be helpful in providing more data about less available thoughts, emotional states, and behaviors. Whereas biologic correlate studies involving the neuroendocrine system, electroencephalographic sleep architectural changes, and neurotransmitter system studies have been used to assess depression in adults, they are not reliable in children.

Prevention

Early detection of depressive symptoms, accurate diagnosis of MDD, and prompt initiation of treatment are key factors in the prevention of more serious sequelae of MDD, such as recurrence and self-injurious behaviors including suicide. This requires wide dissemination of information about MDD to parents and teachers as well as to other healthcare providers. Children whose parents are known to be sufferers of MDD should be screened periodically. Although some sad moments are transient, and depressing events continue to occur, real childhood MDD is a serious illness that can lead to a rapid decline in function, with children falling off their developmental track. Once a child has had a depressive episode, however brief, the risk of recurrence is high—especially with a family history of affective illness. Therefore, any truly depressed child or adolescent with or without self-destructive acts or threats must be taken seriously, followed by prompt referral for psychiatric evaluation and follow-up.

Treatment

1. As the primary care physician, the pediatrician often has a key role as the gatekeeper to mental health services for children. Schools, social service agencies, and parents may all refer worrisome cases to the pediatrician, trusting the pediatrician to identify the psychiatric problem and refer the identified child for further evaluation and possible treatment. Studies suggest that many of the pediatricians who decide not to refer mentally ill children to child psychiatrists base their decisions on protecting the child from the associated stigma of being a "mental case" or on the belief that treatment is simple and straightforward and can be successfully managed without referral. Although this strategy may be effective for some children, it puts others at significant risk.

2. Most children with MDD can be safely managed as outpatients. In general, the comprehensive biopsychosocial approach to treatment of childhood MDD is beyond the expertise of the primary care clinician and should be referred to a child psychiatrist. After recognizing features of MDD in a child or adolescent, and encouraging and preparing appropriate referrals, the primary care clinician may monitor the treatment through his or her ongoing relationship with the family. Urgent psychiatric consultation is indicated whenever the child or adolescent is thought to be psychotic, acutely suicidal, acutely manic, abusing substances, or otherwise difficult to manage safely.

3. The child psychiatrist is uniquely trained to consider biologic, psychosocial, and psychodynamic factors in an integrated schema. He or she can assess the degree of disability considering all aspects of the child's or adolescent's life. When treatment is indicated, the multimodal treatment plan that follows directly from the often multiple diagnoses might include features from several of the following: psychodynamic therapy, play therapy, cognitive therapy, behavioral therapy, family therapy, parent guidance work, environmental interventions, and, when the MDD is found significantly to impair cross-situational functioning, such medications as desipramine, nortriptyline, fluoxetine, sertraline, and lithium.

Outcome

Both chronic illness and treatment resistance increase when MDD is ignored and allowed to become further entrenched in a child's view and expectations of himself or herself. Early recognition, information, and treatment planning can begin to promote self-esteem, improve parent-child relationships, and help siblings cope. Treatment can begin to relieve symptoms within about a month. Further treatment strategies aim to prevent harm and suffering while taking steps to return the child and family to their previous level of functioning. Although outcome studies examining the long-term impact of early recognition and treatment of mood disorders have not yet been conducted, pediatricians can diagnose childhood MDD, alleviate suffering, and help parents to support their child's optimal functioning.

Bibliography

Beardslee W, Keller M, Seifer R, et al: Prediction of adolescent affective disorder: Effects of prior parental affective disorders and child psychopathology. J Am Acad Child Adolesc Psychiatry 1996;35:279–288.

Kashani J, Eppright T: Mood disorders in adolescents. In Wiener J (ed): Textbook of Child and Adolescent Psychiatry. Washington, DC, American Psychiatric Press, 1991.

Reinherz H, Giaconia R, Silverman A, et al: Early psychosocial risks for adolescent suicidal ideation and attempts. J Am Acad Child Adolesc Psychiatry 1995;34:599–611.

Sarles R, Haerian M: Depression and suicide. In Dershewitz R (ed): Pediatric Ambulatory Care. Philadelphia, JB Lippincott, 1993.

Shafii M, Shafii S (eds): Clinical Guide to Depression in Children and Adolescents. Washington, DC, American Psychiatric Press, 1992.

Weller E, Weller R: Mood disorders in children. In Weiner J (ed): Textbook of Child and Adolescent Psychiatry. Washington, DC, American Psychiatric Press, 1991.

50 Anxiety Disorders

Guochuan E. Tsai and *Michael S. Jellinek*

Definition

Anxiety is an essential component of human life. Anxiety provides a stimulus for individual development and a protective mechanism of species survival. However, anxiety can be excessive with fears and worries, phobic avoidance, anticipatory anxiety, generalized vigilance, panic attack with autonomic arousal, or, to the worst extent, overwhelming dread. Anxiety is considered as pathologic when it interferes with achievement of goals, quality of life, or psychologic well-being. Pathologic anxiety usually is intense, recurrent or persists over time, and autonomous with minimal basis in a realistic threat and can proceed to consistent behavior patterns such as avoidance and lifestyle constriction.

Epidemiology

Anxiety disorders are one of the most common adolescent clinical problems. According to community-based epidemiologic studies, 5 to 9 per cent of adolescents have anxiety disorders causing dysfunction and requiring treatment. Panic disorder, agoraphobia, specific phobia, social phobia, obsessive compulsive disorder, posttraumatic stress disorder, or acute stress disorder can have their onset during childhood or adulthood. Three specific anxiety syndromes have been identified in childhood populations: *separation anxiety disorder, avoidant disorder,* and *overanxious disorder.* The prevalence rates of separation anxiety disorder range from 2.0 to 6.8 per cent; the avoidant disorder rate is about 1.6 per cent; overanxious disorder onset ranges from 2.9 to 5.9 per cent; the rate of *social phobia* is about 1 per cent; and *simple phobia* ranges from 2.3 to 9.1 per cent.

Etiology

Multiple and complex theories have been presented concerning the origins of anxiety.

1. Psychodynamic schools postulate anxiety is triggered by external events that activate anxiety associated with unconscious aggressive wishes. The symbolic anxiety manifested by the adolescent serves to disguise the unconscious distortion of unacceptable wishes. For example, anger and the wish to hurt a parent would be manifested by a fear of separating from the parent and the dread that the parent will come to some harm.

2. Behavioral and learning theorists emphasize biologic vulnerability to anxiety is under genetic control. They explain maladaptive behavior through reinforcement such as a mother's fright every time a younger child behaves more autonomously. The correction of maladaptive reinforcement will dictate the success of treatment.

3. For cognitive approaches, anxiety symptoms are the result of cognitive distortions. The disruption of cognitive representations of an individual's environment and experience causes anxiety.

4. Ethologic models consider emotions as adaptive consequences of evolutionary processes resulting from natural selection. Anxiety and fear are protective of naturally occurring dangers and also regulate social bonds that maximize survival and species reproduction.

Overall, psychodynamic, learning, and cognitive theories differ in their identifying the origin of anxiety but consider similar psychologic mechanisms underlying normal and pathologic conditions. In contrast, ethologic views suggest normal fear favors species survival and

Diagnostic Criteria of the Major Adolescent Anxiety Disorders

Separation Anxiety Disorder

Developmentally inappropriate and excessive anxiety concerning separation from home or from those to whom the individual is attached for more than 4 weeks, as evidenced by three or more of the following. The disturbance causes clinically significant distress or impairment in social, academic (occupational), or other important areas of functioning.

1. Recurrent excessive distress when separation from home or major attachment figures occurs or is anticipated
2. Persistent and excessive worry about losing, or about possible harm befalling, major attachment figures
3. Persistent and excessive worry that an untoward event will lead to separation from a major attachment figure (e.g., getting lost or being kidnapped)
4. Persistent reluctance or refusal to go to school or elsewhere because of fear of separation
5. Persistently and excessively fearful or reluctant to be alone or without major attachment figures at home or without significant adults in other settings
6. Persistent reluctance or refusal to go to sleep without being near a major attachment figure or to sleep away from home
7. Repeated nightmares involving the theme of separation.
8. Repeated complaints of physical symptoms (such as headaches, stomach aches, nausea, or vomiting) when separation from major attachment figures occurs or is anticipated.

Generalized Anxiety Disorder (Overanxious Disorder of Childhood)

Excessive anxiety and worry (apprehensive expectation) occurring more days than not for at least 6 months about a number of events or activities (such as work or school performance), and the child finds it difficult to control the worry. The anxiety and worry are associated with one or more of the following six symptoms:

1. Restlessness or feeling keyed up or on edge
2. Being easily fatigued
3. Difficulty concentrating or mind going blank
4. Irritability
5. Muscle tension
6. Sleep disturbance (difficulty falling or staying asleep, or restless unsatisfying sleep)

The anxiety, worry, or physical symptoms cause clinically significant distress or impairment in social, occupational, or other important areas of functioning.

Social Phobia (Social Anxiety Disorder)

The child has the capacity for age-appropriate social relationship with familiar people but he or she has a marked and persistent fear of one or more social or performance situations in which the child is exposed to unfamiliar or to possible scrutiny in a peer setting. The child fears that he or she will act in a way (or show anxiety symptoms) that will be humiliating or embarrassing.

Exposure to the feared social situation almost invariably provokes anxiety, which may take the form of a situationally bound or situationally predisposed panic attack or expressed by crying, tantrums, freezing, or shrinking from social situations with unfamiliar people.

The feared social or performance situations are avoided or else are endured with intense anxiety or distress.

The avoidance, anxious anticipation, or distress in the feared social or performance situation(s) interferes significantly with the person's normal routine, occupational (academic) functioning, or social activities or relationships, or there is marked distress about having the phobia.

The duration is at least 6 months.

From American Psychiatric Association: Diagnostic and Statistical Manual of Mental Disorders, 4th ed (DSM-IV). Washington, DC, American Psychiatric Association, 1994.

pathologic anxiety is qualitatively distinct. However, the ethologic view can account for adaptive behaviors but not the pathologic behaviors that are dysfunctional. These theories are not mutually exclusive, and several may be operative in exacerbating anxiety.

Pathogenesis

1. GABA receptor theories. The development of benzodiazepines and other anxiolytics have advanced neurobiologic theories of anxiety and emotional regulation. Benzodiazepines are high-affinity ligands for the receptor of the inhibitory neurotransmitter γ-aminobutyric acid (GABA). GABA receptors are enriched in the limbic system, a neuronal system that modulates environmental cues and also serves as a relay station for internal affective and visceral signals to the neocortical regions. Animal studies indicate this limbic GABAergic system may play a role in modulating arousal, alertness, and behavioral inhibition. Lesion studies in nonhuman primates on the amygdala, an important limbic structure, provide compelling evidences for its involvement in emotional and social behavior.
2. The noradrenergic locus ceruleus. Fear responses can be elicited by stimulation of the locus ceruleus. The importance of the noradrenergic system is supported by the clinical efficacy of β-adrenergic antagonists in treating anxiety disorders.
3. Cholecystokinin (CCK). Data have accumulated over the past decade supporting the hypothesis that CCK plays a role in the neurobiology of anxiety and panic attacks. CCK is a normal central nervous system endogenous anticipatory stress modulator; enhanced sensitivity to CCKB receptor agonists can result in anxiety and panic attacks.
4. Role of temperament. The neurobiologic theory is complemented by the temperament theory popular from the

past decade. Temperament studies indicate inhibited children have increased risk for anxiety disorders. Inhibited temperament can be the result of genetically determined hypersensitivity of external cues due to the lowered limbic activity threshold. Theoretically, benzodiazepines are therapeutic by reducing the hypervigilance accompanied by the autonomic arousal, and the effect is mediated by correcting the threshold through the inhibitory GABA system.

Clinical Findings

1. Mixed symptoms. Adolescent anxiety disorders, as in other medical diagnosis, are diagnosed by clustering of a symptom complex. There is no single symptom diagnostic for a specific anxiety disorder. For example, school refusal is a major presentation of multiple disorders: simple phobia for school, social phobia, conduct disorder, or depression. At times, dual or triple diagnoses present simultaneously.

2. Transient anxiety. Adolescent anxieties are common, and most resolve spontaneously. Transient anxiety about meeting new friends, a first date, varsity tryouts, or other developmental steps toward autonomy is expectable. Clinicians should pay attention to developmental differences and severity in the presentation of anxiety disorders. For generalized anxiety disorder with childhood onset, adolescents endorse more symptoms than younger children. However, almost all children with generalized anxiety disorder have unrealistic worry about future events as their key symptoms.

3. Degrees of severity

   a. The spectrum of symptomatology ranges from mild worry to incapacitating panic attacks. Some children have little residual symptoms, whereas others can relapse and exacerbate throughout childhood and into adulthood. Because children with anxiety disorders who do not receive treatment sometimes develop chronicity, it is important to have clinical assessment and intervention whenever the anxiety symptoms cause dysfunction of the child, even when the child does not meet the threshold criteria for a specific DSM-IV diagnosis of anxiety disorders. Pediatricians will have to act more quickly when the anxiety interferes with school or peer relationships or causes serious personal suffering.

   b. In clinical practice, anxiety syndromes overlap considerably. For example, panic attack and excessive distress are the major components of panic disorder and separation anxiety disorder. Social phobia is characterized by a persistent fear of situations in which the patient is subjected to public scrutiny; the patient fears in a way that will be humiliating and embarrassing. The social phobia may be well circumscribed (e.g., standing in front of a class) or generalized (e.g., going out with parents).

   c. Co-morbidity is a common rule of childhood anxiety disorder. About one third of children meet criteria for two or more anxiety disorders. Major depression is also a common co-morbidity, ranging from 28 to 69 per cent, of anxiety disorder. Between 15 and 24 per cent of children with separation anxiety disorder

or generalized anxiety disorder also meet criteria for attention-deficit/hyperactivity disorder.

Key Clinical Findings

- Refusal to attend school
- Panic attacks

Differential Diagnosis

Physical conditions, including hypoglycemic episodes, hyperthyroidism, cardiac arrhythmias, caffeinism, pheochromocytoma, seizure disorders, migraine, and other central nervous system disorders (e.g., delirium or brain tumors) can mimic anxiety symptoms. Reactions to medications, including antihistamines, antiasthmatics, sympathomimetics, corticosteroids, haloperidol, pimozide (neuroleptic-induced separation anxiety disorder), other antipsychotics (akathisia), and fluoxetine; diet pills; and cold medicines can result in symptoms of anxiety. The treatment for the anxiety symptoms associated with physical condition or medication is to correct the underlying illness or remove the offending agents.

Prevention and Treatment

When developing a treatment plan, overall adaptation is as important as focal symptoms that define a specific anxiety disorder. A comprehensive focus with long-term perspective in addition to short-term symptom relief is important to modify the maladaptive concomitants and prevent relapse. For example, the comprehensive and long-term perspective emphasizes that separation anxiety disorder can continue in adult life as agoraphobia or panic disorder; social disability and affect constriction are quite common complications of separation anxiety disorder and can persist into adulthood.

1. Integrated approach. Symptom complexity, co-morbidity, and chronicity necessitate an integrated approach in treating an adolescent with anxiety disorder. Both pharmacologic and nonpharmacologic strategies are important in the treatment of childhood anxiety disorder. Multimodal treatment is indicated, as recommended by the *Practice Parameters for the Assessment and Treatment of Anxiety Disorder,* published by the American Academy of Child and Adolescent Psychiatry. A comprehensive treatment plan should take the following components into consideration: cognitive behavioral therapy, pharmacotherapy, psychodynamic psychotherapy, family therapy when indicated, education of parents and child, and communication with school personnel and primary care physicians.

2. Pharmacologic treatment. Research on pharmacologic treatments for adolescent anxiety disorders is in its infancy. Because controlled studies are limited, clinicians treating anxious adolescents often make educated judgments based on information from open trials, case reports, or anecdotal experiences.

   a. Tricyclic antidepressants may be helpful in some cases of separation anxiety disorder and school refusal, but definitive proof is lacking.

   b. Chlordiazepoxide, clonazepam, and alprazolam have been reported effective for separation anxiety disorder.

c. Efficacy of benzodiazepines, serotonin reuptake inhibitors, and buspirone in generalized anxiety disorder with adolescent onset has not been established, although a few open trials suggest these agents may be effective.

d. Many controlled studies have demonstrated that propranolol, benzodiazepines, and antidepressants are effective treatments for panic disorder, but the study is limited in adolescent panic disorder.

e. Similarly, β-adrenergic blockers, benzodiazepines, serotonin reuptake inhibitors, and monoamine oxidase inhibitors are pharmacologic treatment options in adult social phobia, but child psychiatrists have to extrapolate findings from the adult studies for the pediatric population.

3. Cognitive behavior therapy combines a behavior approach with changes in cognition associated with anxiety. It can restructure the adolescent's thoughts into a more positive framework and adaptive behavior. In separation anxiety disorder associated with school refusal, classical conditioning–based systematic desensitization and exposure and operant behavioral techniques were reported to be effective treatments. Improvement of generalized anxiety disorder by cognitive behavioral treatment has also been reported. In the case of simple phobia, behavioral treatment is the treatment of choice. The interventions include modeling and systemic desensitization.

4. Psychoanalysis and psychodynamic psychotherapy see anxiety as a result of maladaptive attempts to cope with internal conflicts. The approaches tie the anxiety symptoms to the adolescent's overall personality structure; in addition to symptom amelioration, modification of the personality structure are the primary goals for this treatment. Choice of different treatment modalities depends on clinical judgment and empirical results. There are no well researched data to support specific treatment for different anxiety disorders. Thus, the pediatrician should consider the spectrum from biologic vulnerability to family dynamics as well as family psychiatric history.

Key Treatment

- Cognitive therapy
- Pharmacologic therapy
- Family therapy

Bibliography

Allen AJ, Leonard H, Swedo SE: Current knowledge of medications for the treatment of childhood anxiety disorders. J Am Acad Child Adolesc Psychiatry 1995;34:976–986.

American Psychiatric Association: Diagnostic and Statistical Manual of Mental Disorders, 4th ed. Washington, DC, American Psychiatric Association, 1994.

Biederman J, Rosenbaum JF, Hirshfeld DR, et al: Psychiatric correlates of behavioral inhibition in young children of parents with and without psychiatric disorders. Arch Gen Psychiatry 1990;47:21–26.

Livingston R: Anxiety disorders. In Lewis M (ed): Child and Adolescent Psychiatry, A Comprehensive Textbook. Baltimore, Williams & Wilkins, 1991, pp 673–685.

Practice parameters for the assessment and treatment of anxiety disorder. J Am Acad Child Adolesc Psychiatry 1993;32:1089–1098.

51 Divorce

Michael S. Jellinek

Although the rate of divorce (after increasing dramatically during the 1950s and 1960s) has stabilized, over 1 million children each year are affected by the divorce process. Many of these divorces occur during the child's infancy and others during adolescence. The average length of marriage ending in divorce is between 6 and 7 years, so that the effects of discord and divorce are of substantial concern to pediatricians.

Most pediatricians will not be aware of parental separation and divorce unless a parent volunteers the information or asks directly about the child's related emotional difficulties. Instead, pediatricians often learn of divorce indirectly, possibly through a change of address, a request to forward records, difficulty in collecting bills as family finances are frozen in negotiations, or a summons to write letters or give testimony (usually indicative of a more hostile divorce).

Impact on Family

The immediate impact of parental separation and pending divorce is a sense of shock or major loss. Early in the process the available time for the child and the quality of that time is less than when the family was intact, and it may decrease further for the noncustodial parent (fathers approximately 90 percent of the time). Both parents are frequently preoccupied by their own mourning of the marriage as well as the divorce process. The child faces the loss of the family unit, a complex social structure that had supported a view of the world that was safe and predictable.

Impact: Financial and Social

Other losses include financial and social ones. Following divorce, mothers generally suffer a substantial drop in disposable income, and many approach or pass below accepted poverty limits, even considering monthly support (the father's disposable income is also reduced but often substantially less so). There is also a financial incentive for men to default on their financial responsibilities, as their standard of living and disposable income will increase by 73 percent without the burden of child support.[1] Only recently has legislation been in effect that encourages court action across state lines to enforce financial agreements. In addition to the financial consequences, children may have to move from the family home with a consequent loss of friends and local social supports, as well as a required change in schools.

Effects on the Child

The short-term clinical consequences of a divorce are dependent on multiple variables.[2] One has to do with the parents and their ability to focus on their children's feelings and needs. A second major factor is the age of the child. A child under the age of 3 years may respond with irritability, whining, crying, fearfulness, separation anxiety, increasing aggressive behavior, sleep problems, and regression in such areas as toilet training. Children at age 4 to 5 years often irrationally blame themselves for the unhappiness of their parents and have doubts about their own worth. School-age children may be moody and preoccupied, may daydream, or may be overtly aggressive (most commonly abusive to their custodial mother, possibly protecting their father from anger so as not to risk a further loss of time with that parent). School performance commonly suffers for the year following the separation/divorce, and loyalty conflicts are common. The adolescent may assume, often prematurely, a greater degree of emotional autonomy as a way of dealing with feelings about the divorce. Angry feelings may emerge as aggressive, antisocial behavior, and the adolescent may worry about the financial and emotional effects of the divorce on the family. Teenagers who seem to have some capacity to withdraw from the crisis, while still deriving emotional support from both parents, may fare best over the short term. Some teenagers accelerate the process of leaving home and invest too quickly or too heavily in peer relationships and sometimes "premature" sexual experience. For all ages, somatization may be an unconscious solution to the deep feelings, including anger, that are inevitable during the divorce process.

Approximately half of children manifest symptoms during the first year of the divorce. Over time the decrease in hostility as well as the adaptive capacities of most children ameliorate the consequences of the divorce. Major risk factors that contribute to the 10 percent or more of children who have difficulty for more than a year after the divorce include ongoing discord and hostility between the parents, maternal depression, other psychiatric disorders in either parent, and poverty. Recent follow-up studies suggest that divorce, especially during later childhood and early adolescence, may impair the young adult's capacity for intimacy and readiness to commit to marriage. Although multiyear follow-up studies of children and families are a complex undertaking, several general findings appear valid. Some effects appear to be linear and immediate, such as school performance; others tend to be "sleeper" effects, in that they reemerge years later, when the child faces intimate adult relationships. Outcome is more favorable if there is a working relationship between parents and if the child's

relationship to the custodial parent is positive.[3] Thus, pediatricians should view their follow-up of divorce as a long-term concern involving parent-parent, parent-child, and an overall review of psychosocial functioning. In later adolescence, divorce follow-up includes asking the teenager about depressive mood and the quality of his or her interpersonal and intimate relationships.

Divorce is a several-year process that includes discord, separation, a lengthy and sometimes hostile court process, a final decree, an initial period of adjustment, and then a long-term stabilization in revised parental roles. As parents adjust, they are able to help their children understand the reasons for the divorce in developmentally appropriate terms, relieve any sense that the children were the key cause of the parents' difficulties, and continue to answer questions. Likewise, children can reconsider the divorce issues either because of increased capacities through maturity or by events such as holidays, school events, illnesses, or beginning to date. A substantial number of children face an additional adjustment as parents begin to date and remarry; thus children may have to integrate parents and stepfamilies.

The Pediatrician's Role

In many pediatric practices, divorce is so common that pediatricians should routinely ask about the quality and status of parental relationships as one of several annual questions in their brief psychosocial review. If there is parental discord prior to separation or divorce, the pediatrician may be able to play a very helpful, preventive role by encouraging a referral for counseling. Once the separation and divorce process has been initiated, the pediatrician can help parents understand their child's need for information, reactions, and fear and serve as advocate for the child's best interests. Parents should discuss in an age-appropriate manner the reasons for divorce and assure as much continuity and stability as possible. Parents should be encouraged to ask on a regular basis during quiet and private moments if the child has any questions, and they should try to maintain an open forum of communication. School-age children feel both insecure and to blame for the divorce and thus need explicit assurance and a rationale for the divorce that eases any guilt. Pediatricians should also help parents understand the potentially serious consequences of withholding visitation and of using the child as a messenger in disputes, for financial leverage, or as a sounding board for harsh criticism of the other parent. Such parental behavior and contentious or lengthy court proceedings are major risk factors to the child's short-term and long-term emotional functioning and adjustment.

In contentious situations, the pediatrician should be careful not to be used by one parent against the other. The pediatrician should avoid taking sides in a divorce dispute unless there is clear evidence that one parent is unfit to care for the child. From a long-term perspective, maintaining a trusted relationship with both parents is the best option.

Separation and divorce should prompt a protocol that is most likely to be successful if initiated early in the process. In the first few weeks following separation, the parents often are still quite focused on their children's well-being and have not yet been faced with complex legal and financial issues that may exacerbate discord. Thus as soon as a potential divorce is in progress and known, the pediatrician should initiate a protocol to assess:

1. The child's acute reaction
2. The parents' level of hostility
3. The parents' capacity to meet the child's physical and emotional needs
4. Indications of parental depression or other serious psychiatric disorder
5. The visitation arrangements and the quality of the relationship between the parents
6. The child's adjustment and functioning at annual intervals after the divorce.

In terms of custody, one must consider both legal and physical custody. Joint custody is designed to keep both parents, more commonly fathers, involved in the child's life. Joint custody means ongoing contact between two, often angry, parents who must be able to separate their feelings about each other as spouses from their feelings as parents. Joint legal custody is relevant to coordinating medical care and assures that both parents must give consent and be informed about their child's medical needs as well as other major life decisions. Joint physical custody necessitates an often complex schedule of visitation between both parents and inevitably includes careful coordination of homework,

sporting events, lessons, and so forth. If joint, physical custody exacerbates ongoing hostility and the child faces a life characterized by tension and hostility between parents, then close monitoring, mediation, and a consideration of sole custody may be necessary.

If the pediatrician sees that the patient is at risk because of poor adjustment, ongoing hostility, dysfunction in major developmental tasks, and difficulty in more intimate relationships, active follow-up and, if indicated, referral to mental health and community services are indicated. Options include court-based or court-ordered counseling, a mental health evaluation, a mediator, psychiatric referral for either parent, and community-based divorce groups.

References

1. Thoreau LC: NY Times, September 3, 1992, Section 4, page 11.
2. Wallerstein JS: The long-term effects of divorce on children: a review. J Am Acad Child Adolesc Psychiatry 1991; 30:3:349–360.
3. Wallerstein JS, Johnston JR: Children of divorce: recent findings regarding long-term effects and recent studies of joint and sole custody. Pediatr Rev 1990;11:7:197–204.

SUGGESTED READING:

Wallerstein JS, Kelly JB: Surviving the Breakup: How Children and Parents Cope with Divorce. New York, Basic Books, 1980.

52 Mental Retardation

Jean A. Frazier

Mental retardation (MR) is a relatively common neuropsychiatric disorder occurring in children of school age. In addition to subaverage cognition, individuals often have physical, sensory, and emotional handicaps that have great impact on daily life. Generally, work with this population, particularly, those persons with psychiatric or behavioral disturbances, requires the effort of a team including pediatricians, child psychiatrists, psychologists, social workers, special education teachers, occupational therapists, and speech and language therapists.

Definition

The American Psychiatric Association (1994) established three criteria necessary to diagnosis an individual with MR:

1. The individual must have significantly subaverage general intellectual functioning, based on the results of a standardized intelligence test.
2. The individual must have concurrent deficits or impairments in adaptive behavior (in at least two of the following areas:
   a. Communication
   b. Self-care
   c. Home living
   d. Social/interpersonal skills
   e. Use of community resources
   f. Self-direction
   g. Functional academic skills
   h. Work
   i. Leisure
   j. Health
   k. Safety
3. The subaverage intellectual and adaptive functioning must be present during the developmental period (< 18 years of age).

In general, *subaverage intelligence* is defined as a full-scale intelligence quotient (IQ) less than 70 (2 standard deviations below the mean). There are four specific diagnostic subtypes that characterize the severity of the disorder: (1) mild: IQ from 50–55 to 70; (2) moderate: IQ from 35–40 to 50–55; (3) severe: IQ from 20–25 to 35–40; (4) profound: IQ less than or equal to 20–25. A child's adaptive functioning must be either equal to or below what would be expected for his or her IQ.

Diagnosis

Cognitive ability for a school-aged child is usually measured by standardized instruments such as the Weschler

Intelligence Scale for Children III (WISC III) and the Stanford Binet (fourth edition). The Leiter International Performance Scale is used to assess the profoundly retarded or the nonverbal children within the population. Because both IQ and deficient adaptive functioning are necessary to diagnose MR, it is important to accurately measure adaptive functioning in individuals with IQs less than 70. The instruments commonly used to measure adaptive functioning are the Vineland Adaptive Behavior Scale and the American Association on Mental Deficiency Adaptive Behavior Scale for Children and Adults. When assessing adaptive functioning, consideration must be given to education and the individual's motivation, personality, sociocultural background, associated handicaps, and cooperation.

Epidemiology

1. MR occurs in 2 to 3 per cent of the school-aged population. Those with mild MR make up approximately 85 to 89 per cent of the MR population. Those rated in the moderate range make up 7 to 10 per cent, and the severely and profoundly retarded groups combined make up 1 to 2 per cent of the total MR population.
2. The lifelong prevalence tends to vary with gender, age, and socioeconomic status. Prevalence increases from preschool to adolescence and decreases in early adulthood.
3. The male:female ratio is 1.9:1 in mild MR and is 1.5:1 in the severe to profound ranges. The increased male predominance might be partially due to cultural tendency to label boys as having MR more readily and/or the overrepresentation of X-linked disorders (e.g., fragile X syndrome).
4. Mild MR is overrepresented in the lower end of socioeconomic status. Children with moderate, severe, and profound MR are more equitably distributed across socioeconomic status.

Etiology

1. A variety of causes can lead to the ultimate manifestation of subaverage IQ and adaptive behavior. Twenty-five per cent of persons with MR have a known biologic cause (either prenatal [25 to 30 per cent of known causes], perinatal [11 per cent], or postnatal [0.8 to 12.8 per cent]). Those in the moderate to profound range are more likely to have a biologic cause.
2. Prenatal factors include infection (e.g., rubella, toxoplasmosis, cytomegalovirus, herpes simplex, hepatitis, human immunodeficiency virus, syphilis), x-ray exposure, drug exposure (e.g., alcohol, heroin), maternal mercury poisoning, genetic abnormalities, maternal medication exposure (e.g., thalidomide, anticonvulsants, chemotherapy) and maternal illness (malnutrition, emphysema, anemia).
3. Perinatal causes include prematurity, asphyxia, and birth injury; and postnatal causes include bacterial infection, head trauma, lead poisoning, and metabolic abnormalities (hypothyroidism).
4. In patients with IQ less than 50, genetic disorders contribute to approximately 50 per cent of the prenatal causes. Genetic disorders can involve either a single gene anomaly, complicated polygenic combinations, or chromosomal abnormalities (Down syndrome [trisomy 21]; trisomies 13, 14, and 15; fragile X syndrome; Turner syndrome; Klinefelter syndrome; and multiple X syndrome).
5. Fragile X is the most common known cause of MR in boys and results from an expansion of a DNA segment in the Xq 27.3 region. Girls with the expanded DNA region are affected to a variable degree or not at all.

Evaluation

1. Evaluation of an individual with MR should include a detailed history about pregnancy, delivery, postnatal health, development, and current social and economic environment.
2. Physical examination to look for stigmata of genetic syndromes and screening for metabolic and chromosomal abnormalities would be indicated.
3. Screening for accompanying handicaps whether physical, sensory, or neurologic is recommended, particularly in the moderately to profoundly retarded individuals because approximately 10 per cent of individuals with moderate MR and 50 per cent of individuals with severe and profound MR have seizure disorders. Blindness and deafness are common particularly in those in the lower IQ range. Physical handicaps are also quite common in those with IQ less than 50 (e.g., spastic quadriparesis).
4. Individuals with MR are at greater risk for behavioral disturbances and emotional difficulties. Those in the mild to moderate range are at increased risk for emotional distress that may arise from a sense of not being like everyone else and from peer rejection and social isolation.
5. Boys with fragile X syndrome have, in addition to mental retardation, macro-orchidism, a long face, and large ears.

Prevention

1. Before pregnancy, genetic counseling is indicated for parents with known genetic disorders (e.g., neurofibromatosis) and for mothers of advanced age, given the increased incidence of Down syndrome with increased maternal years.
2. In the expectant mother, adequate intervention for any substance abuse problem, appropriate monitoring of prescribed medications and medical conditions, and adequate nutrition and prenatal care help to optimize the infant's in utero environment. Once the child is born, active treatment of neonatal infections or metabolic abnormalities (e.g., hypothyroidism) and, in the young child, active treatment of metal intoxication (e.g., lead) are indicated. Also, certain interventions can help ameliorate difficulties found in the mildly retarded individual, in particular, providing appropriate nutrition and infant cognitive stimulation.

Treatment Interventions

1. The individual patient and family of a patient with a subaverage IQ face numerous hurdles during the course of development, including cognitive, physical, emotional, social, and behavioral challenges. These developmental challenges can be satisfactorily addressed by facilitating access to social and educational supports. Additionally, parents as well as siblings have the lifelong task of accepting their child's or sibling's developmental disability. With each milestone that is met or not met comes the family's response, which ranges from joy to ongoing

grief. The way the family system responds to the child and the child responds to the family helps to mold the developmental outcome for the child.

2. Adults and children with MR are at greater risk of medical and psychiatric conditions. There is a known phenomenon called "diagnostic overshadowing" in which changes in mood and behavior are wrongly attributed to the individual's MR rather than to a co-morbid psychiatric condition (e.g., depression, anxiety, bipolar disorder, attention-deficit/hyperactivity disorder, Tourette syndrome, psychotic disorder). The lower the IQ, the greater the tendency toward behavioral disturbance and psychopathology. According to Bregman, between 30 and 60 per cent of the MR population may have a co-morbid psychiatric condition. For example, as many as 50 per cent of noninstitutionalized individuals have been reported to meet criteria for an affective disorder. Some investigators report 25 to 30 per cent of individuals with MR have co-morbid pervasive developmental disorder. Owing to the individual's poor communication skills, the expression of psychopathology may be different from that of a cognitively normal individual (e.g., self-injurious behavior, aggression, rocking). Even minor changes in one's environment can frustrate an individual with MR and result in a behavioral change.

3. It is important to refer a child with a marked change in behavior for a full psychiatric evaluation and for treatment. Common problems in patients with MR that come to the attention of clinicians are self-injury and aggression. The basis of these behavioral changes must be discerned and appropriately treated. Behavioral change may be caused by neurologic, medical, dynamic, and/or psychiatric factors. A physical examination and any indicated medical/neurologic work-up are necessary to rule out underlying treatable conditions. It is also important to assess if there have been any life change events for the individual. If so, either individual psychotherapy (for IQ > 50), behavioral therapy, or family therapy might be indicated.

4. Individual behaviors may represent symptoms of a psychiatric disorder. The patient must be thoroughly evaluated for a psychiatric condition. Often such diagnoses require careful observation over a period of time, owing to the patient's limited ability to express problems verbally, by a psychiatrist with expertise in developmental disabilities. In general, target symptoms of a psychiatric syndrome and not an individual behavior should be the basis of treatment with psychopharmacologic agents. For example, the individual behavior of self-injury may be a symptom of numerous psychiatric disorders (e.g., af-

fective disorders, obsessive-compulsive disorder, psychotic disorders, Tourette syndrome, stereotypical movement disorder). Although neuroleptics are often used to treat self-injury, they are not always indicated and should be used judiciously given their side effect profile. For example, new-onset head banging that occurs within the context of symptoms of depression may in fact represent suicidal behavior in an MR child. This child's symptoms would be best treated with an antidepressant. Another example of self-injury is new-onset hair pulling in a child who also has other symptoms of obsessive-compulsive disorder. In this case, either clomipramine (Anafranil) or a selective serotonin reuptake inhibitor and not a neuroleptic would be the treatment of choice. The cause of a presenting behavior should be determined and viewed within the context of a composite of target symptoms before choosing a psychopharmacologic intervention. As a general rule, individuals with MR require lower doses of psychopharmacologic agents and may be more prone to side effects. Use of multiple medications should be undertaken judiciously.

5. Families often need support and intervention. Additionally, parents and retarded citizens might benefit from support services available through the local chapter of the Association for Retarded Citizens (ARC).

Key Treatment

- Social supports
- Educational supports
- Pharmacotherapy

  When indicated based on psychiatric symptoms

Bibliography

American Psychiatric Association: Diagnostic and Statistical Manual of Mental Disorders, 4th ed. Washington, DC, American Psychiatric Association, 1994, pp 39–46.

Frazier J, Barrett R, Walters A, Feinstein C: Moderate to profound mental retardation. *In* Noshpitz JD, Aless NE (eds): Handbook of Child and Adolescent Psychiatry. New York, John Wiley & Sons, 1997, pp 397–400.

McLaren J, Bryson SE: Review of recent epidemiological studies of mental retardation: Prevalence, associated disorders and etiology. Am J Ment Retard 1987;92:243–254.

Nihira K, Foster R, Hellhaas M, Leland H. AAMD Adaptive Behavior Scale. Washington, DC, American Association on Mental Deficiency, 1975.

Sparrow S, Balla DA, Cicchette DV. Vineland Adaptive Behavior Scales. Circle Pines, MN, American Guidance Service, 1984.

53 Physical Abuse and Neglect; Sexual Abuse

Muriel Sugarman

Physical Abuse and Neglect

Epidemiology

The 1993 study of professional reports of child abuse in 29 counties throughout the United States by the National Center for Child Abuse and Neglect (NCCAN) found over 1.55 million countable reports of child maltreatment, of which almost 25 per cent were of physical abuse and roughly 57 per cent involved neglect. In 1991, a 50-state survey by the National Committee for Prevention of Child Abuse of all reports sent to protective agencies found 2.69 million reported cases, 25 per cent of which were physical abuse and 48 per cent child neglect. Reported and detected deaths from abuse and neglect in 1991 totaled 1383, with 54 per cent involving victims younger than 1 year of age. Approximately 10 per cent of children younger than 5 years of age seen in emergency departments for trauma have inflicted injuries.

There are no identifying characteristics of abusive parents, either demographic or psychopathologic. Physically abusive or neglectful parents come from all social strata, may appear perfectly normal, and may be highly skilled at covering up their behavior. They often show intellectual awareness of what good parenting involves and may participate in treatment without long-lasting effect on their risk of repeat abusive or neglectful behavior once a child is returned to their responsibility.

Physical Abuse

Definitions

Legal definitions of *physical child abuse* vary by statute from state to state. The simplest definition is that of inflicted, rather than accidental, injury. Controversy exists as to whether and at what level of severity physical discipline by parents, causing inflicted injury, constitutes abuse. Children's Hospital of Ohio defines physical abuse as an injury caused to a child by a caretaker for any reason, involving tissue damage beyond erythema, or redness from a slap to any area other than the hand or buttocks. Tissue damage includes bruises, burns, tears, punctures, fractures, ruptures of organs, and disruption of functions. This definition maintains that physical discipline should not be used on any child younger than 12 months of age.

Etiology

1. Child physical abuse is often a reflection of multigenerational parenting failure. Abusive parents prematurely expect and demand performance beyond the developmental capability of a child to achieve. The parent may feel insecure and unloved, expecting the child to love, comfort, and act like a parent to him or her. Such parents are oblivious to and/or resentful of the child's own needs, limited abilities, and helplessness. The abusive parent may have been abusively parented but often believes that the abuse received was necessary discipline.

2. Circumstances that make a parent feel inferior, unloved, needy, angry, or vulnerable, such as loss of a mate, loss of a job, poverty, or isolation, may increase the risks of abusive behavior toward children. Special characteristics of a child, such as hyperactivity, difficult temperament, prematurity, physical disability, mental retardation, or learning disability, may result in that child being singled out for abusive treatment.

3. Abuse of drugs or alcohol, or parental mental illness, including postpartum psychosis, may contribute to physical abuse. A subgroup of abusive parents are sociopathic and sadistic, with histories of violence and abusive behavior toward others and absence of empathy or remorse.

4. It should be kept in mind that children may be physically abused by caretakers other than parents, such as baby sitters, teachers, camp counselors, and so on.

Clinical Findings

1. Presenting problems in physical abuse range from minor bruises to life-threatening battering. Injuries may also be accompanied by signs of physical neglect. Most common are bruises, contusions, and abrasions. The location, stage of healing, and configuration of these injuries are significant. Inflicted injury is suggested by bruises or other skin damage in soft tissue areas not usually vulnerable to falling injuries, such as cheeks, upper arms, thighs, buttocks, and genitals as opposed to forehead, shins, knees, and elbows. Multiple injuries in various stages of healing and marks that are configured to resemble fingermarks, handprints, ropes or cords, belt buckles, or even the adult dental arch may be seen in cases of inflicted injury. Abrasions or lacerations may also be found inside the mouth or other orifices.

2. Burns may also be inflicted, especially those with a suspicious shape. Examples are immersion burns with a water line but no splash marks; burns that are small and circular and result from a lit cigarette; and marks resembling the shape of a hot iron, utensil, or cooking container.

3. Abused children may bear marks of being tied up with wires, belts, or straps. They also may be injured by being pushed, choked, grabbed, shaken, dragged, or pinched as well as by being whipped, slapped, punched, bitten, struck with heavy objects, kicked, or thrown. Inflicted injuries may involve stabbing or shooting.

4. Children may also be abused by being suffocated, being given toxic substances to ingest, being drugged, or being caused to appear ill by a caretaker, resulting in multiple medical procedures and hospitalizations (i.e., Munchausen syndrome by proxy).

5. Clinical presentation may involve external head injuries such as swelling or bruises on two or more sides of the head, traumatic alopecia from hair pulling, or subgaleal hematoma from being lifted by the hair. There may be eye injuries from a black eye to massive eye trauma or retinal hemorrhages secondary to shaking or chest compression.

6. More severe inflicted injuries, or "battering," may involve the following:

   a. Unexplained and/or untreated fractures, especially multiple fractures in various stages of healing

   b. Serious head trauma presenting as skull fracture, intracranial hemorrhage, or brain contusion

   c. Severe chest trauma producing lacerations or contusions of lungs, rib fractures, or intrathoracic hemorrhage

   d. Severe abdominal trauma with intraabdominal hemorrhage, intestinal obstruction from hematoma, perforated intestine, or damage to intraabdominal organs such as kidneys, spleen, or liver.

7. Injuries may result in fatality directly or indirectly, from one or multiple attacks. Twenty-five to 30 per cent of children diagnosed as battered may be dead within months if not protected.

Key Clinical Findings: Physical Abuse

- Bruises in unusual site for usual trauma
- Burns
- Rope or wire marks
- Fractures

Prevention

1. Primary prevention. New evidence suggests that very early parenting support and intervention may decrease the rates of child abuse in a given population. Randomized trials of various home visitation programs with parents of infants suggest that such programs are effective in significantly reducing reports of child abuse, decreasing the use of physical punishment, and improving adequate caregiving capacity in parents. A national initiative, Healthy Families America, modeled on a successful statewide program in Hawaii, has been launched with the goal of reaching all first-time parents with intensive home visitor services on a voluntary basis to ensure that all new parents, particularly those at high risk, get off to a good start.

2. Secondary prevention, involving early identification of families at high risk for child maltreatment and early diagnosis of milder forms of physical abuse, requires entertaining the possibility of inflicted harm and deciding when to report to the proper authorities. This may be a conflicted, difficult process, especially if it involves a family with whom the physician has a long-standing relationship. Reporting suspected child abuse is legally mandated and may be lifesaving or prevent serious physical or psychologic damage to a child. Knowing how to perform and record a careful assessment for abuse is vital to the education of all pediatric caregivers.

Assessment

1. When a child presents with injuries, especially multiple and/or severe ones, the caregiver must entertain a high index of suspicion while maintaining a neutral approach and an open mind about conclusions. The first step is obviously to assess and attend to the child's immediate medical needs. A careful history of the injuries should be obtained from each adult separately and the child interviewed privately if possible.

2. A thorough health history and developmental assessment should be obtained. Special information about the injury that should be gathered includes the time of injury, place, sequence of events, who was present and whether there were actual eyewitnesses, the exact circumstances of the injury (e.g., quantitative estimates of the distance fallen, type of object struck, amount of time in contact with a hot surface), and time lapse before assistance was called for or the child was brought in for care. The examiner should be alert for, and record, any eyewitness account of inflicted injury by a child or adult; a partial or complete confession of inflicted injury by a parent, even if later retracted; failure to explain, denial of, or vague explanation of the injury; an explanation that is implausible or inconsistent with the nature or severity of the injury; allegations of self-inflicted or sibling-inflicted injury inconsistent with a child's developmental stage or known patterns of child behavior; and significant delay in seeking medical care.

3. When the child's condition is stable, a thorough physical examination of the child should be performed, with particular attention to the presence of multiple injuries in different locations and/or stages of healing, injuries in occult sites, and injuries with pathognomonic configurations. Such an assessment may also include radiologic studies, ophthalmologic examination, CT scan, coagulation studies, and so on. The physical examination should be conducted in a gentle manner, with the consent of the child, avoiding use of restraint or force.

4. Whenever possible, photographs of injuries before treatment should be obtained. A discussion of techniques for such photography and specific requirements for legal authorization to take photographs without parental consent are beyond the scope of this chapter but are available in other publications. Photographs, if available, should be supplemented by drawings (or charts) and written descriptions of injuries.

5. In cases of likely severe child physical abuse, the caregiver should arrange if possible, through the proper authorities, for the examination and protection of any other children in the home.

Documentation and Reporting

1. The medical record may be the most tangible and often is the only evidence of physical abuse of a child. The record should be legible, free of jargon, and kept in an organized, professional manner. In addition to a standard thorough pediatric health assessment and medical and relevant social history, it should include statements made by the child and caretakers; observed behaviors; description of the circumstances of the child's injury; and detailed descriptions of all injuries, including type, number, size, degree of healing, possible causes, and location

recorded on a body chart or drawing. The evaluator should give an opinion as to whether the injuries were adequately explained or the likelihood that the injuries were inflicted. The record should also include results of all pertinent laboratory and other diagnostic procedures, any photographs and imaging studies, and any other significant information on the nature, source, and circumstances of the injuries. It may be important for the evaluator to give an opinion of the risk of further harm to the child if returned to the caretakers.

2. The medical caregiver who suspects child abuse must notify the proper authorities and should be aware of the mandatory reporting laws in his or her state. All states provide mandatory reporters with immunity from liability for reports made in good faith and impose criminal penalties for failure to report. Physicians may be required to testify in civil, juvenile, or criminal court, and such participation is an essential part of the physician's responsibility toward a child. In some cases, if the physician has reason to believe that a child will be in imminent danger if released to a caretaker, a legal order for protective custody must be sought by reporting to the appropriate protective, judicial, or law enforcement agencies authorized to handle such cases by state statute.

3. Medical caregivers should obtain information on reporting laws in their own states. The physician who may be called on to testify in court should consider availing himself or herself of written guidelines for such participation and/or taking continuing medical education courses specifically designed for the physician witness.

Treatment

Treatment of child abuse varies with the nature and severity of the abuse. It may range from careful follow-up with supportive services mandated for a family to permanent removal of a child from his or her family. In milder cases, the medical caregiver's role may be to see a child on a regular basis to examine for injuries, assess development, and report parental compliance. In more severe cases, there may be a need for long-term medical care for the consequences of major injuries and referral for long-term mental health treatment for the emotional impact of the maltreatment, separation from family, and/or the impact of foster placement or adoption.

Key Treatment: Physical Abuse

- Stabilize for any serious injuries.
- Document evidence.
- Provide separation followed by either reintroduction or permanent placement.

Child Neglect

Definitions

Child neglect is broadly defined to include all instances in which the major needs of children are not met, regardless of cause. These major needs include adequate nutrition, shelter, protection and supervision, clothing, healthcare, education, and emotional nurturance. According to Dubowitz and Black (Reece, 1994):

1. Neglect is heterogeneous, varying in type, severity, and chronicity.
2. Both actual and potential harm are of concern.
3. The more serious the harm or risk, the more severe the neglect.
4. Neglect may involve a pattern of omissions in a child's care.
5. Neglect may involve single, momentary lapses in care or exposures to harm, particularly when serious risks are involved.

Types of Neglect

Three forms of neglect have been identified: physical neglect, emotional neglect, and educational neglect. The medical caregiver most often is called on to identify and provide treatment for physical neglect but should also be alert to situations of emotional and educational neglect in his or her patients. In the Second National Incidence Study (NIS-2) in 1986, seven forms of physical neglect were examined:

1. Refusal of healthcare
2. Delay in healthcare
3. Abandonment
4. Expulsion of a child from the home
5. Other custody issues, such as repeatedly leaving a child with others for long periods of time
6. Inadequate supervision, such as leaving a young child unsupervised for extended periods of time
7. Other physical neglect, including inadequate nutrition, clothing, or hygiene.

In NIS-2, three forms of educational neglect and seven forms of emotional neglect were also examined. The latter included such issues as inadequate nurturance/affection; exposure to chronic/extreme spouse abuse; permitting drug/alcohol abuse by a child; permitting maladaptive behavior such as chronic delinquency; refusal or delay of psychologic care; and chronically inappropriate expectations in relation to the child's age or developmental level.

Etiology

1. Multiple factors interact to produce child neglect. These include parent characteristics, child characteristics, familial interactions, community circumstances, and societal conditions. Parental characteristics include:
   a. Mental retardation or serious cognitive deficits
   b. Emotional disturbances including serious depression, personality disorder, or psychosis
   c. Chronic or severe physical illness
   d. Substance abuse
   e. Extreme religious, nutritional, or cultural beliefs.

2. The parent of limited intellectual capacity or the parent with significant mental or physical illness may not be capable of providing basic physical and emotional care for children in a consistent, reliable manner. Parental substance abuse almost always compromises caregiving ability and diverts financial resources from ne-

cessities of life to the purchase of drugs and/or alcohol. Parents with extreme beliefs about nutrition, healthcare, child discipline and training, education, and religion may fail to meet their children's needs because of their belief systems.

3. Child characteristics may prove stressful for parents and contribute to neglect. Low birth weight and prematurity have been identified as significant risk factors, but this association may be related to increased surveillance. Chronic physical and/or cognitive disabilities, effects of intrauterine exposure to drugs and alcohol, attention-deficit disorder, and difficult temperament all may result in placing difficult demands on parents to which they may be unable to provide consistent or sustained response.

4. Interactional problems are frequently found in families where there is child neglect. Parents who have been deprived in childhood, exposed to spouse abuse, or lack adequate role models may show disturbances in parent-child attachment; inappropriate and inconsistent or conflicting expectations of children; lack of knowledge about the basic needs of children; inability to nurture; need to control the behavior of the child; family chaos; or marital conflict and violence that may contribute to neglect. Social isolation has long been recognized as a risk factor in child neglect. A high-risk community environment interferes with social support and parental perception of quality of life, which in turn is associated with increased child maltreatment. At the societal level, poverty, in addition to compromising families' abilities to function, results directly in inadequate access to healthcare, insufficient funds for adequate food and housing, exposure to environmental hazards such as lead and violence, and inferior educational opportunities.

Clinical Findings

1. Physical neglect may present in a multitude of forms. Historically, the child may not have had appropriate well-child care, including immunizations and basic dental care. Necessary health aids such as eyeglasses may not have been provided. More serious is a history of failure to obtain appropriate medical care for acute or chronic illness or failure to comply with medical treatment for such illness.

2. Physical findings may include undernutrition on examination or detected on growth curves and/or poor hygiene such as being filthy, having extremely severe diaper rash, or frequent acute or chronic skin infections. Toddlers or preschool children may show signs of lack of physical care, such as dirty, stained clothing, clothing inappropriate to climate or put on improperly by the child, or severely unkempt appearance. The child may exhibit developmental delay, evidence of untreated medical conditions, or rampant dental caries. There may be repeated episodes of gastroenteritis caused by improper preparation or unsanitary handling of formula or food. In some cases, children present with a history of frequent and severe accidental injuries owing to lack of appropriate supervision and care. Great care must be taken to distinguish cultural, ethnic, or lifestyle differences in families

from true neglect of basic needs, but neglect for any cause is still neglect and must be attended to.

3. Behavioral findings may be varied but might include impaired interpersonal relations (lack of cuddliness, gaze avoidance, preference for inanimate objects, or object hunger and intense neediness), apathy, depression, withdrawal, discipline problems, aggressive behavior, poor school performance and/or attendance, "role reversal" in which the child is parentified, inappropriate responsibility for care of younger children, or housekeeping chores.

Key Clinical Findings: Child Neglect

- Lack of basic medical preventive measures
- Undernutrition
- Poor hygiene
- Passivity

Prevention

1. As in child physical abuse, primary prevention may consist of early intervention with parents of infants, providing them with information, social support, parenting education, referral to medical, social, nutritional, and financial services, and so on. Voluntary, culturally sensitive, nonjudgmental home visiting services have an impact on incidence of neglect as well as of physical abuse. Every pediatric caregiver has the opportunity for prevention of neglect in providing anticipatory guidance of new mothers about preventing child accidents, the importance of immunizations and well-baby visits, the developmental stages of children, the effects of noncompliance with care on certain illnesses, and so on.

2. Secondary prevention, that of identifying and treating children already being neglected or at risk of harm because of parents with impaired parenting capacity, suffering from poverty, or overly stressed by life circumstances, depends on recognition by caregivers, assessment of etiology, referral to necessary services, and/or reporting to appropriate agencies and careful follow-up.

Assessment and Reporting

1. In assessing for child neglect, the pediatric caregiver must balance concern for the well-being of the child and therapeutic empathy for the neglectful, but often not deliberately harmful, parents. Neglectful parents love their children and may be oblivious to or suffer deep shame over their failures. Concern for the neglected child may lead the caregiver to be hostile toward the parents, preventing the establishment of rapport and producing noncompliance with follow-up and referrals to services. Too much empathy for an inadequate, deprived, impoverished, or ill parent may prevent interventions that are necessary to the well-being, normal development, or even survival of the child.

2. The first step in assessment is to determine whether a child's major needs are being neglected for whatever cause, to identify clearly the specific harm or risks of harm involved in a particular situation, and to assess the

severity and likelihood of possible future harm. Development of a comprehensive understanding of factors contributing to the neglectful situation is the next step. An interdisciplinary approach, with the assistance of a social worker, is optimal for gathering information about family and community resources. Neurodevelopmental assessment, review of prior medical records, and information from school personnel may also be of importance.

3. Reporting of neglect is mandated by state law, but the decisions about when and in what circumstances to report are often difficult to make. As with child physical abuse, careful recording of data is vital, including such information as missed appointments, emergency department visits about which the caregiver has been contacted, descriptions of hygiene, dental health, nutritional state, body care, and so on.

Treatment

Treatment of neglect obviously varies with the cause, severity, and chronicity of the condition. It is often best accomplished with a team approach that provides support and consultation for the pediatrician from other team members. Interventions should be those whose effectiveness has been proven and targeted toward underlying contributory factors, such as parenting inadequacies or lack of information, environmental stresses, and poverty. Available strengths and resources should be identified and used, including other family members and friends, church support, and peer group support. Multimodal programs that provide training in parenting skills, stress reduction, impulse control, money management, job-finding services, marital counseling, transportation to pediatric appointments, and other such practical, behaviorally oriented services have been shown to be effective. Establishing rapport is critical to effective help. Considering the needs of the entire family, nurturing parents, providing parents respite, home visitor and home help services, and other interventions that assist parents can improve rapport, increase the likelihood of compliance, and enhance parental ability to nurture. Interventions need to be clearly defined and often need to be long term, sometimes for years, because of the multiple, complex, and deeply rooted problems of neglecting families.

Key Treatment: Child Neglect

- Provide needed social services.
- Provide stress reduction.

Bibliography

American Medical Association: Diagnostic and Treatment Guidelines on Child Physical Abuse and Neglect. Chicago, American Medical Association, 1994.

Helfer RE, Kempe CH (eds): The Battered Child, 4th ed. Chicago, University of Chicago Press, 1987.

Reece RM: Child abuse. Pediatr Clin North Am 1990;37(4).

Reece RM (ed): Child Abuse: Medical Diagnosis and Management. Philadelphia, Lea & Febiger, 1994.

Sexual Abuse

Definitions

1. *Sexual abuse* is defined as engaging a child in sexual activities that the child cannot comprehend, for which the child is developmentally unprepared and thus cannot give informed consent, and/or that violate the social and legal taboos of society.

2. Sexual abuse activities may include all forms of oral-genital, genital, or anal contact by or to the child, or nontouching abuses such as exhibitionism, voyeurism, or using the child in child prostitution or the production of pornographic photographs or videotapes. Behaviors include exhibition of genitalia, looking at the victim's genitalia, fondling, frottage (i.e., rubbing the genitalia against a part of the victim's body to climax [including "vulvar" intercourse and interfemoral intercourse]), oral-genital contact (perpetrator to victim and/or victim to perpetrator), anal or vaginal penetration with fingers or objects, and penile penetration of anus or vagina. Harmful genital care practices by parents that are repetitive, intrusive, and/or arousing may be included in the definition of sexual abuse.

3. Sexual abuse among child peers is differentiated from "sexual play" by assessing the frequency and coercive nature of the behavior and determining whether there is developmental, knowledge, or power asymmetry among the participants.

4. Sexual abuse includes a spectrum of circumstances ranging from violent rape to gentle seduction. It commonly involves a progression of behaviors from less to more intrusive, with an engagement phase followed by multiple incidents. Threats, bribery, and/or intimidation may be used to silence the victim.

Epidemiology

Problems in determining incidence and prevalence include serious underreporting due to delayed or no disclosure, failure to report to the proper agencies, methodologic differences in definitions, ages of children included, varied techniques of collecting data, and retrospective nature of studies.

1. *Incidence:* The National Center for Child Abuse and Neglect 1993 study (NIS-3) reported a sexual abuse incidence of 3.2/1000 children, or 217,700 children. The National Committee to Prevent Child Abuse Fifty-State Survey for 1993 found 330,000 reports of child sexual abuse, of which 150,000 were substantiated.

2. *Prevalence:* Taking into account a number of prevalence studies and their methodologies, most reviewers conclude that at least 20 per cent of adult women in North America (range, 19 to 38 per cent) and from 5 to 16 per cent of men have experienced sexual abuse. The male rates are thought to reflect significant underreporting by males.

About one third of victims are under the age of 6 years. Median age for boys is 9.9 years, and for girls it is 9.6 years.

Etiology

1. There is no empirically validated etiology for child sexual abuse. Perpetrators vary in age, occupation, income level, marital status, and ethnic group and may exhibit no de-

tectable characteristics on psychiatric or psychologic evaluation.

2. Perpetrators are male in 90 per cent of cases, but this may be due to underdetection and/or underreporting of female perpetrators. In the majority of cases they are known to the victim and most often are fathers, stepfathers, and surrogate fathers, but they may be teachers, baby sitters, child care workers, scout leaders, or other people who deliberately arrange to come into contact with children.

3. Perpetrators range from those who seek out and form long-term relationships with victims to those who sadistically and violently abuse children they do not know. There are habitual offenders and one-time offenders, intrafamily and extrafamily offenders, offenders who are adults, and offenders who themselves are children or adolescents.

4. A history of physical or sexual abuse may predispose some perpetrators to sexually abuse children, but other factors are also thought to be involved, including substance abuse, social inadequacy, poor impulse control, presence of other sexual deviancy, and sadistic or violent tendencies. It is thought that there exists a continuum of sexual arousal to children, which is in turn influenced by disinhibition of impulses, lack of external supervision, opportunity, victim vulnerability, and so on.

Clinical Findings

Children may present to the pediatric caregiver in several ways:

1. They may be brought in for routine physical examination or an unrelated medical illness without having made a disclosure of sexual abuse, behaviorally asymptomatic, but found to have a sexually transmitted infection or other physical evidence consistent with sexual abuse.

2. They may be children suspected to have been sexually abused because of pertinent physical complaints and/or behavioral conditions who have not made a disclosure of sexual abuse.

3. They may be children whose caretakers, social services personnel, or law enforcement believe have been sexually abused because of a disclosure of sexual abuse, with or without pertinent physical evidence or behavioral symptoms.

4. Some children are seen because of signs of acute genital, anal, or oral trauma.

Key Clinical Findings

- Genital or anal pain and/or trauma
- Dilated hymen
- Scarring of anus
- Semen in mouth, vagina, or anus
- Pregnancy in early puberty without history of sexual activity

---

Signs and Symptoms

1. Physical
   a. Nonspecific symptoms suggestive of sexual abuse include:
      (1) Genital or anal pain or discomfort
      (2) Pain on urination or defecation
      (3) Urinary frequency
      (4) Constipation and/or bowel withholding
      (5) Irritation and/or inflammation of genital or perianal area
      (6) Recurrent nonspecific vulvovaginitis or vaginitis
      (7) Recurrent urinary tract infection without anatomic or hygiene explanation
   b. Specific signs. More specific *physical signs* of sexual abuse are well described and illustrated in other publications and must often be differentiated from physical signs with alternative causes but include:
      (1) Acute evidence of genital/anal trauma (i.e., bleeding, laceration, bruising)
      (2) Dilatation of hymen and/or anus in the prepubertal or nonsexually active child
      (3) Hymenal adhesions, synechiae, irregularities
      (4) Scarring of anus, hymen, or vagina
      (5) Evidence of sexually transmitted infections, including those of the throat
      (6) Presence of semen or sperm in mouth, vagina, or anus
      (7) Pregnancy in early pubertal child who has no history of being sexually active

2. Behavioral
   a. Posttraumatic stress disorder (behavioral symptoms including "flashbacks" or "reexperiencing" the abusive events); avoidant behaviors; mood lability; disorganized, hypermotile, aggressive distractible behavior; easy startling; nightmares and/or night terrors
   b. Traumatic sexualization. Symptoms include sexual preoccupation, compulsive masturbation or other repetitive sexual activities, atypical and/or developmentally sophisticated sexual behaviors, requesting sexual contact from adults, sexually aggressive behavior toward other children, sexually provocative dress and manner, promiscuity, and pregnancy.
   c. Regressive symptoms include enuresis, encopresis, mutism, baby talk, infantile behavior.
   d. Severe anxiety may be manifested by sleep disturbance; appetite disturbance; phobic fears of men or certain situations; nail biting; shortness of breath; stomach aches, vomiting, nervous stomach; anxious facial appearance; and rapid speech.
   e. There may be dissociative symptoms, including "spaciness," staring, seeming dazed, difficulty concentrating, withdrawal, and unresponsiveness.
   f. Other symptoms that may be seen include poor self-esteem; general feelings of shame and guilt; distorted body image; deterioration in school perfor-

mance; running away; and suicidal ideation and/or attempts.

Assessment and Diagnosis

1. A careful history, including current concerns as well as detailed pediatric, developmental, and family information, should be obtained from the nonaccused parent(s). The caregiver should inquire about any physical complaints, behavioral symptoms, or verbal disclosures by the child.

2. The physical examination for sexual abuse involves special techniques often best used by a clinician with experience and expertise in examining children alleged to have been sexually abused. The physician without such experience and expertise who may be called on to perform this examination will be helped by having at hand such aids as one of several excellent pediatric references on this topic; one of several photographic atlases on normal genital/anal anatomy; and one of a number of protocols for such examinations developed by the emergency departments of major hospitals.

3. Goals of the examination are to identify injuries or conditions requiring medical attention; collect and record evidence of abuse; and reassure the child and/or caregivers that the child will be all right.

4. The examination should be explained to the child, conducted with the child's consent in the presence of an adult not suspected to be a party to the abuse and in a gentle sensitive manner, without utilizing restraint or force, and include all aspects of a complete physical examination. The highly resistant child may need to be seen by a mental health consultant before examination or be examined under anesthesia if an immediate evaluation is necessary.

5. For cases of recent sexual assault (less than 48 hours), a rape kit should be used to document presence of sperm, semen, pubic hairs, and so on. All specimens should be collected in the appropriate forensic manner and carefully handled as legal evidence, maintaining the "chain of custody."

6. The child should be examined for bruises; bite marks; suck marks on the skin ("hickeys"); grab marks of hands or fingers; and any other signs of trauma to extremities, skin, head, eyes, ears, nose, mouth, throat, genitalia, and anus. Visual examination of the genitalia and anus should be performed to look for signs of fresh or healed injury. Description of techniques for positioning of the child, traction on surrounding tissues, magnification, and photographing of findings is beyond the scope of this chapter but is discussed in other publications. Cultures of mouth, vagina, and anus for sexually transmitted infections should be performed when indicated.

The Child Interview

1. Sexual abuse, particularly when the victim is a young child, is very difficult to detect and even more difficult to prove, because it usually occurs in secret, without eyewitnesses and there is seldom direct physical evidence. Perpetrators have often spent much of their lives learning to hide their abusive behaviors and often appear normal, respectable, and convincing. The victim is a vulnerable, ingenuous child who may be traumatized, confused, frightened, guilty, and embarrassed. Most people have a negative emotional reaction to sexual abuse and often respond with denial of the credibility of a child's disclosure. Children often conceal, repress, and deny their abuse for long periods of time, even years. When they do disclose the abuse, they often do so hesitantly, partially, and unclearly, giving more details over time, as they "test the waters" to see what response is forthcoming. Retraction of disclosures, followed by redisclosure, is common, especially if the perpetrator or another family member who has colluded in the sexual abuse has access to the child victim.

2. A child may spontaneously disclose details of sexual abuse to the pediatric examiner during the physical examination. The pediatric caregiver may also elect to interview the child before or after the examination. If possible, the interview should be conducted with the child alone, in a child-centered atmosphere, with the interviewer seated at the child's level, and in a gentle, neutral manner. The child should never be examined or interviewed in the presence of a suspected perpetrator.

3. Dolls or drawings may help in demonstrating sexual activities that may be difficult for the child to verbalize, but the use of specialized dolls or drawings should be left to those trained in their use. Using props is best left for clarifying an already-made disclosure rather than trying to elicit one.

4. It is helpful to allow time for building rapport by asking questions about the child's school, friends, activities, or other topics not related to the possible sexual abuse. This also gives the interviewer an opportunity to assess the child's cognitive and linguistic developmental level. Questions should be aimed at matching language to the child's developmental stage, with short, clear, simple sentences using appropriate vocabulary and familiar reference points, such as "lunch time," birthdays, television, and so on. It is important, even for the pediatric caregiver who is not conducting a specialized interview to assess sexual abuse allegations, to avoid (1) pressure or intimidation, (2) use of multiple questions that can only be answered yes or no, and (3) "leading" questions (i.e., those that suggest the answer to the question). The best questions are those that are open ended, that could have multiple answers, and that allow the child to give an expanded answer. However, children who have been traumatized by sexual abuse or threatened and intimidated into silence may be unable to disclose sexual abuse without careful, structured, directed interviewing by a mental health caregiver with experience in such situations.

5. If a child does make a disclosure, the caregiver should respond calmly and in a neutral manner. Questions about details of time, place, person, duration, number of incidents, possible eyewitnesses, whereabouts of supervisory adults, clothing worn or removed, reported comments or behaviors of the perpetrator, and so on, may be very helpful forensically. If the child can give details of the sexual contact without being pressured, these details should be obtained and recorded carefully, using direct quotes as much as possible. The child's expressed feelings, emotional responses, and nonverbal behaviors during the interview and the examination should also be recorded carefully.

Management

1. A clear written record, supplemented with drawings and photographs when indicated, should be made to document physical findings, procedures, specimens collected, observed behaviors, verbalizations by the child and/or caretakers, and any other pertinent information. The medical record should include both the results of physical examination and any medical procedures or tests. Also recorded should be the verbal utterances, behaviors, and emotional responses of the alleged child victim; comments of caretakers; full or partial confessions; descriptions by the child's nonaccused parent(s) of disclosures; behavioral symptoms; and physical complaints. The medical caregiver should give some opinion, if possible, as to whether the information gathered and the examination performed yielded evidence consistent with sexual abuse, the likelihood that sexual abuse did occur, and, if known, the alleged perpetrator. Several pediatric publications give helpful information concerning how to determine the likelihood that particular findings are consistent with sexual abuse.

2. The physician who believes a child has been sexually abused must report to protective services as directed in state statutes. He or she must also be prepared to give evidence to law enforcement officers, to prosecutors, and/or in court. If called on to testify in court, the physician may be helped by reference to publications that detail written guidelines for such participation and/or by attending continuing medical education courses designed for the physician witness.

Treatment

1. For the acutely injured sexually abused child, treatment involves attending to the injuries in a sensitive, gentle manner. The child who has positive cultures for sexually transmitted disease must receive appropriate antibiotic treatment. For the older child, the issue of possible pregnancy must be addressed and attended to.

2. Most sexually abused children do not present with medical problems requiring acute intervention but with emotional problems related to psychic trauma. The nonoffending parents of these children also may present with evidence of posttraumatic psychologic problems. Both children and parents should be referred for assessment to mental health professionals, if possible with expertise in treating victims, and parents of victims, of sexual abuse. The pediatrician, in collaboration with mental health professionals, can provide the child and nonoffending parent(s) with information about the child's physical condition, reassurance about recovery from any injuries or infections, and support in the handling of long-term emotional sequelae.

3. Occasionally, the pediatric caregiver is called on to have contact with the alleged perpetrating parent. It is important that the caregiver try to remain nonjudgmental toward such a parent but continue to support measures that protect a vulnerable child from possible repeat abuse or intimidation until a conclusive decision about the validity of the allegations has been reached.

Key Treatment

- Treatment of infection if present
- Addressing of pregnancy issue if present
- Sensitive, gentle management

Prevention

1. Current efforts at primary prevention of child sexual abuse are directed at education of young children, often in the primary grades of school, in recognizing and resisting attempts by adults to engage them in sexual activity. The efficacy of such educational efforts is still in question, but some studies indicate that certain approaches do empower children to resist sexual abuse attempts and/or to disclose abuse more promptly. Another important preventive intervention is early recognition and treatment of juvenile and adolescent perpetrators, for whom treatment is often much more successful than for adult perpetrators. Currently, very few programs for treatment of juveniles and adolescents are available, and there is a great need for education of all professionals who work with children in recognition and management of juvenile offending by peers and siblings.

2. The pediatrician may play a significant role in educating parents to empower their children to resist suggestions or directions by adults or older children that confuse them, frighten them, seem "wrong," or are forbidden. Providing information for parents on helping children to become "street smart" and having the self-esteem to appropriately resist adult inducements can prevent children from being "easy prey."

3. Secondary and tertiary prevention requires a high index of suspicion in the medical community, to allow for careful assessment of children who present with signs and symptoms of occult sexual abuse. Recognition of sexual abuse often merely requires including it in the differential diagnosis of confusing symptom constellations in children. It is important, however, that, in developing that high index of suspicion, caregivers not "jump to conclusions" about vague comments or "suggestive" behaviors that are not accompanied by physical evidence or a clear, spontaneous disclosure by a child of actual abuse.

 ## Bibliography

American Academy of Pediatrics, Committee on Child Abuse and Neglect: Guidelines for the evaluation of sexual abuse of children. Pediatrics 1991;87:254–260.

American Medical Association: Diagnostic and Treatment Guidelines on Child Sexual Abuse. Chicago, American Medical Association, 1994.

Giardino AP, Finkel MA, Giardino ER, et al: A Practical Guide to the Evaluation of Sexual Abuse in the Prepubertal Child. Newbury Park, CA, Sage, 1992.

Heger A, Emans SJ: Evaluation of the Sexually Abused Child. New York, Oxford University Press, 1992.

Reece RM: Child Abuse: Medical Diagnosis and Management. Philadelphia, Lea & Febiger, 1994.

54 Eating Disorders

David B. Herzog and *Karin M. Nussbaum*

Epidemiology

1. The prevalence of anorexia nervosa and bulimia nervosa in the adolescent female population of this country is approximately 0.5 per cent for anorexia and 2 per cent for bulimia. Ten to 25 per cent of teenage women have substantially disordered eating characterized by occasional binging and self-induced vomiting.
2. Anorexia nervosa and bulimia nervosa are both more common in females than in males. Males represent only 5 to 10 per cent of the eating-disordered population.
3. The age of onset of anorexia nervosa is bimodal, with a peak at 13 to 14 and again at 17 to 18 years, and reports of childhood-onset anorexia nervosa (ages 7–11) are increasing. The onset of bulimia nervosa tends to occur in the middle to late teenage years.
4. Although previously thought to affect primarily upper-class females, eating disorders cut across socioeconomic strata.
5. Risk factors associated with development of an eating disorder include dieting, age at menarche, obesity, and severe weight fluctuation. Specific subgroups at particular risk include persons involved in activities that place undue emphasis on achievement and thinness (i.e., ballet dancing, gymnastics, figure skating, and wrestling).

Pathophysiology

1. Biologic factors
   a. Eating disorders run in families. They are approximately three times more common in relatives of anorexic and bulimic patients than in the general population.
   b. Neurochemically, anorexic and bulimic patients display abnormalities in the noradrenergic, dopaminergic, and serotonergic systems of the brain. Almost all of these abnormalities normalize with weight restoration. The low levels of serotonin in serum and cerebrospinal fluid observed in bulimia nervosa may contribute to understanding the beneficial effect of selective serotonin-reuptake inhibitors in this disorder. Neurochemical abnormalities in weight-recovered anorexics and in bulimics abstinent from binging and purging suggest that these may be trait rather than state markers.
2. Sociocultural factors
   a. The incidence of eating disorders has greatly increased over the past few decades. Western society's emphasis on thinness in women plays an important role in the development of eating disorders.
   b. By adolescence, females are more concerned and dissatisfied with their bodies than are males, and most of teenage girls have dieted in an attempt to lose weight.

3. Psychologic factors
   a. Individuals with certain personality characteristics appear to be at increased risk for development of an eating disorder; these include perfectionism, rigidity, obsessionality, compliance, dependency, cautiousness, competitiveness, impulsiveness, and low self-regard. Social inventory findings typically report feelings of social ineffectiveness and isolation from peers despite a veneer of social competency.
   b. Comorbid psychiatric disorders are common. Almost half of patients with eating disorders meet criteria for major depression. Anxiety disorders are frequently observed in patients with anorexia nervosa, including obsessive-compulsive, social phobic, and simple phobic disorders. In bulimia nervosa, comorbidities include substance abuse, kleptomania, and anxiety disorders.

Clinical Findings

1. Anorexia nervosa most commonly begins in a teenager who is overweight or perceives herself to be overweight. A weight-related comment from a peer or parent precipitates dieting, which then escalates into an obsessive preoccupation with thinness. Significant weight loss may be achieved by restricting caloric intake, engaging in purging behaviors (i.e., vomiting, laxatives, or diuretics), or engaging in excessive physical activity. The anorexic is typically hyperactive and exhibits severe denial of symptoms.
2. Bulimia nervosa commonly begins in a normal-weight or overweight person who has attempted various diets without much success. Through a friend or family member, the individual becomes aware of self-induced vomiting or other compensatory behaviors to control weight, and the cycle of binging and purging begins. Bulimics most often binge in secret, consuming food high in carbohydrates. Bulimics are often embarrassed by their food-related symptoms and report feelings of lack of control, guilt, and shame at their behavior.
3. Specific criteria for anorexia nervosa and bulimia nervosa have been developed by the American Psychiatric Association (1994). The applicability of some of the criteria for adolescents and preadolescents has been questioned. For example, some preadolescents and adolescents may not have lost sufficient weight to be at less than 85 per cent of their ideal body weight even though they meet all the other criteria for anorexia nervosa.
4. Anorexia nervosa and bulimia nervosa often coexist. Many bulimics have a history of anorexia nervosa, and others may lose weight and develop anorexia nervosa. Approximately half of anorexic patients engage in bulimic behaviors. Patients who engage in both anorexic and bulimic behaviors (i.e., low weight and binging and

purging) have more severe medical complications than patients with anorexia nervosa or bulimia nervosa alone.

5. *Differential diagnosis*—Initial medical assessment should be thorough and should include a complete differential diagnosis of presenting symptoms. Patients may also manifest medical conditions in addition to their eating disorder, such as diabetes mellitus, thyroid disorders, inflammatory bowel disorders, or cystic fibrosis. In such cases, the eating disorder can seriously complicate the course and management of the medical disorder.

DSM-IV Diagnostic Criteria for Anorexia Nervosa

1. Refusal to maintain body weight at or above a minimally normal weight for age and height (i.e., weight loss leading to maintenance of body weight <85% of that expected; or failure to make expected weight gain during period of growth, leading to body weight <85% of that expected)
2. Intense fear of gaining weight or becoming fat, even though underweight
3. Disturbance in the way in which one's body weight or shape is experienced, undue influence of body weight or shape on self-evaluation, or denial of the seriousness of the current low body weight
4. In postmenarchal females, amenorrhea (i.e., the absence of at least three consecutive menstrual cycles).

DSM-IV Diagnostic Criteria for Bulimia Nervosa

1. Recurrent episodes of binge eating, characterized by both of the following: (a) eating an unusually large amount of food in a discrete period (i.e., within 2 hours) and (b) a sense of lack of control over eating during the episode
2. Recurrent inappropriate compensatory behavior to prevent weight gain (i.e., self-induced vomiting; misuse of laxatives, diuretics, enemas, or other medications; fasting; or excessive exercise)
3. Binge eating and compensatory behaviors both occur, on average, twice week for 3 months.
4. Self-evaluation is unduly influenced by body shape and weight.
5. The disturbance does not occur exclusively during episodes of anorexia nervosa.

(From Diagnostic and Statistical Manual for Mental Disorders, 4th ed. Washington, DC, American Psychiatric Association, 1994.)

Key Clinical Findings

- Excessive weight loss
- Bulimic behavior (50%)

Medical Complications

1. Medical problems associated with eating disorders are numerous and can be severe (Herzog and Copeland,

---

1985). Malnutrition in anorexia nervosa can cause growth retardation and arrested sexual maturation. Failure to attain bone mineral density, which increases 50 per cent or more during adolescence, and actual loss of bone secondary to malnutrition can lead to osteoporosis. The osteoporosis seen in anorexia nervosa may result from hypoestrogenism, hypercortisolemia, poor calcium intake, or decreased insulin-like growth factor (IGF-I). Although weight restoration is related to increased bone mass, this serious complication may not be reversible in all cases, placing the young woman at risk for bone fractures throughout life.

2. Structural brain abnormalities in anorexics include lateral ventricular and cortical sulcal enlargement, which are strongly associated with severity of weight loss.

3. Cardiac manifestations of anorexia nervosa include decreased cardiac-chamber size and thinning of the left ventricle. These cardiac changes are associated with reduced cardiac output and hypotension. Arrhythmias are common.

4. Renal abnormalities in anorexia nervosa are largely caused by dehydration and a reduced glomerular filtration rate. These factors may lead to renal calculi. With refeeding, peripheral edema is common in anorexia.

Medical Complications of Eating Disorders

Endocrine/metabolic
Amenorrhea
Menstrual irregularities
Osteoporosis
Delayed puberty
Hypercarotenemia
Low T3 syndrome
Cardiovascular
Bradycardia
Hypotension
Arrythmias
Ipecac cardiomyopathy
Renal
Hypokalemia (diuretic-induced)
Increased blood urea nitrogen
Renal calculi
Edema
Gastrointestinal
Decreased gastric emptying
Constipation
Elevated hepatic enzymes
Acute gastric dilatation, rupture
Parotid enlargement
Dental-enamel erosion
Esophagitis
Mallory-Weiss tears, esophageal rupture
Hypokalemia (laxative-induced)
Hematologic
Anemia
Leukopenia
Thrombocytopenia
Pulmonary
Aspiration pneumonia

5. Hematologic changes associated with anorexia nervosa are usually without clinical consequence but may include anemia, leukopenia, and thrombocytopenia.

6. Gastrointestinal complications in anorexia nervosa include delayed gastric motility and constipation.

7. Dermatologic complications of anorexia nervosa consist of brittle hair and nails, the presence of lanugo type hair on the body, dry skin, and sallow complexion.

8. Complications associated with purging behaviors include electrolyte disturbances, parotid enlargement, esophageal rupture, dental enamel erosion (perimolysis) and cavities, gastric and esophageal irritation, and large-bowel dysfunction (secondary to laxative abuse). Ongoing use of ipecac can result in cardiac myopathy. Abrasions on the metacarpophalangeal joints (Russell sign) may be an important diagnostic sign of self-induced vomiting.

Treatment

1. Anorexia nervosa and bulimia nervosa require a multimodal interdisciplinary approach to treatment. Treatment for anorexia nervosa typically takes at least 1 to 2 years, and more complex patients may require extended multidisciplinary care.

2. Patients with eating disorders are known for their resistance to treatment and their denial of the seriousness of the illness. The parents must be encouraged and directed to participate as an integral part of the treatment process, often mandating the necessary treatment for their child, adolescent, or young adult.

3. Inpatient treatment

   a. Anorexia nervosa often requires an initial inpatient admission, whereas bulimia nervosa is commonly managed on an outpatient basis.

   b. Inpatient treatment should be viewed as the first step in a treatment plan that will require outpatient care as well.

   c. Criteria for hospitalization include the following: (1) medical state (i.e., bradycardia, hypotension, hypothermia, or hypokalemia); (2) psychiatric state (i.e., acute depression, suicidal ideation, unsafe home environment, or severity of symptoms causing extreme functional impairment); and (3) failure of outpatient treatment.

   d. Goals of hospitalization include the following: (1) a complete assessment (medical, psychiatric, family, and nutritional); (2) achievement of medical stabilization; (3) confrontation or clarification of denial; (4) treatment of comorbid disorders (e.g., depression), and (5) organization of an outpatient treatment plan (which may initially include partial hospitalization). Establishment of modest and realistic goals is critical.

   e. Inpatient care can take place on a psychiatric or pediatric unit. Patients who are noncompliant, acutely depressed, or in need of more intensive family therapy should have psychiatric hospitalization. Patients who require refeeding may be managed on a pediatric ward.

   f. A nutritional rehabilitation protocol for anorexia is helpful. Patients should be at bed rest initially and particularly after meal times if vomiting is suspected. Activities should be awarded with weight gain and increasing medical safety. Caloric intake should increase by 200 to 300 cal/day every 2 to 3 days. A gain of about one-third pound per day is a safe rate for anorexics.

   g. Although achievement of a medically stable weight must be the primary goal of an anorexic patient's hospitalization, work should be undertaken in the hospital toward making personal changes that will lead to healthy eating behaviors and attitudes.

4. Day treatment

   a. On discharge from an inpatient setting, or in lieu of hospitalization, day treatment may be recommended.

   b. Day treatment offers a less restrictive approach, allowing the patient to participate in a therapeutic group setting while at the same time continuing to attend school and live at home.

   c. These programs include supervised meals, group therapy, nutritional counseling, individual psychotherapy, and pharmacotherapy.

5. Outpatient treatment

   a. Regular medical monitoring, nutritional guidance, family therapy, and individual therapy are important aspects of outpatient treatment for the eating-disordered patient.

   b. Individual psychotherapy should be tailored to the patient's needs and developmental level. It should provide relationship, support, insight, and cognitive behavior instruction.

   c. Cognitive behavior therapy aims to eliminate errors in the patient's thinking and perceptions which result in unrealistic attitudes and unhealthy behaviors. The patient learns and practices new ways of thinking, self-monitors behaviors and attitudes, resumes healthy behaviors at a modest pace, and learns new coping strategies. Family therapy should offer supportive guidance and identify the family dynamics (i.e, separation/individuation issues) that may perpetuate the eating disorder.

   d. Psychopharmacology may be recommended in conjunction with therapy. Selective serotonin-reuptake inhibitors are usually the psychotropic agent of choice in bulimia nervosa and can be helpful in treating comorbid depression. No medication has been shown consistently to be effective in anorexia. However, fluoxetine has shown some promise in weight-recovered anorexics, enabling them to maintain weight, possibly by improving their obsessive-compulsive symptoms.

Key Treatments

- Supportive psychotherapy
- Cognitive behavioral therapy
- Family therapy
- Nutritional support
- Medical monitoring

Course and Outcome

1. Seventy to 80 per cent of both anorexic and bulimic patients improve substantially over time. Bulimics tend to be more responsive to treatment; approximately 60 per cent recover in the first 5 years of follow-up. Anorexics have a lower rate of recovery, approximately 50 per cent at 5-year follow-up.
2. At 5 years after hospitalization, the mortality rate for anorexia nervosa is approximately 4 to 5 per cent. Common causes of death include suicide, malnutrition, and congestive heart failure.
3. No prognostic factor has been found consistently across outcome studies. The most common indicator of poor outcome in anorexia nervosa is the presence of purging. Early age at onset, good premorbid history, friendships, and early intervention are generally considered to be positive predictors. Those patients with a history of sexual abuse, conflictual family environments, comorbid medical or psychiatric conditions, or inability to seek or accept treatment tend to have the most severe course.

Prevention

1. Primary prevention

   a. Primary prevention programs are underway in schools, although there have been no conclusive findings as yet regarding the effectiveness of these programs in preventing eating disorders.

   b. Educators, primary care physicians, and pediatricians in their clinical practices need to provide information to students and parents regarding healthy and pathologic eating attitudes and behaviors.

2. Secondary prevention

   a. Anorexic and bulimic patients often do not seek help or are not brought for help until months or years after the onset of symptoms. The patient or family may feel embarrassed or ashamed, may not recognize the problem, or may think that it will go away without professional help.

   b. Early identification of patients is critical. Inquiring about weight control measures as part of the routine examination of children 10 years of age and older would be a good screening tool.

   c. In concerning cases, a family history of eating disorders and other risk factors can be sought. Those children who are obsessional, who are rigid about food rules, and whose families place great emphasis on high achievement and thinness should be evaluated more closely. Aspiring ballerinas, gymnasts, and ice skaters and their families should be informed of the occupational risk involved in their child's activities.

Bibliography

American Psychiatric Association: Diagnostic and Statistical Manual for Mental Disorders, 4th ed. Washington, DC, American Psychiatric Association, 1994.

Fisher M, Golden NH, Katzman DK, et al: Eating disorders in adolescents: A background paper. J Adolesc Health 1995; 16:420–437.

Harper G: Eating disorders in adolescence. Pediatr Rev 1994; 15:72–77.

Herzog DB, Copeland PM: Eating disorders. N Engl J Med 1985;313:295–303.

55 Attention-Deficit/ Hyperactivity Disorder

Timothy E. Wilens, Thomas J. Spencer, Joseph Biederman, and *David Schleifer*

Definition

Attention-deficit/hyperactivity disorder (ADHD) is a neuropsychological disorder associated with disturbances in attention, impulsivity, and hyperactivity. The disorder was previously known as hyperkinetic reaction of childhood. According to the criteria of the fourth edition of the *Diagnostic and Statistical Manual of Mental Disorders,* it is possible for an individual to meet criteria for the disorder if he or she has symptoms of inattention and/or hyperactivity-impulsivity, depending on the symptoms endorsed (combined, predominantly hyperactive/impulsive, or predominantly inattentive).

Epidemiology

ADHD is estimated to affect 6 to 9 per cent of children and adolescents. Data indicate that children with ADHD are at risk for developing emotional and behavioral problems, such as conduct or antisocial behaviors, substance abuse, depression, and anxiety disorders. Even though follow-up studies show that ADHD persists into adulthood in 10 to 60 per cent of childhood-onset cases, little attention has been paid to the adult form of this disorder, which data suggest may affect up to 2 per cent of adults. The persistence of the disorder appears to be positively associated with the presence of familiarity, other psychiatric disorders, and environmental adversity.

Etiology

Although its etiology remains unknown, data from family-genetic, twin, and adoption studies, as well as segregation analysis, suggest a genetic origin in 20 to 50 per cent of cases. However, other causes are also likely, such as psychologic adversity, perinatal insults, and perhaps other yet unknown biologic causes.

Pathophysiology

ADHD is thought to be related to catecholaminergic dysregulation in general, and more specifically to dopaminergic and noradrenergic neurotransmission. Functional and neuroanatomic studies of the human brain suggest that the frontal-striatal brain pathways appear to be affected.

Diagnostic Considerations

1. Although the symptoms of ADHD may be seen as non-specific, it is important to ascertain the pervasiveness, context, and impairment of each of the symptoms. As in any psychiatric disorder, ADHD symptoms are outside of "normal difficulties" and are both persistent and impairing. Diagnostic information should be gathered from the parents and patient and, whenever possible, from other sources, such as teachers. To facilitate history gathering with the school system, report forms completed by the teacher are commercially available. If ancillary data are not available, information from parents is acceptable for diagnostic and treatment purposes because parent reports have been shown to be reflective of their children's ADHD symptoms at home, socially, and in the school setting.

2. The classic triad of symptoms associated with ADHD—inattention/distractibility, impulsivity, and hyperactivity—may not be present in all children. Whereas preschoolers are frequently referred for hyperactivity, impulsivity, and aggressiveness, school-aged children are often noted to have marked inattention, easy distractibility, impatience, low frustration tolerance, and frequent shifting of activities. In fact, many ADHD children without reading disabilities report difficulties in comprehension, the need to repeat paragraphs because of poor concentration, and the inability to complete a paragraph or page of text. ADHD children and adolescents also commonly report excessive boredom and frequent daydreaming, which, when substantial, may appear to others as a seizure disorder of an absence subtype. Although less defined within ADHD, difficulties with organization, procrastination, and prioritization appear common and may cause the child to feel overwhelmed when faced with multiple tasks to complete. Socially, many ADHD children are noted to talk excessively and intrude into others conversations and "space," exacerbating peer difficulties. Although the majority of children and adolescents with ADHD report difficulties in the school setting, it is not uncommon for ADHD to be more problematic in the home (less structured) or social domains.

3. Children and adolescents with ADHD also commonly manifest other neurologic and psychiatric disorders. Whereas roughly 10 per cent of children with ADHD may have an associated tic disorder, approximately half of children and adolescents with Tourette syndrome appear to manifest ADHD. In many of these cases, ADHD is the major source of distress and disability rather than the tic disorder. There also appears to be an excessive overlap of ADHD and seizure disorders. The presence of other emotional and behavioral problems in ADHD children is significant. For example, a more complicated clinical course and overall poorer outcome is predicted in those ADHD children with conduct disorder.

Key Clinical Findings

- Inattention
- Distractibility
- Impulsivity
- Hyperactivity
- Associated tic (10 per cent)

Treatment

1. Strategies. The treatment of the ADHD patient should consider multimodal intervention attempting to address three main areas of potential dysfunction in the affected individual: biological, psychosocial, and educational. Careful attention should be paid to the onset of symptoms, longitudinal history of the disorder, concurrent psychiatric problems, and differential diagnosis, including coexisting medical or neurologic disorders. Similarly, psychosocial and educational factors contributing to the clinical presentation should be explored. Within the medical spectrum, children and their families should be queried for the presence of neurologic disorders (i.e., tics, seizures), endocrine abnormalities (i.e., thyroid, Wilson disease), cardiovascular perturbations, height/weight stature, and toxic exposure (lead). Patients with substance problems should be referred for further evaluation and treated for ADHD after appropriate addiction treatments have been undertaken. Issues of co-occurring learning disabilities and unspecified academic needs should be addressed. Although children and adolescents with ADHD are predictably underachieving academically, learning difficulties in specific classes or academic delays should signal the need for further assessment (i.e., cognitive testing). Because learning disorders are not drug sensitive, the approximately 30 per cent of ADHD individuals with a learning disorder will require additional education support. Educational support can take the form of tutoring, computer assistance, and placement in special classes and occasionally in specialized schools. Children and adolescents with ADHD often have mild, but troublesome, behavioral problems such as oppositionality, aggressiveness, and intrusiveness. They may also appear immature and poorly coordinated. They often respond poorly to limit setting and frequently have temper tantrums. The chronic underachievement and lack of positive feedback may also predispose these children to develop poor self-esteem and demoralization. Many of these behaviors can be reduced through parental education and behavioral management strategies aimed at increasing the structure and consistency of the child's environment. Diminishing punitive exchanges and increasing positive interactions should be a goal of the family. If problematic behaviors persist, referral to a mental health professional is recommended. Psychotherapeutic efforts found helpful in the management of the ADHD child and adolescent include behavioral and cognitive-behavioral interventions, as well as more traditional forms of psychother-

apy such as family therapy. Cognitive-behavioral interventions used include training in self-instruction, self-evaluation, attribution, social skills, and anger management. Although these procedures have achieved some short-term success in ameliorating the problems of ADHD children and adolescents, they have not been found to generalize to untrained situations or to maintain the gains after treatment ends. The use of medication should follow a careful evaluation of the patient including psychiatric, social, and cognitive domains. Pharmacotherapy of ADHD can help not only abnormal behaviors in school or work but, equally importantly, the individual's social and family life. In concert with pharmacotherapy, educational, cognitive-behavioral, and/or social skills, interventions are useful in tackling difficulties with multiple domains affected by ADHD. The medications most often employed for ADHD include the psychostimulants, antidepressants, and antihypertensives.

2. Medications (Table 55–1)
   a. Stimulants
      (1) Stimulants are sympathomimetic drugs structurally similar to endogenous catecholamines. The most commonly used compounds in this class include methylphenidate (Ritalin), D-amphetamine (Dexedrine), methamphetamine (Desoxyn), and magnesium pemoline (Cylert). These drugs are thought to act both in the central nervous system and peripherally by stimulating catecholaminergic release, preventing reuptake of the catecholamines into presynaptic nerve endings. Methylphenidate and D-amphet-

amine are both short-acting compounds with an onset of action within 30 to 60 minutes and a peak clinical effect usually seen between 1 and 3 hours after administration. Therefore, multiple daily administrations are required for a consistent daytime response. Slow-release preparations, with a peak clinical effect between 1 and 5 hours, are available for methylphenidate and D-amphetamine and can often allow for a single dose to be administered in the morning that will last for the entire school day. Magnesium pemoline is a longer-acting compound, generally allowing for a single daily dose. Although initial studies indicated a delayed onset of action (up to 6 weeks), more recent data indicate a faster onset of action when pemoline is titrated more rapidly.

      (2) The stimulant medications remain the mainstay treatment for children, adolescents, and adults with ADHD, with over 150 controlled studies having documented the efficacy and safety of these medications. Yet, this literature also shows that as many as 30 per cent of individuals treated with stimulants do not improve. Stimulants diminish motor overactivity and impulsive behaviors seen in ADHD and allow the patient to sustain attention. Stimulants can also be effective in patients with ADHD in whom hyperactivity is not a significant problem as well as in the treatment of ADHD patients with mental retardation and developmental delays. The concern that optimal clinical efficacy is attained at

TABLE 55–1. PSYCHOTROPICS USED IN ADHD

AGENT	DAILY DOSE (mg/kg)	DAILY DOSAGE SCHEDULE	COMMON ADVERSE EFFECTS
Stimulants			
Dextroamphetamine (methamphetamine, amphetamine compound)	0.3–1.5	Twice or three times	Insomnia, decreased appetite, weight loss, dysphoria Possible reduction in growth velocity with chronic use Rebound phenomena
Methylphenidate	1.0–2.0		Same as other stimulants
Magnesium pemoline	1.0–3.0	Once	Abnormal results of liver function tests (1–2%)
Antidepressants			
Tricyclics (imipramine, desipramine, nortriptyline)	2.0–5.0 (1.0–3.0 for nortriptyline)	Once or twice	Dry mouth, constipation Weight loss Vital sign and electrocardiographic changes
Bupropion	1–6	Three times	Irritability, insomnia Risk of seizures (in doses > 6 mg/kg) Contraindicated in bulimics
Venlafaxine	0.5–3	Twice	Nausea, gastrointestinal distress Agitation
Antihypertensives			
Clonidine	3–10 μg/kg	Twice or three times	Sedation, dry mouth, depression Confusion (with high dose) Rebound hypertension Localized irritation with patch
Guanfacine	30–100 μg/kg	Twice	Similar to clonidine but less sedation Insomnia, irritability reported

the cost of impaired learning ability has not been confirmed.

(3) Because of their short half-life, the short-acting stimulants should be given in divided doses throughout the day, typically 4 hours apart. The total daily dose ranges from 0.3 mg/kg/day to 2 mg/kg/day. The starting dose is generally 2.5 to 5 mg/day, given in the morning, with the dose being increased if necessary every few days by 2.5 to 5 mg in a divided-dose schedule. Because of the anorexogenic effects of the stimulants, it may be beneficial to administer the medicine after meals. Being longer acting, magnesium pemoline is typically given as a single daily dose in the morning ranging from 1 to 3 mg/kg/day. The typical starting dose of pemoline is 18.75 to 37.5 mg with increments in dose of 18.75 mg every few days thereafter until desired effects occur or side effects preclude further increments.

(4) The most commonly reported side effects associated with the stimulants are appetite suppression and sleep disturbances. The sleep disturbance that is most commonly reported is delay of sleep onset. This usually occurs when stimulants are administered in the late afternoon or early evening. Although less commonly reported, mood disturbances ranging from increased tearfulness to a full-blown major depression–like syndrome can be associated with stimulant treatment. Rebound phenomena between doses can also occur in some patients, creating an uneven, often disturbing, clinical course. In those cases, consideration should be given to alternative preparations or medications. The cardiovascular effects of stimulants are mild, and stimulant-associated toxic psychosis is rare. Administration of magnesium pemoline has been associated with hypersensitivity reactions involving the liver accompanied by elevations in liver function studies (aspartate transaminase) after several months of treatment. Thus, baseline liver function studies and repeat studies are recommended with the administration of this compound.

(5) The precipitation or exacerbation of a tic disorder after stimulant administration is a concern, although stimulants may be used in these individuals with caution. The stimulants may also adversely affect growth velocity in a small number of cases. Careful monitoring of growth is indicated during stimulant therapy; and if a decrease in growth occurs, consideration should be given to a drug holiday or alternative treatment options.

b. Antidepressants

(1) The tricyclic antidepressants (TCAs), including imipramine and desipramine, are commonly prescribed for enuresis and as an alternative treatment for ADHD. TCAs may be particularly useful for ADHD children with tics, severe re-

bound, or weight loss on the stimulants. The mechanism of action appears to be the blocking effects of these drugs on the reuptake of brain norepinephrine. Although superior to placebo, TCAs are less effective than the stimulants.

(2) TCAs are long-acting agents that should be initiated at 10 to 25 mg, with the dose increased every 4 to 5 days until effective or an upper dose of 5 mg/kg for children is reached. Monitoring of baseline and follow-up electrocardiograms and serum TCA levels at higher doses are recommended. Common short-term adverse effects of the TCAs include dry mouth, constipation, headaches, and stomach aches. TCA treatment is also associated with mild elevations in diastolic blood pressure, heart rate, and electrocardiographic evidence of prolongation of cardiac conduction parameters. There have been four cases of sudden death in children aged 12 or younger during treatment with therapeutic doses of desipramine, although the causality remains dubious and absolute risk is minimal.

(3) Bupropion is a novel-structured antidepressant with indirect dopamine agonist effects that has been shown to be superior to placebo. The response of ADHD to bupropion appears to be rapid and sustained. Bupropion should be started at very low doses (i.e., 37.5 mg/day) with dosing for ADHD appearing to be similar to and titrated upward to 450 mg/day divided into three daily doses. Side effects include irritability, rashes, anorexia, tics, and insomnia. It appears to have a somewhat higher (0.4 per cent) rate of drug-induced seizures relative to other antidepressants, particularly in daily doses higher than 6 mg/kg, and in individuals with bulimia or preexisting seizures.

(4) The new generation antidepressants referred to as the serotonin reuptake inhibitors include fluoxetine, fluvoxamine, paroxetine, and sertraline. Although helpful for depression or anxiety, they do not appear helpful for "core" ADHD symptoms. Of interest, venlafaxine, a novel combined serotonergic and noradrenergic reuptake inhibitor, has been reported to be helpful in the treatment of ADHD in both pediatric and adult groups.

c. Antihypertensives

(1) Clonidine is an inhibitory, presynaptic α-adrenergic agonist that has been used in childhood ADHD, particularly in children with marked hyperactivity or aggression at doses of 4 to 5 μg/kg. Clonidine is a short-acting compound with a half-life of 6 hours, necessitating multiple dosings daily. The most common adverse effect of clonidine is sedation, which may be used to treat sleep disturbances commonly reported in ADHD children at baseline or secondary to medication treatment. Clonidine may also produce hypotension, dry mouth, depression,

and confusion. Abrupt withdrawal of clonidine has been associated with rebound hypertension.

(2) Another antihypertensive medication, guanfacine (Tenex) has also been used for ADHD. Like clonidine, guanfacine is an α_2-noradrenergic agonist that has only recently been studied openly for ADHD. Although not well delineated, dosing in school-aged children should be started at 0.5 mg/day and gradually increased as necessary to a maximum of 4 mg/day in two to three divided doses. Guanfacine appears to be longer acting, less sedating, and more effective for attentional problems than clonidine. Somnolence, headaches, and enuresis are among the most common adverse effects.

(3) Combined pharmacotherapy may be necessary in ADHD patients who have multiple disorders, an inadequate response with single agents, or potentially treatable adverse effects in the context of a good clinical response. For instance, the addition of stimulants may improve the anti-ADHD effectiveness of the antidepressants. Clonidine appears to be helpful in ameliorating sleep disturbances often attributed to the stimulants in ADHD children.

Key Treatment

- Educational support
- Stimulants
    Methylphenidate
    Amphetamines
    Magnesium pemoline
- Antidepressants
- Antihypertensives

Bibliography

Barkley RA: Attention Deficit Hyperactivity Disorder: A Handbook for Diagnosis and Treatment. New York, Guilford Press, 1990.

Mannuzza S, Klein RG, Bessler A, et al: Adult outcome of hyperactive boys: Educational achievement, occupational rank, and psychiatric status. Arch Gen Psychiatry 1993;50:565.

Spencer TJ, Biederman J, Wilens TE: Pharmacotherapy of ADHD across the life cycle: A literature review. J Am Acad Child Adolesc Psychiatry 1996;35:409.

Weiss G: Attention-Deficit Hyperactivity Disorder. Philadelphia, WB Saunders, 1992.

Zametkin AJ, Rapoport JL: Neurobiology of attention deficit disorder with hyperactivity: Where have we come in 50 years? J Am Acad Child Adolesc Psychiatry 1987;26:676.

56 Autism, Asperger Syndrome, and Schizophrenia

Jean A. Frazier

Before the 1970s, all psychotic disorders of childhood were diagnosed as childhood schizophrenia. Much diagnostic confusion has existed regarding the different disorders. However, in 1971, Kolvin and colleagues published their landmark studies that helped to clarify that autism (psychosis before the age of 3 years) and schizophrenia (psychosis after the age of 5 years) are separate disorders. Starting with their definitions in the *Diagnostic and Statistical Manual of Mental Disorders,* third edition, autism and schizophrenia with onset in childhood were categorized as distinct disorders.

Autism, Asperger syndrome, and schizophrenia are rare but extremely devastating conditions to the individuals affected and to their families. All three disorders are complex, chronic, and severely debilitating conditions, although Asperger syndrome may have a better prognosis than autism and schizophrenia. Long-term treatment utilizing a multidisciplinary team approach is usually required for all of these conditions.

Autism

Definition

The American Psychiatric Association defines autism as a disorder involving qualitative impairment in social interaction, impairment in social communication, and aberrant behavior (consisting of restrictive repetitive and stereotyped patterns) with the manifestation of delays in at least one of these areas before 3 years of age. The hallmark characteristic of autism is the lack of interest in other persons. The disorder is generally noticed within the first year of life.

Epidemiology

Most studies cite a prevalence of between 2 to 5 in 10,000. The disorder occurs more commonly among boys, with the male:female ratio ranging in studies from 2:1 to 10:1. Girls often have a more severe form of the disorder.

Etiology

1. Although the etiology of the condition still remains elusive, evidence points to an organic cause. This is because autism can be associated with neurologic soft signs, perinatal complications, congenital infection (rubella, tuberculosis), structural brain abnormalities, genetic disorders (fragile X syndrome), and metabolic disorders (phenylketonuria).

2. There may be a genetic component to the disorder because there have been reports of higher rates of learning

disabilities in siblings and a high concordance for the disorder among monozygotic twins (36 per cent).

Evaluation

A careful history (including pregnancy and family history) and thorough physical examination of a child are indicated. There is a higher incidence of medical illness such as upper respiratory tract infections and febrile seizures in children with autism as compared with normal controls. Sight and hearing should be checked. Screening for metabolic disturbances (phenylketonuria) and chromosomal analysis looking for inherited conditions such as fragile X syndrome are indicated. Neurologic consultation and evaluation should be done as necessary. There is a higher rate of seizure disorder in the autistic population (20 to 25 per cent). Cognitive evaluation is indicated (70 to 80 per cent of patients with autism have IQs in the mentally retarded range). A child's adaptive functioning should also be assessed.

Prevention

Genetic counseling for families with a history of autism and conditions such as phenylketonuria and fragile X syndrome is indicated. Optimizing maternal health care during pregnancy is essential.

Treatment

1. The disorder is chronic and often has a poor prognosis. For example, only about one third of adults with autism can achieve some degree of self-sufficiency. Higher intelligence quotient (IQ) and better communication skills are generally indicators of better prognosis.
2. Some interventions can help the child with autism. Early intervention by a multidisciplinary team may decrease the morbidity associated with the condition. The team should work closely with the parents to evaluate the child's cognitive as well as adaptive functioning. Long-term educational interventions with strong emphasis on behavioral approaches and on the acquisition of adaptive skills are indicated.
3. Stereotypical behaviors, or other aberrant behaviors, can be very problematic and should be thoroughly evaluated. New-onset aberrant behaviors may result from a variety of causes, including environmental change or co-morbid medical, neurologic, or psychiatric disorders. Because of the autistic patient's limited communication skills, he or she may not be able to tell a physician what is troublesome and why he or she might have developed a new problematic behavior. Possible medical or neurologic conditions need to be ruled out. If the cause of the new behavior remains elusive, psychiatric consultation should be obtained. Psychopharmacologic intervention may be indicated for inattention, hyperactivity, impulsivity, self-injurious behavior, aggression, affective symptoms, rituals, and so on, depending on the presenting composite of target symptoms. Medications should be used at the lowest possible dose and monotherapy is preferable because autistic children may be more prone to side effects and more sensitive to drug-drug interactions.
4. Families of autistic children need support because these children are often maintained at home. Families can learn how to access resources from advocacy groups such as the Autism Society of America.

Key Treatment: Autism

- Educational support
- Management of co-morbid conditions

Asperger Syndrome

Definition

Asperger syndrome is another disorder of development that is on a continuum with autism. The American Psychiatric Association has included this diagnosis in the fourth edition of its manual. The disorder is characterized by paucity of empathy, naive inappropriate interaction, pedantic speech, egocentrism, poor nonverbal communication, intense absorption in circumscribed topics, and ill-coordinated movements. Although similar to autism in many respects, individuals with Asperger syndrome are less likely to have delayed speech or stereotypical behaviors. They tend to have normal intelligence, and long-term outcome is generally more positive. The disorder may have a later age at onset than autism (> 24 months).

Epidemiology

The prevalence of the disorder is approximately 1 in 10,000. The disorder occurs more often in boys.

Evaluation and Prevention

1. Careful history and physical examination should be done. Neuropsychological, psychological, and language assessments focusing on cognitive, adaptive, motor, and communication skills should be pursued.
2. Genetic counseling in families in which Asperger syndrome exists may be indicated.

Treatment

1. A multimodal approach is indicated. Emphasis on adaptive functioning is important in terms of both evaluation and treatment.
2. Unfortunately these individuals often do not qualify for services because most have a normal full-scale IQ. However, their social skills are deficient and circumscribed interests are marked and can lead to severe impairment, particularly in social situations.
3. The focus of treatment should be on communication skills, social skills, cognitive strategies, physical therapy, and occupational therapy. Supportive psychotherapy can be helpful for some individuals. Pharmacotherapy may be indicated but should be initiated after a full psychiatric evaluation. Children with Asperger syndrome may require medication to help treat symptoms of psychiatric conditions such as major depression, obsessive-compulsive disorder, and anxiety disorders. Additionally, some case reports indicate that these individuals may be at greater risk of developing thought disorder. The presence of a thought disorder would be an indication for treatment with an antipsychotic agent.

Key Treatment: Asperger Syndrome

- Improvement in communication skills
- Physical therapy

Childhood Schizophrenia

Definition

Schizophrenia does occur in childhood. These children have the same signs and symptoms as adults with the disorder. Schizophrenia is characterized by the presence of at least two of the following symptoms: hallucinations, delusions, disorganized speech, disorganized or catatonic behavior, and negative symptoms such as affective flattening, poverty of speech, apathy, asocialty, and inattention. Children with schizophrenia either have a decline in functioning or a failure to achieve expected levels of development. Signs of the disorder should be present for at least 6 months, including at least 1 month of positive and negative symptoms (e.g., hallucinations, delusions, affective flattening). Mood disorder should be ruled out and general medical conditions should not be etiologic.

Epidemiology

1. Childhood-onset schizophrenia (onset of psychotic symptoms before age 12 years) is rare and occurs in 2 per 10,000 persons, 1/50 the prevalence of the adult disorder. Schizophrenia in late adolescence occurs more frequently and begins to approach the prevalence of the adult-onset disorder.
2. Most phenomenologic studies find a male predominance in childhood-onset schizophrenia with the male:female ratio being 2 to 3:1.

Etiology

1. The exact cause of schizophrenia is not clear. The signs and symptoms of the disorder point to a neurobiologic basis that is likely multifactorial.
2. Data support a probable underlying genetic mechanism. For adults with schizophrenia, the risk of siblings developing the disorder is 10 per cent, and that of offspring developing the disorder is 13 per cent. There is a 40 to 50 per cent concordance rate noted in monozygotic twins.
3. Factors such as infection, injury, toxins, nutritional deficiencies, and abnormal hormones during gestation have all been described as potentially having a role in the etiology of the disorder. These epigenetic factors may serve to "trigger" a schizophrenic episode in a genetically vulnerable individual.
4. Many adult studies and one report on children with the disorder indicate numerous brain findings on magnetic resonance imaging, including enlarged lateral ventricles, smaller total cerebral volume, enlarged basal ganglia, reduced medial temporal lobe, and smaller thalamic area. Autonomic dysregulation and abnormal eye tracking have also been reported.

Evaluation

1. Any child who presents with new-onset psychotic symptoms needs to be thoroughly evaluated for medical causes of the presenting problem. A thorough history (including family history, medication history, and possible substance exposure) and physical examination should be done. Neurologic evaluation is indicated, with electroencephalography (to rule out seizure disorder) and magnetic resonance imaging (to rule out tumors, metachromatic leukodystrophy, and so on) as deemed necessary. Toxic causes should be entertained and ruled out through a urine toxic screen. Many infectious and metabolic etiologies (e.g., hyperthyroidism, Wilson disease, mercury poisoning, porphyria, encephalitis, human immunodeficiency virus infection) can also present with such marked behavior disturbances.
2. A psychiatric evaluation is indicated in patients with a new onset of psychotic symptoms.

Prevention

Genetic counseling for families in which the disorder exists should be provided.

Treatment

1. Psychiatric involvement is crucial. Antipsychotic agents are the cornerstone of treatment of schizophrenia. There are only two double-blind studies in the literature that evaluate neuroleptic treatment in children and adolescents with schizophrenia. These studies indicate that neuroleptic agents are efficacious in children and adolescents with schizophrenia. However, side effects such as sedation and extrapyramidal symptoms are problematic. Newer atypical agents such as clozapine, risperidone, and olanzapine hold much promise because these medications not only treat the positive symptoms of schizophrenia (hallucinations and delusions) but they also treat the negative symptoms (affective flattening, poverty of speech), which can be so devastating to social functioning.
2. Once in the mental health system, children and adolescents often do not get the kind of medical and dental care that is necessary. Ongoing routine pediatric and dental checkups are essential for the physical well-being of these children.
3. Appropriate school placement needs to be determined. Often special classrooms or day hospitals are indicated so that the child can learn in a relatively structured environment. Emphasis on adaptive functioning, such as attending to activities of daily living, and on social skills is necessary. For some adolescents, vocational training may be helpful.
4. Prognosis for childhood-onset schizophrenia may be relatively poor.
5. Families may derive support from the National Alliance for the Mentally Ill.

Key Treatment: Childhood Schizophrenia

- Antipsychotic drugs
- School placement
- Family support

Bibliography

American Psychiatric Association: Diagnostic and Statistical Manual of Mental Disorders, 4th ed. Washington, DC, American Psychiatric Association, 1994.

Frazier JA, Giedd JN, Hamburger SD, et al: Brain anatomic magnetic resonance imaging in childhood-onset schizophrenia. Arch Gen Psychiatry 1996;53:617–624.

Klin A: Asperger syndrome. Child Adolesc Psychiatr Clin North Am 1994;1:131–149.

Kolvin I, Ounsted C, Humphrey M, McNay A: The phenomenology of childhood psychoses. Br J Psychiatry 1971; 118:385–395.

Volkmar FR, Cohen DJ: Autism: Current concepts. Child Adolesc Psychiatr Clin North Am 1994;1:43–52.

57 Posttraumatic Stress Disorder

Andrew Clark and *Michael S. Jellinek*

Under extraordinary circumstances in which an individual is faced with an inescapable threat or actual injury, normal coping mechanisms become overwhelmed and the person experiences terror and helplessness. Such a breach of psychological defenses, if contained, may result in moderate symptoms that wane within days or weeks. At other times, more severe symptoms develop that nonetheless remain episodic and do not interfere greatly with overall functioning. In extreme cases, however, the trauma may cause difficulties that reverberate throughout the life span, leading to a wide array of persistent and disabling symptoms, derailing development, and even distorting character formation. The formal psychiatric diagnosis of posttraumatic stress disorder (PTSD) is limited to a restricted constellation of characteristic symptoms that are more or less directly attributable to the traumatic exposure.

Definition

1. Although the disorder has been recognized in combat veterans for over a century as "shell shock" or "battle neurosis," it is only in the last few decades that PTSD has been identified in broader populations, and even more recently that it has been recognized and studied in children and adolescents. Much of the present knowledge in this area has been gained from Terr's longitudinal study of 26 children involved in a 1976 school bus kidnapping in Chowchilla, California, and from Pynoos' study of children exposed to a schoolyard sniper in 1987.

2. The Diagnostic and Statistical Manual IV (DSM-IV) limits the definition of trauma to events that involve an actual threat or injury to oneself or others and that are accompanied by feelings of helplessness, fear, or horror. Such events can be either discrete episodes (such as a kidnapping or a rape) or prolonged and repetitive occurrences (such as ongoing physical or sexual abuse). Traumatic events are not limited to those that the victim experienced directly; posttraumatic symptoms can arise from witnessing an incident (such as a child's witness to domestic violence) and even from indirect exposure to an event (such as in response to a friend's suicide).

3. According to DSM-IV, PTSD symptoms fall into three clusters: those symptoms associated with *reexperiencing* the trauma, such as intrusive memories, nightmares, and flashbacks; those associated with *avoidance and numbing*, such as amnesia for aspects of the events, emotional detachment, and a foreshortened sense of the future; and those associated with *increased arousal*, such as hypervigilance, insomnia, irritability, and an exaggerated startle response.

Etiology and Epidemiology

1. While wars, criminal assaults, and natural disasters stand out as obvious sources of trauma, many children experience trauma in the form of abuse and violence within their own families or through exposure to extraordinary levels of violence within their neighborhoods.

2. The only clearly defined risk factor for the development of PTSD is exposure to the trauma itself. Studies of communities of children exposed to a common trauma such as a natural disaster have found rates of posttraumatic symptoms approaching 100 per cent. However, factors such as social supports, prior history of traumatic exposures, and comorbid psychiatric conditions probably affect long-term outcome, including the development of full-fledged PTSD.

3. Frequently, even a single traumatic exposure brings in its wake additional adversities and losses. For example, abused children are often taken from their parents, and natural disasters can be psychologically and financially devastating for entire families and communities. Those children faced with multiple adversities seem to be at elevated risk of developing not only PTSD but also depressive disorders and separation anxiety.

Pathophysiology

The pathophysiology of PTSD is thought to derive from the massive release of stress hormones in the face of terror and helplessness, with long-term physiologic consequences. Children and adults with PTSD, for example, in addition to their heightened responsiveness to reminders of their trauma, demonstrate an exaggerated startle response, indicating a more global disturbance of stimulus discrimination. It has been suggested that traumatic memories are different in kind from normal ones, registered in different areas of the brain, and lacking the customary modulating influence of the hippocampus. These traumatic memories exist primarily as visceral sensations and visual images rather than as conscious verbal recollections. Furthermore, they can be triggered by any sort of emotional arousal, and they are reexperienced even years later fully as vividly and powerfully as they were initially.

Clinical Findings

1. Children respond to traumatic experiences in a variety of ways, depending in part on the nature and duration of the overwhelming experience and their developmental stage at the time. Indeed, the range of possible outcomes following a trauma spans virtually the entirety of childhood psychopathology, from attachment disorder and depression through attention deficit disorder, conduct disorder, dissociation, and apparent psychosis. Given the diverse nature of the posttraumatic presentation, accurate diagnosis depends on a high index of suspicion coupled with an accurate history.

2. In the immediate aftermath of a traumatic exposure children generally appear still, quiet, and alert. In the following few weeks they may exhibit sleep, attention, and learning difficulties or seem especially irritable or confused. Younger children may suffer a loss of developmental milestones as well. These children may appear fearful, anxious, and vigilant and demonstrate an exaggerated startle response.

3. Classic symptoms of PTSD generally appear within several weeks or months of the event. By this time children's sleep and learning difficulties tend to resolve, but emotional constriction, specific fears related to the trauma, and intrusive memories reach their full force. Such memories are often visual and, remarkably, may even be recreated in the drawings of children who were preverbal at the time of the original event. Children may exhibit repetitive play that has an anxious and driven quality to it, lacking any sense of playfulness. In addition, they may exhibit "reenactments" of the trauma, in which they place themselves in a position to reexperience some aspect of either the trauma or their response. Such reenactments may include victimizing others in some way as well.

4. In the aftermath of a single traumatic exposure, children tend to retain clear and extraordinarily detailed memories of discrete aspects of their experience; those memories, however, are subject to cognitive reworkings and distortions and may not always accurately reflect the complete context of the event. Those children exposed to ongoing or repetitive abuse are more likely to demonstrate amnesia and dissociation (a fracture of the normal integrity of identity, memory, and emotion), which can at times render their narratives fragmented and confusing.

5. Children's long-term response to trauma frequently involves an outward appearance of relatively normal functioning. However, these children are often beset by occult fears, ambushed by anniversary reactions, and limited by their sense of a future that holds little promise, with few expectations of surviving into a productive adult life. They may demonstrate occasional intrusive memories indiscriminately activated by emotional arousal, superimposed onto an emotional style characterized by detachment, constriction, and sadness. For young children, there is a special risk of long-term disruption of attachment capabilities as a result of the traumatic exposure.

Diagnosis

There are no pathognomonic behavioral signs or conclusive test results and no useful laboratory studies to aid in the diagnosis of PTSD. Most helpful is a clear and detailed history of a child's exposure to trauma and any subsequent deviation from his or her baseline level of functioning. For children who were of preschool age at the time of the trauma, play therapy and drawing are often more helpful in reconstructing an accurate picture of their experience than are narrative reports. It is the unusual child who is capable of offering a complete and coherent verbal account of such events, and so clinical data need to be carefully correlated with the known history and with the observations of others. For very small children, modified diagnostic criteria that are more behaviorally based than those of DSM-IV have been developed in an effort to improve diagnostic sensitivity in that age group.

Key Clinical Findings

- Sleep disturbance
- Attention and learning problems
- Regression from developmental milestones

Treatment

1. The essential first step in the treatment of PTSD in children is to ensure that they are provided with a safe environment. Second, helping to elicit and strengthen the support of family and others can go far in minimizing the long-term impact of the trauma. Family members are often in need of reassurance and support themselves, and it is essential that they be capable of actively supporting the child's autonomy in spite of their own anxiety and concern.

2. For traumatized children in need of mental health intervention, psychotherapy is the mainstay of treatment. Indications for referral include posttraumatic symptoms that are distressing, disabling, or persistent. Those children who have suffered multiple adversities or who have suboptimal social supports should be referred early as well. The best time for intervention is in the acute phase of the process, when symptoms seem most amenable to change. Although some children with uncomplicated PTSD can be helped in just a few sessions, others require ongoing treatment for extended periods.

3. The role of medications in treating PTSD is limited to helping manage disabling symptoms, particularly those that interfere with psychotherapy. Although any number of psychotropic medications have been used in some patients with some success, few controlled studies have been done in children, and no medications have demonstrated clear superiority over others. Centrally acting antihypertensives such as clonidine have been shown to be helpful for symptoms of hyperarousal; antidepressants and benzodiazepines have also been found useful in certain cases.

Key Treatment

- Safe environment
- Carefully selected drugs for some

Prevention

1. Although many traumatic events are entirely unpredictable, some reduction in children's exposure to trauma is possible through caregivers' sensitivity to evidence of ongoing abuse or domestic violence and early involvement of the appropriate child protection agencies.
2. Widely experienced events, such as a natural disaster or the suicide of a peer, call for an early response from professionals in order to help minimize the eventual development of PTSD symptoms. Helpful steps under these circumstances include ensuring the dissemination of clear and reliable information in order to quell hysteria and dispel rumors, in addition to realistic reassurance about the children's safety. It is often helpful for professionals to meet in schools with small groups of affected children in an effort to allow each of them to relate their experience of the event. Such expressions may be in the form of pictures, stories, or verbal narratives, depending on the developmental stages of the children involved. These meetings can be helpful in calming unrealistic fears, normalizing responses that might otherwise be thought embarrassing, and providing an acknowledgment that one's experience has been shared by others. Those children who seem especially troubled can be identified though this process and referred for ongoing treatment.

Outcome

Although treatment of PTSD can clearly be helpful, the experience of trauma often leaves children with permanent emotional scars. Even those persons with uncomplicated PTSD who recompensate rapidly may remain vulnerable to subsequent traumas later in life. While research on the neurobiology of trauma and on the effects of trauma on development hold promise for more effective treatments, the most pressing need is in helping to protect children from such experiences in the first place.

Bibliography

Marmar C: An integrated approach for treating posttraumatic stress. Rev Psychiatry 1993;12:239–272.

Scheeringa M: Two approaches to the diagnosis of posttraumatic stress disorder in infancy and childhood. J Am Acad Child Adolesc Psychiatry 1995;34:191–200.

Terr L: Acute responses to external events and posttraumatic stress disorder. In Lewis M (ed): Child and Adolescent Psychiatry. Baltimore, Williams & Wilkins, 1991, pp 755–763.

Terr L: Childhood traumas: An outline and overview. Am J Psychiatry 1991;148:10–20.

van der Kolk B: The body keeps the score: Memory and the evolving psychobiology of posttraumatic stress. In Nicholi A (ed): Harvard Review of Psychiatry. Cambridge, Harvard University Press, 1994, pp 253–263.

58 Death in the Family

Paula K. Rauch

Basic Principles

1. The death of a child or the death of a child's parent is an enormous tragedy.
2. The bereavement process is long and complex. The understanding of a death in the family will be revisited during each successive phase of life development.
3. It is not possible to protect children and families from experiencing the impact of these painful losses, but a developmental understanding permits the most sensitive care in a difficult time.

Infants

Developmental Principles

1. Infancy is characterized by the reciprocal process of attachment between infant and parent. Attachment begins as parental hopes take form during the pregnancy. It is fostered by the infant's dependence (vulnerability) after birth.
2. The degree of attachment is not determined by the length of time a child has been alive. Parents are deeply attached to premature babies and full-term newborns.
3. Attachment is challenged (not negated) by conditions that affect the parents' success in meeting the infant's needs of feeding and soothing.

Death of an Infant

1. The death of an infant is both the loss of the unique baby the family is coming to know and the loss of all the imagined experiences of a lifetime unrealized.
2. Maximizing the quality time a family has with a terminally ill infant offers the precious gift of memories. Separating parents from a dying newborn does *not* prevent deep attachment nor lessen the pain of the impending loss.
3. Respect for the infant's life facilitates the successful grieving of the family.
   a. Always acknowledge the infant's personhood by using his or her name.
   b. Facilitate taking of photographs and religious ceremonies; these are symbols of the infant's place in the family.
   c. Work with parents to create the most loving moment of death possible, such as letting a parent hold the baby when life support is stopped.

Death of an Infant's Parent

1. The immediate needs of the infant are to have as much consistency as possible in caretakers, setting, and daily routine.
2. Acutely, the infant will be most affected by the sadness of the surviving parent and caretakers.
3. If there is time to prepare for the death, the parent may want to write or tape a communication to the infant to be delivered to the child at an appropriate age.
4. Compiling photographs of the infant with the dead or dying parent documents the relationship and provides a vehicle the child can use in later life to ask questions about a parent who is known only through the descriptions of others.

Preschool Children

Developmental Principles

1. Preschoolers understand the world by a seamless interweaving of facts and fantasy.
2. Preschoolers are egocentric, meaning that they imagine events from their own vantage point and envision themselves as the etiologic agent of the events occurring around them.
3. Preschoolers feel vulnerable, as highlighted by concerns about minor scrapes or scratches that require Band-Aids and kisses.
4. The concept of forever is inconceivable to a preschooler, so death is not experienced with the full weight of finality.

Death of a Preschooler

1. Young children rely on parents and caretakers to modulate the scariness of medical settings. Every effort should be made to support parental presence with special attention to treatments, procedures, and sleep time.
2. Treatment plans should be geared to minimizing pain and suffering. If necessary interventions are painful, the child should be forewarned a short time in advance. This preparation may lead to the immediate distress of anticipating the discomfort, but in the long term it diminishes the ambient anxiety of fearing surprise "assaults."
3. Uncomfortable procedures should be performed in a setting other than the child's bed or playroom, because these settings are important safe havens.
4. All interventions should be accompanied by simple explanations of what is to be done to what part of the child's body and what parts will remain untouched.
5. Preschoolers work through difficult experiences by transforming them into play. It is valuable to provide protected play time. The play of ill children may reflect fears of loss, abandonment, or punishment and may be painful for parents to witness. Access to a trained professional can facilitate this important outlet.
6. Preschoolers are likely to believe that the illness is punishment for being bad. Eliciting the child's understanding of the cause of the illness offers an opportunity to correct misconceptions and decrease feelings of guilt. Continuing to remind children that they are not at fault can diminish anxiety.
7. Because young children rely on adults for caretaking in life, some may articulate worries about who takes care of little children in "Heaven." Others may not speak directly about death, but it may appear in play. Many seek the comfort of parental closeness, with heightened distress over separations in anticipation of death.

Death of a Preschooler's Parent

1. A preschooler is likely to feel some responsibility for the death of the parent. Explore the child's understanding and dispel guilt by correcting misconceptions.
2. The child may misinterpret the surviving parent's withdrawal as disappointment in the child's behavior. Help the surviving parent to articulate in simple terms that the child is loved and that the parent is sad about the death.
3. Maintain as much consistency in the child's routine as possible, including preschool, play dates, meal times, and bed time.
4. Creating materials that will help the child maintain the connection to the lost parent, such as special photo albums, is valuable. There are many good children's books on death that may be helpful springboards for further discussion if read to the child some months after the parent's death.

School-Age Children

Developmental Principles

1. School-age children (age 6–12 years) are proud learners of facts, skills, and rules. There is a sense of agency and independence that comes with the mastery.
2. Best friends with whom they share interests, activities, and time are important.

Death of a School-Age Child

1. School-age children both cope by mastery (learning treatment schedules, medication names, and procedures) and regress to more dependency on parents (more characteristic of the preschool years).
2. When the child is ready, she or he may initiate conversations about death, dying, and illness. If family members or medical staff initiate such discussions, it is common for the child to be unwilling to participate.
   a. It is important to communicate that support people are available for these discussions on the child's schedule.
   b. It is neither possible nor helpful to force these conversations. Parents may benefit from talking with a child psychiatric professional to practice articulating what they want to convey to the child about death and their religious beliefs. When parents are more comfortable, children are more likely to initiate discussion.
3. As medical professionals, our job is to listen and to be respectful of different religious and cultural beliefs. We provide information about pain management, educate families about the logistics of medical treatment, and accommodate the wishes and priorities of the family.
4. Children benefit from honesty. It is appropriate to acknowledge that we do not know how it feels to be dead and to invite the child to share his or her own thoughts.

Death of a School-Age Child's Parent

1. School-age children can understand the specific features of a parent's illness. Caretakers must find a balance in providing honest, factual information about the illness without overwhelming the child with too much detail.

2. Communication from the child to the dying parent should be facilitated. Some children and some circumstances permit direct expressions of love to the dying parent. Communications can take the form of speaking, touching, or making cards, tapes, or other gifts.

3. If the medical setting is overwhelming for the child, an adult can deliver the child's communication to the dying parent and report back to the child about the importance of the message to the parent.

4. The guiding principles for preparing a child to visit a critically ill parent or to attend a funeral are similar.

   a. A familiar adult should describe what the child will see and then accompany the child into the room.

   b. It is helpful to describe both the physical setting and the emotional setting (e.g., intubation, an open casket, crying relatives).

   c. A child should not be *forced* to touch a parent (living or dead).

   d. It is helpful to designate a familiar adult for each child, one who is willing to stay or to take the child out according to the child's needs.

5. Surviving parents may worry that their school-age children are not dealing with their grief, because they return to their usual activities so quickly. Being active at school and at play helps children cope. After 4 to 6 weeks, if the grief interferes with school work or leads to withdrawal from friends, child psychiatric referral is warranted.

6. School-age mourners should be invited to share their thoughts and sadness and then be allowed to do so on their own timetables.

7. It is important to assess whether the surviving parent is emotionally able to discuss the dead parent with the child. If the surviving parent is too overwhelmed to bear such discussions or if the child has the perception that the loss is not felt in the same way by the parent (as in the case of divorce), referral to a psychiatric professional is appropriate.

Adolescents

Developmental Principles

1. Adolescents have the abstract thinking capacity of adults. They often think deep thoughts and feel their feelings intensely.

2. Adolescence is a time of dramatic physical change, including appearance of the secondary sexual characteristics. This is associated with tremendous self-consciousness.

3. Teenagers separate from parents by relying on the peer group to define identity. They scrutinize and often challenge parental values and priorities. Conflict between adolescents and their parents is common during this period of growing independence.

Death of an Adolescent

1. As adolescents come to understand their impending deaths, some become philosophical, some articulate the pain they feel by imagining the life experiences they will never have, and a few turn their distress into dangerous risk taking.

2. Serious illness leads to dependency, which runs counter to the adolescent's task of increasing independence. Frailty and baldness can heighten teenage self-consciousness.

3. Adolescents already have established styles of coping. These styles need to be respected. Some adolescents are very verbal and seek opportunities to talk with a broad range of adults and peers; others share their thoughts with a select few; and others thwart any attempts to discuss death.

4. Some teenagers want to and are able to say good-bye directly to loved ones and to share their hopes for what will be after they die. Some communicate their "good-bye" by purchasing or making gifts for loved ones.

5. Children of all ages, but especially adolescents, worry about the capacity of loved ones (including girlfriends and boyfriends) to cope after their death. It is helpful to remind a teenager who voices this concern about the people who will be there to support the most vulnerable mourners.

Death of an Adolescent's Parent

1. The relationships an adolescent has had with the dying parent and the surviving parent may be complex and conflicted. Stresses in preexisting relationships complicate communication and grieving and can lead to feelings of guilt or resentment.

2. Helping an adolescent to communicate the love that underlies the tension, before the parent dies, may decrease guilt and regret after the parent's death.

3. Adolescents may turn to nonparental adults to share their sadness for a number of reasons. Special relationships with adults are a normal component of adolescent development. The teenager may find it uncomfortable to be vulnerable with the surviving parent if the previous relationship was tense, or the teenager may want to spare a grief-stricken and vulnerable parent the additional burden of bearing his or her sadness as well.

4. It is important for the adolescent to have an adult with whom the dead parent can be remembered. This may be the other parent, a family member, teacher, coach, clergyperson, or friend's parent. If there is no such person in the child's life, referral to a professional may be helpful.

5. Many teenagers welcome a brief psychotherapeutic intervention that can focus on the loss from the adolescent's individual vantage point.

6. It is important, and at times difficult, to differentiate grief from depression. It is necessary to follow a teenager's level of functioning over the weeks after the death to see whether symptoms are lessening or increasing. If neurovegetative symptoms are present for more than a couple of weeks, or if the teenager feels guilty or expresses suicidal ideation, psychiatric referral is required.

Recommendations

1. A child who faces death—his or her own or that of a parent—remains first and foremost a child. The child needs support to continue age-appropriate activities whenever possible.
2. The needs of the child and the family are best addressed by a multidisciplinary team of medical, psychological, and school staff in conjunction with well-supported extended family, clergy, and community resources.
3. Families need support before, during, and after a death in the family.
4. It is crucial to identify family members in whom grief has evolved into depression and to refer them for psychiatric treatment. Depression differs from grief in that it is characterized by guilt, a loss of future orientation, a persistent disturbance of sleep, appetite, concentration, and energy, and at times a wish to die.
5. It is helpful to schedule a follow-up meeting 4 to 6 weeks after a death, both to identify family members who may be depressed and to convey the understanding that the grief process is a long one and is certainly not yet over at this juncture.
6. The grieving process of a child for a parent is lifelong. In healthy children and adolescents, it is common to arrive at a sense of the dead parent as a positive presence in the child's life. Many children describe mental dialogues in which they imagine helpful input from the deceased parent.
7. Because parents represent an important piece of a child's identity, children need ongoing assistance in "knowing" the dead parent in new ways as they progress through life development.
8. When a child dies, it is common for the two parents to have different styles of grieving. One may look to work as an essential escape from overwhelming sadness, while the other may seek opportunities to discuss and revisit the events surrounding the child's death. Without education that normalizes these different styles of coping, destructive tensions may arise between the parents about who loved the child most or whose grief is healthier.
9. Grieving parents may believe that the magnitude of their loss separates them from others who have not known this pain. Bereavement groups and informal meetings with other parents who have lost children may be important opportunities to help them overcome isolation.
10. Siblings are too often the forgotten mourners. Commonly, parents have been preoccupied with the needs of the sick child during the illness and then become unavailable again in their grief after the child's death. It is common for siblings to envy the attention lavished on the child who was ill and then to feel guilty after she or he dies. Helping parents become attuned to the needs of the well siblings and offering continuing support may be crucial interventions for the family's future well-being.

Bibliography

Brown MW: The Dead Bird. Reading, MA, Addison-Wesley, 1965.

Silverman PR, Nickman S, Worden JW: Detachment revisited: The child's reconstruction of a dead parent. Am J Orthopsychiatry 1992;62:494–503.

Viorst J: The Tenth Good Thing About Barney. New York, Atheneum, 1971.

59 Triage of Psychiatrically Ill Children

Joseph Shrand

Procedure

Traditionally, psychiatric care for children was limited to two sites: inpatient and outpatient settings. Children and adolescents were frequently discharged from the highly restrictive setting of an intensively staffed inpatient unit to weekly visits in a psychiatrist's outpatient office. Inpatient stays were often weeks or months in duration, with the child expected to make gradual gains in development and stabilization to tolerate the transition to the outpatient world. As hospitalizations have been forced to become brief, measured in days, given the restrictions of managed care and other economic pressures, mental health specialists have been challenged to create intermediate settings to smooth the transition from inpatient to outpatient environments (Table 59–1). These intermediate placements and a smooth transition between them have the goal of decreasing more restrictive inpatient psychiatric hospitalization.

The Emergency Department

Children who are dangerous to themselves (i.e., suicidal), engaging in high-risk behaviors (e.g., runaways, severely anorectic), dangerous to others (e.g., violent, destructive), or gravely disabled (e.g., psychotic, unable to distinguish reality from unreality) are often first sent to an emergency department for a rapid psychiatric evaluation to determine the level

Procedure

TABLE 59–1.   TREATMENT SETTINGS FOR THE PSYCHIATRICALLY ILL CHILD

TREATMENT SETTING	INDICATION
Hospital Based	When office-based/outpatient treatment is not enough to ensure patient safety
Emergency department	High-risk children and adolescents (e.g., psychotic, severely traumatized, suicidal, homicidal, dangerously intoxicated)
Psychiatric inpatient settings	Severity of psychiatric illness requires locked-door setting to ensure patient safety
Psychiatric partial hospital settings	Severity of psychiatric illness and family conflict require both daily structure and monitoring as well as the child temporarily removed from the home (e.g., open-door residential setting)
Psychiatric day-treatment settings	Severity of psychiatric illness requires daily structure and monitoring
Outpatient/Office Based*	When patients can be safely managed in an outpatient setting with one or more members of the treatment team including the psychiatrists, pediatrician, parents, and school personnel
Medical management	Seek organic cause of altered behaviors
Psychopharmacology	Help manage target symptoms
Play therapy	Younger children—nonverbal communication
Insight-oriented therapy	Older children and adolescents—verbal emphasis
Interpersonal psychotherapy	Adolescents, young adults, adults—verbal emphasis
Cognitive-behavioral therapy	Often taught to parents to help with children
Group psychotherapy	Often useful for adolescents with substance abuse, trauma, and interpersonal difficulties; peer support and confrontation can be a powerful group process
Family therapy	Psychoeducation, family conflict
Substance abuse counseling	Substance abuse complicating/interfering with other treatments
Adjustments in the school setting	Difficulty in school, classes too large, school avoidance, school-related problems

*There may be some overlap between these treatments between settings. Usually, many of the outpatient treatments may be started while on an inpatient unit. However, given the short length of inpatient stays, they are usually continued in the outpatient milieu.

of care needed to maintain their safety. Referrals may be from home, school, or a pediatrician's office. These children need a professionally trained mental health staff, preferably a child and adolescent psychiatrist, for rapid assessment and triage to an appropriate treatment setting.

Psychiatric Inpatient Settings

After the emergency department triage, severely ill children and adolescents may need an inpatient level of care, the most "restrictive" being a locked ward, usually with a high staff:patient ratio.

1. Hospital settings—A locked inpatient setting is a 24-hour secure and protected psychiatric treatment environment with the recently defined goal of rapid stabilization of an acute problem. This often includes the use of psychotropic medication to stabilize the child's behavior and intensive social work to design and implement a structured outpatient environment. The children and adolescents who require this level of care are usually suicidal or dangerous to themselves or others, have been severely traumatized, are psychotic, have a substance abuse problem that is critically interfering with their lives, or have

a social situation that poses them imminent and serious danger.

2. Psychiatric residential settings—Some of these children, especially with long-term dysfunction, will move from the inpatient unit to a residential unit where 24-hour psychiatric treatment programs provide supervision in a safe environment. The emotional impairment of these children and adolescents is still so severe that they cannot maintain themselves in the community outside of this setting. A residential program coordinates intensive comprehensive psychiatric evaluation and psychologic treatment.

 Bibliography

Jellinek MS: The outpatient milieu. J Am Acad Child Adolesc Psychiatry 1994;33:277–279.

Kiser LJ, Millsap PA, et al: Results of treatment one year later: Child and adolescent partial hospitalization. J Am Acad Child Adolesc Psychiatry 1996;35:81–90.

Masters KJ: Minimizing child psychiatric hospitalization and bureaucratic inefficiencies by using a coordinated treatment system to minimize child psychiatric hospitalization. J Am Acad Child Adolesc Psychiatry 1997;36:566–568.

Questionnaire Approaches to the Recognition and Assessment of Psychosocial Problems

60

J. Michael Murphy
Michael S. Jellinek

Procedure

Rationale

1. With the increasing prevalence of managed care approaches to medicine, pediatricians and other primary care doctors are being asked to play a larger role in detecting and treating a variety of problems. Psychosocial concerns, "the new morbidity," are increasingly the focus of well-child care. The combination of clearer definitions, better recognition, and rising prevalence of attention-deficit disorder, anxiety, depression, suicide, drug abuse, learning problems, divorce-related concerns, and so on is changing the nature of pediatric practice. Primary care clinicians already treat as many or more children (and adults) with mental health problems as do specialty mental health care providers. However, studies have also shown that psychosocial concerns including psychiatric disorders and stressors (e.g., parental mental health problems, divorce) are present in as many as two thirds of all pediatric visits, but that most are unvoiced by parents or unheard by pediatricians.

2. There is a substantial body of research suggesting that pediatricians recognize only a fraction of the children with psychosocial problems and secure proper treatment for even fewer of them. In general, primary care clinicians cite time constraints, lack of training, parental resistance, and unavailability of mental health resources as the major factors limiting the recognition and management of psychosocial disorders. Most recently, managed care programs have further restricted access for mental health services and controlled care through networks selected and managed by the insurer.

3. Despite these restrictions, many pediatricians want to do more to recognize and address the psychosocial concerns of their patient population. Because time constraints do not allow even brief interview evaluations of every patient, the judicious use of a few basic questionnaires can do a great deal to focus professional time efficiently.

Screening

1. *Who should be screened?* The easy answer is everybody; however, the complexity of the task varies by age. There are no currently available brief, reliable, and valid questionnaires for infants and toddlers. Clinicians must rely on the opportunities afforded by the frequent immunization and well-child care visit schedules to observe and evaluate the development of these very young children. Verbal questions concerning special family stressors or marital discord ("How are things going in the family . . . any special stresses . . . tensions between you and your spouse . . .") and maternal depression ("How has your mood been . . . any feelings of depression . . .") are certainly appropriate on an annual basis. Developmental concerns should be addressed by observation, physical examination, and specialized developmental testing that is beyond the scope of screening.

   a. School-aged children are generally seen by pediatricians for well-child care once a year or less, and each visit represents an important opportunity for pediatricians to screen for psychosocial difficulties in the child's development as well as major family stressors. The potential early recognition of problems in major areas of the child's functioning—with peers, family relationships, activities, the child's mood/self-esteem, and in school—offer unique opportunities to ease the child's suffering and to prevent or limit more serious problems in adolescence or adulthood.

   b. Parents are probably the most important sources of screening information for all children. Parent report is most reliable regarding behavioral symptoms and somewhat less reliable regarding a child's inner mood state. Therefore, especially in adolescence, pediatricians cannot rely on parental report to evaluate their patient's mood and, given the prevalence and risk of adolescent depression, would have to choose a questionnaire specifically designed to screen for adolescent depression or include such questions in a face-to-face, private discussion with the teenager as indicated.

   c. In general, primary care clinicians are usually pressed for time, with limited abilities to pursue secondary sources of information. However, if there is time and interest, for disorders such as attention-deficit/hyperactivity disorder or oppositional disorder, a standardized teacher-report questionnaire (e.g., the Conners or Achenbach questionnaire) can provide objective, valuable information.

2. *What should be screened for?* Pediatricians are accustomed to screening for anemia, diabetes, renal function, and other conditions. The desirable characteristics of a psychosocial screening test include being brief, reliable, and valid and giving an easily interpretable cut-off score. For both general and specific questionnaires the availability of norm-referenced cutoff scores indicating a clinically significant level of dysfunction is extremely helpful. The term *dysfunction* is used as pediatricians appropriately focus on the child's devel-

Procedure *Continued*

opmental tasks and functioning rather than concerning themselves with formal or traditional psychiatric diagnosis. Questionnaires that focus on a specific problem area such as attention-deficit/hyperactivity disorder or depression can, however, be useful in situations in which normative data are desired because these problems are suspected. (A new manual—*"Diagnostic and Statistical Manual–Primary Care"*—developed collaboratively by the American Academy of Pediatrics and a number of mental health organizations is attempting to bridge the gap between primary care and psychiatric diagnostic systems.)

3. *When should screening take place?* Assessing developmental and psychosocial functioning should be a part of all well-child visits and is a specific requirement for Medicaid-eligible children under the EPSDT program. Further or more specific screening is also reasonable after a pediatric visit when a clinician has discovered a potential problem or before the pediatric visit when known risk factors are present (e.g., divorce or if the child has been a witness of violence).

4. *Where should screening take place?* Screening is appropriate as part of an intake process in high-volume settings where time constraints make in-depth interviews impractical. Screening is relevant in poverty settings because, although the positive rate is quite high (20 to 40 per cent), not all children are dysfunctional. Given the limited resources in poverty settings, screening may help focus available services on those who could benefit the most.

5. *How should screening take place?*

   a. Child Behavior Checklist

      (1) CBCL advantages. The single most widely used and studied psychosocial questionnaire is Achenbach's Child Behavior Checklist (CBCL). The

---

PEDIATRIC SYMPTOM CHECKLIST

Please mark under the heading that best describes your child:

	NEVER	SOMETIMES	OFTEN
1. Complains of aches and pains	___	___	___
2. Spends more time alone	___	___	___
3. Tires easily, has little energy	___	___	___
4. Fidgety, unable to sit still	___	___	___
5. Has trouble with a teacher	___	___	___
6. Less interested in school	___	___	___
7. Acts as if driven by a motor	___	___	___
8. Daydreams too much	___	___	___
9. Distracted easily	___	___	___
10. Is afraid of new situations	___	___	___
11. Feels sad, unhappy	___	___	___
12. Is irritable, angry	___	___	___
13. Feels hopeless	___	___	___
14. Has trouble concentrating	___	___	___
15. Less interested in friends	___	___	___
16. Fights with other children	___	___	___
17. Absent from school	___	___	___
18. School grades dropping	___	___	___
19. Is down on him- or herself	___	___	___
20. Visits doctor with doctor finding nothing wrong	___	___	___
21. Has trouble sleeping	___	___	___
22. Worries a lot	___	___	___
23. Wants to be with you more than before	___	___	___
24. Feels he or she is bad	___	___	___
25. Takes unnecessary risks	___	___	___
26. Gets hurt frequently	___	___	___
27. Seems to be having less fun	___	___	___
28. Acts younger than children of his or her age	___	___	___
29. Does not listen to rules	___	___	___
30. Does not show feelings	___	___	___
31. Does not understand other people's feelings	___	___	___
32. Teases others	___	___	___
33. Blames others for his or her troubles	___	___	___
34. Takes things that do not belong to him or her	___	___	___
35. Refuses to share	___	___	___

CBCL is an exceptionally useful instrument and should be in every pediatrician's office for those situations in which a full assessment of overall psychosocial symptomatology is desired. The parent-report CBCL for 4- to 16-year olds is actually just one of a full range of child screening questionnaires that are available from Achenbach at the University of Vermont at a cost of about 50¢ per questionnaire. There are teacher and youth (age 12+) report versions of the original instrument, as well as a teacher instrument for preschool-aged children and a version of the CBCL for 2- to 3-year olds. All of these instruments are available in Spanish, and some of the forms are available in other languages as well.

(2) CBCL disadvantages. Despite its many advantages, when large numbers of children need to be screened routinely in actual primary care settings, the CBCL is not optimal. The standard parent-completed CBCL for 4- to 16-year-old children is made up of 113 behavioral items and an additional 20 social competence items and takes an average of 20 or more minutes for parents to complete and score. If the CBCL is used for routine screening in pediatrics, the result is usually many incomplete questionnaires, which can be worse than no screening at all. Although the basic scoring of the CBCL is relatively simple, tables must be consulted to find out the cutoff scores for "caseness" for six different age/gender groups, and the use of a computer program is recommended if scores on any of the subscales (e.g., depression) rather than a total score are needed.

b. Pediatric Symptom Checklist. Of the shorter instruments, the only one that has been validated and widely used for routine screening in Pediatrics is the Pediatric Symptom Checklist (PSC). A decade of research with the PSC has demonstrated its validity and usefulness in a wide range of pediatric settings including pediatric subspecialties, public health and mental health programs, and low income and minority communities. The PSC is not copyrighted, and there is no charge for its use. The PSC is completed by parents while they sit in the pediatrician's waiting room and takes 3 to 5 minutes to complete and score. Parents rate each of the 35 symptoms as "often," "sometimes," or "never" present. The PSC is scored by assigning 2, 1, or 0 points, respectively, to these ratings and then adding the points for an overall score. Scores of 28 or greater suggest that the child should receive further evaluation.

c. Conners' Rating Scale. Perhaps the second most widely used research questionnaire is Conners' Rating Scales (CRS) for parents and teachers. Although the two parent-completed versions of the Conners scale are somewhat shorter (93 and 48 items) than the CBCL, they are less widely used. However, the 39-item teacher-completed form is widely used and an even shorter 10-item Hyperactivity Index is clinically relevant and has been extensively used in research on attention-deficit/hyperactivity disorder. The brevity of this questionnaire makes it very well suited for pediatric practice, but its exclusive focus on externalizing behaviors and inattention restricts its usefulness to these problems (which are also more easily recognized as noted) and not the broader range of problems that include depression, anxiety, somatization, and so on. In addition, the CRS does not have a cutoff score, which restricts its usefulness as a screening instrument in pediatric settings.

d. PARS III. One other questionnaire that deserves mention is the PARS III, which has been recommended for children with chronic physical illness because of the absence of potentially confounding items about physical illness and a focus on adaptive rather than deviant behaviors. The PARS III is one of the briefer instruments, with only 28 items covering six different areas of functioning, although no cut-off scores are available for total or subscale scores.

e. The best validated age range for the CBCL, PSC, and CRS is 4 to 16 years of age. As noted earlier, there is now a version of the 100+ item CBCL for 2- to 3-year-old children and a slightly revised version of the PSC to include preschoolers as well. Both the parent and teacher forms of the CRS can be used with younger children, although no normative data are available.

6. *Why screen?* The question of why has been left until last because it leads to the question of what to do with children who screen positive. Children with psychosocial problems should be identified because these problems frequently cause emotional pain, interfere with psychosocial development, complicate treatment by limiting compliance, and may result in psychosomatic symptoms leading to subspecialty referrals. Presumably, the patients and their parents who are recognized and treated for psychosocial problems will be more satisfied with treatment and will have better outcomes than children whose problems are not recognized. Although definitive outcome studies have not been done, there are indications that there may be both cost offsets and increased satisfaction when psychosocial problems are targeted more precisely in pediatrics.

7. Use of screening

a. Mild risk. Children who receive scores in the at-

Procedure *Continued*

risk range on the screening questionnaires should be evaluated further during the index visit. If the problem seems relatively mild or if the parent is not overly concerned, the problem may simply be noted in the chart for reference at the next visit. If the problem appears to be more serious or if the parent or child is concerned, then more information should be gathered during the index or follow-up visit. If the pediatrician believes that he or she has expertise in this area, then treatment can be begun. Studies indicate that brief counseling is the most common pediatric intervention, with about 80 per cent of the patients who have an identified psychosocial problem receiving counseling. This kind of counseling can be supplemented by parent education materials or programs that are now available from many health maintenance organizations and in other settings.

b. Serious risks. The next common step is referral to a mental health provider, which occurs following 1 to 4 per cent of all pediatric visits. Every pediatrician should have ready access to and a responsible relationship with a pediatric mental health clinician. In many areas pediatricians should be able to find clinicians who will provide same-day phone consul-

tation as well as evaluations and/or treatment in cases that involve serious mental illness or more complicated problems (e.g., hostile divorce, sexual abuse). For parents with very young children there may be early intervention and/or home visitation programs available to at-risk families at no cost.

Bibliography

Costello EJ, Angold A: Scales to assess child and adolescent depression: Checklists, screens, and nets. J Am Acad Child Adolesc Psychiatry 1988;27:726–737.

Costello EJ, Burns BJ, Costello AJ, et al: Service utilization and psychiatric diagnosis in pediatric primary care: The role of the gatekeeper. Pediatrics 1988;82:435–441.

Jellinek MS, Murphy JM: The recognition of psychosocial disorders in pediatric office practice: The current status of the Pediatric Symptom Checklist. Dev Behav Pediatrics 1990;11:273–278.

Kelleher K, Rickert VI: Management of pediatric mental disorders in primary care. *In* Miranda J, Hoffman AA, Attkisson CC, Larson DB (eds): Mental Disorders in Primary Care. San Francisco, Jossey-Bass, 1994, pp 320–346.

Sturner RA. Parent questionnaires: Basic office equipment? Dev Behav Pediatrics 1991;12:51–54.

Walker DK, Stein REK, Perrin EC, Jessop DJ: Assessing psychosocial adjustment of children with chronic illness: A review of the technical properties of PARS III. Dev Behav Pediatrics 1990;11:116–121.

61 Clinically Important Trisomies

Laurence Finberg

Trisomy 21 (Down Syndrome)

Etiology

1. Meiotic nondysjunction that occurs more commonly in infants of mothers who are nearing the end of their reproductive period. The incidence begins to climb after maternal age 35.
2. Translocation of chromosome 21 material with another chromosome. About half are de novo in the embryo, and half are from a translocation parent. These account for about 4 per cent of trisomy 21 births and 9 per cent of those from mothers under 30 years of age.

Incidence

Once in every 600 to 800 births.

Clinical Findings

Brachycephaly, hypotonia, upward and slanted palpebral fissures, midface hypoplasia, speckled irides (Brushfield spots), simian palmar crease, and mental retardation. Less commonly: cardiac abnormalities, especially endocardial cushion defects, duodenal atresia, pelvic dysplasia, and leukemoid reaction or leukemia.

Key Clinical Findings
• Mental retardation
• Brachycephaly
• Hypotonia
• Slanted palpebral fissures

Treatment

Supportive only, including social and educational support. The degree of mental retardation is variable so that programs must be individually tailored. Mosaicism may occur with diminished abnormalities.

Prevention

When abortion is a parental option, amniocentesis or chorionic villus sampling early in pregnancy. This is routinely advised for mother over 35 years of age.

Trisomy 18 (Edward Syndrome)

Etiology

Meiotic nondysjunction

Incidence

Approximately 1/8000 births.

Key Clinical Findings
• Low birth weight
• Rocker-bottom feet
• Microcephaly
• Closed fist with overlapping index finger over third digit and fifth overlapping the fourth
• Micrognathia
• Mental retardation

Treatment

Supportive only. Ninety five per cent die within the first year.

Prevention

As for trisomy 21.

Trisomy 13 (Patau Syndrome)

Etiology

Meiotic nondysjunction.

Incidence

About 1/20,000 births.

Key Clinical Findings
• Cleft lip
• Flexed fingers with polydactyly
• Microphthalmia
• Cardiac defects

Treatment

None indicated except palliative. Most infants die in the first 6 months; there are rare longer survivors.

Prevention

As for trisomy 21.

62 Disorders of Amino Acid Metabolism

Marc Yudkoff

General

Definition

The term *aminoacidurias* refers to a class of inherited metabolic diseases that are characterized by the abnormal elevation of one or more amino acids in body fluids.

Etiology

In most cases the cause is an inherited deficiency of an enzyme that is necessary for the normal metabolism of an amino acid. This usually is an enzyme that mediates the oxidation of an amino acid or its conversion to CO_2, H_2O, and NH_3. Most aminoacidurias are inherited according to an autosomal recessive pattern.

Epidemiology

The aminoacidurias are a prototypical example of inborn errors of metabolism, a concept introduced by Sir Archibald Garrod in 1908. The cumulative incidence of these diseases is approximately 1/5000 live births. Among the more common disorders is phenylketonuria (1/20,000 live births). It is very important to bear in mind that any aminoaciduria may occur with high frequency in a particular subpopulation.

Infants and children at risk of having an aminoaciduria include:

1. Those with mental retardation or a progressive neurologic syndrome of undetermined cause
2. Those with a positive family history for an aminoaciduria, especially an involved sibling
3. Those with a history of intolerance to dietary protein
4. Those with a history of clinical decompensation in response to an otherwise trivial infection
5. Those with persistent metabolic acidemia and/or growth failure
6. Those with an unusual odor on the urine or perspiration
7. Those with a history of stroke or other thromboembolic phenomena
8. Those with hepatic failure and/or cirrhosis of unexplained origin
9. Those with a history of renal or bladder calculi that are not composed of calcium or urate
10. Those with the renal Fanconi syndrome or hypophosphatemic rickets.

In Table 62–1 are listed those aminoacidurias that affect the central nervous system.

Phenylketonuria

Definition

Phenylketonuria (PKU) refers to an inborn error of phenylalanine metabolism that is characterized by the accumulation of extremely high levels of phenylalanine in body fluids and the excretion of large amounts of phenylalanine metabolites, e.g., phenylacetic acid.

Etiology

1. The cause is a congenital deficiency of phenylalanine hydroxylase, the enzyme that mediates the conversion of phenylalanine to tyrosine. This enzyme, which is coded on chromosome 12, is active primarily in the liver. Brain contains virtually no phenylalanine hydroxylase activity. Frank deletions in the gene are rare. The most common genetic defects, particularly in the northern European population (~40%), are mutations resulting in a truncated enzyme or in a single amino acid substitution.
2. Partial deficiencies of the phenylalanine hydroxylase gene give rise to hyperphenylalaninemia, but not the full-blown PKU syndrome. In addition to the classic deficiency of phenylalanine hydroxylase, PKU can result from a congenital metabolic defect in the handling of pterins, which are obligatory cofactors in the phenylalanine hydroxylase reaction. Infants with the latter metabolic defect may have a form of PKU that is resistant to therapy (see below).

Epidemiology

PKU is most common in the northern European population, in whom the overall incidence is ~ 1/20,000 live births. When PKU first was discovered, in the early 1930s, it was noted that nearly 1 per cent of institutionalized European patients were affected with this disorder. The majority of affected infants are compound heterozygotes for the phenylalanine hydroxylase gene. Infants and children at risk include

1. Those with a history of affected siblings
2. Those whose parents are known to be heterozygotes for this autosomal recessive disorder.

Pathophysiology

1. Phenylalanine is hydroxylated to tyrosine in a complex reaction that requires tetrahydropteridine as a cofactor. The reaction occurs primarily in the liver, with little, if any, activity present in the central nervous system. The mental retardation of untreated PKU therefore appears to be attributable to extreme hyperphenylalaninemia itself rather than an intrinsic enzymatic deficiency in the brain. The majority of youngsters with PKU manifest virtually no residual enzymatic activity.
2. Exposure of the infant's brain to high (>1 mM) levels of phenylalanine early in life results in impaired neuronal maturation and faulty synthesis of myelin. The toxic factor appears to be hyperphenylalaninemia rather than a phenylalanine metabolite or tyrosine deficiency. Very high phenylalanine levels may inhibit the uptake of other neutral amino acids into the brain. If tyrosine transport were compromised the result could be a failure of dopamine synthesis, since tyrosine is precursor to this neurotrans-

TABLE 62–1. DISORDERS OF AMINO ACID METABOLISM AFFECTING THE CNS

DISORDER	BIOCHEMICAL DERANGEMENT	MAIN CLINICAL FINDINGS	THERAPY
Phenylketonuria	Usually phenylalanine hydroxylase deficiency	Mental retardation if untreated	Dietary phenylalanine restriction
Maple syrup urine disease	Branched-chain amino acid decarboxylase deficiency	Coma, seizures, increased intracranial pressure in neonate	Dietary restriction of leucine, isoleucine, and valine
Homocystinuria	Usually cystathionine synthetase deficiency	Stroke, ectopia lentis, mental retardation, thromboembolic diathesis	Diet therapy. Anticoagulant therapy
Urea cycle defects	Congenital enzymopathy of urea cycle. Failure of ureagenesis	Mental retardation, coma, seizures. Often in neonate	Dietary protein restriction. Sodium benzoate and phenylacetate
Nonketotic hyperglycinemia	Deficient glycine cleavage system	Severe seizure disorder in neonate, usually fatal	NMDA receptor blockers helpful in some cases

mitter. Phenylalanine in very high concentration also can inhibit Na^+/K^+ ATPase activity, thereby affecting membrane potential and neurotransmission. It also disaggregates brain polysomes, which may play a role in the dysmyelination that has been associated with PKU.

Clinical Findings

1. It should be emphasized that the affected infant is normal at birth. There are no distinct physical findings that are pathognomonic for PKU. However, a failure to diagnose PKU promptly and to institute appropriate therapy will result in mental retardation in virtually all cases. Although dietotherapy always should be initiated as quickly as possible after birth, there may be grace period of several weeks during which treatment can be deferred and a reasonably good outcome still be obtained.

2. The untreated patient typically manifests a profound degree of mental retardation. A peculiar, musty ("mouselike") odor on the urine often is appreciated. It reflects the presence of a large amount of phenylacetic acid. Autistic features and a tendency to self-mutilation are not unusual. Some patients sit for hours in a cross-legged position ("schneidersalz" or "tailor-like"), rocking back and forth and banging their heads against a wall. The skin is dry and frequently displays a marked eczematoid reaction. Progressive motor dysfunction may occur in long-standing cases.

Key Clinical Findings: Phenylketonuria

- Asymptomatic in neonatal period
- Profound mental retardation if untreated
- Mouse odor to urine

Treatment

The mainstay of treatment is the low-phenylalanine diet. An effort usually is made to maintain blood phenylalanine concentrations <5 mg/dl. This approach, if carefully followed, is compatible with normal intellectual development, although the incidence of learning disabilities may be greater even in ostensibly well-controlled patients. The diet once was thought to be dispensable after 8 years of age, but recent studies have shown a possible deterioration of intellectual function in older individuals in whom the diet was discontinued. It is not clear at present whether the low-phenylalanine diet ever can safely be eliminated.

Prevention

Almost all American neonates are screened routinely for the presence of phenylketonuria. The possibility of obtaining a falsely negative result (~5% in some surveys) has prompted the recommendation that infants be retested at the time of the first well-baby visit. This suggestion may become even more important in light of a recent trend to discharge newborns at an earlier age. Testing of prematures, especially sick infants who have not been fed much dietary protein or who have been treated with antibiotics, also may result in a false negative result with the bacterial inhibition screening test for PKU.

Key Treatment: Phenylketonuria

- Diet low in phenylalanine throughout childhood; possibly lifelong

Maple Syrup Urine Disease

Definition

Maple syrup urine disease is an inborn error of the metabolism of the branched-chain amino acids (leucine, isoleucine, and valine). The accumulation of these amino acids and their cognate α-ketoacids in body fluids is associated with a disabling neurologic syndrome.

Etiology

The cause of this autosomal recessive disorder is a congenital deficiency of branched-chain ketoacid decarboxylase, a very large multienzyme complex that requires thiamine, lipoic acid, NAD, and coenzyme A as cofactors. The decarboxylase is composed of four subunits. Most patients have a mutation that involves the E1-α subunit.

Epidemiology

Maple syrup urine disease is relatively uncommon, occurring with an incidence of 1/250,000 live births in the overall population. It is important to bear in mind that there are population isolates in whom the risk is far greater. Thus, it has been estimated that one in every seven Mennonites carries the MSUD gene.

Infants and children at risk of having MSUD include

1. Those who are known to have affected siblings
2. Those whose parents are known to be carriers
3. Those belonging to populations at risk

4. Newborns with unexplained vomiting, coma, and convulsions
5. Children with a history of recurrent, unexplained coma and ketosis, particularly if associated with intercurrent illness, e.g., infection or surgical procedures.

Pathophysiology

1. The three branched-chain amino acids are readily transaminated to the cognate branched-chain ketoacids. The initial step in the oxidation of the latter to CO_2 and H_2O is decarboxylation, a metabolic transformation that is present to a varying degree in most body tissues, including the brain. Youngsters with the classic form of maple syrup urine disease typically manifest only 2 to 5 per cent of normal enzyme activity. As a consequence, the branched-chain ketoacids accumulate in body fluids. They are readily reaminated to the parent branched-chain amino acid, the level of which rises precipitously in the blood and urine.
2. The probable toxin is the untoward accumulation of the branched-chain ketoacids, which have been shown to impair brain energy metabolism by inhibiting the tricarboxylic acid cycle. In extremely high concentration they also may deplete the concentration of brain glutamate, the major excitatory neurotransmitter of the central nervous system. Finally, some evidence suggests a direct deleterious effect on myelin synthesis.

Clinical Findings

1. The prenatal course is uneventful. At birth the infant appears clinically normal, presumably because during intrauterine life the placenta clears essentially all excess branched-chain ketoacids. However, within a few hours of birth the branched-chain amino acids and ketoacids begin to increase in the blood.
2. The initial symptoms, manifest by 36 to 48 hours of life, include periods of alternating irritability and lethargy. The maple sugar odor frequently is appreciated in the urine, saliva, or ear cerumen. Occasionally the odor is best elicited by freezing a urine sample, which may concentrate the relatively hydrophobic ketoacids on the frozen surface. By the third day of life the infant's comatose state deepens.
3. Convulsions may ensue. Increased intracranial pressure may occur in severe cases.
4. Respiratory embarrassment and a need for mechanical ventilation are common by the end of the first week of life.
5. Brain damage is common in infants who survive the stormy neonatal period, particularly if the diagnosis is delayed beyond the first week. These youngsters may have mental retardation and a neurologic syndrome similar to that of spastic cerebral palsy.
6. A metabolic relapse can occur at any time in the older infant or child. This happens most frequently in association with an otherwise trivial intercurrent infection. Such a stress, which favors the secretion of catabolic hormones and cytokines, elicits so vigorous a rate of breakdown of body protein as to overwhelm the patient's limited ability to oxidize the branched-chain amino acids. These compounds, together with the cognate ketoacids, therefore accumulate in toxic amounts. During the period of relapse the child manifests vomiting, metabolic acidemia with ketosis, mental confusion, and even coma in extreme cases.
7. Occasional patients have a partial deficiency of branched-chain ketoacid decarboxylase. These youngsters first present in later life with ketoacidosis, prostration, and recurrent ataxia. Blood and urine levels of the branched-chain amino acids are elevated during these episodes.

Key Clinical Findings: Maple Syrup Urine Disease

- Odor of maple sugar in urine, saliva, and cerumen
- Alternating irritability and lethargy
- Convulsions

Treatment

1. The dietary restriction of the three branched-chain amino acids should permit adequate metabolic control (plasma levels <5 mg/dl for leucine, isoleucine, and valine) in most instances. Dietotherapy has been greatly simplified by the availability of commercial infant formulas from which the branched-chain amino acids have been removed. Such therapy must be maintained indefinitely. If the diagnosis is made quickly and treatment is promptly instituted, psychomotor development can be nearly normal.
2. Aggressive treatment is indicated in neonates in metabolic crisis. Fluids and glucose must be administered in large amounts in order to minimize endogenous protein catabolism. The infusion of alkali should correct metabolic acidemia in most cases. Vigilance must be exercised in order to anticipate increased intracranial pressure and to initiate prompt treatment for it. Either peritoneal dialysis or hemodialysis has been used increasingly in recent years in order to promote removal of the toxic branched-chain ketoacids. This approach appears to have been useful, even in the affected neonate.

Key Treatment: Maple Syrup Urine Disease

- Restriction of valine, leucine, and isoleucine in diet

Prevention

Newborn screening for MSUD has won increasing acceptance in many localities. Carriers can be detected by measuring enzymatic activity in cultured skin fibroblasts. If the nature of the mutation is known, carriers can be ascertained by the analysis of DNA fragments. Prenatal testing has been performed successfully.

Homocystinuria

Definition

Homocystinuria is a defect of the metabolism of homocystine, a sulfur-containing amino acid. Homocystine is an intermediate in the so-called transsulfuration pathway, or the metabolic sequence that leads from methionine to cystine.

Etiology

The usual cause of this recessive disease is a congenital deficiency of cystathionine synthetase, a vitamin B_6 (pyridoxine)–dependent enzyme that mediates the conversion of homocystine to cystathionine. This enzyme is coded on human chromosome 21. In rare instances, homocystinuria is caused not by a failure to convert homocystine to cystathionine but from a congenital failure to remethylate homocystine to methionine, an essential amino acid that ordinarily is the major source of homocystine in humans.

Epidemiology

Homocystinuria secondary to cystathionine synthetase deficiency occurs in approximately 1/50,000 to 1/100,000 live births. Infants and children at risk include those with a history of affected siblings or with parents who are known to be carriers.

Pathophysiology

1. Numerous mutations have been described, including the synthesis of an unstable enzyme, of a protein that loosely binds pyridoxal phosphate, serine, or homocysteine, or of an enzyme differing in size from the wild strain. Many organs, including brain, have an abundant cystathionine synthetase activity. The congenital enzyme deficiency typically is present in all these tissues.
2. Blood homocysteine levels in homocystinurics usually are 50 to 200 μM (normal <10 μM). The blood methionine may be extremely high, reflecting augmented remethylation of homocysteine that is not converted to cystathionine. A minority of affected children respond to pyridoxine treatment (25 to 100 mg daily) with a reduction of plasma homocysteine and methionine. These individuals tend to have a milder clinical syndrome.
3. The pathologic agent appears to be homocystine itself, which is toxic to platelets and vascular endothelium. This amino acid increases platelet adhesiveness, perhaps by increasing thromboxane synthesis. Homocystine also can cause direct endothelial injury in animals. This may result in diminished platelet survival as the denuded vascular endothelium provides a nidus for clotting. In addition, homocystine may directly activate clotting factor V, thereby increasing conversion of prothrombin to thrombin. Homocystine also favors accumulation of copper in vascular endothelium, leading to the oxidation of ceruloplasmin and the release of a toxic amount of H_2O_2.
4. Brain function is adversely affected by homocystine, which induces convulsions in rats. This may reflect blockade of the GABA receptor or the action of homocysteic acid, which can have an excitatory property. In addition, there may be deleterious effects on methylation reactions, which are essential to the synthesis of lipids and some neurotransmitters.

Clinical Findings

1. The outstanding clinical findings are a thromboembolic diathesis, mental retardation, ectopia lentis, and a marfanoid habitus. The thromboses, which can occur in almost any vessel, are common in peripheral veins and arteries, the cerebral and renal vasculature, and coronary arteries. Almost 25 percent of patients not responsive to pyridoxine will sustain a major vascular insult during childhood. Vascular insults can be precipitated by dehydration or other stress, e.g., major surgery.
2. Children who respond to vitamin B_6 have a median IQ of 78. Nonresponders have an IQ of 56. The mental retardation brings some youngsters to clinical attention. Other neurologic symptoms include convulsions (20%) and psychiatric disease (50%). A common presenting sign is ectopia lentis, which is found in half of affected children by age 5 to 10 years.
3. The marfanoid habitus (arachnodactyly, high-arched palate, tall stature, pes cavus) is common, as are osteoporosis and bony abnormalities such as scoliosis.

Key Clinical Findings: Homocystinuria

- Marfanoid habitus
- Thromboembolism
- Ectopia lentis
- Mental retardation

Treatment

1. The simplest treatment is the administration of vitamin B_6 in high dosage. Folic acid must be given concomitantly in order to avoid a deficiency of this vitamin consequent to pyridoxine administration. Some patients on high doses of pyridoxine may develop a neuropathy or hepatotoxicity.
2. Managing patients who are not pyridoxine-responsive may be quite difficult. Restricting dietary methionine should be helpful, but few children are able to tolerate the stringent diet, especially since it usually is not started until the child is older and more accustomed to a relatively high protein intake. A recent therapeutic innovation is the use of betaine, a naturally occurring amine, which in high dosage (6 to 12 g/day) favors the remethylation of homocystine to methionine, thereby lowering the blood concentration of the former amino acid. This approach appears to be reasonably free from risk except for causing a fishy odor to the urine.
3. Treatments to attenuate the thromboembolic diathesis include the use of salicylate and/or dipyridamole. The latter has been effective in animal studies in restoring platelet survival to a near-normal range. Dietary supplements of L-cystine may be helpful as well.

Key Treatment: Homocystinuria

- High-dosage pyridoxine
- Folic supplement
- Betaine
- Salicylate or dipyridamole

Prevention

A growing number of localities include homocystinuria in the list of genetic diseases that are sought as part of routine newborn screening. Antenatal diagnosis is possible, either with direct enzyme assay of cystathionine synthetase in cultured amniocytes or chorionic villus cells or with mutational analysis of DNA.

Urea Cycle Defects

Definition

The urea cycle defects are a group of disorders characterized by the congenital absence of one of the five enzymes that make up the urea cycle. As a consequence, ammonia is not converted to urea at the normal rate. A syndrome of hyperammonemia occurs. This frequently results in irreparable brain damage.

Etiology

The usual cause is a failure of one of five steps of the urea cycle (ammonia $\rightarrow \rightarrow \rightarrow \rightarrow \rightarrow$ urea). In the most common of the urea cycle defects, ornithine transcarbamylase deficiency, it is the second step of the urea cycle that is congenitally defective. This disease differs from the other inherited enzymopathies of the urea cycle in that it is a sex-linked disorder. All the other defects are inherited according to an autosomal recessive pattern.

Epidemiology

Children at risk of having a urea cycle defect include all those with a positive family history or whose parents are known to be carriers for one of these disorders. The incidence of ornithine transcarbamylase deficiency, the most common disorder, is ~ 1/80,000 live births.

Pathophysiology

1. Essentially all urea is formed in the liver in humans. The severity of a given syndrome will depend upon the completeness of the enzymatic block. In most instances a catalytically inefficient enzyme is synthesized, although the total absence of enzyme protein has been reported.

2. Blood ammonia levels are elevated, often to an extreme degree (normal values: infants and children <50 μM; term neonates <100 μM; premature infants <150 μM). The toxin responsible for some of the neurologic symptoms may not be ammonia itself but glutamine, which many cells, including brain, derive from ammonia and glutamic acid. Depending on the site of the enzymatic defect, there may be extreme elevations of other amino acids that are metabolic intermediates of the urea cycle, e.g., citrulline, argininosuccinic acid, and arginine. The latter finding often is of diagnostic importance.

3. The most prominent symptoms involve the central nervous system. The precise pathophysiology underlying the neurologic symptoms remains uncertain, even after many decades of careful research into the causes of the encephalopathy. However, the available data are consistent with a number of overlapping theories:

   a. Ammonia may lead to a failure of energy metabolism in parts of the brain, e.g., the reticular activating system, which manifests a depletion of the intracellular ATP level. The mechanism may involve a failure of the tricarboxylic acid cycle.

   b. Ammonia may adversely affect ionic homeostasis in the brain, either by inhibiting Na$^+$/K$^+$ATPase or by directly inhibiting brain K$^+$ channels.

   c. Hyperammonemia, perhaps in concert with increased brain glutamine levels, may lead to the breakdown of the blood-brain barrier and the excessive importation into the central nervous system of amino acids that serve as precursors to neurotransmitters. One of these amino acids, tryptophan, also is converted in brain into quinolinic acid, a known neurotoxin that has been shown to be increased in hyperammonemic states.

   d. There may be a failure of myelin synthesis.

Clinical Findings

1. Neonates affected with the classic form of the disease, i.e., with a near-complete enzymatic deficiency, usually become symptomatic within the first few days of life. The initial findings are lethargy, hypotonia, and a failure to feed. The attending physician commonly diagnoses septicemia and institutes antibiotic therapy. However, by the third to fourth day of life the baby will have progressed to frank coma and convulsions. Increased intracranial pressure can occur. Mechanical ventilation will be necessary in many cases by the end of the first week. Brain damage is lamentably common in babies who survive beyond the neonatal period. Many will have mental retardation, spasticity, choreoathetosis, and a profound feeding disorder.

2. Measurement of the blood ammonia always will disclose an extravagantly high value. It usually exceeds 500 μM (nl <100 μM in term infants), and levels >1 mM are not unprecedented. The concentration of blood glutamine and alanine, the major nitrogen carriers of the blood (other than urea), is extremely high. Determination of the blood amino acids is of great importance, since some of the urea cycle defects, e.g., citrullinemia and argininosuccinic aciduria, can be presumptively diagnosed from the plasma aminogram. It also is critical to quantitate urinary orotic acid excretion, since this intermediate of pyrimidine synthesis typically is very high in ornithine transcarbamylase deficiency, the most common of urea cycle defects. The reason is that the liver shuffles nitrogen ordinarily utilized for urea synthesis toward the synthesis of pyrimidines. In contrast, a severe hyperammonemia coupled with normal or low urinary orotic acid is very suggestive of carbamylphosphate synthetase deficiency.

3. Clinical expression of the urea cycle defects is primarily a function of the completeness of the enzymatic defect. In addition to the fulminant neonatal syndrome (see above), many clinical presentations have been described. Thus, a urea cycle defect should be considered in any child with unexplained mental retardation, particularly if there is a history of recurrent hospitalization for prostration and coma in association with an otherwise trivial infection. Some patients may not suffer from mental retardation but may be prone to a syndrome of recurrent nausea and vomiting, sometimes coupled with cerebellar ataxia. These youngsters often are erroneously thought to have a form of migraine. The fact that headache is a frequent finding in hyperammonemia contributes to the diagnostic confusion.

4. Personality changes are not unusual in association with hyperammonemia, and some individuals have been thought to be schizophrenic. In such cases a low-protein diet (see below) commonly ameliorates the psychosis. The affected child commonly learns to avoid foods containing a relatively large amount of protein. Growth fail-

ure therefore is a frequent finding and, on rare occasions, even may be a presenting symptom. Finally, patients with arginase deficiency (argininemia) may manifest a syndrome of spastic diplegia that mimics many of the clinical and radiologic findings of a leukodystrophy.

Key Clinical Findings: Urea Cycle Defects

• Lethargy

• Hypotonia

• Failure to feed

• Convulsions and coma

Treatment

1. The mainstay of therapy is to minimize ammonia production by feeding a low-protein diet. The amount of protein that is tolerated before hyperammonemia develops will vary among patients. A reasonable goal for the infant is 1.5 g protein/kg/day. After 1 year of age this can be reduced to 1.0 g/kg/day. A compromise frequently must be accepted between the avoidance of hyperammonemia, which is toxic to the brain, and the rate of growth, which may be suboptimal in many cases.

2. The treatment of urea cycle defects has been revolutionized by the development of so-called acylation therapy. This involves the administration (usually by mouth) of the salt of an organic acid such as sodium benzoate, sodium phenylacetate, or, more recently, sodium phenylbutyrate. Each of these is conjugated in the liver with an amino acid, e.g., glycine in the case of benzoate and glutamine with respect to phenylacetate and phenylbutyrate. The resulting conjugate—hippurate (when benzoate is given) and phenylacetylglutamine (with either phenylacetate or phenylbutyrate)—is excreted rapidly in the urine, thereby abetting the elimination of waste nitrogen. In effect, the faulty urea cycle is bypassed. If given in sufficiently high dosage (usually 250 to 500 mg/kg/day) this approach actually can normalize whole-body nitrogen homeostasis. There is minimal toxicity, apart from the objectionable odor of sodium phenylacetate (which confers the mousy odor to the urine of untreated patients with phenylketonuria).

3. During an acute hyperammonemic crisis, whether in the newborn or in the older child who has relapsed, the first priority must be the reduction of blood ammonia as rapidly as possible. The long-term outlook for the neonate in crisis is a function of the duration of hyperammonemia rather than the magnitude of this biochemical derangement. Copious amounts of fluid and glucose should be given to minimize endogenous protein catabolism. Both sodium benzoate and sodium phenylacetate or phenylbutyrate can be administered parenterally. Vigilance should be exercised to monitor the patient for possible increased intracranial pressure and convulsions. In recent years the availability of hemodialysis in infants and children has proved to be a great boon to therapy, since this treatment greatly enhances the elimination of ammonia and other nitrogenous compounds from the blood.

4. The long-term outlook is guarded, especially for infants who present during the neonatal period. The majority suffer some degree of brain damage. Care should be taken in all cases to prevent intercurrent infections and to manage them vigorously when they do occur. A few children have been treated with liver transplantation. This approach has been highly successful from a metabolic perspective. It attenuates and even aborts hyperammonemia, although it may not correct all metabolic abnormalities. The availability of cDNA clones for the urea cycle enzymes has focused attention on performing gene transfer with a viral vector. This approach remains experimental.

Key Treatment: Urine Cycle Defects

• Low-protein diet

• Sodium benzoate or phenylacetate

Prevention

1. Prenatal diagnosis of the urea cycle defects now is usually feasible. For the disorders involving the later steps of the urea cycle (citrullinemia, argininosuccinic aciduria, and argininemia) antenatal diagnosis is possible by the measurement of enzymatic activity in cultured amniocytes or chorionic villus cells. For the more proximal steps of the urea cycle (carbamylphosphate synthetase deficiency and ornithine transcarbamylase deficiency) the level of enzymatic activity in amniocytes is normally too low to permit the direct assay of the relevant enzymes. However, the recent development of molecular probes for these gene products has allowed prenatal diagnosis in formerly intractable cases.

2. Mass screening of neonates for urea cycle defects has become feasible in recent years and is now utilized in many communities.

Nonketotic Hyperglycinemia

Definition

Nonketotic hyperglycinemia is caused by a congenital deficiency of the glycine cleavage system, the major route for the conversion of glycine to serine. As a result, glycine accumulates in markedly elevated concentration in body fluids. Affected children suffer a fulminant neonatal course that usually is fatal. Survivors commonly suffer severe brain damage.

Etiology

Affected patients are born with a mutation in one of the several proteins that compose the glycine cleavage system, the primary route of glycine catabolism.

Epidemiology

This autosomal recessive disorder is quite rare, probably affecting <1/200,000 infants in the United States. It has been described in almost all races and nationalities.

Pathophysiology

1. The glycine cleavage system utilizes pyridoxal phosphate (vitamin B_6) and folate as cofactors in order to effect the conversion of C-1 of glycine to CO_2 and C-2 to a folic acid derivative.

$$\text{Glycine} + \text{Tetrahydrofolate} \xrightarrow{B_6} CO_2 + NH_3 + C_1\text{-Folate}$$

The C_1-folate derivative then becomes accessible to the "one-carbon pool" of metabolism, which is essential for the synthesis of a broad variety of compounds, including neurotransmitters, nucleic acids, and other amino acids. Serine is produced in a reversal of this reaction

$$\text{Glycine} + \text{Tetrahydrofolate} \xrightarrow{B_6} CO_2 + \text{Serine}$$

2. The precise pathophysiology underlying the encephalopathy (see below) is not well understood. However, it is likely that one important factor is excessive stimulation in the brain of an excitatory amino acid receptor, the so-called N-methyl-D-aspartate (or NMDA) receptor. The major ligand of this receptor is glutamic acid, the primary excitatory transmitter of the mammalian brain. The NMDA receptor is a complex structure that is potentiated by glycine, a specific binding site for which has been identified in the receptor protein. One hypothesis of the encephalopathy in nonketotic hyperglycinemia is that unchecked stimulation of the NMDA receptor results in a syndrome of excitotoxicity, or the neuronal damage that follows excessive stimulation of glutamatergic neurons.

Clinical Findings

1. The onset of symptoms in the classic, neonatal-onset form of the disease typically occurs on the first or second day of life. The most prominent feature is seizures, which may even occur in utero. In addition to the convulsive disorder, affected infants commonly manifest myoclonic jerks, hiccuping, and a profound hypotonia. When the babies are not suffering seizures they assume a placid appearance. A hypsarrhythmic or burst-suppression pattern commonly is seen in the electroencephalogram (EEG). Few infants will survive past the initial week or two of life. The few who do survive display profound neurologic deficits and mental retardation. Imaging studies of the brain usually disclose severe cortical atrophy and a frank loss of myelin.
2. Occasional patients first become symptomatic in later infancy or even childhood with mental retardation and failure to thrive. A few youngsters have manifested a syndrome of progressive spinocerebellar degeneration. Still others have displayed a period of reasonably normal psychomotor development followed by frank regression.
3. All patients have had a blood glycine concentration that is many times greater than normal (150 to 300 μM). In the cerebrospinal fluid (CSF) the glycine level may be as high as 100 μM, or approximately ten times normal, with a ratio of CSF to blood glycine that typically is five to ten times higher than control (0.02).

Key Clinical Findings: Nonketotic Hyperglycinemia

- Seizures first or second day of life
- Myoclonic jerks
- Hypsarrhythmia on EEG

Treatment

1. Most efforts at treatment have yielded disappointing results. The extremely elevated levels of glycine in the blood can be relieved to an extent by exchange transfusion and/or dialysis, but these therapies do not prevent progressive neurologic deterioration. Nor have other interventions that lower blood glycine, e.g., benzoate treatment or dietary protein restriction, met with much clinical success.
2. A few therapeutic approaches have been developed that seek not to reduce the glycine concentration but to block the physiologic effects of glycine, which is a neurotransmitter with a postsynaptic inhibitory activity in the spinal cord and some central neurons. Treatment with strychnine, an antagonist of glycine action at postsynaptic receptors, has not changed the clinical course, nor has treatment with diazepam, which displaces strychnine from its binding sites.
3. A novel therapy is the administration of antagonists of the NMDA receptor, an excitatory glutamatergic receptor that is potentiated by glycine. Both ketamine and dextromethorphan have been used, but the results have been inconclusive, with diminished irritability and an improved EEG having been observed in a few cases. Treatment with dextromethorphan at the recommended dosage (maximum 5 mg/kg/day) seems to be well tolerated, but additional trials will be needed before the long-term benefit of this therapy can be fully assessed.

Key Treatment: Nonketotic Hyperglycinemia

- Experimental and as yet unsatisfactory

Prevention

The glycine cleavage system is expressed at a very low level in normal amniocytes, a factor that has complicated prenatal diagnosis. However, recent advances in molecular biology have resulted in the cloning of clinically relevant components of the glycine cleavage system and the consequent availability of DNA probes that permit reliable diagnostic testing of most fetuses at risk. It is theoretically possible to screen all newborns for this inherited disorder, but at present this is rarely done.

Bibliography

Eisensmith RC, Woo SL: Phenylketonuria and the phenylalanine hydroxylase gene. Mol Biol Med 1991;8:3.

Kikuchi G: The glycine cleavage system: Composition, reaction mechanism and physiological significance. Mol Cell Biochem 1973;1:169.

Maestri NE, Hauser ER, Bartholomew D, Brusilow SW: Prospective treatment of urea cycle disorders. J Pediatr 1991;119:923.

Nyhan WL: Diagnostic Recognition of Genetic Disease. Philadelphia, Lea & Febiger, 1987.

Scriver CR, Beaudet AL, Sly WS, Valle D: The Metabolic Basis of Inherited Disease. New York, McGraw-Hill, 1989.

Yudkoff M: Disorders of amino acid metabolism. *In* Siegel GJ, Agranoff BW, Albers RW, Molinoff PB (eds): Basic Neurochemistry: Molecular, Cellular and Medical Aspects, 5th ed. New York, Raven Press, 1997, pp 813–839.

63 Disorders of Lipid Metabolism

Richard I. Kelley

Inborn Errors of Mitochondrial β-Oxidation

Etiology

1. Inborn errors of mitochondrial fatty acid β-oxidation constitute a relatively large group of metabolic diseases caused by mutations in 1 of at least 15 different enzymes of the mitochondrial process for the conversion of fatty acids into smaller compounds, largely acetyl-coenzyme A, for the synthesis of citrate in the citric acid cycle and for other synthetic systems.
2. Straight-chain fatty acids of all lengths are oxidized as their coenzyme A (CoA) esters to acetyl-CoA and thence (in the liver) to ketone bodies (acetoacetate and 3-hydroxybutyrate) by a cycle of four oxidative steps that create, in succession, a 2/3-monounsaturated acyl-CoA, a 3-hydroxyacyl CoA, a 3-ketoacyl CoA, and a saturated acyl-CoA shortened by the cleaved two-carbon acetyl-CoA.
3. There are specific enzymes for each of these four steps with various specificities for the chain length. For example, there are at least two acyl-CoA dehydrogenases with overlapping chain-length specificities required for complete β-oxidation of dietary 16- and 18-carbon fatty acid into acetyl-CoA. The longer chain length fatty acids appear to be metabolized by just two enzymes bound to the mitochondrial inner membrane—long-chain acyl-CoA dehydrogenase and "trifunctional enzyme." The latter enzyme consists of two subunits: an α subunit that contains enoyl-CoA hydratase and 3-hydroxyacyl-CoA dehydrogenase activities and a β subunit with long-chain 3-ketoacyl-CoA thiolase activity, which cleaves 3-ketoacyl CoA intermediates to acetyl-CoA and a new saturated acyl-CoA compound shortened by two methylene units.

Epidemiology

1. All genetic defects of mitochondrial β-oxidation are inherited as autosomal recessive diseases which, with one exception, are rare disorders with incidences of <1 in 40,000 births. Collectively, however, these disorders are common causes of treatable metabolic disease in infants and children.
2. One disease, medium-chain acyl-CoA dehydrogenase deficiency, has an incidence as high as 1 in 5000 births in some areas of the United States (e.g., Pennsylvania, West Virginia) and Northern Europe. As such, it is the most common potentially lethal autosomal recessive disease after cystic fibrosis.

Disorders of Mitochondrial Fatty Acid β-Oxidation

Disorders of Primary Fatty Acid β-Oxidation Enzymes

Acyl-CoA dehydrogenase deficiencies—long-, medium-, and short-chain

3-Enoyl-CoA hydratase deficiency—long- and short-chain (crotonase)

3-Hydroxyacyl-CoA dehydrogenase deficiencies—Long- and short-chain; ?medium-chain

3-Ketoacyl-CoA thiolase deficiency—Long- and short-chain (β-ketothiolase deficiency)

Mitochondrial trifunctional enzyme deficiency

Multiple acyl-CoA dehydrogenase deficiency (MADD, type II glutaric aciduria)

Disorders of Carnitine and Acylcarnitine Metabolism

Carnitine palmityltransferase deficiency—type I and type II (outer vs. inner membrane)

Carnitine plasma membrane transporter deficiency

Acylcarnitnine translocase deficiency

Disorders of Ketone Body Synthesis and Metabolism

3-Hydroxy-3-methylglutaryl (HMG)-CoA lyase deficiency

Succinyl-3-ketoacyl-CoA transferase deficiency

Acetoacetyl-CoA thiolase deficiency

Pathophysiology

The oxidation of fatty acids plays a relatively minor role in human metabolism except during fasting and in certain tissues, such as heart and skeletal muscle, for which fatty acids are the preferred fuel. As a result, defects of fatty acid oxidation are often not manifest until a child's first illness associated with prolonged fasting, at which time the failure to supply energy for gluconeogenesis leads to hypoglycemia and encephalopathy. In some deficiencies, however, muscle weakness and cardiomyopathy are the presenting signs. Although the deficient production of acetyl-CoA for ATP synthesis underlies much of the pathology, the abnormal accumulation of fatty acids and fatty acid derivatives in some β-oxidation disorders may be directly toxic to the nervous system and other tissues.

Clinical Findings

1. *Common disorders.* The three most important disorders of fatty acid β-oxidation are the deficiencies of medium-chain and long-chain acyl-CoA dehydrogenase (MCAD and LCAD) and long-chain 3-hydroxyacyl-CoA dehydrogenase (LCHAD). Their clinical pictures are a combination of unique and overlapping features.
   a. *MCAD deficiency.* MCAD deficiency is the most common fatty acid oxidation disorder. It is prevalent among families of Northern European descent but much less common in other ethnic groups. The typical child with MCAD deficiency presents in the

first 18 months at the time of a viral syndrome, surgical procedure, or other fasting stress with signs of progressive lethargy, irritability, vomiting and, ultimately, coma and seizures.

(1) Because birth is also a time when prolonged fasting often occurs, some MCAD patients will develop an encephalopathy in the newborn period but, more often than not, be evaluated for sepsis rather than a metabolic disease.

(2) A less common manifestation of MCAD deficiency is progressive muscle weakness with plasma and muscle carnitine deficiency.

(3) In retrospect, it is also likely that most children under the age of 2 years who died from "Reye syndrome," died from metabolic disease, and of these the most common diagnosis documented is MCAD deficiency. There also appears to be a small proportion (5–10%) of infants dying of sudden infant death syndrome who have MCAD deficiency or a related β-oxidation disorder.

b. *LCAD deficiency*

(1) In contrast to the acute episodic nature of MCAD deficiency, LCAD deficiency typically presents with chronic signs of failure to thrive, hypotonia, cardiomyopathy, or hepatopathy. Nevertheless, the diagnosis of LCAD deficiency may not be made until the chronically ill child, usually a young infant, presents acutely with hypoketotic hypoglycemia and encephalopathy.

(2) At diagnosis, there may be dilated cardiomyopathy, marked hepatomegaly, and advanced hepatocellular disease.

(3) A somewhat less common presentation of LCAD deficiency in young infants and even older children parallels very closely that of MCAD deficiency, i.e., hypoglycemic encephalopathy in a previously normal child or child with mild motor delay. Very commonly, MCAD and LCAD deficiencies at presentation are mistaken for nonmetabolic illnesses such as sepsis, meningitis, or toxic ingestion, causing a critical delay in the diagnosis of a treatable disorder. (Although initially described in the literature as LCAD deficiency, this disorder is now sometimes called very long chain acyl-CoA dehydrogenase (VLCAD) deficiency based on the newly proposed name of the deficient membrane-bound LCAD enzyme, which has slightly longer chain length specificity than the homologous LCAD enzyme in the mitochondrial matrix).

c. *LCHAD deficiency*

(1) The presentation of LCHAD deficiency resembles that of LCAD deficiency except that hepatic involvement is both more common and more severe.

(2) A typical patient with LCHAD deficiency is a 3- to 6-month-old child with mild to moderate failure to thrive who develops jaundice and is found to have severe hepatic disease with marked fibrosis/cirrhosis and macrovesicular fat

infiltration. Because of the hepatic disease, fasting tolerance may be limited to just 3 or 4 hours.

(3) Cardiomyopathy may also be present, and the little understood but not uncommon long-term complications of pigmentary retinopathy and peripheral neuropathy. LCHAD deficiency is also one of the few autosomal recessive diseases in which there are clinically significant manifestations in heterozygotes.

(4) A much greater than expected incidence of *a*cute *f*atty *l*iver of *p*regnancy (AFLP) and of HELLP (*h*emolysis, *e*levated *l*iver enzymes, *l*ow *p*latelets) syndrome occurs in women who are heterozygous for LCHAD deficiency, regardless of whether the fetus is affected with LCHAD deficiency. The fraction of AFLP and HELLP cases attributable to heterozygosity for LCHAD deficiency in mothers without a family history of LCHAD deficiency is not known.

2. *Other fatty acid oxidation disorders*

a. MAD deficiency has been reported under several different names, including type II glutaric aciduria and ethylmalonic adipic aciduria.

(1) The primary defect is in the synthesis or stability of electron transfer flavoprotein (ETF), a flavin acceptor for all acyl-CoA dehydrogenases, or its own dehydrogenase, ETF dehydrogenase. Because ETF is also the acceptor for glutaryl-CoA dehydrogenase and the branched-chain ketoacid dehydrogenases, the urinary organic acid and plasma acylcarnitine profiles characteristic of MADD are more complex than those of the straight-chain fatty acid oxidation disorders and include, for example, metabolites of glutaric acid and isovaleric acid. Primary abnormalities in riboflavin transport and metabolism may also cause a biochemically similar disorder.

(2) Mild forms of the MAD deficiencies may present as lipoid myopathy with ethylmalonic-adipic aciduria or the more complete glutaric aciduria type II organic aciduria. Episodic disease with encephalopathy and hypoglycemia does not occur in all cases. The most severe forms of MADD present as neonates with lethal cerebral dysgenesis, polycystic kidneys, and other internal malformations, not unlike some patients with the severe form of CPT-II deficiency (see below).

b. SCAD deficiency.

(1) Although diagnosed relatively infrequently, SCAD deficiency may be substantially under-recognized because diagnostic urinary organic acid abnormalities are less frequently present. Furthermore, because fatty acid oxidation is only partially blocked in SCAD deficiency, substantial ketonuria and normoglycemia may characterize the sick infant or child with SCAD deficiency.

(2) Failure to thrive, chronic vomiting, and other

gastrointestinal complaints are the most commonly reported abnormalities in SCAD deficiency.

(3) The encephalopathy of SCAD deficiency is most likely caused by the accumulation of butyrate and its CoA ester rather than by hypoglycemia.

c. Deficiencies of carnitine palmityltransferases I and II.

(1) Two forms of carnitine palmityltransferase (CPT), types I and II on the outer and inner mitochondrial membranes, respectively, are required for the transport of free fatty acids from the cytoplasm to the mitochondrial matrix. CPT-I converts a long-chain fatty acyl-CoA into its corresponding carnitine ester, which is then translocated to the mitochondrial matrix by the acylcarnitine translocase. There, CPT-II converts the acylcarnitine back to a fatty acyl-CoA, which serves as the substrate for the mitochondrial long-chain acyl-CoA dehydrogenase.

(2) CPT-I deficiency is a relatively rare fatty acid oxidation disorder that presents with muscle weakness and hypoketotic hypoglycemia with normal or increased plasma carnitine levels. However, because there appear to be several tissue isoforms of CPT-I, a variety of clinical presentations are possible. What is now recognized as CPT-II deficiency was first described in adults as a cause of acute myoglobinuria following prolonged exercise. The disease is characterized by high levels of long-chain carnitine esters and reduced maximal rates of β-oxidation in most tissues. In the classic adult disease, substantial residual activity of CPT-II is found. In contrast, more severe deficiencies of CPT-II deficiency commonly present as hypoketotic hypoglycemia and hyperammonemia in young children or the newborn period with high plasma levels of long-chain carnitine esters.

d. Disorders of carnitine and acylcarnitine transport or synthesis.

(1) Deficiencies of both the plasmalemmal carnitine transporter and the mitochondrial carnitine acyltranslocase, enzymes essential for the movement of free fatty acids from the bloodstream to the inner mitochondrial membrane are associated with dilated cardiomyopathy and fasting intolerance.

(2) Onset of heart failure in carnitine transporter deficiency can occur suddenly in a previously well 1- or 2-year-old child. In carnitine transporter deficiency, plasma carnitine levels are usually <5 μmol/L, whereas in acylcarnitine translocase deficiency, the level of total carnitine may be normal or mildly depressed, but the level of long-chain acylcarnitines is greatly increased.

e. Disorders of ketone body synthesis and metabolism.

(1) There are three principal enzymes associated with the metabolism of ketone bodies, one of the major by-products of fatty acid oxidation. Defects in these enzymes can lead to deficient synthesis of acetoacetate and beta-hydroxybutyrate—key fuels for nonhepatic tissues during the fasting state (HMG-CoA lyase deficiency), or impaired utilization of acetoacetate by peripheral tissues (acetoacetyl-CoA thiolase and succinyl-3-ketoacyl-CoA thiolase deficiencies).

(2) The clinical presentation of HMG-CoA lyase deficiency is nonketotic hypoglycemia or Reye-like syndrome, whereas that of the two thiolases is typically hyperketosis with or without hypoglycemia.

Key Clinical Findings: Mitochondrial Fatty Acid Oxidation Disorders

Recurrent encephalopathy at times of illness or fasting

Motor delay, myopathy, myoglobinuria

Cardiomyopathy, cardiac failure

Acute and chronic hepatic failure, cirrhosis, fibrosis, fatty infiltration

Failure to thrive, recurrent vomiting

HELLP or AFLP syndromes in heterozygote mothers (LCHAD deficiency)

Laboratory Findings

1. Disorders of fatty acid oxidation have a number of diagnostic, often pathognomonic, laboratory abnormalities. With few exceptions, the impaired oxidation of fatty acids leads to inappropriately low levels of ketones in plasma and urine despite often severe hypoglycemia. Unfortunately, this critical clue to the presence of abnormal fatty acid oxidation is often missed because acute urine is not examined.

2. For the majority of β-oxidation defects, acute urine also contains a diagnostic pattern of abnormal fatty acid by-products—largely "dicarboxylic acids" and glycine conjugates of free fatty acids—when examined by gas chromatography–mass spectrometry.

3. In MCAD deficiency, for example, a diagnostic pattern of medium-chain dicarboxylic acids, hexanoylglycine, and suberylglycine is always present during illness.

4. Marked ethylmalonic aciduria in SCAD deficiency and abundant 3-hydroxy mono- and dicarboxylic acids in LCHAD deficiency are strong clues to their respective diagnoses.

5. Analysis of plasma for abnormal levels of specific free fatty acid or acylcarnitine species can also be diagnostic for many of the β-oxidation defects. However, although diagnostic plasma metabolites are usually present, intravenous glucose therapy or high-carbohydrate, low-fat diets can suppress diagnostic metabolite abnormalities.

6. Ultimately, definitive diagnosis usually requires enzymatic assay of leukocytes or cultured fibroblasts or DNA

analysis. For MCAD and LCHAD deficiencies, more than 80 per cent of the patients are homozygous for a common mutation.

Key Laboratory Findings: Mitochondrial β-Oxidation Disorders

Hypoketotic hypoglycemia

Hyperuricemia

Myoglobinuria, increased creatine kinase levels

Dicarboxylic aciduria

Increased plasma acylcarnitine

Increased urinary acylglycine levels

Abnormal plasma free fatty acid species (MCAD, LCAD def.)

Treatment

1. *Acute therapy*
   a. Because biochemical and clinical decompensation in the β-oxidation disorders is precipitated most often by fasting, the acute treatment of disorders of fatty acid requires provision of adequate glucose and rapid reversal of the fasting state with intravenous glucose at a minimum of 8 mg/kg/min (e.g., 10% glucose at 1.5 times maintenance fluid rate). Critical to the success of this therapy is a lowering of the blood free fatty acid levels through the action of insulin. If glucose infusions lead to hyperglycemia, indicating an inadequate insulin response, then insulin must be given together with the glucose infusion.
   b. For the child with marked carnitine depletion, treating with carnitine (50 to 100 mg/kg/day) may be beneficial to restore intramitochondrial free CoA levels, but treatment with pharmacologic doses of carnitine probably has no role in the acute or chronic management of β-oxidation disorders except those associated with chronic and marked carnitine depletion.

2. *Long-term therapy*
   a. Long-term therapy of mitochondrial fatty acid oxidation disorders is largely directed to limiting dietary fat or limiting periods of fasting, or both. Except for the need for essential fatty acids in the diet, long-chain fatty acids (in the form of long-chain triglycerides) can be largely eliminated from the diet for long periods of time, if not indefinitely.
   b. For many children with defects of long-chain fatty acid oxidation, long-chain fat can be partially or almost completely replaced with medium-chain triglycerides, sometimes with considerable improvement.
   c. Although some children with MCAD deficiency have also been maintained on low-fat diets, many others remain healthy and very active consuming normal diets with 40 to 50 per cent fat.
   d. Abnormal levels of essential fatty acids have been noted in LCHAD-deficient patients and may be related to the not infrequent development of pigmentary retinopathy and peripheral neuropathy in this disorder. However, whether supplements of essential fatty acids will affect these problems is not yet known.

Key Treatment: Disorders of Fatty Acid

- Glucose and insulin
- Carnitine for those with depletion
- Limit dietary fat

Prevention

Primary prevention of most β-oxidation disorders is through genetic counseling or prenatal diagnosis. Carrier testing and prenatal diagnosis can be performed for almost all of the known disorders, either by enzymatic assay of cultured cells or, for an increasing number of disorders, by DNA mutational analysis.

Peroxisomal Disorders—General

Classification of Peroxisomal Disorders

Disorders of Peroxisome Assembly
Zellweger syndrome
Neonatal adrenoleukodystrophy
Infantile Refsum disease
Rhizomelic chondrodysplasia punctata
Deficiencies of Single Peroxisomal Enzymes
Peroxisomal thiolase deficiency
Peroxisomal oxidase deficiency
Peroxisomal bifunctional enzyme deficiency
Trihydroxycholestanoyl-CoA oxidase deficiency
Hyperoxaluria type I
DHAP acyltransferase deficiency
Alkyl-DHAP synthase deficiency
Adult Refsum disease
Glutaryl-CoA oxidase deficiency
Acatalasemia

Etiology

1. The peroxisome is a small subcellular organelle bounded by a single membrane and constituted with a large number of both anabolic and catabolic pathways, most notably those of fatty acid and complex lipid metabolism. Although mammalian peroxisomes share a number of oxidative functions with the mitochondria, they also contain many unique enzymatic systems. The clinically most important of these are oxidation of very long chain fatty acids, synthesis of plasmalogens, and oxidation of cholesterol to form bile salts.

2. There are two general categories of peroxisomal disorders: disorders of peroxisomal assembly or enzyme importation (biogenesis) and disorders of the function of a single peroxisomal enzyme. Apart from X-linked adreno-

leukodystrophy, the most common peroxisomal disorders are the defects of peroxisome biogenesis, also called generalized peroxisomal diseases, wherein there is a deficiency of a unique peroxisomal membrane protein or an abnormality of one of the peroxisomal systems for protein targeting and importation.

3. Zellweger syndrome is the prototypical generalized peroxisomal disorder. The other group of peroxisomal disorders, those involving single enzymes or proteins, may closely resemble one of the generalized peroxisomal disorders or differ markedly. For example, single-enzyme defects of peroxisomal β-oxidation, such as peroxisomal thiolase or bifunctional enzyme deficiency, closely resemble Zellweger syndrome, indicating that abnormal metabolism of very long chain fatty acids may be the major factor determining the fetal malformations characteristic of Zellweger syndrome.

Epidemiology

1. All peroxisomal disorders are rare, having individual incidences no greater than 1 in 50,000 births and a collective incidence of only about 1 in 10 to 20,000 births.
2. Except for X-linked adrenoleukodystrophy, all peroxisomal diseases observe autosomal recessive inheritance and are widespread in all ethnic groups.

Pathophysiology

1. Except for X-linked adrenoleukodystrophy, adult Refsum disease, hyperoxaluria type I, and acatalasemia and glutaryl-CoA oxidase deficiency, peroxisomal disorders in their classic forms are characterized by congenital malformations and developmental abnormalities of the central nervous system.
2. Although the specific biochemical mechanisms responsible for the malformations are not known, it is likely that the deficiency of important structural brain lipids, such as plasmalogens, and regulatory factors, such as platelet-activating factor, contribute to the disturbed morphogenesis.
3. The accumulation of possibly toxic metabolites, such as abnormal bile acids, may cause cytotoxicity at critical developmental stages. Indeed, patients with isolated defects of plasmalogen and bile acid biosynthesis demonstrate individually many of the CNS abnormalities, skeletal deformities, and liver disease of generalized peroxisomal diseases.
4. Because the entire peroxisomal organelle is deficient in the generalized peroxisomal diseases, any of more than 100 enzymatic and protein deficiencies may contribute to the complex systemic and CNS pathology of Zellweger syndrome and related clinical disorders of peroxisomal biogenesis.

Specific Peroxisomal Disorders

X-Linked Adrenoleukodystrophy (X-Linked ALD)

Clinical Findings

X-linked ALD is one of the classic leukodystrophies of childhood and also the cause of both isolated Addison's disease and a progressive neurologic disease of adults (adrenomyeloneuropathy).

1. The primary defect is severely deficient peroxisomal oxidation of fatty acids with chain lengths of 22 carbons or more (very long chain fatty acids, VLCFAs). Most children who develop the childhood form of X-linked ALD appear clinically normal until between 5 and 10 years of age, when subtle behavioral changes and gait disturbances first appear.
2. By the time the children are symptomatic, white matter lesions are evident by MRI and progress at a rapid rate such that, within 2 years, most affected children are wheelchair bound, mute, blind, and deaf. Death follows soon after in most cases.
3. Some biochemically affected individuals, even in the same family as children with childhood X-linked ALD, escape the cerebral disease but instead develop a slowly debilitating peripheral neuropathy known as adrenomyeloneuropathy (AMN), sometime after the age of 15 years.
4. Similar symptoms may also occur in some of the older heterozygous women in X-linked ALD families.
5. Another relatively common presentation is addisonian adrenal insufficiency, which may occur in children or adults with or without neurologic disease. A substantial proportion of isolated Addison's disease has now been found to be caused by X-linked ALD.

Key Clinical Findings: X-Linked ALD

- Addison disease
- Behavior and gait disturbances

Laboratory Findings and Radiographic Abnormalities

1. The hallmark of X-linked ALD is the elevated level of VLCFAs in plasma and tissues throughout the body. The VLCFA levels are increased at birth, but the severity of the biochemical abnormality does not correlate with the severity of the clinical disease. Laboratory evidence of adrenal insufficiency, such as elevated levels of ACTH, may also be present. In 1993, the gene for X-linked ALD was identified and shown to be a member of a large group of membrane transporter molecules. As a result, mutational analysis can now be used in most families to identify, in particular, heterozygous carriers of the gene who do not express the biochemical defect.
2. Individuals with the childhood form of X-linked ALD typically develop early CNS white matter changes after 5 years of age. These may at first be limited to relatively subtle density changes by MRI, but the disease rapidly evolves to an inflammatory stage, with enhancing MRI lesions of the central white matter almost indistinguishable from lesions of multiple sclerosis except for their distribution and relentless expansion.

Treatment

1. There is no proven long-term therapy for X-linked ALD.
2. Aggressive dietary management to lower the levels of VLCFAs has not been effective in childhood X-linked ALD, although trials with a combination of triolein and

trierucin (Lorenzo's oil) are still too limited to determine whether dietary treatment will modulate the course of the disease.

3. The same VLCFA-lowering diet used in adults with AMN may have some beneficial effect as measured by nerve conduction velocities.

4. Substantial clinical improvement following bone marrow transplantation (BMT) has been reported in a few cases, but there have also been many failures with BMT, and the long-term outcome after full reconstitution of the successful recipient's immune system is not yet known.

5. Other experimental therapies include thalidomide, which acts to block tumor necrosis factor, and β-interferon therapy, both of which are directed at limiting the white matter inflammatory lesions.

Key Treatment: X-Linked ALD

- Experimental and so far unsuccessful

Prevention

1. There is no prevention of the X-linked ALD other than identification of carriers and all biochemically affected individuals through biochemical and DNA testing and subsequent genetic counseling.

2. Effective prenatal diagnosis, both biochemical and DNA-based, is also available. Because genetic evidence indicates that the manifestation of the same biochemical defect as either childhood X-linked ALD or adult AMN may segregate as a simple autosomal dominant modifying factor, there is an intensive genetic search for the putative modifying gene, possibly one that regulates the immune response to the abnormal CNS lipids.

Zellweger Syndrome, Other Generalized Peroxisomal Disorders, and Single-Enzyme Defects of Peroxisomal Fatty Acid Oxidation

Clinical Findings

1. All the generalized peroxisomal disorders have in common, as in X-linked ALD, abnormal catabolism of VLCFAs.

2. However, unlike children with X-linked ALD, who appear clinically normal for at least several years, children with generalized peroxisomal diseases typically have congenital malformations and serious CNS disease at birth.

3. In the classic peroxisomal disorder, Zellweger syndrome, the most common congenital malformations include relative macrocephaly with very large fontanels, abnormal ears and midfacial structures, epicanthal folds, cataracts, ventricular septal defects, glomerulocystic kidney disease, and rhizomelic dwarfism with punctate cartilage calcifications.

4. The CNS disease is characterized by severe hypotonia, absent neonatal reflexes, seizures, septo-optic dysplasia, abnormal cerebral gyri, heterotopias, agenesis of the corpus callosum, and olivary dysplasia. Milder phenotypes of generalized peroxisomal disease have been reported as neonatal adrenoleukodystrophy (develop-

mental delay, seizures, leukodystrophy) or infantile Refsum disease (developmental delay, pigmentary retinopathy, elevated serum phytanic acid levels), but all three classic presentations are now recognized as elements of a spectrum of severity within a single syndrome.

5. Conversely, there appear to be at least ten different genetic lesions that lead to abnormal peroxisomal biogenesis and the clinical presentation within the Zellweger syndrome–neonatal ALD–infantile Refsum disease spectrum.

   a. The natural history of these conditions varies considerably. Infants with the more severe Zellweger syndrome phenotype usually die of their neurologic abnormalities (e.g., seizures, aspiration) or progressive liver disease before age 6 months.

   b. Among patients classified clinically as neonatal ALD or infantile Refsum disease, survival into the second decade is not uncommon, but death from progressive hepatic disease or neurologic degeneration nevertheless occurs during childhood in most.

6. A special, more limited form of a generalized peroxisomal disease is the rare CNS–skeletal dysplasia syndrome, rhizomelic chondrodysplasia punctata (RCDP). Children with RCDP typically have a severe skeletal dysplasia at birth and have profound growth retardation and lack of neurologic development after birth. In addition to rhizomelic shortening of the bones, there is widespread calcific stippling of cartilage similar to, but more severe than, Zellweger syndrome. Most die in the first year from pulmonary insufficiency or seizures, but rare long-term survival has been described, and a few patients with minimal CNS disease are also known.

Diagnostic Criteria for a Generalized Peroxisomal Disorder

Abnormal peroxisomal enzyme or metabolite level
Characteristic facial appearance
Evidence of cerebral dysgenesis
Hepatic fibrosis/cirrhosis, cholestasis, biliary dysgenesis
Polycystic (cortical) kidney disease
Abnormal electroretinogram, optic atrophy, pigmentary retinopathy
Sensorineural hearing loss
Punctate calcification of cartilage, large fontanels

Laboratory Findings and Radiographic Abnormalities

Because the fundamental defect in the generalized peroxisomal disorders is the failed development of an entire subcellular organelle, there are many biochemical tests that can be used to confirm a clinical diagnosis of Zellweger syndrome and related disorders.

1. Among the most important is the finding of increased levels of VLCFAs in plasma, cultured cells, or solid tissues. This biochemical abnormality is similar to but

more severe than the VLCFA abnormality in X-linked ALD.

2. Other useful diagnostic measures include increased levels of phytanic acid, pipecolic acid, and abnormal bile acids; and decreased levels of plasmalogens, cholesterol, and several isoprenoid compounds.

3. The diagnosis of a generalized peroxisomal disorder can also be confirmed by the assay of various peroxisomal enzymes related to the same catabolic or anabolic pathways.

4. Histologic methods of diagnosis less commonly used today include the demonstration of absent or reduced hepatic peroxisomes in hepatocytes and demonstration of characteristic lipid accumulations in tissues of some of the longer surviving children.

5. Patients with RCDP differ from those with Zellweger syndrome in having a much more restricted abnormality of peroxisomal function. Only four enzymes are known to be abnormal in RCDP: DHAP acyltransferase. alkyl-DHAP synthase, phytanic acid oxidase, and peroxisomal thiolase (incomplete processing). VLCFAs are normal in RCDP.

6. By CT or MRI, infants and children with Zellweger syndrome and its congeners have a variety of abnormalities, including enlarged ventricles, heterotopias, pachygyria, microgyria, and dysmyelination. In older children the dysmyelinating process may become frankly demyelinating terminally. However, even when MRI studies are normal, there may be substantial cerebral dysgenesis with the expected sequelae of seizures and severe mental retardation.

. The demonstration of calcific stippling, especially of the apophyseal cartilages, is an important clue to the diagnosis of a generalized peroxisomal disorder.

Recently, molecular defects responsible for several of the generalized peroxisomal disease complementation groups have been identified. These discoveries will soon lead to more precise genetic diagnosis, prenatal diagnosis, and carrier testing for these disorders.

Laboratory Findings: Major Peroxisomal Diseases

X-linked adrenoleukodystrophy	Increased very long chain fatty acid levels
Zellweger syndrome, infantile Refsum disease, neonatal adrenoleukodystrophy	Increased very long chain fatty acid levels
	Decreased red cell plasmalogen levels
	Hyperpipecolic acidemia/aciduria
	Abnormal serum/urine bile acids
	Increased serum phytanic acid levels
	Abnormal cellular catalase distribution
Rhizomelic chondrodysplasia punctata	Decreased red cell plasmalogen levels
	Increased serum phytanic acid levels
Peroxisomal oxidase deficiency	Increased very long chain fatty acid levels
Peroxisomal bifunctional enzyme deficiency	Increased very long chain fatty acid levels
Peroxisomal thiolase deficiency	Abnormal serum/urine bile acids

---

Treatment

As in X-linked ALD, there is no definitive treatment for the generalized peroxisomal disorders, only supportive therapy. However, because of the many different metabolic disturbances present in patients with these disorders, various empiric therapies designed to decrease elevated metabolite levels or restore deficiencies have been attempted. These included:

1. VLCFA-lowering diets for Zellweger syndrome and related disorders (especially those associated with deficiencies of single peroxisomal β-oxidation enzymes).

2. Supplementation with batyl alcohol, a precursor of plasmalogens.

3. Bile acid supplementation for the peroxisomal disorders with deficient bile acid biosynthesis.

4. Unfortunately, as yet no empirical therapy has been proved effective. Moreover, apart from X-linked ALD, these disorders are associated with congenital malformations and, in particular, cerebral dysgenesis, for which only supportive care can be offered.

Key Treatment: Peroxisomal Diseases

• Experimental and so far unsuccessful

Prevention

Prenatal diagnosis and identification of carriers for these genetic disorders remain the only effective means of prevention.

 ## Bibliography

Kelley RI: Peroxisomal disorders. *In* Walker WA, Durie P, Hamilton R, et al (eds): Pediatric Gastrointestinal Disease. Toronto, BD Decker, 1996, pp 1246–1290.

Lazarow P, Moser HW: Disorders of peroxisomal biogenesis. *In* Scriver CR, Beaudet AL, Sly WS, Valle D (eds): The Metabolic Basis of Inherited Disease, 6th ed. New York, McGraw-Hill, 1995, pp 2287–2345.

Taubman B, Hale DE, Kelley RI: Familial Reye syndrome: a presentation of medium-chain acyl-CoA dehydrogenase deficiency. Pediatrics 1987;76:382–385.

Vockley J: The changing face of disorders of fatty acid oxidation. Mayo Clin Proc 1994;69:249–257.

64 Disorders of Carbohydrate Metabolism

James B. Gibson

Inborn errors are known that affect the metabolism of simple sugars as well as complex carbohydrates. In this chapter the focus is on the disorders of galactose, fructose, and glycogen metabolism. The disorders of glucose metabolism are covered in the chapters on diabetes and the lactic acidosis disorders (see Chapters 266 through 269).

Galactosemias

Definition

The galactosemias refer to the three inherited disorders of the catabolic pathway of galactose. Most often the term is used to refer to the most common of these disorders, galactose-1-phosphate uridyl transferase deficiency. All of the disorders present as toxicity syndromes.

Etiology

1. Galactose is found in naturally occurring foodstuffs. It is a major component of mammalian milks, where it is found in the disaccharide lactose. Galactose accounts for 40 per cent of the energy from human milk. It is also present in the simple and complex sugars of many plants.
2. The diseases are the result of deficiencies in each of the three enzymes that catalyze the normal conversion of galactose to glucose. The majority of galactose metabolism occurs in the liver, but the effects of inborn errors of galactose metabolism can affect many of the organ systems. Galactokinase (GALK) catalyzes the reaction of adenosine triphosphate (ATP) with galactose to form galactose-1-phosphate. This compound is reacted with uridine diphosphate glucose by galactose-1-phosphate uridyltransferase (GALT) to yield uridine diphosphate galactose and glucose-1-phosphate. Uridine diphosphate galactose can then be converted into uridine diphosphate glucose by uridine diphosphate galactose-4-epimerase (GALE). The net catabolic reaction is galactose + ATP → glucose-1-phosphate + ADP.
3. Alternative metabolic pathways exist for galactose. Galactitol can be formed by aldose reductase in an irreversible pathway. Galactitol cannot be further metabolized in humans. Some galactose can be metabolized by a minor alternative pathway, which leads to the pentose pathway. The role of this pathway in altering the consequences of GALT deficiency is unknown.
4. All three disorders are autosomal recessive conditions whose genes have been localized to chromosomes 17 (GALK), 9 (GALT), and 1 (GALE). The sequencing of the GALT gene has shown that there are many mutations; however, a common mutation is responsible for about 70 per cent of the disease alleles in individuals of Northern European ancestry.

Epidemiology

Galactosemia occurs worldwide. From screening of newborns, the following incidences are estimated:

1. GALK deficiency occurs in 1 in 500,000 births.
2. Complete or nearly complete GALT deficiency occurs in 1 in 40,000 to 60,000 births. A compound heterozygote for a low-activity allelic variant and GALT deficiency (Duarte/galactosemic) is more common, with an estimated incidence of 1 in 3000 to 4000 births.
3. Severe GALE defects are very rare; the disease has been reported in only two patients. A milder form (so-called peripheral epimerase deficiency) has been found throughout the world.

Pathophysiology

1. Galactose is an essential component of many glycoproteins and hormones. It is synthesized and catabolized by the body with a daily turnover estimated in adults to be 1 to 2 g/day. Galactose is not an essential component of adult diets, as shown by the large proportion of the world's adult population who have lactase deficiency, preventing the breakdown of lactose to glucose and galactose in the intestinal tract. Whether this monosaccharide is essential during some part of prenatal or postnatal life is controversial. Galactose is synthesized in large quantities during lactation when gram quantities are used for the formation of lactose.

   a. In the absence of GALK activity, a portion of the excess galactose is metabolized to the sugar alcohol galactitol by aldose reductase. Galactitol is toxic to the lens of the eye, causing osmotic injury and denaturation of lens proteins. The consequences are the formation of cataracts. In some individuals younger than the age of 40 who develop cataracts, lower than normal GALK activity may be present.

   b. Liver, kidney, and brain damage is not seen in GALT deficiency.

2. The pathophysiology of GALT deficiency (classic galactosemia) may be due in part to synthetic defects as well as the intoxication produced by galactose metabolites.

3. Defects in GALT lead to two types of toxicities.

   a. An acute toxicity due to untreated disease usually manifests in the first days to weeks of life. Hepatic dysfunction, renal disease, and cerebral edema can occur. Infants can die of sepsis due to *Escherichia coli* without the presence of other symptoms. Inanition and liver or kidney failure can also cause death. The compound(s) responsible for this acute toxicity are not clearly identified. The concentrations of galactose-1-phosphate can be extraordinarily high and the excretion of galactitol an order of magnitude higher than in treated patients. The liver may have fatty changes and fibrotic changes. Edema and ascites can occur, perhaps as a result of hepatic dysfunction and malnutrition. The risk of death from sepsis rapidly diminishes with removal of galactose from the diet.

b. A chronic toxicity syndrome occurs owing to the accumulation of galactose-1-phosphate, the shunting of galactose into galactitol, the failure of the production of appropriate glycoproteins, alterations in intracellular reducing potential, or a combination of these processes. Poor growth and chronic hepatic disease are the usual manifestations. In some patients, the constant exposure to high levels of galactitol results in cataract formation.

4. Despite appropriate and lifelong treatment there are sequela in GALT deficiency. The organ systems at risk are the central nervous system and, in females, the ovaries. The ovarian dysfunction is a form of hypergonadotropic hypogonadism with very few follicles present in the few sampled gonads. The end organs are responsive to exogenous sex hormones. Central nervous system dysfunction is most often noted as cognitive rather than motor dysfunction. The mechanisms underlying these late consequences are unknown. Cataracts do not occur in individuals who are on diets of galactose restriction.

5. Systemic epimerase deficiency presents a clinical picture similar to that of GALT deficiency. These patients are unable to synthesize galactose from glucose and are galactose dependent. This dependency results in the impaired synthesis of galactosylated compounds.

6. Patients with mild GALE deficiency have an incomplete enzyme defect. Alterations in the stability of the protein and a greater than normal requirement for the nicotinamide adenine dinucleotide cofactor have been demonstrated.

Clinical Findings

1. Patients with GALK defects can be detected by newborn screening in a presymptomatic stage. Symptomatic GALK deficiency causes cataracts.

2. In those individuals whose GALT deficiency is detected by newborn screening, no symptoms of acute toxicity may be present.

a. Acute toxicity often manifests with feeding difficulties, hepatotoxicity, vomiting, jaundice, and poor weight gain. Hepatomegaly, diarrhea, anemia, proteinuria, renal Fanconi syndrome, pseudotumor cerebri, and cataracts can also occur. The most common reason for hospital admission is jaundice. Approximately 15 per cent of all newborns with GALT deficiency die of their disease and its complications in the neonatal period. Sepsis can be the presentation in the neonatal period.

b. Chronic toxicity of untreated galactosemia presents as calorie malnutrition, hepatic enlargement, and liver dysfunction. Lethargy and renal dysfunction similar to that of the more acute presentation are also seen.

c. Patients with treated galactosemia may have overt evidence of their disease despite strict adherence to diet. These long-term consequences of galactosemia occur regardless of the age at onset of treatment. They can even be present in individuals treated

with maternal dietary restriction. The affected organ systems are the central nervous system and ovary.

(1) The majority of patients with GALT defects have one or more of the following: a specific speech disorder, verbal dyspraxia; difficulties in cognition; and/or below-normal mental development. In the second or third decades, some patients develop progressive ataxias.

(2) Ovarian dysfunction, occurring in over 80 per cent of females, ranges from failure to enter puberty to premature menopause. Very few women with classic galactosemia have become pregnant. Pregnancies are carried to term with the birth of normal infants.

(3) Bone hypomineralization has been reported in many treated galactosemics who have not had calcium supplementation from nondairy sources.

Key Clinical Findings: GALT Deficiency

- Hepatic dysfunction with jaundice, hepatomegaly, vomiting, feeding difficulties
- Sepsis in acute toxicity phase
- Failure to thrive
- Cerebral edema/pseudotumor cerebri
- Ovarian dysfunction (not recognizable in neonate)
- Cataracts

Laboratory Findings

1. Newborn screening is performed in a majority of the states. Elevations of erythrocyte galactose or of galactose-1-phosphate are detected by a variety of techniques from dried blood spots. These elevations will suggest GALK or GALT deficiencies. GALT defects can also determined from the newborn blood filter paper as a direct assay of enzyme activity.

2. Non–glucose-reducing substances in the urine may represent galactose, thus suggesting GALK or GALT deficiencies.

3. GALT defects in the untreated state can result in elevations of hepatic enzymes and of bilirubin, hemolytic anemia, and proximal renal dysfunction.

4. Definitive diagnosis in each of the diseases is made by specific assays for the presence of the appropriate enzyme in erythrocytes. Tissue specimens can also be used. Blood transfusions may make erythrocyte assays unreliable for up to 120 days. Several of the alleles of GALT such as the Duarte allele can be phenotypically identified by isoelectric focusing of the protein.

5. Alterations in the concentrations of uridine diphosphate glucose and uridine diphosphate galactose may occur in GALT and GALE defects. Such alterations should not be used for diagnosis.

6. Elevations of erythrocyte galactose-1-phosphate and urinary galactitol are always present in GALT, even in the treated state. Prognosis cannot be based on the magnitude

of the abnormal compound accumulations, but their concentrations do increase with dietary indiscretions.

7. Identification of the mutation is possible in many instances of GALT deficiency. A common point mutation is found in over 70 per cent of the abnormal alleles in individuals of Northern European ancestry.

Key Laboratory Findings: GALT, GALE, or GALK Deficiency

- Elevated levels of aspartate and alanine transaminases and bilirubin (GALT, possibly GALE)

- Nonglucose urinary reducing substances (GALK, GALT)

- Elevated levels of erythrocyte galactose-1-phosphate (GALT) or galactose (GALK, GALT)

- Abnormal erythrocyte enzyme assays

Radiographic Findings

There are no specific changes seen on plain films. Osteopenia can be seen in individuals with GALT deficiency who do not have adequate calcium intake.

Differential Diagnosis of Galactosemia

- Sepsis
- Hepatic dysfunction: such as fructosemias, tyrosinemia, cystic fibrosis, a_1-antitrypsin defects, structural defects in bile ducts, bile dysmetabolism
- Gastroesophageal reflux
- Infectious hepatitis
- Other reasons for failure to thrive, including psychosocial factors
- Abnormal blood flow bypassing the liver with resultant hypergalactosemia

Treatment

The mainstay of treatment for GALK and GALT deficiencies is a galactose-free diet.

1. This is easily done in infancy with the use of available formula. Early dietary elimination of galactose (and lactose) results in the resolution of the acute toxicity syndrome. Dietary restriction should not be relaxed in older children because there is no evidence for a later ability to handle galactose.
2. The absolute elimination of galactose from the diet of those eating table foods is impossible. However, by the elimination of all foods labeled as having galactose or lactose, strict avoidance of dairy products, and selection of lower galactose-containing fruits and vegetables, an older galactosemic can reduce his or her intake to 0.5 to 1 mg/kg/day. Endogenous production (1 mg/kg/hr) is much greater than this.
3. Ovarian dysfunction is treated with exogenous estrogen and progesterone.
4. Regression of cataracts in GALT deficiency can occur with elimination of galactose from the diet.
5. Verbal dyspraxia is amenable to intensive speech therapy.

Prevention

1. The disorders cannot be prevented, but the life-threatening consequences of GALT deficiency can be eliminated with treatment.
2. Newborn screening can reduce the incidence of acute toxicity.

Key Treatment: GALT Deficiency

- Galactose-free diet

Fructose Dysmetabolism

Definition

The most widely recognized disorder of fructose catabolism is hereditary fructose intolerance, which is due to a deficiency in fructose-1,6-bisphosphate aldolase. A benign disorder, essential fructosuria, results from a deficiency of hepatic fructokinase. Several disorders of gluconeogenesis such as fructose-1,6-bisphosphatase also involve the metabolism of this sugar.

Etiology

1. Fructose is ingested as the disaccharide sucrose and as the monosaccharide from fruits and vegetables.
2. Fructose-1,6-bisphosphate aldolase catalyzes the conversion of fructose-1-phosphate to glyceraldehyde and droxyacetone phosphate as well as that of fructose-1,6-diphosphate to glyceraldehyde-3-phosphate and dihydroxyacetone phosphate. The enzyme is located in hepatic, renal cortical, and small intestinal tissues.
3. Several isozymes are known with different catalytic properties and tissue distributions. In hereditary fructose intolerance, the activity of aldolase B, which is found in the liver, kidney, and intestine, is less than 10 to 15 per cent of normal.

Epidemiology

1. It is an autosomal recessive disorder with the gene for the hepatic aldolase B localized to chromosome 9q. The true incidence is not known. Estimates have ranged as high as 1 in 20,000 for a Swiss population.
2. Symptoms can be recognized in individuals of all ages. Diagnosis in those other than infants often takes place during evaluations for failure to thrive, storage disorders, anomalous behaviors, or as the result of no dental caries. A number of individuals have been identified as adults after the discovery of a younger affected relative. Other patients are identified after they have received infusions of the offending sugars.

Pathophysiology

1. The pathophysiologic effects are an exaggeration of the untoward effects of fructose in normal individuals, including hyperuricemia, lactic acidosis, and a lowering of blood glucose. The consequences of aldolase deficiency include decreased intracellular concentrations of ATP and of inorganic phosphate. As a result of the lowered concentration of inorganic phosphate, adenylate deaminase is deinhibited and inosine monophosphate accumulates.

This compound, in turn, inhibits the residual hepatic aldolase activity. Secondary inhibition of fructokinase and phosphorylase also occurs.

2. Hypoglycemia results from both impaired glycogenolysis as a result of the elevated concentrations of fructose-1-phosphate and inhibited gluconeogenesis. Both glucose 6-phosphate isomerase and liver aldolase are inhibited by fructose-1-phosphate. The depletion of ATP may also explain the lowered gluconeogenesis.

3. The chronic ingestion of fructose can lead to hepatopathy with increased aspartate transaminase, lipid accumulation, and hepatomegaly as well as cirrhotic changes.

4. Fructose is not responsible for the toxic effects because individuals with essential fructosuria have no symptoms.

Clinical Findings

1. Symptoms are present only after the ingestion of fructose. Acute manifestations are hypoglycemia, dizziness, sweating, nausea, tremors, disorientation, vomiting, and lethargy. If the hypoglycemia is severe or prolonged, coma and convulsions can occur. Hypoglycemia characteristically occurs rapidly. Clotting disorders and hypocomplementemia can occur. Hemorrhage is seen in some patients.

2. Chronic symptoms lead to signs and symptoms similar to GALT deficiency galactosemia: poor feeding, failure to thrive, irritability, jaundice or hyperbilirubinemia, hepatomegaly, recurrent vomiting, aminoaciduria, and proteinuria.

3. Symptoms tend to be more severe in infants. Many older children develop a strong aversion to fruits, sweets, and other foods containing fructose or sucrose.

4. Recurrent exposure to the sugar can lead to hepatic or renal failure and death.

Key Clinical Findings: Fructose Dysmetabolism

- Acute: Present only after the ingestion of fructose, sucrose, or sorbitol with vomiting, sweating, lethargy, hypoglycemia, and coma
- Chronic: Failure to thrive, hepatomegaly, abdominal distention, and acquired avoidance behaviors

Laboratory Findings

1. Characteristic findings are hypoglycemia, fructosuria, which yields a positive non–glucose-reducing substance test, and aminoaciduria.

2. Serum potassium and phosphorus levels may be low, whereas serum urate and magnesium levels may be high. Elevations in lactate with lowered pH are often seen in the acute setting.

3. Laboratory abnormalities resolve with avoidance of the offending compounds.

4. Fructose challenges may cause prolonged and severe hypoglycemia. Intravenous fructose challenges should be performed only in closely monitored situations. Oral challenges may produce more acute gastrointestinal symptoms than intravenous challenges.

5. The enzyme can be assayed in liver tissues. Several mutations have been described that may lead to the use of molecular diagnostic techniques without the risk of fructose challenges.

6. Liver biopsy samples can show steatosis and patchy necrosis with resultant fibrosis or cirrhosis.

7. Renal tissues may show dilated proximal tubules and vacuolization of the epithelium.

8. Molecular analysis of aldolase B mutations are possible using a panel of allele-specific oligonucleotides.

Differential Diagnosis

- Pyloric stenosis
- Gastroesophageal reflux
- Infectious causes of hepatitis
- Acute intoxication, such as with oral hypoglycemic agents
- Chronic disease: causes of failure to thrive; resembles GALT deficiency, hepatitis, storage disorders, and other inborn errors of metabolism

Treatment

1. All sources of fructose, sucrose, and sorbitol are excluded from the diet.

2. Acute incidents are treated with intravenous glucose. Supportive measures are used for alleviation of coagulopathy.

3. Treated individuals grow normally and have normal intellectual outcomes. Catch-up growth occurs.

Prevention

As a recessive disorder, there is no a priori determination of decreased aldolase activity.

Key Treatment: Fructose Dysmetabolism

- Eliminate all sources of fructose, sucrose, and sorbitol from diet.
- For acute incidents, administer glucose infusion.

Glycogen Storage Diseases

Definition

The glycogen storage diseases (GSDs) are a group of inherited diseases characterized by deficiencies, or abnormal function, of the enzymes involved in breakdown of glycogen (glycogenolysis) or its synthesis (glycogenesis). They are characterized by the accumulation of abnormal amounts or types of glycogen in the affected tissues.

Etiology

These disorders can be broadly grouped into the hepatic and muscular glycogenoses. This division is artificial because some of the hepatic disorders also cause muscle symptoms.

1. The hepatic group includes types I (von Gierke disease), III (debrancher defects), IV (branching enzyme defect), and VI (liver phosphorylase and phosphorylase kinase defects).

2. The muscle disorders include types II (Pompe disease), V (McArdle or muscle phosphorylase disease), and VII

(phosphofructokinase deficiency). An additional related disorder, sometimes referred to as GSD type 0, does not cause glycogen storage because the defect is in the synthesis of glycogen.

3. Because of the differing roles of hepatic and muscle glycogen, the diseases that are associated with defects in its metabolism present differently. Liver disease tends to present as hepatomegaly and hypoglycemia, whereas muscle glycogenoses present as generalized weakness (as in infantile GSD type II) or with fatigability, cramps, exercise intolerance, and myoglobinuria (type V).

4. All of the glycogenoses are autosomal recessive disorders except for liver phosphorylase kinase defects (the most common form of type VI disease) and muscle phosphoglycerate kinase disease, which are X-linked.

Epidemiology

The GSDs are relatively rare, with a combined incidence of 1 in 20,000 to 25,000. Types I, II, III, and VI are the most common and represent over 90 per cent of the recognized cases. The incidence of muscle glycogenoses is probably underestimated.

Pathophysiology

1. Glycogen consists of glucose residues, which are joined in straight chains by $\alpha 1$–4 linkages. At intervals of 4 to 10 residues, branches occur as the result of $\alpha 1,6$ linkages. Muscle glycogen forms spherical particles that can contain up to 60,000 glucose residues. In addition to spherical particles, rosette aggregates can occur in the liver. Each spherical particle is covalently attached to a 37-kd protein called glycogenin that serves as the nucleation site for the formation of the glucose polymer.

2. Glycogen serves as the primary storage form of glucose. In muscle it provides a fuel source for short-term, high-consumption states. Glycogen in the central nervous system is an emergency supply to buffer brief periods of hypoglycemia or hypoxia. Liver glycogen is used to prevent the fall of blood sugar and to supply energy to tissues that cannot make significant amounts of glucose.

    a. Two to 8 per cent of liver mass is glycogen. In normal individuals, despite the access to food, glycogen is constantly being degraded and synthesized. The release of glucose from the liver is under endocrine regulation, with epinephrine and glucagon as examples of glycemic hormones.

    b. The amount of glycogen in muscle is 0.5 to 1 per cent of its mass. It is not depleted rapidly by fasting, in contrast to hepatic glycogen. Epinephrine causes the enhancement of phosphorylase activity, which causes glucose-6-phosphate production. This compound cannot be hydrolyzed to glucose in muscle. Glycolysis occurs with the diffusion of lactate and pyruvate from the muscle.

    c. In the liver, the pyruvate and lactate of muscle origin are taken up and used as the substrates for gluconeogenesis or glycogenesis.

3. There are four different disorders within category of GSD type I. All of the disorders are due to defects in the function of glucose-6-phosphatase.

    a. Type Ia is due to a primary defect in the phosphatase.

    b. Type Ia disease is the prototype for the hepatic glycogenoses.

    c. Type Ib is due to defective transport of glucose-6-phosphatase into hepatic microsomes.

    d. Type Ic is a disorder of microsomal transport of phosphate.

    e. Type Id results from defects in the transport of glucose out of the microsomes.

4. In a hepatic glycogenosis such as type Ia, profound hypoglycemia occurs when the exogenous sources of glucose are exhausted. Glucose production from both gluconeogenesis and glycogenolysis are blocked by defects in glucose-6-phosphatase.

    a. The degradation of glycogen to pyruvate is intact and results in the formation of lactate.

    b. Additional pyruvate is converted to acetyl-coenzyme A and malonyl-coenzyme A, which leads to formation of fatty acids. In turn, these processes lead to lactic acidemia and hyperlipidemia.

    c. Hyperuricemia occurs because of the excess of glucose-6-phosphate.

5. Type II (Pompe disease) is the result of a lysosomal disorder due to a defect in production or intracellular processing of acid α-glucosidase. Infantile, juvenile, and adult forms of the disease are recognized.

    a. In its severe (infantile) form, the enzyme activity is missing from all tissues. As a result, glycogen accumulates in muscle, liver, kidney, heart, Schwann cells, neurons, and smooth muscle.

    b. The juvenile form of the disease presents as muscle weakness and pseudohypertrophy. It is a later manifesting form of the infantile disease. Death occurs by 5 to 6 years as a result of respiratory muscle failure. Cardiac function is generally not compromised, although myocardial glycogen is increased.

    c. A form of the disease (type IIc) is found in adults and presents as a slowly progressive myopathy of striated muscle. No organomegaly or cardiac involvement occurs. Residual activity of the enzyme is often greater than 10 per cent of normal.

6. In type V (McArdle disease), impaired glycogen degradation alters the ability of the muscle to sustain energy needs. Resting muscle relies on oxidation of fatty acids. Early into exercise, muscle shifts to glycogen breakdown and anaerobic glycolysis. In continued exercise, blood glucose and, finally, fatty acids supply larger shares of the energy demand. Over half of these patients demonstrate a "second wind phenomenon" when nonglycogen energy sources are used. Muscle damage occurs with rhabdomyolysis. In a significant number of cases, the myoglobinuria is intense enough to cause acute renal failure. Short periods of rest often alter exercise tolerance.

Clinical Findings (Table 64–1)

1. In type I disease, poor growth with marked hepatomegaly occurs.

    a. Symptomatic hypoglycemia is characteristic, but it

TABLE 64–1. SELECTED FEATURES OF GSDs ORGANIZED BY TISSUE INVOLVEMENT

TYPE	ENZYME	ORGANS	GLYCOGEN STRUCTURE	CLINICAL SYMPTOMS
I	Glucose-6-phosphatase	Liver, kidney, intestinal mucosa	Normal	Organomegaly, hypoglycemia, hyperlipidemia, acidosis, dwarfism
III	Amylo-1,6-glucosidase	Liver, heart, muscle	Outer chains missing or very short	Hepatomegaly, hypoglycemia, hyperlipidemia, abnormal electrocardiogram, growth retardation; improvement after puberty
IV	Amylo-(1,4→1,6)-transglycosylase	Generalized amylopectin deposition	Abnormal with long inner and outer unbranched chains	Hepatosplenomegaly, ascites, cirrhosis, liver failure, neuromuscular involvement, cardiomyopathy
VI	Liver glycogen phosphorylase	Liver	Normal	Hepatomegaly, normal spleen, often normal glucose and lipids, no acidosis, improves with age
II	α-1,4-Glucosidase	All organs	Normal	Hepatomegaly, cardiomegaly, electrocardiographic changes; muscle changes
V	Muscle glycogen phosphorylase	Skeletal muscle	Normal	Weakness and cramps without lactate rise, second wind phenomenon, myoglobinuria
VII	Phosphofructokinase	Skeletal muscle	Normal	Weakness, cramps without lactate rise, hemolysis, hyperuricemia
VIII	Hepatic phosphorylase kinase	Liver	Normal	Hepatomegaly that resolves by puberty, mild retardation of growth, hypoglycemia is rare

may not be prominent in the neonatal period. Hypoglycemic seizures can occur.

b. Typical physical features include doll-like facies with excessive fatty tissue in the cheeks, very protuberant abdomen due to a massively enlarged liver, relatively thin extremities, accentuated lumbar lordosis, as well as the short stature.

c. Muscle hypotonia can occur at a relatively young age.

d. Xanthomas and retinal changes may occur as a result of the hyperlipidemia.

e. Spleen and heart are of normal size.

f. The typical age at presentation is after 3 to 4 months with hepatomegaly or hypoglycemia. One contributing factor for presentation at this age may be increased spacing between meals.

g. Recurrent bacterial infection suggest type Ib. Enteritis may be very significant. Infections cause significant morbidity and may be the cause of death in these patients.

h. Long-term complications (second or third decade) in type I disease include hepatic adenomas, chronic renal disease, and gout. The renal disease is preceded by glomerular hyperfiltration and microalbuminuria. Puberty is often delayed.

2. Infantile type II disease presents as muscle weakness, hypotonia, and often symptoms of cardiac or respiratory failure.

a. Whereas in some infants the disorder is recognized at or shortly after birth, in others the signs and symptoms are often noticed during an acute respiratory tract infection.

b. Unlike spinal muscular atrophy, the diaphragm is involved in infantile type II.

c. Enlargement of the tongue, liver, and kidneys can be demonstrated.

d. Electrocardiographic abnormalities occur with massive QRS complexes and shortened PR intervals.

e. Death occurs within the first 2 years as a result of respiratory tract infection, cardiac compromise, and bulbar paralysis.

f. Later presentations of type II disease are more variable, with muscle involvement and less rapid cardiac involvement. Delays in motor milestones have been reported with loss of skills as the disease progresses. Hypoventilation as a result of diaphragmatic disease may occur.

3. Type V disease is restricted to muscle findings or the consequence of muscle breakdown. Progressive signs are easy fatigability in childhood, stiffness or cramps on exertion, and myoglobinuria with minimal to moderate exercise. Later signs include weakness and wasting of the proximal muscles. Discomfort on exertion that responds to short rest should always raise the possibility of type V disease. A forearm ischemia test, performed by exercising the muscles after inflation of an occluding cuff, may reproduce the muscle cramps.

Laboratory Findings

1. Typical findings for GSD type I include: hypoglycemia 4 to 6 hours after a meal, lactic acidemia, and increased plasma fatty acids. Hypertriglyceridemia and hypercholesterolemia with milky serum and hyperuricemia are typical. Platelet aggregation is faulty and factor VIII levels are decreased as secondary phenomena.

2. Unique to type Ib are neutropenia and neutrophil dysfunction with altered chemotaxis and decreased oxidative activity.

3. Liver transaminase levels are usually normal or only slightly elevated. Although adenomas are common, cirrhosis does not occur.

4. Liver biopsy demonstrates the glycogen accumulation and the specific enzyme defect.

5. Glucagon will increase blood lactate but not blood glucose in either the fasting or fed states.

6. Type II disease is generally diagnosed based on clinical suspicion and muscle biopsy, which shows decreased

enzyme activity. Blood glucose levels are normal, and the other laboratory features seen in type I disease are absent.

7. In type III, blood lactate elevations are not a prominent finding. The serum creatine kinase level can be elevated because of the muscle disease. Glucagon can cause an increase in blood glucose in the fed but not fasting state.

8. Patients with type V disease will not have lactate elevations after ischemic exercise.

   a. Blood ammonia concentrations are elevated in the ischemic bed. The definitive diagnosis is made on muscle tissue in which absence of the phosphorylase can be demonstrated histologically and biochemically.

   b. Myoglobinuria is another clue.

   c. Ischemic testing will also be abnormal in debrancher diseases when performed in the fasted state and in other metabolic myopathies.

Radiographic Findings

1. In GSD type 1, the hepatomegaly can be confirmed. Ultrasound examinations in the second or third decade will show the adenoma. Malignant transformation occurs rarely, so follow-up examinations are indicated.

2. In type II GSD, echocardiography and ultrasonography demonstrate the involvement of the heart, liver, and kidneys.

3. Bone disease is not a prominent part of the GSDs.

Treatment

1. The treatment of GSD Ia involves the maintenance of blood glucose concentrations and the suppression of hyperlacticacidemia by dietary means.

   a. Goals are providing glucose: 8 to 10 mg/kg/min in infants and 5 to 7 mg/kg/min in school-aged children. Caloric distribution is 65 to 70 per cent carbohydrate, 10 to 15 per cent protein, and the rest from fats. A third of the calories are provided at night. During infancy, frequent feedings are essential. With increasing age, nocturnal glucose-containing feeds by nasogastric tube are used. Uncooked cornstarch has been shown to be effective in providing a slowly released source of glucose in older patients. It provides a means of achieving normal glycemia for 6 to 8 hours when the equivalent amount of glucose would maintain normal blood sugar levels for 3 hours.

   b. Fructose and galactose (as well as lactose) are restricted because these sugars cannot be converted to free glucose. These sugars contribute to lactate production.

   c. Therapy is monitored by determining blood glucose concentrations before meals and during continuous caloric supplementation. Lactate measurements are also useful to gauge the adequacy of therapy.

   d. Liver transplantation has been performed in a few cases with resolution of the dysmetabolism. Because metabolic control can be achieved without the risks of the transplant, it is not considered a first-line therapy.

2. No specific treatment exists for type II GSD presenting in infancy. Late forms of the disease may be treated with a high-protein diet with some success.

3. Type V GSD is most often treated by avoiding strenuous exercise. Exercise tolerance can be increased by oral glucose or fructose as well as by glucagon injection. Some patients benefit from a high-protein diet. Coenzyme Q (ubiquinone) may provide subjective relief.

 ## Bibliography

Chen YT, Burchell A: Glycogen storage diseases. *In* Scriver CR, Beaudet AL, Sly WS, Valle D (eds): The Metabolic and Molecular Bases of Inherited Disease, 7th ed. New York, McGraw-Hill, 1995, pp 935–966.

Fernandes J: The glycogen storage diseases. *In* Fernandes J, Saudubray J-M, Tada K (eds): Inborn Metabolic Diseases: Diagnosis and Treatment. Berlin, Springer-Verlag, 1990, pp 69–88.

Gitzelmann R: Disorders of galactose metabolism. *In* Fernandes J, Saudubray J-M, Tada K (eds): Inborn Metabolic Diseases: Diagnosis and Treatment. Berlin, Springer-Verlag, 1990, pp 95–106.

Gitzelmann R, Steinmann B, Van de Berghe G: Disorders of fructose metabolism. *In* Scriver CR, Beaudet AL, Sly WS, Valle D (eds): The Metabolic and Molecular Bases of Inherited Disease, 7th ed. New York, McGraw-Hill, 1995, pp 905–934.

Odievre M, Gentil C, Gautier M, Alagille D: Hereditary fructose intolerance in childhood: Diagnosis, management and course in 55 patients. Am J Dis Child 1978;132:605–608.

Segal S, Berry GT: Disorders of galactose metabolism. *In* Scriver CR, Beaudet AL, Sly WS, Valle D (eds): The Metabolic and Molecular Bases of Inherited Disease, 7th ed. New York, McGraw-Hill, 1995, pp 967–1000.

65 Lysosomal Storage Disorders

Carol L. Greene

General Discussion

Definition

Lysosomal storage disorders are caused by failure to degrade one or more molecules in lysosomes.

Etiology

1. For each biochemical step in the lysosome, the possibility exists for a lysosomal storage disorder. An authoritative text on inborn errors of metabolism has 17 chapters on the various categories of lysosomal storage disorders, describing at least 34 unique enzyme defects.
2. The etiology may be autosomal recessive, with some being X-linked (Hunter syndrome and Fabry disease).

Epidemiology

1. Frequency of all lysosomal storage disorders in the general population is unknown, but most individual disorders apparently affect ≤1/100,000. Since these conditions are often undiagnosed, true frequency is likely to be higher than currently estimated.
2. Ethnicity is an important risk factor for some conditions, with frequency of a specific disorder more than 1/10,000 births in certain populations. However, each disease may still appear in any population.
3. Specific population increased risks include
   a. Tay-Sachs disease in Ashkenazi Jews, French-Canadians, Acadians (Louisiana), and Pennsylvania Dutch; additionally, in Switzerland and Japan.
   b. Gaucher disease in Ashkenazi Jews.
   c. Niemann-Pick type C disease in Nova Scotia and in the southern Colorado Hispanic population.

Pathophysiology

1. Lysosomes are intracellular organelles in which certain biochemical functions are localized in a unique microenvironment. Molecules metabolized in the lysosome are typically large and found in membranes (e.g., mucopolysaccharides [MPS, aka glycosaminoglycans], sphingolipids, glucocerebrocides, gangliosides, and glycoproteins). The lysosome is also the location for metabolism of some small molecules, such as sialic acid. Type of material stored is an important criterion for classification of lysosomal disorders.
2. Varying mutations have been observed in different families with each disorder. In some lysosomal storage diseases with ethnic predilection, specific mutations may be common. However, even in these populations, many different mutations may be seen. This variability in type of mutation (genotype) causes differences in the nature and severity of the biochemical defect and thereby contributes to the variability in clinical findings (phenotype).

3. The term *lysosomal storage disorders* connotes the diagnostic and pathophysiologic importance of the accumulated material that proved to contain undigested large molecules in lysosomes (also see Laboratory Findings).
   a. The amount of stored material varies from tissue to tissue.
   b. In a few lysosomal disorders, characteristic pathology does not include stored material within the membrane-bound lysosome.
4. Biochemical and cellular mechanisms by which lysosomal storage disorders cause the clinical phenotype are not well understood. Membrane function may be altered by changes in membrane components due to failure of degradation of macromolecules or from incorrect handling of small molecule components of membrane macromolecules.
5. Some typical patterns of organ involvement are observed for individual disorders or classes of disorders. Some conditions appear to affect only a single organ system during the individual's natural life span, and some disorders affect multiple organ systems.
   a. Most lysosomal disorders may affect the central nervous system (CNS). Some individual disorders invariably affect the brain (e.g., Tay-Sachs, Sanfilippo), while some invariably affect the peripheral nervous system (e.g., Fabry). For some disorders (e.g., Gaucher), the same enzyme defect may be observed with or without neurologic involvement. Neurologic presentation is determined by the portion of the nervous system most affected, that is, gray or white matter, central or peripheral.
   b. Some lysosomal disorders always have an evident and often clinically significant effect on bones (e.g., mucopolysaccharidosis [MPS]), whereas some appear to have no bone findings.
   c. Skin and soft tissue involvement in some conditions leads to coarse features (described below) and upper airway obstruction.
   d. Some lysosomal storage diseases significantly affect hematopoietic tissues.
   e. Other important organs that may be affected include kidney, eye, heart and lower respiratory system (also see Clinical Findings).
   f. If overwhelming multiple organ system involvement is present before birth, nonimmune hydrops may be present.
6. For each condition, there is a wide range for the age of onset and the severity of symptoms. Siblings usually have similar presentation, but variation may be seen within families.

Clinical Findings

1. Presentation and course vary widely. Some general features found in more than one condition are described below.
2. All lysosomal disorders are progressive.
3. For most, there is a period of normal growth, development, and health before the onset of symptoms. This may vary from months (e.g., classic Tay-Sachs) to decades (adult Tay-Sachs).
   a. Some individuals have no recognizable period of normal development.
   b. Prenatal onset may be seen. Presentation may include bone disease and coarse features; may resemble intrauterine infection with hepatosplenomegaly and evidence of peripheral hematopoiesis; or may be nonspecific with nonimmune hydrops or intractable seizures.
4. For conditions altering neurologic function and behavior:
   a. Loss of developmental milestones, generally described as regression, occurs only when the progress of the disease is faster than normal development. In late-onset disease, development slows and plateaus for months or years before regression is apparent.
   b. Isolated behavioral and/or psychiatric presentation may be the first finding at any age in disorders affecting the neurologic system, with neurologic and developmental problems evident only later.
5. For most conditions, careful physical and neurologic evaluation will reveal clues to the presence of a lysosomal storage disorder. *However, findings may be subtle or restricted to one organ system, and not all features associated with lysosomal storage disorders are present in all conditions.* Important clinical presentations include
   a. Neurodevelopmental abnormality may include regression in developmental or intellectual function; hypotonia, hypertonia, or dystonia; seizures; ataxia; pain or paresthesias; and behavioral or psychiatric disturbance. Secondary neurologic dysfunction may also result from bone disease compromising nerve roots.
   b. Hepatomegaly or splenomegaly is invariably present in some classes of lysosomal storage disease and ranges from dramatic to subtle.
   c. Coarse features usually develop with variable severity in MPS and the disorders of glycoprotein metabolism. A fullness in the appearance of the area between upper lid and brow may be the earliest change, progressing to fullness and thickening of lips and facies. Coarse features may be difficult to distinguish from the appearance of prolonged exposure to phenytoin.
   d. Bone and joint changes (also see Radiology)
      (1) In some conditions, dysostosis multiplex may be subtle or obvious on physical examination. Subtle findings are widened metaphyses and decreased range of motion of joints. Later, spine and joint changes may severely limit function, with severe restriction of range of motion of chest and proximal joints. Bone disease may present as short stature.
      (2) Atlanto-occipital instability is present in some conditions (especially Hunter syndrome) and may cause paresis or death with fairly mild hyperextension. Other spine changes may cause damage to spinal column or spinal roots.
      (3) Pathologic fractures due to osteoporosis are seen in later stages of Gaucher disease, along with bone pain and occasionally "aseptic osteomyelitis."
   e. Cardiac disease is important in some lysosomal diseases, with valvular disease, cardiomyopathy, or endomyocardial fibroelastosis. When the respiratory system is compromised, cor pulmonale may cause or contribute to mortality.
   f. Many lysosomal conditions produce eye findings. Some cause changes in the retina; the classic "cherry red spot," virtually pathognomonic for lysosomal storage disease, describes the appearance of macular pallor and a prominent fovea centralis. Some conditions cause corneal clouding, cataracts, or other retinal findings.
   g. Deafness resulting primarily from a combination of decreased motion of ossicles and recurrent otitis is common in some lysosomal disorders.
   h. Acute or chronic respiratory failure is the most common cause of death in most lysosomal storage disorders. Lung parenchyma may be directly involved, with evidence of storage compromising function. Upper airway obstruction is important in MPS and some disorders of glycoprotein metabolism, presenting with chronic rhinorrhea and noisy or labored breathing. Anesthesia is highly risky in these patients because of extreme difficulty with intubation. Some conditions cause restrictive pulmonary disease because of spine and chest wall configuration. Recurrent pneumonia, due to failure to cough and/or aspiration, is the most common cause of death in any of the lysosomal disorders affecting the neurologic system.
   i. Altered growth velocity is found with both tall stature (some Sanfilippo patients) and short stature; short stature may be the first clinical clue to important bone changes.
   j. Altered head growth is important in a few disorders, with both macrocephaly (e.g., Tay-Sachs) and microcephaly (e.g., Krabbe) possible.
   k. Skin findings are present in some disorders, ranging from thickened or sometimes "pebbly" skin (some MPS) to ichthyotic changes (neonatal presentation of Gaucher disease) or angiokeratoma (telangiectasias seen in Fabry disease).
   l. Hydrops fetalis may be the presentation of several lysosomal storage disorders.

- All lysosomal disorders are progressive.

- Age of onset ranges from prenatal to adult years.

- Lysosomal diseases may involve almost any organ system.

- Neurologic disease may first present as behavior disturbance.

Laboratory Findings

1. Light and electron microscopy shows storage material in almost every lysosomal storage disorder, and in most the evidence is seen in skin and conjunctival specimens as well as clinically affected tissue and organs. White blood cells may show a characteristic appearance. Pathologic specimens may give the first laboratory evidence of lysosomal storage disease. However, usually diagnosis can be pursued with less invasive testing designed to give a specific biochemical diagnosis.

2. Excretion in urine of partially metabolized substrate can be shown in most conditions and is used for clinical diagnostic evaluation in some categories of disease. In other conditions, measurement of urine excretion is not suitable for rapid diagnostic testing.

   a. In most individuals with MPS, the amount of mucopolysaccharide in urine is increased and the pattern is altered. Most laboratories offering MPS assay begin with a spot or screening test that may be positive in normal individuals. Analysis of type of MPS is required. Urine mucopolysaccharide may be falsely negative in a dilute sample, and in one of the disease types, no mucopolysaccharide is excreted.

   b. Analysis of amount and pattern of smaller molecules in urine, such as oligosaccharides, or specific assay for one molecule associated with a particular disease suspected on clinical grounds, may be considered and discussed with a biochemical genetics laboratory or consultant.

3. Enzyme assay to demonstrate deficiency or, when possible, search for a specific mutation in DNA is required to prove diagnosis of disease or carrier state.

   a. Enzyme assay must be performed in samples properly handled to preserve activity of lysosomal enzymes. Protocol for the reference laboratory must be followed.

   b. For some conditions, pseudodeficient genes (gene for enzyme that has no activity in the test tube but has sufficient activity in the individual to prevent disease) complicate the interpretation of results of enzyme assays.

   c. Most conditions can be diagnosed using white blood cells, with serum useful in a few (e.g., Tay-Sachs). In some conditions, fibroblasts or other tissues are necessary to make the diagnosis or to clarify ambiguous results.

   d. Carrier testing by enzyme assay is available only when the typical carrier can be distinguished from noncarriers in the population. Accuracy of carrier identification varies with factors such as the tissue type tested, the population tested, and, for some conditions, whether the individual is tested while pregnant.

   e. For carrier tests utilizing DNA diagnosis, accuracy depends upon the correct identification of the disease causing mutation in the family being tested. When the mutation is known, carrier testing may be highly accurate. When DNA tests are used for individuals identified only as members of an at-risk population, results are expressed as statistical risk of being a carrier.

- Urine screening tests are available for some lysosomal disorders.

- Diagnosis is made by demonstration of specific enzyme defect or DNA change.

- Carrier tests and prenatal tests are usually, but not always, available.

Radiographic Findings

1. Bone changes may be diagnostic for some of the lysosomal storage disorders.

   a. Dysostosis multiplex is characteristic of MPS and some of the disorders of glycoprotein metabolism. Earliest changes of dysostosis are often found most easily on examination of a lateral spine film. Changes may include alteration of the intervertebral space, "beaking" of vertebrae, loss of lumbar lordosis, and development of lumbothoracic kyphosis.

   b. Infiltration of bone marrow with storage material in some conditions causes osteoporosis beginning in tubular bones and vertebrae, followed by loss of concavity above the femoral condyles. In later stages, thinning of cortex is seen and periostitis may be present; finally, destruction of femoral and humeral head and sclerosis are seen in severe disease.

2. Head imaging is invaluable in the diagnosis and monitoring of many lysosomal disorders. For conditions that cause both chronic atrophy and risk for acute and chronic increased intracranial pressure, there is controversy over the use of routine CT or MRI for monitoring in the absence of new symptoms. Either may fail to identify signs of increased intracranial pressure; MRI is the more accurate test but has significantly higher risk in patients in whom upper airway disease increases the likelihood of morbidity or mortality from sedation.

Treatment

1. Research now in progress may lead to rapid changes in treatment, and it will always be appropriate to inquire whether new clinically validated or research therapies are available.

2. Gene therapy is expected to be the optimal treatment. For some lysosomal disorders, efforts to develop gene

therapy are already under way, but no human trials have begun.

3. Currently the most powerful approach to treatment of lysosomal storage disease is delivery of functioning enzyme to affected cells. Two general strategies are employed:

    a. Enzyme infusion requires targeting and uptake of the infused enzyme into lysosomes of appropriate cells and tissues. For Gaucher disease, clinically effective enzyme infusion is now available.

    b. Bone marrow transplantation is the most commonly considered method to introduce cells with normal production of enzyme into the affected individual. Outcome varies with the disease and with timing of intervention. For diseases whose primary effect is on the reticuloendothelial system, bone marrow transplantation is highly successful. For conditions with more involvement of other tissues, ongoing studies in animals and humans show evidence for delay of development of systemic symptoms, and studies to determine whether symptoms are prevented are in progress. Clinical evidence in humans and animals also shows better developmental outcome in some conditions, but not in others.

4. Most therapy is supportive and involves monitoring for symptoms found in a specific condition; intervention is designed to decrease the effect of the disease on function. Important examples of intervention include:

    a. For conditions causing upper airway obstruction, monitoring by ENT with appropriate use of tonsillectomy and adenoidectomy is standard in order to slow the development of chronic hypoxia and cor pulmonale. In later stages, oxygen may be used at night, and more aggressive therapy may be considered (see below).

    b. Orthopedic problems must be closely followed and treated aggressively to preserve function as long as possible. For some conditions, surgery protects joint function and prevents or decreases compromise of spinal cord and nerve roots.

    c. Cardiac status must be monitored in some disorders; treatment may include endocarditis prophylaxis and treatment for heart failure.

    d. Neck hyperextension must be avoided in conditions with unstable atlantoaxial joint. This affects recreational activity, physical therapy, and anesthesia.

    e. Eye examination provides clues to function and to intracranial pressure. When present, cataracts or corneal opacity may be treated.

    f. Deafness that may be caused by lysosomal storage disease will often be amenable to augmentation. Many affected individuals can effectively use alternative communication, and speech and language therapy is appropriate.

    g. Splenectomy may be needed to control hypersplenism; splenectomy should be avoided, if possible, in Gaucher disease while medical treatment is begun (see below). Transfusions may be required in conditions affecting the hematopoietic system.

    h. Ventricular shunting will alleviate symptomatic increased intracranial pressure. Prophylaxis is not appropriate, since most patients do not develop symptoms.

    i. Anesthesia requires special precautions in individuals with upper or lower airway compromise, neck instability, or heart disease.

    j. More invasive and possibly extraordinary supportive interventions exist and must be considered. A nasogastric or gastrostomy tube permits delivery of fluids and nutrients to the individual who is no longer able to swallow adequately. Tracheostomy may be considered when upper airway obstruction is part of the pathophysiology. Tracheostomy may also be considered in late stages of any of the conditions affecting the neurologic system, in order to better control clearance of secretions. In some cases, positive pressure ventilation may be considered. Patients and families may have or develop strong opinions about whether such interventions prolong life or prolong dying. Clear presentation of facts and alternatives is necessary, followed by support for the decision of the patient and family.

Key Treatment: General Lysosomal Disorders

- Supportive treatment for airway
- Enzyme replacement where possible

Prevention

1. Since these conditions are present from conception, approaches to prevention are limited to reproductive options when there is reason to suspect risk of disease, usually in a family with a previously affected member or in certain populations at significant risk. Currently, reproductive options available for most lysosomal conditions range from simply accepting known risk, to carrier testing and prenatal diagnosis. Genetic counseling is the process by which health care providers and families acquire and evaluate the information that permits informed choices.

2. Accuracy of carrier testing varies (see Laboratory Findings, above). For certain disorders, such as Tay-Sachs, voluntary population carrier testing is offered worldwide to at-risk individuals; for other conditions, however, no carrier test is currently possible.

3. Prenatal testing is available for most lysosomal storage disorders by appropriate enzyme assay, and for some conditions DNA diagnosis may contribute. For most of these disorders, a sample for assay may be collected either by amniocentesis or by chorionic villus sampling; however, exceptions are important, and it is always necessary to obtain the most current information for each disorder.

Specific Lysosomal Disorders

Hurler Syndrome (MPS I)

Mild or late-onset disease is called Scheie disease or MPS I-S.

Etiology

1. Caused by decreased activity of the enzyme α-L-iduronidase, with storage in lysosomes primarily of dermatan sulfate and heparan sulfate
2. Autosomal recessive.

Clinical Findings

1. Bone, soft tissue, and heart are invariably affected, and the CNS is clinically affected in early-onset but not late-onset disease.
2. Moderate dysostosis multiplex and development of coarse features are usual presenting features. Changes are subtle but evident by age 6 months in the childhood form, and obvious by age 2 years. In the milder form, bone changes are milder and of later onset.
3. Spinal disease may cause myelopathy in either form. In the childhood form, the CNS is invariably involved, with plateau and loss of milestones usually evident by age 2 years. Acute and chronic increased intracranial pressure may develop and contribute to clinical neurologic presentation.
4. Deafness is progressive.
5. Corneal opacity is progressive and other eye findings may be present.
6. Cardiorespiratory disease is the usual cause of death, with heart failure usually due to a combination of cardiac valve disease and cor pulmonale.
7. Life expectancy for the classic early-onset presentation is ≤10 years. For the later onset form, life expectancy varies but is measured in decades and may be normal in the most mildly affected individuals.

Laboratory and Radiographic Findings

1. Dermatan and heparan sulfate are present in urine.
2. Dysostosis multiplex is evident on radiologic study.
3. Diagnosis is made by demonstrating decreased α-L-iduronidase activity.
4. Head imaging shows loss of volume of cerebral cortex.

Treatment

1. Supportive treatment is offered, including monitoring hearing and providing aids and alternative communication when needed; monitoring vision; monitoring cardiac status and using medical therapy for congestive failure; monitoring neurologic status and providing shunting, if required. Tonsillectomy and adenoidectomy, used with caution because of the high anesthesia risks, provide temporary relief of some upper airway obstruction, and tracheostomy is considered.
2. Bone marrow transplant, performed early in the course of the disorder, delays or prevents development of many of the systemic symptoms. In some early cases, decreased mucopolysaccharide was seen in spinal fluid. A systematic program of ongoing monitoring of patients post transplant is in progress to determine the effect of transplantation on long-term neurologic outcome.

Prevention

Carrier testing and prenatal diagnosis by enzyme assay are available.

Hunter Syndrome (MPS II)

Etiology

1. Caused by decreased activity of the enzyme iduronate sulfatase, with storage in lysosomes of primarily dermatan sulfate and heparan sulfate
2. X-linked recessive.

Clinical Findings

Features are similar to Hurler syndrome except for

1. Slower progress of both the somatic and the neurologic features, with life expectancy varying from death before age 15 years in the early-onset severe form to survival to the twenties to sixties in the milder presentation.
2. Similar dysostosis multiplex and coarse features but with more severe cervical instability, which may be the cause of death or disability
3. There is no corneal clouding.

Laboratory and Radiographic Findings

1. Dysostosis multiplex is evident on radiologic study.
2. Heparan and dermatan sulfate are excreted in urine (same as in Hurler syndrome).
3. Diagnosis is made by demonstration of decreased iduronate sulfatase activity.
4. Head imaging shows loss of volume of cerebral cortex.

Treatment

Treatment is essentially the same as for Hurler syndrome.

Prevention

1. Carrier testing is available by enzyme assay in blood or other tissue but is complicated by X-chromosome inactivation. If a specific mutation is known, DNA diagnosis improves accuracy.
2. Prenatal diagnosis by enzyme assay is available. In families with a known mutation, prenatal diagnosis by DNA analysis is possible.

Sanfilippo Syndrome (MPS III)

Etiology

1. Caused by deficient activity of any one of four enzymes required for the metabolism of the mucopolysaccharide heparan sulfate, resulting in storage of heparan sulfate. Types A, B, C, and D are recognized and correspond to each of the four enzyme deficiencies observed.
2. Autosomal recessive.

Clinical Findings

1. The CNS is the primary organ affected. Bone is involved with mild dysostosis radiologically and late development of mild clinical findings of bone and soft tissue.
2. The typical initial presentation is behavioral with hyperactivity and aggressive behavior developing in a toddler or preschool child, but presentation may be earlier or later. Although some children have no apparent period of normal development, most show early normal development followed by plateau for months or years before evidence of regression. Presentation in early childhood resembles autism.

3. Seizures develop and severe neurologic degeneration leads to death after a course lasting years or decades.

Laboratory and Radiographic Findings

1. Heparan sulfate is usually excreted in the urine in amounts sufficient to be detected on examination of mucopolysaccharides in urine. False negative tests may be observed, however, especially in dilute samples.
2. Diagnosis is made by demonstration of deficiency of activity of one of the four enzymes required for metabolism of heparan sulfate.
3. Mild dysostosis is evident, especially on examination of the lateral spine.
4. Mild to moderate cortical atrophy is usually evident on CT or MRI studies.

Treatment

Supportive treatment addresses the severe behavioral and sleep disturbances, but pharmacologic management is usually not very successful.

Prevention

1. Carrier testing may be available by assay of appropriate enzyme.
2. Prenatal diagnosis by enzyme assay is available.

Tay-Sachs Disease

Etiology

1. Caused by deficient activity of hexosaminidase A, with resulting storage of gangliosides and related glycolipids
2. Autosomal recessive.

Epidemiology

1. Frequency is increased in several populations, including Ashkenazi Jews, French-Canadians, Acadians (Louisiana), and Pennsylvania Dutch; additionally in Switzerland and Japan. The carrier frequency in Ashkenazi Jews is estimated at 1/27.
2. Some common mutations have been identified in specific populations.

Clinical Findings

1. The classic presentation is the infantile form, with clinical onset in the first months of life and death expected by age 4 years. Infants appear normal at birth, with mild motor weakness and exaggerated startle response appearing at age 3 to 5 months.
2. Weakness is progressive, with developmental plateau and regression at age 6 to 10 months, sometimes with visual inattentiveness and/or unusual eye movements.
3. Seizures are typical by 1 year of age, and neurologic deterioration progresses until the child develops swallowing difficulties, demonstrates decerebrate posturing, and finally becomes completely unresponsive.
4. Head circumference increases across percentiles over time, with macrocephaly usual in the second year of life.
5. By the onset of symptoms, a "cherry red spot" is usually present on ophthalmologic examination.
6. Onset may be later, with survival into later childhood or adult life. In childhood onset, typical initial symptoms are ataxia and incoordination, followed by developmental regression and dementia and progressive spasticity. Seizures and blindness develop, and death is usual in adolescence.
7. Adolescent and later onset disease is characterized by a more variable presentation. Psychiatric symptoms, including acute-onset schizophrenia, may precede or accompany progressive dystonia, spinocerebellar degeneration, or a presentation resembling lower motor neuron disease.

Laboratory Findings

Hexosaminidase A deficiency must be demonstrated in serum, white blood cells, or fibroblasts. Pseudodeficiency alleles may occasionally complicate diagnostic testing.

Treatment

Supportive treatment addresses feeding and respiratory problems.

Prevention

1. Carrier testing is available by enzyme assay on serum, white blood cells, or other cultured cells. Pseudodeficiency alleles are sufficiently common in the general population to complicate the interpretation of carrier testing in individuals from populations that are not at high risk for Tay-Sachs disease. DNA analysis for specific known mutations or pseudodeficiency alleles may be used for clarification.
2. Prenatal diagnosis by enzyme assay is available.

Metachromatic Leukodystrophy

Etiology

1. Caused by deficiency of arylsulfatase A, resulting in storage of sulfatides
2. Autosomal recessive.

Clinical Findings

1. The most common age of onset is infancy or early childhood; it is manifested as difficulty in walking. Peripheral neuropathy usually leads to decreased or absent reflexes. Dementia and spastic paraplegia are followed by death, usually in the first 6 years of life.
2. Childhood onset is usually noted in early school years, with retrospective recognition of poor coordination and slow development over previous years. Ataxia, spasticity, and decreased tendon reflexes are followed by dementia, spastic quadriplegia, and sometimes dystonia over the next few years. In adolescent or adult presentation, psychiatric symptoms resembling schizophrenia are often the initial feature.
3. Primarily affects the central and peripheral nervous systems. The kidney may also be involved, with renal tubular acidosis observed, but this has little impact on the clinical course.

Laboratory Findings

1. Spinal fluid protein is elevated.
2. CT and MRI show central demyelination, and there may be cerebellar atrophy.
3. Diagnosis is made by demonstration of decreased activity of arylsulfatase A in blood or other tissue. A pseudodeficient allele is found in .05 to 1 per cent of the general population.

Treatment

1. Bone marrow transplantation may slow the course of the neurodegeneration. However, since the disease progresses rapidly once symptomatic, and any potential benefit of transplantation will not be seen for several months, risks of the treatment are usually considered to outweigh benefit except in those individuals in whom diagnosis can be made before any symptoms are observed.
2. Supportive therapy is offered.

Prevention

1. Carrier testing is available on blood or other tissue. The pseudodeficient allele complicates carrier testing, and further biochemical or DNA analysis may be needed.
2. Prenatal diagnosis by enzyme assay is available. The pseudodeficient allele is sufficiently common that enzyme assay of both parents is necessary in order to be certain that prenatal test results are interpretable.

Krabbe Disease

Etiology

1. Caused by deficient activity of galactosylceramidase, resulting in storage of ceramide
2. Autosomal recessive.

Epidemiology

Worldwide incidence estimated at 1/100,000 to 200,000 births, with possible higher frequency in Scandinavian countries.

Clinical Findings

1. Early-onset disease presents in the first 6 months of life with extreme irritability, hypertonicity, and exaggerated response to stimuli. Vision and hearing are lost rapidly. The infant develops opisthotonus, seizures, and microcephaly. Peripheral neuropathy is present.
2. Hypotonia develops later in the course, and loss of brainstem function may be accompanied by unexplained fevers. Death usually occurs from respiratory complications at around 1 year of age.
3. Later onset disease may begin in infancy with loss of vision, ataxia, irritability, and motor regression with hypertonia. Later in childhood, loss of vision is the most common presenting symptom, but hemiparesis may be the first feature. Peripheral neuropathy is variable.

Laboratory and Radiographic Findings

1. Spinal fluid protein is elevated.
2. Nerve conduction velocities are delayed.
3. Diagnosis is made by demonstration of deficiency of galactosylceraminidase activity.
4. White matter degeneration is seen on CT and MRI, and calcifications may be present in basal ganglia or white matter.

Treatment

No specific treatment is available. For the early infantile form, treatment must especially address the severe irritability. Bone marrow transplantation has been attempted in late-onset disease, without conclusive evidence of effectiveness.

Prevention

1. Carrier testing is available by enzyme assay on blood or other tissue but is not completely reliable, since some carriers have enzyme activity measured in the normal range.
2. Prenatal diagnosis by enzyme assay is available.

Fabry Disease

Etiology

1. Caused by deficiency of α-galactosidase A, resulting in storage of glycosphingolipids
2. X-linked recessive.

Epidemiology

Incidence is estimated at 1/40,000, and all races may be affected.

Clinical Findings

1. Affected males typically present in late childhood or early adolescence with episodic or chronic severe pain in extremities. Abdominal painful crises may resemble appendicitis or renal colic. Pain crisis is usually accompanied by low-grade fever and increased erythrocyte sedimentation rate, which may lead to a misdiagnosis of conditions such as rheumatic fever or collagen vascular disease.
2. The course is characterized early by variable development of angiectases of skin, especially around the groin and buttocks, and by a characteristic lens opacity.
3. With increasing age, the vascular disease leads to cardiac dysfunction ranging from arrhythmias to hypertrophy, infarction, and heart failure.
4. Renal involvement may begin in childhood, presenting with proteinuria and hypertension, with progression to renal failure by middle age.
5. Episodic diarrhea, nausea, and vomiting may be present at any age.
6. A few affected males have virtually no symptoms, or only cardiac findings, at ages well past the usual age of onset in their family members.
7. Hemizygous females may have significant symptoms or may be completely asymptomatic. Corneal changes are eventually present in more than half the carrier females, and isolated skin angiectases may be seen. Intermittent pain may be present, renal involvement may be evident, and cardiac disease may develop over time.

Laboratory Findings

Diagnosis is made by demonstration of decreased activity of α-galactosidase A.

Treatment

1. Experimental studies in progress include chronic plasmapheresis or repeated phlebotomy to deplete the levels of unmetabolizable substrate; efforts to develop enzyme infusion treatment; and transplantation with fetal liver.
2. Phenytoin and carbamazepine have proved fairly effective for control of pain.
3. Renal transplantation is used to correct kidney failure.

Prevention

1. Carrier testing is complicated by random X-inactivation, and enzyme activity in carriers may also change with age. DNA diagnosis is used to clarify diagnosis of carrier status; it first requires identification of the mutation in each family, since no common mutations are observed. Closely linked DNA markers may aid in diagnosis if the mutation is unknown.
2. Prenatal diagnosis is possible by enzyme assay.

Gaucher Disease

Etiology

1. Caused by deficient activity of glucocerebrocidase, resulting in storage of glucosylceramide
2. Autosomal recessive.

Epidemiology

1. Increased frequency in Ashkenazi Jews, with carrier frequency ≥1 in 20
2. Much is known about the various mutations that cause decreased enzyme activity, with some correlation between the type of mutation and the clinical presentation.

Clinical Findings

Current classification divides Gaucher disease into three types. Type 1 is the most common over all ages. Types 2 and 3 always present in childhood. Definition of the types of Gaucher disease depends upon the presence or absence and the nature of neurologic disease.

1. Bone disease due to infiltration of the bone marrow is present and in late stages causes disability due to pathologic fractures and degeneration of large joints. Painful bone crises and recurrent aseptic osteomyelitis, when present, are also debilitating. When vertebrae are involved, spine disease may progress rapidly in puberty. Vertebral disease at any age may compromise spinal cord or nerve roots.
2. Lung parenchyma may be affected in any form of Gaucher disease and may cause clinically significant compromise of oxygenation, especially in individuals with childhood onset.
3. Neurologic disease is seen in types 2 and 3 Gaucher disease. In type 2, onset is in early infancy, with rapid progression and death in early childhood due to aspiration and inanition. Type 3 presents in childhood. It is distinguished from childhood onset of type 1 by the presence or development of subtle neurologic findings beginning with abnormal eye movement, followed by development of ataxia and slow progression of neurologic disease.
4. Fetal onset of symptoms is seen in some individuals with Gaucher disease who are born with massive hepatosplenomegaly resembling in utero infection. Usually, but not always, these babies have severe neonatal ichthyosis.

Laboratory and Radiographic Findings

1. "Gaucher cells" are monocyte-macrophage line cells with a characteristic striated or tubular appearance to the cytoplasm; these are seen in bone marrow aspirates or other tissue samples and may be observed in the peripheral blood. These cells resemble storage cells seen in other conditions, and diagnosis must be made by enzyme assay or DNA studies.
2. Diagnosis is made by demonstration of deficient glucocerebrocidase activity.
3. Bone films show osteoporosis. "Erlenmeyer flask deformity" of the distal femur is common. Chest x-ray may show infiltrative lung parenchymal disease.

Treatment

1. Gaucher disease is one of the few lysosomal storage disorders for which currently available treatment is known to be effective. However, the treatment is effective only in individuals without neurologic disease. The enzyme glucocerebrocidase has been both isolated from human placenta and synthesized using recombinant DNA technology. From either source, the enzyme must be appropriately modified to ensure uptake by affected cells. The modified enzyme is periodically infused by vein. Controversies exist about appropriate dose, and studies are ongoing with respect to risk of long-term complications, including development of antibodies against the infused enzyme. Clear improvement in existing symptoms, including resolution of hepatosplenomegaly and anemia as well as some healing of bone disease, is expected in the treated patient. Development of further symptoms is prevented, but existing joint deformity does not resolve. Growth improves in children with type 1 disease treated before puberty.
2. Splenectomy is now avoided when possible but is still occasionally necessary.
3. Supportive treatment, such as transfusion for anemia and management of neurologic symptoms, is the only strategy available for individuals with types 2 and 3 disease.

Prevention

Carrier testing and prenatal diagnosis are available by enzyme assay or, if the mutation is known, DNA testing.

Niemann-Pick Disease

Etiology

1. Types A and B are caused by deficient activity of sphingomyelinase, resulting in storage of sphingomyelin in lysosomes.
2. Type C is caused by a defect in metabolism of cholesterol, resulting in storage of unesterified cholesterol in lysosomes.
3. Autosomal recessive.

Epidemiology

Niemann-Pick disease is panethnic, with observed increased frequency of types A and B in Ashkenazi Jews, and type C in a Colorado Hispanic population and in Nova Scotia.

Clinical Findings

1. Type A typically presents in early infancy with hepatosplenomegaly, feeding problems, and failure to thrive.
   a. Moderate lymphadenopathy is usually present.
   b. Development plateaus, then regresses.
   c. Cherry red spot is present on ophthalmologic examination in about half the patients.

d. Seizures are unusual, and head circumference remains normal. Neurodegeneration progresses to unresponsiveness, and death is usual by age 3 years.

2. Type B typically presents in childhood or adolescence with mild or moderate hepatomegaly and/or splenomegaly. Neurologic status is usually normal, but some patients with cherry red spot on ophthalmologic examination or ataxia have been reported. Clinical symptoms are due primarily to primary parenchymal lung disease, with death usually in late childhood to adult years due to respiratory failure.

3. Type C typically presents in childhood with behavior problems and loss of intellectual function as well as and clumsiness. Ataxia and dystonia progress, and seizures may develop. Hepatosplenomegaly is mild, and some patients have no hepatosplenomegaly noted. Death occurs in adolescence,and is usually due to swallowing difficulties leading to aspiration.

Laboratory and Radiographic Findings

1. "Foam cells" or "Niemann-Pick cells" are seen for all types in bone marrow aspirates or biopsy of other involved tissue and occasionally in peripheral blood. These cells are histiocytes with numerous, uniform-sized lipid droplets in the cytoplasm. Observation of foam cells is useful, but diagnosis depends upon enzyme assay, since similar cells are seen in other conditions.

2. Diagnosis is made by demonstration of specific biochemical defects.

a. In types A and B, decreased sphingomyelinase activity is demonstrable.

b. In type C, the specific biochemical defect can be demonstrated only in fibroblasts.

3. Chest x-ray reveals diffuse reticular or finely nodular infiltration, especially in type B.

Treatment
No specific treatment is currently available. Supportive treatment addresses the nutrition and respiratory problems of types A and C and the pulmonary disease of type B.

Prevention
1. Carrier testing by enzyme assay is not completely reliable. If the specific mutation is known, carrier tests may be performed by DNA analysis.
2. Prenatal testing by enzyme assay is available for all types of Niemann-Pick disease. If the specific mutation is known, DNA diagnosis may be available.

Bibliography

Aicardi J: The inherited leukodystropies: A clinical overview. J Inher Metab Dis 1993;16:733–743.

Grabowski GA: Clinical and therapeutic perspectives on Gaucher disease. Int Pediatr 1993;(1):22–29.

Muenzer J: Mucopolysaccharidoses. Adv Pediatr 1986;33:269–302.

Scriver CR, et al (eds): The Metabolic and Molecular Bases of Inherited Disease, 7th ed. New York, McGraw-Hill, 1995, pp 2427–2882.

Tager JM: Inborn errors of cellular organelles: an overview. J Inher Metab Dis 1987;10(Supp1):3–10.

66 Metabolic Bone Disorders

Laurence Finberg

Etiology
This group of disorders produces a failure to calcify osteoid in children (rickets) because of a disorder in the pathway of either vitamin D or phosphate metabolism. Seven of these nine disturbances are of genetic origin, and one is secondary to acquired disease. An additional condition is included because of similarity of clinical findings. Four other ways in which rickets develops are discussed in Chapter 8 on nutritional rickets.

Pathophysiology
The calcification of osteoid is dependent on adequate levels of ionized calcium and phosphate in the extracellular fluid. These levels are influenced by vitamin D (cholecalciferol) which must be hydroxylated at the 25 position in the liver to calcitriol and the one position in the kidney to calcitriol. If the enzyme controlling either of these steps is deficient because of mutation, vitamin D function will be subnormal or absent. Phosphate metabolism may be altered by a renal tubular defect, reducing reabsorption. Finally, if the receptor for calcitriol should be absent on a genetic basis, the calcification will be deficient. Disorders of parathyroid hormone and calcitonin may also cause skeletal pathology simulating rickets (see Chapter 264).

Clinical and Laboratory Findings
The clinical picture and laboratory findings vary somewhat with each disorder. All of them result in some or all of the features of rickets described in Chapter 8. The variations are mentioned with each entity along with recommended management.

Clinical Types
1. Familial hypophosphatemia (formerly called vitamin D–resistant rickets)

The physiologic disorder is a failure by the kidney to

reabsorb sufficient phosphate, leading to very low levels of this ion after about 6 to 10 months of age. Prior to this, the low glomerular filtration rate (GFR) sustains an adequate PO_4 level. Once renal maturity is reached, PO_4 levels are below 3.5 mg/dl, often below 2.5. The molecular basis has not been elucidated (1997) but presumably involves a defect in a phosphate transporter system. Most of the families exhibit an X-linked dominant inheritance. The same phenotype has been found as an autosomal dominant and as an autosomal recessive. About a third of patients have a new mutation. The clinical findings are similar to those of nutritional rickets though usually occurring at a later age so that the infantile skull defects are not seen. Because calcium levels remain normal there is no tetany, no myopathy, no secondary hyperparathyroidism, and therefore no aminoaciduria. Optimal therapy consists of calcitriol 0.5 to 1.5 µg/day plus a sodium/potassium phosphate mixture to provide 1 to 3 g of elemental P per day in divided dosage. The addition of growth hormone therapy to this regimen is undergoing clinical trial (1997) to see if it produces increased linear growth in these patients, most of whom exhibit short stature.

Key Clinical Findings: Metabolic Bone Disease (Familial Hypophosphatemia)

- Tibial and femoral bowing after weight bearing
- Marfan sign ("double malleolus")

Key Treatment: Metabolic Bone Disease (Familial Hypophosphatemia)

- Calcitriol
- Na/K phosphate mixture

WARNING!

- **Very minor changes in calcitriol dose may produce hypercalcemia and renal damage. The Ca/creatinine (mg/mg) ratio in urine must be monitored closely at first, and then every 3 to 6 months. The ratio should remain below 0.25; over 0.4 is dangerous.**
- **Too high a PO_4 intake may produce secondary hyperparathyroidism.**
- **These patients should therefore be managed by experienced therapists only.**

---

2. Vitamin D dependent–rickets, type I

This disorder results from a genetic deficiency (variable) in the enzyme to convert calcidiol to calcitriol in the kidney. Inheritance is autosomal recessive of a gene carried on chromosome 12. The clinical and laboratory findings are those of nutritional rickets with a more variable phosphate concentration. The treatment is calcitriol

0.5 to 1.5 µg/day. These patients also respond to pharmacologic doses of vitamin D (5000 to 10,000 U/day).

Key Clinical Findings: Vitamin D–Dependent Rickets

- Same as for other rickets

Key Treatment: Vitamin D–Dependent Rickets

- Calcitriol

---

3. Receptor defect rickets (formerly vitamin D–dependent rickets, type II)

This disorder results from a recessively inherited lack of calcitriol receptor sites. This variety may be properly called vitamin D resistant. About half the patients also have alopecia, sometimes complete. Since there are calciferol receptors in many tissues, there may be other more subtle dysfunctions. The patients are hypocalcemic and usually normophosphatemic. There are several mutant forms and a wide range of severity and of response to calcitriol therapy, including some totally resistant. Intravenous calcium has helped some patients as has high oral calcium intake plus calcitriol.

Key Treatment: Receptor Defect Rickets

- Calcitriol plus high calcium intake

---

4. Defective 25-hydroxylase

A single family in the United States and possibly one in Germany have been reported as having deficiency of 25-hydroxylase. The inheritance probably is autosomal recessive.

The clinical picture resembles that of nutritional rickets with a later age of onset. Treatment with calcidiol in physiologic dosage is sufficient.

5. Fanconi syndrome

In this group of disorders, which includes cystinosis and tyrosinemia, there is renal phosphate wasting along with aminoaciduria and glycosuria.

The causes may be genetic as in the above disorders or acquired from a variety of toxins, including heavy metals (e.g., mercury and lead) and drugs. The clinical picture varies with age and cause. Most are responsive to a combination of managing the underlying cause, when possible, and to either vitamin D or calcitriol. Renal tubular acidosis may also cause rickets through phosphate wasting.

6. Oncogenous

Several mesenchymal tumors of bone or connective tissue, including those called nonossifying fibromas, fibroangioma, and giant cell tumors, secrete a phosphaturic substance that results in rickets (or osteomalacia in young adults.) The age of onset has been late childhood, adolescence, or young adulthood. The clinical characteristics are those of familial hypophosphatemia. The treatment is surgical removal of the tumor, with excellent results.

7. Renal osteodystrophy (renal rickets)

In end-stage renal disease the 1-hydroxylase function is diminished or lost, and there is defective excretion of phosphate. This leads to hypocalcemia and failure of osteoid calcification; this is the only variety of rickets with a high serum phosphate level. Recently it has been discovered that there are calcium receptors in various tissues, including bone, that are regulated by growth hormone. Thus management of these patients includes a low phosphate intake, calcitriol, and perhaps injection of growth hormone.

8. Hypophosphatasia

This autosomal recessive condition resulting in absence of alkaline phosphatase causes rickets without disturbance of calcium and phosphate metabolism. There is a range of clinical expression from a severe, even lethal, form to mild disturbance. There is currently no useful treatment.

The following disorder is not rickets pathologically but is indistinguishable in most of its radiographic characteristics.

9. Metaphyseal dysplasia (Schmid variety)

A dominant genetic disorder of collegen with the gene locus on chromosome 6. The appearance of the metaphyses on radiographs cannot be distinguished from changes seen in rickets; however, there is disproportionate disturbance at the proximal femur to that seen in rickets of comparable severity. There is no medical treatment. Osteotomies, if needed, should be deferred until growth is complete.

Bibliography

Casella SJ, Reiner BJ, Chen TC, et al: A possible genetic defect in 25-hydroxylation as a cause of rickets. J Pediatr 1994; 124:929–932.

Glorieux FH (ed): Rickets. Nestle Nutrition Workshop Series, vol 21. New York, Raven Press, 1991.

Harrison HE, Harrison HC: Disorders of Calcium and Phosphate Metabolism in Childhood and Adolescence. Phildelphia, WB Saunders, 1979.

Scriver CR, Blaudet AL, Sly WS, Valle D (eds): The Metabolic and Molecular Bases of Inherited Disease. New York, McGraw-Hill, 1995.

67 Hypoglycemia

Steven M. Willi

General Considerations

The definition of hypoglycemia, simply stated, is low blood glucose. This concept has generated a good deal of controversy over the past 30 years, as pediatricians differ on "how low is low," particularly in the newborn period. Classic studies in the 1960s demonstrated that a certain proportion of normal newborns will have blood glucose measurements in the range of 30 to 40 mg/dl (1.7–2.2 mM). Similar studies that surveyed blood glucose readings in preterm infants frequently discovered readings of 20 to 30 mg/dl (1.1–1.7 mM). These population-based observations were made at a time when standard nursery management included caloric restriction for a 24- to 48-hour period. As the clinical signs of hypoglycemia are nonspecific in the newborn period, it may be erroneous to define hypoglycemia on the basis of such a statistical argument. More recent studies of breast-fed premature infants have seldom revealed plasma glucose levels <45 mg/dl (2.5 mM). Furthermore, neurodevelopmental impairment has been reported in infants with recurrent episodes of even moderate hypoglycemia (i.e., blood glucose levels <2.6 mM). Although blood glucose levels <50 mg/dl (2.8 mM) may be "abnormal," maintaining the plasma glucose concentration >40 mg/dl (2.2 mM) is advisable.

Etiology

The causes of hypoglycemia are many, and they vary with the age and mode of presentation. Blood glucose measurements reflect the balance between the supply of and the demand for metabolic substrates in the body. In the case of hypoglycemia, the supply of glucose (and other substrates) is outstripped by the body's demand for energy. Thus, hypoglycemia occurs as a result of an abnormally increased demand for glucose, or limitations in the body's ability to provide for basic demands, or a combination of both. When considering the etiology of hypoglycemia, a distinction should be drawn between transient and persistent forms.

1. Transient reductions in blood glucose are not uncommon, particularly in the newborn period, and generally reflect a maladaptation to extrauterine life. The normal fetus, in utero, can be viewed as being constantly in a fed state. Glucose is provided via the placenta through facilitated transport. Birth represents the child's first introduction to the fasted state.

2. The maintenance of glucose homeostasis during fasting is a complex process that depends upon adequate hepatic glucose output from glycogenolysis and/or gluconeogenesis. Euglycemia requires an ample supply of gluconeogenic substrates and alternative fuels (for tissues not obliged to utilize glucose) as well as intact endocrine modulation of homeostatic mechanisms.

3. During the newborn period, glucose demands are prodigious owing to the relative abundance of brain tissue in proportion to body size. A number of critical enzymes

in gluconeogenesis and ketone body production are immature and respond sluggishly to hormonal signals. These idiosyncrasies frequently result in hypoglycemia whenever glycogen stores are depleted. A number of clinical conditions may predispose infants to transient forms of hypoglycemia.

Causes of Transient Hypoglycemia

Decreased Supply of Substrates
Very low birth weight infants
Small for gestational age infants
Increased Demand for Glucose
Infant of a diabetic mother
Erythroblastosis fetalis
Asphyxia
Cold stress
Septicemia

---

4. The persistence of hypoglycemia beyond the perinatal period suggests a fixed enzymatic or endocrine abnormality. Congenital defects generally present in the first year of life. Insulin excess, the most common cause of persistent hypoglycemia in infancy, leads to an inability to release liver glycogen in the face of increased peripheral glucose utilization. The enzymatic deficiencies most frequently associated with hypoglycemia impair hepatic glucose production. However, defects in fatty acid metabolism and/or ketone body generation may also cause excessive glucose utilization, owing to the unavailability of alternative fuels. Finally, inborn abnormalities of the counterregulatory hormones (e.g., hypopituitarism, congenital adrenal insufficiency) may result in hypoglycemia because of a failure in substrate mobilization.

5. The initial presentation of hypoglycemia beyond infancy suggests the possibility of acquired disease. A number of drugs (salicylates, β blockers, sulfonylureas, and ethanol) are known to impair gluconeogenesis.

6. Acquired hormone deficiencies (e.g., growth hormone deficiency and Addison disease) may present at almost any age. Congenital hyperinsulinism can rarely present beyond the first year of life, but factitious insulin administration or islet cell tumors should also be considered in this clinical setting.

7. Severe liver disease often results in hypoglycemia, as the liver's ability to produce adequate glucose is impaired.

8. A number of the milder inborn errors of metabolism (e.g., glycogen storage disease, type III and MCAD) may not present until the child undergoes sufficient stress or becomes able to articulate the symptoms of moderate hypoglycemia.

9. Ketotic hypoglycemia is the most common form of hypoglycemia between the ages of 1 and 5 years. This condition typically results from a limited substrate supply during a prolonged fast or intercurrent illness; it resolves spontaneously by 9 years of age. While ketotic hypoglycemia is generally considered a diagnosis of exclusion, its occurrence is especially likely when a child is underweight for height.

10. The clinical entity of reactive hypoglycemia is particularly uncommon in pediatrics. To date, reactive hypoglycemia has been consistently described only in children with prior gastrointestinal surgery and the "dumping syndrome."

Differential Diagnosis of Persistent Hypoglycemia in Infancy and Childhood

Hyperinsulinism
1. Idiopathic congenital hyperinsulinism
2. Beckwith-Weidemann syndrome
3. Early juvenile diabetes mellitus
4. Islet cell adenoma
Counterregulatory Hormone Deficiency
1. Hypopititarism (combined)
2. Growth hormone deficiency
3. Glucocorticoid deficiency (CAH, Addison disease)
4. Catecholamine deficiency
5. Glucagon deficiency(?)
Defective Gluconeogenesis
1. Glucose-6-phosphatase deficiency (GSD, type I)
2. Fructose-1,6-diphosphatase deficiency
3. Phosphoenol pyruvate carboxykinase deficiency
4. Pyruvate carboxylase deficiency
5. Organic acidemias (methylmalonic, propionic)

Carbohydrate Intolerance Syndrome
1. Hereditary fructose intolerance (fructose-1-phosphate aldolase deficiency)
2. Galactosemia (galactose-1-phosphate uridyl transferase deficiency)
Defective Glycogenolysis
1. Glycogen synthetase deficiency (GSD, type 0)
2. Debrancher enzyme deficiency (GSD, type III)
3. Phosphorylase phosphorylase kinase deficiency (GSD VI)
Defective Alternative Substrate Metabolism
1. Fatty acid oxidation defects (MCAD, LCAD)
2. Ketogenesis defects (HMG CoAlyase deficiency)
3. Glutaric acidemia, type II
Miscellaneous Disorders
1. Drugs (ethanol, sulfonylureas, salicylates, β blockers, insulin)
2. Liver disease (hepatitis, cirrhosis)
3. Extrapancreatic tumors (neuroblastoma, Wilms' tumor)
4. Ketotic hypoglycemia

Pathophysiology

1. In the fed state, glucose and other nutrients are absorbed via the gastrointestinal (GI) tract. Through the action of insulin, they are metabolized or shunted into storage materials (triglycerides, glycogen, protein). Upon fasting, blood glucose levels fall, leading to an inhibition of insulin release. If this fall in serum glucose remains unchecked, counterregulatory hormone secretion ensues. This combination of events (decreased insulin secretion and counterregulatory hormone production) causes a shift in metabolism toward the breakdown of available substrates.

2. In the earliest stages of fasting, hepatic glycogen provides the majority of glucose for the bloodstream. Glucagon and epinephrine stimulate glycogenolysis through a cascade of phosphorylation reactions, eventually leading to glucose-6-phosphate. This substrate may enter glycolysis directly, but the majority is then converted to glucose for utilization in distant sites. With more prolonged fasting (i.e., 8–12 hours), gluconeogenesis, the de novo synthesis of glucose from noncarbohydrate sources, predominates. This process is stimulated by growth hormone, glucagon, and cortisol. The precursors of gluconeogenesis are amino acids (derived from muscle protein), lactate (from blood cell glycolysis), and glycerol (from triglycerides). Gluconeogenesis occurs primarily in the liver and requires considerable energy, which is provided by hepatic fatty acid oxidation.

3. Maximal rates of gluconeogenesis in infants are in the range of 5 to 8 mg/kg/min, which provides only 35 to 50 per cent of the basal metabolic requirement of some neonates. The remaining energy requirements during fasting are met through the metabolism of fats. Lipolysis, the breakdown of triglycerides into fatty acids and glycerol, is stimulated by glucagon, epinephrine, and growth hormone. Fatty acids provide a direct and efficient energy source for a variety of tissues; such as muscle, kidney, and heart. Circulating free fatty acids are also converted to ketone bodies in the liver. These ketone bodies, acetoacetate and β-hydroxybutyrate, are small molecules that readily cross the blood-brain barrier and therefore represent alternative substrates for brain metabolism. Thus, normal fatty acid metabolism has a significant glucose-sparing effect and may protect the central nervous system (CNS) from the effects of hypoglycemia.

4. An understanding of the physiology of fasting adaptation is essential in the diagnostic evaluation of hypoglycemia, as the mode of presentation may provide some clues as to the underlying cause. For example, the timing of low blood sugar in relation to meals may suggest a specific diagnosis. While insulin excess can present at any time, most other defects in the metabolic or endocrine systems will result in hypoglycemia at a time when these functions are most critical. Glycogen storage diseases may present within 4 to 6 hours of a meal, as patients are incapable of glycogenolysis. In contrast, disorders of lipid metabolism or mobilization (e.g., acyl-CoA dehydrogenase deficiencies, hypopituitarism, and "ketotic" hypoglycemia) typically present after more prolonged fasting. Carbohydrate intolerance syndromes (e.g., hereditary fructose intolerance, galactosemia) will provoke hypoglycemia soon after a feeding of the offending sugar.

Clinical Findings

The clinical signs and symptoms of hypoglycemia are divided into two major categories: adrenergic and neuroglycopenic.

1. The adrenergic signs result from increased epinephrine secretion in response to hypoglycemia. These symptoms may predominate in older children and adults, especially in the presence of mild hypoglycemia. However, young children, and particularly neonates, do not reliably manifest these signs before CNS depression becomes evident. The neuroglycopenic signs result from the lack of substrate for brain metabolism, and they demonstrate a progression from irritability to mental confusion and finally convulsions, coma, and death.

2. The manifestations of hypoglycemia in the neonate may be nonspecific and are frequently confused with sepsis. Poor feeding, irritability, cyanosis, hypotonia, and apnea should prompt the astute clinician to consider testing the blood glucose, before the child is exposed to the potential hazards of neuroglycopenia. The lack of specific clues to the diagnosis of hypoglycemia, particularly in this age group, underscores the importance of accurate documentation of blood sugar readings. Bedside blood glucose monitors should serve only in a screening capacity and cannot be substituted for laboratory measurements. Ideally, the diagnosis of hypoglycemia should be established in the presence of Whipple triad:

   a. Signs or symptoms of hypoglycemia

   b. A well-documented low blood glucose level at the time of symptoms

   c. Disappearance of symptoms in response to the correction of hypoglycemia.

3. A number of clinical findings may, by their coexistence with hypoglycemia, suggest a specific diagnosis.

   a. Hyperinsulinism may be present in an infant who is particularly large for gestational age.

   b. Hepatomegaly is evident in many of the enzymatic defects of gluconeogenesis and glycogenolysis but may take several months to develop. A midline defect, such as cleft palate, or microphallus may accompany hypopituitarism. Ketotic hypoglycemia is readily recognized by the presence of decreased subcutaneous fat in a child between the ages of 18 months and 5 years.

   c. When specific facial anomalies (hypoplastic philtrum, thinned upper vermilion) and developmental delay coexist with ketotic hypoglycemia, fetal alcohol syndrome should be suspected.

Key Clinical Findings

Adrenergic	Neuroglycopenic
Pallor	Headache, visual disturbance
Diaphoresis	Irritability
Tachycardia	Mental confusion, psychosis
Palpitations	Convulsions
Weakness	Coma

Laboratory Findings

1. The diagnosis of hypoglycemia is never based solely on rapid, bedside detection techniques, as these methods are not particularly accurate below the level of 60 mg/dl (3.3 mM).

2. Rather, when hypoglycemia is suspected, sufficient blood should be collected for precise measurement of glucose as well as other substrate levels. In the absence of a preservative, such as sodium fluoride, red blood cells rapidly metabolize glucose. Therefore, dilatory processing of samples will result in falsely depressed readings.

3. The "critical" blood sample, collected prior to therapy, is the single most useful, and often overlooked, diagnostic measure in the evaluation of the hypoglycemic patient. This serum can be analyzed for glucoregulatory hormones (insulin, cortisol, growth hormone) and substrate levels (lactate, alanine, ketones, free fatty acids).

4. If an organic acidopathy or fatty acid oxidation defect is suspected, the laboratory investigation can be facilitated by determining the level of carnitine and its esters in the serum.

5. While carnitine deficiency is not entirely specific to this class of disorders, a low total carnitine or an elevated esterified:free ratio should prompt the examination of urine for abnormal organic acids or blood for unusual carnitine esters.

6. If a "critical" blood sample was not obtained, a formal fasting study may be necessary but only after adequate resuscitation and in the presence of experienced medical personnel.

   a. The previous pattern of hypoglycemia should be determined, so that the fast can be timed in a manner that assures that the acute hypoglycemic episode occurs when adequate medical attention is available (typically, between 0900 and 1600 hours).

   b. Glucose levels should be monitored at least every 3 hours, and with greater frequency as the level drops. At a minimum of two to three times throughout the period of fasting, blood is collected for metabolic substrate levels.

   c. The fast is terminated with oral or intravenous glucose, after the collection of a comprehensive blood sample analogous to the "critical" sample described previously.

   d. Criteria for termination of the diagnostic fasting study include hypoglycemia (confirmed laboratory glucose level ≤40 mg/dl), profound symptoms in the presence of a marginal glucose level, or the presence of significant ketosis at 24 to 36 hours into the fast.

   e. When hypoglycemia occurs within 12 hours and ketones are absent from the urine, hyperinsulinism should be suspected. In this case, the fast can be terminated with a dose of intravenous glucagon (0.03 mg/kg), which prompts a glycemic increment of >40 mg/dl. In any case, blood glucose levels should be monitored after resuscitation to ensure an adequate response.

7. Within 12 to 18 hours of fasting, serum insulin levels typically fall <10 μIU/ml. An insulin:glucose ratio of ≥0.3 in the face of a blood glucose <60 mg/dl is distinctly unusual and suggests the diagnosis of hyperinsulinism. Provocative testing with insulin secretagogues (e.g., tolbutamide, leucine) is hazardous and offers no advantage over a well-controlled fasting study. Hypoglycemia is a potent stimulus to cortisol and growth hormone release, and failure to produce adequate amounts of these counterregulatory hormones will be apparent from limited substrate mobilization. Growth hormone levels <10 ng/dl or cortisol <20 μg/dl suggest the presence of a hormonal abnormality but should always be followed by more definitive provocative testing.

8. The development of lactic acidosis during fasting should prompt the careful consideration of a defect in hepatic gluconeogenesis. These disorders also demonstrate an accelerated ketotic response, as fatty acids are quickly mobilized to spare the available glucose. Hyperlipidemia and hyperuricemia also result from the recurrent hypoglycemia. When a defect in gluconeogenesis is suspected, definitive diagnosis can be established via liver biopsy. A number of laboratories will perform enzyme studies on snap frozen or, preferably, fresh tissue.

9. Prolonged fasting may be required to uncover the diagnosis of defective fatty acid metabolism.

   a. In these disorders, fatty acids are mobilized appropriately but are inefficiently metabolized to ketone bodies. In normal children, the ratio between fatty acids and β-hydroxybutyrate rarely exceeds 1:1.

   b. In contrast, most of the children with fatty acid oxidation disorders will demonstrate high free fatty acid levels but low serum ketones (ratio ≥2:1), when fasted to the point of hypoglycemia.

   c. Extreme caution should be exercised whenever one is fasting patients with suspected fatty acid oxidation defects, as blood glucose levels do not provide an adequate guide to the degree of illness. Several sudden deaths have been reported during provocative fasting studies, in the presence of only modest hypoglycemia.

Radiographic Findings

1. Diagnostic imaging techniques are of limited utility in the diagnosis of hypoglycemia. Once a diagnosis of hyperinsulinism has been established, imaging of the pancreas can be undertaken. Abdominal CT and MRI studies are rarely helpful, because the size of the organ, much less an adenoma, would be below the level of resolution for these techniques. Pancreatic ultrasonography, especially as an intraoperative procedure, has been found useful in identifying adenomas in children and adults. Islet cell adenomas have a characteristic echopenic appearance on ultrasound and may guide the surgical approach.

2. When hypopituitarism is suspected, MRI or CT frequently reveals abnormalities of the hypothalamus and/or pituitary. In children with abnormalities of the gluconeogenic enzymes (fructose-1-phosphate aldolase, fructose-1,6-bisphosphatase, glucose-6-phosphatase), hepatic ste-

atosis may be evident from a large, echogenic liver pictured on ultrasound. The glycogen storage diseases have been associated with the development of adenomatous nodules in the liver (visible with ultrasonography or liver scan) and osteoporosis (evident with x-rays or bone densitometry).

Treatment

1. After appropriate diagnostic blood tests have been collected, intravenous dextrose (3–4 ml/kg of $D_{10}W$) should be administered immediately. If intravenous access is not readily available, an intraosseous line can be used for treatment and often provides sufficient blood for diagnostic studies.

2. Solutions of 25 and 50 per cent dextrose are contraindicated in neonates, as they may cause rapid osmotic shifts or sclerosis of tiny veins. Such high concentrations of dextrose also may perpetuate hyperinsulinemia, leading to "rebound hypoglycemia."

3. Oral feedings can be used in the presence of mild to moderate hypoglycemia but should be avoided in any child with altered consciousness.

4. After initial resuscitative efforts, serum glucose should be promptly monitored to determine the effectiveness of treatment. Neuroglycopenic symptoms may persist, despite a normal serum glucose, but are not an indication for repeated boluses of dextrose.

5. To avoid recurrent hypoglycemia, a continuous infusion of dextrose is essential. When treating children with hypoglycemia, the consideration of glucose requirements takes precedence over fluid requirements. Glucose should be administered at a rate that supports the blood sugar >50 mg/dl (2.8 mM). The infusion rate may somewhat exceed that of normal hepatic glucose production (i.e., 5–8 mg/kg/min for infants, 3–6 mg/kg/min for older children). However, hypoglycemia unresponsive to an infusion rate of 10 to 12 mg/kg/min is pathognomonic of hyperinsulinism.

6. Transient hypoglycemia, as the name implies, will generally resolve spontaneously if rebound hypoglycemia can be averted. Adequate oral or parenteral nutrition will gradually replenish glycogen stores, and the gluconeogenic hormones quickly mature under the chronic stimulation of counterregulatory hormones. However, persistent hypoglycemia often requires more aggressive therapy, which should be specific to the diagnostic entity under consideration.

7. Within the spectrum of hypoglycemic disorders, the management of congenital hyperinsulinism presents perhaps the greatest therapeutic challenge to clinicians. During the acute care of hyperinsulinism, extraordinary rates of glucose infusion (i.e., 15–20 mg/kg/min) may be required to maintain even marginal blood glucose levels. Although glucagon and glucocorticoids may be used to temper the acute effects of insulin, they are not well suited to long-term use.

8. To date, the most effective medical therapy for hyperinsulinism is diazoxide. Since its introduction in 1965, over half of reported cases of hyperinsulinism have been controlled without requiring surgery. The initial dose of diazoxide is 10 to 15 mg/kg/day divided into three equal portions. If hyperglycemia is encountered, the dose can be decreased to 5 mg/kg/day, in order to minimize the fluid retention and hypertrichosis that are frequent side effects. Maximal response to diazoxide may be delayed for 48 to 72 hours, so hydrocortisone (5mg/kg/day) and/ or glucagon may be necessary as temporizing adjuncts.

9. Octreotide, a long-acting analog of somatostatin, suppresses insulin secretion and can be added if diazoxide alone is not effective. A subcutaneous trial dose of 5 µg/kg is recommended, followed by hourly blood sugars. As tachyphylaxis to octreotide is common, rapid upward dose titration is frequently required. If not effective, the dosage can be increased to a maximum of 40 µg/kg/day, divided into three to six doses. Based on available information in the literature, concerns about the widespread inhibitory effects of octreotide on pituitary peptide hormones seem unwarranted. Transient steatorrhea, from exocrine pancreatic insufficiency, appears to be the only consistent side effect of this drug.

10. If the combination of octreotide, diazoxide, and frequent feedings is unsuccessful in controlling hyperinsulinism, subtotal (90–95%) pancreatectomy is inevitable. Whenever possible, diazoxide should be discontinued several days prior to surgery, as the procedure is complicated by fluid retention. The need for an aggressive surgical approach toward congenital hyperinsulinism has been called into question for two reasons. First, spontaneous remission of this disease in later childhood is not uncommon. Second, several recent reports have noted the occurrence of insulin-dependent diabetes mellitus at puberty in children who previously underwent subtotal pancreatectomy. If surgery is imperative, 90 per cent pancreatectomy combined with aggressive postoperative medical treatment seems the most prudent course of action.

11. Other endocrine disorders are treated with hormone replacement protocols that especially avoid deficiencies during times of stress or fasting. Adrenal insufficiency should be treated with oral hydrocortisone (12–15 mg/ m^2/day ÷ tid). During significant stress this dose is tripled, and daily intramuscular administration of the drug may avoid the need for hospitalization when the child is vomiting. Recombinant human growth hormone (0.04 mg/kg/day) given at bedtime will prevent hypoglycemia and promote normal growth in deficient children.

12. Therapy for the inborn errors of metabolism is primarily nutritional. Frequent carbohydrate feedings are the cornerstone of treatment for the gluconeogenic enzyme deficiencies as well as for ketotic hypoglycemia. In the more severe gluconeogenic defects (e.g., GSD, type I), this treatment is combined with the nighttime administration of uncooked cornstarch or a constant nasogastric glucose infusion. In the case of carbohydrate intolerance syndromes (e.g., hereditary fructose intolerance, galactosemia), the offending substrates are scrupulously eliminated from the diet. Most fatty acid oxidation disorders respond favorably to a low-fat diet in combination with the avoidance of fasting. When the defect involves only long-chain fatty acids, medium-chain triglyceride oil provides a nontoxic form of dietary fat. Frequent carbohydrate feedings or parenteral glucose is indicated during any catabolic stress. If carnitine deficiency exists, it

can be treated with 75 to 100 mg/kg/day of oral L-carnitine.

Key Treatment

- Glucose infusion
- Diazoxide
- Octreotide

Prevention

Hypoglycemia in the high-risk neonate can be readily prevented through the liberal administration of metabolic substrates.

1. The early institution of feedings is indicated for any child at significant risk for developing transient hypoglycemia, unless respiratory or abdominal symptoms preclude them. If feedings are contraindicated, IV dextrose should be administered at rates that simulate hepatic glucose production (i.e., 5–8 mg/kg/min).
2. Blood sugar should be monitored frequently and the rate of glucose delivery calibrated to the infant's requirements.

Weaning of the infusion should proceed slowly to prevent recurrent hypoglycemia.

3. In the event of a recurrence, a small bolus of 10 per cent dextrose (1–2 ml/kg) can be followed by resumption of the previous infusion rate. A composed, systematic approach will avoid perpetuating hyperinsulinism.
4. Neonatal hypoglycemia has been linked to excessive rates of maternal glucose administration prior to delivery. High doses of glucose are frequently given during active labor to suppress maternal ketosis or to act as a vehicle for oxytocin administration. A number of studies suggest that neonatal hypoglycemia can be prevented by avoiding rates of maternal glucose administration that exceed 12 g/hour.

Bibliography

Bier DM, Leake RD, Haymond MW, et al: Measurement of "true" glucose production rates in infancy and childhood with 6,6-dideuteroglucose. Diabetes 1977;26:1016–1023.

Bonham JR: The investigation of hypoglycemia during childhood. Ann Clin Biochem 1993;30:238–247.

Cahill G: Starvation in man. N Engl J Med 1970;282:668–672.

Haymond MW: Hypoglycemia in infants and children. Endocrinol Metab Clin North Am 1989;18(1):211–252.

68 Host Defense Systems

Mark Ballow

Definition

The host defense systems are composed of the plasma proteins, cellular elements, and cell-derived soluble mediators. They work together to protect the host against foreign substances that may be infectious or toxic by eliminating them before they can cause tissue injury and disease.

Components of the Defense Systems

1. Innate immunity (native or natural immunity) describes the defense mechanisms that are present prior to exposure to an infectious agent or foreign macromolecule. It does not discriminate between foreign substances and is not enhanced by prior exposure.

   a. The natural barriers of the skin and mucosal surfaces offer the first line of defense. The ciliated epithelia of the upper and lower airways are particularly important in eliminating large foreign particles entering through the nose and mouth. Enzymes found in the saliva and gastrointestinal tract also play an important role in "neutralizing" foreign substances.

   b. The complement system is a cascade of specialized plasma proteins whose components have a number of biologic functions to enhance the movement of cells (e.g., chemotaxis) or enhance the phagocytosis of bacteria, a process known as opsonization.

   c. Phagocytic cells are of hematopoietic origin. They protect the host by eliminating microbial organisms through phagocytosis, or engulfment of foreign particles (neutrophils and macrophages), and by killing virus-infected or malignant cells (natural killer cells). Many of these cells produce mediators or cytokines that enhance the inflammatory process.

2. Specific (adoptive or acquired) immunity describes the host defense mechanisms that are induced or stimulated by exposure to foreign substances.

   a. Antibodies, the secreted products of B lymphocytes and plasma cells, are capable of specific recognition and elimination of foreign substances or antigens.

   b. Lymphocytes make up the cellular components of the specific immune system.

   (1) B lymphocytes are those cells that produce immunoglobulin upon differentiating into plasma cells. Antibodies participate in the defense against extracellular microbes and their secreted toxins.

   (2) T lymphocytes are the central cells of the cellular immune system whose principal task is to destroy intracellular microbial agents. Different subsets of T cells have various biologic functions ranging from cytotoxicity and suppressor activities to helping B cells produce antibodies. The latter is accomplished, in part, by the secretion of soluble mediators called cytokines or interleukins, which regulate the immune response.

Key Components of the Host Defense Systems

Innate
- Skin and mucous membranes

- Complement

- Phagocytic cells
  Neutrophils
  Macrophages

- Cytotoxic cells
  Natural killer cells

- Cytokines

Specific
- Immunoglobulin and antibodies

- Lymphocytes
  B cells and plasma cells
  T cells
    CD4+ T cells

- Interleukins

---

   c. Characteristics of specific immunity

   (1) Specificity: Immune responses are specific for an antigen or component of an antigen; the latter is often referred to as a determinant or epitope.

   (2) Diversity: The specific immune system is capable of responding to a large number of antigens. The repertoire of the immune system has been estimated at 10^9 distinct antigenic determinants. This property is essential if the immune system is to defend itself against the many microbes and other foreign agents in the environment. Failure to generate diversity in the immune response could lead to immune deficiency.

   (3) Memory: Upon a second exposure to a given antigen, the immune system can produce a more rapid and more prolonged immune response. Two important components of this memory response are clonal proliferation, or the expansion of specific lymphocytes capable of responding to a specific antigen, and the development of memory lymphocytes.

   (4) Self-limitation: The host's immune response to a specific antigen is limited. Regulatory mechanisms provide a feedback system to prevent the immune system from overreacting. Abnormalities of this function could lead to hypersensitivity disease or allergies.

(5) Discrimination of self from non-self: This property is extremely important in maintaining protection of the host against foreign invaders but at the same time in preventing the immune system from reacting against itself. Breakdown of this important function of unresponsiveness (tolerance) to our own tissues or cellular components can lead to autoimmune disease.

Key Characteristics of the Specific Immune Response

- Specificity
- Diversity
- Memory
- Self-limitation
- Discrimination

3. The interplay of the cellular and plasma or serum elements of the nonspecific and specific immune systems and their secreted molecules provides the stage for an extraordinarily complex but coordinated orchestration of all the components of the immune system. This operates for the protection of the host against potentially harmful environmental factors.

Bibliography

Abbas AK, Lichtman AH, Pober JS: General properties of immune responses. *In* Abbas A, Lichtman A, Pober J (eds): Cellular and Molecular Immunology. Philadelphia, WB Saunders, 1994, pp 3–13.

Janeway C, Travers P: Basic concepts in immunology. *In* Janeway J, Travers P (eds): Immunobiology. New York, Garland Publishing, 1994, pp 1:1–1:43.

Male D, Roitt I: Adaptive and innate immunity. *In* Roitt I, Brostoff J, Male D (eds): Immunology, 2nd ed. St. Louis, CV Mosby, 1989, pp 1.1–1.10.

69 Disorders of the Complement System

Mark Ballow

Genetic Deficiencies of the Early Complement Components

Definition

The complement system is an important component of the innate immune system. Complement proteins form an integrated amplification system of functionally linked plasma proteins. Their interactions result in important biologic functions to enhance inflammation and the humoral immune response. In the classical complement pathway, antibody molecules complex with specific antigens that sequentially bind and activate the early complement components. The initial or early steps of this cascade consist of sequentially activated C1, C4, C2, and C3. C3 is an important pivotal complement component between the classical and the alternative complement pathways that leads to activation of the late-acting complement components, C5 through C9.

Etiology and Epidemiology

Genetic deficiencies of the early complement components have been reported for C1q, C1r, C4, C2, and C3. These deficiencies are inherited as autosomal recessive traits. The genes for complement components C4 and C2 are found on chromosome 6 within the major histocompatibility complex (MHC) between the class I HLA-B loci and the class II HLA-DR loci. C2 is the most common homozygous complement deficiency, with a prevalence of 1:10,000 to 1:30,000 individuals.

Pathophysiology

1. Homozygous deficiencies of the early complement components are associated with immune complex disease. The classical complement pathway is required for clearance and solubilization of circulating immune complexes. Abnormalities of this function predispose patients to immune complex disease.

2. The persistence of circulating immune complexes leads to the deposition of complexes in blood vessel walls and tissues and activation of the complement cascade with the release of biologically activated complement fragments:

   a. Chemotaxis—C5a

   b. Anaphylatoxins—C3a.

Clinical Findings

1. The inability to clear immune complexes leads to autoimmune disease and vasculitis.
2. More than 50 per cent of patients with C2 and C4 deficiencies have systemic lupus erythematosus (SLE).
3. Glomerulonephritis is another common disease in patients with deficiencies of the early complement components, especially C3.
4. Occasionally, patients with early complement deficiencies have increased susceptibility to pyogenic infections. In particular, patients with C3 deficiency are susceptible to pyogenic infections, especially with gram-negative organisms.

Laboratory Findings

1. The single most important screening test is the CH50, or total hemolytic complement. The CH50 should be zero in patients with a homozygous genetic deficiency in one of the early complement components.
2. Analysis of the serum for individual complement components requires specialized testing laboratories.
3. Patients who present with SLE-like disease often have low antinuclear antibody (ANA) titers and do not have antibodies to double-stranded DNA. These laboratory findings identify those lupus patients without genetic complement deficiencies who present with high ANA titers and antibodies to double-stranded DNA.

Treatment

1. There is no satisfactory treatment for correction of the underlying complement defect in patients with genetic complement deficiencies.
2. Treatment is directed at the underlying autoimmune disease and, if present, the bacterial infections.

Genetic Deficiencies of the Alternative and Late Complement Components

Definition

Enzyme complexes of both the classical and the alternative pathways initiate the activation of the terminal complement components that ends in a lytic sequence of the target cell, e.g., bacterium or red cell. The late or terminal complement components are C5, C6, C7, C8, and C9. The components C5b, C6, C7, C8 together form a complex known as a membrane attack complex (MAC) that initiates the lysis of bacteria or cells. This activity is enhanced by the binding of C9 to the complex. The fully mature MAC, which includes C9, forms pores in the plasma membrane, ultimately permitting the passive exchange of small soluble molecules, ions, and water, leading to lysis of the cell.

Etiology and Epidemiology

Although deficiencies of the late complement components are unusual, they are more common than deficiencies of the early complement components. Absence of C6 is the second most frequent component deficiency, with an estimated prevalence of 1:60,000.

Pathophysiology

1. Patients with a genetic absence of a terminal complement component cannot generate the MAC and are thus poorly capable of lysing organisms or cells. These patients are particularly susceptible to disseminated infections with *Neisseria* organisms, which suggests that complement-mediated lysis of this class of bacteria is especially important for host defense.
2. Deficiencies in the components of the alternative complement pathway, such as properdin and factor D, are mainly associated with increased susceptibility to *Neisseria* infections, such as meningococcal meningitis and gonococcal septicemia. Properdin deficiency is inherited as an X-linked trait.

Clinical Findings

1. Patients with the genetic absence of one of the terminal complement components have an increased susceptibility to infections with *Neisseria* organisms. Typical infections include recurrent meningococcal meningitis or disseminated gonococcal disease. Infections are often caused by unusual serotypes of meningococcus.
2. A deficiency of C5, C6, C7, or C8 should be suspected in any patient who has had recurrent *Neisseria* infections or has had more than one family member with *Neisseria* infections, such as meningococcemia or meningococcal meningitis.
3. These disorders are inherited as an autosomal recessive trait.

Key Clinical Findings: Congenital Complement Deficiencies

- Early Complement Deficiencies
  Lupus-like disease with low-titer ANA
  Pyogenic infections

- C3 Deficiency
  Glomerulonephritis
  SLE-like disease
  Susceptibility to infection, expecially gram-negative bacteria

- Late Complement Deficiencies
  Susceptibility to *Neisseria* infections

- Alternative Complement Deficiencies
  Susceptibility to *Neisseria* infections

Laboratory Findings

1. The total hemolytic complement (CH50) is unmeasurable in patients with C5, C6, C7, or C8 deficiency.
2. The CH50 in patients with C9 deficiencies is only partially reduced.
3. Patients with C9 deficiencies do not have increased susceptibility to infection as seen in patients with C5, C6, C7, or C8 deficiencies.

Treatment

Treatment consists of penicillin prophylaxis of the patient with increased susceptibility to *Neisseria* infection.

Deficiencies of the Regulatory Complement Proteins

Definition

A number of serum proteins play an important regulatory role in the activity of the classical and alternative pathways. The best-characterized regulatory abnormality of the complement cascade is the deficiency of the C1 esterase inhibitor—a serum glycoprotein that is a member of the serum protease inhibitor family. Other members of this protease inhibitor family are α_1-antitrypsin, angiotensinogen, and antithrombin II.

Etiology and Epidemiology

A deficiency of C1 inhibitor is associated with hereditary angioedema. This complement abnormality is inherited as an autosomal dominant trait with variable penetrance. The estimated prevalence of this genetic disease is 1:50,000. An acquired form of C1 inhibitor deficiency can occur in patients with lymphoproliferative disease or other malignancy and in persons with collagen vascular diseases.

Pathophysiology

1. The C1 inhibitor inhibits the ability of C1r and C1s to cleave their respective substrates, which results in impaired activation of C4. C1 inhibitor also inactivates kallikrein, plasmin, and Hageman factor. Most of the C1 in the plasma is bound to the C1 inhibitor, which prevents the spontaneous activation of the early components of the classical pathway. In the absence of the C1 inhibitor there is spontaneous activation of the classical pathway with the release of mediators, which causes edema of the skin and mucous membranes. A proteolytic fragment of C2, called C2 kinin, and bradykinin are thought to be the principal mediators of edema in patients with this disease.
2. Two genetic types of C1 inhibitor deficiency exist. Eighty-five per cent of patients have a defective gene, which leads to absent or markedly reduced plasma levels of the protein. In the other 15 per cent of patients, C1 inhibitor protein levels are normal, but the protein does not function.

Clinical Findings

1. The patients with hereditary C1 inhibitor deficiency or hereditary angioedema have intermittent acute episodes of edema of the skin and mucosal tissues lasting from 24 to 72 hours. Initial episodes often occur in childhood. The skin of the face and extremities, the larynx, and the intestinal mucosa are the sites most frequently involved. The cutaneous edema is not pruritic or pitting. Urticaria does not occur in this disease; patients do not respond to antihistamine, steroid, or epinephrine therapy.
2. Edema of the bowel wall leads to recurrent abdominal pain, nausea, vomiting, and diarrhea. Patients may present with an acute abdomen and have unnecessary exploratory surgery.
3. The most life-threatening component of this disease is edema of the larynx, which can lead to fatal airway obstruction. Before effective prophylactic treatment was available, the mortality was 20 to 30 per cent.
4. Acute episodes of edema can be triggered by many factors. Trauma (50%) and emotional stress (25%) are common initiating events. Females usually have more attacks around the time of their menstrual period and during estrogen therapy.
5. There is a high incidence of autoimmune disease in patients with C1 inhibitor deficiency.

Key Clinical Features: Hereditary Angioedema

- Nonpruritic and nonpitting edema
- Edema of face and larynx is life-threatening
- Edema of bowel wall presenting as an acute abdomen
- Trauma is the most common initiating factor
- Nonresponsive to antihistamines and epinephrine
- Preventive therapy with anabolic steroids
- Acute therapy with fresh frozen plasma

Laboratory Findings

1. Approximately 85 per cent of patients have low to absent C1 inhibitor protein in their plasma or serum.
2. Fifteen per cent of patients have normal plasma levels of the protein but have a dysfunctional protein.
3. C2 and C4 levels of the classical complement pathway are low, especially during an attack. C1 and C3 levels are normal. In the acquired form of the disease, C1q levels are low.

Key Laboratory Features: Hereditary Angioedema

- Absent C1 inhibitor protein—85%
- Dysfunctional C1 inhibitor protein—15%
- Low C2 and C4 but normal C1 and C3
- Acquired type C1 inhibitor deficiency has low C1q

Radiographic Changes

In association with the abdominal symptoms and edema of the bowel wall, contrast radiographs of the small bowel may show the "stacked-coin" appearance or signs of bowel obstruction.

Treatment

1. The principal treatment in this disease is the avoidance of trauma, if possible, including such things as the extraction of teeth, accidental trauma, and surgery.
2. If an episode of angioedema is initiated, prompt medical care is necessary, particularly for the observation of life-threatening laryngeal edema.
3. The control of acute symptoms is possible with fresh frozen plasma at a dose of 10 ml/kg given twice, approximately 6 to 8 hours apart. In the future, C1 inhibitor protein concentrates may be available to give to patients both prophylactically and for the treatment of acute episodes.
4. Long-term preventive therapy is possible with the use of anabolic steroids or antifibrinolytic agents (ϵ-aminocaproic acid). The latter agents have severe side effects. Danazol (50 to 600 mg/day) and stanozolol are highly effective and have been reported to control symptoms in 90 per cent of users. Caution needs to be exercised in children, and these drugs should be avoided in preadolescent females.

Key Treatment: Hereditary Angioedema

- Avoid trauma
- Maintain airway
- Fresh frozen plasma 10ml/kg

Bibliography

GENETIC DEFICIENCIES OF THE EARLY COMPLEMENT SYSTEM

Abbas AK, Lichtman AH, Pober JS: The complement system. *In* Abbas A, Lichtman A, Pober J (eds): Cellular and Molecular Immunology. Philadelphia, WB Saunders, 1994, pp 293–316.

Ballow M, Shira JE, Harden L, et al: Complete absence of the third component of complement in man. J Clin Invest 1975;56:703–710.

Frank MM: Complement in the pathophysiology of human disease. N Engl J Med 1987;16:1525–1530.

Roord JJ, Daha M, Kuis W, et al: Inherited deficiency of the third component of complement associated with recurrent pyogenic infections, circulating immune complexes and vasculitis in a Dutch family. Pediatrics 1983;1:81–87.

Ross SC, Densen P: Complement deficiency states and infection: epidemiology, pathogenesis and consequences of neisserial and other infections in an immune deficiency. Medicine 1984;63:43–273.

GENETIC DEFICIENCIES OF THE ALTERNATIVE AND LATE COMPLEMENT COMPONENTS

Abbas AK, Lichtman AH, Pober JS: The complement system. In Abbas A, Lichtman A, Pober J (eds): Cellular and Molecular Immunology. Philadelphia, WB Saunders, 1994, pp 293–316.

Densen P, Weiler JM, Griffiss JM, Hoffman LG: Familial properdin deficiency and fatal meningococcemia: correction of the bactericidal effect by vaccination. N Engl J Med 1987;316:922–926.

Frank MM: Complement in the pathophysiology of human disease. N Engl J Med 1987;316:1525–1530.

Rasmussen JM, Brandslund I, Teisner B: Screening for complement deficiencies in unselected patients with meningitis. Clin Exp Immunol 1987;68:437–445.

Ross SC, Densen P: Complement deficiency states and infection: epidemiology, pathogenesis and consequences of neisserial and other infections in an immune deficiency. Medicine 1984; 63:243–273.

DEFICIENCIES OF THE REGULATORY COMPLEMENT PROTEINS

Agostoni A, Cicardi M: Hereditary and acquired C1-inhibitor deficiency: biological and clinical characteristics in 235 patients. Medicine 1992;71:206–215.

Cicardi M, Bisiani G, Cugno M, et al: Autoimmune C1 inhibitor deficiency: report of eight patients. Am J Med 1993;95:169–175.

Sim TC, Grant JA: Hereditary angioedema: its diagnostic and management perspectives. Am J Med 1990;88:656–664.

Stoppa-Lyonnet D, Tosi M, Laurent J, et al: Altered C1 inhibitor genes in type 1 hereditary angioedema. N Engl J Med 1987; 317:1–6.

70 Disorders of the Phagocytic System

Mark Ballow

The second major innate or native immune system that works in concert with the complement system is the phagocytic system, which constitutes the first line of defense against infectious organisms. In general, disorders of phagocytic function result in recurrent pyogenic infections. Any one of several phagocytic functions may be affected, which can lead to abnormalities in the host response to foreign microbes: adherence to vascular endothelium, recognition and movement toward a chemical gradient (chemotaxis), phagocytosis, and intracellular killing of microbes. Abnormalities of leukocyte phagocytic or chemotactic function are listed in Table 70–1.

Key Abnormalities of Phagocytic Function

- Adherence to vascular endothelium
- Chemotaxis
- Phagocytosis
- Intracellular killing of microbes

Chronic Granulomatous Disease

Definition

Chronic granulomatous disease (CGD) is a genetically heterogeneous disorder in which the respiratory burst is not activated owing to several defects in the NADPH oxidase system. Neutrophils, eosinophils, monocytes, and macrophages from CGD patients fail to generate superoxides and oxygen radicals by a membrane-bound cytochrome system that is part of the respiratory burst oxidase system (NADPH oxidase). The defect in the production of superoxide radicals results in defective microbial killing of phagocytosed bacteria. The disease is characterized by recurrent bacterial and fungal infections.

Epidemiology

The estimated prevalence of this disease is about 1:250,000 to 1 in 1 million individuals. Only two thirds of patients exhibit an X-linked recessive pattern of inheritance.

TABLE 70–1. DISORDERS OF THE LEUKOCYTIC AND PHAGOCYTIC SYSTEMS

Congenital neutropenia
Cyclic neutropenia
Leukocyte adhesion deficiency (types 1 and 2)
Leukotactic disorders
    Shwachman syndrome
    Juvenile periodontitis
    Actin deficiency
    Tuftsin deficiency
Chronic granulomatous disease
Myeloperoxidase deficiency
Glucose-6-phosphate dehydrogenase deficiency, severe
Chédiak-Higashi syndrome
Transcobalamin II deficiency

In other patients with CGD the abnormality is inherited as an autosomal recessive trait.

Pathophysiology

1. The molecular basis for CGD is a defective neutrophil cytochrome b_{558} system, which is responsible for the generation of antimicrobial oxidants by the enzyme NADPH oxidase, which catalyzes the reduction of oxygen to superoxide radicals (O_2^-).
2. In addition to the superoxide radical (O_2^-), other antimicrobial products are generated as a result of this metabolic pathway, including hydrogen peroxide, hypochlorous acid, and free OH radicals. These oxygen metabolites form the basis for the intracellular killing mechanism of phagocytes.
3. The X-linked forms of CGD have defects in the membrane portion of the cytochrome b system. The majority of patients with X-linked CGD (55%) have abnormalities of the gene encoding the 91kD cytochrome b peptide subunit, which is located on the X chromosome at Xp 21.1. In contrast, patients with the autosomal recessive form of CGD (approximately 42%) have abnormalities of two cytosolic proteins involved in the NADPH oxidase system.
4. Abnormalities of the NADPH oxidase system with failure of superoxide generation lead to severe impairment in the ability of phagocytic cells to kill phagocytosed intracellular microbial organisms.

Clinical Findings

1. Catalase-positive organisms commonly cause infections in patients with CGD. Interestingly, these patients do not have problems with catalase-negative organisms, such as *Streptococcus pneumoniae* and *Haemophilus influenzae* type b. There is no increase in viral infections.
2. The most common bacterial pathogens are *Staphylococcus aureus, Serratia, Pseudomonas, Escherichia coli, Klebsiella, Proteus, Salmonella,* and fungal agents such as *Aspergillus*. Infections with *Pseudomonas cepacia* are characteristic of CGD. Approximately 80 per cent of the deaths are related to infections with this gram-negative bacterium and by fungal infections caused by *Aspergillus*. Problems with recurrent infections can start early in life and range from mild skin infections to more severe infections involving the major organ systems.
3. The clinical hallmark of this disorder is enlarged lymph nodes, which can be seen in 75 per cent of patients. The cervical node region is commonly involved, and the condition can progress to chronic lymphadenitis. Eczematoid skin lesions are often the first sign of disease. Recurrent infections usually begin in the first year of life. A dermatitis with pyoderma is very frequent, occurring with a frequency of approximately 68 per cent. Adenopathy and hepatosplenomegaly develop in more than half the patients.
4. Eventually, bacterial pulmonary infections occur in almost all patients. Although most lung infections are related to *S. aureus* or gram-negative bacteria, fungal infections with *Aspergillus* and *Nocardia* species are also seen.
5. Perianal abscess and fistula formation are other common problems in CGD patients. Those who have poor wound healing may experience fistula formation following trauma or surgery. Hepatic abscesses may occur in a third of patients.
6. Another important clinical characteristic is noncaseating granuloma formation at the sites of infection. Granulomas may cause gastric outlet obstruction as well as obstructive uropathies.
7. Osteomyelitis occurs in a third of CGD patients and commonly involves the small bones of the hands and feet. The most common bacterial organism associated with bone infections is *Serratia marcescens*.

Key Clinical Findings: CGD

- Onset of infections in the first year of life
- Skin and lymph nodes are common infection sites
- Lymphadenopathy
- Infections with catalase-positive bacteria
- Perianal abscess and fistula formation
- Osteomyelitis
- Noncaseating granulomas at the site of infection

Laboratory Findings

1. The most widely used laboratory test for the diagnosis of CGD is the neutrophil nitroblue tetrazolium dye reduction test (NBT). Today there are many variations on this assay, but essentially they all measure the ability of neutrophils to undergo an oxidative burst through the cytochrome oxidative system. In normal neutrophils the formazan dye is reduced to an insoluble blue-black product that precipitates within the cell and denotes an intact NADPH oxidase cytochrome b system. The neutrophils of CGD patients are unable to reduce the dye with stimulation.
2. Functional measurements examine intracellular bactericidal killing using peripheral blood neutrophils and *Staphlyococcus*. Flow cytometry using monoclonal antibodies to components of the cytochrome b system and special fluorescent dyes is a newer method for diagnosing CGD.
3. The NBT test can also be used to detect female carriers of the X-linked form of the disease. Since there is random inactivation of one of the X chromosomes (Lyon hypothesis), approximately half the neutrophils will be able to reduce the NBT dye while the other half of the cells with the defective cytochrome b component will not be able to reduce the NBT dye.

Radiographic Changes

1. Because of the frequent involvement of the lungs, older children usually have an abnormal chest radiograph showing evidence of recurrent infections involving segmental portions of the lungs and even late changes of pulmonary fibrosis.
2. Radiocontrast studies may be important when gastrointestinal (GI) or urogenital obstruction is suspected. Liver-spleen scans can be helpful in diagnosing hepatic abscesses. Intravenous pyelograms may be necessary in CGD patients with dysuria and may reveal areas of granuloma and chronic inflammation. Patients with persistence

of vomiting should have GI contrast studies done for the evaluation of gastric outlet obstruction. Ultrasound examination may also be helpful in looking for an obstructive component to the gastric antrum.

Treatment

1. The first line of therapy is good skin care to reduce skin colonization with staphylococci in addition to the use of prophylactic antibiotics. Sulfamethoxazole-trimethoprim has become the drug of choice for CGD patients. Studies on the efficacy of this prophylactic antibiotic have shown a prolongation of the mean infection-free period from 3.7 months to 10.7 months. There is some evidence that this agent stimulates bactericidal activity of neutrophils. Dicloxacillin has been used in patients who have allergies to sulfa antibiotics.

2. Corticosteroids have been used when there is danger of obstruction by granuloma formation in the GI or urogenital tract.

3. Gamma interferon (IFN-γ) has more recently been shown to be clinically effective in most patients with CGD. Gamma interferon is administered subcutaneously three times per week at a dosage of 50 $\mu g/m^2$ when the patient's body surface area is greater than 0.5 m^2. If the surface area is less than 0.5 m^2, IFN-γ is administered at 1.5 $\mu g/kg$. This medication is well tolerated, although a few side effects, including fever, headaches, chills, and erythema, can occur at the site of the injection. The mechanisms by which IFN-γ improves clinical responsiveness to infection in CGD patients is not clear. Increases in superoxide generation with improvement of phagocytic function can be demonstrated in some cases.

4. Although white blood cell transfusions have been done in some patients with CGD, this is not an acceptable mode of therapy. Matching for blood components should include antigens associated with the Kell series, since a significant number of patients with X-linked CGD do not have Kell antigens on their erythrocytes. White cell transfusions potentially may sensitize patients to the Kell blood group antigen, which could cause future difficulties in cross matching blood components and potential transfusion reactions.

5. Two other approaches to the treatment of patients with CGD are bone marrow transplantation and, in the future, gene therapy.

Key Treatment: CGD

- Good skin care
- Sulfamethoxazole-trimethoprim prophylaxis
- Corticosteroids for obstructive granulomas
- Gamma interferon

Leukocyte Adhesion Deficiencies

Definition

Leukocyte adhesion deficiencies (LAD) are a group of inherited abnormalities characterized by impaired adhesion-dependent function of leukocytes, which leads to recurrent bacterial and fungal infections.

Etiology and Epidemiology

1. These abnormalities are inherited as an autosomal recessive disorder.
2. Leukocyte adhesion deficiencies are a group of rare disorders, with fewer than 100 patients described.

Pathophysiology

1. Patients with leukocyte adhesion deficiency-1 (LAD-1) have absent or deficient expression of the β-2 integrins of the CD11/CD18 family of glycoproteins, which are expressed on a wide variety of cell types. These leukocyte integrins are heterodimers in which a unique α subunit present on the cell membrane is noncovalently complexed to a common β subunit (CD18). Deficiencies of the common β subunit result in the absence of, or decreased expression of, the intact cell membrane adhesion molecule. This adherence abnormality results in defective leukocyte mobility, cell-cell communication, cytotoxicity, and leukocyte trafficking to lymphoid compartments. An important ligand for these adhesion molecules is the intercellular adhesion molecule-1 (ICAM-1), which is expressed on a variety of cell types, including vascular endothelial cells. Five subtypes of LAD-1 exist based on the expression of a variable gene defect that results in a heterogeneous clinical phenotype.

2. A second type of disorder has been described—leukocyte adhesion deficiency-2 (LAD-2). Clinically indistinguishable from LAD-1, it has a different molecular basis. In LAD-2 there is absence of the sialyl-Lewis x determinant on neutrophil membranes, a carbohydrate ligand that is required for binding to specialized ligand receptors on activated endothelium, e.g., E-selectin. In LAD-2, the expression of CD11/CD18 on leukocytes is normal.

3. Neutrophils cannot accumulate at the site of inflammation because they cannot exit from the vascular space across the endothelium. This abnormality results in poor pus formation and impaired wound healing.

Clinical Findings

1. Patients with LAD present with delayed separation of the umbilical cord. Normally, the cord should separate in 2 to 4 weeks. In these patients the cord does not separate until after the sixth to eighth week of life.

2. Patients have an increased susceptibility to skin infections, commonly with *Staphylococcus aureus* and *Pseudomonas aeruginosa*. Skin lesions start out as small, erythematous nodules and progress to ulceration and cellulitis. Healing, often with scar formation, is impaired.

3. The most common infections include recurrent otitis media, sinusitis, pneumonia, skin abscesses, and severe periodontal disease. Gingival proliferation and loss of teeth may occur in untreated patients. Skin infections may present with rapidly spreading, necrotizing lesions (pyoderma gangrenosum). These patients may also have pneumonia and fungal skin infections with *Candida*.

4. Patients with LAD-2 deficiency have similar problems with recurrent infections but are also mentally retarded and have distinctive facies, short-limbed dwarfism, and the Bombay (LL) erythrocyte phenotype.

Laboratory Findings

1. Characteristically, the absolute neutrophil count in the peripheral blood is persistently elevated ($>15,000$ cells/mm^3).
2. Adherence-dependent assays of cell movement are abnormal.
3. Flow cytometry using monoclonal antibodies to the α and β subunits of the β-integrin complex shows absent or markedly deficient activity.
4. Other biologic functions that require cell adherence may also be abnormal, such as cytotoxic T-cell responses, natural killer cell activity, and phagocytosis of complement-coated target cells. Adhesion-independent functions, such as intracellular bacterial killing and degranulation, are normal.

Key Clinical and Laboratory Findings: LAD

- Delayed separation of the umbilical cord
- Skin infections with *Staphylococcus aureus*
- Severe periodontal disease
- Leukocytosis
- Absent or deficient leukocyte membrane integrins—CD11/CD18

Treatment

1. Treatment of this disease is largely supportive.
2. Granulocyte transfusions may be necessary in life-threatening infections.
3. As in CGD patients, prophylactic antibiotics directed against *Staphylococcus* may be beneficial.

4. Bone marrow transplantation and, in the future, gene therapy may become modalities for treatment.

Key Treatment: LAD

- Supportive
- Granulocyte infusions for serious infections

Bibliography

CHRONIC GRANULOMATOUS DISEASE

Ezekowitz RAB: The International CGD Cooperative Study Group: A controlled trial of interferon gamma to prevent infection in chronic granulomatous disease. N Engl J Med 1991;324:509–516.

Malech HL, Gallin JI: Neutrophils in human diseases. N Engl J Med 1987;317:687–694.

Margolis DM, Melnick DA, Alling DW, Gallin JI: Trimethoprim-sulfamethoxazole prophylaxis in the management of chronic granulomatous disease. J Infect Dis 1990;162:723–726.

Quie PG, Mills EL, Roberts RL, Noya FJD: Disorders of the polymorphonuclear phagocytic system. In Stiehm ER (ed): Immunologic Disorders in Infants and Children, 4th ed. Philadelphia, WB Saunders, 1996, pp 443–468.

Smith RM, Curnutte JT: Molecular basis of chronic granulomatous disease. Blood 1991;77:673–686.

LEUKOCYTE ADHESION DEFICIENCIES

Quie PG, Mills EL, Roberts RL, Noya FJD: Disorders of the polymorphonuclear phagocytic system. In Stiehm ER (ed): Immunologic Disorders in Infants and Children, 4th ed. Philadelphia, WB Saunders, 1996, pp 443–468.

Ross GD: Clinical and laboratory features of patients with an inherited deficiency of neutrophil membrane complement receptor type 3 (CR_3) and the related membrane antigens LFA-1 and p150,95. J Clin Immunol 1986;6:107–113.

Schmalstieg FC: Leukocyte adherence defect. Pediatr Infect Dis J 1988;7:867–872.

71 Disorders of the B-Cell Immune System

Mark Ballow

X-Linked Agammaglobulinemia (Bruton's Disease)

Definition

This disorder, identified by Bruton in 1952, describes children with recurrent severe life-threatening infections who have absent serum immunoglobulins. The differential list of B-cell immune disorders is shown in Table 71–1.

Etiology

X-linked agammaglobulinemia (XLA), or Bruton's disease, is an inherited immunodeficiency of males in which there is a defect in the maturation of pre–B cells into B cells. The abnormal gene is located on the midportion of the long arm of the X chromosome at Xq22. The gene has been identified as a tyrosine kinase that is expressed only in B cells.

Epidemiology

Family history often reveals an X-linked inheritance pattern.

Pathophysiology

1. The primary defect in XLA is the failure of precursor or early B cells to differentiate into mature B lymphocytes. This block in differentiation results in the absence of plasma cells and a severe agammaglobulinemia.
2. The gene responsible for this defect in B-cell maturation is a tyrosine kinase gene called *Btk*, or Bruton's/B-cell tyrosine kinase gene. A number of mutations have been described in the *Btk* gene. This gene is expressed at all stages of B-cell development and is unique for the B-cell lineage; T cells do not express this particular tyrosine kinase and thus XLA patients have normal T-cell immunity.

TABLE 71–1. THE B-CELL IMMUNE DEFICIENCY DISORDERS

X-linked agammaglobulinemia (Bruton's disease)
Transient hypogammaglobulinemia of infancy
Common variable immunodeficiency
Immunodeficiency with thymoma
X-linked hyper-IgM syndrome
Selective IgA deficiency
Selective IgM deficiency
IgG subclass deficiency
Antibody deficiency with normal immunoglobolins

3. The *Btk* gene functions during the process of early B-cell differentiation. The mechanism by which the defective *Btk* gene in XLA is related to the failure of B-cell maturation has not yet been defined.
4. The block in B-cell differentiation results in few or no circulating B cells that express surface immunoglobulin.
5. The fact that 45 per cent of cases are nonfamilial suggests that a spontaneous mutation of the X chromosome in the *Btk* gene leads to XLA.

Clinical Findings

1. Patients are usually well until 7 to 9 months of age, when the transplacentally acquired maternal IgG decreases to below protective levels, leaving the child susceptible to pyogenic infections.
2. Patients have recurrent pyogenic infections with otitis media, sinusitis, sepsis, meningitis, conjunctivitis, pneumonia, and pyoderma. Urinary tract infections and osteomyelitis are less common.
3. Organisms responsible for these infections commonly include *Haemophilus influenzae, Streptococcus pneumoniae, Staphylococcus aureus,* and *Pseudomonas* species. Infections with *Salmonella* and *Campylobacter* may also be a problem.
4. Patients with XLA are particularly at risk for enteroviral infections (echovirus and coxsackievirus) that are associated with chronic meningoencephalitis, a disease complex resembling dermatomyositis, and hepatitis.
5. Infection with *Giardia lamblia* causes chronic diarrhea and malabsorption.
6. XLA patients are at risk for acquiring paralytic poliomyelitis from the live oral polio vaccine.
7. Arthritis of the large joints occurs in 25 to 35 per cent of the patients and may be caused by a *Mycoplasma* infection (*Ureaplasma urealyticum*).

Key Clinical Findings: XLA

- Onset of recurrent infections at 7 to 9 months of age
- Absent or small lymphoid tissues
- Infections with encapsulated bacterial organisms
- Susceptibility to enteroviral infections
  Meningoencephalitis
  Dermatomyositis-like syndrome
- Susceptibility to live viral vaccines, especially polio
- Arthritis

Laboratory Findings

1. Serum quantitative immunoglobulins show agammaglobulinemia with marked reduction or absence of all immunoglobulin isotypes.
2. Patients are incapable of making specific antibodies in response to antigen exposure or vaccine challenge. Isohemagglutinins (blood group antibodies to ABO blood group determinants) are absent.
3. Circulating mature B cells are absent as assessed by flow cytometry.
4. Cell-mediated immunity is normal in patients with XLA. Circulating T-cell numbers are normal, and peripheral blood lymphocyte responses to mitogens and specific antigens are also normal.
5. Adenoids, tonsils, and peripheral lymph nodes are small and hypoplastic; germinal centers are absent; and plasma cells are few, if present at all, in the lymphoid tissues.
6. Pre–B cells are normal or high in the bone marrow, and a small number of B-cell precursors may circulate in the blood.
7. A subset of patients have growth hormone deficiency.

Key Laboratory Findings: XLA

- Absent serum immunoglobulins
- Absent production of specific antibodies
- Absent circulating mature B cells
- Normal T-cell function

Radiographic Changes

1. Changes in chest x-ray reflect the frequency or chronicity of lower respiratory tract infections.
2. Sinus x-rays usually show evidence of sinusitis.
3. Lateral x-rays of the nasopharynx usually show absence of the adenoidal tissues.

Treatment

1. A standardized form of therapy is supportive, with pulmonary hygiene and appropriate antibiotic use to prevent or treat infections.
2. Replacement therapy with intravenous immunoglobulin (IVIG) at a dose of 300 to 400 mg/kg/month has allowed patients to lead a fairly normal life.
3. Doses of IVIG may need to be modified to maintain a trough level in serum of IgG at 500 mg/dl to control the frequency or severity of infections.
4. Both intravenous and intraventricular routes may be necessary in XLA patients with meningoencephalitis.
5. The dermatomyositis-like clinical picture and arthritis usually respond to replacement gamma globulin therapy.
6. Since IVIG replaces only IgG, the gastrointestinal manifestations of immune deficiency may not respond.
7. Live-virus vaccines are contraindicated in patients with immune deficiency.

Key Treatment: XLA

- Antibiotics
- Pulmonary hygiene
- No live virus vaccines
- Replacement intravenous immune serum globulin (IVIG)

Prevention

1. This disease being an X-linked disorder, female carriers can be identified because mothers exhibit nonrandom inactivation of the X chromosome. Only maternal B cells with the normal X chromosome that has the normal *Btk* gene survive.
2. Female carriers of XLA can be evaluated by DNA methylation patterns, X-chromosome inactivation patterns, and linkage analysis to polymorphic DNA markers (DXS178).
3. Prenatal diagnosis can be made by linkage analysis of amniotic fluid cells or by the enumeration of B cells in fetal cord blood.

Transient Hypogammaglobulinemia of Infancy

Definition

Transient hypogammaglobulinemia of infancy (THI) is characterized by a prolongation and accentuation of the physiologic hypogammaglobulinemia that normally occurs during the first 3 to 6 months of life and that resolves with increasing age to reach normal values.

Epidemiology

The prevalence of this disease is not known. In one study this diagnosis was present in 5.2 per cent of children referred for the immunologic evaluation of recurrent infection. In a study from Japan, this diagnosis was present in 18.5 per cent of patients diagnosed with primary immunodeficiency disorders.

Pathophysiology

1. Infants have a physiologic period of hypogammaglobulinemia between 4 and 6 months of age, when the serum levels of IgG placentally transferred from the mother start to decrease. Thereafter, the child independently produces substantial amounts of immunoglobulin, resulting in increased plasma immunoglobulin levels at 7 to 9 months of age.
2. Children with THI have prolongation and accentuation of their physiologic hypogammaglobulinemia to approximately 3 years of age, with full resolution usually by age 5 years. A few patients may have persistent low values of IgA beyond 5 years of age.
3. The pathophysiology of THI is not known, although early investigations suggested that these patients have a transient deficiency of T-helper cells.

Clinical Findings

1. Patients with THI have problems with recurrent sinopulmonary tract infections during the period of persistent hypogammaglobulinemia.

2. The mean age of presentation is usually 10 months. More males than females are affected.
3. The most frequent infections are otitis media and sinusitis. Pneumonia and impetigo may also occur.
4. Atopic disease is frequent, including asthma (54%), formula intolerance (46%), infantile colic (31%), and eczema (15%).
5. Patients have increased frequency of gastrointestinal problems, including lactose intolerance, chronic diarrhea, and infections with *G. lamblia* and *Clostridium difficile*.
6. These patients usually do not have life-threatening infections. The frequency of infections becomes less with age, as the hypogammaglobulinemia resolves by age 5 years.

Laboratory Findings

1. Typically, patients have reduced serum levels of more than 2 standard deviations (S.D.) below age-matched normal children of one or more immunoglobulin isotypes. Patients generally have low serum IgG levels, with a mean of 270 mg/dl at 10 months of age. Serum IgA levels are commonly low as well. All patients have normal serum IgM; a few patients may subsequently develop selective IgA deficiency.
2. Antibody production following immunization with tetanus toxoid, diphtheria, and other vaccine glycoproteins is normal. Antibodies to the ABO blood group determinants (isohemagglutinins) are normal.
3. The ability to produce specific antibodies to the respiratory viruses, such as parainfluenza, influenza A and B, adenovirus, and respiratory syncytial virus, is usually delayed in 80 per cent of patients. Specific antibody to the respiratory viruses appears before the serum IgG levels return to age-appropriate normal levels in the majority of patients.
4. T-cell function as measured by lymphocyte proliferative responses is normal. B- and T-cell numbers and subsets as measured by flow cytometry are also normal.

Key Clinical and Laboratory Findings: THI

- Recurrent sinopulmonary tract infections
- Atopic disease frequent
- Do not have life-threatening infections
- Low serum IgG and IgA, but normal IgM
- Resolution by age 5 years

Treatment

1. Supportive measures, including appropriate antibiotic use, are the mainstay of therapy.
2. Prophylactic antibiotics may be useful in some patients who have recurrent upper respiratory tract infections.
3. Occasionally patients may need supplemental gamma globulin replacement for short periods (9 months), particularly if the individual does not respond well to prophylactic antibiotics. The dose of gamma globulin is as follows: (a) intramuscular gammaglobulin—0.6 ml/kg on a monthly basis, or (b) intravenous immune serum globulin therapy (IVIG)—200 to 300 mg/kg on a monthly basis. However, therapy with gamma globulin is usually

not necessary, since patients with THI do not have life-threatening infections.

Key Treatment: THI

- Support measures
- Gamma globulin supplementation

Common Variable Immunodeficiency

Definition

This disorder is a heterogeneous group of humoral immune abnormalities that present with increased susceptibility to pyogenic infections and hypogammaglobulinemia.

Etiology and Epidemiology

1. Several patterns of inheritance have been identified, including autosomal recessive and autosomal dominant with variable penetrance. Sporadic cases have also been reported.
2. Common variable immunodeficiency (CVI) is one of the most common types of humoral immune abnormalities affecting males and females equally. Although patients usually present in the second and third decades of life, symptoms may be traced back to childhood or adolescence, predating the diagnosis. The interval between the onset of symptoms and diagnosis can be as long as 10 years. The older literature often refers to this group of patients as having late-onset hypogammaglobulinemia, adult-onset hypogammaglobulinemia, or acquired hypogammaglobulinemia.

Pathophysiology

1. The immune abnormalities in patients with CVI are extremely variable and complex. A number of mechanisms have been proposed for the pathogenesis, including a defective interaction between T and B cells, increased T-suppressor activity, defective T-helper function, and a variety of immunomodulatory cytokine abnormalities.
2. Studies have shown that if B cells from individuals with CVI are incubated with the appropriate mitogen and soluble T-cell factors, patients can be divided into three subgroups based on in vitro immunoglobulin synthesis: those who make little or no immunoglobulin, those in whom IgM synthesis is normal but not IgG production, and those who can produce normal levels of IgM and IgG. These studies indicate that most CVI patients have an intrinsic B-cell defect but that, in a few, the B cells can function normally if given the appropriate stimuli and cytokine mixture. The latter suggests a primary T-cell defect.

Clinical Findings

1. The most common presenting clinical feature is recurrent pyogenic sinopulmonary infections. Approximately 25 per cent of patients may have gastrointestinal disturbances as their principal clinical presentation. If patients are not diagnosed early in their clinical course, bronchiectasis and chronic lung disease may develop. The most common organism responsible for these pyogenic infections are the encapsulated bacteria, such as *S. pneumoniae* and *H. influenzae*. In patients with bronchiectasis, *S. aureus* and *Pseudomonas aeruginosa* are a problem. Rarely, echovirus meningoencephalitis occurs in CVI patients, as in XLA. Persistent *Mycoplasma pneumoniae* can also occur. Patients may have recurrent exacerbations of herpes simplex, and herpes zoster develops later in life in 20 per cent.

2. Unusual infections include infestation of the gastrointestinal tract with enteropathogens such as *Campylobacter, Salmonella,* or *Shigella* organisms or with the parasite *G. lamblia*. Patients present with a malabsorption syndrome characterized by chronic diarrhea, steatorrhea, lactose intolerance, and protein-losing enteropathy. Opportunistic infections with *Pneumocystis carinii* and various fungal infections have been reported. Aggressive forms of hepatitis B and C are also seen in patients with CVI.

3. This group has an unusually high incidence (8 to 13%) of malignancy. Cancers include lymphoreticular malignancy, e.g., lymphoma and adenocarcinoma of the gut. The incidence of gastric carcinoma is 50 times greater in CVI patients than in the general population. These cancers affect women more frequently than men and usually have their onset in the fourth or fifth decade of life.

4. In contrast to patients with XLA, CVI patients have diffuse lymphadenopathy and splenomegaly. Their lymphoid organs show follicular hyperplasia. These findings are due to hyperplasia of the reticuloendothelial system in the absence of opsonic antibodies. The gastrointestinal tract is commonly involved in this process, which is called nodular lymphoid hyperplasia. Noncaseating granuloma of the lungs, liver, and spleen has been reported.

5. Patients with CVI have an increased prevalence of autoimmune disease involving the hematopoietic and endocrine systems. Approximately 20 per cent of patients will develop autoimmune disease, with autoimmune hemolytic anemia (Coombs' positive) and idiopathic thrombocytopenic purpura being the most frequent. Ten per cent of patients develop pernicious anemia. A rheumatoid arthritis–like disease is also seen.

6. Relatives commonly have immune disorders with an unusually high incidence of IgA deficiency. Family members also have an increased incidence of autoimmune disease and malignancy.

7. A subgroup of patients with CVI have thymoma. These patients can develop a pure red cell aplasia. Thymectomy usually resolves the problem, but the hypogammaglobulinemia persists.

Clinical Findings: Common Variable Immunodeficiency

- Hypogammaglobulinemia
- Recurrent pyogenic infections of the sinopulmonary tract
    Encapsulated virulent bacteria
- Gastrointestinal infections with enteropathogens
    Symptoms of malabsorption
- Increased incidence of malignancy
- Diffuse lymphadenopathy and splenomegaly
- Autoimmune disease

Laboratory Findings

1. Patients have hypogammaglobulinemia ranging from a profound agammaglobulinemia to a dysgammaglobulinemia with two or more immunoglobulin isotypes being reduced more than 2 or 3 S.D. below normal for age. All patients have low IgG; the serum IgM and IgA may be low or undetectable.
2. CVI patients have poor specific antibody production both to natural infections and following immunization with vaccines.
3. Most patients have normal or elevated numbers of circulating B cells. However, a subset of CVI patients (12%) have markedly diminished or even absent circulating B lymphocytes.
4. B cells differentiate poorly into plasma cells in vitro. Stimulation of peripheral blood B cells with polyclonal B-cell activators shows a markedly impaired in vitro synthesis of immunoglobulins, particularly IgG and IgA.
5. Approximately 50 per cent of CVI patients have T-cell abnormalities. These abnormalities include moderately reduced numbers of peripheral blood T cells and T-cell subsets. Patients also have diminished lymphocyte proliferative responses to mitogens, specific antigens, and allogeneic cells. They may also be anergic on skin testing with recall antigens, such as tetanus toxoid, *Candida*, mumps, purified protein derivative (PPD), and *Trichophyton*.

Radiographic Changes

1. Small bowel radiographic contrast studies show nodular lymphoid hyperplasia, particularly in the jejunum and ileum.
2. A history of repeated lower respiratory tract infections leads to bronchiectasis and pulmonary fibrosis, which may be detected on chest x-ray or CT scans of the lung.

Treatment

1. Supportive therapy includes the appropriate use of antibiotics and pulmonary hygiene; the latter is especially important in patients with bronchiectasis.
2. Patients with gastrointestinal symptoms should be evaluated for infection with *G. lamblia* and treated, as needed, with metronidazole.
3. Patients need close follow-up and evaluation for autoimmune disease. In older patients, close follow-up for malignancies is important.
4. Replacement therapy with IVIG has been very effective in preventing infections. A dose of 300 to 400 mg/kg monthly is recommended. Patients with chronic bronchitis or sinusitis may require higher doses to maintain a serum trough level of 500 mg/dl.

Key Treatment: CVI

- Supportive therapy with antibiotics and pulmonary hygiene
- Evaluation for GI parasitic disease
- Replacement IVIG therapy
- Surveillance for autoimmune disease and malignancies

IgA Deficiency

Definition

IgA deficiency is a B-cell immune deficiency in which patients have absence of serum (<5 mg/dl) and secretory IgA.

Epidemiology

IgA deficiency is the most frequent type of immune deficiency, with an incidence of approximately 1:600 in the general population. This disorder is found predominately in Caucasians and occurs almost twice as often in males as in females.

Pathophysiology

1. The absence of serum and secretory IgA appears to be derived from a block in B-cell differentiation from IgA-bearing B cells into IgA-secreting plasma cells.
2. IgA-deficient patients have normal numbers of IgA-bearing lymphocyte precursors, which suggests a normal constant region immunoglobulin α heavy-chain gene locus and the genetic machinery for B cells to undergo isotype switching.
3. There is no evidence that T-cell deficiency plays a role in IgA deficiency. The T cells of IgA-deficient individuals support the differentiation of IgA B cells from normal subjects. These findings suggest an inherent B-cell defect and/or some subtle T-cell signal deficiency.
4. IgA deficiency is associated with certain HLA haplotypes (HLA-A1,B8,DR3), suggesting an association with immunoregulatory genes within the major histocompatibility complex (MHC). Recent data indicate that a gene or genes contributing to the development of IgA deficiency may be located between the HLA B and D loci, e.g., the MHC class III region. However, a structual gene defect for IgA deficiency has not been delineated.
5. The administration of certain drugs can also be associated with the development of IgA deficiency. This association has been seen with phenytoin, D-penicillimine, gold salts, sulfasalazine, and antimalarial agents. Reversal of the IgA deficiency occurs with discontinuation of the drug.

Clinical Findings

1. Clinical problems of patients with IgA deficiency can be quite variable. Many of the IgA-deficient individuals have no significant medical problems, whereas others have recurrent sinopulmonary infections and still others have gastrointestinal disorders.
2. Patients with recurrent infections have recurrent or persistent sinusitis and pneumonia. The latter may lead to bronchiectasis.
3. Allergic disorders occur with a high frequency in patients with IgA deficiency and include rhinitis, eczema, asthma, and food allergies. The absence of secretory IgA at the mucosal surface is thought to allow increased penetration of potential allergens into the tissues, leading to an IgE response.
4. Autoimmune diseases are associated with IgA deficiency. Rheumatoid arthritis and systemic lupus erythematosus occur in 5 to 7 per cent of IgA-deficient individuals. Other autoimmune disorders of both hematopoietic and endocrine systems can be seen with IgA deficiency.

5. Gastrointestinal problems are frequent and manifest as chronic diarrhea and malabsorption. Specific disorders include celiac disease, disaccharidase deficiency, and inflammatory bowel disease. Young patients have a high incidence of IgG antibodies to cow's milk, which may produce symptoms of milk allergy.

Laboratory Findings

1. Serum IgA is extremely low (<5 mg/dl) or absent. However, IgA-bearing B lymphocytes in the peripheral blood are normal.
2. Patients with IgA deficiency can make antibodies to IgA if given tranfusions of blood products. The production of IgE anti-IgA antibodies can predispose these patients to severe anaphylactic transfusion reactions.
3. Patients who tend to have fewer infections at the mucosal surface frequently have higher concentrations of IgM in their secretions as a compensatory host defense measure in the absence of secretory IgA. In contrast, symptomatic patients have absent secretory IgA in their secretions and frequently (15 to 18%) have IgG_2 and IgG_4 subclass deficiency. Patients with recurrent sinopulmonary tract infections tend to have more frequent IgG subclass deficiencies.

Key Clinical and Laboratory Findings: IgA Deficiency

- Serum IgA levels < 5 mg/dl
- Recurrent sinopulmonary tract infections
- Frequent gastrointestinal disorders
- Increased prevalence of allergies
- Autoimmune disease
- Associated with IgG subclass abnormalities (15%)

Treatment

1. Treatment of the IgA deficiency is principally supportive, with appropriate antibiotics for bacterial infections.
2. IgA-deficient patients with IgG subclass deficiency and specific antibody deficiencies may benefit from intravenous immune serum globulin replacement therapy. IVIG preparations containing low quantities of IgA should be used to minimize the risk of patients' developing anti-IgA antibodies, which can result in transfusion reactions or even anaphylaxis.

Key Treatment: IgA Deficiency

- Antibiotics as indicated
- IVIG infusions
- Avoid blood/plasma products to prevent sensitization to IgA
- Wear Medical Alert bracelet

IgG Subclass Deficiencies

Definition

Four subclasses of IgG exist: IgG_1, IgG_2, IgG_3, and IgG_4. These are based on the uniqueness of the constant region of the immunoglobulin heavy-chain gene locus on chromosome 14. Subjects with an IgG subclass deficiency (>2 S.D. below normal for age) can have increased susceptibility to recurrent infections.

Epidemiology

1. IgG subclass deficiency may be one of the most common types of B-cell immune abnormalities; however, the exact prevalence of IgG subclass deficiency is not known.
2. The IgG subclasses have different rates of maturity, with IgG_2 serum levels not reaching adult levels until approximately age 10 years. Children between the ages of 3 and 6 years may have low serum levels of IgG_2. This does not represent an immune deficiency but rather a developmental delay in the production of this particular IgG subclass.
3. IgG subclass deficiencies have been associated with other primary immune deficiencies, including ataxia-telangiectasia, complement deficiencies, and IgA deficiency.

Pathophysiology

1. The pathogenesis for a deficiency in an IgG subclass has not been defined.
2. Genetic factors that influence IgG subclass serum levels have been reported. The Gm immunoglobulin allotypic alleles control the expression of serum IgG levels. Individuals homozygous for the Gm(n) allele have higher levels of IgG_2; similarly, individuals homozygous for the G3m(b) allele have higher levels of IgG_3. In contrast, individuals who have the G2m(n) negative allotype can have a sevenfold decrease in vaccine success following administration of *H. influenzae* type b polyribose phosphate polysaccharide vaccine. Individuals with the G2m(n) negative allotype may also not respond to other polysaccharide vaccines, such as Pneumovax for *S. pneumoniae*.

Clinical Findings

1. A low IgG_2 subclass level has been associated with recurrent respiratory tract infections, sinusitis, otitis media, and invasive diseases caused by *S. pneumoniae* and *H. influenzae* type b.
2. However, a healthy individual with selected IgG subclass deficiency due to a deletion of a specific immunoglobulin heavy-chain constant region gene has been described. In addition, IgG_2-deficient children identified by random screening showed no evidence of increased susceptibility to infection. Thus, the ability of the patients to produce specific antibodies following either natural exposure or vaccine immunization is a better criterion for immunodeficiency than the protein quantitation of IgG subclasses in the serum.
3. IgG_3 deficiency occurs most often in adults, whereas IgG_2 deficiency is more common in children. IgG_2 deficiency is often associated with low serum levels of IgG_4.
4. The IgG_2 and IgG_4 deficiencies can be associated with IgA deficiency (15 to 20% of patients). Interestingly, IgA-deficient patients without IgG_2 subclass deficiencies usually have fewer clinical problems.
5. Ten per cent of the normal population have absent IgG_4. Therefore, the clinical significance of an isolated deficiency of serum IgG_4 is minimal.

Laboratory Findings

1. Subclass deficiency is defined as serum levels >2 S.D. below normal for age, using age-appropriate methods, such as enzyme-linked immunosorbent assays (ELISA). Laboratory methods can be a problem in quantifying IgG subclasses, as studies have shown widely discrepant results among laboratories using a common serum panel.
2. Since IgG$_1$ makes up the majority of the total serum IgG (65%), individuals with low IgG$_1$ usually have low total serum IgG.
3. The assessment of the ability of an individual to respond to specific glycoproteins, e.g., tetanus toxoid, and capsular polysaccharides, e.g., Pneumovax, is important in evaluating the clinical significance of IgG subclass abnormalities.

Key Clinical and Laboratory Findings: IgG Subclass Deficiency

- Recurrent respiratory tract infections
- IgG$_2$ and IgG$_4$ deficiencies associated with IgA deficiency
- IgG$_2$ deficiency is commonly developmentally delayed
- Measurement for functional or specific antibodies is important

Treatment

1. Supportive measures with appropriate antibiotic therapy for infection, prophylactic antibiotics, and supportive therapy such as chest physiotherapy is first-line treatment in patients with subclass abnormalities.
2. Patients should be immunized with conjugate *H. influenzae* type b (Hib) vaccine and, when available, the conjugate *S. pneumoniae* vaccine.
3. Patients with IgG subclass abnormalities and selective antibody deficiency who have recurrent infections and are poorly responsive to medical management are candidates for replacement IVIG therapy. The initial dose of intravenous immune serum globulin is 300 mg/kg on a monthly basis.

Key Treatment: IgG Subclass Deficiency

- Antibiotics for infection
- Immunize for *H. influenzae* type b and pneumococcus
- Regular replacement of IV gamma globulin

Bibliography

X-LINKED AGAMMAGLOBULINEMIA (BRUTON'S DISEASE)

Buckley RH: Humoral immunodeficiency. Clin Immunol Immunopathol 1986;40:13–24.

Buckley RH: Breakthroughs in the understanding and therapy of primary immunodeficiency. Clin Immunol 1994;41(4):665–690.

Huston DP, Kavanaugh AF, Rohane PW, Huston MM: Immunoglobulin deficiency syndromes and therapy. J Allergy Clin Immunol 1991;87:1–16.

Ochs HD, Winkelstein J: Disorders of the B-cell system. *In* Stiehm ER (ed): Immunologic Disorders in Infants and Children, 4th ed. Philadelphia, WB Saunders, 1996, pp 296–338.

Rosen FS, Cooper MD, Wedgwood RJP: The primary immunodeficiencies. N Engl J Med 1995;333(7):431–440.

TRANSIENT HYPOGAMMAGLOBULINEMIA OF INFANCY

Cano F, Mayo DR, Ballow M: Absent specific viral antibodies in patients with transient hypogammaglobulinemia of infancy. J Allergy Clin Immunol 1990;85:510–513.

McGeady SJ: Transient hypogammaglobulinemia of infancy: Need to reconsider name and definition. J Pediatr 1987;110:47–50.

Ochs HD, Winkelstein J: Disorders of the B-cell system. *In* Stiehm ER (ed): Immunologic Disorders in Infants and Children, 4th ed. Philadelphia, WB Saunders, 1996, pp 296–338.

Wood RA, Sampson HA: The child with frequent infections. Curr Probl Pediatr 1989;19:235–284.

COMMON VARIABLE IMMUNODEFICIENCY

Buckley RH: Humoral immunodeficiency. Clin Immunol Immunopathol 1986;40:13–24.

Huston DP, Kavanaugh AF, Rohane PW, Huston MM: Immunoglobulin deficiency syndromes and therapy. J Allergy Clin Immunol 1991;87:1–16.

Ochs HD, Winkelstein J: Disorders of the B-cell system. *In* Stiehm ER (ed): Immunologic Disorders in Infants and Children, 4th ed. Philadelphia, WB Saunders, 1996, pp 296–338.

Rosen FS, Cooper MD, Wedgwood RJP: The primary immunodeficiencies. N Engl J Med 1995;333(7):431–440.

Sneller MC, Strober W, Eisenstein E, et al: New insights into common variable immunodeficiency. Ann Intern Med 1993;118:720–730.

IgA DEFICIENCY

Buckley RH: Humoral immunodeficiency. Clin Immunol Immunopathol 1986;40:13–24.

Huston DP, Kavanaugh AF, Rohane PW, Huston MM: Immunoglobulin deficiency syndromes and therapy. J Allergy Clin Immunol 1991;87:1–16.

Ochs HD, Winkelstein J: Disorders of the B-cell system. *In* Stiehm ER (ed): Immunologic Disorders in Infants and Children, 4th ed. Philadelphia, WB Saunders, 1996, pp 296–338.

Schaffer FM, Monteiro RC, Volankis JE, Cooper ME: IgA deficiency. Immunodefic Rev 1991;3:15–44.

Wood RA, Sampson HA: The child with frequent infections. Curr Probl Pediatr 1989;19:235–284.

IgA SUBCLASS DEFICIENCIES

Herrod HG: Management of the patient with IgG subclass deficiency and/or selective antibody deficiency. Ann Allergy 1993;70:3–11.

Huston DP, Kavanaugh AF, Rohane PW, Huston MM: Immunoglobulin deficiency syndromes and therapy. J Allergy Clin Immunol 1991;87:1–16.

Jefferis R, Kumaratne DS: Selective IgG subclass deficiency: quantification and clinical relevance. Clin Exp Immunol 1990;1:357–367.

Ochs HD, Winkelstein J: Disorders of the B-cell system. *In* Stiehm ER (ed): Immunologic Disorders in Infants and Children, 4th ed. Philadelphia, WB Saunders, 1996, pp 296–338.

Wood RA, Sampson HA: The child with frequent infections. Curr Probl Pediatr 1989;19:235–284.

72 Disorders of the T-Cell Immune System

Mark Ballow

Severe Combined Immune Deficiency Disease (SCID)

Definition

Patients with combined immunodeficiencies present with similar clinical findings but have a variety of genetic etiologies. Some cases are X-linked, whereas others are autosomal recessive or even sporadic without known heritable delineation.

Etiology and Epidemiology

1. SCID occurs three times more frequently in males than in females; 50 to 60 per cent of the reported cases are X-linked.
2. The most common cause of the autosomal recessive variety of SCID is an inherited deficiency of the purine salvage pathway enzymes—adenosine deaminase (ADA) and nucleoside phosphorylase.
3. The list of T-cell immunodeficiencies is shown in Table 72–1.

Pathophysiology

1. The X-linked form of SCID has been mapped to Xq13.1. The defect occurs within the γ chain of the IL-2 receptor, which is also a component of other interleukin receptors such as IL-4, 7, 9, 11, and 15. This receptor component appears to be important in the cell growth and differentiation of T cells and in the late stages of B-cell differentiation.

TABLE 72–1. THE T-CELL IMMUNE DEFICIENCY DISORDERS

Severe combined immunodeficiency
  common γ chain of IL2 receptor
  JAK3 gene mutations
  STAT gene mutations
  ZAP70 gene mutations
Bare lymphocyte syndrome
  MHC class I and class II deficiencies
    TAP2 gene defects
Immunodeficiency with enzyme deficiency
  Adenosine deaminase deficiency
  Purine nucleoside phosphorylase deficiency
DiGeorge anomaly
Wiskott-Aldrich syndrome
X-linked hyper-IgM syndrome
Natural killer cell deficiency
Omenn syndrome (combined immunodeficiency with eosinophilia)
X-linked lymphoproliferative syndrome
Ataxia-telangiectasia
Autoimmune lymphoproliferative syndrome
  Fas deficiency immune disorder
Interferon gamma receptor deficiency
Cartilage-hair hypoplasia; short-limbed dwarfism with immune deficiency
Hyper-IgE syndrome
Chronic mucocutaneous candidiasis

2. Gene defects of the enzyme ADA, which maps to chromosome 22q13.4, lead to the accumulation of adenosine and deoxyadenosine. The accumulation of these two substrates produces elevated levels of adenosine triphosphate (ATP) that are toxic to lymphocytes. The production of elevated levels of S-adenosylhomocysteine (SAH) inhibits DNA methylation pathways.
3. A second enzyme deficiency of the purine pathway, purine nucleoside phosphorylase deficiency, results in a combined immunodeficiency by similar mechanisms as for ADA deficiency.
4. Rarer forms of SCID have been described in patients with T-cell activation defects. These patients present with similar clinical features. A variety of defects in T-cell responsiveness to mitogens or activation signals and the capacity to produce cytokines have been described.
   a. A deficiency of the CD3γ subunit results in the defective surface expression of the T-cell receptor/CD3 complex.
   b. Other patients have abnormal membrane or cytoplasmic components, resulting in defective activation of the T-cell receptor/CD3 complex and the intracellular signal transduction pathways.
   c. Abnormal cytokine generation has been linked to defects in the NFAT-1 transcriptional complex.
   d. Patients with CD8 deficiency (ZAP-70 defect) have a selective absence of CD8+ T cells, which is thought to be due to a block in the development of mature CD8+ cells from double-positive thymocytes. The gene defect responsible for this immune deficiency is the ZAP-70 kinase gene, which is associated with the ζ chain of the CD3-TCR complex.
   e. Defective genes of the signal transduction pathway of several cytokines have also been discovered. Mutations in the JAK3 gene, a member of the Janus family of protein tyrosine kinases, leads to an autosomal-recessive SCID.
5. Another cause of SCID is defective expression of class I and/or class II major histocompatibility complex (MHC) determinants on cells. The class II MHC components are expressed on antigen-presenting cells, such as B cells, dendritic cells, macrophages, and thymic epithelial cells. These molecules are critical for presenting antigen to the T-cell receptor of CD4+ helper T cells, which are important in cell-mediated immunity and humoral immune responses. MHC class I molecules are important in cytotoxic reactions and immunity to viruses in conjunction with CD8+ T cells. A transcriptional defect results in a deficiency in the expression of MHC class II molecules on cell surface membranes. In patients with MHC class I deficiency, a

defect in a transporter gene (TAP 2) has been reported. The protein product of the TAP gene is necessary to transport the MHC class I molecule to the cell surface.

Clinical Findings

1. The most common clinical phenotype of patients with SCID is early onset of recurrent infections, candidiasis, infection with opportunistic organisms, and chronic diarrhea, often leading to failure to thrive. Symptoms usually begin within the first 8 months of life.
   a. Oral candidiasis is a common finding in patients with T-cell deficiency. It responds poorly to topical therapies.
   b. Of all the opportunistic infections, *Pneumocystis carinii* is most common, with atypical mycobacteria appearing with increasing frequency.
   c. Systemic viral infection with complications, particularly with the DNA viruses such as varicella, cytomegalovirus (CMV), and adenovirus, are also characteristic of patients with SCID.
2. Patients with severe defects in T-cell immunity are at risk for graft-versus-host (GVH) reactions either from the transplacental passage of maternal lymphocytes or from immunocompetent lymphocytes from the transfusion of blood products.
3. Patients often develop failure to thrive from gastrointestinal disease manifesting as chronic diarrhea and malabsorption. An underlying infectious cause for the chronic diarrhea should be sought.
4. Hematologic abnormalities characterized by neutropenia, red blood cell aplasia, and megaloblastic anemia may occur. *P. carinii* may be associated with peripheral blood eosinophilia as can GVH reactions.
5. Neurologic disease, ranging from mental retardation to a chronic encephalomyelopathy, is common in SCID patients.

Key Clinical Findings: SCID

- Early onset of recurrent infections—virus, bacteria, and mycobacteria
- Oral candidiasis and infections with opportunistic pathogens
- Failure to thrive
- Risk of GVH disease from transfused blood products

Laboratory Findings

1. A complete blood count with differential shows lymphopenia (for age). Delayed hypersensitivity skin responsiveness to recall antigens is abnormal (anergy).
2. Enumeration of T cells and T-cell subsets in the peripheral blood shows low numbers of total T cells (CD2 + and CD3 + T cells). There is also a deficiency of the T-cell subsets—CD4 + and CD8 + cells. However, absolute counts can be variable, ranging from absent T cells to a variable pattern of T-cell subset deficiency.
3. Peripheral blood lymphocyte proliferative responses to mitogens, specific antigens, and allogeneic cells are usually abnormal but can be variable. Patients may also have a deficiency in cytokine production.
4. Serum immunoglobulin levels and specific antibody responses are also low because of the deficiency in T-cell helper function.
5. Patients with abnormalities of the purine metabolic pathway have a deficiency of cell and tissue ADA or purine nucleoside phosphorylase (PNP) enzymes.
   a. Patients with ADA deficiency have increased amounts of adenosine and deoxyadenosine in their plasma, and they excrete large amounts of deoxyadenosine in the urine. Inside cells, the accumulated deoxyadenosine is phosphorylated to deoxy ATP, which not only is trapped inside the cells, especially T cells, but also inhibits ribonucleotide reductase, which is important in DNA replication. In addition, the enzyme SAH hydrolase is inactivated, which results in the inhibition of DNA methylation pathways.
   b. There are two biochemical abnormalities in ADA and PNP deficiency.
      (1) A low level of serum uric acid is characteristic of PNP deficiency.
      (2) There is accumulation of deoxy ATP in cells as well as increased concentrations of adenosine and deoxyadenosine in the plasma, with the excretion of large amounts of deoxyadenosine in the urine.
6. In patients with MHC class I and class II deficiency (the bare lymphocyte syndrome), the lymphocyte count is typically normal or only moderately reduced. The number of circulating T and B cells is normal, but the number of CD4 + cells is low, particularly in patients who lack the expression of MHC class II determinants. By flow cytometry, mononuclear cells have markedly diminished or absent expression of class I and/or class II MHC determinants. As in other patients with SCID, humoral immunity is severely diminished.

Key Laboratory Findings: SCID

- Severe lymphopenia
- Low T-cell numbers
- Poor T-cell function; skin anergy
- Low serum immunoglobulins and poor antibody responses

Radiographic Changes

1. In the newborn period (only) the thymic shadow in the superior mediastinum of the chest is absent or very small. Stress alone can shrink the thymus, making radiographic interpretation of the thymic shadow difficult.
2. Fifty per cent of patients with ADA deficiency have characteristic x-ray findings of cupping and flaring of the costochondral junctions. Radiographic abnormalities of the transverse processes of the vertebrae and of the scapula are also found.

Treatment

1. Supportive therapy with prophylactic antibiotics for *P. carinii* and replacement therapy with intravenous immune serum globulin (IVIG) can diminish infections with bacterial pathogens.
2. All blood products should be irradiated (3000 rads) to reduce the risk of GVH disease.
3. In patients with failure to thrive and gastrointestinal symptoms, nutritional support with hyperalimentation is important. Gastrointestinal disturbances should be evaluated further for the presence of bacterial or parasitic infections.
4. Reconstitution of the cellular deficiency requires a more complex solution. The treatment of choice is bone marrow transplantation, particularly if an HLA/MLC tissue match is available. Haploidentical T-cell depleted bone marrow transplantation has become more widely available for persons without a sibling HLA/MLC tissue match.
5. In patients with ADA deficiency, treatment with ADA derived from calf intestine conjugated to polyethylene glycol (PEG-ADA) has been utilized as a direct replacement for the deficient enzyme. PEG-ADA is given by either intramuscular or subcutaneous injections once or twice weekly to maintain a plasma level of ADA enzyme activity. This reduces the toxic by-products and the accumulation of the substrates, e.g., adenosine and deoxyadenosine.
6. As more genetic defects are delineated in patients with SCID, gene therapy may become a possible option. Preliminary success of ADA-deficient patients has been reported.

Key Treatment: SCID

- Prophylactic antibiotics for *Pneumocytis carinii*
- IVIG replacement therapy
- Irradiation of all blood products
- Nutritional support
- Evaluation of gastrointestinal disturbances for infection
- Bone marrow transplantation
- Gene therapy

DiGeorge Anomaly or Thymic Hypoplasia

Definition

DiGeorge anomaly or thymic hypoplasia is an embryologic abnormality of the third and fourth pharyngeal pouches that occurs during early embryogenesis. The embryogenic defect results in hypoplasia or aplasia of the thymus and parathyroid glands, congenital heart disease, and abnormalities of the facies.

Etiology and Epidemiology

1. DiGeorge anomaly occurs equally in males and females. The estimated frequency in the general population is 1:66,000. However, in autopsies of children with congenital heart disease, 3 per cent had DiGeorge anomaly.

2. Patients frequently have abnormalities on chromosome 22 with microscopic deletions at 22q11.2. Most cases represent a sporadic event. Familial cases are associated with deletions on chromosome 22.

Pathophysiology

1. This clinical entity comprises a broad spectrum of malformations related to disturbed embryogenic development of tissues from the third and fourth pharyngeal pouches. Timing of the insult is thought to occur during the fourth through the seventh weeks of gestation. Severity and timing cause a varying picture of clinical defects.
2. Embryologists have proposed that the embryonic abnormalities associated with DiGeorge anomaly are related to a field defect. The neural crest tissue abnormality (neurocristopathy) can be associated with a number of etiologies, such as teratogens including alcohol, retinoids, and chromosomal defects, particularly those on chromosome 22.

Clinical Findings

1. The facial features of DiGeorge anomaly are very characteristic. Findings consist of hypertelorism, micrognathia, short philtrum of the upper lip, fish-shaped mouth, and low-set and posteriorly rotated ears.
2. Neonatal tetany occurs from hypocalcemia within the first 24 to 48 hours of life secondary to the hypoparathyroidism.
3. Congenital cardiac lesions involving conotruncal cardiac malformations are common. There is a high frequency (50%) of interrupted aortic arch type B and truncus arteriosus. Other cardiac defects include tetralogy of Fallot, right-sided aortic arch, and ventricular septal defects.
4. Patients usually present in the newborn period with symptoms of hypocalcemia and congenital heart disease. Problems with recurrent infections and candidiasis may not start until the seventh month of age, and then only depending on the severity of the immune defect.

Laboratory Findings

1. Involvement of the parathyroid gland leads to hypocalcemia, particularly in the newborn period. Parathyroid hormone levels are low to absent.
2. Chromosome abnormalities are common and can be seen in 90 per cent of patients. Involvement of chromosome 22 (22q11) is common. Monosomy 10p13, monosomy 18q21.33, and trisomy 18 have also been reported.
3. The degree of T-cell deficiency is related to the extent of the thymic hypoplasia and can be quite variable. T-cell numbers should be evaluated by flow cytometry, and tests of T-cell function by in vitro lymphoproliferative responses to mitogens and specific antigens should be performed.
4. Low CD4+ T-cell counts (<400 cells/mm^3) and/or poor phytohemagglutinin (PHA) proliferative responses ($\leq 10 \times$ background) suggest a degree of T-cell deficiency that will persist and require correction by immune reconstitution.
5. Most patients with DiGeorge anomaly have partial thymic hypoplasia with variable T-cell defects (partial DiGeorge anomaly). These patients have a good prognosis with regard to their immune function. Humoral immune re-

sponses are often normal in patients with partial DiGeorge anomaly but are usually abnormal in patients with complete DiGeorge anomaly.

Key Clinical and Laboratory Findings: DiGeorge Anomaly

- Aplasia or hypoplasia of the thymus
- Neonatal tetany secondary to hypocalcemia
- Abnormalities of the facies
- Congenital heart disease—conotruncal defects
- T-cell deficiency
- Abnormalities on chromosome 22

Radiographic Changes

1. Chest x-rays will be abnormal in patients with congenital heart disease; the findings will depend on the type of cardiac defect.
2. Often the thymic shadow is very prominent at birth but is absent or very small in patients with DiGeorge anomaly. Unfortunately, this is not a reliable indicator of T-cell deficiency.

Treatment

1. Hypoparathyroidism is managed with calcium supplements and vitamin D.
2. The congenital cardiac lesions need to be corrected, particularly if cyanotic congenital heart disease is present.
3. No live viral vaccine should be used in patients with T-cell deficiencies; patients with complete DiGeorge anomaly should receive trimethoprim-sulfamethoxazole antibiotic prophylaxis for the risk of infection with *P. carinii*.
4. Several approaches have been used to correct the thymic hypoplasia. Both thymic hormones and thymus transplantation have been employed.
5. In patients with complete DiGeorge anomaly and severe immune defects, IVIG may be required to supplement the humoral immunodeficiencies.
6. Bone marrow transplantation has been used in a few patients with DiGeorge anomaly to correct the immune defect.

Key Treatment: DiGeorge Anomaly

- Vitamin D
- Correct cardiac defects
- IVIG, if inadequate antibody responses
- If complete anomaly: PcP prophylaxis; thymic transplantation

Hyper-IgM Syndrome

Definition

1. In this immunodeficiency, patients have elevated serum levels of IgM but no IgA and very low concentrations of IgG, resulting in increased susceptibility to pyogenic infections. This disease is inherited as an X-linked disorder in approximately 70 per cent of patients.
2. Female patients with the same clinical findings have been described.
3. The gene defect for this X-linked form of hyper-IgM syndrome has been defined and mapped to Xq26 on the long arm of the X chromosome.

Pathophysiology

1. The gene defect for the hyper-IgM syndrome encodes for a membrane determinant called CD40 ligand on activated T cells. Mutation in the CD40 ligand gene results in a dysfunctional protein, while gene deletions result in the absence of the ligand expression on activated T cells.
2. The CD40 ligand on activated T cells provides an activation signal to B cells that induces memory B-cells and the switch from IgM to other immunoglobulin isotypes. Thus, patients with this defect fail to switch their B cells from making IgM to making other immunoglobulin isotypes. This occurs because the T cells of these patients cannot provide the appropriate switch signal to the CD40 receptor on B cells.
3. B cells from hyper-IgM patients can be stimulated to produce IgG, IgA, and IgE when given the appropriate cell membrane signal through the CD40 receptor and certain cytokines. This suggests that the major defect in these patients is in the T-cell population. CD40 is expressed on the surface of other cells, such as monocytes, dendritic cells, and thymic epithelial cells, which indicates that other cell-cell interactions mediated by the CD40 ligand/CD40 receptor interaction may be abnormal.
4. Since the CD40 ligand molecule is not required for normal T-cell development, female obligate heterozygote carriers of the X-linked hyper-IgM syndrome do have random inactivation (Lyon hypothesis) of the X chromosome in T lymphocytes.

Clinical Findings

1. Patients with hyper-IgM syndrome have a clinical history of pyogenic infections, including otitis media, sinusitis, and pneumonia.
2. Unlike the case with many of the humoral immunodeficiencies, patients are susceptible to opportunistic infections with *P. carinii* and *Cryptosporidium*. The latter has been associated with protracted diarrhea.
3. These patients are prone to a variety of autoimmune processes mainly of the hematopoietic system, such as autoimmune neutropenia, hemolytic anemia, and thrombocytopenic purpura. Autoimmune neutropenia may be seen in 50 per cent of patients, causing persistent stomatitis and recurrent oral ulcers.
4. Patients with hyper-IgM syndrome have an increased risk of abdominal cancers. In the second decade of life, proliferation of IgM plasma cells invading the gastrointestinal tract and liver has been associated with early death.
5. Lymphoid hyperplasia can be marked, with lymphadenopathy and hepatosplenomegaly.

Laboratory Findings

1. Patients with hyper-IgM syndrome have elevated serum IgM levels, ranging from high-normal to ≥1000 mg/dl.

IgD levels are also elevated. Serum IgA and IgE levels are usually undetectable, and the serum IgG is very low (<150 mg/dl). Patients have the ability to make a primary IgM antibody response, but they fail to make specific IgG antibodies.

2. B lymphocytes circulate in normal numbers but express only IgM and IgD on their cell surface.

3. The number of T cells and T-cell subsets is normal, but the cells lack expression or have diminished expression of the CD40 ligand (gp39). In vitro lymphocyte proliferative responses to mitogens and antigens are normal in most patients.

Key Clinical and Laboratory Findings: Hyper-IgM Syndrome

- Recurrent pyogenic infection
- Infections with opportunistic organisms
- Autoimmune neutropenia
- Lymphoid hyperplasia
- Increased risk of abdominal cancers
- Markedly elevated serum levels of IgM
- Low or absent IgG and IgA
- Absent or decreased expression of the CD40 ligand on T cells

Prevention

1. Although the X chromosome exhibits random X-inactivation, a polymorphic region at the 3′ end of the gene allows prenatal diagnosis of the X-linked form of hyper-IgM syndrome.

2. Carriers of the X-linked abnormality can also be diagnosed by this polymorphic region of the CD40 ligand gene.

Treatment

1. Treatment is the same as for patients with X-linked agammaglobulinemia (XLA).

2. Prophylaxis with trimethoprim-sulfamethoxazole for *P. carinii* infections is helpful.

3. Patients with neutropenia have responded to cytokine therapy with granulocyte-colony stimulating factor (G-CSF).

4. Patients must be carefully followed for the development of malignancies.

Key Treatment: Hyper-IgM Syndrome

- Antibiotics
- IVIG

Wiskott-Aldrich Syndrome

Definition

Wiskott-Aldrich syndrome is an X-linked recessive disorder in which affected males have thrombocytopenia, eczema, and recurrent infections.

Etiology

The gene defect in Wiskott-Aldrich syndrome is located on chromosome Xp11.23 on the short arm. Obligate female heterozygous carriers have nonrandom inactivation of their X chromosome, which facilitates carrier detection in females.

Pathophysiology

1. The defective gene for Wiskott-Aldrich syndrome has recently been identified; it encodes a proline-rich protein (WASP) that is involved in cytoskeleton actin organization.

2. A platelet-leukocyte surface molecule defect involving a sialophorin (CD43) was reported. CD43 is expressed early in thymocyte ontogeny, suggesting its importance in lymphocyte differentiation. CD43 is part of the cytoskeletal structure of cells and is thus involved in cell activation and proliferation. The gene for CD43 is located on chromosome 16; in these patients this cell surface molecule is unstable on in vitro culture of lymphocytes. This CD43 cell surface determinant can be used as a marker to help diagnose the disorder.

Clinical Findings

1. Patients have increased susceptibility to pyogenic and opportunistic infections.

2. The early onset of thrombocytopenia is associated with the risk of a severe bleeding disorder. Infections often exacerbate the bleeding, which can be severe and life-threatening.

3. Most patients have moderate to severe eczema.

4. Autoimmune disease is common, particularly autoimmune hemolytic anemia.

5. Patients have increased risk for malignancies such as lymphomas, especially beyond the age of 8 years. These malignancies are frequently found in the brain.

Key Clinical and Laboratory Features: Wiskott-Aldrich Syndrome

- X-linked disorder
- Eczema
- Recurrent infections
- Petechiae and thrombocytopenia with small platelets
- Autoimmune hemolytic anemia
- Lymphomas of the brain
- Low serum levels of IgM
  Normal or elevated serum concentrations of IgG, IgA, and IgE
- Poor antibody responses to polysaccharide antigens

Laboratory Findings

1. Patients with Wiskott-Aldrich syndrome have small platelets. The presence of thrombocytopenia plus small platelets is diagnostic for the syndrome.

2. Serum quantitative levels of IgG are normal; IgA and IgE are elevated, and IgM is low.

3. Patients have absent antibody responses to polysaccharide antigens and poor responses to protein antigens. Isohemagglutinins to blood ABO groups are often absent.
4. T-cell function as measured by in vitro lymphocyte proliferative responses to mitogens and specific antigens is poor.
5. The number of B cells circulating in the peripheral blood may be elevated, while the number of T cells gradually diminishes with age.

Treatment

1. Supportive therapy with antibiotics and IVIG is important.
2. Splenectomy may be necessary for patients with thrombocytopenia and severe bleeding problems and in those with life-threatening autoimmune hemolytic anemia.
3. Bone marrow transplantation has successfully been used in a few patients. The survival of matched bone marrow transplants is quite good, whereas the survival of haploidentical (from mother or father) bone marrow transplants is poor (20 to 25%). A high incidence of B-cell lymphoma and GVH disease accounts for the poor outcome.

Prevention

1. Since the obligate carrier has nonrandom X-chromosome inactivation, the carrier state can be identified in females.
2. Polymorphism in the DNA regions close to the Wiskott-Aldrich gene allows prenatal diagnosis.

Ataxia-Telangiectasia (AT)

Definition

Ataxia-telangiectasia is a multisystem disorder characterized by recurrent infection, telangiectasia, and progressive ataxia.

Etiology

It is inherited as an autosomal recessive disorder.

Pathophysiology

1. The multisystem involvement in and the complexity of the clinical presentation suggests that the gene defect is a nuclear regulatory factor. Recent genetic analysis has identified a possible candidate gene region on chromosome 11q 22–23 in AT families. The gene responsible for AT has been named ATM and is related to known signal transduction factors involved in cell cycle control, mammalian PI-3 kinase, and DNA repair from ionizing radiation damage.
2. The defect in cell growth may be linked to chromosomal integrity and difficulty in repairing DNA damage. These observations have been associated with an increased sensitivity to ionizing radiation.
3. An elevated serum α-fetoprotein level suggests a defect in tissue differentiation.

Clinical Findings

1. The cerebellar ataxia develops in infancy in most patients but can be delayed until age 4 or 5 years. The ataxia progresses slowly, eventually leading to severe disability. In addition to the ataxia, patients develop chorioathetosis as well as myotonic and oculomotor abnormalities.
2. Telangiectasia appears between ages 2 and 8 years, initially on the bulbar conjunctivae and later on the surfaces of the nose and ears and dorsa of the hands and feet. Other skin lesions include skin atrophy, hypopigmentation, hypertrichosis, eczema, and cutaneous malignancies.
3. The immunodeficiency leads to recurrent sinopulmonary infections, most of which are bacterial. Opportunistic infections are uncommon despite the T-cell abnormalities in AT. Persistent infections of the lower respiratory system may lead to bronchiectasis.
4. Numerous malignancies have been reported in patients with AT, including lymphosarcoma, Hodgkin's disease, adenocarcinoma, reticulum cell carcinoma, and medulloblastoma. In addition, family members of patients with AT have an increased risk for malignancy.
5. Endocrine abnormalities occur frequently. Over 50 per cent of patients have metabolic glucose abnormalities, including hyperinsulinemia, insulin resistance, and hyperglycemia. Female patients have delayed or absent secondary sex characteristics. Male patients have hypogonadism.
6. Liver dysfunction occurs in 40 to 50 per cent of patients. Histopathology shows fatty infiltration and an inflammatory cell infiltrate.

Key Clinical Findings: Ataxia-Telangiectasia

- Cerebellar ataxia
- Telangiectasia
- Recurrent infections
- Malignancies
- Endocrine abnormalities
- Liver dysfunction

Laboratory Findings

1. Serum IgA deficiency is frequently found (70%), and 80 per cent have IgE deficiency. Most patients have reduced IgG$_2$ and IgG$_4$ subclass serum levels. Specific antibody responses are impaired.
2. About 60 per cent of patients have T-cell deficiencies. Mitogen responses and specific antigen responses are abnormal. Lymphopenia may be present, and reduction in total T cells and T-cell subsets occurs. The thymus gland histology often shows hypoplasia.
3. Chromosome analysis reveals excessive chromosomal breaks. Chromosomal rearrangements and translocations are 40 times higher in AT patients than in normal subjects. These translocations usually involve chromosomes 7 and 14 at the sites of the T-cell receptor and the immunoglobulin heavy-chain genes.
4. Patients have elevated α-fetoprotein in their serum.

Key Laboratory Findings: Ataxia-Telangiectasia

- IgA and IgE deficiency
- Elevated serum levels of α-fetoprotein
- Excessive chromosomal breaks
- T-cell deficiency

Radiographic Changes

1. Scans of the brain show enlarged ventricles and diffuse cerebral atrophy.
2. MRI of the brain often shows marked cerebellar atrophy.

Treatment

1. Supportive therapy with pulmonary hygiene and appropriate antibiotics for the treatment of recurrent sinopulmonary infections is important.
2. Treatment of the degenerative CNS cerebellar ataxia is not available.
3. Immune reconstitution is difficult in AT patients. IVIG has not proved to be of benefit except perhaps in those patients with IgG subclass and specific antibody deficiencies.

Bibliography

SEVERE COMBINED IMMUNODEFICIENCY DISEASE (SCID)

Fischer A: Primary T-cell immunodeficiencies. Curr Opin Immunol 1993;5:569–578.

Hershfield MS: PEG-ADA replacement therapy for adenosine deaminase deficiency: An update after 8.5 years. Clin Immunol Immunopathol 1994;76(3):228–232.

Hirschhorn R: Adenosine deaminase deficiency: molecular basis and recent developments. Clin Immunol Immunopathol 1995;76(3):219–227.

Hong R, Clement LT, Gatti RA, Kirkpatrick CH: Disorders of the T-cell system. In Stiehm ER (ed): Immunologic Disorders in Infants and Children, 4th ed. Philadelphia, WB Saunders, 1996, pp 339–408.

Stephan JL, Vlekova V, Le Deist F, et al: Severe combined immunodeficiency: A retrospective single-center study of clinical presentation and outcome in 117 patients. J Pediatr 1993;23:64–572.

DIGEORGE ANOMALY OR THYMIC HYPOPLASIA

Bastian J, Law S, Vogler L, et al: Prediction of persistent immunodeficiency in the DiGeorge anomaly. J Pediatr 1989;115:391–396.

Hong R: The DiGeorge anomaly. Immunodefic Rev 1991;3:1–14.

Hong R, Clement LT, Gatti RA, Kirkpatrick CH: Disorders of the T-cell system. In Stiehm ER (ed): Immunologic Disorders in Infants and Children, 4th ed. Philadelphia, WB Saunders, 1996, pp 339–408.

Junker AK, Driscoll DA: Humoral immunity in DiGeorge syndrome. J Pediatr 1995;127:231–237.

HYPER-IgM SYNDROME

Conley ME: X-linked severe combined immunodeficiency. Clin Immunol Immunopathol 1991;61:94–99.

Hong R, Clement LT, Gatti RA, Kirkpatrick CH: Disorders of the T-cell system. In Stiehm ER (ed): Immunologic Disorders in Infants and Children, 4th ed. Philadelphia, WB Saunders, 1996, pp 339–408.

Noelle RJ: The role of gp39 (CD40L) in immunity. Clin Immunol Immunopathol 1995;76(3):203–207.

Ochs HD, Aruffo A: Advances in X-linked immunodeficiency diseases. Curr Opin Pediatr 1993;5:684–691.

Rosen FS, Cooper MD, Wedgwood RJP: The primary immunodeficiencies. N Engl J Med 1995;333(7):431–440.

WISKOTT-ALDRICH SYNDROME

Hong R, Clement LT, Gatti RA, Kirkpatrick CH: Disorders of the T-cell system. In Stiehm ER (ed): Immunologic Disorders in Infants and Children, 4th ed. Philadelphia, WB Saunders, 1996, pp 339–408.

Ochs HD, Aruffo A: Advances in X-linked immunodeficiency diseases. Curr Opin Pediatr 1993;5:684–691.

Rosen FS, Cooper MD, Wedgwood RJP: The primary immunodeficiencies. N Engl J Med 1995;333(7):431–440.

ATAXIA-TELANGIECTASIA

Hong R, Clement LT, Gatti RA, Kirkpatrick CH: Disorders of the T-cell system. In Stiehm ER (ed): Immunologic Disorders in Infants and Children, 4th ed. Philadelphia, WB Saunders, 1996, pp 339–408.

Rosen FS, Cooper MD, Wedgwood RJP: The primary immunodeficiencies. N Engl J Med 1995;333(7):31–440.

Waldmann TA, Misiti J, Nelson DL, Kraemer KH: Ataxia-telangiectasia: A multisystem hereditary disease with immunodeficiency, impaired organ maturation, x-ray hypersensitivity, and a high incidence of neoplasia. Ann Intern Med 1983;99:367–379.

73 Asthma

James N. Moy

Definition

Asthma can be classified as a reversible obstructive airway disease with chronic inflammation and hyperreactivity of the airways.

Etiology

Almost all children with asthma are sensitized to inhalant allergens. Genetically susceptible individuals inhale common allergens, such as pollens, mold spores, and animal or insect proteins, and their allergen-sensitive T lymphocytes produce cytokines (e.g., IL-4) that lead to IgE production by B lymphocytes. Mast cells in the airways are then sensitized by the allergen-specific IgE antibodies. Upon reexposure to the allergen, the mast cells are activated by the cross-linking of IgE Fc receptors, and mediators are released that cause the signs and symptoms of asthma.

Epidemiology

In the United States, the prevalence of asthma has been reported to be from 4 to 8 per cent of the general population. Mortality rates among 5- to 34-year-olds increased by 6.2 per cent a year (from the 1977 low to slightly over 4 per million population in 1987) and seem to have stabilized at this level. However, mortality among African Americans is three to four times higher than among white Americans.

1. The prevalence of asthma is greater in blacks than in Caucasians. The asthma prevalence in inner-city African American children might be as high as 12 to 15 per cent.
2. Boys have a higher prevalence than girls by a 2:1 ratio before 14 years of age.
3. A positive family history of asthma or atopy among first-degree relatives is associated with an increased risk of asthma.
4. The relative risk for the development of asthma is four times higher in children with a family history of atopy who are exposed to high levels of dust mite allergen during infancy.
5. Exposure to passive cigarette smoke is a risk for the development of asthma in children.

Pathophysiology

1. In 50 per cent of asthmatics there are two phases to an asthma episode: the early asthmatic response (EAR) and the late asthmatic response (LAR).
   a. Activation of mast cells and the resultant effects of mast cell mediators within the first 20 to 30 minutes is known as the early phase of asthma, or EAR. The early phase is characterized by bronchospasm.
   b. Upon inhalation of the offending allergen, mast cells in the airways are activated and release mediators that give rise to the initial bronchoconstriction. These mediators include preformed mediators such as histamine and newly synthesized mediators such as leukotrienes (LTC_4, LTD_4, LTE_4), prostaglandin D_2, and platelet-activating factor (PAF). In addition to causing bronchoconstriction, these mediators cause increased microvascular permeability and increased mucus secretion.
   c. A second, prolonged inflammatory state often follows the immediate phase and is referred to as the late-phase response (LAR). The early phase usually resolves within an hour after the individual is removed from the allergen. However, over the next few hours the LAR develops, and the symptoms can be more severe than in the early phase. The late phase may last from hours to days.
   d. The late phase results from the recruitment of inflammatory cells, such as eosinophils, basophils, and T lymphocytes, by mediators released in the early phase. PAF is a potent chemotactic agent for eosinophils.
   e. Eosinophils, T lymphocytes, and monocytes also release mediators, cytokines, and chemokines that can damage the bronchial epithelium and propagate the inflammation in the airways.
2. Mediators of IgE-mediated reactions are from mast cells during the immediate phase. In the late phase, mediators are released by eosinophils, T lymphocytes, respiratory epithelial cells, basophils, monocytes/macrophages, and neutrophils. Table 73–1 lists the mediators that are involved in IgE-mediated asthma.
3. The histopathology of asthma consists of desquamation of respiratory epithelium and eosinophilic infiltration of the airway walls. There is bronchial smooth muscle

TABLE 73–1. MEDIATORS IN ASTHMA

CELL OF ORIGIN	MEDIATOR	ACTIONS
Early Phase		
Mast cells (preformed)	Histamine	Bronchoconstriction
		Increased vascular permeability
	TNF-α	Activation of other cells
Mast cells (newly synthesized)	LTC_4, LTD_4, LTE_4	Bronchoconstriction
		Increases vascular permeability
	PGD_2	Bronchoconstriction
	Platelet-activating	Bronchoconstriction
		Increases vascular permeability
		Chemotaxis of eosinophils and neutrophils
Late Phase		
Eosinophils	Major basic protein	Epithelial cell damage
		Activation of basophil histamine release
		Activation of neutrophils and platelets
Basophils	Histamine, $LTC_4/D_4/E_4$	Same as above
T lymphocytes	IL-3, GM-CSF	Together with IL-5, prolongs survival of eosinophils
	IL-4	Promotes IgE synthesis
	IL-5	Promotes eosinophil survival and chemotaxis
Macrophages	LTD_4/E_4	Same as above
	TNF-α	
	GM-CSF	
Epithelial cells	Endothelin-1	Bronchoconstriction
	IL-8	Neutrophil chemotaxis
	GM-CSF	Same as above
	RANTES	Eosinophil chemotaxis and activation
	MCP-1	Basophil chemotaxis and activation
Neutrophils	Superoxide anion and proteases	Host tissue damage
	Elastase	Increases mucus secretion

hypertrophy and thickening of the basement membrane. The airway lumen is frequently filled with mucous plugs.

Clinical Findings

1. The most common symptom of asthma is wheezing. However, a dry cough, chest tightness, chest pain, and shortness of breath with exertion are regularly seen. The earliest sign of bronchospasm may be cough. Nocturnal symptoms of wheezing and cough are often seen in poorly controlled asthma.
2. In addition to wheezing, physical examination may reveal retractions, tachypnea, poor air entry, and a prolonged expiratory phase. Children with poorly controlled, long-standing asthma may have an increased diameter of the chest.
3. Many children will have signs and symptoms of atopy, such as allergic rhinitis, atopic dermatitis, and a history of food allergy. Although children are often atopic, viral infections are the most frequent triggers of asthma in the young child.
4. Children with chronic asthma can be classified as mild, moderate, or severe in order to enable optimal management of the disease (Table 73–2).
5. The severity of an acute exacerbation of asthma may be estimated using the parameters in Table 73–3.

TABLE 73–2. CLASSIFICATION OF SEVERITY IN CHRONIC ASTHMA

MILD

Symptoms <2 times/week
No symptoms in between episodes
Exercise-induced asthma (EIA) only with strenuous exercise
Nocturnal symptoms <2 times/month
No acute episodes necessitating medical appointments or hospitalizations for asthma in the past year
PEFR ≥80% of predicted
PEFR variability ≤20%

MODERATE

Symptoms >2 times/week
Occasional symptoms in between episodes
EIA with mild exercise
Nocturnal symptoms 4 to 5 nights per month
Three or fewer acute episodes necessitating medical appointments and no hospitalizations for asthma in the past year
PEFR 60–80% of predicted
PEFR variability 20–30%

SEVERE

Symptoms almost daily
EIA even with medication; activity limited
Nocturnal symptoms almost nightly
More than 3 acute episodes necessitating medical appointments or 1 or more hospitalizations for asthma in the past year
PEFR <60% of predicted
PEFR variability >30%

Adapted from NHLBI Expert Panel Report.

6. Severe complications of status asthmaticus include

  a. Pneumothorax or pneumomediastinum

  b. Acute mucous plugging of the airways with atelectasis

Differential Diagnosis of Wheezing (from common to rare)

- Bronchiolitis in infants ≤18 months of age
- Foreign body
- Recurrent aspiration
- Cystic fibrosis
- Left ventricular failure
- Vascular anomalies of the great vessels
- Mediastinal masses
- Tracheoesophageal fistula

7. Clinical variations of asthma include exercise-induced asthma (EIA), nocturnal asthma, and gastroesophageal reflux–induced wheezing.

  a. Patients with EIA wheeze within 5 minutes after exercise. EIA can be prevented by using 2 puffs of a β_2 agonist, cromolyn sodium, or nedocromil sodium 20 minutes before exercise. Exercise such as running in cold, dry air is more likely to provoke EIA than swimming in an indoor pool.

  b. Patients with poorly controlled asthma tend to have more nocturnal symptoms of wheezing and/or cough. However, some asthmatics will have only nocturnal symptoms. The usual period for nocturnal symptoms is between 1 A.M. and 4 A.M. Clinical studies looking at cell counts in bronchoalveolar lavage fluids of patients with nocturnal asthma have demonstrated an increase in inflammatory cells, such as eosinophils, at 4 A.M. Nocturnal asthma can be treated with a 24-hour release (Uniphyl) or, in the younger child, a 12-hour release (Slo-bid) theophylline preparation at 7 mg/kg to be taken between 5 and 7 hours before the usual time of night asthma symptoms. Some patients may also benefit from a long-acting β_2 agonist.

  c. Gastroesophageal reflux may cause wheezing or worsen existing asthma. However, there are few studies that clearly demonstrate a role for reflux in the pathogenesis of asthma. If the patient's asthma is recalcitrant despite optimal management, a workup for reflux is warranted. Gastroesophageal reflux should also be considered in patients with nocturnal asthma symptoms.

 Key Clinical Findings: Asthma

- Dry cough
- Chest tightness
- Shortness of breath
- Cough with exercise
- Cough during sleep
- Wheezing
- Signs and symptoms of atopy

TABLE 73–3. EVALUATION OF ACUTE EXACERBATION OF ASTHMA

SIGN/SYMPTOM	SEVERITY OF ACUTE EXACERBATION OF ASTHMA		
	Mild	Moderate	Severe
Alertness	Normal	Normal	Decreased
Dyspnea	Absent, speaks complete sentences	Speaks phrases	Speaks short phrases or words only
Pulsus paradoxicus (mmHg)	<10	10–20	20–40
Accessory muscle use	None	Sternocleidomastoid	All accessory muscles, nasal flaring
Color	Good	Pale	Cyanotic
Auscultatory findings	End-expiratory wheezing	Inspiratory and expiratory wheezing	Decreased breath sounds
O$_2$ saturation (%)	>95	90–95	<90
Pco$_2$ (mmHg)	<35	<40	>40
PEFR (% of predicted or % of best)	70–90	50–70	<50

Laboratory Findings

1. Pulmonary function testing is paramount in the diagnosis of asthma. In asthma, the airway obstruction should be reversible, as evidenced by a 15 per cent improvement in the forced expiratory volume (FEV_1) in 1 second with administration of an inhaled β_2 agonist. Specific features on spirometry testing include

    a. Forced vital capacity (FVC) is usually normal or slightly decreased in asthma.

    b. FEV_1 is decreased.

    c. FEV_1/FVC ratio is 0.7 or less.

    d. Peak expiratory flow rate (PEFR) is decreased.

    e. Forced expiratory flow (FEF_{25-75}) is decreased.

2. Many children with asthma will have positive IgE skin test results to inhalant allergens, indicating underlying atopy.

3. In an acute episode of asthma exacerbation, the Po_2 is decreased. The Pco_2 is also initially decreased because of hyperventilation. If the asthma episode persists, the Pco_2 may become normal or elevated. Even a Pco_2 of 40 mm in an asthmatic with hyperventilation indicates pending respiratory failure.

Key Laboratory Finding: Asthma

- Diminished peak flow rates
- Decreased FEV_1 with 15% improvement after β_2-agonist
- Hyperinflation with flat diaphragms on chest x-ray
- Positive immediate skin tests, indicating atopy

Radiographic Changes

1. Children with chronic, poorly controlled asthma may have chest radiographs that show increased anteroposterior (AP) diameter.

2. In the acute exacerbation of asthma, there may be hyperinflation of the lungs with flattened diaphragms.

    a. Areas of atelectasis may be present.

    b. The presence of pneumothorax and pneumomediastinum should always be determined on the radiograph.

Treatment

Treatment is divided into the management of chronic asthma and the management of acute episodes.

1. For chronic management, the goal of therapy is to optimize daily activity with minimal medication side effects. Physicians caring for asthmatics should provide their patients with a written asthma management plan.

    a. Spacer devices should always be used with metered-dose inhalers for optimal delivery of the medications to the airways.

    b. Patients with moderate to severe asthma should perform and record PEFR readings every morning and evening. The asthma management plan should include instructions for medication use and for contacting the physician when the PEFR readings fall below predetermined values. Usually, the patient and the parents are instructed to use an inhaled β_2 agonist when the PEFR falls below 80 per cent of baseline and to contact the physician when the PEFR falls below 50 per cent of baseline.

2. Medications used include preventive medications and rescue medications. Preventative medications are anti-inflammatory drugs and should be used on a regular basis.

    a. Cromolyn sodium prevents both the EAR and the LAR.

    b. Nedocromil also prevents both the EAR and the LAR.

    c. Inhaled corticosteroids prevent the LAR only.

3. Rescue medications are short-acting β_2 agonists, which provide prompt bronchodilation and should be used on an as-needed basis. They prevent the EAR only. The β_2 agonists include

    a. Albuterol

    b. Metaproterenol

    c. Pirbuterol

4. Other bronchodilators include ipratropium bromide and theophylline, but these should not be used as rescue medicines because they have a slower onset of action. Salmeterol is a long-acting β_2 agonist and should not be used as a rescue medication.

5. Systemic corticosteroids are used for severe asthmatics and for chronic asthma; the lowest dose on an alternate-day regimen that provides optimal control should be used.

6. Chronic management can be guided by the severity of the asthma as outlined above.

    a. Mild—Inhaled β_2 agonists as needed and inhaled b2 agonists or cromolyn or nedocromil 20 minute before exercise for EIA.

    b. Moderate—Inhaled cromolyn or nedocromil, 2 puffs q.i.d., and inhaled β_2 agonists as needed. If the cromolyn or nedocromil is ineffective, an inhaled corticosteroid should be used. A long-acting theophylline preparation may be added at bedtime for nocturnal symptoms.

    c. Severe—Inhaled corticosteroids with or without the addition of nedocromil on a regular basis. Theophylline may be added, as may inhaled ipratropium bromide. A short-acting β_2 agonist is to be used as needed for symptoms of bronchospasm, but the patient may find that it is needed three to four times a day. Salmeterol may decrease the frequency of short-acting β_2 agonist use, but the patients and parents must be reminded that for immediate relief of bronchoconstriction, a short-acting β_2 agonist must be used.

7. Immunotherapy may be also be given a trial, but the effects of immunotherapy for asthma are not as clearly beneficial as for allergic rhinitis.

8. For mild to moderate acute exacerbation of asthma at home, an inhaled β_2 agonist should be given up to three times every 20 minutes until a good response is achieved. If the child is in a medical facility, he or she

should be placed on supplemental oxygen. The child should then be started on oral prednisone 1 mg/kg up to 60 mg/ day for 5 to 7 days. Beta-2 agonists should be given three to four times a day for the next 2 to 3 days and then on an as-needed basis.

9. If there is poor response after three β_2 agonist treatments, the patient should go to an emergency room or a physician's office to be evaluated.

   a. In the emergency room, supplemental oxygen should be started. Beta-2 agonist inhalation may be given every 20 minutes or continuously, and corticosteroids (2 mg/kg prednisone equivalent) given orally or intravenously.

   b. The severity of the asthma should be assessed using the guidelines listed in Table 73–2. An arterial blood gas measurement may be avoided if O_2 saturation monitoring is available. A chest radiograph is necessary if pneumothorax, pneumomediastinum, or pneumonia is suspected.

   c. If treatment is required past 4 hours, the patient may need to be hospitalized.

   d. If the patient responds, prednisone should be continued for at least 5 to 7 days and may need to be tapered over 2 weeks. The patient and parents should be instructed to stay in touch with the physician by phone over the next several days.

Prevention

1. Prevention of acute exacerbation of asthma consists of

   a. Avoiding triggers such as cigarette smoke and known allergens.

Key Treatment: Asthma

- Allergen and cigarette smoke avoidance
- Prevention with anti-inflammatory medications
- Rescue with short-acting β_2 agonists
- Spacer devices for metered-dose inhalers
- Asthma monitoring with peak flow meters
- Asthma education for parents and child

   b. Using medication as prescribed on a regular basis.

   c. If possible, avoiding contact with persons with known viral respiratory infections.

2. Prevention of the development of asthma has been demonstrated in a cohort of children with positive family histories for atopy when these infants were raised in an environment with strict dust mite control measures.

Bibliography

Barnes PJ: Cytokines as mediators of chronic asthma. Am J Respir Crit Care Med 1994;150:S42–S49.

Middleton E, Reed CE, Elliot FE, et al (eds): Allergy: Principles and Practice, 4th ed. St. Louis, CV Mosby, 1993.

Shapiro GG: Childhood asthma: update. Pediatr Rev 1992;13:403–412.

Tinkelman DG, Naspitz KN (eds): Childhood Asthma: Pathophysiology and Treatment, 2nd ed. New York, Marcel Dekker, 1993.

U.S. Department of Health and Human Services, Public Health Service: International Consensus Report on Diagnosis and Management of Asthma. Publication No. 92-3091. Washington, DC, National Institutes of Health, 1992.

74 Angioedema/Urticaria

James N. Moy

Definition

Urticarial lesions, or hives, are pruritic, erythematous, cutaneous elevations that blanch with pressure. Angioedema is swelling that occurs in the deep dermis and subcutaneous tissue. In contrast to urticaria, angioedema has little or no associated pruritis.

1. Acute urticaria is self-limited.
2. Chronic urticaria is arbitrarily classified as lasting longer than 6 weeks.

Etiology

Urticaria/angioedema may be allergic (IgE-mediated), immunologic, or nonimmunologic. Allergic causes may be foods, medications, and, rarely, inhalant allergens. Immunologic causes are usually medications or perhaps infection. Physical urticarias fall under the nonimmunologic classification. Examples of physical urticarias are cold urticaria, pressure urticaria, and solar urticaria.

Epidemiology

More than 20 per cent of the general population have suffered an eruption of urticaria or an episode of angioedema at some point in their lives. Chronic urticaria is much more common in adults than in children.

Pathophysiogy

1. The pathology in urticaria and angioedema is caused by vasoactive mediators that lead to the dilation of small venules and capillaries in the superficial dermis (urticaria) or in the deeper dermal layers (angioedema). There is widening of the dermal papillae, flattening of the rete pegs, and swelling of collagen fibers.

Common Causes of Urticaria and Angioedema

Reactions to Ingestants
Foods
Food additives
Drugs
Inhalant Allergens
By inhalation or contact (e.g., cat allergen)
Infections
Viral
Hepatitis
Bacterial
Group A streptococcal pharyngitis
Urinary tract infection
Parasitic
Systemic Diseases
Thyroid dysfunction
Collagen vascular diseases
Malignancy
Physical Urticarias
Dermatographism
Cholinergic urticaria
Cold urticaria
Pressure urticaria/angioedema
Solar urticaria
Vibratory angioedema
Urticaria Pigmentosa and Systemic Mastocytosis
Hereditary Disorders
Hereditary angioedema
Familial cold urticaria
Urticaria with amyloidosis, deafness, and limb pain

2. The mediators include histamine; leukotrienes C_2, D_2, and E_2; prostaglandin D_2; and platelet-activating factor from activation of mast cells and bradykinin from autoactivation of Hageman factor.

Clinical Picture

1. Urticarial lesions can appear on any part of the body where there is skin. The lesions are usually multiple but rarely can appear as a single hive. Each lesion should last less than 24 hours. Urticarial lesions do not result in discoloration of the skin. There may be areas of excoriation of skin due to pruritus.
2. Angioedema usually involves the face, tongue, distal extremities, and sometimes genitalia. Angioedema does not involve dependent areas, as opposed to edema from hypo-

Key Clinical Findings: Urticaria

- Skin pruritus
- A lesion persisting ≤24 hours
- No discoloration of the skin
- Common causes include
  Viral infections
  Antibiotic hypersensitivity

proteinemia or congestive heart failure. As in the case with urticaria, angioedema swellings tend to be transient and nonsymmetric.
3. The most common cause of urticaria and angioedema in children is a viral infection; the second most common cause is a hypersensitivity reaction to antibiotics.

Laboratory Findings

1. There are no laboratory findings that confirm that diagnosis of urticaria/angioedema. However, a skin biopsy should be obtained if another process, such as vasculitis, is suspected.
   a. The findings in biopsies of lesions of acute urticaria and most physical urticaria demonstrate increased vascular permeability and edematous tissue, without a cellular infiltrate.
   b. A biopsy of a lesion from a patient with chronic urticaria will reveal a non-necrotizing perivascular mononuclear cell infiltrate in addition to the findings in acute urticaria.
2. Laboratory tests may be helpful in determining the underlying cause of acute urticaria/angioedema.
   a. A child with acute urticaria/angioedema secondary to an IgE-mediated reaction should easily be identified by history. An in vitro blood test (e.g., RAST) for specific IgE antibodies to food antigens may be obtained to confirm the diagnosis. Skin tests for suspected foods in a patient with angioedema or severe urticaria is not recommended because even a small amount of antigen in the skin test extracts might cause a severe reaction (even anaphylaxis) in a food-allergic patient.
   b. Except for penicillin, diagnostic in vitro testing or skin testing for drug allergies has not been well established.
   c. Evaluation of suspected ingestants as the cause of chronic urticaria is more difficult. Skin testing with food antigens in chronic urticaria is rarely useful. The skin tests tend to have a high incidence of false positive reactions. Patients with daily hives (or at least every other day) may be placed on an elimination diet for 5 days. The diet consists of water, rice, and lamb or chicken. If the urticaria resolves on this regimen, a new food is added to the diet every 2 to 3 days. Thus, if the hives recur, the last food added is implicated as the culprit. However, food allergy is best diagnosed by double-blind, placebo-controlled food challenges.
   d. In the evaluation of chronic urticaria/angioedema when the cause is not obvious, the tests listed in the following box are recommended. However, in over 70 per cent of cases of chronic urticaria/angioedema an etiology is never determined.
   e. Cold urticaria can be diagnosed by placing an ice cube on the patient's forearm for 4 minutes and observing for urticaria at the site over the next 10 minutes.
   f. The characteristic small punctuate wheals of cholinergic urticaria can be elicited by having the patient run in place for 10 minutes.

g. Testing for pressure urticaria/angioedema is performed by placing a sling containing a 5- to 15-pound weight over the forearm or shoulder for 10 to 20 minutes.

Laboratory Tests for the Evaluation of Chronic Urticaria and Angioedema

Initially
Complete blood count with differential
Urinalysis
Erythrocyte sedimentation rate

Additional Tests
Screening for hepatitis
Stool for ova and parasites
Antinuclear antibodies
Thyroid function tests
Complement C4 level

Prevention

1. Persons with known IgE-mediated allergies to foods or medications must avoid ingesting these substances.
2. Patients with aspirin sensitivity should be given a list of all known medications containing nonsteroidal anti-inflammatory drugs (NSAIDs).
3. Physical urticarias may be prevented by specific measures.
   a. Persons with cold urticaria should cover all skin surfaces in the winter. They should never swim in large, cold bodies of water that may not warm up significantly even in the middle of summer. They should avoid directly holding cold drink containers.
   b. Individuals with pressure urticaria should wear loose-fitting clothing and avoid carrying heavy packs with shoulder straps.
   c. Sun screen can be effective for persons sensitive to light in the 2800 to 3200 Å range but not for the visible light spectrum. These persons should avoid sunlight as much as possible and wear protective garments when in the sunlight.

Treatment

1. It should be emphasized that if a cause of the urticaria/angioedema is known, the best treatment is avoidance of the inciting agent or condition. If the cause is unknown, symptomatic relief may be achieved with antihistamines for urticaria and non–life threatening angioedema.
   a. For acute urticaria, diphenhydramine at 1 mg/kg, up to 50 mg per dose every 6 hours is very effective. Because of the sedative side effects of diphenhydramine, nonsedating antihistamines may be used if the child can swallow a tablet. Both terfenadine 60 mg and loratadine 10 mg are effective in acute urticaria. However, none of the nonsedating antihistamines is approved by the FDA for children under 12 years of age.
   b. Cyproheptadine 0.25 to 0.5 mg/kg/24 hours, up to 12 to 16 mg per day in three divided doses is recommended for cold-induced urticaria.

c. The antihistamine of choice for cholinergic urticaria is hydroxyzine 2 mg/kg/24 hours up to 200 mg/24 hours.
d. Antihistamines have little effect on pressure urticaria. Patients with severe disease may need to be treated with systemic corticosteroids. Treatment should start with 1 mg/kg per day of prednisone and the dose should be decreased to the lowest dose given on alternate days that allows adequate control of the symptoms.
e. Life-threatening angioedema, such as upper airway compromise, should be treated with subcutaneous epinephrine.

2. Chronic idiopathic urticaria, although rare in children, will require chronic antihistamine regiments.
   a. Hydroxyzine is very effective. Again, a nonsedating antihistamine should be used, if possible, since the child might need to be on daily medication. Astemizole is a better nonsedating antihistamine for chronic urticaria than are terfenadine and loratadine. However, patients on long-term astemizole tend to gain a significant amount of weight. The reason for this side effect is unknown. In addition, because astemizole has a very long half-life, the potential for adverse reactions (life-threatening cardiac arrhythmias) is increased when astemizole is taken in conjunction with a macrolide antibiotic, ketoconazole, or itraconazole. This interaction has also been reported for terfenadine.
   b. If the use of H_1 antihistamines does not give satisfactory relief of symptoms, the addition of an H_2 antihistamine may prove beneficial.
   c. Tricyclic antidepressants, such as doxepin and amitriptyline, may also be tried in place of H_1 antihistamines because they also have potent antihistaminic properties.
   d. In severe cases of chronic urticaria/angioedema, systemic corticosteroids will need to be used. A short (5 to 7 day) course of 1 mg/kg per day usually brings the symptoms under control. Rarely, patients will require long-term corticosteroid therapy. In this case, the corticosteroid dose should be tapered to the lowest alternate-day dose that provides relief of symptoms.

Key Treatment: Urticaria/Angioedema

- Antihistamines
  Diphenhydramine
  Cyproheptadine
  Hydroxyzine

Bibliography

Middleton E, Reed CE, Elliot FE, et al (eds): Allergy: Principles and Practice, 4th ed. St. Louis, CV Mosby, 1993.
Monroe EW: Nonsedating H1 antihistamines in chronic urticaria. Ann Allergy 1993;71:585–591.
Orfan N, Kolski GB: Physical urticarias. Ann Allergy 1993; 71:205–212.

75 Anaphylaxis and Serum Sickness Reactions

Anita Gewurz

Definition

Anaphylaxis and serum sickness are systemic, immune-mediated hypersensitivity reactions to exogenous agents.

1. Anaphylaxis is an acute, fulminant, and sometimes fatal reaction characterized by urticaria and angioedema together with airway obstruction due to angioedema or bronchospasm, gastrointestinal hypermotility, hypotension, and/or cardiorespiratory arrest.

   a. "Anaphylaxis" may be used to describe an IgE-mediated systemic reaction, while "anaphylactoid" may used to refer to a non–IgE mediated systemic reaction with similar features.

   b. Since the clinical manifestations of IgE-mediated anaphylaxis and non–IgE mediated anaphylactoid reactions do not differ, it is appropriate to describe either process as anaphylaxis regardless of etiology.

2. Serum sickness, by contrast, is a delayed-onset reaction characterized by acute vascular and perivascular inflammation of skin and other organs, fever, and lymphadenopathy.

Etiology

Anaphylaxis and serum sickness are inflammatory responses caused by different immunologic mechanisms.

1. Anaphylaxis results from intense activation of mast cells and basophils, induced by agents with the following properties:

   a. Antigens that bind to multiple IgE antibodies on the surface membranes of sensitized mast cells or basophils (type I hypersensitivity). This mechanism is described for Hymenoptera venoms (see Chapter 79) and also applies to food, drug, and latex allergens.

   b. Agents that generate circulating C3a and C5a (complement-derived histamine-releasing factors or anaphylatoxins) by activating serum complement, either directly (as in dextran anaphylaxis) or via formation of immune complexes (see below).

   c. Substances that interact directly with mast cells or basophils, including codeine and other opiates, macrolide antibiotics, aspirin and other nonsteroidal antiinflammatory drugs (NSAIDs), and radiocontrast media.

   d. Endogenous histamine-releasing factors and unknown factors (in exercise-induced and idiopathic anaphylaxis) that may cause or predispose to anaphylaxis.

   e. Anaphylaxis can be triggered by minute (μg-to-ng) amounts of activating agent.

Mast Cell/Basophil Activators Involved in Anaphylaxis

- IgE to foods, drugs, latex, or stinging insect venoms
- Complement activation
- Direct activators of mast cells and basophils (opiates, NSAIDs, radiocontrast media)
- Endogenous and unknown histamine-releasing factors

---

2. Serum sickness results from the formation of immune complexes containing IgG (and possibly IgM) antibodies to circulating exogenous antigens.

   a. Antigens that trigger serum sickness are usually therapeutic agents or their metabolites.

   b. The prototype antigens are foreign protein(s); examples include horse serum antithymocyte globulin or antitoxins and nonhuman monoclonal antibodies, such as mouse anti–T cell OKT3 antibody.

   c. "Neoantigens" created by the interaction of hapten derivatives from penicillin and other β-lactams, notably cefaclor, or other drugs with blood and tissue proteins can also stimulate a humoral immune response.

   d. Unlike anaphylaxis, serum sickness reactions are unlikely to occur unless the antigen concentration is fairly high.

   e. When antigens and antibodies are both present in high concentrations, with a slightly higher proportion of antigen, they form intravascular immune complexes that deposit in small blood vessels of the skin, in large joints (knees, ankles, wrists), and, less often, in peripheral nerves and renal glomeruli.

   f. Tissue inflammation results from activation of complement, via C1q, and phagocytes by the immune complexes (type III hypersensitivity).

Antigens Involved in Serum Sickness

- Foreign proteins (antitoxins, antilymphocyte globulin, monoclonal antibodies)
- Neoantigens formed by binding of drug haptens to tissue proteins

---

3. Certain antigens, such as penicillin, Hymenoptera venom, or foreign protein, can elicit anaphylaxis and/or serum sickness, depending upon the host's immune response to the antigen.

Epidemiology

The incidence of either anaphylaxis or serum sickness is difficult to estimate accurately.

1. Both types of reaction are infrequent and probably occur in less than 0.1 per cent of patients exposed to agents that are capable of provoking anaphylaxis or serum sickness.

2. Anaphylaxis is generally more common among individuals who are atopic (see Chapter 301) and is estimated to occur in 1 of every 3000 inpatients.

   a. Anaphylactic reactions to allergens frequently involve foods (peanut, tree nuts, fish, and shellfish as well as cow milk and egg [in infants]), drugs, Hymenoptera stings, allergen extracts for skin testing or immunotherapy and latex; relative risk varies with the allergen and dose.

   b. Reactions to penicillin affect atopic and nonatopic patients equally.

   c. Fatalities occur in 3 to 9 per cent of reported cases, and it is estimated that anaphylaxis causes more than 500 deaths annually in the United States.

   d. Fatal anaphylaxis is more likely to occur in adults, possibly owing to greater exposure to causative agents, underlying cardiopulmonary disease, and the use of β blockers, which may exacerbate anaphylaxis.

   e. Latex allergy is highly prevalent among children and adults with spina bifida or other congenital neurologic or urogenital abnormalities (up to 60%) as well as medical, dental, and laboratory personnel with occupational exposure to latex (up to 18%); latex-allergic individuals are at considerable risk of latex anaphylaxis during medical, diagnostic, surgical, and dental procedures.

   f. Allergy to latex also predisposes to anaphylaxis from cross-reacting allergens in avocado, banana, chestnut, and kiwi fruit.

3. Serum sickness reactions were first described in patients treated with foreign serum proteins, but other drugs are currently the most frequent cause.

   a. In the general population, penicillin (and other β-lactam drugs) are the most common cause of serum sickness–like reactions.

   b. Among patients treated with antithymocyte globulin the incidence of serum sickness reactions is up to 1 per cent per milliliter infused.

   c. Other drugs reported to produce serum sickness include sulfonamides, thiouracils, cholecystographic radiocontrast media, and phenytoin.

Pathophysiology

1. The mechanism of IgE-mediated anaphylaxis is described in Chapter 79.

2. Complement-mediated anaphylaxis results from activation of C3 and C5 via the classical or alternate pathway.

   a. Classical pathway activation by aggregates of IgG is responsible for anaphylaxis from the inadvertent intravenous administration of intramuscular gamma globulin.

   b. Alternate pathway activation is involved in anaphylaxis secondary to dextran, radiocontrast media, or cuprophane hemodialyzer membranes.

3. Mechanisms of direct mast cell and basophil activation are less well understood; only a very small percentage of people exposed to these agents experience anaphylaxis from them.

4. Upon activation, mast cells and basophils release preformed and newly synthesized mediators.

   a. Preformed mediators include histamine and tryptase, a trypsin-like protein in mast cell granules that activates kinin and complement; they are responsible for the early (0 to 1 hour) phase of anaphylaxis.

      (1) Histamine, via binding to histamine (H_1, H_2, and H_3) receptors, is responsible for most of the early symptoms of anaphylaxis.

      (2) Plasma histamine rises during anaphylaxis; levels of 12 ng/ml or more have been detected in severe reactions.

      (3) Tryptase is released only by activated mast cells; therefore, elevated (>5 ng/ml) levels of serum tryptase are uniquely associated with anaphylaxis or mastocytosis.

   b. Severe anaphylactic reactions may also involve a late (>4 hour) phase due to the continuing release of mediators, including prostaglandins and leukotrienes, from activated mast cells and basophils.

      (1) Mediators released during the initial reaction recruit and activate seven other leukocytes, including eosinophils, and platelets.

      (2) Arachidonic acid metabolites and other mediators intensify and prolong the acute episode, producing biphasic and protracted anaphylaxis in approximately 7 per cent of cases.

5. Mechanisms of serum sickness reactions have been modeled in animals, but there are limited data on the pathogenesis of serum sickness in humans.

   a. Serum sickness requires the accumulation of circulating immune complexes that have C1q-binding activity. Predisposing factors include

      (1) Excessive rate of formation

      (2) Reduced clearance due to decreased binding to reticuloendothelial cell receptors for IgG (Fc receptor) or complement (C receptor)

   b. Primary serum sickness typically begins 7 to 14 days following initial administration of the causative agent.

      (1) The latent period reflects the time required to synthesize sufficient quantities of antibodies.

      (2) Symptoms persist, on the average, for 1 week or more but resolve completely.

   c. Accelerated serum sickness begins within 1 to 4 days of exposure to the agent.

      (1) Accelerated reactions follow prior sensitization to the agent (anamnestic response).

      (2) Atopic patients with IgE, as well as IgG, to the sensitizing antigen ($\cong$1%) may experience anaphylaxis as well as serum sickness.

Clinical Findings

1. Anaphylaxis and serum sickness share certain clinical features, namely pruritus, erythema, urticaria, and angioedema, but have different time courses reflecting different immunologic mechanisms.

2. Anaphylaxis is generally defined by its signs, symptoms, and time course (see under *Definition* and *Pathophysiology*), as there are currently no standard criteria for diagnosis.

   a. The most frequently reported findings are dermatologic signs including urticaria and/or angioedema (up to 90%)), hypotension (72%), and symptoms of upper or lower respiratory tract obstruction (70%) or gastrointestinal hypermotility (30%).

   b. Anaphylaxis typically begins within 30 minutes (85%) to 1 hour (92%) of exposure to the causative agent (diagnostic or therapeutic agents in 73 per cent, foods and additives in 14 per cent, and insect stings in 7 per cent of reported cases).

   c. Fatal reactions are associated with irreversible shock or respiratory failure.

   d. Idiopathic anaphylaxis is self-limited and rarely fatal; psychosomatic factors are frequently implicated.

   e. In anesthetized surgical patients the signs of anaphylaxis are easily confused with other events such as myocardial infarction, pulmonary embolus, or, in surgical patients, hypovolemia or anesthetic complication; hence, the diagnosis is frequently missed or the condition is misattributed to other causes. This is particularly true of latex anaphylaxis in intraoperative (medical or dental) and intrapartum patients, which is misdiagnosed as drug reaction in more than 10 per cent of cases.

   f. Confirmation of the diagnosis is provided by the detection of IgE to allergens (by skin or RAST tests), if involved, and elevated serum tryptase (see under *Laboratory Findings*).

   g. Differential diagnoses include mastocytosis, C1 esterase inhibitor deficiency and Munchausen's syndrome (particularly in cases of recurrent anaphylaxis), scombroid intoxication from ingested histamine, carcinoid, pheochromocytoma, idiosyncratic reaction to angiotensin-converting enzyme (ACE) inhibitors, and other causes of shock.

Differential Diagnosis of Anaphylaxis

- Systemic mastocytosis
- C1 esterase inhibitor deficiency
- Munchausen syndrome (in cases of recurrent anaphylaxis)
- Scombroid intoxication
- Carcinoid
- Pheochromocytoma
- Idiosyncratic reaction to ACE inhibitor
- Other causes of shock

---

3. Serum sickness is also defined by clinical criteria and characteristic chronology.

   a. Cardinal manifestations include two or more of the following: skin eruptions (100%), fever, joint symptoms, and lymphadenopathy; proteinuria may be associated.

      (1) Dermatologic findings include pruritus, erythema, urticaria, angioedema, and morbilliform or other rashes.

      (2) A characteristic, serpiginous, palmar-plantar rash of the hands and feet has been observed coincident with the onset of serum sickness in patients undergoing treatment with antithymocyte globulin for bone marrow failure.

   b. Intensity of symptoms correlates with the serum concentration of circulating immune complexes and consumption of complement.

   c. Time of onset varies with the extent of prior sensitization (see under *Etiology* and *Pathogenesis*).

   d. The duration of symptoms is highly variable; urticaria may persist for weeks after other symptoms have cleared.

   e. Confirmation of the diagnosis is provided by detection of IgM or IgG to the causative agent, positive tests for immune complexes in blood or tissue, and complement activation in symptomatic patients (see under *Laboratory Findings*).

   f. Differential diagnoses include IgE-mediated urticarial reactions, other circulating immune complex diseases (viral infection, cryoglobulinemia), and connective tissue diseases including hypocomplementemic urticarial vasculitis syndrome (HUVS), systemic lupus erythematosus (SLE), and rheumatic fever.

Key Clinical Findings: Anaphylaxis

- Acute, fulminant, concurrent, and life-threatening symptoms (as follows) closely following exposure to a food, drug, or insect sting
- Urticaria and/or angioedema
- Angioedema of the oral cavity, pharynx, or largynx
- Signs of bronchial obstruction
- Syncope, hypotension
- Gastrointestinal signs (emesis, cramping, diarrhea)

Key Clinical Findings: Serum Sickness

- Persistent symptoms (see below) beginning 1 or more days after the initiation of treatment with foreign proteins or other drugs
- Pruritic rash
- Fever
- Arthralgia ± arthritis
- Diffuse lymphadenopathy
- Proteinuria (±)

> ## Differential Diagnosis of Serum Sickness
> - IgE-mediated urticarial reactions
> - Other circulating immune complex diseases (viral infection, cryoglobulinemia)
> - Connective tissue diseases (HUVS, SLE, rheumatic fever)

Laboratory Findings

1. Laboratory tests are useful for confirming a clinical diagnosis of anaphylaxis or serum sickness, but negative tests do not necessarily rule out either diagnosis.

2. Severe anaphylaxis, particularly when accompanied by hypotension, is associated with evanescent increases in plasma histamine and serum tryptase $\geq$5 ng/ml) levels.

   a. Plasma histamine levels peak within minutes of onset of anaphylaxis and then rapidly decay.

   b. Exogenous histamine from food sources may elevate the concentration of plasma histamine in patients with acute scromboid intoxication.

   c. In contrast, elevated serum tryptase levels ($\geq$5 ng/ml) are specific for mast cell activation and may persist for up to 4 hours post onset of anaphylaxis.

   d. Similar elevations are found in 50 per cent of patients with systemic mastocytosis, including asymptomatic patients, and this should be considered when interpreting positive results.

   e. Positive tests for allergen-specific IgE, in the appropriate setting, support a diagnosis of anaphylaxis from immediate hypersensitivity.

   f. Other diagnostic tests should be performed, when necessary, to exclude diseases that could be confused with anaphylaxis (see under *Clinical Findings*).

3. The following in vitro tests are useful to confirm a diagnosis of serum sickness, if one or more is positive when the patient is symptomatic:

   a. Elevated erythrocyte sedimentation rate

   b. Positive test(s) for circulating immune complexes, such as the C1q binding assay and Raji cell assay (or its equivalent)

   c. Decreased levels of serum C4, with or without decreased C1q and/or C3

   d. Otherwise unexplained proteinuria.

> ### Key Laboratory Findings: Anaphylaxis
>
> - Anaphylaxis is characterized by acute elevation of serum tryptase due to release of this enzyme from activated mast cells.
>
> - Positive tests for allergen-specific IgE, in the appropriate setting, support a diagnosis of anaphylaxis from immediate hypersensitivity to insect stings, foods, drugs, latex, or other allergens.

> - Other diagnostic tests should be performed, when necessary, to exclude diseases that could be confused with anaphylaxis.
>
> - Serum sickness is characterized by the presence in serum of immune complexes and decreased C4 and C3, which normalize when symptoms resolve.

Treatment and Prevention

1. Anaphylaxis

   a. Treatment should begin with a rapid history (including causative factors, cardiovascular disease, and use of β blockers) and physical examination and measurement of vital signs, together with immediate administration of epinephrine (1 mg/ml), 0.01 mg/kg up to 0.3 mg given subcutaneously.

   b. For persistent symptoms, injections should be repeated at 15-minute intervals, two or three times. For patients at risk of cardiac arrhythmia, reduced doses may be given at more frequent intervals. If it is suspected that the inciting agent is a drug that is being administered or contact with latex, exposure should be halted.

   c. Depending upon the extent of circulatory and respiratory tract compromise, initial treatment may be supplemented with oxygen delivered nasally or via intubation or cricothyroidectomy and ventilation; hypotensive patients should be placed supine with the legs elevated and given intravenous fluids (normal saline, Ringer's lactate) to maintain venous access and blood pressure.

   d. Additional treatment, as indicated, includes

   (1) Diphenhydramine 1 mg/kg up to 50 mg PO or IM q 4–6 hr

   (2) Corticosteroid, either as hydrocortisone or methylprednisolone 1–2 mg/kg IV or IM q 4–6 hr, or prednisone 1 mg/kg (up to 60 mg) PO daily in single or divided doses

   (3) Nebulized albuterol 5 mg/ml, 0.05 mg/kg in children, and up to 2.5–5.0 mg in adults, in normal saline to a total volume of 3 ml, continuously over 20-minute intervals

   (4) Dopamine 5–20 ug/kg/min IV drip infusion or other pressors as per Advanced Cardiac Life Support protocols for children and adults

   (5) Glucagon 1 mg IV bolus for protracted anaphylaxis, particularly in patients on β blockers; the initial dose may be followed by IV infusion of glucagon at 5–15 μg/min, but nausea and vomiting may limit therapy

   (6) Ranitidine up to 50 mg IV or IM may be helpful if epinephrine and diphenhydramine without H_2 blocker is unsuccessful.

   e. Prevention requires identification and avoidance of the inciting agent.

   (1) In nonhospitalized patients, particular attention should be given to contact with allergens or NSAIDs; in hospitalized patients, to medications or latex (see under *Laboratory Findings*).

   (2) Identification, such as the Medic-Alert tag (1-800-922-3320), and self-injectable epinephrine,

such as EpiPen Jr. (0.15 mg) or EpiPen (0.3 mg), should be made available to the patient.

(3) The use of venom immunotherapy for allergy to Hymenoptera venoms is discussed in Chapter 79. Allergen immunotherapy should be administered only by persons who are familiar with this technique, who are trained in resuscitation for anaphylaxis, and who have equipment and supplies for treating anaphylaxis.

(4) Consultation with an allergist/immunologist may be helpful in special situations, such as the administration of egg-containing vaccines or drugs such as penicillin to patients at risk of anaphylaxis from these agents.

(5) It is not yet possible to desensitize patients with IgE antibodies to foods. Instructions regarding strict avoidance of allergenic food(s) and the use of self-injectable epinephrine must be given.

(6) Latex-allergic patients should also be instructed to inform all their physicians and dentists about the need for strict latex avoidance.

2. Serum sickness

a. Once the diagnosis is established, the causative agent (usually a medication) should be identified and discontinued.

b. Treatment is symptomatic, as the reaction is generally self-limited, and includes antihistamines, NSAIDs for arthralgia, and low-to-moderate doses of corticosteroids until symptoms subside.

c. Desensitization is not possible.

Key Treatment and Prevention

- Treatment of anaphylaxis should include rapid assessment of vital signs and cardiorespiratory status, together with administration of subcutaneous epinephrine 0.15–0.3 mg.

- Prevention of anaphylaxis requires thorough patient education about avoidance of causative agents, together with medical identification tags and self-injectable epinephrine; it should include consultation with an allergist/immunologist.

- Serum sickness is treated symptomatically with antihistamines and antiinflammatory drugs.

- Serum sickness can be prevented only by avoidance of antigen.

Bibliography

ANAPHYLAXIS

Apter AJ, LaVallee HA: How is anaphylaxis recognized? Arch Fam Med 1994;3:717–722.

Sampson HA, Mendelson L, Rosen JP: Fatal and near-fatal anaphylaxis to food in children and adolescents. N Engl J Med 1992;27:380–384.

Yuninger JW: Anaphylaxis. Ann Allergy 1992;69:87–96.

SERUM SICKNESS

Hebert AA, Sigman ES, Levy ML: Serum sickness–like reactions from cefaclor in children. J Am Acad Dermatol 1991;5:805–808.

Lawley TJ, Bielory L, Gascon P, et al: A prospective clinical and immunologic analysis of patients with serum sickness. N Engl J Med 1984;311:1407–1413.

76 Allergic Rhinitis

James N. Moy

Definition

Rhinitis is an inflammatory disease of the nasal mucous membrane. Allergic rhinitis is caused by an IgE-mediated hypersentivity response to inhalant allergens.

Etiology

Exposure to inhaled antigens in susceptible children leads to the development of IgE antibodies, which upon reexposure causes degranulation of mast cells in the nasal mucosa.

Epidemiology

About 20 to 30 per cent of the general population has allergic rhinitis.

Pathophysiology

1. Similar to asthma, IgE-mediated allergic reactions in the nose can result in two phases of pathology: the early phase and the late phase.

a. Upon exposure to an allergen, T lymphocytes of susceptible individuals produce IL-4, which promotes class switching of B lymphocytes from IgG to IgE synthesis. The IgE then binds to high-affinity Fc receptors on mast cells.

b. Upon subsequent exposure to the allergen, the mast cells are activated and release mediators such as histamine, leukotrienes, and cytokines, which gives rise to the initial signs and symptoms of allergic rhinitis.

c. Activation of mast cells and the resultant effects of mast cell mediators within the first 20 to 30 minutes is known as the early phase of an IgE-mediated hypersensitivity reaction. The early phase of allergic rhinitis is characterized by sneezing, itching, and rhinorrhea with a thin nasal discharge.

d. A second, prolonged inflammatory state often follows the early phase and is referred to as the late phase. The late phase of allergic rhinitis is characterized by severe nasal congestion and tenacious nasal mucus.

2. In the late phase, mediators are released by eosinophils, T lymphocytes, respiratory epithelial cells, basophils, monocytes, and neutrophils.

Clinical Findings

1. Nasal congestion and itching, rhinorrhea, and sneezing are the most prominent symptoms of allergic rhinitis. Common signs are infraorbital dark circles (allergic shiners), Dennie's lines of the lower eyelids, a transversal nasal crease resulting from repeated upward rubbing of the nose (allergic salute), mouth breathing, and a high-arch palate with dental malocclusion and overbite.

2. Upon examination, the nasal turbinates will be swollen with a pale or violaceous mucosa. There may be a copious clear nasal discharge. Tenacious mucus may be seen on the posterior pharynx, indicating postnasal drainage. A cobblestone appearance of the posterior pharyngeal wall represents hyperplasia of lymphoid tissue from mucous irritation.

3. In many children, there is also accompanying eye symptoms of itching, watering, and swelling.

4. Thick greenish yellowish nasal discharge and foul-smelling breath suggest sinusitis. The clinician should consider sinusitis when patients respond poorly to optimal therapy for allergic rhinitis.

5. Nasal polyps should also be considered when patients continue to have signs and symptoms of rhinitis despite optimal medical therapy and following environmental control measures. In childhood, nasal polyps are mainly associated with cystic fibrosis. Although nasal polyps are usually seen in young adults, they have been reported in children without cystic fibrosis. A history of loss of smell and/or taste is commonly elicited with nasal polyps. When nasal polyps are found, a detailed history of wheezing or worsening of existing asthma with aspirin (or other nonsteroidal antiinflammatory drugs) ingestion should be obtained.

Key Clinical Findings

- Nasal congestion
- Nasal pruritus
- Rinorrhea (clear, watery)
- Throat clearing
- Infraorbital congestion (dark circles)
- Sneezing

Differential Diagnosis of Rhinitis

- Adenoidal hypertrophy
- Foreign body
- Congenital choanal atresia
- Sinusitis
- Nasal polyps
- Tumors of the nose and paranasal sinuses

Laboratory Findings

1. Skin tests to common inhalant allergen extracts will be positive, and symptoms should correlate with the history of exposure. Although not as sensitive as skin testing, an in vitro blood test (RAST, FAST, or MAST) for specific IgE antibodies to allergens may be performed when skin testing is not possible.

2. A nasal smear will show eosinophils.

Common Inhalant Allergens

Perennial
Dust mite
Molds (indoor)
Cockroach
House pets (dogs, cats)

Seasonal
Pollens
Trees
Grasses
Ragweed (and other weeds)
Molds (outdoor)

Radiographic Changes

1. If sinusitis is present, there may be air-fluid levels in the sinuses, or opacification of the sinuses may be seen. Mucosal thickening is seen in sinusitis and allergic rhinitis.

2. Coronal CT scans are more sensitive than plain radiographs in the diagnosis of sinusitis, especially for ethmoidal and sphenoidal disease.

Treatment

1. Paramount is avoidance of the allergen plus environmental controls.

2. Antihistamines, nasal cromolyn, and nasal steroids are all effective pharmacologic options (Table 76–1).
   a. For seasonal allergic rhinitis, pharmacologic agents should be started 1 to 2 weeks prior to the beginning of the pollen season.
   b. In perennial allergic rhinitis, one should start with the maximal recommended doses and try to taper to the minimal doses needed for control of symptoms.

3. Eye drops that contain an antihistamine or mast cell stabilizer may be used if oral antihistamines do not adequately control ocular symptoms.

4. Immunotherapy (allergy injections) is reserved for patients with severe symptoms that respond poorly to pharmacologic therapy and environmental controls.

Prevention

Prevention of symptoms is achieved by avoidance of the allergen(s).

TABLE 76–1. ANTIHISTAMINE CLASSES AND DOSAGES IN YOUNG CHILDREN

CLASS	NONPROPRIETARY NAME (TRADE NAME)	DOSAGE FOR CHILDREN <12 YEARS
Ethanolamines	Diphenhydramine (Benadryl)	5 mg/kg/d in 3–4 divided doses
	Clemastine (Tavist)	0.34–0.67 mg bid
Ethylenediamines	Pyrilamine (in Rynatan, Atrohist)	6.25 mg to 25 mg bid
	Tripelennamine	5 mg/kg/d in 3–4 divided doses
Alkylamines	Chlorpheniramine (Chlor-Trimeton)	<2 y, 1.25 mg, 2–3 times daily
		>2 y, 0.4 mg/kg/d in 3–4 divided doses
	Brompheniramine (in Dimetane, Bromfed)	0.4 mg/kg/d in 3–4 divided doses
Piperazines	Hydroxyzine (Atarax, Vistaril)	2 mg/kg/d in 4 divided doses
Piperidines	Cyproheptadine (Periactin)	0.25 mg/kg/d in 3–4 divided doses
Nonsedating antihistamines	Terfenadine (Seldane)	<12 y, not FDA approved
		>12 y, 60 mg bid
	Astemizole (Hismanal)	<12 y, not FDA approved
		>12 y, 10 mg daily
	Loratadine (Claritin)	<12 y, not FDA approved
		>12 y, 10 mg daily

Key Treatment

- Allergen avoidance
- Antihistamines
- Nasal cromolym
- Nasal steroid sprays
- Allergen immunotherapy

1. During specific pollen or mold spore seasons, patients should stay indoors in an air-conditioned building whenever possible.
2. For children with dust mite sensitivity, mattress and pillow encasements that are allergen-impermeable should be used. Bedding should be washed once a week in 130°F water. Stuffed toys should not be kept on the bed. Carpets should be removed if possible, especially in the bedroom. Remaining carpets should be vacuumed once a week with vacuum cleaners fitted with multilayer dust bags. The room should not be overhumidified, as dust mites grow best at 75 to 85 per cent relative humidity.
3. If the child is allergic to a house pet, the pet should never be allowed into the bedroom; nor should the pet be replaced when it dies or runs away. Cats are the most allergenic of all pets because the allergen sticks to all surfaces for up to 9 months after the cat has been away from a home. In addition, when the cat allergen becomes airborne, it stays suspended in the air.

Bibliography

Meltzer EO: An overview of current pharmacotherapy in perennial rhinitis. J Allergy Clin Immunol 1995;95:1097–1110.

Middleton E, Reed CE, Elliot FE, et al (eds): Allergy: Principles and Practice, 4th ed. St. Louis, CV Mosby, 1993.

Mygind N, Maclerio RM (eds): Allergic and Non-allergic Rhinitis: Clinical Aspects. Philadelphia, WB Saunders, 1993.

Simons FER, Simons KJ: The pharmacology and use of H1-receptor-antagonist drugs. N Engl J Med 1994;330:1663–1670.

77 Food Allergies

James N. Moy

Definition

The American Academy of Allergy, Asthma, and Immunology recommends *adverse food reaction* as the term to be used for an untoward response to an ingested food.

Etiology

Adverse food reactions can be divided into food hypersensitivity (immune-mediated) and food intolerance. The term *food allergy* should be used to describe an immune-mediated reaction. Food hypersensitivity is immune-mediated, and all four types of Gell and Coombs reactions to foods have been described.

1. In type I IgE-mediated reactions, food proteins are presented to T lymphocytes in the gastrointestinal mucosa of the susceptible child, leading to production of IL-4. IL-4 promotes IgE production by B lymphocytes, and the IgE binds to Fc receptors on mast cells in the gut mucosa. Upon subsequent ingestion of the food, the mast cells are activated with release of mediators that can lead to wheezing, urticaria/angioedema, exacerbation of atopic

dermatitis, or anaphylaxis. Other adverse food reactions that are thought to be IgE-mediated include allergic eosinophilic gastroenteritis, infantile colic, gastrointestinal anaphylaxis, food-induced enterocolitis syndrome, and oral allergy syndrome.

2. An example of a type II antibody-dependent cytotoxicity reaction is milk-induced thrombocytopenia.

3. Disorders involving a type III antigen-antibody complex reaction include cow's milk–induced intestinal blood loss, celiac disease, and food-induced pulmonary hemosiderosis (Heiner syndrome).

4. A type IV cell-mediated reaction is also implicated in celiac disease and food-induced pulmonary hemosiderosis.

5. Food intolerance includes enzyme deficiencies and idiopathic reactions to food additives and dyes.

Epidemiology

1. The prevalence of IgE-mediated food allergy is approximately 6 per cent in infants and 2 per cent in children. The distribution is even between males and females. The most common foods causing IgE-mediated reactions in children are milk, egg, soy, wheat, peanut, and fish.

2. Food hypersensitivity is implicated in 15 per cent of infants with colic.

Pathophysiology

1. In IgE-mediated hypersensitivity reactions, mast cell activation via cross-linking of IgE Fc receptors by food antigens results in the release of mediators that cause bronchospasm, urticaria/angioedema, and anaphylaxis.

2. Food allergy as a cause of atopic dermatitis is controversial. However, double-blind oral challenges have demonstrated increased itching and erythema of lesions after ingestion of foods to which the child has demonstrated positive skin tests. The itching and vasodilatation (resulting in erythema) is probably secondary to release of histamine from mast cells.

Clinical Findings

Most IgE-mediated food reactions occur within minutes after the ingestion. Common reactions are urticaria/angioedema, wheezing, rhinoconjunctivitis, nausea, abdominal pain, diarrhea, and anaphylaxis with hypotension.

1. Oral allergy syndrome is pruritus and edema of the lips, tongue, palate, and throat after eating a food. This can be an isolated syndrome, or it may herald a more severe reaction. This syndrome usually occurs in individuals with pollen allergies, and it occurs after eating fresh fruits and uncooked vegetables.

2. Patients with allergic eosinophilic gastroenteritis present with postprandial nausea and vomiting, abdominal pain, and diarrhea. Infants will have failure to thrive, and older children will have weight loss.

3. Food-induced enterocolitis syndrome usually presents in infants between 1 week and 3 months of age. Infants will have protracted vomiting and diarrhea with dehydration. Cow's milk and soy protein are the most common offending foods.

4. Infants with Heiner syndrome will have pulmonary infiltrates on a chest radiograph, hemosiderosis, gastrointesti-

nal blood loss, iron-deficiency anemia, and failure to thrive.

5. Celiac disease presents with malabsorption and steatorrhea. Malabsorption syndrome can also be a manifestation of hypersensitivity to food proteins. The infant will have protracted diarrhea, vomiting, and failure to thrive.

6. The ingestion of foods such as celery or shellfish prior to exercise has been associated with exercise-induced anaphylaxis. In these patients, eating the food without exercise and exercise without eating did not result in anaphylaxis. Exercise-induced anaphylaxis is discussed in Chapter 75.

7. Fatal and near-fatal anaphylactic reactions to foods have been reported in a group of 13 children aged 2 to 17 years. Of the 13 children, 12 had a history of well-controlled asthma. Five of the six patients who died had onset of symptoms that were later (10 to 30 minutes after the ingestion of the food) when compared with the seven patients who survived (1 to 5 minutes after ingestion). The offending foods were peanut (four patients), nuts (six patients), eggs (one patient), and milk (two patients).

Key Clinical Findings

- Urticaria or angioedema
- Rhinorrhea and nasal congestion
- Abdominal pain and diarrhea
- Wheezing
- Anaphylaxis with hypotension

Unusual Presentations of Food Allergy

- Oral allergy syndrome
- Allergic eosinophilic gastroenteritis
- Heiner syndrome
- Celiac disease
- Exercise-induced anaphylaxis

Laboratory Findings

1. Type I hypersensitivity reactions to foods can be diagnosed with puncture skin tests or in vitro testing (RAST) for serum-specific IgE to food proteins. If a patient has a history of anaphylaxis or respiratory symptoms after ingestion of a food, skin tests should not be performed because of the risk of a systemic reaction.

2. Because food extracts do not necessarily contain the protein antigens that the body's immune system sees after a food is ingested, skin tests and in vitro IgE testing may be falsely negative. In this case, if a food allergy is suspected and the history of the reaction is not severe, a double-blind, placebo-controlled food challenge (DBPCFC) can be performed by an allergist.

3. If the foregoing tests are negative and a food is still suspected as the culprit, an elimination diet as described in Chapter 74 should be instituted.

4. Patients with allergic eosinophilic gastroenteritis will usually have peripheral eosinophilia along with eosinophils

in the stool. Gastric or intestinal biopsy samples will demonstrate infiltration of the mucosal, muscular, and/or serosal layers with eosinophils.

5. Patients with Heiner syndrome will have pulmonary infiltrates on chest radiograph, hemosiderosis, and iron-deficiency anemia. Stool samples should be tested for occult blood.

6. IgA antibodies to gliadin are positive in celiac disease. There is villous atrophy of the small bowel and lymphocytic infiltration of the intraepithelial space.

Treatment

1. Treatment should be aimed at the signs and symptoms that follow accidental ingestion of the offending food. Anaphylactic reactions should be treated aggressively with epinephrine, intravenous fluids, diphenhydramine, and corticosteroids. Airway patency must be ensured if laryngeal edema develops. Bronchospasm should be treated with inhaled β_2 agonists. Antihistamines may be used for urticaria.

2. Persons with a history of life-threatening food allergies should have on hand at all times subcutaneous epinephrine in the form of EpiPen or Ana-Kit.

3. Patients with celiac disease should be placed on a gluten-free diet.

Key Treatment

- Epinephrine
- Antihistamines

Prevention

1. Once the immune response has been established, prevention of reactions can be accomplished only by avoiding ingestion of the offending food.

   a. Several drugs have been studied for use in food allergy. These include H_1 and H_2 antihistamines, corticosteroids, and oral cromolyn sodium. None of these has proved to be consistently effective.

   b. Immunotherapy for food allergy has also been tried and also has not been proved to be effective.

2. For foods such as milk, soy, or eggs, children might outgrow their allergies or develop a tolerance. This is more likely to occur if the allergy developed early in life and the food was eliminated from the diet after the diagnosis of food allergy was made. Most children become tolerant after 3 years of avoiding the offending food. Older children and adults who develop a food allergy are less likely to lose their allergies. In addition, patients with allergies to peanut, nuts, fish, or shellfish almost never lose these allergies.

3. Avoidance of milk, eggs, and other "allergenic" foods by the mother during pregnancy and while breast feeding has been advocated as a strategy to prevent the development of IgE-mediated food allergies in the offspring. However, there are few well-controlled studies to support this hypothesis.

4. Except for a few positive studies on atopic dermatitis, delaying the introduction of foods such as eggs, peanut butter, fish, and citrus fruits until after the first year of life probably only delays the onset of food allergies.

Bibliography

Metcalfe DD, Sampson HA, Simon RA (eds): Food Allergy: Adverse Reactions to Foods and Food Additives. Cambridge, MA, Blackwell Scientific Publications, 1991.

Middleton E, Reed CE, Elliot FE, et al (eds): Allergy: Principles and Practice, 4th ed. St. Louis, CV Mosby, 1993.

Moon A, Kleinman RE: Allergic gastroenterology in children. Ann Allergy Asthma Immunol 1995;74:5–12.

Sampson HA, Mendelson L, Rosen JP: Fatal and near-fatal anaphylactic reactions to food in children and adolescents. N Engl J Med 1992;327:380–384.

78 Adverse Drug Reactions

Anita Gewurz

Definition

Adverse drug reactions (ADR) are untoward effects of substances used in the diagnosis, therapy, or prevention of disease.

Etiology

The causes and mechanisms of ADR are complex and sometimes idiopathic. They include the following:

1. Pharmacologic, pathologic, genotoxic (DNA-altering), or other reactions

2. Direct or indirect results of treatment (e.g., neutrophilia vs. thrush during treatment with high-dose prednisone)

3. Local or systemic effects (e.g., skin atrophy from chronic topical triamcinolone vs. osteoporosis from chronic oral triamcinolone)

4. Immune or non–immune mediated reactions (e.g., lip edema from an IgE-mediated reaction to penicillin vs. from the ACE inhibitor captopril)

5. Drug-drug interactions

   a. Pharmacokinetic (altered absorption, distribution, or clearance of one drug by another drug)—e.g., elevation of serum theophylline concentration by concurrent treatment with erythromycin

b. Pharmacodynamic (altered effect of one drug by the action of another drug on the same or different tissues)—e.g., antagonism of β_2 agonists by β blockers

6. Infection or altered immunity
   a. Multiple antibiotic sensitivity in HIV-positive patients
   b. Reactivation of tuberculosis by prednisone
   c. Ampicillin rash with Epstein-Barr virus infection or chronic lymphocytic leukemia

7. Pseudoreactions
   a. Vasovagal or other nonspecific responses to therapeutic intervention
   b. Latex sensitivity, masquerading as allergy to anesthetic or other drugs administered intraoperatively or intravenously
   c. Microbial or endotoxin contamination of multiple-dose vials or blood products.

Epidemiology

1. ADRs are less common among pediatric outpatients than inpatients, presumably because the latter are sicker and treated with more drugs. Up to 30 per cent of inpatients may experience an ADR.
2. Susceptibility to ADR depends on the interplay of multiple endogenous and exogenous factors, as in hemolytic anemia from sulfonamides in a patient with glucose-6-phosphate dehydrogenase deficiency or a phototoxic reaction to sulfonamides in a patient exposed to sunlight.
3. Atopy does not appear to increase the risk of IgE-mediated ADR. Whether genetic factors play a role in IgE- or other immune-mediated ADR has not been determined.

Pathophysiology

1. The majority of ADRs are nonimmunologic. They are reviewed elsewhere (see *Bibliography*).
2. Immune-mediated mechanisms account for approximately 5 to 10 per cent of ADR. They produce inflammation by one or more of the following mechanisms:
   a. Interaction of an allergenic drug with mast cells sensitized by antidrug (hapten) IgE antibody (type I or immediate hypersensitivity)
      (1) In the absence of cross-reacting antibody, symptoms rarely occur in less than 1 week of continuous treatment with a new drug. Drugs that have been used for several months or longer are unlikely to cause type I hypersensitivity.
      (2) IgE-mediated reactions tend to develop rapidly, often within minutes to hours, following reexposure to a sensitizing drug.
      (3) Reactions may be localized to skin or may be systemic (anaphylaxis).
      (4) Blood and tissue eosinophilia may be present.
      (5) Complement is not activated, and vasculitis does not occur.
      (6) Examples include IgE-mediated reactions to penicillin, allergen extracts, other protein drugs, or latex; IgE to other drugs is rare.

   b. Direct activation of mast cells
      (1) Symptoms are indistinguishable from type I hypersensitivity, except that they may occur on initial as well as repeat exposure to a drug.
      (2) Examples include opiates, macrolide antibiotics, thiopental, muscle relaxants, and NSAIDs.
   c. IgG antibody to cell-bound drug (hapten) or drug-induced cellular neoantigen and activation of complement involving specific tissues, as in drug-induced hemolytic anemia (type II hypersensitivity).
   d. Nonspecific deposition of circulating immune complexes (IgG-CIC) containing IgG antidrug antibodies and activated complement, as in a serum sickness reaction to antilymphocyte globulin (type III hypersensitivity).
      (1) In the absence of cross-reacting antibody, symptoms rarely occur in less than 1 week of continuous treatment with a new drug.
      (2) IgG-CIC form rapidly after reexposure to a sensitizing drug but generally require hours to days to become clinically significant.
      (3) Complement activation by IgG-CIC may produce hypocomplementemia (low C4, CH50) and mast cell activation by C3a and C5a.
      (4) Perivasculitis and vasculitis may occur.
   e. Direct activation of complement, as by radiocontrast media or endotoxin
   f. Cutaneous cell-mediated immunity, as in contact dermatitis to parabens (type IV hypersensitivity)
      (1) Activation of hapten-specific CD4+, T helper-1 (Th-1) cells in skin
      (2) Occurs 10 to 14 days after first use of a new topical agent or within 36 to 72 hours of its reapplication
   g. Idiopathic
      (1) Phenytoin-induced IgA deficiency
      (2) Drug-induced autoimmunity (e.g., antihistone antibodies)
      (3) Stevens-Johnson syndrome, other inflammatory reactions.

Clinical Findings

1. Signs and symptoms of ADR depend on the drug, dose, rate and route of administration, mechanism(s), and numerous independent host variables.
2. Clinical signs of ADR due to types I to IV immunologic hypersensitivity are outlined below; other reaction patterns are reviewed elsewhere (see *Bibliography*).
   a. *Type I hypersensitivity, mast cell activation:* flushing, pruritus, urticaria/angioedema, upper and/or lower airway obstruction, activation of gastrointestinal or genitourinary tract smooth muscle, and hypotension associated with vasodilation and increased capillary permeability
   b. *Type II hypersensivity:* one or more hematologic cytopenias
   c. *Type III hypersensitivity:* fever, rash (urticaria/

angioedema, palpable purpura or palmar-plantar sign), adenopathy, arthralgia, glomerulonephritis and/or mononeuritis multiplex

d. *Type IV hypersensitivity:* pruritic, inflammatory eczema confined to areas of skin previously (36 to 72 hours) in contact with topical agents.

Key Diagnostic Criteria

- ADR may be nonimmunologic or immunologic (antibody- or cell-mediated).

- Antibody-mediated, type I (IgE), II (IgG), or III (IgG-CIC) hypersensitivity generally does not occur during the first week of treatment with a new drug or from drugs that have been given continuously for several weeks or longer.

- Cell-mediated, type IV (Th-1) hypersensitivity involves skin that was previously (36–72 hours) in contact with medication.

- Drugs that activate mast cells or complement directly mimic type I hypersensitivity.

Laboratory Findings

1. Type I hypersensitivity is confirmed by positive skin or in vitro tests for IgE to

   a. Penicillin (major or minor determinants)

   b. Cephalosporin-specific determinants

   c. Protein drugs (insulin, chymopapain, streptokinase, protamine, psyllium)

   d. Egg-cultured vaccines or vaccine components (egg white or gelatin)

   e. Latex

2. Type I hypersensitivity is frequently accompanied by blood eosinophilia.

3. Levels of serum tryptase, a mast cell enzyme, may be elevated in systemic reactions as a result of mast cell activation.

4. Type II hypersensitivity is suggested by acute leukopenia, hemolytic anemia, and/or thrombocytopenia during drug therapy, confirmed by a positive serologic test for IgG or complement on (or complement fixation by) patient cells when exposed to a drug.

5. Type III hypersensitivity is revealed by positive tests for

   a. IgG antidrug antibody, CIC, or hypocomplementemia (low C4) in serum

   b. IgG and C1q or C4 deposition in biopsy of skin or other tissue biopsy

   c. Red blood cells or protein casts in urine

   d. Elevated erythrocyte sedimentation rate

   e. Circulating immune complexes (C1q-binding, Raji cell assays)

6. Type IV hypersensitivity is confirmed by a positive patch test to the drug or to another chemical ingredient of the topical preparation that was used.

Key Laboratory Findings

- Drug (vaccine or latex)-specific IgE

- Drug-specific IgG

- Positive patch test to drug or related compound

Treatment

1. Therapy of immunologic hypersensitivity to drugs includes

   a. Stopping the drug (if possible)

   b. β_2 Adrenergic drugs, such as subcutaneous epinephrine, to reverse anaphylaxis

   c. Symptomatic treatment and supportive care

   d. Corticosteroids

2. Whether a drug that has caused an ADR may be safely readministered depends upon the circumstances.

   a. Drugs that have induced immunologic hypersensitivity reactions should be avoided, unless there is no satisfactory alternative *and* an effective "desensitization" or modified treatment protocol is available.

   b. The patient must understand the risks as well as benefits of retreatment, and informed consent should be obtained (see DeSwarte, 1993).

3. All serious adverse events and product problems should be reported to the Food and Drug Administration (1-800-FDA-1088, or submit a MedWatch form).

Key Treatment and Prevention

- Avoid unnecessary drugs, particularly antibiotics, especially in hospitalized patients.

- Maintain a high index of suspicion and discontinue drugs that may be causing ADRs.

- Justify, use a modified protocol, and obtain informed consent before administering any drug that previously caused an ADR.

- Report all serious ADRs to the FDA.

Prevention

No drug has a single effect. To minimize ADR, physicians and patients must avoid unecessary drugs, particularly antibiotics.

Bibliography

DeSwarte RD: Drug allergy. *In* Patterson R, Grammer LC, Greenberger PA, Zeiss CR (eds): Allergic Diseases: Diagnosis and Management. Philadelphia, JB Lippincott, 1993, pp 395–552.

Klaassen CD: Principles of toxicology. *In* Gilman AD, Rall TW, Nies AS, Taylor P (eds): Goodman and Gilman's The Pharmacological Basis of Therapeutics. New York, Pergamon Press, 1990, pp 49–61.

Nies AS: Principles of therapeutics. *In* Gilman AD, Rall TW, Nies AS, Taylor P (eds): Goodman and Gilman's The Pharmacological Basis of Therapeutics. New York, Pergamon Press, 1990, pp 62–74.

79 Insect Allergies

Anita Gewurz

Definition

Insect allergy is an IgE-mediated inflammatory reaction to allergens introduced by contact with insects, including arthropods and arachnids (mites and ticks), that is associated with cutaneous or systemic involvement.

Etiology

Allergic reactions to insects result from type I (immediate) hypersensitivity and binding of IgE on mast cells and other cells of sensitized individuals to allergens in the following:

1. Saliva of biting insects, including flies, mosquitos, fleas, reduviids, and ticks
2. Venoms of stinging insects (Hymenoptera), including bees, vespids (wasps, hornets, yellow jackets), fire ants, and harvester ants
3. Inhalants (body or fecal proteins) from domestic mites, cockroaches, Chironomid midges, and other insects
4. Honeybee proteins in honey
5. In addition to allergenic proteins, Hymenoptera venoms contain vasoactive amines, including histamine, and mast cell–activating peptides that can produce nonspecific inflammatory reactions closely resembling IgE-mediated allergic reactions. Most local and large local cutaneous reactions and some systemic reactions to venoms are caused by these toxins, rather than IgE.

Epidemiology

Up to 25 per cent of the general population, including persons with no history of insect sting reactions, have IgE antibodies that are reactive with Hymenoptera venom allergens, as determined by skin tests for immediate hypersensitivity to venoms or blood tests for venom-specific IgE.

1. Individuals who are atopic (i.e., who have IgE to inhalant and food allergens and allergic rhinitis, asthma, or eczema) are twice as likely to experience allergic sting reactions, but the majority of reactions occur in persons who are nonatopic.
2. The prevalence of sting allergy varies by region: in the South and Southwest, reactions to fire ants and harvester ants predominate; elsewhere, yellow jackets are the major cause, followed by wasps.
3. IgE antibodies to airborne proteins of domestic insects, including dust mites and cockroaches, can be detected in up to 20 per cent of the general population and indicate the presence of atopy.
4. The prevalence and role of IgE in allergy to other insects have not been established.

Pathophysiology

1. *Sensitization:* Following initial contact with insect allergens, certain individuals produce allergen-specific IgE that binds to (sensitizes) cells with IgE receptors, including mast cells and basophils.

    a. The major allergens of bee, vespid, and stinging ant venoms are phospholipases and other glycoprotein enzymes.

    b. Multiple (>50) stings are more likely to sensitize for venom anaphylaxis.

    c. Homologous Hymenoptera allergens may produce cross sensitization following the sting of one species to the venom of another species.

    (1) Sensitization by yellow jacket venom may produce immediate hypersensitivity reactions to both yellow jacket and hornet stings.

    (2) First-sting anaphylaxis may involve cross-reacting venom allergens and/or factors other than IgE.

    d. The major allergens of dust mites are digestive enzymes excreted with feces and disseminated into surrounding air by domestic activity.

    e. Other insect allergens have not been fully characterized.

2. *Reexposure:* Subsequent interaction with allergen activates IgE-sensitized cells to release mediators that produce an immediate hypersensitivity reaction with early and late phases of inflammation corresponding to release of preformed and newly formed mediators (as discussed in Chapters 73 and 76). Typically, reactions begin within minutes.

    a. Reexposure to Hymenoptera venom (re-sting) may produce local cutaneous reactions, generalized urticaria/angioedema, or systemic anaphylaxis, as described under *Clinical Findings*.

    b. Re-sting reactions are usually similar to, and rarely more severe than, the initial reaction.

    (1) In children with previous local reactions to Hymenoptera stings, only 2 per cent developed systemic reactions during re-stings, and these reactions were mild.

    (2) In persons with previous anaphylaxis to Hymenoptera stings and positive venom skin tests, re-sting reactions produced systemic reactions in only 14 per cent of children and less than 60 per cent of adults.

    c. The clinical course of stinging insect allergy is generally self-limited (see under *Clinical Findings*), suggesting that antiidiotypic antibody or other immunoregulatory factors are involved.

    d. Significant exposure to dust mite and cockroach allergens is associated with increases in specific IgE and allergic skin disease (eczema) and/or respiratory tract disease (rhinoconjunctivitis, asthma) among atopic individuals.

3. Aypical reactions associated with insect stings include delayed urticaria, vasculitis, nephrosis, neurologic

involvement, and serum sickness. Mechanisms of these reactions are not well defined, although IgE may play a role.

Clinical Findings

1. The clinical picture and natural history of insect allergy are highly variable, depending upon the insect species involved; route and extent of allergen exposure; the patient's age, allergic sensitivity, history of previous anaphylaxis, other diseases, and immunotherapy; and other as yet undefined factors. The clinical picture of Hymenoptera venom allergy is outlined below.

2. Up to 90 per cent of Hymenoptera reactions involve the skin only.

   a. Local reactions

      (1) Involve immediate pain, erythema, angioedema, and induration at the sting site

      (2) Are generally benign and self-limited

      (3) Do not predispose to systemic reactions.

   b. Large local reactions extend beyond the immediate sting site to involve portions of, or an entire, extremity or side of the face.

      (1) They persist for several days.

      (2) The prognosis is the same as for local reactions.

   c. IgE to Hymenoptera venom(s) can be detected in up to 80 per cent of local and large local reactors, but its role in these limited reactions is unclear.

   d. Acute urticaria/angioedema without other signs of anaphylaxis has special clinical significance.

      (1) In children, urticarial reactions are generally benign and self-limited; they recur following re-sting in up to 20 per cent but do not predispose to anaphylaxis or warrant preventive therapy.

      (2) In adults, urticaria and angioedema are risk factors for systemic reactions to re-stings; venom skin testing and preventive immunotherapy are indicated (see under *Prevention* and *Treatment*).

3. Systemic reactions to stings occur in less than 1 per cent of individuals.

   a. Signs and symptoms include immediate flushing, generalized pruritus, urticaria/angioedema, sneezing, upper airway obstruction, asthma, gastrointestinal hypermotility (nausea, cramps, urgency, and involuntary defecation), uterine cramps, a premonition of impending doom, and/or circulatory collapse.

   b. Severe reactions may occur at any age.

   c. Most nonfatal systemic reactions occur in male children, presumably because they have more contact with stinging insects.

   d. Fatal reactions ($\approx$ 40/year) usually involve adults. Risk factors include underlying cardiovascular or respiratory disease, including asthma; mastocytosis, and possibly therapy with β blockers.

   e. Allergic reactions to fire ant and harvester ant stings are rarely fatal.

Key Features of Hymenoptera Sting Reactions

Classification by type and extent of inflammation:
- Local
- Large local
- Generalized urticaria/angioedema
- Systemic anaphylaxis, including airway obstruction (oropharyngeal or laryngeal edema, asthma) and/or vascular collapse

4. Information about allergic reactions to biting insects is limited. Most cases involve the skin only; anaphylaxis is rare. The role of IgE is not well studied.

   a. Whealing of the skin frequently occurs at sites of mosquito, flea, or tick bites in atopic individuals.

   b. Flea bites may cause papular urticaria and vesicular eruptions.

   c. Scabies infection may be mistakenly diagnosed as urticaria or impetigo.

5. The clinical picture of insect allergy caused by inhalants (e.g., dust mites and cockroaches) is described in Chapters 73 and 76.

6. Allergic reactions to honey have occurred in children and adults. Clinical characteristics include oral itching and angioedema alone or with systemic involvement. Honey contains bee- and pollen-derived proteins that bind IgE from patient sera. In a recent report, 10 per cent of honey-allergic persons were also allergic to bee venom, and 70 per cent of persons with bee venom allergy had IgE, but not clinical reactions, to honey proteins.

Key Clinical Findings

- Ninety per cent of allergic reactions to stinging insects involve non–life threatening cutaneous inflammation, with localized induration or generalized urticaria/angioedema.

- The majority of systemic reactions to stinging insects involve children, who are at increased risk because of a greater likelihood of being stung.

- Sting reactions are rarely fatal in childhood; even without preventive therapy, most children do not develop systemic reactions to re-stings.

- Atopy does not increase the risk of allergic reactions to stinging insects.

Laboratory Findings

1. Accurate diagnosis of insect allergy is based on the history and physical findings, confirmed by positive immediate hypersensitivity skin tests or serology (radioallergosorbent test or RAST) for specific IgE, using well-characterized allergens.

2. Satisfactory allergen preparations include commercially available Hymenoptera venoms, standardized dust mite extracts, and cockroach extracts.

3. Tests for IgE to Hymenoptera venoms require careful interpretation.

   a. Nonspecific inflammation may produce false positive skin tests, particularly when venom is used at 1 µg/ml.

   b. A positive venom skin test or RAST is not by itself an indication for venom immunotherapy; appropriate clinical history is required as well.

   c. Positive tests for inhalant (dust mite, cockroach) allergy indicate atopy and correlate with allergic rhinitis, eczema, and asthma in children.

   d. Whole-body extracts of ants and other insects may yield invalid results.

4. Patients receiving insect or venom immunotherapy show changes in serum levels of allergen-specific IgE and IgG.

   a. During the first months of therapy, levels of IgE as well as IgG increase.

   b. Subsequently, IgE levels decrease and may become undetectable.

   c. IgG levels decline rapidly after therapy is discontinued and do not correlate with protection against re-sting reactions.

Key Laboratory Findings

- Positive tests for IgE to inhalant (dust mite, cockroach) insect allergens correlate with atopic disease in children.

- Positive tests for venom-specific IgE require careful interpretation to exclude false positive findings.

- Testing with whole-insect body extracts may be unreliable.

- Venom immunotherapy produces a decrease in venom-specific IgE and transient increases in venom-specific IgG.

Prevention

Patients with insect allergy should minimize exposure by means of environmental control or avoidance, as indicated.

1. Control measures for dust mite and cockroach exposure are discussed in Chapters 73 and 76.

2. Reasonable avoidance measures to minimize insect sting reactions in children include

   a. Wearing socks and shoes and not eating when out of doors

   b. Not using odorant-containing preparations for the hair and skin

   c. Professional extermination of Hymenoptera nests adjacent to the home.

3. In addition, all children at risk of venom anaphylaxis (or their caretakers) should

   a. Obtain identification tags (Medic-Alert Foundation, 800-922-3220)

   b. Receive a treatment plan and instruction in the use of self-injectable subcutaneous epinephrine (EpiPen Jr., 0.15 mg for children ≤15 kg, or EpiPen, 0.3 mg if >15 kg)

   c. Consult an allergist/immunologist regarding venom allergy testing and immunotherapy (see *Bibliography* for references regarding patient selection, venom selection, dosages, treatment regimens (conventional vs. rush immunotherapy) and duration of therapy. Special consideration is required for patients who are pregnant or on β blocker therapy.

Treatment

Therapy for acute allergic reactions to insects depends upon the extent of organ involvement.

1. Cutaneous reactions may be treated symptomatically with cold packs and antihistamines.

   a. If a bee's stinger remains in the skin, it should be removed promptly.

   b. Corticosteroids are of unproven benefit for local or large local reactions to Hymenoptera, but prednisone (1 mg/kg/day) or methylprednisolone may be helpful for urticaria/angioedema.

2. Systemic reactions to insects should be treated according to standard guidelines for management of anaphylaxis (see Chapter 75). Patients should be monitored prospectively for protracted and biphasic anaphylaxis, which would warrant more aggressive treatment.

3. Secondary bacterial infection may complicate cutaneous reactions.

Key Treatment and Prevention

- Contact with allergenic insects should be minimized.

- Minor cutaneous reactions should be treated symptomatically.

- Urticaria/angioedema and systemic reactions should be treated promptly with antihistamines, epinephrine, and corticosteroids as well as supportive therapy.

- Patients at risk for systemic reactions should have a treatment plan that includes self-injectable epinephrine and consultation with an allergist/immunologist regarding skin testing and immunotherapy.

 ## Bibliography

Essayan DM, Kagey-Sobotka A, Lichtenstein LM: Nearly fatal anaphylaxis following an insect sting. Ann Allergy 1994; 73:297–300.

Levine MI, Lockey RF (eds): Monograph on insect allergy (American Academy of Allergy and Immunology, Committee on Insects), 3rd ed. Pittsburgh, Dave Lambert Associates, 1995.

Reisman RE: Insect stings. N Engl J Med 1994;331:523–527.

Stafford CT: Fire ant allergy. Allergy Proc 1992;13:11–16.

80 Juvenile Arthritis

K. M. O'Neil

Definition

Juvenile arthritis (JA) is a group of conditions causing chronic (≥ 6 weeks' duration) inflammation of synovial joints that has onset before 16 years of age. JA was commonly known as juvenile rheumatoid arthritis in the United States, but the designation "rheumatoid" has been dropped because only 5 to 6 per cent of children have true rheumatoid arthritis as seen in adults. In the United Kingdom, it is known as juvenile chronic arthritis and at least 3 months' duration of disease is a criterion for diagnosis.

Subtypes

Initially, the conditions were grouped into three categories (systemic, polyarticular, and pauciarticular) based on pattern of joint involvement in the first 6 months. Currently, several patterns are recognized based on differences in disease onset and course, among which variations in disease duration, severity, and pattern of complications produce different prognoses and outcomes (Table 80–1).

Etiology

Most forms of rheumatic disease, including JA, are of unknown etiology.

1. *Genetics.* Evidence exists to support the role of genetic predisposition in most forms of JA, with certain major histocompatibility complex antigens overrepresented in children with oligoarthritis in comparison to population controls and with other antigens prevalent in those with polyarticular forms of JA. In particular, HLA-B27 is prevalent in individuals with enthesitis (inflammation of insertions)-related arthritis.

2. *Environmental factors. Infectious agents* have been implicated in a variety of inflammatory arthropathies.

   a. Rheumatic fever is a result of infection with *Streptococcus pyogenes.* Reactive arthritis follows enteritis due to *Yersinia enterocolitica* and related enteric pathogens.

   b. HLA-B27 molecules share certain epitopes found on *Klebsiella* species, and these homologies may play a role in the pathogenesis of enthesitis-related arthritis.

   c. Rubella and parvovirus have been implicated in some children with JA.

Epidemiology

The best estimates on the prevalence of JA in the pediatric population indicate that 1.1/1000 to 1/1500 children are affected with chronic joint inflammation. JA is more common in children of European whites than those of African or Asian heritage. Estimates of relative prevalence rates of the different forms of JA vary somewhat with the referral patterns in the region. General trends for gender and age data are outlined in Table 80–1.

Pathophysiology

1. *Histopathology.* Lesions in early arthritis show proliferation of macrophage-like and fibroblastoid synoviocytes to produce early pannus. Subsequent infiltration with neutrophils and lymphocytes, with eventual accumulation of B and T lymphocytes in chronic lesions, ensues.

2. *Autoimmunity.* Evidence of autoimmunity is common in JA, but classic IgM rheumatoid factors (anti-IgG autoantibodies) are seen in a minority of patients (i.e., 5 to 10 per cent who have adult-type polyarticular rheumatoid disease). "Hidden rheumatoid factors" of low titer are frequent in other forms of the disease, and antinuclear antibodies are common.

3. *Cytokine production.* Inflammatory cytokines including tumor necrosis factor-α, interleukin-1, interleukin-2, and interleukin-6 have been demonstrated to be produced in inflamed joints. In systemic JA, plasma levels of these cytokines are elevated during periods of active disease.

Clinical Findings

1. *Arthritis.* Joint inflammation is present in all children with JA.

   a. *Stiffness.* Stiffness of involved joints, which is worst in the morning and after rest, is a characteristic finding. Pain that is worse after exercise and improves with rest is usually mechanical/traumatic in mechanism, not inflammatory. Examples are tendinitis of the quadriceps tendon related to torsional deformity (excess femoral anteversion) and patellofemoral joint disease or chondromalacia patellae.

TABLE 80–1. JUVENILE ARTHRITIS SUBTYPES

JA SUBTYPE	MALE : FEMALE	PEAK AGE	% OF JA CASES
Systemic arthritis	1.2 : 1	Throughout childhood	10–15
Polyarthritis: RF negative	1 : 9	Throughout childhood	15–20
Polyarthritis: RF positive	1 : 9	≥8 years old	5–10
Oligoarthritis	1 : 4	Early childhood	50–60
Extended oligoarthritis	F > M	Early childhood	10–15
Enthesitis-related arthritis	9 : 1	≥8 years old	10–15
Psoriatic arthritis	1 : 5	Early to mid childhood	5–10

b. *Pain.* Joint pain is usually mild to moderate and aching (severe pain that wakes a child suggests other causes, e.g., infection and malignancy).

c. *Physical findings.* Physical signs of joint inflammation are required for a definite diagnosis of arthritis. Without these, the child has arthralgia.

Key Physical Findings

- Heat found locally over inflamed joints

- Swelling due to effusion and/or thickening of the synovial membrane (doughy texture)

- Tenderness along the joint line—must be differentiated from tender tendons, ligaments, muscles, etc.

- Loss of range of motion and function of the joint

d. *Posture.* The child will typically hold the affected joint(s) in slight flexion to decrease pressure on the inflamed tissues and may walk with a limp.

e. *Ocular disease.* Some children will have chronic inflammation of the uveal tract of the eye, called iritis, iridocyclitis, or uveitis. This is usually asymptomatic but can result in visual loss. Routine ophthalmologic consultation should be obtained for slit lamp examination (Table 80–2).

2. *Differential Diagnosis.* JA is a diagnosis of exclusion. Many other clinical conditions may present with joint pain, swelling, or limp, with or without rash and fever. Other conditions must be carefully excluded, particularly infections, malignancy, and inflammatory bowel disease.

Differential Diagnosis

Trauma
Infection
Septic arthritis
Toxic synovitis
Postinfectious arthritis (rheumatic fever, postenteritic arthritis)
Serum sickness
Inflammatory bowel disease
Hematologic disorder (sickle cell disease, hemophilia)
Malignancy (leukemia, lymphoma, neuroblastoma, and bone or cartilage tumors)
Other rheumatic disease (e.g., systemic lupus erythematosus, Sjögren syndrome, mixed connective tissue disease)

3. *Clinical Subsets of JA*

a. *Systemic Arthritis.* In this form of JA, which is also known as Still disease, joint inflammation is seldom the presenting complaint. It may be delayed for weeks, months, or occasionally years after the onset of systemic symptoms. This subtype of JA may present at any age, and it occurs slightly more often in boys than girls (M:F = 1.2:1).

(1) *Fever.* Spiking daily fevers with one to two

TABLE 80–2. RECOMMENDATIONS FOR UVEITIS SCREENING

SUBTYPE	UVEITIS FREQUENCY	SCREENING FREQUENCY
Systemic arthritis	5%	Every 6 months
Polyarthritis: RF negative	5%	Every 6 months
Polyarthritis: RF positive	<5%	Every 6 months
Oligoarthritis	15–20%	Every 3 months if ANA positive Every 4 months if ANA negative
Extended oligoarthritis	15–20%*	As for oligoarthritis
Enthesitis-related arthritis	5–10% acute uveitis	Every 6 months
Psoriatic arthritis	15–20%	As for oligoarthritis

*Because the classification is new, prevalence is estimated and not based on epidemiologic studies. True prevalence may be somewhat lower, as in polyarthritis.

daily peaks of 39°C or higher are present in all affected children. The child with a few febrile days every month is unlikely to have systemic JA.

(2) *Rash.* An evanescent pale pink macular rash is seen in over 90 per cent of children. The rash is most prominent during febrile periods and on warmer regions of the body (e.g., trunk).

(3) *Lymphoid hypertrophy.* Diffuse adenopathy and hepatosplenomegaly are seen in 75 to 80 per cent of children with systemic JA. This finding may suggest malignancy.

(4) *Hematologic abnormalities.* Anemia that may be severe at times (5 g/dl Hb) and prominent leukocytosis are typical. Thrombocytosis may be prominent, and the degree of thrombocytosis correlates with serum interleukin-6 levels.

(5) *Liver.* Mild to moderate elevation of serum transaminase levels may occur. Liver biopsy, when done, shows only nonspecific periportal infiltration. An uncommon complication of systemic JA, the "macrophage activation syndrome" or "hematophagocytic syndrome" may occur either with infection or when medications are changed. This syndrome is often heralded by an abrupt drop in the erythrocyte sedimentation rate and can lead to multiorgan system failure, shock, disseminated intravascular coagulation, and death. Impressive rises in serum transaminase levels occur in children with this complication. The mortality is high, with 25–50 per cent dying of their disease.

(6) *Metabolic.* Weight loss with wasting of muscle and fat may occur, and linear growth may be arrested.

(7) *Articular involvement.* Joint involvement may not be present at disease onset and can be delayed for months or occasionally years after fevers begin.

(a) The arthritis in most children pursues a polyarticular course.

(b) Up to 45 per cent develop joint space narrowing (loss of cartilage) or erosions, with median time to these destructive changes being 2.2 years.

(c) At 10 years after disease onset, approximately 50 per cent have active synovitis, and many of these patients have significant functional limitations.

(8) *Renal disease.* Renal involvement is uncommon and usually relates to toxicity of the medications used to control inflammation.

b. *Polyarthritis, RF Negative.* Polyarticular JA without a classic rheumatoid factor (RF) occurs in about 20 per cent of children with JA. Onset may be at any age, with girls outnumbering boys in a ratio of 9:1. The principal manifestation is joint inflammation; but with more severe arthritis or poor inflammatory control, affected children may have mild to moderate systemic involvement.

(1) *Articular disease.* Polyarticular involvement is defined as arthritis of five or more synovial joints. As with other forms of arthritis, morning or rest stiffness is characteristic, and physical signs of joint inflammation are present in the form of warmth, tenderness, swelling, synovial thickening, and loss of joint function (range of motion).

(a) Among all children with polyarticular disease, 45 per cent have persistent synovitis at 10 years after disease onset.

(b) Radiographic studies in polyarticular disease demonstrate that over 50 per cent of children have joint space narrowing or erosions, with a median time to destructive changes of 2.4 years.

(c) Joints involved in juvenile polyarthritis include the cervical spine, the temporomandibular joint (which may lead to micrognathia and dental malocclusion), shoulders, elbows, small joints of the hands and wrists, hips, knees, ankles, and small foot joints. The sacroiliac joints and the thoracolumbar spine tend to be spared.

(2) *Extraarticular manifestations.* These are usually milder than in systemic arthritis.

(a) Mild anemia of chronic disease usually relates to the severity of inflammation and often improves with control of the arthritis.

(b) Adenopathy and hepatosplenomegaly may occur, especially with active disease, and are usually mild.

(c) Weight loss and slowing of linear growth may occur and reflect periods of high disease activity.

(d) Serum transaminase levels may be elevated during flares and especially at diagnosis, but this usually resolves with antiinflammatory treatment.

(e) Chronic uveitis occurs in approximately 5 per cent of children with this form of JA, so periodic screening is required.

c. *Polyarthritis, RF Positive.* The older child who is approaching or has achieved puberty and develops chronic arthritis of five or more joints may have a positive RF.

(1) *Articular disease.* Joint involvement is similar to RF-negative juvenile polyarthritis, except

(a) It produces more erosive changes and seldom resolves.

(b) Half of the patients have functional disability 5 years after disease onset.

(2) *Nodules.* As in adult-onset rheumatoid arthritis, RF-positive polyarthritis may be associated with subcutaneous nodules over extensor surfaces.

(a) Nodules correlate with high-titer RF.

(b) Histopathologic examination reveals palisading granuloma.

(c) These nodules occur and remit spontaneously.

(3) *Systemic disease.* Systemic manifestations are similar to that seen in RF-negative disease, including mild to moderate anemia, hepatosplenomegaly and adenopathy, and growth disturbances.

d. *Oligoarthritis.* Inflammation of one to four joints with morning stiffness, joint warmth, and swelling from synovial proliferation with or without effusion is the usual presentation for children with juvenile oligoarthritis. Because knees and ankles are most commonly affected, limp may be an early finding. Children with oligoarthritis tend to be young (<8 years old), and there is a female predominance. Antinuclear antibody is present in approximately half of these children.

(1) *Systemic symptoms.* These are rare and are usually limited to mild anemia during periods of active arthritis.

(2) *Articular manifestations.* These are less likely to be erosive than those of the other subtypes of JA.

(a) In 60 to 80 per cent of affected children, clinical resolution of the arthritis occurs by 10 years after disease onset.

(b) Limb length discrepancies may occur, because overgrowth can result from the growth-promoting effects of inflammatory cytokines. Advanced epiphyseal age may result in eventual limb shortening.

(c) Functional disability tends to be mild.

(3) *Ocular involvement.* Approximately 15 per cent of children with oligoarticular disease will develop inflammation of the uveal tract. It is most commonly ascertained on screening ophthalmologic examinations, which may demonstrate a flare (light scattering caused by protein and inflammatory cells) in the anterior chamber on slit lamp examination.

(a) The presence of antinuclear antibody and

early onset ($<$ 4 years old) of oligoarthritis correlate with increased risk of uveitis.

(b) The eye inflammation usually causes no symptoms until visual impairment has occurred due to scar formation.

(c) Eye involvement is temporally unrelated to joint disease and may occur before arthritis or up to 4 decades or more later. Life-long eye examinations by a trained ophthalmologist are essential.

e. *Extended Oligoarthritis.* Of children with oligoarticular presentation, those most likely to progress to a polyarticular course (20 to 30 per cent) are those with involvement of three or four joints in the first 6 months.

(1) *Time course.* Progression to polyarthritis occurs from 1 to 6 years after onset, with a mean of 2.5 years.

(2) *Systemic symptoms.* Manifestations of systemic inflammation are mild, as in oligoarthritis, and eye disease occurs nearly as often as in oligoarthritis without extension to polyarticular course.

(3) *Outcome.* Risk of joint erosion, persistently active arthritis, and functional disability is much greater in children with extended oligoarthritis than in classic oligoarthritis.

f. *Enthesitis-Related Arthritis.* The disorder formerly known as pauciarticular onset type 2, or childhood spondyloarthropathy, represents a group of clinically related conditions characterized by joint inflammation, inflammation at sites of insertion of fascia or tendons (enthesitis), and spine arthritis (spondylitis). The acronym SEA syndrome has been used to denote *s*pondylitis, *e*nthesitis, and *a*rthritis. There is strong association with HLA-B27, and the majority of these children are male. Family history is often positive. Many children develop ankylosing spondylitis, inflammatory bowel disease (Crohn disease or ulcerative colitis), or psoriasis. Children should be monitored for growth pattern and abnormal bowel habits. Similar joint involvement can occur after genitourinary infections or enteritis (see under Infection-Related Arthritis). This is given the eponym Reiter syndrome.

(1) *Enthesitis.* The most common sites for enthesitis are the insertions of the Achilles and quadriceps tendons and the calcaneal insertion of the plantar fascia. Involvement of the insertions of the paravertebral muscles is also common and contributes to the back pain and limited spine mobility seen in this disorder. There are often asymptomatic periods of months between episodes early in the disease course.

(2) *Arthritis.* Asymmetric inflammation of the joints of the extremities, frequently involving the ankles, knees, hips, and metatarsophalangeal and toe joints is characteristic of this disease. Costovertebral involvement may lead to loss of chest expansion, which is measured at maximal inspiration at the nipple line.

(3) *Spondylitis.* Back or buttock pain, sacroiliac pain and tenderness, and restricted range of motion of the lumbar spine may be present at onset or may occur later. Flattening of the normal lumbar lordosis is frequent. Impaired flexion of the spine occurs. Cervical involvement tends to occur later in the disease.

(4) *Acute, symptomatic uveitis.* In contrast to other forms of JA, 5 to 10 per cent of children with enthesitis-associated arthritis develop acute, painful, and photophobic iritis with prominent erythema of the sclera and conjunctiva. The uveitis may be unilateral, it tends to recur, and it may be seen before any joint involvement.

(5) *Cardiopulmonary involvement.* Aortic insufficiency has been reported in children with juvenile ankylosing spondylitis but is rare.

g. *Psoriatic Arthritis.* Juvenile psoriatic arthritis is defined as arthritis occurring before age 16 in individuals with dermal psoriasis. Arthritis may precede the rash by many years. The ratio of girls to boys is approximately 2.5:1. Onset is often in early childhood, with a mean age of 6 years (4.5 for girls, 10 for boys).

Diagnostic Criteria for Psoriatic Arthritis

Arthritis with typical psoriatic rash or three (definite) or two (probable) of the following:
- Dactylitis (sausage digit)
- Nail pitting or onycholysis
- Psoriasis in first- or second-degree relative
- Psoriasis-like rash (location or appearance atypical)

---

(1) *Joint involvement.* The most common pattern is asymmetric arthritis of large and small joints.

(a) Sacroiliac involvement occurs occasionally.

(b) Dactylitis with flexor tenosynovitis can present as a "sausage digit," with red-violet color of the skin overlying the swollen digit.

(c) Distal interphalangeal joint involvement, which is uncommon in JA, is seen in psoriatic arthritis, often in association with nail pitting of the affected digit.

(d) Cervical spine involvement may occur.

(2) *Dermatitis.* Only 50 per cent of affected children have characteristic papulosquamous skin changes of psoriasis at onset of arthritis.

(a) Nails pits are common, with 20 or more found on all fingers and toes. Involved fingers may have distal interphalangeal arthritis.

(b) Periungual flaking and onycholysis may be seen.

(c) Extensor surfaces, behind the auricles, and

the scalp should be checked carefully for psoriatic scales and plaques.

(3) *Eye disease.* Children with juvenile psoriatic arthritis have chronic, asymptomatic uveitis identical to that of oligoarthritis but often more resistant to treatment.

Key Clinical Findings of JA Subsets

Systemic Arthritis
- Fever
- Rash
- Hepatosplenomegaly
- Adenopathy
- Growth failure
- Polyarticular arthritis
- Uveitis in 5 per cent

Polyarthritis RF-negative
- Mild systemic symptoms
- Polyarthritis may involve neck and jaw
- Uveitis in 5 per cent

Polyarthritis RF-positive
- Symmetric hand involvement
- Often destructive polyarthritis
- Rheumatoid nodules
- Rare uveitis

Oligoarthritis
- Arthritis of knees and/or ankles
- Limb-length discrepancy
- Chronic uveitis in 15 per cent

Extended Oligoarthritis
- Involvement of three to four joints early in disease
- Persistent polyarthritis

Enthesitis-related JA
- Hip and lumbar spine arthritis
- Acute uveitis in 5 to 10 per cent
- Occasional aortic outlet or valve disease

Psoriatic Arthritis
- Skin psoriasis
- Nail pits
- Distal interphalangeal arthritis
- Sausage digits
- Chronic uveitis in some

Laboratory Findings

Laboratory findings in JA vary somewhat according to subtype and disease severity. Most abnormalities reflect the presence and degree of chronic inflammation.

1. *Hematology.* In mild disease such as oligoarthritis, or in other forms of arthritis during periods of quiescence, the complete blood cell count is usually normal or may show only mild thrombocytosis. With moderate disease activity, the hemoglobin falls but red blood cell indices are normal. This anemia of chronic disease reflects inefficient iron utilization resulting from the action of inflammatory cytokines. With severe polyarticular disease or active systemic arthritis, more profound anemia and thrombocytosis occur and leukocytosis may be seen. In active systemic arthritis, the leukocyte count may be in the range of 30 to $100,000/mm^3$ and the hemoglobin may be as low as 5 g/dl.

2. *Acute-phase reactants.* Erythrocyte sedimentation rates are normal in mild disease, but in active polyarthritis or systemic disease they may be extremely high, sometimes exceeding 100 mm/hr. Fibrinogen is high in active disease, and C-reactive protein value may be elevated. Serum immunoglobulins may be high in children with severe inflammation, owing to polyclonal B-lymphocyte stimulation, particularly during systemic flares. These findings are largely the effect of interleukin-6, which is produced in high quantities in children with active systemic arthritis.

3. *Serum chemical analyses.* These studies are usually normal except in children with systemic symptoms, who may have depression of albumin with secondary falls in serum calcium but preserved ionized calcium.

4. *Serology.* Antinuclear antibody is positive in 25 to 88 per cent of children with JA, depending on the subtype. Rheumatoid factor is found in only 5 per cent, in those with polyarthritis of adult type. Serum complement levels are normal.

Key Laboratory Findings: JA

- *Hemoglobin:* Normal, or low with chronically active disease

- *White blood cell count:* Abnormal only in systemic arthritis; leukocytosis through leukemoid reactions may be seen during active systemic disease

- *Platelet count:* Usually elevated in proportion to severity of arthritis; low platelet count should raise suspicion of leukemia

- *Erythrocyte sedimentation rate:* Normal in oligoarthritis and mild polyarticular disease; moderate elevation (20–40 mm/hr) seen with moderate joint inflammation; very high in active systemic disease and inflammatory bowel disease

- *Antinuclear antibody:* Present in 25 to 75 per cent, depending on subtype; correlates with risk for eye disease

- *Rheumatoid factor:* Present in 20 to 30 per cent of children with polyarthritis; usually seen when disease onset is after age 8

Radiographic Changes

1. *Plain radiographs*

   a. *Early radiographic changes.* Radiographs of affected joints early in JA may demonstrate soft tissue swelling and effusion but may be normal.

   b. *Late radiographic findings.* As disease progresses, juxta-articular osteopenia occurs.

      (1) After 2 years of active synovitis, cartilage loss may produce joint space narrowing.

      (2) Particularly in polyarticular disease, joint erosions occur, leading to laxity within the joint, and dislocations.

      (3) In enthesitis-associated JA, ankylosis may occur as a late finding, most prominently in the tarsal joints, the sacroiliac, and, later still, the spine in juvenile ankylosing spondylitis.

c. *Corticosteroid-related radiographic findings.* Bony changes may be seen on radiographs in children treated with corticosteroids.

(1) Osteopenia, particularly of trabecular bone, may be seen in children treated with corticosteroids. Risk of osteopenia relates to the duration and dose of agent used.

(2) Vertebral collapse may be seen on lateral chest or lumbosacral spine films in children treated with long courses of corticosteroids.

(3) Osteonecrosis of the femoral head may be detected by plain radiography as a subcortical crescent of lucency adjacent to the articular cartilage. Deformities of the femoral head may occur as later findings.

2. *Technetium bone scans*

a. *Early disease.* With early active synovitis, bone scans may show increased flow of isotope to the affected joints in the immediate images. Later static images may show increased uptake at the epiphyses of involved joints.

b. *Aseptic necrosis of the hip.* Avascular necrosis of the hip can occur in children with severe hip arthritis or corticosteroid therapy, and there may be decreased blood flow to the femoral head.

3. *Magnetic resonance imaging.* Magnetic resonance studies can demonstrate changes in synovium and cartilage, including erosions, that are not evident on clinical or standard radiographic examinations, so they may be helpful in early disease before plain radiographic changes. Cost prohibits its routine use.

Key Radiographic Findings: JA

- Soft tissue swelling of area surrounding inflamed joint
- Juxta-articular osteopenia
- Narrowing of joint space (articular cartilage loss)
- Cystic changes of subchondral bone
- Erosion, subluxation, and deformities

Treatment

Therapy for JA is aimed at controlling inflammation and its symptoms (i.e., pain, stiffness, and swelling) and preventing damage to joint structures, thereby preventing permanent disability. Unfortunately, definitive or curative treatment is not available. Aggressive suppression of inflammation is the current trend in therapy for JA, particularly in the more severe and destructive forms of the disease. Treatment to alleviate symptoms without full suppression of inflammation does not alter disease course or progression to erosions. Many antiinflammatory medications are available for the treatment of JA. The major classes include

1. *Nonsteroidal antiinflammatory drugs (NSAIDs).* Most children with JA will show improvement in symptoms and signs of inflammation with NSAID treatment. The prototype agent of this class is aspirin. The NSAID medications approved for use in children younger than

the age of 12 and dosing recommendations are outlined in Table 80–3. Most children with oligoarthritis respond to an NSAID.

a. *Mechanisms of action.* These drugs produce analgesia at a lower dose than that required for antiinflammatory effect. At higher doses, inhibition of cyclooxygenase, and thereby the production of prostaglandins, inhibition of phospholipase C and oxygen radical formation, and the transcription of inflammatory cytokine messenger RNA occur.

b. *Onset of action.* Pain relief is rapid (1 to 3 days). Antiinflammatory response is usually seen by 1 to 3 months.

c. *Side effects.* Toxicity includes anorexia, gastritis, and gastrointestinal bleeding and, less frequently, hepatic and renal impairment or central nervous system symptoms (irritability, headache).

d. *Gastric protection.* Children should take these medications with food, but often such agents as sucralfate, misoprostol, antacids, or histamine-2 blockers may be necessary.

e. *Monitoring.* Patients treated with high doses of NSAIDs should be closely monitored: fecal blood, urinalysis, and transaminase and creatinine levels should be checked every 3 to 6 months.

2. *Sulfasalazine.* Uncontrolled trials suggest that this agent is effective in treating JA, particularly oligoarthritis and enthesitis-associated JA.

a. *Mechanism.* The drug and its metabolites appear to exhibit inhibitory activity on prostaglandin formation, transcription of inflammatory cytokines, and mild inhibition of 5-lipoxygenase, the enzyme required for the formation of leukotrienes.

b. *Onset of action.* Improvement may be seen within several weeks.

c. *Toxicity.* Side effects include allergic reactions, marrow suppression, gastrointestinal complaints, reversible oligospermia, and hepatic and renal dysfunction.

d. *Dosing recommendations.* Treatment usually starts

TABLE 80–3. NONSTEROIDAL MEDICATIONS APPROVED FOR CHILDREN

MEDICATION	DOSE	COMMON (SERIOUS) TOXICITY
Aspirin*	80–100 mg/kg/day (qid)	Platelet dysfunction, gastrointestinal ulceration, anorexia, tinnitus, salicylism, hepatic injury, decreased glomerular filtration rate (Reye syndrome)
Ibuprofen	30–40 mg/kg/day (tid–qid)	Milder gastrointestinal toxicity, reversible platelet effects, occasional hepatic and renal dysfunction
Tolmetin*	20–30 mg/kg/day (tid)	Similar to ibuprofen
Naproxen	10–20 mg/kg/day (bid)	Similar to ibuprofen; (photosensitive bullous skin eruption that can scar, most common in fair-skinned children)

*Not available as a liquid.

at 10 to 20 mg/kg/day; doses may be increased weekly to 30 to 50 mg/kg/day.

    e. *Monitoring.* Blood cell counts and liver enzyme levels should be monitored within 1 to 2 weeks, 4 to 6 weeks later, and then every 3 to 6 months.

3. *Methotrexate.* Methotrexate has been added to the treatment regimen in severe JA in the past decade based on its efficacy in controlling refractory rheumatoid arthritis in adults. Its use is primarily in children with polyarticular or systemic disease, and it can be effective in psoriatic disease as well. At 10 mg/M²/wk, it is effective in suppression of JA; and in adults, it can slow or halt radiographic progression of erosive changes.

    a. *Mechanism.* At low doses (i.e., in the antiinflammatory range), interleukin-1 production is decreased and a variety of cellular inflammatory functions are inhibited.

    b. *Onset of action.* Methotrexate shows relatively rapid onset of action, with some benefit noted within 2 to 4 weeks in most children.

    c. *Dosing recommendations.* Usual starting dose is 5 mg/M²/wk. The dose is gradually advanced by 2.5 mg/wk until adequate control of arthritis is achieved, usually in the range of 10 to 15 mg/M²/wk. Absorption is best if the drug is taken on an empty stomach. Subcutaneous or intramuscular injections may be used for doses above 15 mg/M²/wk to prevent nausea and limit first-pass metabolism in the liver.

    d. *Adverse effects.* Toxic reactions include nausea, oral ulcers, mild hair loss, and marrow suppression; these are lessened or prevented by folate supplementation (1 mg/day). The risk of hepatic injury mandates careful monitoring and the avoidance of alcohol intake but is relatively uncommon in children. Restrictive lung disease may occur in some individuals. Impaired fertility can occur while on the medication but usually reverses a few months after discontinuing the medication. There is a risk of teratogenicity. Contraception is recommended in sexually active teens.

    e. *Monitoring.* Liver transaminases, albumin levels, and prothrombin times should be checked routinely; and persistent abnormalities, even when mild, are an indication for liver biopsy. Complete blood cell counts should be monitored every 4 to 6 weeks initially; every 8- to 12-week monitoring may be sufficient after several months.

4. *Corticosteroids.* Corticosteroids are among the most potent antiinflammatory medications currently in use, but side effect profile and inability to prevent erosive joint disease limit their routine use as systemic therapy in JA.

    a. *Intraarticular agents.* For disease limited to one or two joints, the use of local therapy may avoid systemic medication. Triamcinolone hexacetonide is most commonly used owing to its long duration of action.

        (1) *Efficacy.* A single injection of corticosteroid can control signs and symptoms in most children with monoarticular arthritis.

        (2) *Time course of response.* Onset is fairly rapid, with improvement in signs and symptoms noted within a week or so. Remission of knee arthritis exceeds 6 months in the majority of children with oligoarthritis.

        (3) *Toxicity.* Systemic side effects can occur (see later) but are seldom clinically significant. Concern about effects on growth limit use of repeated injections in children. Small children may tolerate joint injection poorly.

    b. *Systemic agents.* Oral or parenteral corticosteroids can be very useful in controlling systemic manifestations that do not respond to nonsteroidal medication in children with systemic arthritis. Such therapy can be life-saving when severe heart or lung involvement is present.

        (1) *Efficacy.* Although findings of inflammation (heat, swelling, tenderness) may be suppressed in most patients treated with prednisone or an equivalent agent, the erosive process is unaffected. Corticosteroids are effective in suppressing disease-associated carditis, hepatitis, and pulmonary manifestations and can relieve the systemic manifestations of fever, cachexia, and anemia.

        (2) *Toxicity.* Systemic side effects include growth impairment, glucose intolerance, weight gain, hirsutism, osteopenia with risk of vertebral collapse and other pathologic fractures, ocular cataract formation, hyperlipidemia, hypertension, immune suppression, affective changes, and myopathy. The risk of most side effects is related to dose and duration of therapy.

        (3) *Dose.* The dose used in systemic disease depends on the severity of the disease manifestations and the urgency of disease control. With carditis and congestive failure or pericarditis with tamponade, for example, methylprednisolone at a dose of 1 to 2 mg/kg/day may be required. Most other manifestations can be controlled at doses of less than 1 mg/kg/day using oral prednisone. Rarely, pulse methylprednisolone (30 mg/kg/dose) may be required for extreme manifestation of systemic arthritis.

    c. *Mechanism of action.* The mechanisms of action of corticosteroids are complex. Corticosteroids are potent in vitro inhibitors of many lymphocyte functions at suprapharmacologic doses, including mitogen and antigen responses, antibody production, and phagocyte respiratory burst. At doses used in vivo, there is down-regulation of adhesion molecule expression on inflammatory cells and endothelium, which prevents migration into tissue. In addition, it has been shown that these agents induce production of a peptide that binds to and inhibits NFκB, a transcription factor important in production of inflammatory cytokines including tumor necrosis factor-α and interleukin-6. Consequently, corticosteroids impair the production of these cytokines after an inflammatory stimulus.

5. Hydroxychloroquine, D-penicillamine, and gold salts are seldom used in children.

Prevention

Because these diseases are idiopathic, prevention is not currently available. Preventive efforts are focused on averting joint destruction and disability and on early detection of ocular inflammation.

Key Issues in Management of Juvenile Arthritis

- Preventive management:
  Routine slit lamp examinations for uveitis
  Periodic laboratory examination for medication toxicity
  Physical and occupational therapy

- Therapeutic goals:
  Minimize discomfort with medication, rest, splinting if needed
  Maintain full joint range and function
  Limit or prevent erosion, destruction, and deformity
  Limit physical and psychological disability

Bibliography

Fink CW, Fernandez-Vina M, Stastny P: Clinical and genetic evidence that juvenile arthritis is not a single disease. Pediatr Clin North Am 1995;42:1155–1169.

Giannini EH, Cawkwell GD: Drug treatment in children with juvenile rheumatoid arthritis: past, present and future. Pediatr Clin North Am 1995;42:1099–1125.

Wallace CA, Levinson JE. Juvenile rheumatoid arthritis: outcome and treatment for the 1990s. Rheum Dis Clin North Am 1991;17:891–905.

81 Systemic Lupus Erythematosus

K. M. O'Neil

Definition

Systemic lupus erythematosus (SLE) is an idiopathic inflammatory condition affecting many organ systems that is characterized by polyclonal B-lymphocyte activation and autoantibody and immune complex formation.

Etiology and Pathogenesis

The etiology is unknown, but several epidemiologic factors are known to play a role in pathogenesis.

1. *Genetics.* Approximately 20 per cent of children with SLE have a first-degree relative with the disease, and 5 to 10 per cent of adults with the disease have a positive family history. Fifty-seven per cent of monozygotic twins are concordant for SLE.

   a. *HLA associations.* The HLA-DR antigens DR2 and DR3 correlate with risk ratios of 2.8 and 3.8 in comparison to the general population.

   b. *Complement deficiencies.* Complement deficiencies, particularly of the early classical pathway components, are strongly associated with SLE. In adults, 1 per cent of SLE patients have complement deficiencies (1/10,000 in the normal population), but these may be more common in children with lupus, as high as 42 per cent in one study.

2. *Environmental factors.* Genetics alone does not account for all cases of SLE. A variety of environmental factors are associated with disease expression.

   a. *Hormonal influence.* Over the age of 10 years, SLE is ninefold more common in females and is often precipitated by menarche, pregnancy, or oral contra-

ceptive use. In children younger than the age of 10, the female:male ratio is 3:1. In animal models, ovariectomy can prevent or ameliorate disease expression.

   b. *Climate.* Incidence is seasonal, with peaks during the summer months in temperate climates; in tropical climates, no seasonal incidence variation is found. Ultraviolet light can induce lupus, particularly in C2-deficient patients.

   c. *Infectious agent(s).* Flares of lupus activity can be precipitated by infection. Viral agents are most often implicated. Vertical or horizontal transmission of a presumed viral agent has been suggested by some family studies. Spouses of individuals with SLE have increased rates of antinuclear antibody (ANA) positivity, as do technicians with frequent exposure to serum from SLE patients.

   d. *Drugs.* Certain medications, notably hydralazine and procainamide, can induce lupus in individuals with the slow acetylator phenotype.

Pathophysiology

1. *Polyclonal B-lymphocyte activation.* A variety of immunologic defects have been hypothesized, documented, and disputed in SLE. The most prominent immunologic abnormality in most individuals with SLE is the production of numerous autoantibodies.

   a. *Autoimmunity.* True autoimmunity, per se, as is seen in processes such as myasthenia gravis (where antibody directed against the acetylcholine receptor produces the disease manifestations) is not the pathophysiologic defect in SLE.

b. *B-lymphocyte hyperactivity.* The basic defect in lupus is believed by most investigators to be nonspecific activation of B lymphocytes, with resulting polyclonal hypergammaglobulinemia. Under normal conditions, clones of B cells capable of producing autoantibodies are suppressed and do not undergo expansion (proliferation) or activation to antibody secretion. This normal suppression is not seen in people with lupus. Consequently, autoantibody formation ensues.

c. *Defective apoptosis.* In some animal models of SLE, defects in apoptosis (programmed cell death) affecting B lymphocytes prominently have been described. Similar abnormalities in humans are a rare cause of SLE.

2. *Immune complex formation and clearance.* Abnormal immunoglobulin production leads to the formation of immune complexes (ICs). These ICs then produce a variety of inflammatory effects that result in the clinical phenomena seen in SLE.

a. *Macrophage activation.* ICs can directly activate macrophages through Fc and complement receptors, leading to lymphocyte recruitment through the production of inflammatory cytokines and subsequent tissue damage.

b. *Complement activation.* ICs activate the complement system, releasing inflammatory complement peptides, further promoting tissue inflammation.

c. *Complement receptor abnormalities.* Complement-mediated IC clearance is abnormal in active lupus, with impaired expression and function of the erythrocyte CR1 receptor for C3b. CR1 is important in transport of circulating ICs to the liver and spleen. The receptor also functions as a cofactor in the cleavage of C3b to iC3b. This reaction generates the ligand (iC3b) for avid binding to CR3 receptors on liver and splenic macrophages and the ingestion and elimination of the ICs.

d. *Immune complex disease in complement deficiency.* The traffic of ICs is impaired in children with early complement component deficiencies; this is probably related to the high risk of SLE in C2-deficient children.

3. *Inflammation.* ICs are deposited widely in the tissues of people with SLE. Inflammation is triggered by the ICs, leading to activation of mononuclear and polymorphonuclear phagocytes, lymphocytes, and so on. Endothelium in blood vessels undergoes inflammatory changes that produce the clinical picture of vasculitis in many organs and leads to ischemic damage.

Clinical Findings

1. Systemic lupus erythematosus manifestations

a. *Diagnostic criteria.* There is no specific test for SLE and no one sign or symptom that is pathognomonic. Eleven diagnostic criteria have been developed that yield 98 to 99 per cent specificity but somewhat lower (90 per cent) sensitivity when four criteria are present.

Key Factors in the Pathophysiology of SLE

- Autoantibody formation is universal in patients with lupus.

- Autoantibodies are not produced in an antigen-specific fashion.

- Polyclonal activation of B lymphocytes is seen.

- The normal suppression of autoreactive B-cell clones does not occur.

- Animals with defective apoptosis have an SLE-like illness.

- Immune complexes are abundant, and clearance may be impaired.

- These defects lead to a generalized inflammatory state resulting in immune damage to numerous organ systems.

Diagnostic Criteria for SLE

- *Malar rash:* Maculopapular or fixed erythema of skin over cheeks and bridge of nose, sparing nasolabial folds. Telangiectatic elements may be present.
- *Discoid rash:* Inflammatory changes deeper in the dermis, producing follicular plugging, hypopigmentation and hyperpigmentation, and scarring.
- *Photosensitivity:* Rash is exacerbated by ultraviolet radiation exposure.
- *Oral or nasopharyngeal ulcers:* Shallow palatal ulcers; may occur on the uvula.
- *Serositis:* Pericarditis, pleuritis, or peritonitis. Pericardial tamponade may occur. Aseptic meningitis occasionally seen.
- *Arthritis:* Symmetric joint inflammation, often with effusion; synovial thickening is rare, and erosions do not occur.
- *Nephritis:* Proteinuria or casts in urine. Hematuria and hypertension may occur. Diffuse proliferative glomerulonephritis may lead to hyperkalemia and renal failure. Poor outcome with high-titer anti-DNA antibody, low C3.
- *Central nervous system lupus:* Seizures and psychosis early in course. Cranial or peripheral neuropathies. Stroke with antiphospholipid antibody. Memory or calculation disorders common. Laboratory values may be normal.
- *Hematologic disorder:* Leukopenia or thrombocytopenia is evident. Recurrent or persistent idiopathic thrombocytopenic purpura may precede other manifestations by years.
- *Positive ANA:* ANA is seen in nearly all children with SLE. Discoid lupus erythematosus may have a negative ANA but often a positive anti-SS-A (Ro).
- *Immunologic abnormality:* Antibodies to dsDNA, anti-SM antibody, or biologic false-positive serologic test for syphilis.

b. *Symptoms.* In addition to the 11 diagnostic criteria, numerous less specific problems are seen in affected children. Arthritis and dermatitis are most common, with lethargy, low-grade fever, headache, myalgia (occasionally with myositis), depression, and memory problems or dyscalculia frequent. Weight loss or growth impairment may occur. Less common are alopecia and Raynaud syndrome (white, then blue color change of extremities in cold, with red on rewarming). Digital ulceration may result. Pancreatitis may be seen and may be the presenting finding. Cardiovascular involvement includes verrucous endocarditis (Libman-Sacks endocarditis) and pericarditis. Pulmonary atelectasis, interstitial pneumonitis, hemorrhage, and pulmonary hypertension are rare.

Key Common Nonspecific Findings: SLE

- *Systemic symptoms:* Fever, myalgia, weight loss, poor growth
- *Skin disorders:* Rashes including bullous eruptions
- *Vascular problems:* Raynaud phenomenon, digital ulcers
- *Neurologic disorders:* Headache, memory problems, dyscalculia

c. *Disease course.* A single complaint may predominate for months or years, or onset may be multisystemic. Eventually, the disease usually affects several organ systems in most individuals. Children with SLE are at higher risk for renal involvement. Ten-year survival is approximately 90 per cent. The most common cause of death is infection, whereas renal disease was the primary cause of death before the 1980s.

(1) *Systemic symptoms.* Fever, weight loss, and poor energy occur in most patients at the time of presentation. These features may recur with exacerbations in disease activity and may herald upcoming flares. Fever must always be considered to be infection until proved otherwise, especially in individuals on high doses of corticosteroids and/or immunosuppressive agents.

(2) *Neurologic symptoms.* Headache and lethargy are common early symptoms. Major neurologic manifestations (e.g., seizures and psychosis) are most common during the first 2 years after diagnosis and decrease over time. Serologic evidence of disease activity (complement consumption, high erythrocyte sedimentation rate, elevation in anti-DNA titer) may not be present, even with severe central nervous system disease. Milder organic brain syndromes, memory defects, and dyscalculia occur throughout the course and may be cumulative. An acute change in personality or school performance should raise concern about central nervous system involvement with lupus or infection.

(3) *Renal disease.* Hematuria, proteinuria, or casts on urinalysis may be present at onset or may occur months later. Children must be monitored for hypertension, electrolyte changes, and high serum creatinine or urea nitrogen levels indicating a fall in glomerular filtration rate. A fall in serum complement levels or a rise in anti-DNA antibody titer may provide evidence of worsening lupus nephritis. Renal biopsy may indicate mesangial glomerulonephritis, focal or diffuse proliferative glomerulonephritis, membranous nephritis, or interstitial disease with minimal or no glomerular pathology. Diffuse proliferative glomerulonephritis has the least favorable prognosis.

(4) *Cardiovascular disease.* Pericarditis may occur at any time. Large effusions can cause congestive failure and symptoms of dyspnea and orthopnea. Cardiac valvular disease is present at autopsy in most individuals with SLE but is much less commonly symptomatic. New murmurs and onset of congestive heart failure may indicate valvular insufficiency due to verrucous endocarditis or rupture of chordae tendineae. Late in disease course, there is a high risk of arteriosclerotic disease related to both the use of corticosteroid medication and to the presence of SLE itself. Stroke, peripheral thrombophlebitis, and peripheral arterial disease can occur at any time in the disease course and are more common in children and adults with antiphospholipid antibodies and lupus anticoagulant.

2. *Neonatal lupus erythematosus.* Infants born to mothers with preclinical, asymptomatic, or active SLE may develop illness due to transplacental passage of IgG antibodies.

a. *Hematologic disease.* Thrombocytopenia or a Coombs-positive hemolytic anemia may be seen in infants of mothers with overt or preclinical SLE who have autoantibodies to platelets or erythrocytes. Thrombocytopenia may produce severe hemorrhagic complications in the neonate, and hemolytic anemia can produce prenatal heart failure and hydrops fetalis.

b. *Neonatal lupus syndrome*

(1) Discoid skin lesions usually disappear by 6 months of age.

(2) Heart block is associated with maternal anti-SS-A (Ro) or, somewhat less commonly, anti-SS-B (La) or anti-RNP antibodies. Permanent pacemakers are required.

c. *Disease course.* Manifestations disappear as maternal antibody wanes except heart block, which is due to permanent immune destruction of the developing cardiac conduction system.

3. *Mixed connective tissue disease.* A variant of SLE, mixed connective tissue disease (MCTD) combines features of other rheumatic syndromes, notably juvenile dermatomyositis, juvenile arthritis, and scleroderma, with those of SLE. This syndrome is rare in childhood. Many patients have Raynaud syndrome, esophageal

dysmotility, and sclerodactyly in addition to arthritis and myositis. Up to 30 per cent of children with MCTD have recurrent parotid swelling and sicca syndrome. Renal disease, initially believed to be uncommon in MCTD, occurs in up to 27 per cent of one pediatric series, with pathology similar to lupus nephritis.

4. *Sjögren syndrome.* This variant of SLE is rare in childhood. It usually presents as recurrent episodes of parotid swelling, with the development of progressive sicca syndrome. Leukopenia is common, but anemia and thrombopenia are less prominent than in SLE. There is usually polyclonal hypergammaglobulinemia and high titer autoantibody formation. ANA is present in nearly all patients, and antibodies to SS-A (Ro) and/or SS-B (La) are present in most. In addition to the B-lymphocyte hyperreactivity, there appears to be hyporesponsiveness of T cells, and skin test anergy may be present. Pathologically, there is infiltration of lymphocytes into lacrimal and salivary glands and other organs. In the salivary glands, ductal lining cells proliferate and form epimyoepithelial islands, a finding typical of Sjögren syndrome. There is an increased risk of lymphoreticular malignancy and macroglobulinemia with prolonged disease. Treatment is supportive for sicca syndrome, and systemic symptoms are treated as in patients with SLE.

Key Findings: Sjögren Syndrome

- Sicca complex
  Bilateral parotid swelling
  Lymphoid myositis
  Pancreatitis
  Hepatomegaly

- Rheumatic disease
  Systemic lupus erythematosus
  Vasculitis
  Raynaud phenomenon

- Autoantibodies

- Lymphoreticular malignancy

Laboratory Findings

1. *Hematology.* Usual nonspecific findings of inflammation include elevated erythrocyte sedimentation rate, mild normochromic normocytic anemia, and thrombocytosis. Coombs-positive hemolytic anemia with reticulocytosis may raise the mean corpuscular volume and cause anemia. Thrombocytopenia, leukopenia, or lymphopenia may occur.

2. *Urinalysis.* With renal involvement, proteinuria is the most common finding. Sediment may be bland or may contain erythrocytes and casts. This must be followed frequently in all patients with SLE.

3. *Serum chemical analyses*
   a. *Protein abnormalities.* Abnormalities of serum proteins are the most characteristic laboratory findings in SLE.
      (1) *Hypergammaglobulinemia.* Elevated total protein, with a high globulin fraction, and high

IgG, IgA, and IgM are found in most patients with SLE.
      (a) IgA deficiency ($<$ 5 mg/dl) is seen occasionally.
      (b) Kidneys are rarely if ever involved in IgA-deficient children.
   (2) *Complement depletion.* During active disease, immune complexes activate complement and components are consumed, so C3 and C4 are low. C4 is usually more severely depressed than C3, because C3 is an acute-phase protein whose production is increased in inflammation. In occasional patients, C3 may be depressed and C4 may be normal. Complement activation through the alternative pathway may be involved in this type of consumption. C3 depression correlates with the occurrence of renal disease. The CH50 is depressed during active disease. A CH50 near 0 is unusual from depletion alone and usually represents a classical complement deficiency. Deficiency of C1 is rare but is strongly associated with SLE. In these patients, no activation of C4 or C3 occurs despite active immune complex disease.

   b. *Metabolic changes.* Depending on the organs involved in each patient, varying patterns of metabolic abnormalities may be seen.
      (1) *Renal disease*
         (a) Azotemia, hyperkalemia, and high serum creatinine levels may occur.
         (b) In nephrosis, cholesterol is high and albumin is low.
         (c) Creatinine clearance is best measured after cimetidine loading for 2 days, because glomerular filtration rate may be overestimated up to 48% by creatinine clearance.
      (2) *Enzymes*
         (a) *Transaminases.* Mild elevations of aspartate and alanine transaminases may reflect liver inflammation or muscle disease.
         (b) *Amylase.* Elevation of serum amylase is seen in pancreatitis, often in conjunction with high levels of triglycerides. Pancreatitis may be associated with corticosteroid-induced hypertriglyceridemia or a primary manifestation of SLE.

4. *Serology*
   a. *ANA.* The presence of antibodies reacting with nuclear components is seen in more than 95 per cent of patients with SLE.
   b. *Anti-DNA antibody.* Antibody that binds to native (double-stranded) DNA is highly specific for lupus (95%) but only 70 per cent sensitive. Such autoantibodies are common in renal disease. Comparison of sequential anti-DNA titers may be used as an index of disease activity.
   c. *Antibody to Sm.* These autoantibodies are seen in 30 per cent of patients with SLE, but their occurrence is highly specific for SLE.

d. *Anti-SS-A and anti-SS-B antibodies.* Antibodies to these nuclear components usually are not detected with the usual ANA techniques. These antibodies are found in 15 to 20 per cent of people with SLE but are not specific for the disease. They are common in Sjögren syndrome and are present in half of patients with "ANA-negative" lupus.

e. *Antibodies to histone.* This antibody is found in drug-induced lupus.

f. *Antibodies to ribonucleoprotein.* Antibodies to ribonucleoprotein may be seen in low titer in a small proportion of patients with SLE. They are seen in high titer in MCTD.

g. *Antiphospholipid antibodies.* This class of autoantibodies is seen in a minority of children with SLE. Some of these autoantibodies have clinical importance.

   (1) *Lupus anticoagulant.* This antiphospholipid antibody reacts with clotting factors, activating thrombosis and prolonging the prothrombin time. Lupus anticoagulants have been implicated in stroke, other thromboembolic diseases, and fetal loss. Patients with serious thromboembolic disease require anticoagulation.

   (2) *False-positive test for syphilis.* The presence of an antibody that reacted with antigens from the syphilis spirochete was identified as a common finding in patients with SLE decades ago. It represents another example of an antiphospholipid antibody.

   (3) *Anticardiolipin antibodies.* The presence of anticardiolipin antibodies in SLE correlates with cardiac valvular disease, stroke, chorea, and thrombocytopenia.

5. *Cerebrospinal Fluid (CSF) Analysis.* Even with active central nervous system disease, CSF is often normal. Only 1 in 3 with lupus cerebritis will have abnormalities of CSF, with mild protein elevation being the most common finding. Mild to moderate leukocytosis may occur. CSF pressure may be elevated.

Key Laboratory Findings: SLE

- *Hematology:* Hemolytic anemia, leukopenia, thrombopenia
- *Coagulation:* Prolonged partial thromboplastin time, lupus anticoagulant
- *Chemistry:* Complement consumption, renal dysfunction
- *Urinalysis:* Hematuria, proteinuria, casts
- *Serology:* antinuclear, anti-DNA, anti-Sm, anti-RNP, anti-SS-A and anti-SS-B antibodies; false-positive serologic test for syphilis.

6. *Pathology*

   a. *Skin biopsy.* Immunoglobulin deposits on skin biopsy suggest the diagnosis of SLE but can be seen in unaffected relatives of patients with lupus. These deposits are seen in skin affected by vasculitis and other rashes but also in unaffected skin.

   b. *Renal biopsy.* Histologic examination of kidney tissue is essential in the management of significant renal disease. Important factors evaluable only by direct examination of a renal biopsy specimen include severity and chronicity.

   (1) *Severity:* The extent of disease (diffuse or focal glomerular involvement), the extent of damage to glomeruli done by the disease, and the type of pathologic lesion is important in predicting risk of progression to renal failure and response to medication.

   (2) *Chronicity:* If disease has progressed to the point that diffuse glomerular sclerosis is present, then little response to therapy can be expected. In that case, aggressive therapy may not be warranted.

Radiographic Changes

No radiographic changes are characteristic of SLE; the findings in the disease reflect the organ system involvement. For example, pericarditis may produce an enlarged cardiac silhouette on chest radiograph. With central nervous system involvement, radiographic studies may be normal or abnormal. If focal findings are present on neurologic examination, CT of the brain may reveal infarcts or other focal defects. Magnetic resonance imaging is more sensitive in the evaluation of children with presumed lupus cerebritis, demonstrating focal or diffuse cerebral edema in 20 to 30 per cent of patients with central nervous system symptoms and nonfocal neurologic examinations.

Treatment

1. *Standard therapy.* Treatment is dictated by the disease manifestations. Generally, one uses the least toxic agent(s) that effectively controls the disease. Corticosteroids, when used, have their dose tapered carefully with close monitoring of complete blood cell count, erythrocyte sedimentation rate, and urinalysis. Falls in complement concentrations or rises in anti-DNA antibody titer can predict flares before clinical symptoms in many patients.

   a. *Arthritis and serositis.* Nonsteroidal antiinflammatory drugs (NSAIDs) suffice for most children. NSAIDs decrease the glomerular filtration rate and so must be used with caution in children with nephritis. Acute renal compromise can occur in patients with SLE treated with NSAIDs. Pleuritis and pericarditis that is severe or not responding to NSAID therapy may require corticosteroids.

   b. *Skin manifestations.* Hydroxychloroquine (3 to 7 mg/kg/day) controls many dermatologic manifestations and also may be helpful for malaise associated with the disease.

   c. *Thrombopenia and hemolytic anemia.* Cytopenias usually require moderate doses of corticosteroid (0.5 to 1 mg/kg/day prednisone or equivalent), which is then tapered as tolerated. High-dose intravenous immunoglobulin (2 g/kg) may be an effective though expensive corticosteroid-sparing agent; cyclophosphamide or splenectomy may be required in severe or persistent disease.

d. *Cardiac and pulmonary manifestations.* Inflammation of heart or lungs may be life threatening and often demands high corticosteroid doses (1 to 2 mg/kg/day prednisone or the equivalent), depending on severity. Mild pericarditis or pleuritis may respond to NSAID therapy.

e. *Renal disease*

(1) *Mild nephritis:* Proteinuric children with normal blood pressure, glomerular filtration rate, blood urea nitrogen, and creatinine usually receive a 1- to 2-month trial of corticosteroid with close monitoring of urinalysis, serum chemistries, and glomerular filtration rate. Those failing this regimen undergo renal biopsy and subsequent treatment based on the findings.

(2) *Diffuse proliferative glomerulonephritis:* Cyclophosphamide treatment preserves renal function better than corticosteroids alone or even corticosteroids in combination with azathioprine.

(a) Monthly intravenous pulse cyclophosphamide therapy (500 mg/M^2) for 6 to 7 months followed by infusions every 3 months for 10 cycles has been shown to be effective and limits the bladder toxicity of oral cyclophosphamide.

(b) Close monitoring of the leukocyte count and differential are required during cyclophosphamide treatment.

(c) Dose is decreased for leukopenia or neutropenia at nadir and held for persistent abnormality in leukocyte counts.

(d) This regimen allows for tapering of corticosteroid and preservation of renal function in most children.

f. *Neurologic involvement.* Infection, metabolic abnormalities, hypertension, and drug toxicity must be eliminated from diagnostic consideration when neurologic symptoms occur. Seizures should be treated with appropriate anticonvulsants. Thrombotic events in children with antiphospholipid antibody should be treated with anticoagulation. Psychosis or cerebritis usually require high doses of intravenous or oral corticosteroids or pulse cyclophosphamide therapy, often in combination with a corticosteroid.

Prevention

1. *Primary prevention.* Prevention of SLE is not yet possible.

2. *Minimizing risk of flares.* Preventive efforts are focused on avoiding flares, disease complications, and organ damage, especially renal injury, through careful control of the inflammation and uncontrolled antibody production.

a. *Ultraviolet radiation.* Sun exposure should be avoided, and use of sunscreens is mandatory. Skin disease may be photosensitive, and sun exposure can cause flares of systemic manifestations of SLE also.

b. *Medication risks.* When oral contraceptives are indicated, a low estrogen preparation should be used, because formulations containing higher doses of this hormone may cause flares of inflammatory disease.

3. *Prevention of drug side effects*

a. *Corticosteroids.* Most physicians reserve corticosteroids and other toxic medication for severe disease. To avoid toxicity of these potent antiinflammatory medications, one should use the minimum dose that controls disease manifestations. Alternate-day dosing regimens are desirable but not always achievable.

b. *Cyclophosphamide.* The use of intravenous pulse cyclophosphamide rather than daily oral administration in severe nephritis and cerebritis helps to minimize risk of cystitis and subsequent urogenital malignancies associated with the drug.

Key Treatment and Prevention: SLE

- Use sunscreens and avoid ultraviolet radiation.
- Avoid high-estrogen contraceptives.
- Follow complete blood cell count, erythrocyte sedimentation rate, complement, and serologies for signs of flares.
- Treat with least toxic medication regimen that controls disease manifestations in the patient and prevents organ damage.

 Bibliography

Jacobs JC: Systemic lupus erythematosus. *In* Pediatric Rheumatology for the Practitioner. New York, Springer Verlag, 1992, pp 409–526.

Lehman TJA: A practical guide to systemic lupus erythematosus. Pediatr Clin North Am 1995;42:1223–1238.

Lockshin MD: Therapy for systemic lupus erythematosus. N Engl J Med 1991;324:189–191.

Mills JA. Systemic lupus erythematosus. N Engl J Med 1994;330:1871–1879.

82 Juvenile Dermatomyositis and Polymyositis

K. M. O'Neil

Definition

Juvenile dermatomyositis (JDMS) is a multisystem disease characterized by small vessel vasculitis whose primary manifestations are inflammatory myopathy and dermatitis. It presents as symmetric proximal muscle weakness and characteristic rashes involving any site, but with a predilection for the face and hands. *Juvenile polymyositis* has similar muscle disease, but the skin is spared.

Diagnostic Criteria

The diagnosis of definite JDMS is made when four criteria (see box) are present; probable JDMS is diagnosed when three of these criteria are present. Polymyositis is confirmed when three of the four muscle-related criteria are present, although histopathologic differences between the two diseases exist.

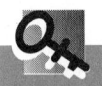

Key Diagnostic Criteria for Childhood Inflammatory Myopathy

- *Juvenile Polymyositis:* A definite diagnosis is made when three criteria are present
  Symmetric proximal muscle weakness
  Elevated levels of muscle-derived enzymes
  Histology demonstrating inflammatory myositis
  Electromyographic changes showing inflammatory myopathy

- *Juvenile Dermatomyositis:* The diagnosis is definite when three, or probable when two, of the four muscle disease criteria above are present in conjunction with the characteristic rash

Epidemiology

Peak age at onset for dermatomyositis and polymyositis is 5 to 14 years, but these diseases may occur throughout childhood. JDMS is rare (1 to 3 per million whites and 7.7 per million African Americans). Polymyositis is 10- to 20-fold less common. Between 3000 and 5000 children are affected in the United States, where onset is slightly more common during the summer.

Etiology

No single etiology has been identified, but several factors appear to play a role.

1. *Infection.* A variety of viruses (e.g., picornaviruses, including coxsackievirus B2 and A9, and hepatitis B), bacteria, and parasites have been implicated in children with inflammatory myopathy.
2. *Genetics.* Sporadic familial cases of JDMS have been reported. HLA associations include B8, DR3, and DQα1*0501.

Pathophysiology

1. *Histopathology*
   a. *Muscle.* Biopsy of muscle shows perivascular lymphocytic infiltrate of predominantly CD4+ cells, with immunoglobulin and complement C5b-9 deposited on vascular endothelial cells. Vessels involved are small arterioles, capillaries, and small venules.
   b. *Skin.* Skin biopsy reveals vessel dropout, loss of dermal papillae, and varying degrees of fibrosis.
2. *Autoimmunity.* There is no evidence of generalized immune hyperreactivity in the inflammatory myopathies of childhood. Antinuclear antibodies (ANAs) are present in about 80 per cent. PM-1 is present in some children; other autoantibodies are absent.
3. *Muscle damage.* Muscle cells undergo ischemic damage, with injury to both type I and type II fibers. Injury is patchy, with individual fibers affected, whereas neighboring fibers may be spared.

Clinical Findings

1. *Onset.* Muscle weakness and rash begins acutely in 50 per cent; subacute disease with rash and mild or minimal muscle weakness may delay diagnosis in the remainder. Rarely, children will present with the late findings of calcinosis or ulceration of the skin.
2. *Disease manifestations*
   a. *Cutaneous findings*
      (1) *Heliotrope rash.* A violaceous eruption may occur in a heliotrope (sun seeking) pattern on the face and chest. On the face, the rash usually involves eyelids with accompanying periorbital edema, forehead, cheeks, and chin. Capillary telangiectasia of the lids is seen in the majority. The rash may be brought on by sun exposure (i.e., it may be photosensitive).
      (2) *Gottron papules.* The finding of erythema with induration followed by atrophy, often with hypopigmentation of the skin overlying the dorsum of the metacarpophalangeal and interphalangeal joints of the hands, is almost pathognomonic of juvenile dermatomyositis. Similar skin changes involving the extensor surfaces of the knees, elbows, or medial malleoli may be found.
      (3) *Maculopapular scaly rash.* A more diffuse maculopapular eruption that may involve the upper torso and extensor surfaces of the extremities can be seen.
      (4) *Brawny edema of extremities.* Nonpitting edema of the extensor surfaces of the extremities may occur.
      (5) *Skin vasculitis.* Eyelid and nail bed telangiecta-

sia, livedo reticularis, and ulceration of skin, digits, or oral mucosa may be seen. Lesions of the nail beds may be better seen with an ophthalmoscope at +15 to +40 diopters, after coating the nail bed with immersion oil.

b. *Muscle disease*

(1) *Proximal weakness.* The child may have difficulty rising from a chair, climbing stairs, or even lifting his or her head or extremities off a bed. Onset may be rapid or indolent. Gower sign (the child must climb up his or her legs using the arms to stand from a seated position on the floor) is common.

(2) *Oropharyngeal involvement.* Nasal speech is common; dysphagia may be seen that can progress to difficulty handling secretions. Aspiration into the lungs may occur in severe cases.

c. *Systemic involvement*

(1) *Gastrointestinal tract.* Vasculitis of the bowel may lead to malabsorption (including medications), to ischemia, or to hemorrhage.

(2) *Lungs.* Pneumonic infiltrates with interstitial vasculitis, pulmonary hemorrhage, and fibrosis occurs uncommonly.

(3) *Cardiovascular.* Myocarditis may be seen, and, rarely, diffuse vasculitis may lead to hypotension and shock.

(4) *Other organ system involvement.* Cerebritis is occasionally seen, and renal involvement with hematuria and proteinuria may occur. Cardiac, brain, and kidney disease usually respond promptly to corticosteroid. In severe cases, myoglobinuria may damage the kidneys.

3. *Disease course.* Disease may be monocyclic and resolve completely, may be polycyclic, or may be persistent. Outcome depends on prompt identification of the disorder and early, aggressive antiinflammatory treatment. Long-term disability may result from muscle damage by severe myositis, from weakness due to persistent myositis, or from calcinosis limiting joint and muscle function.

Key Clinical Findings: JDMS

- Muscle Disease
  Proximal muscle weakness, usually symmetric
  Nasal voice
  Difficulty chewing and swallowing
  Muscle pain and tenderness ± swelling

- Skin Changes
  Periorbital edema
  Eyelid telangiectasia
  Scaly maculopapular rash of trunk and proximal arms
  Livedo reticularis ± ulcerations (digits, skin, oral mucosa)
  Gottron papules on knuckles, extensor surfaces of joints

Laboratory Findings

1. *Serum chemical analyses*

a. *Muscle enzymes.* Creatine phosphokinase and aldo-

lase are usually elevated, reflecting injury to muscle cells. Levels of aspartate transaminase (AST) and alanine transaminase (ALT) may also be elevated (AST > ALT), but levels of γ-glutamyl transferase are usually normal. The pyruvate kinase level may be elevated as well. All muscle enzyme levels may be abnormal; in more indolent disease, only one enzyme (usually the aldolase) level may be abnormal.

b. *Von Willebrand antigen.* Endothelial injury may lead to high factor VIII antigen levels, and the degree of elevation reflects activity of vasculitis in many patients.

c. *Serum complement components.* With very active vasculitis, complement consumption may be reflected in low C4 and C3. CH50 is usually normal.

2. *Immunologic markers of disease*

a. *Lymphocyte abnormalities.* Peripheral lymphopenia may occur, with CD4+ cells most affected, whereas B cells (CD19+) are increased in number.

b. *Autoantibodies.* ANA is commonly positive (>60 per cent), but other autoantibodies are usually absent. Anti-Jo1 is seen in a minority of children with JDMS and is more common in those with pulmonary involvement.

3. *Hematology.* The complete blood cell count is usually normal, although the white blood cell count may be elevated in acute fulminant disease; the erythrocyte sedimentation rate may be normal or elevated. With severe or protracted disease, platelet counts may be elevated and anemia of chronic disease may occur.

4. *Electromyography (EMG).* EMG often shows insertional irritability, spontaneous activity at rest, and abnormal full recruitment of muscle fibers with moderate effort. High-frequency discharges may be seen. EMG findings indicate myopathy but are not specific for JDMS. The site used for EMG should not be used for biopsy. Several sites may need to be tested to demonstrate myopathic changes in mild disease.

Key Laboratory Findings: JDMS

- Elevated muscle enzymes
  Creatine phosphokinase
  Aldolase
  Aminotransferases (ALT > AST)

- Serologic findings
  ANA in 60 to 80 per cent
  Anti-PM-1 in minority
  Anti-Jo-1 rarely (lung vasculitis)

Radiographic Changes

1. Magnetic resonance imaging can identify edema in inflamed regions of muscles and may be useful to help target sites for EMG or biopsy. It may also be useful in differentiating between persistent disease activity and corticosteroid myopathy or residual weakness.

2. Plain radiographs may demonstrate calcinosis in subcutaneous tissues, in surrounding joints, or in fascial planes that occur as a consequence of vasculitis in up to 30 per cent of children as a late finding.

Treatment

1. *Activity.* Excessive activity is avoided during acute inflammation to limit metabolic demands on poorly perfused muscle cells. Proper positioning is important and may require splinting. Careful attention to the avoidance of pressure points, which can lead to skin breakdown, is important. When inflammation is controlled, active rehabilitation through physical therapy is critical to optimal functional outcome.

2. *Nutrition.* If swallowing is impaired, soft foods or liquid nutritional supplements may be needed. With severe dysphagia, feeding through a nasogastric tube or parenteral nutrition may be required. If gut vasculitis causes malabsorption, bleeding, or ischemia, children commonly need parenteral nutrition or hyperalimentation.

3. *Supportive measures.* If respiratory muscles are compromised, assisted pulmonary toilet and air movement through mechanical ventilation may be required. Pulmonary hemorrhage or vasculitis may produce a diffusion defect, requiring supplemental oxygen or mechanical ventilation.

4. *Antiinflammatory therapy*
   a. *Corticosteroids*
      (1) *Classic therapy.* Usual recommendations are for 2 mg/kg/day prednisone or equivalent in four divided doses daily to control the disease acutely. The drug is maintained at high dose for several months and tapered slowly with the aim to be on alternate-day dosing by 6 months, if disease is controlled. Note that oral drug may be poorly absorbed in the presence of gut vasculitis; intravenous therapy may be needed.
      (2) *Pulse therapy.* In acute active disease, pulse therapy with methylprednisolone, 30 mg/kg/day up to 1 g intravenously every 24 to 48 hours until muscle enzymes and other indicators of inflammation improve, may be the treatment of choice. Lower-dose oral corticosteroids may then be used to sustain control ($\leq$ 0.5 mg/kg/day) and then tapered. Pulses may be stretched to greater intervals (1, 2, 3, and 4 weeks), allowing daily corticosteroid dose to be minimized and side effects of high dose prednisone to be limited.
   b. *Methotrexate.* This potent antiinflammatory agent can be effective as a corticosteroid-sparing agent and in the treatment of disease that responds poorly to corticosteroids. Efficacy begins in the same dose range used for juvenile arthritis (10 mg/M²/wk), but higher doses may be required in refractory cases.
   c. *Intravenous immunoglobulin (IVIG).* High-dose IVIG (2 g/kg divided over 2 days) has been used with anecdotal success as a corticosteroid-sparing agent in children with disease refractory to corticosteroids or in children with severe corticosteroid toxicity. Controlled trials are in progress. Insufficient data are available at this time to assess whether this agent will be effective as first-line therapy.
   d. *Hydroxychloroquine.* The antimalarial agent hydroxychloroquine (3–7 mg/kg/day) is often effective in controlling the dermal vasculitis of juvenile dermatomyositis, but efficacy of this agent in the muscle or visceral disease has not been proved.
   e. *Other agents for refractory disease.* Cyclosporine has been used successfully in a limited number of patients in conjunction with standard therapy to control resistant disease. In adults with Jo-1 positive inflammatory myopathy, FK506 has shown some efficacy, but there is little experience in childhood dermatomyositis. Cyclophosphamide has been used with efficacy in severe disease, generally given as monthly pulses to limit bladder toxicity.
   f. *Rehabilitation.* When active disease has ceased, physical therapy to improve motor strength, range of motion, and posture is critical in the attempt to minimize disability.

Prevention

Preventive efforts are aimed at the prevention of flares through the avoidance of ultraviolet light exposure, the prevention of calcinosis by early diagnosis of the disease and aggressive treatment, and the preservation of skin integrity during periods of active vasculitis. Treatment aims at avoiding disability from persistent myositis, weakness due to extensive muscle damage, and calcinosis. Long-term high-dose corticosteroid therapy can cause significant disability, however, if osteopenia ensues and compression fractures of the vertebrae or aseptic necrosis of the femoral heads occur. Care should be taken to monitor dietary intake of calcium and bone density, and therapy should be formulated to minimize demineralization.

Key Treatment and Prevention

- Rest inflamed muscles to limit metabolic demands.
- Monitor for impaired chewing and swallowing, pulmonary toilet, or ventilation and support as needed.
- Provide corticosteroid therapy at high daily doses or as pulses.
- Administer hydroxychloroquine for dermatitis.
- Provide adjunctive therapy with methotrexate, intravenous immunoglobulin, or other agents as required.
- Avoid sun exposure and use sunscreens.
- Prescribe physical and occupational therapy.

Bibliography

Ansell BM: Juvenile dermatomyositis. Rheum Dis Clin North Am 1991;17:931–942.

Laxer RM, Stein LD, Petty RE: Intravenous pulse methylprednisolone treatment for juvenile dermatomyositis. Arthritis Rheum 1987;30:329–334.

Pachman LM: Juvenile dermatomyositis: Pathophysiology and disease expression. Pediatr Clin North Am 1995;42:1071–1098.

Roifman CM: Use of intravenous immune globulin in the therapy of children with rheumatological diseases. J Clin Immunol 1995;15(suppl):42S–51S.

83 Scleroderma

K. M. O'Neil

Definition

Scleroderma means "hard skin." Scleroderma syndromes include several rare idiopathic diseases causing prominent skin hardening through collagen deposition, sometimes with involvement of internal organs. Several scleroderma syndromes are recognized in childhood, the most common being the localized forms: morphea and linear scleroderma. The manifestations of the systemic sclerodermas are discussed first and those of the limited forms second.

Classification of Scleroderma

- Systemic Scleroderma
  Diffuse: Diffuse skin fibrosis; early prominent organ involvement
  Limited: Distal skin involvement with late/no organ involvement (CREST syndrome)
  Overlap: Scleroderma skin disease with features of other rheumatic diseases (e.g., systemic lupus erythematosus and juvenile dermatomyositis) in children
- Localized scleroderma
  Morphea
  Generalized morphea
  Linear scleroderma
- Eosinophilic fasciitis
- Secondary sclerodermas
- Pseudoscleroderma

Etiology

Scleroderma is idiopathic, although major insights into the pathophysiology of scleroderma have been made in the past two decades.

Pathophysiology

Numerous factors are believed to be involved in the genesis of fibrosis in scleroderma.

1. *Vascular abnormalities.* Vascular damage leads to increased expression of adhesion molecules on endothelial cells and to the recruitment of neutrophils, monocytes, and platelets.
2. *Immunologic abnormalities.* Inflammatory cells become activated and secrete inflammatory cytokines such as interleukin-1 and platelet-derived growth factor. These, in turn, activate endothelium, increase adhesion molecule expression, and stimulate fibroblast growth and activation. T-lymphocyte activation is reflected in increased serum interleukin-2 receptor in active disease. Autoantibodies to nucleolar antigens are produced by B lymphocytes. Mast cells, increased in number in the skin of patients with scleroderma, may contribute to the sclerotic process by secreting heparin, which promotes further fibroblast growth.
3. *Excess collagen deposition in skin and other organs.* Collagen is synthesized in abnormal quantities by fibroblasts and is deposited in the intimal layer of arteries, causing increased vascular resistance and organ ischemia. Ischemic damage then activates inflammatory cell adhesion, migration, and activation, promoting further collagen synthesis and deposition.

Clinical Findings

1. *Systemic sclerodermas*
   a. *Skin.* All forms of scleroderma involve skin tightening and hardening. In the systemic forms of the disease, painless nonpitting edema of the hands and feet progresses to gradual tightening and thickening of the skin, leaving it shiny. Dermal appendages disappear, and sweating decreases. Thickening progresses to subcutaneous tissues, resulting in a woody texture. Pruritus may be present as the skin tightens, and the child may complain of stiffness.
      (1) *Face.* The face becomes progressively tightened, with loss of expression. Mouth opening or closure may be difficult. In limited systemic scleroderma, the face and distal extremities are usually involved, but it does not generalize. Telangiectasia may occur.
      (2) *Fingers.* Pitting of finger pads from ischemia and resorption of the digital tufts may occur from progressive vascular deprivation. Calcium deposits in subcutaneous tissues over the fingers and joints may cause disabling joint restriction. Raynaud phenomenon is present in most patients and may precede fibrosis by months to years. In severe cases, ulcers or even gangrene may develop. Nail bed capillary changes (disorganization, dropout, and neovascularization) may be seen with an ophthalmoscope at +15 to +40 diopters and immersion oil.
   b. *Gastrointestinal tract.* Any portion of the gastrointestinal tract may be involved in systemic sclerosis. Facial fibrosis may limit mouth opening. Dry mouth may result from fibrosis of salivary glands. There may be lingual atrophy, diminished taste sensation, gingivitis, and loss of teeth. Esophageal dysmotility is common in children with systemic sclerosis, resulting from fibrosis of the distal two thirds of the esophagus. Incompetence of the gastroesophageal sphincter causes reflux esophagitis. This often requires therapy with agents that treat esophageal dysmotility (e.g., cisapride and metoclopramide) and inhibition of acid production. Small bowel fibrosis may result in bowel dilatation, dysmotility, and mal-

absorption. Bacterial overgrowth may occur. The colon is rarely involved in children.

c. *Kidneys.* Renal disease may be life threatening in systemic sclerosis. Kidney involvement correlates with rapidly progressive skin disease and usually occurs early in the disease course. Proteinuria may be isolated or may herald the onset of renal crisis. Hypovolemia or cold-induced vasospasm can cause renal vessels that have been compromised by intimal hyperplasia to lose perfusion, triggering massive renin and angiotensin release and malignant hypertension. Oliguria and acute renal failure may develop. Angiotensin-converting enzyme inhibitors may be lifesaving.

d. *Cardiovascular system.* Pulmonary hypertension due to intimal thickening of pulmonary arteries may cause dyspnea. The myocardium and conduction system may develop fibrosis, leading to myocarditis, congestive heart failure, and arrhythmias. Coronary arteries may undergo spasm with resulting ischemia. Pericardial effusions may occur. Fibrosis of the conducting system may cause arrhythmias.

e. *Lungs.* Pulmonary involvement may occur early in the disease, usually in the form of interstitial lung disease. Inflammatory interstitial pneumonitis may be seen in diffuse scleroderma, sometimes at onset. Cor pulmonale may result from fibrotic lung disease. In limited systemic scleroderma, pulmonary hypertension may be a late finding. Symptoms of pulmonary involvement include dry cough, fatigue, and dyspnea on exertion. Reduced diaphragmatic excursion, basilar crackles, or signs of cor pulmonale may be present on physical examination. Young males of African descent are at increased risk for lung involvement.

f. *Other.* Arthralgia is common, but arthritis is rare. Recurrent ischemia may cause bony resorption of the distal finger tufts. Muscle inflammation and fibrosis is seen in 20 to 40 per cent of children with systemic scleroderma. Cerebral vasculitis is rare. Peripheral neuropathy is uncommon, but fibrosis may compress the sensory portion of the fifth cranial nerve.

2. *Localized scleroderma.* The localized scleroderma syndromes all share skin fibrosis, a typical period of disease activity of 2 to 5 years, and the possibility of remission in a large number of affected individuals. The mean age at onset in pediatric series is 6 to 8 years. This disorder may be seen in infants.

a. *Morphea.* Morphea accounts for approximately 10 per cent of children with localized scleroderma. It is characterized by the appearance of well-demarcated patches of indurated skin, often on the trunk, which range in diameter from less than 1 cm to 20 cm. The border is often violaceous, with a hypopigmented center. After several years, the lesions soften and may be hyperpigmented or hypopigmented. Some lesions condense and become firm.

b. *Generalized morphea.* Morphea is said to be generalized when large areas of skin are involved with a single lesion or with numerous, or confluent, lesions.

c. *Linear scleroderma.* Hyperpigmented fibrotic bands of skin occurring on the extremities or on the face ("scleroderma en coup de sabre") are classified as linear scleroderma. Morphea on the trunk and linear scleroderma on an extremity may occur in the same patient. At onset, inflammation occurs in the skin, progressively extending to subcutaneous tissue, underlying muscle, and bone as inflammation gives way to fibrosis. Limb size and function may be impaired with large or severe lesions. Rarely, seizures and fibrotic lesions of brain have been described in children with coup de sabre lesions overlying the cranium. Spinal cord abnormalities have been described. Progression to systemic scleroderma is rare (<2%).

3. *Scleroderma-like syndromes*

a. *Eosinophilic fasciitis.* This disease is extremely rare in children. Skin thickening and induration develops rapidly, but no other organ system involvement is seen. The skin appearance is described as "peau d'orange" or orange peel–like. Skin biopsy is diagnostic but must be full thickness, including fascia. Infiltration with eosinophils and mononuclear cells is characteristic. Peripheral blood eosinophilia accompanies the dermal eosinophilic infiltrate. The disease usually responds well to oral prednisone at moderate doses (0.5 to 1 mg/kg/day) within 1 to 2 months.

b. *Secondary scleroderma.* Several drugs and chemical occupational exposures have been reported to cause skin hardening with or without pulmonary fibrosis. These include bleomycin (skin and lung), pentazocine (skin), vinyl chloride, and silica.

c. *Pseudoscleroderma.* Endocrine and metabolic diseases can cause skin thickening not associated with rheumatic conditions. Included in this group are scleromyxedema and phenylketonuria.

Laboratory Findings

1. *Hematology.* The complete blood cell count and erythrocyte sedimentation rate are usually normal. Anemia may reflect gastrointestinal bleeding, nutritional deficiency, or malabsorption.

2. *Serology* (Table 83–1)

a. *Systemic scleroderma.* Polyclonal hypergammaglobulinemia may be seen. Most (90 per cent) have antinuclear antibodies. Anti-Scl 70 (topoisomerase-1) is seen in 20 to 40 per cent of patients with systemic sclerosis and correlates with diffuse disease, lung involvement, and poorer prognosis. Antihistone antibodies also correlate with diffuse systemic scleroderma and lung disease; they are seen in one third of patients. Anticentromere antibodies are seen in limited systemic scleroderma (CREST syndrome [calcinosis–*R*aynaud phenomenon–*e*sophageal dysmotility–*s*clerodactaly–*t*elangiectasia]). Von Willebrand factor antigen elevation may signal increased vascular disease activity.

b. *Localized scleroderma syndromes.* Antinuclear anti-

TABLE 83–1. SEROLOGIC MARKERS IN SCLERODERMA

TYPE OF SCLERODERMA	ANA	DsDNA	ssDNA	SCL 70	HISTONES	CENTROMERE
Systemic scleroderma						
Diffuse	+ + +			+ +	+ +	
Limited	+ + +					+ + +
Overlap	+ + +	+ +				
Localized scleroderma						
Morphea	+ + +		+ +		+ +	
Generalized morphea	+ + +		+ + +		+ +	
Linear scleroderma	+ + +		+ +		+ +	

bodies are seen commonly and are more frequent with more extensive involvement. Anti-ssDNA and antihistone antibodies correlate with more severe disease and may fluctuate with disease activity. Anti-Scl 70 is not seen in localized scleroderma, and anticentromere antibody is rare.

3. *Plethysmography.* This technique may be used to measure digital artery closure after cold challenge in individuals suspected of having Raynaud phenomenon, particularly in children with limited systemic scleroderma (CREST syndrome), although this is usually unnecessary.

4. *Pathology.* Biopsy of salivary glands in children with xerostomia reveals fibrosis, rather than the lymphocytic infiltration seen in Sjögren syndrome.

5. *Pulmonary function testing.* Pulmonary function tests may show decreased carbon monoxide diffusion capacity early and reduced forced vital capacity later in individuals with systemic scleroderma and lung disease. These findings may be more sensitive than history, physical examination, or plain radiography.

Radiographic Changes

1. *Plain radiograms.* Calcinosis may be noted on plain radiographs of affected regions in limited systemic scleroderma (CREST syndrome). Resorption of finger tufts (acro-osteolysis) may be seen with long-standing systemic scleroderma affecting the fingers. Chest radiographs may show interstitial infiltrates, usually in a bibasilar distribution. High-resolution thin-section computed tomography demonstrates early lung lesions at the bases, which progress to a characteristic subpleural reticulonodular pattern. Gallium or diethylenetetraminepentaacetic acid (DTPA) radionuclide scans may demonstrate lung inflammation before plain film and computed tomography.

2. *Contrast studies.* Barium swallow studies are abnormal in the majority of patients with systemic sclerosis, demonstrating poor motility, dilatation, gastroesophageal reflux, or reflux esophagitis.

3. *Echocardiography.* Echocardiography may detect pericardial effusions, ventricular thickening, and decreased compliance.

4. *Nuclear medicine.* Ventilation-perfusion scans of the lungs may show decreased alveolar capillary permeability. Gallium scans may reveal early lung involvement before it is clinically suspected. Radioisotope scans allow assessment of myocardial perfusion and function.

5. *Computed tomography.* High-resolution thin-slice computed tomography of the lung can demonstrate early pneumonic infiltrates or juxtapleural inflammatory lesions in patients with systemic scleroderma.

Treatment

1. *Vascular disease*
   a. *Raynaud phenomenon.* For treatment of Raynaud phenomenon, prevention of cold exposure is essential. Vasodilators or calcium channel blockers, especially nifedipine, are used. Topical nitroglycerine paste may improve digital blood flow. When ischemia occurs, prostaglandin E_1 given intravenously for 3 consecutive days or iloprost may be helpful.
   b. *Pulmonary hypertension.* Because severe lung disease can be fatal, aggressive therapy with corticosteroids and immunosuppression is often attempted. Pulmonary hypertension may respond to calcium channel blockers (verapamil), angiotensin-converting enzyme inhibitors (captopril), and serotonin antagonists (ketanserin).
   c. *Renal disease.* Early identification and use of angiotensin-converting enzyme inhibitors can dramatically reduce mortality of this complication of systemic scleroderma.

2. *Inflammation suppression.* Arthralgia or arthritis can be improved with nonsteroidal antiinflammatory drugs (NSAIDs). During the early, edematous phase of skin involvement, low dose (10 mg/day) prednisone therapy may be of some benefit, but this is not proved. In overlap syndromes, high doses of corticosteroids may be needed to control myositis or lupus manifestations. Cytotoxic agents have been used in severe progressive disease but are of unproved benefit. In localized scleroderma, anecdotal reports suggest that active fasciitis may respond to oral low-dose corticosteroids. Rapidly progressing lesions are often treated with D-penicillamine at 2 to 5 mg/kg/day with or without prednisone, until the disease has been in remission for 3 or more months.

3. *Fibrotic phase.* D-Penicillamine has been used extensively in rapidly progressive skin fibrosis. No adequately controlled trials have been published, however. This agent inhibits cross-linking of the collagen fibers, reducing collagen formation. Toxicities include marrow suppression and renal tubular injury, which presents as proteinuria. Colchicine and methotrexate may have some efficacy as well, but experience with these agents in children with systemic sclerosis is limited. T cell–

directed therapies including cyclosporine and antithymocyte globulin have failed to affect organ damage, although skin may be improved. With antithymocyte globulin, morbidity was high. Interferon-γ and interferon-α have the ability to inhibit collagen synthesis in vitro, but clinical trials of these agents have failed to demonstrate significant improvement of disease, whereas toxicity is significant.

4. *Experimental therapies.* Reports of significantly greater improvement in skin disease with extracorporeal photochemotherapy than with D-penicillamine suggests that this treatment may have a role to play in systemic scleroderma syndromes in the future.

5. *Supportive measures.* Physical therapy is important in prevention of joint contractures. Passive stretching, muscle strengthening, and resting splints can help maintain function. Psychosocial support may be important when body image is impaired.

Key Treatment: Vascular Disease

- Vasodilator (Raynaud phenomenon)
- Corticosteroid (pulmonary hypertension)
- Angiotensin-converting enzyme inhibitors (renal disease)

Prevention

No prevention of disease is available. Some complications may be amenable to preventive interventions, however.

1. *Smoking prevention.* Tobacco consumption should be prohibited, because it can worsen vascular, cardiac, and pulmonary disease.
2. *Cold exposure.* Protection of extremities from cold exposure is important in preventing peripheral vascular spasm and distal ischemia.
3. *Hypertension.* Close blood pressure monitoring and surveillance for proteinuria in individuals with systemic sclerosis is critical for the early identification of renal disease and its treatment.

Bibliography

Cassidy JT, Sullivan DB, Dabich L, Petty RE: Scleroderma in children. Arthritis Rheum 1977;20(suppl 2):351–354.
Clements PJ: Clinical aspects of localized and systemic sclerosis. Curr Opin Rheumatol 1992;4:843–850.
Uziel Y, Krafchik BR, Sliverman ED, et al: Localized scleroderma in childhood: A report of 30 cases. Semin Arthritis Rheum 1994;23:328–340.
Uziel Y, Miller ML, Laxer RM: Scleroderma in children. Pediatr Clin North Am 1955;42:1171–1203.

84 Vasculitis Syndromes of Childhood
K. M. O'Neil

Definition

Vasculitis is an inflammatory process of arteries, capillaries, and/or veins that damages the vessels and consequently causes damage to the organs supplied by the involved vessels. Pathologically, inflammatory cells infiltrate vessel walls, often producing destruction of the vessels.

Etiology

In most cases, vascular inflammation is idiopathic. In some cases of vasculitis, however, a drug or virus can be linked to the vasculitis syndrome, and there is evidence that immune complexes are involved in the process. The classification of vasculitis syndromes of childhood is based on clinical characteristics of the disease produced and pathologic features of the involved vessels (size of vessel; whether arteries, veins, or capillaries are involved; and nature of the inflammatory infiltrate). Typically, vasculitis syndromes affect many organ systems, but, in some cases, only skin or a few internal organs may be involved. Because a clear etiology is absent in the majority of cases, classification of the vasculitis syndromes is, of necessity, imprecise. Moreover, evolution from one clinical syndrome to another through spread to other tissues or organs makes strict boundaries difficult to define.

Epidemiology

There were approximately 172 new patients with vasculitis referred to academic pediatric rheumatologists in the United States in 1992, representing about 4 per cent of the children evaluated in those centers. A large number of children with vasculitis are not seen by rheumatologists, however, because pediatricians are generally comfortable with the care of Kawasaki disease and Henoch-Schönlein purpura, two of the more common vasculitis syndromes occurring in childhood. Consequently, data for incidence and prevalence of these diseases are unavailable.

Pathophysiology

Just as the vasculitis syndromes are variable, so are the pathophysiologic processes recognized as important in these diseases. Several mechanisms that appear to be active in clinical vasculitis syndromes are described in this chapter. It is likely, however, that research will uncover even more variation in the mechanisms of vascular injury in the near future.

1. *Direct immune attack on vessels.* One particular vasculitis syndrome, Goodpasture syndrome, has been shown to be related to the formation of antibodies to vascular basement membrane. In this syndrome, antibody reacts with glomerular and pulmonary vascular basement membranes, causing glomerulonephritis and pulmonary hemorrhage.

2. *Immune complex–related vasculitis.* In serum sickness, a form of vasculitis that has been extensively studied in animals as well as humans, soluble immune complexes have been shown to play a central role in pathogenesis of vascular damage.

   a. *Initiation of the process.* Immune complexes deposit in vessel walls at sites of high vascular permeability, where they activate complement.

   b. *Mechanism of inflammation.* The release of chemotactic and anaphylatoxic complement peptides bring activated inflammatory cells to the region. Cytokines such as tumor necrosis factor-α and interleukin-1 and interleukin-8 further promote the localization of inflammatory cells in the region of immune complex deposition by increasing the expression of adhesion molecules on both inflammatory cells and endothelium.

   c. *Mechanism of vascular damage.* The activated cells in the inflammatory infiltrate subsequently release enzymes and toxic oxygen species that damage the vessel wall, leading to ischemic injury to the tissue supplied by the damaged vessel.

3. *Activation of neutrophils by antibody.* Antibodies reacting with cytoplasmic proteins have been identified in the serum of patients with Wegener granulomatosis and, subsequently, other forms of vasculitis. These antineutrophil cytoplasmic antibodies (ANCAs) have been demonstrated to activate neutrophils from normal individuals, stimulating adhesion, migration, respiratory burst activity, and release of lysosomal granules. It is hypothesized that neutrophil stimulation by ANCAs may be involved in the pathogenesis of some vasculitis syndromes.

   a. *c-ANCA.* Because the antigen with which these antibodies react is located in the neutrophil cytoplasm, they are referred to as c-ANCAs. In Wegener granulomatosis, the majority of these antibodies are directed against proteinase-3. c-ANCAs are seen in other forms of vasculitis as well and are not, as was originally thought, specific for Wegener granulomatosis, nor are they present in all patients with Wegener granulomatosis.

   b. *p-ANCA.* In other vasculitis syndromes (and in some patients with inflammatory bowel disease) ANCAs do not react with proteinase-3, and if exposed to alcohol-fixed neutrophils, they produce a perinuclear staining pattern. These are referred to as p-ANCAs (perinuclear) in distinction to the c-ANCAs (cytoplasmic) seen in Wegener granulomatosis. The majority of the p-ANCAs react with myeloperoxidase, but the specificity may be to other as yet unidentified proteins.

Clinical Findings

Several distinct vasculitis syndromes are recognized in childhood. Classification is based on the pattern of vessels involved, the organs affected, and the clinical features of the disease. Some signs and symptoms common to many vasculitis syndromes are outlined in the box below, and the more important pediatric vasculitis syndromes are then discussed individually.

Key Signs and Symptoms of Vasculitis

- *General:* Fever, fatigue, weight loss, anorexia, lethargy

- *Skin:* Urticaria, livedo reticularis, palpable purpura, nodules, ischemic lesions, gangrene

- *Neurologic:* Headache, seizures, peripheral neuropathy, cerebritis, stroke

- *Eyes:* Iritis, retinal vasculitis, cotton-wool spots, retinal hemorrhage

- *Respiratory:* Sinusitis, otitis, pulmonary infiltrates, hemorrhage, nodules, pulmonary cavities

- *Cardiovascular:* Congestive heart failure, rhythm disturbances, infarction

- *Renal:* Hypertension, hematuria

- *Musculoskeletal:* Arthralgia, arthritis, myalgia

1. *Hypersensitivity Vasculitis Syndromes.* Leukocytoclastic vasculitis involving small vessels that is frequently precipitated by drugs or viral infection, especially penicillin and sulfa antibiotics, anticonvulsants, or serum infusion (e.g., antithymocyte globulin in transplant rejection), is classified as hypersensitivity vasculitis. Clinical characteristics of this group of syndromes includes prominent skin involvement, with palpable purpura and/or maculopapular rash. Biopsy shows neutrophils in the wall of arterioles or venules and an eosinophilic component in the infiltrate. The two most common hypersensitivity vasculitis syndromes are Henoch-Schönlein purpura (HSP) and serum sickness.

   a. *Henoch-Schönlein purpura.* The characteristic findings of HSP, the most common vasculitis syndrome of childhood, include palpable purpura, arthritis, colicky abdominal pain, and nephritis. Other organ systems may be involved in the vasculitic process, but with lower frequency. The presenting symptom may be rash; however, an acute arthritis or abdominal pain may be seen without purpura. The rash and other manifestations may not occur for days to a few weeks after the first symptoms. The typical course lasts from 2 weeks to 3 months, with recurrences up to 1 year seen in approximately 10 per cent of children. Rash is present in all patients with definite HSP. It is possible, however, that some individuals with acute arthritis, nephritis, and/or gut involvement but no skin vasculitis have the same pathologic process as classic HSP.

Key Diagnostic Criteria: Henoch-Schönlein Purpura

- *Characteristic rash:* Palpable purpura of legs and buttocks
- *Abdominal pain:* Colicky pain, usually periumbilical
- *Arthritis:* Transient periarthritis of knees, ankles
- *Nephritis:* Proteinuria, hematuria, hypertension, or azotemia

(1) *Skin vasculitis.* Palpable purpura affecting primarily the lower extremities and the buttocks is a required diagnostic criterion of HSP. The rash may involve trunk, face, and upper extremities in severe cases. Angioedema may be the first skin manifestation, beginning one to a few days before purpura. Purpuric lesions often resolve with ecchymosis, and in most cases last from 3 days to 1 month. One or more recurrences are seen in 10 per cent of cases, usually within the first 3 months, but may occur for up to 1 year. Platelet count and coagulation studies are normal. In very young children, an urticarial vasculitis may be seen. In this case, there is little or no pruritus, and histamine-1 antihistamines are of no benefit. The vasculitis may precede or follow any of the other manifestations. Once it appears, the diagnosis can easily be made.

(2) *Gastrointestinal involvement.* A variety of gastrointestinal manifestations of HSP are seen, the most common complaint being abdominal pain. Symptoms of partial obstruction with vomiting may reflect ileus from mucosal edema, pancreatitis, intussusception (usually ileoileal), or duodenal hematoma. Diarrhea and malabsorption from mucosal vasculitis may occur. Gastrointestinal bleeding may be occult, overt with currant-jelly stools typical of intussusception, or massive and life threatening.

(3) *Arthritis.* Joint inflammation with warmth, swelling, and often erythema overlying inflamed joints may be an early manifestation of HSP. Synovial thickening is not seen, and effusions are uncommon. Edema and tenderness often extend beyond the synovial space, producing a periarthritis in many children. The arthritis tends to be migratory, with a predilection for knees and ankles. Antiinflammatory medication may alleviate symptoms but may not be required. Concern about platelet dysfunction and gastrointestinal bleeding due to therapy with nonsteroidal antiinflammatory drugs (NSAIDs) limits their use.

(4) *Nephritis.* Approximately 10 per cent or less children develop renal involvement, a potentially serious complication of HSP. Proteinuria is the most common abnormality, with hematuria, hypertension, and renal compromise less frequent. Isolated proteinuria or hematuria usu-

ally resolves completely; overt nephritis or nephrosis may persist or progress to renal failure. Biopsy reveals glomerular IgA deposits, with variable degrees of glomerular damage. Renal disease typically occurs within 3 months of onset of HSP. Close monitoring of urinalysis and blood pressure during the first few months after onset is recommended.

(5) *Other manifestations.* Pulmonary infiltrates or hemorrhage, cerebritis with seizures, mental status changes, aseptic meningitis, peripheral neuropathy, pancreatitis, scrotal pain and swelling from testicular and epididymal vessel vasculitis, and, rarely, ovarian vasculitis may occur.

(6) *Management issues.* Treatment is supportive, with care given to hydration and electrolyte balance. Pain control with acetaminophen is usually sufficient. Testing for intestinal bleeding is important in children with abdominal pain. Urinalysis and blood pressure should be closely monitored for evidence of significant renal disease during the acute phase of HSP. Corticosteroids do not affect nephritis once it is established, but conflicting evidence about their role in prevention of significant renal damage exists. In severe abdominal pain or severe incapacitating arthritis, corticosteroids may be useful in shortening the duration of symptoms.

Key Treatment: Henoch-Schönlein Purpura

Skin
- No specific care is needed.

Gut Involvement
- Monitor hydration status.
- Provide nutrition support as indicated.
- Monitor for gastrointestinal blood loss.
- Prescribe corticosteroids for severe disease.

Renal Involvement
- Monitor blood pressure.
- Treat hypertension.
- Monitor urine for blood and protein.
- Provide supportive care for renal failure.

Arthritis
- Prescribe analgesic and NSAID use as needed.

b. *Serum sickness.* This systemic vasculitis syndrome was seen commonly in the preantibiotic era, when diphtheria and tetanus were treated with horse antiserum. The most common precipitants currently are antibiotics and viral infections. Immune complexes containing antibody and foreign protein begin to form 4 to 5 days after the inciting event and initiate the vasculitic process.

(1) *Symptoms.* Rash, myalgia and arthralgia, and fever begin 2 to 3 days after immune complexes can first be detected, with expression of the full syndrome by day 10 to 12 in most children. Urticaria or diffuse morbilliform rash with involvement of the skin at the junction of the palmar or plantar and dorsal skin of the hands

and feet may occur. Arthritis, nephritis, lymphadenopathy, carditis, and neuropathy may be found.

(2) *Laboratory findings.* Erythrocyte sedimentation rate rises, and C3 and C4 levels may fall at the peak of symptoms. The leukocyte count may be normal or elevated, and the differential may be normal or show a left shift. Eosinophilia may be found. Circulating immune complexes can sometimes be detected using C1q binding, Raji cell, or other assay systems.

(3) *Treatment.* The first principle in management is to eliminate any identifiable trigger, such as medications. The disease is usually self-limiting. Therapy is supportive, based on symptoms. Arthritis, myalgia, and fever usually respond to NSAIDs. Corticosteroids may be indicated for severe symptoms, but data on efficacy are variable.

Key Clinical Findings: Serum Sickness

- History of antiserum, infectious, or medication exposure 5 to 10 days before onset of illness
- Fever, adenopathy, myalgia, and arthralgia ± arthritis
- Urticarial or morbilliform rash
- Erythema of the skin at the junction of the palmar or plantar and dorsal skin of the hands and feet
- Nephritis, carditis, and neuropathy may be found
- Variable findings on complete blood cell count; may be normal
- High erythrocyte sedimentation rate, low C4 ± C3, detectable circulating immune complexes, occasional hematuria and proteinuria

2. *Vasculitis of medium-sized vessels.* The vasculitis syndromes involving medium-sized vessels (small and medium-sized muscular arteries) that are seen in childhood fall into the broad category of the polyarteritis syndromes. The two more common forms in childhood are Kawasaki disease, which occurs primarily in children, and polyarteritis nodosa (PAN), which is significantly more common in adults. In the pediatric age group, PAN is quite rare.

a. *Kawasaki disease* (see Chapter 186)

b. *Polyarteritis nodosa.* PAN is a systemic vasculitis involving medium-sized muscular arteries and producing disease in the kidneys, central nervous system (CNS), skin, muscle, and gastrointestinal tract. Coronary vasculitis with myocardial ischemia and infarction may occur. Pulmonary involvement is rare. Up to 30 per cent of PAN in adults is related to infection with hepatitis B virus. This association is rare in children, but streptococcal infection has been implicated more commonly. Evidence of autoimmunity is uncommon, but some patients have ANCAs (usually p-ANCA) in their serum.

(1) *Clinical manifestations.* Fever, weight loss, and

skin lesions are the most common findings in children with PAN. Skin findings include painful subcutaneous nodules, ulcers, livedo reticularis (a mottled reticular rash with cyanotic regions), ischemic areas, and gangrene. The usual renal lesion is necrotizing glomerulonephritis, but involvement of medium-sized renal vessels may produce hyperreninemic hypertension and aneurysms of the intrarenal or extrarenal arteries. Muscle pain is common, often accompanied by muscle weakness, tenderness, or swelling. Acute testicular pain and tenderness may occur.

Key Diagnostic Criteria: Polyarteritis Nodosa

Three or more of the following are diagnostic of PAN in adults, with 82 per cent sensitivity and 86 per cent specificity (1990 American College of Radiology criteria):
- Weight loss of 4 kg or more, or over 5 per cent body weight
- Livedo reticularis
- Unexplained testicular pain or tenderness
- Myalgia, muscle weakness, or tenderness of legs
- Mononeuropathy or polyneuropathy
- Hypertension
- Elevated blood urea nitrogen or creatinine levels not due to other causes
- Hepatitis B virus infection
- Arteriographic abnormality
- Polymorphonuclear leukocytes in artery walls on biopsy

(2) *Cutaneous PAN variant.* Cutaneous PAN is more common than systemic PAN in children. Major organ involvement is not seen. Fever, arthralgia, myalgia, and tender subcutaneous nodules are the predominant clinical manifestations. Prognosis is better than for the systemic form of the disease.

(3) *Laboratory findings.* No laboratory test is diagnostic of PAN, although biopsy of involved vessels is most specific.

(a) *Hematology.* The erythrocyte sedimentation rate is usually very high, and there may be prominent leukocytosis.

(b) *Chemistry.* Hematuria, proteinuria, or elevations of blood urea nitrogen and creatinine signal renal vasculitis. Stools may be positive for occult blood if there is mesenteric artery involvement.

(c) *Serology.* Many individuals may have positive ANCA. p-ANCAs are most common. Other autoantibodies are rare.

(d) *Pathology.* Biopsy of skin or involved organs reveals longitudinal inflammation of medium-sized vessels with fibrin plugging and leukocytic infiltration of the intima. Full-thickness involvement of the media and destruction of the elastic layer ensue, which may lead to aneurysm formation, often at vessel branch points.

(e) *Angiography.* Arteriography of cerebral or abdominal vessels shows arterial narrowing or occlusion, frequently with aneurysm formation.

(f) *Neurology.* Electromyography and nerve conduction studies may confirm mononeuritis or polyneuritis.

(4) *Management.* High-dose corticosteroids, usually using a pulse regimen (30 mg/kg/day up to three times in a 5-day period not to exceed 1 g/dose), often in conjunction with immunosuppressive agents such as cyclophosphamide, may be required for severe systemic disease. Cutaneous PAN may respond adequately to oral corticosteroids. Hydroxychloroquine may be useful in the treatment of livedo reticularis and other skin manifestations.

Key Treatment: Polyarteritis Nodosa

• High doses of corticosteroids

• Hydroxychloroquine

3. *Granulomatous Vasculitis.* Granulomatous vasculitis is characterized by granuloma formation in inflamed tissues and poor response to corticosteroids. In most cases, cyclophosphamide is required for adequate therapeutic response.

a. *Wegener granulomatosis.* Wegener granulomatosis is a clinical syndrome of disseminated granulomatous vasculitis of small and medium-sized vessels, with necrotizing focal glomerulonephritis and upper and lower airway granulomatous vasculitis. Males with the disorder outnumber females by 2:1.

Key Clinical Findings: Wegener Granulomatosis

• Sinusitis, sometimes with bony erosion of the sinus walls

• Pulmonary infiltrates, often with hemorrhage

• Necrotizing focal glomerulonephritis

• Disseminated granulomatous vasculitis of small and medium-sized vessels

(1) *Clinical findings.* Fever, anorexia, skin purpura, muscle pain, chest pain, and dyspnea are the usual symptoms. Upper airway symptoms including obstruction, epistaxis, sinusitis, and otitis are common. Hematuria and findings of renal compromise occur in many patients. Arthritis and arthralgia may be noted. Uveitis and conjunctival and corneal lesions are the most common ocular manifestations. Mononeuritis multiplex and other neurologic lesions including intracranial granulomas may be seen.

(a) *Upper airway disease.* The sinusitis may be destructive, with ulcerations of the nasal mucosa and erosion of the bone in the sinus walls or the nasal septum. Saddle-nose deformity may result.

(b) *Pulmonary involvement.* Dyspnea and cough may be accompanied by hemoptysis and pulmonary infiltrates on chest radiograms. Massive pulmonary hemorrhage may be fatal in some children. Pulmonary function testing may reveal restrictive disease and impaired diffusing capacity.

(c) *Renal disease.* Glomerulonephritis is rapidly fatal without cytotoxic therapy.

(d) *Midline granuloma.* A limited form of Wegener granulomatosis may occur in children in which upper and lower airway disease occurs but kidneys are spared. The mortality is lower than with the systemic form of the disease.

(2) *Laboratory findings*

(a) *Nonspecific findings of inflammation.* Elevated erythrocyte sedimentation rate, leukocytosis with anemia of chronic disease, and hypergammaglobulinemia are common.

(b) *Serology.* Serum from the majority of individuals with Wegener granulomatosis demonstrates the presence of ANCA. The usual staining pattern is c-ANCA, whereas the majority of ANCA-positive patients with other forms of vasculitis have p-ANCA. The primary antigen in c-ANCA is the neutrophil protease-3.

(c) *Pathology.* Biopsy of upper airway lesions usually confirms the diagnosis. Granulomatous lesions with foci of necrosis and giant cells are characteristic. Biopsy of skin and renal lesions demonstrate vasculitis, but findings are often not specific for this disorder.

(3) *Therapy.* It is important to treat Wegener granulomatosis aggressively and quickly. Without such an approach, mortality is over 90 per cent. After remission, treatment is tapered slowly, with withdrawal of therapy possible in many patients after a few years.

(a) *Cyclophosphamide.* Daily oral cyclophosphamide is usually used, beginning with doses between 1 and 2 mg/kg/day. The dose is then adjusted as required to maintain a total leukocyte count above 3000/mm³ and neutrophil count between 1000 and 1500/mm³. This regimen provides clinical results superior to the intravenous pulse regimens used in systemic lupus erythematosus. In the presence of aggressive, life-threatening disease, induction with doses of 4 mg/kg/day intravenously for the first 3 days then tapered to standard daily doses is recommended.

(b) *Corticosteroids.* Although corticosteroids may produce improvement in symptoms, they produce little long-term benefits if used alone. Corticosteroids may be added to cyclophosphamide in doses of 2 mg/kg/day in four divided doses. Pulse therapy at 30 mg/kg/day given up to three times on an every-other-day schedule may be needed in extreme cases or when cerebritis is present. Single corticosteroid pulses should not exceed 1 g each.

(c) *Sulfamethoxazole-trimethoprim.* There is some evidence that long-term treatment with this combination antimicrobial drug may be effective in treating some individuals with Wegener granulomatosis.

Key Management Issues: Wegener Granulomatosis

- Diagnosis is suggested by a constellation of clinical signs and symptoms, radiographic findings of airway or sinus involvement, and presence of c-ANCA.

- Biopsy of airway lesions usually confirms the diagnosis.

- Cyclophosphamide is the drug of choice: 1–2 mg/kg/day.

- Maintain white blood cell count more than 3000/mm³ and polymorphonuclear leukocyte count between 1000 and 1500/ mm³.

- Corticosteroids are not effective as isolated therapy.

- Corticosteroids may be useful in acute fulminant disease for symptom relief.

b. *Primary vasculitis of the CNS.* Primary angiopathy of the CNS presents as a broad range of neurologic symptoms. Radiographic studies usually identify the process as vasculitic. There is no extracranial disease.

(1) *Clinical manifestations.* Changes in mental status or school performance are usual early complaints. Headache, diplopia or blurred vision, nausea or vomiting, and cranial nerve defects are common. Seizures, hemiparesis, and stroke syndromes may be the first manifestations of CNS disease.

(2) *Laboratory diagnosis.* Serologic examination is usually normal, including erythrocyte sedimentation rate, antinuclear antibody, and so on. Cerebrospinal fluid analysis usually shows few mononuclear cells and elevated protein. Computed tomography and magnetic resonance imaging may show microinfarcts, edema, or stroke. Magnetic resonance arteriography may demonstrate aneurysmal changes of the CNS vessels but is not sufficiently sensitive in most cases. Arteriograms show beading of small to medium-sized arteries, saccular aneurysms, or areas of occlusion. Meningeal biopsy may demonstrate granulomatous vasculitis.

(3) *Therapy.* Controlled studies have not been done. Patients often improve with dexamethasone given for intracranial hypertension. Deterioration seen with tapering of the corticosteroid implies therapeutic efficacy. Cytotoxic agents such as cyclophosphamide are effective in most children when corticosteroid response is poor or corticosteroid toxicity is unacceptable.

4. *Other Rare Forms of Vasculitis.* A variety of other vasculitis syndromes may be seen rarely in children and adolescents.

a. *Takayasu arteritis.* This rare, large-vessel vasculitis involves the aorta and proximal major large elastic arteries deriving from it. Takayasu arteritis usually affects adolescent and young adult (11 to 30 years of age) females. Only 15 per cent are male. It is more common in Asians, particularly Japanese. Affected vessels rely on the vasa vasorum for nutrition. Tuberculosis has been implicated in some cases, and Takayasu arteritis is more prominent in regions where tuberculosis is endemic.

(1) *Clinical manifestations.* Failure to thrive, malaise, and fatigue are usual early symptoms. Joint pain and low-grade fever may occur. As arterial flow is compromised, claudication, heart failure, hypertensive syncope, chest pain, dysphagia from aortic arch dilatation, or hypertensive encephalopathy and seizures develop. Decreased peripheral pulses, vascular bruits, and hypertension may be found on examination.

(2) *Laboratory findings.* Polyclonal hypergammaglobulinemia and high erythrocyte sedimentation rate may be early findings. Radiographs may show aortic dilatation. Diagnosis is confirmed by magnetic resonance imaging or angiography, which show arterial stenosis, dilatation, or aneurysms and arterial irregularity. Pathology reveals granulomatous inflammation with giant cells in the vasa vasorum, medial inflammation with granuloma formation, and areas of necrosis. Later, fibrosis of the media, then adventitia and intima, may occur.

(3) *Management.* Aggressive therapy for hypertensive and ischemic complications is required. The vasculitis usually responds to daily high doses of a corticosteroid, which are then tapered to alternate-day regimens based on the erythrocyte sedimentation rate and immunoglobulin levels. Cyclophosphamide may be required in corticosteroid-resistant cases. Arterial bypass or valve replacement surgery may be required. Five-year survival approaches 95 per cent in the United States.

b. *Corticosteroid-responsive encephalomyelitis.* A variant of isolated CNS vasculitis is an encephalomyelitis-like illness with deterioration of mental status to coma, severe brainstem dysfunction, and possible hemiparesis. In some patients, there has been antecedent viral or leptospiral illness. Dramatic response to corticosteroids with tapering to alternate-day regimens and return to normal within 2 to 6 months is reported.

c. *Churg-Strauss vasculitis.* Vasculitis with primarily pulmonary involvement and eosinophilia occurs rarely in children with asthma.

Key Clinical Findings: Churg-Strauss Vasculitis

- Child with history of asthma and allergic disease

- Fever, cough, and pulmonary infiltrates

- Prominent peripheral eosinophilia

- Skin vasculitis, painful subcutaneous nodules

- Pericarditis, congestive heart failure, peripheral neuropathy, arthritis, and intestinal vasculitis may occur.

- Renal and central nervous system involvement is rare.

- Biopsy shows necrotizing granulomatous vasculitis or pulmonary eosinophilic infiltrates.

- p-ANCA may be positive.

- Responds to corticosteroid treatment but may require cyclophosphamide

d. *Goodpasture syndrome.* Goodpasture syndrome, which presents as acute glomerulonephritis and pulmonary hemorrhage, is rarely seen in children. Its importance stems from its pathophysiology, where vessel inflammation and destruction occur as a direct consequence of autoantibodies that bind through their antigen binding region with vascular basement membrane. This is recognized in the clinical situation as homogeneous basement membrane staining of renal tissue with fluorescence-tagged antiimmunoglobulin reagents.

e. *Behçet Syndrome.* The clinical triad of recurrent oral and genital ulceration, ocular inflammation, and arthritis constitute Behçet syndrome, an idiopathic vasculitic syndrome that is rare in childhood. It is more common in Turkey, its neighboring countries, and in Japan than it is in the Western hemisphere.

(1) *Clinical manifestations.* Behçet syndrome usually presents as recurrent, severe aphthous oral ulcers, but it may progress to involve numerous organ systems. Genital and intestinal ulcerations, ocular and nonerosive large joint inflammation, CNS or systemic vasculitis, and, less commonly, recurrent peripheral or caval venous thromboses are seen. Ocular inflammation may involve the uveal tract, vitreous, or retina. The most common form of CNS involvement with Behçet disease is aseptic meningitis, which may be recurrent. Neurologic symptoms may range from isolated cranial nerve palsies to cerebellar ataxia, cavernous sinus thrombosis, vasculitic cerebritis, or hemiparesis or quadriparesis from corticospinal tract involvement.

Key Findings: Behçet Syndrome

- Severe, recurrent aphthous ulcers of oral and genital mucosa

- Gastrointestinal ulcers of esophagus or small or large bowel

- Hematuria from urethritis or bladder ulcers

- Ocular inflammation

- CNS vasculitis

- Venous thrombosis

- Recurrent, nonerosive arthritis

(2) *Laboratory findings.* No test is diagnostic of Behçet syndrome. The pathergy sign is the formation of a pustule with red halo at the site of skin puncture by a needle, 24 hours after the puncture occurs. It is commonly found in Behçet syndrome in Turkey and Japan. In the United States, however, fewer than 20 per cent of individuals with Behçet syndrome demonstrate the typical findings.

(3) *Therapy.* A broad variety of agents have been used with variable success in the treatment of Behçet syndrome. Corticosteroids in an oral cream base may be useful for aphthous stomatitis. NSAIDs, particularly indomethacin, can be of benefit in treating arthritis, fevers, and mucocutaneous lesions. Colchicine can decrease recurrences in some patients. Methotrexate (10 mg/M²/wk) has been effective in some patients. Severe gut or mucosal lesions and ocular or CNS disease may require systemic corticosteroids. Thalidomide may prevent disease manifestations in some patients but is not routinely available in the United States. With severe CNS or ocular disease, chlorambucil (0.1–0.16 mg/kg/day) may be required. Cyclosporine appears to be useful in ocular disease.

Laboratory Findings

1. *Nonspecific indicators of inflammation.* The most common laboratory abnormalities in vasculitis syndromes are nonspecific and are the consequence of cytokine production in systemic inflammation. Elevation in the erythrocyte sedimentation rate, C-reactive protein, and immunoglobulin concentration is characteristic of inflammatory diseases in general but may be particularly dramatic in vasculitis. These parameters tend to follow disease activity and may be useful as guides to therapy. Other nonspecific inflammatory findings include thrombocytosis, particularly in Kawasaki syndrome, anemia of chronic disease, and leukocytosis. Eosinophilia is present in Churg-Strauss vasculitis.

2. *Metabolic abnormalities.* Because the kidney is often involved in vasculitis syndromes, particularly polyarteritis nodosum, Wegener granulomatosis, HSP, and Takayasu disease, hematuria, proteinuria, and biochemical markers of renal dysfunction may be seen. Abnormalities of serum

urea nitrogen, creatinine, or potassium may result. Muscle involvement in PAN may cause a rise in the serum alanine and aspartate transaminases (ALT and AST) and in creatine kinase. Liver disease in Kawasaki disease may cause elevation of liver enzymes. Stool guaiac may be positive with gut involvement.

3. *Serologic findings.* In most vasculitis syndromes, true autoimmunity is not found. The most notable exception is the presence of ANCAs. p-ANCA is found in most patients with PAN and may be found in many other vasculitis syndromes. c-ANCA, which stains a cytoplasmic antigen, is most common in Wegener granulomatosis, but it is not specific for this disease. ANCAs have been shown to activate neutrophils and may play an active role in the pathogenesis of vasculitis. In some patients with vasculitis of medium-sized vessels, cryoglobulins are present. Complement depletion may be seen during acute flares, with depression of C4 and/or C3.

Key Laboratory Investigation of Suggested Vasculitis

Hematology
- Complete blood cell count, with evidence of leukocytosis, anemia of chronic disease, and thrombocytosis
- Erythrocyte sedimentation rate and C-reactive protein
- Prothrombin time and partial thromboplastin time

Chemistry
- Urinalysis for blood, protein
- Assessment of renal and hepatic function and other indicators of end-organ damage (muscle enzymes, amylase, cerebrospinal fluid analysis)
- Complement
- Immunoglobulins
- Cryoglobulins

Serology
- Antineutrophil cytoplasmic antibody
- Anti–glomerular basement membrane antibody
- Antinuclear antibody
- Anti-DNA
- Antibody to extractable nuclear antigens
- Rheumatoid factor
- Antiphospholipid antibody

Pathology
- Biopsy of skin lesions, muscle, kidney, liver, meninges, or other affected tissues

4. *Biopsy.* The single most valuable test in the diagnosis of most vasculitic syndromes (except where the clinical syndrome makes the diagnosis obvious, as in Kawasaki disease and HSP) is biopsy of involved vessels. This can often be performed using skin, but in the absence of dermal involvement, muscle or organ biopsy may be required. In Wegener granulomatosis, biopsy of airway lesions usually is most informative.

Radiographic Findings

1. *Plain films.* Radiographs aid in the diagnosis of Churg-Strauss vasculitis, where pulmonary infiltrates are seen. Sinus pathology and erosion of the bony walls of the sinuses may be seen in Wegener granulomatosis. Pulmo-

nary interstitial infiltrates indicate lower respiratory tract involvement in Wegener granulomatosis. Similar infiltrates may be seen in HSP, PAN, and Kawasaki disease. Cardiomegaly may be seen on a chest radiograph; and in Takayasu arteritis, aortic widening may be diagnostic. With gastrointestinal vasculitis in HSP, PAN, Takayasu disease, or Kawasaki disease, nonspecific ileus, bowel wall edema, or signs of perforation may occur. Intussusception with mass effect in the right upper quadrant can be observed on plain film in HSP and Kawasaki disease and confirmed when needed with contrast medium–enhanced studies.

2. *Angiography.* Direct visualization of vessel anatomy may be needed to confirm the diagnosis of vasculitis, but it is most useful in disease of medium or large vessels. Echocardiography is usually employed in Kawasaki disease to evaluate coronary vessels for aneurysms; angiography may be required. In the evaluation of CNS vasculitis, angiography is often the one diagnostic study.

3. *Computed tomography and magnetic resonance imaging.* CT and MRI may define the extent of organ damage from vasculitis. In CNS disease, MRI may suggest the diagnosis of vasculitis because of multiple foci of edema or may define small infarcts not seen on CT. With the use of contrast agents, the vessels can be digitally reconstructed in a technique called MR angiography, sometimes avoiding the need for a more risky classic angiogram.

Key Radiographic Studies in Vasculitis

Plain Films
- Chest radiographs
- Sinus films
- Contrast studies of the gastrointestinal tract

Ultrasonography
- Renal and gallbladder ultrasonography
- Echocardiography

Computed Tomography
- Sinus, pulmonary and brain CT
- Thoracic or abdominal CT of large vessels

Magnetic Resonance Imaging
- MRI of brain and sinuses
- MR angiography may define vascular lesions (insensitive)

Angiography
- Examination of medium- to large-vessel disease
- Venography for venous thrombosis

Treatment

With the exception of HSP, in which treatment is symptomatic, vasculitis requires prompt and aggressive therapy to prevent permanent damage or death. In general, treatment with antiinflammatory agents such as systemic corticosteroids is required for major organ system involvement. Cyclophosphamide and other cytotoxic agents may be required to control corticosteroid-unresponsive disease or as corticosteroid-sparing agents. In Wegener granulomatosis, cyclophosphamide is required for good outcome.

1. *Corticosteroids.* Prednisone or methylprednisolone at

doses up to 2 mg/kg/day in divided doses and then tapered to alternate-day regimens is the mainstay of antiinflammatory therapy in many forms of vasculitis. Pulse therapy using doses of 30 mg/kg/dose to a maximum of 1 g/dose given up to three times at 48-hour intervals may be used for severe or resistant disease. Toxicity is significant (see Chapter 80). Corticosteroids are associated with worse outcomes in Kawasaki disease and are therefore avoided in this syndrome. They are reserved for severe complications of HSP and appear to have little or no efficacy in the renal disease seen in this disorder.

2. *Intravenous immunoglobulin (IVIG)*. High doses (2 g/kg body weight over 2 to 5 days) of IVIG can produce a variety of antiinflammatory effects, including interference with complement activation, suppression of autoantibody formation possibly through anti-idiotype networks, and suppression of cytokine production. In Kawasaki disease, IVIG decreases the risk of coronary aneurysms, death, and symptoms within a few days of administration. Preliminary studies suggest IVIG may be effective in suppressing ANCA titers and symptoms in ANCA-positive vasculitis. Toxicity is minimal, confined primarily to rate-related reactions. Hepatitis C transmission has been reported with IVIG product purified by a process that is no longer licensed in the United States. Financial cost is significant, however.

3. *NSAIDs*. For the arthritis accompanying Behçet disease, HSP, and serum sickness, usual doses of NSAIDs may be used. In self-limited illnesses such as the latter two, however, this may not be required. Colchicine is useful in some individuals with Behçet disease.

4. *Immunosuppressive and cytotoxic drugs*. Azathioprine may be useful in ocular involvement in Behçet disease. Cyclophosphamide is usually the drug of choice in se-

vere, life-threatening vasculitis, particularly with granulomatous diseases. It is also useful as a corticosteroid-sparing agent in protracted disease when corticosteroid toxicity is unacceptable. Its side effects include marrow suppression, infertility, hemorrhagic cystitis, and long-term risk of genitourinary malignancy. In cerebral vasculitis associated with Behçet disease, chlorambucil is the most efficacious agent but carries with it the risk of later malignancy, sterility, and marrow suppression.

Key Treatment: Vasculitis

- Corticosteroids
- IVIG
- NSAIDs
- Immunosuppressive drugs
- Cytotoxic agents

Bibliography

American College of Rheumatology: 1990 criteria for the classification of vasculitis. Arthritis Rheum 1990;33:1065–1144.

Athreya BH: Vasculitis in children. Pediatr Clin North Am 1995;42:1239–1261.

Fauci AS, Leavitt RY: Systemic vasculitis. *In:* Current Therapy in Allergy, Immunology and Rheumatology—3. Philadelphia, BC Decker, 1988, pp 149–155.

Jacobs JC: Systemic vasculitis syndromes. *In:* Pediatric Rheumatology for the Practitioner. New York, Springer Verlag, 1992, pp 556–640.

Shulman ST, De Innocencio J, Hirsch R: Kawasaki disease. Pediatr Clin North Am 1995;42:1205–1222.

85 Infection-Associated Rheumatic Syndromes

K. M. O'Neil

Definition

A variety of rheumatic syndromes have been associated with infections. These syndromes encompass a range of symptoms and physical findings but have in common inflammation that is not limited to the infected tissue and that occurs as a result of the infectious trigger. Most of these syndromes were initially presumed to be idiopathic rheumatic conditions and were subsequently found to be due to infection.

Etiology

After infection of a susceptible host, an immune response is initiated. Cytokines are generated that promote the inflammatory process and enhance host defense. Specific antibody binds microbial antigens, producing immune com-

plexes; complement is activated, and inflammation is initiated. Important examples of postinfectious rheumatic syndromes include rheumatic fever, Lyme arthritis, and reactive (postenteritis) arthritis. In addition, a number of viruses commonly incite similar reactions, usually during the convalescent phase of illness (see box). Often, arthralgia or serum sickness–like syndromes may be seen with influenza, enterovirus infections, adenovirus infection, infectious mononucleosis, and a variety of other viral syndromes. These are usually self-limiting and improve spontaneously within days to a few weeks.

Clinical Findings

1. *Acute rheumatic fever and poststreptococcal arthritis* (see Chapter 188)

Key Viral Infections Associated with Arthritis

Rubella
- Arthritis usually accompanies characteristic rash
- Adolescent and adult women affected most commonly
- Spontaneous resolution in 2 weeks in most
- Immune response to viral antigens occurs in joints

Parvovirus B19
- Serum sickness–like arthritis
- Affects adolescent females > males > young children
- Arthritis occurs soon after rash begins
- Self-limiting 7- to 10-day course, with occasional recurrences

Hepatitis B
- Acute polyarthritis; urticaria or maculopapular rash
- Occurs during anicteric prodrome
- Resolves with onset of jaundice
- Low complement, immune complexes in serum
- May be seen with hepatitis A and C

Key Findings: Reactive Arthritis

- History of genitourinary or gastrointestinal infection 1 to 4 weeks before onset of joint disease
- Oligoarticular arthritis, usually involving knees and ankles
- Asymmetric joint involvement
- Acute keratoconjunctivitis or uveitis
- Occasional circinate balanitis or keratoderma blennorrhagicum
- High frequency of HLA-B27 antigen
- Frequent asymptomatic intestinal inflammation
- Response to indomethacin and/or sulfasalazine

3. *Reactive Arthritis.* This term is usually reserved for arthritis syndromes appearing 1 to 4 weeks after infection of the gastrointestinal or genitourinary tracts. Pathogens include *Yersinia*, *Salmonella* and other enteric bacteria, and *Chlamydia* in the urethra. Reactive arthritis may be associated with extraarticular disease (i.e., urethritis and conjunctivitis, keratitis or iritis); if so, it is called Reiter syndrome. In general, the clinical syndromes share significant overlap with the subset of juvenile arthritis known as enthesitis-associated arthritis (see Chapter 80).

a. *Clinical manifestations.* Clinical manifestations are variable, but enthesitis (inflammation of tendinous and ligamentous insertions) is common. Carditis similar to that seen in the enthesitis-associated arthritis subset of children with juvenile arthritis is uncommon.

(1) *Arthritis.* Reactive arthritis usually begins as large joint oligoarthritis but may present as an acute polyarthritis. It is self-limited in many individuals but may recur and remit. In some, continuous disease may be present. In long-term studies of children with reactive arthritis, as many as 42 per cent may have some long-term joint complaints, usually mild persistent peripheral arthritis. Some have sacroiliitis evident on radiographs.

(2) *Eye disease.* Ten to 15 per cent of children with reactive arthritis will have uveitis, conjunctivitis, or keratitis at some time in their course. The eye disease is symptomatic, with pain, photophobia, and redness.

(3) *Skin manifestations.* Circinate balanitis, or psoriasiform lesions of the tip of the penis, are uncommon in children with Reiter syndrome and related postenteritic arthritis. They may be seen in adolescents and are reported in 25 per cent of adults. Keratoderma blennorrhagicum typically affects the palms and soles, with presence of papulovesicular lesions that crust and may become hyperkeratotic.

b. *Laboratory findings.* Elevated erythrocyte sedimentation rate may be noted. As many as 80 per cent of individuals with Reiter syndrome express the HLA-B27 antigen. The presence of this marker increases the risk of arthritis after infection with an arthritogenic agent by 5- to 20-fold compared with HLA-B27–negative persons. The B27 antigen is present in 8 to 15 per cent of normal individuals, however, and is absent in 20 per cent or more of affected children.

c. *Radiographic findings.* In acute disease, periarticular soft-tissue swelling is the only radiographic finding. Calcification of involved insertions may be seen in chronic disease. With persistent joint disease, progression to ankylosing spondylitis may occur, along with the characteristic radiographic findings of that disease: vertebral ankylosis and sacroiliitis.

d. *Management issues.* Management principles are similar to those used in the care of children with juvenile arthritis. Joint inflammation and enthesitis often respond to therapy with nonsteroidal antiinflammatory agents. Tolmetin or naproxen may be somewhat more efficacious than aspirin in the young child, and indomethacin may be most effective in the adolescent. Patients with chronic arthritis who do not respond to therapy with nonsteroidal antiinflammatory agents may benefit from sulfasalazine, 30 to 40 mg/kg/day given in two to three divided doses. Three months of doxycycline may be indicated in adolescents with chlamydial urethritis. Better functional outcome and pain control are seen with vigorous physical therapy. A life-long exercise program is important in the management of children with chronic reactive arthritis.

Bibliography

Arnett FC: The seronegative spondyloarthropathies. Bull Rheum Dis 1987;37:1–12.

Dajani A, Taubert K, Ferrieri P et al: Treatment of acute streptococcal pharyngitis and prevention of rheumatic fever: a statement for health professionals. Pediatrics 1995;96:758–764.

Hughes RA, Keat AC: Reiter's syndrome and reactive arthritis: a current view. Semin Arthritis Rheum 1994;24:190–210.

Shapiro ED: Lyme disease in children. Am J Med 1995;98:69S–73S.

86 Symptoms of Infectious Disease

| Symptom | **Fever in Infants Less than 3 Months of Age** | *Robert H. Pantell* |

Definition

Temperature varies during the course of the day and may be a full degree centigrade higher at 4 P.M. than at 4 A.M. The method of temperature taking will also influence the reading obtained; rectal temperatures are most accurate and axillary temperatures are also useful when taken properly, whereas skin strips are unacceptable and digital ear thermometers vary in accuracy. A temperature of 38.0°C in an infant is 2 standard deviations above mean infant temperature and empirically considered the threshold for a fever.

Etiology

1. An elevated body temperature in an infant may represent external factors such as overbundling or excessive room heat.
2. Most commonly, infectious agents result in the release of interleukins, tumor necrosis factor, and interferon, which stimulate sites near the hypothalamus to release prostaglandins, which in turn cross the blood-brain barrier and stimulate fever.
3. In rare circumstances, severe brain disturbances may result in hypothalamic dysfunction and inability to regulate temperature properly.

Epidemiology

1. Neonates. Fevers occurring in the newborn nursery may be seen in 1%–5% of infants. Because of a different set of potential bacterial organisms, such as staphylococci and group B streptococci, these infants are treated according to current nursery policies and epidemics but closely resemble the usual management and treatment suggested for infants in the first few months of life.
2. Infants 0–3 months. Fever >38.0°C is seen with increasing frequency as infants become older, and occurs in 1 to 5 per cent in the first month and in up to 10 per cent of 2–3 month olds. Temperature >38.3°C is less common, occurring in only 1 to 2 per cent of this age group.

Differential Diagnosis

1. External factors—Excessive clothing or ambient temperature
2. Measurement factors—Inaccurate recording device or human error
3. Infections—See Table 86–1.

Clinical Findings

1. History
   a. Perinatal events: Maternal group B streptococcal colonization, fevers
   b. Perinatal exposures: Antibiotics, toxins, medications, illicit drugs
   c. Nursery course and exposure to outbreaks
   d. Recent family illness
   e. Daycare exposure
   f. Immunization within past 72 hours
   g. Home treatment: Acetaminophen, ibuprofen, other available medications
   h. Recent behavioral changes (feeding, sleeping, eating, interactions)
   i. Parental experiences, expectations, concerns, and cultural beliefs about fever (see further on).
2. Physical Findings
   a. Rectal temperature >38°C
   b. Global clinical appearance: Well or minimally ill, somewhat ill, moderately or severely ill
      (1) Social interaction: Ability to engage, make eye contact
      (2) Exhibits different states: Quiet, active, appropriately upset during examination
      (3) Ability to be quieted if disturbed
      (4) Quality and intensity of crying

TABLE 86–1. COMMON INFECTIONS CAUSING FEVER IN INFANTS

TYPE OF INFECTION	FREQUENCY IN FEBRILE INFANTS (%)
Undetermined	27
URI	34
LRI (bronchiolitis, wheezing, pneumonia)	17
Otitis media	16
Urinary tract infection	6.5
Gastroenteritis (with and without dehydration)	7.5
Bacteremia/sepsis	3
Organism	**% of Bacteremia**
Group B streptococcus	35–45
E. coli	20–30
Salmonella	5–10
Staphylococcus aureus/epidermidis	25–35
S. pneumoniae	<5
Enterobacter	<5
Enterococcus	<5
Klebsiella	<5
N. meningitides	<5
H. influenzae	
M. catarrhalis	
Streptococcus pyogenes	
Streptococcus viridans	
Pseudomonas	
Listeria	
Viral meningitis	5
Bacterial meningitis	.3–.5
Other meningitis (e.g., *Listeria*)	<<.1
Cellulitis	2.5
Osteomyelitis	<0.1
Septic arthritis	<0.1

(5) Color: Pink, mottled, ashen, pale

(6) Hydration

(7) Respiratory effort and frequency.

  c. Specific findings:

    (1) Fontanel: Check for fullness

    (2) Skin: Evaluate elasticity and capillary refill for dehydration

    (3) Respiration: Rate should be <60

    (4) Abdomen: Check cord and surrounding area for omphalitis.

Key Clinical Findings

Otitis Externa	Otitis Media
• Pain, itching, exquisite tenderness of pinna • External skin is edematous and red	• Ear tugging, irritability • Fever, lethargy • Redness and fluid behind the tympanic membrane with distortion of normal architecture

Laboratory Findings

1. Specific symptom/physical finding complexes: In many cases a diagnosis will be apparent and tests will be used for confirmatory purposes. For example, a child with diarrhea and suspected enteritis should have a stool smear for WBC and culture and a urinalysis for specific gravity and serum electrolytes; a wheezing child might prompt RSV antigen, while a child with severe cough should have a chest x-ray and testing for pertussis and *Chlamydia.*

2. Nonspecific symptoms/findings: Because young infants may not exhibit the behavioral repertoire of older infants to indicate the precise nature and severity of their illness, there has been a tendency in recent years to minimize uncertainty and risks by maximizing testing and costs. Because extensive laboratory testing has its own potential harms, more recent efforts have been directed toward a selective testing approach. The guidelines in Table 86-2 can be modified based on the clinician's special knowledge of a particular case.

3. Special tests for partially treated meningitis: Antigen tests

TABLE 86-2. SUGGESTED LABORATORY EVALUATION

	CLINICAL APPEARANCE		
		Well/Minimally Ill	
	Sick	0-4 Weeks	>4 Weeks
CBC/differential	+	+	+
Blood culture	+	+	+/−
Urinalysis	+	+	+
Urine culture (suprapubic tap or catheterized)	+	+	+
CSF examination	+	+	+/−
Chest x-ray (respiratory symptoms)	+	+/−	+/−
Stool WBC culture (GI symptoms)	+	+/−	+/−

are available for group B *Streptococcus, E. coli,* K1, *H. influenzae,* and *S. pneumoniae.* For viral meningitis, herpes and enteroviruses can be cultured in most laboratories, while some laboratories have the capacity for PCR on these organisms.

Management

1. Disposition

  a. Home: Infants may be managed at home if they are older than 4 weeks, have parents who are cognitively and emotionally capable of competent assessment of changes and able to return promptly if required, and do not need treatment requiring hospitalization.

  b. Hospital: Infants <4 weeks requiring antibiotics or requiring closer supervision than can be provided at home should be hospitalized.

2. Treatment

  a. Antipyretics: Either acetaminophen or ibuprofen can be given in doses of 10 mg/kg q 4-6h.

  b. Antibiotic indications: Specific antibiotics may be suggested based on a clinical diagnosis or Gram stain or antigen test. Otherwise the following guidelines are suggested.

Key Treatment

Sick	0-4 Weeks	Well/Minimally Ill >4 Weeks
Antibiotics	Antibiotics	Antibiotics optional if WBC >5000 and <1500 Urinalysis negative No other abnormal laboratory findings

  c. Antibiotic choices

    (1) Ampicillin and aminoglycoside

    (2) Ampicillin and cephalosporin (cefotaxime/ceftazidime)

    (3) Ceftriaxone: Although this agent is convenient and daily IM dosing may prevent hospitalization, ceftriaxone is not effective against all pathogens (e.g., *Listeria*). In vitro sensitivity should guide choices.

  c. Antivirals

    (1) Acyclovir: Should be given in viral meningitis if there is any suspicion of herpes

    (2) Ribavirin: For moderately ill infants with bronchiolitis when RSV is identified or suspected.

3. Follow-up: Infants discharged home before a diagnosis is cleared should be monitored on a daily basis. Once the episode of illness is over, clinicians should ask about the impact of the illness on the parents' perception of the child's health and vulnerability. A febrile illness in the first few months of a child's life can have a long-lasting impact on the parents that is out of proportion to the seriousness of the illness.

Bibliography

Baraff LJ, Bass JW, Fleisher GR, et al: Practice guidelines for the management of infants and children 0 to 36 months of age with fever without source. Pediatrics 1993; 92:1–12.

Dagan R, Powell KR, Hall CB, et al: Identification of infants unlikely to have serious bacterial infection although hospitalized for suspected sepsis. J Pediatr 1985; 107:855–860.

Hoberman A, Chao HP, Keller DM, et al: Prevalence of urinary tract infection in febrile infants. J Pediatr 1993; 123(1):17–23.

McCarthy PL, Sharpe MR, Spiesel SZ, et al: Observation scales to identify serious illness in febrile children. Pediatrics 1982; 70:802–809.

McCarthy PL: The febrile infant. Pediatrics 1994; 94(3):397–399.

Pantell R, Bergman D: Epidemiology of fever in infants and young children in the evaluation and management of febrile children. *In* McCarthy P (ed): Dialogues in Pediatric Management. Norwalk, CT, Appleton-Century-Crofts, 1985.

| Symptom | Earache | *Robert Finberg* |

Definition

A child who complains of ear pain may be suffering from either inflammation of the external auditory canal (otitis externa) or inflammation of the middle ear (otitis media). Otitis media is said to be the most common diagnosis made by physicians who care for children.

Etiology

1. Otitis externa
   a. Otitis externa can be either localized or diffuse. A furuncle, often a hair follicle infected with *Staphylococcus aureus*, or localized erysipelas caused by group A streptococcus may produce severe pain, with or without localized adenopathy.
   b. Children with diffuse otitis externa may present with swimmer's ear, a syndrome typically associated with hot, humid weather in which *Pseudomonas aeruginosa* is the usual pathogen. The presentation consists of itching and redness in the canal.
2. Otitis media
   a. Otitis media is an inflammation of the middle ear. Acute otitis media (AOM) is defined by the presence of fluid in the middle ear in the face of a compatible clinical presentation. It is an extremely common diagnosis in pediatric practice and accounts for more than 40 per cent of all antibiotic use in children. Otitis media is most common in children between 6 months and 3 years of age. By age 3, more than two thirds of children have had one or more episodes of otitis media, and one third have had more than three episodes. The incidence declines with increasing age (except for a blip at the age of school entry—age 5 to 6 years).
   b. Early development of AOM predisposes to the development of recurrent otitis media or chronic/persistent otitis media with effusion (sometimes referred to as OME). Controversy has surrounded the treatment of this entity; surgery, antibiotics (see below), and watchful waiting are all widely touted as being cheap and efficacious.

Pathophysiology

1. Otitis externa, when it is a localized infection, is often the result of a furuncle, as may be found in any other area of the skin. The external canal runs between the concha of the auricle and the tympanic membrane. As expected for an epithelialized surface, the normal micro-biologic flora of the skin is similar to that of skin in other parts of the body. The flora consist primarily of *Staphylococcus epidermidis*, *S. aureus*, corynebacteria, and *Propionibacterium acnes*. In situations in which the normal skin layer is denuded, particularly if there is persistent moisture in the canal, other microorganisms (including gram-negative organisms) may invade. Particularly common in this circumstance is invasion with *P. aeruginosa*. Superficial colonization with this organism can be the first stage before invasion of deeper tissues resulting in vasculitis and osteomyelitis of the temporal bone in immunocompromised patients and diabetics. The diffuse form, swimmer's ear, often results from growth of bacteria, such as *P. aeruginosa*, that favor a moist environment. Invasion is enhanced by maceration of the skin, which may occur with prolonged moisture.

Common Etiologic Organisms for Ear Infection

Otitis Externa	Otitis Media
Pseudomonas aeruginosa	*Streptococcus*
Staphylococcus aureus	*pneumoniae*
Streptococcus pyogenes	*Haemophilus influenzae*
	Moraxella catarrhalis

---

2. Otitis media occurs as a result of bacterial growth in mucous secretions adjacent to the tympanic membrane. The growth of bacteria, with resulting disease, is often a result of blockage of the eustachian tube, which prevents clearing of both bacteria and mucus. Any condition that predisposes to either eustachian tube blockage or a failure to eliminate bacteria based on immune dysfunction results in a predisposition to otitis media. Therefore, children whose anatomy does not lead to rapid drainage of mucus and those with low immunoglobulin levels or an inability to make antibodies to polysaccharides are predisposed to develop otitis media.

Clinical Findings

1. The patient with otitis externa typically presents with an itchy or painful external ear. The pinna is usually exquisitely tender to touch. There may be a purulent area or diffuse hemorrhagic bullae on the canal walls and tympanic membrane.
2. Children younger than 3 years of age with otitis media

may present with nonspecific signs and symptoms, including irritability, poor feeding, ear tugging, and sleep disturbances. Nystagmus, vertigo, tinnitus, and ear pain may be present but are not reliably seen. Because associated upper respiratory infection occurs in most cases, coryza, eye discharge, and other upper respiratory symptoms are common in this age group, but the diagnosis often cannot be made on history alone. Older children are more likely to present with ear pain and fever.

3. The diagnosis of otitis media is based on detection of a middle ear effusion by pneumatic otoscopy (using an instrument that assesses the mobility of the tympanic membrane) or by visualization of a red, bulging tympanic membrane with loss of normal landmarks.

4. Otitis media is accompanied by hearing loss. Because the effusions of otitis media are persistent (approximately 40% have effusions 1 month after infection, and 10% have fluid 3 months after infection), the occurrence of several infections in the same child (a common event) can result in a hearing problem for a prolonged period. Children with recurrent otitis tend to score lower on tests than their peers.

Laboratory Findings

Although cultures of middle ear fluid (obtained by tympanocentesis) are diagnostic, this technique is seldom used in routine clinical settings. Bacteremia is not common, and therefore blood cultures are not usually of value. No convincing association has been demonstrated between cultures of the nasopharynx and the middle ear, so nasopharyngeal cultures are not of much value. Tympanocentesis, a safe and useful technique in experienced hands, is not commonly performed in routine settings; its use is usually reserved for critically ill or immunocompromised patients and those who have not responded to conventional therapy.

Radiographic Changes

X-ray changes are not expected in uncomplicated otitis media or otitis externa. Malignant otitis externa, a disorder of immunocompromised hosts and diabetics, may cause invasion of the temporal bone with accompanying changes. Mastoiditis, a common complication of otitis media in the era before the availability of antibiotics, can lead to radiographic abnormalities including bony demineralization and abnormalities in pneumatization. Computed tomography or magnetic resonance imaging can define the anatomy in these cases.

Differential Diagnosis

1. Otitis externa is usually caused by staphylococcus or streptococcus when it is localized (and commonly presents as a furuncle). Diffuse disease is usually caused by gram-negative rods, especially *P. aeruginosa.* Unusual causes of otitis externa include tuberculosis, syphilis, yaws, leprosy, and sarcoidosis.

2. Otitis media is caused by *Streptococcus pneumoniae* in 30 to 40 per cent of cases in the United States, by *Haemophilus influenzae* (usually not type B) in 20 to 30 percent, and by *Moraxella catarrhalis* in 20 to 30 per cent. In most large series in which microbiologic data are reported, approximately one third of middle ear fluid cultures obtained by tympanocentesis grow no organism.

Viral cultures have revealed the presence of respiratory syncytial virus, influenza, enteroviruses, and rhinoviruses in middle ear fluids. Epidemiologic data indicate a coincidence of viral infection and otitis media. In many cases it is assumed that secondary bacterial infection develops in the face of antecedent viral infection. Some studies have revealed the presence of both virus and bacteria in the same middle ear fluid. Other organisms that have been isolated from middle ear fluids include *Mycoplasma pneumoniae* and *Chlamydia trachomatis* (from infants). Uncommon causes of otitis include *Corynebacterium diphtheriae,* *Mycobacterium chelonei,* *Ascaris* spp., and Wegener granulomatosis.

Treatment

1. Otitis externa

   a. Localized otitis externa—A combination of systemic antibiotics (such as oral dicloxacillin, or intravenous oxacillin in severe cases) and local incision and drainage (if necessary) should lead to rapid resolution of the problem.

   b. Diffuse otitis externa—Cleansing of the area and application of topical antibiotic ear drops may be used. (A neomycin-polymycin combination otic solution is marketed with hydrocortisone and may help relieve inflammation.) The vehicle is acetic acid, which is probably the active agent, because *Pseudomonas* will not grow in an acid medium. The combination of local antibiotics and cleansing of the area (with removal of debris if necessary) is usually sufficient to cure the infection. Systemic antibiotics are necessary only if there is tissue destruction or invasive disease (commonly seen only in diabetics and immunocompromised hosts).

2. Otitis media

   a. It is perhaps symptomatic of the state of the art that although every medical student is taught that it is very important to treat otitis media, controlled trials of placebo versus antibiotic for AOM and of antibiotic versus placebo versus tubes for chronic effusions are still being undertaken. Part of the problem concerns the definition: Otitis media is a symptom, not an etiologically defined disorder. Even the presence of classic physical findings does not make an etiologic diagnosis, and microbiological diagnoses are also not commonly made in clinical practice or even in research settings. Therefore, any study will consist of a mixed bag of disorders, only a fraction of which may be treatable by antibacterial agents.

   b. AOM is usually treated with oral amoxicillin. Although resistant *S. pneumoniae* and *H. influenzae* are fairly common (currently 20–30% and growing) and almost all *M. catarrhalis* are resistant to amoxicillin, the drug is still effective against most *S. pneumoniae* and *H. influenzae*, is palatable (important in this age group), is relatively inexpensive, and has few serious side effects. Routine treatment with antibiotics is credited with decreasing the serious complications of otitis media (mastoiditis, sinusitis, meningitis) that were common in the preantibiotic era. Since most cases of uncomplicated otitis media, particularly those caused by *H. influenzae* and *M. catarrhalis*, would be anticipated to resolve spontaneously anyway, the failure rate for any given episode of AOM in a normal child is anticipated to be less than 10 per cent. Trimethoprim-sulfamethoxazole (TMP-SMX) is an alternative first-line therapy for children allergic to penicillin.

Key Treatment: Otitis Media

Initial treatment for acute otitis media
- Amoxicillin—40 mg/kg/day in three divided doses ×7–10 days

Alternatives or secondary antibiotics
- Trimethoprim-sulfamethoxazole—8 mg of TMP and 40 mg of SMX per kilogram per day in two doses ×7–10 days
- Erythromycin-sulfisoxazole—40 mg of erythromycin and 150 mg of sulfisoxazole per kilogram per day in two doses ×7–10 days

"Prophylaxis" for recurrent disease
- Amoxicillin—20 mg/kg/day in one or two doses ×3–6 mo
- Sulfisoxazole—75 mg/kg/day in one or two doses ×3–6 mo

c. Because of the possibility of drug resistance based on production of β-lactamases (common in the case of *H. influenzae* or *M. catarrhalis*), patients who fail initial therapy with amoxicillin can be treated with TMP-SMX, erythromycin-sulfisoxazole, or an oral cephalosporin. Sequential administration of amoxicillin and another antibiotic (in either order) has the advantage that TMP-SMX and erythromycin-sulfisoxazole is effective against most β-lactamase–producing organisms. Amoxicillin, on the other hand, is excellent treatment for *Streptococcus pyogenes,* which may not be optimally treated with TMP-SMX.

d. If the child appears ill or has a bulging tympanic membrane, myringotomy (by an experienced practitioner) enables the clinician to obtain a culture of the organism.

e. There is no evidence that decongestants offer any benefit, and topical ear drops are avoided by most authorities because of the risk of damaging the tympanic membrane and introducing foreign material into the inner ear.

f. Approximately 50 per cent of children have some persistence of middle ear effusion lasting 1 month after antibiotic therapy; only about 10 per cent have effusions 3 months after therapy.

g. Although steroid therapy has been advocated for patients with persistent effusions, convincing data documenting its efficacy are lacking.

h. Many authorities recommend antibiotic prophylaxis with amoxicillin (20 mg/kg/day in one or two doses per day) or sulfisoxazole (75 mg/kg/day in one or two doses) for 3 to 6 months in patients with recurrent otitis (more than three episodes in a 6-month period).

i. Ventilating tubes should be considered in patients with persistent effusions for at least 4 months who have a documented bilateral hearing loss of 20 dB or more. Tubes are placed to restore hearing.

Prevention

1. The 23-type pneumococcal polysaccharide vaccine includes most of the strains of *S. pneumoniae* that are responsible for otitis media. Unfortunately, young children do not respond well to polysaccharide vaccines. Many clinicians, particularly in view of the increased incidence of antibiotic resistance among pneumococcal strains, recommend the use of the available pneumococcal vaccine in children older than 2 years of age who have recurrent otitis media; younger children are thought to be unlikely to respond to the vaccine. The *H. influenzae* type B conjugate vaccine is capable of eliciting good immune responses in young children but it has no efficacy against non-typable strains of *H. influenzae,* which are the overwhelming majority of the strains of *H. influenzae* seen in the setting of acute otitis.

2. In the future, it is likely that the pneumococcal conjugate vaccines, now in clinical trials, will have a role in this setting.

Bibliography

Balen FAM, de Melker RA, Touw-Otten FWMM: Double-blind randomised trial of co-amoxiclav versus placebo for persistent otitis media with effusion in general practice. Lancet 1996;348:713–716.

Barnett ED, Klein JO: The problem of resistant bacteria for the management of acute otitis media. Pediatr Clin North Am 1995;42:509–517.

Berman S: Otitis media in children. N Engl J Med 1995;332:1560–1565.

Rosenfeld RM: What to expect from medical treatment of otitis media. Pediatr Infect Dis J 1996;14:731–738.

Williams RL, Chalmers TC, Stange KC, et al: Use of antibiotics in preventing recurrent acute otitis media and in treating otitis media with effusion: A meta-analytic attempt. JAMA 1991;270:1344–1351.

87 Congenital Infections

Sandra K. Burchett

Viral infections of the fetus and newborn are transmitted congenitally (in utero) or perinatally (intrapartum or immediately postpartum). Those with the highest prevalence are described.

Cytomegalovirus (CMV)

Epidemiology

One per cent of all newborn infants in the United States are infected with CMV, and 10 per cent are symptomatic; 4000 infants are severely affected by or die from CMV yearly.

1. *Congenital infection*—In 30 to 40 per cent of pregnancies with primary maternal infection, fetal infection ensues; 15 per cent have significant disease. Maternal recurrent or reactivation infection can result in fetal infection, but these infants rarely show clinical symptoms. One third of newborn infants with symptomatic disseminated CMV infection die.
2. *Perinatal infection*—The probable incubation period is 4 to 12 weeks, and the infection is acquired by
   a. Intrapartum exposure to the virus within the maternal genital tract,
   b. Postnatal exposure to infected breast milk, or
   c. Exposure to infected blood or blood products (unusual).

Clinical Findings

1. *Symptomatic infants*—Congenitally infected infants may have petechiae (79%), hepatosplenomegaly (74%), jaundice (63%), microcephaly (50%), small for gestational age (41%), prematurity (34%), inguinal hernia in males (26%), chorioretinitis (12%), and intracranial calcification (anywhere, but often periventricular). Infants in long-term follow-up may show developmental abnormalities and neurologic dysfunction (mental retardation, hearing deficits, language and learning disabilities, motor abnormalities, and visual disturbances). Perinatally infected preterm infants may have hearing abnormalities or pneumonitis (tachypnea, cough, coryza, nasal congestion, intercostal retractions, hypoxemia, apnea with hyperinflation, diffuse increased pulmonary markings, thickened bronchial walls, and focal atelectasis).

Key Laboratory Findings: CMV

- Jaundice
- Petechiae
- Hepatosplenomegaly
- Microcephaly
- Periventricular calcification

2. *Asymptomatic infants*—Whereas congenitally infected infants in this group show no mortality, 5 to 15 per cent have developmental abnormalities (hearing loss, mental retardation, motor spasticity, and microcephaly). Perinatally infected term infants remain asymptomatic.

Laboratory Findings

Elevated hepatic transaminases and bilirubin are seen, as are anemia and thrombocytopenia.

Key Laboratory Findings: CMV

- Abnormal liver test
- Hematologic abnormalities

Diagnosis

Identification of virus from urine or saliva of infants (defined as congenital infection if <2 weeks of life) is diagnostic. Specimens are kept at 4°C for transport and storage to optimize viral recovery. Standard tissue culture requires weeks; rapid detection using specific antibodies, which recognize CMV antigens that are present early in viral cultures, requires 2 days. Serum antibody titers to CMV, if negative, exclude congenital CMV infection; CMV-specific immunoglobulin M (IgM) has limitations but may identify infant infection.

Treatment

1. Ganciclovir (9-13-dihydroxypropoxymethyl guanine) is in trial for infants with CNS involvement associated with congenital CMV infection.
2. Monoclonal antibody to a segment of CMV is in early trials.
3. Passive immunization with hyperimmune anti-CMV immunoglobulin has not been found highly effective.

Key Treatment: CMV

- Ganciclovir

Human Immunodeficiency Virus (HIV)

Epidemiology

By the end of 1995, there were 500,000 people (12% female and 2% children) with the acquired immunodeficiency syndrome (AIDS) in the United States. In Africa and Asia, heterosexual spread is dramatically increasing and up to 50 per cent of pregnant women are infected. By the year 2000, there will be 7000 children with AIDS in the United States, >90 per cent of whom will have acquired HIV by perinatal transmission. In 25 to 30 per cent of untreated pregnancies in HIV-infected mothers, fetal/neonatal infection results. Infection occurs congenitally (in utero) in approximately one third of cases, peripartum in the remaining cases, and may occur neonatally through breast feeding.

1. *Maternal Factors*—Women with higher cell-associated or cell-free HIV viral load, lower number of CD4+ lymphocytes, more advanced HIV disease, or concomitant sexually transmitted disease, and women who use illicit substances are more likely to transmit HIV to their offspring.
2. *Delivery Factors*—Some studies have suggested that cesarean section may be preventive in perinatal transmission; however, prolonged rupture of membranes, which is less likely in delivery by cesarean section, is probably a stronger correlate than delivery mode itself.

Clinical Findings

Infants infected in utero may have lymphadenopathy and/or hepatosplenomegaly at birth but are usually asymptomatic.

1. Far too often, infected infants who were previously not known to be at risk for HIV infection present with *Pneumocystis carinii* pneumonia (PCP), which shows a peak onset at 3 to 5 months of age, accounts for 37 per cent of AIDS-defining illnesses in pediatrics and is often fatal.
2. Lymphoid interstitial pneumonitis is found with an AIDS-defining illness in one third of children who present at approximately 2 years of age.
3. Developmental delay, loss of milestones, and overt HIV encephalopathy may present at any age.
4. Refractory thrush or wasting may occur.
5. Disseminated infection with CMV (including retinitis) or with *Mycobacterium avium* intracellularis infection are also possible presentations.

Key Clinical Findings: HIV

- Most asymptomatic
- Hepatosplenomegaly (<10%)
- Lymphadenopathy (<10%)

Laboratory Findings

1. Viral detection is the mainstay of diagnosis in an infected infant, because passively acquired maternal antibody precludes serology as a means of diagnosing infection with (rather than exposure to) HIV. Tests include detection of HIV by viral culture, polymerase chain reaction (PCR) for viral DNA by reverse transcription, or by HIV p24 antigen detection (if older than 1 month of age). If the culture or PCR is positive in samples obtained during the first 48 hours of life, the infant is defined as having been infected in utero. If tests are negative in the first few days of life and positive thereafter, the infant is assumed to have been infected at the time of birth. There may be some prognostic association with timing of infection.
2. Serology is diagnostic if an HIV-positive enzyme-linked immunosorbent assay (ELISA) is confirmed by Western blot as HIV-specific in infants older than 18 months of age; by that time, maternally derived antibody is no longer present, and a positive test represents the infant's own host response to infection.

Key Laboratory Tests: HIV

- Viral detection
- Serology

Treatment

Infants may be offered antiretroviral therapy as neonates to decrease early viral load or as older infants and children based on clinical symptomatology or decline in CD4+ lymphocyte number or percentage. Monotherapy and combination therapy with a variety of nucleoside analog reverse transcriptase inhibitors (zidovudine [AZT], didanosine, stavudine, lamivudine, zalcitabine), non-nucleoside reverse transcriptase inhibitors (nevirapine, delavirdine), and protease inhibitors (saquinavir, indinavir, ritonavir, nelfinavir) are available or in current trials. The antiretroviral regimen is tailored to each child's needs.

Key Treatments: HIV

- Reverse transcriptase inhibitors (AZT)
- Protease inhibitors

Prevention

1. Vertical transmission can be dramatically reduced (to ≤8%) by the use of AZT: 500 mg/day during pregnancy, 2 mg/kg load and 1 mg/kg/hr IV to the mother peripartum, and 2 mg/kg orally every 6 hours in the infant for 6 weeks). Other reverse transcriptase inhibitors and protease inhibitors are currently under study to further reduce transmission. In countries with adequate formula preparations, such as the United States, breast feeding is contraindicated.
2. AIDS-defining illnesses are prevented by offering prophylaxis to infants known to be infected with HIV. This includes trimethoprim-sulfamethoxazole therapy to prevent PCP and rifabutin or macrolide therapy to prevent *Mycobacterium avium* complex infection.

Herpes Simplex Virus (HSV)

Epidemiology

The vast majority (95%) of HSV-infected infants acquire infection at the time of birth, although congenital infection can occur. Infection occurs in approximately 1 of every 1500 to 3000 live births. Women with primary genital HSV infection during pregnancy may transmit HSV to their infants as often as 33 to 50 per cent of the time. Women with prior infection with HSV type 1 but new onset of HSV type 2 during pregnancy transmit HSV at a rate of approximately 33 per cent, whereas women with a previous clinical history or serologically confirmed HSV infection prior to pregnancy transmit HSV rarely (approximately 2–3%). The latter group, however, contributes the majority of infants infected with HSV since approximately one third of the delivery population is infected with HSV type 2. Neonatal infection is usually acquired by exposure to HSV types 1 and 2 in the maternal birth canal but can occasionally result from exposure to orolabial HSV type 1. Of infected infants, 80 per cent have HSV type 2.

Clinical Findings

Neonatal HSV infection is grouped into three descriptive and prognostic categories:

1. Skin, eye, or mucocutaneous (SEM) infection accounts for approximately 50 per cent of HSV-infected infants, with vesicles appearing on day 2 to 12 (usually day 7). There is no mortality, but skin lesions may recur even with appropriate treatment in the neonatal period. Of infants infected with type 2 HSV, 10 per cent may progress to CNS involvement.
2. Central nervous system (CNS) infection accounts for 33 per cent of HSV infected infants, and the mortality rate may be 30 per cent. Clinical signs are seen at day 7 to 28 (usually day 12) of life. Presenting signs may include seizures, temperature instability (usually hypothermia), lethargy, or poor feeding. As many as 40 per cent of affected infants have no skin lesions, making diagnosis more difficult. The morbidity rate in survivors is 60 per cent and includes microcephaly, hydranencephaly, blindness, chorioretinitis, and learning disabilities.
3. Disseminated infection accounts for 17 per cent of HSV-infected infants and has a mortality rate of >80 per cent. Presentation is on day 3 to 14 (usually day 5). This presentation involves multiple organs and may manifest with hepatitis, adrenal insufficiency, pneumonia, enteritis, or disseminated intravascular coagulation. The majority (two thirds) also have CNS involvement; vesicles are absent in 80 per cent. Morbidity is higher in survivors of type 2 infection.

Key Clinical Findings: HSV

- Vesicular lesions on skin or mucosa
- Seizures

Laboratory Findings

1. Cultures of vesicles and/or the nasopharynx are positive in 1 to 21 days (usually <3 days if from a vesicle).
2. Antigen detection by staining of cells obtained from lesions with antibodies specific to HSV antigens is rapid and highly sensitive.
3. PCR of HSV is diagnostic of CNS infection if a positive result is obtained from the cerebrospinal fluid.
4. Serology is not particularly useful since passively acquired antibodies from the maternal circulation reflect the maternal status; generally, routine serology cannot differentiate type 1 from type 2.

Key Laboratory Tests: HSV

- Culture of virus
- Antigen detection
- PCR

Treatment

Treatment is with intravenous acyclovir (10–15 mg/kg per dose every 8 hours) for 10 to 14 days for SEM infection and for 21 days for CNS or disseminated disease. Trials are being conducted to determine whether, after the initial intravenous course of therapy, additional benefit would accrue to infants receiving oral suppressive therapy for the first 6 months after infection.

Key Treatment: HSV

- Acyclovir

Prevention

Many obstetric providers offer cesarean section if a woman has had onset of primary HSV infection during pregnancy, and most offer cesarean section if lesions are seen at the time of delivery in women with a long-standing history of HSV. Clinical trials are being conducted to determine whether administration of acyclovir reduces the incidence of lesions (and thus the rate of cesarean section) in the latter group. Parents of infants born to women with HSV infection should be fully advised as to the possible signs and symptoms associated with neonatal HSV and requested to alert the care provider immediately should they occur.

Rubella

Epidemiology

Thirty years ago, rubella accounted for 11,000 fetal deaths and 20,000 cases of congenital rubella syndrome (CRS). Childhood immunization has dramatically reduced the number of cases of rubella in the United States; however, 12 to 24 per cent of postpubertal individuals are susceptible. The rate of CRS depends on the timing of primary maternal infection, and fetuses are generally symptomatic if infected before 16 weeks' gestation:

1. 0 to 12 weeks: 81 per cent symptomatic
2. 13 to 16 weeks: 54 per cent symptomatic
3. 17 to 22 weeks: 36 per cent symptomatic
4. 23 to 30 weeks: 30 per cent symptomatic
5. 37 to ≥40 weeks: 100 per cent asymptomatic

Clinical Findings

Manifestations of CRS can include cataracts, sensorineural hearing loss, congenital heart disorders (patent ductus arteriosus and pulmonary artery stenosis), intrauterine growth retardation, retinopathy, microphthalmia, meningoencephalitis, electroencephalographic abnormalities, mental retardation, behavioral disorders, hypotonia, dermatoglyphic abnormalities, hepatosplenomegaly, thrombocytopenic purpura, radiographic bone lucencies, and diabetes mellitus.

Key Clinical Findings: Rubella

- Cataracts
- Hepatosplenomegaly
- Petechiae
- Congenital heart disorders

Laboratory Findings

1. Antenatal diagnosis

   a. Specific IgM in fetal blood from percutaneous umbilical blood sampling

   b. Direct detection of rubella antigen and RNA in a chorionic villous biopsy

2. Postnatal diagnosis

   a. Isolation of rubella virus (oropharynx, urine)

   b. Detection of rubella-specific IgM in cord or neonatal blood

   c. Persistent rubella-specific titers over time (i.e., no decline in titer as expected for transplacentally derived maternal IgG). If, in addition, there are congenital defects present, the diagnosis of CRS is made.

Key Treatment: Rubella

- IgM therapy

- Serology (persistent titer)

Treatment

There is no specific therapy for either maternal rubella or CRS.

Prevention

Seronegative women with recognized or suspected exposure for whom interruption of pregnancy is not an option may be offered high-dose immune serum globulin; however, the efficacy is unknown. Women who are exposed in the first 16 weeks of pregnancy and who go on to seroconvert (3 weeks apart) should be informed of the likelihood of symptomatic fetal infection.

Bibliography

Connor EM, Sperling RS, Gelber R, et al: Reduction of maternal-infant transmission of human immunodeficiency virus type 1 with zidovudine treatment. N Engl J Med 1994;331:1173–1180.

Oxtoby MJ: Vertically acquired HIV in the United States. *In* Pizzo PA, Wilfert CM (eds): Pediatric AIDS: The Challenge of HIV Infection in Infants, Children, and Adolescents, 2nd ed. Baltimore, Williams & Wilkins, 1994, pp 3–20.

Stagno S: Cytomegalovirus. *In* Remington JS, Klein, JO (eds): Infectious Diseases of the Fetus and Newborn Infant, 4th ed. Philadelphia, WB Saunders, 1995, pp 312–353.

Whitley RJ: Neonatal herpes simplex virus infections. J Med Virol (Suppl)1993;1:13–21.

88 Congenital Syphilis

Laurence Finberg

Definition

Congenital syphilis is an infection of the newborn contracted from a mother with active syphilis.

Etiology

The cause is *Treponema pallidum,* a spirochetal bacterium.

Epidemiology

1. Women with untreated early syphilis (first 2 years) have a 95 per cent chance of transmitting the disease to the fetus transplacentally or during passage through the birth canal.

2. Even during later years, if remaining untreated, the disease may be transmitted.

Clinical Findings

1. Early syphilis

   a. If the fetus is infected early in gestation, a stillbirth usually occurs.

   b. Most infected infants are asymptomatic at birth.

   c. Occasionally, a rash is present at birth, and bullous lesions of palms and soles uncommonly occur.

   d. Typically the rash appears at 6 to 10 weeks with copper-colored macules and papules.

   e. There is generalized lymphadenopathy, including epitrochlear node enlargement.

   f. Condylomata lata may appear perigenitally and periorally in subsequent eruptions.

   g. Hepatosplenomegaly is common, and obstructive liver disease with jaundice may occur.

Key Clinical Findings: Early Syphilis

- Recurrent copper-colored maculopapular rash

- Generalized lymphadenopathy, including epitrochlear

- Hepatosplenomegaly

- Condylomata lata in genitorectal region

   h. Nephrotic syndrome, though uncommon, accounts for 50 per cent of this disorder in infants.

   i. Symmetric lesions of the long bones are nearly universal if there is no treatment.

j. In severe fetal infection, pneumonia alba may occur, usually in stillborn or moribund neonates.

k. Neurosyphilis is usually silent in infancy (see under *Laboratory Findings*).

2. Late congenital syphilis

a. Stigmata

These are changes or activities found after the age of 2 years, and usually later, from damage done in untreated early syphilis.

(1) Hutchinson teeth—Second dentition peg-shaped, carious central incisors, occasionally with a central notch

(2) Eighth nerve deafness—Rare

(3) Interstitial keratitis—Inflammation of the cornea and uvea manifesting between 6 and 18 years. Untreated, it leads to severe scarring and blindness.

(4) Saber shin from early tibial periosteal disease

(5) Clutton joints—Painless, usually symmetric swelling of knee joints

(6) Rhagades—Radial spoke scarring of the perioral region.

b. Neurosyphilis

(1) Meningovascular syndromes

(2) Paresis

(3) Tabes dorsalis

c. Gummata in virtually all tissues. Perforation of the palate and nasal septum is relatively common.

Key Clinical Findings: Late Congenital Syphilis

- Hutchinson teeth—second dentition
- Interstitial keratitis
- Clutton joints (painless swelling)
- Rhagades

Laboratory Findings

1. Serology

a. The rapid plasma reagin test (RPR), now in use instead of the VDRL, Kahn, and similar tests, measures a nonspecific antibody. In infants a significant titer may occur both from passive transfer from the mother and from active production.

(1) Passively transferred antibody diminishes over several weeks to being undetectable by 12 weeks or sooner.

(2) The infant's own antibody may be present at birth or, more often, rises in titer during the first several weeks after birth and will be present by 9 weeks.

b. A specific antibody, the fluorescent treponemal antibody (FTA), may also be passively transferred.

2. Darkfield examination of serum from skin and genital lesions will demonstrate *T. pallidum*.

3. Hematologic findings (not constant) include hemolytic anemia and leukocytosis.

4. Cerebrospinal fluid—Increase in white blood cells (lymphocytes) and in protein concentration diagnoses neurosyphilitic activity. After treatment, the cell count should fall to zero over a few months.

Radiologic Findings

1. Periostitis of the long bones, especially the tibia and humerus but often also the ulna, radius, and femur. These changes are nearly universal prior to treatment and heal spontaneously even without treatment.

2. Osteomyelitis, particularly the medial aspect of the tibiae (Wimberger sign).

Key Radiologic Findings

- Symmetric periostitis
- Wimberger sign (osteomyelitis of tibiae)

Treatment

1. Treatment for early congenital syphilis, as recommended by the Centers for Disease Control and Prevention (CDC), is a 10- to 14-day course of penicillin: aqueous penicillin G, 100,000 U/kg/day IV in two or three divided doses; or procaine penicillin, 50,000 U/kg/day IM daily. It is probable that two doses of 300,000 units of procaine penicillin IM 2 days apart will suffice for asymptomatic newborns. Even neural invasion will probably be adequately treated by this regimen, though some recommend a full 10- to 14-day course.

2. Infants born to mothers adequately treated for syphilis prior to or early in pregnancy probably do not require treatment. Maternal treatment during pregnancy with a drug other than penicillin, or treatment that is not followed by at least a fourfold decline in serologic titers, cannot be presumed to be adequate in protecting the fetus from infection.

3. Infants with clinical, radiologic, or serologic evidence of congenital syphilis, as well as those born to mothers with untreated or inadequately treated syphilis during pregnancy, require a full course of penicillin therapy.

Key Clinical Treatment

- Penicillin, dose appropriate to age and stage
- Interstitial keratitis—local hydrocortisone installation in eye

4. In cases in which the risk of congenital syphilis is low or follow-up uncertain, a single intramuscular injection of 50,000 U/kg of benzathine penicillin may be adequate treatment. This approach must be used with caution, as a rare treatment failure has been reported.

5. All infants at risk for congenital syphilis require careful

follow-up, to ensure that they do not develop serlogic or clinical evidence of active infection.

6. Late congenital syphilis is treated by a full course of penicillin.

7. If found after 3 months of age, neurosyphilis is treated by a full course of penicillin. Repeated CSF examinations are required until there are no white cells for at least a year after therapy.

8. Interstitial keratitis is treated with local corticosteroids.

Prevention

The risk of congenital syphilis can be eliminated by the identification and treatment of infected women prior to pregnancy, using sufficient dosage to cross the placenta and thus treating the fetus in utero.

Bibliography

Evans GE, Frenkel LD: Congenital syphilis. Clin Perinatol 1994; 21:149–162.

Hammerschlag MR, Rawstrom SA: Sexually transmitted diseases. *In* Krugman S, Katz SL, Gershon AA, Wilfert CM (eds): Infectious Diseases of Children. St. Louis, Mosby–Year Book, 1992.

Rawstrom SA, Jenkins S, Blanchard S, et al: Maternal and congenital syphilis in Brooklyn, NY: Epidemiology, transmission, and diagnosis. Am J Dis Child 1993; 147:727–731.

89 Sore Throat, Cervical Adenitis, and Mumps

Robert Finberg

Definition

Sore throat, defined as self-reported pain on swallowing, is one of the most common problems in pediatric practice. The differential diagnosis of this entity is broad and includes some very common and some rare infectious causes (see below). Of importance to the clinician is the differentiation of acute epiglottitis, a true ear/nose/throat emergency, from routine sore throat. Cervical adenitis may or may not be related to the infection causing a sore throat but is a common pediatric problem often associated with infectious agents.

Etiology

1. Although a large list of organisms may be associated with sore throat, in most series group A *Streptococcus* is the most common isolate associated with sore throat.

2. The association between non–group A streptococci and sore throat is less clear. However, both group C and group G streptococci express M proteins (an important streptococcal virulence factor), and both have been documented to be associated with foodborne outbreaks of pharyngitis. Therefore, many authorities recommend treatment of these organisms if they are isolated from a symptomatic patient.

3. *Arcanobacterium haemolyticus* (previously referred to as *Corynebacterium haemolyticum*) may also be associated with acute pharyngitis sometimes accompanied by a rash (and thus mimicking scarlet fever), particularly in adolescents and young adults.

4. Although some serologic studies have suggested a role for *Mycoplasma* and *Chlamydia* spp., the evidence that either agent is a common cause of pharyngitis is not compelling.

5. Despite a grab bag of other, rarely diagnosed causes of pharyngitis, in most cases of patients presenting with sore throat no etiologic agent is isolated. Whether this is because viruses are not isolated, as assumed by some, or because other undefined agents are causing the disorder, or because the cause is not infectious has yet to be clarified.

CAUSES OF SORE THROAT

Bacterial Causes	Nonbacterial Causes
Streptococcus pyogenes (group A *Streptococcus*)	*Chlamydia* spp. (especially *C. pneumoniae*)
Non–group A streptococci (groups C, G)	*Mycoplasma* spp.
Neisseria gonorrhoeae	Coxsackievirus A
Vincent angina (mixed anaerobes)	Herpes simplex virus
Corynebacterium diphtheriae	Epstein-Barr virus
Arcanobacterium hemolyticus	Human immunodeficiency virus (HIV-1)
Yersinia pestis	"Common cold" agents (rhinovirus, coronavirus, adenovirus, parainfluenza virus)
Yersinia enterocolitica	
Francisella tularensis (oral tularemia)	Aphthous stomatitis
Treponema pallidum (secondary syphilis)	

---

6. Certain unusual infections are worth mentioning.

   a. Postanginal sepsis (or Lemierre syndrome) is a disorder seen most commonly in adolescents who present with a sore throat (often accompanied by neck pain). Throat cultures are likely to be negative, but blood cultures are often positive for fusobacteria, since the illness involves a thrombophlebitis of the internal jugular vein. The diagnosis can be suggested by the physical examination, which reveals pain, swelling, and/or induration below the angle of the mandible and/or the lateral regions of the neck. Confirmatory evidence can be obtained by magnetic resonance imaging or computed tomography scan. Complications include septic pulmonary emboli (often accompanied by pleural effusions) and other metastatic septic foci.

b. The diagnosis of *Corynebacterium diphtheriae* (suggested by the presence of a membranous exudate in the posterior pharynx) requires use of a special culture medium. Vincent angina is a mixed anaerobic infection associated with gingivitis, often with a pseudomembranous exudate and malodorous breath. This may be the dreaded "trench mouth," which the author's mother-in-law warned one can get from eating food from the floor. The author is unaware that one can get any disease from eating food off the floor, but he doesn't make a habit of the practice.

Pathophysiology

1. The symptom of sore throat can be caused by infection with many different organisms, and in some cases it is difficult to relate the presence of the symptom to the colonizing organism (for example, although *Haemophilus influenzae* clearly causes epiglottitis, it is uncertain whether it causes sore throats; similarly, group A streptococci commonly colonize the throat without causing disease).

2. Both viruses and bacteria may invade the pharynx, leading to tissue destruction with or without a polymorphonuclear leukocyte response. However, it is now hypothesized that the "scratchy" feeling of a sore throat precipitated by the common cold (often a rhinovirus or coronavirus) is the result of bradykinin and lysylbradykinin stimulation of pain-sensing nerves. Infections with adenovirus and coxsackievirus, on the other hand, appear to be associated with tissue destruction.

Clinical Findings

1. The classic streptococcal sore throat is a disorder of children 3 to 12 years of age. It classically presents as a clinical triad of fever, vomiting, and sore throat.

2. Younger children are prone to different disorders caused by the same organism.

   a. Infants younger than 6 months are described as having "streptococcosis," a syndrome consisting of nasopharyngitis with a mild temperature elevation, sometimes accompanied by excoriations around the nose. The diagnosis is by culture of streptococci from the nasal discharge.

Key Clinical Findings

- Fever, adenopathy, and exudates suggest bacteria or infectious mononucleosis
- Pseudomembranes suggest *C. diphtheriae*
- Unilateral neck swelling suggests Kawasaki disease or several different infectious agents

b. In children between 6 months and 3 years of age, a symptom complex consisting of low-grade fever, cervical adenopathy, and nasopharyngitis with or without otitis and sinusitis may be associated with streptococcal infection.

Laboratory Findings

1. A specific diagnosis of the infectious cause of a sore throat rests on the laboratory findings. The controversy as to which patients should have cultures taken is a complex one, and the specifics of the patient population, the clinical setting, and the epidemiologic setting (e.g., whether there is an ongoing epidemic) should all be considered.

2. Both the Committee on Rheumatic Fever, Endocarditis, and Kawasaki Disease of the American Heart Association and the American Academy of Pediatrics recommend that clinicians consider relevant clinical as well as epidemiologic facts in determining whether cultures should be obtained. It is difficult to apply hard and fast rules to all patients.

3. A key issue is to try to culture group A *Streptococcus* from patients who are at risk for development of rheumatic fever or are sufficiently ill that secondary complications (soft tissue cellulitis, sinusitis, or local abscess) is suggested. In addition, most authorities would agree that obtaining cultures from all patients with a sore throat, without compelling epidemiologic reason to do so, would be needlessly expensive.

4. The suspicion of diphtheria, yersinial infection, or other unusual causes of sore throat should lead to institution of the relevant procedures for culture of these organisms.

Key Laboratory Findings

- Complete blood count: elevated leukocyte count with a left shift suggests bacterial infection
- Gram staining of the pharyngeal exudate may reveal gram-positive cocci (streptococci) or Chinese letters (*C. diphtheriae*)
- Culture of *C. diphtheriae* requires special medium—Loeffler's or tellurite selective medium

Radiographic Changes

X-ray changes are not anticipated with routine sore throats. Epiglottitis may be diagnosed by lateral neck films that reveal an enlarged hypopharynx and swollen epiglottis.

Differential Diagnosis

1. Lymphadenopathy of the neck can be either bilateral, in which case it is likely to be a component of a systemic response, or unilateral, in which case localized bacterial infection or a small number of other infectious agents account for most infectious causes.

2. Most cases of acute cervical lymphadenitis in children are caused by streptococcal or staphylococcal infection.

3. The differential diagnosis of a unilateral mass in the neck includes malignancies (especially rhabdomyosarcoma, thyroid tumor, sternocleidomastoid tumor, and metastatic carcinoma) and a variety of cysts (cystic hygroma, bronchial cleft cyst, thyroglossal cyst, epider-

moid cyst). Among the infectious causes of unilateral neck swelling are *Staphylococcus aureus* (often associated with abscesses), atypical mycobacteria, tularemia, and bacteria or viruses found in the mouth and throat.

4. Patients with Kawasaki disease (formerly called mucocutaneous lymph node syndrome) often present with cervical adenopathy. The diagnosis of this disorder is made on the basis of the occurrence of fever, conjunctival injection, mouth changes (erythema, fissuring, strawberry tongue), changes in the peripheral extremities (including induration of the hands and feet and desquamation of the skin of the fingers and toes), an erythematous rash, and an enlarged lymph node.

5. Among viral infections, herpes simplex may present with cervical swelling, although gingivostomatitis and/or pharyngitis is a more likely presentation.

6. Mumps, a paramyxovirus, presents with swelling of the parotid glands. Although the disorder usually involves the parotids (and often other salivary glands) on both sides, a unilateral presentation is common.

   a. Mumps is spread by droplets and by direct contact with the saliva of infected persons. It has been isolated from saliva 6 to 7 days before and up to 9 days after the development of parotitis. The average incubation period is 18 days. Nonimmune exposed persons are considered infectious from the twelfth through the twenty-fifth day after exposure.

   b. One third of mumps infections are clinically asymptomatic, but asymptomatic infection may be communicable. The natural history in symptomatic cases is a febrile illness with parotid swelling that peaks at 48 hours and resolves at approximately 1 week after infection.

Causes of Unilateral Cervical Adenopathy or Swelling

Bacterial Causes
Group A *Streptococcus*
Staphylococcus aureus
Atypical mycobacteria
Cat-scratch bacillus
Actinomycosis
Other anaerobic bacteria
Diphtheria
Tularemia

Viral Causes
Herpes simplex virus
Mumps virus

Other Causes and Unknown Agents
Toxoplasma gondii
Kawasaki disease

---

   c. Complications of mumps include pancreatitis (in approximately 4 per cent of cases) and orchiditis (often unilateral and seen in approximately 25 per cent of infected postpubertal males). Central nervous system abnormalities are also seen. An aseptic meningitis (without sequelae) is common, whereas deafness (usually unilateral) and encephalitis are rare. The mortality of mumps is approximately 1 per 10,000 cases.

Treatment

1. Despite a voluminous literature and a reasonable amount of hard data, opinions still vary from treating everyone with a red throat to treating no one. The academicians (the American Heart Association and the American Academy of Pediatrics) have indicated that obtaining microbiologic confirmation of clinical impressions is desirable.

2. Many series demonstrate that clinicians cannot reliably predict who has group A *Streptococcus*.

3. The use of the rapid streptococcal antigen test is desirable, particularly for office practitioners, because a positive result can be reported in minutes, allowing for therapy to be given. The drawback of the rapid tests is that although they are specific, they are not as sensitive as culture techniques; therefore, a negative result cannot be relied on.

4. Culture on blood agar of properly obtained swabs (i.e., including swabbing of the posterior pharynx and tonsils and avoiding the tongue) still misses 10 per cent of potential positive cases. The significance of this fact is doubtful, because many of these cases may represent colonization and/or low-virulence organisms. Since the prevalence of positive cultures exceeds the prevalence of clinical disease, it seems likely that many positive cultures are not important. This fact affects the approach of most clinicians to diagnosis as well as treatment of sore throats.

5. Because streptococci have continued to be sensitive to penicillin, it remains the standard therapy for streptococcal sore throat. A single dose of benzathine penicillin G (600,000 U IM for children older than 1 month who weigh less than 27 kg and 1.2 million U, an adult dose, for children who weigh more than 27 kg) is an excellent, if somewhat painful, treatment. Oral penicillin V (250 mg PO two or three times per day for children younger than 12 years of age and 500 mg PO two or three times per day for children older than 12 years) is a reasonable treatment if given for a full 10-day course. Weight-based dosing, recommended for very young children, is 15 to 62.5 mg/kg or 0.5 to 1 g/m^2 given in three to six divided doses. Follow-up cultures (at 2 to 7 days after treatment) are indicated only for patients with persistent or recurrent symptoms and those with a history of rheumatic fever. Failure rates are high if the treatment is not continued for a full 10-day course.

6. Several studies suggest that cephalosporins may achieve better results (fewer failures), and azithromycin requires only 5 days of therapy. These treatments have not been tested for their ability to prevent rheumatic fever.

7. Erythromycin can also be given to patients over 1 week of age with serious penicillin allergy (40 mg/kg/day given in three divided doses).

8. Treatment of cervical adenitis depends on the etiologic agent. Treat as for pharyngitis, and test for tuberculosis.

Prevention

1. Preventive efforts are directed at diphtheria and group A streptococcal disease. Although a vaccine for group A

streptococci was first produced in 1937, no efficacious product exists today.

2. Patients with a history of rheumatic fever should receive continuous prophylaxis against streptococcal infection. A single intramuscular injection of 1.2 million U of benzathine penicillin G monthly is recommended. However, levels drop to zero by the end of the month. An alternative regimen is penicillin V, 250 mg PO twice daily.

3. Most authorities recommend continued prophylaxis at least until the age of 18 years in patients who have had rheumatic fever. However, adolescents with a history of rheumatic fever should receive prophylaxis for at least 5 years after an episode of acute rheumatic fever, and those at high risk for contacting streptococci (e.g., school teachers) are advised to continue prophylaxis into early adulthood.

4. Mumps is prevented by the administration of the mumps vaccine (a live attenuated virus).

Bibliography

Bisno AL: Acute pharyngitis: Etiology and diagnosis. Pediatrics 1996;97:949–954.

Blumer JL, Goldfarb J: Meta-analysis in the evaluation of treatment for streptococcal pharyngitis: A review. Clin Ther 1994;16:604–620.

Kline JA, Runge JW: Streptococcal pharyngitis: A review of pathophysiology, diagnosis, and management. J Emerg Med 1994;12:665–680.

Little PS, Williamson I: Are antibiotics appropriate for sore throats? Costs outweigh benefits. BMJ 1994;309:1010–1011.

Todd JK: The sore throat: Pharyngitis and epiglottitis. Infect Dis Clin North Am 1988;2:149–162.

90 Approach to the Child with Fever and Rash

Robert Finberg

A child with a fever and a skin eruption is likely come to medical attention sooner or later. Rashes related to infection can be caused by (1) primary invasion of the skin by bacteria (see Chapter 94); (2) vascular invasion by bacteria, viruses, fungi, rickettsiae, mycoplasmas, or chlamydiae; (3) emboli from a bacterial or fungal endovascular focus; (4) immune vasculitis with immune complex formation; or (5) the distant effects of toxins produced by a localized infection (as in the skin findings of toxic shock syndrome). Crucial to diagnosis is a history that explores previous travel, exposure to ill persons, and especially drug history. This review focuses on North American infections that lead to presentation with fever and a rash.

Differential Diagnosis

1. Traditionally, childhood exanthems were listed by number (e.g., first, second, third). Despite the fact that the etiologic agent of sixth disease has now been defined, most authorities have lost interest in the numbering schema. Nevertheless, an understanding of the various patterns of rashes in children is of use in differentiating the skin manifestations of infections (Table 90–1).

2. Measles in a vaccinated host may appear as a modified measles with a less severe rash. Atypical measles is seen in patients who received the killed measles vaccine (given in the United States in 1967 and in other countries for a longer period), but similar cases have been described in patients receiving the live attenuated vaccine. Atypical measles is characterized by high fever, myalgia, a rash that begins on the extremities, and papular or papulovesicular lesions that may resemble chickenpox and a segmental pneumonia. Koplik spots, if present, precede the rash and are virtually diagnostic of measles; they are not seen in atypical measles. Typical measles has high fever, marked coryza, and pneumonitis. Complications in order of frequency include bacterial otitis media, bacterial pneumonia, and, uncommonly, an encephalitis that can be devastating.

3. The rash of sixth disease (roseola or exanthem subitum), caused by human herpesvirus 6, is characterized by a febrile prodrome in a child between 6 months and 3 years of age. A typical presentation is that the rash develops as the fever abates. Recent series using culture methods have suggested that acquisition or reactivation of the virus may be a common cause of fever in children who present to emergency rooms.

4. In addition to the numbered childhood exanthems, a variety of viruses cause skin rashes. Children who have chickenpox (caused by varicella-zoster virus) typically present with macules and papules over the face and trunk which rapidly evolve into vesicles on an erythematous base (Table 90–2). The important diagnostic finding is the presence of vesicles.

5. Infections with adenovirus, echovirus, lymphocytic choriomeningitis virus, and dengue virus; viral hemorrhagic fevers; and Colorado tick fever are all viral illnesses causing fever and a rash (see Table 90–2).

6. Children who have Lyme disease, an illness caused by a tickborne bacterium (*Borrelia burgdorferi*), present with an annular expanding erythematous rash (erythema chronicum migrans) that surrounds the tick bite. The disorder, which is associated with a chronic arthritis and may involve neurologic or cardiac complications, is usually diagnosed on the basis of the rash and a history of exposure to ticks.

7. Children with disseminated fungal infections may pre-

TABLE 90–1. CHILDHOOD EXANTHEMS

TRADITIONAL NAME*	COMMON NAME	CHARACTERISTIC EXANTHEM	ASSOCIATED ENANTHEM	ETIOLOGIC AGENT	DIAGNOSTIC TEST
First disease	Measles	Erythematous macules and papules	Koplik spots (blue-white spots on a red base on buccal mucosa and gingiva)	Paramyxovirus (measles)	Fluorescent antibody of nasal secretions
Second disease	Scarlet fever	Sunburn-like eruption, increased intensity of skin folds	Red pharynx, petechiae on palate, white to strawberry tongue	β-Hemolytic streptococcus	Bacterial culture of throat
Third disease	German measles	Rose or pink macules, often evanescent in character	Petechiae or red macules on soft palate	Togavirus (rubella)	Serology
Fifth disease	Erythema infectiosum	"Slapped face" appearance of cheeks, macules and papules in a "lacy" pattern	None	Parvovirus B19	Serology
Sixth disease	Roseola	Discrete, red macules, predominantly on the trunk	Macules and streaks on the soft palate	Human herpesvirus 6	Culture, serology

*Fourth or Duke disease is not currently thought to define a distinct exanthum.

sent with macular rashes, as may those infected by *Chlamydia* or *Mycoplasma.*

8. Of immediate concern to the clinician should be the diagnosis of a life-threatening illness in a child presenting with fever and a rash. The presence of petechiae suggests certain diagnoses. Meningococcemia (caused by *Neisseria meningitidis*) is perhaps the most worrisome illness, because it can be rapidly fatal. However, a number of other bacteria, including *Streptobacillus moniliformis* (a cause of rat bite fever), *Borrelia* species, *Capnocytophaga canimorsus* (often associated with dog bites), *Staphylococcus aureus* (particularly in the case of endocarditis or high-grade sepsis), and *Neisseria gonorrhoeae,* may all cause petechial rashes.

9. Illnesses caused by several rickettsial species are associated with petechial rashes. These include Rocky Mountain spotted fever, which should be considered in patients with any potential exposure to ticks, and epidemic typhus. Rocky Mountain spotted fever, a potentially fatal disease if untreated, can be rapidly diagnosed by fluorescent antibody staining of a cutaneous biopsy.

10. Vesicular and vesiculobullous lesions are more unusual and tend to better define an infection. Among the bacteria, *Vibrio vulnificus* causes vesicular lesions. This organism is found in salt water in warm areas and should be included in the differential diagnosis if there is a history of contact with salt water or with animals living in these areas. *Rickettsia akari,* the etiologic agent of rickettsialpox, is a rickettsia known to be associated with a vesicular rash. The presence of a papule that ulcerates and a history of contact with mice (the organism is carried by a mite of mice) is suggestive.

Clinical Findings

1. History
   a. Almost any medicine is capable of causing an allergic response that may manifest as fever and rash. Certain drugs, like diphenylhydantoin, may be associated with fever and adenopathy as well. Drug fever, although usually a diagnosis of exclusion, is easy to exclude in most cases.
   b. A travel history is important in the diagnosis of rashes associated with fever. A history of travel to areas where certain rickettsiae or viral hemorrhagic fevers are endemic should be carefully obtained.

2. Physical examination
   a. Careful determination of the type of rash (macular/papular, nodular, vesiculobullous, petechial, or diffuse erythema) should be obtained, because certain infections as well as noninfectious disorders are associated with characteristic findings on presentation (see Table 90–1).

TABLE 90–2. RASHES CAUSED BY VIRAL INFECTIONS

MACULAR RASHES

HIV-1
Rubella
Lymphocytic choriomeningitis
Dengue virus
Rubella
Colorado tick fever
Cytomegalovirus
Hepatitis B virus
Parvovirus B19
Human herpesvirus 6

VESICULAR RASHES

Varicella-zoster (chickenpox)
Varicella-zoster (shingles)
Herpes simplex

PETECHIAL RASHES (usually seen in association with a macular rash)

Viral hemorrhagic fevers
Measles
Adenovirus
Rubella
Epstein-Barr virus

MACULAR, VESICULAR, AND PETECHIAL RASHES (alone or in combination)

Echoviruses
Coxackieviruses

TABLE 90–3. COMMON EXANTHEMS

DISEASE AND ETIOLOGIC AGENT	INCUBATION PERIOD	DURATION OF RASH AND INFECTIVITY	MAJOR CLINICAL FEATURES	COMPLICATIONS	PREVENTION
Measles RNA virus	8–12 days to coryza, 14 days to rash	Rash, 3–5 days Infectivity, onset of coryza until fading of rash	Fever, coryza, cough, photophobia, Koplik spots, disseminated maculopapular rash beginning in neck region (morbilliform), brawny desquamation.	Otitis media, pneumonia, thrombocytopenia, encephalitis, SSPE	Vaccination (MMR at 12–15 mo and 11–12 yr) Gamma globulin for passive immunity
Rubella RNA virus (German measles)	2–3 wk (infection, 17 days)	Rash, 1–3 days Infectivity, during febrile period	Fever, maculopapular rash, lymphadenopathy (especially posterior auricular)	Arthralgia; polyarthritis, especially in adolescent and adult females; encephalitis (rare)	MMR at 12–15 mo
Exanthem subitum Roseola Herpesvirus 6 DNA virus	9 days	Rash, 4–5 days Infectivity, during febrile period (?)	High fever 3–4 days, generalized macular rash with disappearance 2–3 hr to 36 hr, suboccipital lymphadenopathy, marked polymorphonuclear leukopenia	Convulsions, encephalitis (rare)	None
Erythema infectiosum Slapped cheek Parvovirus DNA virus	4–20 days	Rash, 2–3 days Infectivity, variable	Fever; rash predominantly on cheeks, may appear on arms, trunk, and thighs	Arthralgias	None
Chickenpox Varicella Herpesvirus Varicella-zoster	14–21 days (average, 16–17 days)	Rash, 3–7 days Infectivity, duration of rash until crusted	Vesicular rash in cross over entire body; pruritus, fever; zoster lesions after primary infection follow dermatomes; painful	Encephalitis (usually cerebellitis), pneumonia (rare in children)	Vaccine at 1 yr VZIG for passive immunity
Scarlet fever β-hemolytic (group A) *Streptococcus*	48 hr	Rash, 2–4 days Infectivity, until 24 hr after antibiotic is given	Maculopapular erythema (sandpaper), circumoral pallor, Pastia lines, desquamation in sheets	As with any group A streptococcal infection	No recommended vaccine

MMP, measles-mumps-rubella; SSPE, subacute sclerosing panencephalitis; VZIG, varicella-zoster immunoglobulin.

309

b. The presence of adenopathy, nuchal rigidity or signs of abnormalities of the central nervous system, hepatosplenomegaly, or lesions of the conjunctival, oral, or anogenital mucosa should be carefully sought and may be helpful in diagnosing the disorder.

c. The presence of a heart murmur or any prosthetic device should suggest the possibility of disseminated bacterial infection in a patient presenting with fever and rash. Extensive culturing with special attention to fastidious and/or slow-growing bacteria is indicated (Table 90–3).

Key Clinical Findings

- Type of rash
- Adenopathy present or absent

Laboratory Examinations

1. The determination of the complete blood count (with an assessment of the platelet count) is helpful in determining whether an underlying disorder (e.g., leukemia) is present and may give clues as to the diagnosis.
2. Blood cultures are mandatory in cases in which bacterial sepsis is suspected on the basis of the toxic appearance of the child or the presence of indwelling hardware.
3. Fluorescent antibody staining of cutaneous biopsies is a rapid and reliable way to diagnose Rocky Mountain spotted fever and several other rickettsial infections.
4. Fluorescent antibody staining of cells scraped from the base of a vesicle is the optimal method to diagnose herpes simplex and herpes zoster (see Chapter 93).
5. Laboratory serologic tests may make diagnosis of certain rashes (e.g., syphilis, rubella) that cannot be made in any other way.
6. Enteroviruses are best diagnosed by culture of stool or throat swab specimens. The use of polymerase chain reaction techniques should make possible the identification of enteroviruses that have been difficult to grow and characterize by routine culture methods.

Key Laboratory Tests

- Leukocyte count
- Platelet count
- Blood cultures (toxic-appearing patients)
- Fluorescent antibody staining
- Throat and stool culture
- Serology

Treatment

1. The major problem in approaching patients with a fever and a rash is to define whether this is a presentation of a life-threatening illness (e.g., meningococcemia, toxic

TABLE 90–4. COMMON ILLNESSES PRESENTING WITH FEVER AND A RASH THAT REQUIRE IMMEDIATE TREAMENT

TYPE OF INFECTION	COMMON ETIOLOGIC AGENTS	TREATMENT
Bacterial Infections		
Unknown bacteremia/ sepsis	*N. meningitidis, S. pneumoniae, S. aureus, H. influenzae*	Cefotaxime 50 mg/kg IV q 8h or ceftriaxone 100 mg/kg q 24h
Toxic shock syndrome (*S. aureus*–associated)	*S. aureus* toxin producing strain, especially vaginal (tampon-associated) or wound infection	Nafcillin or oxacillin 150 mg/kg/day—up to 12 g/day given in six divided doses
Toxic shock syndrome (*Streptococcus*-associated)	*Streptococcus* (groups A, B, C) associated with erysipelas, cellulitis	Penicillin G 200,000–300,000 units/kg given in six divided doses—up to 24 million units/day
Lyme disease	*Borrelia burgdorferi*—the rash of erythema migrans following a tick bite is the diagnostic feature	Amoxicillin 25–50 mg/kg/day in 3 divided doses Adults—doxycycline 100 mg po bid × 14–21 days
Rickettsial Infections		
Rocky Mountain spotted fever	*R. rickettsii*	Neonates—25 mg/kg in one daily dose
Murine typhus	*R. typhi*	Infants—50 mg/kg/day in two divided doses
Scrub typhus	*R. tsutsugamushi*	Children—chloramphenicol 50–100 mg/kg/day in four doses (max 3 g/day)
Rickettsialpox	*R. akari*	Adults—doxycycline, 100 mg po bid

shock) or of a self-limited disorder (e.g., hand-foot-and-mouth disease caused by a coxsackievirus). Considerable care and as much time as necessary should be devoted to this determination. Laboratory tests may be helpful (see above).

2. Treatment of the patient obviously depends on the diagnosis. Too often clinicians muddle the problem by substituting one iatrogenic disorder for another. Careful consideration should be given to diagnostic tests before empirical therapy is begun (Table 90–4).

Bibliography

Cherry JD: Contemporary infectious exanthems. Clin Infect Dis 1992;16:199–207.

Frieden IJ, Resnick SD: Childhood exanthems old and new. Pediatr Clin North Am 1991;38:859–887.

Kingston ME, Mackey D: Skin clues in the diagnosis of life-threatening infections. Rev Infect Dis 1986;8:1–11.

Morens DM, Katz AR: The fourth disease of childhood: Reevaluation of a nonexistent disease. Am J Epidemiol 1991;134:628–640.

Weber DJ, Cohen MS: The acutely ill patient with fever and rash. *In* Mandell GL, Bennett JE, Dolin R (eds): Principles and Practice of Infectious Diseases, 4th ed. New York, Churchill Livingstone, 1995.

91 Upper Respiratory Infections

Robert Finberg and
Jeffrey Bergelson

Infections of the upper respiratory tract are among the most common illnesses for which children are brought to the pediatrician. Most of these are self-limited viral infections that do not require specific treatment. However, infections of the larynx or epiglottis may cause obstruction of the airway and require immediate intervention. A diagnosis of sinusitis may lead to treatment for a possible bacterial infection. The following types of upper respiratory infections are considered here: the common cold, laryngotracheobronchitis (croup), herpangina, epiglottitis, pertussis, and sinusitis.

The Common Cold

Etiology

1. The common cold is a mild illness caused by a wide variety of viruses. These include rhinoviruses, respiratory syncytial virus, parainfluenza virus, influenza, enteroviruses, and adenoviruses.
2. Thirty to 40 per cent of colds are caused by rhinoviruses. There are approximately 100 rhinovirus serotypes. Because immunity appears to be serotype specific, the opportunity for repeated infections is apparent.

Epidemiology

1. Respiratory viral infections occur in the colder months in temperate climates and in the rainy season in the tropics, for reasons that are not well defined.
2. Young children are thought to be the major reservoir of respiratory viruses. Adults with children at home have more colds than those without children at home.

Pathophysiology

1. The symptoms of the common cold (see below) appear to result from a combination of local irritation to the nasal passages and release of inflammatory mediators with systemic effects.
2. The incubation period for the common cold varies from 24 to 72 hours, with a median duration of 1 week. However, one fourth of illnesses last up to 2 weeks.

Clinical Findings

1. Clinical findings include malaise, sneezing, watery nasal discharge, and mild sore throat. Fever may or may not be present, but the child does not seem very ill, and there is no evidence of respiratory distress.
2. Physical examination is remarkable only for inflammation of the nasal passages and nasal discharge.
3. Most children with runny noses have either colds or allergies.
4. In young infants, chronic nasal congestion and discharge may be caused by streptococci or by congenital syphilis, and in older children prominent purulent discharge may be a symptom of sinusitis. Foreign bodies may cause chronic discharge from one nostril.

Key Clinical Findings: Common Cold

- Watery nasal discharge
- Fever (usually)

Laboratory Findings

1. No abnormalities in the complete blood count or other routine tests are expected in patients with colds.
2. Microbiologic studies are not routinely performed. Rapid viral techniques such as direct fluorescent antibody (DFA) staining of secretions are available to diagnose adenovirus, respiratory syncytial virus (RSV), influenza virus A and B, and parainfluenza 1 and 3. These diagnostic tests are usually reserved for patients who are immunocompromised or have serious lung disease.

Radiographic Changes

X-ray studies are not recommended for diagnosis of patients with cold symptoms.

Treatment

No treatment is currently available for the common cold. Although antihistamines and decongestants provide some symptomatic relief for adolescents and adults, there is little evidence that they are helpful for young children. Even though viral upper respiratory infection may predispose to bacterial pneumonia, the bulk of the evidence does not favor routine use of antibiotics (which may be toxic and may lead to antibiotic resistance) to prevent lower respiratory tract disease.

Prevention

1. Rhinovirus replication peaks approximately 48 hours after infection, but virus may persist in the nasal mucosa for up to 3 weeks.
2. Clinical studies demonstrate that rhinoviruses and RSV are spread on hands. Airborne spread of influenza and other respiratory viruses may also occur. Therefore, attention to handwashing and containment of coughs and sneezes are required to prevent spread.

Laryngotracheobronchitis

Definition

Inflammation of the larynx may result in a mild illness with hoarse voice or a more severe illness with fever, inspiratory stridor, and the barking cough typical of croup. The trachea and bronchi may also be inflamed.

Etiology

1. Croup is almost invariably caused by viruses. Parainfluenza virus type 1 is the most common cause in winter epidemics. A range of other viruses (including parainfluenza viruses 2 and 3, influenza A and B, adenoviruses,

rhinoviruses, enteroviruses, herpes simplex, and reoviruses) have been associated with croup.

2. In some cases, bacterial infections of the trachea, most often caused by staphylococci, have produced similar obstructive symptoms. The diagnosis of bacterial tracheitis is usually made when a patient with severe symptoms requires intubation and a purulent discharge is observed.

3. Diphtheria and tuberculosis may also involve the larynx.

Epidemiology

1. Croup is primarily a disease of children aged 7 to 36 months. Very few cases are seen in patients older than 6 years.

2. In temperate climates, croup occurs in epidemics during the fall and winter, in association with community epidemics of parainfluenza or influenza viruses.

Pathophysiology

Inflammation of the larynx causes swelling and airway obstruction, leading to inspiratory stridor. In milder cases, vocal cord edema may lead to a hoarse voice.

Clinical Findings

1. Patients with croup present with inspiratory stridor, which may be dramatic and alarming for both child and adult. Stridor usually follows several days of milder cold symptoms, typically worsens at night, and may be accompanied by cough and hoarseness.

2. The most important alternative diagnosis is epiglottitis (see below).

3. Retropharyngeal abscesses, foreign bodies, acute allergic reactions, and hemangiomas may also cause airway obstruction and stridor and should be considered in the differential diagnosis.

Key Clinical Findings: Croup

- Gradual onset of symptoms (1–2 days)
- Hoarseness
- Barking cough
- Stridor
- Retractions
- Worse at night (lower relative humidity)

Laboratory Findings

Laboratory tests usually are not necessary to make the diagnosis of croup. In some cases, if croup is suspected but epiglottitis is still a concern, a lateral neck x-ray study showing a normal epiglottis may be helpful. Laryngeal diphtheria should be ruled out with appropriate cultures if it is considered likely.

Treatment

1. Therapy is directed at reducing airway edema and obstructive symptoms. Allowing the child to breathe moist air in a steamy bathroom may be a helpful approach at home; mist tents are sometimes used for hospitalized patients.

2. Nebulized epinephrine is effective, although symptoms

may rebound after several hours. Corticosteroids (administered parenterally, orally, or by inhalation) can also reduce subglottic edema and have a more prolonged effect. Their use in hospitalized patients is now widely accepted, but there is continuing debate about whether and how they should be used in patients with milder symptoms, since the disorder usually resolves with no therapy.

3. Antibiotics are not indicated in typical cases of croup.

Prevention

As noted previously for colds, prevention of spread involves handwashing and containment of coughs and sneezes. No vaccines are currently available.

Herpangina

Etiology

Herpangina is caused by enteroviruses of the coxsackievirus or echovirus group.

Clinical Findings

Clinical findings include high fever and vesiculoulcerative lesions on the pharynx, palate, and tonsils. Occasionally, the buccal mucosa and gingiva are also involved. The process lasts 3 to 4 days.

Key Clinical Findings: Herpangina

- High fever
- Ulcers on soft palate, tonsils, and pharynx

Laboratory Findings

There are no specific laboratory findings.

Treatment

Treatment is symptomatic only.

Hand-Foot-and-Mouth Disease

Etiology

This disorder is caused by an enterovirus and is often said to be associated with coxsackievirus A16.

Clinical Findings

Clinical findings include vesicular lesions on hands, feet, and oropharynx after an incubation period of 4 to 5 days. Mild fever usually is present.

Laboratory Findings

There are no specific laboratory findings.

Treatment

No treatment is required. Lesions may last 6 to 7 days.

Epiglottitis

Definition and Etiology

Epiglottitis is a life-threatening infection of the epiglottis that may result in acute airway obstruction. Epiglottitis is caused by *Haemophilus influenzae* type b and has virtually disappeared in North America as a result of widespread immunization. The disease may rarely be caused by group A streptococci.

Clinical Findings

1. Epiglottitis is characterized by fever, dysphagia, and respiratory distress.
2. The symptoms of epiglottitis may overlap those of croup, but toxicity, severe sore throat, drooling, absence of hoarseness, and the child's insistence on sitting forward with the neck hyperextended all suggest epiglottitis.

Key Clinical Findings: Epiglottitis

- Fever
- Stridor
- Drooling
- Dysphagia

Laboratory Findings and Treatment

1. Laboratory investigation of the child with presumed acute epiglottitis should be approached with caution, because acute airway obstruction may be provoked by disturbing the patient. In some patients believed to have viral croup, a lateral neck x-ray to exclude the diagnosis of epiglottitis may be helpful.
2. Rapid intervention to secure the airway is essential. In clinical settings in which epiglottitis is considered a likely diagnosis, the child should not be disturbed until experienced personnel, ready to perform intubation or tracheotomy, are present. Direct examination of the epiglottis to confirm the diagnosis can then be attempted.
3. Once the airway is secured, routine blood tests, blood cultures, and surface culture of the epiglottis can be performed.
4. Antibiotic therapy with ceftriaxone or cefotaxime should be continued for 7 to 10 days.

Key Treatment: Epiglottitis

- Intubation or tracheostomy
- Antibiotics

Prevention

1. The best preventative strategy is the employment of the *H. influenzae* conjugate vaccine.
2. In households with unvaccinated children younger than 4 years of age, all household members (including the index patient) should receive treatment with rifampin to eliminate nasopharyngeal carriage of the organism. Rifampin is given once a day (20 mg/kg per dose; maximum, 600 mg) for 4 days.

Pertussis

Etiology

1. Pertussis is caused by *Bordetella pertussis* and *Bordetella parapertussis*.
2. *Chlamydia trachomatis* and adenovirus may produce a similar symptom complex.

Epidemiology

1. Pertussis is spread by close contact with an infected individual. This is often a sibling or a young parent whose symptoms are minimal.
2. The incubation period is 4 to 10 days.

Clinical Findings

1. The early phase is that of an upper respiratory infection.
2. The next phase is paroxysmal coughing, often followed by an inspiratory "whoop" and vomiting. Infants may not whoop but often have posttussive apnea.
3. The cough may persist for 6 to 10 weeks and may recur during intercurrent upper respiratory infections.
4. Secondary bacterial pneumonia occurs in 30 to 40 per cent of patients.
5. Encephalopathy, secondary to hypoxia and to increased vascular pressure and hemorrhage during paroxysms, occurs rarely.

Key Clinical Findings: Pertussis

- Paroxysmal cough
- Inspiratory whoop
- Vomiting
- Apnea
- Secondary pneumonia

Laboratory Findings

1. Marked lymphocytosis is characteristic but not invariably present, especially not in infants.
2. Organism may be cultured on specific media.
3. DFA (direct fluorescent antibody test) of nasopharyngeal secretions.

Key Treatment: Pertussis

- Oxygen for cyanosis and apneic spells
- Refeeding
- Antibiotics for pneumonia
- Erythromycin 40–50 mg/kg/d × 14 days for eradication of organism

Sinusitis

Definition

Sinusitis, an inflammation of one or more paranasal sinuses, is often associated with infection. Complications of bacterial sinusitis include osteomyelitis of the frontal bone (Pott puffy tumor) and extension to the brain and meninges.

Epidemiology

1. Sinusitis is more common in the fall, winter, and spring, and is associated with upper respiratory infections.

2. The disease is more common in adolescents and adults because full development of the sinuses does not occur until adolescence.

Pathophysiology

1. In most cases, sinusitis is thought to result from a bacterial superinfection of the paranasal sinuses, occurring after a viral upper respiratory infection (with rhinovirus, RSV, influenza, or other cold-causing viruses—see above). The virus leads to inflammation, swelling, and sinus obstruction with consequent secondary bacterial infection.
2. Approximately 5 to 10 per cent of cases of maxillary sinusitis are thought to be the result of ascending dental infection.
3. Allergic rhinitis/sinusitis may predispose to the development of bacterial sinusitis, as may obstructive foreign bodies or tumors. Indwelling nasal tumors may also predispose to bacterial sinusitis.

Clinical Findings

1. The classic clinical presentation of sinusitis occurs in a child who does not recover from a cold and presents with persistent, severe symptoms of nasal congestion and discharge more than 10 days after infection.
2. The combination of a history of a maxillary toothache, poor response to nasal decongestants in a child with a low-grade fever, an abnormal sinus transillumination examination, and colored nasal discharge is very suggestive of bacterial infection of the sinuses.
3. Sinusitis is often associated with otitis media in children and can present insidiously. Unlike the picture seen with adults, the classic complaint of a severe, localized headache is uncommon in children.

Key Clinical Findings: Sinusitis

- Pain in area of sinuses
- Purulent discharge
- Headache

Laboratory Findings

1. Definitive diagnosis of infectious sinusitis is obtained by sinus aspiration. A skilled otolaryngologist can perform this procedure in an ambulatory setting.
2. The most likely bacterial organisms to be cultured from the sinuses of children are *Streptococcus pneumoniae*, *H. influenzae* (unencapsulated strains), and *Moraxella catarrhalis*.
3. Anaerobic bacteria (e.g., *Bacteroides* spp., fusobacteria, and spirochetes) are found in adults, presumably on the basis of less dental-associated disease in children.

Radiologic Findings

1. Although sinus x-rays may be of some help in diagnosing acute sinusitis (by the presence of air-fluid levels), computed tomography scans are much more sensitive and specific.
2. The mere presence of an abnormal x-ray does not mean that treatment is indicated. In a recent study, most healthy adults with colds were found to have dramatic abnormalities (including sinus opacification) that were evident on computed tomography scans but required no intervention. Studies of children presenting with persistent respiratory symptoms also reveal that the sinuses are markedly abnormal. Not all of these children need antibiotic therapy for bacterial pathogens. Therapeutic decisions should be based on clinical criteria, not on x-ray findings alone.

Treatment

1. Bacterial infection of the orbit and the frontal and sphenoid sinuses may require surgical intervention.
2. Medical therapy for bacterial sinusitis is conventionally begun with amoxicillin, 40 mg/kg/day in three divided doses.
3. In patients with high fever or periorbital swelling, many clinicians employ a broad-spectrum agent such as amoxicillin-clavulanate, using the same dose of amoxicillin. This combination has activity against *Moraxella* and *Staphylococcus*, organisms unlikely to be sensitive to amoxicillin.
4. Alternative therapies for patients with penicillin allergies are trimethoprim-sulfamethoxazole (8 mg trimethoprim and 40 mg sulfamethoxazole per kilogram per day in two divided doses), erythromycin-sulfisoxazole (50 mg erythromycin and 150 mg sulfisoxazole per kilogram per day in four divided doses), cefaclor (40 mg/kg/day in three divided doses), or cefuroxime axetil (30 mg/kg/day in two divided doses).
5. Nasal decongestants (0.25 or 0.5% phenylephrine nose drops or similar preparations) may provide symptomatic relief in older children and adolescents.

Prevention

1. Since most cases of sinusitis are believed to follow infections by cold viruses or influenza, prevention of these illnesses in the future will probably have a major impact on the incidence of sinusitis.
2. Good dental hygiene and treatment of infected teeth should help prevent maxillary disease related to tooth infection.

Bibliography

Gadomski AM: Antibiotic treatment for URI does not prevent pneumonia. Pediatr Infect Dis J 1993;12:115–120.

Gwaltney JM Jr: Rhinovirus infection of the normal human airway. Am J Respir Crit Care Med 1995;152:S36–S39.

Gwaltney JM Jr, Phillips CD, Miller RD, Riker DK: Computed tomographic study of the common cold. N Engl J Med 1994;330:25–30.

Smith MB, Feldman W: Over-the-counter cold medications: A critical review of clinical trials between 1950 and 1991. JAMA 1993;269:2258–2263.

Wald ER: Sinusitis in children. N Engl J Med 1992;326:319–323.

Williams JW, Simel DL: Does this patient have sinusitis? Diagnosing acute sinusitis by history and physical examination. JAMA 1993;270:1242–1246.

92 Lower Respiratory Infections

Jeffrey Bergelson and
Robert Finberg

Infection of the lower respiratory tract in children can be divided into four major groups: bronchiolitis, pneumonia, empyema, and lung abscess. In this chapter, empyema and lung abscess are considered as complications of pneumonia. Croup and epiglottitis are discussed in Chapter 91.

Bronchiolitis

Definition
1. Bronchiolitis is an inflammation of the small airways that results in expiratory obstruction and wheezing.
2. The term "bronchiolitis" is usually applied to an illness of young infants and children, characterized by respiratory distress and hypoxemia. Older children may also have wheezing with viral infections.

Etiology
1. Bronchiolitis is typically caused by respiratory syncytial virus (RSV).
2. Other agents that have been associated with bronchiolitis include adenoviruses, parainfluenza viruses, rhinoviruses, and *Mycoplasma pneumoniae*.

Epidemiology
1. Bronchiolitis is a disease of infants; the peak incidence is between 2 and 6 months of age.
2. The disease may be seen in older children, but 80 per cent of cases occur in children younger than 1 year old.
3. Epidemic bronchiolitis caused by RSV (the most common etiologic agent) peaks between January and April in the temperate climates of North America, with essentially no disease between August and October.

Clinical Findings
1. The illness begins with common cold symptoms, but, as small airways become obstructed, the symptoms become more severe.
2. On examination, the infant with severe bronchiolitis may be cyanotic and tachypneic. Respiratory distress may be evidenced by flaring of the nostrils and by intercostal and subcostal retractions. Expiration is prolonged, and wheezes are audible.

Key Clinical Findings: Bronchiolitis

- Tachypnea
- Nasal flaring
- Retractions
- Prolonged expiration and wheezing
- Cyanosis

Differential Diagnosis
1. Children with asthma may wheeze in response to viral upper respiratory infections.

2. Other diagnostic considerations in a child with respiratory distress and wheezing include pneumonia, foreign bodies, anatomic abnormalities of the airway, congestive heart failure, and gastroesophageal reflux.

Laboratory Findings
1. In infants with moderately severe bronchiolitis, pulse oximetry or arterial blood gas analysis reveals hypoxemia. Retention of carbon dioxide may indicate impending respiratory failure.
2. Specific diagnosis of RSV and other common respiratory viruses can be made rapidly by immunofluorescence analysis of nasal wash specimens.

Key Laboratory Findings: Bronchiolitis

- Hypoxemia
- Relative hypercarbia
- RSV antigen in nasal secretions

Radiographic Changes
The chest x-ray shows evidence of hyperinflation, with increased lucency and depressed diaphragms. Typically, there is no infiltrate, although areas of atelectasis may be present.

Treatment
1. Supportive care for patients with bronchiolitis includes administration of oxygen, monitoring for apnea, and, if necessary, mechanical ventilation.
2. Bronchodilators are often used but have limited efficacy.
3. Treatment with nebulized ribavirin, an antiviral agent with activity against RSV, was found in some but not all studies to improve oxygenation and to reduce duration of illness. Indications for its use are not certain at this time. It may be considered primarily for severely ill patients and for those with underlying conditions (e.g., prematurity, bronchopulmonary dysplasia, congenital heart disease, immune deficiencies) that put them at risk for severe infection.

Key Treatment: Bronchiolitis

- Oxygen
- Bronchodilators (?)
- Steroids (?)
- Assisted ventilation
- Ribavirin (?)

Prevention
1. Passive immunization with RSV immune globulin has been shown to protect high-risk infants from severe RSV disease and has recently been licensed for this indication.

2. Research on the use of monoclonal antibodies and new vaccines for prevention of RSV disease is in progress.

Pneumonia

In adults, it is common practice to distinguish bacterial pneumonia—characterized by productive cough, purulent sputum, and lobar consolidation on chest x-ray—from atypical pneumonia caused by nonbacterial agents. In children, the distinction is harder to make: most pneumonia is caused by agents other than bacteria, cough is often absent from the clinical presentation, and young children do not produce sputum.

Etiology

1. The etiologic agents causing pneumonia vary tremendously depending on the age of the patient (Table 92–1).
2. Adenovirus, influenza, RSV, parainfluenza viruses, rhinoviruses, and some enteroviruses are common causes of pneumonia in children. Pneumonia can also be seen with measles, rubella, human immunodeficiency virus, varicella-zoster, cytomegalovirus, Epstein-Barr virus, and herpes simplex virus.
3. Beyond the neonatal period, *Streptococcus pneumoniae* is the most common cause of bacterial pneumonia in children. *Haemophilus influenzae*, *Staphylococcus aureus*, and group A streptococci—and, in cases of nosocomial pneumonia, gram-negative bacilli—must also be considered.
4. Viral pneumonia may be complicated by a secondary bacterial infection, most commonly caused by *S. aureus*, *S. pneumoniae*, or *H. influenzae*. Postviral pneumonia is most common during influenza epidemics.
5. Pneumonia caused by *Mycoplasma pneumoniae* is common in school-age children. *Chlamydia pneumoniae* (the TWAR agent) also causes atypical pneumonia. Another chlamydia species, *Chlamydia trachomatis*, causes pneumonia in infants between the ages of 1 and 3 months; tachypnea, staccato cough, absence of fever, eosinophilia, and hyperinflation on chest x-ray are characteristic. *Chlamydia psittaci* is an unusual cause of pneumonia that is associated with exposure to birds.
6. Pneumonia caused by endemic fungi (such as histoplasmosis, blastomycosis, or coccidioidomycosis) occurs in both normal and immunocompromised patients. *Aspergillus* pneumonia occurs primarily in patients with abnormal leukocyte function (e.g., neutropenia, chronic granulomatous disease). For more detail, see Chapter 108.
7. *Coxiella burnetii* (a rickettsia that causes Q fever) can cause primary pneumonia and is usually acquired from animal exposure.
8. In immunocompromised patients, pneumonia due to *Pneumocystis carinii* is common, and *Toxoplasma gondii* is seen (see Chapter 110).
9. Pneumonia caused by *Toxocara canis* is a consideration in the child who eats (handles) dirt.
10. Pulmonary infections with mucoid strains of *Pseudomonas aeruginosa* are typical in patients with cystic fibrosis.
11. Pulmonary tuberculosis should be considered in patients with undiagnosed pneumonia that does not respond to antibiotic therapy.

Clinical Findings

1. In adults and older children, symptoms of pneumonia include fever, cough, chest pain, and respiratory distress. Characteristic physical findings—crackles, decreased breath sounds, bronchial breath sounds, or egophony—may be evident. Absent breath sounds or dullness to percussion may indicate the presence of a significant pleural effusion.
2. Infants and young children with pneumonia may present with fever alone. Specific respiratory symptoms and signs may be absent or subtle; auscultatory findings such as rales may be absent, and an increased respiratory rate may be the only clue to the diagnosis. Nasal flaring, expiratory grunting, or intercostal retractions suggest respiratory compromise.
3. Prolonged and paroxysmal cough, particularly if associated with vomiting, suggests pertussis (whooping cough).
4. Complications of pneumonia include lung abscess and pleural empyemas.
   a. Lung abscess is a circumscribed, purulent process that is a consequence of bacterial infection. Abscesses may occur when necrotizing pneumonia, caused by pyogenic bacteria, fails to resolve completely. *S. aureus* is an important cause of lung abscess in this setting. Alternatively, lung abscess may follow aspiration of bacteria; oral flora, including anaerobes, can cause abscesses after aspiration.
   b. Pleural empyemas usually occur by direct extension of a bacterial pneumonia into the pleural space. *S. aureus*, pneumococcus, and *H. influenzae* are the

TABLE 92–1. COMMON CAUSES OF PNEUMONIA IN DIFFERENT POPULATIONS

INFANTS (0–3 mo)

Bacteria: Group B streptococci, enteric gram-negative bacilli, *Staphylococcus aureus*
Viruses: RSV and other respiratory viruses; herpes simplex; cytomegalovirus
Chlamydia trachomatis
Ureaplasma urealyticum

INFANTS AND YOUNG CHILDREN (2 mo–5 yr)

Respiratory viruses: RSV, influenza, parainfluenza, adenovirus
Pyogenic bacteria: *Streptococcus pneumoniae*, *Haemophilus influenzae* type b, *Staphylococcus aureus*, group A streptococcus *Mycoplasma pneumoniae*

SCHOOL-AGE CHILDREN AND ADOLESCENTS

Mycoplasma pneumoniae
Chlamydia pneumoniae (TWAR)
Respiratory viruses
Pyogenic bacteria: *Streptococcus pneumoniae*
Mycobacterium tuberculosis

LESS COMMON INFECTIONS ASSOCIATED WITH PARTICULAR EXPOSURES OR CLINICAL SETTINGS

Mycobacterium tuberculosis
Fungi: histoplasmosis, coccidioidomycosis, paracoccidioidomycosis, and blastomycosis in endemic areas; cryptococcus and aspergillus in immunocompromised patients
Nocardia and actinomycosis
Pneumocystis carinii in immunocompromised patients

common pathogens. Empyemas are characterized by purulent fluid, with low pH and high lactate dehydrogenase. Drainage is important and may require placement of a chest tube as well as prolonged treatment with antibiotics.

Key Clinical Findings: Pneumonia

- Fever
- Tachypnea
- Nasal flaring
- Retractions
- Cough
- Decreased breath sounds over affected region
- Crackles

Laboratory Findings

1. A markedly elevated leukocyte count with a predominance of immature neutrophils suggests bacterial infection, most typically caused by *S. pneumoniae.*
2. Although examination and culture of sputum are valuable in older children and adults, young children rarely, if ever, provide a sputum specimen. Since pneumococci and other potential bacterial pathogens are normal flora in the upper respiratory tract, bacterial cultures of the nasopharynx are not helpful diagnostically.
3. Nasal wash specimens are valuable for rapid viral diagnosis.
4. Blood cultures may provide the bacteriologic diagnosis.
5. Bronchoalveolar lavage is valuable in the diagnosis of *Pneumocystis carinii* pneumonia in immunocompromised patients.
6. Transcutaneous oximetry is helpful in assessing hypoxemia.

Key Laboratory Tests: Pneumonia

- Leukocyte count (elevated)
- Blood culture
- Sputum culture and Gram stain
- Bronchoalveolar lavage

Radiographic Changes

1. The chest x-ray is the most important diagnostic procedure. In young children with fever, x-rays may reveal pneumonia that was not suspected on the basis of symptoms or physical examination.
2. Lobar or segmental consolidation is the classic pattern in bacterial pneumonia; more diffuse, "atypical" infiltrates are characteristic of nonbacterial pneumonia but do not exclude the possibility of bacterial infection.
3. Bullae or pneumatoceles suggest pneumonia caused by *S. aureus*, although other bacteria may also cause these findings.

Treatment

1. Optimal treatment of bacterial pneumonia depends on both the organism causing disease and the resistance pattern in the community. Penicillin-resistant pneumococci have become increasingly prevalent throughout the United States, and strains resistant to multiple antibiotics are a significant problem.
2. Most children who are only moderately ill can be treated with an oral antibiotic.
   a. Amoxicillin is commonly used for outpatient therapy; however, as pneumococci become more resistant, use of this antibiotic may have to be reassessed.
   b. Clindamycin is a possible alternative oral agent when resistant pneumococci are likely.
   c. In school-age children, among whom mycoplasma pneumonia is common, clarithromycin or erythromycin is often used. Both agents are effective against *Mycoplasma* and *Chlamydia,* but clarithromycin (15 mg/kg/day divided in two doses; maximum dose 1 g/day) is better tolerated.
3. Although high-dose penicillin is effective in treating pneumonia caused by moderately resistant pneumococci, the situation is less clear for organisms with high-level resistance. Because of the possibility of staphylococcal or *Haemophilus* pneumonia, we suggest that the hospitalized child be treated with cefuroxime or cefotaxime, although these agents are not necessarily more effective than penicillin against resistant pneumococci. In critical cases, or if pneumonia is complicated by meningitis, vancomycin should be added.
4. Nosocomial pneumonia is often caused by resistant strains of gram-negative bacilli. Empiric therapy should include an aminoglycoside as well as a third-generation cephalosporin.
5. If *S. aureus* is a likely pathogen (as with empyema, pneumatoceles, or postviral pneumonia) a specific antistaphylococcal agent (oxacillin or vancomycin) should be added.
6. Large pleural effusions necessitate examination of pleural fluid to rule out empyema.

Key Treatment: Pneumonia

- Antibiotics, varying with presumed or verified cause

Prevention

1. Vaccination of all children with the *H. influenzae* vaccine has already dramatically reduced the number of *H. influenzae* pneumonias seen in this country.
2. Pneumovax should be given to all patients with underlying pulmonary or cardiovascular disease and to those with diabetes, renal disease, or immune deficits, all of whom are susceptible to severe illness.
3. Annual vaccination of high-risk patients against influenza is an important preventive measure against seasonal disease.
4. Amantadine and rimantadine have antiviral activity

against influenza A and are used both for prophylaxis and for therapy.

Bibliography

Block S, Hedrick J, Hammerschlag MR, et al: *Mycoplasma pneumoniae* and *Chlamydia pneumoniae* in pediatric community-acquired pneumonia: Comparative efficacy and safety of clarithromycin and erythromycin ethylsuccinate. Pediatr Infect Dis J 1995;14:471–477.

Committee on Infectious Diseases, American Academy of Pediatrics. Reassessment of the indications for ribavirin therapy in respiratory syncytial virus infections. Pediatrics 1996;97:137–140.

Foy HM: Infections caused by *Mycoplasma pneumoniae* and possible carrier state in different populations of patients. Clin Infect Dis 1993;17:S37–S46.

Friedland IR, McCracken GH Jr: Management of infections caused by antibiotic-resistant *Streptococcus pneumoniae*. N Engl J Med 1994;331:377–382.

Grayston JT: Chlamydia pneumonia (TWAR) infections in children. Pediatr Infect Dis J 1994;13:675–684.

93 Herpes Virus Infections

Robert Finberg

Etiology

The herpes viruses are a group of large, double-stranded DNA viruses that are grouped together on the basis of the characteristic architecture of their virions. Herpes viruses have been described in many species, from fish to fowl, and eight are currently recognized as causing disease in humans (Table 93–1).

Epidemiology

1. Herpes simplex virus type 1 (HSV-1) is usually acquired in childhood; the child may present with pharyngitis, or the infection may be clinically silent. It is spread through contact with infected oral secretions.
2. Herpes simplex type 2 (HSV-2) is usually congenital (see Chapter 28) or sexually acquired, and primary infection is often associated with local adenopathy. It is usually spread by direct contact with genital secretions.
3. Varicella infection causes chickenpox, a viral exanthem characterized by a diffuse vesicular eruption. It is spread by direct contact or airborne droplets from virus found in skin lesions or from respiratory tract secretions.
4. Epstein-Barr virus (EBV) may be acquired in early childhood, where it is asymptomatic, or in adolescence or early adulthood, where it causes infectious mononucleosis. By adulthood, 90 to 95 per cent of people are seropositive. The disease is usually spread by direct contact with infectious secretions.
5. Cytomegalovirus (CMV) typically manifests at presentation as generalized lymphadenopathy and is acquired with sexual activity.
6. Human herpesvirus 6 (HHV-6) causes a macular rash after a prodrome characterized by high fever in a child between 6 months and 3 years of age.
7. Human herpesvirus 7 (HHV-7) may cause an illness similar to that associated with HHV-6.
8. A serologic study suggests that HHV-8 is sexually acquired.

Pathophysiology

1. Common to the herpes viruses is an ability to produce a large number of virus-specific proteins (some of which are homologous to host proteins important in cellular regulation).

TABLE 93–1. HUMAN HERPES VIRUSES

VIRUS	VIRUS TYPE	COMMON NAME	PRIMARY ILLNESS	REACTIVATION DISEASE	COMPLICATIONS
Human herpesvirus 1	Alpha	Herpes simplex virus 1	Pharyngitis and adenopathy	"Cold sores"	Encephalitis, meningitis
Human herpesvirus 2	Alpha	Herpes simplex virus 2	Genital sores and adenopathy	Recurrent genital sores	Meningitis, encephalitis
Human herpesvirus 3	Beta	Varicella-zoster virus	Chickenpox (vesicular rash)	Shingles (dermatomal rash and pain)	Encephalitis
Human herpesvirus 4	Gamma	Epstein-Barr virus	Infectious mononucleosis	EBV lymphoproliferative disease	B-cell lymphoma, Hodgkin disease?
Human herpesvirus 5	Beta	Cytomegalovirus	Mononucleosis-like illness	Fever, retinitis, pneumonia	—
Human herpesvirus 6	Beta	—	Roseola	Pneumonitis? bone marrow failure?	—
Human herpesvirus 7	Beta	—	—	—	—
Human herpesvirus 8	Alpha	KS virus	—	—	Kaposi sarcoma

2. Herpes viruses have the ability to exist in two entirely different states relative to the host environment: a replicative phase, during which progeny virus are produced and the cell is irreversibly damaged, and a latency phase (characterized by host cell viability), during which the viral genome assumes a circular structure and only a small subset of viral proteins are made.

3. The ability of these viruses to remain in a latent, nonreplicating form, producing few viral proteins, makes them dangerous for immunocompromised patients, because they retain their ability to cause cellular destruction when reactivated.

Clinical Findings

1. Although primary infection with herpes viruses is usually self-limited in normal hosts, neonates are uniquely vulnerable to HSV, varicella, and CMV, all of which cause severe disease in this age group (see Chapter 28).

2. Outside the neonatal period, the herpes group viruses are usually acquired, as primary infections, in childhood or at the onset of sexual activity.

3. HSV-1 usually manifests in young children as mild or asymptomatic illness. In young adults, pharyngitis with or without fever is a common presentation of primary HSV-1. The prevalence of the disease varies with socioeconomic status, being much higher and with earlier acquisition in patients from underdeveloped countries and from low-income families in industrialized nations.

   a. Children with symptomatic primary HSV-1 present with signs of fever, sore throat, gingivostomatitis, and fever. The infection has an incubation period of 2 to 12 days (mean, 4 days), and a febrile illness persisting for 2 to 3 weeks is possible even in an entirely normal host. In neonates and immunocompromised patients, the virus may be cultured from the blood, indicating the possibility of a viremic phase.

   b. Recurrent HSV-1 is most commonly characterized by the presence of vesicles on the vermilion border of the lip. The pain is usually most severe at the onset of disease and decreases over the next 3 to 4 days with resolution of the lesions. Factors leading to reactivation include fever (hence the term, fever blisters) and exposure to ultraviolet light. HSV may also involve the cornea (herpes keratitis) and can cause serious damage if untreated.

   c. Erythema multiforme, round or oval macules and papules which often appear with rings of erythema (to form target lesions), is associated with HSV-1 or HSV-2. Recurrent attacks often precede the development of the rash.

   d. Encephalitis is a rare complication of HSV, but HSV is one of the most common causes of sporadic viral encephalitis. The virus presumably follows the nerve cells into the brain, where it causes destruction of brain matter, most commonly involving the temporal lobes. It is fatal if untreated.

4. HSV-2 is usually a sexually acquired disease.

   a. Primary illness is heralded by the development of macules and papules which may progress to vesicles, pustules, or ulcers over genital organs. Local pain and adenopathy is characteristic, and systemic signs and symptoms are seen in up to 70 per cent of cases. Extragenital lesions are seen in approximately 20 per cent of cases and aseptic meningitis in 10 per cent. Severe pain at the site of the lesions is common, and urinary retention is seen in 10 to 15 per cent of women. In primary disease, virus shedding lasts approximately 2 to 3 weeks.

   b. Recurrent HSV-2 is associated with less severe, localized disease. The incidence of recurrence varies among patients, with one third having more than 8 to 9 episodes per year, one third having 4 to 7, and one third having 2 to 3. Cultivable (and therefore infectious) virus is present in asymptomatic patients with either HSV-1 or HSV-2. Therefore, physicians cannot justifiably assure an HSV carrier that he or she will not transmit disease even if no lesions or symptoms are present.

5. Varicella is a highly communicable illness (with a secondary attack rate of approximately 90%) which previously (before widespread use of the varicella vaccine) occurred predominantly among children of early school age (5 to 9 years old). The illness is characterized by a maculopapular rash that becomes vesicular and usually heals within 3 to 4 days. The lesions tend to develop in crops and are often found in greatest concentration on the trunk. They may occur in areas of irritation such as diaper rash, sunburn, or poison ivy rash. The disease may be infectious up to 5 days (more commonly, 1 to 2 days) before the rash appears but is not usually contagious beyond 5 days after the rash develops in a normal host.

   a. Children, with the exception of neonates, usually have mild illness with primary varicella infection. The most common complication of disease is bacterial superinfection of vesicles. The case-fatality rate in the United States is approximately 2 per 100,000 cases overall, but it rises to 30 per 100,000 in adults because of a higher incidence of primary viral pneumonia.

   b. Among school-age children, in addition to bacterial superinfection of the vesicles, central nervous system abnormalities are the most common complication. Cerebellar ataxia is estimated to occur in 1 of every 4000 cases of chickenpox in children younger than 15 years old. The syndrome consists of ataxia, vomiting, altered speech, vertigo, and tremor. It usually occurs within 1 week after the rash but may occur up to 21 days later. Cerebrospinal fluid examination reveals a lymphocytosis and elevated protein. The syndrome usually resolves within 2 to 4 weeks without sequelae. Encephalitis (characterized by headaches, seizures, and depression of consciousness) is a much less common complication but it may be life-threatening, especially in adults.

   c. Neonates of susceptible mothers (those who develop disease 5 days before or 2 days after delivery) have a fatality rate as high as 30 per cent, mandating treatment.

6. EBV is the cause of infectious mononucleosis. Although the virus typically does not cause disease when

acquired at a very early age, in the United States primary infection often occurs in the 13- to 24-year-old age group, with 12 per cent of susceptible students seroconverting every year in college studies.

a. The classic presentation of infectious mononucleosis is the triad of sore throat, fever, and adenopathy in an adolescent. Physical examination is likely to be remarkable for a red pharynx with an exudative tonsillitis, sometimes with petechiae. A small number of patients may have a rash on presentation, but almost all will develop a maculopapular rash if they are treated with ampicillin. Laboratory examination is remarkable for a lymphocytosis with a large percentage of atypical lymphocytes. A heterophile test, such as the monospot test, is positive. Complications of infectious mononucleosis include autoimmune hemolytic anemia, splenic rupture, and rare neurologic complications (including encephalitis, meningitis, Guillain-Barré syndrome, Bell palsy, and transverse myelitis). The overwhelming number of patients with neurologic complications recover completely.

b. Primary EBV infection in young children is likely to be asymptomatic, and even clinically apparent infections may be heterophile-negative (monospot-negative).

c. In most patients with adolescent-acquired EBV, the disorder resolves in 2 to 3 weeks. An overwhelming fatal syndrome of EBV infection is associated with a rare X-linked genetic predisposition.

7. CMV is usually acquired at birth (see Chapter 28) or in association with sexual activity. Adolescents and adults with CMV usually present with fever and generalized lymphadenopathy. Mild elevations of liver function tests and an atypical lymphocytosis are expected, as in primary EBV infection; pharyngitis or tonsillitis, on the other hand, is rare. Guillain-Barré syndrome, meningoencephalitis, myocarditis, thrombocytopenia, and hemolytic anemia are all complications of CMV in normal hosts. The spectrum of disorder is broader and more varied in the immunocompromised patient (see Chapter 110).

8. HHV-6 and HHV-7 infect children younger than 3 years of age. Acquisition of both viruses may be asymptomatic, but both have been associated with roseola or exanthem subitum (see Chapter 90). HHV-6 infections are associated with febrile seizures. Reactivation disease can be associated with fever, rash, and bone marrow suppression (see Chapter 110).

9. Serologic data indicate that HHV-8, which is associated with the development of Kaposi sarcoma (KS), is acquired through sexual activity. It is probably asymptomatic in most cases.

Laboratory Findings

1. HSV and varicella-zoster viruses can be diagnosed on the basis of fluorescent staining of cells in a skin lesion. Both can be readily isolated in tissue culture as well.

2. Although conventional culture methods require 1 to 2 weeks, a newer combination of culture and fluorescent

---

Key Clinical findings

Virus	Primary Infection	Recurrent Disease	Complications
HSV-1	Pharyngitis, gingivostomatitis	"Fever blisters" on vermilion border	Encephalitis, keratitis
HSV-2	Genital lesions, fever, adenopathy	Genital lesions	Meningitis
Varicella	Disseminated vesicles	Dermatomal vesicles (zoster)	Ataxia, encephalitis
EBV	Adenopathy, membranous pharyngitis, hepatosplenomegaly	Associated with tumors	Hepatitis, splenic rupture
CMV	Adenopathy	Pneumonitis, fever, bone marrow suppression in immunocompromised hosts	Multiple congenital anomalies
HHV-6	Roseola infantum, fever	Pneumonitis, fever, bone marrow suppression in immunocompromised hosts	—
HHV-7	Roseola, other febrile illnesses, central nervous system syndromes	Undefined	—
KS virus (HHV-8)	Undefined, sexually transmitted	Associated with Kaposi sarcoma in immunocompromised hosts	—

diagnosis allows for the identification of CMV within 1 to 2 days.
3. A diagnosis of EBV infection is usually made using serologic techniques. The monospot, a hemagglutination test, allows for rapid diagnosis of acute infectious mononucleosis and is used by many laboratories. Measurement of other EBV-specific antibodies is required for diagnosing prior infection.
4. HHV-6 and HHV-7 can be cultured, and specialty laboratories can do fluorescent analysis of tissue specimens (e.g., bone marrow biopsies).
5. HHV-8 can be isolated in tissue culture.

Treatment
1. HSV encephalitis can be treated with 10 mg/kg IV acyclovir every 8 hours for 14 to 21 days.
2. Herpes keratitis is usually treated with a 1% solution of trifluridine (Viroptic) given every 2 hours up to 9 times per day for a maximum of 21 days.
3. Primary genital herpes can be treated with acyclovir (400 mg PO t.i.d. is a conventional dose). The symptoms may be attenuated by treatment, but treatment does not prevent the development of a latent state.
4. Varicella in normal children (2 to 12 years) can be treated with 20 mg/kg PO qid of acyclovir for 5 days (starting within 24 hours of a rash). Adolescents or young adults can be treated with 800 mg acyclovir PO five times/day. IV therapy can be given for patients who are pregnant or have pneumonia (10 mg/kg every 8 hours).
5. Treatment of CMV, EBV, HHV-6, HHV-7, and HHV-8 is indicated only for immunocompromised hosts (see Chapter 110).

Prevention
1. A varicella vaccine (consisting of a live attenuated virus) is available and should be used to prevent varicella.
2. Vaccines for both HSV and CMV are currently under study but none are licensed.

Bibliography

Benenson AS: Control of Communicable Diseases Manual, 16th ed. Washington, DC, American Public Health Association, 1995.

Jones CA, Isaacs D: Human herpevirus-6 infections. Arch Dis Child 1996;74:98–100.

Kedes DH, Operskalski E, Busch M, et al: The seroepidemiology of human herpesvirus 8 (Kaposi's sarcoma–associated herpesvirus): Distribution of infection in KS risk groups and evidence of sexual transmission. Nat Med 1996;2:918–924.

Miller CS: Viral infections in the immunocompetent patient. Dermatol Clin 1996;14:225–241.

Nathwani D, Wood MJ: Herpesvirus infections in childhood: 2. Br J Hosp Med 1993;50:301–308.

94 Cellulitis

Robert Finberg

Definition
1. The skin can be primarily infected by an organism (cellulitis), or a systemic infection may lead to a skin manifestation (see Chapter 90).
   a. Cellulitis is an inflammation of the subcutaneous tissue and dermis without involvement of the epidermis. A break in the skin is the usual predisposing condition leading to invasion by a microorganism.
   b. Facial cellulitis is a disorder of children that is often divided on the basis of whether the infection involves the preseptal space (periorbital cellulitis), the orbit (orbital cellulitis), or the buccal mucosa (buccal cellulitis).
      (1) Periorbital (preseptal) cellulitis is an infection of the area between the eyelid skin and the orbital septum. Infection in this space involves the periorbital area.
      (2) Orbital cellulitis involves the area bounded by the bony cavity that surrounds the eye, the eye socket.
      (3) Buccal cellulitis is characterized by swelling and pain in the cheeks.

Etiology
1. Cellulitis of most skin surfaces is the result of organisms that colonize the skin. For this reason, *Staphylococcus* and *Streptococcus* spp. are prominent as etiologic agents. Penetrating wounds may result in infections with organisms not usually carried on the skin surface (e.g., sneaker injuries are associated with *Pseudomonas aeruginosa*).
2. Periorbital and buccal cellulitis are likely to be caused by *Haemophilus influenzae* type b or pneumococcus. In cases of trauma, skin flora such as *Staphylococcus* or *Streptococcus* are likely pathogens. Orbital cellulitis is likely to be caused by agents that cause cellulitis. Recent series have suggested that *Streptococcus milleri* should be considered in addition to *Staphylococcus aureus* and *H. influenzae*.

Pathophysiology
1. The epidermis usually provides a protective covering for the skin that is not penetrable to microorganisms. Group A streptococcus are thought to bind specifically to fibronectin exposed as a consequence of trauma. *S. aureus* colonizes the nares and is thought to spread from that site. Anaerobic organisms such as *Clostridium perfringens* grow in devitalized tissues.

2. The orbit shares common walls with the ethmoid, maxillary, and frontal sinuses. Although it has a rich, valveless venous circulation (leading to spread of infection to the cavernous sinuses), lymphatic drainage is poor, so any bacteria that penetrate are able to grow.

Clinical Findings

1. Children with infections of the skin usually present with fever, pain, and erythema over the involved area.

   a. Erysipelas is a spreading cellulitis characterized by a sharply demarcated area of erythema and induration. In its classic form the rash is hot, shiny, and bright red. There is an elevated margin that stands out from the rest of the skin and is often described as peau d'orange in appearance. Erysipelas is classically seen on the face and extremities and is usually caused by group A streptococcus.

   b. Impetigo, although also most often caused by group A streptococci, is characterized by initially vesicular lesions which later become crusted, producing the characteristic honey-colored crusts. Impetigo is a highly infectious illness seen predominantly in preschool-aged children.

   c. Necrotizing fasciitis or streptococcal gangrene is a rare but deadly entity often associated with a portal of entry (puncture wound or minor laceration) but sometimes occurring without any obvious break in the skin. The disorder begins as a cellulitis but progresses to necrosis of both skin and muscle with spread along fascial planes. The skin progressively becomes dusky or blue. Vesicles or bullae frequently appear, and these may progress from containing yellowish fluid to reddish-black fluid.

   d. Bullous impetigo and staphylococcal scalded skin syndrome are disorders associated with the production of an exfoliative toxin produced by *S. aureus* of phage group II.

   e. Involvement of the subcutaneous tissues with *C. perfringens* leads to anaerobic cellulitis and involvement of the muscles leads to gas gangrene. Clostridial infections typically occur in devitalized tissue, and the clinical presentation is usually characterized by a foul serous discharge from an extremity or other area where circulation may have been compromised after trauma. Anaerobic cellulitis may have relatively few polymorphonuclear leukocytes at presentation and little focal pain or edema. Gas gangrene is a rapidly progressive infection involving the muscle with secondary changes to the overlying skin. The disease has a rapid, potentially fatal course beginning with pain followed by necrosis of areas of the skin and a shock-like picture with high fever and hypotension. The presence of plump, gram-positive rods strongly suggests the diagnosis.

   f. Bacteremic infections, particularly endocarditis, commonly show skin lesions at presentation. The appearance of multiple pustules with or without purpura suggests *S. aureus* bacteremia. Janeway lesions (nontender erythematous lesions on the palms and soles) and Osler nodes (tender lesions on the digital tufts) are a manifestation of the vasculitis that occurs in endocarditis and may be caused by a variety of organisms. Blood cultures are usually diagnostic in these settings.

2. The presentation of facial cellulitis depends on the location of the infection.

   a. Periorbital cellulitis is characterized by the acute onset of unilateral eyelid edema and tenderness. It is not associated with pain on eye motion or visual disturbances. In approximately 50 per cent of the time, patients with periorbital cellulitis have a predisposing cause of infection (trauma, upper respiratory tract infection, and sinusitis are most common). Blood cultures are positive approximately half the time, and *H. influenzae*, *Staphylococcus pyogenes* and other *Staphylococcus* spp., and *Streptococcus*

Key Clinical Findings

Skin Infection	Physical Findings	Clinical Setting	Microbiology
Impetigo	Crusted, superficial lesions	Preschool-age children	Group A streptococcus
Bullous impetigo	Vesicles develop into flaccid bullae containing clear fluid	Usually seen in newborns	*S. aureus* phage group II
Erysipelas	Well-defined, often raised area of erythema, peau d'orange appearance	Any age, seen on extremities and face, often follows a "nick" or laceration	Predominantly group A streptococcus
Cellulitis	Pain and erythema of skin	Often follows trauma or breaks in the epidermis	Many organisms, both gram-negative and gram-positive, depending on the setting
Necrotizing fasciitis	Edema and pain progressing to gangrene	Often seen in patients with underlying diseases (diabetes, immunocompromised hosts), but also occurs in normal hosts	Group A streptococci are common; mixed anaerobic infection may cause a similar picture, particularly after trauma

pneumoniae are the most common isolates. A history of trauma suggests *Streptococcus* or *Staphylococcus,* whereas an upper respiratory tract infection suggests *H. influenzae* or *S. pneumoniae.*

b. Orbital cellulitis is characterized by severe edema of the lid with proptosis. Ocular motion may be decreased, and vision may be affected. This condition is likely to occur either as a result of trauma to the eye or with extension from an adjacent sinus. Likely pathogens again depend on whether the infection is associated with trauma, but *S. milleri* and anaerobes should be considered in addition to *Staphylococcus* and *Streptococcus.*

c. Buccal cellulitis is defined as swelling, tenderness, induration, and warmth of the buccal soft tissues in the absence of an adjacent skin lesion. It is sometimes, but not always, associated with otitis media. Blood cultures are positive in most cases, and *H. influenzae* and *S. pneumoniae* are likely pathogens.

Key Laboratory Findings

- A leukocytosis is common with bacterial cellulitis.
- The yield of cultures of skin in cellulitis is debated. Blood cultures are often valuable. If lesion cultures are obtained, maximal yield is from aspirates of the advancing (or leading) edge of the erythema.

Radiographic Changes

1. The appearance of gas in the tissues suggest the possibility of *C. perfringens.* However, other anaerobic organisms (including *Bacteroides* spp. and anaerobic streptococci) may be associated with gas formation, and *Escherichia coli* and *Klebsiella* are aerobes that can produce gas in tissues.
2. Computed tomography or magnetic resonance imaging of the orbits and sinuses is invaluable for delineating the involvement of the sinuses in cases of orbital cellulitis.

Treatment

Treatment obviously varies according to the type of cellulitis being treated.

1. Unknown cellulitis of the skin is usually treated with a semisynthetic penicillin to provide good antibacterial activity against both staphylococci and streptococci. If the patient is not systemically ill and the disorder is not rapidly progressive, oral therapy is satisfactory.
2. Bullous impetigo and erysipelas are usually empirically treated with a semisynthetic penicillin with activity against both staphylococci and streptococci.
3. Gas gangrene is usually treated with a combination of high-dose penicillin plus a clindamycin or metronidazole, pending culture results. The involvement of surgeons immediately on diagnosis is mandatory.
4. Impetigo with a small number of superficial lesions may be treated with topical mupirocin alone. In the presence of multiple lesions or a clinically ill patient, systemic treatment is recommended. In areas without a significant amount of resistance, erythromycin (30 to 40 mg/kg/day, maximum 2 g/day, given PO in three to four divided doses) is a convenient treatment. Alternative drug regimens include dicloxacillin, clindamycin, amoxicillin-clavulanate combinations, and a cephalosporin.

Key Treatment

- Semisynthetic penicillin for staphylococci and streptococci
- High-dose penicillin plus clindamycin for gas gangrene

Prevention

Application of local antibacterial ointments (mupirocin) may be helpful in limiting person-to-person spread of impetigo caused by group A streptococcus, a highly contagious disorder.

Bibliography

Chartrand SA, Harrison CJ: Buccal cellulitis reevaluated. Am J Dis Child 1986;140:891–893.

Dagan R: Impetigo in childhood: Changing epidemiology and new treatments. Pediatr Ann 1993;22:235–240.

Darmstadt GL, Lane AT: Impetigo: An overview. Pediatr Dermatol 1994;11:293–303.

Fleisher G, Ludwig S: Cellulitis: A prospective study. Ann Emerg Med 1980;9:246–249.

Spires JR, Smith RJH: Bacterial infections of the orbital and periorbital soft-tissues in children. Laryngoscope 1996;7:763–767.

95 Enteritis

Robert Finberg

Food poisoning and gastritis, in which the predominant presentation is with upper gastrointestinal (GI) tract symptoms, are discussed separately from diarrhea, in which lower GI symptoms predominate.

Upper Gastrointestinal Tract Infections

Definition

Gastritis is an inflammation of the gastric mucosa. Food poisoning refers to the development of illness, usually nausea and vomiting, after ingestion of food. Although ingestion of toxins (e.g., *Amanita phalloides* poisoning associated with mushroom ingestion, or scombroid associated with ingestion of fish) can cause toxin-mediated GI distress, so can preformed toxins produced by several bacteria.

Etiology

1. Infectious gastritis is most commonly associated with *Helicobacter pylori*, a short, gram-negative bacterium. Persistent infection with this organism is associated with the development of peptic ulcer disease.
2. Food poisoning is typically divided into different categories based on how long after ingestion symptoms occur (Table 95–1).

Pathophysiology

1. Gastritis induced by *H. pylori* is associated with the production of several bacterial proteins that damage the stomach mucosa.
2. Rapidly acting food poisoning caused by infectious organisms is associated with the production of preformed toxins by the bacteria. Both *Bacillus cereus* and *Staphylococcus aureus* produce neurotoxins that act on the host to cause vomiting. Ingestion of large amounts of bacteria containing the toxin leads to the rapid onset of symptoms. In addition, *Clostridium perfringens* and *B. cereus* can produce disease when ingested spores are able to grow in the host and produce toxins.

Clinical Findings

1. Acute infectious gastritis associated with *H. pylori* may be asymptomatic or associated with abdominal pain and cramping.
2. Food poisoning caused by *S. aureus* or ingestion of preformed toxin of *B. cereus* is associated with severe vomiting and cramps. Diarrhea may be present, but fever is unusual. A short time (1 to 6 hours) between ingestion of contaminated food and appearance of symptoms is expected.
3. When food poisoning is caused by the ingestion of spores that release bacteria that in turn produce toxin in the GI tract (commonly seen with *B. cereus* and *C. perfringens*), severe abdominal cramps and diarrhea are common but vomiting is rare. A longer postingestion history (8 to 16 hours) is likely.
4. Physical examination is often positive for dehydration with or without abdominal tenderness but is otherwise unlikely to be revealing.

Key Clinical Findings: Upper GI Tract Infections

- Nausea, vomiting
- Abdominal cramps
- Diarrhea

Laboratory Findings

1. *H. pylori* infection can be diagnosed on the basis of gastric biopsy or a breath test for urea produced by this organism.
2. It is difficult to diagnose *S. aureus*, *B. cereus*, or *C. perfringens* food poisoning unless the contaminated food itself is cultured for bacteria. These examinations are usually performed by state health departments.

Key Laboratory Findings: Upper GI Tract Infections

- Breath test (*H. pylori*)
- Culture of contaminated food

Treatment

1. *H. pylori* is usually treated with a combination of antibiotics. Optimal regimens for children are still under study.
2. Food poisoning from *S. aureus*, *C. perfringens*, or *B. cereus* is self-limited when careful attention is paid to hydration with uncontaminated foods and fluids.

TABLE 95–1. UPPER GASTROINTESTINAL TRACT INFECTIONS

ORGANISM	SYMPTOMS	TIME AFTER INGESTION FOR DEVELOPMENT OF SYMPTOMS	FOODS ASSOCIATED WITH DISEASE
Staphylococcus aureus	Nausea, vomiting	1–6 h	Ham, poultry, potato and egg salads, mayonnaise, pastries
Bacillus cereus	Nausea, vomiting	1–6 h	Fried rice
Clostridium perfringens	Abdominal cramps, diarrhea	8–16 h	Beef, poultry, legumes, gravies
Bacillus cereus	Abdominal cramps, diarrhea	8–16 h	Meats, vegetables, dried beans, cereals

Lower Gastrointestinal Tract Infections

Definition

The major manifestation of lower GI infection is diarrhea, the passage of liquid stool.

Etiology

1. Bacterial causes of diarrhea
    a. *Campylobacter*, *Salmonella*, and *Shigella* are the most common causes of bacterial diarrhea in children in the United States. *Campylobacter* and *Shigella* are organisms that invade the bowel wall. *Salmonella typhi*, also an invasive organism, usually invades the small bowel but does not usually cause diarrhea. Most non-*typhi* *Salmonella* tend to be less invasive.
    b. *Yersinia enterocolitica* has been associated with several foodborne outbreaks of diarrhea. Affected persons may present with mesenteric adenitis mimicking appendicitis.
    c. *Vibrio* spp., including *Vibrio cholera* (the El Tor strain is found in the United States) are causes of diarrheal illness often associated with the ingestion of seafood.
    d. *Escherichia coli*, in addition to being a common commensal organism found normally in all stools, is the causative agent for a variety of diarrheal illnesses.
        (1) Enterotoxigenic *E. coli* (ETEC) produces enterotoxins that lead to a secretory diarrhea. This pathogen is associated with most cases of travelers' diarrhea. It should be suspected as a cause of diarrhea in the returning traveler.
        (2) Enteropathogenic *E. coli* (EPEC) is a bowel-invasive organism (like *Campylobacter* or *Shigella*). This organism is also associated with diarrhea in infants in underdeveloped countries.
        (3) Enterohemorrhagic *E. coli* (EHEC) is associated with hemorrhagic colitis and the development of the hemolytic-uremic syndrome. These *E. coli* are often of the serotype O157 and produce a toxin that causes the endovascular hemolytic-uremic syndrome.
    e. *Aeromonas* and *Plesiomonas* are both associated with the development of diarrhea in children but are less common than those mentioned above.
    f. *Clostridium difficile* produces a toxin that causes diarrhea and/or pseudomembranous colitis. This organism is seen in patients treated with antibiotics and is a common cause of antibiotic-associated colitis.
2. Viruses are the most common causes of diarrhea in children.
    a. Rotavirus is primarily a winter illness that is seen most often in children between 6 and 24 months of age.
    b. Adenoviruses types 40 and 41 are common causes of sporadic diarrhea in children younger than 2 years of age.
    c. The Norwalk agent and related caliciviruses (Hawaii agent, Snow Mountain agent, W-Ditching agent) cause year-round epidemics in both children and adults.
    d. The astroviruses have occasionally been associated with diarrheal disorders. Although other viruses, including coronaviruses and enteroviruses, may be isolated from the stool, their role in causing diarrhea is not established.
3. Several parasites, including *Giardia* spp., *Cryptosporidium* spp., and amebas, are common causes of diarrhea (see Chapter 107).

Pathogenesis

Acute dehydration from diarrheal illness is thought to be the most common cause of death in children younger than 3 years of age (predominantly in underdeveloped countries).

Clinical Findings

1. Physical examination of the child with diarrhea should include a careful assessment of the degree of dehydration.
2. Aside from fever and abdominal tenderness, physical examination is unrevealing in most cases of infectious diarrhea.

Laboratory Findings

1. Examination of the stool is helpful in assessing the probable etiologic agent and is important to determine whether antibiotics should be given. However, stool examination is positive for fecal leukocytes in only 60 to 70 per cent of cases of bacterial diarrhea and does not make an etiologic diagnosis.

TABLE 95–2. LOWER GASTROINTESTINAL TRACT INFECTIONS

ORGANISM	STOOL EXAMINATION	METHOD OF IDENTIFICATION
Bacteria		
Campylobacter, Salmonella, Shigella	Fecal polymorphonulear leukocytes are common because these organisms are invasive	Use CampBA-selective media (at 42°C) and *Salmonella-Shigella* medium
Yersinia enterocolitica	PMNs may be seen	Use CIN (cefsulodin-ingrasan-novobiocin) agar with cold enrichment
Vibrio species	No fecal leukocytes in cases of cholera or other secretory diarrheas	TCBS (thiosulfate citrate bile salts sucrose) agar is required
Escherichia coli	EPEC and EHEC are associated with leukocytes on stool examination; ETEC is a secretory diarrhea	*E. coli* O157:H7 (cause of EHEC) can be isolated with sorbitol-MacConkey medium; notify laboratory
Clostridium difficile	PMNs in the stool are expected in cases of colitis	Diagnosis is routinely made by identification of the *C. difficile* toxin
Viruses		
Rotavirus	No PMNs are seen; lymphocytes or monocytes may be present	Diagnosis is by ELISA of stool
Adenovirus	No PMNs; lymphocytes or monocytes may be present	Diagnosis is by ELISA of stool
Norwalk and other caliciviruses	No PMNs; lymphocytes or monocytes may be present	No commercial test (ELISA under development)

PMNs, polymorphonuclear neutrophils.

2. Many bacterial pathogens require special culture conditions for identification. Certain viruses can often be identified by enzyme-linked immunosorbent assay (ELISA) of the stool (Table 95–2)

Treatment

1. Diarrhea caused by invasive bacteria (such as *Campylobacter* and *Shigella*) should always be treated.
2. *S. typhi*, the causative agent of typhoid fever, a potentially lethal invasive infection, should be treated with antibiotics. Non-*typhi Salmonella* are usually treated in very young children (<1 year), because of a fear of osteomyelitis and disseminated disease, and in very old patients, because of the association of *Salmonella* with vascular disorders and aneurysms. Healthy adolescents and young adults need not be treated for non-*typhi Salmonella* in a stool culture. Follow-up cultures to ensure eradication of the organism are recommended.
3. No treatment is currently available for viral diarrheas aside for supportive care; most noninvasive bacterial and viral diarrheas resolve if the patient receives adequate food and drink from an uncontaminated source.
4. Treatment of other diarrheal pathogens depends on the resistance pattern from the area where the organism was acquired. Some general guidelines are listed in Table 95–3.

Key Treatments: Lower GI Tract Infections

- Correct dehydration and metabolic disturbances, if any
- Antimicriobial therapy for selected bacteria

Prevention

1. Because most infectious diarrheas are spread by the fecal-oral route, good hygienic practices and attention to handwashing are key to limiting spread. In daycare, food-handling, and hospital settings, removal of the index case until the patient is no longer infectious is the first step in preventing epidemics.
2. *C. difficile* diarrhea is associated with antibiotic use and may resolve after withdrawal of antibiotics.
3. Two new typhoid vaccines. a purified polysaccharide and an oral attenuated *S. typhi* vaccine, are now available for children older than 2 and older than 6 years of age, respectively. Vaccination is currently recommended only for travelers to areas in which there is a high risk of infection with *S. typhi*.

Bibliography

Butterton JR, Calderwood SB: Acute infectious diarrheal diseases and bacterial food poisoning. *In* Isselbacher KJ, Braunwald E, Wilson JD, et al (eds): Harrison's Principles of Internal Medicine, 13th ed. New York, McGraw-Hill, 1994.

TABLE 95–3. ANTIMICROBIAL THERAPY FOR DIARRHEAL PATHOGENS

BACTERIUM	ANTIMICROBIAL	DOSE
Salmonella, Shigella, Yersinia, Aeromonas, and *Plesiomonas*	Trimethoprim-sulfamethoxasole	5 mg/kg of trimethoprim (maximum 160 mg) and 25 mg/kg of sulfamethoxasole (maximum, 800 mg) given twice daily
Campylobacter	Erythromycin	10 mg/kg (maximum, 750 mg) PO four times daily
Clostridium difficile	Metronidazole	7 mg/kg (maximum, 500 mg) PO three times daily

Hoshiko M: Laboratory diagnosis of infectious diarrhea. Pediatr Ann 1994;23:570–574.
Laney DW, Cohen MB: Approach to the pediatric patient with diarrhea. Gastroenterol Clin North Am 1993;22:499–516.
Stutman HR: Salmonella, Shigella, and Campylobacter: Common

bacterial causes of infectious diarrhea. Pediatr Ann 1994; 23:538–543.
Thompson SC: Infectious diarrhoea in children: Controlling transmission in the child care setting. J Pediatr Child Health 1994;30:210–210.

96 Osteomyelitis and Septic Arthritis

Robert Finberg

Definition

Bone and joint infections are common causes of morbidity in children. Osteomyelitis is an inflammation of bone that is almost always associated with an infectious microbe, and septic arthritis is an infection of the joint space. Although in some cases (particularly in very young children) an infected bone may discharge bacteria into the joint space, leading to the development of a septic arthritis, these two entities are usually entirely separate disorders. Although viruses may be associated with joint disease, the term septic arthritis usually refers to synovial disease caused by bacteria or fungi.

Etiology

1. Osteomyelitis may be caused by hematogenous spread of bacteria through the bloodstream, by direct invasion from contiguous structures infected by a microorganism, or by direct inoculation (through surgery or trauma).

   a. Acute hematogenous osteomyelitis in children is overwhelmingly a disorder of the lower extremity. Approximately 70 per cent of all cases occur in either the femur or tibia (with almost equal representation by each).

   b. In children younger than 5 years of age, approximately 50 per cent of all osteomyelitis is caused by *Staphylococcus aureus*. Group A streptococci and *Haemophilus influenzae* account for an additional 10 per cent each, and the remaining causes include a variety of gram-positive and gram-negative organisms and occasionally fungi.

   c. Children older than 5 years of age are even more likely to be infected with *S. aureus* (approximately 80% of cases).

   d. Children with hemoglobinopathies (including not only patients with hemoglobin SS phenotype but those with SC, S-Thal, and others) are particularly prone, at ages 18 to 48 months, to the development of recurrent osteomyelitis with gram-negative bacteria—especially *Salmonella* but also *Shigella*, *Escherichia coli*, and *Serratia* spp.

2. Septic arthritis may also be caused by hematogenous seeding, local spread from a contiguous source of infection, or traumatic or surgical introduction of organisms.

   a. Septic arthritis in children is a disorder of large joints: the knee is most commonly involved (38%), followed by the hip (32%), the ankle (11%), the elbow (8%), the shoulder (5%), and the wrist (4%).

   b. Most cases of septic arthritis are caused by *S. aureus*.

   c. Group A streptococci and *Streptococcus pneumoniae* together account for approximately 30 per cent of cases.

   d. *H. influenzae* is a major pathogen in young children who have not been vaccinated with the *H. influenzae* vaccine. Before the widespread use of the vaccine, *H. influenzae* accounted for almost 50 per cent of cases in children younger than 2 years of age and 25 per cent of cases of suppurative arthritis in children younger than 5 years of age. With the use of the *H. influenzae* vaccine, this entity is vanishing.

Epidemiology

1. Group B streptococcus and other nursery pathogens should be considered in neonates.
2. *Neisseria gonorrhoeae* may be seen in neonates and in sexually active adolescents.
3. Adolescent intravenous drug users are at risk for gram-negative septic arthritis.
4. Puncture wounds in patients with sneakers suggest *Pseudomonas,* and cat bites are associated with *Pasteurella multocida* osteomyelitis.

Pathophysiology

1. Osteomyelitis usually results from bacteria deposited in the metaphysis because of the relatively slow blood flow through the capillary bed in this area.

   a. The growing bacteria and accompanying inflammatory exudate usually migrate through the haversian system to the periosteal space.

   b. The increased pressure in the periosteal space may lead to compromise of the vascular system with necrosis of bone: the development of a sequestrum. New bone formed in this site produces an involucrum.

   c. In a few locations the metaphysis lies within the adjacent joint capsule (the proximal femur-hip joint, proximal humerus-shoulder joint, lateral distal tibia,

Acute Osteomyelitis

Fever

Bone pain: in neonates there may be swelling, edema and discoloration over the bone; toddlers or young children may have joint tenderness; most will not walk

Neonates may present with fulminant sepsis or irritability and poor feeding

Septic Arthritis

Fever

Local erythema, swelling, and severe pain on motion of the involved joint

The differential diagnosis includes juvenile rheumatoid arthritis, rheumatic fever, and reactive arthritis (including postinfectious arthritides)

---

ankle joint, and radial neck in the elbow joint). If infection breaks through the metaphyseal cortex in these locations, it will involve the adjoining joint.

2. Septic arthritis, occasioned by the entry of bacteria into the synovial space, results in an influx of inflammatory cells into the joint space. The synovial fluid has glucose and electrolyte concentrations similar to those of plasma and a rich vascular system to supply the synovial membrane, all of which allow for growth of the organism in the joint space.

Clinical Findings

1. The clinical presentation of osteomyelitis varies according to the age of the patient.
   a. Infants or neonates are likely to present with poor feeding or loss of movement of a limb (pseudoparalysis).
   b. Infants may also present with an erythematous, edematous, or discolored limb as a result of injury to the epiphysis.
   c. Toddlers and young infants may be able to describe point tenderness. Osteomyelitis in the lower extremity is often associated with a failure to walk.
   d. Adolescents are likely to present with point tenderness but may present with only a limp in some cases of lower extremity disease.
   e. Chronic osteomyelitis, a disorder usually seen in adults, may be seen in children who are not adequately treated with antibiotics for acute osteomyelitis. This illness is characterized clinically by recurrent episodes of fever with purulent drainage and pathologically by dead or poorly vascularized bone. It is difficult to cure this disease without surgery to remove all dead and infected bone.
   f. Tuberculosis should be considered in patients with an exposure history and a chronic presentation.
2. Patients with septic arthritis present with fever, malaise, and arthralgias.
   a. Physical examination is remarkable for erythema, warmth, and swelling over the involved joint.
   b. Exquisite pain on motion of the joint is the hallmark of the disorder.
   c. Tuberculosis should be considered in patients with chronic disease and a history of exposure or other findings of tuberculosis.

Laboratory Findings

1. Osteomyelitis
   a. An elevated leukocyte count with a left shift, a high erythrocyte sedimentation rate, and a high C-reactive protein value are expected.
   b. Culture of the involved area is usually obtained by a surgical procedure in neonates.
   c. In older children, needle aspiration may be attempted.
   d. Drilling of bone or needle aspiration in older patients is controversial because of the risk of damage to the growing bone.
   e. Blood cultures should be drawn on all children suspected of having osteomyelitis; cultures are positive approximately 60 per cent of the time.
2. Septic arthritis
   a. A joint aspirate for cell count, Gram stain, and culture should be obtained in all case of septic arthritis.
   b. Expected findings in patients with septic arthritis are joint fluid leukocyte counts higher than 10,000 cells/mm³ with a polymorphonuclear leukocyte predominance, a synovial fluid/blood glucose level less than 0.5, and a positive mucin clot test.
   c. Blood cultures should be obtained in all cases of septic arthritis but are positive only about 30 per cent of the time.
   d. Polymerase chain reaction diagnosis of organisms such as *Borrelia* (Lyme disease) or *N. gonorrhoeae* looks promising for the future.

Radiographic Changes

1. Plain films of patients with acute osteomyelitis are usually negative (it takes 7 to 10 days to see bony changes and 3 to 7 days to see abnormalities of intermuscular fat planes).
   a. Technicium scans are positive during the first 24 to 48 hours of infection and are able to define multiple sites of infection. These scans are not useful for neonates or for patients with sickle cell disease.
   b. Magnetic resonance imaging is able to define edema in the marrow and soft tissue and, with the use of gadolinium enhancement, areas of necrotic bone.
   c. Computed tomography scans are useful for defining cortical destruction and bony sequestrations.

Key Laboratory Findings

Osteomyelitis

Positive technicium scan or characteristic findings on magnetic resonance imaging

Needle aspiration or surgical drainage may reveal the organism

Blood cultures positive 60%

Elevated erythrocyte sedimentation rate

Septic Arthritis

No specific x-ray changes aside from swelling

Organism may be seen on aspirate of joint

Blood cultures positive 30%

Elevated erythrocyte sedimentation rate

2. Plain radiographs of septic joints reveal evidence of soft-tissue swelling, such as loss of normal fat lines.

Differential Diagnosis

1. Differential diagnosis of osteomyelitis includes tumors of bone, leukemia, and toxic synovitis (an ill-defined synovitis of unknown cause). Chronic recurrent multifocal osteomyelitis causes chronic recurrent bone lesions which are visible on x-ray studies, do not reveal a microorganism by conventional techniques, and disappear spontaneously. Approximately 20 per cent of cases are associated with palmar pustulosis. Nonsteroidal antiinflammatory agents provide relief of pain.

2. The differential diagnosis of septic arthritis includes viral arthritis (including parvovirus B19 and enteroviruses), leukemia, metabolic disorders that may affect joints (e.g., ochronosis), serum sickness, villonodular synovitis, toxic synovitis, juvenile rheumatoid arthritis, rheumatic fever, and arthritides associated with bowel disorders (ulcerative colitis or granulomatous colitis).

    a. Examination of the joint fluid and appropriate culture is usually necessary to make an etiologic diagnosis.

    b. Arthritis in the knee in a patient exposed to ticks should suggest a diagnosis of Lyme arthritis. This disorder is treated with either doxycycline or amoxicillin (in children younger than 12 years of age).

Treatment

1. Osteomyelitis should be treated with an antibiotic that is effective against the organism diagnosed.

    a. Surgical debridement may be necessary if pus is found on aspiration of bone.

    b. It is essential that any abscess, intramedullary debris, or sequestra be removed. Any contiguous process should also be drained.

    c. Chronic osteomyelitis may be caused by untreated acute disease. Surgery is essential to remove avascular bone. Multiple procedures may be necessary to prevent development of an untreatable process that cannot be cured with antibiotics.

    d. Because failure to eradicate disease initially may lead to poor outcomes (abnormal bone, chronic infection), acute osteomyelitis is usually treated with a prolonged course of antibiotics.

    (1) Convential treatment involves 4 to 6 weeks of therapy. The patient with osteomyelitis caused by *S. aureus* is treated with a semisynthetic penicillin (IV oxacillin or nafcillin at 200 to 300 mg/kg/day in six divided doses) until the patient is afebrile and ambulatory and able to reliably take oral medicines. The remainder of the course is completed with an oral preparation of cephalexin (25 to 50 mg/kg/day) or dicloxacillin (12 to 25 mg/kg/day). In patients younger than 5 years of age (particularly if they have not been vaccinated against *H. influenzae*), treatment with an agent with activity against *H. influenzae* (e.g., cefuroxime) should be considered until culture results are available.

    (2) Measurement of serum bactericidal levels (if available) has predictive value in determining which patients will relapse and is helpful to ensure that the patient is taking the medicine. Early experience with unmonitored oral treatment of osteomyelitis in children was marked by an high failure rate (19%), stressing the importance of ensuring compliance with any oral regimen.

    (3) Abbreviated courses of therapy (<4 weeks) have been recommended by some authorities for patients whose erythrocyte sedimentation rate returns to normal on treatment.

    (4) Home IV therapy should be considered for noncompliant patients and those unable to take oral medicines.

2. Septic arthritis in infants and young children is usually diagnosed by an open surgical procedure. Because this is a rapidly progressive illness that can cause permanent damage to the joint, a diagnostic procedure should be performed without delay.

    a. Antibiotics are usually given immediately after a diagnostic procedure has been performed.

Key Treatments

• Antibiotics

• Surgical drainage

    b. Treatment with an agent active against *Staphylococcus* is mandatory until final culture data are available. In children younger than 5 years of age, an antibiotic with activity against *H. influenzae* should be included until final culture results are available.

c. Antibiotic treatment should be geared to the sensitivities of the organism involved.

d. Failure rates in acute septic arthritis are lower than those for osteomyelitis (using the drug regimens outlined above), but most patients are treated with a combination of intravenous followed by oral antibiotics, as described for osteomyelitis.

Prevention

The use of the *H. influenzae* vaccine should result in fewer cases of septic arthritis caused by this organism.

Bibliography

Dagan R: Management of acute hematogenous osteomyelitis and septic arthritis in the pediatric patient. Pediatr Infect Dis 1993;12:88–93.

Jaramillo D, Treves ST, Kasser JR, et al: Osteomyelitis and septic arthritis in children: Appropriate use of imaging to guide treatment. Am J Radiol 1995;165:399–403.

Nocton JJ, Dressler F, Rutledge BW, et al: Detection of *Borrelia burgdorferi* DNA by polymerase chain reaction in synovial fluid from patients with Lyme arthritis. N Engl J Med 1994;330:229–234.

Sonnen GM, Henry NK: Pediatric bone and joint infections: Diagnosis and antimicrobial management. Pediatr Clin North Am 1996;43:933–947.

Syrogiannopoulos GA, Nelson JD. Duration of antimicrobial therapy for acute suppurative osteoarticular infections. Lancet 1988;1:37–40.

97 Meningitis

Jeffrey Bergelson

Inflammation of the meninges can have variety of causes. *Bacterial* meningitis is diagnosed by routine culture of the cerebrospinal fluid (CSF) and is most often characterized by a neutrophilic inflammatory response. *Aseptic* meningitis, with negative bacterial cultures and most often a lymphocytic response, may be caused by a variety of infectious agents, including mycobacteria, viruses, and fungi, or it may be noninfectious. Because of its potential to cause lasting neurologic damage, meningitis must be recognized and treated promptly.

Etiology

1. Bacterial meningitis
   a. Newborns: group B streptococcus; *Escherichia coli* and other enteric gram-negative rods; *Listeria monocytogenes*
   b. Infants and young children (2 months to 4 years): *Haemophilus influenzae* type b; *Streptococcus pneumoniae*; *Neisseria meningitidis*
   c. School-age children and adolescents: *S. pneumoniae* and *N. meningitidis*
2. Viral meningitis: enteroviruses (echovirus, poliovirus, coxsackievirus), herpes simplex virus, adenoviruses, lymphocytic choriomeningitis virus, arboviruses
3. *Mycobacterium tuberculosis*
4. Spirochetes: *Treponema pallidum* (syphilis); *Borrelia burgdorferi* (Lyme disease); *Leptospira interrogans*
5. Fungi: *Cryptococcus neoformans*; *Coccidioides immitis*; *Histoplasma capsulatum*
6. Rickettsiae: Rocky Mountain spotted fever; typhus; Q fever
7. Parasites: Amebas (*Naegleria fowleri*, *Acanthamoeba*); *Angiostrongylus cantonensis*

8. Parameningeal infection: A clinical picture suggesting meningitis may also result from brain abscess, spinal epidural abscess, or sinusitis
9. Noninfectious
   a. Systemic disorders: lupus, sarcoidosis
   b. Tumors
   c. Intracranial thrombosis or embolism
   c. Chemical irritation: intrathecal injections; epidermoid cysts
   d. Drugs: nonsteroidal antiinflammatory agents; trimethoprim-sulfa; high-dose intravenous immunoglobulin.

Epidemiology

The primary agents of bacterial meningitis—pneumococci, meningococci, and *H. influenzae* type b—colonize the upper respiratory tract and are transmitted from person to person by respiratory droplets. Invasive disease is most common in young children, who fail to mount protective antibody responses to polysaccharide antigens in the bacterial capsule. Patients with defects of humoral immunity or with splenic dysfunction are also at increased risk of meningitis caused by these organisms.

History

1. *Age of the patient*—The incidence of bacterial meningitis is highest in infants and young children. Although adults and older children with meningitis often complain of headache and stiff neck, young children are likely to present with less specific symptoms such as irritability or lethargy. Symptoms in newborns may be nonspecific (e.g., poor feeding, abnormal cry) or potentially misleading (e.g., isolated tachypnea or vomiting).

2. *Duration of symptoms*—Bacterial and viral meningitis are acute in onset, and subacute or chronic presentations should lead to consideration of other causes, including *M. tuberculosis* or fungi. Tuberculous meningitis evolves over 1 to 3 weeks, beginning with headache and low-grade fever, progressing to lethargy and vomiting, then culminating in coma and death.

3. *Other illnesses and medications*—Patients with cellular immunodeficiency secondary to steroid use, organ transplantation, or acquired immunodeficiency syndrome are likely to have meningitis caused by *Cryptococcus* spp. (subacute) or by *Listeria* spp. (acute). Patients with antibody deficiency, complement deficiency, or splenic dysfunction have increased risk of sepsis and meningitis from *S. pneumoniae, N. meningitidis,* and *H. influenzae.* Recurrent bacterial meningitis may suggest a CSF leak, whereas recurrent aseptic meningitis may be caused by an epidermoid cyst. Specific inquiries about antibiotic use should be made, since such use may lead to falsely negative bacterial cultures and a mistaken diagnosis of aseptic meningitis.

4. *Specific exposures*—Most children with tuberculosis have been infected by a family member, so it is important, in cases of aseptic meningitis, to identify family members with a history of tuberculosis, skin test conversion, or chronic cough. Lyme disease and rickettsial infection may be suggested by exposure to ticks, and arboviral infection by exposure to mosquitoes. Residence or travel in particular geographic regions may be clues to coccidioidomycosis (southwestern United States) or histoplasmosis (central or southeastern United States). In unusual cases, swimming in fresh water has been associated with acute meningitis caused by *Naegleria.*

Clinical Findings

1. Classic signs of meningitis include fever, headache, photophobia, nausea and vomiting, confusion, and stiff neck. These reflect both meningeal irritation and increased intracranial pressure. Kernig sign (resistance to extension of the knee by the examiner when the patient's leg is held flexed at the hip) and Brudzinski sign (involuntary flexion of the leg and knee when the neck is flexed by the examiner) may be present. Not all patients (and particularly infants) with meningitis have signs of meningeal irritation, and some patients may be afebrile.

2. Younger children are less likely show specific signs of meningeal irritation. In young infants, a bulging fontanelle or high-pitched cry may be evident.

3. The clinical picture may be dominated by signs of sepsis, such as hypotension and disseminated intravascular coagulation.

4. Seizures are common early in the course of bacterial meningitis.

5. Focal neurologic findings may represent intracranial complications of meningitis (including subdural effusion or empyema, venous thrombosis, and brain abscess) and warrant further evaluation. Patients with increased intracranial pressure due to space-occupying lesions may suffer cerebral herniation after lumbar puncture; therefore, patients with focal findings and papilledema should be evaluated by computed tomography (CT) or magnetic resonance imaging (MRI) before lumbar puncture is performed. Antibiotics should be given even if CSF samples have not been obtained.

6. Focal neurologic findings may also result from damage to cranial nerves caused by inflammation, vasculitis, or increased pressure. Bacterial meningitis is a common cause of acquired hearing loss in children. Tuberculous meningitis causes intense inflammation at the base of the brain and may affect multiple cranial nerves.

7. Evaluation of skin lesions may be helpful in diagnosis. Petechial or purpuric lesions are associated typically with *N. meningitidis,* or uncommonly with *H. influenzae,* but may also suggest rickettsial infection such as Rocky Mountain spotted fever. Skin lesions or conjunctivitis in a young infant with aseptic meningitis should lead to consideration of herpes simplex virus.

8. Bacterial meningitis may be accompanied by other focal bacterial infections, including pneumonia and septic arthritis. Noninfectious arthritis resulting from immune complexes may be seen in *H. influenzae* or meningococcal meningitis.

Key Clinical Findings

- Fever
- Nuchal rigidity
- Headache
- Vomiting
- Confusion
- Seizures
- Kernig and Brudzinski signs

Laboratory Findings

1. Examination and culture of the CSF (Table 97–1) are the most important diagnostic tests. In every case, CSF samples should be sent for bacterial culture and Gram stain, cell count, and determinations of glucose and protein. Additional samples may be sent for viral culture, stains and cultures for mycobacteria, and testing for cryptococcal antigen. In some cases, if focal neurologic findings or papilledema is present, it may be prudent to administer antibiotics but to delay lumbar puncture until an intracranial mass lesion has been ruled out by CT scan.

2. Typically, bacterial meningitis is characterized by a marked CSF pleocytosis with a neutrophil predominance, although early in the illness cells may be absent. In viral meningitis (most often caused by enteroviruses), there are typically several hundred lymphocytes, but neutrophils may predominate in the first few hours.

3. CSF profiles in enteroviral meningitis may resemble findings in aseptic meningitis from other causes. Therefore, patients who fail to improve as expected must be evaluated further to exclude treatable disorders such as sinusitis, brain abscess, or meningitis caused by mycobacteria or fungi. In tuberculous meningitis, the CSF profile may be confused with that of viral meningitis;

TABLE 97–1. CEREBROSPINAL FLUID IN MENINGITIS

TYPE OF MENINGITIS	LEUKOCYTES	GLUCOSE	PROTEIN	GRAM STAIN
Bacterial	Neutrophils: hundreds or thousands	Low	High	Often positive
Viral	Lymphocytes: hundreds	Normal	Slightly high	Negative
Tuberculous	Lymphocytes: hundreds	Low	High	Negative
Cryptococcal	Lymphocytes: few or hundreds	Low	Normal or high	Negative
Brain abscess (parameningeal)	Lymphocytes: few	Normal	High	Negative

however, as the illness progresses, repeated CSF examination often shows decreasing glucose and increasing protein. Although CSF glucose may be decreased in viral meningitis, very low values suggest tuberculous or fungal infection or carcinomatous invasion of the meninges. In very young infants, herpes simplex encephalitis may initially be mistaken for enteroviral meningitis; in some cases, other findings suggestive of herpes infection (skin lesions, conjunctivitis) have been dismissed with devastating consequences.

4. Some nonbacterial infections may cause a CSF pleocytosis with neutrophil predominance. These include eastern equine encephalitis (caused by an arbovirus) and meningitis caused by *N. fowleri* (an ameba).

5. Specific antigen tests are available for *H. influenzae* and other bacterial pathogens, although some lack sensitivity and specificity. They may be helpful in cases of partially treated meningitis. The latex agglutination test for cryptococcal antigen is specific and more sensitive than the India ink test. Latex tests for *H. influenzae* and group B streptococcus are helpful if positive.

6. Polymerase chain reaction (PCR) tests are available for enteroviruses and may prove useful in aseptic meningitis. PCR tests for herpes simplex virus are now used commonly. PCR tests for *M. tuberculosis* are being evaluated.

Key Laboratory Tests

- CSF examination for cells
- CSF culture
- CSF chemical analysis
- Viral studies when indicated

Radiographic Changes

1. Conventional radiographs are not helpful in the diagnosis of meningitis.
2. CT or MRI should be performed to evaluate suspected focal complications (e.g., infarction, subdural empyema) or worsening intracranial hypertension. Imaging should be considered in patients with focal neurologic findings, depressed level of consciousness, or persistent fever, and in neonatal meningitis caused by *Citrobacter diversus*, which is frequently associated with formation of brain abscesses.

Treatment

1. *Antibiotic treatment*—Presumptive antibiotic treatment for suspected bacterial meningitis is based on the likely pathogens in each age group (Table 97–2). Antibiotics are then adjusted after culture results are available (Table 97–3). In most cases, patients with suspected aseptic meningitis are treated with antibiotics until the bacterial culture results are reported to be negative.

2. For infants <2 months old, ampicillin plus an aminoglycoside is appropriate therapy for meningitis caused by group B streptococci. Cefotaxime may be substituted for the aminoglycoside if gram-negative meningitis is suspected.

3. In the past several years, immunization of young infants against *H. influenzae* type b has significantly reduced the incidence of meningitis caused by this organism. However, penicillin- and cefotaxime-resistant pneumococci have become an increasing concern. In children older than 2 months, when bacterial meningitis is strongly suspected, vancomycin is recommended for empiric treatment. If resistant pneumococci are not isolated, vancomycin should be discontinued.

4. *Steroids*—Early administration of dexamethasone (preceding or within hours of the initiation of antibiotic therapy) has been shown to decrease hearing loss associated with *H. influenzae*, and its use is recommended by many experts when bacterial meningitis is strongly suspected in children older than 6 weeks. The recommended dosage is 0.6 mg/kg/day divided in four doses (0.15 mg/kg per dose) for the first 2 days of antibiotic treatment. The most likely complication of dexamethasone therapy is gastrointestinal bleeding. Because dexamethasone may interfere with antibiotic penetration into the CSF, and may mask signs of inflammation, a repeat lumbar puncture after 24 to 48 hours should be considered when dexamethasone is used in treatment of pneumococcal meningitis.

5. Patients must be monitored carefully, and physical and neurological examinations must be repeated regularly. Management in an intensive care unit may be necessary to control increased intracranial pressure and ensure ade-

TABLE 97–2. EMPIRICAL ANTIBIOTICS FOR BACTERIAL MENINGITIS

AGE	LIKELY PATHOGEN	EMPIRICAL ANTIBIOTIC
0–2 mo	Group B streptococcus *E. coli* Listeria	Ampicillin + aminoglycoside or ampicillin + cefotaxime
2 mo–5 yr	*H. influenzae* Pneumococcus Meningococcus	Vancomycin + cefotaxime
>5 yr	Pneumococcus Meningococcus	Vancomycin + cefotaxime

TABLE 97–3. RECOMMENDED ANTIBIOTICS BY ORGANISM

ORGANISM	ANTIBIOTIC	COMMENTS
Group B streptococcus	Ampicillin or penicillin ± aminoglycoside	14–21 days
E. coli	Cefotaxime ± aminoglycoside	At least 21 days
Listeria	Ampicillin ± aminoglycoside, trimethoprim-sulfa	14 days
H. influenzae	Ampicillin (if sensitive), cefotaxime or ceftriaxone, chloramphenicol	7–10 days
Pneumococcus	Penicillin, cefotaxime or ceftriaxone, vancomycin, chloramphenicol	10–14 days
Meningococcus	Penicillin, cefotaxime or ceftriaxone, chloramphenicol	5–7 days
M. tuberculosis	Isoniazid + rifampin + pyrazinamide + streptomycin ± others	For fully susceptible organisms, 2 mo of four-drug combination followed by 10 mo of isoniazid + rifampin
Cryptococcus	Amphotericin ± 5-flucytosine	

quate cerebral perfusion. Fluid and electrolyte balance must be monitored, with attention to the possibility of hyponatremia due to inappropriate antidiuretic hormone secretion.

Key Treatments

- IV antibiotics appropriate to age and circumstances
- Consider dexamethasone, 0.6 mg/kg/day

Prevention

1. *N. meningitidis*—Persons closely exposed to patients with meningococcal meningitis may be at risk of infection. Patients with suspected meningococcal infection admitted to the hospital should be placed in respiratory isolation until antibiotics have been administered for 24 hours. The local public health department should be notified early. Household, daycare, and nursery school contacts should receive prophylactic antibiotic treatment. Other candidates for chemoprophylaxis include those who have contacted the patient's oral secretions through kissing, sharing eating utensils, or performing certain medical procedures. The recommended agent is oral rifampin (10 mg/kg per dose every 12 hours for four doses; maximum, 600 mg); a single dose of ceftriaxone (125 mg IM in children, 250 mg in teenagers and adults) is an effective alternative. The index patient should receive chemoprophylactic antibiotics before discharge.
2. *H. influenzae*—Young, unvaccinated children exposed to patients with *H. influenzae* may be at increased risk of invasive infection. The risk is greater in household than in daycare or nursery school contacts. If an unvaccinated child <4 years old has been exposed to a sibling with *H. influenzae* meningitis, all household members, including the index patient, should receive chemoprophylaxis. Rifampin (20 mg/kg per dose; maximum, 600 mg) is given once daily for 4 days. Prophylaxis may be indicated in other circumstances, and additional specific recommendations have been made by the Committee on Infectious Diseases of the American Academy of Pediatrics.
3. *Immunization*—All infants should receive *H. influenzae* type b conjugate vaccine. Children 2 years and older with underlying conditions that put them at particular risk for pneumococcal infections (e.g., sickle cell disease, or functional or anatomic asplenia, nephrotic syndrome, immunosuppression, CSF leaks) should be immunized with 23-valent pneumococcal vaccine. Children 2 years and older with functional or anatomic asplenia, or with deficiencies of properdin or terminal complement components, should receive meningococcal vaccine; unfortunately, the vaccine does not protect against infection by serogroup B meningococci, which are common pathogens in the United States.

Outcome and Follow-up

Children who have recovered from bacterial meningitis may have significant or subtle neurologic sequelae that require later intervention; audiometric evaluation should be performed at the time of discharge from the hospital, and all children should be monitored carefully. In enteroviral meningitis, complete recovery is the rule.

 ## Bibliography

Ashwal S, Perkin RM, Thompson JR, et al: Bacterial meningitis in children: Current concepts of neurologic management. Curr Probl Pediatr 1996;24:267–284.

Peter G (ed): 1997 Red Book: Report on the Committee on Infectious Diseases. Elk Grove, IL, American Academy of Pediatrics, 1997.

Rorabaugh ML, Berlin LE, Heldrich F, et al: Aseptic meningitis among infants less than two years of age: Acute illness and neurologic complications. Pediatrics 1993;92:206–211.

98 Poliomyelitis

Laurence Finberg

Etiology

The cause of poliomyelitis is an enterovirus. There are three types: types 1, 2, and 3.

Epidemiology

1. Spread is fecal-oral. In the recent past, almost universal infection occurred.
2. Incubation period is 3 to 7 days.

Clinical Findings

1. At least 90 per cent of infected individuals are asymptomatic.
2. Low-grade fever and sore throat occur in 5 to 8 per cent of patients.

Key Clinical Findings

- Fever
- Stiff neck
- Head drop
- Tripod sign
- Paralysis

3. Paralytic disease occurs in about 1 in 1000. These patients have fever, stiff neck, head drop, tripod sign (placing hands behind the back on sitting up in bed), and paralysis.
   a. Limb and abdominal muscles may be affected.
   b. Muscles of respiration may be affected.
   c. Bulbar paralysis may occur.
   d. Combinations of the above.

Laboratory Findings

1. Cerebrospinal fluid pleocytosis (10 to 150 cells, polymorphonuclear cells or lymphocytes, depending on stage of illness).
2. Culture of virus from stool or cerebrospinal fluid.
3. Serology.

Treatment

Treatment is supportive and may include use of a ventilator for respiratory muscle paralysis and constant suction for bulbar paralysis.

Prevention

Vaccine (see Chapter 2). There is the prospect for total elimination of the virus in 4 to 5 years.

99 Encephalitis

Jeffrey Bergelson

Encephalitis refers to inflammation involving the brain. In many instances, both brain and meninges are involved, and the term *meningoencephalitis* is appropriate. *Encephalopathy* is a term used to describe cerebral dysfunction, whether or not there is evidence of inflammation.

Etiology

1. Patients with viral encephalitis typically present with a history of fever, headache, vomiting, and altered mental status or convulsions evolving over several days.
2. In most cases, a diagnosis cannot be established on clinical grounds, and often no specific agent is implicated. Almost all of the agents that cause meningitis can cause disease with an encephalitic component. In addition, many cases of "postinfectious" encephalitis follow a seemingly insignificant viral or mycoplasma infection.
3. It is also important to consider noninfectious causes of encephalopathy, including cerebral vasculitis, metabolic abnormalities, Reye syndrome, mass lesions, and intoxications.
4. Discussed below are encephalitides that are clinically distinct or for which specific therapy is available.
   a. Herpes simplex virus is the most common treatable cause of encephalitis. Therapy with acyclovir is effective in reducing mortality and neurologic sequelae. Herpes encephalitis in adults (but not in newborns) characteristically involves the temporal lobes, with focal electroencephalographic (EEG) findings; hypodense lesions are evident on computed tomography (CT) scan but may not be seen early in the illness. Cerebrospinal fluid (CSF) is almost always abnormal, with lymphocytes and red blood

cells present, and with increased protein. In infants, virus is sometimes isolated from the CSF, and characteristic skin lesions may suggest the diagnosis. In adults and older children, CSF viral cultures are almost never positive, and the presence of skin or mucosal lesions has no diagnostic value. Polymerase chain reaction (PCR) analysis of CSF has been shown in some laboratories to be both sensitive and specific in diagnosing herpes encephalitis and is supplanting culture of biopsy material as the definitive diagnostic test.

b. Acute disseminated encephalomyelitis (ADEM) is a postinfectious inflammatory disorder that may follow viral, bacterial, or mycoplasma infections and has been associated with a variety of immunizations. Onset occurs several weeks after the inciting event. Symptoms include fever, headache, vomiting, stiff neck, changes in mental status, and focal neurologic signs. Diagnosis is made by magnetic resonance imaging (MRI), which shows evidence of focal demyelination. Recognition of ADEM is important, because many patients respond to steroid therapy.

c. Cat scratch disease is caused by a rickettsia, *Bartonella* (formerly *Rochalimaea*) *henselae*. Cat scratch encephalitis caused by this organism is uncommon but is distinctive because of its rapid onset and rapid resolution. CSF is often acellular. The diagnosis is suggested by a history of contact with kittens and sometimes by the presence of typical regional lymphadenopathy. Serologic testing for *B. henselae* is available through the Centers for Disease Control.

d. Arboviruses are a heterogeneous group of insect-borne viruses that, in the United States, typically cause encephalitis in the late summer. St. Louis, California, and western and eastern equine encephalitis viruses are transmitted by mosquitoes; Colorado tick fever is transmitted by ticks. In endemic areas, public health authorities survey mosquito populations and sentinel animals such as horses for arboviral infection. In most viral encephalitides, CSF shows a moderate number of lymphocytes. Eastern equine encephalitis is unique in that it causes neutrophilic pleocytosis. Although there are no clinical data, this virus shows in vitro sensitivity to ribavirin.

e. Cysticercosis is caused by encysted larvae of the pork tapeworm, *Taenia solium*. The infection is rare in the United States but common in Mexico, Central and South America, India, and Southeast Asia. Symptoms depend on the locations of the cysts. Seizures are most common, but hydrocephalus and mass effects are also frequently seen. On CT or MRI scan, multiple cysts may be evident, with areas of surrounding inflammation; with time, these shrink and calcify. Specific serologic tests are available, but they are most sensitive when multiple cysts are present. Therapy with praziquantel or albendazole is effective but may transiently cause exacerbation of inflammation and symptoms.

f. Toxoplasmosis causes subacute focal encephalitis in patients with cellular immunodeficiency. Patients present with headache, altered mental status, and focal neurologic signs. Typically, CT scans show multiple lesions that are enhanced with the use of contrast medium. Specific diagnosis requires biopsy, but in a patient who shows serologic evidence of *Toxoplasma* infection, response to a 10- to 14-day therapeutic trial of pyrimethamine plus sulfadiazine or clindamycin may obviate the need for invasive procedures.

g. Progressive multifocal leukoencephalopathy is a demyelinating disease seen in immunocompromised patients (usually adults) infected with the JC virus. Clinical signs include visual changes, motor weakness, and dementia. Lesions typically involve the periventricular white matter.

h. Subacute sclerosing panencephalitis is a rare sequela of measles. Its hallmarks are intellectual deterioration, behavioral changes, and seizures. Isoprinosine and intraventricular interferon-α have shown therapeutic effect.

i. Rabies may present with characteristic signs including agitation, bizarre behavior, and pharyngeal spasm, or it may appear as a paralytic disorder resembling poliomyelitis or Guillain-Barré syndrome. In the United States, human rabies is so unusual that the diagnosis may not be considered, and several recent cases have been mistaken for more routine viral encephalitis. Although no specific therapy is available, antemortem diagnosis—by immunofluorescence analysis of skin or brain biopsy specimens—may be important for decisions about prophylaxis for persons exposed to infectious saliva.

History

1. Inquire about insect exposures (arboviruses, Lyme disease, rickettsiae), contact with cats, or animal bites.
2. Was there a preceding illness suggestive of mycoplasma or a respiratory virus? A recent vaccination?
3. Consider any recent travel. A camping trip to the Rockies may suggest Colorado tick fever; a recent visit to Asia could suggest malaria or Japanese encephalitis.
4. Does the patient have the acquired immunodeficiency syndrome or another immunosuppressive illness? In this setting, opportunistic infections such as *Cryptococcus*, cytomegalovirus, toxoplasmosis, and progressive multifocal leukoencephalopathy become important considerations.
5. Is there a history of animal bite or contact with bats?

Clinical Findings

1. In many cases the patient is febrile and obtunded.
2. The neurologic examination should specifically assess the level of consciousness, evidence of increased intracranial pressure, and focal neurologic signs.
3. The general physical examination should look for evidence of systemic illness, including skin rashes and lymphadenopathy.

Key Clinical Findings

- Fever
- Disturbance of consciousness
- Focal neurologic signs

Laboratory Findings

1. Examination and culture of the CSF, as in meningitis, are important to exclude treatable bacterial and fungal infections. Samples should also be sent for viral culture and for PCR detection of herpes simplex and enteroviruses.
2. The need for brain biopsy to confirm the diagnosis of herpes encephalitis has been controversial. Many clinicians have chosen to use empiric acyclovir rather than subject patients to the low but demonstrated risk of biopsy. However, in some cases, other treatable illnesses—including bacterial, fungal, and tuberculous infections—have mimicked herpes encephalitis and have been diagnosed only after biopsy. The availability of a sensitive and specific PCR-based diagnostic test for herpes may suggest a role for biopsy in the management of patients with focal encephalitis with negative PCR results.
3. In the proper setting, serologic testing for other viral pathogens may be useful. For many of the arboviruses, specific immunoglobulin M can be detected approximately 1 week after symptoms begin.
4. A tuberculin skin test (purified protein derivative, PPD) should be performed in all patients who are encephalopathic and febrile.

Key Laboratory Tests

- CSF examination
- Serologic test
- CT/MRI scans
- Tuberculin skin test (PPD)

Radiographic Changes

1. CT and MRI imaging are important to exclude brain abscess and mass lesions, demonstrate focal lesions suggestive of herpes, and detect evidence of demyelination.

A normal CT scan early in the disease does not exclude the possibility of herpes encephalitis, and repeat scans may be necessary.
2. EEG is more sensitive than CT for demonstrating focality early in the course of herpes encephalitis.

Treatment

1. Most patients with encephalitis are treated with antibiotics until bacterial cultures are negative, and with acyclovir unless the diagnosis of herpes encephalitis has been excluded.
2. In infants, the acyclovir dose for herpes encephalitis is 15 to 20 mg/kg every 8 hours. In older children and adults, the dose is 500 mg/m^2 every 8 hours. Because relapses have been reported after a 10-day course, acyclovir therapy is continued for 14 to 21 days.
3. Supportive care includes control of seizures, therapy for cerebral edema, and airway management in comatose patients.

Key Treatment

- Acyclovir for herpes simplex
- Supportive

Bibliography

Deresiewicz RL, Thaler SJ, Hsu L, et al: Clinical and neuroradiographic manifestations of eastern equine encephalitis. N Engl J Med 1996;336:1867–1874.

Peter G (ed): 1997 Red Book: Report on the Committee on Infectious Diseases. Elk Grove, IL, American Academy of Pediatrics, 1997.

Lakeman FD, Whitley RJ, and the National Institute of Allergy and Infectious Diseases Collaborative Antiviral Study Group: Diagnosis of herpes simplex encephalitis: Application of polymerase chain reaction to cerebrospinal fluid from brain-biopsied patients and correlation with disease. J Infect Dis 1995;171:857–863.

100 Brain Abscess

Jeffrey Bergelson

Brain abscess is a suppurative infection within the brain parenchyma. Brain abscesses can arise from spread of a local infection, particularly sinusitis or otitis; after trauma or surgery; or by hematogenous spread from another focus of infection. In patients with cyanotic congenital heart disease, bacteria in the bloodstream may reach the brain after bypassing the normal filtering activity of the pulmonary circulation. Because its clinical presentation is varied, brain abscess must be considered in children with neurologic symptoms, particularly in those with predisposing conditions.

Etiology

1. The organisms most often isolated from brain abscesses are microaerophilic and anaerobic streptococci and anaerobic gram-negative rods.
2. Brain abscesses occurring after trauma or surgery are likely to involve *Staphylococcus aureus,* and those associated with otitis often involve gram-negative rods.

Pathophysiology

Predisposing factors can be identified in most children with brain abscess. Recognition of these may lead the clinician to consider the correct diagnosis. The following conditions predispose to the development of brain abscess in children:

1. *Cyanotic congenital heart disease*—This is the most common underlying condition in children. It is presumed that bacteria in the bloodstream reach the brain after bypassing the filtering effect of the lungs. Intrapulmonary arteriovenous fistulas (as seen in hereditary hemorrhagic telangiectasia) also predispose to brain abscess.
2. Chronic sinusitis, otitis, or mastoiditis.
3. Penetrating head trauma or recent craniotomy.
4. Pulmonary infection (abscess, bronchiectasis, cystic fibrosis).
5. Bacterial endocarditis.
6. *Meningitis*—Brain abscess may complicate meningitis, particularly in neonates. In older children, subdural empyema is more common.
7. *Cellular immune defect*—Patients with cellular immune defects may have abscesses caused by opportunistic organisms, including *Cryptococcus*, *Listeria*, and *Toxoplasma*.

Clinical Findings

1. The classic triad is fever, headache, and focal neurologic deficit, but all three features are present in only a minority of patients. Vomiting and seizures are common. Papilledema is seen in some but not all patients.
2. Meningitis may be suspected in patients in whom neck stiffness is a prominent finding and encephalitis in those with acutely altered mental status or seizures.
3. Epidural abscess or subdural empyema may cause fever and neurologic deficits; like brain abscess, they are seen as complications of sinusitis or otitis.
4. If fever is absent, particularly when symptoms have developed slowly, brain abscess can be mistaken for tumor.

Key Clinical Findings

- Disturbance of consciousness
- Fever
- Headache
- Vomiting
- Focal neurologic signs

Laboratory Findings

1. Lumbar puncture should not be performed when brain abscess is suspected, because of the well-documented risk of herniation. Cerebrospinal fluid findings are not diagnostic.

Key Laboratory Test

- Culture of abscess fluid

2. Bacteriologic diagnosis is made by culture (anaerobic and aerobic) of abscess fluid or, sometimes, by blood cultures.

Radiographic Changes

1. Computed tomography (CT) and magnetic resonance imaging (MRI) studies are the essential diagnostic tests. The characteristic CT finding is a spherical hypodense lesion with a contrast-enhancing rim and surrounding edema. Delayed scanning after administration of contrast material may help distinguish the early lesions of cerebritis from a mature encapsulated abscess.
2. Radiologic evaluation of the sinuses, as well as chest x-ray films, are helpful to identify contributing foci of infection.

Treatment

1. Treatment includes administration of antibiotics, surgery, and management of increased intracranial pressure.
2. Presumptive therapy combines penicillin G in high doses (250,000 to 400,000 U/kg/day, divided in six daily doses) with chloramphenicol (75 to 100 mg/kg/day divided in four doses). In some centers, metronidazole (30 mg/kg/day, divided in three doses) is substituted for chloramphenicol. Prolonged antibiotic courses are given, often combining a month or more of intravenous therapy with several months of oral therapy.

    a. In brain abscesses associated with otitis, gram-negative aerobic rods—particularly *Proteus* spp.—have often been isolated. For this reason, some experts recommend an empiric regimen of cefotaxime and metronidazole.

    b. After trauma or neurosurgery, infections are often caused by *S. aureus.* In these cases, oxacillin or nafcillin should be added.

3. Most patients with brain abscess are treated surgically, with aspiration, drainage, or excision. However, patients are also treated successfully with antibiotics alone. The decision to intervene surgically is influenced by the clinical presentation and the number, size, and locations of the lesions. Large abscesses causing increased intracranial pressure may necessitate emergency surgery. Early cerebritis, or abscesses that are small, numerous, or not easily accessible, may warrant a trial of antibiotics alone. Whether or not surgery is performed, patients must be monitored clinically and with repeated CT scans until the lesions have resolved.

Key Treatments

- Antibiotics
- Surgical drainage (selective)

Bibliograpy

Peter G (ed): 1997 Red Book: Report on the Committee on Infectious Diseases. Elk Grove, IL, American Academy of Pediatrics, 1997.

101 Endocarditis

Jeffrey Bergelson

Infectious endocarditis is initiated when microorganisms present in the bloodstream adhere to the endocardial surfaces of the heart. Most organisms adhere only where mechanical stress—induced most commonly by turbulent blood flow—has led to the deposition of a thrombus composed of platelets and fibrin. Once such a thrombus has formed, transient bacteremia, even with nonvirulent organisms, may result in infection.

Etiology

Infectious endocarditis is caused by a variety of bacterial and fungal pathogens (Table 101–1).

Epidemiology

1. In adults, valves damaged by rheumatic fever or athero-sclerotic disease are commonly involved. In children, most cases of endocarditis occur in patients with congenital heart malformations, including tetralogy of Fallot, ventricular septal defect, and aortic stenosis. Prosthetic valves and graft material are highly susceptible to infection, and many cases occur after surgical repair.
2. Bacteremia occurring after dental procedures or instrumentation of the genitourinary or gastrointestinal tract, or secondary to a remote focus of infection, may result in infection of susceptible valves.
3. Central venous catheters may traumatize the valvular endothelium and serve as a nidus for bloodstream infection.
4. Intravenous drug abuse predisposes to infection, particularly of the right heart valves.

Clinical Findings

1. *Presentation*—Symptoms in endocarditis are related to sepsis, valvular incompetence, embolic phenomena, and the generation of immune complexes.
   a. In *subacute* endocarditis, patients may be ill for a month or longer, with low-grade fever and fatigue. There may be slowly worsening congestive failure, or there may be no symptoms referable to the heart; most patients have an underlying valvular disorder, and changing murmurs are rarely evident. The clinical picture may be dominated by a sudden embolism or by arthritis or nephritis.
   b. In *acute* endocarditis, fulminant sepsis may bring patients to medical attention within a few days of the onset of symptoms. Rapid destruction of a valve may result in a new regurgitant murmur.
   c. In intravenous drug abusers, infection often involves the right heart (tricuspid valve); these patients may present with pulmonary symptoms related to emboli.
2. *Specific signs and symptoms*
   a. Fever, often low-grade, is present in most but not all patients with endocarditis and is accompanied by malaise, anorexia, and night sweats. High fever, chills, and toxicity are more typical in acute disease.
   b. Cardiac signs and symptoms include congestive failure, chest pain, and arrhythmias.
   c. Neurologic complications include stroke, cerebritis, meningitis, vasculitis, mycotic aneurysms, and brain abscess.

TABLE 101–1. MICROBIOLOGY OF ENDOCARDITIS

ORGANISM	FREQUENCY	CLINICAL SETTING
Viridans streptococci	Common	Subacute disease
		Abnormal valve
		After dental procedure
Staphylococcus aureus	Common	Acute disease
		Normal or abnormal valve
		After bacteremia associated with soft-tissue infection
		After cardiac surgery
		In drug addicts
Staphylococcus epidermidis	Common	Prosthetic valve
		Otherwise uncommon
Enterococcus	Uncommon	Acute or subacute
		Normal or abnormal valve
Fastidious gram-negative organisms: HACEK*	Uncommon	Subacute, abnormal valve
Gram-negative bacilli	Uncommon	Prosthetic valve after cardiac surgery
		Drug addicts, burn patients
Pneumococcus, group A streptococcus	Rare	Acute disease
Fungi (*Candida, Aspergillus*)	Uncommon	Intravenous drug abuser
		Prosthetic valve
		Immunocompromised patients
		Central venous catheter
		Prolonged antibiotic therapy

HACEK, *Haemophilus* species, *Actinobacillus actinomycetemcomitans, Cardiobacterium hominis, Eikenella corrodens, Kingella kingae.*

d. Skin manifestations are common. *Petechiae,* involving the extremities, conjunctivae, and oral mucosa, and *splinter hemorrhages,* red-brown lines visible beneath the distal nails, are common but are also seen in normal people. *Osler nodes,* small, painful red-blue nodules on the tufts of the fingers, and *Janeway lesions,* painless purple macules on the soles of the feet, are less frequently seen but are quite specific.

e. Musculoskeletal complaints include back pain, arthralgias, and synovitis.

f. Splenomegaly is common in patients with prolonged symptoms.

g. Nephritis is common but usually asymptomatic.

Key Clinical Findings

- Fever
- Heart failure
- Petechiae
- Osler nodes
- Janeway lesions
- Splenomegaly

Laboratory Evaluation

1. The hallmark of endocarditis is sustained bacteremia, and blood culture is the essential diagnostic tool. Unless antibiotics have been administered in the preceding 2 weeks, one of the first two blood cultures will be positive for the causative organism in 95 to 100 per cent of culture-proven cases.

   a. In nontoxic patients, three or four sets of blood cultures can be drawn over 24 hours. If the patient has received antibiotics, it is desirable to draw additional cultures on subsequent days before beginning therapy.

   b. In acute endocarditis, three or four independent blood cultures should be drawn 10 to 20 minutes apart before antibiotic treatment is begun.

   c. Some of the bacteria that cause endocarditis are slow-growing and fastidious and may require prolonged incubation or subculturing onto special media; the microbiology laboratory should therefore be informed whenever endocarditis is a diagnostic possibility.

2. Echocardiography is helpful to demonstrate vegetations, assess cardiac function, and diagnose complications such as perivalvular abscess. Transesophogeal echocardiography is more sensitive than transthoracic studies for detecting both vegetations and abscesses, and it is particularly useful for evaluation of prosthetic valves. The absence of vegetations on an echocardiogram does not exclude the diagnosis of endocarditis.

3. Electrocardiography may reveal arrhythmias or conduction defects.

4. Chest radiography is routinely performed. Cranial computed tomography or magnetic resonance imaging may be indicated in patients with neurologic symptoms.

5. Anemia and increased sedimentation rate are very common. Rheumatoid factor may be present in adults. Microscopic hematuria or proteinuria is often seen.

Key Laboratory Findings

- Blood cultures
- Hematuria
- Anemia
- Increased erythrocyte sedimentation rate

Treatment

1. Empiric therapy is directed against the most likely pathogens. After culture results are available, decisions about definitive therapy can be made. Prolonged therapy with bactericidal antibiotics is required to cure endocarditis. Combination therapy is often used to obtain synergistic bactericidal activity.

   a. In subacute endocarditis, empiric therapy with ampicillin plus gentamicin is directed against viridans streptococci and enterococci.

   b. In acute endocarditis or in drug addicts, *Staphylococcus aureus* is a common pathogen, and oxacillin or nafcillin is added to the regimen.

   c. In prosthetic valve endocarditis, vancomycin plus gentamicin is used because of the high incidence of *Staphylococcus epidermidis* infection.

2. Published consensus recommendations for treatment of endocarditis are referred to in the bibliography and should be consulted. A summary of recommendations is presented in Table 101–2.

3. In some cases of endocarditis, blood cultures remain negative. This is usually the result of previous antibiotic therapy or inadequate culture technique.

   a. In some cases, unusual organisms cause endocarditis. These include fungi, *Coxiella burnetii* (the agent of Q fever), *Brucella* spp., *Chlamydia psittaci,* and *Legionella.* Fungal endocarditis should be suspected, in the clinical situations outlined in Table 101–1, if patients fail to respond to empiric antibiotic therapy. Serologic tests and antigen tests may be helpful in diagnosing the other rare diseases.

   b. Occasionally, endocarditis is not caused by infection. Nonbacterial thrombotic endocarditis (marantic endocarditis), a disorder characterized by embolic events, is often associated with malignancies.

Key Treatments

- Antibiotics
- Surgery on indication

4. Surgery may be necessary in some cases. Surgery is clearly indicated if valvular damage leads to congestive

TABLE 101–2. TREATMENT OF INFECTIOUS ENDOCARDITIS

ORGANISM	ANTIBIOTICS	DURATION
Viridans streptococci (penicillin MIC ≤0.1 μg/ml)	Penicillin* *or*	4 wk
	Penicillin *plus* gentamicin	2 wk 2 wk (uncomplicated cases)
(penicillin MIC >0.1 and <0.5 μg/ml)	Penicillin *plus* gentamicin	4 wk 2 wk
Staphylococcus aureus (methicillin sensitive)	Oxacillin* ± gentamicin for MIC >0.1	4–6 wk (gentamicin used only for first 3–5 days)
Staphylococcus epidermidis, prosthetic valve (methicillin resistant)	Vancomycin + rifampin *plus* gentamicin	≥6 wk 2 wk
Enterococci† (or viridans streptococci with penicillin MIC ≥0.5 μg/ml)	Ampicillin + gentamicin (if sensitive to ampicillin) Vancomycin + gentamicin (if resistant to ampicillin)	4–6 wk
HACEK organisms‡	Ceftriaxone or cefotaxime	4 wk
Culture-negative, native valve	Ampicillin + gentamicin	4–6 wk
Culture-negative, prosthetic valve	Vancomycin + gentamicin	≥6 wk
Fungal endocarditis	Amphotericin Surgery	

MIC, minimal inhibitory concentration.
*Vancomycin may be used instead of penicillin in penicillin-allergic patients.
†Many enterococci are now resistant to ampicillin, vancomycin, and aminoglycosides. Therapy for these organisms is not well defined and may depend on surgery.
‡*Haemophilus* species, *Actinobacillus actinomycetemcomitans, Cardiobacterium hominis, Eikenella corrodens,* and *Kingella kingae.*

heart failure or if sepsis cannot be controlled with antibiotics. Fungal infections require surgical treatment. Whether surgery is indicated to prevent embolic events when large vegetations are demonstrated by echocardiography remains controversial.

Prevention

1. Antibiotics are administered to patients at high risk for bacterial endocarditis (primarily those with congenital malformations of the heart, postrheumatic valve disease, or prosthetic valves) to reduce the likelihood of bacteremia after dental or medical procedures. Specific oral and intravenous regimens, depending on the specific procedure and the specific cardiac lesion, have been recommended (see Bibliography).

2. For routine dental procedures likely to cause gingival bleeding in patients at risk, the standard prophylactic regimen is to administer amoxicillin (50 mg/kg PO to a maximum of 2 g) 1 hour before the procedure. No additional dose is necessary. Clindamycin (20 mg/kg PO to a maximum of 600 mg), cephalexin or cefadroxil (50 mg/kg PO to a maximum of 2 g), or azithromycin or clarithromycin (15 mg/kg PO to a maximum of 500 mg) all given 1 hour before the procedure are alternatives for penicillin-allergic patients. Patients unable to take oral medicines can be treated with either clindamycin (20 mg/kg to a maximum of 600 mg) or cefazolin if there is no history of immediate type hypersensitivity to penicillins (25 mg/kg to a maximum of 1 g) given IV 30 minutes before the procedure.

3. Other oral or intravenous regimens may be appropriate for patients undergoing gastrointestinal or genitourinary procedures and for patients considered to be at especially high risk, such as those with prosthetic valves or previous episodes of endocarditis.

Bibliography

Dajani AS, Taubert KA, Wilson W, et al: Prevention of bacterial endocarditis: Recommendations by the American Heart Association. JAMA 1997;277:1794–1801.

Saiman L, Prince A, Gersony WM: Pediatric infective endocarditis in the modern era. J Pediatr 1993;122:847–853.

Starke JR: Infective endocarditis. *In* Feigin RD, Cherry JD (eds): Textbook of Pediatric Infectious Diseases. Philadelphia, WB Saunders, 1992.

Wilson WR, Karchmer AW, Dajani AS, et al: Antibiotic treatment of adults with infective endocarditis due to streptococci, enterococci, staphylococci, and HACEK microorganisms. JAMA 1995;274:1706–1713.

102 Myocarditis

Jeffrey Bergelson

Myocarditis is inflammation of the cardiac muscle. In many cases the pericardium is also involved, and the combined term *myopericarditis* is appropriate. *Cardiomyopathy* refers to myocardial dysfunction with or without inflammation.

Etiology

1. Myocarditis in children is most often associated with viral infections, but many infectious agents can involve the heart. In addition, there are many noninfectious causes of cardiac inflammation.
2. Viral myocarditis is commonly caused by enteroviruses, particularly coxsackieviruses. Because virus is rarely recovered directly from the heart, diagnosis of viral myocarditis is often based on isolation of virus from a stool or throat culture or is made presumptively based on a prodromal respiratory illness. Recent studies using the polymerase chain reaction to detect viruses in myocardial specimens suggest that adenoviruses, as well as enteroviruses, are important causes of this disorder. Myocarditis is associated with many other viral infections, including human immunodeficiency virus.
3. Many nonviral agents may infect the heart, including bacteria, fungi, rickettsiae, and protozoa. In South and Central America, Chagas disease (*Trypanosoma cruzi*) is the most common cause of myocarditis. Myocarditis is an important but uncommon manifestation of Lyme disease.
4. Systemic inflammatory diseases, in particular juvenile rheumatoid arthritis, may cause cardiac dysfunction. Inherited metabolic disorders, such as the glycogen storage disorders, may also cause cardiomyopathy without inflammation.

Epidemiology

1. Viral myocarditis is usually sporadic.
2. Enterovirus epidemics in the late summer and fall are associated with an increased incidence of myocarditis caused by these viruses. The incidence of idiopathic myocarditis shows the same seasonal variation, suggesting that enterovirus infections may go undiagnosed.

Pathophysiology

1. Although cytolytic viruses may damage the heart directly, an ongoing inflammatory response triggered by viral infection appears to be at least as important. Inflammation causes myocardial dysfunction and disturbances of conduction.
2. Pyogenic bacteria and fungi may cause focal infections of the myocardium.
3. In diphtheria, a toxin elaborated by the organism is responsible for myocardial damage.

Clinical Findings

1. Children with acute myocarditis are often febrile, and most have had a flu-like viral prodrome.
2. Decreased cardiac output is reflected by fatigue, dyspnea, pulmonary edema, and, in fulminant cases, shock. The acutely ill child may appear septic. In other cases, onset of congestive failure is more insidious. Chest pain may be ischemic or may suggest pericardial inflammation. Arrhythmias may be clinically silent, or the patient may experience palpitations, syncope, or sudden death.
3. Physical examination typically reveals tachycardia, indistinct heart sounds, and gallop rhythm. Poor peripheral perfusion, pulmonary rales, and hepatomegaly are common in more severe cases.

Key Clinical Findings

- Fatigue
- Tachycardia
- Arrhythmias
- Muffled heart sounds
- Gallop rhythm

Laboratory Findings and Radiographic Changes

1. The chest radiograph may show an enlarged heart and evidence of pulmonary edema.
2. The electrocardiogram most often shows sinus tachycardia, but a variety of arrhythmias, ischemic changes, and voltage abnormalities are seen.
3. The echocardiogram may show dilated chambers and decreased ventricular contractility.
4. The diagnosis is confirmed histologically by endomyocardial biopsy demonstrating lymphocytic infiltration and myocyte damage. It is important to recognize that inflammation is spotty and that evaluation of multiple specimens may be required.
5. Polymerase chain reaction analysis of myocardial specimens is used for identification of viral agents. Viruses may also be cultured from the nasopharynx or from stool.

Key Laboratory Tests

- Chest x-ray
- Electrocardiogram
- Echocardiogram

Differential Diagnosis

1. Myocarditis may not be the first consideration when a febrile patient presents in shock, but it should be suspected if cardiomegaly and pulmonary edema are present.
2. A variety of metabolic and genetic disorders cause cardiomyopathy and myocardial dysfunction in the absence of inflammation.
3. In young infants, congenital malformations of the heart (in particular, anomalous origin of the left main coronary

artery) can cause acute myocardial failure and must be excluded.

Treatment

1. Treatment is supportive. Bed rest is recommended even in mild cases, because exercise has been shown to worsen cardiac damage in animal models. Management of congestive failure, control of arrhythmias, and maintenance of cardiac output often necessitate monitoring and treatment in an intensive care setting.
2. Available antiviral agents are not known to be effective. Although a variety of immunosuppressive regimens have been tried in an attempt to control inflammation and are used in some centers, they have not been shown to provide significant benefit. High-dose immunoglobulin

appeared promising in a preliminary study but has yet to be tested in a randomized clinical trial.

Key Treatment

- Supportive

Bibliography

Gajaarski RJ, Towbin JA: Recent advances in the etiology, diagnosis, and treatment of myocarditis and cardiomyopathies in children. Curr Opin Pediatr 1995;7:587–594.

Lewis AB: Myocarditis. *In* Emmanouilides GC, Riemenschneider TA, Allen HD, Gutgesell HP (eds): Moss and Adams' Heart Disease in Infants, Children, and Adolescents, 5th ed. Baltimore, Williams & Wilkins, 1995.

103 Pericarditis

Jeffrey Bergelson

Definition and Etiology

1. Pericarditis, inflammation involving the visceral or parietal pericardium, has a variety of infectious and noninfectious causes.
2. Infectious pericarditis is most commonly caused by viruses, by pyogenic bacteria, or by *Mycobacterium tuberculosis*.
3. Bacterial (purulent) pericarditis in children is most often caused by *Staphylococcus aureus*, *Haemophilus influenzae*, *Streptococcus pneumoniae*, or *Neisseria meningitidis*. Gram-negative infections occur after cardiac surgery.
4. Noninfectious causes of pericarditis include rheumatic fever, collagen vascular disorders, drug reactions, uremia, and the postpericardiotomy syndrome.

Pathophysiology

1. Infectious agents may reach the pericardium by way of the bloodstream or by direct extension from the lung or mediastinal lymph nodes.
2. The inflammatory response to the infectious agent may result in accumulation of fluid within the pericardial sac. Cardiac tamponade occurs when fluid accumulates rapidly and intrapericardial pressure restricts ventricular filling, resulting in decreased cardiac output.
3. During normal inspiration, expansion of the chest increases the capacitance of pulmonary vessels, leading to decreased cardiac filling and a small decrease in cardiac output and systolic blood pressure (<10 mm Hg). Cardiac tamponade further reduces cardiac filling, exaggerating the inspiratory decrease in blood pressure (paradoxical pulse).

Clinical Findings

1. The most common symptoms of infectious pericarditis are chest pain (often exaggerated by inspiration or motion) and fever.

2. Tachycardia is typical. The pathognomonic auscultatory finding is the pericardial friction rub, which is scratchy, sometimes biphasic or triphasic, and best heard with the patient sitting up and leaning forward.
3. Paradoxical pulse or respiratory distress suggest tamponade.

Key Clinical Findings

- Chest pain
- Tachycardia
- Friction rub
- Distant heart sounds

Laboratory and Radiographic Findings

1. Cardiomegaly on chest radiograph is typical but is not always present. A pulmonary infiltrate may suggest a bacterial cause.
2. Pericardial effusion is most easily demonstrated by echocardiography.

Key Laboratory Tests

- Chest x-ray
- Echocardiogram
- Examination of pericardial fluid
- Blood culture

3. In purulent pericarditis, blood cultures often reveal the bacterial pathogen.
4. Pericardial fluid should be examined and cultured for bacteria, mycobacteria, fungi, and viruses. Viral cultures of the nasopharynx and stool should be performed. In bacterial pericarditis, there is a neutrophil predominance; in viral and tuberculous disease, mononuclear cells are more typical.

Differential Diagnosis

1. Pericarditis should be considered in children with chest pain or cardiomegaly, especially when fever is present.
2. The echocardiogram is important to distinguish pericardial effusion from cardiac chamber enlargement caused by myocarditis or cardiomyopathy.

Treatment

1. Drainage of the pericardial effusion is essential if tamponade is present and in cases of purulent pericarditis.
2. Empiric therapy for bacterial pericarditis should include an antistaphylococcal agent, such as oxacillin, plus a third-generation cephalosporin to treat other likely pathogens. Narrow-spectrum therapy is used once the organism

and its sensitivities have been identified. Antibiotic treatment is usually continued for 3 to 4 weeks.
3. Viral pericarditis is treated with nonsteroidal antiinflammatory agents (NSAIDs).
4. Antituberculous therapy is discussed in the chapter on tuberculosis.
5. All patients with infectious pericarditis should be monitored carefully because of the risk of tamponade.

Key Treatments

- Antibiotics for bacterial cause
- NSAIDs for viral cause
- Drainage for tamponade

Bibliography

Rheuban KS: Diseases of the pericardium. *In* Emmanouilides GC, Riemenschneider TA, Allen HD, Gutgesell HP (eds): Moss and Adams' Heart Disease in Infants, Children, and Adolescents, 5th ed. Baltimore, Williams & Wilkins, 1995.

104 Hepatitis

Robert Finberg

Etiology

1. Although a number of systemic infections may involve the liver, at least five viruses (hepatitis A through E) have been shown to manifest disease primarily in the liver. Hepatitis G virus, a virus identified by molecular techniques, is not clearly associated with clinical hepatitis or carcinoma. The existence of one or more yet unidentified agents is postulated.
2. None of the currently defined viruses (A through E and G) is thought to be responsible for the majority of the

cases of posthepatitis aplastic anemia, suggesting that an as yet undefined agent is responsible for these sporadically occurring cases.

Epidemiology

See the following box for mode of transmission.

Pathophysiology

1. Although the mechanisms by which they enter and spread vary among the different viruses, destruction of liver

Epidemiology of Hepatitis

Type of Hepatitis	Method of Transmission	Incubation Period	Clinical Presentation
A	Fecal-oral, water-based epidemics	25 days	Acute illness, low mortality
B	Blood exposure, sexual contact	75 days	Acute and chronic illness
C	Blood, sexual contact, perinatal, undefined	50 days	Chronic illness
D	Blood products in hepatitis B–carrying patient	35 days	Severe disease in patients with hepatitis B
E	Fecal-oral	40 days	Acute disease usually of mild to moderate severity
G	?	?	Not defined

hepatocytes seems to be key to the pathogenesis of infection.

2. In the case of fulminant hepatitis or chronic viral hepatitis, the host T-cell response may actually result in damage to the liver as well.

Clinical Findings

1. Hepatitis A is an illness spread by the fecal-oral route; it is caused by a picornavirus and has an incubation period of 15 to 45 days. Clinical presentation of disease, as with many picornaviruses, is very dependent on age. In endemic areas (Africa, Central and South America, and central and southeast Asia), virtually all of the population has become infected by age 5 to 10 years, and there is very little clinically manifest illness. In the United States, Scandinavia, and other developed countries, illness is seen in older children and adults. The disorder can be sporadic (accounting for up to 30% of cases of clinically reported hepatitis in the United States) or associated with epidemics (a massive epidemic of hepatitis A in Shanghai in 1988 was attributed to ingestion of raw or undercooked shellfish). It usually has a preicteric stage characterized by malaise and fever, followed by an icteric phase that brings the patient to medical attention. High fevers and flulike illness are typical of the preicteric but not the icteric phase (the patient may actually feel better at the time that jaundice and elevated liver enzymes are manifest). Fulminant disease is uncommon (mortality of 0.2% or less), and the disease does not become chronic, although virus may be shed for as long as 6 months in neonates.

2. Hepatitis B is usually acquired by parenteral exposure to blood or blood products. It has an incubation period of 30 to 180 days. Unlike hepatitis A, it is a chronic disorder, but again age of onset is important in the clinical outcome. More than 90 per cent of newborns who acquire disease develop chronic (usually asymptomatic) infection, but this incidence decreases progressively, so that by age 6 the adult pattern exists (2 to 7% develop chronic, symptomatic illness). Chronic disease is associated with a variety of serum sickness–like illnesses and autoimmune disorders (including periarteritis nodosa and cryoglobulinemia). It is also associated with the development of liver cancer.

3. Hepatitis C is acquired through blood transfusion and has an incubation period of 15 to 150 days. Before the hepatitis C virus (HCV) was identified and screening techniques were developed, this disorder was the major cause of transfusion-related hepatitis after screening for hepatitis B virus (HBV) was initiated in the United States. Despite the importance of transfusion as a means of acquiring hepatitis, more than 40 per cent of hepatitis C cases in the United States today are acquired by some other (unknown) route. Although acute disease has a low mortality (<1%), a high percentage of patients (up to 50% in some series) develop a chronic infection which can be associated with cryoglobulinemia and the development of B-cell lymphomas.

4. Hepatitis D is an incomplete virus; coinfection with HBV is necessary for disease to occur, so the incubation period is not well defined. Infection is usually through needle exposure (parenteral exposure to blood).

5. Hepatitis E is usually acquired through fecal-oral exposure. It has an incubation period of 15 to 60 days and is endemic in central and southeast Asia, northern and western Africa, and parts of Mexico. Hepatitis E carries a mortality rate of 0.2 to 1 per cent (and as high as 20% in the third trimester of pregnancy). Waterborne epidemics have been well described, but sporadic disease also occurs in endemic areas.

6. Hepatitis G was defined on the basis of an isolate from a human with non-ABCDE hepatitis that infected a nonhuman primate. Its epidemiology and clinical features have yet to be defined.

7. Other systemic infections may lead to presentation with liver function abnormalities with or without jaundice.

   a. Epstein-Barr virus (the etiologic agent of infectious mononucleosis) can cause mild elevations in the serum aminotransferases (two to five times normal). Patients usually present with high fever, with or without typical lymphadenopathy. The presence of atypical lymphocytosis should suggest the diagnosis, which can be confirmed with a heterophile or monospot test.

   b. Abnormal liver function tests can be seen in adolescents with cytomegalovirus. A lymphocytosis would be expected, and the diagnosis can be confirmed by culture of urine, blood, or oropharyngeal secretions or by serologic conversion to cytomegalovirus.

   c. A large number of systemic viral infections may be associated with liver function test abnormalities. These viruses, which include rubella, rubeola, mumps, and coxsackieviruses, do not cause jaundice or liver failure outside the newborn period, but they may cause elevations of the serum aminotransferases.

   d. Herpes simplex virus has, rarely, been associated with fulminant hepatitis even in normal individuals (immunosuppression and pregnancy appear to predispose to this illness). Since this disorder is treatable, a high index of suspicion is warranted. Liver biopsy reveals characteristic intranuclear inclusions in this disorder, which are not necessarily associated with herpes infection elsewhere in the body. Severe hepatitis has also been reported with cytomegalovirus and varicella-zoster virus.

   e. Yellow fever, a mosquito-borne virus in which severe disease is marked by the development of jaundice, is seen in tropical America and Africa. The disorder is often epidemic in the savanna regions, where epidemics (spread by *Aedes* mosquitoes) occur toward the end of the rainy season.

8. Many bacterial illnesses (particularly pneumococcal pneumonia and bacterial sepsis) are associated with mild jaundice and/or liver function test abnormalities (elevated serum enzymes).

a. Pulmonary and miliary tuberculosis are associated with liver abnormalities, and liver biopsy may be diagnostic in many cases. Infections such as brucellosis, tularemia, plague, and legionnaires disease are all routinely associated with abnormal liver chemistries.

b. Syphilis (especially secondary syphilis) is associated with liver function abnormalities, and a diagnosis with a VDRL test should be sought.

c. Leptospirosis typically causes a biphasic illness and may be accompanied by central nervous system abnormalities as well as jaundice. Severe muscle tenderness and fever are common. A history of exposure to animals (rats, dogs, cattle, and swine carry the various serotypes) or their excreta should be sought. The diagnosis is usually made on the basis of serology.

d. Q fever, a disease caused by a rickettsia, *Coxiella burnetii*, is uncommon in the United States, but patients may present with jaundice. A history of exposure to animals is usually present.

9. A variety of medicines can cause liver damage. Elevations of liver function tests, particularly without other systemic symptoms, mandate an investigation of the possibility of drug-related liver toxicity.

Key Clinical Findings

- Jaundice

- Right upper quadrant tenderness with or without splenomegaly is expected

- Signs of chronic liver failure (palmar erythema, spider angiomata) are not expected in acute viral hepatitis and should suggest another cause of jaundice

Laboratory Findings

1. Acute viral hepatitis is characterized by elevations in the hepatic transaminases, alanine aminotransferase (ALT) and aspartate aminotransferase (AST), usually to more than eight times normal values.

Key Laboratory Findings: Acute Viral Hepatitis

- Marked elevations of ALT and AST

- Mild elevations of LDH and alkaline phosphatase

- Elevated bilirubin (both direct and indirect)

- Normal or low leukocyte count (a mild lymphocytosis may occur)

2. Only mild elevations of enzymes seen with obstructive disorders (alkaline phosphatase, gamma-glutamyltransferase, and 5′-nucleotidase) are characteristic of acute viral hepatitis. Lactate dehydrogenase (LDH) is also routinely only mildly elevated. Chronic liver injury may be associated with recurrent elevations of transaminases and a progressive downhill course that eventually results in cirrhosis with its accompanying loss of synthetic function. Loss of liver synthetic function (low albumin, inadequate production of proteins important in the coagulation cascade) is an ominous sign.

3. Marked elevations of alkaline phosphatase and 5′-nucleotidase, out of proportion to the elevations in transaminases, suggest a cholestatic picture. In addition to biliary obstruction, such an enzyme profile is characteristically found in cases of bacterial hepatic abscess and amebic abscess.

Radiographic Changes

No characteristic x-ray findings are helpful in diagnosis.

Differential Diagnosis

Differentiating between the various causes of hepatitis is routinely done by serologic techniques.

Differential Diagnosis of Acute Viral Hepatitis	
Diagnosis Viral Hepatitis	**Other Diseases That Could Mimic Viral Hepatitis**
Hepatitis A: Diagnosis is based on an IgM anti-HAV	Other viruses: EBV, CMV, HSV, VZV, yellow fever, rubella, rubeola, mumps, Coxsackievirus
Hepatitis B: Diagnosis is based on an anti–hepatitis B core IgM with or without HBSAg	Bacteria: Sepsis (particularly *Legionella*, other gram-negative bacteria, and pneumococcus), plague, tularemia, leptospirosis, syphilis, tuberculosis
Hepatitis C and D: Diagnosed by the presence of anti-C or anti-D antibodies in the patient	
Hepatitis E: Current diagnosis is one of exclusion (negative serologies for hepatitis A–D) in a patient with a history of travel to an endemic area	Rickettsiae: Q fever (others may also be associated with transient abnormalities in liver function tests)

CMV, cytomegalovirus; EBV, Epstein–Barr virus; HAV, hepatitis A virus; HBSAg, hepatitis B surface antigen; HSV, herpes simplex virus; IgM, immunoglobulin M; VZV, varicella-zoster virus.

Treatment

1. Hepatitis A and E are usually self-limited illnesses.
2. Interferon-α has been used successfully in the treatment of chronic hepatitis caused by hepatitis B and C, but relapse is common when it is stopped. Reverse transcriptase and polymerase inhibitors look promising as future therapies for chronic hepatitis B.
3. Fulminant hepatitis can be treated successfully with liver transplantation. The determination of who should get a transplant is difficult, because two thirds of patients who develop grade 4 encephalopathy survive even without transplantation. Current selection criteria used by transplantation centers include the presence of a long history

of jaundice, rapid onset of encephalopathy, and a poor coagulation profile, all of which are ominous features.

Key Treatments

- Hepatitis A and E—self-limited, no treatment
- Hepatitis B and C—interferon for chronic disease
- Liver transplantation for fulminant disease

Prevention

1. All children should be immunized with the hepatitis B vaccine (a three-injection series is currently recommended).
2. Unimmunized children exposed to HBV (by blood or sexual contact) and infants born to hepatitis B– seropositive mothers should receive hepatitis B immunoglobulin (HBIG) and the first dose of vaccine.
3. The hepatitis A vaccine is recommended for children traveling in endemic areas.

Bibliography

Alter MJ, Gallagher M, Morris TT, et al: Acute non A–E hepatitis in the United States and the role of hepatitis G virus infection. N Engl J Med 1997;336:741–746.

Alter MJ, Nakatsu Y, Melpolder J, et al: The incidence of transfusion associated hepatitis G virus infection and its relation to liver disease. N Engl J Med 1997;336:747–750.

Gregoria GV, Mieli-Vergani G, Mowat AP: Viral hepatitis. Arch Dis Child 1994;70:343–348.

O'Grady J: Management of acute and fulminant hepatitis A. Vaccine 1992;10(Suppl 1):21–23.

Purcell RH: Heptatis viruses: Changing patterns of human disease. Proc Natl Acad Sci USA 1994;91:2401–2406.

105 Sexually Transmitted Diseases

Tamar Barlam

Etiology

1. Gonorrhea (GC), caused by *Neisseria gonorrhoeae*, is often asymptomatic in women but can cause cervicitis, urethritis, and pelvic inflammatory disease (PID). Men are symptomatic with dysuria and urethral discharge. Disseminated infection can occur.
2. *Chlamydia trachomatis* infection is also often asymptomatic in women but can be associated with cervicitis, dysuria, and vaginal discharge. It is the main cause of PID in teenage women. Men have symptoms of urethritis.
3. Herpes simplex virus type 2 (HSV-2) is a common cause of recurrent genital or perirectal ulcers. The primary infection can range from being asymptomatic to causing severe systemic symptoms, extensive genital ulcerations that coalesce, sacral paresthesias, urethral discharge, acute urinary retention, and inguinal lymphadenopathy. Recurrences are characterized by localized, painful vesicles and ulcers without systemic symptoms. HSV-2 proctitis has additional symptoms of tenesmus, rectal pain, constipation, and anal discharge.
4. Human papillomavirus (HPV) serotypes 6 and 11 cause exophytic warts or condyloma acuminata. HPV serotypes 16, 18, 31, 33, and 35 are usually subclinical but are associated with cervical cancer and are the serotypes most common in adolescents. The relative risk of carcinoma in situ secondary to HPV is highest in young women.
5. Syphilis is sexually transmitted when mucocutaneous lesions of primary or secondary disease are present. The primary chancre is painless unless superinfected. Secondary syphilis occurs 6 to 8 weeks after the primary stage, and systemic flulike symptoms, generalized lymphadenopathy, and hepatosplenomegaly may be present in association with cutaneous or mucocutaneous findings. The disease then usually enters a latent phase.

Epidemiology

1. One third of all sexually transmitted diseases (STDs) occur in adolescents. More than 50 per cent of teens are sexually active, and one fourth will acquire an STD before they graduate from high school.
2. GC and chlamydial infections have the highest rates in the 15- to 19-year age group and are the most common STDs in this age period.
3. Adolescent females have cervical ectopy, with columnar endothelial cells located on the exocervix. *N. gonorrhoeae* and chlamydia have a predilection for this tissue. In addition, the squamous metaplasia at the transformation zone increases susceptibility to HPV.
4. Adolescents do not consistently use barrier protection that can prevent STD transmission.

Clinical Findings

1. Genitourinary
   a. Genital ulcers
      (1) Painless ulcerations
         (a) *Syphilis*—Common sites are shaft and glans of penis, labia, and introitus of vagina.
         (b) *Chlamydia*—Lymphogranuloma venereum is caused by *C. trachomatis* serotypes L1, L2, and L3, and the primary papule or herpetiform ulcer is often missed. Painful, enlarged inguinal nodes are the classic presentation.

(2) Painful ulcerations

    (a) HSV-2 causes vesicles as well as ulcers.

    (b) Chancroid, caused by *Haemophilus ducreyi*, begins as a tender, red papule and progresses to a sharply demarcated ulcer with ragged, undermined edges. One third are associated with tender inguinal nodes that can suppurate.

b. Genital growths

    (1) HPV causes acuminate, filiform, or verrucous papules and plaques.

    (2) Molluscum contagiosum, caused by a member of the Poxviridae family, produces asymptomatic growths with umbilicated centers.

c. Vaginitis

    (1) *Trichomonas*—Trichomonal infection is more often symptomatic in women, causing a diffuse, malodorous, yellow-green discharge and vulvar irritation.

    (2) Bacterial vaginosis is caused by the replacement of lactobacilli in the vagina with anaerobes such as *Gardnerella*. White, adherent vaginal discharge with a fishy odor is characteristic.

    (3) *Candida*–Candidiasis causes vaginal itching and a cheesy discharge.

d. *Mucopurulent cervicitis*—Most often caused by GC or chlamydia, it produces a yellow, purulent cervical discharge.

e. *Urethritis*—Patients present with a mucoid or purulent urethral discharge caused by GC or chlamydia in 23 to 55 per cent of cases, by *Ureaplasma* urealyticum in 20 to 40 per cent, and by *Trichomonas* in 2 to 5 per cent.

f. *Epididymitis*—This is a common STD in young men and is most frequently caused by GC or chlamydia.

g. *PID*—One fifth of PID occurs in adolescents. Symptoms are lower abdominal pain, adnexal pain, and cervical motion tenderness caused by endometritis, salpingitis, and/or tubo-ovarian abscess. Etiologic organisms are GC (cultured in 36%), chlamydia (cultured in 45%), anaerobes, group B streptococci, enteric gram-negative rods, and possibly genital mycoplasmas. Tubal scarring, infertility, and ectopic pregnancies are serious sequelae. Inpatient therapy for severe PID should be considered in adolescents, because teens are noncompliant with antibiotic regimens more than half the time.

2. Oral

a. Mucosal lesions

    (1) GC can cause lip ulcerations, gingivitis, glossodynia, and mucosal ulcers.

    (2) Chlamydial infection occasionally causes painless mucositis with erythema.

    (3) HPV can cause multiple small, pink, nodular areas or flat condylomas.

    (4) Syphilis can cause chancres (on lips, tongue, and tonsils), mucocutaneous lesions (in association with the skin rash of secondary syphilis), and gummas.

b. Pharyngitis

    (1) GC pharyngitis occurs in 25 per cent of infected homosexual men, 20 per cent of women, and 7 per cent of heterosexual men. In 5 per cent of patients, it is the only site of GC. There are three syndromes, which produce an exudative pharyngitis resembling streptococcal infection, a viral pharyngitis with erythema, or a normal throat on pharyngeal examination. Most people are asymptomatically infected.

    (2) *Chlamydia* has been reported to cause a mild pharyngitis.

    (3) HSV-2 causes an exudative pharyngitis during primary infection acquired by oral-genital contact.

3. Cutaneous

a. *Syphilis*—During secondary syphilis, a roseolar rash is followed by a papular or maculopapular rash that has a predilection for the palms and soles. Another cutaneous manifestation is condyloma lata—broad, flat papules that are extremely infectious. They are usually found on the labia, anus, and scrotum and in the oral cavity.

b. *Scabies*—Scabies causes pruritus, excoriations, and burrowing lesions. Pruritis occurs secondary to sensitization to the ectoparasite and can take several weeks with first infestation, but it can develop in days with reinfection.

4. Systemic

a. Disseminated gonorrhea

    (1) *Tenosynovitis-dermatitis*—Patients have fever and chills, maculopapular petechial lesions that form pustules, polyarthralgia and erythema, swelling, and pain in the affected tendon group.

    (2) *Suppurative arthritis*—only 30 to 40 per cent of patients have fever; about one third have skin lesions and tenosynovitis. It can be a migratory arthritis, or it can affect a single joint.

b. *Reiter syndrome*—Chlamydia and GC are the most common venereal causes. The syndrome includes arthritis, urethritis, and conjunctivitis.

c. *Fever and adenopathy*—Primary herpes infection, lymphogranuloma venereum, and secondary syphilis can all cause fever and adenopathy. If the patient has a mononucleosis-type syndrome with negative serology for Epstein-Barr virus, acute seroconversion to human immunodeficiency virus should be considered.

Key Clinical Findings

- Genital ulcerations
- Vaginitis
- Cervicitis
- Oral mucosal lesions
- Rash
- Lymphadenopathy

TABLE 105–1. TREATMENT OF STDS OF PROVEN CAUSE

ORGANISM	THERAPY	ALTERNATIVE
Syphilis		
Primary, secondary, early latent (<1 yr duration)	Benzathine penicillin, 2.4 million U IM × 1	Doxycycline, 100 mg b.i.d. × 14 days
Latent syphilis (>1 yr)	Benzathine penicillin, 2.4 million U IM q wk × 3	Doxycycline, 100 mg b.i.d. × 28 days
Gonorrhea*	Ceftriaxone, 125 mg IM × 1	Cefixime, 400 mg × 1, or azithromycin, 2 g × 1
Chlamydia	Doxycycline, 100 mg b.i.d. × 7 days	Azithromycin, 1 g × 1, or erythromycin, 500 mg q.i.d. × 7 days
Herpes simplex virus type 2		
Primary episode	Acyclovir, 200 mg 5 times a day for 7–10 days	
Suppression of recurrences	Acyclovir, 400 mg b.i.d.	
Human papilloma virus	Cytodestructive therapy	
Chancroid	Azithromycin, 1 g PO × 1, or ceftriaxone, 250 mg IM × 1	Augmentin, 500 mg t.i.d. × 7 days, or erythromycin, 500 mg q.i.d. × 7 days
Lymphogranuloma venereum	Doxycycline, 100 mg b.i.d. × 21 days	Erythromycin, 500 mg q.i.d. × 21 days
Trichomonas	Metronidazole, 2 g × 1	
Bacterial vaginosis	Metronidazole, 500 mg b.i.d. × 7 days or 2 g × 1	Clindamycin cream or metronidazole cream intravaginally × 7 days
Scabies	Permethrin 5%, wash off after 8 hr	Lindane 1%, wash off after 8 hr

*Always consider therapy for *Chlamydia* infection.

Laboratory Findings

1. *Ulcers*—Ulcers should be scraped to make a diagnosis. The material can be used to diagnose syphilis by a dark-field examination or by a direct fluorescent antibody test and to diagnose herpes by culture and a direct antigen test. Culture for chancroid can also be sent, although *H. ducreyi* is difficult to isolate.
2. *Cervical/vaginal secretions*—Cervical/vaginal secretions can be tested for *Chlamydia* by culture and nonculture techniques (direct fluorescent antibody, enzyme immunoassay, DNA hybridization assays) and for GC by culture. Vaginal secretions can be examined for *Trichomonas* by looking for motile, pear-shaped, flagellated organisms, and for bacterial vaginitis by checking for the presence of clue cells (epithelial cells dotted with adherent bacteria) and a pH greater than 4.5.
3. *Urethritis/epididymitis*—Urethral exudate should be examined by Gram stain to look for gram-negative diplococci diagnostic of GC and polymorphonuclear leukocytes (five per high-power field is consistent with urethritis). A leukocyte esterase test on the urinalysis supports the diagnosis of urethritis. Urethral exudate culture should be sent. Urine can be used for nonculture techniques to diagnose *Chlamydia* in males and females.

Torsion of the testes, more common in adolescents, must be excluded.

4. Serology for syphilis should always be sent during evaluation for an STD. A nontreponemal test such as the rapid plasma reagin (RPR) test is useful for screening and reflects disease activity. It can be negative early in primary syphilis. A specific treponemal test such as the fluorescent treponemal antibody absorption (FTA-ABS) test should be done to confirm a positive RPR result.

Key Laboratory Tests

- Darkfield examination or DFA test (syphilis)
- Culture of urethral and vaginal secretions
- Serology–RPR for syphilis

Treatment

1. *Documented cause*—Fluoroquinolone alternatives are not included because they are not recommended in people younger than 17 years of age (Table 105–1).
2. *Presumptive therapy* (Table 105–2).

TABLE 105–2. TREATMENT FOR STDS OF PRESUMPTIVE CAUSE

PRESENTATION	CAUSES	THERAPY	COMMENT
Urethritis or mucopurulent cervicitis	Gonorrhea, chlamydia, *Ureaplasma*	Ceftriazone, 125–250 mg IM × 1, then doxycycline, 100 mg bid × 7 days	Azithromycin, 2 g × 1, is an alternative.
Epididymitis	Gonorrhea, chlamydia	Ceftriaxone, 250 mg IM × 1, and doxycycline, 100 mg bid × 10 days	If no pyuria, rule out other diagnoses such as torsion of the testes.
Pelvic inflammatory disease	Gonorrhea, chlamydia, anaerobes, enteric gram-negative rods, group B streptococci	Clindamycin and gentamicin IV, or cefoxitin IV and doxycycline IV or PO	Treatment should continue for 14 days; after defervescence, the course can be completed with doxycycline.

3. *Preventive measures*—Physicians caring for adolescents must be alert to the possibility of STDs. Barrier methods (i.e., condoms) and contraception must be discussed to encourage early and consistent use. In women, pelvic examination should be done regularly. Screening for chlamydia and GC and Papanicolaou (Pap) smears to diagnose carcinoma in situ from HPV are essential. Physicians should have a high suspicion for PID and treat it early to avoid sequelae. Always rule out syphilis with appropriate serology when treating for other STDs.

Key Treatments

- Proven cause—see Table 105–1
- Presumptive cause—see Table 105–2

Bibliography

Beach RK, and the Committee on Adolescence: Sexually transmitted diseases. Pediatrics 1994;94:568–572.

Beck-Sague C, Alexander ER: Sexually transmitted diseases in children and adults. Infect Dis Clin North Am 1987;1:277–304.

Centers for Disease Control: 1993 Sexually Transmitted Diseases Treatment Guidelines and Prevention. MMWR Morb Mortal Wkly Rep 1993;42(RR-14):1–102.

Martin DH, Mroczkowski TF: Dermatologic manifestations of sexually transmitted diseases other than HIV. Infect Dis Clin North Am 1994;8:533–582.

Shafer MA, Sweet RL: Pelvic inflammatory disease in adolescent females. Pediatr Clin North Am 1989;36;513–532.

106 Tuberculosis and Atypical Mycobacteria

Robert N. Husson

Tuberculosis

Definition

Tuberculosis is clinically or radiographically evident disease caused by infection with *Mycobacterium tuberculosis.* Only a small proportion of tuberculous infection results in disease. *M. tuberculosis* infection without disease is defined by a positive tuberculin skin test, without clinical or radiographic evidence of disease.

Etiology

Tuberculosis is usually caused by *M. tuberculosis* and rarely by *M. bovis.* These are closely related, slow-growing, aerobic, acid-fast bacilli that require specialized laboratory procedures for their isolation from clinical specimens.

Epidemiology

1. Following decades of steady decline, the incidence of tuberculosis in the United States began to rise in the late 1980s. This increase has occurred primarily in young adults and children and is the result of three changes that occurred during that decade: decreased public health resources for tuberculosis control, the increased incidence of AIDS, and increased immigration from countries where tuberculosis is prevalent.

2. Tuberculosis remains a major cause of morbidity and mortality in less developed countries. In populations in which HIV and TB are endemic, co-infection is common. The incidence of active tuberculosis is much higher in HIV-infected children and adults infected with *M. tuberculosis* than in those who are *M. tuberculosis*–infected but HIV-uninfected.

3. Multidrug-resistant tuberculosis (MDR-TB) has emerged as a major factor in the resurgence of tuberculosis. In some urban areas, MDR strains have become prevalent and have been responsible for outbreaks in several settings, including hospitals, homeless shelters, and prisons. MDR strains remain uncommon in much of the United States.

4. Risk factors for tuberculous infection:
   a. Exposure to a person with infectious tuberculosis
   b. Residence in a high-prevalence community
   c. Immigration from, or residence in, a household with immigrants from countries with high rates of tuberculosis
   d. Frequent exposure to adults at increased risk for tuberculosis (e.g., HIV-infected persons, homeless persons, IV drug users).

5. Risk factors for tuberculosis following *M. tuberculosis* infection:
   a. HIV infection
   b. Young age (<4 years and especially <1 year of age)
   c. Pharmacologic immunosuppression (e.g., steroids, cancer chemotherapy)
   d. Other causes of immunosuppression (e.g., malnutrition, chronic renal failure, lymphoma)
   e. Clinical or radiographic findings suggestive of tuberculosis.

Pathophysiology

1. Infection by *M. tuberculosis* most often occurs via inhalation of droplet nuclei containing viable bacilli that reach the terminal air spaces of the lung. Gastrointestinal and mucocutaneous sites of infection occur but are rare. Local replication of bacilli and ingestion by macrophages take place at the primary site of infection, followed by lym-

phatic spread to regional lymph nodes and hematogenous spread throughout the body.

2. With the onset of tuberculin skin test positivity (delayed type hypersensitivity) 3 to 10 weeks following infection, cell-mediated immunity and local inflammation result in bacterial killing. This inflammatory response is associated with low-grade fever and may result in the appearance of radiographic abnormalities. In most cases, the host immune response controls the infection at the primary and secondary foci of infection. Viable bacilli may remain in these foci and are the source of reactivation tuberculosis that may occur in later life. When the infection is not controlled by immunity, the primary infection progresses to take any of several courses resulting in disease.

Clinical Findings

1. Most pediatric tuberculosis is the result of progression from the primary infection. Reactivation of latent tuberculosis occasionally occurs in adolescents. *M. tuberculosis* can infect every organ system in the body.

2. Primary tuberculosis
   a. Symptoms are usually mild, with low-grade fever and mild (or absent) cough.
   b. Pleuritis and pleural effusions are common and typically are asymptomatic, though they may result in clinical findings of dullness to percussion and diminished breath sounds.
   c. Intrathoracic adenopathy is more prominent than the lung parenchymal abnormalities on chest radiograph, and pleural abnormalities are often not visible.

3. Endobronchial tuberculosis and collapse-consolidation
   a. Bronchial obstruction may result from granuloma formation within the bronchus or compression from enlarged hilar or mediastinal lymph nodes.
   b. This manifestation is most common in infants and decreases with age.
   c. Cough is often a prominent symptom.
   d. Examination may reveal decreased breath sounds, wheezing, or rales, depending on the extent of obstruction.
   e. Lymphadenopathy and collapse-consolidation are apparent on chest radiograph. Obstructive hyperaeration may occur but is less common.

4. Progressive primary tuberculosis
   a. Failure of host immunity to limit bacterial replication results in enlargement, caseation, and liquefaction of the primary focus, resulting in cavity formation.
   b. Systemic illness—fever, cough, weight loss—is prominent.
   c. Drainage from the primary focus into adjacent bronchi may result in dissemination to other parts of the lung.
   d. Chest radiograph shows consolidation, and cavitation may occur at the primary site of infection; infiltrates may also be present in other lobes of the lung.

5. Tuberculous meningitis
   a. Typically occurs within several months of infection
   b. More common in children <4 years of age
   c. Gradual onset with irritability, malaise, and fever progressing over 1 to 3 weeks to meningismus, somnolence, cranial nerve abnormalities (especially III, VI, VII), vomiting, seizures, and ultimately coma and death if untreated
   d. CT or MRI scan findings include hydrocephalus, basilar enhancement, and infarcts.

6. Tuberculosis of the bone and joints
   a. Seeding occurs at the time of initial dissemination; disease becomes evident within the first few years following infection.
   b. Bone involvement is more common in young children.
   c. The spine is most commonly involved, followed by lower extremity bones and joints (knees and hips).
   d. Tuberculosis of the spine may be associated with abscess of adjacent tissues; neurologic deficits occur in a substantial minority of patients.
   e. Clinical signs include fever, abnormal gait or posture, and waking from sleep because of pain associated with movement.
   f. Radiographic findings may be limited to disk space narrowing in early disease, progressing to involvement of multiple vertebrae, with anterior collapse (wedging) in advanced disease of the spine.

7. Tuberculosis of superficial lymph nodes
   a. Enlargement of lymph nodes resulting from the lymphatic spread of bacilli is a hallmark of tuberculosis in any location.
   b. Intrathoracic lymph nodes are not visible on examination but are detected radiographically.
   c. Spread of tuberculosis beyond the lung may result in infection of lymph nodes in any location. Those most commonly involved include the cervical, supraclavicular, and inguinal lymph nodes.

8. Miliary tuberculosis
   a. Typically occurs within first 6 months following infection but may be a manifestation of reactivation disease.
   b. More common in young infants
   c. Onset often gradual but may be abrupt; manifestations include fever, weight loss, and fatigue.
   d. Eye (choroidal) lesions may be visible, and skin lesions occur in some cases.
   e. The characteristic chest radiograph shows multiple small lesions present in all lung fields. Lesions in liver and spleen may be detected by CT or MRI scan.

9. Other sites of tuberculosis that are less common in children include the heart and pericardium, skin, eyes, kidneys, gastrointestinal tract, genital tract, and middle ear. Infection at these sites is often associated with pulmonary or disseminated disease but may be isolated. Infection at these sites is often indolent, and there is frequently significant delay in diagnosis.

Key Clinical Findings: Tuberculosis

- Fever
- Hilar adenopathy or mediastinal widening
- Infiltrate with pleural effusion

Key Clinical Findings: Tuberculous Meningitis

- Fever
- Meningismus
- Somnolence
- Cranial nerve signs
- Coma and seizures (late)

Laboratory Findings

1. General laboratory findings of pulmonary tuberculosis are nonspecific. Anemia and hypoalbuminemia may be present if there is long-standing disease.
2. The cerebrospinal fluid (CSF) in tuberculous meningitis typically is under increased pressure and shows moderate pleiocytosis (<100 to 500 cells). A polymorphonuclear predominance is present in early disease; it evolves to the lymphocyte predominance characteristic of late disease. The CSF protein concentration may be mildly elevated early in the course but subsequently rises to very high levels. Similarly, the CSF glucose may be near-normal early in the course but falls steadily to very low levels in untreated disease. Serum hyponatremia and hypochloremia are common.
3. Fluid from pleural or pericardial space infections will have a high protein and a low glucose content and moderate cell count, usually with lymphocytes predominating, unless the fluid is obtained early during the course of infection.
4. Microbiologic evaluation of samples for *M. tuberculosis* includes acid-fast stain and mycobacterial culture, both of which require specific expertise.
5. Nucleic acid amplification tests (recently licensed) for direct identification of *M. tuberculosis* in sputum.
6. Culture in liquid medium has replaced solid media–based methods in many mycobacteriology laboratories as the method of choice for initial isolation of *M. tuberculosis* from clinical specimens because of increased speed of isolation. Once a pure culture has been obtained, rapid speciation is performed using nucleic acid probes.
   a. More rapid broth-based methods for susceptibility testing have been developed and are coming into widespread use in place of traditional agar-based methods.
   b. Because mycobacterial culture requires special expertise as well as BL3 level containment, many clinical microbiology laboratories send specimens for mycobacterial culture to reference laboratories.
7. Polymerase chain reaction has been developed to identify *M. tuberculosis* in clinical specimens other than sputum and is available in some centers; this test is not well standardized at present, however.

Key Laboratory Findings: Tuberculous Meningitis

- Positive PPD (unless very sick)
- CSF
  Cell count 8–100 wbc
  Very low glucose
  High protein
  Culture AFB
- Electrolytes
  Hyponatremia and hypochloremia without acidosis

Treatment

Table 106–1 lists commonly used drugs for the treatment of tuberculosis in children.

1. For drug-sensitive pulmonary tuberculosis, a 6-month course consisting of isoniazid, rifampin, and pyrazinamide for the first 2 months followed by 4 months of isoniazid and rifampin is recommended.
2. For tuberculosis of the central nervous system, bone and joint tuberculosis, and miliary tuberculosis, 1 year of therapy is recommended. Four drugs (isoniazid, rifampin, pyrazinamide, and streptomycin or ethambutol) are administered for the first 1 to 2 months, followed by isoniazid and rifampin for the remaining course. Other forms of extrapulmonary tuberculosis may be treated with the 6-month course used to treat pulmonary disease.
3. In areas where there is a substantial prevalence (>4%) of isoniazid-resistant tuberculosis, initial therapy with four drugs (isoniazid, rifampin, pyrazinamide, and streptomycin or ethambutol) is indicated until specific drug susceptibilities for the patient's isolate are known.
   a. Additional agents may be indicated based on the susceptibility pattern of the isolate of the source case, if known.
   b. Patients with isolates that are resistant to both isoniazid and rifampin require prolonged therapy and tend to respond poorly to treatment. Consultation with an expert is recommended.
4. Treatment of tuberculosis in HIV-infected children is similar to that in non–HIV-infected children, except that an increased duration of therapy is recommended, e.g., 12 months' total duration for pulmonary tuberculosis.
5. Directly observed therapy to assure compliance with the treatment regimen is recommended for all patients. The use of two or three times per week therapy, in place of daily therapy, after the first 2 months of treatment facilitates the use of directly observed therapy for all patients.

Prevention

1. Approaches to prevention of tuberculosis include treatment of infectious cases and preventive therapy of

TABLE 106–1. COMMONLY USED DRUGS FOR THE TREATMENT OF TUBERCULOSIS IN CHILDREN

DRUGS	DOSAGE FORMS	DAILY DOSE (MG/KG/D)	TWICE WEEKLY DOSE (MG/KG PER DOSE)	MAXIMUM DOSE	ADVERSE REACTIONS
Ethambutol	Tablets: 100 mg 400 mg	15–25	50	2.5 g	Optic neuritis (reversible), decreased visual acuity, decreased red-green color discrimination, gastrointestinal disturbance, hypersensitivity
Isoniazid	Scored tablets: 100 mg 300 mg Syrup: 10 mg/mL	10–15†	20–30	Daily: 300 mg Twice weekly: 900 mg	Mild hepatic enzyme elevation, hepatitis,* peripheral neuritis, hypersensitivity
Pyrazinamide	Scored tablets: 500 mg	20–40	50	2 g	Hepatotoxicity, hyperuricemia
Rifampin	Capsules: 150 mg 300 mg Syrup: formulated in syrup from capsules	10–20	10–20	600 mg	Orange discoloration of secretions/urine, staining of contact lenses, vomiting, hepatitis, "flu-like" reaction, and thrombocytopenia; may render birth-control pills ineffective
Streptomycin‡ (IM administration)	Vials: 1 g 4 g	20–40	20–40	1 g	Ototoxicity, nephrotoxicity, skin rash

*When used in combination with rifampin, an increased risk of hepatotoxicity is associated with doses of isoniazid in excess of 10 mg/ml.

Adapted from Committee on Infectious Diseases, American Academy of Pediatrics. Tuberculosis. Report of the Committee on Infectious Diseases. Elk Grove Village, IL, American Academy of Pediatrics, 1994, pp 480–500.

persons with infection but no disease. This approach relies on public health measures of effective source and contact tracing. Vaccination with bacille Calmette-Guérin (BCG) is rarely used in the United States, though it is widely used in countries where tuberculosis is prevalent.

2. Tuberculin skin testing is the means to diagnose tuberculosis infection.
   a. Testing should be performed by intradermal injection of 5 tuberculin units of purified protein derivative (PPD), with the largest diameter of induration (not erythema) read at 48 to 72 hours post injection (Mantoux method).
   b. Interpretation depends on the extent of induration and the risk factors of the person being tested (Table 106–2).
   c. Routine testing of all children is no longer recommended; tuberculin testing should be performed on children with risk factors for tuberculosis, as described above.
   d. Multiple puncture tests are unreliable because of inconsistent administration and interpretation and should not be used.
3. Preventive treatment with isoniazid for 6 to 9 months is recommended for children with positive tuberculin skin tests who do not have active tuberculosis. Evaluation for active tuberculosis, including a chest radiograph, must be completed before preventive therapy with isoniazid is begun.

Atypical Mycobacteria

Etiology

Nontuberculous mycobacteria are traditionally grouped and speciated on the basis of pigment production and growth and biochemical characteristics. Although many species may cause disease in children, the majority of nontuberculous mycobacterial (NTM) infections in immunocompetent children are caused by organisms of the *Mycobacterium avium-intracellulare* complex (MAC). Commonly identified species isolated in specific disease settings are listed in Table 106–3.

Epidemiology

1. Most NTM live free in the environment; some are major pathogens of animals (e.g., *M. avium*).
2. Based on skin testing with antigens derived from several NTM and the geographic distribution of reactivity to these antigens and to PPD, it is believed that a large proportion of the United States population becomes infected by adulthood with one or more NTM. The vast majority of these infections do not cause clinical disease.
3. Clinical disease caused by NTM is uncommon; one national survey in the early 1980s found an annual incidence of 1.8/100,000 in the United States.
4. Person-to-person transmission is rare, if it occurs at all; contaminated solutions and instruments have been implicated in nosocomial outbreaks.
5. In HIV-infected children with advanced immunosuppression, disseminated *M. avium* infection is an important cause of morbidity and is associated with early mortality.

Pathophysiology

The presumed portal of entry is reflected in the clinical manifestations of disease.

1. Cervical/submandibular lymphadenitis is thought to result from ingestion of bacilli, lung disease from inhalation of bacilli, and skin disease from infection of breaks in the skin by contaminated water or other sources.

TABLE 106–2. DEFINITION OF A POSITIVE MANTOUX SKIN TEST*

REACTION ≥ 5 MM

Children in close contact with persons who have known or suspected infectious cases of tuberculosis:

    Households with active or previously active cases if (1) treatment cannot be verified as adequate before exposure, (2) treatment was initiated after period of child's contact, or (3) reactivation is suspected

Children suspected to have tuberculosis disease:

    Chest roentgenogram consistent with active or previously active tuberculosis

    Clinical evidence of tuberculosis

Children with immunosuppressive conditions† or HIV infection

REACTION ≥ 10 MM

Children at increased risk of dissemination from:

    Young age: <4 y of age

    Other medical risk factors, including Hodgkin's disease, lymphoma, diabetes mellitus, chronic renal failure, and malnutrition

Children with increased environmental exposure:

    Born, or whose parents were born, in regions of the world where tuberculosis is highly prevalent

    Frequently exposed to adults who are HIV infected, homeless, users of intravenous and other street drugs, poor and medically indigent city dwellers, residents of nursing homes, incarcerated or institutionalized persons, and migrant farm workers

REACTION ≥ 15 MM

Children ≥4 y of age without any risk factors

*These interpretive criteria apply only to skin testing performed by injection of 5 TU of purified protein derivative intradermally. Reaction is read as millimeters of induration after 48 to 72 hours. These criteria apply regardless of whether BCG has been previously administered.

†Including immunosuppressive doses of corticosteroids.

¶Adapted from Committee on Infectious Diseases, American Academy of Pediatrics. Tuberculosis. Report of the Committee on Infectious Diseases. Elk Grove Village, IL, American Academy of Pediatrics, 1994, pp 480–500.

2. The primary portal of entry resulting in disseminated MAC infection in patients with AIDS is not known; ingestion and inhalation may both play a role.
3. Local replication of bacilli at the site of disease, without dissemination, is the rule in nearly all NTM infections in immunocompetent patients.
4. Dissemination with replication in macrophages and macrophage-like cells throughout the reticuloendothelial system occurs in AIDS patients and in these with other causes of immunodeficiency, resulting in organomegaly and very large bacterial burdens.

TABLE 106–3. MOST COMMON MYCOBACTERIAL SPECIES FOUND IN SPECIFIC CLINICAL SETTINGS

DISEASE	MOST COMMONLY ISOLATED SPECIES*
Lymphadenitis	MAC, *M. scrofulaceum, M. kansasii*
Pulmonary disease	MAC, *M. kansasii, M. fortuitum, M. chelonae, M. xenopi*
Skin infection	*M. marinum, M. fortuitum, M. chelonae, M. leprae, M. haemophilum* (in immunocompromised patients), *M. ulcerans* (Africa, Australia)
Disseminated infection	MAC, *M. kansasii*

*Several other species may cause each of the diseases less commonly than those included in the table.

MAC, *Mycobacterium avium* complex.

Clinical Findings

The major clinical syndromes caused by NTM are lymphadenitis, pulmonary disease, skin disease, and disseminated infection with constitutional symptoms.

1. Lymphadenitis is most commonly caused by *M. avium*, followed by *M. scrofulaceum* and *M. kansasii*. This disease occurs almost exclusively in young children; *M. tuberculosis* is a more common cause of mycobacterial lymphadenitis in adolescents and adults. Lymphadenitis typically occurs as a unilateral swelling in the high anterior cervical or submandibular areas, usually with little pain, tenderness, or fever. Mediastinal and other locations occur rarely. Early in the course, the mass is firm but will progress to discoloration of the overlying skin, fluctuance, and spontaneous drainage in the absence of treatment. The inflammatory mass usually consists of several adjacent nodes and surrounding soft tissue.
2. Pulmonary disease is uncommon in children and may be caused by MAC, *M. kansasii, M. fortuitum, M. chelonae,* and other species. When lung disease does occur, cough is a prominent symptom and hemoptysis may occur; fever is often not present. In patients with cystic fibrosis and associated lung disease, NTM can be isolated from sputum from a substantial minority. The role of these organisms in causing pulmonary disease in these cases is uncertain and must be evaluated on an individual basis.
3. Skin disease may be caused by *M. marinum, M. fortuitum, M. chelonae,* and others. Lesions may be papular or nodular with crusting and drainage; ulceration may be present, though large ulcers are rare. Postoperative wound infections and central venous line exit site infection may be caused by NTM, particularly *M. fortuitum* and *M. chelonae*.
4. Disseminated NTM infection occurs almost exclusively in immunocompromised patients. MAC is the most common cause of disseminated mycobacterial infection in AIDS patients as well as in those with other forms of immunodeficiency. *M. kansasii* as well as several other mycobacteria that are uncommon pathogens (e.g., *M. gordonae, M. haemophilum, M. malmoense*) also cause infection in AIDS patients. Constitutional symptoms are prominent, with fever and weight loss occurring in most. Other common symptoms in patients with AIDS and disseminated MAC infection are abdominal pain caused by enlarged mesenteric lymph nodes and diarrhea. MAC is not a common cause of acute pneumonia in these patients.

Key Clinical Findings: Atypical Mycobacteria

- Unilateral lymphadenopathy, cervical or submandibular
- Immunocompromised host: disseminated disease

Radiographic Picture

1. CT scanning may be useful to determine the extent of lymphadenitis caused by NTM and to guide the surgeon performing excision of the infected nodes. Involvement of multiple superficial and deep nodes is typical. Central

necrosis, even when clinical findings of fluctuance are not present, is commonly seen.

2. Chest radiography of patients with NTM pulmonary disease often reveals hilar/mediastinal lymphadenopathy. Infiltrates may be localized, diffuse, or absent. Pleural effusions and cavitation are usually not present.

3. Radiography of NTM skin disease is nonspecific unless there is infection of adjacent bone. Soft tissue swelling may be visible.

4. Radiography of disseminated NTM disease is also nonspecific. Enlargement of liver and spleen and of mesenteric lymph nodes may be seen on ultrasound or CT scan. The organ enlargement associated with disseminated MAC infection typically has a homogeneous appearance without focal abnormalities in these imaging studies.

Laboratory Findings

1. Routine laboratory findings in NTM disease are nonspecific. In disseminated NTM disease in AIDS, infiltration of bone marrow may contribute to the anemia and leukopenia that is often present in advanced AIDS. Mineral and electrolyte abnormalities may be present in patients with severe diarrhea.

2. Microbiologic identification is essential in NTM disease in order to design an appropriate therapeutic regimen. Acid-fast stain of biopsy material may be positive in lymphadenitis, pulmonary disease, or skin disease, although in the absence of immunosuppression the number of organisms is often small. Culture and speciation as well as susceptibility testing require specialized procedures and are typically performed in reference laboratories. Molecular probes are available for the rapid identification MAC isolates.

Key Laboratory Findings: Atypical Mycobacteria

• Culture of aspirate

Treatment

1. The newer macrolides (clarithromycin, azithromycin) are active in vitro against many but not all NTM; evaluation of these drugs in clinical disease treatment is limited, but indications are that they are effective in treating infections caused by several mycobacterial species. Important pharmacokinetic interactions have been observed between these agents and several other drugs that are metabolized by the liver. The potential for such interactions should be determined before these macrolides are prescribed.

2. Many NTM are resistant to most available antimicrobials, so that treatment regimens should always be based on knowledge of the mycobacterial species causing the disease and, if possible, on the susceptibilities of the patient's isolate. Consultation with an expert in infectious diseases is recommended to develop a treatment plan for NTM infection that is based on the infecting mycobacterial species, the site of infection, and the immune status of the host.

3. The standard treatment for NTM lymphadenitis is surgical excision, with cure rates of >90 per cent without adjunctive antimicrobial chemotherapy. Regimens containing clarithromycin or azithromycin have been used successfully to treat lymphadenitis caused by MAC without surgery; at present there are inadequate data to indicate whether this approach will have a cure rate comparable to that of surgical excision.

4. Disseminated MAC infection in children with AIDS is treated with at least three drugs. Most experts recommend a regimen that includes one of the new macrolides (clarithromycin or azithromycin) plus ethambutol and one or more of the following: rifampin, rifabutin, amikacin, and ciprofloxacin. Multidrug therapy in these patients is often limited by drug intolerance. Painful uveitis has occurred in patients taking high doses of rifabutin in combination with a macrolide.

5. Surgical excision in combination with antimicrobial therapy may be necessary for cure of skin disease when the lesions are extensive or have been injected with steroids; the infection is associated with a foreign body, e.g., a central venous catheter or prosthetic heart valve; the patient is immunocompromised; or the organism is resistant to available antimicrobial agents.

Key Treatment

• Macrolide antibiotics
• Surgery

Prevention

1. There are no known risk factors for NTM disease in immunocompetent children, although certain species more commonly cause disease in specific geographic regions. Person-to-person transmission of NTM infection is extremely rare, if it occurs at all, so that no preventive measures or prophylactic medications are recommended.

2. In patients with AIDS and advanced immunosuppression, prophylactic therapy with rifabutin, clarithromycin, or azithromycin has been demonstrated to decrease the incidence of disseminated MAC infection. Clarithromycin or azithromycin prophylaxis is recommended for children and adults with <100 CD4 cells/mm^3, although some experts prefer to start prophylaxis only when the CD4 count has fallen below 50 to 75 cells/mm^3.

3. There is no known vaccine to prevent NTM disease, though it has been speculated that BCG may provide some protection.

Bibliography

TUBERCULOSIS

American Thoracic Society: Treatment of tuberculosis and tuberculosis infection in adults and children. Am J Respir Crit Care Med 1994;149:1359–1374.

Committee on Infectious Diseases, American Academy of Pediatrics: Tuberculosis. Report of the Committee on Infectious Diseases. Elk Grove Village, IL, American Academy of Pediatrics, 1994, pp 480–500.

Iseman M: Treatment of multidrug-resistant tuberculosis. N Engl J Med 1993;329:784–791.

Starke J: Tuberculosis. Semin Pediatr Infect Dis 1993;4(4):203–319. [This entire issue is devoted to pediatric tuberculosis.]

Starke J, Correa A: Management of mycobacterial infection and disease in children. Pediatr Infect Dis J 1995;14:455–470.

ATYPICAL MYCOBACTERIA

Dalovisio J, Pankey G: Dermatologic manifestations of nontuber-culous mycobacterial diseases. Infect Dis Clin North Am 1994;8:677–688.

Margileth A: Nontuberculous (atypical) mycobacterial disease. Semin Pediatr Infect Dis 1993;4:307–315.

Public Health Service Task Force on Prophylaxis and Therapy for *Mycobacterium avium* Complex: Recommendations on prophy-laxis and therapy for disseminated *Mycobacterium avium* complex disease in patients infected with the human immunodeficiency virus. N Engl J Med 1993;329:898–904.

Wallace R, Tanner D, Brennan P, Brown B: Clinical trial of clarithromycin for cutaneous disseminated infection due to *Mycobacterium chelonae*. Ann Intern Med 1993;119:482–486.

Wolinsky E: Mycobacterial lymphadenitis in children: a prospective study of 105 nontuberculous cases with long-term follow-up. Clin Infect Dis 1995;20:954–963.

107 Selected Parasitic Diseases

Peter F. Weller

This chapter considers the specific parasitic infections and infestations that are likely to be encountered in pediatric practice.

Giardiasis

Definition

Giardiasis is an infection caused by the common protozoan parasite, *Giardia lamblia*.

Etiology

G. lamblia exists in two forms, the environmentally hardy cyst form and the replicating trophozoite form. Infections usually arise from ingestion of fecally derived cysts.

Epidemiology

Because cysts are immediately infectious when passed, person-to-person transmission is likely in settings with impaired hygiene, including childcare centers. The risk is greatest for young children not yet toilet trained, who also may be a source of secondary transmission within families. Foodborne transmission may occur when cysts contaminate previously cooked foods. Waterborne transmission accounts for the majority of infections and involves mostly surface water (not deep well water), including mountain streams and some reservoirs.

Pathophysiology

1. Trophozoites derived from ingested cysts replicate and live in the proximal small intestine.
2. Parasites are not invasive, and the mechanisms by which they cause intestinal symptoms in some but not all infected individuals are uncertain.
3. Malabsorption, which results in part from altered brush border enzyme activities (including lactase deficiency), accounts for some symptoms.
4. In a minority of infected children, sufficient malabsorption may lead to cessation of weight gain and even failure to thrive. Patients with hypogammaglobulinemia, secretory immunoglobulin A deficiency, or cystic fibrosis are at risk for development of persistent infection, which often is more difficult to treat.

Clinical Findings

1. The clinical manifestations of an acute phase of giardiasis may develop after an incubation of about 7 to 10 days but do not occur in all infected persons.
2. Diarrhea, abdominal cramping, midepigastric discomfort, heightened flatus and eructation, foul-smelling stools, and fatigue often persist for longer than 1 week.
3. A chronic phase of giardiasis may follow the acute phase or may develop without an antecedent acute illness. Stools are often loose but are not diarrheic in chronic giardiasis. Increased abdominal gaseousness with cramping, borborygmi, flatulence, and burping occurs. Symptoms may be remitting and episodic. For some, moderate to marked malabsorption may develop with persistent infection.

Key Clinical Findings: Giardiasis

- Diarrhea
- Abdominal pain
- Eructation

Laboratory Findings

1. Leukocytosis and eosinophilia are not typical of giardiasis.
2. Tests for lactase deficiency often are positive, and in more severe infections there may be additional laboratory evidence of malabsorption. The diagnosis is made by detection of parasites on stool examinations or examinations of small-bowel aspirates or biopsies. Newer assays to detect parasite antigens in stools are as sensitive and specific as conventional microscopic stool examinations.

Key Laboratory Finding: Giardiasis

- Detection of *Giardia*

Radiographic Findings

An upper gastrointestinal radiographic series may show evidence of mucosal edema but often is normal.

Treatment

Metronidazole is the principal treatment; it is given at 15 mg/kg/day in three doses for 5 days. For young children intolerant of the bitter taste of metronidazole, furazolidone (6 mg/kg/day in four doses for 7 to 10 days) is an effective alternative.

Key Treatment: Giardiasis

• Metronidazole–15 mg/kg/day × 5 days

Prevention

Attention to hygiene is necessary to prevent person-to-person transmission of giardiasis. The risks and benefits of treating asymptomatic children in daycare centers have not been fully ascertained.

Pinworm Infestation

Definition

Pinworm infection is caused by the parasite, *Enterobius vermicularis,* and is termed enterobiasis.

Etiology

The cause is ingestion of pinworm eggs.

Epidemiology

Eggs may be present on the hands of infected children who scratch their perirectal areas, and eggs at times may contaminate bedding and other household items.

Pathophysiology

1. Adult female worms migrate from the colon to the perirectal area, usually in the morning, to deposit eggs on the perirectal skin.
2. Inflammatory responses to the eggs lead to local irritation and pruritus.
3. Less commonly, eosinophilic colitis may be elicited by larger numbers of larvae or adult worms.

Clinical Findings

1. The cardinal symptom of pinworm infestation is perianal pruritus, but some infected patients remain asymptomatic. The pruritus often worsens at night, when the worms tend to migrate.
2. Infrequently, migration of adult worms into or through the female genital tract results in vaginitis or peritoneal inflammation.

Key Clinical Finding: Pinworm

• Perianal itching

Laboratory Findings

1. Because pinworm eggs are deposited by female worms on the perianal skin, stool examinations usually are negative.
2. Pinworm infestations are diagnosed by applying cellulose acetate tape to the perianal skin in the morning and microscopically examining the tape on a slide to detect the eggs.
3. Adult pinworms may be visualized by anoscopy or colonoscopy.

Key Laboratory Finding: Pinworm

• Demonstration of worms or eggs

Radiographic Findings

Barium enemas are rarely done and are not indicated.

Treatment

1. Pinworm infestation may be treated with either pyrantel pamoate (11 mg/kg once) or mebendazole (single 100-mg dose). With either agent, therapy should be repeated in 2 weeks.
2. Because household members are often infected and can provide a source for reinfection, simultaneous treatment of all household members is indicated.

Key Treatment: Pinworm

• Pyrantel pamoate–11mg/kg once

Prevention

Hygienic measures such as frequent baths and the clipping of fingernails may reduce both the opportunity for reinfection and the spread of infection to others.

Visceral Larva Migrans

Definition

Visceral larva migrans refers to infestations that develop when nematode parasites of animals invade humans.

Etiology

1. The principal cause of visceral larva migrans is the canine ascarid, *Toxocara canis* or, less commonly, the feline ascarid, *Toxocara cati.*
2. Occasionally other nematodes, including the raccoon ascarid, *Baylisascaris procyonis,* may cause the syndrome of visceral larva migrans with eosinophilic meningoencephalitis.

Epidemiology

1. Eggs of ascarid parasites passed in animal feces become infectious after about 3 weeks on the ground and may remain infectious for many months.
2. Humans acquire infestation principally by ingesting eggs in soil. Direct contact with infected animals is not a major source of infestation because of the time required for eggs to activate.
3. A history of eating soil increases the risk, and visceral larva migrans is most likely to develop in children with geophagia; soil from public playgrounds may contain *Toxocara* eggs.

Pathophysiology

1. After infectious *Toxocara* eggs are ingested, the larvae hatch, migrate into the circulation, and are carried hematogenously into various tissues.
2. The manifestations of visceral larva migrans are the result of damage caused by migrating larvae and the induced eosinophilic granulomatous reaction to the larvae.

Clinical Findings

1. Many infestations are mild and subclinical.
2. Clinically apparent infestations may present in one of two distinct patterns: visceral and ocular.
   a. In the visceral form, patients are usually aged 1 to 5 years and generally have a history of geophagia.
      (1) Malaise, irritability, weight loss, wheezing, cough, fever, hepatomegaly, and pruritic rashes are common.
      (2) Neurologic involvement may cause seizures and behavioral disorders.
      (3) Rarely, death occurs from severe neurologic or myocardial involvement.
   b. In the ocular form, patients are older, with a mean age of 7.5 years and a range that includes young adults. A history of antecedent visceral form of the disease is rare.
      (1) Patients with ocular larva migrans often present with strabismus and failing vision. The characteristic ocular lesion is a whitish, elevated granuloma measuring one to two disk diameters that is located in the posterior pole of the retina.
      (2) Less commonly, uveitis or endophthalmitis occurs.

Key Clinical Findings: Visceral Larva Migrans

- Malaise
- Weight loss
- Cough
- Hepatomegaly

Laboratory Findings

1. In mild cases of visceral larva migrans, the only finding may be elevated blood eosinophilia.

2. In heavier infestations, leukocytosis, prominent blood eosinophilia, and hypergammaglobulinemia, often with elevated titers of anti-A and anti-B isohemagglutinins, are common.
3. In the ocular form of larva migrans, these findings are rare. In both the visceral and ocular forms, an enzyme-linked immunosorbent assay (ELISA) serologic test is sensitive and specific.

Key Laboratory Finding: Visceral Larva Migrans

- Eosinophilia

Radiographic Changes

Transient pulmonary infiltrates are found in about one half of patients with pulmonary symptoms.

Treatment

The efficacy of the anthelminthic drugs diethylcarbamazine and thiabendazole remains uncertain for both the visceral and ocular forms of larva migrans. In patients with prominent systemic or ocular inflammation, corticosteroids help suppress the inflammatory manifestations.

Key Treatment: Visceral Larva Migrans

- Corticosteroids for suppression of inflammation

Prevention

Prevention is aimed at diminishing the opportunities for children to ingest soil contaminated by feces of dogs, cats, or other animals. Preventing dogs from defecating in public parks helps prevent contamination of soil that might be ingested by children.

Bibliography

Drugs for parasitic infections. Med Lett 1995;37:99.

Gluckman LT, Magnaval JF: Zoonotic roundworm infections. Infect Dis Clin North Am 1993;7:717.

Hotez PJ: Visceral and ocular larva migrans. Semin Neurol 1993;13:175.

Lengerich EJ, Addiss DG, Juranek DD: Severe giardiasis in the United States. Clin Infect Dis 1994;18:760.

Overturf GD: Endemic giardiasis in the United States: Role of the daycare center. Clin Infect Dis 1994;18:764.

108 Fungal Infections

Robert Finberg

Definition

Although children become infected with many different fungal organisms, this chapter describes only systemic fungal infections that are endemic to North America.

Etiology and Epidemiology

1. Most fungal infections are not spread from person to person. Infection with certain fungi is limited to areas of the country where the environment supports the growth of the fungus (Table 108–1).

   a. Histoplasmosis (caused by *Histoplasma capsulatum*) is found in areas with moderate temperatures. The causative agent grows particularly well in fertile river valleys, and most cases in the United States cluster around the land supplied by the Mississippi and Missouri river valleys (the midwest and southeast regions). The disorder is not commonly seen in either the northeast, southwest, or northwestern parts of the country. Point source outbreaks are well described and often involve urban renewal or construction projects.

   b. Coccidiodomycosis (caused by *Coccidioides immitis*) is a disorder of low deserts and is found in the southwestern portion of the United States.

   c. Blastomycosis (caused by *Blastomyces dermatitidis*) is found in the United States in the areas bordering the Mississippi and Ohio river valleys. The largest number of cases occur in the states of Kentucky, Arkansas, Mississippi, North Carolina, Tennessee, Louisiana, Illinois, and Wisconsin. Point source epidemics have been described, and the organism can be isolated from bird droppings, dirt, and rotting wood.

2. Several species of fungi have a wide distribution throughout the world and are found in all regions of the United States (Table 108–2).

   a. *Candida* causes thrush, an infection of the tongue and oral cavity characterized by creamy white patches on the tongue (they may be curd-like in nature) which, when removed by scraping, may result in bleeding. This syndrome is normal in neonates but when seen in older children suggests immunosuppression (or use of local or systemic steroids).

   b. *Candida* diaper rash and vaginitis are commonly seen in infants and reflect the abundance of *Candida* in normal stool. They may be seen in older children as well.

   c. Both *Aspergillus* and *Candida* species may cause invasive disease in drug abusers and other people who use intravenous lines and in immunocompromised patients (see Chapter 110).

   d. Colonization of airways by *Aspergillus*, particularly in asthmatics, may lead to an allergic form of lung disease characterized by an eosinophilic response to *Aspergillus* antigens.

   e. Sporotrichosis is caused by *Sporothrix schenckii*. This microorganism is found in soil and plant material in most of the world, and source outbreaks have been reported. Most commonly, this agent causes localized disease of the skin and cutaneous lymph nodes and is associated with contact with soil or plants. Sporotrichosis is an occupational disorder of florists.

   f. *Cryptococcus neoformans* is a fungus associated with meningitis and pulmonary infection in normal individuals and is a common cause of meningitis in patients with the acquired immunodeficiency syndrome or lymphoreticular malignancies.

   g. Zygomycosis is a term used for all fungal infections caused by members of the class Zygomycetes, which includes the genera *Mucor*, *Rhizomucor*, and *Rhizopus*. Invasive disease caused by this class of organisms (often referred to previously as mucormycosis) occurs in patients with uncontrolled diabetic ketoacidosis, hematologic malignancies, burns, trauma, or other causes of immunosuppression or immunodeficiency.

   h. *Malassezia furfur*, a lipophilic fungus that causes the superficial infection termed pityriasis versicolor (or tinea versicolor), can also cause systemic infections in patients receiving intravenous lipids for nutrition.

TABLE 108–1. ENDEMIC FUNGI

TYPE OF FUNGAL INFECTION	GEOGRAPHIC LOCATION (UNITED STATES)	USUAL PRESENTATION	POTENTIAL COMPLICATIONS
Histoplasmosis	Midwest	Fever, pulmonary symptoms	Chronic pneumonia, mediastinitis
Blastomycosis	Midwest	Weight loss, fever	Skin and bone involvement, chronic pneumonia
Coccidiodomycosis	Southwest	Dry cough, pleuritic chest pain	Skin and bone involvement, meningitis, chronic pulmonary disease

TABLE 108–2. NONGEOGRAPHICALLY LOCALIZED FUNGI

TYPE OF FUNGUS	PRESENTATION IN NORMAL HOSTS	PRESENTATION IN IMMUNOCOMPROMISED HOSTS
Candida	Thrush (neonates), vaginitis, diaper rash, catheter infections	Disseminated infection (especially liver and spleen)
Aspergillus	Allergic disease in asthmatics	Pneumonia, brain abscesses
Zygomycetes genera	—	Rhinocerebral disease
Cryptococcus	Meninigitis, pulmonary disease	Meningitis, pulmonary disease, disseminated infection (including fungemia)
Sporothrix schenckii	Subcutaneous infection, adenopathy	Pneumonia, disseminated disease

i. A number of other fungi, including *Bipolaris*, *Trichosporon beigelii*, and *Pseudallescheria boydii*, cause infections in immunocompromised patients. Their appearance reflects the local flora to which the patient is exposed.

Pathophysiology

1. Host defenses against fungi involve polymorphonuclear leukocytes as well as T cells and macrophages.
2. The geographically defined fungal infections (histoplasmosis, blastomycosis, coccidioidomycosis) usually cause mild or self-limited disease in normal hosts. *Aspergillus* and *Candida* species do not routinely cause disease in normal hosts (except for the local skin infection associated with *Candida* vaginitis or diaper rash). All these organisms cause serious, invasive infections in immunocompromised hosts (see Chapter 110).

Clinical Findings

For the geographically defined fungi, the presentation depends on the specific fungus.

1. *Histoplasmosis*—Patients usually present with fever and pulmonary symptoms.
   a. The symptoms associated with histoplasmosis are thought to depend on the size of the inoculum of fungus, with only 1 per cent of people exposed to a low inoculum, but 50 to 100 per cent of those exposed to a large inoculum, developing disease.
   b. Most patients develop acute, self-limited disease, which if symptomatic is characterized by fever, myalgias, headache, chest pain, and cough.
   c. Progressive disseminated histoplasmosis is said to occur in 1 of every 2000 to 5000 cases. Progressive disseminated disease is likely to occur in infants and in patients with underlying immunodeficiency disorders.
      (1) Disseminated disease is characterized by fever, pancytopenia, and hepatosplenomegaly. Adrenal involvement is not an uncommon finding at autopsy.
      (2) Renal failure and subcutaneous nodules are reported in disseminated cases, but bone and joint disease is rare.
   d. Chronic pulmonary histoplasmosis is characterized by an interstitial pneumonitis (possibly related to an allergic reaction) accompanied by cough, weight loss, fever, dyspnea, and chest pain.
   e. Mediastinal granulomata, which occurs as a result

of *Histoplasma* infection, can lead to compression of the superior vena cava, large airways, or pulmonary vessels.
   f. Fibrosing mediastinitis is a rare complication of histoplasmosis, but histoplasmosis is one of the more common causes of this disorder. It may be the result of a host response to the *Histoplasma* organism. Most patients are initially unaware of the progression of the disease and present later with superior vena cava or tracheobronchial obstruction.
2. *Blastomycosis*—Patients most commonly present with pulmonary symptoms (fever, productive cough), but bone involvement (particularly of the vertebrae, pelvis, sacrum, skull, ribs, or long bones) is seen in 25 to 50 per cent of cases. Genitourinary tract infection and central nervous system infection are also reported.
3. *Coccidiodomycosis*—Patients typically present with pulmonary symptoms.
   a. Patients with acute disease most often have a dry cough and/or pleuritic chest pain that may be accompanied by symptoms such as fever, night sweats, and headache. Arthralgias, erythema nodosum, and erythema multiforme are also reported.
   b. Chronic disease can be characterized by progressive disease of the chest or by organ dissemination. The most common sites for disseminated disease are the skin, bone, and meninges.

Laboratory Findings

1. Laboratory diagnosis of most fungal infections is made on the basis of culture of the organism. This usually requires special media and often requires tissue samples.
2. Histoplasmosis, blastomycosis, and coccidioidomycosis can all be cultured from lung aspirates. Characteristic morphologic identification is helpful if cultures are not obtained.
3. *Candida* is easy to grow on routine media.
4. Antigen tests for *Cryptococcus* and *Histoplasma* make diseases caused by these organisms easy to diagnose on the basis of tests of serum (or of secretions). Serial antigen levels may allow decisions concerning the duration of therapy.

 Key Laboratory Tests

- Culture
- Antigen levels

Radiologic Findings

1. Most of the endemic fungi produce radiographic abnormalities in the lungs. All can result in presentation with nodules as well as diffuse infiltrates, making diagnosis difficult without culture or antigen analysis. A miliary appearance on chest x-ray is characteristic of histoplasmosis. Chest x-rays of patients with old histoplasmosis (after calcification of many small nodules) have the appearance of lung fields sprayed with buckshot.
2. *Aspergillus* in immunocompromised patients often leads to cavitary disease. The scooped-out area of a cavity with a residual rim is sometimes referred to as the crescent sign of *Aspergillus*.

Treatment

1. Endemic fungi have traditionally been treated with amphotericin B, a toxic drug that is difficult to administer. Recent data in adults indicate a use for azoles, which are given orally. In children, experience with fluconazole has been promising, but itraconazole has not been used extensively.

    a. Blastomycosis can be treated with itraconazole; an adult dose is 200 to 400 mg daily. Itraconazole is also efficacious for the treatment of coccidioidomycosis and histoplasmosis. Coccidiodomycosis can be treated with fluconazole as well. In cases of meningitis, fluconazole is preferred to itraconazole or amphotericin B because of its central nervous system penetration.

    b. Cryptococcus is usually treated with amphotericin B (0.5 to 0.8 mg/kg) as an initial agent with or without flucytosine. After a response has been obtained, the patient can be switched to fluconazole.

    c. Fluconazole in doses of 3 to 6 mg/kg/day has been given safely to children. Single daily doses of 400 to 800 mg are well tolerated in adults with serious infections.

    d. Although itraconazole is well tolerated by adults (and adolescents), few studies of pediatric dosing are available. A few children have been treated with 100-mg doses without obvious side effects. As of 1996, concerns related to bone and tooth pulp abnormalities in rats that received high doses have prevented approval of the routine use of itraconazole in patients younger than 18 years old.

2. Despite earlier literature suggesting that candidemia in a normal host is usually a benign event, most authorities treat candidemia even in nonimmunocompromised patients because of the risk of organ involvement (especially endophthalmitis).

    a. Recent data indicate that fluconazole may be as effective as amphotericin B in this setting. Most authorities recommend treatment for candidemia for at least 2 weeks in the absence of complicating issues.

    b. Itraconazole, but not fluconazole, has activity against *Aspergillus*.

    c. The addition of lipids makes amphotericin less toxic to the kidneys and allows higher doses of the drug to be administered without serious toxicity. Recently, several different preparations of liposomal amphotericin have been licensed. Currently these are recommended as therapy only in patients with nephrotoxicity, but studies are underway to compare them for efficacy against the standard amphotericin B preparation.

    d. Whether azoles should be added to amphotericin B in difficult-to-treat cases is still a matter of controversy. Most authorities would reserve combining the drugs (which could theoretically lead to antagonism rather than synergism) for difficult-to-treat illnesses.

Key Treatments

- Amphotericin B
- Itraconazole
- Fluconazole
- Flucytosine

Prevention

1. No vaccines have been shown to be protective against any fungal illness.
2. Immunocompromised patients are advised to avoid exposure to fungi during their periods of maximum vulnerability (see Chapter 110).

Bibliography

Bradsher RW: Histoplasmosis and blastomycosis. Clin Infect Dis 1996;22:S103–S111.

Como JA, Dismukes WE: Oral azole drugs as systemic antifungal therapy. N Engl J Med 1994;330:263–272.

Leenders ACAP, de Marie S: The use of lipid formulations of amphotericin B for systemic fungal infections. Leukemia 1996;10:1570–1575.

Ng PC: Systemic fungal infections in neonates. Arch Dis Child 1994;71:130–135.

Sugar A: Use of amphotericin B with azole antifungal drugs: What are we doing? Antimicrob Agents Chemother 1995;39:1907–1912.

Wheat LJ: Histoplasmosis: Recognition and treatment. Clin Infect Dis 1994;19:S19–S27.

109 Human Immunodeficiency Virus

William L. Marshall

Definition

1. The human immunodeficiency viruses HIV-1 and HIV-2 are human retroviruses of the lentivirus family that infect CD4-positive T lymphocytes and macrophages, leading to lymphoid organ destruction and to depletion and dysfunction of CD4+ T cells.
2. These events are accompanied by dysfunction and dysregulation of B lymphocytes. As the plasma HIV RNA level rises and the number of CD4+ T cells (CD4 count) falls, immune derangement gives rise to opportunistic infections and malignancies.
3. The presence of low CD4 count or defined pathologic processes define development of the acquired immunodeficiency syndrome (AIDS). Disease also closely correlates with the level of HIV viremia; for example, the presence of >100,000 copies of HIV RNA per milliliter of plasma predicts sixfold greater mortality from AIDS.
4. Prevention of HIV infection requires prevention of parenteral or sexual exposure, and several steps can be taken to prevent mother-to-infant transmission (see below). Treatment and prophylaxis in the HIV-infected child may prolong disease-free life.

Epidemiology

1. The peripartum period accounts almost 90 per cent of HIV transmission to infants and children.
2. The remainder of HIV transmission to children is through use of blood products or sexual abuse.
3. Although breast feeding is a known mode of HIV transmission, this rarely occurs in the United States owing to substitution of bottle feeding by HIV-positive mothers.
4. Mother-to-child transmission rates vary from 13 to 40 per cent, depending on country examined and maternal disease stage.
5. Partial prevention of transmission (the rate decreases from 25% to 8%) is achieved with zidovudine (ZDV). The dose is 100 mg ZDV 5 times per day, initiated at 14 to 34 weeks' gestation. During delivery, a 2 mg/kg 1-hour loading dose is administered, followed by 1 mg/kg continuous infusion until delivery. This is followed by 2 mg/kg PO ZDV every 6 hours administered to the infant for 6 weeks post partum. Side effects include nausea, anemia, and leukopenia. There is no known teratogenicity or embryotoxicity in humans, but risks and benefits should be explained to the mother.
6. Other factors also affect HIV transmission: prematurity, higher maternal viremia, and delivery >4 hours after rupture of membranes all increase the risk.
7. New treatments utilizing a combination of three antiretroviral drugs are highly effective for decreasing viral load and increasing CD4 number in adults and therefore are likely to be used in pregnant women. Their teratogenicity and their impact on transmission of HIV to infants are not yet defined.

Postpartum Management of Children Born to HIV+ Mothers

1. Diagnosis by polymerase chain reaction (PCR) or viral culture approaches 100 per cent sensitivity by 6 months. The immune-complex-dissociated p24 HIV antigen test is specific but not so sensitive.
2. By 15 months, most infants have lost circulating maternal immunoglobulin G (IgG), and therefore HIV serologic testing becomes more specific.
3. Because severe disease may be present before a virologic diagnosis is made, clinical judgment and judicious use of PCR and viral culture may need to be used along with CD4 number and the percentage of CD4+ lymphocytes (CD4 percentage). HIV infection can reasonably be excluded among children who have had two or more negative HIV diagnostic tests (i.e., PCR or HIV culture) since 1 month of age, if one was performed at ≥4 months of age. Alternatively two or more negative HIV IgG antibody tests performed at >6 months of age in children who have no clinical evidence of HIV disease can serve to dismiss HIV-1 and -2 infection by serotypes present in United States children.
4. Immunologic category is based on age-specific CD4+ count and CD4+ per cent (Table 109–1). Evidence of severe (and, in some experts' opinion, mild) immune suppression should prompt antiretroviral treatment, regardless of clinical status. Because mortality and disease progression correlate most closely with plasma HIV copy number, it may be prudent to consider prophylaxis and treatment for those with >100,000 copies of HIV/ml, regardless of CD4+ counts or clinical parameters. The goal of antiretroviral therapy is suppression of viral RNA to below detectable levels. The primary rationale for this goal, beyond increasing survival of the immune system, is prevention of viral resistance that is driven by replication-induced changes

TABLE 109–1. IMMUNOLOGIC CATEGORY BASED ON AGE-SPECIFIC CD4+ T LYMPHOCYTE NUMBER AND PERCENTAGE

| IMMUNOLOGIC CATEGORY | AGE OF CHILD | | | | | |
| | <12 mo | | 1–5 yr | | 6–12 yr | |
	Cells/μl	%	Cells/μl	%	Cells/μl	%
No evidence of suppression	≥1500	≥25	≥1000	≥25	≥500	≥25
Evidence of moderate suppression	750–1499	15–24	500–999	15–24	200–499	15–24
Severe suppression	<750	<15	<500	<15	<200	<15

From Centers for Disease Control and Prevention: 1995 Revised guidelines for prophylaxis against *Pneumocystis carinii* pneumonia for children infected with or perinatally exposed to human immunodeficiency virus. MMWR Morb Mortal Wkly Rep 1995;44:(RR-4).

in the viral genome. Therapy should be switched if (1) the patient is intolerant of the drug's side effects; (2) the viral load increases >0.5 log in a compliant patient; or (3) more effective therapy is available. Those choosing alternate drugs need to consider cross resistance between antiretrovirals, e.g., between the protease inhibitors indinavir and ritonavir. It is unclear at this time whether HIV can be routinely eradicated from individuals by antiretroviral therapy. It is prudent not to stop prophylaxis against opportunistic infections, even in the face of increased CD4+ counts following antiretroviral therapy.

5. In children <13 years of age, treatment of HIV infection currently incorporates didanosine (ddI) alone 90 mg/m² q12h or the therapeutically equivalent combination of ZDV and ddI dosed as ZDV 90 mg/m² q6h and ddI 90 mg/m² q12h. Recent studies in infants have shown a significant (up to 1.5 log decrease in plasma HIV RNA) virologic response to triple therapy with ZDV 180 mg/m² every 8 hours, ddI 120 mg/m² q12h, and the non-nucleoside reverse transcriptase inhibitor nevirapine at 120 to 200 mg/m². Combination therapy including ZDV with another reverse transcriptase inhibitor, e.g., 3TC, and protease inhibitors is extremely effective in reducing HIV viremia in adults and is being investigated in children at this time (see Table 109–2 for some dosages and common side effects).

In children 13 years and older, combination therapy with ZDV 200 mg tid and indinavir 800 mg tid (or, presumably, another protease inhibitor), and 3TC 150 mg bid is recommended, based upon the excellent virologic response and improved longevity in adults.

Newer regimens under consideration include combinations of protease inhibitors as well as combinations of non-nucleoside reverse transcriptase inhibitors and protease inhibitors.

6. *Pneumocystis carinii* pneumonia (PCP) is the first AIDS opportunistic infection in up to 40 per cent of children, and it results in substantial morbidity and mortality. It is caused by a silver stain–positive fungal microorganism. Prophylaxis is indicated if the CD4 number or percentage falls below a certain age-specific level (Table 109–3), for all children of HIV+ mothers in whom HIV infection cannot be excluded, and after an episode of PCP. Dosing of prophylactic anti-PCP medications is outlined in Table 109–4.

7. Primary prophylaxis of non-PCP opportunistic infections depends on the particular organism. (The organisms are described and secondary prophylaxis measures are detailed in the next section.)
   a. *Mycobacterium tuberculosis*—For a positive (5-mm) tuberculin skin test or contact with someone known or suspected to have tuberculosis (TB), prophylaxis should begin with 10 mg/kg (maximum 300 mg) PO or IM isoniazid (INH) daily for 12 months. An alternative is rifampin 20 mg/kg (maximum 600 mg) PO or IV daily for 12 months; this regimen is also indicated for INH-resistant TB. For multidrug-resistant (MDR) TB, contact local public health authorities.
   b. *Varicella-zoster virus (VZV)*—For exposure without infection, give varicella-zoster immune globulin

(VZIG), 1 vial (1.25 ml) per 10 kg (maximum, 5 vials) IM, within 96 hours after exposure, and ideally within 48 hours.

   c. *Toxoplasmosis*—Although rarely necessary owing to its low incidence in children in most of the United States, the Centers for Disease Control and Prevention (CDC) recommends that children with IgG antibody to *Toxoplasma gondii* and severe immunosuppression (see Table 109–1) receive prophylaxis with trimethoprim-sulfamethoxazole (TMP-SMX). An alternative is dapsone (in children >1 month old) 2 mg/kg or 15 mg/m² (maximum 25 mg) PO daily, plus pyrimethamine 1 mg/kg PO daily, plus leucovorin 5 mg PO every 3 days.

   d. *Mycobacterium avium* complex (MAC)—Prophylaxis for MAC disease is indicated in patients with CD4 counts <75 cells/μl. Azithromycin, 20 mg/kg

TABLE 109–2. DRUGS USED IN TREATMENT OF HIV INFECTION

GENERIC DRUG NAME	DOSAGE	MAJOR SIDE EFFECTS
Nucleoside Analogs		
Didanosine (ddI)	<13 y/o (see text) ≥13 y/o <60 kg 125 mg q12h >60 kg 250 mg q12h	Pancreatitis, LFT elevation, neuropathy, decreased dapsone absorption
Lamivudine (3TC)	3 mos.–12 y/o 4 mg/kg q12h ≥13 y/o 150 mg q12h	Cytopenia, HA, high amylase
Stavudine (d4T)	<13 y/o 1 mg/kg q12h ≥13 y/o 30 mg q12h	Peripheral neuropathy, N/V, rarely pancreatitis
Zalcitabine (ddC)	<13 y/o 0.01 mg/kg q8h >0.75 mg q8h	Peripheral neuropathy, oral ulcers, pancreatitis
Zidovudine (ZDV)	<13 y/o (see text) ≥13 y/o 200 mg tid	Cytopenia, esp. anemia, myopathy, HA, N/V
Non-nucleoside Reverse Transcriptase Inhibitors		
Nevirapine (NVP)	<13 y/o 120 mg/m² qd × 28d, then 200 mg/m² bid >13 y/o 200 mg qd × 14d, then 200 mg bid	Rash, fever, myalgia
Protease Inhibitors		
Nelfinavir	<13 y/o (see package insert) ≥13 y/o 750 mg tid	Diarrhea
Ritonavir (RTV)	2*–13 y/o 350 mg/m² q12h ≥13 y/o 600 mg q12h	Drug interactions, high CPK, N/V
Indinavir (IND)	<13 y/o undetermined ≥13 y/o 800 mg q8h	Nephrolithiasis (decreased with hydration), high bilirubin
Saquinavir (SQV)	<13 y/o undetermined ≥13 y/o 600 mg q8h	N/V/diarrhea

*Safety <2 y/o not established at time of FDA approval.
N/V, nausea, vomiting.
Source: 1997 Red Book: Report of the Committee on Infectious Diseases, pp 289–294.

TABLE 109–3. RECOMMENDATION FOR PCP PROPHYLAXIS AND CD4+ MONITORING FOR HUMAN IMMUNODEFICIENCY VIRUS (HIV)–EXPOSED INFANTS AND HIV-INFECTED CHILDREN, BY AGE AND HIV-INFECTION STATUS

AGE AND HIV-INFECTION STATUS	PCP PROPHYLAXIS	CD4+ MONITORING
Birth to 4–6 wk, HIV exposed	No prophylaxis	1 mo
4–6 wk to 4 mo, HIV exposed	Prophylaxis	3 mo
4–12 mo		
HIV infected or indeterminate	Prophylaxis	6, 9, and 12 mo
HIV infection reasonably excluded	No prophylaxis	None
1–5 yr, HIV infected	Prophylaxis if CD4+ count is <500 cells/μl or if CD4+ percentage is <15%†‡	Every 3–4 mo*
6–12 yr, HIV infected	Prophylaxis if CD4+ count is <200 cells/μl or if CD4+ percentage is <15%‡	Every 3–4 mo*

*Monthly monitoring is recommended for children whose CD4+ counts or percentages are approaching the threshold at which prophylaxis is recommended.
†Children 1–2 yr of age who were receiving PCP prophylaxis and had a CD4+ count of <750 cells μl or a percentage of <15% at <12 mo of age should continue prophylaxis.
‡Prophylaxis should be considered on a case-by-case basis for children who might otherwise be at risk for PCP, such as children with rapidly declining CD4+ counts or children with "severe" C conditions (Table 109–2). Children who have had PCP should receive lifelong PCP prophylaxis.
From Centers for Disease Control and Prevention: 1995 Revised guidelines for prophylaxis against *Pneumocystis carinii* pneumonia for children infected with or perinatally exposed to human immunodeficiency virus. MMWR Morb Mortal Wkly Rep 1995:44:(RR-4).

(maximum, 1200 mg) PO weekly is favored by many experts. An alternative is clarithromycin, 5 to 12 mg/kg PO daily. A third choice for prophylaxis in children 6 to 12 years old is rifabutin, 300 mg PO daily (in children <6 years old, 5 mg/kg PO daily).

   e. *Cytomegalovirus (CMV)*—No recommendations exist for children. In adults with CD4 counts <50 cells/μl and positive CMV antibodies, ganciclovir (1 g PO tid) is given as prophylaxis.

Specific AIDS-Associated Syndromes

1. *Pneumocystis carinii* pneumonia
     a. Symptoms of PCP include tachypnea, fever, and cough. Chest radiographs display diffuse interstitial changes. There is often a large alveolar-arterial gra-

TABLE 109–4. DRUG REGIMENS FOR PCP PROPHYLAXIS FOR CHILDREN ≥4 WEEKS OF AGE

RECOMMENDED REGIMEN

• Trimethoprim/sulfamethoxazole (TMP-SMX) 150 mg TMP/m²/day with 750 mg SMX/M²/day administered orally in divided doses b.i.d. 3 times per week on consecutive days (e.g., Monday-Tuesday-Wednesday)

ACCEPTABLE ALTERNATIVE TMP-SMX DOSAGE SCHEDULES

• 150 mg TMP/m²/day with 750 mg SMX/m²/day administered orally as a single daily dose 3 times per week on consecutive days (e.g., Monday-Tuesday-Wednesday)
• 150 mg TMP/m²/day with 750 mg SMX/m²/day orally divided b.i.d. and administered 7 days per week
• 150 mg TMP/m²/day with 750 mg SMX/m²/day administered orally divided b.i.d. and administered 3 times per week on alternate days (e.g., Monday-Wednesday-Friday)

ALTERNATIVE REGIMENS IF TMP-SMX IS NOT TOLERATED

• Dapsone*
  2 mg/kg (not to exceed 100 mg) administered orally once daily
• Aerosolized pentamidine* (children ≥5 yr of age)
  300 mg administered via Respirgard II inhaler monthly

*If neither dapsone nor aerosolized pentamidine is tolerated, some clinicians use intravenous pentamidine (4 mg/kg) administered every 2 or 4 weeks.
From Centers for Disease Control and Prevention: 1995 Revised guidelines for prophylaxis against *Pneumocystis carinii* pneumonia for children infected with or perinatally exposed to human immunodeficiency virus. MMWR Morb Mortal Wkly Rep 1995;44:(RR-4).

dient in partial pressure of oxygen that increases with exercise.

  b. Bronchioalveolar lavage reveals pneumocysts on silver stain or toluidine blue stain. Disease often represents primary infection with a poor outcome (<12 months' median survival time).

  c. Treatment consists of respiratory support and TMP-SMX 15 mg/kg divided every 8 hours and continuing for 21 days. Complications are rash and cytopenias. As an adjunct to therapy for moderate to severe PCP (partial pressure of oxygen, 70 mmHg), consider prednisone 2 mg/kg PO or IV divided b.i.d. × 5 days, then 1 mg/kg PO or IV divided b.i.d. × 5 days, then 0.5 mg/kg PO or IV divided b.i.d. × 11 days. Alternative anti-PCP therapies include pentamidine (3 to 4 mg/kg IV daily), which carries significant toxicities of hypoglycemia, hypotension, renal insufficiency, and cytopenias.

  d. Treatment is followed by lifetime prophylaxis (see Table 109–4).

2. Lipoid interstitial pneumonitis (LIP) was diagnosed in 20 per cent of CDC-recorded cases in 1990.

  a. Patients present, as with PCP, with bilateral infiltrates on chest x-ray, dyspnea, and hypoxia.

  b. Digital clubbing, parotitis, lymphadenopathy, and hypergammaglobulinemia are often present simultaneously.

  c. LIP may represent polyclonal activation of lymphocytes caused by Epstein-Barr virus (EBV) and HIV.

  d. LIP can be diagnosed on bronchoalveolar lavage with biopsy, or presumptively with 2 months of unchanged pulmonary infiltrates.

  e. Treatment is 2 mg/kg prednisone per day followed by rapid tapering.

3. Fungal infections
     a. *Candida*—Persistent oral whitish plaques, vaginitis, or esophagitis may be caused by *Candida* species, and such infections are common. Milder disease can be treated with Mycostatin, clotrimazole troches, oral fluconazole (3 mg/kg/day, or 6 mg/kg/day for

systemic *Candida* or *Cryptococcus*), or ketoconazole. With more severe immunosuppression, extensive mucocutaneous candidiasis can develop. Esophagitis that does not respond to azole antifungals can be treated with amphotericin B (0.6 mg/kg IV daily).

b. Cryptococcosis is rare in children, but cryptococcal antigen should be monitored in meningitis. Therapy is with amphotericin B, which is followed by fluconazole, 6 mg/kg/day for 8 to 10 weeks, and maintenance fluconazole, 2 to 8 mg/kg/day for life.

c. Histoplasmosis is present in endemic areas (e.g., Ohio River Valley); patients present with pulmonary or bone marrow involvement. Therapy is with amphotericin B; maintenance is with itraconazole, 2 to 5 mg/kg PO every 12 to 24 hours for life.

d. Coccidioidomycosis is present in endemic areas (e.g., southwestern United States); patients present with pulmonary and often extrapulmonary involvement. Therapy is with amphotericin B, but meningitis may require intracisternal therapy or the use of fluconazole, 6 mg/kg/day; maintenance is with fluconazole, 2 to 8 mg/kg/day for life.

e. Bacterial infections can also define AIDS illness. The presence of recurrent sepsis, pneumonia, meningitis, osteomyelitis, septic arthritis, or abscess of an internal organ (excluding otitis media, superficial skin or mucosal abscesses, and indwelling catheter-related infections) also defines AIDS in children.

(1) *Otitis/sinusitis*—These infections initially occur as often in HIV+ children as in uninfected children, but they are much more likely to be recurrent and to persist beyond 3 years of age in the HIV+ child.

(2) *Pneumonia*—In one study of patients with respiratory failure, 42 per cent had PCP and 29 per cent had bacterial pneumonia; 55 per cent of the latter group had *Pseudomonas aeruginosa*, and 10 per cent each had *Klebsiella pneumoniae*, *Staphylococcus aureus*, *Haemophilus influenzae*, or *Streptococcus pneumoniae*. Treatment should be based on knowledge of local antibiotic susceptibilities for this range of organisms.

(3) *Tuberculosis*—MDR TB can be problematic in certain parts of the United States and must be considered in management of cases of TB. Consultation with local public health authorities is frequently helpful in designing a treatment regimen tailored to local strains of MDR TB.

(a) HIV+ patients with *M. tuberculosis* infection typically present with extrapulmonary involvement, and the organism may be widely disseminated. Therapy for presumed non-MDR TB is typically begun with INH, 10 mg/kg (maximum 300 mg) PO daily; rifampin, 20 mg/kg (maximum 600 mg) PO daily; pyrazinamide 30 mg/kg (maximum 2 gm) PO daily; and streptomycin 20 to 30 mg/kg (maximum, 1 g) PO daily. (Ethambutol 15 mg/kg/day can be used as an alternative to streptomycin in children old enough to report signs of optic neuritis.) Once sensitivity to INH/rifampin is established, 9 months of therapy is sufficient for TB in cases without central nervous system (CNS) involvement.

(b) Constitutional symptoms associated with MAC may be alleviated by treatment with clarithromycin (15 mg/kg PO b.i.d.) combined with at least one of the following drugs ethambutol, 15 mg/kg PO daily (see caution above); clofazimine, 2 mg/kg (maximum, 100 mg) PO daily; rifabutin in children 6 to 12 years old, 300 mg PO daily (in children <6 years old, 5 mg/kg PO daily); or ciprofloxacin, 20 to 30 mg/kg in two divided doses PO daily. (According to the CDC, use of ciprofloxacin in HIV+ children older than 6 years of age is reasonable in light of the risks and benefits.)

(4) *Bacteremia/sepsis*—The microbial cause of bacteremia is *S. pneumoniae* in 30 per cent of cases, *Salmonella* species in 14 per cent, *Staphylococcus* in 14 per cent, *Pseudomonas* in 6 per cent, and *Enterobacter* in 6 per cent. Likely sites for infection in one study were lung, skin, and catheter sites. Children with recurrent bacterial infection, documented antibody deficiency (IgG <250 mg/dl), failure to form antibodies to common antigens, or failure to form antibodies to measles after two vaccinations with MMR 1 month apart should also receive 400 mg/kg of monthly IVIG (which should be considered for children with recurrent bacterial infection on TMP-SMX prophylaxis). *Salmonella* bacteremia should be followed by several months of TMP-SMX therapy.

4. Viral infection

a. *VZV and herpes simplex virus (HSV)*—Infections can be prolonged in the presence of an HSV ulcer for weeks. Both HSV and VZV are prone to disseminate and may be more likely to cause bronchitis or pneumonia in HIV+ children. Therapy for VZV is with acyclovir, 500 mg/m² every 8 hours, whereas HSV is treated with acyclovir, 250 mg/m² every 8 hours.

b. *Cytomegalovirus*—Patients may present with viremia and fever, pancreatitis, acalculous cholecystis, bone marrow suppression, necrotizing adrenalitis, upper and lower gastrointestinal or respiratory tract infection, chorioretinitis, and CNS infection. Therapy is with ganciclovir, 5 mg/kg every 12 hours; this regimen carries significant hematologic toxicity that may be limited by granulocyte colony-stimulating factor, 5 μg/kg SC three times per week. Maintenance is required for retinitis with ganciclovir, 6 mg/kg/day 5 days/week; intraocular implants of drug are sometimes necessary. Foscarnet, 60 mg/kg every 8 hours for 14 days with maintenance of 90 mg/kg/day, may be used for virologic or clinical ganciclovir resistance. Complications include interstitial nephritis, seizures, and hypocalcemia. Some experts recommend use of both anti-CMV agents in combination for CNS disease.

c. *Adenoviruses*—Patients present with pneumonia (which can be fatal), gastrointestinal involvement (including hepatitis), myocarditis, and conjunctivitis.

d. *Respiratory viruses*—Respiratory syncytial virus (RSV) infection in HIV+ children is associated with increased pneumonia, prolonged excretion, and higher incidence of coinfection or superinfection. Mortality is high, similar to what is observed in other immunocompromised hosts. Therapy in symptomatic cases is with aerosolized ribavirin for 5 days, given via nebulizer either as 20 mg/ml of reservoir over 16 hours (protocol approved by United States Food and Drug Administration) or as 60 mg/ml of reservoir over 2 hours q8 hours (not approved).

e. *JC virus*—JC virus is a papovavirus that is thought to cause the untreatable disorder progressive multifocal leukoencephalopathy, which is characterized by ataxia, weakness, and altered mentation. Computed tomography and magnetic resonance imaging reveal nonenhancing hypodense lesions of the brain. There is no approved therapy.

f. *Parasitic infection*—*Toxoplasma gondii* is rare in children and is associated with encephalitis, brain abscess, chorioretinitis, and myocarditis. Treatment is with pyrimethamine (2 mg/kg divided b.i.d. for 3 days), followed by pyrimethamine (1 mg/kg divided b.i.d.) for 4 weeks along with sulfadiazine (100 to 200 mg/kg/day, to a maximum of 8 g, in two to four divided doses). Steroids may be necessary to treat increased intracranial pressure. Maintenance or secondary prophylaxis is with pyrimethamine (1 mg/kg or 15 mg/m^2 daily) and oral leucovorin (5 mg every 3 days), combined with sulfadiazine (100 mg/kg/day in two to four divided doses) or clindamycin (20 to 30 mg/kg in four divided doses).

Organ System Involvement

1. CNS HIV encephalopathy is manifested by the presence of the following for at least 2 months:

   a. Failure to attain or loss of developmental milestones or loss of intellectual ability, determined by standard developmental scale or neuropsychologic tests

   b. Impaired brain growth or acquired microcephaly demonstrated by head circumference measurements, or brain atrophy demonstrated by computed tomography or magnetic resonance imaging (serial imaging is required for children <2 years of age)

   c. Acquired symmetric motor deficit manifested by two or more of the following: paresis, pathologic reflexes, ataxia, or gait disturbance

   d. Treatment with ZDV or ddI ameliorates some of these findings. Progressive multifocal leukoencephalopathy, CNS toxoplasmosis, cryptococcosis, and lymphoma, which are often seen in adults, are rare (but increasing with longer life expectancies of children with HIV), whereas CMV and *Candida* menin-

gitis with microabscesses have been reported to occur more commonly in HIV+ children.

2. *Pulmonary*—Many of the manifestations of AIDS are pulmonary: RSV pneumonia, PCP, fungal disorder, bacterial pneumonia, and LIP are described under specific syndromes.

3. *Renal*—Renal failure in AIDS is caused by acute tubular necrosis, glomerular disease or HIV nephropathy characterized by proteinuria, focal glomerulosclerosis, and rapid renal failure. Primary renal disease occurs in <10 per cent of HIV+ children; it progresses more slowly in children than in adults, and death usually results from another AIDS-related condition.

4. Gastrointestinal

   a. Parotitis may be an early symptom of disease in HIV+ patients. Esophagitis may be caused by *Candida*, HSV, or, less commonly, CMV. Sometimes the only clue to disease in the child is poor food intake. Therapy is based on identification of the organism and is instituted as described above.

   b. Hairy leukoplakia, a whitish raised proliferation of EBV+ cells on the tongue, responds to acyclovir (reserve for symptomatic cases). Idiopathic esophageal ulceration may develop in children; in adults, it responds to therapy with prednisone for 4 weeks (use prednisone 2 mg/kg in children). In refractory cases of aphthous ulceration in HIV+ children, some experts recommend thalidomide at 5 to 10 mg/kg.

   c. Diarrhea is a common AIDS-related symptom and may be caused by a host of enteric pathogens, such as *Salmonella, Shigella, Campylobacter, Clostridium difficile*, or atypical mycobacteria. Viruses (CMV, adenovirus, and rotavirus), parasites, and fungi are also associated with infectious diarrhea. *Cryptosporidium* appears in stool as an acid-fast–staining oocyte that causes a prolonged noninflammatory diarrhea (untreatable). *Isospora belli* is a coccidian parasite with large acid-fast cysts (treat with TMP-SMX for 1 month and consider continuous prophylaxis). *Microsporidia* is a unicellular obligate intracellular parasite (which may respond to albendazole) that also contributes to diarrheal syndromes.

   d. The biliary tree, the eye, and the respiratory tract can all be a site for invasion by *Microsporidia*. Hepatosplenomegaly also occurs early in HIV disease. Involvement of the liver with viral, mycobacterial, and bacterial pathogens is seen occasionally.

5. *Cardiac*—Cardiomyopathy, pericarditis, and arteritis are all seen in HIV+ patients. The cause is unknown, and therapy is supportive. Some experts suggest antiretroviral treatment for HIV+ children with severe cardiac disease.

6. *Hematology/oncology*—Cytopenias are extremely common in HIV infection.

   a. Anemia exists at presentation in 5 to 95 per cent of patients examined, depending on disease stage. Removal of offending drugs is usually followed by a trial of erythropoietin before transfusion for severe

TABLE 109–5. CLINICAL CATEGORIES FOR CHILDREN WITH HIV INFECTION

MODERATELY SYMPTOMATIC (PARTIAL LISTING)

- Anemia (<10 g/dl), neutropenia (<1000/mm³), or thrombocytopenia (<100,000/mm³) persisting ≥30 days
- Bacterial meningitis, pneumonia, or sepsis (single episode)
- Candidiasis, oropharyngeal (thrush), persisting (>2 mo) in children >6 mo of age
- Cardiomyopathy
- Cytomegalovirus infection, with onset before 1 mo of age
- Diarrhea, recurrent or chronic
- Hepatitis
- Herpes simplex virus (HSV) stomatitis, recurrent (more than two episodes within 1 yr)
- HSV bronchitis, pneumonitis, or esophagitis with onset before 1 mo of age
- Herpes zoster (shingles) involving at least two distinct episodes or more than one dermatome
- Varicella, disseminated (complicated chickenpox)
- Leiomyosarcoma
- Lymphoid interstitial pneumonia (LIP) or pulmonary lymphoid hyperplasia complex
- Nephropathy
- Nocardiosis
- Persistent fever (lasting >1 mo)
- Toxoplasmosis, onset before 1 mo of age

SEVERELY SYMPTOMATIC

- Serious bacterial infections, multiple or recurrent (i.e., any combination of at least two culture-confirmed infections within a 2-yr period)
- Candidiasis, esophageal or pulmonary (bronchi, trachea, lungs)
- Coccidioidomycosis, disseminated (at site other than or in addition to lungs or cervical or hilar lymph nodes)
- Cryptococcosis, extrapulmonary
- Cryptosporidiosis or isosporiasis with diarrhea persisting >1 mo
- Cytomegalovirus disease with onset of symptoms at age >1 mo (at a site other than liver, spleen, or lymph nodes)
- Wasting syndrome in the absence of a concurrent illness other than HIV infection
- Encephalopathy
- Herpes simplex virus infection causing a mucocutaneous ulcer that persists for >1 mo; or bronchitis, pneumonitis, or esophagitis for any duration affecting a child >1 mo of age
- Histoplasmosis, disseminated (at a site other than or in addition to lungs or cervical or hilar lymph nodes)
- Kaposi sarcoma
- Lymphoma, primary, in brain
- Lymphoma, small, noncleaved cell (Burkitt), or immunoblastic or large cell lymphoma of B-cell or unknown immunologic phenotype
- *Mycobacterium tuberculosis,* disseminated or extrapulmonary
- *Mycobacterium,* other species or unidentified species, disseminated (at a site other than or in addition to lungs, skin, or cervical or hilar lymph nodes)
- *Mycobacterium avium* complex or *Mycobacterium kansasii,* disseminated (at site other than or in addition to lungs, skin, or cervical or hilar lymph nodes)
- *Pneumocystis carinii* pneumonia
- Progressive multifocal leukoencephalopathy
- Salmonella (nontyphoid) septicemia, recurrent
- Toxoplasmosis of the brain with onset at >1 mo of age

Adapted from MMWR 1994:43(RR-12).

anemias. Parvovirus B19 is a potentially treatable cause of acquired anemia. Diagnosis can be made by serology, if positive, or by PCR. Therapy with immune globulin is effective

b. Leukopenia associated with HIV can be severe and is exacerbated by common therapies such as ZDV and TMP-SMX. Treatment with granulocyte colony-stimulating factor, 5 μg/kg SC 2 to 4 times per week, can be effective.

c. Thrombocytopenia is also common and is an early sign of HIV infection. Treatment of severe disease progressively with antiretrovirals, intravenous immunoglobulin, prednisone, or splenectomy may be successful.

d. Kaposi sarcoma is rare in children.

e. CNS lymphomas, which appear as more or less enhancing lesions on computed tomography or magnetic resonance imaging, are also rare (<1% patients at referral centers), but the incidence may increase with longer life spans on antiretroviral therapy.

7. Skin

a. In addition to viral disease, HSV, and VZV, fungal agents such as *Malassezia* and *Pityrosporon* may cause folliculitis, seborrheic dermatitis, and dandruff, which respond to topical ketoconazole.

b. Norwegian scabies may develop as the result of infestation with the scabetic mite in an immunocompromised host. Symptoms include pyoderma, alopecia, hyperpigmentation, and pruritic vesiculopapular eruption mimicking psoriatic dermatitis with thousands of mites in the skin. Treatment is with lindane (Kwell) or permethrin (Elimite).

c. Drug eruptions are quite common in AIDS.

d. Nutritional deficiencies may also cause skin eruption, as in the dermatitis of niacin deficiency (part of the symptom complex known as pellagra) or the seborrheic-like facies of pyridoxine (B6) deficiency.

8. Constitutional symptoms may lead to the diagnosis of AIDS in the absence of an alternative explanation.

a. Symptoms of wasting illness include (1) persistent weight loss >10 per cent of baseline; (2) downward crossing of at least two of the following percentile lines on the weight-for-age chart in a child ≤1 year of age: 95th, 75th, 50th, 25th, 5th; or (3) <5th percentile on weight-for-height chart on two consecutive measurements more than 30 days apart.

b. Finally, documented fever (intermittent or constant) for ≥30 days also defines a criterion for constitutional symptoms consistent with AIDS (see list of severe symptoms, Table 109–5).

Immunizations

1. The potential benefits of immunization outweigh the theoretical risks of HIV activation when killed vaccines such as diphtheria-pertussis-tetanus, *Haemophilus influenzae* type b, hepatitis B, and inactivated poliomyelitis vaccine are used (live poliovirus vaccine is contraindicated).
2. Use of influenza vaccine is currently recommended annually before influenza season. Children >2 years old should receive the 23-valent pneumococcal vaccine.
3. The use of measles-mumps-rubella vaccine is currently recommended by the CDC in healthy HIV+ patients because of the risk of severe measles pneumonia (which has been fatal in some cases) in unvaccinated HIV+ patients. However, in the case of severely immunosuppressed patients (see Table 109–1), risks (including a

recent fatal case of vaccine-associated pneumonia) must be balanced on an individual basis.
4. Immune globulin should be given to all HIV+ patients exposed to measles cases.
5. Bacille Calmette-Guérin should not be given to HIV+ children.

Bibliography

American Academy of Pediatrics: HIV infection. *In* Peter G (ed): 1997 Red Book: Report of the Committee on Infectious Diseases, 24th ed. Elk Grove Village, IL, American Academy of Pediatrics, 1997, pp 289–294.

Gulick RM, Mellors JW, Havlir D, et al: Treatment with a combination of indinavir, zidovudine, and lamivudine in HIV-infected adults with prior antiretroviral use. N Engl J Med (in press).

Bach MC, Howell DA, Valenti A, et al: Aphthous ulceration of the gastrointestinal tract in patients with the acquired immunodeficiency syndrome (AIDS). Ann Intern Med 1995;112:465–467.

Frickofen N, Abkowitz JL, Safford M, et al: Persistent B19 parvovirus infection in patients infected with human immunodeficiency virus type 1 (HIV-1): A treatable cause of anemia in AIDS. Ann Intern Med 1990;113:926–933.

Working Group on Antiretroviral Therapy: National Pediatric HIV Resource Center. Antiretroviral therapy and management of the human immunodeficiency virus-infected child. Pediatr Infect Dis 1993;12:513–522.

110 Infection in the Immunocompromised Host

Robert Finberg

Definition

A patient can be immunocompromised by anything that prevents a normal response to infection. Either lack of a particular defense mechanism (lack of ability to initiate a T-cell or B-cell response) or a paucity of cells (neutropenia) may result in infections. Some prediction as to the type of infection a patient may acquire can be made based on the type of host defense defect (see below).

Etiology (Table 110–1)

Epidemiology

1. Traditionally, immunocompromised patients were those who were born with inborn errors of metabolism or specific deletions of proteins important in host defense; recently, the clinician is more likely to be confronted with patients who have acquired an immunosuppressive disease (e.g., human immunodeficiency virus infection) or are receiving medicines that cause immunosuppression (e.g., organ transplant recipients).
2. Patients with hemoglobinopathies (e.g., sickle cell anemia) are particularly likely to be predisposed to systemic infections because of autoinfarction of the spleen.

Pathophysiology

1. Lack of a cell type (e.g, T cells, polymorphonuclear leukocytes [PMNs]) clearly leads to loss of the immunologic function important to those cells.
2. Chronic use of medicines designed to prevent graft rejection (e.g., steroids, cyclosporin) leads to impairment of host responses, which results in susceptibility to viruses and intracellular bacteria.

Clinical Findings

1. Infection in the face of neutropenia after chemotherapy for cancer has a characteristic presentation, and the outcome is dramatically affected by the clinician's response.
   a. Fever in a neutropenic patient should always be considered to indicate infection.
   b. Infections in neutropenic patients are rapidly fatal if untreated. It is essential to treat from the beginning for a broad spectrum of organisms.
   c. In general, neutropenic patients develop bacterial infections early in the course of their neutropenia. Later, after some days of treatment for bacterial infections, they are predisposed to develop fungal infections (Table 110–2).

TABLE 110–1. TYPES OF IMMUNODEFICIENCY

DEFICIENCY STATE	EXAMPLE	CONSEQUENCE	SPECIFIC INFECTIONS
Abnormalities in PMNs	Cytotoxic chemotherapy for cancer Lazy leukocyte or Chédiak-Higashi syndrome	PMNs kill extracellular organisms; lack of PMNs leads to serious systemic and local infections	Infections by many extracellular bacteria, particularly gram-positive cocci and aerobic gram-negative rods, fungi (*Aspergillus* and *Candida*)
Abnormalities of antibody production	X-linked agammaglobulinemia, SCIDS	Antibodies are particularly important in "opsonizing" encapsulated bacteria	*Streptococcus pneumoniae, Haemophilus influenzae, Neisseria meningitidis*
Abnormalities of T-cell function	AIDS, SCIDS, chronic steroid therapy, or immunosuppression	T cells are crucial in the defense against intracellular pathogens after organ or bone marrow transplantation, DiGeorge syndrome	Herpes group viruses, intracellular bacteria (*Mycobacterium* spp.), *Nocardia, Actinomyces, Listeria*), fungi (especially *Cryptococcus, Histoplasma capsulatum, Coccidioides immitis, Pneumocystis carinii*)
Loss of spleen	Sickle cell (S-S) or other hemoglobinopathies, postsplenectomy patients (includes both trauma and patients undergoing staging for Hodgkin disease)	The spleen serves as a bacterial filter; its absence allows organisms (especially encapsulated bacteria) to survive in the bloodstream	*S. pneumoniae, H. influenzae, N. meningitidis*

AIDS, acquired immunodeficiency syndrome; PMNs, polymorphonuclear leukocytes; SCIDS, severe combined immunodeficiency syndrome.

d. Because such patients remain susceptible to infection with endogenous organisms for as long as they remain neutropenic, standard practice is to continue broad-spectrum antimicrobial treatment for the entire period.

2. Patients who are recipients of solid organ transplants are predisposed to certain infections based on the time after transplantation.

   a. Early, during the first weeks after transplantation, patients are most likely to develop infections related to the complications of surgery (e.g., gram-negative rods causing urinary tract infections, pyelonephritis in renal transplant recipients, mediastinitis after heart and lung transplantation).

   b. Because of the administration of steroids and other immunosuppressive agents that are necessary to prevent graft rejection, organ transplant recipients become susceptible to intracellular pathogens. Prime among these, approximately 1 month after transplantation, is cytomegalovirus (CMV). The infection has different manifestations depending on the transplant (ranging from coronary artery disease to vanishing bile ducts), but in almost all settings the presence of CMV seems to lead to a higher risk of complications and impaired graft survival.

   c. Even after all the scars of surgery have healed and the patient is leading a normal life, he or she remains susceptible to intracellular organisms by virtue of continued immunosuppressive therapy.

3. Skin lesions are a key sign of infection in immunocompromised patients. A skin biopsy is often revealing, especially in settings (such as fungal infections) in which blood culture may be negative despite progressive infection.

4. Many immunocompromised patients have long-term intravenous catheters in place. Such catheters are a major cause of infectious complications. Both blood cultures and careful attention to the sites is important in caring for these patients.

 Key Clinical Findings

- Skin lesions
- Catheter site involvement

Laboratory Findings

1. The critical evaluation of an immunocompromised host includes measurement of the number of circulating

TABLE 110–2. TIMING OF TYPICAL INFECTION IN IMMUNOCOMPROMISED HOST

ORGANISM	EARLY (<1 MO)	MIDDLE (1–5 MO)	LATE (>6 MO)
Bacteria	Surgical infections related to type of operation	Intracellular organisms (*Nocardia, Mycobacteria, Salmonella, Listeria*)	Intracellular organisms (*Nocardia, Mycobacteria, Salmonella, Listeria*)
Viruses	Herpes simplex	Cytomegalovirus	Human papillomaviruses, Epstein-Barr virus, varicella-zoster virus
Fungi	*Candida*	*Cryptococcus, Histoplasma capsulatum, Coccidioides immitis*	*Cryptococcus, H. capsulatum, C. immitis*
Parasites	*Toxoplasma gondii, Strongyloides stercoralis*	*Pneumocystis carinii*	*T. gondii, P. carinii*

PMNs, antibody levels, and the number of circulating T cells.

2. In assessing the presence of infection, routine cultures and antigen tests (especially cryptococcal antigen) are usually of value. Serologic tests (such as antibody rises after infection), may be falsely negative.

Radiographic Changes

1. Radiologic techniques are crucial to diagnosis of infections in immunocompromised patients. Computed tomography (CT) and/or magnetic resonance imaging (MRI) studies should be performed in patients with central nervous system findings to evaluate mass lesions of the brain, which in this group of patients include tumors as well as infections (e.g., toxoplasmosis, CMV infection).

2. Whereas gallium scanning and indium-labeled leukocyte scanning are often helpful in defining occult infection in normal hosts, these techniques can be difficult in neutropenic patients, in whom MRI may be superior.

3. Although conventional chest radiographs are often helpful in defining pneumonias in immunocompromised patients (even those without conventional clinical signs of pneumonia), high-resolution CT scans (or MRI) may be required to define nodules or cavities characteristic of patients in this setting.

Differential Diagnosis

1. Although it is usually wise to avoid administration of antibiotics (particularly broad-spectrum agents) to normal hosts unless the suspicion of infection is high, neutropenic patients presenting with fever should be assumed to be infected and treated immediately.

2. Immunocompromised patients with severe T-cell and/or B-cell deficiencies should be evaluated seriously for *Pneumocystis carinii* infection unless they have been reliably receiving prophylaxis.

3. It is a good general rule to assume that immunocompromised patients presenting with signs of infection (e.g., fever, infiltrates on chest x-ray) are likely to have more than one infection. For example, the patient who presents with *P. carinii* pneumonia may well have underlying CMV disease also. For this reason, it may be preferable to perform an invasive procedure (e.g., lung biopsy) early in the evaluation of a sick patient rather than waiting for a response to therapy—at which time the patient may be too sick to tolerate a procedure.

Treatment

1. Approach to treatment of neutropenic patients with infection

   a. Febrile neutropenic patients should be treated with antibacterial agents that are effective against both aerobic gram-positive and gram-negative organisms, considering the local resistance pattern of the hospital or care setting.

   b. Antibiotics should be adjusted on the basis of culture results without sacrificing spectrum.

   c. In general, antibiotics are continued until the patient's PMN counts increase.

   d. It is standard practice to add antifungal coverage empirically (without culture data).

2. Approach to treatment of transplantation recipients with infection

   a. In the early period (first month) after transplantation, treatment should be directed toward infections related to the transplantation procedure.

   b. After the initial early period, CMV (in patients who were CMV seropositive or who received a transplant from a seropositive individual) becomes one of the major causes of fever and should be seriously considered as a cause of many infectious complications.

   c. Late transplant infections are likely to be associated with intracellular organisms such as *Listeria*, *Toxoplasma*, *Mycobacterium* spp., and *P. carinii*. Prophylaxis with trimethoprim-sulfamethoxazole (TMP-SMX) is efficacious in preventing *Pneumocystis* and *Toxoplasma gondii* infection and should be given to all patients who continue to receive immunosuppressive treatments.

Prevention

1. The administration of CMV immune globulin has been shown to decrease CMV-related disease in solid organ transplant recipients, especially renal transplant recipients who are CMV seronegative before transplantation.

2. If possible, solid organ transplant recipients should receive all necessary vaccines before the transplantation procedure. Siblings of severely immunocompromised patients should not receive oral polio vaccine because of the risk of spreading the virus, but immunization of siblings (not patients) with measles, mumps, rubella, and varicella vaccines is recommended.

3. Surgically splenectomized or autosplenectomized patients should be vaccinated against *Haemophilus influenzae*, *Streptococcus pneumoniae*, and *Neisseria meningitidis*. Penicillin prophylaxis is recommended in patients with sickle cell (S-S) disease. Other splenectomized patients should be warned about the risk of overwhelming bacteremias and instructed to report signs of fever to a physician at once. Some clinicians recommend giving patients or their parents antibiotics to keep at home in case of infection.

4. Prophylactic antibiotics, especially TMP-SMX to prevent *P. carinii* infection, should be considered in patients who will remain immunosuppressed for long periods.

5. Immunocompromised patients who are seronegative for varicella-zoster virus and are exposed to someone with chickenpox should receive varicella-zoster immune globulin (VZIG). Treatment of exposed people (with 40 or 80 mg/kg of acyclovir in four divided doses beginning 7 days after exposure) has been shown to modify disease and is a reasonable course of action in a susceptible immunocompromised patient. Similarly, patients who have not been vaccinated against measles should receive globulin after an exposure to attenuate this disease.

6. In addition to routine infection-control procedures, patients who are neutropenic for extended periods (e.g., bone marrow transplant recipients), should be housed in

facilities with high-efficiency particulate air filters (HEPA filters) for the duration of their neutropenia.

Bibliography

Asano Y, Yoshikawa T, Suga S, et al: Postexposure prophylaxis of varicella in family contact by oral acyclovir. Pediatrics 1993;92:219–222.

Bodey GP: Dermatologic manifestations of infections in neutropenic patients. Infect Dis Clin North Am 1996;8:655–675.

Chanock SJ, Pizzo PA: Fever in the neutropenic host. Infect Dis Clin North Am 1996;10:777–796.

Green JN: Catheter-related complications of cancer therapy. Infect Dis Clin North Am 1996;10:255–295.

Molrine D, Ambrosino DA: Vaccinations in immunocompromised patients. Infect Med 1996;13:259–275.

111 Animal Exposures

Robert Finberg

By virtue of sharing the same space, humans come into contact with animals and animal microbes. Some of the interactions have undesirable outcomes. The same can be said of human-human interactions.

Etiology

1. Dog and cat exposures
   a. The organisms causing infections after bites by mammals reflect the flora in the mouth of the animal. Dog bites are the most common animal bite wounds treated in the United States.
      (1) *Pasteurella multocida* is carried in the mouths of most dogs, and this organism is found in 25 per cent of dog bites.
      (2) *Staphylococcus aureus* and *P. multocida* are isolated together in 20 to 30 per cent of cases.
      (3) *Staphylococcus intermedius*, a coagulase-positive staphylococcus, is also seen in approximately one fourth of cases. This organism, unlike *S. aureus*, is usually sensitive to penicillin.
      (4) Aerobic organisms that are associated with dog bites include *Micrococcus*, β-hemolytic streptococci, α-hemolytic streptococci (and enterococci), and coagulase-negative staphylococci.
      (5) Gram-negative organisms such as *Haemophilus aphrophilus*, *Proteus mirabilis*, *Enterobacter cloacae*, *Pseudomonas fluorescens*, and *Pasteurella* spp. have been reported in dog bite wounds.
      (6) *Capnocytopaga canimorsus* (formerly called DF-2) is a facultatively anaerobic gram-negative rod that has been associated with fulminant sepsis after dog bites.
      (7) Anaerobes that have been isolated from dog bite wounds include *Fusobacterium*, *Bacteroides*, *Veillonella*, *Proprionibacterium*, and *Peptococcus* spp. and anaerobic streptococci.
   b. Cat bites are the second most common bite wounds reported.
      (1) Approximately 80 per cent of cats carry *P. multocida* in their mouths. *Pasteurella* is the most common organism cultured from cat bite wounds (including lion, cougar, and tiger bites).
      (2) Because of the sharp teeth of cats, puncture wounds are common and resultant osteomyelitis and septic arthritis with *P. multocida* is common.
      (3) Contact with cats can also lead to cat scratch disease, an illness caused by *Bartonella henselae* that usually occurs after a scratch wound.

2. Exposures to other animals
   a. Snakes are common causes of toxin-induced disease. The venom is sterile, but organisms may be introduced during procedures designed to remove the venom.
   b. Ants are capable of both biting and stinging children. The fire ant (*Solenopsis invicta* or *Solenopsis xyloni*) produces an intensely painful wheal with a sting.
   c. The presence of small puncture wounds (especially two close together) should suggest the possibility of a spider bite. Both the black widow and the brown recluse spider can cause serious injury to small children. Brown recluse spiders tend to cause local damage (with necrotic skin lesions), whereas black widow bites may lead to serious systemic illness in infants or small children.
   d. In cases of exotic animal bites, the mouth flora of the animal involved should be considered. In part, the mouth flora is a function of the animal's environment. For example, alligator bites have been associated with *Aeromonas hydrophilia* (a freshwater organism); *Vibrio* species (saltwater organisms) may be associated with shark bites.
   e. The normal flora of the human mouth includes *S. aureus*, *Eikenella corrodens*, *H. influenzae*, and oral anaerobes (some of which are β-lactamase producing).
   f. Monkey mouth flora is similar to that of humans

with the exception that some species (especially old world *Macaca*) carry simian B virus (cercopithecine herpesvirus 1).

Epidemiology

1. The lifetime incidence of animal or human bites to Americans is approximately 50 per cent.
2. The incidence of mammalian bites is reported to be as high as 15 per cent in children by 1 year of age.
3. The peak age of dog bite wounds is 5 to 14 years, and most (50 to 75%) of all dog bites occur in persons younger than 20 years old.
   a. Fifteen to 20 per cent of the sites become infected.
   b. Pathogenic organisms can be cultured from most wounds.
4. Most bite wounds seen in emergency departments occur in boys in the summer months.

Pathophysiology

1. The mouth flora of mammals is a polymicrobial soup. Inoculation of these organisms into skin and subcutaneous tissue is likely to lead to abscess formation and may lead to sepsis with naturally invasive organisms.
2. Although pathogenic mouth organisms can be cultured from most wounds, estimates for the rate of clinical infection range from 2 to 30 per cent for dog bites and 16 to 50 per cent for cat bites.
3. Puncture wounds may lead to osteomyelitis and/or septic arthritis, and devitalized tissue is subject to infection, especially with anaerobes.

Clinical Findings

1. Persons with bite wounds from dogs or cats usually present with a limited cellulitis, often accompanied by a gray, foul-smelling discharge.
2. Patients with *P. multocida* infection typically develop intense pain, swelling, and erythema, often within hours of the injury. Rapid development of an intense response is characteristic of *P. multocida* infection.

Expected Microorganisms

Dog and Cat Bites	Human Bites
Pasturella multocida	Streptococci
Staphylococcus aureus	*S. aureus*
Haemophilus species	*Haemophilus*
Bacteroides species	species
Capnocytophaga canimorsus	*Bacteroides* species

---

3. Human bites are said to be more serious than those produced by most animal exposures.
   a. Part of the seriousness of human bites may relate to the occurrence of the "clenched fist" injury.
   b. The "clenched fist" injury occurs when the fist of one person strikes the teeth of another. The wound is usually ignored by the involved party, who presents late; the infection may have a poor outcome. *Eikenella corrodens* infection is commonly seen in this setting.

4. Spider bites are characterized by single or closely paired puncture wounds.
   a. Black widow *(Lactrodectus hesperus)* bites present with a punctate wound with surrounding pallor. The child may present with muscular rigidity and muscle spasms.
   b. Brown recluse *(Lactrodectus reclusa)* bites produce necrotic lesions that may become large and painful.

Key Clinical Findings

- Cellulitis
- Intense pain

Laboratory Findings

An elevated leukocyte count may be present, but the physical examination is usually key in making a diagnosis.

Radiographic Changes

1. It is important to look for evidence of gas, which may suggest infection with a gas-producing organism and/or devitalized tissue necessitating surgical intervention.
2. X-ray studies are particularly important in the case of large animal bites, which are commonly associated with bone fractures.

Differential Diagnosis

1. Small children and infants may not be able to describe animal exposures. A thorough history to define the child's contacts is important in terms of diagnosis and treatment.
2. Most spider bites go unseen, and it is rare to recover the actual spider. The presence of paired small, punctate lesions suggests a spider bite.
   a. Black widow bites are characterized by a punctate wound with surrounding pallor.
   b. Brown recluse spider bites are characterized by necrotic lesions.

Treatment

1. Thorough irrigation of the wound (without damaging sensitive tissues) is recommended. High-pressure irrigation (using normal saline forced through a small opening such as an 18- or 19-gauge needle) is more effective than low-pressure irrigation.
2. If the host is immunocompromised (has no spleen, has neutropenia, is receiving chemotherapy, or has an immunodeficiency syndrome), antibiotics should be given to prevent serious infection.
3. The risks of rabies and tetanus should be considered.
   a. Tetanus immunization is recommended if the patient has not had a booster within the last 5 years.
   b. In the United States, rabies is predominantly a disease of wild animals (raccoons, skunks, and bats). Care providers should check with state health departments to obtain the latest information concerning the presence of rabies in a given animal population. If the animal can be found, many health departments can analyze brain tissue for the pres-

Issues to Consider in Treatment

Therapy	When Recommended
Irrigation, avoiding damage to tissues	Always
Tetanus prophylaxis	If >5 yr has lapsed since a booster, another immunization is needed; for unimmunized persons, tetanus immune globulin and a complete series is indicated
Rabies prophylaxis	In the United States, wild animals are the most common vectors; consult local authorities
Antibiotics	Recommended when there are signs of cellulitis; prophylaxis for severe injuries, especially for cat and human bites, is recommended

ence of rabies, and unnecessary prophylaxis may be avoided.

4. Although it is not clear that all bites need to be treated with antibiotics (most do not result in clinical infection), many authorities give prophylactic antibiotics to bite victims. Because higher infection rates and more serious infections have occurred after cat or human bites, these issues should be considered in the decision about whether to treat. The presence of cellulitis, especially with a purulent discharge, should suggest the need to add antibiotics.

5. Antibiotic treatment with a drug with activity against staphylococcus, streptococcus, *P. multocida*, and anaerobes should be considered in dog, cat, and human bites. For this reason, amoxicillin with clavulanate (250 to 500 mg tid) is recommended. Alternative PO therapies include second-generation cephalosporins (e.g., cefuroxime). In older children or adults, a fluroquinolone plus clindamycin or tetracycline could be given. For serious infections, intravenous therapy with ampicillin and sulbactam is recommended.

6. Antibiotic treatment of bites from other animals varies according to the mouth flora of the animal involved.

7. Specific antivenom can be given for bites of certain snakes and black widow spiders.

Key Treatments

- Irrigation of wound
- Tetanus prophylaxis
- Antibiotics
- Rabies prophylaxis for wild animal bites (United States)

Prevention

1. Parents should be cautioned about leaving small children alone with any animal.
2. Certain species, such as ferrets, although kept as pets, are particularly vicious and may kill infants if left alone with them.

Bibliography

Dire DJ: Emergency management of dog and cat bite wounds. Emerg Med Clin North Am 1992;10:719–736.

Fang G, Araujo V, Guerrant RL: Enteric infections associated with exposure to animals or animal products. Infect Dis Clin North Am 1991;5:3:681–701.

Feder HM, Shanley JD, Barbera JA: Review of 59 patients hospitalized with animal bites. Pediatr Infect Dis J 1987;6:24–28.

Goldstein EJC: Bite wounds and infection. Clin Infect Dis 1992;14:633–638.

Griego RD, Rosen T, Orengo IF, Wolf JE: Dog, cat, and human bites: A review. J Am Acad Dermatol 1995;33:1019–1029.

Weber DJ, Hansen AR: Infections resulting from animal bites. Infect Dis Clin North Am 1991;5:663–701.

112 Symptoms of Hematologic Disorders

Symptom | **Pallor**   *Sreedhar P. Rao*

An infant or child is considered to have pallor when the skin or mucous membrane is pale. Although the two most common causes of pallor are severe anemia and asphyxia, lack of sufficient exposure to sunlight or edema may also produce skin pallor.

Differential Diagnosis
1. Severe anemia
2. Hypovolemic shock
3. Asphyxia, particularly in a newborn
4. Edema.

History
1. Determine if there is a history of trauma or blood loss, e.g., epistaxis, menorrhagia, or blood in stools.
2. Obtain detailed nutritional history: breast feeding or formula feeding with or without supplemental iron; age at the time of introduction of whole cow's milk; intake of iron-fortified food and meat.
3. Inquire about episodes of jaundice or enlarged spleen as well as dark urine following accidental mothball ingestion, which suggest a diagnosis of hemolytic anemia.
4. Inquire about a family history of anemia or gallbladder disease.
5. Obtain perinatal history with specific reference to delivery, evidence of fetal distress before delivery, and Apgar score at birth.
6. Investigate history of rapid weight gain, swelling of eyelids, decreased urinary output, or renal disease.

Clinical Findings
1. If pallor is due to anemia, both skin and mucosa will be pale.
2. Hypotension, tachycardia, rapid shallow respirations, and drop in hemoglobin favor significant blood loss.
3. Jaundice, hepatomegaly, and splenomegaly in a patient with pallor support a diagnosis of hemolytic anemia.
4. Petechiae/ecchymosis together with pallor suggest that the patient may be thrombocytopenic in addition to being anemic.
5. An asphyxiated infant may manifest retractions, tachy-

pnea or slow breathing, tachycardia or bradycardia, and cyanosis. The hemoglobin concentration may be normal.

Tests
1. Complete blood count and reticulocyte count. If the patient is anemic, appropriate investigations are performed (see *Evaluation of a Patient with Anemia*) to determine the cause of anemia.
2. If the patient is anemic and thrombocytopenic, perform a direct Coombs test; autoimmune hemolytic anemia and immune thrombocytopenia will constitute Evans syndrome. A bone marrow aspiration and biopsy are done for evidence of leukemia, aplastic anemia, or infiltrative disorders of the bone marrow.
3. A newborn with asphyxia may or may not be anemic; if the infant is anemic, appropriate diagnostic tests are obtained (see *Evaluation of a Newborn with Anemia*).
4. In a child who is pale because of edema, evaluate for renal disease (nephrotic syndrome), liver disease, or cardiac disease.

Management
1. If the patient is anemic, treat the underlying cause of the anemia, e.g., with administration of iron. Depending on the patient's age and history, an investigation for blood loss may be required (See Chapter 113 for details).
2. If a patient is severely anemic and exhibiting signs of impending or overt heart failure, cautious packed red blood cell transfusion or partial red blood cell exchange transfusion is indicated. While awaiting blood transfusion, the patient should be administered oxygen to improve the oxygen-carrying capacity of blood.
3. A patient who is pale owing to severe acute blood loss is managed by supportive measures (fluids management to restore circulation) and by red blood cell transfusion.
4. Asphyxia in a newborn or pallor due to edema is managed accordingly.

 ## Bibliography

Oski FA: Pallor. *In* Kaye R, Oski FA, Barness LA (eds): Core Textbook of Pediatrics. Philadelphia, JB Lippincott, 1978, pp 79–80.

Symptom | **Jaundice**   *Sreedhar P. Rao*

Definition
Jaundice, defined as yellowish discoloration of sclerae and/or skin, is due to increased serum levels of bilirubin. Normal serum bilirubin in older infants and children is ≤ 1 mg/dl with ≤ 0.2 mg/dl of conjugated (direct) bilirubin.

Jaundice is frequently seen in the neonatal period, when etiology and management are quite different (see Chapter 16) from those in older infants and children. The following discussion will be limited to the evaluation and management of an older infant or a child with jaundice.

Differential Diagnosis

It is essential to determine if a child has unconjugated (indirect) hyperbilirubinemia or hyperbilirubinemia with elevated conjugated bilirubin (≥ 2 mg/dl) because of differences in etiology and management. The causes of hyperbilirubinemia are listed in Table 112–1.

History

1. Family history of hemolytic anemia or metabolic disease is important for an early diagnosis of these conditions.
2. History of prior blood transfusion suggests delayed hemolytic transfusion reaction or viral hepatitis, depending on the time interval.
3. History of ingestion of drugs known to produce jaundice.

Physical Examination

1. Determine the liver span for accurate assessment of the size of the liver. Many conditions causing jaundice are associated with an enlarged liver.
2. Palpate the abdomen for evidence of splenomegaly or other abdominal masses. Splenomegaly in a patient with jaundice, particularly unconjugated hyperbilirubinemia, is suggestive of hemolytic anemia. Splenomegaly may also be seen in patients with infiltrative (storage) disorders.

Tests

1. Liver tests
   a. Serum bilirubin, total and direct
   b. Serum alanine aminotransferase (ALT) and aspartate aminotransferase (AST)—these are increased in hepatocellular injury (hepatitis).
   c. Serum albumin, prothrombin time, partial thromboplastin time; these are abnormal in liver disease because of decreased protein synthesis.
   d. Serum alkaline phosphatase is increased in biliary obstruction.
2. Tests for hepatitis; serology for Epstein-Barr virus (EBV), cytomegalovirus (CMV), and hepatitis A, B, C if ALT or AST is abnormal.
3. Complete blood count with reticulocyte count and blood smear evaluation. Anemia and reticulocytosis indicate hemolytic anemia. If hemolytic anemia is a likely diagnosis, appropriate studies are done (e.g., hemoglobin electrophoresis).
4. Abdominal ultrasound is helpful in evaluating for

choledocholithiasis, choledochal cyst, or any mass compressing the biliary tree.
5. Measurements of appropriate enzymes when metabolic or storage disease is a diagnostic consideration.
6. Liver biopsy when other tests have failed to reveal a diagnosis.

Management

Treatment of these patients will depend on the diagnosis; for example, patients with Crigler-Najjar syndrome (type II) will respond to phenobarbital administration.

Bibliography

Thaler MM: The liver and bile ducts. *In* Rudolph AM (ed): Rudolph's Pediatrics, 19th ed. East Norwalk, CT, Appleton and Lange, 1991, pp 1054–1065.

TABLE 112–1. CAUSES OF HYPERBILIRUBINEMIA

UNCONJUGATED

Hemolytic Anemias

Hemoglobinopathies
Thalassemia syndrome
Hereditary spherocytosis and elliptocytosis
Red cell enzyme deficiency disorder, e.g., G6PD deficiency
Autoimmune or alloimmune hemolysis
Schistocytic hemolytic anemia, e.g., HUS

Inherited Enzyme Disorders

Crigler-Najjar syndrome
Gilbert syndrome

Parasitic Infestations

Leptospirosis
Schistosomiasis

Miscellaneous

Reye syndrome
Wilson disease
Malaria

CONJUGATED

Hepatitis

Viral
Drug-induced

Extrahepatic Biliary Obstruction

Choledocholithiasis
Choledochal cyst
Extrahepatic biliary atresia
Tumor or enlarged nodes compressing the biliary tract
Kawasaki disease

Metabolic Disorders

Dubin-Johnson syndrome
Rotor syndrome
α_1-antitrypsin deficiency
Galactosemia*
Total parenteral nutrition

Infiltrative Disorders

Familial or viral hemophagocytic syndrome
Langerhan cell histiocytosis
Gaucher disease*
Neimann-Pick disease*

*Only rarely have conjugated hyperbilirubinemia.

Symptom | **Anemia in Children** — *Sreedhar P. Rao*

Definition

Anemia is defined as decreased concentration of hemoglobin or red blood cell count, or both. Since the normal hemoglobin concentration is dependent on age and gender, one needs to take into account these factors in deciding if a child is anemic. Table 112–2 lists the mean values as well as the lower limit of normal values for hemoglobin, hematocrit, and mean corpuscular volume (MCV). The hemoglobin level rises shortly after birth, returns to birth values at age 2 weeks, and then drops approximately 1 g/week to the physiologic values of 9.5 to 11.5 g/dl at age 2 months. Note that the lower limit of normal for MCV from age 6 months to 10 years is approximately 70 plus age in years.

Classification

Anemia may be classified according to physiologic basis or red cell size (MCV), as shown in Tables 112–3 and 112–4.

Evaluation

A detailed history and physical examination are very important first steps in the evaluation of a child with anemia.

TABLE 112–2. VALUES (NORMAL MEAN AND LOWER LIMITS OF NORMAL) FOR HEMOGLOBIN, HEMATOCRIT, AND MCV DETERMINATIONS

AGE (yr)	HEMOGLOBIN (g/dL)		HEMATOCRIT (%)		MCV (μ³)	
	Mean	*Lower Limit*	*Mean*	*Lower Limit*	*Mean*	*Lower Limit*
Birth (cord blood)	16.5	13.5	51	42	108	98
2 mos	11.2	9.4	35	28	96	77
0.5–1.9	12.5	11.0	37	33	77	70
2–4	12.5	11.0	38	34	79	73
5–7	13.0	11.5	39	35	81	75
8–11	13.5	12.0	40	36	83	76
12–14						
Female	13.5	12.0	41	36	85	78
Male	14.0	12.5	43	37	84	77
15–17						
Female	14.0	12.0	41	36	87	79
Male	15.0	13.0	46	38	86	78
18–49						
Female	14.0	12.0	42	37	90	80
Male	16.0	14.0	47	40	90	80

Modified from Oski FA: Differential diagnosis of anemia. *In* Nathan DG, Oski FA (eds): Hematology of Infancy and Childhood, 4th ed. Philadelphia, WB Saunders, 1993.

These are followed by complete blood count (CBC) and evaluation of the blood smear. Establishing a definitive diagnosis may require additional laboratory tests.

1. History

   a. Age—Anemia in the early newborn period is usually due to blood group isoimmunization (Rh and ABO hemolytic disease), infection, blood loss, or inherited hemolytic anemia. Nutritional iron deficiency anemia has become unusual in the United States, thanks to the WIC program, but when present is typically seen in infants between 9 and 24 months of age. Occasionally adolescents, and especially women, may become iron deficient owing to increased needs and capricious diet. Infants born prematurely may manifest iron deficiency anemia by 6 months of age.

   b. Gender—Anemia in male infants may suggest an X-linked disorder (e.g., G6PD deficiency).

   c. Race—Sickle hemoglobinopathy and C-hemoglo-

TABLE 112–3. PHYSIOLOGIC CLASSIFICATION OF ANEMIA

DECREASED RED CELL PRODUCTION

Marrow failure
  Aplastic anemia
  Malignancies infiltrating bone marrow
  Pure red cell aplasia (Diamond-Blackfan anemia)
  Transient erythroblastopenia of childhood
Impaired erythropoietin production
  Chronic renal insufficiency
  Chronic infection/inflammation

DISORDERS OF ERYTHROID MATURATION AND INEFFECTIVE ERYTHROPOIESIS

Iron deficiency
Thalassemia syndromes
Lead poisoning
Folic acid deficiency
Vitamin B₁₂ deficiency

HEMOLYTIC ANEMIAS

Hemoglobin disorders
  Structural mutation—sickle hemoglobin, hemoglobin C
  Synthetic mutation, e.g., thalassemia syndromes
Red cell membrane disorders—spherocytosis, elliptocytosis, pyropoikilocytosis
Defects of red cell metabolism—G6PD deficiency, pyruvate kinase deficiency
Antibody-mediated hemolysis
Isoimmune hemolytic anemia
Autoimmune hemolytic anemia
Schistocytic injury to the red cell
Microangiopathic hemolytic anemia

BLOOD LOSS

Modified from Oski FA: Differential diagnosis of anemia. *In* Nathan DG, Oski FA (eds): Hematology of Infancy and Childhood, 4th ed. Philadelphia, WB Saunders, 1993.

TABLE 112–4. CLASSIFICATION OF ANEMIA BASED ON RED CELL SIZE (MCV)

MICROCYTIC ANEMIAS

Iron deficiency
Thalassemia syndromes
Chronic lead poisoning
Chronic infection/inflammation
Hemoglobin SC disease, sickle thalassemia, and hemoglobin C disease

MACROCYTIC ANEMIAS

Vitamin B₁₂ deficiency
Folic acid deficiency
Aplastic anemia
Diamond-Blackfan anemia
Myelodysplastic syndromes
Drug therapy—hydroxyurea, AZT

NORMOCYTIC ANEMIAS

Hemolytic anemias
  Sickle cell anemia
  Red cell enzyme defects
  Antibody-mediated hemolyis
Acute infection
Acute blood loss
Chronic renal disease

Modified from Oski FA: Differential diagnosis of anemia. *In* Nathan DG, Oski FA (eds): Hematology of Infancy and Childhood, 4th ed. Philadelphia, WB Saunders, 1993.

binopathy are mainly seen in blacks. Cooley anemia is usually seen in Caucasians of Mediterranean ancestry.

  d. Nutritional history—Infants fed iron-containing formula in the first year of life generally do not develop iron deficiency. In contrast, infants fed non–iron containing formula or those with early introduction of whole cow milk (before 6 months of age) are likely to develop iron deficiency. Breast-fed infants whose mothers are strict vegetarians may become vitamin B_{12} deficient. Infants who are fed exclusively goat milk may develop folate deficiency.

  e. Drug or chemical exposure—Infants or children presenting with anemia a few days after exposure to naphthalene mothballs or oxidant drugs are probably G6PD deficient. Prolonged phenytoin therapy may produce folate deficiency. Prior history of jaundice, pallor, cholecystectomy, and/or splenectomy in the patient or a family member is suggestive of hemolytic anemia.

  2. Physical examination
Abnormal physical findings and their clinical significance are depicted below.

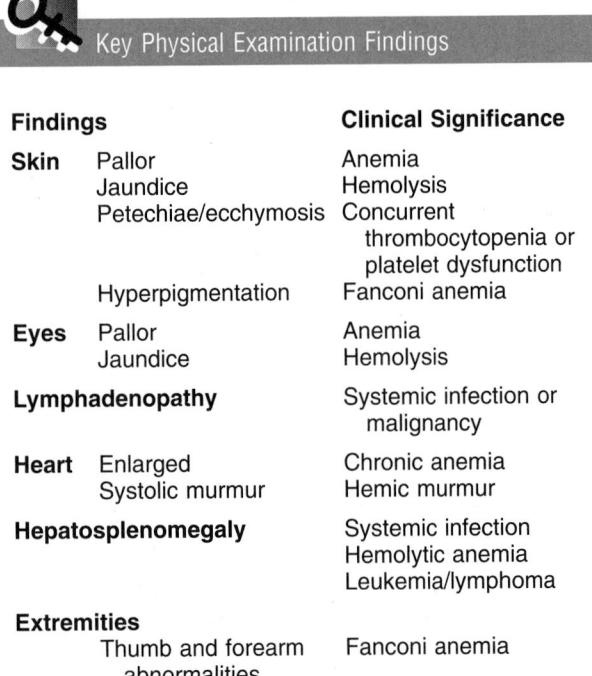

Key Physical Examination Findings

Findings		Clinical Significance
Skin	Pallor	Anemia
	Jaundice	Hemolysis
	Petechiae/ecchymosis	Concurrent thrombocytopenia or platelet dysfunction
	Hyperpigmentation	Fanconi anemia
Eyes	Pallor	Anemia
	Jaundice	Hemolysis
Lymphadenopathy		Systemic infection or malignancy
Heart	Enlarged	Chronic anemia
	Systolic murmur	Hemic murmur
Hepatosplenomegaly		Systemic infection Hemolytic anemia Leukemia/lymphoma
Extremities	Thumb and forearm abnormalities	Fanconi anemia

Laboratory Evaluation

  1. Most laboratories use electronic counters for performing a CBC, which provides the following information:

  a. Hemoglobin

  b. Red blood cell count

  c. Mean corpuscular volume (MCV)

  d. Mean corpuscular hemoglobin concentration (MCHC)

  e. Mean corpuscular hemoglobin (MCH)

  f. Red cell distribution width (RDW)

  g. WBC count with differential

  h. Platelet count.

  2. Two additional tests, reticulocyte count and peripheral blood smear, are essential for evaluation of a patient with anemia.

  3. Once a child is found to be anemic, it should be determined if there is concomitant leukopenia/neutropenia and/or thrombocytopenia. The major diagnostic considerations in a child with pancytopenia are leukemia, aplastic anemia, severe megaloblastic anemia, and systemic lupus. If a child has isolated anemia, one must determine if the MCV is low, normal, or increased. This is followed by careful examination of the peripheral blood smear for red cell size; central pallor; presence of target cells, spherocytes, elliptocytes, or sickle cells; variation in red cell size (anisocytosis) and shape (poikilocytosis); and red cell fragmentation, blister cells, basophilic stippling, and inclusions in the red cells (e.g., Howell-Jolly bodies). RDW measures variability in red cell size. In a patient with microcytic anemia, an elevated RDW (>16) is suggestive of iron deficiency; a normal RDW suggests thalassemia trait.

  4. Based on a CBC, reticulocyte count, and smear evaluation, it is possible to characterize a child's anemia as microcytic, normocytic, or macrocytic as well as whether it is a hypoproliferative anemia or due to hemolysis or bleeding. Combined with history, physical examination, and the test results, one can arrive at a preliminary diagnosis that can be confirmed by appropriate diagnostic tests. The following case histories will illustrate the diagnostic approach listed above.

  a. *Case 1.* A 1-year-old boy has a hemoglobin of 8g/dl, MCV 65 fl, reticulocyte count 1%, with normal white cell and platelet count. He has a history of consumption of large quantities of whole cow milk since the age of 6 months. Based on a probable diagnosis of iron deficiency anemia, one may give a therapeutic trial of iron without additional investigations or confirm the diagnosis by documenting low serum ferritin or low transferrin saturation before therapy with oral iron. It is essential to recommend dietary changes to prevent recurrent anemia in those with nutritional iron deficiency anemia.

  b. *Case 2.* A 2-year-old with history of pallor and jaundice of 1 day's duration and history of exposure (inhalation or vapor may be sufficient) to naphthalene mothballs is pale and icteric. A CBC reveals a hemoglobin of 5 g/dl, normal MCV, normal white cell and platelet count, reticulocyte count 12%, and indirect bilirubin 4 mg/dl. A blood smear reveals numerous bite cells, blister cells, and polychromatophilia. A supravital stain reveals Heinz bodies. Most probable diagnosis is G6PD deficiency–associated acute hemolytic anemia, precipitated by exposure to naphthalene. A quantitative G6PD assay may give a normal value because of destruction of old red cells with lower concentration of G6PD and the presence of a large number of reticulocytes with a higher content of G6PD. Investigation of the mother may reveal that she is a carrier. After the child has fully recovered from anemia, a quantitative assay for G6PD should be repeated.

5. A child with normocytic anemia and a low reticulocyte count has hypoproliferative anemia, which may be due to chronic disease (infection/inflammation), renal insufficiency, or transient erythroblastopenia. A history of fever and high erythrocyte sedimentation rate favor a diagnosis of chronic infection/inflammation or malignancy. An elevated serum urea nitrogen and creatinine are indicative of anemia of renal insufficiency. The following laboratory studies may be needed in some patients with anemia in addition to CBC, reticulocyte count, and blood smear evaluation.

  a. Serum ferritin

  b. Serum chemical analyses; bilirubin, LDH, K, BUN, creatinine

  c. Serum B_{12} and folic acid, red cell folic acid

  d. Direct and indirect Coombs tests

  e. Hemoglobin electrophoresis

  f. Screening for unstable hemoglobin disorder

  g. Red cell osmotic fragility.

When evaluating a child for probable inherited anemia, hematologic evaluation of the parents is extremely useful and should be done whenever possible. When a diagnosis cannot be made by standard laboratory tests, a bone marrow aspiration is indicated.

Symptom | **The Child with a Bleeding Tendency** | *Andrea Hagani* and *James Bussell*

Definition

Symptoms of a bleeding tendency include purpura (both ecchymoses and petechiae), epistaxis, and other types of prolonged bleeding, e.g., prolonged bleeding after dental extraction, circumcision, and tonsillectomy and adenoidectomy.

Differential Diagnosis

1. Petechiae (without extensive ecchymosis)

  a. Thrombocytopenia

    (1) Immunologic

      (a) Immune thrombocytopenic purpura

      (b) Drug-induced immune thrombocytopenia

      (c) Neonatal immune thrombocytopenia

    (2) Nonimmune

      (a) Infectious (concurrent with, not after, the infection)

        1. Viral (rubella, varicella, EBV, CMV, herpes, measles, HIV)

        2. Bacterial sepsis

      (b) Microangiopathic: hemolytic uremic syndrome, thrombotic thrombocytopenic purpura, Kasabach-Merritt syndrome, DIC

      (c) Drug-induced (nonimmune): valproic acid, heparin, G-CSF, amiodarone, thiazide diuretics (?), alcohol, chemotherapy

      (d) Hypersplenism: congestive, infiltrative (Gaucher disease), sequestrative (sickle cell disease), rheumatologic (Felty syndrome)

      (e) Leukemia, other infiltrative malignancies

      (f) Miscellaneous: ionizing radiation

    (3) Congenital thrombocytopenia

      (a) Infection: bacterial sepsis, syphilis, CMV, HSV, rubella, HIV, toxoplasmosis

      (b) Immunologic: alloimmunization, maternal autoantibody induced (SLE, ITP)

      (c) Bone marrow abnormality: amegakaryocytic thrombocytopenia, thrombocytopenia-absent radius (TAR) syndrome, phocomelia syndrome, Fanconi anemia, aplastic anemia, trisomy syndromes (13 and 18), osteopetrosis, congenital leukemia

      (d) Maternal drugs: tolbutamide, hydralazine, hydantoin, azathioprine

      (e) Intravascular coagulation syndromes: DIC, major vessel thrombosis (renal vein, aorta), NEC

      (f) Peripheral consumption: giant hemangioma, hyperviscosity syndrome, erythroblastosis fetalis, congenital heart disease

      (g) Hereditary thrombocytopenias: Wiskott-Aldrich syndrome, May-Hegglin anomaly, miscellaneous familial

      (h) Miscellaneous causes: post–exchange transfusion syndrome, maternal hyperthyroidism, metabolic disorders (mucolipidosis), maternal toxemia, neonatal neuroblastoma, neonatal cold injury, perinatal pulmonary syndromes

    (4) Qualitative platelet abnormalities

      (a) Acquired

        (1) Drug induced

          (i) Cyclooxygenase inhibitors such as aspirin-containing compounds or NSAIDS, e.g., ibuprofen (Motrin)

          (ii) High-dose intravenous antibiotics, e.g., Timentin

        (2) Uremia

        (3) Severe liver disease, alcohol

      (b) Congenital

        (1) Glanzmann thrombasthenia

        (2) Bernard-Soulier syndrome

        (3) Gray platelet syndrome

        (4) Storage pool disorders

        (5) Abnormalities of platelet release reaction

        (6) Disorders associated with platelet dys-

function: type Ib glycogen storage disease, cyanotic congenital heart disease

2. Prolonged bleeding, including epistaxis
    a. Inherited coagulation factor deficiencies
        (1) Hemophilias A and B and less common entities such as factors XI, II, V, X, and XIII deficiency
        (2) von Willebrand disease
    b. Acquired coagulopathies
        (1) Acquired hemophilia A or von Willebrand disease (autoantibody)
        (2) Consumption coagulopathy (DIC)
        (3) Hemorrhagic disease of the newborn (vitamin K deficiency)
    c. Angiofibroma, other tumors of the nasopharynx
    d. Scurvy and other dietary deficiencies

History

If there is only one isolated symptom, i.e., any one of the above types of prolonged bleeding, it is less likely that a major clinical bleeding tendency is present, but in no way does it exclude it.

1. Bruises are normally present on the shins of small children. However, multiple large and, especially, palpable bruises in areas not readily exposed to trauma are abnormal.

2. Petechiae may be present on the face with prolonged crying or vomiting and may be scattered diffusely with a viral infection, although meningococcemia must be considered in the latter case. However, marked thrombocytopenia may present with diffuse petechiae as the only symptom (p in petechiae = p in platelet).

3. Oral cavity petechiae and, particularly, large black areas or blood blisters typically indicate a platelet count <10,000/μl.

4. Questions to ask about epistaxis illustrate the general approach to the bleeding child:
    a. Was the nosebleed unilateral or bilateral?
    b. Was there a history of trauma (including nose picking)?
    c. How long did the episode last?
    d. Did the bleeding stop with pressure alone?
    e. Is there a family history of bleeding?
    f. Has this occurred before and, if so, how often?
    g. Does it occur only in the winter, when the heat is turned on in the house?
    h. Finally (and perhaps most definitive of a bleeding tendency if answered positively): Were interventions such as packing and cautery required?

5. Prolonged bleeding can be difficult to define, but usually any bleeding that continues such that medical attention is required should be considered significant. Some examples include
    a. Bleeding after a circumcision that requires a physician's attention and/or hospitalization
    b. Bleeding after tooth extraction requiring a return to the dentist and/or suturing
    c. Menstrual periods heavy enough to result in significant anemia
    d. Bleeding after tonsillectomy, either early or late.

Physical Examination

1. Petechiae—Can be distinguished from angiomas because petechiae do *not* blanch with pressure
    a. Search for other bruises or purpura, including in the mouth and the fundi.
    b. Hepatosplenomegaly and adenopathy are usually absent in immune causes of thrombocytopenia but are common findings when the cause is infectious or malignant.
    c. Check the radial x-rays for abnormalities indicative of congenital causes.

2. Epistaxis and prolonged bleeding
    a. The presence of petechiae, ecchymoses, or other signs and symptoms with epistaxis would imply a more global problem.
    b. In the case of epistaxis, the nares should be examined for evidence of a bleeding vessel or prominent vasculature.

Tests

1. Petechiae: The initial triage requires a CBC with platelets.
    a. If *isolated thrombocytopenia* is present
        (1) Coombs direct and indirect tests to rule out Evans syndrome (anemia may not be apparent early in the illness)
        (2) Antiplatelet antibodies are not yet diagnostic of ITP.
        (3) Blood type for potential usage of anti-D
    b. If thrombocytopenia is *not isolated* and/or hepatosplenomegaly and/or adenopathy is present), systemic work-up is required, including a bone marrow examination according to the clinical picture based upon the differential diagnosis above.
    c. If the *platelet count is normal*, consider PT and PTT, von Willebrand work-up, and platelet aggregation studies.

2. Epistaxis or prolonged bleeding: Triage with a CBC including platelets, PT, and PTT if the history and/or PE are considered significant by the criteria above.
    a. If *PT and PTT are normal*, work-up for von Willebrand disease is indicated and possibly for factor XIII deficiency if the bleeding tendency is severe.
    b. Abnormal PT and/or PTT
        (1) Mixing studies to distinguish a factor deficiency from a circulating inhibitor*
        (2) If mixing studies are normal and
            (a) Only the PT is abnormal: levels of factors II, V, VII and X
            (b) Only the PTT is abnormal: levels of factors VIII, IX, XI, and XII

---

*Except for rare cases of a true circulating inhibitor, a mixing study consistent with an inhibitor is not usually associated with a bleeding tendency (despite, for example, the prolonged PTT).

(c) Both the PT and the PTT are abnormal: levels of factors II, V, and X. Can be either hereditary deficiency or secondary to vitamin K deficiency or warfarin therapy.

  (i) Thrombin and reptilase times to rule out heparin effect and low or dysfunctional fibrinogen

  (ii) Fibrinogen and fibrin degradation products to rule out DIC and/or liver disease as well as other causes of low fibrinogen.

Management

1. The management must be tailored to the specific diagnosis reached with the above work-up and is outlined in the relevant chapters.
2. In all instances, patient and parent education is extremely important in order to anticipate situations that put the patient at risk for bleeding (e.g., dental work) as well as to recognize the early signs of a bleed (e.g., knee pain without swelling in a hemophiliac).
3. Genetic counseling and testing of family members are strongly recommended for cases of hereditary abnormalities.

B Bibliography

Casella JF: Disorders of coagulation. *In* Oski FA, DeAngelis RD, McMillan JA, Warshaw JB (eds): Principles and Practice of Pediatrics, 2nd ed. Philadelphia, JB Lippincott, 1994, pp 1685–1699.

Hathaway WE: Bleeding disorders in the newborn infant. *In* Hathaway WE, Bonnar J (eds): Hemostatic Disorders of the Pregnant Woman and Newborn Infant. New York, Elsevier Science, 1987, pp 104–150.

Symptom **Lymphadenopathy**   *Sreedhar P. Rao*

Definition

Lymphadenopathy is defined as painless enlargement of the lymph nodes measuring ≥10 mm in diameter. It can be local (one area or two contiguous areas) or generalized (more than two contiguous regions). Enlargement of lymph nodes is a common finding in children and adolescents. In most cases, lymphadenopathy results from a transient illness that resolves without specific therapy. Malignancy or a serious infection may also present with isolated lymphadenopathy, which can be diagnosed by careful history, physical examination, and appropriate diagnostic studies. The causes of lymphadenopathy are listed in Table 112–5.

History

1. Determine the duration of lymphadenopathy and if the nodes are increasing in size.
2. Inquire about symptoms of fever, malaise, pain, or redness over the area of enlarged nodes; the latter symptoms suggest infection or inflammation.
3. Obtain history of weight loss. Significant weight loss suggests serious underlying illness, e.g., disseminated tuberculosis, HIV infection, lymphoma, or metastatic malignancy.
4. History of seborrheic dermatitis, recurrent otitis media, and skin rash, particularly in infants, suggests a diagnosis of Langerhans cell histiocytosis.
5. Determine if there is a history of infection in the area drained by the enlarged nodes, exposure to cats (cat scratch disease), and drug history (phenytoin-associated adenopathy).

Physical Examination

1. Determine if lymphadenopathy is localized or generalized, if the nodes are discrete or matted, and if the nodes are tender. Tender lymph nodes with or without inflammation of the overlying skin suggest infection as the cause of lymph node enlargement.
2. Look for skin rash, which may be seen in Kawasaki disease, rheumatoid arthritis, systemic lupus, Langerhans cell histiocytosis, leukemia, AIDS, and infectious mononucleosis.
3. Determine if supraclavicular nodes are enlarged. Supraclavicular adenopathy usually indicates a serious underlying illness, e.g., lymphoma, metastatic malignancy (neuroblastoma), tuberculosis, sarcoidosis, or histoplasmosis.
4. Thyroid enlargement in a child with cervical adenopathy suggests thyroid carcinoma with metastasis to the nodes.

Tests

1. CBC with differential leukocyte count and erythrocyte

TABLE 112–5. CAUSES OF LYMPHADENOPATHY

INFECTION	
Bacterial	Streptococcosis, staphylococcosis, mycobacteriosis, brucellosis, tularemia, syphilis
Viral	Especially Epstein-Barr virus, cytomegalovirus, human immunodeficiency virus, rubella
Fungal	Histoplasmosis, coccidioidomycosis
Protozoon	Toxoplasmosis and malaria
AUTOIMMUNE DISEASE	Rheumatoid arthritis, systemic lupus erythematosus, serum sickness Autoimmune hemolytic anemia
STORAGE DISEASE	Niemann-Pick and Gaucher disease
DRUG REACTIONS	Phenytoin and others
MALIGNANCY	Lymphoma, leukemia Metastatic rhabdomyosarcoma, neuroblastoma, thyroid carcinoma, other carcinomas Langerhans cell histiocytosis, familial erythrophagocytic Lymphohistiocytosis, malignant histiocytosis, sinus histiocytosis with massive lymphadenopathy
MISCELLANEOUS	Sarcoidosis Kawasaki disease Cat scratch fever

From Link MP, Donaldson SS: The lymphomas and lymphadenopathy. *In* Nathan DG, Oski FA (eds): Hematology of Infancy and Childhood. 4th ed. Philadelphia, WB Saunders, 1993.

sedimentation rate (ESR): An elevated WBC count, anemia, and thrombocytopenia suggest a diagnosis of leukemia or infectious mononucleosis. Increased numbers of atypical lymphocytes are frequently seen in patients with infectious mononucleosis. An elevated ESR may be seen in patients with inflammatory disorders, infection, or malignancy, less commonly in viral illness.

2. When cytopenias are present, bone marrow aspiration/ biopsy is indicated to confirm the diagnosis of leukemia or metastatic lymphoma or to differentiate between leukemia/lymphoma and infectious mononucleosis. Only a small proportion of patients with lymphadenopathy will need a bone marrow examination.

3. Serologic testing for evidence of infection with EBV, CMV, toxoplasmosis, and possibly HIV (if clinically indicated).

4. Serum lactate dehydrogenase (LDH): Markedly elevated serum LDH favors a diagnosis of leukemia, lymphoma, or metastatic malignancy.

5. Serum ALT, AST, and bilirubin for evidence of hepatitis, which may be seen in patients with CMV, EBV, or hepatitis A, B, or C virus infection.

6. Tuberculin test

7. X-ray of chest to look for enlarged nodes in the mediastinum or hilum and for evidence of lung disease. Pulmonary infiltrates with hilar adenopathy favor a diagnosis of tuberculosis or sarcoidosis, whereas anterior or middle mediastinal adenopathy suggests a diagnosis of leukemia/ lymphoma.

8. Lymph node biopsy: If a diagnosis cannot be made based on the above tests and the lymphadenopathy is persistent or progressive, a lymph node biopsy is indicated. The largest lymph node should be biopsied and the material appropriately processed to look for infections and neoplasia.

Management

The main objective of management is to make an appropriate diagnosis and administer therapy based on the diagnosis.

1. If the patient has evidence of bacterial adenitis, antibiotic therapy is started after appropriate cultures (blood culture and/or throat culture) are obtained. Node aspirate should be done if there is no improvement on antibiotics.

2. If the patient is asymptomatic and the diagnosis is not obvious, appropriate diagnostic tests are performed and the patient is closely followed. It is important to measure and document the size of the nodes.

3. Lymph node biopsy is indicated if the adenopathy does not resolve in 4 to 6 weeks or if there is progressive enlargement of the nodes. Early biopsy is indicated in patients with supraclavicular adenopathy. Lymph node biopsy will reveal a definite diagnosis in only about 50 per cent of the patients. The patients whose biopsy is nondiagnostic should be followed until the problem is resolved. Some patients may need a second biopsy if nodes continue to grow. Rarely, patients with non-Hodgkin lymphoma present with compression of the superior vena cava and/or upper airway. These patients are at risk for respiratory arrest when subjected to general anesthesia. Diagnosis should be attempted by bone marrow aspiration/biopsy or thoracentesis or by performing biopsy of the node under local anesthesia, if possible.

Bibliography

Knight PJ, Mulbine AF, Vassy LE: When is lymph node biopsy indicated in children with enlarged peripheral nodes? Pediatrics 1982;69:321.
Link MP, Donaldson SS: The lymphomas and lymphadenopathy. *In* Nathan DG, Oski FA (eds): Hematology of Infancy and Childhood, 4th ed. Philadelphia, WB Saunders, 1993, pp 1345–1347.

| Symptom | **Neck Mass** | | *Sreedhar P. Rao* |

Neck mass is a common presenting symptom in children. A thorough history and physical examination are essential to differentiate between various benign and malignant conditions that present with a neck mass. In addition, some tests are needed to confirm a particular clinical diagnosis.

Differential Diagnosis

Neck masses in children can be classified into five broad categories, each of which includes several clinical conditions.

1. Congenital neck mass
   a. Thyroglossal duct cyst
   b. Second branchial cleft cyst
   c. Cystic hygroma
   d. Hemangioma
   e. Congenital muscular torticollis
2. Lymphadenopathy
   See preceding section for causes of lymphadenopathy.

3. Malignant tumors presenting with neck mass
   a. Hodgkin and non-Hodgkin lymphoma
   b. Rhabdomyosarcoma and fibrosarcoma
   c. Neuroblastoma
   d. Thyroid carcinoma
4. Posttraumatic neck mass
   a. Hematoma
   b. Subcutaneous emphysema
5. Antigen mediated
   a. Bee sting
   b. Other allergies

History

A mass that is noted at birth or within a few months after birth and is growing slowly is likely to be a congenital and benign lesion. However, a mass that does not have signs of inflammation/infection and grows rapidly is likely to be malignant. A mass that appears shortly after trauma may be due to hematoma or subcutaneous emphysema.

Physical Examination

Generally, masses in the anterior triangle of neck are benign, except for a thyroid mass, which is likely to be malignant. Posterior triangle masses are more likely to be malignant, as are the masses occupying anterior and posterior triangles.

1. A midline mass that retracts when the tongue is protruded is probably a thyroglossal duct cyst.
2. A mass in the anterior triangle of neck, anterior to the middle third of sternocleidomastoid, particularly if it retracts with swallowing, is likely to be a second branchial cleft cyst.
3. Cystic hygromas and hemangiomas present as spongy masses; cystic hygromas usually transilluminate. The hemangiomas may have bluish coloration of the overlying skin and do not transilluminate.
4. If a mass feels like lymph node(s), determine the size of the node(s) and whether they are tender, matted, or fixed to the overlying skin or underlying tissues. A fixed node or group of nodes is more likely to be due to tuberculosis or malignancy.

Tests

1. X-ray of neck may demonstrate soft tissue mass or subcutaneous emphysema.
2. X-ray of chest to look for mediastinal or hilar adenopathy.
3. Ultrasound or CT scan of the neck (and upper chest, if indicated) if the mass appears to be a congenital lesion. Generally, a cystic lesion is likely to be either a thyroglossal duct cyst or a branchial cleft cyst. However, small cysts may appear solid on imaging studies. CT scan will also be useful to determine the extent of cystic hygroma prior to planned surgical excision. See preceding section for laboratory evaluation of patients with lymphadenopathy.
4. Radionuclide scan if a thyroid mass is palpated. A cold nodule in the thyroid is suggestive of malignant tumor.
5. Platelet count and coagulation studies for hemangioma.

Management

1. Surgical excision is performed for thyroglossal duct cyst or branchial cleft cyst. If the cyst is infected, antibiotic therapy should precede the surgery.
2. Cystic hygroma—Periodic observation unless there are signs and symptoms of obstruction, in which case surgical excision is advised.
3. Hemangiomas—Periodic observation if patient is asymptomatic. If symptomatic, consider treating with prednisone, interferon, or surgery.
4. Biopsy if mass is persistent or progressively enlarging. Subsequent treatment is based on the diagnosis.
5. Subcutaneous epinephrine, antihistamines with or without systemic steroids if swelling is an allergic response to a bee sting or other allergies.

Bibliography

Zitelh BJ: Evaluating the child with a neck mass. Contemp Pediatr 1990;7:90–112.

| Symptom | **Abdominal Mass** | *Sreedhar P. Rao* |

Any abdominal mass in a child requires immediate evaluation because some malignant tumors present with only an abdominal mass. Common conditions that may present with an abdominal mass are listed in Table 112–6. Nearly half the abdominal masses detected in the newborn period represent malformations of the genitourinary tract. The others are masses connected with liver, biliary tract, gastrointestinal tract, ovary, and adrenal gland. Neuroblastoma, hepatoblastoma, or mesoblastic nephroma may present with an abdominal mass in the newborn period. In older infants and children, other malignant tumors are more likely.

History

1. History of maternal diabetes mellitus in a newborn with a renal mass suggests a diagnosis of renal vein thrombosis.
2. History of fever, bone pain, and weight loss suggests neuroblastoma with bone metastasis or lymphoma.
3. Chronic diarrhea, history of abnormal eye movements, and unsteady gait are rare manifestations of ganglioneuroblastoma/ganglioneuroma.
4. History of intermittent abdominal pain followed by gelatinous bright red blood in stools (currant jelly stools) strongly suggests intussusception.
5. History of constipation suggests the mass to be either stool or a tumor compressing the bowel.

Physical Examination

1. Hypertension may be seen in patients with neuroblastoma, Wilms tumor, hydronephrosis, multicystic kidney, and other renal abnormalities.
2. Hemihypertrophy or nonfamilial aniridia or genitourinary tract abnormalities are associated with an increased incidence of Wilms tumor.
3. Hemangiomas of the skin in a patient with a hepatic mass are suggestive of hemangioma of the liver.
4. Rectal examination—Rectum filled with stool suggests that the abdominal mass may be a stool mass.
5. Imperforate hymen with an abdominal mass is suggestive of hydrocolpos or hematocolpos.

Tests

1. CBC with differential leukocyte count. Patients with neuroblastoma are frequently anemic and have thrombocytosis. Anemia may also be seen in patients with Wilms tumor if there is bleeding into the tumor (usually after trauma). Anemia with leukopenia or leukocytosis and thrombocytopenia is suggestive of leukemia/lymphoma.
2. Hematuria is occasionally seen in patients with Wilms tumor or renal cell carcinoma.

TABLE 112–6. ABDOMINAL MASS

NEWBORN

Renal

Hydronephrosis
Multicystic kidney
Renal vein thrombosis
Mesoblastic nephroma

Hepatic

Hematoma of the liver
Hemangioma of the liver
Hepatic cyst

OLDER INFANTS AND CHILDREN

Renal

Hydronephrosis
Wilms tumor
Renal cell carcinoma (rare)

Adrenal and Sympathetic Chain

Ganglioneuroma/neuroblastoma

Hepatic

Hepatoma
Metastatic tumor of the liver
Hemangioma
Hepatic abscess or cyst

Lymphatic System

Hodgkin and non-Hodgkin
lymphoma

Gastrointestinal Tract

Duplication of the small intestine
Mesenteric cyst

Adrenal

Adrenal hemorrhage
Neuroblastoma

Genitourinary Tract

Hydro- or hematocolpos
Ovarian cyst
Distended urinary bladder

Gastrointestinal Tract

Gastrointestinal duplication
Intussusception
Volvulus
Stool mass

Ovary

Ovarian cyst
Ovarian tumor

Miscellaneous

Rhabdomyosarcoma
Teratoma
Appendiceal abscess

3. Serum lactate dehydrogenase (LDH), uric acid, potassium, calcium, phosphate, urea nitrogen, and creatinine. Elevated levels of LDH are seen in patients with leukemia, lymphoma, or neuroblastoma. Evidence of tumor lysis syndrome (elevated serum uric acid, potassium, and phosphate) before initiation of therapy is occasionally seen in patients with Burkitt (non-Hodgkin) lymphoma.

4. Plain x-ray of abdomen, abdominal ultrasound and/or CT scan, MRI. These studies will determine the origin and extent of the mass, if there is invasion into blood vessels (renal vein, inferior vena cava), size of the abdominal lymph nodes, calcification in the mass, and any evidence of metastasis in other structures (e.g., liver and spleen).

5. Barium enema if intussusception is suspected

6. Chest x-ray for evidence of mediastinal adenopathy (lymphoma), posterior mediastinal mass (neuroblastoma), pulmonary metastases (Wilms tumor, rhabdomyosarcoma)

7. Additional radiologic studies. Skeletal survey, bone scan, gallium scan, or MIBG scan is done if clinically indicated.

8. Bone marrow aspiration/biopsy. Leukemia can be confirmed by bone marrow examination. Bone marrow metastasis from lymphoma or neuroblastoma may be seen. A negative bone marrow aspiration/biopsy does not rule out bone marrow infiltration by these tumors; some recommend several examinations to increase the likelihood of detecting metastatic disease.

Management

1. If a stool mass is suspected, the patient should be reexamined after an enema.

2. Laparotomy—Most patients with an abdominal mass will undergo laparotomy for diagnosis and surgical management. Further treatment will be based on the diagnosis.

3. Sometimes a parent or caregiver may bring a child to a physician with complaint of an abdominal mass, but the mass is not palpated by the physician. It is nonetheless prudent to obtain an abdominal sonogram, a noninvasive test without radiation exposure. A delay in the diagnosis of an abdominal mass may result in distant metastasis of a potentially curable tumor or further loss of renal function in a patient with obstructive uropathy.

Bibliography

Oski FA: Abdominal mass. In Kaye R, Oski FA, Barness LA (eds): Core Textbook of Pediatrics. Philadelphia, JB Lippincott, 1978, pp 118–123.

Symptom | **Hepatosplenomegaly**   *Sreedhar P. Rao*

Enlargement of the liver and spleen occurs in many conditions. This chapter addresses conditions associated with hepatomegaly *and* splenomegaly, but in some only the liver or spleen may be enlarged. The liver edge is usually palpable 1 to 2 cm below the right costal margin in normal infants and children. The best way to determine hepatomegaly is to measure the liver span, the distance between the upper margin of the liver (determined by percussion at the right midclavicular line) and lower margin of the liver by palpation. Normally the upper margin of the liver is within 1 cm of the fifth intercostal space. The normal mean liver span in children is 8 cm and ranges from 6 to 10 cm. Any palpable spleen beyond 2 years of age is considered, with rare exceptions, to be an enlarged spleen.

Differential Diagnosis

The causes of hepatosplenomegaly are listed in Table 112–7.

History

1. History of fever is suggestive of infectious, inflammatory, or neoplastic disease.

2. History of pallor, jaundice, splenectomy, or cholecystectomy at an early age in the patient or family is suggestive of hemolytic anemia. However, history of jaundice alone suggests hepatitis due to any one of the infections listed in Table 112–7.

3. History of arthralgia or arthritis with or without skin rash would suggest collagen vascular disorder or hepatitis.

Physical Examination

1. Jaundice and pallor are indicative of hemolytic disease.
2. Generalized adenopathy and petechial rash/ecchymosis are suggestive of leukemia or SLE with thrombocytopenia or Langhans cell histiocytosis.
3. Coarse facial features, cloudy cornea, mental retardation, and short stature are suggestive of mucopolysaccharidosis.
4. Ascites suggests a diagnosis of severe malnutrition or cirrhosis.

Tests

1. CBC, reticulocyte count and differential leukocyte count, examination of the blood smear for morphology and parasites if clinically indicated (e.g., malaria)
2. Urinalysis for bile, urobilinogen (hepatobiliary disease), proteinuria, and hematuria (SLE)
3. Tuberculin test
4. Blood culture
5. Liver function studies—If evidence of hepatitis is found, do serologic tests for hepatitis A, B, C; EBV; and CMV infection.
6. Indirect hyperbilirubinemia, reticulocytosis, and high LDH are indicative of hemolytic disease and warrant appropriate diagnostic studies.
7. Antinuclear antibodies, anti-DNA antibodies, and serum complement, when collagen vascular disease is suspected
8. Bone marrow aspiration/biopsy when leukemia is suspected
9. Appropriate biochemical studies when a storage disorder is suspected

Radiologic Studies

Chest x-ray for evidence of mediastinal or hilar adenopathy, pulmonary infiltrates (lymphoma, tuberculosis); ultrasound and/or CT scan of the abdomen for primary or metastatic tumor of the liver or when an abscess in the liver or spleen is a diagnostic consideration (*Candida, Aspergillus*).

TABLE 112–7. CAUSES OF HEPATOSPLENOMEGALY

INFECTIONS	NEOPLASTIC DISORDERS
Bacterial	Leukemia
Salmonellosis	Lymphoma
Brucellosis	Langhans cell histiocytosis
Tuberculosis	Hepatoblastoma and hemangiomas (only hepatomegaly)
Viral	Metastatic neuroblastoma, Wilms tumor, gonadal tumors (only hepatomegaly)
Epstein-Barr virus	
Cytomegalovirus	**COLLAGEN VASCULAR DISORDERS**
Hepatitis A, B, C	
Human immunodeficiency virus 1	Systemic lupus erythematosus
	Juvenile rheumatoid arthritis
Parasitic	**HEMOLYTIC ANEMIAS**
Malaria	
Toxoplasmosis	Erythroblastosis fetalis
Syphilis	Thalassemia major
Pneumocystis carinii	Hemoglobinopathies
	Hereditary spherocytosis and elliptocytosis
Leishmaniasis	Autoimmune hemolytic anemia
Fungal	**MISCELLANEOUS DISORDERS**
Systemic candidiasis	
Aspergillosis	Cirrhosis with portal hypertension
Storage Disorders	Congestive heart failure (mainly hepatomegaly)
Glycogen storage disease	Malnutrition
Mucopolysaccharidosis	
Gaucher disease	
Niemann-Pick disease	
Gangliosidosis	
Alpha₁-antitrypsin deficiency	
Amyloidosis	

Management

Therapy will be based on the diagnosis.

Bibliography

McMillan JA, Neiburg PI, Oski FA (eds): The Whole Pediatrician Catalog. Philadelphia, WB Saunders, 1977, pp 2–26.

Symptom | **Neutrophilic Leukocytosis (Neutrophilia)** | *Marc S. C. Cheah*

Definition

Neutrophilic (granulocytic) leukocytosis or neutrophilia refers to an increase in the total number of neutrophils in the peripheral circulation $\geq 7.5 \times 10^9$/L. However, the normal mean absolute neutrophil count (ANC) for preterm newborns is 7×10^9/L and 13×10^9/L for the term neonate. These return to the adult values within the first few weeks of life and are sustained thereafter.

Pathophysiology

1. Increased neutrophil granulopoiesis in bone marrow
2. Increased release of neutrophils from marrow
3. Increased mobilization from marginating to circulating pool
4. Decreased neutrophil egress into tissues

Conditions Associated with Neutrophilia

1. Physiologic
   a. Newborn
   b. Exercise
   c. Stress
   d. Hypoxia
2. Down syndrome
   a. Down syndrome infants may develop a leukemoid reaction that is transient and self-limiting.
   b. The mechanism is an intrinsic defect in regulating neutrophil proliferation and maturation.
3. Leukocyte adhesion deficiency (LAD)
   a. Autosomal recessive inheritance
   b. Repeated bacterial infections
   c. Persistent neutrophilia up to 12 to 100×10^9/L
   d. Severe gingivitis or periodontitis
   e. Slow wound healing with delayed umbilical cord separation

TABLE 112–8. LEUKEMIA VS. LEUKEMOID REACTION

	LEUKEMIA	LEUKEMOID REACTION
General condition	Sick-looking child	Underlying sepsis or Down syndrome
Hepatosplenomegaly	Often present	Often absent
Lymphadenopathy	Often present	Often absent
Anemia	Present	Infrequent
Thrombocytopenia	Present	Infrequent
Peripheral blood smear	Blasts and mature forms may be present; few intermediates (leukemic hiatus)	Shift to the left, presence of intermediate forms; white cells may have toxic granules
Bone marrow aspirate	Presence of leukemic blasts; hypercellular; decreased erythroid precursors or megakaryocytes	Myeloid hyperplasia and normal maturation; may be hypercellular
Leukocyte alkaline phosphatase (LAP) score	Absent	High
Cytogenetics	Often abnormal	Normal except in patients with Down syndrome (trisomy 21)

f. Defect in surface membrane glycoprotein, β_2 integrin, Mac-1 (CD11b/CD18)

4. Disorders of neutrophil motility, e.g., actin dysfunction. The mechanism relates to decreased neutrophil circulatory egress.

5. Hereditary neutrophilia
   a. Autosomal dominant inheritance
   b. ANC between 14 and $164 \times 10^9/L$
   c. Hepatosplenomegaly, Gaucher type histiocytes

6. Infections
   a. Bacterial: *Staphylococcus aureus, Streptococcus pneumoniae, Mycobacterium tuberculosis*
   b. Viral: Epstein-Barr virus (EBV), herpes simplex, varicella, cytomegalovirus (CMV), rabies, and poliovirus
   c. Systemic mycotic, protozoal, leptospiral, and rickettsial infections

7. Drugs
   a. Corticosteroids
   b. Epinephrine
   c. Lithium

8. Chronic inflammatory diseases
   a. Juvenile rheumatoid arthritis
   b. Inflammatory bowel disease: ulcerative colitis
   c. Kawasaki disease

9. Hematologic disorders
   a. Myeloproliferative disorders
   b. Following splenectomy or functional asplenia
   c. Leukemia
   d. Postneutropenia rebound
   e. Acute hemolytic reaction
   f. Metastatic bone marrow disease

Leukemoid Reaction vs. Leukemia

Leukemoid reaction refers to a reactive leukocytosis in which all stages of neutrophil maturation populate the blood; there is a shift to the left, with the appearance of immature myeloid precursors (Table 112–8). Leukemoid reactions have been associated with bacterial sepsis, tuberculosis, histoplasmosis, vasculitis, and Down syndrome (trisomy 21).

 Bibliography

Curnutte JT: Neutrophilia. *In* Nathan DG, Oski FA (eds): Hematology of Infancy and Childhood, 4th ed. Philadelphia, WB Saunders, 1993, pp 951–953.

113 Iron Deficiency Anemia and Other Microcytic Anemias

Sreedhar P. Rao

Iron Deficiency Anemia

Definition

Anemia is usually a late manifestation of iron deficiency and is best defined by demonstration of a therapeutic response to iron.

Etiology and Epidemiology

1. Iron deficiency may result from decreased dietary iron intake and/or increased iron requirements during periods of rapid growth. Both infants between 6 and 24 months of age and adolescents are at risk of developing iron deficiency because of increased requirements during rapid

TABLE 113–1. CAUSES OF IRON DEFICIENCY

INCREASED IRON REQUIREMENT

Infants, adolescents

BLOOD LOSS

Gastrointestinal blood loss
    Peptic ulcer disease
    Polyposis
    Meckel's diverticulum
    Milk-induced enteropathy
    Inflammatory bowel disease
    Chronic salicylate use
Iatrogenic blood loss
Intravascular hemolysis with hemosiderinuria
    Heart valve replacement
    Intense exercise and hemoglobinuria
Idiopathic pulmonary hemosiderosis

DECREASED IRON ASSIMILATION

Iron-poor diet
Iron malabsorption
Gastric resection, sprue
Pica

growth unless adequate amounts of iron are provided in the diet.

2. Conditions associated with high iron demand, such as cyanotic congenital heart disease, iron loss from gastrointestinal tract or pulmonary bleeding, menorrhagia, iatrogenic blood loss, and chronic intravascular hemolysis (due to urinary iron loss), may result in iron deficiency (Table 113–1).

3. Whole cow's milk introduced to infants before 6 months of age may produce iron deficiency; it is a poor source of dietary iron and may cause gastrointestinal blood loss.

4. There is a dramatic increase in the need for iron in adolescents, particularly in girls because of concomitant menstrual blood loss. If the diet includes foods low in iron and foods that interfere with iron absorption, iron deficiency is likely to develop.

Pathophysiology

Iron is needed for the production of heme proteins, which function in the transport and utilization of oxygen. The iron-containing proteins hemoglobin, myoglobin, and cytochromes account for 70 to 90 per cent of the total iron in the body. The remainder is stored as ferritin and hemosiderin in the liver, spleen, and bone marrow. During periods of decreased iron intake, iron is mobilized from the storage compounds to maintain normal production of hemoglobin and related proteins. Storage iron depletion is usually followed by iron-limited erythropoiesis and ultimately anemia (Table 113–2).

Clinical Findings

1. Patients are usually asymptomatic if the anemia is mild. As the anemia becomes severe, patients may manifest fatigue, irritability, loss of appetite, pallor, decreased physical activity, and loss of interest in the surroundings. In very severe cases, congestive heart failure may develop.

2. Several nonhematologic consequences are detected in patients with iron deficiency, including pica, koilonychia (spoon-shaped nails), angular stomatitis, and exercise in-

TABLE 113–2. STAGES OF IRON DEFICIENCY

TEST	STORAGE IRON DEFICIENCY	IRON-LIMITED ERYTHROPOIESIS	IRON DEFICIENCY ANEMIA
Hemoglobin	Normal	Normal	Decreased
Serum iron	Normal	Decreased	Decreased
Serum iron-binding capacity	Normal	Increased	Increased
Transferrin saturation	Normal	Decreased	Decreased
FEP	Normal	Increased	Increased
Serum ferritin	Decreased	Decreased	Decreased

tolerance. Behavioral changes, such as apathy and short attention span, improve early after initiation of iron therapy and are probably not due to anemia.

Key Clinical Findings

- Pallor
- Fatigue
- Apathy
- Heart failure—if severe

Laboratory Findings

1. The diagnosis of mild iron deficiency anemia is difficult. There is a considerable overlap in the laboratory values between mildly iron-deficient and iron-sufficient subjects. Characteristic laboratory findings in children with moderate to severe iron deficiency anemia are shown in Table 113–3. It is important to recognize that infection and/or inflammation and recent iron administration may alter the results of these and that any or all of these tests may be normal in iron-deficient individuals.

2. Differential diagnosis of disorders that are commonly confused with iron deficiency anemia is shown in Table 113–4. Microcytosis is more severe compared with the degree of anemia in patients with thalassemia trait; patients with iron deficiency do not become microcytic before becoming anemic. Patients with thalassemia trait are usually microcytic even when the hemoglobin level is normal or only slightly decreased. It is uncommon to see microcytic anemia in patients with lead intoxication unless it is severe or there is concurrent iron deficiency. When evaluating an infant between 6 and 18 months of age for iron deficiency anemia, appropriate history, complete blood count, including MCV and RDW, and a

TABLE 113–3. BIOCHEMICAL VALUES INDICATIVE OF IRON DEFICIENCY

TEST	CUTOFF VALUE	AGE (yr)
Transferrin saturation (%)	<12	0.5–4
	<14	5–10
FEP (μg/dl of whole blood)	>80	0.5–4
	>70	5–10
Serum ferritin (μg/L)	<10	1–10

Modified from Dallman PR, Yip R, Oski FA: Iron deficiency and related nutritional anemias. *In* Nathan DG, Oski FA (eds): Hematology of Infancy and Childhood, 4th ed. Philadelphia, WB Saunders, 1993.

TABLE 113–4.   DIFFERENTIAL DIAGNOSIS OF CONDITIONS CONFUSED WITH IRON DEFICIENCY ANEMIA

TEST	IRON DEFICIENCY ANEMIA	THALASSEMIA TRAIT (α or β)	CHRONIC INFECTION/ INFLAMMATION	LEAD POISONING
Hb	Reduced	Normal/Reduced	Normal/Reduced	Normal/Reduced
MCV	Reduced	Reduced	Normal/Reduced	Normal/Reduced
RDW	Increased	Normal	Increased	Normal
FEP	Increased	Normal	Increased	Increased
Serum iron	Reduced	Normal	Reduced	Normal
TIBC	Increased	Normal	Normal/Reduced	Normal
Serum ferritin	Reduced	Normal	Increased	Normal

Modified from Lukens JN: Iron metabolism and iron deficiency. *In* Miller DR, Baehner RL (eds): Blood Diseases of Infancy and Childhood, 7th ed. St. Louis, CV Mosby, 1995.

trial of iron therapy are usually adequate. If inadequate dietary intake cannot be documented in an iron-deficient individual, investigations for gastrointestinal, pulmonary, or renal blood loss should be done.

3. Red cell distribution width is an indicator of degree of anisocytosis. The normal value of RDW in children is from 11.5 to 14.0. It is elevated early in iron deficiency. A combination of low MCV and high RDW is highly suggestive of iron deficiency. In patients with thalassemia, RDW is usually normal.

Key Laboratory Findings

- Low hemoglobin and HCT
- Microcytosis; low MCV
- Anisocytosis; high RDW
- Low reticulocyte count
- Reticulocyte and hemoglobin response to iron therapy

Treatment

A therapeutic trial of iron may be given to any infant suspected of having iron deficiency anemia. A response to the trial confirms the diagnosis of iron deficiency anemia and avoids expensive laboratory tests. Oral iron is administered (as ferrous sulfate) in a dose of 3 mg/kg in one or two divided doses daily for 1 month. A therapeutic response is defined as an increase in hemoglobin level of 1 g/dl or more; iron should be continued an additional 2 or 3 months in patients who respond. A sharp rise in reticulocytes (>5%) in 4 to 7 days is also a good response. There is no need to continue iron administration beyond 1 month in the absence of a therapeutic response, and the differential diagnosis should be pursued. Patients with hemoglobin level as low as 3 g/dl due to iron deficiency anemia may be managed with oral iron therapy unless signs and symptoms of impending or overt heart failure are evident. In such patients, small volume packed red cell transfusion or partial exchange transfusion is recommended. Parenteral iron (intramuscular or intravenous) is recommended for patients with documented iron malabsorption or noncompliance with oral iron. The rate of increase in hemoglobin level is similar with oral or parenteral iron administration and maximally is approximately 0.4 g/dl/day. The more severe the anemia, the more rapid the reticulocyte response and increase in hemoglobin level.

Key Treatment

- Iron, orally, 3 mg/kg/day × 1 month as trial
- Continue 2–3 months if successful

Prevention

The following are the guidelines for prevention of iron deficiency in infants.

1. Encourage breast milk feeding until 5 to 6 months of age. If an infant receives only breast milk beyond 6 months of age, iron should be supplemented in a dose of 1 mg/kg/day.
2. Infants who are not breast-fed should receive iron-fortified formula (12 mg of iron/L) for the first 12 months of life.
3. When solid foods are introduced into the diet, iron-enriched cereal should be among the first foods provided.
4. Avoid feeding whole cow's milk at least until 9 to 12 months of age because of the risk of occult gastrointestinal blood loss. Commercial milk formulas or evaporated milk do not appear to cause gastrointestinal blood loss; if the latter is used, supplemental iron should be given.

Other Microcytic Anemias

In addition to iron deficiency anemia, the following conditions may be associated with microcytic anemia:

1. Hemoglobinopathies
   a. Hemoglobin CC, C-β-thal
   b. Hemoglobin SC, S-β-thal
2. Red cell membrane disorders
   a. Hereditary pyropoikilocytosis (HPP)
   b. Hereditary spherocytosis
3. Sideroblastic anemia
4. Pyridoxine deficiency

Bibliography

Lukens JL: Iron metabolism and iron deficiency. *In* Miller DR, Baehner RL (eds): Blood Disease of Infancy and Childhood. St. Louis, CV Mosby, 1995.

Oski FA: Iron deficiency in infancy and childhood: N Engl J Med 1993;329:190–193.

114 Megaloblastic Anemia in Infants and Children

Sheldon P. Rothenberg

Definition

Megaloblastic anemia is a disorder of hematopoiesis that results from impaired synthesis of deoxyribonucleic acid (DNA). This perturbation slows cell replication and, as a consequence, developing hematopoietic cells become large and contain the fragmented and dispersed chromatin that characterizes the megaloblast. Hematopoiesis is "ineffective" and results in macrocytic anemia, which, in severe cases, may be accompanied by leukopenia and thrombocytopenia. Depending on the underlying cause, the central and/or peripheral nervous system may also be affected.

Etiology

1. The most common cause of megaloblastic anemia and associated clinical disturbances is deficiency of vitamin B_{12} (cobalamin, Cbl) or of folic acid (pteroylglutamic acid, folate), or of both.
2. Rare but important causes of megaloblastic hematopoiesis are genetic defects that selectively impair the cellular uptake of either vitamin or impair the synthesis of the respective active cofactor form that is necessary for intracellular metabolism.

Physiology and Pathophysiology

In order to develop a diagnostic and therapeutic strategy to manage a patient with an apparent megaloblastic disorder, it is necessary to understand the physiology and pathophysiology that underlies Cbl or folate deficiency.

1. Physiology
   a. Cbl is assimilated from a diet containing meat and meat-derived products. There is little Cbl in vegetarian diets. Cbl is released from complexes with food protein by enzymic and acid hydrolysis in the stomach and is bound primarily in the duodenum to intrinsic factor (IF), a glycoprotein secreted by gastric parietal cells. The IF-Cbl complex binds to a surface receptor in the distal ileum and is internalized by endocytosis. In the cell the Cbl is released and appears in the portal blood bound to transcobalamin II (TCII). TCII is a plasma protein that delivers Cbl to tissues, where the TCII-Cbl complex binds to receptors on the plasma membrane of cells and is internalized by receptor-mediated endocytosis. Within the endocytic vesicle, the Cbl is released and moves to the mitochondria, where it is converted to deoxyadenosyl-Cbl, and to the cytosol, where it is converted to methyl-Cbl. These two forms of Cbl are the metabolically active cofactors of Cbl.
   b. Folate is obtained from both meat and vegetables and is absorbed from the proximal small intestine. No carrier protein is required, but a membrane protein on the brush border of the epithelial mucosa appears necessary for absorption. Folate in food (unlike the nutrient vitamin) is in the form of folyl

polyglutamates (i.e., several additional molecules of glutamic acid). Hydrolysis to the monoglutamate is required for absorption of the vitamin.

Folate is absorbed into the portal blood and is not transported by any specific plasma protein. It is distributed to the liver for storage and other cells for immediate metabolic processes. The major circulating form of folate is N^5methyltetrahydrofolate (methyl-FH_4). Other folate cofactors are derived from methyl-FH_4 in cells. Polyglutamation of the cofactors occurs, and they all function as carbon and methyl group donors for pyrimidine and purine synthesis and for the interconversion of some amino acids. An important metabolic pathway where Cbl and folate function coordinately is for the methylation of homocysteine to form methionine, as shown below.

$$\text{methyl-}FH_4 + \text{homocysteine} \xrightarrow[\text{methionine synthase}]{\text{methyl-Cbl}} \text{methionine} + \text{tetrahydrofolate}$$

A deficiency of either Cbl or folate will impair methionine synthesis, and this will result in an accumulation of cellular and plasma homocysteine. Methionine, in the form of S-adenosylmethionine, is the major source of methyl groups for most methylation processes (DNA, RNA, neurotransmitters).

2. Pathophysiology of Cbl deficiency
   a. Impaired absorption
      (1) Juvenile pernicious anemia (PA) is similar to the adult form of PA with atrophic gastritis, achlorhydria, and lack of intrinsic factor (IF). The serum usually contains antibodies to gastric parietal cells and to IF. It appears to be an autoimmune disorder and may also occur with hypothyroidism, idiopathic hypoparathyroidism, or Addison disease. It is sometimes also associated with hypogammaglobulinemia.
      (2) *Diphyllobothrium latum* infestation is a fish tapeworm that interferes with the transit of the IF-Cbl to the terminal ileum by sequestering the vitamin.
      (3) Bacterial overgrowth in the small intestine occurs with multiple diverticula as well as motility and malabsorption disorders.
      (4) Enteroenteric or enterocolic fistulas in which the terminal ileum is bypassed, or inflammatory disorders of the small intestine that affect the terminal ileum (Crohn disease)
      (5) Malabsorption syndromes (celiac disease and tropical sprue)
   b. Dietary deficiency occurs if the diet lacks all meat or meat products. Human and cow milk contain

sufficient Cbl, although Cbl in human milk may be low if the mother is Cbl deficient.

   c. Inborn errors of metabolism—In general, these patients present in early infancy.

     (1) Lack of a functional IF protein is a genetic disorder, and the stomach is structurally and functionally normal.

     (2) Lack of the IF-Cbl receptor on the terminal ileum is associated with proteinuria (Imerslund-Gräsbeck syndrome).

     (3) Congenital TCII deficiency

     (4) Congenital failure to synthesize the active cofactor, methyl-Cbl.

3. Pathophysiology of folate deficiency—Usually dietary or from a folate-deficient nursing mother

   a. Premature infants—Usually the mother is folate deficient.

   b. Infancy

     (1) Inadequate dietary intake and often in association with kwashiorkor or marasmus in underdeveloped countries

     (2) Occurs with a marginal folate intake with an increased requirement for folate (e.g., chronic hemolytic anemia or infection)

     (3) Goat milk anemia: Cbl and folate are both low in this milk, but folate deficiency is the major cause of the megaloblastic anemia.

   c. Infancy and childhood

     (1) Disease of the small intestine—Celiac disease and tropical sprue; in sprue, Cbl deficiency may also occur.

     (2) Inadequate intake to meet an increase in the requirement for folate as occurs with chronic hemolytic anemias.

   d. In vitamin C (ascorbic acid) deficiency; may be prescorbutic. Occurrence of megaloblastic anemia indicates associated deficiency or impaired metabolism of folate.

   e. Drugs

     (1) Anticonvulsants—Usually phenytoin or primidone and often in association with phenobarbital.

     (2) Folate antagonists

   f. Inborn errors of metabolism—Rare causes of megaloblastic anemia; frequently associated with a neurologic disorder and mental retardation because folate cofactors are essential for the development of the nervous system during fetal life and for rapid growth in infancy.

     (1) Congenital malabsorption and cellular uptake

     (2) Methionine synthase deficiency (very rare).

Clinical Findings

1. Cbl deficiency

   a. Macrocytic anemia with megaloblastic erythropoiesis, usually accompanied by abnormal myeloid cells (giant metamyelocytes) and abnormal megakaryocytes

   b. Leukopenia and thrombocytopenia usually occur when the anemia is severe.

   c. Neurologic disease may also occur secondary to demyelinization of the posterior and lateral columns (combined system disease), peripheral neuropathy, psychiatric disturbances, or any combination of such disorders.

   d. In advanced cases, the tongue may be painful, lack papillae, and appear red.

   e. Early cases may be identified even without anemia when macrocytosis is observed in the blood smear or indicated by the blood count.

   f. Inborn errors (congenital IF or TCII deficiency or impaired synthesis of methyl-Cbl). Such infants may present with failure to thrive, neurologic dysfunction, or mental retardation before the anemia is observed.

2. Folate deficiency

   a. The anemia is morphologically indistinguishable from that observed in Cbl deficiency.

   b. The associated clinical findings depend on the underlying cause of the deficiency.

     (1) Early in infancy if the mother is folate deficient, especially with prematurity

     (2) In children, poor diet or malnutrition is most common, but malabsorption syndromes may also occur. Usually there is diarrhea and steatorrhea.

     (3) Chronic hemolytic anemia increases the daily requirement of folate, especially during periods of growth.

     (4) Chronic anticonvulsant therapy for treatment of epilepsy

     (5) Neurologic disorders of the central nervous system may occur with the inborn errors of folate metabolism but rarely occur with acquired deficiency in childhood.

Key Clinical Findings

Cbl Deficiency
- Macrocytic anemia with megaloblastic hematopoiesis
- Disorder of the central or peripheral nervous system
- Presentation is usually earlier with inborn errors of Cbl metabolism

Folate Deficiency
- Similar hematologic findings
- Nutritional deficiency is more apparent than in Cbl deficiency
- Presentation occurs earlier with inborn errors of folate metabolism

---

Laboratory Findings

1. General findings for Cbl and folate deficiency

   a. Macrocytic anemia—High mean corpuscular volume (MCV), elevated mean corpuscular hemoglobin

(MCH), and high red cell distribution width (RDW). Leukopenia and thrombocytopenia occur in severe cases.

b. Peripheral smear shows macrocytosis, small fragmented red cells, and multilobed neutrophils (three cells with >5 lobes; one cell with >6)

c. Megaloblastic bone marrow

d. Indirect hyperbilirubinemia due to intramedullary destruction of erythroblasts (in the bone marrow)

e. Elevated serum lactate dehydrogenase (LDH)

f. Elevated serum homocysteine

The above laboratory findings occur in both Cbl and folate deficiency and with inborn errors resulting in intracellular deficiency of Cbl or folate.

2. Specific for Cbl deficiency

a. Low serum Cbl in acquired deficiency

b. Serum antibodies to gastric parietal cells and to IF in juvenile PA but absent in other Cbl malabsorption syndromes or in association with hypogammaglobulinemia

c. Elevated MMA in serum and urine

d. Inborn errors of metabolism

(1) Congenital absence or abnormality of gastric IF or IF receptor: low serum Cbl, *no* serum antibodies to IF or gastric parietal cells

(2) Congenital TCII deficiency or impaired methyl-Cbl synthesis: *normal* serum Cbl

e. Elevated MMA in serum and urine.

3. Specific for folate deficiency

a. Low serum (<3 ng/ml) and red cell (<150 ng/ml) folate. (Red cell folate may be low in Cbl deficiency but serum folate should be normal or elevated.)

b. Normal serum and red cell folate in hereditary oroticaciduria, a disorder characterized by megaloblastic anemia because of impaired DNA synthesis.

Key Laboratory Findings

Megaloblastic hematopoiesis (Cbl or folate deficiency)
- Macrocytic anemia with or without leukopenia and thrombocytopenia

- Elevated serum LDH

- Indirect hyperbilirubinemia (variable)

In Cbl deficiency
- Low serum Cbl in PA and congenital absence or nonfunctional IF

- Elevated plasma homocysteine

- Elevated plasma and urine MMA

- Normal serum Cbl in congenital TCII deficiency and inborn error of methyl-Cbl synthesis

In folate deficiency
- Low serum and red cell folate

- Elevated plasma homocysteine (not MMA)

c. Low serum and red cell folate in congenital malabsorption of folate.

4. Special laboratory studies

a. Measurement of plasma TCII if serum Cbl is normal with elevated homocysteine and MMA and with normal serum folate

b. Radio-Cbl absorption test (Schilling test) can distinguish PA from intestinal malabsorption if serum Cbl is low and there are no serum antibodies to IF.

c. Gastric analysis for HCl and IF when the Schilling test confirms absence of IF and there are no serum antibodies to IF (this will identify congenital absence of IF or abnormal form of IF protein).

d. Small bowel barium contrast studies for malabsorption due to sprue. If the study is abnormal, a small bowel biopsy will be diagnostic.

e. Stool examination for fat or parasites if malabsorption is the problem

f. Analysis of cultured skin fibroblasts for methyl-Cbl cofactor synthesis with megaloblastic anemia, elevated serum homocysteine, and normal serum and urine MMA (special laboratories do such studies).

Management and Treatment

1. Cbl deficiency

a. Correct any intestinal disorder if the cause of deficiency is not PA (e.g., bacterial overgrowth, diverticula, distal ileal disease) and replenish stores as indicated below.

b. If the cause is PA, administer weekly parenteral vitamin B$_{12}$, 10 to 100 μg for infants and young children and 1000 μg for older children and adolescents for a minimum of 10 weeks to replenish tissue stores. Alternatively, ten doses can be given in a shorter time period. Monthly injections of 100 to 1000 μg are given regularly if there is a noncorrectable disorder (e.g., juvenile PA, congenital malabsorption of Cbl, congenital absence of TCII).

c. Hydroxycobalamin should be given instead of cyanocobalamin for patients with an inborn defect of methyl-Cbl synthesis.

d. Folate should *never* be given to a patient with Cbl deficiency unless there is associated folate deficiency. Folate may accelerate neurologic deterioration in Cbl deficiency.

e. Following the correction of *severe* anemia with Cbl, substantial iron may be consumed from stores, resulting in iron deficiency. Iron supplements should be prescribed for such patients.

2. Folate deficiency

a. Correct any intestinal disorder (e.g., celiac disease, sprue).

b. To treat the deficiency, administer parenteral folate (0.5–1 mg) to infants and (2–3 mg) to older children and adolescents twice weekly for 3 to 4 weeks to replenish stores. Oral folic acid (0.5 mg–1.0 mg) is an adequate maintenance dose if the underlying cause is not corrected or if an increase in daily intake is required (e.g., chronic hemolytic anemia).

Key Treatment

- **PA**
  Vitamin B_{12} weekly × 10 weeks (dosage by age)
- **Folate**
  Folic acid—0.5–3 mg twice weekly

Bibliography

Chanarin I: The Megaloblastic Anemias. London, Blackwell Scientific Publications, 1979.

Cooper BA, Rosenblatt DS, Whitehead VM: Megaloblastic anemia. *In* Nathan DG, Oski FA (eds): Hematology of Infancy and Childhood. Philadelphia, WB Saunders, 1993, pp 354–390.

Wickramasinghe SN (ed): Megaloblastic Anemia, Vol 21, no 3. London, Bailliere Tindall, 1995.

115 Aplastic Anemia

Sreedhar P. Rao

Definition

Aplastic anemia is a condition in which there is peripheral blood pancytopenia (anemia, neutropenia, and thrombocytopenia) caused by decreased production of blood cells in the bone marrow. It may be inherited or acquired.

Pathophysiology

The following mechanisms have been suggested in the pathogenesis of aplastic anemia.

1. *Quantitative or qualitative defect of stem cells.* Hematologic recovery after bone marrow transplantation supports the concept of stem cell abnormalities.
2. *Immunosuppression of hematopoiesis.* Immunosuppression as a possible cause of marrow failure is supported by the observations that (a) nearly 50 per cent of twin-to-twin bone marrow transplants require cytotoxic conditioning therapy to permit engraftment; (b) about 50 per cent of patients with acquired aplastic anemia respond to immunosuppressive therapy with antithymocyte globulin; and (c) autologous marrow recovery is seen following matched or mismatched marrow transplantation in patients prepared with antilymphocyte sera or cyclophosphamide.
3. *Defective microenvironment in the bone marrow.* Stromal cell abnormality may not be an independent or a sole etiologic factor in the pathogenesis of aplastic anemia, since most patients recover following allogeneic bone marrow transplantation.

Etiology

Although there are multiple causes for acquired aplastic anemia, a cause may not be found in some cases. Table 115–1 lists the causes of aplastic anemia.

1. *Epstein-Barr virus (EBV).* Although reversible pancytopenia is seen in ≤1 per cent of patients with infectious mononucleosis, at least a dozen cases of aplastic anemia are reported in patients with EBV infection, with a 50 per cent mortality.

2. *Hepatitis.* Most cases of aplastic anemia associated with hepatitis do not appear to be caused by any of the known hepatitis viruses.
3. *B19 parvovirus.* B19 parvovirus produces transient aplastic crisis in patients with hemolytic anemia; mild leukopenia and thrombocytopenia have been observed in these patients as well as in healthy individuals following the infection. However, a clinical course resembling that of aplastic anemia has been described following B19 parvovirus infection in immunodeficient patients.
4. *Human immunodeficiency virus (HIV).* Cytopenias (including pancytopenia) are common in patients with advanced HIV infection. Some of these patients have hypo-

---

TABLE 115–1. CLASSIFICATION OF APLASTIC ANEMIAS

INHERITED

Fanconi anemia
Dyskeratosis congenita
Reticular dysgenesis
Shwachman-Diamond syndrome
Amegakaryocytic thrombocytopenia

ACQUIRED

Infection
    Epstein-Barr virus
    Hepatitis
    B19 parvovirus
    Human immunodeficiency virus
Radiation
Drugs
    Cytotoxic drugs
    Chloramphenicol
    Nonsteroidal antiinflammatory drugs and gold
Immunologic disorders
    Hypogammaglobulinemia
    Thymoma
    Pregnancy
    Paroxysmal nocturnal hemoglobinuria

Modified from Alter BP, Young NS: The bone marrow failure syndromes. *In* Nathan DG, Oski FA (eds): Hematology of Infancy and Childhood, 4th ed. Philadelphia, WB Saunders, 1993.

cellular bone marrow. Whether marrow failure is due to HIV infection alone or also to concurrent opportunistic infections is not known.

5. *Chloramphenicol.* This is known to produce both dose-related and idiosyncratic aplasia of the bone marrow. Idiosyncratic marrow aplasia, with an estimated incidence of 1 in 40,000, usually occurs following oral administration and may be seen up to 1 year after the drug administration. Familial cases have been reported. It carries a very high mortality rate.

6. *Paroxysmal nocturnal hemoglobinuria (PNH).* This is a rare clonal stem cell disorder characterized by hemolytic anemia and hemoglobinuria. Twenty to 30 per cent of patients with PNH have evidence of aplastic anemia at the time of initial presentation. Blood cells of these patients bind complement and lyse. The diagnosis is made by acidified serum lysis test or sucrose hemolysis test.

Epidemiology

There is a wide geographic variation in the incidence of aplastic anemia that may be related to exposure to drugs and infection. In the United States and Europe, incidence is estimated to be 2 to 6 cases per million per year, whereas in Asia it may be as high as 30 per million per year.

Clinical Findings

Most patients present with pallor, tiredness, petechiae, ecchymosis, gum bleeding, or epistaxis. Fever is an uncommon initial presenting symptom. Hepatosplenomegaly is uncommon; significant hepatosplenomegaly suggests that aplastic anemia is secondary to an infection or leukemia.

Key Clinical Findings: Aplastic Anemia

- Pallor
- Fatigue
- Petechiae and ecchymosis
- Epistaxis

Laboratory Findings

1. Complete blood count reveals anemia, usually macrocytic, reticulocytopenia, leukopenia/neutropenia, and thrombocytopenia. Platelet size is normal (giant platelets are observed in patients with increased platelet turnover). Fetal hemoglobin concentration and red cell i antigen expression are often increased.

2. If serum ALT, AST, and bilirubin are abnormal, appropriate serologic studies for hepatitis should be done.

3. Peripheral blood and bone marrow chromosomes are abnormal in Fanconi's aplastic anemia and myelodysplastic syndrome, respectively.

4. Documentation of bone marrow hypocellularity is essential to a diagnosis of aplastic anemia and may require several bone marrow biopsies. There will be reduction in erythroid and myeloid precursors and megakaryocytes, but lymphocytes, plasma cells, and histiocytes are normal in number. There may be dyserythropoiesis and megaloblastoid changes.

Key Laboratory Findings: Aplastic Anemia

- Anemia, usually macrocytic
- Reticulocytopenia
- Neutropenia
- Thrombocytopenia
- Bone marrow, hypocellular with normal lymphocytes, plasma cells, and histiocytes

Prognosis

Prognosis depends on the severity of aplastic anemia and the therapy administered. Patients with severe aplastic anemia have ≤20 per cent survival at 6 months from diagnosis with supportive care alone. Spontaneous recovery may occur in some patients with moderate aplastic anemia, but it is rare in those with severe aplastic anemia.

Criteria for Severe Aplastic Anemia

- Blood findings (at least two abnormalities)
  Neutrophils < 0.5 × 10^9/L
  Platelets < 20 × 10^9/L
  Reticulocytes < 1% (corrected for hematocrit)
- Bone marrow findings (at least one abnormality)
  Severely hypocelluar
  Moderately hypocelluar with <30% hematopoietic cells

Treatment

1. *Bone marrow transplantation (BMT).* Allogeneic BMT is the treatment of choice for patients with severe aplastic anemia. Untransfused or minimally transfused patients have the best outcome. A 10-year survival rate of 90 per cent is expected in untransfused patients with severe aplastic anemia who receive BMT. When a histocompatible sibling is unavailable, transplantation using bone marrow from matched unrelated donors or partially matched relatives is a consideration. Preparative regimens consist of high-dose cyclophosphamide alone or cyclophosphamide and low-dose total-body or lymphoid irradiation. Standard regimens to prevent graft-versus-host disease (GVHD) are used.

2. *ATG and cyclosporine* in combination have recently been shown to give results superior to those seen with either treatment alone. This is the treatment of choice if a BMT donor is not available.

3. *Corticosteroids.* High-dose corticosteroids (30–100mg/kg methylprednisolone) are reported to produce hematologic response in nearly 40 per cent of patients in small series. This therapy, because of considerable toxicity, may be employed only in patients when ATG is unavailable.

4. *Androgens.* Androgens were shown to be no more efficacious than supportive care alone in the management of patients with severe aplastic anemia in a prospective multicenter study.

5. *Hematopoietic growth factors (IL-3 and GM-CSF).* May be a useful adjunct to immunosuppressive therapy.

Key Treatment: Severe Aplastic Anemia

- Bone marrow transplantation
- Immunosuppressive therapy
- Hematopoietic growth factors

Fanconi Anemia (FA)

Definition

The term is used to describe patients who have characteristic chromosomal abnormalities following clastogenic stress regardless of the presence or lack of physical abnormalities and/or aplastic anemia. Until recently, a diagnosis of FA was made only in the presence of aplastic anemia in a patient with characteristic physical abnormalities; obviously, several cases were not diagnosed.

Epidemiology

FA is an autosomal recessive disorder and has been reported in all races and ethnic groups.

Clinical Findings

Hematologic abnormalities are first evident between the ages of 5 and 10 years. However, many cases can be diagnosed using chromosomal studies before the development of hematologic abnormalities if there is a positive family history.

The usual physical abnormalities are short stature, broad nasal base, thumb and forearm abnormalities, epicanthal folds, café-au-lait spots, and hypopigmented areas. In addition, affected individuals have genitourinary, gastrointestinal, and cardiopulmonary abnormalities.

Key Clinical Findings: Fanconi Anemia

- Short stature
- Forearm and thumb abnormalities
- Café-au-lait spots

Laboratory Findings

These are similar to the findings in other types of aplastic anemia. Most patients present with anemia or thrombocytopenia before manifesting pancytopenia. Macrocytosis precedes anemia. There is also evidence of stress "erythropoiesis" with elevated levels of fetal hemoglobin and red cell i antigen.

Pathophysiology

The basic defect that results in bone marrow failure is not known. Furthermore, the relationship between physical abnormalities, marrow failure, and propensity to develop malignant tumors is also unexplained. There is a suggestion that blood cells in patients with FA have decreased capacity for DNA repair, which may be due in part to free radicals of oxygen.

Treatment

1. Androgens are the first line of therapy for patients with Fanconi aplastic anemia. Fifty to 75 per cent of the patients respond to androgens but ultimately become refractory to them. Usually, there is complete resolution of anemia and some improvement in neutropenia and thrombocytopenia. There is clear evidence that androgens prolong survival in patients with FA. Oxymethalone is used in a dose of 2 to 5 mg/kg/day; prednisone, in a dose of 5 to 10 mg on alternate days, is often used to counteract the growth-promoting effect of androgens and to improve the capillary stability.

2. Bone marrow transplantation is reserved for patients who initially fail to respond to androgens or who become refractory after initial response. Because of increased toxicity from preparative regimens consisting of high-dose cyclophosphamide and total-body irradiation, several modifications to the regimen are made, consisting of a lower dose of cyclophosphamide and reduction in radiation dose and field. It is important to fully investigate the potential sibling donor for occult aplastic anemia. This is done by physical examination, CBC with particular attention to MCV, fetal hemoglobin concentration, and, finally, chromosome studies using DEB or mitomycin C.

3. Immunosuppressive therapy has not been useful in these patients. The precise role of hematopoietic growth factors is not defined.

4. Supportive care. Red cell and platelet transfusions are used sparingly and should be administered using a leukocyte filter to minimize febrile reactions and HLA sensitization. Bone marrow transplant candidates should not receive transfusion of blood products obtained from blood relatives.

Key Treatment: Fanconi Anemia

- Androgens

Complications

Acute leukemia, predominantly acute myelocytic or myelomonocytic types, is reported in 10 to 20 per cent of patients with FA at a median age of 10 years. These patients also have an increased incidence of gastrointestinal, gynecologic, and hepatic malignant tumors.

Bibliography

Bacigalupo A, Podesta M, Van Lint MT, et al: Severe aplastic anemia: Correlation of in vitro tests with clinical response to immunosuppression in 20 patients. Br J Hematol 1981;47:423.

Rosenfeld SJ, Kimball J, Donna V, Young NS: Intensive immunosuppression with antithymocyte globulin and cyclosporine as treatment for severe acquired aplastic anemia. Blood 1985; 85:3058.

Saunders JE, Storb R, Anasetti C, et al: Marrow transplant experience for children with severe aplastic anemia. Am J Pediatr Hematol Oncol 1994;16:43.

116 Hypoplastic Anemias

Sreedhar P. Rao

These are characterized by decreased production of red cells alone (pure red cell aplasia, transient erythroblastopenia of childhood, transient aplastic crisis) or red cells, neutrophils, and platelets (aplastic anemia).

Pure Red Cell Aplasia

Definition

Pure red cell aplasia is characterized by anemia and reticulocytopenia; the platelet count is normal and the white blood cell count is normal to moderately decreased. Although there are many causes of pure red cell aplasia, the three conditions that account for most episodes of pure red cell aplasia in children are Diamond-Blackfan anemia (DBA), transient erythroblastopenia of childhood (TEC), and transient aplastic crisis.

Diamond-Blackfan Anemia

Definition

An inherited form of anemia that manifests in early infancy and is characterized by selectively impaired production of red cells.

Etiology

DBA is often an inherited disorder; transmission may be dominant or recessive or X-linked.

Pathophysiology

The disease may have multiple etiologies based on the variable inheritance pattern; age at presentation and physical abnormalities are present in only some patients.

1. Humoral and/or cell-mediated inhibition of erythropoiesis has been described in some children; adults with pure red cell aplasia often have humoral inhibition of erythropoiesis and associated thymoma.
2. The consensus is that the erythroid progenitor cell is intrinsically defective in most pediatric patients.

Clinical Findings

1. Most patients have a history of pallor at birth or in early infancy and may present with pallor, lethargy, irritability, and sometimes heart failure.
2. About a third of the patients have physical abnormalities, such as short stature unrelated to steroid therapy, triphalangeal thumbs, absent or subluxed thumbs, short neck, and eye and renal anomalies.

Laboratory Findings

1. All patients are anemic and reticulocytopenic; macrocytosis is seen in most patients.
2. White blood cell count is usually normal but may be low.
3. The platelet count is normal or increased.

4. Fetal hemoglobin concentration is usually elevated with heterocellular distribution, i.e., only some cells have fetal hemoglobin.
5. Bone marrow aspiration is essential to the diagnosis. Marrow cellularity is normal with normal numbers and maturation of myeloid precursors and megakaryocytes. The erythroid precursors are markedly decreased or absent in 90 per cent, normal in 5 per cent, and increased in 5 per cent of patients.

Key Laboratory Findings: Diamond-Blackfan Anemia

- Low hemoglobin
- Low reticulocyte count
- High MCV
- Normal or low white cell count
- Normal or elevated platelet count
- Elevated fetal hemoglobin concentration
- Bone marrow with markedly reduced numbers of erythroid precursors, normal myeloid series, and normal megakaryocytes

Differential Diagnosis

Diamond-Blackfan anemia needs to be differentiated from transient erythroblastopenia of childhood. The differentiating features are listed in Table 116–1.

Treatment

1. Corticosteroids
   Approximately 50 per cent of patients respond to steroid

TABLE 116–1. CLINICAL AND LABORATORY FEATURES OF DIAMOND-BLACKFAN ANEMIA (DBA) AND TRANSIENT ERYTHROBLASTOPENIA OF CHILDHOOD (TEC)

	DBA	TEC
Mean age at dx (months)	5–6	26–28
Etiology	Inherited	Acquired
Antecedent history	None	Viral illness
Physical abnormalities	30%	None
Hemoglobin at dx (g/dl)	1.5–10	2.4–11
WBC ≤5000/μl(%)	20	20
Platelet count ≥400,000/μl(%)	20	20
Elevated MCV at dx (%)	80	5
During recovery (%)	100	90
In remission (%)	100	0
Hb F elevated at dx (%)	100	20
During recovery (%)	100	100
In remission (%)	85	0

Modified from Alter BP, Young NS: The bone marrow failure syndromes. *In* Nathan DG, Oski FA (eds): Hematology of Infancy and Childhood 4th ed. Philadelphia, WB Saunders, 1993.

administration. Prednisone, 2 mg/kg/day, should be given in divided doses. Once hemoglobin concentration reaches a level of 10 to 11 g/dl, prednisone should be tapered. The goal is to administer the smallest dose of prednisone in a single dose on alternate days that maintains hemoglobin around 10 g/dl, in order to minimize long-term side effects; some patients require a very small dose of prednisone on alternate days, and attempts should be made periodically to discontinue steroid therapy.

If a patient fails to respond to 2 mg/kg/day of prednisone, a dose of 4 to 6 mg/kg/day for 2 to 4 weeks or very high dose methylprednisolone, 30 to 100 mg/kg/day, IV, for 3 to 7 days followed by rapid tapering has been used. In a recent report, three of eight patients who failed 30 mg/kg/day of methylprednisolone responded to a 100 mg/kg/day dose. Treatment options for patients not responsive to steroids include the following:

2. Anabolic steroids

A rare patient may respond to oxymethalone or danazol.

3. Chronic blood transfusion

Nearly 30 to 40 per cent of the patients may need chronic transfusion and chelation therapy.

4. Bone marrow transplantation

Allogeneic marrow transplantation should be considered if a histocompatible sibling is available. Ideally, transplantation should be done before the patient has received multiple blood transfusions, although a history of chronic transfusion is not a contraindication for marrow transplantation.

5. Hematopoietic growth factors

In a recent report, 4 of 18 patients had clinically significant erythroid response following interleukin-3 (IL-3) administration. Other growth factors, either singly or in combination, may be useful as they become available.

Key Treatment

- Corticosteroids
- Repeated transfusion
- Bone marrow transplant
- Growth factors
- Hematopoietic

Prognosis

Eighty per cent of patients responding to steroids have long-term survival. For the others, the long-term prognosis is not clear. Deaths may occur as a result of transfusional iron load or infection. Leukemia is a rare complication in these patients.

Transient Erythroblastopenia of Childhood

Definition

Transient erythroblastopenia of childhood (TEC) is an acquired anemia with reticulocytopenia in previously healthy children. As the name implies, it is a transient disorder.

Pathophysiology

Viral infection is the most likely cause, since more than 50 per cent of children have a history suggestive of anteced-

ent viral illness; parvovirus B19 has been implicated in a very small proportion of patients with TEC. Most patients have reduced erythroid colony forming units in the bone marrow owing, in most cases, to serum inhibitors of erythropoiesis.

Clinical Findings

The mean age at diagnosis is 26 months (boys) to 29 months (girls), with a slight male preponderance. Nearly 90 per cent of the patients are ≥1 year of age. Most patients present with pallor. Seizures and/or transient ischemic episodes are rarely reported. TEC has been reported in twins and siblings, suggesting genetic and/or environmental predisposition. Physical examination is usually normal except for pallor in patients with severe anemia.

Laboratory Findings

1. Hemoglobin levels may be very low or only slightly decreased. Reticulocyte count is decreased in ≥90 per cent of patients. Nearly 20 per cent of the patients may have low WBC (≤5000/μl) or elevated platelet count (≥400,000/μl).

2. Bone marrow examination reveals marked erythroblastopenia in nearly 90 per cent of the patients; it may reveal normal or increased erythroid precursors with erythroid maturation arrest in others.

3. During the recovery phase of TEC, many patients have evidence of "stress erythropoiesis," characterized by an elevated MCV, fetal hemoglobin concentration, and i antigen on red cells. However, these characteristics are constant in DBA.

Treatment

Blood transfusion is recommended if the patient is severely anemic and symptomatic. Almost all patients recover in 4 months from the time of diagnosis and have an excellent prognosis.

Transient Aplastic Crisis

Definition

Transient reticulocytopenia and worsening anemia in patients with chronic hemolytic anemia.

Etiology

B19 parvovirus infection, the cause of erythema infectiosum (fifth disease), is the most common cause of transient aplastic crisis.

Pathophysiology

Patients with compensated hemolytic anemia (e.g., sickle cell anemia) maintain their hemoglobin at a certain level because of increased erythropoiesis characterized by reticulocytosis. Infection of erythroid precursors with B19 parvovirus results in cell lysis, marked reticulocytopenia, and worsening of anemia. Once antibodies are produced by the patient, the viremia resolves and erythropoiesis returns. Reticulocytopenia usually lasts 7 to 10 days.

Clinical Findings

These include fever, malaise, abdominal pain, arthralgia, pallor, and lethargy. Skin rash, while common in otherwise healthy children, is rare in infected patients with sickle cell disease.

Laboratory Findings

1. There is a rapid decline in hemoglobin concentration from baseline values, and reticulocytopenia is usually profound (<1%). WBC count and platelet counts are usually normal but may be reduced.
2. Bone marrow aspiration is rarely needed but, if done early in the clinical course, may show erythroid hypoplasia, a few giant erythroblasts, and otherwise normal findings.

Treatment

Packed red cell transfusion is given to severely anemic or symptomatic patients. Patients should be isolated from other patients with hemolytic anemia, immunosuppressed patients, and pregnant staff.

Bibliography

Alter BP, Young NS: The bone marrow failure syndromes. *In* Nathan DG, Oski FA (eds): Hematology of Infancy and Childhood, 4th ed. Philadelphia, WB Saunders, 1993, pp 262–270.

Bernini JC, Carillo JM, Buchanan GJ: High dose intravenous methylprednisolone therapy for patients with Diamond-Blackfan anemia refractory to conventional doses of prednisone. J Pediatr 1996; 27:654–659.

Gillio AP, Faultrer LB, Alter BP, et al: Treatment of Diamond-Blackfan anemia with recombinant human interleukin 3. Blood 1993;82:744–751.

117 Glucose 6-Phosphate Dehydrogenase Deficiency

Sreedhar P. Rao

Deficiency of the red cell enzyme glucose 6-phosphate dehydrogenase (G6PD) is one of the most commonly inherited metabolic disorders and may affect 3 per cent of the world's population. G6PD deficiency is an example of "balanced polymorphism," in which there is an evolutionary advantage of resistance to falciparum malaria in carrier females. The majority of people with G6PD deficiency are normal with minimal or no hemolysis in steady state. They develop acute hemolytic anemia when the red cells are exposed to oxidant stress from drugs or infection.

Pathophysiology

Hemolysis in G6PD deficiency is precipitated when the red cells and hemoglobin are exposed to oxidant stress, which results in damage to hemoglobin and the red cell membrane. The mechanism by which infections cause oxidant stress is not well understood.

1. The oxidant drugs convert reduced glutathione (GSH) to oxidized glutathione (GSSG). The glutathione peroxidase and glutathione reductase are normally responsible for converting the glutathione to a reduced state, which will remove harmful peroxides. Because of G6PD deficiency there is inadequate generation of NADPH, which in turn will adversely affect the glutathione peroxidase and glutathione reductase system.
2. In the presence of oxidant drugs, the hemoglobin is oxidized to methemoglobin and sulfhemoglobin. The oxidized heme is dissociated from methemoglobin and leaves behind free globin, which may undergo further oxidation. The denatured hemoglobin precipitates as intracellular inclusions (Heinz bodies), which are removed when these cells pass through the spleen. This will result in a fragmented red cell, or a spherocyte.
3. Oxidant drugs also damage the red cell membrane and enzymes, resulting in irreversible damage and eventually intravascular hemolysis.

Terminology

Normal G6PD is designated B (or B+). A fast-moving normal variant that is seen in some blacks is designated A (or A+). There are at least four major variants that are associated with acute drug- or infection-induced hemolytic anemia and/or chronic hemolytic anemia. These are A− (blacks, Africans, and African Americans); Mediterranean (Greeks, Sardinians, Israelis); Canton (Chinese); and Chicago (persons of North European descent). The major differences between G6PD A− and G6PD Mediterranean are listed in Table 117–1.

Clinical Findings

Three distinct clinical syndromes are related to G6PD deficiency. These are acute hemolytic anemia, neonatal jaundice, and chronic nonspherocytic hemolytic anemia.

1. Acute hemolytic anemia may develop following an infection or after exposure to one of the drugs (Table 117–2) or ingestion of fava beans. The child may be in the usual

TABLE 117–1. DIFFERENCES BETWEEN G6PD A− AND G6PD MEDITERRANEAN

MEASURE PARAMETER	G6PD A−	G6PD MEDITERRANEAN
Degree of enzyme deficiency	Mild	Severe
Deficiency seen in	Old red cells	All red cells
Clinical severity	Mild to moderate	Severe
G6PD levels immediately after hemolysis	May be normal	Always low
Hemolysis after fava beans	Rare	Common

TABLE 117–2. DRUGS TO BE AVOIDED IN G6PD DEFICIENCY

Drugs listed below in **bold** type should be avoided by people with all forms of G6PD deficiency.
Drugs in regular type should be avoided, in addition, by G6PD-deficient persons of Mediterranean, Middle Eastern, or Asian origin.
Items in regular type and within square brackets apply only to people with the African ($-$) variant.

Antimalarials
Primaquine [people with the African ($-$) variant may take it at reduced dosage, 15 mg daily or 45 mg twice weekly under surveillance]
Pamaquine naphthoate
Chloroquine (may be used under surveillance when required for prophylaxis or treatment of malaria)

Sulfonamides and Sulfones
Sulfanilamide
Sulfapyridine
Sulfadimidine
Sulfacetamide (albucid)
Sulfafurazole (Gantrisin)
Salicylazosulfapyridine (Azulfidine)
Dapsone*
Sulfoxone*
Glucosulfone sodium (Promin)
Septrin

Other Antibacterial Compounds
Nitrofurans—Nitrofurantoin
Furazolidone
Nitrofurazone
[Nalidixic acid]
Chloramphenicol
p-Aminosalicylic acid

Analgesics
Acetylsalicylic acid (aspirin): moderate doses can be used
Acetophenetidin (acetaminophen)
Safe alternative: paracetamol

Anthelminthics
Betanaphthol
Stibophen
Niridazole

Miscellaneous
Vitamin K analog (1 mg of menadione can be given to infants)
Naphthalene* (mothballs)
Probenecid
Dimercaprol (BAL)
Methylene blue
Arsine*
Phenylhydrazine*
Acetylphenylhydrazine*
Toluidine blue
Mepacrine

*These drugs may cause hemolysis in normal individuals if given in large doses. Many other drugs may produce hemolysis in particular individuals.
From WHO Working Group: Glucose-6-phosphate dehydrogenase deficiency. Bull WHO 1989; 67:601.

steady state for between a few hours and up to 1 to 3 days, when symptoms of irritability or decreased activity may develop. Other symptoms are pallor, jaundice, dark urine (tea or cola-colored), abdominal or back pain, and fever.

2. Physical examination reveals pallor, jaundice, tachycardia, or, rarely, heart failure/hypovolemic shock. There may be moderate enlargement of the liver and/or spleen.

3. In most patients, the hemolytic episode is self-limited and resolves spontaneously. However, severely anemic patients may need red cell transfusion.

Key Clinical Findings

- Sudden onset
- Pallor
- Jaundice
- Abdominal or back pain
- Dark urine

Laboratory Findings

These are characterized by evidence of intravascular hemolysis.

1. CBC reveals anemia (moderate to severe), reticulocytosis with normal or elevated WBC count and normal platelet count. Blood smear typically reveals fragmented red cells (bite cells), blister cells, microspherocytes, polychromasia, and normoblasts. Supravital stain will reveal increased numbers of reticulocytes and inclusions (Heinz bodies) representing denatured hemoglobin.

2. Serum chemical analysis will reveal elevated indirect bilirubin, lactate dehydrogenase (LDH), and decreased or absent haptoglobin. Plasma hemoglobin is increased.

3. Dark urine is usually due to free hemoglobin, as demonstrated by few or no red cells in the urine sediment after centrifugation.

Key Laboratory Findings

- Anemia
- Reticulocytosis
- Fragmented red cells
- Heinz bodies
- Hemoglobinuria
- Elevated serum bilirubin and LDH

Diagnosis

Acute intravascular hemolysis in an otherwise healthy child with a history of exposure (inhalation or ingestion) to naphthalene, fava beans, or primaquine is highly suggestive of G6PD deficiency. Because of the higher content of the enzyme in reticulocytes and young red cells in the A$^-$

variant, diagnosis is difficult to establish immediately after a hemolytic episode. Investigation of the patient's mother (in the case of boys) or both parents (in the case of girls) may reveal evidence of heterozygosity or hemizygosity. Once the patient returns to steady state, the diagnosis can be established by quantitative assay of the enzyme.

The following tests are available for diagnosis of G6PD deficiency:

1. Enzyme assay based on the rate of generation of NADPH using spectrophotometry. This is a functional assay, and normal activity is between 7 and 10 IU/g Hb.
2. Several semiquantitative screening tests are available that are useful in evaluating a patient in steady state. These tests will not identify all the heterozygotes because of variation in the enzyme levels. The three most common screening tests are
   a. Dye decolorization test
   b. Methemoglobin reduction test
   c. Fluorescence spot test.

   Any individual who is found to be enzyme deficient by screening should have confirmation by quantitative assay.
3. It is well known that only some G6PD-deficient neonates develop hyperbilirubemia. There is a considerable variation in the incidence of hyperbilirubinemia in G6PD-deficient babies in different parts of the world, even among populations with the same genetic variant of the enzyme. The incidence is very high in Greek and Chinese newborns. Environmental factors are considered among the reasons for the discrepancy. In some babies, the triggering factor could be infection in the baby or a drug ingested by the mother or baby.
4. A small proportion of individuals with severe variants of G6PD manifest chronic nonspherocytic hemolytic anemia. Virtually all patients are male, and most have a history of neonatal jaundice. Most patients are of northern European extraction, Mediterranean, or Asiatic; about 5 per cent are black. The degree of anemia ranges from mild to moderately severe with reticulocytosis. The red cell morphology is unremarkable except for polychromasia. There are other changes of chronic hemolysis, e.g., hyperbilirubinemia, elevated LDH, and decreased haptoglobin level. Rarely, patients may develop large spleen and secondary hypersplenism.

Treatment

1. General supportive measures for treating acute hemolytic anemia consist of close monitoring of vital signs and urine output and of oxygen administration while waiting for blood transfusion.
2. Generally 60 to 75 per cent of patients with acute hemolytic episode receive transfusion. The decision to transfuse depends on the hemoglobin concentration and if the patient has evidence of ongoing hemolysis, namely persistent hemoglobinuria. Packed red cell transfusion is recommended in all patients with hemoglobin level ≤6 g/dl or between 6 and 9 g/dl if associated with ongoing brisk hemolysis. Large-volume transfusion should be avoided in severely anemic patients; instead, it can be administered in small aliquots.
3. Renal failure is very rare in children, but when it is present, appropriate management should be instituted.
4. Management of patients with neonatal hyperbilirubinemia or chronic hemolytic anemia due to G6PD deficiency is similar to that due to other reasons, namely, phototherapy or exchange transfusion, blood transfusion, folic acid supplementation, and splenectomy in selected cases.

Key Treatment: Acute Hemolytic Anemia

• Packed RBC transfusion

Prevention

Once a child is diagnosed with G6PD deficiency, a list of drugs should be provided to the family (see Table 117–2). The list should be made available to the treating physician whenever a medication is prescribed. Patients are advised not to eat fava beans; naphthalene (mothballs) should not be kept in the house. When primaquine has to be given to eradicate a certain type of malaria, it should be given at a lower dose for a longer period of time with close monitoring of the patient. Obviously, it is not possible to prevent hemolysis following infection.

Bibliography

Arese P, DeFlora A: Pathophysiology of hemolysis in glucose 6-phosphate dehydrogenase deficiency. Semin Hematol 1990;27:1.

Babior BM, Stossel TP: Hemolytic anemias: Intravascular destruction of red cells. *In* Hematology: A Pathophysiological Approach, 3rd ed. New York, Churchill Livingstone, 1994, pp 121–134.

Beutler E: Glucose 6-phosphate dehydrogenase deficiency. N Engl J Med 1994;324:169.

Luzzato L: G6PD deficiency and hemolytic anemia. *In* Nathan DG, Oski FA (eds): Hematology of Infancy and Childhood, 4th ed. Philadelphia, WB Saunders, 1993, pp 674–695.

118 Pyruvate Kinase Deficiency

Sreedhar P. Rao

Hemolytic anemia due to pyruvate kinase (PK) deficiency is the first described enzyme abnormality of the Embden-Meyerhof pathway. It is inherited as an autosomal recessive disorder, with evidence of clinical disease in homozygotes and compound heterozygotes. Simple heterozygotes are normal clinically. Although cases have been described worldwide, most cases have been in persons of North European extraction, with few cases in blacks, Japanese, Mexicans, and Chinese.

Pathophysiology

Pyruvate kinase catalyzes the conversion of phosphoenolpyruvate to pyruvate. At the same time, ADP is converted to ATP. The enzymatic block at the PK level results in a decrease in overall glycolysis and increased concentration of several glycolic intermediates proximal to PK. The level of 2,3-diphosphoglycerate (DPG) is increased two to four fold. Increased levels of 2,3-DPG will increase oxygen delivery to the tissues by lowering the oxygen affinity of hemoglobin. Elevated levels of 2,3-DPG also decrease hexokinase and phosphofructokinase as well as the activity of pentose-phosphate shunt. ATP depletion in the red cells from PK deficiency leads to increase in the cation permeability, resulting in loss of potassium, gain of sodium, loss of water, and formation of rigid red cells. Finally, decreased deformability of the red cells will lead to hemolysis.

Clinical Findings

1. The symptoms are typically those of chronic hemolytic anemia, consisting of anemia and hyperbilirubinemia in the newborn period (in some patients only) and anemia, jaundice, and splenomegly in older children.
2. The degree of anemia ranges from mild to severe, with some patients requiring repeated blood transfusions. Few patients have normal hemoglobin levels, with evidence of compensated hemolytic anemia (elevated LDH and indirect bilirubin). There may be episodes of worsening anemia due to transient aplastic crisis or increased hemolysis.

Key Clinical Findings

- Anemia
- Jaundice
- Splenomegaly

Laboratory Findings

1. Hemoglobin levels range from 6 to 12 g/dl, with normal WBC and platelet count.

2. Reticulocyte count may range from 5 to 10 per cent presplenectomy to 30 to 90 per cent post splenectomy despite an increase in hemoglobin level.
3. Blood smear presplenectomy may be normal or reveal macrocytes and spiculated red cells.
4. Osmotic fragility of fresh and incubated red cells is normal.

Key Laboratory Findings

- Low Hgb/HCT
- High reticulocyte count
- Macrocytosis (sometimes) and spiculated RBCs

Diagnosis

1. In vitro enzyme assay
2. Characterization of PK mutants is possible by determining the kinetics and electrophoretic mobility. The enzyme mutants with unfavorable kinetics are usually associated with severe hemolysis.

Treatment

1. No specific therapy is recommended for patients with mild to moderate hemolytic anemia other than to provide folic acid supplementation (1 mg/day).
2. Splenectomy is recommended for patients with severe hemolytic anemia. Although the degree of clinical benefit is not predictable, most patients have a moderate increase in hemoglobin level with a decrease in bilirubin level.
3. Large doses of salicylates are known to inhibit oxidative phosphorylation and result in depletion of intracellular ATP and increase in the rate of hemolysis. If patients do need high-dose salicylate therapy, they should be observed closely for an increase in hemolysis; alternatively, other therapy should be chosen for these patients.

Key Treatment

- Folic acid supplementation
- Splenectomy (severe cases)

 Bibliography

Mentzer WC Jr: Pyruvate kinase deficiency and disorders of glycolysis. *In* Nathan DG, Oski FA (eds): Hematology of Infancy and Childhood, 4th ed. Philadelphia, WB Saunders, 1993, pp 634–673.

119 Microangiopathic Hemolytic Anemia

Sreedhar P. Rao

Definition

Microangiopathic hemolytic anemia refers to hemolytic anemia resulting from mechanical damage to red cells due to pathology in the small blood vessels (e.g., vasculitis). However, this term has also been used to describe mechanical hemolysis resulting from abnormal heart valves or a synthetic graft used to repair intracardiac defects. An appropriate term to describe these two types of hemolytic anemias is schistocytic hemolytic anemia, which is characterized by the presence of schistocytes (fragmented red cells) and spherocytes in the blood smear. Some of the common causes of schistocytic hemolytic anemia in children are as follows:

1. Cardiac abnormalities
   a. Repair of intracardiac defect
   b. Diseased or prosthetic heart valve
2. Hemolytic uremic syndrome (HUS)
3. Thrombotic thrombocytopenic purpura (TTP)
4. Acute renal allograft rejection
5. Microangiopathy associated with cancer
6. Localized or disseminated intravascular coagulation, e.g., Kasabach Merritt syndrome, fulminant meningococcemia

Cardiac hemolytic anemia and hemolytic uremic syndrome, two of the common causes of schistocytic hemolytic anemia, are described below.

Cardiac Hemolytic Anemia

Definition

A hemolytic anemia seen in some patients with congenital or acquired disease of the heart or aorta; usually due to mechanical damage to the red cells.

Pathophysiology

Intravascular hemolysis results when red cells are damaged by increased shear forces due to abnormal blood flow and red cell contact with abnormal surfaces in the heart or aorta. Improvement or resolution of hemolysis is seen after covering the prosthetic surface with endothelium.

Clinical Findings

1. Pallor and/or jaundice and dark urine develop in a patient soon after or within a few days of cardiac surgery.
2. The above symptoms may improve in some patients without any intervention but may also worsen as the patient becomes ambulatory with increase in cardiac output.

 Key Clinical Findings

- Pallor
- Jaundice
- Dark urine

Laboratory Findings

1. Complete blood count reveals anemia, reticulocytosis, and normal WBC and platelet count.
2. Urinalysis usually reveals hemoglobinuria and may reveal hemosiderinuria if hemolysis persists.
3. Serum chemical analysis reveals elevated LDH, indirect bilirubin, plasma hemoglobin, and decreased or absent serum haptoglobin.
4. Blood smear reveals characteristic schistocytes (fragmented red cells) and spherocytes.
5. Evidence of iron deficiency, i.e., low serum iron and elevated TIBC in patients with persistent intravascular hemolysis due to urinary iron loss.

 Key Laboratory Findings

- Anemia
- Reticulocytosis
- Elevated LDH
- Schistocytes

Treatment

1. Blood transfusion if anemia is severe
2. Surgical correction of the underlying hemodynamic abnormality; generally, surgery is delayed for a few weeks to months to determine if hemolysis will resolve or decrease.
3. Supplemental iron and folic acid if hemolysis is persistent.

Hemolytic Uremic Syndrome

Definition

The hemolytic uremic syndrome is a triad of microangiopathic hemolytic anemia, consumptive thrombocytopenia, and renal failure in infants and young children. It encompasses a spectrum of diseases with variable renal and platelet involvement as well as intravascular hemolysis. While the typical HUS is associated with diarrhea, atypical or sporadic cases also occur. Furthermore, systemic lupus erythematosus and drugs such as mitomycin C have been associated with HUS (see Chapter 223).

 Bibliography

Steward CL, Tina LU: Hemolytic uremic syndrome. Pediatr Rev 1993;14:218.

120 Autoimmune Hemolytic Anemia

Sreedhar P. Rao

Definition

It is a hemolytic anemia in which there is immune destruction of red cells due to antibodies directed against the patient's own red cell antigens. In children, antibodies of the IgG class are usually responsible for hemolytic anemia and usually appear to be of complex specificity directed against antigens of the Rh complex. Generally, these present as panagglutinins reacting with all except Rh null cells. Less often, the IgM class of antibodies, usually cold agglutinins, are the cause of autoimmune hemolytic anemia (AIHA) in children.

Etiology

Infections, particularly viral, are the most common cause of AIHA in children. Disorders commonly associated with AIHA in children are as follows:

1. Epstein-Barr virus (EBV), cytomegalovirus, and HIV are among the common viruses associated with AIHA.
2. Pneumonia due to mycoplasma is another common cause.
3. Autoimmune disorders that may be associated with AIHA are systemic lupus erythematosus (SLE), rheumatoid arthritis, inflammatory bowel disease, and chronic active hepatitis.
4. Immunodeficiency syndromes, both inherited and acquired
5. Malignancies such as acute lymphoblastic leukemia, lymphoma (Hodgkin and non-Hodgkin) are rarely associated with AIHA in children.

Pathophysiology

1. Antibodies of the IgG class are frequently the cause of AIHA. These are directed against antigens of the Rh complex; they have maximal activity at 37°C and thus result in warm antibody-induced hemolytic anemia. Antibody or antibody-complement complex or complement alone may coat the red cell surface. These antibody-coated red cells are ingested by macrophages mainly in the spleen and to a lesser degree in the liver. There is usually loss of a portion of red cell membrane, resulting in the formation of a microspherocyte, a cell with markedly decreased survival because of decreased deformability. Alternatively, the macrophages may ingest and lyse the entire cell, resulting in hemolysis.
2. In cold hemagglutinin disease, IgM antibody interacts with red cell membrane and activates the complement pathway, resulting in the generation of C3b. There is moderate intravascular hemolysis with a very high level of IgM- and C3b-induced hemolysis. Cold hemagglutinin disease is usually due to reaction with antigen of the I/i system. *Mycoplasma pneumoniae*–associated hemolysis is characterized by anti-I antibody, whereas anti-i antibody is usually found in patients with EBV-induced infectious mononucleosis.
3. The Donath-Landsteiner cold hemolysin, an uncommon IgG antibody with an anti-P specificity, is rarely found in children with viral infections. This antibody usually produces mild intravascular hemolysis.

Clinical Findings

1. The usual presenting symptoms are pallor, jaundice, dark urine, abdominal pain, and fever. Patients with mild anemia may present with fatigue, while those with severe anemia (Hb ≤5 g/dl) may be acutely ill with tachycardia and tachypnea.
2. Physical examination reveals pallor, jaundice, and usually hepatomegaly and splenomegaly. Patients with AIHA secondary to systemic diseases such as SLE or lymphoma will manifest symptoms and signs of the disorder in addition.

Key Clinical Findings

- Pallor
- Jaundice
- Abdominal pain
- Hepatosplenomegaly

Laboratory Evaluation

1. Complete blood count will reveal anemia, reticulocytosis with normal or elevated WBCs, and normal platelet count. Peripheral blood smear typically reveals microspherocytes, polychromatophilia, and normoblasts. Clumping of the red cells may be seen in patients with cold agglutinin disease.
2. Serum chemical analysis shows indirect hyperbilirubinemia, elevated levels of lactate dehydrogenase (LDH) and plasma hemoglobin, and decreased concentration of serum haptoglobin.
3. A positive direct antiglobulin test (DAT or Coombs test) establishes the diagnosis of AIHA. In this test, red cells of the patient are mixed with an antiglobulin reagent; detection of red cell agglutination indicates a positive test. A positive direct antiglobulin test (DAT) with antibody against IgG is described as a positive gamma Coombs test; agglutination with anti C3 is referred to as positive non-gamma Coombs test. The red cells of patients with IgG-induced hemolytic anemia demonstrate IgG and often demonstrate complement. In IgM-induced hemolytic anemia, neither IgG nor IgM is found on red cell membrane, but C3 will be detected.
4. Cold agglutinin titers are very high in children with cold hemagglutinin disease.

Key Laboratory Findings

- Anemia
- Reticulocytosis
- Positive direct Coombs test

Treatment

1. Many patients with mild disease have self-limited disease and do not require any therapy.

2. *Corticosteroids.* These are given to patients with IgG-induced hemolytic anemia of moderate to severe degree (Hb ≤8 g/dl). The mechanism of action of steroids is by inhibition of phagocytosis of antibody-coated red cells. The dose of prednisone ranges from 2 to 8 mg/kg/day in divided doses for 2 to 4 weeks. Once adequate clinical response is seen, the dose may be tapered and eventually discontinued. Some patients may need a low to moderate dose of prednisone on alternate days to maintain hemoglobin in the 8 to 10 g/dl range. Patients with IgM-induced AIHA usually do not respond to steroids. Fortunately, most patients have a clinically mild disease.

3. *Blood transfusion.* Severely anemic and symptomatic patients require red cell transfusion. It is important to rule out the presence of alloantibodies, which may be obscured by autoantibodies. For transfusion, it is important to choose red cell units negative for antigens corresponding to any significant alloantibodies identified. It is not often possible to obtain completely compatible blood, since IgG autoantibodies usually are panagglutinins reacting with almost all red cells and with broad specifity for antigens of the Rh complex. It is practical to obtain the least incompatible red cell unit and transfuse very slowly while the patient is closely monitored for increase in hemolysis (e.g., by serial gross observation for increase in hemoglobin in supernatant plasma).

4. *Intravenous immune globulin (IVIG).* It may be useful in selected patients with AIHA who respond poorly to at least 2 weeks of steroids. Generally, a dose of 0.5 to 1.0 g/kg/day for 5 days is recommended. Approximately 40 per cent of patients, many receiving concomitant steroids, respond to IVIG. Most responses are transient. Patients with pretreatment hemoglobin of <7 g/dl have the highest response rate.

5. *Splenectomy.* This is reserved for patients who fail to respond to steroids or who require fairly large doses to keep the disease under control or those with steroid toxicity. Nearly 50 to 75 per cent of patients respond to splenectomy, although it may not be a complete response.

6. Other modalities

   a. Rarely, plasmapheresis or exchange transfusion is done for temporary improvement in severe AIHA unresponsive to steroids and IVIG. This procedure may be transiently effective in IgM-induced AIHA.

   b. Immunosuppressive agents work by decreasing the production of autoantibody. Because of long-term toxicity, particularly in children, they are recommended for patients who fail to respond to steroids, IVIG, and splenectomy. The drugs most commonly used are azathioprine and cyclophosphamide. About 50 per cent of patients show some response to these drugs.

Key Treatment

- Corticosteroids
- Transfusion
- IVIG
- Splenectomy

Prognosis

Most patients with acute AIHA have resolution of their disease within 6 months of diagnosis. These patients are generally between 2 and 12 years of age and have acute onset of symptoms with less prominent reticulocytosis as well as normoblastemia and normal platelet count. Patients with a chronic course are generally below 2 or above 12 years of age, have slow onset of disease with marked reticulocytosis, and are often thrombocytopenic. These latter patients have a higher morbidity and mortality.

Bibliography

Flores G, Cunningham Rundles C, Newland AC, Bussel JB: Efficacy of intravenous immunoglobulin in the treatment of autoimmune hemolytic anemia. Am J Hematol 1993; 44:237–242.

Heisel MA, Ortega JA: Factors influencing prognosis in childhood autoimmune hemolytic anemia. Am J Pediatr Hematol Oncol 1983;5:147.

Schreiber AD, Gull FM, Manno CS: Autoimmune hemolytic anemia. *In* Nathan DG, Oski FA (eds): Hematology of Infancy and Childhood, 4th ed. Philadelphia, WB Saunders, 1993, pp 495–506.

121 Hereditary Spherocytosis and Hereditary Elliptocytosis

Joel M. Schwartz

Hereditary Spherocytosis

Definition

Hereditary spherocytosis (HS) is a hereditary hemolytic disorder of variable severity characterized by osmotically fragile spheroidal erythrocytes that become trapped, by virtue of their geometry, in the red pulp of the spleen. Surgical removal of the spleen improves erythrocyte survival and permits the anemia to remit, although the underlying molecular defects of the cell membrane persist.

Etiology

HS red cells assume spheroidal shapes as their surface area is reduced through the conjoint loss of cholesterol, phospholipid, and integral membrane proteins. The propensity to lose these components results from mutations affecting the synthesis, stability, or function of proteins that normally stabilize the surface membrane.

The stabilizing proteins are of two types (Fig. 121–1):

1. Cytoskeletal components such as ankyrin (band 2.1), spectrin, or pallidin (band 4.2) that underlie the lipid bilayer and laminate to it.
2. Band 3, the anion exchange channel, which is the major protein traversing the lipid bilayer.

Epidemiology

The HS phenotype may be inherited as an autosomal dominant trait (approximately 75 per cent of HS families) or an autosomal recessive disorder (about 25%). Rarely, it arises as the result of de novo mutation. The disease has been reported among many ethnic groups and races. Most commonly it occurs in individuals of Northern European extraction, in whom its prevalence approximates 1 in 5000.

Pathophysiology

1. Relevant aspects of normal RBC membrane structure and function:

   a. The external surface of the red cells consists of a lipid bilayer formed predominantly of phospholipids and cholesterol in both its inner and outer halves. The bilayer is traversed by integral membrane proteins—mainly band 3 and the glycophorins. The bilayer configuration is stabilized, in part, by hydrophobic interactions in its core among the fatty acid tails of phospholipids and the transmembrane segments of integral proteins (see Fig. 121–1).

   b. The bilayer provides the red cell with a fluid surface with which to interact with plasma components and other blood cells in the course of rapid flow. The mechanical strength required to survive turbulent flow in the heart and great vessels and the deformability needed to maintain integrity while negotiating narrow capillary and splenic channels are imparted to the lipid bilayer by a network of interacting skeletal proteins applied to its inner surface and laminated to it.

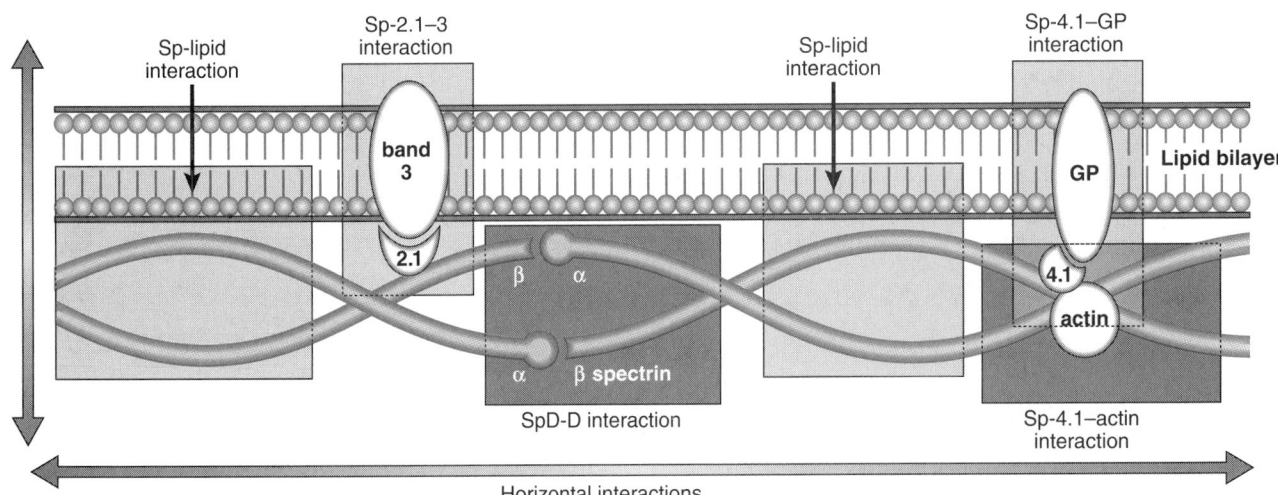

Figure 121–1 Molecular defects in the pathogenesis of HS and HE. HS arises as a result of loss of surface membrane due to disruption of vertical interactions that join the RBC skeleton to the overlying lipid bilayer and integral membrane proteins. HE results from weakened horizontal interactions between spectrin dimers or spectrin tetramers that destabilize the cytoskeleton when HE cells are subjected to shear stress. Pallidin (band 4.2), not shown in the diagram, is believed to strengthen the interaction between band 3 and ankyrin (band 2.1). (Modified from Palek J: Disorders of red cell membrane skeleton: an overview. *In* Erythrocyte Membrane 3: Recent Clinical and Experimental Advances. New York, Alan R. Liss, 1984.)

c. The skeletal network occupies more than half the inner surface of the lipid bilayer. It is composed of spectrin, actin, band 4.1, ankyrin (band 2.1), pallidin (band 4.2), and other proteins. Spectrin accounts for 50 to 75 per cent of the skeletal mass. Beta-spectrin binds vertically to band 3, the major integral protein, via ankyrin and pallidin; to glycophorin C via band 4.1; and to aminophospholipids in the inner bilayer leaflet directly (see Fig. 121–1). The linkage of the cytoskeleton to band 3 is believed to restrict band 3's lateral movement and thus limit the formation of lipid membrane domains devoid of band 3 and its stabilizing influence.

2. RBC abnormalities in HS

a. The hallmark of HS is the microspherocyte, a hyperchromic RBC of narrow diameter with reduced surface-to-volume ratio. Formation of microspherocytes requires that congenitally defective HS cells be "conditioned" as they are diverted through the slow-flow compartments of the red pulp of the spleen. Limited supply of glucose, local accumulations of lactic acid and oxygen radicals, and close proximity to hyperplastic macrophages are features of the congested red pulp, which may damage RBCs predisposed to accelerated loss of lipid bilayer because of inherent defects. Conditioned cells become progressively more spherocytic and less deformable. Many are detained in the splenic cords and destroyed. Cells that manage to escape between sinusoidal endothelial cells into the venous circulation are recaptured and destroyed by the spleen.

b. The primary molecular defects in HS and their respective patterns of inheritance are given in Table 121–1. According to one estimate (Eber et al, 1996), primary deficiency of ankyrin accounts for roughly 50 per cent of all HS, and deficient β-spectrin or protein 3 for 20 to 25 per cent, respectively, of all HS; deficient pallidin (band 4.2) or α-spectrin accounts for the remaining 5 to 10 per cent. The diverse molecular defects give rise to cells that have in common a weakening of the vertical interactions between the RBC skeleton and the overlying integral proteins and lipid bilayer. This results in loss of membrane material, which in turn leads to deficient surface area and spherocytosis.

(1) Most HS is caused by primary deficiency of ankyrin. Since ankyrin provides the major site for the assembly of β-spectrin on the membrane,

ankyrin deficiency is accompanied by approximately equal spectrin loss. Spectrin/ankyrin deficiency (70 to 90% of normal) and hemolysis are generally mild in dominant HS and more severe in recessively inherited HS.

(2) Deficiencies of band 3 or of β-spectrin are fairly common dominant disorders of mild severity.

(3) Deficiencies of pallidin (band 4.2) or α-spectrin are uncommon, recessively inherited, and of mild to moderate clinical severity.

Clinical Findings

1. Hemolytic anemia with spherocytosis, intermittent jaundice, and splenomegaly are the principal features of HS. The disease may present at any age. In newborns, severe jaundice may predominate and may require phototherapy or exchange transfusion to prevent kernicterus. Progressive anemia may develop over the next few months of life because of sluggish marrow response to hemolysis. Thereafter, the course of the disease is determined by the relationship established between RBC production and splenic destruction.

2. *Mild HS:* In about 20 per cent of patients, RBC production compensates for the destruction, and the patients have little or no anemia. The disorder may remain subclinical unless it is complicated by

a. Parvovirus infection causing transient red cell aplasia

b. Folate deficiency—especially during pregnancy—causing ineffective marrow erythropoiesis

c. Splenic enlargement by viral or other illness causing hyperhemolysis.

3. *Typical HS:* In about 70 per cent of patients, enhanced red cell production compensates only partially for hemolysis, and mild to moderate anemia persists throughout life. The spleen is palpable in half the patients during infancy and in nearly all by late childhood. Jaundice fluctuates in degree depending on the rate of hemolysis and the intermittent passage of small bilirubin stones.

4. *Severe HS:* In about 10 per cent of patients, anemia is severe, skeletal growth is retarded and aberrant, and iron overload results from frequent transfusion.

Key Clinical Features

- Hemolytic anemia

- Splenomegaly

- Intermittent jaundice due to hemolysis or biliary obstruction

- Aplastic, megaloblastic, or hyperhemolytic crises

- Dominant or recessive inheritance

- Remission of the disease after splenectomy

Laboratory Findings

1. Anemia, reticulocytosis, and erythroid hyperplasia in the bone marrow occur in varying degree.

TABLE 121–1. MOLECULAR ABNORMALITIES OF RBC MEMBRANE PROTEINS IN HS

PRIMARY DEFICIENCY	MODE OF INHERITANCE
Ankyrin	AD and AR
Beta-spectrin	AD
Band 3	AD
Pallidin (band 4.2)	AR
Alpha-spectrin	AR

AD, autosomal dominant; AR, autosomal recessive.

2. Spherocytes and microspherocytes are observed in the blood smear; they may be sparse in clinically mild HS.

3. The MCHC is increased in half the patients.

4. The Coombs test is negative, which helps to distinguish HS from immune hemolytic anemia.

5. Since HS cells have reduced surface-to-volume ratios, they tolerate less swelling than normal when suspended in salt solutions of decreasing tonicity. HS cells are therefore said to be osmotically fragile. The osmotic fragility test may be rendered more sensitive for the diagnosis of HS by preincubating whole blood for 24 hours at 37°C.

6. Proteins known to be primarily deficient in the various forms of HS may be quantified. These measurements are performed in research laboratories and are not generally available.

Key Laboratory Findings

- Reticulocytosis
- Spherocytosis
- Elevated MCHC
- Increased osmotic fragility
- Negative Coombs test
- Decreased concentration in HS cells of ankyrin and spectrin or spectrin or band 3 or band 4.2

Treatment

1. Splenectomy cures the hemolytic anemia and jaundice of typical HS. In the 10 per cent of patients with severe HS, splenectomy is beneficial but corrects the hemolysis only partially.

2. Fulminant sepsis and other serious bacterial infections in splenectomized infants and children occur more often than normal, particularly in the first few years after surgery. Splenectomy should therefore be delayed in most patients until the age of 3 to 5 years or more, even if the infants require repeated transfusions during the interval.

3. Immunizations against pneumococcal strains, *H. influenzae,* and meningococcus are given before surgery. Antibiotic prophylaxis against pneumococcus is practiced for several years or indefinitely after surgery. Both measures aim to reduce the rate and morbidity of postsplenectomy infection.

4. Lux (1995) recommends splenectomy for

   a. All patients with severe HS

   b. Patients with moderate HS (Hb 8 to 11 g/dl, reticulocytes >8%) and reduced stamina attributable to anemia

   c. Patients with extramedullary hematopoietic tumors

   d. Patients whose anemia compromises the delivery of oxygen to vital organs.

5. Folic acid 1 mg PO per day is provided to HS patients with active hemolysis.

Hereditary Elliptocytosis

Definition

Hereditary elliptocytosis (HE) is a heterogeneous group of congenital disorders characterized by the presence of an excessive number of elliptocytes on the peripheral blood film. In the hemolytic forms of HE, poikilocytes, red cell fragments, or spherocytes may supplement or even supplant the elliptocytes. Hereditary pyropoikilocytosis (HPP), a rare syndrome related clinically and genetically to HE, is characterized by extraordinary fragmentation and poikilocytosis and moderate to severe hemolytic anemia.

Etiology

HE is conventionally classified into three major groups:

1. Common HE, by far the most prevalent, is caused by dysfunctional mutations of α- or β-spectrin or by deficiency of protein 4.1.

2. Southeast Asian ovalocytosis is due to a deletion within the cytoplasmic portion of band 3 at the boundary between the cytoplasmic and the transmembrane domains.

3. Spherocytic HE is a rare disorder of uncertain molecular cause.

Epidemiology

The HE shape defect with minimal or no hemolysis (common mild HE), spherocytic HE, and Southeast Asian ovalocytosis are inherited as autosomal dominant traits. HPP and the chronic hemolytic forms of common HE excepting neonatal poikilocytosis are usually inherited as autosomal recessive disorders (Table 121–2). HE is found among all races. The frequency of the disorder is highest in malarial zones of Africa, where the prevalence may reach 1:160. The prevalence of HE in the United States is about 1:2500.

Pathophysiology

1. Relevant aspects of normal membrane structure and function:

   a. Spectrin consists of two long polypeptide chains with a high degree of homology. The chains are composed of a series of repeating subunits (22 in

TABLE 121–2. CLINICAL FORMS OF HEREDITARY ELLIPTOCYTOSIS

	FREQUENCY	MODE OF INHERITANCE
Heterozygous common HE syndromes		
Silent carrier state		
Elliptocytic shape defect with minimal or no hemolysis (mild common HE)	Common	AD
Mild common HE with transient episodes of hemolytic anemia		
Common HE with chronic hemolytic anemia	10–15% of heterozygotes for common HE	AR and AD
Common HE with neonatal poikilocytosis		
Homozygous or compound heterozygous common HE	Rare	AR
Hereditary pyropoikilocytosis	Rare	AR
Spherocytic HE	Rare	AD
Southeast Asian ovalocytosis	Common	AD

AD, autosomal dominant; AR, autosomal recessive.

the α chain and 17 in the β chain)—each of them in the form of an alpha triple helix. The α- and β-spectrin chains align side by side in an antiparallel fashion to form firm flexible heterodimers. The dimers self-associate head to head into tetramers and, in the presence of protein 4.1, bind at their distal ends to actin. Junctional complexes formed by spectrin, actin, and protein 4.1 bind the cytoskeleton to glycophorin C and serve as branch points for the two-dimensional spectrin-actin skeletal network (see Fig. 121–1).

b. RBCs assume an ellipsoidal shape when they are propelled by the hydrostatic pressure through terminal arterioles and capillary beds. They revert to their normal biconcave disk shape upon entering the venous circulation. The ability of the RBC to tolerate tens of thousands of deformations without undergoing fragmentation depends on several variables. Among these are

(1) The normal redundancy of the cell membrane (bilayer and cytoskeleton) conferred by the discoid shape. The extra surface area permits normal RBCs to stretch when they deform—a luxury that is not shared by cells that have lost surface membrane, e.g., the microspherocytes in HS and HPP.

(2) The capacity of the membrane cytoskeleton of RBCs to change in geometric shape without change in surface area. This is accomplished by skeletal rearrangements discussed below.

c. The helical subunits of individual spectrin molecules are tightly coiled in the resting state. Upon deformation of the cell in the normal circulation, some of the spectrin molecules become uncoiled and extended, whereas others become more compressed and folded. Deformation has produced no net change in surface area, and withdrawal of the deforming force permits the skeleton to spring back to its normal shape. However, when normal RBCs are deformed in a diseased microcirculation or when excessive force is applied in vitro, some spectrin molecules may exceed their maximal linear extension, leading to an increase in cell surface area and rupture of critical horizontal and vertical interactions of the RBC skeleton. Tolerable stretching of the membrane allows the skeleton to reorganize by forging new connections that produce permanent deformation of the cell. Excessive stretching leads to membrane fragmentation and hemolysis.

2. RBC abnormalities in HE

The shape defects and the cell fragmentation that characterize HPP and the various common HE disorders may be explained by weakened horizontal interactions that render the membrane intolerant of shear stresses generated in the *normal* circulation. Repeatedly deformed cells fail to recover their normal shape, becoming fixed instead in elliptocytic or poikilocytic configurations. Severe disruption of horizontal junctions adds an element of mechanical instability to the membrane, resulting in membrane budding and fragmentation.

The molecular defects in HE are of several types.

a. *Spectrin defects that impair head-to-head self-association of dimers to form tetramers.* These mutations occur close to the contact sites between α- and β-spectrin chains of opposed heterodimers; they are more commonly due to mutations of the α than the β chains and account for about 60 to 80 per cent of common HE. The clinical severity of any α-spectrin defect correlates with the proportion of dimeric spectrin accumulated by the cell. The latter is determined by several factors:

(1) The degree of the impairment in self-association caused by the mutation

(2) The mutant spectrin gene dose

(3) The presence *in trans* of other gene defects that reduce the synthesis of normal α chains.

The most important of these is α LELY, a polymorphism affecting 20 to 30 per cent of α-spectrin alleles in certain populations. α LELY specifies an internally deleted α-spectrin chain that is not able to pair with β-spectrin. Of itself, it is harmless, since α chains are made in 3-fold excess. However, when co-inherited *in trans* with a mutant spectrin allele, the loss of normal chains favors the incorporation of mutant chains into mixed heterodimer, greatly increasing the clinical severity of any given α-spectrin defect.

b. Deficiency (or rarely dysfunction) of protein 4.1. Loss of protein 4.1 removes an essential component required for the formation of the spectrin-actin-protein 4.1 junctional complex. Protein 4.1 deficiency accounts for about 20 to 40 per cent of all common HE. Fifty per cent levels in deficient heterozygotes cause mild HE, while complete absence of the protein in deficient homozygotes causes a severe hemolytic anemia.

Clinical Findings

The clinical subtypes of HE, their mode of inheritance, and estimates of their frequency are given in Table 121–2.

1. *Heterozygous common HE* is an autosomal dominant trait that usually presents as an elliptocytic shape defect with little or no hemolysis and, less often, as a silent carrier state with normal red cell morphology. However, 10 to 15 per cent of individuals with this disorder have conspicuous elliptocytosis and moderately severe chronic hemolytic anemia associated with RBC budding and poikilocytosis. The chronic hemolysis is most often due to co-inheritance of a mutant α-spectrin gene and an α LELY allele, although it may be caused on occasion by simple heterozygous inheritance of a grossly dysfunctional mutant α chain.

a. Sporadic episodes of hemolytic anemia in the course of otherwise mild HE or worsening of chronic hemolysis may occur in response to spleen enlargement, microangiopathic disorders (especially DIC), pregnancy, or deficiency of vitamin B_{12}.

b. Neonatal poikilocytosis is a moderately severe hemolytic anemia of newborn infants that resembles HPP clinically and morphologically. It can present as neonatal jaundice requiring exchange transfusion. Unlike HPP, which is a lifelong disorder, neonatal poikilocytosis reverts to mild common HE as the proportion of hemoglobin F declines during the first 1 to 2 years of life. The syndrome has been attributed to superimposition of destabilized spectrin-actin-4.1 junctional complexes on a mild underlying defect in spectrin self-association. The destabilizing factor is assumed to be free erythrocyte 2,3-diphosphoglycerate (2,3-DPG), a metabolite that weakens spectrin-actin-protein 4.1 interactions in vitro and that binds much less completely to hemoglobin F than to hemoglobin A. The self-limited nature of neonatal poikilocytosis may reflect progressive reduction in the concentration of unbound 2,3-DPG as hemoglobin F is replaced by hemoglobin A. The factors that dispose some but not all infants with α-spectrin defects to neonatal poikilocytosis are not known.

2. *Homozygous or compound heterozygous common HE:* Occasional cases have been reported of homozygous deficiency of protein 4.1 or of homozygous or doubly heterozygous defects of α- or β-spectrin. The clinical syndrome associated with these autosomal recessive disorders is chronic hemolytic anemia of mild to life-threatening severity, depending on the underlying molecular defects. Many cases resemble HPP clinically and morphologically as well as in their dramatic response to splenectomy.

3. *Hereditary pyropoikilocytosis:* HPP is a rare, recessively inherited severe hemolytic anemia characterized by extraordinary poikilocytosis with RBC fragmentation and budding, microspherocytosis, and variable number of elliptocytes. Other salient features include extreme microcytosis, thermal instability, and partial spectrin deficiency (about 70 per cent of normal). Most HPP patients are double heterozygotes for a mutant α-spectrin chain that markedly impairs self-association *and* a defect in spectrin biosynthesis caused by α LELY. Typically, one parent has common HE, while the parent who transmits the α LELY allele has normal red cells and skeletal proteins. HPP may also result from homozygosity for one dysfunctional α-chain variant or from double heterozygosity for two such variants. The partial spectrin deficiency in the latter groups is presumably due to instability of one of the mutant α-spectrin chains.

4. *Spherocytic HE* is a rare disorder characterized by mild to moderate hemolytic anemia, rounded elliptocytes, and excellent response to splenectomy. The molecular defect is largely unknown, but truncated β-spectrin chains with defective spectrin self-association have been identified in a few cases.

5. *Southeast Asian ovalocytosis (SAO)* is a very frequent autosomal dominant disorder within its endemic area. It is characterized by rounded elliptocytes with a transverse bar through the area of central pallor. The RBCs are rigid and resistant to invasion by malarial parasites. Their survival is near-normal. The rigidity is ascribed to enhanced associations among the cytoplasmic tail of mutant band 3, ankryin, and the underlying spectrin network that inhibit the uncoiling and stretching of spectrin tetramers required for membrane extension.

Key Clinical Features: HPP and the Hemolytic Forms of HE

- Hemolytic anemia
- Splenomegaly
- Neonatal jaundice
- Jaundice due to hemolysis or biliary obstruction
- Aplastic and megaloblastic crises
- Recessive or dominant inheritance
- Good response to splenectomy

Laboratory Findings

1. Elliptocytosis (>15% and usually >30% of the RBC, normal <5%) may be the only morphologic abnormality on the blood smear of patients with HE. The diagnosis of HE is strengthened by demonstrating similar findings in a parent and by excluding other known causes of elliptocytosis such as iron deficiency, thalassemia, megaloblastic anemia, myelofibrosis, myelophthisis, and myelodysplasia. A finding of red cell budding and fragmentation on an elliptocytic smear suggests a hemolytic form of HE, whereas fragmentation and microspherocytosis suggest HPP.

2. Osmotic fragility is increased in the hemolytic forms of HE and in HPP because of the presence of cell fragments and microspherocytes with low surface-to-volume ratios. The RBC fragmentation in these disorders is also reflected by microcytosis with MCV as low as 50 μm^3.

Key Laboratory Findings: Common Hemolytic HE and HPP

Common Mild HE
- Elliptocytosis
- No anemia, 1–3% reticulocytes
- Normal MCV and osmotic fragility

HPP and Hemolytic Variants of Common HE
- Anemia
- Reticulocytosis
- Cell fragments, poikilocytes, ± elliptocytes, ± microspherocytes
- Low MCV and increased osmotic fragility
- Partial spectrin deficiency (HPP only)

HPP and All Forms of Common HE
- Increased thermal and mechanical instability
- Deficiency (or rarely dysfunction) of protein 4.1 *or* qualitative mutations of spectrin that impair self-association

3. Thermal instability is tested by incubating RBCs for 10 to 15 minutes at 45° to 50°C. Denaturation of the spectrin in normal cells occurs at 50°C and leads to

cell fragmentation. The mutant spectrins in HPP and in common HE are characterized by increased instability; HPP cells typically fragment at 45 to 46°C.

4. Mechanical instability of RBC ghosts or isolated cytoskeletons can be demonstrated by shaking them or by exposing them to shear stresses in the ektacytometer. HPP cells are highly fragile. Nonhemolytic common HE cells demonstrate instability that is intermediate between normal cells and HPP cells.

5. A variety of tests, some of them available only in research laboratories, may be used to detect impaired spectrin self-association and to identify the specific skeletal protein abnormalities and genetic mutations that give rise to common HE.

Treatment

1. Exchange transfusion may be required for jaundiced neonates with HPP, neonatal poikilocytosis, and other forms of severe hemolytic HE.

2. The RBCs in HPP and in the chronic hemolytic forms of HE are sequestered in the engorged red pulp of the spleen. Splenectomy is indicated for patients with moderate to severe hemolytic anemia but should be delayed, if possible, until the age of 3 to 5 years or more in order to reduce the very high risk of postsplenectomy sepsis in infants and young children. An additional benefit of delaying surgery is the avoidance of splenectomy of neonatal poikilocytosis, a self-limited condition that is difficult to distinguish from HPP in the first year or so of life. The immunization of young children before splenectomy and the management thereafter have been outlined under *Treatment* in the section on HS. The response to splenectomy is often dramatic but not complete. In HPP, the hemoglobin concentration typically rises to the 10 to 14 g/dl range, and the need for RBC transfusions is abolished. However, reticulocytosis (3–10%) and morphologic evidence of RBC fragmentation persist.

Key Treatment: Common Hemolytic HE and HPP

- Exchange transfusion (neonates)
- Splenectomy (after 3 years of age)

Bibliography

HEREDITARY SPHEROCYTOSIS

Becker PS, Lux SE: Disorders of the red cell membrane. *In* Nathan DG, Oski FA (eds): Hematology of Infancy and Childhood, 4th ed, vol 1. Philadelphia, WB Saunders, 1993, pp 529–633.

Eber SW, Gonzalez JM, Lux ML, et al: Ankyrin-1 mutations are a major cause of dominant and recessive hereditary spherocytosis. Nature Genet. 1996;13(2):214–218.

Lux SE, Forget BG, Platt OS: Inherited disorders of the red cell membrane. *In* McArthur JR, Kaushansky K (eds): Hematology—1995. The Education Program of the American Society of Hematology, Dec. 1995, pp 1–9.

Palek J, Jarolim P: Clinical expression and laboratory detection of red blood cell membrane mutations. Semin Hematol 1993;30:249–283.

HEREDITARY ELLIPTOCYTOSIS

Benz EJ Jr: The erythrocyte membrane and cytoskeleton: structure, function and disorders. *In* Stamatoyannopoulos G, Nienhuis AW, Majerus PW, Varmus H (eds): The Molecular Basis of Blood Diseases, 2nd ed. Philadelphia, WB Saunders, 1994, pp 257–292.

Lux SE, Palek J: Disorders of the red cell membrane. *In* Handin RI, Lux SE, Stossel TP (eds): Blood: Principles and Practice of Hematology. Philadelphia, JB Lippincott, 1995, pp 1701–1818.

Mohandas N, Chassis JA: Red blood cell deformability, membrane material properties and shape: regulation by transmembrane, skeletal and cytosolic proteins and lipids. Semin Hematol 1993;30:171–192.

122 Sickle Cell Disease

Scott T. Miller

Definition

Production of abnormal hemoglobin (Hb S) causes hemolytic anemia and acute and chronic organ damage.

Etiology and Epidemiology

1. Origins in Africa and Asia
   a. β-Globin haplotypes differ among populations and influence severity.
   b. Individuals with sickle *trait* are protected from meningitis caused by falciparum malaria; individuals with *disease* are not protected.
      (1) Individuals with trait have one normal and one abnormal gene.
      (2) Individuals with disease are largely asymptomatic—may have hematuria, complications of traumatic hyphema, splenic infarct in unpressurized aircraft; sudden death possible under very strenuous environmental stress.
   c. Homozygous sickle cell anemia (Hb SS) is the prototype; other double heterozygotes can have disease (Table 122–1).
      (1) Definitive diagnosis is critical; newborn screening is not diagnostic.
      (2) Parental studies are helpful.
   d. Concurrent alpha-thalassemia (α-thal) affects clinical course.

TABLE 122–1. SICKLE CELL DISORDERS

GENOTYPE	NAME	CLINICAL SEVERITY
AS	Sickle cell trait	0 (minimal clinical impact)
SS	Sickle cell anemia	+ + + + (but variable)
S-HPFH	Sickle-hereditary persistence of fetal hemoglobin	0 (? mild hemolysis)
S-β^0 thal	Sickle-beta^0 thalassemia	+ + +
S-β^+ thal	Sickle-beta$^+$ thalassemia	+
SC	Sickle-hemoglobin C disease	+ +
SD, SO, or SC$_{Harlem}$	Sickle-hemoglobin D, O$_{Arab}$, or C$_{Harlem}$ disease	+ + + +
SE	Sickle-hemoglobin E disease	0/ +

(1) Twenty to 30 per cent of blacks are "silent carriers" (single α-globin gene deleted from normal four) 2 to 3 per cent have α-thal trait (two-gene deletion).

(2) Associated with higher Hb concentration, less organ damage, stroke; *more* avascular necrosis.

Pathophysiology

1. Polymerization of sickle Hb
   a. Mutation in β-globin gene results in substitution of valine for glutamic acid at sixth amino acid position and instability of Hb molecule with tendency to polymerize.
      (1) Polymerization is enhanced by hypoxia, hypercarbia, (i.e., postcapillary bed, spleen, renal medulla), hyperthermia.
      (2) Polymerization lessened by reduction of intracellular Hb S concentration is due to increased fetal hemoglobin (Hb F) concentration, concurrent thalassemia, iron deficiency(?).
   b. Mutation of β-globin gene also results in shortened red cell survival.
      (1) Anemia and need for increased red cell production
      (2) Impaired oxygen delivery to tissues
      (3) Increased cytokine production?
   c. Mutation also results in membrane damage, reduced deformability.
      (1) Likelihood of ischemia/infarction of tissues increased due to "sludging," further polymer formation (vicious circle)
      (2) Vascular damage due to abnormal red cell adherence to endothelium; intimal proliferation with luminal narrowing and further potential for tissue damage

2. Specific pathologic syndromes and their clinical manifestations
   a. Acute anemia
      (1) Transient aplastic crisis (TAC)
         (a) Severe anemia, profound reticulocytopenia (<1%), often well compensated
         (b) 70 to 100 per cent due to parvovirus B19 infection
            (i) Can cause marrow necrosis
            (ii) Association with acute chest syndrome (ACS)
            (iii) Agent of erythema infectiosum in non–sickle cell children; rarely, a rash with TAC
      (2) Acute splenic sequestration crisis
         (a) Rapid pooling of blood in spleen results in splenomegaly and hypovolemia with cardiovascular compromise.
         (b) Usually reticulocytosis and thrombocytopenia
         (c) High recurrence rate (see under *Prevention*)
      (3) Hyperhemolysis
         (a) Often associated with febrile illness
         (b) Look for associated G6PD deficiency
   b. Splenic infarction, hypofunction
      (1) Thirty to 50 per cent of infants with Hb SS have diminished to absent splenic function by age 1 year; high risk of infection and mortality due to infections by encapsulated organisms, especially *S. pneumoniae* and especially prior to age 3 years.
      (2) Spleen function better preserved in Hb SC
   c. Lung disease
      (1) Acute chest syndrome
         (a) Defined as new pulmonary findings (tachypnea, chest pain, rales, hypoxemia, infiltrate on x-ray)
         (b) Infectious etiologies
            (i) Bacterial infection (*S. pneumoniae* now uncommon)
            (ii) Atypical most common (*Mycoplasma* and *Chlamydia pneumoniae*)
            (iii) Viral pathogens include respiratory syncytial virus (RSV) and parvovirus
         (c) Noninfectious etiologies
            (i) Sickle cell sludging (ischemia/infarction, thrombosis)
            (ii) Pulmonary fat embolism is often associated with bone pain and a severe clinical course.
            (iii) Hypoventilation
               (I) Postoperative
               (II) Splinting due to thoracic bone infarction
               (III) Respiratory depression due to narcotic analgesia
      (2) Chronic sickle cell lung disease
         (a) Fibrosis and vasculopathy (intimal hyperplasia)
         (b) Association with recurrent ACS in adults —not clear in children
         (c) Hypoxemia, pulmonary dysfunction common in steady state

d. Neurologic

(1) Cerebrovascular accident (CVA)

(a) Thrombosis most common in children; intracranial hemorrhage occurs in all age groups.

(b) Most (70–90%) have vasculopathy of large and mid-size cerebral vessels (circle of Willis) with stenosis/occlusion; often "watershed infarcts"

(c) Hemiparesis most common presentation (i.e., painless limp, weakness)

(d) Recurrence rate of 49 to 90 per cent without intervention

(e) Equivocal neurologic symptoms should prompt careful neurologic examination, possibly search for vasculopathy (e.g., magnetic resonance angiography [MRA])

(2) Several studies have shown diminished performance on neuropsychologic testing.

e. Skeletal

(1) Acute pain episodes due to bone/bone marrow infarction may be associated with impressive inflammatory signs (e.g., fever, elevated white cell count, swelling, warmth, tenderness, erythema).

(2) Avascular necrosis of femoral or humeral head sometimes occurs and is symptomatic in childhood.

(3) Increased risk of osteomyelitis

(a) Common organisms are *Salmonella, S. pneumoniae*, other gram-negative organisms, *Staphylococcus*.

(b) Difficult to distinguish from bone infarction

f. Hepatobiliary

(1) Jaundice common, but serum bilirubin should not exceed 4 mg/dl due to hemolysis alone.

(2) Gallstones, "sludge" present in 50 per cent of adolescents; occasionally acute/chronic cholecystitis, choledocholithiasis, and gallstone pancreatitis occur.

(3) Viral hepatitis due to hepatitis C (especially in older children, adults), EBV, others associated with high ALT; AST and LDH may be elevated owing to hemolysis alone.

(4) "Extreme benign hyperbilirubinemia" is associated with high (often >40 mg/dl) bilirubin, mostly conjugated, and resolves without sequelae. Severe hepatic dysfunction is uncommon in children.

g. Renal

(1) Infarction of medulla and tubular dysfunction cause isosthenuria, natriuresis, and often enuresis.

(2) Hyperfiltration (high GFR) common in children; may ultimately be associated with proteinuria, diminished GFR/renal failure in adults, with focal sclerosis on biopsy.

h. Growth/sexual development

(1) Normal growth through late first decade; 1 to 2 year delay in adolescent growth spurt, sexual maturation

(2) Increased fetal loss during pregnancy, small babies

(3) Priapism common in males

(a) Ischemic, "low-flow" more common in postpubertal males. Permanent impotence common after episodes lasting >24 hours.

(b) "High-flow," especially recurrent, brief "stuttering" episodes, may have better prognosis but may also culminate in a prolonged episode.

(c) Cavernosal infarction/fibrosis; vasculopathy described. Tricorporal episodes associated with severe disease.

Clinical Findings

1. Survival through childhood >80% even before uniform recommendation for penicillin prophylaxis. Median adult survival at least to mid-forties in Hb SS; survival to sixties in Hb SC.

2. Morbidity variable

a. Higher Hb F concentration generally associated with milder course

b. β-Globin haplotypes have clinical correlates; Saudi, Senegal, Cameroon tend to be mild; Benin moderate; Central African Republic (CAR) severe.

c. Most children do have complications; there is a need for a severity index to predict clinical course before severe organ damage has occurred (Table 122–2).

d. See previous section for clinical manifestations of damage to specific organ systems.

Laboratory Findings

1. Hemoglobin electrophoresis

a. Must have [Hb A] > [Hb S] in trait

b. Only two β-globin genes; no such thing as Hb SC trait

c. Definitive diagnosis critical; research laboratory may be needed, especially for uncommon heterozygotes.

TABLE 122–2. FREQUENCY OF CLINICAL EVENTS (DATA FROM THE COOPERATIVE STUDY)

OUTCOME	INCIDENCE*
Adult death	Median survival: Male 42 years, Female 48 years
Pediatric death	1.1
CVA (infarctive)	1.2
Acute chest	27.0
Pain rate	27.6
Avascular necrosis	2.5 (ages 5–9 years)
Bacteremia	4.5

*Data from a number of manuscripts from the Cooperative Study of Sickle Cell Disease. Unless otherwise indicated, incidence figures are cumulative for a pediatric cohort of patients followed over the first decade of life and are for children with Hb SS without concurrent α-thalassemia. Numbers reflect rates per 100 patient-years of observation.

2. Hematologic measures

a. Important to establish steady-state values for each patient; norms for sickle cell disease have been reported by the Cooperative Study of Sickle Cell Disease (CSSCD) for ages birth through 5 years (Table 122–3).

b. Increased WBC and platelets may be due to cytokines, loss of splenic reservoir

Radiographic Findings

1. Chronic radiographic findings

a. Avascular necrosis of femur, humerus (bone scan and MRI more sensitive to early changes)

b. "Fish-mouth" vertebrae, may collapse

c. "Hair-on-end" appearance of skull due to marrow hyperplasia, seen in older children

d. Cardiomegaly due to chronic anemia

2. Acute findings

a. Acute chest syndrome

(1) Generally cannot distinguish infection from other causes of ACS

(2) Perfusion (VQ scan) may be misleading unless baseline exists (not recommended)

(3) Findings may lag behind clinical picture

(a) Initial x-ray sometimes normal

(b) X-ray worsens as patient improves

b. Acute splenic sequestration

(1) May show decreased uptake of sulfur colloid even when enlarged

(2) Uptake may normalize after transfusion.

c. Neurologic

(1) CT scan may miss new CVA but should be done urgently to rule out hemorrhage.

(2) MRI more sensitive for infarction/ischemia, but abnormal in ~15 per cent of children without stroke

(3) MRA usually abnormal in stroke patients; incidence of abnormality in nonstroke under study

(4) Conventional angiography may be indicated if neurologic symptoms, signs, and/or noninvasive imaging are equivocal.

TABLE 122–3. CSSCD INFANT COHORT HEMATOLOGIC REFERENCE VALUES BY AGE GROUP, SS INFANTS*

MEASUREMENT	STATISTIC	AGE, MO										
		2–3.9	4–5.9	6–8.9	9–11.9	12–14.9	15–17.9	18–23.9	24–29.9	30–35.9	36–47.9	48–60
Hemoglobin level, g/dl	5%	7.0	7.0	7.1	7.2	7.2	7.2	7.1	6.9	6.7	6.4	6.6
	50%	9.3	9.2	9.2	9.2	9.1	9.0	8.9	8.6	8.3	8.1	8.3
	Mean	9.3	9.2	9.2	9.2	9.1	9.1	8.9	8.7	8.5	8.2	8.1
	95%	11.4	11.3	11.4	11.5	11.5	11.5	11.3	11.1	10.9	10.5	10.4
RCB count, ×10¹²/L	5%	2.53	2.50	2.46	2.41	2.37	2.34	2.29	2.26	2.21	2.14	2.03
	50%	3.44	3.42	3.39	3.35	3.31	3.25	3.17	3.04	2.92	2.79	2.68
	Mean	3.39	3.40	3.41	3.40	3.38	3.35	3.27	3.12	3.00	2.86	2.80
	95%	4.48	4.54	4.59	4.63	4.65	4.64	4.57	4.42	4.29	4.19	4.24
Mean corpuscular volume, fL	5%	72	69	68	67	67	67	67	68	69	71	72
	50%	84	81	81	82	82	83	84	85	86	88	90
	Mean	84	81	81	81	82	82	83	84	86	88	88
	95%	96	94	94	95	95	96	96	97	97	98	100
Fetal hemoglobin level, %	5%	14.6	12.3	10.8	9.1	7.8	6.7	5.6	4.8	4.5	4.4	3.3
	50%	43.5	34.1	29.1	24.3	20.6	17.7	14.8	12.8	12.4	12.4	9.0
	Mean	40.4	31.8	28.1	24.6	21.8	19.5	17.1	15.2	14.2	13.1	9.0
	95%	68.5	59.0	53.0	47.3	42.7	39.1	35.3	32.5	31.2	29.6	21.9
Reticulocyte count, %	5%	1.0	1.1	1.2	1.3	1.4	1.6	1.9	2.3	2.6	2.7	1.8
	50%	4.0	5.1	5.9	6.7	7.4	8.0	8.7	9.3	9.8	10.4	11.8
	Mean	5.4	6.7	7.5	8.4	9.1	9.7	10.4	11.0	11.4	11.7	12.4
	95%	15.5	17.9	19.4	20.7	21.8	22.5	23.2	23.5	23.6	23.6	25.8
Packed RBC count, %	5%	0.0	0.0	0.0	0.0	0.1	0.4	0.7	0.8	0.8	0.8	1.8
	50%	1.0	1.0	1.0	1.1	2.2	3.6	5.6	7.7	9.3	11.2	14.1
	Mean	1.4	1.7	2.2	3.0	3.9	5.0	6.5	8.2	9.8	11.9	14.3
	95%	4.8	6.0	8.1	10.9	13.7	16.3	19.0	20.2	20.0	19.7	26.4
WBC count, ×10⁹/L	5%	6.0	6.0	6.3	6.6	6.9	6.9	6.9	6.8	7.0	7.8	7.8
	50%	9.5	9.4	10.2	11.3	12.2	12.9	13.4	13.7	13.7	13.5	13.6
	Mean	10.3	10.3	11.2	12.6	13.6	14.1	14.3	14.0	13.8	14.2	14.3
	95%	15.7	15.8	18.6	22.1	24.1	24.8	24.2	22.4	21.9	23.9	21.2
Platelet count, ×10⁹/L	5%	224	216	207	199	192	186	182	181	182	187	198
	50%	419	405	390	376	366	361	361	374	387	405	423
	Mean	432	417	400	385	374	368	368	380	394	410	424
	95%	683	649	615	586	572	571	596	667	719	743	674

*Values are smoothed longitudinal data. CSSCD, Cooperative Study of Sickle Cell Disease; SS, sickle cell anemia; RBC, red blood cell; WBC, white blood cell.
From Brown AK, Sleeper LA, Miller ST, et al: Reference values and hematologic changes from birth to 5 years in patients with sickle cell disease. Arch Pediatr Adolesc Med 1994;146:796–804.

(a) Reduce Hb S to <30 per cent before procedure.

(b) Use low osmolal medium.

(5) Transcranial Doppler sonography often abnormal in stroke patients; may be useful as screening tool to predict first stroke (under study)

(6) Radioisotope scans (SPECT, PET) are sensitive to detect hypoperfusion.

d. Acute bone pathology; differentiation of infection (osteomyelitis) from infarction (pain episode)

(1) X-rays rarely indicated acutely (normal); may be abnormal and similar after 7 to 10 days

(2) Bone scans usually show increased uptake in both infection and infarction, but uptake may be diminished in either. Bone scans are indicated to look for osteomyelitis in children with *Salmonella* bacteremia or persistent fever.

(3) Bone marrow scans nearly always show decreased uptake in infarction; clinical findings of inflammation with normal uptake suggest osteomyelitis.

(4) Gallium uptake increased or diminished in infarction; markedly increased uptake suggests osteomyelitis

(5) MRI often very abnormal and similar in both.

e. Abdominal (right upper quadrant)

(1) Sonograms often show stones or sludge (only 10 per cent are radiopaque) in gallbladder but may miss common duct stones; look for thickening of gallbladder wall, pericholic fluid, intra- or extrahepatic duct dilatation to correlate symptoms.

(2) Radionuclide scans (e.g., DISIDA) may show biliary tree with serum bilirubin as high as 30 mg/dl.

(a) Delayed or absent excretion suggests partial or complete obstruction.

(b) Nonvisualization of gallbladder suggests cholecystitis or cystic duct stone.

f. Renal sonogram often shows large echogenic kidneys.

g. Radionuclide penile scans and Doppler sonography have been used in priapism to assess penile perfusion.

Treatment

1. Supportive—general

a. Establish baseline hematologic values (Hb, WBC, reticulocyte, bilirubin). Pulmonary function, neuropsychologic testing, MRI scan may be useful. Hepatitis B immunization series should be given (see under *Prevention*).

b. Transfusion often given for acute complications to improve oxygen delivery and/or to dilute sickle cells.

(1) Simple transfusion of 5 to 20 ml/kg of packed erythrocytes will accomplish both in an anemic patient.

(a) Smaller volumes are required for extremely anemic patients who have expanded intravascular volume.

(b) Larger volumes may be split into two aliquots from a single donor; transfusions of aliquots are separated by several hours.

(2) Partial exchange transfusion of packed cells and/or whole blood will achieve low Hb S concentration and reduce risk of hyperviscosity.

(3) Posttransfusion Hb should always be <12 g/dl.

(4) Try to use full units if possible; ask for aliquots.

(5) Use of non–Hb S and genotypically matched (at least for C, E, and Kell antigens) units is recommended, especially for chronic transfusion patients.

2. Management of specific complications

a. Aplastic crisis usually necessitates transfusion.

(1) Use small (5 to 7.5 ml/kg) volume packed cells to prevent congestive heart failure.

(2) Isolate patient (respiratory) from other Hb SS children, immunocompromised patients (may have chronic viremia and hypoplastic anemia), and pregnant staff (fetal hydrops) until reticulocytes increase.

b. Acute splenic sequestration may be associated with hypovolemia, requiring a more rapid infusion of packed cells or whole blood.

(1) Cells trapped in spleen recirculate; do not over-transfuse.

(2) Splenectomy or chronic transfusion (infants <age 2 years) indicated after recurrence

c. Acute chest syndrome mandates hospitalization.

(1) Antibiotic coverage to include "atypical" pathogens (*Mycoplasma* and *Chlamydia pneumoniae*); *S. pneumoniae* and *H. influenzae* less common; consider antiviral agents for RSV.

(2) Supplemental oxygen; 1½ maintenance fluids (monitor output, avoid overload); cautious analgesia for pain; continuous monitoring of oxygen saturation

(3) Transfuse for significant respiratory distress with hypoxemia; elevated (>30 mmHg) arterial/alveolar oxygen gradient may predict severe course.

d. Urgent transfusion to reduce Hb S to <30 per cent of total recommended for newly diagnosed CVA

(1) Indefinitely prolonged chronic transfusion therapy indicated to reduce recurrence risk to <10 per cent; may reduce intensity of transfusion to maintain Hb S <60 per cent after 4 years. Iron chelation therapy mandatory

(2) Consider bone marrow transplantation if histocompatible donor available.

(3) Role of transfusion in preventing first stroke in children with abnormal TCD screening under study

(4) No data re intervention for neuropsychologic defects, "silent infarcts" on MRI

e. Outpatient management of pain includes encouraging fluids, oral analgesics (e.g., acetaminophen/codeine); hospitalize patients if relief inadequate.

   (1) Fluids at 1½ maintenance (twice basal requirements); monitor output, serum sodium. Maintain good hydration, do not overload.

   (2) Standing orders for analgesic with prn rescue; use a quantitative pain assessment scale.

   (3) Non-narcotic preferable (e.g., ketorolac) if effective to avoid risk of respiratory depression

   (4) When needed, narcotics should be given at a dose appropriate to half-life; some prefer patient-controlled analgesia (PCA).

   (5) Narcotic tolerance after several days expected; may have to increase dose. Addiction unusual, placebo administration inappropriate

f. Gallstones usually asymptomatic; cholecystectomy not recommended for incidental stones. Consider surgery (laparoscopic may be preferred) for symptoms of chronic cholecystitis or following an episode of obstruction or acute cholecystitis.

g. "Prophylactic" transfusion not helpful during pregnancy; if transfusion required, genotyping desirable to prevent alloimmunization and potential hemolytic disease of newborn

h. Hospitalization indicated for priapism episodes lasting >2 to 3 hours for hydration and analgesia

   (1) If no resolution within 24 hours, transfusion; cavernosal aspiration; cavernosal injection or irrigation with solutions containing an α-adrenergic agent; or shunt procedure (Winter glans-cavernosal) indicated

   (2) Frequently recurrent "stuttering" episodes have been treated with chronic transfusion, patient-administered injection of epinephrine or other adrenergic agent, pseudoephedrine, hydralazine, stilbestrol.

i. For elective surgery, give parenteral fluids preoperatively while patient is NPO (ambulatory surgery not generally appropriate).

   (1) Simple packed cell transfusion preoperatively to raise Hb to 9 to 11 g/dl; more aggressive transfusion does not reduce sickle cell complications but does increase risk of transfusion-related complications.

   (2) Minor surgery may be safe without transfusion.

   (3) Aggressive pulmonary toilet, spirometry postoperatively to reduce risk of ACS (most common serious perioperative complication)

3. Specific therapy

  a. Bone marrow transplant curative but high-risk; sterility expected

   (1) Safer when done early, but patient selection controversial owing to variability of natural course of disease

   (2) Currently requires histocompatible sibling donor; often not available.

TABLE 122–4. REASONS FOR ASSIGNMENT TO THE PRIMARY HIGHER-RISK GROUP

EXCLUSION CRITERION	NO. (%) OF EPISODES
Seriously ill appearance	1 (1)
Severe pain	11 (13)
Temperature >40°C	29 (34)
Hemoglobin level, white cell count, platelet count*	12 (14)
Pulmonary infiltrate	20 (23)
Poor fluid intake, decreased urine output	8 (9)
Previous sepsis	5 (6)

*A hemoglobin level below 5 g per deciliter; a white cell count below 5000 per cubic millimeter or above 30,000 per cubic millimeter; or a platelet count below 100,000 per cubic millimeter.

From Wilimas JA, Flynn PM, Harris S, et al: A randomized study of outpatient treatment with ceftriaxone for selected febrile children with sickle cell disease. N Engl J Med, 1993;329:472–476.

b. Pharmacologic increase in Hb F may be of clinical benefit. Hydroxyurea (15 to 25 mg/kg/day) reduces acute pain episodes and ACS in adults with moderate to severe disease; role in children and effect on other acute and chronic complications unknown.

c. Potential for gene therapy is reason for optimism.

 Key Treatment

- Transfusion
- Penicillin prophylaxis
- Bone marrow transplant

Prevention

1. Antenatal testing should include CBC, Hb electrophoresis, Hb A₂ level for both parents in groups at risk; prenatal diagnosis possible by chorionic villous sampling (8 to 11 weeks' gestational age) or amniocentesis

2. Universal newborn hemoglobinopathy screening is recommended; infants with disease must be seen by age 4 months for confirmation of diagnosis and initiation of comprehensive care.

3. Prophylaxis against *S. pneumoniae* infection reduces infection rate and mortality.

  a. Penicillin VK 125 mg po bid to begin by age 4 months in Hb SS infants and severe double heterozygotes; increase to 250 mg po bid at age 3 years, and discontinue in most patients after pneumococcal booster immunization at age 5 years.

  b. Give 23-valent pneumococcal vaccine at ages 2 and 5 years; consider continued booster doses every 3 to 5 years.

   (1) Antibody response not durable

   (2) Conjugated vaccine may permit earlier administration and better response (under study).

  c. Educate parents concerning the need to seek urgent evaluation of fever by medical personnel.

   (1) Prompt administration of parenteral antibiotic

required; choice depends upon local sensitivity of *S. pneumoniae.*

    (2) Some can be managed on an ambulatory basis, i.e., with administration of long-acting cephalosporin; adequate follow-up is mandatory and high-risk patients require hospitalization (Table 122–4).

4. Teaching caretakers splenic palpation and signs of anemia reduces mortality from acute sequestration; splenectomy or chronic transfusion is indicated for recurrent episodes.

5. Incentive spirometry reduces risk of ACS in patients with thoracic bone pain; may be recommended in all patients with pain, especially those requiring narcotic analgesia.

Bibliography

Brown AK, Sleeper LA, Miller ST, et al: Reference values and hematologic changes from birth to 5 years in patients with sickle cell disease. Arch Pediatr Adolesc Med 1994;146:796–804.

Embury SH, Hebbel RP, Mohandas N, Steinberg MH (eds): Sickle Cell Disease: Basic Principles and Clinical Practice. New York, Raven Press, 1994.

Gill FM, Sleeper LA, Weiner SJ, et al: Clinical events in the first decade in a cohort of infants with sickle cell disease. Blood 1995;86:776–783.

Reid CD, Charache S, Lubin B (eds): Management and Therapy of Sickle Cell Disease, 3rd ed. Washington, DC, U.S. Department of Health and Human Services, Public Health Service, National Institutes of Health, NIH Publication #95-2117, revised December 1995.

123 Thalassemias

Scott T. Miller

Definition

Genetic alterations lead to diminished or absent globin production, accumulation of abnormal globin tetramers, and thus ineffective erythropoiesis.

Etiology and Epidemiology

1. Mediterranean, African, Asian populations affected (Fig. 123–1)
2. Heterozygous states extremely common
   a. Incidence of β-thal trait >20 per cent in some Greek villages; 0.5 to 1 per cent in American blacks
   b. α-Thal incidence 5 to 10 per cent in Mediterranean; 20 to 30 per cent in West Africa (and American blacks); up to 60 per cent in SW Pacific
   c. Apparently thal trait protects against malaria; mechanisms not entirely understood.

Pathophysiology

1. Diminished synthesis of α- or β-globin chains results in impaired production and survival of red cells.
   a. Fewer complete hemoglobin molecules ($\alpha_2\beta_2$) result in hypochromia and microcytosis.

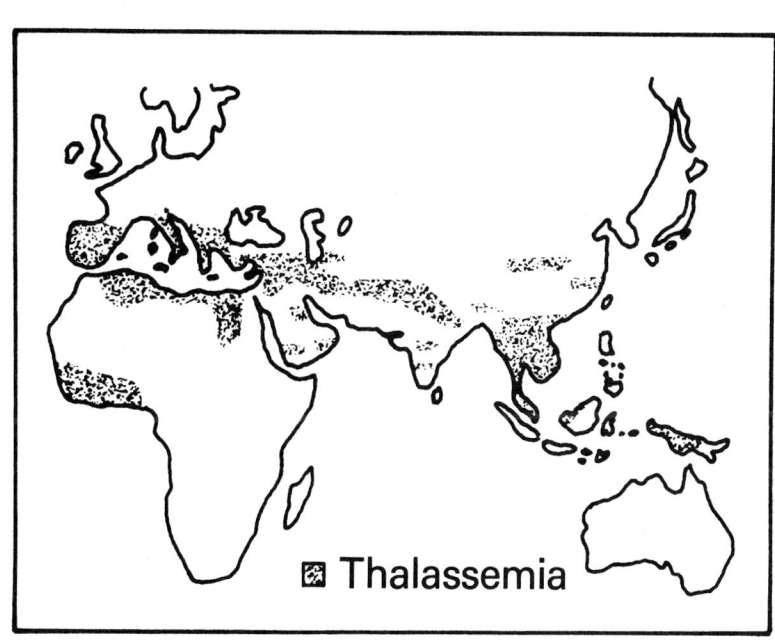

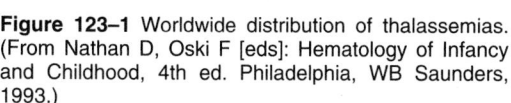

Figure 123–1 Worldwide distribution of thalassemias. (From Nathan D, Oski F [eds]: Hematology of Infancy and Childhood, 4th ed. Philadelphia, WB Saunders, 1993.)

b. Abnormal tetramers formed

    (1) In β-thal, α_4 tetramers are very insoluble and precipitates interfere with erythroblast maturation (impaired cell division) and cause oxidative damage to precursor membranes (ineffective erythropoiesis); membrane injury also shortens red cell survival.

    (2) β_4 tetramers (Hb H) more soluble but unstable; if present in significant concentration will shorten red cell survival.

2. Over 150 mutations described for β-thal

  a. Normally one β-globin gene present on each of two chromosomes 11

  b. β° mutations result in absent β-globin production; some residual production with β⁺ mutations

  c. Five broad categories of mutations

    (1) Transcriptional mutations in the promoter region of the gene result in β⁺ lesions.

    (2) Mutations that affect posttranscriptional modification of RNA also lead to β⁺-thal.

    (3) RNA processing mutations result in splicing being abolished, interfered with, or rerouted and can cause β⁺ or β⁰-thal depending on the site of mutation.

    (4) Mutations causing nonfunctional RNA, nonsense mutations, or frameshift mutations lead to β°-thal.

    (5) Mutations resulting in unstable β-globin are associated with significant clinical problems even in heterozygotes (dominant β-thalassemia)

    (6) Thalassemia intermedia may result if one or both thalassemia mutations are mild, β⁺ lesions; if concurrent α-thal is present; if δβ-thal is present; or with "dominant" β-thal.

3. Most α-thalassemias are due to mutations that result in gene deletions.

  a. Normally two α-globin genes on each chromosome 16 (total four genes)

  b. Unequal or nonhomologous recombination results in deletion of one or both genes from a chromosome.

    (1) Blacks generally have a single gene deletion from a chromosome; both genes are generally deleted in Asians. Blacks therefore rarely have the severe forms of α-thal (Hb H disease and hydrops fetalis), which are prevalent in Asians.

    (2) The clinical syndromes related to gene α deletions are presented in Table 123–1.

4. Other thalassemia syndromes

  a. Deletion mutations in the β-globin gene cluster cause hereditary persistence of fetal hemoglobin (HPFH), δβ-thal.

  b. Unequal crossover in the β-globin gene cluster results in Hb Lepore, Kenya, and others.

  c. Some α-thal individuals have Hb Constant Spring, an elongated hemoglobin resulting from a termination codon mutation.

TABLE 123–1. ALPHA-THALASSEMIA SYNDROMES

GENOTYPE	CLINICAL	% BARTS (BIRTH)
$\dfrac{\alpha -}{\alpha\ \alpha}$	"Silent carrier" (α-Thal-2)	1–2
$\dfrac{\alpha -}{\alpha -}$ or $\dfrac{\alpha\alpha}{-\ -}$ (Blacks) (Asians)	Microcytosis ± anemia (α-Thal-1)	2–6
(Blacks) (Asians) $\dfrac{\alpha -}{-\ -}$	Thal intermedia (Hb H disease)	20–40
$\dfrac{-\ -}{-\ -}$	Hydrops fetalis (stillbirth)	80

Clinical Findings

1. β-thalassemia trait

  a. Largely asymptomatic

  b. Ten to 19 per cent of Mediterraneans have hepatosplenomegaly.

  c. "Silent carriers" appear normal and are heterozygous for a mild β⁺ mutation.

2. Thalassemia major (Cooley anemia)

  a. Pallor, poor growth and development, enlarged abdomen, usually by 6 months of age

  b. Untreated

    (1) Bony abnormalities (prominent maxillary bones, tooth deformities, prominent forehead—"thalassemia facies"; shortening of long bones; joint deformities)

    (2) Hepatosplenomegaly, jaundice

    (3) Extramedullary hematopoiesis can cause paravertebral masses and spinal cord compression.

  c. Chronic transfusion can attenuate/eliminate bone changes and extramedullary hematopoiesis but results in pathologic hemosiderosis.

    (1) Hemosiderosis due to increased gastrointestinal absorption of iron

    (2) Further iron loading from chronic transfusion resulting from lack of intrinsic mechanism for iron excretion

    (3) Cardiac toxicity major cause of death

      (a) Recurrent pericarditis, arrhythmias, congestive heart failure

      (b) Dilation and thickening of atria and ventricles because of iron deposition in myocardium and later in conductive tissues

    (4) Liver enlargement formerly due to extramedullary hematopoiesis, now due to hemosiderosis

      (a) Viral hepatitis may worsen function and contribute to fibrosis and cirrhosis.

      (b) Iron chelation retards and/or reverses damage.

    (5) Endocrinopathies due to hemochromatosis

(a) Growth retardation now unusual in first decade, occurs later; associated with diminished production of growth hormone, somatomedin, androgens in some patients.

(b) Sexual maturation delay in majority of patients due to hypothalamic–pituitary dysfunction; delayed menarche, secondary amenorrhea, or lack of virilization in males

(6) Chemical hypothyroidism, usually not clinical

(7) Abnormal glucose tolerance in 50 per cent; diabetes mellitus due to both decreased production of and resistance to insulin

(8) Other transfusion complications

(a) Febrile, allergic, hemolytic transfusion reactions

(b) Alloimmunization

(c) Viral infection (hepatitis B and C, HIV)

3. β-Thalassemia intermedia is of variable severity; some have minimal symptoms, others have growth retardation, bone disease, extramedullary hematopoiesis, and hemochromatosis.

4. α-Thalassemias

a. "Silent carriers" and heterozygotes for Hb Constant Spring have no clinical manifestations.

b. α-thal trait largely asymptomatic

c. Hb H disease results in moderate anemia; course variable but usually of moderate severity (thal intermedia–like syndrome).

(1) Hepatosplenomegaly, jaundice common; bone abnormalities rare

(2) Folate deficiency, gallstones, leg ulcers, and hypersplenism occur.

d. Infants lacking all four α globin genes are generally stillborn at 30 to 40 weeks' gestation and have hydrops fetalis (edema due to congestive heart failure).

Key Clinical Findings: Thalassemia Major

- Poor growth
- Hepatosplenomegaly
- Skeletal deformities (acquired)

(1) Pathology shows extensive extramedullary hematopoiesis and placental hypertrophy.

(2) Reports of premature infants surviving but transfusion dependent

(3) High incidence of toxemia and postpartum hemorrhage in mothers

Laboratory Findings

1. Hb values, MCV, electrophoresis findings are presented in Table 123–2.

2. Hypochromia, microcytosis, target cells on peripheral smear

3. Prominent Heinz bodies in Hb H disease

4. Bone marrow shows erythroid hyperplasia; degree correlates with severity of the clinical syndrome.

5. For the differential diagnosis from iron deficiency, see Chapter 113.

6. In chronically transfused or thal intermedia patients

a. Serum iron elevated, transferrin variable, transferrin saturation (Fe/TIBC) high

b. Serum ferritin elevated

(1) Variable correlation with iron load, especially when liver disease is present

(2) Liver biopsy with quantitation of hepatic iron more indicative of iron load but invasive

(3) Hepatic transaminases minimally elevated, serum bilirubin <2 mg/dl (mostly unconjugated) unless there is concurrent hepatitis

Radiographic Changes

Changes due to disease can be prevented/attenuated with transfusion therapy.

1. Small bones of hands and feet are tubular; the trabecular pattern is coarse; and cystic abnormalities are present.

2. Long bones show thinning cortices and dilation of medullary cavities; there is proneness to pathologic fracture.

3. "Hair-on-end" appearance of skull, delayed pneumatization of maxillary sinuses; maxillary overgrowth leads to overbite, prominent upper incisors, and separation of orbits.

4. Widening of ribs, masses of extramedullary hematopoesis in chest

5. Echocardiography, radionuclide cineangiography, electrocardiography with continuous monitoring show the effect of iron accumulation on the heart (Table 123–3).

6. CT scan or MRI can detect iron loading of liver, spleen, lymph nodes; not quantitative.

TABLE 123–2. LABORATORY FINDINGS IN CHILDREN WITH THALASSEMIA SYNDROMES

DISORDER	Hb	MCV	ELECTROPHORESIS
β-Thal trait	10–12 g/dl	61 ± 5 fl	↑ Hb A$_2$ (nearly always) ↑ Hb F (50% of patients)
β-Thal major	3–7 g/dl	50–60 fl	Hb F 20–100% Hb A$_2$ 2–7% Hb A 0–80%
α-Thal trait	10–12 g/dl	65 ± 3 fl	Hb A$_2$, F normal 2–6% Hb Barts at birth
Hb H disease	7–10 g/dl	50–60 fl	Hb H 5–30% Hb Constant Spring (small amount in 50% of SE Asians)

TABLE 123–3. CARDIAC DISEASE IN PATIENTS WITH IRON OVERLOAD

STAGE I (<100 UNITS TRANSFUSION)

Asymptomatic
Echocardiogram: slight left-ventricular wall thickening
Radionuclide cineangiogram: normal
24-hour ECG: normal

STAGE II (100–400 UNITS TRANSFUSION)

Asymptomatic or mild fatigue
Echocardiogram: left-ventricular wall thickening; left ventricular dilatation but normal ejection fraction
Radionuclide cineangiogram: normal at rest but no increase or fall in ejection fraction with exercise
24-hour ECG: atrial and ventricular premature beats

STAGE III

Palpitations and/or congestive heart failure
Echocardiogram: decreased ejection fraction
Radionuclide cineangiogram: normal or decreased ejection fraction at rest but a fall in ejection fraction during exercise
24-hour ECG: atrial and ventricular premature beats, often in pairs or runs

Adapted from Nienhuis AW, Griffith P, et al.: Ann NY Acad Sci 1980; *344*:384.

7. Good assessment of hepatic iron using superconducting quantum interference device susceptometer (SQUIDS); limited availability

Key Radiographic Findings: Thalassemia Major

- Dilation of marrow cavities
- "Hair-on-end" skull
- Coarse trabecular pattern

Treatment

1. β-Thalassemia intermedia
   a. Avoid meat; drink tea to reduce GI absorption of iron.
   b. Consider chronic transfusion (see below) if Hb <7 gm/dl or bone abnormalities or complications of extramedullary hematopoiesis occur.
   c. Splenectomy may be indicated for cytopenias (hypersplenism), early satiety, splenic pain; usually accompanied by improved red cell survival and Hb level.
   d. Chelation therapy in patients with pathologic iron overload
   e. Use of medications to improve Hb F level may be useful in some patients (see below)
2. β-Thalassemia major
   a. Most recommend a chronic transfusion regimen to maintain nadir hb level >9 to 10 gm/dl if endogenous level <7 gm/dl.
      (1) Usually 10 to 15 ml/kg packed red cells q2 to 4 weeks; small, more frequent transfusions reduce total iron load but are less convenient.
      (2) Use of white cell–depleted packed cells appropriate (filtration, saline washing). Frozen, de-glycerolized cells may be needed for alloimmunized patients.
      (3) New patients should have complete red cell phenotyping performed in the event that significant alloimmunization occurs. Provision to all patients of phenotypically matched cells will reduce alloimmunization and should be considered.
   b. No intrinsic mechanism to remove iron; chelation therapy with deferoxamine required
      (1) Begin program age 3 to 4 years; growth retardation in children <age 3 years.
      (2) Usual dose is 20 to 40 mg/kg/day SQ by infusion pump over 8 to 12 hours nightly.
         (a) Noncompliance a major problem
         (b) Higher doses (6 to 12 g/day IV over 12 to 24 hrs) may increase iron excretion but also toxicity and inconvenience. Need for central venous catheter is also associated with risks of thrombosis and infection.
      (3) Reduced risk of cardiac disease, improved survival in well-chelated patients. Survival into fourth decade likely in compliant patients.
      (4) Toxicity of deferoxamine
         (a) Local erythema, pain, SQ nodules may be reduced by adding hydrocortisone (5 to 10 mg) to deferoxamine solution.
         (b) Neurosensory toxicity
            (i) Thirty to 40 per cent may have high-frequency hearing loss; can progress to symptomatic loss.
            (ii) Night and color blindness and visual field defects may occur.
            (iii) Toxicity may be reversible and is more likely with higher doses, lower iron burdens; patients should routinely have vision and hearing examinations.
            (iv) Some bacteria are siderophilic; deferoxamine may potentiate growth. Hold chelation in patients with acute infections and consider empirical anti-*Yersinia* therapy for diarrheal disease to prevent severe ileocolitis and potential bowel perforation.
      (5) Orally administered iron chelators, notably deferiprone (L1), are alternatives under study.
   c. Splenectomy generally required; delayed in aggressively transfused patients.
      (1) No longer believed to increase risk of early hepatic disease
      (2) Recommended if cytopenias significant because of hypersplenism
      (3) If transfusion requirement >200 to 250 ml/kg/year, significant reduction anticipated post splenectomy.
      (4) Pneumococcal vaccine should be given. Penicillin prophylaxis and expectant treatment of fever with parenteral antibiotics are recommended by many.

(5) Postsplenectomy thrombocytosis has been associated with pulmonary vascular disease; monitor lung function, consider low-dose (0.5–1.0 mg/kg day) aspirin therapy.

d. Other conventional treatment recommendations

(1) Vitamin C deficiency common in iron-loaded patients; supplementation in low doses (50–100 mg/day or 3 mg/kg/day) may improve efficacy of chelation. High doses are associated with cardiac toxicity.

(2) Vitamin E replacement may reduce iron-induced oxidative damage to cell membranes.

(3) Folate deficiency can occur as a result of poor absorption and markedly increased requirements. Supplementation (1 mg/day) recommended, although deficiency is less likely in well-transfused patients.

(4) Patients with abnormal hepatic transaminase levels should be screened for hepatitis C infection. Patients with antibody to hepatitis C should be considered for liver biopsy; those with chronic active hepatitis may benefit from α-interferon therapy, although concurrent hemosiderosis may reduce likelihood of therapeutic effect.

e. Bone marrow transplantation is curative and a reasonable option for those with a histocompatible donor.

(1) Original prognostic groups based on hepatomegaly, portal fibrosis on liver biopsy, and compliance with chelation therapy; with current preparative regimens, survival >80 per cent anticipated even in higher risk patients. Young, well-chelated patients without liver disease have a projected survival of 92 per cent.

(2) Risk of peritransplant mortality, graft-versus-host disease, sterility, perhaps other long-term problems

(3) No prospective studies comparing marrow transplant with transfusion/chelation

f. Other potential therapies

(1) Pharmacologic increases in Hb F

(a) 5-Azacytidine increases Hb F but is mutagenic.

(b) Hydroxyurea has associated risks of myelosuppression, teratogenesis; modest increase in Hb F is seen in some patients.

(c) Butyrate therapy encouraging in some patients, but administration unpleasant (foul-smelling) and difficult (continuous intravenous infusion).

(d) Erythropoietin increases Hb F in some patients; may be synergistic with hydroxyurea.

(2) Cord blood stem cell transplantation may be associated with lower risk of GVHD; under investigation.

(3) Gene therapy to insert either a normal β-globin gene or a gene to increase Hb F production into stem cells has been hampered by difficulties in achieving substantive globin production and concern over risk of viral vectors.

3. Most individuals with Hb H disease require supportive care alone.

a. Folate supplementation is recommended.

b. Avoid oxidant drugs, which may worsen hemolysis.

c. Splenectomy for unequivocal hypersplenism; postsplenectomy thrombocytosis may worsen a hypercoagulable state and increase potential for pulmonary emboli.

Key Treatment

- Low iron intake
- Repeated transfusion
- Deferoxamine
- Splenectomy (selective)
- Bone marrow transplantation

Prevention

1. Nondirective counseling of potential parents with thal trait has resulted in substantial reduction in β-thal major; screening for trait (MCV, Hb A$_2$ levels) is appropriate in populations at risk.

2. Spouses of known thal trait individuals should also be screened for hemoglobinopathies (e.g., Hb E or S).

a. Sickle β-thalassemia can be a severe sickle cell disease (see Chapter 122).

b. Hb E β-thalassemia is a common cause of transfusion-dependent anemia in Southeast Asia.

3. Racial differences in α-thal counseling

a. Blacks generally have a *trans* deletion of α-globin genes (see Table 123–1) and are not at risk for severe forms of α-thal.

b. Asians generally have a *cis* deletion and thus require counseling re risks of hydrops fetalis and Hb H disease; latter will require restriction enzyme analysis to diagnose a silent carrier.

4. Antenatal diagnosis available for α-thal, most β-thal; diagnosed by chorionic villus sampling (8–11 weeks) or by amniocentesis at 16 to 20 weeks.

Bibliography

Brittenham GM, Griffith PM, Neinhuis AW, et al: Efficacy of deferoxamine in preventing complications of iron overload in patients with thalassemia major. N Engl J Med 1994;331:567–573.

Lucarelli G, Galimberti M, Polchi P, et al: Marrow transplantation in patients with thalassemia responsive to iron chelation therapy. N Engl J Med 1993;329:840–844.

McDonagh KT, Neinhuis AW: The thalassemias. *In* Nathan DG, Oski FA (eds): Hematology of Infancy and Childhood, 4th ed. Philadelphia, WB Saunders, 1993, pp 783–879.

Olivieri NF, Brittenham GM: Iron-chelating therapy and the treatment of thalassemia. Blood 1997;89:739–761.

Perrine SP, Ginder GD, Faller DV, et al: A short-term trial of butyrate to stimulate fetal-globin-gene expression in beta-globin gene disorders. N Engl J Med 1993;328:81–86.

124 Hemorrhagic Disease of the Newborn

Mary Kaufman

Definition

A newborn who presents with prolonged bleeding after venipuncture or circumcision, large cephalhematoma, bleeding from umbilical cord, gastrointestinal bleeding, central nervous system bleeding, petechiae or ecchymosis has hemorrhagic disease. Inherited or acquired bleeding disorders may manifest bleeding in the neonatal period.

Etiology

Common causes of bleeding in the newborn
1. Platelet disorders
   a. Thrombocytopenia
      (1) Autoimmune (passive)
      (2) Alloimmune (or isoimmune)
      (3) Infections
      (4) Disseminated intravascular coagulation (DIC)
   b. Platelet dysfunction
      (1) Inherited
      (2) Acquired
2. Coagulation abnormalities
   a. Inherited—hemophilia and related disorders
   b. Acquired
      (1) Vitamin K deficiency
      (2) Liver disease
      (3) DIC

Clinical Findings

Bleeding in infants who are otherwise well is likely to be due to inherited coagulation disorders (e.g., hemophilia), immune thrombocytopenia (auto- or allo-), or vitamin K deficiency. In contrast, bleeding in sick neonates is due to thrombocytopenia secondary to infection, liver disease (infection or metabolic), or DIC (infection, hypoxia, hypothermia, shock).

Diagnosis

Diagnosis is based on appropriate history, physical examination, and laboratory studies (see Evaluation of a Patient with Bleeding, Chapter 112).

Treatment

Treatment depends on the underlying disease. For a discussion of DIC, see Chapter 131; for a discussion of thrombocytopenia see Chapter 128; for a discussion of hemophilia, see Chapter 125.

Vitamin K Deficiency

Definition

The bleeding diathesis in vitamin K deficiency is due to a quantitative lack of one or more of the procoagulant proteins (factors II, VII, IX, and X) that depend on vitamin K for their conversion to an active form.

Etiology and Epidemiology

1. The deficiency can be due to a systemic lack or pharmacologic antagonism of vitamin K.
   a. The deficiency can develop when there is prolonged unsupplemented parenteral nutrition, antibiotic suppression of intestinal flora, and decreased absorption of this fat-soluble vitamin due to biliary obstruction or intestinal disease (e.g., cystic fibrosis, colitis, sprue).
   b. In the newborn, it may be due to lack of stores, lack of intake and intestinal synthesis, or pharmacologic antagonism by warfarin or, rarely, phenytoin or salicylates.
2. This condition occurs worldwide and has no ethnic or gender preponderance. It can be seen at any age.

Pathophysiology

1. Vitamin K is one of a group of naphthoquinone derivatives that act as a hepatic microsomal enzyme cofactor. Vitamin K_1 is the major form in the diet. It is taken in via leafy green vegetables and legumes. It is an essential fat-soluble vitamin and needs bile salts and normal fat absorption to maintain the blood level; its storage pool only lasts 1 week.
2. Hepatocytes synthesize the involved procoagulant proteins in a nonfunctional form. Vitamin K is an essential cofactor for carboxylation in the hepatocyte. If there is no vitamin K, the proteins are secreted as abnormal (decarboxy) forms that are nonfunctional.
3. The daily requirement for vitamin K is about 0.1 mg. It is stored in the liver. Intestinal bacterial synthesis is important in newborns, since they have virtually no intake. Vitamin K content in milk is as follows: human milk, 2 to 15 μg/ml; cow's milk, 10 to 20 μg/ml; cow's milk formulas, 55 to 60 μg/ml.
4. Bacteria in the proximal colon and ileum are rich sources of intestinal synthesis of vitamin K in young children. Because intestinal flora supply 100 to 200 μg/day, dietary deficiency alone does not cause vitamin K deficiency unless some intestinal problems are present, e.g., absent bile salts. In older children, most vitamin K is absorbed in the proximal small intestine. In young children, vitamin K decreases after broad-spectrum antibiotics, which alter normal intestinal flora. When vitamin K is decreased, multiple factor deficiencies result.

Clinical Findings

Vitamin K deficiency causes mild to moderate bleeding with bruising, ecchymoses, and oozing from intravenous sites. Although uncommon, it may cause gastrointestinal or intracranial bleeding. In the newborn a hemorrhagic diathesis can occur in two forms, early or late, owing to a deficiency of vitamin K. Affected infants can bleed from many sites, including GI bleeding, bleeding into skin and mucous membranes, and intracranial bleeding.

1. Very early disease (first day) occurs when the mother is on medications (e.g., anticonvulsants) that interfere with vitamin K.
2. The usual form is seen at 2 to 5 days of age and is due to low intake and a relatively sterile gut. Bleeding diatheses due to vitamin K deficiency were seen in 1 in 200 to 1 in 400 newborns prior to the use of prophylactic vitamin K.
3. Late evidence of vitamin K deficiency (after the first weeks) can occur in infants on antibiotics or those with chronic diarrhea.

Medication history, dietary history, and family history are all important. Except in the newborn, malabsorption is the most common cause of vitamin K deficiency.

Key Clinical Findings

- Prolonged bleeding
- Ecchymoses

Laboratory Findings

Screening tests: Activated partial thromboplastin time (APTT) and prothrombin time (PT) are prolonged.

Specific factor assays (factors II, VII, IX, and X) for both coagulant activity and antigen level; assays for decarboxylated forms of these proteins (PIVKA—proteins induced by vitamin K absence); and direct vitamin K levels (normal adult 0.5 mg/ml, cord 0.2 mg/ml to nonmeasurable) are also helpful in establishing the diagnosis.

Key Laboratory Findings

- Prolonged PT
- Prolonged APTT

Treatment

1. Vitamin K$_1$ or K$_2$ (1 to 2 mg) is administered SC or slow IV when hemorrhagic disease of the newborn (HDN) is a strong consideration.
2. In patients with mild to moderate bleeding, fresh frozen plasma is administered, since vitamin K alone may take 2 to 4 hours to increase the levels of vitamin K–dependent factors.
3. Administration of prothrombin complex concentrates is recommended in patients with life-threatening bleeding despite the increased risk of viral transmission and risk of thrombosis.
4. Rodenticide poisoning causes severe, prolonged bleeding. These patients need daily doses of 100 to 150 mg K$_1$ orally.
5. Vitamin K is not useful for patients with hereditary metabolic problems in the vitamin K cycle or with severe liver disease. In patients with vitamin K deficiency, other drugs that interfere with hemostasis (e.g., aspirin) should be avoided.

Key Treatment

- Vitamin K$_1$ or K$_2$—IV or SC
- Fresh frozen plasma

Bibliography

Furie BC: Vitamin K deficiency. *In* Hoffman R, Benz EF Jr, Shattil SJ, et al (eds): Hematology: Basic Principles and Practice. New York, Churchill Livingstone, 1995, pp 1758–1769.

Mammen EF: Vitamin K deficiency. Clin Lab Med 1994;1:769–789.

Montgomery RR, Scott JP: Hemostasis: Disorders of the fluid phase. *In* Nathan DG, Oski FA (eds): Hematology of Infancy in Childhood, 4th ed. Philadelphia, WB Saunders, 1993, pp 1637–1638.

Ratnoff OD: Vitamin K deficiency. *In* Ratnoff OD, Forbes CD (eds): Disorders of Hemostasis, 2nd ed. Philadelphia, WB Saunders, 1991, pp 459–479.

125 Hemophilia

Mary Kaufman, Andrea Hagani, and *James Bussell*

Definition

A severe, hereditary bleeding disorder due to a quantitative deficiency or qualitative defect in the activity of a plasma protein required in the first phase of normal clotting. Hemophilia A is due to a deficiency of or abnormal function of the procoagulant protein factor VIII. Hemophilia B is due to a similar problem with factor IX. The genes for both these proteins are on the X chromosome; both disorders are inherited as sex-linked recessive and are clinically identical. Hemophilia C is due to a lack of factor XI activity. This is inherited as an autosomal trait and is a milder disease.

Epidemiology

1. Hemophilia is the most common severe congenital bleeding disorder and has been recognized for nearly 2000 years.

2. It is seen worldwide and in all ethnic groups. In the United States, the incidence of hemophilia A is 1 in 10,000 males; hemophilia B occurs in 1 in 40,000 males. As an X-linked recessive, all daughters of a hemophiliac male are obligate carriers and all sons are normal. Carrier females have 50 per cent sons with hemophilia, and 50 per cent daughters are carriers.

Physiology of Coagulation

1. Clotting is a physiologic response to injury, with procoagulant substances being released from tissues and/or platelets or activation of contact factors (XI, XII). Platelets, vascular endothelium, phospholipids, and a series of plasma proteins circulating in inactive form are involved. Primary hemostasis involves platelets adhering to subendothelial tissues (especially collagen) and sticking to one another. A platelet plug is formed, accompanied by vasoconstriction. In secondary hemostasis the process continues with sequential activation of a series of circulating procoagulant proteins (serine proteases and their cofactors), mostly by proteolytic cleavage resulting in the generation of thrombin and the conversion of soluble fibrinogen to insoluble fibrin. The entire process is controlled and modulated by naturally occurring anticoagulants (ATIII, protein C and protein S) and inhibitors (tissue factor pathway inhibitor). There are many feedback loops, with some accelerating and others inhibiting the process. Calcium ions and phospholipids are essential. Once traces of thrombin are generated, there is increased activation of platelets and factors VIII, V, and XI.

2. The series of reactions is divided for convenience into an intrinsic (surface-activated) and an extrinsic (tissue factor–activated) segment. These paths are not independent. Of interest, a recent revised pathway of coagulation incorporates all the known factors in coagulation into a single pathway initiated by factors VIIa and tissue factor; in this, contact factors (XII, kallikrein, and HMWK) are not required. A deficiency of any major component in either pathway (except for factor XII, PK, or HMWK) will lead to a bleeding disorder. Lack of factor VIII or IX produces a profound abnormality, since factor Xa generated by VIIa/TF is insufficient because of TFPI, and these factors (VIII and IXa) are required to amplify the production of factor Xa.

Pathophysiology

Factor VIII and factor IX are critical in the intrinsic pathway and accelerate the activation of factor X in the presence of calcium ions and phospholipids. Factor IXa and factor VIIIa interact on a phospholipid surface (or cell surface), and a conformational change occurs in the enzyme that permits it to act. This is critical for effective thrombin formation. This step cannot be bypassed by tissue factor. Thrombin is critical for platelet aggregation, clot retraction, and factor XIII activation. In hemophilia, there is delayed formation of thrombin, resulting in slow formation of an abnormal clot. Because of friable clot, rebleeding is common in these patients, especially with inadequate treatment. The half-life of factor VIII is only 2 to 4 hours without von Willebrand factor and 10 to 12 hours with it. When von Willebrand factor binds to platelet GP Ib, it brings factor VIII to the area of injury. Mutations at the binding site for factor VIII on von Willebrand factor will profoundly decrease factor VIII levels. The concentration of factor VIII in plasma is 0.1 to 0.2 ng/ml.

Genetics

1. The factor VIII gene is 186kb and is one of the largest genes discovered. Both factors VIII and IX show a wide variety of genetic defects consisting of DNA deletions, insertions, and point mutations. Many are family specific. Mutations at cleavage and binding sites may result in normal amounts of a nonfunctional protein.

2. The factor IX gene is much smaller (34 kb) than factor VIII gene. It has also been completely sequenced. Its molecular weight is 56,000. It is synthesized and stored in the liver and has a half-life of 24 hours. Ten to 30 per cent of patients with factor IX deficiency hemophilia have normal antigen level (CRM positive) but decreased coagulant activity (i.e., dysfunctional molecule), whereas only 5 to 10 per cent of factor VIII deficiency hemophiliacs have this.

3. Although factor VIII and IX deficiencies are X-linked recessive, females can manifest the disorder if homozygous (carrier mother and affected father), or if due to extreme lyonization. Likewise, a phenotypic female with an abnormal genotype (Turner phenotype) or autosomal dominant disease due to an abnormal von Willebrand factor with abnormal binding to factor VIII and resultant accelerated degradation of factor VIII may manifest the condition.

Clinical Findings

The disorder is clinically heterogeneous and may be severe, moderate, or mild with involved coagulation factor level ≤1 per cent, between 1 and 5 per cent, and ≥5 per cent, respectively.

Bleeding into muscles and joints is the predominant problem. Delayed bleeding is common, since the platelet plug forms but is not reinforced by fibrin clot. Patients with mild hemophilia may go undiagnosed for many years and bleed only after major trauma. Patients with moderate disease bleed after mild to moderate trauma, while patients with severe hemophilia bleed with minimal trauma or sometimes without history of trauma.

1. Age of onset—Thirty per cent of affected males bleed at circumcision, but only 1 to 2 per cent may develop intracranial hemorrhage if full term. As the patient becomes mobile, bruising will be evident. Eruption of teeth or intramuscular injections can cause bleeding. The more severe the case, the earlier the bleeding manifestations.

2. Sites
   a. Bleeding into muscles and joints is classic—hemarthroses start in the toddler stage. Swelling, pain, and decreased movements are seen. Recurrent bleeding leads to cartilage erosion, joint space narrowing, chronic arthritis, and fibrosis. Decreased mobility leads to muscle weakness and disuse atrophy. Joints are boggy and deformed and may fuse. Knees, ankles, elbows, shoulders, and hips are the most frequently involved joints. Deep hematomas may cause compression damage, pain, fever, and leukocytosis.

b. Intracranial bleeding is a common cause of death (25%) and only half the patients have a history of trauma. Rebleeding within 1 year is common. Though mortality has decreased, nearly half of survivors have serious neurologic sequelae.

c. Oral bleeding following torn frenulum in infants or after dental extraction is a frequent problem.

d. Genitourinary bleeding (gross hematuria) or gastrointestinal bleeding may also bring these patients to medical attention.

3. Hemophilia carriers are rarely asymptomatic. They run factor VIII levels of 25 to 40 per cent. Some carriers of factor IX deficiency may bleed excessively after trauma, surgery, or childbirth. This is rarely seen with factor VIII deficiency.

Key Clinical Findings

- Bleeding into joints and muscles
- Oral bleeding, frenulum and tongue
- Hematuria

Laboratory Findings

1. Diagnostic tests should include a bleeding time for platelet and vascular function, APTT and PT for all protein procoagulant factors, and a thrombin time. The typical hemophilic pattern is normal bleeding time, abnormal PTT, and normal PT and TT. Specific assays are then done for factors VIII, IX, and XI.

2. Inhibitors are tested for by incubating equal volumes of patient's plasma with normal plasma and noting whether factor VIII is neutralized.

3. Carrier identification: The ratio of factor VIII coagulant activity to von Willebrand factor antigen (normally 1:1) is significantly less than 1 in carriers. In addition, detailed studies of DNA from patients with hemophilia and their family help in detecting the carriers.

Key Laboratory Findings

- Normal bleeding time
- Normal PT
- Prolonged PTT
- Reduced factor VIII or factor IX

Radiographic Changes

1. Ultrasound, CT, and routine x-ray studies are used to determine the location and extent of bleeding as well as to follow response to therapy.

2. Intravenous pyelogram to localize site and extent of obstruction after hematuria. If there is ureteral dilation, it should be followed.

3. Joint changes: Loss of cartilage, loose flakes in joints, osteoporosis and cysts, changes in joint space, and osteophytes. Evaluate the need for surgical intervention or joint replacement.

Treatment

Factor replacement is the mainstay of therapy for most patients with the exception of mild hemophiliacs, who are treated with desmopressin (DDAVP). Currently several plasma-derived concentrates of factor VIII and IX as well as recombinant factor VIII concentrates are available for clinical use. The dose and frequency of administration depend on the size, severity of the bleed, and half-life of the factor and whether the patient has inhibitors. Home therapy (self-administered or parent-administered) has become the standard of care for acute bleeding episodes and has the advantage of prompt treatment, decreased long-term morbidity, decreased cost, and independence for the patient and family. Each unit of factor VIII/kg body weight results in an increase in plasma level of 2 per cent with a half-life of 8 to 12 hours; each unit of factor IX/kg of body weight results in an increase in plasma level of 1 to 1.5 per cent with a half-life of 15 to 24 hours.

1. *Desmopressin (DDAVP).* Patients with mild hemophilia A and mild to moderate bleed (e.g., hemarthrosis) may be treated with intravenous or nasal DDAVP (Stimate). This should be done only if a significant increase in factor VIII level has been demonstrated previously. The dose may be repeated in 12 to 24 hours. The dose of IV desmopressin is 0.3 μg/kg given as IV infusion over 15 minutes; the nasal preparation dose is 75 μg in each nostril for patients weighing >50 kg and 75 μg in one nostril for patients <50 kg.

2. Mild to moderate hemorrhage

   a. Joint bleeds

      (1) Factor VIII 20 to 40 U/kg

      (2) Factor IX 25 to 30 U/kg

   b. Muscle bleeds

      (1) Factor VIII 20 U/kg

      (2) Factor IX 15 U/kg

   Prednisone 1 mg/kg/day is given for patients with joint bleed for 3 to 5 days to decrease inflammation in the joint.

   c. Oral bleeding

      (1) 30 to 50 U/kg of factor

      (2) Amicar (epsilon aminocaproic acid) 100 mg/kg q 6h × 5–7d or Cyclokapron 25 mg/kg q 6h × 5–7d.

      (3) Restrict diet to clear liquids until area is healed and avoid the use of a straw.

   d. Hematuria

      (1) The most important goal is to prevent the formation of clots in the kidneys and ureters by maintaining adequate hydration. Vigorous activity should be avoided for 2 weeks after the hematuria resolves.

      (2) Prednisone 0.5 mg/kg at onset and then BID × 48 hr.

      (3) If hematuria persists or is severe, infuse 40 U/kg.

3. Severe or life-threatening bleeding

   a. Retroperitoneal or retropharyngeal bleed: 50 U/kg STAT; repeat as needed.

   b. Head trauma—Head injuries should be taken very

seriously and should be treated with an infusion even if there are no signs of intracranial bleeding. Injuries in the neck and throat area can also be serious because swelling in these areas can obstruct the airway. A HEAD CT OR MRI IS MANDATORY IF THERE IS ANY SUGGESTION OF HEAD TRAUMA, EVEN IF SYMPTOMS ARE MINIMAL.

(1) Loss of consciousness or amnesia of event requires a neurology consult and CT scan.

   (a) CT NEG: 50 U/kg BID × 1d, then QD × 7d

   (b) CT POS: 50 U/kg TID × 2 days, then BID × 12 days, then QD × 21 d; surgical intervention as indicated. Future prophylaxis (e.g., 40–50 U/kg QOD) should be considered.

(2) Vomiting, nuchal rigidity, unexplained fever or sleepiness, irritability, or persistent headache mandates a CT scan.

   (a) CT NEG: 50 U/kg QD × 3d

   (b) CT POS: as above

(3) Lumbar puncture can be performed safely after factor infusion as indicated.

(4) Witnessed head trauma on a soft surface with crying but no headache, vomiting, or other sequelae: Treat with 50 U/kg × 1 and observe.

Specific factor levels should be followed in patients with severe or life-threatening bleeding.

4. Management of patients with inhibitors—Ten to 15 per cent of patients with hemophilia A and 2 to 4 per cent of patients with hemophilia B develop inhibitors. These are alloantibodies of IgG class, mostly IgG4. Choice of replacement therapy depends on the level of inhibitor, degree of anamnestic response, and severity of the bleed. Mild hemorrhage can be treated with appropriate doses of factor VIII or IX. Patients with low-level inhibitors but with a serious hemorrhage may be treated with human or porcine factor VIII depending on the cross reactivity. Patients with high-titer inhibitors to human and porcine factor are treated with bypass products such as activated prothrombin complex concentrates (PCC), which contain varying amounts of factors II, VII, IX, X and protein C, or recombinant VIIa (not approved by FDA as of 4/97). Patients receiving PCC should be monitored for thrombotic complications (DIC or myocardial infarction). Long-term management of these patients consists of immune tolerance induction by daily administration of factor for 6 to 12 months or plasma exchange followed by IVIG and immunosuppression with cyclophosphamide. These latter therapies are very expensive and have a success rate of 30 to 50 per cent.

5. Gene therapy—Studies are in progress to introduce normal cDNA and a promoter sequence into a patient's genome using a retroviral vector. To date, more progress has occurred for hemophilia B than for hemophilia A.

6. Prophylaxis—Administration of factor three times a week in a dose sufficient to maintain the factor levels at about 2 to 3 per cent at all times can prevent most bleeding episodes with excellent performance status. This form of treatment is quite costly and is done in very few countries.

Complications

HIV infection and hepatitis are major problems for older patients. A large proportion of patients who received commercial concentrates prior to 1985 were infected with HIV and hepatitis. Current viral inactivation methods have practically eliminated the risk of HIV, hepatitis A and B, and, to a lesser extent, hepatitis C. All patients with hemophilia should receive hepatitis A and B immunization.

Prevention

Total prevention is not possible because of the high rate of spontaneous mutation of the gene. However, careful identification of carrier and prenatal testing of fetal blood using molecular methods combined with genetic counseling could significantly decrease the incidence of hemophilia.

Bibliography

Broze GT Jr: The role of tissue factor pathway inhibitor in a revised coagulation cascade. Semin Hematol 1962;29:159–169.

Forbes CD, Madhock R: Genetic disorders of blood coagulation: Clinical presentation and management. *In* Ratnoff OD, Forbes CD (eds): Disorders of Hemostasis, 2nd ed. Philadelphia, WB Saunders, 1991, pp 141–202.

Kaufman RJ, Antonarakis SE, Brettler D, et al: Structure, biology and genetics of factor VIII. *In* Hoffman R, Benz EF Jr, Shattil SJ, et al (eds): Hematology: Basic Principles and Practice. New York, Churchill Livingstone, 1995, pp 1633–1648.

Montgomery RR, Scott JP: Hemostasis: Disease of the fluid phase. *In* Nathan DG, Oski FA (eds): Hematology of Infancy and Childhood, 4th ed. Philadelphia, WB Saunders, 1993, pp 1605–1650.

Thompson AR: Molecular biology of the hemophiliacs. Prog Hemost Thromb 1991;10:175–214.

126 Von Willebrand Disease

Mary Kaufman

Definition

Von Willebrand disease is a heterogeneous group of hereditary bleeding disorders caused by quantitative or qualitative abnormality of a specific circulatory protein, von Willebrand factor (vWf), which is required for normal adherence of platelets to subendothelial substances at areas of endothelial injury. This disorder is associated with mucocutaneous bleeding and bleeding after trauma. Most cases are mild to moderate in clinical severity, and many cases are undiagnosed.

Epidemiology

These disorders are extremely common and may affect up to 1 per cent of the population worldwide.

Pathophysiology

1. Von Willebrand factor is a large, multimeric glycoprotein synthesized in megakaryocytes and endothelial cells. It is stored in granules of the Weibel-Palade body of endothelial cells and the α-granules of platelets. Following injury to endothelium, local concentration of vWf is markedly increased. Von Willebrand factor adheres to exposed collagen (specific binding site) at these areas of injury and undergoes a conformational change that permits binding to platelet GPIb (another specific binding site). This activates the platelets, resulting in platelet aggregation, platelet plug formation, activation of plasma clotting factors, and production of fibrin clot (secondary hemostasis). Von Willebrand factor also binds to platelet receptor GP IIb/IIIa. In the absence of functional vWf, platelets are not targeted to the area of damage, and there is poor plug formation and delayed fibrin formation. Von Willebrand factor is an essential carrier of factor VIII and is required for its normal survival. In the absence of vWf, there is decreased plasma level of factor VIII. Thus deficiency of vWf, quantitative or functional, results in a bleeding disorder.
2. The autosomal dominant gene for vWf is on the short arm of chromosome 12, band 21. It spans 178 kb. Various protein interactions, such as binding sites for platelet GPIb, GPIIb/IIIa, factor VIII, and collagen, are localized to specific regions of the molecule. It is first synthesized as pre/pro von Willebrand factor, which is cleaved into two molecules: mature vWf and von Willebrand antigen II. Von Willebrand factor then assembles as multimers of varying sizes. The largest multimers are functionally most active with regard to platelet function. Von Willebrand factor binding to platelet GPIb brings factor VIII to the platelet. Mutations at the vWf binding site for factor VIII give rise to apparently autosomal hemophilia.
3. More than 20 genetic variants have been reported since the vWf gene was cloned and sequenced in 1985 (Fig. 126–1). Large gene deletions are the basis for some of the rare but severe von Willebrand disease known as type

III. Smaller deletions, missense mutations, and nonsense mutations result in quantitative decreases.

Clinical Findings

Von Willebrand disease is seen in both sexes.

1. Mucous membrane bleeding (epistaxis, menorrhagia) easy bruising, and excessive posttraumatic and postsurgical bleeding are characteristic. A history of ecchymosis over legs and forearms is not so significant as bruises on the trunk, upper arms, and thighs. Menorrhagia can be a serious problem. Nearly a third of females may experience delayed postpartum bleeding. Hemarthroses are rare.
2. The severity of the disease in terms of both bleeding manifestations and laboratory abnormalities varies considerably among members of the same family—sometimes in the same patients. Therefore, repeated testing may be required to establish the diagnosis. Von Willebrand factor levels also vary with the individual's blood type; the levels are lowest in persons with blood group O.
3. Acquired von Willebrand disease is seen, rarely, late in life and in association with another illness such as lymphoproliferative/myeloproliferative disease, SLE, or Wilms tumor. It may be due to inhibitors inactivating vWf or proteolysis of vWf.
4. Rarely, patients with severe disease may develop inhibitors similar to those seen in patients with hemophilia.
5. Pseudo–von Willebrand disease is an autosomal dominant bleeding disorder with an abnormal platelet receptor (GP Ib) having an increased affinity for vWf. It resembles type IIb disease with increased platelet aggregation to low-dose ristocetin.

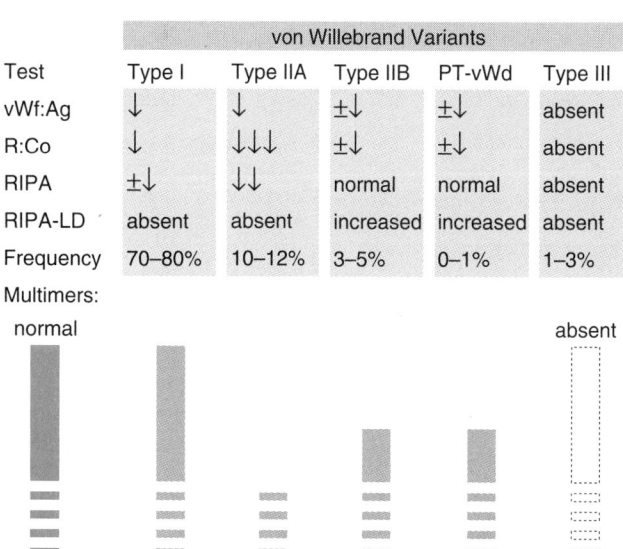

| Test | von Willebrand Variants | | | | |
	Type I	Type IIA	Type IIB	PT-vWd	Type III
vWf:Ag	↓	↓	±↓	±↓	absent
R:Co	↓	↓↓↓	±↓	±↓	absent
RIPA	±↓	↓↓	normal	normal	absent
RIPA-LD	absent	absent	increased	increased	absent
Frequency	70–80%	10–12%	3–5%	0–1%	1–3%
Multimers:					

Figure 126–1 Von Willebrand variants. (From Nathan DG, Oski FA [eds]: Hematology of Infancy and Childhood, 4th ed. Philadelphia, WB Saunders, 1993.)

Key Clinical Findings

- Epistaxis
- Menorrhagia
- Easy bruising

Treatment

Treatment depends on the type of disease and severity of bleeding.

1. *Desmopressin acetate (DDAVP)*—It is the treatment of choice for patients with mild type I disease. It can be given by IV infusion (dose 0.3 μg/kg over 15 minutes) and may be repeated in 12 to 24 hours. Repeated administration may result in tachyphylaxis. Recently, a nasal preparation of desmopressin (1.5 mg/ml) was approved for these patients. It is important to do a therapeutic trial (repeat bleeding time and vWf level 30 minutes to 1 hour after DDAVP) with IV or nasal preparation of desmopressin in all newly diagnosed patients with type I disease. Monitor serum sodium levels in infants and young children if multiple doses are given.

Key Laboratory Findings

Test	Result
Bleeding time	Usually prolonged, may be normal
aPTT	Abnormal only in severe cases
vWf Ag	Usually decreased
vWf (ristocetin cofactor)	Decreased
Factor VIII clotting activity	Usually decreased
Ristocetin-induced platelet aggregation (RIPA)	Decreased, may be normal
Low-dose RIPA	Absent or increased
vWf multimers	Absent or decrease in large multimers only or decrease in large and small multimers

2. *Plasma-derived von Willebrand factor*—Cryoprecipitate or factor concentrates with vWf are indicated for the treatment of type I patients who fail to respond adequately to desmopressin and for patients with type IIa, IIb, and III disease. Solvent detergent–treated cryoprecipitate is preferable to the usual cryoprecipitate to minimize the risk of viral transmission. Some factor VIII concentrates, in particular humate P, have adequate concentration of vWf multimers and may be used in place of cryoprecipitate.
3. Platelet transfusion is recommended for patients with platelet type disease.
4. Local measures such as nasal pressure, nasal packing to control epistaxis, and ε-aminocaproic acid for patients with oral bleeding are helpful.

Key Treatment

- Desmopressin (DDAVP)
- Cryoprecipitate

Prevention

Since most cases of von Willebrand disease are mild to moderate, appropriate care is even more important than prevention. For severe cases, counseling as to hereditary pattern is vital. Since the gene has been sequenced and restriction fragment length polymorphism (RFLP) with polymerase chain reaction (PCR) augmentation is available, carrier identification and prenatal diagnosis are possible. Chorionic villus sampling or amniocentesis can provide material for fetal diagnosis, and the parents will have a chance to make an informed decision based on the severity of disease.

Bibliography

Gralnick HR: von Willebrand disease. *In* Ratnoff OD, Forbes CD (eds): Disorders of Hemostasis, 2nd ed. Philadelphia, WB Saunders, 1991, pp 203–244.

Montgomery RR, Scott JO: Congenital factor deficiencies. *In* Nathan DG, Oski FA (eds): Hematology of Infancy and Childhood, 4th ed. Philadelphia, WB Saunders, 1993, pp 1605–1650.

Rick ME: Laboratory diagnosis of von Willebrand disease. Clin Lab Med 1994;1:781–794.

Wagner DD, Ginsburg D, White GC, Montgomery RR: Structure, biology and genetics of von Willebrand factor and clinical aspects of and therapy of von Willebrand disease. *In* Hoffman R, Benz EF Jr, Shattil SJ, et al (eds): Hematology: Basic Principles and Practice, 2nd ed. New York, Churchill Livingstone, 1995, pp 1717–1736.

127 Polycythemia

Marc S. C. Cheah

Definition

Polycythemia is defined as an increase in the red blood cell mass. This usually means a hemoglobin in excess of 17 g/dl or a hematocrit of 50 per cent or more in a child. In the newborn, a venous hemoglobin exceeding 22.0 g/dl or a hematocrit greater than 65 per cent during the first week of life is evidence of polycythemia.

Childhood: Primary Polycythemia, Polycythemia Vera

Physiology

Increase in red cell mass

Pathophysiology

Intrinsic abnormality of hematopoietic stem cell

Clinical Findings

Exceedingly rare in children
Plethora

Childhood: Secondary Polycythemia

Physiology

Increase in red cell mass

Pathophysiology

1. Increased erythropoietin (EPO) production
2. Decreased tissue oxygenation
   a. High altitudes
   b. Chronic lung disorders
   c. Sleep apnea
   d. Congenital heart disease (right-to-left shunt)
   e. Abnormal hemoglobins (methemoglobinemia, high-affinity hemoglobins)
3. Inappropriate EPO secretion
   a. Wilms tumor
   b. Pheochromocytoma
   c. Renal cysts, hydronephrosis
   d. Uterine leiomyoma
   e. Renal cell carcinoma
   f. Hepatoma
   g. Cerebellar hemangioblastoma (von Hippel–Lindau disease)

Clinical Findings

1. Asymptomatic
2. Flushed complexion
3. Fatigue, headaches
4. Shortness of breath
5. Elevated hemoglobin, hematocrit
6. Normal white cell count and platelets

Childhood: Relative Polycythemia, Stress Erythrocytosis

Physiology

Normal red cell mass, reduced plasma volume

Pathophysiology

Carbon monoxide (CO) in tobacco smoke implicated in pathogenesis

Clinical Findings

Exclusively in middle-aged persons

Neonatal Polycythemia

Etiology

1. Hypertransfusion: Fetal-fetal (monozygotic twins), maternal-fetal transfusion, delayed cord clamping
2. Placental insufficiency with intrauterine hypoxia, placenta previa, preeclampsia
3. Endocrine and metabolic disorders
   a. Congenital adrenal hyperplasia
   b. Neonatal thyrotoxicosis

Pathophysiology

1. Increase in blood viscosity; decreased blood flow to major organs results in symptoms
2. Increased red cell mass breakdown results in hyperbilirubinemia.

Clinical Findings

1. Asymptomatic
2. Respiratory distress
3. Cyanosis
4. Congestive heart failure
5. Seizures
6. Jaundice
7. Tetany
8. Renal vein thrombosis

Key Clinical Findings

- Florid complexion
- Fatigue

Laboratory Findings

1. Elevated hemoglobin and hematocrit
2. Thrombocytopenia
3. Hyperbilirubinemia
4. Hypocalcemia
5. Hypoglycemia

Key Laboratory Findings

• Elevated Hgb, HCT
• Normal WBC and platelets

Treatment

Partial exchange transfusion with fresh frozen plasma or 5 per cent albumin (respiratory, cardiac, or central nervous system symptoms) to decrease the blood viscosity by lowering hematocrit to about 55 per cent.

Key Treatment

• Partial exchange transfusion

Bibliography

Berlin NI: Diagnosis and classification of the polycythemias. Semin Hematol 1976;12:339.

128 Platelet Disorders (Thrombocytopenia)

Andrea Hagani and *James Bussell*

Definition

The normal platelet count ranges from 150,000 to 400,000/μl; a count lower than 150,000/μl indicates thrombocytopenia.

Etiology

Congenital and acquired forms occur, with the acquired forms being much more prominent. Thrombocytopenia can be caused by either decreased production or excessive destruction of platelets.

1. Inadequate production results from bone marrow dysfunction as evidenced by decreased or abnormal megakaryocytes.
2. Excessive destruction, on the other hand, is accompanied by normal or increased numbers of megakaryocytes.

Epidemiology

1. *Inherited.* Inherited thrombocytopenias are manifestations of several relatively rare syndromes. The inheritance pattern is both X-linked and autosomal recessive. Examples include the Wiskott-Aldrich syndrome and thrombocytopenia with absent radius (TAR).
2. *Acquired.* Idiopathic (immune) thrombocytopenic purpura (ITP) is by far the most common cause of acquired thrombocytopenia in childhood. In approximately 70 per cent of cases there is a history of an antecedent viral illness 1 to 4 weeks before the onset of symptoms. Viral antigens may trigger the production of antibodies that cross react with glycoproteins on the platelet membrane. Acute ITP predominantly occurs between the ages of 2 and 5 years, and it occurs equally in both sexes. Chronic ITP, on the other hand, is more common in children older than 7 to 10 years, and it is more common in girls.

Differential Diagnosis

Thrombocytopenia can be the result of a variety of pathologic conditions but can be broken down into the following categories:

1. Decreased production—Megakaryocytes are decreased or function abnormally in a number of illnesses with various etiologies.
   a. Bone marrow failure syndromes—Aplastic anemia, Fanconi anemia, Wiskott-Aldrich syndrome, TAR syndrome, trisomy syndromes, dyskeratosis congenita, histiocytosis, osteopetrosis
   b. Drug-induced—G-CSF, chloramphenicol, alcohol, chemotherapy
   c. Infections can result in bone marrow suppression manifested as an isolated thrombocytopenia, neutropenia, anemia, or any combination of the three. Examples include viruses (rubella, varicella, EBV, CMV, HSV, measles, HIV, hepatitis), toxoplasmosis, malaria, syphilis, tuberculosis, and overwhelming sepsis.
2. Increased consumption
   a. Immunologic causes—Thrombocytopenia results from antibody-mediated destruction of platelets. The spleen is presumed to be the major site of consumption.
   b. Microangiopathy—Thrombocytopenia results from shortened platelet survival secondary to a local microangiopathic process involving fibrin deposition as seen in the hemolytic-uremic syndrome and thrombotic thrombocytopenic purpura (TTP). The primary etiologies of these disorders are speculative but include bacterial and viral infections, toxins, drugs, and prostaglandin abnormalities.
   c. Sequestration and destruction of platelets in giant hemangiomas (Kasabach-Merritt syndrome) or in the spleen (hypersplenism) can also be found.

Clinical Findings

1. Regardless of the cause, the risk of bleeding in a thrombocytopenic child is directly related to the degree of thrombocytopenia, with the highest risk present if the platelet count is ≤20,000/μl.

2. Spontaneous bruising and metromenorrhagia (in menstruating adolescent females) will occur with platelet counts from 10,000 to 50,000/μl.
3. If the platelet count is ≤10,000/μl, the patient is at risk for mucosal and life-threatening bleeding (including the central nervous system).
4. ITP usually has an abrupt onset, with petechiae, purpura, and mucosal bleeding the most prominent symptoms. Remarkably, the children generally appear well. The acute phase associated with spontaneous hemorrhages usually lasts for only 1 to 2 weeks, but the bleeding risk is defined by the platelet count more than by the time from onset of the thrombocytopenia.
5. Chronic ITP, defined by its persistence for more than 6 months, develops in 10 to 20 per cent of patients.
6. Recurrent ITP, with intervals of at least 3 months between episodes, will develop in 1 to 4 per cent.
7. The liver, spleen, and lymph nodes are usually not enlarged.

Key Clinical Findings

- Petechiae
- Purpura
- Mucosal bleeding
- Metromenorrhagia

Laboratory Findings in Destructive Thrombocytopenia

1. Isolated thrombocytopenia is the hallmark of ITP. Platelet counts vary from mildly to severely decreased and tend to be lower in the acute form of the illness. The few platelets observed on blood smear are large, reflecting increased marrow production.
2. The CBC is otherwise normal.
3. Abnormal coagulation studies point to disseminated intravascular coagulation (DIC), hemolytic uremic syndrome, or TTP.
4. Bone marrow aspiration, if performed, reveals normal or increased numbers of megakaryocytes. The myeloid and erythroid series are normal. Abnormal appearance of marrow cells suggests myelodysplasia.
5. Direct Coombs test will be positive in Evans syndrome.
6. Blood typing should be performed in anticipation of possible anti-D globulin treatment.

Key Laboratory Findings

- Thrombocytopenia
- Normal or increased megakaryocytes in bone marrow

Treatment

1. ITP
   a. Because the spontaneous remission rate is high, no therapy is necessary if the disease is mild (i.e., platelet count >20,000/μl, no bleeding other than purpura).
   b. Platelet counts ≤10,000/μl and extensive mucosal hemorrhage imply a higher risk for internal hemorrhage and warrant treatment. Treatment goals are the cessation of bleeding and the increase of platelet count to >20,000 to 30,000/μl. In the past, when steroids were the mainstay of treatment, bone marrow examinations were performed routinely. However, now that other treatments are available and studies have shown that leukemia essentially never presents with isolated thrombocytopenia and a normal physical examination, therapy can be instituted without performing this study. The following therapies are given in the order that they should be attempted.
      (1) IV gamma globulin 0.5 to 1.0 gm/kg/day and IV methylprednisolone 30 mg/kg/day. This regime can be tried for up to 3 days, depending upon response, with no steroid taper needed. Oral prednisone can also be used at doses of 1 to 4 mg/kg/day.
      (2) Anti-D immune globulin: Immune gamma globulin preparation of antibodies directed against the Rh antigen. It is useful in patients with ITP who are Rh positive (85%) and have not had a splenectomy. The dose is 50 μg/kg/dose as an IV infusion over 3 minutes. The peak response is not seen for 3 to 7 days. Anemia is the dose-limiting toxicity.
      (3) Platelet transfusions should be reserved for acute, ongoing, life-threatening bleeding that cannot be controlled by other means.
      (4) Treatment of chronic ITP is more complicated and less successful (except for splenectomy). In addition to splenectomy, high-dose dexamethasone, vincristine, danazol, interferon, and other agents may be of use.
      (5) Treatment is continued with single infusions on a prn basis for platelet counts <20,000/μl. Platelet counts should be measured about once per week until stable. Infusions can be continued indefinitely as long as the patient responds. A rule of thumb is to try to wait for at least 1 year from diagnosis before considering splenectomy; it is best not to perform splenectomy in a child ≤5 years of age.
      (6) For the other causes of thrombocytopenia, the underlying cause must be treated. Drug withdrawal usually reverses the thrombocytopenia in cases of drug-induced effects. Platelet transfusions (leukocyte-depleted only) should be reserved for severe or life-threatening bleeding to avoid refractoriness, particularly in patients who may ultimately require bone marrow transplantation (e.g., aplastic anemia, Fanconi anemia, Wiskott-Aldrich syndrome). Fresh frozen plasma may be needed in patients with DIC, whereas plasma exchange is usually required in TTP.
2. Platelet functional disorders
Some platelet disorders result from a defect in platelet function with a normal platelet number.

TABLE 128–1. CONGENITAL PLATELET ABNORMALITIES

NAME	PATHOPHYSIOLOGY	SYMPTOMS
Glanzmann thrombasthenia	Failure of platelet aggregation in response to adenosine diphosphate, collagen, epinephrine, and thrombin, but they do aggregate in the presence of ristocetin and von Willebrand factor (vWF). Caused by the partial or complete absence of glycoprotein IIb/IIIa from the platelet membrane. Inherited as an autosomal recessive trait.	Life-threatening hemorrhages can occur
Bernard-Soulier syndrome	Platelet agglutination does not occur in the presence of ristocetin, even with vWF, although they do aggregate in the presence of adenosine diphosphate, collagen, epinephrine, and thrombin. Platelets appear large and bizarre and can be reduced in number. The primary defect is an absence of glycoproteins Ib, V, and IX from the platelet surface. The lack of glycoprotein Ib leads to the inability to bind vWF or ristocetin.	Severe hemorrhagic complications
Gray platelet syndrome	Suspected deficiency of α granules as evidenced by a reduction in platelet levels of their constituents, such as fibrinogen, vWF, factor V; high molecular weight kininogen, fibronectin, thrombospondin, β-thromboglobulin, platelet factor 4, and platelet-derived growth factor.	Bleeding diathesis usually apparent at birth. Platelets appear washed out or gray-appearing on peripheral blood smears.
Storage pool disorders	Deficiencies of the adenine nucleotide–containing dense granules or their contents. Diminished response to collagen, which depends on the release of endogenous platelet nucleotides (second phase) for completion of aggregation.	Bleeding symptoms usually not severe
Abnormalities of the platelet release reaction	Abnormalities of arachidonic acid metabolism in some, defects of calcium metabolism in others, results in the defective release of platelet granular contents.	Bleeding usually not severe
Congenital disorders associated with platelet dysfunction	Type I glycogen storage disease, cyanotic congenital heart disease, pseudoxanthoma elasticum, May-Hegglin anomaly, Epstein's syndrome	Bleeding usually not severe

a. Acquired abnormalities are most common after taking drugs that affect platelet function, such as aspirin-containing drugs or other cyclooxygenase inhibitors. Valproic acid can also cause a prolongation of the bleeding time.

b. Congenital platelet abnormalities are a diverse group of disorders that share the traits of purpura, abnormal platelet aggregation, and prolonged bleeding times. Platelet morphology is also abnormal in some cases. These disorders, which are quite rare, are summarized in Table 128–1. The work-up of these disorders often includes platelet aggregation studies that evaluate platelet agglutination in response to epinephrine, collagen, adenosine diphosphate, and arachidonic acid. Other studies are available on a research basis.

3. The use of desmopressin (DDAVP) in other than Glanzmann thrombasthenia and Bernard-Soulier syndrome, and of Amicar if there is mouth or nose bleeding, may be helpful in other than proven, serious bleeding.

4. Platelet transfusion is the only highly effective therapy for these disorders, but it may lead to refractoriness as a result of the development of antibodies directed against the deficient glycoproteins that are present on the transfused platelets; this is less likely with leukocyte-depleted platelets (irradiation should be used for immunodeficiency states and impending marrow transplantation). It is therefore vital that platelet transfusions be reserved for truly life-threatening or uncontrolled bleeding emergencies.

Key Treatment

- IV gamma globulin
- Prednisone

Bibliography

Behrman RE, Vaughan VC, Nelson WE: Hemorrhagic diseases. *In* Behrman RE, et al (eds): Nelson Textbook of Pediatrics, 13th ed. Philadelphia, WB Saunders, 1987, pp 1065–1075.

Casella JF: Disorders of coagulation. *In* Oski FA, DeAngelis RD, McMillan JA, Warshaw JB (eds): Principles and Practice of Pediatrics, 2nd ed. Philadelphia, JB Lippincott, 1994, pp 1685–1699.

Hathaway WE: Bleeding disorders in the newborn infant. *In* Hathaway WE, Bonnar J (eds): Hemostatic Disorders of the Pregnant Woman and Newborn Infant. New York, Elsevier Science, 1987, pp 104–150.

Imbach P: Immune thrombocytopenia in children: The immune character of destructive thrombocytopenia and the treatment of bleeding. Semin Thromb Hemost 1995;21(3):305–312.

129 Childhood Neutropenia

Marc S. C. Cheah

Definition

Neutropenia is defined as a reduction in the number of circulating neutrophils in the peripheral blood. The absolute neutrophil count (ANC) is computed as the percentage of neutrophils and bands in the total white blood cell count. Normal neutrophil levels should be correlated with age and race. For whites, the lower limit for normal neutrophil counts is 1.5×10^9/L. Blacks have a somewhat lower neutrophil count, their lower limit being 1.0×10^9/L.

Risk of Infection

Individual patients may be characterized as having mild, moderate, or severe neutropenia, with the severe cases showing counts generally $\leq 0.5 \times 10^9$/L. This stratification is useful for predicting the risk of pyogenic infections, since only patients with severe neutropenia have significantly increased susceptibility to life-threatening infections (Table 129–1).

Pathophysiology

1. Bone marrow
   a. Production failure
   b. Maturation arrest
   c. Release failure.
2. Peripheral circulation
   a. Accelerated utilization
   b. Reduced survival
   c. Marginal pool shifts.

Disorders Associated with Neutropenia

1. Congenital neutropenias
   a. Kostmann syndrome (infantile agranulocytosis)
      (1) Autosomal recessive, sporadic inheritance
      (2) Patients present during the first month of life with disseminating infections (blood, CNS, peritoneum) and recurrent fevers, stomatitis, cellulitis, and perianal abscesses.
      (3) Absolute neutrophil counts usually $<0.2 \times 10^9$/L
      (4) Bone marrow reveals maturational arrest at the promyelocyte or myelocyte stage with depletion of mature neutrophils.
      (5) Defect: Mutation in G-CSF (granulocyte colony stimulating factor) receptor results in inability to transmit intracellular signals required for granulocytic maturation.
      (6) Treatment: G-CSF
   b. Fanconi anemia
      (1) Autosomal recessive inheritance
      (2) May present as isolated leukopenia or anemia, although usually pancytopenic
      (3) Multiple congenital anomalies: Short stature, hypogonadism; skeletal, CNS, renal, and cardiac anomalies
      (4) Cytogenetics: Chromosomal breakages, gaps, and other structural anomalies with chromatid exchanges and endoreduplications. These anomalies are induced or increased by mutagens such as diepoxybutane (DEB) and are required for the diagnosis of Fanconi anemia.
      (5) Treatment: Prenatal diagnosis possible; steroid and androgen therapy; bone marrow transplantation
   c. Shwachman-Diamond syndrome
      (1) Exocrine pancreatic insufficiency
      (2) Neutropenia
      (3) Metaphyseal chondrodysplasia—short stature
      (4) Chemotactic defect
   d. Cartilage hair hypoplasia
      (1) Autosomal recessive inheritance
      (2) Short-limb dwarfism
      (3) Fine hair
      (4) Moderate neutropenia
   e. Dyskeratosis congenita
      (1) X-linked inheritance
      (2) Leukoplakia, nail dystrophy
      (3) Reticulated hyperpigmentation
      (4) Marrow hypoplasia
      (5) Neutropenia
2. Cyclic neutropenia
   a. Autosomal dominant inheritance
   b. Periodic variations of hematopoietic cells, mostly neutrophils, usually cycling every 21 days
   c. Defect of early hematopoietic precursor cells
   d. Treatment: G-CSF
3. Drug-induced neutropenia
   a. Toxins inducing marrow injury
      (1) Heavy metals, benzene
      (2) Chemotherapy
      (3) Irradiation, radiation therapy
      (4) Drugs: idiosyncratic, hypersensitive hapten-antibody

TABLE 129–1. ANC INDICATOR OF RISK OF INFECTION

	ANC	RISK OF INFECTION
Mild	$>1.0 \times 10^9$/L	None
Moderate	$0.5–1.0 \times 10^9$/L	Minimal (skin, mucous membranes)
Severe	$<0.5 \times 10^9$/L	Pulmonary infection, severe overwhelming sepsis

b. Drugs inducing marrow suppression
   (1) Phenothiazines
   (2) Sulfonamides
   (3) Phenylbutazone
   (4) Chloramphenicol
   (5) Aminopyrine.

4. Neutropenia in infections
   a. Viral infections—Respiratory syncytial virus (RSV), influenzas A and B, measles, rubella, varicella (for HIV infection, see below)
   b. Bacterial infections—Typhoid and paratyphoid fever, rickettsial disease, staphylococcal and pneumococcal infection
   c. Neutropenia may develop during first 24 to 48 hours and persist for 3 to 6 days or longer.
   d. Mechanism
      (1) Margination of neutrophils on endothelial surfaces
      (2) Increased utilization, especially bacterial infections
      (3) Decreased production.
   e. Treatment—Self-limiting; treatment of underlying infection.

5. Autoimmune neutropenia
   a. Primary from antibodies directed at neutrophil-specific antigens, including ND1, NE1
      (1) Usually occurs in children ≤2 years of age
      (2) Resembles autoimmune thrombocytopenia (ITP)
      (3) Usually asymptomatic or mild infection.
      (4) Treatment—Steroids for severe neutropenia with recurrent infection or intravenous immune globulin (IVIG).
   b. Secondary to diseases such as collagen vascular disease, Graves disease, Hashimoto thyroiditis, chronic active hepatitis, lymphoproliferative disease

6. Neutropenia with B- and T-cell abnormalities
   a. Congenital—Dysgammaglobulinemia, X-linked agammaglobulinemia
   b. Acquired—Acquired immunodeficiency disease (AIDS); HIV (human immunodeficiency virus) infection.

Clinical Findings

1. History
   Fever—Degree, duration, regularity, associated symptoms, e.g., chills, rigor
   Symptoms of an acute pyogenic infection: pulmonary or urinary tract infection
   Drug ingestion, including chemotherapy, radiation therapy
   Recent history of viral or bacterial infections
   Family history of recurrent infections, neutropenia.
2. Physical examination
   General—Dwarf, short stature, dysmorphic features
   Skin—Furunculosis, nail dystrophy, hyperpigmentation, fine hair

Ulcerations of mucous membranes: Oral, rectal, vaginal
Evidence of an acute pyogenic infection, including mastoiditis and pharyngitis.

Laboratory Tests

1. Complete blood count with differential and ANC, repeated two to three times a week for at least 8 weeks, if cyclic neutropenia is suspected
2. Bone marrow aspirate and biopsy to evaluate cellularity and maturation of the myeloid cells as well as erythroid precursors
3. Evaluation of immunologic status: humoral and cell-mediated immunity, including CD4/CD8
4. Evaluation of pancreatic function (Shwachman-Diamond syndrome)
5. Chromosome karyotype (Fanconi anemia)
6. Skeletal survey (cartilage hair hypoplasia, Shwachman-Diamond syndrome, Fanconi anemia)
7. Assays for antineutrophil antibodies (autoimmune neutropenia)
8. Steroid mobilization tests help define storage pool size.
9. Miscellaneous: HIV screening, sucrose hemolysis test (paroxysmal nocturnal hemoglobinuria), urine and serum amino acids (metabolic disorders).

Key Laboratory Findings

- Low WBC
- Low neutrophil count (ANC)

Management

Depends on the cause and degree of neutropenia and associated diseases, including the immune status of the patient. Patients with severe neutropenia and little or no marrow reserve have decreased marrow cellularity with early myeloid arrest and tend to have severe pyogenic infections. However, since these patients cannot respond to infection, many of the inflammatory signs of infection may not be present. Management guidelines for patients with neutropenia with fever are given below.

Key Treatment

With Fever	Management
Chemotherapy-induced neutropenia Kostmann syndrome	Broad-spectrum antibiotics initially, with addition of amphotericin if fever and neutropenia persist for >1 week
Without Fever	
Cyclic neutropenia Kostmann syndrome	G-CSF 5–20 μg/kg/dose SC daily for patients with Kostmann syndrome and on alternate days for patients with symptomatic cyclic neutropenia

Bibliography

Baehner RL: Neutropenia. *In* Rakel RE (ed): Conn's Current Therapy. Philadelphia, WB Saunders, 1995, pp 327–329.
Bonilla MA, Gillio AP, Ruggiero M, et al: Effects of recombinant human granulocyte colony–stimulating factor on neutropenia in patients with congenital agranulocytosis. N Engl J Med 1989;320:1574–1580.
Hammond WP, Price TH, Souza LM, Dale DC: Treatment of cyclic neutropenia with granulocyte colony stimulating factor. N Engl J Med 1989;320:1306–1311.

130 Thrombophilia

Andrea Hagani and *James Bussell*

Critical State

Definition
Thrombosis is localized, unregulated hemostasis.

Epidemiology
1. Thrombosis is an underrecognized entity in the pediatric age group.
2. It may occur in a child with several coexisting predispositions, e.g., a congenital abnormality, inflammation (vasculitis), stasis, trauma, and/or a central catheter.
3. Thrombosis is
   a. A major problem in the neonatal period, most commonly associated with central catheters
   b. Relatively uncommon in the first decade of life
   c. More common in the second decade and during adulthood.

Etiology
1. Acquired causes
   a. Central catheters
   b. Shock, dehydration
   c. Cyanotic congenital heart disease
   d. Vascular injury (Kawasaki disease, infection, vasculitis, trauma)
   e. Flow disturbances (A-V shunts, AVMs)
   f. Hyperviscosity (sickle cell disease, polycythemia)
   g. Drugs (estrogen, L-asparaginase, prothrombin complex concentrates)
   h. Immobility
   i. Neoplasms: direct effect and paraneoplastic syndromes
   j. Abortion
   k. Pregnancy (increased c4b binding protein decreases free protein s levels)
   l. Acquired antithrombin III deficiency (liver disease, nephrotic syndrome, DIC, apheresis, neonate, L-asparaginase)
   m. Trauma
   n. Lupus anticoagulant
2. Inherited causes
   a. Antithrombin III deficiency or dysfunction
   b. Protein C deficiency—autosomal recessive trait
      (1) Homozygous patients have more severe thrombotic complications including purpura fulminans, may die in utero, and often present with "neonatal DIC." They are at high risk for deep vein thrombosis (DVT) if they survive.
      (2) Heterozygous patients are at increased risk for thrombosis, especially when coupled with other prothrombotic risk factors, many of which are unknown.
   c. Activated protein C resistance is also called factor V Leiden: most common predisposition to thrombosis; may function as a critical cofactor for other thrombophilic tendencies, e.g., heterozygote protein C deficiency
   d. Protein S deficiency
      (1) More likely to cause arterial thrombosis (especially stroke) than protein C deficiency, but venous thrombosis is still more common.
      (2) Venous thrombosis also occurs as in protein C–deficient patients.
      (3) Free protein S level is crucial—dependent on equilibrium with c4b binding protein.
   e. Homocysteinuria heterozygote: arterial embolic disease in adolescents (female>male); may not be detectable without loading.
   f. Rarer causes
      (1) Heparin cofactor II deficiency
      (2) Plasminogen deficiency
      (3) Increased plasminogen activator inhibitor
      (4) Dysfibrinogenemia—Autosomal dominant inheritance. Depending upon the mutation, pa-

Critical State *Continued*

tients may be at risk for either bleeding or thrombosis (thrombosis much less common).

Pathophysiology

Naturally occurring anticoagulant pathways are present to keep the coagulation cascade in check and prevent thrombosis. When any of the important elements is deficient, clotting can proceed in an unregulated fashion and result in thromboses.

1. Protein C anticoagulant pathway
   a. Thrombin binds to thrombomodulin, which in turn activates protein C.
   b. Proteins C and S form a complex that binds to the activated forms of factors VIII and V on the platelet surface, thereby inactivating them. If factors V and VIII were to remain activated, i.e., in factor V Leiden, a mutation that renders factor V insensitive to activated protein C, clotting would continue, resulting in thrombosis.
   c. Protein C also inhibits platelet and fibrin deposition and therefore helps prevent arterial thrombosis (e.g., in grafts or catheters).
   d. Factor V Leiden occurs in as many as 3 per cent of Caucasians and may be a common cofactor for other tendencies to thrombosis.
2. Anti–thrombin III pathway
   a. Its efficiency of inhibition of serine proteases, e.g., thrombin, is catalyzed (accelerated) by heparin; little fluid phase efficacy
   b. Naturally occurring glycoaminoglycans on intact endothelial cell contributes to nonthrombotic nature of endothelial cells
   c. Many clotting factors are serine proteases, e.g., X, IX, VII.
3. Stasis due to immobilization, hyperviscosity, polycythemia, congestive heart failure, vascular damage, or occlusion is a major cause of thrombosis.
4. Abnormal intravascular surfaces due to indwelling catheters, artificial heart valves, vasculitis (e.g., Kawasaki disease, SLE), or homocysteinuria can also lead to thrombosis. Different entities can mediate their effects by different pathways (e.g., stimulation of coagulation, activation of platelets, or inhibition of fibrinolysis).

Clinical Findings

1. Venous thromboses
   a. Deep vein thrombosis
      (1) Tenderness, warmth, and swelling of the affected extremity with positive Homans sign
      (2) Flow Doppler ultrasound demonstrates decreased flow in the affected vessel. Venograms are required in very selected cases only. Can be used only when the vessel in question is accessible to sonography; limited use for superior vena cava syndrome.
      (3) Careful studies in adults have documented a limited ability to make a precise diagnosis on physical examination *alone*.
   b. Renal vein thrombosis
      (1) Associated with asphyxia, dehydration, shock, infant of diabetic mother, and sepsis in newborns and infants.
      (2) Sudden onset of gross hematuria and unilateral or bilateral flank masses. Hypertension may also be present.
      (3) Patients also have a microangiopathic hemolytic anemia and (consumptive) thrombocytopenia.
      (4) Radiologic evaluation
         (a) Ultrasound—renal enlargement, abnormal blood flow
         (b) Radionuclide studies—decreased function of the affected kidney
         (c) CT scan or MRI may be needed to distinguish from intraabdominal tumor or from adrenal hemorrhage.
   c. Cerebral venous thrombosis
      (1) Presents with abnormal neurologic findings depending on the site of occlusion, including the sagittal sinus, lateral sinus, and cavernous sinus. Symptoms can include signs of increased intracranial pressure (headache and vomiting), seizures, paresis, chills, fever, and altered mental status.
      (2) Radiologic evaluation
         (a) CT scan may reveal swelling, infarct or hemorrhage.
         (b) MRI, MRA, or, if necessary, cerebral angiography can confirm the diagnosis and localize the site of obstruction.
   d. Purpura fulminans
      (1) Can be a presentation of severe protein C or S deficiency in the neonatal period
      (2) Diffuse cutaneous thrombotic lesions are present, similar to those seen in DIC; may progress to blackish lesions and loss of digits or even parts of extremities.
      (3) May be associated with an otherwise typical acute infectious (viral) episode resulting in acquired (transient) severe protein C deficiency.
2. Arterial thromboses
   a. Cerebrovascular
      (1) Patients present with focal neurologic signs related to the site of infarction or with signs of increased intracranial pressure.
      (2) CT scan and MRI are helpful, as in venous thromboses.

Critical State *Continued*

b. Renal artery thrombosis

(1) Usually associated with umbilical artery catheters, this entity often presents with hematuria, proteinuria, oliguria or anuria, and azotemia. Hypertension may be present but is more common with renal vein thrombosis. Renal failure can occur if the obstruction is bilateral.

(2) Radiologic evaluation includes ultrasound with flow studies and radionuclide imaging.

Key Clinical Findings

- Deep vein thrombosis
- Purpura fulminans

Evaluation

1. Both patient and family histories as well as the type of thrombosis are extremely important in determining the extent of the work-up indicated in an individual with thrombosis. However, in children with thromboses, a systemic work-up, detailed below, is usually warranted. This work-up must pursue multiple predisposing factors and should not be satisfied by only one explanation for thrombosis. This is true also for patients with polycythemia and SLE or other collagen vascular disorders. It remains unclear whether neonates and children with predisposing factors, one episode of thrombosis, and no significant family history require a work-up for these additional causes of thrombosis and, if so, which ones. Similarly, it is unclear if children without a clear etiology require additional investigation by a particularly experienced hematologist if the initial work-up (ATIII, proteins C *and* S, *and* factor V Leiden) fails to reveal an etiology.

a. In general, arterial thromboses without other predisposing factors, such as catheters, mandate a systemic work-up as well.

b. Patients with recurrent venous thromboses or those with family members who have suffered similar complications also require a systemic work-up that pursues an etiology.

2. Systemic work-up

a. PT, aPTT, Staclot test (looking for a lupus type anticoagulant)

b. Thrombin time, fibrinogen

c. Proteins C and S and antithrombin III levels

d. Factor V Leiden

Additional work-up could be performed when the index of suspicion for a predisposition to thrombophilia is high and the above work-up fails to reveal such an etiology. It could include functional assays for the above factors, urine for homocysteine and/or a homocysteine loading test, plas-

minogen level or function, and other tests depending upon the clinical picture.

Urgently needed ongoing studies helping to define this field may alter these recommendations, especially in newborns.

Treatment

1. General principles guiding treatment

a. The presence of a clot (especially in conjunction with a catheter) does not in itself mandate any therapy.

b. The critical reason to treat thrombosis is either ongoing organ damage or high risk of such damage. This is more apparent in arterial than in venous thrombosis. Over time, however, venous insufficiency may result in substantial morbidity.

c. Different imaging studies provide optimal information for therapy decisions depending upon the type and site of the thrombosis.

2. Neonatal thrombosis

a. If the thrombosis is catheter-related, the catheter should be immediately removed unless it is required for diagnostic imaging studies or targeted infusion of fibrinolytic agents.

b. Surgical thrombectomy may be an option depending on the site and on surgical expertise but typically cannot be performed owing to the small vessel size. It also impedes postoperative anticoagulation, allowing re-formation of thrombosis and progression of microthrombi.

c. If the thrombosis is progressive with evidence of organ dysfunction (e.g., renal failure in the case of renal vessel involvement), anticoagulant and especially thrombolytic therapy should be strongly considered. *A head ultrasound is a mandatory part of the decision process in order not to exacerbate a preexisting intracranial hemorrhage, especially in a premature infant.*

d. Heparin therapy

(1) Higher doses of heparin are required in the neonate owing to increased clearance and lower AT III levels.

(a) Preterm—50 U/kg bolus; 20 to 30 U/kg/h maintenance. Adjust to prolong PTT.

(b) Full-term—100 U/kg bolus; 25 U/kg/hr maintenance.

(2) Platelet transfusions should be given to keep the count >50,000/μl. Plasma should be given to keep the fibrinogen >100 mg/dl and the PT <15 seconds. It may also increase AT III levels as would the plasma in platelet concentrates.

(3) Continue heparin until the clot has cleared or is significantly decreasing in size. This usually takes about 7 to 21 days.

(4) Long-term (oral) anticoagulation is rarely indicated, in part because of difficulties in dosing. Subcutaneous heparin may be used (70 unit/kg q 8–12 hours) The efficacy and dosing of low molecular weight heparin in the newborn is incompletely defined.

(5) Antithrombin III concentrate is under investigation as a way to optimize heparinization.

e. Fibrinolytic therapy

(1) Efficacy in neonates has not been well established and is currently undergoing evaluation.

(2) Much higher doses of urokinase (> 4400 U/kg/hr) or streptokinase are required in neonates because their plasminogen is more resistant to lysis.

(3) The risk of bleeding is high if thrombocytopenia or hypofibrinogenemia is present. Therefore, transfusion therapy is vital.

(4) There are currently no data favoring urokinase over tPA and vice versa.

3. Thrombosis in older children

a. Anticoagulant therapy

(1) Heparin bolus 50 to 100 U/kg IV, then 15 to 25 U/kg/hr continuous infusion. Adjust rate every 4–8h until aPTT is 1.5 to 2.0 × the upper limit of normal.

(2) For prophylactic heparin in patients at high risk for thrombosis (e.g., immobilized patients), give subcutaneous heparin 70 U/kg every 8 to 12 hours. The PTT will not be prolonged and does not need to be followed.

(3) Warfarin (Coumadin) therapy—Because the effect of warfarin is not reached until after 4 to 5 days, heparin and warfarin are given together until the warfarin is therapeutic, at which point the heparin can be discontinued.

(a) Start with a dose of 0.1 mg/kg/day po with a maximum of 10 mg/day; a single loading dose to speed the onset of the effect is useful, e.g., 10 to 20 mg.

(b) The PT will not be prolonged until after about 2 days. Adjust the dose to achieve a PT 1.5 to 2 × control. *Remember:* The dose given today affects the PT in 48 to 72 hours. You actually need to use international normalized ratios (INRs) to correct for the different reagents in use in different laboratories. Usually the INR should be 2 to 3× control. *Note:* The INR can be used only in the steady state.

(c) Maintenance for infants is usually 1 to 2 mg/day.

(d) Patients with heterozygous protein C defi-ciency may experience warfarin-induced skin necrosis, which requires continued use of heparin therapy or protein C replacement until stable coumadinization is achieved (approximately 1 week).

b. Thrombolytic therapy

(1) Urokinase—Loading dose = 4400 U/kg IV in 15 ml over 30 min, then 4400 U/kg/hr for 12 to 48 hours if for pulmonary embolus and for 24 to 72 hours if for DVT or peripheral arterial occlusion.

(2) Streptokinase—Loading dose = 250,000 U IV over 30 min, then 100,000 U/hr for 12 to 48 hours if for pulmonary embolism and for 24 to 72 hours if for DVT or peripheral arterial occlusion.

(3) To monitor both these therapies, follow thrombin time, PT, aPTT, and platelet count. The thrombin time should be 2 to 5 × normal.

(a) If this has not been achieved after 4 to 8 hours, stop the infusion and start heparin.

(b) If the thrombin time is >7 to 8 × normal, hold the infusion until it is back to 5 × normal and then restart at half the dose.

(4) Start heparin 4 hours after completion of thrombolytic therapy. Often, low-dose heparin (10 U/kg/hr) is used simultaneously with fibrinolytic therapy to prevent rethrombosis.

(5) Contraindications to thrombolytic therapy

(a) Surgery within past 10 days (including biopsy, thoracentesis, paracentesis)

(b) Intraarterial diagnostic procedure within 10 days

(c) Active GI bleeding

(d) Abnormal hemostasis

(e) Recent CVA or predisposing condition

(f) Intracranial tumor

(g) Severe diastolic hypertension

(h) Active cavitary lung disease

(i) Acute or chronic renal or hepatic insufficiency other than that due to current thrombosis

(j) Ulcerative cutaneous lesion

(k) Pregnancy or within 10 days post partum.

(6) Precautions

(a) Avoid invasive procedures and excessive handling of patient.

(b) Avoid anticoagulants and antiplatelet agents other than low-dose heparin.

(7) Adverse reactions

(a) Bleeding, fever, allergic reaction

(b) If bleeding occurs, give Amicar 5 g po or

Critical State

IV over 1 hour load, then 1 g q 2–4 hr. Then follow thrombin time and when <2 × normal, start heparin.

4. Severe, homozygous protein C deficiency (purpura fulminans)

   a. In the acute setting, treatment consists of fresh frozen plasma and prothrombin complex concentrates, both sources of protein C. Currently, a protein C product is not available but should be soon and will be the treatment of choice.

   b. After the acute illness has been controlled, warfarin therapy should be instituted to prevent recurrences.

Key Treatment

- Heparin
- Fibrinolytic therapy
- Surgery

Bibliography

Schmidt B, Andrew M: Neonatal thrombosis: report of a prospective Canadian and international registry. Pediatrics 1995;96(5, Pt 1):939–943.

131 Disseminated Intravascular Coagulation

Mary Kaufman

Critical State

Definition

Disseminated intravascular coagulation (DIC) is a profound hemorrhagic disorder associated with activation of procoagulant, anticoagulant, and fibrinolytic mechanisms by trigger events such as severe gram-negative sepsis, hypotensive shock, massive trauma, leukemia, malignancies, or release of tissue factor; it can be acute, subacute, or chronic. A list of disorders that may be associated with DIC is given in Table 131–1. Diffuse activation of clotting factors results in fibrin formation, depletion of multiple clotting factors, and activation of fibrinolysis.

Epidemiology

Disseminated intravascular coagulation occurs worldwide without any gender, age, or ethnic predilection.

Pathophysiology

1. In DIC there is massive activation of the coagulation system that results in increased thrombin and fibrin production. Common triggers are intravascular release of tissue factor, endotoxin, immune complexes, and diffuse endothelial damage. This is aggravated by hypoxia, acidosis, and slowing of the microcirculation, which favors thrombosis. There are deficiencies of procoagulant, anticoagulant, and fibrinolytic factors. There is both microvascular hemorrhage and thrombosis depending on the balance between proteolytic enzymes, enzyme cofactors, and inhibitors. Gross thrombi are not often seen, but platelet-fibrin thrombi are found in the smallest blood vessels, especially in lung, liver, and kidney.

2. Immune complexes activate FXII and/or FXI and platelets and damage endothelium and so start the process. The increase in clotting leads to activation of fibrinolysis, with resultant biodegradation of factors I, V, VIII, IX, and XI via plasmin. Complement is also activated, generating kinins, which increase vascular permeability and slow the blood flow.

3. The neonate is at an increased risk for DIC because of poor splenic clearance of activated coagulant factors and low levels of antithrombin III (AT III) and proteins C and S, decreased plasminogen, poor ability to compensate by increasing platelet production, and decreased response to fibrinolysis. Infections, respiratory distress syndrome (RDS), severe liver disease, or severe cold stress will aggravate all of these.

4. The bleeding seen in DIC may be due to thrombocytopenia, decreased concentration of clotting factors, inhibition of fibrin polymerization by fibrin degradation products (FDPs), and increased fibrinolysis. In acute DIC the process is so rapid that there is little time for compensation, and bleeding is prominent. In chronic DIC, thrombosis may be more frequent than bleeding because of compensation or even overcompensation.

Clinical Findings

1. The clinical picture will depend on the primary underlying disease. The patient is usually profoundly ill. Fever,

TABLE 131–1. CONDITIONS ASSOCIATED WITH DIC

I. INFECTIONS

Bacterial
Gram-positive (group B
Streptococcus)
Gram-negative
meningococcemia
Haemophilus,
Pseudomonas
Viral—varicella, CMV
Parasitic—malaria
Fungal
Rickettsial—
Rocky Mountain spotted
fever

II. TISSUE INJURY

Severe head injury
Crush injury
Profound shock, hypoxia
Hypothermia
Burns

III. MALIGNANCY

Acute promyelocytic
leukemia
Acute myeloblastic or
monoblastic leukemia
Disseminated tumors

IV. VENOM OR TOXIN

Snake bite, insect bite

**V. MICROANGIOPATHIC
HEMOLYTIC ANEMIA**

Hemolytic uremic syndrome
Thrombotic thrombocytopenic
purpura
Giant hemangioma (Kasabach-
Merritt syndrome)

**VI. HEREDITARY
THROMBOTIC
DISORDERS**

Homozygous protein C
deficiency
Antithrombin III deficiency

NEWBORN

Infections
Maternal trauma
Severe respiratory distress
Abruptio placentae
Necrotizing enterocolitis

MISCELLANEOUS

Hemolytic transfusion reaction
Infusion of activated prothrombin
complex concentrates
Severe collagen vascular disease

TABLE 131–2. LABORATORY FINDINGS IN DIC

TEST	RESULTS
Platelet Count	Decreased
Coagulant Factors	
Factor I (fibrinogen)	Decreased
Factor II (prothrombin)	Decreased
Factor V	Decreased
Factor VIII	Decreased
Anticoagulant Factors	
Proteins C, S; AT III	Decreased
Fibrinolytic System	
Plasminogen	Decreased
α_2-Antiplasmin	Decreased
Fibrin split products	Increased
Blood Smear	Decreased platelets, red cell fragmentation, spherocytes, toxic changes in neutrophils in severe sepsis

hypotension, acidosis, and hypoxia are common. Petechiae, purpura, acral cyanosis, hemorrhagic bullae, oozing from puncture sites, and even peripheral gangrene may be seen. There may be evidence of cardiac, pulmonary, renal, hepatic, and central nervous system dysfunction. All these manifestations are in addition to the clinical picture of the primary disease.

2. Obstetric catastrophes in the mother can also cause DIC in neonates, with massive bleeding leading to shock and death.

Key Clinical Findings

- Petechiae

- Oozing from puncture sites

Laboratory Diagnosis

1. Screening tests usually reveal thrombocytopenia and prolonged PT, PTT, and thrombin time.
2. Coagulation factor assays reveal decreased levels of fibrinogen, prothrombin, and factors V and VIII.
3. Fibrinopeptides A and B, FDPs, and fibrin monomer, indicative of breakdown of fibrinogen and fibrin, are usually present in the plasma of patients with DIC (Table 131–2).

Treatment

1. Since DIC is a secondary complication, first efforts must be directed at aggressive treatment of the primary disease. Tissue perfusion, oxygen delivery, and acid-base balance must be improved along with administration of appropriate antimicrobials.
2. Replacement of deficient clotting factors via cryoprecipitate or fresh frozen plasma and platelets is only an adjunct. Exchange transfusion can also accomplish this and is used when practical, especially in newborn infants.
3. Heparin is usually recommended in patients with purpura fulminans to prevent further thrombosis and tissue necrosis as well as in some patients with chronic DIC. An initial loading dose of 50 to 100 U/kg is given as IV push followed by 10 U/kg/hr as continuous infusion. Response to therapy is demonstrated by increase in plasma fibrinogen and platelet count and decrease in fibrin split products. There must be adequate levels of AT III for heparin to be effective. This can be achieved by infusion of fresh frozen plasma.
4. Finally, the effectiveness of therapy for DIC depends on how well the underlying process is controlled.

Key Treatment

- Treatment of primary conditions

- Replacement of clotting factors and platelets

- Heparin (purpura fulminans)

Purpura Fulminans

1. It is an acute illness that is potentially fatal and is characterized by rapid development of large ecchymotic areas, with eventual necrosis of skin and subcutaneous tissues. Cutaneous lesions are frequently seen in lower extremi-

ties, although they can be seen over the entire body. Infections that may be associated with purpura fulminans are varicella, scarlet fever, meningococcemia, pneumococcal sepsis, and gram-negative sepsis. There is frequently laboratory evidence of DIC.

2. In addition to appropriate treatment of the underlying disease, heparin therapy should be started as soon as possible. Administration of platelets and fresh frozen plasma is often required. Neonatal purpura fulminans is usually caused by homozygous protein C deficiency. Therapy consists of administration of protein C concentrate or fresh frozen plasma when protein C concentrate is not available.

Bibliography

Bick RL: Disseminated intravascular coagulation: Clin Lab Med 1994;1:729–768.
Ratnoff OD: Disseminated intravascular coagulation. *In* Ratnoff OD, Forbes CD (eds): Disorders of Hemostasis, 2nd ed. Philadelphia, WB Saunders, 1991, pp 292–326.
Scott JP, Montgomery RR: Disseminated intravascular coagulation. *In* Nathan DG, Oski FA (eds): Hematology of Infancy and Childhood, 4th ed. Philadelphia, WB Saunders, 1993, pp 1605–1650.
Williams EC, Mosher DF: Disseminated intravascular coagulation. *In* Hoffman R, Benz EJ Jr, Shattil SJ, et al (eds): Hematology: Basic Principles and Practice, 2nd ed. New York, Churchill Livingstone, 1995, pp 1758–1769.

132 Blood Transfusion

Elizabeth Gloster

Definition

Blood transfusion is the intravenous infusion of whole blood and blood components and derivatives, i.e., plasma, packed red cells, platelets, leukocytes, cryoprecipitate, albumin, and factor and/or immunoglobulin concentrates.

Blood Groups/Antigen Systems

1. The most important antigen system in red cell transfusion is the ABO system. ABO antigens are weakly expressed at birth but usually reach almost full expression by 18 months of age. Concurrently, as a result of stimulation by substances in the environment, possibly bacteria and food, naturally occurring plasma antibodies develop against those ABO antigen specificities lacking on the red cells (Table 132–1). Red cell transfusions must be compatible with, i.e., lack the antigens corresponding to, recipient ABO antibodies. An immediate hemolytic transfusion reaction with intravascular hemolysis may follow an ABO-incompatible transfusion.

2. The Rh system is next in importance. Its antigens (C, D, E, c, e) are fully developed at birth. The most immunogenic of these is the D antigen. Rh antibodies are not naturally occurring. D and the other Rh antigens can alloimmunize, or stimulate irregular antibodies in, antigen-negative recipients during transfusion or during pregnancy and delivery. These may cause hemolysis that is predominantly, though not exclusively, extravascular.

   a. Individuals lacking the D antigen, commonly referred to as Rh negative, should be transfused with red cells and red cell–containing components (e.g., platelet and granulocyte concentrates) from Rh-negative donors.

   b. If Rh-negative red cell–containing components are unavailable and transfusion is necessary, it may be possible to prevent alloimmunization by the administration of Rh immune globulin (a preparation of high-titer anti-D), with dose, timing, and mode of administration recommended by the blood bank physician.

3. Other significant red cell antigens, such as those of the Kell, Kidd, and Duffy families, also may stimulate irregular antibodies in a manner similar to the Rh system. These can cause variable degrees of hemol-

TABLE 132–1. ANTIGEN AND ANTIBODY CHARACTERISTICS OF THE MAJOR ABO GROUPS

BLOOD GROUP	RED CELL ANTIGEN	PLASMA ANTIBODY
O	—	Anti-A, -B, -AB
A	A	Anti-B
B	B	Anti-A
AB	AB	—

Procedure *Continued*

ysis—usually, but not exclusively, extravascular hemolysis.

Indications and Special Considerations for Component Transfusion

1. Current medicolegal opinion favors full and documented discussion by the transfusing physician with patients or their surrogates about the indications for, risks and benefits of, and alternatives to elective transfusion. The worst known adverse effects should be mentioned as well as the possibility that there may be other, as yet unknown, ill effects.

2. It is prudent to follow local law and hospital guidelines for this discussion and its documentation. If none exist, a chart note, signed and dated by the transfusing physician and including the elements mentioned above, is advisable.

3. The effects of transfusion should be documented, i.e., clinical and/or laboratory evaluation. Although some authorities recommend counts before and 1 hour after platelet transfusion, prothrombin times (PT) and activated partial thromboplastin times (APTT) before and after fresh frozen plasma transfusion, and hematocrits before and within 24 hours after red cell transfusions, this may not always be necessary, may be impractical for small children, and may increase transfusion requirements in sick infants.

4. The Transfusion Practices Quality Assurance Committee of the American Association of Blood Banks has issued and updated guidelines for auditing pediatric transfusions. Audit guidelines are not identical to indications or standards of care; i.e., physicians may wish to transfuse in situations not covered by the audit guidelines or may elect to withhold transfusions in situations that meet audit criteria for component administration. Also, each hospital has the right and responsibility to set up its own guidelines. However, the published and periodically updated audit guidelines offer insight into the current consensus regarding appropriate indications for transfusion.

   a. *Whole blood or reconstituted whole blood* (red cells reconstituted with fresh frozen plasma). Whole blood is generally unavailable, and its use is discouraged in modern transfusion practice. Red cells reconstituted with fresh frozen plasma are offered instead by many transfusion services. Isotonic (0.9%) saline or 5 per cent albumin may be used instead of fresh frozen plasma for some exchange transfusions, depending upon the indication, the number of exchanges required, and the age and coagulation status of the child. The dose generally reflects the volume of blood to be replaced. For large-volume transfusions, red cells that are negative for hemoglobin S, no older than 7 days, and

preferably collected in CPDA-1 or CPD should be used, if available. They should be CMV seronegative for intrauterine transfusions, for infants weighing <1200 g at birth (when either the recipient or the mother is CMV seronegative or that information is unknown), and for other categories of immunodeficient patients. Leukocyte depletion reduces the risk of CMV transmission by seropositive red cells. Finally, the red cells should be irradiated for intrauterine transfusion, for selected immunocompetent or immunocompromised recipients, for patients with Hodgkin disease, for patients who have received bone marrow or peripheral stem cell transplantation, and if the donor is a blood relative of the transfusion recipient. Some authorities also recommend irradiation of red cells to be used for exchange transfusion for newborns who previously have received intrauterine transfusion (Table 132–2).

   b. *Red cells.* There are separate guidelines for infants <4 months of age, reflecting the normally high hemoglobin in the first day of life and the impact of phlebotomy losses in very young sick infants (Table 132–3). For older infants and children, the guidelines are similar to those for adults (Table 132–4). The standard dose is 10 to 15 ml/kg and

---

TABLE 132–2. PEDIATRIC AUDIT GUIDELINES FOR WHOLE BLOOD OR RECONSTITUTED WHOLE BLOOD (RED CELLS RECONSTITUTED WITH FRESH FROZEN PLASMA) TRANSFUSION

Some institutions may wish to consider making whole blood (or its equivalent) available for neonates for the following circumstances:
Exchange transfusion
Extracorporeal membrane oxygenation and cardiopulmonary bypass
Replacement of >1 unit blood volume in 24 hours

From Stehling L, Luban NLC, Anderson KC, et al: Guidelines for blood utilization review. Transfusion 1994;34:438–448.

TABLE 132–3. PEDIATRIC AUDIT GUIDELINES FOR RED CELL TRANSFUSION TO CHILDREN YOUNGER THAN 4 MONTHS OF AGE

Hemoglobin <130 g/L (<13 g/dl) and severe pulmonary or cyanotic heart disease or heart failure
Acute loss of ≥10 per cent of blood volume or phlebotomy for laboratory testing when cumulative amount exceeds 10 per cent of blood volume in a 1-week period
Hemoglobin <80 g/L (<8 g/dl) in a stable newborn infant with clinical manifestations of anemia

From Stehling L, Luban NLC, Anderson KC, et al: Guidelines for blood utilization review. Transfusion 1994;34:438–448.

TABLE 132–4. PEDIATRIC AUDIT GUIDELINES FOR RED CELL TRANSFUSION TO CHILDREN OLDER THAN 4 MONTHS OF AGE

Preoperative hemoglobin <80 g/L (<8 g/dL) when alternative therapy is not available or postoperative hemoglobin <80 g/L (<8 g/dl) with signs or symptoms of anemia

Acute loss of ≥15 per cent of blood volume or signs and symptoms of hypovolemia that is not responsive to fluid administration

Hemoglobin <130 g/ (<13 g/L) and severe cardiopulmonary disease

Hemoglobin <80 g/L (<8 g/dl) in patients receiving chemotherapy and/or radiotherapy

Hemoglobin <80 g/L (<8 g/dl) in patients with chronic anemia without expected response to medical therapy and signs or symptoms of anemia

Complications of sickle cell disease, such as cerebrovascular accident, acute chest syndrome, or for preoperative preparation

Chronic transfusion regimen for thalassemia or other red cell–dependent disorder

From Stehling L, Luban NLC, Anderson KC, et al: Guidelines for blood utilization review. Transfusion 1994;34:438–448.

TABLE 132–6. ADULT AND PEDIATRIC (FULL-TERM INFANTS AND ALL OTHER CHILDREN) GUIDELINES FOR PLATELET TRANSFUSION

Platelet count <10–20 $\times$ 10^9/L (<10,000–20,000/μl) in a nonbleeding patient with failure of platelet production

Platelet count <50 $\times$ 10^9/L (<50,000/μL) and impending surgery or invasive procedure

Diffuse microvascular bleeding in a patient with documented disseminated intravascular coagulation or transfusion ≥1 unit blood volume and platelet count <50 $\times$ 10^9/L (<50,000/μl) or laboratory values not yet available

Diffuse microvascular bleeding following cardiopulmonary bypass or with intraaortic balloon pump and platelet count not yet available or <100 $\times$ 10^9/L (<100,000/μl)

Bleeding in a patient with a qualitative platelet defect, regardless of platelet count

From Stehling L, Luban NLC, Anderson KC, et al: Guidelines for blood utilization review. Transfusion 1994; 34:438–448.

may vary within that range, depending upon the hematocrit of the packed cells. The recommendations for CMV seronegativity and irradiation (see above) apply for red cells.

c. *Platelets.* There are separate guidelines for premature infants because they may have hemostatic abnormalities and are felt to be at increased risk for intracranial hemorrhage (Table 132–5). For other infants and older children, the guidelines are similar to those for adults (Table 132–6). The standard dose to raise the platelet count of a newborn infant above 100 $\times$ 10^9/L is 10 ml/kg. For older, nonbleeding thrombocytopenic children, 1 unit (U) per 10 to 15 kg of platelets prepared from conventional blood donation may be sufficient to prevent bleeding, whereas larger doses (e.g., 1 U/5 kg) may be necessary for bleeding patients. The recommendations for CMV seronegativity, leukocyte depletion of CMV seropositive concentrates, and irradiation (see above) apply for platelets. In addition, HLA-matched platelets should be irradiated.

(1) Platelets should not be administered for autoimmune thrombocytopenia unless there is life-threatening bleeding. Such disorders should be treated with intravenous IgG and steroids.

TABLE 132–5. PEDIATRIC AUDIT GUIDELINES FOR PLATELET TRANSFUSION TO PREMATURE INFANTS (GESTATIONAL AGE LESS THAN 37 WEEKS)

Platelet count <50 $\times$ 10^9/L (<50,000/μl) in a stable infant

Platelet count <100 $\times$ 10^{9}L (<100,000/μl) in a sick infant

Institutions performing extracorporeal membrane oxygenation may wish to develop specific guidelines for this procedure.

From Stehling L, Luban NLC, Anderson KC, et al: Guidelines for blood utilization review. Transfusion 1994;34:438–448.

(2) *Neonatal alloimmune thrombocytopenia* is caused by transplacental passage of maternal alloantibody directed against an antigen on fetal (but not maternal) platelets, most commonly P1^{A1}. If the infant is severely thrombocytopenic, bleeding, or at risk of bleeding, either maternal platelets or platelets from a known antigen-negative donor should be transfused. If maternal platelets are used, their antibody-containing plasma should be removed; platelets from the mother or any other close relative should be irradiated prior to transfusion.

(3) *Qualitative platelet defects* may be inherited (e.g., Bernard-Soulier syndrome) or acquired as a result of uremia, myeloproliferative disorder, cardiopulmonary bypass, and exposure to aspirin-containing drugs. Platelet transfusions should be given in response to significant bleeding. They should not be given prophylactically, unless there is an additional risk factor for bleeding or an invasive procedure is scheduled and bleeding is a concern. Desmopressin acetate (DDAVP) may enhance platelet function, especially in uremia, and lessen the need for platelet transfusion.

d. *Fresh frozen plasma.* Fresh frozen plasma is appropriate for deficiencies of multiple coagulation factors. The standard dose is 15 ml/kg. It has been used also for C1 esterase inhibitor deficiency if specific concentrate is unavailable. The indications are similar for adults and children (Table 132–7). There are several additional indications, most of them specific to neonates.

(1) Reconstitution of red cells to a whole-blood equivalent, usually for exchange transfusion, as mentioned above

Procedure *Continued*

TABLE 132–7. ADULT AND PEDIATRIC AUDIT GUIDELINES FOR FRESH FROZEN PLASMA TRANSFUSION

PT and PTT >1.5 × the mean normal value in a nonbleeding patient scheduled for surgery or invasive procedure

Diffuse microvascular bleeding in a patient given ≥1 blood volume and PT and PTT >1.5 × the mean normal value or not yet available

Warfarin overdose with major bleeding or impending surgery

Other indications may include thrombotic thrombocytopenic purpura, emergency reversal of warfarin, and treatment of plasma anticoagulant deficiencies such as protein C, protein S, or antithrombin III when specific therapy is not available or advisable

From Stehling L, Luban NLC, Anderson KC, et al: Guidelines for blood utilization review. Transfusion 1994; 34:438–448.

TABLE 132–9. PEDIATRIC AUDIT GUIDELINES FOR GRANULOCYTE TRANSFUSION

Bacterial sepsis in an infant <2 weeks of age with neutrophil count <3 × 10^9/L (<3000/μl)

Bacterial sepsis or disseminated fungal infection that is unresponsive to antibiotics in a patient >2 weeks of age with neutrophil count <0.5 × 10^9L (<500/μl)

Infection that is unresponsive to antibiotics and the presence of a qualitative neutrophil defect, regardless of neutrophil count

From Stehling L, Luban NLC, Anderson KC, et al: Guidelines for blood utilization review. Transfusion 1994; 34:438–448.

(2) Hemorrhage secondary to vitamin K deficiency

(3) Disseminated intravascular coagulation (DIC)

(4) Hemorrhage secondary to congenital coagulation factor deficiency, if more specific therapy is unavailable or inappropriate.

e. *Cryoprecipitate.* The indications are similar for adults and children (Table 132–8). For hypofibrinogenemia, therapy should be directed toward achieving a fibrinogen level of 100 mg/dl. Two units of cryoprecipitate/10 kg of body weight will generally raise the fibrinogen level by 100 mg/dl, except in instances of consumptive coagulopathy. A baseline fibrinogen level should be obtained prior to deciding upon a dosage. Often 1 U/7–10 kg of body weight is adequate. The treatment of choice for patients with hemophilia or von Willebrand disease who are unresponsive to DDAVP or for whom it is inappropriate (von Willebrand disease, type III; type IIB currently is being reevaluated) is a factor VIII concentrate. At this time, only Humate-P and possibly Alphanate contain von Willebrand factor. Similarly, cryoprecipitate may be used to treat factor XIII deficiency, if specific factor concentrate is unavailable (see also Chapters 125 and 126).

f. *Granulocytes.* Currently, granulocyte transfusions are not as popular for neutropenic infected adults or children as they were a decade or two ago. This is because of the efficacy of antibiotics and marrow recovery in resolving infection, the difficulty in obtaining adult therapeutic doses of granulocytes, and

TABLE 132–8. ADULT AND PEDIATRIC AUDIT GUIDELINES FOR CRYOPRECIPITATE TRANSFUSION

Diffuse microvascular bleeding and fibrinogen <100 mg/dl (1.0 g/L)

von Willebrand disease or, in selected patients, hemophilia unresponsive to 1-deamino-8-D-arginine vasopressin (DDAVP)

Dysfibrinogenemias

Factor XIII deficiency

Modified from Stehling L, Luban NLC, Anderson KC, et al: Guidelines for blood utilization review. Transfusion 1994; 34:438–448.

conflicting reports regarding their usefulness. There is some evidence that apheresis granulocyte concentrates may be useful in conjunction with antibiotics for neutropenic septic neonates in the first few weeks of life as well as for selected older children (Table 132–9). Neonates and infants weighing <10 kg should receive 1–2 × 10^9 neutrophils/kg/infusion. Larger infants and children should receive at least 1 × 10^{10} neutrophils and adolescents 2–3 × 10^{10} neutrophils/infusion if possible. Granulocytes should be administered daily until either the infection resolves or the neutrophil count rises to greater than 0.5 × 10^9/L (>500/μl). Granulocyte concentrates generally are contaminated with red cells and therefore must be ABO- and crossmatch-compatible with the recipient. The recommendations for CMV seronegativity (*but not for leukocyte depletion*) and irradiation (see above) apply for granulocytes, and some authorities feel that all granulocyte concentrates should be irradiated. Granulocytes should *not* be transfused through microaggregate depth (20–40 μm) or leukocyte-removal filters.

Adverse Reactions to Blood Transfusions

1. Hemolytic transfusion reactions can be divided into immune and nonimmune etiologies and acute and delayed presentations.

   a. Immune hemolysis is that caused by antibodies, usually alloantibodies.

      (1) The most common cause of acute immune hemolytic transfusion reaction is ABO mismatching secondary to identification errors at the time of specimen collection or initiation of transfusion.

         (a) Neonates lack ABO antibodies, and red cell alloimmunization is extremely uncommon during the first few months of life.

         (b) Older children have ABO antibodies and may acquire irregular antibodies (alloantibodies).

Procedure *Continued*

(c) Acute hemolytic transfusion reactions present as intravascular hemolysis, manifest within minutes to hours of transfusion, and may cause fever, chills, tachycardia, shock, back pain, cyanosis, hemoglobinuria, and gastrointestinal symptoms. In a neonate, such a reaction might be subtle but probably would include hypotension and abnormality in pulse rate and/or rhythm.

(d) In the face of *any* of these, the transfusion must be stopped immediately, the intravenous access maintained, and the blood bag, tubing, and intravenous fluids sent to the blood bank with the appropriate documentation and specimens.

(e) A urinalysis also should be requested, including a microscopic examination. It is important to distinguish hematuria, i.e., the presence of free red cells in urine, from hemoglobinuria, the presence of free hemoglobin. Both, as well as myoglobin, can cause red urine and a positive dipstick result, but only hemoglobinuria is suggestive of hemolysis.

(f) If hemolytic transfusion reaction is confirmed, baseline and follow-up coagulation and renal function studies should be obtained. Renal function should be preserved by alkalinization of the urine, administration of fluids, and furosemide, if necessary, in dosages appropriate to the patient's hydration. Such patients should be moved to intensive care areas if possible.

(2) Delayed hemolytic transfusion reactions are not uncommon among adults and older children but are rare in neonates. They are noted from days to weeks after transfusion and generally are caused by an anamnestic rise in titer of a previously absent or undetected alloantibody. The hemolysis usually is extravascular.

(a) Manifestations include fever, dark urine, hyperbilirubinemia, unexplained anemia or inadequate response to the recent transfusion, and a newly positive direct Coombs test. This is accompanied by appearance of a significant alloantibody in the serum, which also can be eluted, i.e., removed from the red cells.

(b) Often a serologic delayed transfusion reaction may be present without significant clinical findings.

(c) Very rarely, delayed hemolytic transfusion reactions result in renal failure and/or disseminated intravascular coagulation (DIC).

b. Nonimmune hemolysis is not caused by antibodies and may be secondary to intrinsic or extrinsic red cell defects. It usually is characterized by intravascular hemolysis. It is important to identify it as nonimmune so that the cause can be discovered quickly and the condition corrected, if possible.

(1) Intrinsic red cell defects (in either donor or recipient) may cause hemolysis. They include sickle cell disease, G6PD deficiency, and paroxysmal nocturnal hemoglobinuria.

(2) Extrinsic red cell defects, which may cause hemolysis, can result from overheating, freezing without cryopreservative, dilution with inappropriate intravenous solution, addition of medication to the blood bag, and excessive infusion pressure through small-gauge needles, leukocyte depletion filters, or electromechanical pumps not approved for red cell infusion. Occasionally, infusion tubing may be kinked or compressed within mechanical infusion devices, resulting in damaged red cells.

(3) Massive nonimmune hemolysis, particularly that secondary to the extrinsic red cell defects mentioned above, occasionally may cause renal failure. Therefore, such episodes should be reported to the blood bank, investigated to rule out an immune etiology, and treated as described for acute immune hemolytic reactions.

2. Febrile nonhemolytic transfusion reactions consist of rises in temperature of >1°C or >1.8°F, often accompanied by chills and rigors, occurring during or within 2 hours after a transfusion, in 1 per cent of adult red cell transfusions. These rarely are identified in neonates, perhaps because of their decreased capacity for leukocyte alloimmunization, the tendency to use fresher red cells for them, and the transience and relative subtlety of most of these reactions. Originally they were thought to be secondary to interaction between white cells and recipient (or sometimes donor) leukocyte antibodies. Leukodepletion filters are used following repeat reactions and prophylactically for chronic transfusion recipients. More recently, it has been suggested that they are caused by cytokines released by donor leukocytes during storage. Research is under way on the possible efficacy of prestorage leukodepletion. Febrile nonhemolytic transfusion reaction is a diagnosis of exclusion, after hemolytic reaction has been excluded by serologic work-up and septic transfusion reaction by history and/or culture.

3. Transfusion-associated lung injury (TRALI) is an uncommon type of noncardiogenic pulmonary edema. It is believed to be caused most commonly by the interaction of transfused donor granulocyte or HLA antibodies with recipient leukocytes, resulting in the release and

activation of cytokines injurious to the lung. A febrile nonhemolytic reaction or chills may precede the pulmonary symptoms. Within 1 to 8 hours post transfusion, the recipients demonstrate cyanosis and dyspnea, accompanied by bilateral interstitial infiltrates, without elevation of central venous pressure. This is a life-threatening type of reaction, which has occurred in neonates as well as in older children and adults. Recommendations for treatment include high doses of intravenous steroids and ventilatory support. Since this is occasionally caused by interaction between recipient antibody and donor leukocytes, leukodepletion filters may be useful for prevention in some patients. Also, the transfusion service may want to inform the blood supplier, since the donor, often a multiparous female, may not be appropriate for plasma-containing components for transfusion.

4. Allergic reactions occur in 1 per cent of transfusions and consist of urticaria, wheezing, and sometimes signs of angioneurotic edema. They are assumed to be allergic reactions to soluble plasma allergens. Usually they respond to antihistamines.

5. Metabolic adverse effects are of concern usually for (large-volume transfusion of) neonates and/or patients with preexisting metabolic imbalance, e.g., hyperkalemia secondary to renal failure.

    a. Hyperkalemia is avoided by the use of relatively fresh (<7 days old) red cells for large-volume or exchange transfusions. Washed or frozen deglycerolized red cells also may be useful for minimizing potassium.

    b. Citrate toxicity can result from the chelation of calcium by citrate in the anticoagulant of large-volume blood transfusion, potentiated by rapid infusion, hypothermia, and hepatic and renal dysfunction. It can be avoided by careful monitoring of ionized calcium and administration of calcium if ionized hypocalcemia occurs.

    c. Hyperglycemia is a concern primarily for large-volume transfusions to neonates. Currently, there are insufficient data to support the use of blood preservative solutions containing larger concentrations of dextrose than CPDA-1, for exchange transfusion, extracorporeal membrane oxygenation (ECMO), and cardiac bypass surgery.

    d. Hypoglycemia may occur in neonates if parenteral nutrition with high-concentration glucose solutions is stopped or slowed during transfusion or exchange transfusion. Glucose levels should be monitored during and after exchange transfusion.

6. Hypothermia may occur, especially in neonates receiving relatively large volumes of blood rapidly. Use of a blood warmer with visible thermometer and audible alarm is desirable for large-volume and exchange transfusions. Smaller volume transfusions to infants should be warmed by leaving the blood at room temperature or in a temperature-controlled isolette for 30 minutes prior to transfusion.

7. Graft-versus-host-disease (GVHD) may be caused by donor T lymphocytes in immunosuppressed or immunoincompetent recipients or in recipients whose HLA type is similar to that of the donor. Irradiation of all cellular components for transfusion with a dose of 2500 rads is suggested for intrauterine transfusion, for patients with Hodgkin disease, for selected categories of immunosuppressed recipients, for patients who have received bone marrow or peripheral stem cell transplantation, for directed donations (especially from blood relatives), and for HLA matched components. Cell concentrates for transplantation should *not* be irradiated.

8. Infectious diseases may be transmitted by transfusion. The risks for this will vary, depending upon disease prevalence and the sensitivity of donor testing. Current risks of transmission per unit transfused in the United States are 1:420,000 to 1:640,000 for HIV; 1:200,000 for hepatitis B; 1:50,000 for HTLV-I/II; <1:6000 for hepatitis C; and <1:1,000,000 for other, rare infections (personal communication, C. Bianco, M.D., New York Blood Center, 1995).

Practical Considerations

1. A filter should be used with every transfusion. The standard filter has a 170 μm pore size.

    a. When available, a special components infusion set with shorter tubing and a filter with smaller surface area and identical pore size may be used.

    b. Special leukocyte-depletion filters for platelet and red cell transfusions may be used to reduce CMV transmission and to eliminate at least some reactions caused by leukocyte antibodies and/or cytokines.

2. Isotonic saline, fresh frozen plasma, and 5 per cent albumin are the only acceptable diluents for blood components. Other intravenous fluids may cause hemolysis or clotting. Medications should never be added.

3. Wide-bore (18- or 19-gauge) needles should be used for older children. In neonates and younger children, 23- to 25-gauge needles or 22- to 24-gauge vascular catheters may be used for blood component infusion.

    a. Constant rate syringe delivery pumps approved for the use are satisfactory for red cell infusion through small-gauge needles, although hemolysis increases with cells stored longer than 7 days and with slow rates of infusion.

    b. Concomitant use of a leukocyte-removal filter and a pressure infusion device may result in hemolysis, may impair the function of the filter, and should be avoided.

Procedure

4. The following infusion rates are commonly used, with no transfusion to exceed 4 hours.

   a. Red cells may be infused at 3 to 5 ml/kg/hour.

   b. Fresh frozen plasma may be infused within 30 minutes, if the volume does not exceed 5 to 10 ml/kg.

   c. Platelets may be infused within 30 minutes. Volume reduction should not be a concern if the dose does not exceed 5 to 10 ml/kg. If volume is a concern, because of the small size or cardiovascular status of the recipient, volume reduction may be considered.

   d. Transfusions under 10 ml may be given without a pump, administered with a syringe by intermittent small bolus.

5. Care should be exercised in patient identification at the times of specimen drawing and transfusion and in ensuring that tags and paperwork accompanying units are consistent with each other, with previous documentation in the chart, and with the patient identification bracelet, prior to starting a transfusion.

Bibliography

Blanchette VS, Hume HA, Levy GJ, et al: Guidelines for auditing pediatric blood transfusion practice. Am J Dis Child 1991;145:787–796.

Guidelines for the Administration of Cryoprecipitate. Albany, New York State Council on Human Blood and Transfusion Services, New York State Department of Health, 1995.

Guidelines for Transfusion Therapy of Infants from Birth to Four Months of Age. Albany, New York State Council on Blood and Transfusion Services, New York State Department of Health, 1993.

Neonatal and obstetrical transfusion practice. *In* Walker RH (ed): American Association of Blood Banks Technical Manual, 11th ed. Bethesda, American Association of Blood Banks, 1993, pp 435–469.

Stehling L, Luban NLC, Anderson MH, et al: Guidelines for blood utilization review. Transfusion 1994;34:438–448.

---

133 Examination of Peripheral Blood

Sreedhar P. Rao

Procedure

Examination of the peripheral blood smear is a simple but extremely useful laboratory procedure in hematology.

Indications

1. Evaluation of a patient with anemia
2. Evaluation of a patient with leukocytosis, leukopenia, or reported abnormal leukocytes regardless of leukocyte count
3. Evaluation of a patient with thrombocytopenia
4. Evaluation of a patient for parasitic infestation (e.g., malaria, filariasis).

Preparation of Blood Smear

1. Place a small drop of blood from capillary, needle tip, or well-mixed EDTA anticoagulated blood in the center of a clean glass slide, about 1.5 inch away from the clear end of frosted slide.
2. The slide should be on a flat surface and held in place by two fingers of one hand.
3. Using another clean slide as a spreader slide, back the spreader slide into the drop at an angle of 30 degrees, and quickly move the spreader slide to the opposite end with an even motion.
4. A proper push-wedge blood smear is 1 to 1.5 inch in length and has smooth margins with smooth transition from thick to thin area without any holes or ridges.

Staining the Blood Smear

1. Wright's stain is one of the most commonly used stains for routine morphology of the blood and bone marrow. Many laboratories currently use an automatic staining device.
2. The following special stains are used for enumeration of reticulocytes, Heinz bodies, and detection of fetal hemoglobin-containing red cells.

   a. Supravital stain (methylene blue or brilliant cresyl blue) for reticulocytes and Heinz bodies.

   b. Kleihauer–Betke stain to detect fetal hemoglobin-containing red cells.

Examination of the Peripheral Blood Smear

1. Examine the smear with a low-power objective (10–25 ×) to locate appropriate area of the smear. This is usually about 0.5 inch away from the tip of the smear. An experienced examiner may be able to detect very high or

Procedure

TABLE 133–1. COMMON CELLULAR ABNORMALITIES

TERMS	APPEARANCE	CLINICAL SIGNIFICANCE
White Blood Cells		
Toxic neutrophils	Dense nuclear chromatin, dark cytoplasmic granules, blue or gray inclusions (Döhle body), cytoplasmic vacuolization	Bacterial infection Viral infection
Hypersegmented neutrophils	5 or more nuclear lobes	Megaloblastic anemia Post chemotherapy
Atypical lymphocytes	Large lymphocytes with abundant blue cytoplasm, nuclear membrane indented by red cells. May have nucleoli	Infectious mononucleosis Other viral infections
Lymphoblast	Normal to increased in size. Scanty cytoplasm, loose nuclear chromatin, occasional nucleoli	Acute lymphoblastic leukemia
Myeloblast	Large cell, abundant cytoplasm, irregular nuclear membrane, prominent nucleoli, may contain Auer rods	Myelogenous leukemia, leukoerythroblastic reaction
Platelets		
Giant platelets	Larger than normal (normal ⅓–¼ of RBC size)	Increased platelet turnover, immune thrombocytopenia, May-Hegglin anomaly, Bernard-Soulier syndrome
Small platelets	Smaller than normal	Wiskott-Aldrich syndrome
Gray platelets	Gray-appearing platelets	Gray platelet syndrome, a mild bleeding disorder

low white blood cell count or platelet count and the presence of rouleau formation.

2. Examination of the smear using $100\times$ oil objective: This is most useful for red cell morphology, red cell inclusions, leukocyte differential, estimation of platelet number, and morphology.

Table 133–1 lists the common cellular abnormalities and their clinical significance. Table 133–2 lists the types of red blood cells by appearance and significance.

TABLE 133–2. RED BLOOD CELLS

TERMS	APPEARANCE	CLINICAL SIGNIFICANCE
Normocyte, discocyte	Normal round RBC	Normal
Spherocyte	Small round RBC with no central pallor	Hereditary spherocytosis, autoimmune hemolytic anemia, ABO hemolysis, other hemolytic anemias
Elliptocyte, ovalocyte	Elongated or oval	Hereditary elliptocytosis, thalassemia, iron deficiency anemia
Target cell	Hemoglobin in center and periphery (bull's-eye)	Thalassemia, hemoglobinopathies (hemoglobin S, C), liver disease
Macrocyte	Large oval red cell	Megaloblastic anemia, aplastic anemia, Diamond-Blackfan anemia
Microcyte	Small, usually with increased central pallor	Thalassemia, iron deficiency
Teardrop cell	Pear-shaped or hand-mirror cell	Extramedullary hematopoiesis
Schistocyte, fragmented RBC	Small RBC with at least one irregular edge	Hemolysis, HUS, TTP
Bite cell, helmet cell	One or more pointed projections with loss of cell membrane	Hemolysis
Blister cell	Red cell with clear area on one side and hemoglobin on other side	Hemolysis
Sickle cell	Crescent-shaped cell with dense center	Sickle hemoglobinopathy
Acanthocyte, spiculated RBC	Few, irregularly placed spiny projections on membrane of a small RBC	Liver disease, abetalipoproteinemia, pyruvate kinase deficiency
Howell-Jolly body	Small round inclusion, usually at the periphery	Splenic hypofunction, post splenectomy
Basophilic stippling	Multiple small fine inclusions	Thalassemia, lead poisoning, unstable hemoglobin disorders
Hypochromic red cells	Increase in central pallor	Thalassemia, iron deficiency anemia

RBC, red blood cell; HUS, hemolytic uremic syndrome; TTP, thrombotic thrombocytopenic purpura.

134 Examination of Bone Marrow

Sreedhar P. Rao

Procedure

Aspiration and biopsy of bone marrow are very useful tools in the evaluation of children with hematologic disorders. Bone marrow aspiration alone is adequate in most instances. However, a bone marrow biopsy is essential to accurately determine the marrow cellularity, marrow fibrosis, and presence of granulomas in the bone marrow. Some consider that a bone marrow biopsy is superior to aspiration to demonstrate metastatic tumor in the bone marrow.

Indications

1. Bone marrow aspiration
   a. Evaluation of a patient with pancytopenia
   b. Evaluation of a patient with macrocytic anemia, e.g., megaloblastic vs. nonmegaloblastic anemia, Diamond-Blackfan anemia
   c. Evaluation of a patient with unexplained moderate to severe normocytic anemia with reticulocytopenia
   d. Evaluation of a patient with severe and/or persistent leukopenia/neutropenia
   e. Evaluation of a patient with thrombocytopenia, e.g., amegakaryocytic thrombocytopenia vs. thrombocytopenia due to increased platelet turnover
   f. To confirm or rule out leukemia, myelodysplastic syndrome, or congenital dyserythropoietic anemia
   g. To determine the response to therapy in patients with leukemia or metastatic bone marrow disease
   h. Cytogenetic and immunophenotic analysis in patients with leukemia, myelodysplastic syndrome, or metastatic tumor
   i. Bone marrow for culture when a diagnosis of tuberculosis or *Mycobacterium avium-intracellulare* (MAI) infection is a consideration and blood culture is negative
2. Bone marrow biopsy
   a. To diagnose aplastic anemia
   b. To demonstrate tumor, fibrosis, or granulomas in the bone marrow.

Technique

1. Bone marrow aspiration
   a. Optimal sites are anterior or posterior iliac crests; less common sites are at the lower thoracic and lumbar vertebral spinous processes. There is tibial tuberosity in the first few months of life (<6 months).
   b. Patients may undergo the procedure using conscious sedation with parenteral ketamine or pentobarbital or other drugs along with appropriate monitoring of the patient.
   c. Skin at the site is prepared using a topical antiseptic (e.g., Betadine).
   d. Local analgesic (1% lidocaine) using a 25-gauge needle. Infiltration of the skin is followed by the subcutaneous tissue and finally the periosteum.
   e. A 16- or 18-gauge, 1 to 1.5 inch long needle is used in most children. The point of needle entry should be 1 cm below and posterior to the anterior superior iliac spine, or the midpoint of the superior spine of the posterior iliac crest, 1 cm below the lip of the ilium or the midpoint of the spinous process. Care should be taken to prevent slippage of the needle. The needle direction is perpendicular to the iliac crest or spinous process. A steady, circular motion with moderate force is used to advance the needle through the periosteum. A firmly fixed needle in the bone is usually indicative of needle in the marrow space. Using a 10 ml plastic syringe, 0.2 to 0.3 ml bone marrow is aspirated into the syringe. Before removing the bone marrow needle, the suction

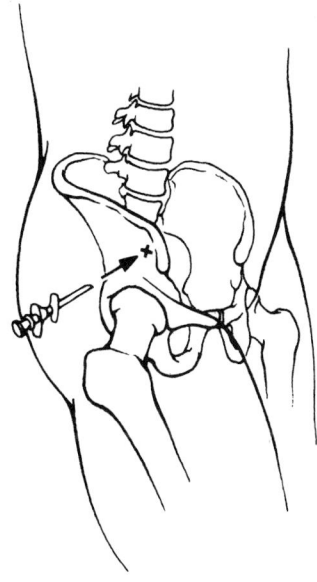

Procedure *Continued*

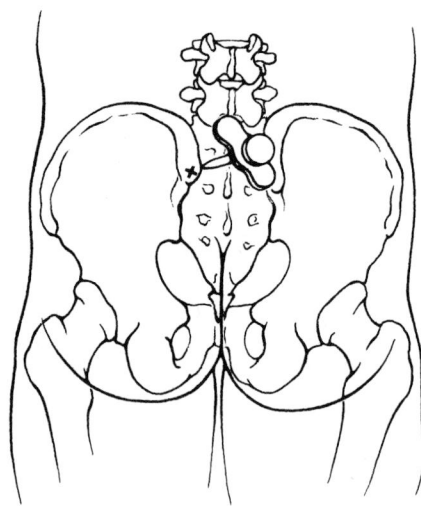

should be released. Additional 1 to 2 ml bone marrow aspiration is required for special studies in patients with leukemia and aplastic anemia. Bonemarrow is expelled onto a clean glass slide in a tilted position. This allows the marrow particles to settle on the slide. Using a different slide, marrow particles are used to prepare multiple smears.

2. Bone marrow biopsy

Posterior iliac crest is the preferred site for bone marrow biopsy. Jamshidi bone marrow biopsy needle has an outer tapered cutting edge and an inner stylet that projects beyond the cutting edge. After periosteum is entered, the inner stylet is taken out and the needle is advanced farther. This would provide a piece of the bone marrow along with bone. Touch preparations are made on glass slides, and the core is placed in 10 per cent formalin for appropriate processing.

Examination of the Bone Marrow Aspirate Smear

1. A Wright-stained smear is evaluated for the following:
   a. Cellularity (biopsy is more reliable)
   b. Megakaryocyte numbers and morphology
   c. Numbers and maturation of myeloid cells, features suggestive of dysmyelopoiesis or megaloblastosis
   d. Numbers and maturation of erythroid cells, evidence of dyserythropoiesis or megaloblastic anemia
   e. Myeloid to erythroid ratio (M:E)
   f. Number of blasts (myeloid vs. lymphoid)
   g. Presence of tumor cells
   h. Presence of storage cells, e.g., Gaucher cells
   i. Hemo- or erythrophagocytosis

2. Other stains

The following stains may be used for bone marrow smears depending on the diagnosis.

   a. Sudan black B, peroxidase, periodic acid–Schiff, specific and nonspecific esterase to distinguish between lymphoblastic and myeloid leukemia
   b. Iron stain to evaluate marrow iron stores and the presence of ringed sideroblasts.

Bibliography

Miller DR: Normal blood values from birth through adolescence. *In* Miller DR, Baehner RL (eds): Blood Diseases of Infancy and Childhood, 7th ed. St. Louis, CV Mosby, 1995, pp 40–58.

135 Acute Lymphoblastic Leukemia

Peter G. Steinherz

Etiology

Acute lymphoblastic leukemias (ALL) are biologically and clinically heterogeneous malignancies of the lymphoid progenitor cells. The disease begins as a random, clonal change in a single cell. The abnormal cells

1. Proliferate uncontrolled

2. Fail to respond to normal growth inhibition mechanisms
3. Do not undergo apoptotic changes
4. Inhibit growth of normal hematopoietic cells
5. Infiltrate normal organs.

If untreated, the disease leads to pancytopenia and organ

failure. Death results from infection or bleeding in 100 per cent of cases within 9 months.

Epidemiology

1. Of all pediatric malignancies, 31 per cent are leukemias.
2. Of childhood leukemias, 86 per cent are ALL.
3. Approximately 2500 new cases of ALL are diagnosed annually in the United States in children <15 years of age, with an incidence rate of 31/1 million (or 1/3226) children <15 years of age.
   a. Males 34/mill/yr
   b. Females 28/mill/yr
   c. Whites 33/mill/yr
   d. Blacks 17/mill/yr
4. Males constitute 57 per cent of the cases.
5. Caucasians constitute 89 per cent of the cases.
6. Peak age incidence occurs at 2–3 years, with age-specific incidence of
   a. <1 yr old—20/mill/yr
   b. 1 yr old—38/mill/yr
   c. 2 yr old—77/mill/yr
   d. 3 yr old—73/mill/yr
   e. 4 yr old—55/mill/yr
   f. 5 yr old—42/mill/yr
   g. 6 yr old—33/mill/yr
   h. 7 yr old—26/mill/yr
   i. 8–15 yr old—13–18/mill/yr
7. Seventy-seven per cent of patients are 1 to 9 years; 3 per cent ≤1 year; 20 per cent are >10 years old.

Pathophysiology

Random mutations are believed to cause most cases. At least two mutations around a regulatory gene or an oncogene in proliferating lymphoid cells are required. The first event is a genetic rearrangement or mutation; the second event is the loss of heterozygosity of the gene. Interaction of host, environment, and genetic factors may play a significant role.

1. Increased risk factors (account for only 1 per cent of cases)
   a. Genetic
      (1) Concordant ALL in monozygotic twins (20%)
      (2) Three- to four-fold increased risk in siblings 1:720 vs. 1:2500
      (3) Infants of mothers with leukemia
      (4) Parental consanguinity.
   b. Host
      (1) Damaged bone marrow (aplastic anemia)
      (2) Chromosome fragility syndromes: Bloom syndrome 1:8; Fanconi anemia 1:12; Ataxia telangiectasia 1:8.
      (3) Down syndrome 1:200
      (4) Neurofibromatosis
      (5) Immunodeficiency (common, X-linked, IgA deficiency)
      (6) Shwachman syndrome
      (7) Wiskott-Aldrich syndrome.
   c. Environmental
      (1) Radiation
      (2) Hydrocarbons
      (3) Viral: EBV, HTLV-1
      (4) Parental occupation: Hydrocarbon, chemical, solvent-related industries
      (5) Maternal smoking
      (6) Alkylating agents.
2. Classification
   a. Morphologic—French-American-British (FAB)
      (1) L_1—Variable cell size, little cytoplasm (occasional vacuoles), nuclear clefts, rare nucleolus.
      (2) L_2—Large cell—Abundant cytoplasm, prominent nucleoli, irregular nuclear outline.
      (3) L_3—Large cell—Small to moderate basophilic cytoplasm, prominent vacuoles.
      (4) FAB L_1 = > 90% L_1 (78% of cases)
          FAB L_1/L_2 = 10–25% L_2 (12% of cases)
          FAB L_2/L_1 = 26–50% L_2 (6% of cases)
          FAB L_2 = > 50% L_2 (3% of cases)
          FAB L_3 = > 25% L_3 (1% of cases).
   b. Immunophenotypic
      B-lineage markers—CD19, CD20, CD22
      T-lineage markers—CD2, CD5, CD7
      Myeloid markers—CD13, CD14, CD33
      Nonlineage-associated markers CD10, CD34, HLA-DR.
      (1) Early pre-B CD19+, CD10±, frequency of 64%
      (2) Pre-B CD19+, CD20+, CD10+, frequency of 14%
      (3) Transitional pre-B CD19+, CD20+, cytoplasmic immunoglobulin+, frequency of 1%
      (4) B cell CD19+, CD20+, surface immunoglobulin+, frequency of 1%
      (5) T cell CD7±, CD2+/CD4+, CD5+, CD8+, frequency of 15%
      (6) Mixed lineage/biphenotypic/unclassifiable, frequency of <5%
   c. Cytogenetic
      (1) Hypodiploid (<46 chromosomes), frequency of 7%
      (2) Diploid (46 chromosomes), frequency of 8%
      (3) Hyperdiploid (47–50 chromosomes), frequency of 15%
      (4) Hyperdiploid (>50 chromosomes), frequency of 27%
      (5) Triploid (>65 chromosomes), frequency of 1%
      (6) Pseudoliploid (46 chromosomes with abnormalities), frequency of 42%
   d. Nonrandom chromosomal translocation associated with
      (1) B cell: t(8;14), t(8;22), t(2;8)
      (2) T cell: t(11;14), t(10;14), t(1;14), t(8;14), t(7;9), t(7;19), t(1;7)

(3) Pre-B/early pre-B: t(1;19), t(4;11), t(5;14), t(11;19), t(9;11), t(17;19)

(4) All lineages: t(9;22)

(5) Mixed lineage: t(4;11)

Clinical Findings

1. Symptoms
   a. Fatigue or malaise, 92%
   b. Bone pain, 79%
   c. Fever, 66%
   d. Purpura, 51%
2. Physical findings
   a. Splenomegaly, 86%
   b. Lymphadenopathy, 76%
   c. Hepatomegaly, 74%
   d. Bone tenderness, 69%
   e. Ecchymosis or petechiae, 50%
   f. Down syndrome, 2%
3. Minimum work-up
   a. History and physical examination
      (1) History—Immunodeficiency, preexisting chromosomal or genetic abnormalities, e.g., Down syndrome, ataxia-telangiectasia
      (2) Previous malignancy, allergy, infection (e.g., varicella), and immunizations
      (3) Family history—Family cancer syndrome, insulin-dependent diabetes mellitus
      (4) Environmental exposures
      (5) Social history
      (6) Physical examination—Retinal lesions, lymph node size, liver size, spleen size, testes, neurologic deficits, signs of bleeding or infection, height (cm), weight (kg), and body surface area (m^2).
   b. Laboratory studies
      (1) Complete blood counts plus differential
      (2) Blood chemical analyses—Bilirubin, SGPT or SGOT, total protein, albumin, BUN, creatinine, uric acid, calcium, phosphorus, sodium, potassium, chloride, bicarbonate, glucose fibrinogen, amylase.
4. Differential diagnosis
   a. Nonmalignant
      (1) Viral infections
      (2) Mononucleosis/Epstein-Barr virus
      (3) AIDS
      (4) Congenital infections (TORCH, syphilis)
      (5) Rheumatoid arthritis
      (6) Multiple iron/vitamin deficiency
      (7) Immune cytopenia
      (8) Congenital cytopenia
      (9) Bone marrow hypoplasia/aplasia (postinfectious, drug, toxin)
      (10) Pertussis
      (11) Infectious lymphocytosis
      (12) Leukemoid reaction (Down syndrome)
      (13) Osteopetrosis
      (14) Hypereosinophilia
   b. Malignant
      (1) Myelodysplastic syndrome
      (2) Nonlymphoid leukemia
      (3) Small cell sarcoma metastatic to marrow
         (a) Lymphoma
         (b) Neuroblastoma
         (c) Rhabdomyosarcoma
         (d) Ewing sarcoma
         (e) Primitive neuroectodermal tumor
         (f) Retinoblastoma
         (g) Medulloblastoma
5. Prognostic factors (Table 135–1)

Key Clinical Findings

- Fever
- Bone pain
- Malaise
- Hepatosplenomegaly
- Petechiae, ecchymoses
- Lymphadenopathy

6. Criteria of response to therapy
   Patient must have >25 per cent blast in marrow for diagnosis of leukemia.
   During therapy

TABLE 135–1. PROGNOSTIC FACTORS AT DIAGNOSIS OF ALL

	FAVORABLE	UNFAVORABLE
At Diagnosis		
WBC	<10,000/μl	>100,000/μl
Age	<2–10 yrs	<1 yr, >10 yrs
Sex	Female	Male
Hemoglobin	<10 g/dl	>10 g/dl
Platelet count	Normal	<100,000/μl
Organomegaly	Minimal	Marked
Mediastinal mass	None	Present
Lymphadenopathy	Minimal	Marked
Extramedullary disease	Absent	Present
FAB morphology	L$_1$	L$_2$, L$_3$
Immunoglobulins	Normal	Depressed
Surface immunoglobulin	Absent	Present
CALLA	Positive	Negative
Diploidy	Hyperdiploid	Hypo/pseudodiploid
DNA index	>1.16	<1.16
Translocation	None	t(4–11), t(8–14), t(9–22)
Rare	Caucasian	Black
Infection	Absent	Present
Hemorrhage	Absent	Present
Response to Therapy		
Marrow day 7	<25% blasts	>25% blasts
Marrow day 14	<5% blasts	>5% blasts

M_1 marrow $= < 5\%$ blasts
M_2 marrow $= 5\text{–}25\%$ blasts
M_3 marrow $= > 25\%$ blasts
For complete response, or to be called "in remission," a patient must have <5 per cent blasts in the marrow, with normal hematopoietic elements present, and a recovering normal peripheral blood count.

Laboratory Findings

1. WBC
   a. <10,000/μl: 50% frequency
   b. 10,000–50,000/μl: 35% frequency
   c. 50,000–100,000/μl: 8% frequency
   d. >100,000/μl: 7% frequency
2. Hemoglobin
   a. <10 g/dl: 80% frequency
   b. >10 g/dl: 20% frequency
3. Platelets
   a. <20,000/μl: 28% frequency
   b. 20,000–100,000/μl: 47% frequency
   c. >100,000/μl: 25% frequency
4. Mediastinal mass
   a. Yes: 5%
   b. No: 95%
5. CNS disease
   a. Yes: 4%
   b. No: 96%
6. Bone marrow blasts (25% needed for diagnosis)
   a. 25–64%: 25%
   b. 65–94%: 50%
   c. >95%: 25%

Key Laboratory Findings

- Normal WBC: 50%
- Increased WBC: 15–20%
- Anemia
- Thrombocytopenia

Radiographic Changes

At diagnosis

1. Osseous manifestations in 50 to 100 per cent
   a. Long bones
      (1) Multiple punctate osteolytic areas: 60–90%
      (2) Diffuse demineralization/collapsed vertebrae: 30%
      (3) Metaphyseal lucent bands: 10–40%
      (4) Periosteal reaction: 5–30%
      (5) Osteosclerotic involvement: 2%
      (6) Mixed lesions: 18%
   b. Skull: <10%
      (1) Small lytic areas or focal rarefaction
      (2) Separated sutures (infants)

2. Chest
   a. Mediastinal/hilar lymphadenopathy (7%)
   b. Pulmonary infiltrates (infectious vs. leukemia)
   c. Pleural effusion
   d. Extrapleural density
   e. Interstitial pattern/cardiomegaly (severe anemia)
3. Abdomen
   a. Hepatosplenomegaly
   b. Renal enlargement

Advanced disease

With uncontrolled disease the osseous manifestations progress. Pulmonary changes due to infection and/or hemorrhage increase in frequency. Intracranial abnormalities due to disease, treatment complications, and hemorrhage or thrombosis become evident.

Key Radiographic Findings

- Punctate osteolytic areas in long bones
- Osteopenia, collapsed vertebrae

Treatment

1. Risk group categories

   The uniform age and WBC criteria for separation of B-precursor ALL patients into standard and high-risk cohorts as adopted at the CTEP/NCI workshop are shown in Table 135–2. There is no uniform risk group definition for the 15 per cent of patients who have T-cell immunophenotype. The Children's Cancer Group considers those (25%) with WBC < 50,000/μl and age < 10 years as being at standard risk, whereas the Pediatric Oncology Group considers all T cell patients as being at high risk.

2. Strategy for disease control

   a. Prompt, complete remission induction with combination chemotherapy
   b. Intensive supportive care to prevent tumor lysis and hemorrhagic and infectious complications
   c. Disease prophylaxis and/or treatment for the central nervous system and other sanctuaries
   d. Combination chemotherapy tailored to the patient's risk group based on initial prognostic factors and early response to therapy
   e. Therapy of sufficient duration to minimize risk of posttherapy relapse

TABLE 135–2. RISK CATEGORIES FOR B-PRECURSOR ALL PATIENTS

RISK	DEFINITION	4-YEAR EFS (%)	B-PRECURSOR PATIENTS (%)
Standard	WBC <50,000 *and* Age 1.00–9.99 yrs	80.3	68
High	WBC ≥ 50,000 *or* Age ≥ 10.00 yrs	63.9	32

f. Monitoring of organ functions to minimize late effects of therapy.

3. Specific disease control steps

a. Induction
Vincristine, glucocorticoid, and asparaginase are the minimum + daunorubicin ± cyclophosphamide for the higher risk group.

b. Supportive care (Table 135–3)

c. Sanctuaries

(1) Central nervous system

(2) Testes

(3) Anterior chamber of eye

(4) Skin

d. Risk group–directed therapy

(1) Lower risk ALL

(a) Remission induction (3 to 4 drugs) for 4 weeks—A glucocorticoid (prednisone 40 mg/m²/day) PO in three divided doses for 28 days, followed by a 9-day taper. Vincristine (1.5 mg/m², maximum 2 mg) weekly for four doses. L-Asparaginase (6000 to 10,000 U/m²/dose IM) thrice weekly for 6 to 9 doses ± daunorubicin (25 to 45 mg/m²) for two to four doses.

(b) Consolidation/intensification or reinduction (similar to induction) treatment may be added

(c) Continuation treatment for 2 to 3 years—6-Mercaptopurine (50 to 75 mg/m²/day) PO. Methotrexate (20 to 40 mg/m²/week) PO, IV, or IM; reinforced with high-dose methotrexate (0.5 g to 2 g/m² IV) for 6 to 12 courses with leucovorin

rescue, and/or a glucocorticoid (prednisone 40 mg/m²/day × 5) plus vincristine (1.5 mg/m²/week × one to two doses) pulses, every 4 to 6 weeks.

(d) Sublinical CNS treatment (prophylaxis)—Intrathecal treatment for 1 to 2 1/2 years.
Methotrexate (6, 8, 10, or 12 mg for ages <1, 1 to 2, 2 to 3, and >3 years, respectively) or methotrexate plus hydrocortisone plus cytarabine (age-adjusted dosage; hydrocortisone and cytarabine in doses generally equivalent to 2 to 3 times that of methotrexate), two to three times during induction, 4 weekly doses during consolidation, and then every 6 to 12 weeks during continuation treatment.

(2) Intermediate risk ALL

(a) Remission induction (four to seven drugs) for 4 to 6 weeks—A glucocorticoid (prednisone 40 to 60 mg/m²/day, or dexamethasone 8 mg/m²/day) PO in three divided doses for 28 days, followed by a 9-day taper. Vincristine (1.5 mg/m², maximum 2 mg) IV weekly for 4 doses. L-Asparaginase (6000 to 10,000 U/m²/dose) IM thrice weekly for 9 doses. Daunorubicin (25 to 60 mg/m²) for two to four doses ± high-dose cyclophosphamide, high-dose methotrexate, and/or teniposide (or etoposide) plus cytarabine.

(b) Consolidation/intensification and/or reinduction (similar to induction) treatment generally will be added during the first 6 months of treatment and may be repeated one more time.

(c) Continuation treatment for 2 to 3 years—6-Mercaptopurine (75 mg/m²/day) PO. Methotrexate (20–40 mg/m²/week), reinforced with: High-dose methotrexate (1 to 5 gm/m² IV) for 6 to 12 courses with leucovorin rescue; and/or a glucocorticoid (prednisone 40 mg/m²/day × 5) plus vincristine (1.5 mg/m² for one to two doses) every 4 weeks; and/or high-dose asparaginase (25,000 U/m² weekly) plus doxorubicin (30 mg/m² every 3 weeks) for 20 weeks; and/or alternating drug pairs with teniposide (150 mg/m²) or etoposide (300 mg/m²) plus cyclophosphamide (300 mg/m²) or cytarabine (300 mg/m²).

(d) CNS treatment—Intrathecal methotrexate (age-adjusted) or triple intrathecal (age-adjusted) three times during induction (weekly × 4 for patients with CNS leukemia at diagnosis), 4 weekly doses during consolidation and then every 6 to 8 weeks or every 4 weeks (for cases of CNS leukemia at diagnosis). Cranial irradiation (12 Gy to 18 Gy) for selected group of patients (e.g., B-lineage ALL with WBC ≥ 50 × 10/L). Cranial irradiation (18 Gy to 24 Gy) for those with CNS leukemia at diagnosis.

TABLE 135–3. SUPPORTIVE THERAPY FOR COMPLICATIONS OF ALL

COMPLICATION	THERAPY
Metabolic	
Hyperuricemia	Allopurinol, hydration, alkalinization
Hyperkalemia	No IV K⁺, alkalinization, glucose/insulin, Kayexalate, dialysis
Hyperphosphatemia	Low-phosphate diet, Amphojel
Hypocalcemia	Replacement
Hypercalcemia	Fluids, calcitonin, pamidronate
Lactic acidosis	Fluids, electrolyte replacement
Hematologic	
Hyperleukocytosis	Hydration, do not correct anemia, leukophoresis/exchange transfusion
Anemia	Transfusion (all blood products should be filtered and irradiated)
Thrombocytopenia	Platelets, aminocaproic acid
Hypofibrinogenemia	Fresh frozen plasma, cryoprecipitate
Prolonged PT	Vitamin K, factor replacement
Granulocytopenia	Broad-spectrum antibiotics if febrile
Thrombosis	Heparin, fresh frozen plasma
Infectious	
Bacterial	Broad-spectrum antibiotics if febrile
Fungal	Nystatin, fluconazole, amphotericin
Viral (VZ)	Acyclovir, zoster immune globulin
Opportunistic	Trimethoprim/sulfa, pentamidine

Intrathecal treatment may be discontinued after cranial irradiation.

(3) High-risk ALL

(a) Remission induction for 4 to 7 weeks (four to eight drugs)—Glucocorticoid (prednisone 40 to 60 mg/m²/day or dexamethasone 8 to 15 mg/m²/day IV or PO in three divided doses for 21 to 28 days followed by a 7- to 14-day taper). Vincristine (1.5 mg/m²/dose, maximum 2 mg, IV weekly for four to five doses). L-Asparaginase (*E. coli* 6000 U/m² thrice weekly for nine doses IM, or 10,000 to 25,000 U/m²/dose IM weekly or PEG asparaginase 2500 U/m²/dose IM q 2 to 4 weeks. Daunorubicin (25 to 60 mg/m²/dose for two to four doses IV push or continuous infusion) ± cyclophosphamide high-dose methotrexate/citrovorum factor (CF) rescue, prolonged asparaginase, epipodophilotoxin, cytarabine ± brief investigational window to evaluate newer approaches.

(b) For slow early responders, early intensification may be added with high-dose cytarabine, induction drugs not already used, and/or alternative anthracyclines and steroids.

(c) Consolidation and periodic reinduction/reintensification (similar to induction) treatment cycles follow remission induction for the first 6 to 12 months.

(d) New modalities of therapy to decrease or eliminate minimal residual disease, such as immune modulation, monoclonal antibody therapy, or allogeneic bone marrow transplant in first complete remission may be tried.

(e) Continuation treatment for 2 to 3 years post remission; induction with doses adjusted to keep absolute neutrophil count 1000 to 2000/μl. 6-Mercaptopurine (75 mg/m²/day PO). Methotrexate (25 to 40 mg/m²/week PO or IM). Vincristine/pred-

nisone pulses q 3 to 4 weeks reinforced with periodic high-dose methotrexate/CF and/or periodic or cyclic reintensification cycles.

(f) CNS treatment

Intrathecal therapy (age-adjusted dose schedule) Cytarabine or methotrexate or triple therapy at diagnosis, twice during induction, weekly × 4 during consolidation with cranial irradiation (1200–1800 cGy), and periodically during the reinduction/reintensification/continuation cycles of therapy. For those with CNS disease at diagnosis, the frequency of intrathecal therapy and irradiation dose and field may be increased.

e. Duration of therapy

(1) Two years for girls

(2) Two to three years for boys.

Key Treatment

- Antineoplastic agents
- Corticosteroids
- Supportive metabolic, hematologic, and infection control measures

Bibliography

Bleyer WA: Acute lymphoblastic leukemia in children—Advances and prospects. Cancer 1990;65:689–695.

Greaves M: A natural history for pediatric acute leukemia. Blood 1993;82:1043–1051.

Gurney JG, Severson RK, Davis S, Robison LL: Incidence of cancer in children in the United States. Sex-, race-, and 1-year age specific rates by histologic type. Cancer 1995;75:2186–2195.

Miller DR: Hematologic malignancies: leukemia and lymphoma. *In* Miller DR, Baehner RL, Miller LP: (eds): Blood Diseases of Infancy and Childhood, 7th ed. St Louis, CV Mosby, 1995, pp 660–804.

Pui C-H, Crist WM: Biology and treatment of acute lymphoblastic leukemia. J Pediatr 1994;124:491–503.

136 Acute Myeloid Leukemia

Robert J. Wells and *Robert J. Arceci*

Definition

Acute myeloid leukemia (AML) can be defined as replacement of the bone marrow with more than 25 per cent blasts that are of a nonlymphocytic (myeloid, erythroid, or megakaryocytic) phenotype.

Epidemiology

AML, formerly known as acute nonlymphocytic leukemia, accounts for 15 to 20 per cent of all childhood (age < 15 years) leukemia. In contrast, in adults it accounts for almost 80 per cent of acute leukemia. AML is associated with radiation exposure, syndromes that have abnormalities of chromosomal repair (Fanconi anemia, Bloom syndrome, and ataxia-telangiectasia), chromosomal anomalies (Down syndrome), and hydrocarbon and pesticide exposures. In addition, it is one of the more common second malignant neoplasms seen in patients treated with chemotherapy (particularly alkylating agents and topoisomerase inhibitors) and radiation therapy.

Etiology

Up to 80 per cent of patients with AML have an associated cytogenetic abnormality in the leukemia cell line. In many cases, specific genetic alterations such as a chromosomal translocation results in the generation of "chimeric" molecules that often involve transcription factors. Thus, a translocation may produce a new "chimeric" protein with the DNA binding site from one transcription factor attached to a different regulatory protein binding site from another transcription factor. For example, the *AML1* gene is a chimeric protein of two transcription factors (PEPP2/CBFαB) associated with the t(8;21) translocation. The inv(16) oncoprotein, found in the M_{4eo} subtype of AML is the result of the fusion of regions CBFβ with MYH11. The t(15;17) translocation found in promyelocytic AML (M_3) generates a chimeric protein containing the *PML* protooncogene and the retinoic acid receptor RARα. In addition, mutations that activate the *NRAS* protooncogene are frequently observed in AML.

Pathophysiology

1. At the molecular level, presumably, chance events generate an abnormal but persistent clone as just described. Underlying genetic predisposition including the specific conditions listed earlier and/or environmental stimuli increase the probability of such an event. Key characteristics for the new clone are the ability to reproduce and a lack of inhibition of reproduction by factors that normally control growth.

2. At the systemic level
   a. Uncontrolled growth of an abnormal clone in the bone marrow gradually results in the displacement of cells normally found there. The lack of a normal number of red blood cells causes the symptoms of anemia; the lack of platelets results in an increase in the risk for bleeding; and the lack of white blood cells results in increased susceptibility to infection.
   b. The leukemia cell population also has the capability to proliferate in sites other than the bone marrow similar to normal blood cells (extramedullary hematopoiesis). Tissues that are commonly infiltrated include the liver, spleen, and lymph nodes. Less commonly, the kidneys, lungs, and central nervous system are involved. Autopsy studies of patients who died of AML indicate that almost all tissues can be involved with leukemia cells.

Clinical Findings

1. *Signs and symptoms.* The presenting signs and symptoms of AML are similar to those of other diseases that result in the failure of the bone marrow to produce normal cells (acute lymphocytic leukemia or aplastic anemia). These are usually some combination of anemia (fatigue, pallor, or weakness), thrombocytopenia (bruising, bleeding), and infection (fever, pneumonia, cellulitis). Less common are organomegaly, lymphadenopathy, chloromas (collections of myeloblasts forming a tumor; also referred to as granulocytic sarcoma), seizures or obtundation (central nervous system leukemia), and respiratory failure (pulmonary leukostasis). Depending on their location, chloromas may constitute a medical emergency such as when they involve epidural sites, cranial nerves, or spinal cord or when they compress the airway. Another medical emergency associated with AML is leukostasis, which usually occurs when cell numbers are so high in the peripheral blood (usually >150,000/mm³) that they lead to blood flow sludging, infarction, and hemorrhage. These patients may experience somnolence and symptoms related to stroke as well as tachypnea and respiratory insufficiency.

2. *Differential diagnosis.* The main disorders to differentiate from AML are aplastic anemia, myelodysplastic disorders (preleukemic syndromes), acute lymphocytic leukemia, chronic myeloid leukemia, and megaloblastic anemias such as folic acid or vitamin B_{12} deficiencies. In the neonatal period a variety of disorders can mimic AML.

3. *Problems with newborns.* The newborn bone marrow response to infection, hypoxemia, or hemolysis can result in the so-called leukemoid reaction, which can be quite difficult to differentiate from congenital leukemia. Usually, careful study of the trends in the blood cell counts and physical findings over time is required to differentiate these conditions. In addition, in infants with Down syndrome, an enigmatic myeloproliferative disorder is seen. This condition mimics both AML and the leukemoid reaction seen in normal infants, may be associated with anemia and thrombocytopenia, and may include cytogenetic abnormalities. However, most of these patients have their hematologic status return to normal over several weeks to months. The long-term outcome for these patients is variable, with most surviving without any subsequent episodes of hematologic problems. However, some of these patients (about 25 per cent) develop leukemia that does not resolve spontaneously.

Key Clinical Findings

- Fatigue
- Pallor
- Bruising
- Infections

Laboratory Findings

1. *Clinical.* An abnormal hemogram is present in almost all patients with leukemia at presentation. About 10 per cent of patients will have a white blood cell count greater than 100,000/mm³, but 20 per cent will have a count of less than 5,000/mm³. Key findings are abnormalities of two or all three cell lines, blasts, or leukoerythroblastic changes that suggest the need for a bone marrow aspirate/biopsy. Other findings seen frequently include an elevated lactate dehydrogenase level. Abnormalities of the coagulation system, metabolic disturbances (electrolyte and uric

TABLE 136–1. FRENCH-AMERICAN-BRITISH CLASSIFICATION OF ACUTE MYELOID LEUKEMIA

CLASS	MORPHOLOGY	HISTOCHEMISTRY	% CASES	CYTOGENETICS	SURFACE ANTIGENS
M₁	Myeloblasts	MP+	14	t(8;21)	CD15,33,34
M₂	Myeloblasts	MP+	23	t(8;21)	CD15,33,34
M₃	Promyelocytes	MP+	11	t(15;17)	CD15,33,34
M₄	Myelo/monoblasts	MP+/NSE+	21	t(1;11),t(9;11)	CD14,15,33,34
M₅	Monoblasts	NSE+	13	t(1;11),t(9;11)	CD14,15,33,34
M₆	Abnormal erythro/myeloblasts	MP+/PAS+	<2	—	CD33,34 GPIIb/IIIa,GPIb
M₇	Megakaryoblasts	PP+	10	Abnormal 21	CD33,34
MDS	Myelodysplasia	—	6	Monosomy 7	Variable

MP, myleoperoxidase; NSE, nonspecific esterase; PAS, periodic acid–Schiff; PP, platelet peroxidase; GPIb and GPIIb/IIIa, platelet specific antigens; GPA, glycophorin A. Information about the frequency of subtypes is taken from CCG 2891/2911 protocols.

acid), and renal function problems are also found but generally represent complications of the leukemia and are usually important from the standpoint of supportive care of a patient with leukemia rather than suggesting the diagnosis.

2. *Diagnosis.* The diagnosis of leukemia is confirmed by finding more than 25 per cent blasts in the bone marrow. Identification and differentiation of the blasts from lymphoblasts is accomplished by use of light microscopy morphology using various histochemical stains, by immunophenotype, and by cytogenetics. The type of AML is classified into more than seven types using the French-American-British (FAB) classification system (Table 136–1).

3. *Prognosis.* Unlike in acute lymphoblastic leukemia, it has been very difficult to identify reliable prognostic factors in AML. Only very recently has a high white blood cell count at diagnosis (>100,000/mm³) and some specific cytogenetic abnormalities (e.g., monosomy 7) and AML as a second malignancy been identified as predicting adverse outcome. Down syndrome has been identified as an extremely favorable indicator allowing a reduction in the intensity of therapy. FAB classification and immunophenotype have been of only limited value in this regard.

 Key Laboratory Findings

- Decreased WBC 20 per cent
- Increased WBC 10 per cent
- Blast cells in bone marrow

Radiographic Changes

There are no typical radiographic changes for AML. The changes that do occur are usually the result of leukemic infiltrates of specific organs.

Treatment

The treatment of AML is in almost all cases intense, near-myeloablative chemotherapy. Therapy is usually divided into the induction, consolidation/intensification, and maintenance phases. The goal of induction is to achieve a remission (<5 per cent blasts in the bone marrow and a normal hemogram). The most effective drugs have been daunorubicin, cytarabine, etoposide, and thioguanine. Idarubicin is being tested

as a potential replacement for daunorubicin. Generally, induction therapy results in prolonged hospitalization requiring supportive care measures, such as the treatment of infection (>50 per cent in many series), blood product replacement, and complications of mucositis. The one exception to this may be in promyelocytic leukemia where all-*trans*-retinoic acid may "ease" the patient into remission and allow the intense therapy to be given at a time when the patient is less vulnerable to its effects. Retinoic acid seems to work by causing the differentiation of the leukemia cells rather than by killing them.

Once a patient achieves a remission, consolidation (giving more of the same drugs that achieved the remission) or intensification (giving new drugs or the same drugs at a markedly increased dose) or both are done. This phase may include bone marrow transplantation or cord blood from a variety of donors (HLA identical, mismatched, or autologous). In recent years, maintenance therapy has come into disfavor because if intensification therapy is aggressive enough there is no advantage for it.

Currently, the best AML therapies have remission induction rates of between 75 and 85 per cent with about half of the patients not achieving a remission succumbing to complications (usually infection or bleeding) during induction and the other half being resistant to the therapy. Of the patients achieving a remission, 40 to 50 per cent remain in remission and are apparently cured whereas the remainder relapse or succumb to toxicity of further therapy.

 Key Treatment

- Myeloablative chemotherapy

Prevention

Not enough is known about the cause of leukemia to allow an effective preventive strategy to be applied.

 Bibliography

Choi SI, Simone JV: Acute nonlymphocytic leukemia in 171 children. Med Pediatr Oncol 1976;2:119–146.
Creutzig U, Ritter J, Zimmerman M, Schellong G: Does cranial radiation reduce the risk of bone marrow relapse in acute my-

elogenous leukemia? Unexpected results of the childhood acute myelogenous leukemia study BFM-87. J Clin Oncol 1993; 11:279–286.

Grier HE, Gelber RD, Camitta BM, et al: Prognostic factors in childhood acute myelogenous leukemia. J Clin Oncol 1987; 5:1026–1032.

Ravindranath Y, Abella E, Krischer JP, et al: Acute myeloid

leukemia in Down's syndrome is highly responsive to chemotherapy: Experience of Pediatric Oncology Group AML study 8498. Blood 1992;80:2210–2214.

Rubin CM, Arthur DC, Woods WG, et al: Therapy related myelodysplastic syndrome and acute myeloid leukemia in children: Correlation between chromosomal abnormalities and prior therapy. Blood 1991;78:2982–2988.

137 Chronic Myelogenous Leukemia

Farid Boulad

Definition

Chronic myelogenous leukemia (CML) is a myeloproliferative disorder that occurs rarely in childhood. It is a clonal disorder that results from the malignant transformation of the earliest hematopoietic stem cell and therefore involves all the subsequent hematopoietic cell lines and elements. Clinically, CML is usually characterized by an enlarged spleen, a high white blood cell count, and a high platelet count. Its hallmark is the presence of the cytogenetic marker known as the Philadelphia chromosome.

Etiology

The only factor that has been associated with an increased incidence of CML is radiation, for example, in survivors of the atomic bomb explosions and in people who have been exposed to excessive doses of radiation. No other chemical or physical carcinogen and no infectious agents have been associated with this disease. In most cases, especially in children, the etiology remains unknown.

Epidemiology

CML is rare in childhood and accounts for 3 to 5 per cent of all childhood leukemias. Although described as early as in the first year of life, it is usually seen in children older than age 2 years, with 80 per cent of cases presenting after 4 years of age. There is no difference in the incidence of CML with regard to race or gender. As mentioned, radiation has been associated with an increased incidence of CML.

Pathophysiology

1. The Philadelphia chromosome (Ph¹) is the cytogenetic marker of CML and is intimately linked to its pathophysiology. Described in 1960, it represents the first specific abnormality associated with a human malignancy. It was initially described as a chromosome 22 with a shorter long arm. It actually represents the result of the breaks on chromosomes 9 and 22, with a reciprocal translocation of the distal genetic material resulting in a t(9;22)(q34;q11). The translocation transposes the c-*abl* proto-oncogene from its normal location on chromosome 9 to a new position on chromosome 22, in proximity to the breakpoint cluster region (bcr). A new hybrid *bcr-abl* oncogene is formed that produces an abnormal RNA that itself encodes for a 210-kd (p210) fusion protein that

is presumed to change normal hematopoietic cells into multilineage-involved CML cells. The Ph¹ chromosome is found in approximately 90 per cent of patients with CML. In the remaining 10 per cent of Ph¹-negative patients there is a variant translocation or a break at the 9q34 region without the reciprocal break on chromosome 22. Lastly, a subtype of acute lymphoblastic leukemia (ALL) may be associated with the Ph¹ chromosome. In this Ph¹-positive ALL, the breakpoint on chromosome 22 is proximal to the bcr region and usually results in a smaller RNA and a smaller 190-kd protein (p190). This change is associated with a lymphoid lineage-specific involvement.

2. CML is an acquired disorder of unicellular origin. The target of its neoplastic transformation is a multilineage stem cell that generates all the hematopoietic cells (erythrocytes, megakaryocytes, neutrophils, basophils, eosinophils, and monocytes). The clonality of this initial single cell involvement has been demonstrated specifically in patients who are heterozygous for the X-linked glucose-6-phosphate dehydrogenase (G6PD) enzyme, in whom all the Ph¹ cells express a single isoenzyme pattern while the rest of the cells from somatic tissues are heterozygous for the enzyme.

3. Because of molecular abnormalities, CML cells lose their adherence to the marrow stroma and therefore remain longer in a late progenitor proliferative phase before differentiation. This translates into the proliferation of myeloid cells at all different stages of maturation in the marrow and peripheral blood. In addition, there is a growth advantage of CML cells over normal cells. CML cells appear to live longer than normal cells and do not undergo programmed cell death or apoptosis to the same degree. However, at some time in the course of the disease, there appears to be a maturation/differentiation arrest with production of immature blasts that give rise to the blastic phase of the disease.

Clinical Course

The natural course of CML usually involves three phases. It usually presents with a *chronic phase* that is indolent and easily controlled with therapy. With conventional treatment, it lasts approximately 3 years but eventually progresses into an *accelerated phase* that lasts less than 1 year. It is then followed by a *blastic phase* that results in patient death within 3 to 6 months. In rare instances, patients may present de novo in blastic phase.

1. *Chronic phase*

   a. Clinical findings

      (1) Normal hematopoietic cells proliferate in all stages of maturation in the marrow, blood, and reticuloendothelial system. This translates into symptoms or signs of organ infiltration and high blood cell counts.

      (2) Patients usually present with nonspecific complaints such as fever, malaise, night sweats, weakness, or left upper quadrant pain. One third of patients with CML are asymptomatic at presentation, with their diagnosis made after a blood cell count or a routine test. On rare occasions, patients may present with very high white blood cell counts and symptoms or signs associated with hyperleukocytosis (i.e., neurologic problems, priapism).

      (3) On physical examination, low-grade fever and pallor may be found as well as ecchymoses and petechiae. Splenomegaly can be found in half of the patients and can actually be used to monitor the patients' response to treatment. Less frequently, hepatomegaly can be palpated.

      (4) In the rare patients with hyperleukocytosis, signs relating to leukostasis, such as papilledema or neurologic abnormalities, can be found.

Key Clinical Findings

- Asymptomatic (one third)
- Fever
- Night sweats
- Weakness
- Splenomegaly

   b. Laboratory findings

      (1) A marked leukocytosis and thrombocytosis are the most common laboratory findings. The white blood cell count at diagnosis may vary from 8,000 to 800,000/mm^3 and is actually $\geq$ 100,000/mm^3 in half of the patients.

      (2) The peripheral smear reveals myeloid cells at all stages of differentiation with a "left shift" (cells in the early stages of maturation, i.e., promyelocytes, myelocytes, metamyelocytes, and bands). In contrast to the acute leukemias, there is no "hiatus leukemicus" in chronic-phase CML. There is an increase in eosinophils and basophils.

      (3) A mild normochromic, normocytic anemia can usually be seen at presentation.

      (4) The platelet count is usually elevated, with an approximate mean platelet count of 500,000/

mm^3 and sometimes platelet counts $\geq 1 \times 10^6$/mm^3.

      (5) In addition to the hematologic findings, there can be an increase in lactate dehydrogenase, uric acid, and vitamin B$_{12}$. A decrease in the leukocyte alkaline phosphatase activity is classically found.

      (6) The bone marrow is hypercellular with a striking myeloid hyperplasia at all stages of maturation. Again, basophils and eosinophils are increased, as are megakaryocytes. Histiocytes that resemble Gaucher cells can sometimes be seen in the marrow. Cytogenetic studies performed on the marrow reveal the pathognomonic presence of Ph^1 with the translocation of chromosome 9 and 22 and the *bcr-abl* gene rearrangement.

Key Laboratory Findings

- High white blood cell count (over 100,000 in 50 per cent)
- Mild anemia
- High platelet count
- Hypercellular bone marrow with myeloid hyperplasia
- Cytogenetics: t(q22)

   c. Differential diagnosis. The differential diagnosis includes leukemoid reactions and juvenile CML. In leukemoid reactions, no splenomegaly is found on examination and cytogenetic studies as well as leukocyte alkaline phosphatase activity are normal. Patients with juvenile CML are usually younger ($<$ 2 years), have lymphadenopathy, and may have a massively enlarged spleen. They usually present with a white blood cell count lower than 100,000/mm^3 and a markedly decreased platelet count. Monocytosis is a typical finding of juvenile CML. In addition, these patients have elevated levels of fetal hemoglobin associated with ineffective erythropoiesis. They typically have normal cytogenetic studies.

2. Accelerated phase. Well-defined criteria exist for the definition of the accelerated phase of CML

   a. Peripheral blasts $\geq$ 15 per cent

   b. Peripheral blasts plus promyelocytes $\geq$ 30 per cent

   c. Peripheral basophils $\geq$ 20 per cent

   d. Thrombocytopenia with $<$ 100,000/mm^3

   e. The presence of new cytogenetic abnormalities

   f. In addition, other criteria are sometimes used in common practice and include the need for higher drug dosage to keep the white blood cell count under control, the development of splenomegaly that is unresponsive to therapy, the development of collagen fibrosis in the marrow, persistent unexplained fever, unexplained anemia and thrombocytopenia, and blasts $\geq$ 10 per cent in marrow or blood.

3. Blastic phase
   a. *Clinical picture.* The blastic phase occurs in most instances after a chronic phase but can also rarely occur de novo. The clinical picture is that of an acute leukemia with anemia and thrombocytopenia and their subsequent signs of pallor, ecchymoses, and petechiae. White blood cell counts may be elevated and sometimes accompanied by signs of hyperleukocytosis, or they may be decreased and possibly associated with bacterial infections.
   b. *Laboratory findings.* Anemia and thrombocytopenia are usually present. White blood cell counts may be elevated or less often decreased. Typically, as in acute leukemias, blasts can be seen in the peripheral smear. Bone marrow examination reveals a blast count greater than 30 per cent with the presence of a hiatus leukemicus and absence of maturation. In two thirds of patients the transformation is myeloblastic, and in one third it is lymphoblastic. The Ph[1] chromosome can be found on these blasts sometimes together with additional cytogenetic abnormalities.
   c. *Differential diagnosis.* The diagnosis of de novo acute leukemia or blastic-phase CML can sometimes be difficult to make because 3 to 10 per cent of childhood acute leukemias can be associated with the Ph[1] chromosome. These two entities cannot be distinguished clinically. Because the initial treatment is the same, one usually treats patients who present with this picture whereas the final differential diagnosis is usually one made at the cytogenetic and molecular levels.

Treatment

A number of therapeutic approaches are available for disease control in CML. Intensive chemotherapy as used in acute leukemias has not been shown to be effective in the treatment of this disease.

1. Three agents have been most frequently used for disease control.
   a. Busulfan was used in the early 1960s and has brought long periods of disease control but has also been associated with unpredictable prolonged myelosuppression. The median survival with busulfan was 42 months.
   b. Hydroxyurea has brought comparable results with less toxicity. Both these agents have produced hematologic responses in 75 per cent of patients with chronic-phase CML. However, cytogenetic studies

have shown the persistence of Ph[1]-positive cells in most cells.
   c. Interferon alfa, used more recently, has brought longer median survivals, up to 62 months. Therapy with interferon α has produced hematologic responses in 75 per cent of patients but has also been associated with cytogenetic responses with a decrease in the number of Ph[1] cells and, in 8 to 20 per cent of cases, with a complete resolution of the Ph[1] chromosome.

2. Allogeneic bone marrow transplantation has been the only curative approach for this disease. The transplant cytoreduction regimens used have included total-body irradiation and cyclophosphamide or busulfan and cyclophosphamide. In patients receiving marrow transplants from human leukocyte antigen (HLA)-matched siblings, the disease-free survivals have been 65, 35, and 15 per cent for patients in first chronic phase, accelerated phase, or blastic phase, respectively. For patients receiving marrow transplants from unrelated donors, early results have been lower, with 45 and 25 per cent for patients in first chronic or accelerated phase, respectively. Unrelated donor transplants in blastic phase have not been successful.

   Recently, an exciting approach for patients who relapse post transplant is the use of donor-derived leukocyte infusion.

Key Treatment

- Hydroxyurea
- Busulfan
- Interferon α
- Bone marrow transplantation

Bibliography

Altman AJ: Chronic leukemias of childhood. *In* Pizzo P, Poplack D (eds): Principles and Practice of Pediatric Oncology. Philadelphia, JB Lippincott, 1989, pp 383–396.

Gamis AS, Haake R, McGlave P, Ramsay NK: Unrelated-donor bone marrow transplantation for Philadelphia chromosome–positive chronic myelogenous leukemia in children. J Clin Oncol 1993;11:834–838.

Kantarjian HM, Deisseroth A, Kurzrock R, et al: Chronic myelogenous leukemia: A concise update. Blood 1993;82:691–703.

Kurzrock R, Gutterman JU, Talpaz M: The molecular genetics of Philadelphia chromosome–positive leukemias. N Engl J Med 1988;319:990–998.

138 Hodgkin Disease

Sharon Gardner and *Jonathan L. Finlay*

Definition

Hodgkin disease is a disorder of the lymphoid system first described by Thomas Hodgkin in 1832.

Etiology and Epidemiology

1. There is a bimodal age peak in the incidence of Hodgkin disease.
   a. The first peak occurs in children younger than 5 years of age in developing countries and in young adults between 15 and 40 years of age in industrialized societies. Hodgkin disease is very rare in children younger than 5 years of age in industrialized countries.
   b. The second peak occurs in adults older than age 55 years.
2. In industrialized societies, teenagers are often of higher socioeconomic status.
3. There is a male predominance, particularly in children younger than 12 years of age.
4. Hodgkin disease is rare in blacks, and there is no peak in the teenage years.
5. Hodgkin disease is more common in individuals with an underlying immunodeficiency disorder.
6. Epstein-Barr virus has been suggested as an etiologic agent in some patients.

Pathophysiology

1. Histologically, a mixture of Reed-Sternberg cells and normal reactive cells including lymphocytes, plasma cells, eosinophils, neutrophils, and macrophages is seen. Reed-Sternberg cells are large cells with abundant cytoplasm and two or more nucleoli. These cells are usually but not always present and are not pathognomonic for Hodgkin disease.
2. The Rye classification is the scheme used to subdivide Hodgkin disease histologically into four categories.
   a. Lymphocyte predominant: Reed-Sternberg cells are sparse, and eosinophils, plasma cells, and neutrophils are often absent.
   b. Mixed cellularity: Reed-Sternberg cells are plentiful. Eosinophils, plasma cells, and lymphocytes are numerous. Patients may have "skip" areas of nodal involvement.
   c. Lymphocyte depleted: There are predominantly malignant cells (usually more than 15 per high-power field) and few lymphocytes remaining in the lymph nodes. Fibrosis and necrosis are common and diffuse. Prior to modern therapy, this histologic subtype was usually associated with a poor prognosis.
   d. Nodular sclerosing: This is distinct from the other three subtypes. Usually a thickened capsule is present with a proliferation of collagenous bands that divide the node into nodules. Often seen are lacunar cells, which are variants of Reed-Sternberg cells with abundant cytoplasm, hyperlobate nuclei, and multiple small nucleoli. This is the most common subtype seen in pediatric patients and usually involves lymph nodes in the cervical, supraclavicular, and mediastinal regions.

Clinical Findings

1. The most common presentation is painless adenopathy in the middle to lower neck.
2. At least half of the patients have mediastinal disease at diagnosis.
3. Splenomegaly, hepatomegaly, or both are found in up to 30 per cent of patients at diagnosis. This may be due to disease or may represent reactive cellular infiltration.
4. Systemic features including fever, night sweats, weight loss, and pruritus may be present. Although Pel-Epstein fever rarely occurs, it is considered characteristic of Hodgkin disease and is defined as cyclical periods of fever lasting several days to weeks followed by afebrile periods of similar duration.

Key Clinical Findings

- Fever
- Painless adenopathy
- Hepatosplenomegaly, 30 per cent at onset

Diagnosis

1. A complete history and physical examination with particular attention to all nodal areas is essential. All enlarged lymph node areas must be measured.
2. Blood studies should include a complete blood cell count, erythrocyte sedimentation rate, liver and renal function studies, and thyroid-stimulating hormone and free thyroxine studies. Acute-phase reactants such as serum copper, iron, and iron-binding capacity may also be abnormal but are of limited clinical value.
3. Biopsy (most often of a lymph node) is required to confirm the diagnosis of Hodgkin disease.
4. A chest radiograph with anteroposterior and lateral views should also be performed. If a mediastinal mass is present, its size should be measured in comparison with the intrathoracic diameter. In addition, the patency of the airway must be noted.
5. Computed tomography (CT) of the chest is often helpful in further evaluating disease above the diaphragm. CT of the neck should be performed in patients with disease in high cervical nodes. CT of the abdomen and pelvis is often performed to evaluate disease below the diaphragm; however, this technique is not ideal for evaluating disease

in children who lack retroperitoneal fat or for determining involvement of the spleen or upper abdominal lymph nodes.

6. Bone marrow biopsies should be performed from two different sites, especially in patients with stage III or IV disease or with systemic symptoms.

7. Bipedal lymphangiography is one of the most accurate techniques for detecting disease in lymph nodes below the renal hila; however, this study is difficult to perform, particularly in children, and the false-positive rate may be as high as 25 per cent. In addition, it is contraindicated in patients with respiratory compromise because the contrast medium may accumulate in the lungs.

8. Gallium scanning may be helpful in screening patients at diagnosis and after therapy is completed, particularly in patients with systemic symptoms or abnormal laboratory studies but normal physical examination.

9. Staging laparotomy (i.e., splenectomy and biopsies of periaortic [upper and lower], mesenteric, celiac, and splenic hilar lymph nodes as well as biopsy of both lobes of the liver) should be performed *only* in patients who are at least 4 to 6 years of age and in whom radiation therapy is being considered as the sole treatment.

Staging

The Ann Arbor staging system is used to classify the extent of disease based on the location of disease and the presence or absence of systemic symptoms.

1. The stage of disease is identified by a roman numeral as described below:

   I. Involvement of a single lymph node region or of a single extralymphatic organ or site.

   II. Involvement of two or more lymph node regions on the same side of the diaphragm or localized involvement of an extralymphatic organ or site and of one or more lymph node regions on the same side of the diaphragm (II$_E$).

   III. Involvement of lymph node regions on both sides of the diaphragm that may also be accompanied by involvement of the spleen (III$_S$) or by localized involvement of an extralymphatic organ or site (III$_E$) or both (III$_{SE}$).

   IV. Diffuse or disseminated involvement of one or more extralymphatic organs or tissues, with or without associated lymph node involvement.

2. The presence of systemic symptoms is denoted by the letter "B"; if no symptoms are present, the letter "A" is used. "B" symptoms include

   a. Unexplained fever greater than 38°C during the previous month

   b. Unexplained loss of 10 per cent or more of body weight in the 6 months preceding diagnosis

   c. Night sweats

   d. Pruritus is *not* a systemic symptom that leads to "B" designation at the present time, although originally this was the case.

Treatment

Radiation therapy was the initial treatment for Hodgkin disease. However, more recently, multiagent chemotherapy has been found to be effective, particularly in combination with low-dose involved-field irradiation. Two chemotherapy combinations that have formed the backbone of drug therapy for Hodgkin disease include MOPP (nitrogen mustard, Oncovin [vincristine], procarbazine, and prednisone) and ABVD (doxorubicin [Adriamycin], bleomycin, vinblastine, and dacarbazine). Therapy is tailored based on the patient's age and extent of disease, with the goal of curing patients with the least long-term toxicity.

1. Low-dose involved-field irradiation in combination with multiagent chemotherapy is the treatment of choice for most children with Hodgkin disease.

2. In adolescents and fully grown adults with limited disease defined by staging laparotomy, high-dose extended-field irradiation alone is still used in some countries.

3. Patients with advanced disease are most often treated with multiagent chemotherapy with irradiation to sites of bulky disease.

 Key Treatment

- Multiagent chemotherapy

- Radiation

Late Effects

1. Second malignancies are becoming increasingly prevalent as survival after therapy for Hodgkin disease is prolonged.

   a. Hematologic malignancies (specifically acute non-lymphocytic leukemia and non-Hodgkin lymphoma) are the most common secondary malignancies and occur with increasing frequency until approximately 10 years after therapy when the incidence plateaus.

   b. Solid tumors often occur within sites of radiation therapy and include tumors such as breast cancer, thyroid carcinoma, and basal cell carcinoma. The incidence of solid tumors begins to increase approximately 10 years after diagnosis of Hodgkin disease.

2. There is an increased risk of cardiac disease, particularly in patients treated with mediastinal radiation with or without chemotherapy.

3. Endocrine sequelae consist primarily of thyroid abnormalities and gonadal dysfunction.

   a. Thyroid abnormalities including hypothyroidism and hyperthyroidism, thyroid nodules, and thyroid cancer have been described.

   b. Gonadal dysfunction is more prevalent in males than in females both before and immediately after therapy. Gonadal function in males ranges from complete azoospermia to full recovery of spermatogenesis, depending on the age of the patient at the time of treatment and the type of therapy used. The hormone-producing cells of the testis appear to be more resistant to therapy, and therefore normal growth and development patterns may be maintained. Although many women regain regular menses after treatment, these women may experience early menopause.

 Bibliography

Hancock SL, Donaldson SS, Hoppe RT: Cardiac disease following treatment of Hodgkin's disease in children and adolescents. J Clin Oncol 1993;11:1208–1215.

Leventhal BG, Donaldson SS: Hodgkin's disease. *In* Pizzo PA, Poplack DG (eds): Pediatric Oncology, 2nd ed. Philadelphia, JB Lippincott, 1993, pp 577–594.

Meadows AT, Obringer AC, Marrero O, et al: Second malignant neoplasms following childhood Hodgkin's disease: Treatment and splenectomy as risk factors. Med Pediatr Oncol 1989;17:477–484.

Thompson EI: Hodgkin's disease. *In* Fernbach DJ, Vietti TJ (eds): Clinical Pediatric Oncology, 4th ed, pp 355–375. St. Louis, Mosby–Year Book, 1991.

139 Non-Hodgkin Lymphoma

Norma Wollner and *Jonathan L. Finlay*

Non-Hodgkin lymphoma (NHL) is an uncommon disease in the pediatric age group. It ranks third in order of frequency of childhood tumors and it shares this ranking with Hodgkin disease. As in leukemia, it has a bimodal age distribution curve with a first peak at age 5 to 7 years and a second peak at 12 to 14 years of age. As with most pediatric tumors, it has a male preponderance with a male:female ratio of 2:1.

Definition
NHL is a malignancy of the lymphoid tissue that is present is most organs and systems in the human body.

Etiology
Little is known of the cause of NHL in children. Association with Epstein-Barr virus (EBV) is known for small non–cleaved cell lymphomas mostly in Africa, with some in Europe and South and North America as well. The association of B-cell lymphomas, either large cell or small non–cleaved cell disease, with human immunodeficiency virus is also well known. Differences exist between the African Burkitt lymphoma (called also endemic Burkitt lymphoma [BL]) and Burkitt lymphoma elsewhere (sporadic Burkitt lymphoma). A viral etiology has been postulated for the endemic variety; 95 per cent of all patients with BL in Africa express the EBV genome in their tumor cells, but no more than 20 per cent of American BL tumors express EBV. It is unknown if EBV exposure predisposes to BL formation or is an essential aspect of BL development. The high incidence of BL in the equatorial belt, coinciding with areas of malarial endemicity, has raised speculation that exposure to malaria at a young age may heighten the predisposition to BL development through the effects on the immune system.

There is increased incidence of BL and certain types of large cell lymphomas, known as immunoblastic lymphomas, in children with inherited immunodeficiency disorders, such as the Wiskott-Aldrich syndrome and ataxia-telangiectasia, as well as in patients with acquired immunodeficiency states, such as those that develop after organ (heart, lung, liver, or bone marrow) transplantation or in association with the acquired immunodeficiency syndrome. In these cases, EBV is usually detected in association with the tumors and may reflect B-cell proliferation of EBV-infected cells unrestrained by the immunoincompetent host.

Clinical Findings
1. *Primary sites.* Any tissue or organ system in the body can be affected. The primary presentation can be nodal or extranodal. The nodal primary sites (45 per cent of all lymphoma cases) are the peripheral (about 20 per cent), mediastinal (22 per cent), and intraabdominal (3 per cent) nodes. Fifty-five per cent of all lymphomas present in extranodal sites such as the gastrointestinal tract, nasopharynx, skeleton, subcutaneous and cutaneous skin, kidneys, liver, spleen, ovaries, testes, epidural region, central nervous system (brain and epidural region), thyroid, breasts, gallbladder, and pancreas, in order of frequency.
2. *Symptomatology.* The features vary with each primary site (Table 139–1). Most of the patients present with a history ranging from 1 day to 1 month, with few patients presenting with symptoms of a few hours' duration (primary gastrointestinal tract) and, rarer still, with durations from 6 months to a year (some primary nodal, primary skeletal, and cutaneous lymphomas).
3. *Staging.* Because NHL is one of the fastest growing tumors, the majority of the patients present with disseminated disease. It is also a disease that quickly spreads beyond the primary sites to bone marrow and central

TABLE 139–1. STAGING FOR ALL PRIMARY SITES EXCEPT INTRAABDOMINAL AND NASO-OROPHARYNGEAL

STAGE	CRITERIA
I	Localized disease (nodal or extranodal)
II	Two extranodal primary lesions or two nodal areas on the same side of the diaphragm
III	Disseminated disease above and below diaphragm
IV	Only those with initial bone marrow or central or epidural nervous system disease

For those with bone marrow involvement, there are two subgroups:

IVA	Involvement is ≤25% of total marrow cells
IVB	Involvement is >25% of total marrow cells (leukemia/lymphoma)

nervous system. The staging systems are simple (see Tables 139–1 through 139–3).

Key Symptoms for Most Frequent Primary Sites

- *Nodal:* Large nodes, neck swelling, fever—about 45 per cent

- *Mediastinum:* Cough, chest pain (50 per cent), difficulty breathing (50 per cent)

- *Intraabdominal:* Pain, swelling, and mass (60 to 80 per cent)

- *Naso-oropharynx:* Neck swelling (45 per cent); facial swelling, facial edema on awakening, or stuffy nose (20 per cent)

- *Skeletal:* Bone pain, difficulty using limb, local swelling

Diagnostic Tests

Because NHL in children usually presents as an emergency, because of either syncope caused by upper airway obstruction, vascular compromise, or intestinal obstruction, the work-up of this disease has to be extremely expeditious and completed within a few hours (for emergencies) or within 48 hours (for all other patients). It consists of

1. Computed tomography (CT) of the head and neck for oropharyngeal tumors, central nervous system primary tumors, and cervical lymph node primary tumors
2. CT scan of the chest, abdomen, and pelvis for all primary lesions
3. Bone scan (can be delayed for 1 week even if treatment has started)

TABLE 139–2. STAGING FOR INTRAABDOMINAL PRIMARY SITE

STAGE/ VOLUME	CRITERIA
I	Disease limited to one organ; no regional node involvement; tumor completely resectable
II	Disease extends to regional nodes; completely resectable; disease involving two organs → surgically resectable
III	Extensive intraabdominal tumor surgically unresected, or if resected, distant disease unresected; resectable primary intraabdominal tumor with extraabdominal extension
IV	Involvement of central nervous system, peripheral nervous system, or epidural space
IVA	Marrow involvement with ≤25% blasts in one or more of the marrow sites examined
IVB	Marrow involvement with >25% blasts in one or more of the marrow sites examined

Intra-abdominal disease is further refined by measuring volume of disease, since prognosis is determined not only by initial stage but also by volume of disease present at diagnosis:

A	Primary tumor 5 cm or less, with or without extraabdominal tumor <5 cm
B	Primary tumor 6–15 cm, with or without extraabdominal or intraabdominal tumor <5 cm
C	Very large intraabdominal (>15 cm) tumor with or without ascites, with or without marrow involvement, with or without small (<5 cm) or large (>5 cm) extraabdominal disease

TABLE 139–3. STAGING FOR PRIMARY NASO-OROPHARYNGEAL

TUMOR		
	T1	Tumor 2 cm or less in greatest diameter
	T2	Tumor >2 cm, but not >4 cm in greatest diameter
	T3	Tumor >4 cm in greatest diameter
	T4	Massive tumor >4 cm in diameter with invasion of bone, soft tissues of neck, or root (deep musculature) of tongue, base of skull, or cranial nerves depending on primary site
NODES		
	N0	No clinically positive node
	N1	Single node clinically positive <3 cm
	N2	Single clinically positive homolateral node 3 to 6 cm or multiple homolateral nodes not >6 cm
	N3	Massive homolateral nodes, bilateral nodes, or contralateral nodes
METASTASES		
	M0	No known metastasis
STAGE GROUPING		
	Stage I	T1, N0, M0
	Stage II	T2, N0, M0
	Stage III	T3, N0, M0 or T1 or T2 or T3, N1, M0
	Stage IV	T4, N0 or N1 or any T, N2 or N3, M0

From American Joint Commission on Staging of Nasopharyngeal Tumors (1977; 1988).

4. Gallium scan
5. Bone marrow aspirates and biopsies. We recommend four bone marrow aspirates and two bone marrow biopsies because involvement of the bone marrow is patchy and irregular.
6. Spinal tap with cell count, protein, sugar, and cytocentrifugal examination of cerebrospinal fluid cells
7. Complete blood cell count
8. Liver and renal function studies
9. Lactate dehydrogenase, electrolytes
10. Eight-hour creatinine clearance, if indicated.

Pathology

The four present histologic classifications are being slowly recognized as incomplete and insufficient for most NHL, especially that affecting the adult population. We recommend the Working Formulation, which recognizes four major subtypes in children. All of the lymphomas in children are of the diffuse type. Nodular lymphomas are rare.

1. Lymphoblastic lymphoma is encountered most often in nodal and mediastinal primary lesions, skeletal tumors, and some of the cutaneous and subcutaneous disease. A few cases have been described in intraabdominal lymphomas. It usually is of the T-cell immunophenotype, some (rare) B cell, and some non-T, non-B.
2. Large cell lymphoma is found in most primary sites such as mediastinal, intraabdominal, skeletal, central nervous system, breast, and testis. There is a new subtype of large cell lymphoma—the large cell anaplastic Ki-1 lymphoma—of difficult diagnosis that is thought to be a transitional form between Hodgkin disease and NHL. These cells can present as B-cell, T-cell, or inconclusive immunophenotype.
3. Small non–cleaved cell lymphomas occur most often in the gastrointestinal tract, liver, naso-oropharynx, central

nervous system, and epidural and peripheral nodes. They all have a B-cell immunophenotype.

4. Other rarer histologic subtypes include small cell cleaved lymphoma, diffuse mixed lymphocytic plasmacytic disease, and diffuse small cell cleaved and large cell immunoblastic lymphomas.

Treatment

1. The treatment of NHL consists mostly of chemotherapy. Radiation therapy, which was used in the past, is no longer recommended in a disease that can be cured by chemotherapy alone. Radiation therapy in growing children will cause permanent muscle and skin atrophy when given with chemotherapy and has added long-term effects on the heart, lungs, and thyroid gland. Radiation therapy, even in low dosages, when combined with chemotherapy can cause second tumors in 5 to 7 per cent of the surviving patients.

2. The drugs most effective in this disease, in order of importance, are cyclophosphamide, vincristine, doxorubicin, methotrexate (high, moderate, or low dose), cytarabine (high, moderate or low dose), 6-mercaptopurine, thioguanine, L-asparaginase, etoposide, corticosteroids, and cisplatin. Combinations and dose variations are the basis for different protocols for the different histologies and stages. The intent today is to be able to treat all histologies with a common protocol with minor modification depending on the immunophenotype (B or T cell). The only variance would be the duration of therapy, which would be different whether it is a lymphoblastic lymphoma (duration of therapy 18 months) or large B-cell type (6 months), large T-cell type (12 to 18 months), or small non–cleaved cell (3 to 4 months).

Patients whose disease is stage I and II except for lymphoblastic lymphomas do very well with a milder treatment for 6 months. Any other stage requires a very intensive treatment, and the length of time for treatment will depend on histology and whether it is a B- or T-cell lymphoma. The intensity of chemotherapy for small non–cleaved cell lymphoma has markedly increased over the past 10 years, particularly for those patients with disseminated disease. As a result, children with localized, low-stage disease (stages I through III with normal serum lactate dehydrogenase levels) achieve high cure rates (about 85 per cent) with just 3 to 6 months of fairly simple chemotherapy (CHOP: cyclophosphamide, doxorubicin [Adriamycin], Oncovin [vincristine], and prednisone; or COMP: cyclophosphamide, Oncovin, methotrexate, and prednisone) as well as intrathecal methotrexate to "mop up" tumor cells that may have infiltrated the brain.

Patients with disseminated, high-stage BL (stage III with elevated lactate dehydrogenase or stage IV with bone marrow and/or nervous system involvement) now enjoy very high cure rates (about 80 per cent) with 3 to 5 months of intensified chemotherapy using the same drugs as just listed, usually with higher doses of cyclophosphamide, in addition to high-dose intravenous methotrexate and/or cytarabine, drugs that penetrate the brain efficiently and so eradicate tumor in that location. If lymphomas do recur despite initial chemotherapy, it is rare for further treatment to result in cure. However, if a second remission can be achieved with further chemotherapy, then a small proportion of such patients can be cured through the use of a single cycle of very high-dose (marrow ablative) chemotherapy with either autologous or allogeneic bone marrow rescue.

Key Treatment

• Chemotherapy

Bibliography

Fisher RI, Dahlberg S, Nathwani BN, et al: A clinical analysis of two indolent lymphoma entities: mantle cell lymphoma and marginal zone lymphoma (including the mucosa-associated lymphoid tissue and monocytoid B-cell subcategories): A Southwest Oncology Group Study. Blood 1995;85:1075–1082.

Kadin ME: Primary Ki-1–positive anaplastic large-cell lymphoma: A distinct clinicopathologic entity. Ann Oncol 1994;5(Suppl 1):S25–S30.

Magrath I: Malignant non-Hodgkin's lymphoma. In Pizzo PA, Poplack DG (eds): Principles and Practices of Pediatric Oncology, 2nd ed. Philadelphia, JB Lippincott, 1993, pp 537–575.

Wollner N, Lane JM, Marcove RC, et al: Primary skeletal non-Hodgkin's lymphoma in the pediatric age group. Med Pediatr Oncol 1992;20:506–513.

Wollner N, Mandell L, Filippa D, et al: Primary nasal-paranasal-oropharyngeal lymphoma in the pediatric age group. Cancer 1990;65:1438–1444.

140 Wilms Tumor

Peter G. Steinherz

Epidemiology

1. About 460 new cases of Wilms tumor occur annually in the United States in children younger than age 15 years.
2. The tumor occurs in 1 in 10,000 births (7 per million per year).
3. Fifty-five per cent of tumors occur on the left; the male:female ratio is 1.2:1; the black:white incidence is 3:1.
4. Three to 5 per cent are bilateral; 21 per cent of familial cases are bilateral.
5. One to 2 per cent of patients have positive family history.
6. Peak onset is age 2 to 3 years; 90 per cent are diagnosed before 7 years of age.
7. Bilateral or familial cases or those associated with other congenital anomalies occur at a younger age.
8. Later age at onset is associated with higher stage at presentation.
9. Associated anomalies
   a. Genitourinary—horseshoe kidney, double collecting systems, ambiguous genitalia, cryptorchidism, hypospadias, Danys-Drash syndrome
   b. Hemihypertrophy (1 in 14,000 live births); 1 of 32 develop Wilms tumor
   c. Visceromegaly syndrome, Beckwith-Wiedemann syndrome
   d. Hamartomas
   e. Mental retardation
   f. Aniridia (1 in 70,000 live births)—25 per cent develop Wilms tumor
      (1) 1 in 1287 (1 per cent) patients have aniridia
      (2) Deletion at 11p13 locus, near proto-oncogene c-*HRAS1*, near catalase gene (30 to 50 per cent have low red blood cell catalase)
   g. Cardiopulmonary abnormalities
   h. Musculoskeletal abnormalities
   i. Nephroblastomatosis
   j. Neurofibromatosis
10. Eighty per cent due to somatic causes, 20 per cent germline mutation
   a. Dominant gene with 63 per cent penetrance
   b. For sporadic cases, risk to offspring is 6 per cent; for known familial case, risk to offspring or siblings is 32 per cent.

Etiology

1. Possible involvement of multiple genes
2. Due to germline or somatic mutation
3. Two-stage mutation model

a. First event—in prezygotic (hereditary, present in all cells) or postzygotic (sporadic, only in one cell line)
   (1) Deletion at 11p13-WT1 (Wilms tumor suppressor gene and aniridia) locus
   (2) *WT1* gene produces four distinct messenger RNAs indicating two alternative splice sites; it is a transcription factor that regulates the expression of other genes during normal kidney development.
   (3) *WT1* gene also plays a role in gonadal development
   (4) *WT2* gene at chromosome 11p15: second Wilms tumor suppressor gene (cytomegaly syndromes)
   (5) Additional Wilms tumor locus at chromosome 16q; loss of heterozygosity in this region is also associated with hepatocellular carcinoma.
   (6) Maternal allele was lost in 52 of 53 cases studied
b. Second event—in postzygotic cell: loss of second allele

Pathophysiology

1. Unicentric or multicentric (7 per cent), unilateral tumor with pseudocapsule
2. Three to 5 per cent bilateral
3. Rarely extrarenal
4. Arises from primitive metanephric blastema
5. Triphasic: blastemal, epithelial, and stromal elements, rarely skeletal muscle, cartilage, or squamous epithelium in addition
   a. Favorable histology (89 per cent)
   b. Unfavorable histology (11 per cent)
      (1) Anaplasia (nuclear atypia), focal or diffuse
      (2) Sarcomatous—clear cell sarcoma
      (3) Rhabdoid tumor
6. Associated with nephroblastomatosis (precursor lesions) (25 per cent)
   a. Intralobar
   b. Perilobar

Clinical Findings

1. Initial symptoms
   a. Asymptomatic mass (62 per cent)
   b. Pain (25 per cent)
   c. Hematuria (21 per cent)
   d. Fever
   e. Vomiting, anorexia (5 per cent)
   f. Polycythemia—rare
   g. Anemia—sudden, subcapsular hemorrhage—rare
   h. Hypertension—rare

2. Diagnostic work-up
   a. Preoperative period
      (1) Careful physical examination to rule out congenital anomalies
      (2) Blood pressure
      (3) Complete blood cell count
      (4) Urinalysis, mucin
      (5) Calcium, blood urea nitrogen, creatinine, bilirubin, transaminases
      (6) Abdominal ultrasonography, visualization of the vena cava
      (7) Posteroanterior and lateral chest radiographs
      (8) Computed tomography (CT) of chest and abdomen with contrast medium enhancement
   b. Postoperative period
      (1) Bone scan for those patients with clear cell sarcoma
      (2) CT or magnetic resonance imaging of head for those with rhabdoid tumor and clear cell sarcoma
      (3) Bone marrow aspiration—clear cell sarcoma only
   c. Monitoring during and after therapy
      (1) Posteroanterior and lateral chest radiographs every 3 months during and for 2 years after therapy, then every 6 months for third and fourth year
      (2) Chest CT at end of therapy (more frequent for those with disease in the chest).
      (3) Abdominal ultrasonography or CT midway through therapy (more frequent for those with known residual disease) every 6 months for 2 years after therapy discontinuation for stage III kidney lesions
      (4) Abdominal ultrasonography every 4 months for 5 years for those with nephrogenic rests.
      (5) Abdominal ultrasonography or CT every 4 months for 5 years after therapy discontinuation for all bilateral cases.
   d. Monitoring of siblings of familial cases or offspring of patients
3. Differential diagnosis
   a. Benign
      (1) Renal—hydronephrosis, cystic disease, hamartoma, mesoblastic nephroma
      (2) Hepatic—hemangioma, hamartoma, cyst, cirrhosis, infestation
      (3) Splenic—hemangioma, blood dyscrasias
      (4) Bowel—duplication, cyst
      (5) Pancreatic pseudocyst
   b. Malignant
      (1) Renal—renal cell carcinoma
      (2) Adrenal—neuroblastoma, pheochromocytoma
      (3) Liver—hepatoblastoma, hepatocarcinoma, metastatic disease
      (4) Abdominal—lymphoma, teratoma, germ cell

(5) Retroperitoneal—sarcoma
   c. Most common differential problem—neuroblastoma vs. Wilms tumor. Helpful diagnostic hints:
      (1) Tumor crosses the midline—neuroblastoma more likely
      (2) Multiple bone lesions—neuroblastoma more likely
      (3) Perirenal calcifications (10 to 15 per cent of Wilms tumor)—neuroblastoma more likely
      (4) Intrarenal mass—Wilms tumor more likely
      (5) Kidney displaced inferiorly and lateral—neuroblastoma more likely
      (6) Intraparenchymal pulmonary lesions—Wilms tumor more likely
      (7) Pleural lesions—neuroblastoma more likely
      (8) Normal complete blood cell count or polycythemia—Wilms tumor more likely
4. Staging

Staging of Wilms Tumor

I—Tumor limited to the kidney and completely resected, capsule intact (35 per cent)

II—Tumor penetration of the capsule but completely resected, tumor biopsied or local spillage (30 per cent)

III—Residual nonhematogenous tumor in the abdomen (20 per cent)
   (a) Resection margins positive for tumor
   (b) Lymph nodes are positive
   (c) Diffuse peritoneal contamination by tumor spillage
   (d) Peritoneal, implants found

IV—Hematogenous metastasis—lung, liver, bone, brain (12 per cent)

V—Bilateral involvement (3–5 per cent) each side needs to be separately staged I to IV

---

5. Pattern of spread
   a. Direct extension: pseudocapsule, renal sinus, perinephric fat, soft tissues
   b. Lymphatic: perinephric, paraaortic nodes
   c. Hematogenous: renal vessels, vena cava, right atrium
   d. Metastatic at diagnosis (10 to 20 per cent)
      (1) Lung (80 per cent)
      (2) Liver (15 per cent)
      (3) Lymph node
   e. Metastasis after diagnosis (10 to 20 per cent)
      (1) Lung (14 per cent)—66 per cent of relapses with good histology, 40 per cent of those with unfavorable histology
      (2) Abdomen (6 per cent)—18 per cent of relapses with good histology, 48 per cent of those with poor histology
      (3) Liver (2 per cent)—10 per cent of relapses with good, 20 per cent with poor histology

(4) Other kidney (1 per cent)—10 per cent of those with good histology

(5) Bones (< 1 per cent)—4 per cent of those with poor histology

(6) Nodes (peripheral)

(7) Testis

(8) Brain

6. Prognostic factors

   a. Stage

   b. Histology

   c. Age

   d. Size of tumor

   e. Positive nodes

   f. Therapy

Key Clinical Findings

- Asymptomatic mass
- Pain
- Hematuria
- Fever
- Vomiting, anorexia

Laboratory Findings

Nonradiologic laboratory findings associated with Wilms tumor are rare.

1. Elevated renin
2. Anemia (usually with intratumor hemorrhage)
3. Polycythemia (increased erythropoietin activity)
4. Increased protein-mucopolysaccharide complex or mucin (hyaluronic acid) in plasm and urine

Key Laboratory Findings: Wilms Tumor

- Hematuria
- Elevated renin
- Hypertension (uncommon)

Radiologic Findings

1. Chest radiograph

   a. Single or multiple pulmonary nodules (8 to 15 per cent)

   b. Pleural effusion, rare

   c. Pleural or mediastinal lesions, uncommon

2. CT of chest will pick up nodules missed on plain films

3. Abdominal radiograph

   a. Bulging in the flank

   b. Soft tissue mass with indistinct border in the region of the kidney

   c. Obliterated psoas outline

   d. Air in colon, draped over mass

   e. Perirenal calcification (10 to 15 per cent) spotlike

or ringlike calcification as opposed to stippled or flaky densities with neuroblastoma

   f. Abdominal ultrasonography

      (1) Solid vs. cystic mass—Wilms usually solid with echoes within the mass. Tumor may contain areas of hemorrhage or necrosis or cause hydronephrosis producing echo-free zones.

      (2) Visualize renal vein and inferior vena cava to the right atrium.

      (3) Visualize contralateral kidney.

   g. Abdominal CT with contrast medium enhancement

      (1) Intrarenal vs. suprarenal mass

      (2) Function of contralateral kidney

      (3) Metastatic disease in liver or peritoneal cavity

   h. Skeletal survey or bone scan for patients with clear cell sarcoma

   i. CT or magnetic resonance imaging of head for patients with clear cell sarcoma or rhabdoid tumor

Treatment

1. Preoperative treatment. Preoperative chemotherapy or radiation therapy should be reserved for the rare case in which the tumor is so large that the surgical risks are too great.

2. Surgery. Biopsy of tumor before removal should be avoided.

   a. Transabdominal, transperitoneal incision needed for adequate exposure.

   b. Thoracic extension may be necessary.

   c. Visualization and palpation of contralateral kidney before nephrectomy can rule out bilateral tumor.

   d. Suspicious areas of contralateral kidney should be sampled and marked with titanium clips.

   e. Presence or absence of hilar and regional nodes and extrarenal peritoneal disease noted and sampled.

   f. Before mobilization of primary tumor, an attempt should be made to dissect, expose, and ligate the renal vessels to lessen the chance of hematogenous spread.

   g. Renal vein and vena cava should be palpated before ligation to rule out tumor extension into the vein.

   h. Partial nephrectomy only for patients with

      (1) Solitary kidney

      (2) Bilateral disease

      (3) Syndromes at risk of multiple neoplasms

   i. Peritoneum should be considered contaminated if the tumor is sampled, spilled, or ruptured.

3. Radiation therapy—when needed must begin as soon after surgery as possible to be maximally effective. A delay of more than 10 days has been shown to adversely effect survival. The patient should be scheduled for simulation and radiation therapy right after surgery. This can be canceled if inappropriate because of stage or histology.

   a. Dose fraction

      (1) 180 cGy per day, five times a week

      (2) 150 cGy per day, five times a week if very large volume is treated

b. Field
    (1) Positive hilar or paraaortic nodes or residual disease confined to flank: tumor bed and flank, crossing the midline to include the entire spinal column and bilateral paraaortic nodes
    (2) Peritoneal seeding, preoperative rupture, gross operative spill or gross residual disease: whole abdomen
    (3) Liver metastases: include at least a 2-cm margin of uninvolved liver
    (4) Pulmonary metastasis: both lungs
c. Dose—favorable histology
    (1) Abdomen or flank
        (a) Stage I—no radiation therapy
        (b) Stage II—no radiation therapy
        (c) Stage III—1080 cGy
        (d) Stage IV—as per abdominal stage of the removed kidney tumor
    (2) Liver—1980 cGy to total liver, or 3060 cGy if less than 75 per cent of liver volume is irradiated. Remaining kidney must be shielded to receive less than 1440 cGy.
    (3) Pulmonary—1200 cGy in eight fractions. Infants younger than 18 months old with pulmonary metastases receive 900 cGy, only if less than total resolution with chemotherapy.
    (4) Nodes, bone, brain—3060 cGy
d. Dose—unfavorable histology anaplastic
    (1) Abdomen
        (a) Stage I—no radiation therapy
        (b) Stages II, III, and IV—1080 cGy with additional 1080 cGy to areas of bulk disease. Remaining kidney must not receive more than 1440 cGy.
    (2) (3) (4) As in c. (2) (3) (4)
e. Dose—unfavorable histology—clear cell sarcoma
    (1) Abdomen. Stages I, II, III, and IV—1080 cGy with additional 1080 cGy to areas of bulk disease with remaining kidney shielded to 1440 cGy.
    (2) (3) (4) As in c. (2) (3) (4)
f. Unfavorable histology—rhabdoid tumor
    (1) Abdomen
        (a) Stages I and II—no radiation therapy
        (b) Stage III—1080 cGy with additional 1080 cGy to area of bulk disease and remaining kidney shielded to 1440 cGy
        (c) Stage IV—according to abdominal stage of removed tumor (I to III)
    (2) (3) (4) As in c. (2) (3) (4)
4. Chemotherapy—should begin as soon after surgery as possible (fewer than 5 days). Doses are per body surface area. Infants younger than 12 months of age receive one half of the recommended dose of all chemotherapeutic agents on the basis of body weight, not surface area. Doses should be escalated to full dose as tolerated, and full doses should be given when the child is older than 12 months of age. Dose conversion:

Dose/kg = dose/m^2 ÷ 30 (30 mg/m^2 = 1 mg/kg)

a. Favorable histology—stages I and II, anaplastic tumor stage I
    (1) Dactinomycin, 1.35 mg/m^2/dose (2.3 mg maximum), 0.045 mg/kg/dose intravenously on weeks 0, 3, 6, 9, 12, 15, and 18
    (2) Vincristine, 1.5 mg/m^2/dose, 0.05 mg/kg/dose (maximum 2.0 mg) intravenously, 10 weekly doses beginning day 7 after surgery; 2.0 mg/m^2/dose (maximum 2.0 mg) IV on weeks 12, 15, and 18.
    (3) It is possible that patients with favorable histology stage I disease who are younger than 24 months of age with a tumor that weighed less than 550 g may not need any therapy other than surgical excision.
b. Favorable histology—stages III and IV (focal anaplastic tumor stages II, III, or IV and focal anaplasia stage IV)
    (1) Dactinomycin, 1.35 mg/m^2 (maximum 2.3 mg) administered intravenously on weeks 0, 6, 12, 18, and 24. The week 6 dose should be decreased by 50 per cent if whole lung or abdomen radiation therapy was given.
    (2) Vincristine, 1.5 mg/m^2 (maximum 2.0 mg) per week intravenously for 10 doses beginning day 7; 2.0 mg/m^2 (maximum 2.0 mg) intravenously on weeks 12, 15, 18, and 24
    (3) Doxorubicin, 45 mg/m^2 IV on weeks 3 and 9; dose on week 3 should be reduced by 50 per cent if whole lung or abdomen radiation therapy was given; 30 mg/m^2 to be given intravenously on weeks 15 and 21
c. Favorable histology—stage V. Chemotherapy as in a., followed by reevaluation with second-look laparotomy 5 weeks after diagnosis. Switch to chemotherapy as in b. if viable tumor is present. Use renal parenchymal sparing surgery, if possible.
d. Clear cell carcinoma stages I through IV or diffuse anaplasia II through IV. Standard effective therapy has not yet been found. Chemotherapy in 1997 is with vincristine, doxorubicin, etoposide, and cyclophosphamide/mesna.
e. Rhabdoid tumor stages I through IV. Standard effective therapy has not yet been found. Chemotherapy is with carboplatin, etoposide, and cyclophosphamide/mesna.

Key Treatment

• Surgery
• Radiation therapy
• Chemotherapy

Prognosis

1. Prognostic factors
    a. Stage
        (1) Stage I favorable histology

(a) Chance of relapse: 8 per cent

(b) Two-year survival: 96 per cent

(2) Stage II favorable histology

(a) Chance of relapse: 10 per cent

(b) Two-year survival: 92 per cent

(3) Stage III favorable histology

(a) Chance of relapse: 19 per cent

(b) Two-year survival: 87 per cent

(4) Stage IV favorable histology

(a) Chance of relapse: 16 per cent

(b) Two-year survival: 80 per cent

(5) Unfavorable histology

(a) Chance of relapse: 28 per cent

(b) Two-year survival: 53 to 68 per cent

b. Tumor weight

(1) Less than 250 g: chance of relapse, 6 per cent

(2) 250 to less than 499 g: chance of relapse, 8 per cent

(3) 500 to less than 999 g: chance of relapse, 12 per cent

(4) More than 1000 g: chance of relapse, 15 per cent

c. Age

(1) Birth to 23 months: chance of relapse, 5 per cent

(2) 24 to 47 months: chance of relapse, 10 per cent

(3) More than 48 months: chance of relapse, 16 per cent

2. Time of relapse

a. Within 6 months from diagnosis: 45 per cent of those destined to relapse

b. 6 to 12 months from diagnosis: 28 per cent of those destined to relapse

c. During second year after diagnosis: 21 per cent of those destined to relapse

d. More than 2 years after diagnosis: 6 per cent of those destined to relapse

Bibliography

D'Angio GJ, Evans AE, Beckwith JB, et al: The treatment of Wilms' tumor: Results of the Third National Wilms' Tumor Study. Cancer 1989;64:466–479.

Green DM, Beckwith JB, Breslow NE, et al: Treatment of children with Stages II–IV anaplastic Wilms' tumor: A report from the National Wilms' Tumor Study Group. J Clin Oncol 1994; 12:2126–2131.

Holland P: Clinical and biochemical manifestations of Wilms' tumor. *In* Pochedly C, Miller D (eds): Wilms' Tumor. New York, John Wiley & Sons, 1976, pp 11–30.

Tournade MF, Cam-Naugue C, Vaute PA, et al: Results of the Sixth International Society of Pediatric Oncology Wilms' Tumor Trial & Study: A risk-adapted therapeutic approach in Wilms' tumor. J Clin Oncol 1993;11:1014–1023.

141 Neuroblastoma

Nai-Kong V. Cheung and *Brian H. Kushner*

Etiology and Epidemiology

1. *Incidence.* Neuroblastoma (NB) is the most common extracranial pediatric solid tumor and the most common neoplasm of infants. It occurs in 1 in 10,000 births. More than 90 per cent of the more than 500 cases diagnosed yearly in the United States occur in children 5 years old or younger.

2. *Etiology.* NB probably results from random genetic mutations. Environmental causative factors have not been identified, nor has NB been significantly associated with any other disease or condition. Familial aggregations of NB occur very rarely.

3. *Prognosis.* Cure rates of patients diagnosed at 1 year of age or older with metastases to bone or bone marrow (the majority of patients) are less than 20 per cent. In contrast, patients with localized disease and infants with widespread disease are highly curable, often with little or no cytotoxic therapy. Biologic markers can identify patients who, despite a favorable clinical profile (e.g., localized tumor), are likely to develop lethal metastatic disease.

Clinical Findings

1. Diagnosis

a. Characteristic histopathologic findings, or

b. Tumor-cell clumps (syncytia) in bone marrow, plus elevations in urine of vanillylmandelic acid (VMA), homovanillic acid (HVA), or other catecholamines.

2. Presenting signs and symptoms

a. *Local effects of primary or metastatic tumor.* NBs arise (in order of decreasing frequency) in the celiac axis and suprarenal area, posterior mediastinum, pelvis, and neck and metastasize to bone marrow, bone, liver, lymph nodes, and skin; spread to lung or brain parenchyma is rare. NBs can cause genitourinary tract obstruction, respiratory impairment (from pleural effusion or from airway obstruction), Horner syndrome, orbital proptosis and ecchymosis ("raccoon eyes"), bone pain with limp, or paralysis (intervertebral extension by "dumbbell" tumor). Infants may have skin nodules or massive liver invasion.

b. *Paraneoplastic syndromes.* Less than 3 to 5 per cent of NBs (usually prognostically favorable forms) cause paraneoplastic syndromes, that is, symptoms unrelated to local mass effect. Watery diarrhea (sometimes mistaken for intestinal malabsorption disease) results from vasoactive intestinal peptide production by tumor cells and resolves after complete tumor removal. Ataxia or opsoclonus-myoclonus ("dancing eyes, dancing feet") is of uncertain etiology; encephalopathy may develop after tumor resection. Long-term neurodevelopmental deficits have been documented in up to 50 per cent of these patients.

c. *Unsuspected disease.* Asymptomatic NBs are detected by routine physical examination, by screening neonates for elevations in urinary catecholamines, or by studies performed for other reasons (e.g., antenatal ultrasonography or radiography for suspected pneumonia).

Key Clinical Findings

- Mass in abdomen, chest, or neck
- Limp or bone pain
- Orbital proptosis
- Horner syndrome
- Opsoclonus/myoclonus

Laboratory Findings

1. Anemia and thrombocytopenia or thrombocytosis
2. Elevated serum levels of lactate dehydrogenase, ferritin, and/or neuron-specific enolase
3. Elevated urinary levels of catecholamines (VMA, HVA, and/or dopamine)

Key Laboratory Findings

- Anemia
- Elevated lactate dehydrogenase level
- Elevated catecholamine levels

Radiographic Findings

1. *Computed tomography.* Soft tissue mass with calcifications and often with associated adenopathy. Differential diagnosis includes teratoma (presence of fat or teeth), Wilms tumor (intrarenal origin with calyceal distortion plus crescentic calcifications), primitive neuroectodermal tumor, and sarcomas.
2. *Spine magnetic resonance imaging.* Epidural invasion by direct extension of primary or metastatic tumor.
3. *Bone scan.* Uptake occurs in primary tumor or in one or more distant bones.
4. *Skeletal survey.* Lytic lesions
5. *MIBG scan.* Metaiodobenzylguanidine (an analog of catecholamine precursors) is taken up by primary and metastatic NB (not restricted to any organ).

Staging

Clinical Staging: International Neuroblastoma Staging System (INSS)

Stage 1: Localized tumor with complete gross excision

Stage 2A: Localized tumor with incomplete excision (gross residual disease)

Stage 2B: Localized tumor with or without complete gross excision, with ipsilateral nonadherent lymph nodes positive for tumor

Stage 3: Unresectable tumor infiltrating across the midline, or localized tumor with contralateral lymph node involvement

Stage 4: Any primary tumor with dissemination to distant lymph nodes, bone, bone marrow, liver, and/or other organs

Stage 4S: Localized primary tumor (stage 1 or 2), with other involvement limited to skin, liver, and/or bone marrow (<10 per cent of nucleated cells deemed malignant on biopsy or aspirate); limited to infants younger than 1 year of age

---

Prognosis

Adverse findings for various prognostic factors include

1. *Clinical features*
   a. Age: older than 1 to 2 years
   b. Pattern of disease: bone metastases, extensive bone marrow involvement
2. *Tumor cell features*
   a. N-*myc* proto-oncogene: amplified
   b. Chromosomal ploidy: near diploid or near tetraploid
   c. Chromosome 1p36 region: loss of heterozygosity
   d. Nerve growth factor receptor (TrkA): not expressed
   e. CD44: not expressed
   f. In vitro growth: cell line established
   g. Histopathology: unfavorable by Shimada criteria or by Joshi criteria
3. *Biochemical markers*
   a. Serum ferritin: more than 142 ng/mL (or greater than upper limit of normal)
   b. Serum lactate dehydrogenase: greater than 1500 U/L
   c. Serum neuron specific enolase: greater than 100 ng/mL
   d. Urine: $\dfrac{VMA \times ULN_{HVA}}{HVA \times ULN_{VMA}} < 1$

Treatment

1. *Chemotherapy.* Combined use of cyclophosphamide/ifosfamide, doxorubicin, cisplatin/carboplatin, and etoposide is the standard. High-risk tumors require higher dose intensity (i.e., larger doses of drugs given over the same treatment period).
2. *Surgery*
   a. *At diagnosis.* Gross total resection (GTR) of the

TABLE 141–1. TREATMENT RESULTS BY STAGE

INSS STAGE	INCIDENCE	TREATMENT	SURVIVAL AT 5 YEARS
1	14	S	>90%
2A, 2B	16	S ± CT ± RT	70–80%
3	11	S ± CT ± RT	40–70%
4	52	CT + S ± RT	>60% if <1 year
		CT + S ± RT ± ABMT	20% if 12–24 months
		CT + S ± RT ± ABMT	10% if >2 years
4S	7	± S ± CT	>80%

ABMT, myeloablative therapy followed by autologous bone marrow transplantation or peripheral stem cell rescue; CT, chemotherapy; RT, radiotherapy; S, surgical resection.

primary tumor is undertaken if risk of surgical complications is small.

b. *Second-look surgery.* Chemotherapy-induced shrinkage of tumor may facilitate GTR. GTR may prolong the survival of stages 3 and 4 patients receiving intensive therapies.

c. *Emergency.* Surgical intervention may be used to relieve epidural compression.

3. *Radiation therapy*

a. *Local radiation.* For residual disease: 2100 to 3000 cGy. For life-threatening/major organ complications or for palliation, smaller doses of radiation can relieve acute symptoms.

b. *Total body irradiation:* 1000 to 1200 cGy as part of myeloablative regimen

c. Targeted radiotherapy using radiolabeled MIBG or antitumor monoclonal antibodies.

4. *Biologic therapy*

a. Retinoic acid to induce tumor cell differentiation

b. Anti–ganglioside G_{D2} monoclonal antibodies to tar-

get serum complement and leukocytes selectively to achieve tumor cell lysis

Key Treatment

- Chemotherapy
- Surgery
- Radiation therapy
- Biologic therapy

Outcome (Table 141–1)

Although age and stage are strong prognostic factors, biologic prognostic markers have further refined risk group classifications. For example, intensive therapy is given to some patients with localized but N-*myc*-amplified tumors and to infants with advanced-stage diploid tumors.

Bibliography

Brodeur GM, Castleberry RC: Neuroblastoma. *In* Pizzo PA, Poplack DG (eds): Principles and Practice of Pediatric Oncology. Philadelphia, JB Lippincott, 1993, p 739.

Brodeur GM, Pritchard J, Berthold F, et al: Revisions of the international criteria for neuroblastoma diagnosis, staging, and response to treatment. J Clin Oncol 1993;11:1466.

Cheung NK: Biological and molecular approaches to diagnosis and treatment: I. Principles of immunotherapy. *In* Pizzo PA, Poplack DG (eds): Principles and Practice of Pediatric Oncology, 3rd ed. Philadelphia, JB Lippincott, 1995.

Cheung NK, Kushner BH, LaQuaglia M, Lindsley K: Treatment of advanced-stage neuroblastoma. *In* Reghavan D, Scher HI, Leibel SA, Lange P (eds): Principles and Practice of Genitourinary Oncology. Philadelphia, JB Lippincott, 1996, p 1101.

Kushner BH, LaQuaglia M, Cheung NKV: Therapeutic approach to low risk and intermediate risk neuroblastoma. *In* Reghavan D, Scher HI, Leibel SA, Lange P: Principles and Practice of Genitourinary Oncology. Philadelphia, JB Lippincott, 1996, p 1085.

142 Brain Tumors

Ira J. Dunkel and Jonathan L. Finlay

Brain tumors are heterogeneous in histopathology and location.

Etiology

In most cases, we do not understand why a given child develops a brain tumor. In a small percentage of cases an underlying genetic predisposition exists, and obtaining a good family history is important.

1. Patients with *neurofibromatosis type 1* have an increased incidence of optic pathway gliomas and other astrocytomas.

2. Patients with *neurofibromatosis type 2* have a very high likelihood of developing acoustic neuromas and meningiomas.

3. Patients with *Li-Fraumeni syndrome*, who have a germline abnormality of one *p53* gene allele, may develop brain tumors, usually gliomas, among their spectrum of other cancers in children and/or young adults.

4. Patients with *bilateral retinoblastoma*, who have a germline mutation of one *RB1* gene allele, have an increased risk of developing pineoblastomas, the "trilateral" retinoblastoma syndrome.

5. Patients with *Turcot syndrome*, a rare autosomal recessive

disorder, develop both gastrointestinal polyps and malignant brain tumors (medulloblastoma and glioblastoma multiforme).

Epidemiology

1. In contrast to brain tumors in adults, the majority of pediatric brain tumors arise below the tentorium.
2. Astrocytic tumors are the most common type of brain tumors in children, with supratentorial low-grade and high-grade astrocytomas contributing 25 and 11 per cent; cerebellar astrocytomas, 12 per cent; brainstem gliomas, 9 per cent; ependymomas, 8 per cent; and optic gliomas, about 5 per cent. Medulloblastomas make up about 23 per cent, and other primitive neuroectodermal tumors (PNETs) another 2 to 3 per cent. Other rare tumors such as choroid plexus tumors and germ cell tumors comprise most of the remainder.
3. Most brain tumors occur roughly as often in males as in females, although medulloblastomas and germ cell tumors may be more common in boys.

Pathophysiology

1. Cancer is the uncontrolled proliferation of undifferentiated cells. Astrocytic cells, neuronal cells, oligodendroglia, and microglia all normally form the structures of the central nervous system, and precursors of these cells are presumed to be the cell of origin of brain tumors. The molecular genetic mechanisms underlying this in pediatric brain tumors are under intense investigation, but our current understanding of the process is still very incomplete.
2. Although the histopathologic appearance of a tumor is very important in determining prognosis and treatment, it is important to realize that low-grade tumors, which might be considered to be histologically benign in other parts of the body, are still potentially life-threatening problems in the brain if their location makes resection impossible.

Clinical Findings

The site of the tumor is largely responsible for the presenting symptoms.

1. Hydrocephalus may be present if the tumor is obstructing the normal flow of the cerebrospinal fluid (CSF), as in many posterior fossa tumors, and may produce signs such as morning headache, emesis, and lethargy. Fatigue, poor school performance, and personality changes may also be seen.
2. Posterior fossa tumors may also present as signs referable to brain structures in the area of the tumor. Tumors invading the brainstem may cause cranial nerve palsies and long-tract signs. Ataxia is also common.
3. Supratentorial tumors may present as headache, seizures, and/or paresis. Seizures are more common in the slow-growing, low-grade astrocytomas of the cerebral hemispheres.
4. Although metastasis outside the central nervous system is very rare, tumors such as medulloblastomas, PNETs, and germ cell tumors have a predilection to spreading through the cerebrospinal fluid pathways, depositing tumor clumps and growing along the leptomeninges that cover both the brain and spinal cord. Back pain, spine tenderness, extremity weakness, and bowel and/or bladder dysfunction may be signs of spinal cord compression from "drop" metastases, situations that represent medical emergencies. The neurologic dysfunction may be reversible with rapid diagnosis and treatment but irreversible if of longer standing.

Key Clinical Findings

- Ataxia
- Headache
- Craniomegaly
- Seizures

Laboratory Findings

The usefulness of laboratory studies is limited in brain tumors.

1. Cytologic examination of the CSF is important in the patient with tumors that spread along the leptomeninges, including medulloblastomas, PNETs, and germ cell tumors.
2. Patients with certain subtypes of germ cell tumors may have elevated levels of certain proteins in their serum or CSF that are useful as a diagnostic aid or to monitor disease status: endodermal sinus tumors (also known as yolk sac tumors) produce α–fetoprotein, and choriocarcinomas and embryonal tumors produce the β subunit of human chorionic gonadotropin.

Key Laboratory Findings

- Usually normal
- CSF cytology
- CSF α–fetoprotein

Radiographic Changes

Radiographic studies are very important in the diagnosis and follow-up of children with suspected or known brain tumors.

1. Magnetic resonance imaging (MRI), with and without intravenous gadolinium contrast material, is the preferred modality for imaging brain tumors. A disadvantage is that MRI takes more time to perform than computed tomography (CT), and the young child often requires general anesthesia for optimal images to be obtained. CT scanning can be performed rapidly; and when the specific questions to be addressed are whether hydrocephalus or hemorrhage is present, it may be the preferred modality.
2. Spine MRI is performed to image the spine as part of the staging evaluation in patients with tumors (medulloblastomas, PNETs, germ cell tumors) that have a propensity to

metastasize through the CSF along the leptomeninges. Myelography, the injection of contrast material into the subarachnoid space by means of a lumbar puncture and subsequent visualization via x-ray fluoroscopy, is an alternative modality that is being performed less frequently since the introduction of spine MRI.

Differential Diagnosis by Tumor Location

Posterior Fossa
- Medulloblastoma
- Cerebellar low-grade astrocytoma
- Ependymoma
- Brainstem glioma

Supratentorial
- Astrocytoma (low-grade or high-grade)
- Ependymoma
- Primitive neuroectodermal tumor

Treatment

1. Neurosurgery
   a. Neurosurgery is performed in most children in whom a brain tumor is suspected, both to provide a histopathologic diagnosis and to resect as much of the tumor mass as can be safely done without incurring permanent, serious neurologic deficits. Radical surgical resection may be curative in itself, as in low-grade astrocytomas, or may at least diminish the tumor bulk that adjuvant irradiation or chemotherapy will need to treat.
   b. The ability to resect the tumor completely depends largely on its location. Complete resections may often be performed in the posterior fossa or some superficial supratentorial locations. On the other hand, locations such as the brainstem, thalamus, and motor cortex often preclude radical surgery. Some locations may prohibit even a biopsy: diffuse, intrinsic pontine tumors are routinely diagnosed and treated based on their radiographic appearance. Optic pathway gliomas in patients with neurofibromatosis type 1 are also often diagnosed radiographically, without the need for surgical confirmation.
   c. Another important role for the neurosurgeon is to insert a ventriculoperitoneal shunt if significant hydrocephalus is present to relieve the increased intracranial pressure.
2. Radiation therapy
   a. Radiation therapy is an important component in the treatment of many types of brain tumors, including incompletely resected low-grade astrocytomas, high-grade astrocytomas, brainstem tumors, ependymomas, and medulloblastomas, among others. Standard doses and fields of irradiation depend on the tumor type, site, and the patient's age, but in many cases the primary tumor site is treated to a total dose of about 5400 cGy. When extended fields, such as whole brain or the cranial spinal axis are treated, lower doses such as 2400 to 3600 cGy are administered and the primary site is boosted to the higher dose. Such craniospinal irradiation is reserved for tumors with a known propensity to disseminate throughout the neuraxis such as medulloblastomas and PNETs.
   b. Radiation therapy is clearly effective treatment; however, the toxicity of large fields of irradiation, especially in the developing brain of infants and young children, is a major concern. Significant loss of IQ points, memory deficits, and neuroendocrine deficits have all been clearly documented as side effects. This has led most pediatric oncologists to try to avoid, or at least delay, the administration of irradiation to the brain of young children through the use of chemotherapy.
3. Chemotherapy

   Chemotherapy is a mainstay of treatment in almost every childhood malignancy outside the central nervous system, but its role in the treatment of pediatric brain tumors is still evolving. Tumors such as medulloblastomas, PNETs, and germ cell tumors are clearly sensitive to several commonly used chemotherapeutic agents, such as cyclophosphamide, platinum agents, etoposide, and vincristine. Astrocytic tumors are also sensitive to chemotherapy, although on a less consistent basis. Whether this chemosensitivity provides clear survival benefits is not always clear, and many pediatric multiinstitutional clinical research trials in the past 10 to 15 years have treated children with combination chemotherapy to try to answer this question. Table 142–1 is a summary of our current management of the most common types of tumors.

Key Treatment

- Surgery
- Radiation therapy
- Chemotherapy

TABLE 142–1.   TREATMENT OF PEDIATRIC BRAIN TUMORS

DISEASE	SURGERY	RADIATION THERAPY*	CHEMOTHERAPY*
Low-grade astrocytoma	Yes	Involved field (if incomplete resection)	No
High-grade astrocytoma	Yes	Involved field	Yes
Brainstem glioma	No	Involved field	Unproven
Ependymoma	Yes	Involved field	If incomplete resection
Medulloblastoma	Yes	Craniospinal	Yes
PNET	Yes	Craniospinal	Yes

*For children older than 6 years old. For younger children, chemotherapy is often used to try to avoid or delay radiation therapy.

Prevention

1. Although prevention would certainly be preferable to treatment of established brain tumors, the vast majority of children who develop brain tumors have no known risk factors.
2. Radiation causes brain tumors to develop as a second malignancy in a small percentage of children treated for primary cancers such as leukemia, brain tumors, or retinoblastoma; and avoidance of irradiation, if possible, could prevent a very small number of brain tumors.
3. Some data suggest that the introduction of folic acid supplementation during pregnancy has been associated with a decreased incidence of medulloblastoma in Great Britain and Ireland.

Bibliography

Bailey CC, Gnekow A, Wellek S, et al: Prospective randomised trial of chemotherapy given before radiotherapy in childhood medulloblastoma. International Society of Paediatric Oncology (SIOP) and the (German) Society of Paediatric Oncology (GPO): SIOP II. Med Pediatr Oncol 1995;25:166–178.

Cohen ME, Duffner PK: Brain Tumors in Children: Principles of Diagnosis and Treatment, 2nd ed. New York, Raven Press, 1994.

Duffner PK, Horowitz ME, Krischer JP, et al: Postoperative chemotherapy and delayed radiation in children less than three years of age with malignant brain tumors. N Engl J Med 1993;328:1725–1731.

Finlay JL, Boyett JM, Yates AJ, et al: Randomized phase III trial in childhood high-grade astrocytoma comparing vincristine, lomustine, and prednisone with the eight-drugs-in-1-day regimen. J Clin Oncol 1995;13:112–123.

143 Rhabdomyosarcoma

Fereshteh Ghavimi

Rhabdomyosarcoma (RMS) is the most common soft tissue sarcoma in children younger than 15 years of age. It was first described in 1854 by Weber.

Classification

1. The first histologic classification of RMS in 1958 recognized three morphologic subtypes: embryonal (botryoid was considered a subtype of it), alveolar, and pleomorphic. The Intergroup Rhabdomyosarcoma Study (IRS), consisting of three pediatric cancer study groups, collected nearly 2000 patients, recognized embryonal RMS in 51 per cent, alveolar RMS in 21 per cent, botryoid in 6 per cent, pleomorphic in 1 per cent, undifferentiated sarcoma in 7 per cent, and other subtypes in 14 per cent.
2. The most acceptable new classification scheme is that of the National Cancer Institute. Immunohistochemical, electron microscopic, and cytogenetic discoveries have delineated structural abnormalities of the two cell types of embryonal and alveolar RMS, each characterized by specific genetic changes.
3. RMS and normal fetal skeletal muscles share muscle specific gene *MyoD* expression, and its restriction to cells of the myogenic origin is useful in distinguishing RMS from other small cell sarcomas. Alveolar RMS has translocation involving chromosomes 2 and 13, t(2;13)(q35;q14) which has led to development of a specific molecular diagnostic assay. Embryonal RMS is characterized by loss of heterozygosity for multiple loci at chromosome 11p15.5.
4. Among prognostic factors, undifferentiated sarcoma and alveolar RMS are associated with unfavorable survival outcome whereas embryonal RMS has intermediate survival and botryoid has a favorable outcome.

Clinical Findings

1. Approximately 70 per cent of cases present before the age of 10 years. The primary sites of the tumor are head and neck area in 35 per cent; extremities, 17 per cent; genitourinary tract, 23 per cent; and trunk and other sites, 25 per cent.
2. Signs and symptoms of the disease vary according to location of the primary tumor. In the head and neck area the most frequent tumor site is the orbit. Orbital tumors usually present as proptosis. Nasopharyngeal tumors may present as sinusitis, airway obstruction, or dysphagia. Middle ear tumors may present as polyps in the ear canal, chronic otitis media, and hemorrhagic discharge. Due to the proximity of head and neck tumors, particularly in parameningeal sites (middle ear, nasal cavity, nasopharynx, paranasal sinuses, infratemporal fossa) to the base of the skull and with opportunity for direct extension of the tumor to this area and to the central nervous system, cranial nerve palsies are often present at the time of diagnosis. Urinary tract symptoms are usually produced when the tumor causes obstruction of the urinary or fecal pathway. Frequency, dysuria, urinary retention, constipation, and hematuria are the symptoms of bladder and prostate tumors. Vaginal, cervical, and uterine tumors present as mucosanguineous discharge or protruding perineal mass. Paratesticular tumors produce painless unilateral scrotal enlargement. Extremity tumors usually present as painless mass and swelling.
3. The most common sites of metastases are lungs, bones,

Key Clinical Findings

- According to site
  Proptosis
  Sinusitis
  Urinary tract symptoms

liver, bone marrow, regional lymph nodes, and central nervous system (usually by direct extension).

Laboratory Findings

Diagnosis of RMS is made by biopsy and histopathologic and, when possible, cytogenetic examination of the tumor. For planning treatment and determining prognosis, staging of the tumor at diagnosis is necessary. Determination of stage is derived by clinical, hematologic, radiologic, and isotopic examinations of the patients for evidence of metastases. Pretreatment evaluation should include complete medical history; physical examination; documentation of measurable disease, complete blood cell count with differential, hepatic and renal chemistries, bilateral anterior and posterior iliac bone marrow aspirations, and bilateral posterior iliac crest biopsies; examination of CSF in patients with primary tumor of the head and neck; and appropriate radiologic studies, including chest radiography, computed tomography (CT) of the chest, CT and magnetic resonance imaging (MRI) of specific sites of primary tumor or metastases, bone scan, and gallium-67 scan. Radiologic examination allows the presumed site of origin and extension of the tumor to be defined. CT scan reveals the tumor, gives guidance for the surgical biopsy, and contributes to determining the extent of the tumor. MRI is complementary to CT but provides better visualization of the tumor and its adjacent structures and vessels. After completing the work-up and determining the site and size and invasiveness of the primary tumor and sites of metastases to regional nodes or distant organs the stage of the disease is established.

Staging

A surgicopathologic staging system known as Clinical Grouping has been used in IRS studies to design treatment and evaluate the prognosis. The TNM system has been used in other studies. A combination of the two is now being evaluated in the IRS-IV study. IRS studies have demonstrated that 60 to 70 per cent of patients have advanced disease at diagnosis (unresectable tumor or metastatic disease) (Table 143–1).

Treatment

During the 1960s only 20 to 30 per cent of children with early-stage operable RMS survived. During 1970s the institution of a multidisciplinary approach by surgery, radiation therapy, and multiple drug cycles of chemotherapy for the treatment of childhood RMS resulted in marked improvement in the outcome of therapy. Refinement of the coordinated multimodal treatment plans according to stage, site, and histology of the tumor in 1980s resulted in a 70 per cent 5-year survival rate.

1. *Chemotherapy*

   a. Chemotherapy has significantly altered the outcome of the therapy in RMS and has increased the survival rate of the patients. All patients with RMS should receive chemotherapy. The justification for chemotherapy has been based on the assumption that even in the early stages of tumor, occult metastases are present and chemotherapy can arrest their growth. The efficacy of chemotherapy can be increased by concurrent administration of several drugs with different mechanisms of action and minimal overlapping toxicity. Chemotherapy given before radiation or surgery may shrink large tumor masses, permit complete excision of the tumor in a previously unresectable case, or make definitive surgery much easier. It may also be possible to use a smaller radiation field after a tumor has been shrunk with chemotherapy.

   b. The standard agents used for chemotherapy for early stages of disease are vincristine, dactinomycin, cyclophosphamide, and doxorubicin (Adriamycin) given in combination of two to four drugs for an average period of 1 year. In addition to the same drugs given at high doses and frequent intervals, ifosfamide and etoposide are used to intensify therapy for advanced stages of disease.

   c. Although significant progress has been made in survival of the patients with nonmetastatic disease, patients with metastatic disease continue to have low survival rate (Table 143–2). Programs using new combinations of existing drugs at high doses and utilizing hematopoietic growth factors and stem cell rescue are being tried that may improve the outcome for these patients.

2. *Surgery.* The initial treatment of RMS in most locations is radical surgical excision of the tumor. An attempt at wide resection of the primary tumor and/or metastases with an adequate margin of normal surrounding tissue should be made when feasible and without sacrifice of vital organs or loss of function. During therapy, it may be beneficial to obtain tissues to determine the histopathologic response to therapy. For orbital tumors, simple biopsy followed by radiation therapy and chemotherapy is the current surgical treatment. For head and neck tumors, accessible tumors that can be re-

TABLE 143–1. TNM STAGING SYSTEM FOR RHABDOMYOSARCOMA

CLINICAL STAGE	SITES	INVASIVENESS	SIZE	STATUS OF NODES	STATUS OF METASTASIS
I	Orbit, head and neck (nonparameningeal), genitourinary (non–bladder/prostate)	T1	a or b	N0	M0
II	Bladder/prostate, extremity, parameningeal trunk, retroperitoneal	T2	a or b	N0	M0
III	Same as II	T1 or T2	a or b	N1	M0
IV	All sites	T1 or T2	a or b	N0 or N1	M1

T1, tumor confined to anatomic site of origin; T2, tumor extends beyond site of origin; N1, regional nodes not involved; N2, regional nodes involved; M0, no distant metastases; M1, distant metastases.
Size a < 5 cm; size b ≥ 5 cm.

TABLE 142–2. PERCENTAGE OF FIVE-YEAR SURVIVAL ACCORDING TO STAGE AND SITE, RESULTS OF IRS I, IRS II, AND IRS III

SITE	IRS I	IRS II	IRS III
Orbit	89	92	95
Head and neck	55	81	78
Parameningeal	47	69	74
Genitourinary non–bladder/prostate	74	80	89
Genitourinary bladder/prostate	—	73	81
Extremities	47	70	74
Other sites	45	53	67
Group I	83	87	93
Group II	70	73	81
Group III	52	66	73
Group IV	20	26	30
All patients	60	63	71

moved without creating any major cosmetic defects should be excised. For extremity tumors, wide local excision of the tumor mass and surrounding normal tissue is required. Gross removal of the tumor is often impossible, but attempts should be made to excise as much tumor as possible and still have a functionally viable extremity. Amputation is rarely recommended unless other modalities have failed. Radical surgical removal of pelvic RMS is no longer necessary for the majority of patients with pelvic tumors. Surgical assessment of regional lymph nodes by multiple node biopsies or by dissection should be done at the time of initial diagnosis in patients with pelvic soft tissue, retroperitoneal, perineal, and extremity tumors.

3. *Radiation therapy*

   a. To eradicate the residual tumor at primary site or gross metastatic sites radiation therapy is necessary. The dose and field of radiation is planned according to the stage and bulk of disease. For patients with localized, completely resected tumor without microscopic residual, radiation therapy is not necessary. Radiation therapy can be omitted in this group and delayed side effects of radiotherapy avoided

   b. For patients with microscopic residual disease, 4000 to 4500 cGy may be sufficient to achieve local control in 90 per cent of patients. For patients with gross tumor who receive intensive chemotherapy, the dose of 5000 cGy is necessary. Control of the primary tumor with conventional radiation therapy

in patients with unresectable or metastatic tumor remains a problem, and local control is achieved in only 60 to 70 per cent of patients. Hyperfractionated radiation therapy to a dose of 6000 cGy has resulted in (limited experience) improved local control in the majority of patients with unresectable RMS. Radiation therapy to involved lymph node areas is given when histologic involvement of the nodes is demonstrated.

Survival

Integrating rational, multidisciplinary, risk-oriented therapy has increased the overall survival rate of patients with RMS from a historical 20 to 30 per cent to 70 per cent. This improvement in survival rate of patients according to site of tumor and Clinical Groups in the three IRS studies is summarized in Table 143–2. Patients with orbital primary or those in groups I and II who have resectable localized tumor have excellent prognosis. Patients with primary tumors of extremities or trunk, paraspinal region, or abdomen or in groups III and IV with unresectable or metastatic disease have not fared as well. Clearly, innovative therapies are needed to improve the outcome in these groups.

Key Treatment

- Chemotherapy
- Surgery
- Radiation therapy

Bibliography

Crist W, Gehan E, Ragab A, et al: The third Intergroup Rhabdomyosarcoma Study. J Clin Oncol 1995;13:610–630.

Donaldson S, Asmar L, Breneman J, et al: Hyperfractionated radiation in children with rhabdomyosarcoma—results of an Intergroup Rhabdomyosarcoma pilot study. Int J Radiat Oncol Biol Phys 1995;15:903–911.

Maurer HM, Gehan EA, Beltangady M, et al: The Intergroup Rhabdomyosarcoma Study—II. Cancer 1993;71:1904–1922.

Regine W, Fontanesi J, Kumar P, et al: Phase II trial evaluating selective use of altered radiation dose and fractionation in patients with unresectable rhabdomyosarcoma. Int J Radiat Oncol Biol Phys 1995;31:799–805.

Tsokos M, Webber BL, Praham DM, et al: Rhabdomyosarcoma: A new classification scheme related to prognosis. Arch Pathol Lab Med 1992;116:847–855.

144 Soft Tissue Sarcomas

Michael P. LaQuaglia

Fibrosarcoma

Epidemiology

1. Fibrosarcomas, although rare, are the most common non-rhabdomyomatous sarcomas of infancy, childhood, and adolescence.
2. A biphasic age incidence similar to that observed with rhabdomyosarcoma is characteristic, with one peak in children younger than age 5 years and the second in the 10- to 15-year age group.
3. These tumors are most frequently encountered on extremities, with 70 per cent of congenital fibrosarcomas occurring distally.
4. Cases are equally distributed between males and females. Most reports suggest that prognosis is better in younger children.

Pathology

1. Fibrosarcomas are spindle cell tumors characterized by a herringbone or interweaving pattern of tumors cells with a large amount of stromal collagen putatively arising from a fibroblastic lineage.
2. The tumor must be distinguished from undifferentiated rhabdomyosarcomas, neurofibrosarcoma, nodular fasciitis, myositis ossificans, and inflammatory pseudotumor.

Clinical Findings

1. Congenital fibrosarcomas and those diagnosed in early childhood are usually on the distal upper or lower extremity. The trunk is a less common site. A hard, often infiltrating mass is appreciated, and there may be skin or deep fixation.
2. Fibrosarcomas in the head and neck, associated with swallowing and airway problems, are also occasionally observed and may require lifesaving tracheostomy.
3. High-grade lesions may invade bony or neural structures and metastasize to lung and/or liver.
4. Multifocal lesions with multiple primary lesions affecting an extremity are sometimes seen.
5. Bone marrow metastases do not develop.

Key Clinical Findings: Fibrosarcoma

- Mass on hand or foot
- Other possible sites include neck, trunk, and head

Staging

The TNM schema is used, although lymph node metastases from fibrosarcoma are very uncommon except with very high-grade lesions. An adequate incisional or excisional biopsy depending on the extent and invasiveness of the primary lesion should be obtained.

Treatment

1. At present the primary treatment of fibrosarcoma is a surgical resection with negative microscopic margins if this can be done without significant debilitation or deformity.
2. Occasionally, patients will present with rapidly progressive or extensive lesions. Under these circumstances an initial trial of systemic chemotherapy may result in gratifying tumor regression.
3. In very young children (usually younger than 5 years) these tumors can be very indolent and may sometimes regress spontaneously. In these cases in which a complete resection requires mutilating surgery such as amputation or laryngectomy a plan of simple observation may be best.
4. Heroic resections should only be done if the tumor is progressive or otherwise causing severe symptoms.

Outcome

The survival for low-grade nonmetastatic fibrosarcomas occurring in infancy is above 90 per cent. Patients with metastatic disease have a guarded prognosis and require multidisciplinary therapy.

Tenosynovial Sarcoma

Epidemiology

1. Tenosynovial sarcoma is the third most common malignant pediatric soft tissue tumor. In large combined adult and pediatric series tenosynovial sarcomas comprise approximately 8 per cent of all soft tissue sarcomas. In a report of nonrhabdomyomatous soft tissue sarcomas from St. Judes Research Hospital this histology was identified in 29 per cent of patients.
2. The male:female distribution is 1:1.2 to 1.6.
3. Most patients present in the early teenage years, but there is also a small incidence spike centered on 5 years of age, giving the familiar bimodal age distribution observed with other sarcomas.

Pathology

1. Tenosynovial sarcomas arise from the synovial tissue that is ubiquitous in the body and helps compose tendons, joint membranes, and bursae. Synonyms include synovioma or tenosynovioma, pseudoglandular synovial sarcoma, clear cell sarcoma, and chordoid sarcoma.
2. The lower extremity is the most common site of origin with an equal distribution between the thigh, foot, and posterior knee. The shoulder and forearm are also common areas of involvement. Tenosynovial sarcomas close to bone may incite a periosteal reaction. Other possible primary sites include the abdominal wall and trunk. The head and neck are also sites of occurrence, with the tongue and retropharyngeal or hypopharyngeal areas being the most common.

3. The most common metastatic sites are lungs and pleura. Tenosynovial sarcomas are known to relapse in lungs even decades after a resection of the primary tumor. Metastases to regional lymph nodes and subcutaneous sites have been described but are rare. Terminally, metastases to diffuse organs are possible.

4. Microscopically, tenosynovial sarcoma is divided into two subtypes: monophasic and diphasic. In the diphasic form epithelioid cells and stromal spindle cells are observed. The epithelioid component is arranged in glandlike structures resembling true epithelial cells but without basement membrane. Usually the stromal element is much more abundant than the pseudoglandular. The diphasic subtype has been associated with a better prognosis, but more recent studies have not verified this finding. The monophasic variant is the most common and consists of sheets and parallel cords of spindle-shaped cells with little cytoplasm and cigar-shaped nuclei.

Clinical Findings and Diagnostic Evaluation

Most patients present with an enlarging mass on an extremity. Pain may be prominent if bony or neural invasion is present. Regional lymph node metastases occur in 3 per cent and distant metastases (lung) occur in 6 per cent of patients at diagnosis. Adequate radiographic imaging of the primary site is crucial because of the impact of a complete resection on outcomes.

Treatment

1. Chemotherapy has historically been ineffective, and the primary treatment of tenosynovial sarcoma is surgical. The goal is clear microscopic margins, and every effort should be made to accomplish this, including use of amputation.

2. Limb-sparing procedures are acceptable if a complete resection is accomplished.

3. Incomplete removal results in a high rate of local recurrence.

Key Treatment: Tenosynovial Sarcoma

• Surgery

Outcome

1. Overall survival rates are between 43 and 75 per cent.

2. Important prognostic indicators are large primary tumor size and high nuclear grade with extensive tumor necrosis (high grade), as well as the presence of metastases at diagnosis.

3. Worsened survivals are correlated with tumors greater than 10 cm in diameter at diagnosis compared with those less than 5 cm: 86 vs. 22 per cent 5-year survival. Recent series have shown no effect of monophasic versus biphasic histology on outcome.

Primitive Neuroectodermal Tumor

Epidemiology, Pathology, and Clinical Presentation

1. Primitive neuroectodermal tumors (PNETs) (peripheral neuroepithelioma, Askin tumor, peripheral neuro-

blastoma) is a small, round blue cell malignancy only recently distinguished from Ewing sarcoma by ultrastructural and immunocytochemical features.

2. This tumor shares the t(11;22)(q24;q12) translocation with Ewing sarcoma and esthesioneuroblastoma.

3. The incidence is low. Approximately two thirds of patients are 19 years of age or younger at diagnosis, and 57 per cent are male. The disease affects predominantly white patients, and 82 per cent of tumors are localized at diagnosis.

4. Common sites of involvement include chest wall (33 per cent), pelvis (22 per cent), paraspinal region (13 per cent), retroperitoneum (11 per cent), limbs (9 per cent), and abdomen (7 per cent). Epidural extension from the primary is reported in 24 per cent of patients at diagnosis, and 18 per cent had distant metastases.

5. Urinary catecholamines are *not* elevated in peripheral primitive neuroectodermal tumor.

6. There is no familial or sex predilection.

7. Light microscopic criteria include fairly uniform, poorly differentiated round cells arranged in cords, nests, or clusters; no spindle cells with fine reticular or collagenous processes; no ganglionic or schwannian differentiation; and positive immunostaining for neuron-specific enolase. Ultrastructurally, neurosecretory-like granules and tapering ("neuritic") cytoplasmic processes are evident.

Treatment

1. It is recommended that the diagnosis be established by incisional biopsy and the patient quickly started on an intensive multiagent chemotherapy regimen.

2. Occasionally, the tumor can be completely resected before chemotherapy, and this should be done if feasible.

3. In most cases, definitive resection should be deferred until after administration of several cycles of systemic treatment.

4. External-beam radiation therapy (4500–6000 cGy) can shrink but not cure macroscopic tumors. Radiation may be effective in improving local control after resection, especially if margins are microscopically positive.

5. Outcome with PNETs has been historically poor whereas survival in Ewing sarcoma, which is a related neoplasm sharing the typical t(11;22) translocation, has approached 60 to 65 per cent in reported series of patients presenting without distant metastases. In patients with localized PNET at diagnosis, complete resection of all gross disease within 3 months resulted in an improved progression-free survival ($p = 0.0003$).

Key Treatment: Primitive Neuroectodermal Tumor

• Chemotherapy

• Surgery

• Radiation therapy

Desmoplastic Small Round Cell Tumor

Definition

The desmoplastic small round cell tumor (DSRCT) is a recently identified, distinctive malignant neoplasm.

Epidemiology

1. Eighty per cent of patients present before the age of 30, and approximately half will be 5 to 20 years at diagnosis.
2. There is a striking male predominance (male:female ratio = 4.1:1), and most of the patients are white.

Pathology

1. The vast majority of patients are found to have tumor localized to the abdominal cavity often with multiple peritoneal implants. In some cases a major tumor mass in the retroperitoneum, pelvis, omentum, or peripancreatic region was identified.
2. There have been two reports of extraabdominal disease: one in lung and another in the anterior mediastinum. In both cases the tumor was in contact with pleura.
3. Initially, the tumor remains localized to the abdominal cavity but distant metastases may occur with progression.
4. A striking feature is the frequent occurrence of divergent, multilineage differentiation with expression of epithelial, neural, and myogenic immunophenotypes. On light microscopy, variably sized and shaped and sharply outlined nests of tumor cells are separated by a cellular desmoplastic stroma.

Biology

Cytogenetic analyses of these tumors have shown a t(11;22)(p13;q11.2–12) translocation. Band 22q12 is the site of the *EWS* (Ewing sarcoma) gene, and 11p13 contains the *WT1* (Wilms tumor gene) site. It has been determined that the *EWS* and *WT1* genes are fused in DSRCT. The consequences of this translocation and the mechanism by which it might contribute to the malignant phenotype remain to be elucidated.

Clinical Findings

1. Common presenting complaints include abdominal or back pain, abdominal distention or mass, acute abdomen, and bowel, biliary, or ureteral obstruction.
2. Small nodules found in hernia sacs during repair have been the first indication of a DSCRT.
3. Computed tomography (CT) of the chest and abdomen using both gastrointestinal and vascular contrast media is the most useful diagnostic procedure. Initial laparoscopic biopsy is adequate to establish the diagnosis and assess the extent of abdominal disease.
4. Small serosal nodules not detected by imaging studies can be identified using laparoscopic magnification. A careful pelvic and serosal inspection should be carried out.

Key Clinical Findings: Desmoplastic Small Round Cell Tumor

- Back pain
- Abdominal mass
- Ureteral obstruction

Treatment

1. Because DSCRT is a diffuse serosal malignancy, systemic chemotherapy using a dose-intense sarcoma regimen is the initial treatment. Serial abdominal CT scans can be followed to judge response, remembering that small mucosal implants may escape detection with imaging studies.
2. After four to seven cycles, exploratory laparotomy with resection of all gross disease is attempted. Consolidation chemotherapy and external-beam radiation therapy to the primary site are then employed.
3. If diffuse peritoneal seeding is identified either at diagnostic or second-look laparotomy/laparoscopy, total abdominal irradiation is required. Myeloablative chemotherapy with autologous marrow reconstitution may also be necessary.

Key Treatment: Desmoplastic Small Round Cell Tumor

- Chemotherapy
- Surgery

Outcome

Of 19 reported patients with adequate follow-up only two were disease-free 2 and 3.5 years after diagnosis. The other 17 died of progressive disease within 6 months to 4 years after presentation. Prognosis may improve with more aggressive multidisciplinary regimens.

Neurofibrosarcoma

Epidemiology

1. Neurofibrosarcomas (neurogenic sarcomas, malignant schwannomas, malignant nerve sheath tumor, malignant neurilemoma) comprise 5 to 10 per cent of nonrhabdomyomatous soft tissue sarcomas in childhood.
2. About 20 per cent of all patients (children and adults) with neurofibrosarcoma have von Recklinghausen disease (neurofibromatosis type I [NF1]) and 5 to 16 per cent of patients with NF1 develop a neurofibrosarcoma. The incidence of NF1 in children with neurofibrosarcomas is as high as 66 per cent.
3. Neurofibrosarcomas have been reported as secondary tumors after external-beam radiation therapy.

Pathology

1. The most common sites in children are extremity (42 per cent), retroperitoneum (25 per cent), and trunk. Primary neurofibrosarcoma of skin and subcutaneous tissues has also been described.
2. Less than 10 per cent of patients present with metastatic disease.
3. Microscopically, the tumor resembles fibrosarcoma but is differentiated by the presence of schwannian elements.

Clinical Findings

1. Two thirds of patients will have associated NF1, and aggressive diagnostic procedures including biopsy are warranted when enlarging extremity or truncal masses are observed.
2. Pain may be prominent depending on location. Radicular

or sciatic pain is reported with paraspinal or retroperitoneal tumors causing sciatic pressure.

3. Spontaneous hemothorax has been reported with chest wall primary lesions.

4. Pelvic tumors may present as a perineal or perianal mass.

Key Clinical Findings: Neurofibrosarcoma

- Associated neurofibromatosis

Treatment

The primary treatment of neurofibrosarcoma is wide local excision. In one series of 20 patients (14 with neurofibromatosis), local recurrence developed in 8 of 12 patients undergoing local tumor excision plus radiation therapy or chemotherapy but only 1 of 6 treated with radical excision as well as chemotherapy or irradiation. Unfortunately, a significant proportion developed distant metastases despite local control.

Key Treatment: Neurofibrosarcoma

- Radical excision
- Chemotherapy
- Radiation

Leiomyosarcoma

Epidemiology and Pathology

1. This tumor accounts for 7 per cent of soft tissue sarcomas in adults but less than 2 per cent of childhood sarcomas.

2. The gastrointestinal (oropharynx to anus) or genitourinary tract, retroperitoneum, lungs, pulmonary artery, vascular wall (i.e., middle third of the inferior vena cava, saphenous or femoral vein), popliteal artery, sinonasal area, and peripheral soft tissue (extremities) are reported sites of involvement. The great majority of cases are gastrointestinal in origin.

3. The lungs are the most common site for metastases. Regional lymph node involvement occurs in 14 per cent of gastric (perigastric nodes) and 5 per cent of small intestinal leiomyosarcomas at diagnosis. Dissemination to liver and brain has also been reported.

4. Tumors arising from gastrointestinal structures can disseminate throughout the peritoneal cavity.

5. Leiomyosarcoma has been reported in patients with von Recklinghausen disease and coincident with the occurrence of neurofibrosarcoma.

Clinical Findings

1. True leiomyosarcomas are derived from smooth muscle and are often pseudoencapsulated and cytologically demonstrate uniform elongated cells with cigar-shaped nuclei. An epithelioid variant with more aggressive behavior is reported to arise in up to 40 per cent of cases. Leiomyosarcoma may arise diffusely and can be accompanied by areas of leiomyoblastoma that are benign smooth muscle tumors.

2. Usual criteria for determination of malignancy include cellular atypia, necrosis, gross tumor size, the presence of one mitosis per two high-power fields (one per five high-power fields in cases of epithelioid leiomyosarcoma), or the finding of lymph node, peritoneal, or parenchymal metastases.

3. Bone marrow metastases are not reported.

4. The usual presentation is pain (up to 80 per cent) or gastrointestinal bleeding (60 per cent). There are also reports of presentation with intussusception and perforation of a Meckel diverticulum. Some authors state that intussusception does not occur in childhood. Congenital leiomyosarcoma associated with hydrops has also been reported.

5. Double-contrast CT scans, gastrointestinal contrast studies, and endoscopy may aid in diagnosis.

Key Clinical Findings: Leiomyosarcoma

- Abdominal pain
- Gastrointestinal bleeding

Treatment and Outcome

1. At present the most effective treatment of leiomyosarcoma is complete surgical resection. This should be accomplished even when resection requires amputation or results in other disability because chemotherapy and radiation are ineffective. There are reports of long-term survival with resection for cases with hepatic and cerebral metastases.

2. It is recommended that, for gastrointestinal tumors, a 10-cm margin of bowel be obtained along with a wide mesenteric resection. For gastric primary lesions omentectomy is advised as well.

3. Overall, about 50 per cent of patients with gastrointestinal primary lesions can be resected for cure at diagnosis; and of these, survival is 50 per cent at 5 years and falls to 35 per cent at 10 years.

4. Pediatric colorectal leiomyosarcomas, although extremely rare, are reported to have a relatively favorable prognosis.

Key Treatment: Leiomyosarcoma

- Surgery

Liposarcoma

Epidemiology and Pathology

Liposarcomas are one of the most common soft tissue sarcomas in adults but are extremely rare in childhood. The peak incidence is in the second decade of life, and there is equal distribution between the sexes. Most pediatric tumors are of the myxoid histopathologic subtype and are low grade.

Clinical Findings

1. The most common sites are, in order, the lower extremity, upper extremity, and retroperitoneum. Head and neck and genitourinary primary lesions have also been described.

2. The usual presenting complaint is a mass that is often painless.
3. Metastases are uncommon but, when present, the lung is the most common site. Lymph node metastases are possible but extremely rare, and their presence casts doubt on the diagnosis.

Key Clinical Findings: Liposarcoma

• Painless mass

Treatment and Outcome

The treatment of choice is complete surgical excision with negative microscopic margins. External-beam radiation may be useful for control of residual microscopic disease. Patients with gross residual disease after resection have a very poor prognosis.

Key Treatment: Liposarcoma

• Surgical excision

Alveolar Soft Part Sarcoma

Epidemiology and Pathology

1. Alveolar soft part sarcoma is a rare tumor; only 102 cases have been reported in the literature over a 50-year period. Because the cell of origin is unknown this malignancy has sparked considerable interest.
2. The thigh and buttocks are the most common sites of presentation (39.5 per cent), followed by abdominal and chest walls.
3. Approximately one third will have metastases at diagnosis, with the most common metastatic sites being lung, bone, and brain in that order. Microscopically, the tumor comprises a mass or ball of cells with a necrotic center that mimics an alveolar space.

Key Clinical Findings: Alveolar Soft Part Sarcoma

• Mass, often on thigh or buttocks

• Sometimes abdominal or chest wall occurrence

Treatment and Outcome

The primary treatment is surgical, and the role of chemotherapy or radiation remains undefined. Unfortunately, most patients will subsequently develop relapse in distant sites and die of progressive disease, although this may take 20 years or more.

Key Treatment: Alveolar Soft Part Sarcoma

• Surgery

Hemangiopericytoma

Epidemiology and Pathology

1. Hemangiopericytomas are rare in childhood, comprising approximately 3 per cent of all soft tissue sarcomas in this group. In a report from St. Judes Research Hospital, 5 of 62 (8 per cent) nonrhabdomyogenic soft tissue sarcomas were classified as hemangiopericytomas. The tumor arises from pericytes, which in themselves are multipotent and can be precursors of endothelial cells, smooth muscle, rhabdomyoblasts, or fibroblasts.
2. Hemangiopericytoma may exhibit a benign or malignant phenotype. Histologic criteria of malignancy include hypercellularity, high mitotic index, and intratumoral hemorrhage and necrosis.
3. Hemangiopericytomas may arise anywhere in the body including the head and neck (especially tongue), lacrimal glands, chest wall, retroperitoneum, prostatic area and pelvis, liver, central nervous system, temporal bone, and extremities (thigh, hand). The most common sites are the extremities, followed by the retroperitoneum.
4. Metastases are bloodborne and usually affect lungs and bone.
5. Infantile hemangiopericytomas have histologic characteristics that are similar to the adult form but follow a more benign course. These tumors are usually localized to the subdermal layers, although extensive local infiltration may be noted.

Key Clinical Findings: Hemangiopericytoma

• Mass—many sites

Treatment and Outcome

1. The mainstay of therapy is complete surgical resection with negative microscopic margins. Resection alone controls disease in 30 per cent of patients.
2. External-beam radiation therapy has been effective against microscopic residual disease and may also cause regression of gross tumor deposits. In general, external-beam radiation is more effective against microscopic levels of tumor.
3. Some tumors have also responded to systemic chemotherapy, although a standard regimen has not been employed and response rates have been variable.
4. Standard treatment for a malignant tumor includes complete local excision if possible or excision plus external-beam radiation therapy for residual tumor. This is usually followed by a course of adjuvant chemotherapy because of the observation that 50 per cent of patients develop subsequent recurrence.
5. Benign tumors are curable with complete surgical resection. Most infantile hemangiopericytomas follow this course and are adequately treated by wide local excision. The reported survival for malignant forms of the disease ranges from 30 to 70 per cent, and at least 50 per cent of patients will develop a recurrence.

Key Treatment: Hemangiopericytoma

• Surgical excision

Malignant Fibrous Histiocytoma

Epidemiology and Pathology

1. Malignant fibrous histiocytoma (MFH) is the most common soft tissue sarcoma observed in adults but comprises 8 to 10 per cent of nonrhabdomyomatous sarcomas in childhood.
2. Microscopically, the tumor resembles fibrosarcoma but can be differentiated by the absence of a herringbone pattern and by the presence of cellular pleomorphism and a variety of cell types.
3. Certain childhood recurrent fibrosarcomas and sometimes aggressive fibromatosis can have the appearance of MFH.
4. MFH is one of the most common radiation-induced sarcomas, and orbital occurrence after radiation therapy for retinoblastoma has been reported on several occasions.
5. The extremities (lower more often than upper) are most frequently affected, followed by the trunk, scalp, and viscera. Pulmonary metastases are observed most often, followed by brain and other sites. Systemic symptoms including fever, chills, weight loss, hypergammaglobulinemia, and amyloidosis may occur.

Key Clinical Findings: Malignant Fibrous Histiocytoma

- Mass, various sites

Treatment and Outcome

The accepted primary treatment of MFH is wide surgical excision. Limb salvage is feasible in certain small extremity lesions with close margins by the addition of external-beam radiation to the tumor bed. In a series of nine patients with MFH from the Children's Hospital of British Columbia there were six survivors 20 months to 8 years after surgical resection. The authors note that two children developed pulmonary metastases and died despite the use of adjuvant multiagent chemotherapy and radiation therapy. Poor outcome was associated with large, deep, and proximal tumors as well as the storiform-pleomorphic histologic subtype with atypical mitoses.

Key Treatment: Malignant Fibrous Histiocytoma

- Surgical excision

Rhabdoid Tumor

Epidemiology and Pathology

1. Rhabdoid tumors are rare, highly malignant neoplasms usually observed in the kidney and once thought of as a variant of Wilms tumor.
2. Presently, rhabdoid tumors, although the cell of origin remains unidentified, are considered sarcoma-like in their biologic behavior and are usually treated with chemotherapy protocols designed for soft tissue sarcomas. Other primary sites include brain, mediastinum, forehead, liver, and paravertebral region.
3. The Intergroup Rhabdomyosarcoma Study identified 26 rhabdoid tumors among 3000 childhood sarcomas. Eleven of the patients were infants younger than 1 year of age. The tumors affected predominantly the soft tissues of the proximal extremities, trunk, and retroperitoneum/abdomen/pelvis.
4. Histologically, the growth pattern is predominantly solid or solid-trabecular and the cells are polygonal with vesicular nuclei and prominent nucleoli.

Key Clinical Findings: Rhabdoid Tumor

- Mass often in kidney

Treatment and Outcome

The tumor is both chemotherapy and radiation resistant and has a very poor outcome. Most treatment regimens combine all surgery, chemotherapy, and radiation therapy. Overall survival is 20 per cent or less.

Key Treatment

- Surgery
- Chemotherapy
- Radiation therapy (poor prognosis)

Secondary Sarcomas

Epidemiology and Pathology

1. As the survival of pediatric malignancies has improved with the use of multidisciplinary therapy the incidence of secondary malignancies has increased.
2. These secondary tumors are associated with the use of mutagenic treatments (radiation therapy, chemotherapy) and predisposing genetic traits in the patient (i.e., retinoblastoma gene or *p53* deletions or mutations). Tucker and colleagues reported on 9170 cancer patients with a 2-year or more follow-up and mean age at diagnosis of 7 years. They identified 48 cases of *secondary* bone cancer in this cohort with an expected incidence that was calculated to be 0.4 case. This risk was highest among patients with retinoblastoma and Ewing sarcoma. The risk of a second primary lesion rose with time. The most commonly observed secondary soft tissue sarcoma is malignant fibrous histiocytoma.

Treatment

Treatment should follow guidelines established for primary tumors of the same phenotype.

145 Osteosarcoma

Paul A. Meyers

Definition

An osteosarcoma is a pleomorphic spindle cell tumor of bone that produces the extracellular matrix osteoid.

Etiology

Like virtually all childhood cancers, there is almost nothing known about the etiology of this tumor. A dramatically increased incidence of osteosarcoma has been noted in survivors of retinoblastoma, both within the field of radiation therapy and at distant sites. Osteosarcoma occurs in the field of radiation after treatment of other malignancies. Most osteosarcomas arise with no predisposing factors.

Epidemiology

Osteosarcoma, like all childhood cancers, is extremely rare. There are only 600 cases of osteosarcoma each year in the United States, not all of which occur in children. Osteosarcoma occurs at all ages. The disease in older adults usually arises in areas of previously abnormal bone, such as long-standing Paget disease. Osteosarcoma in children and young adults has a peak incidence in the years after puberty. Therefore, the median age of diagnosis is approximately 16 in girls and 18 in boys. Osteosarcoma is more common in boys than in girls, with a roughly 60:40 male:female ratio. Osteosarcoma arises with equal frequency in all races and ethnic groups.

Pathophysiology

1. Osteosarcoma arises in a primary site in a single bone. It is not entirely clear which cell type undergoes malignant transformation to initiate the disease, but the osteoblast is the most likely candidate. The cells proliferate and are insensitive to the normal feedback signals that limit growth. They cause local destruction of bone, eroding normal bone. Eventually, the tumor breaks through the cortex into the surrounding soft tissue.
2. Like all sarcomas, osteosarcoma becomes metastatic extremely early in its evolution. This is in stark contradistinction to the carcinomas, the more common tumors of adults. Carcinomas become large and clinically apparent before they develop metastasis and are amenable to cure by surgical resection if detected early. Sarcomas are metastatic before they are clinically detectable and can almost never be cured by surgery alone.
3. Osteosarcoma spreads through hematogenous metastasis. The most common site of metastasis for osteosarcoma is the lungs. Other sites that can be involved include distant bony sites, locoregional nodes, and soft tissues.
4. Without treatment the primary tumor will continue to grow, causing increasing pain and loss of mobility. The metastatic disease will continue to grow, ultimately leading to pulmonary failure and death.

Clinical Findings

1. The classic presentation of osteosarcoma is a painful mass in an extremity. The bones of the axial skeleton can be involved, but this is much less frequent. The single most common site of involvement is the distal femur, followed by the proximal tibia and the proximal humerus. The pain is variable in intensity.
2. Osteosarcoma is almost always initially suspected by the appearance of the tumor on a plain film of the mass. The tumor both destroys preexisting healthy bone and creates new tumor bone by ossification of the extracellular matrix osteoid secreted by the tumor cells. This results in a picture of mixed lysis and sclerosis of the bone. Osteosarcoma is distinguished from possible benign tumors of bone by the lack of a sharp zone of transition to surrounding normal bone.
3. Osteosarcoma grows rapidly. When it penetrates the cortex, it elevates the periosteum, tearing this tough membrane away from the underlying bone. This results in bleeding into a newly created space. This phenomenon is visible on plain film as an elevated periosteum and is referred to as a Codman triangle.
4. All patients with osteosarcoma have metastatic disease; a subset have metastatic disease that is big enough to detect by plain film or computed tomography (CT) of the chest. Even these patients will have no symptoms referable to the metastases. Lung metastases can grow to a large size before they interfere with respiration enough to cause symptoms.

Key Clinical Finding

- Painful mass in an extremity

Diagnostic Work-Up

At a minimum the initial evaluation of the patient with osteosarcoma should include

1. History
   a. Duration of symptoms
   b. Pain at sites distant from primary lesion; respiratory symptoms
   c. History of previous malignancy
   d. Family history of cancer
2. Physical examination
   a. Lymph node examination
   b. Chest examination
   c. Size and extent of primary tumor mass
3. Laboratory
   a. Complete blood cell count
   b. Tests of liver function
   c. Assessment of renal function
   d. Serum lactate dehydrogenase and alkaline phosphatase levels

e. Baseline echocardiogram or radionuclide heart scan
f. Baseline audiogram
4. Radiology
  a. Posteroanterior and lateral chest radiographs
  b. CT of the chest
  c. Radionuclide bone scan
  d. Plain films of the primary site
  e. Magnetic resonance imaging (preferred) or CT of the primary site

Laboratory Findings

There are no laboratory abnormalities that are pathognomonic for osteosarcoma. Most patients have an increased serum alkaline phosphatase value, sometimes to dramatically elevated levels. Many patients have an elevation of the serum lactate dehydrogenase level.

Key Laboratory Findings

- No consistent findings
- Elevated serum alkaline phosphate value

Radiographic Changes

1. The diagnosis of osteosarcoma is almost always suggested by an initial plain film. The tumor exhibits a mixture of lytic and sclerotic changes. There is no clear zone of transition between the tumor and surrounding normal bone. The tumor breaks through the cortex and does not respect the physis. There is often a Codman triangle as the result of rapid tumor growth with disruption of the periosteum. There is usually a soft tissue mass, but this may be difficult to see on a plain film.
2. Evaluation of the primary tumor requires cross-sectional imaging with either CT or magnetic resonance imaging. This is essential to define the extent of the tumor within the bone as well as the soft tissue extension and the relation of the tumor to adjacent neurovascular structures.
3. Further evaluation of the patient includes a search for clinically detectable metastatic disease. At a minimum, this should include a bone scan to evaluate the entire skeleton and a CT scan of the chest. Clinical studies have proven that CT can detect metastatic nodules that are not seen on a plain film of the chest.

Treatment

1. Before the introduction of chemotherapy, the only treatment for osteosarcoma was surgery. Osteosarcoma was treated as a surgical emergency, with amputations carried out immediately. Despite this aggressive surgical approach, 80 to 90 per cent of patients developed lung nodules within a median of 5 months after amputation. This proves that the great majority of patients already had microscopic metastases in their lungs at initial clinical presentation.
2. Current treatment of osteosarcoma involves the combined use of chemotherapy and surgery. Many treatment centers employ a period of initial chemotherapy before definitive surgical removal of the primary tumor. This period of initial chemotherapy is intended to shrink the tumor to a point where surgical removal can be carried out more easily.
3. Osteosarcoma is treated with a combination of several different chemotherapeutic agents. The use of a combination of drugs has several rationales. First, no single agent is effective against all tumors; the use of several agents increases the chances that an individual tumor will respond. Second, the spectrum of toxicities of the drugs differ, and toxicities need not be additive, whereas efficacy may be additive or even synergistic. Most current treatment approaches for osteosarcoma employ some combination of doxorubicin, cisplatin, high-dose methotrexate, and ifosfamide.
4. Despite the activity of chemotherapy, drugs alone cannot permanently control osteosarcoma. There are simply too many cells in even a small primary tumor for chemotherapy to eradicate all of them. Surgical removal of all tumors that are large enough to see by conventional imaging technique is essential for long-term control of the disease.
5. Control of the primary tumor in the extremity requires removal of the tumor-bearing bone and soft tissues with an adequate margin of resection. In tumors of the extremity this can be achieved by amputation. Orthopedic oncologists have devised a number of surgical techniques designed to preserve limbs and allow adequate removal of the tumor. The ability to carry out limb-sparing surgery depends on the location and size of the primary tumor and its relation to surrounding neurovascular structures. It is necessary to be able to preserve blood supply and innervation to the extremity distal to the resection and to have adequate skin and soft tissue to close the surgical site over the resection.
6. In patients who present with clinically detectable metastatic disease, it is necessary to remove the visible tumors by surgery. The most common site of metastasis is the lung. These patients require thoracotomy. Osteosarcoma metastatic to lung is very firm and gritty. By collapsing the lung, the surgeon is able to identify more and smaller nodules than can be seen on CT scan. Even if imaging studies identify metastatic disease in only one lung, it is strongly recommended to perform thoracotomy with careful surgical examination of *both* lungs.

Key Treatment

- Chemotherapy
- Surgery

Prognosis

1. Several factors are helpful in predicting the success of therapy for osteosarcoma:
  a. Favorable
    (1) Distal primary site (distal femur, proximal tibia)
    (2) Low serum lactate dehydrogenase level
    (3) Low serum alkaline phosphatase level
    (4) Necrotic tumor after initial chemotherapy
    (5) No clinically detectable metastases
  b. Unfavorable

(1) Proximal primary site (axial skeleton, proximal femur)
(2) High serum lactate dehydrogenase level
(3) High serum alkaline phosphatase level
(4) Viable tumor after initial chemotherapy
(5) Clinically detectable metastases

2. Patients who present without clinically detectable metastases have a probability of between 65 and 75 per cent to be alive, well, and continuously free of osteosarcoma more than 5 years from diagnosis. Presentation with clinically detectable metastases confers a much worse prognosis: fewer than 25 per cent of patients will be expected to remain well and free of disease 5 years from diagnosis.

Bibliography

Horowitz SM, Glasser DB, Lane JM, et al: Prosthetic and extremity survivorship after limb salvage for sarcoma: How long do the reconstructions last? Clin Orthop Rel Res 1993;293:280–286.

Meyers PA, Heller G, Healey J, et al: Chemotherapy for non-metastatic osteogenic sarcoma: The Memorial Sloan-Kettering Cancer experience. J Clin Oncol 1992;10:5–15.

Meyers PA, Heller G, Healey J, et al: Osteogenic sarcoma with clinically detectable metastasis at initial presentation. J Clin Oncol 1993;11:449–453.

Rougraff BT, Simon MA, Kneisl JS, et al: Limb salvage compared with amputation for osteosarcoma of the distal end of the femur: A long-term oncological, functional, and quality-of-life study. J Bone Joint Surg Am 1994;76:649–656.

146 Ewing Sarcoma

Paul A. Meyers

Definition

Ewing sarcoma is a small, round, blue-cell sarcoma of bone (and more rarely, of soft tissue).

Etiology

Like virtually all childhood cancers, there is almost nothing known about the etiology of this tumor. The great majority of tumors (approximately 85 per cent) exhibit a consistent chromosomal translocation between the q24 band of chromosome 11 and the q12 band of chromosome 22 [t(11;22)]. This translocation juxtaposes a portion of the *FLI1* gene, a member of the ETS proto-oncogene family from chromosome 11 with a portion of the *EWS* gene from chromosome 22. The new, abnormal gene that results from this translocation encodes a protein that makes normal cells behave in a malignant fashion. This strongly suggests that the translocation has a role in the pathogenesis of this tumor.

Epidemiology

Ewing sarcoma, like all childhood cancers, is extremely rare. There are only 450 cases of Ewing sarcoma each year in the United States. Over 90 per cent of Ewing sarcoma arises in patients 21 years old or younger. There is no obvious peak of incidence at any age, but the tumor is extremely rare before age 5. The condition occurs slightly more often in males. Ewing sarcoma is striking for its virtual absence in African Americans and Asian Americans.

Pathophysiology

1. Ewing sarcoma arises in a primary site in a single bone (or more rarely, soft tissue). It is not entirely clear which cell type undergoes malignant transformation to initiate the disease. Expression of surface markers related to neural differentiation has led to suspicion of a neural crest origin for this tumor. The cells proliferate and are insensitive to the normal feedback signals that limit growth. They cause local destruction of normal tissue. Bony primary tumors erode through the cortex of the bone into the surrounding soft tissues.

2. Like all sarcomas, Ewing sarcoma is metastatic long before it is clinically evident. This is in contradistinction to the behavior of carcinomas, the common form of cancer in adults. Carcinomas typically become large and clinically apparent before they develop metastasis. Therefore they are amenable to cure by surgical resection if detected early. Sarcomas are metastatic from their earliest evolution and can almost never be cured by surgery alone.

3. Ewing sarcoma spreads by hematogenous metastasis. The most common site for metastasis of Ewing sarcoma is the lung. Other sites of involvement include distant bony sites, locoregional nodes and soft tissues, and the bone marrow.

4. Without treatment, the primary tumor will grow, causing increasing pain and disability. Metastatic disease will continue to grow, ultimately leading to pulmonary failure and death.

Clinical Findings

1. The classic presentation of Ewing sarcoma is a painful mass. When bones of the axial skeleton are involved, pain may be the only symptom. Tumors of the extremities typically present as pain and a mass. The single most common site of involvement is the femur, followed by the pelvis and the lower leg, but Ewing sarcoma has been reported in every bone and soft tissue in the body.

2. The diagnosis of Ewing sarcoma is almost always initially suggested by the appearance of a mass on plain films of the involved bone. In areas that are difficult to visualize on plain film, such as the pelvis and spine, the tumor is sometimes first recognized on a radionuclide bone scan.

In long bones, the tumor typically arises in the midshaft. The presentation of a painful lesion in the midshaft of a long bone with increased uptake on radionuclide bone scan is also compatible with the diagnosis of osteomyelitis. Ewing sarcoma must be included in the differential diagnosis of any patient with suspected osteomyelitis.

3. Ewing sarcoma typically arises in the medullary cavity of the bone. It permeates through the cortex to the subperiosteal space. The tumor typically grows very quickly and penetrates to surrounding soft tissues.

4. All patients with Ewing sarcoma have metastatic disease. A subset have metastatic disease that is advanced enough to detect by radionuclide scan, plain film, or CT scan of the chest or examination of the bone marrow.

Key Clinical Finding

- Painful mass in an extremity

Diagnostic Work-up

At a minimum, the initial evaluation of the patient with Ewing sarcoma should include

1. History
    a. Duration of the symptoms
    b. Pain at sites distant from the primary lesion; respiratory symptoms
    c. Family history of cancer
2. Physical examination
    a. Size and extent of the primary tumor mass
    b. Lymph node examination
    c. Chest examination
3. Laboratory
    a. Complete blood cell count
    b. Tests of liver function
    c. Assessment of renal function
    d. Serum lactate dehydrogenase
    e. Baseline echocardiogram or radionuclide heart scan
4. Radiology
    a. Posteroanterior and lateral chest radiographs
    b. Computed tomography (CT) of the chest
    c. Radionuclide bone scan
    d. Plain films of the primary site
    e. Magnetic resonance imaging or CT of the primary site

Laboratory Findings

There are no routine laboratory abnormalities that are pathognomonic for Ewing sarcoma. Most tumors exhibit the t(11;22) translocation. This can be detected by classic cytogenetics or by polymerase chain reaction examination of the primary tumor biopsy specimen. Most patients have an elevated level of serum lactate dehydrogenase.

Key Laboratory Finding

- No consistent abnormalities

Radiographic Changes

1. The diagnosis of Ewing sarcoma is usually considered on a plain film of the affected area. Bone tumors exhibit permeative, moth-eaten changes, typically in the metaphysis. Permeation of the tumor through the cortex leads to a lamellated or onion-skin appearance of the cortex. There is usually a soft tissue mass, but this may be difficult to see on a plain film.

2. Evaluation of the primary tumor requires cross-sectional imaging with either CT or magnetic resonance imaging. This is essential to define the extent of the tumor within the bone as well as the soft tissue extension and the relation of the tumor to adjacent normal structures.

3. Further evaluation of the patient requires a search for clinically detectable metastatic disease. At a minimum, this should include a radionuclide bone scan to evaluate the entire skeleton and a CT scan of the chest.

Treatment

1. Before the introduction of chemotherapy, Ewing sarcoma was treated by surgical resection and/or radiation therapy. Over 95 per cent of patients who presented without apparent metastatic disease developed overt metastases within 6 months after initial presentation. This demonstrates that virtually all patients with Ewing sarcoma have metastases at initial presentation.

2. Current treatment of Ewing sarcoma involves the use of systemic chemotherapy and therapy aimed at controlling the primary tumor. Local control of the primary tumor can be accomplished with surgical resection and/or radiation therapy. Many treatment centers employ a period of initial chemotherapy before definitive local control therapy is applied. This period of initial therapy is intended to shrink the primary tumor to allow greater preservation of normal tissue and function.

3. As for pediatric sarcomas, Ewing sarcoma is treated with a combination of several different chemotherapeutic agents. The use of a combination of drugs has several rationales. First, no single agent is effective against all tumors; the use of several agents increases the chances that an individual tumor will respond. Second, the spectrum of toxicities of the drugs differ, and toxicities need not be additive, whereas efficacy may be additive or even synergistic. Most current treatment approaches for Ewing sarcoma employ some combination of doxorubicin, cyclophosphamide, vincristine, ifosfamide, and etoposide.

4. Despite the activity of chemotherapy, drugs alone cannot permanently control Ewing sarcoma. There are simply too many cells in even a small primary tumor for chemotherapy to eradicate all of them. Local control of all tumors that are large enough to be detected by conventional imaging technique is essential for long-term control of disease.

5. Control of the primary tumor in a bone requires either removal of the tumor-bearing bone and soft tissues with an adequate margin of resection or the use of radiation therapy. There is no information about which approach is superior for a given tumor. The choice of modality is based on the size and location of the primary tumor and the age of the patient. Age is an important factor, because a young child will lose significant growth of a bone from either surgery or radiation therapy to that bone.

Key Treatment

- Chemotherapy
- Surgery

Prognosis

1. Several factors are helpful in predicting the success of therapy for Ewing sarcoma:
   a. Favorable
      (1) Distal primary site (tibia, fibula, radius)
      (2) Low serum lactate dehydrogenase level
      (3) Small primary tumor
      (4) Necrotic tumor after initial chemotherapy
      (5) No clinically detectable metastases
   b. Unfavorable
      (1) Proximal primary site (axial skeleton)
      (2) High serum lactate dehydrogenase level
      (3) Large primary tumor
      (4) Viable tumor after initial chemotherapy

      (5) Clinically detectable metastases

2. Patients who present without clinically detectable metastatic disease have a probability of between 60 and 65 per cent to be alive, well, and continuously free of Ewing sarcoma more than 3 years from diagnosis. Presentation with clinically detectable metastasis confers a much worse prognosis: fewer than 25 per cent of patients will be expected to remain well and free of disease 3 years from diagnosis. Ewing sarcoma sometimes recurs many years after initial treatment. Patients successfully treated for Ewing sarcoma have a significant incidence of second malignancies, including leukemia.

Bibliography

Burgert EO, Nesbit ME, Garnsey LA, et al: Multimodal therapy for the management of nonpelvic, localized Ewing's sarcoma of bone: Intergroup Study IESS-II. J Clin Oncol 1990;8:1514–1524.

Dunst J, Sauer R, Burgers JMV, et al: Radiation therapy as local treatment in Ewing's sarcoma. Cancer 1991;67:2818–2825.

Scully SP, Temple HT, O'Keefe RJ, et al: Role of surgical resection in pelvic Ewing's sarcoma. J Clin Oncol 1995;13:2336–2341.

147 Retinoblastoma

David Abramson

Etiology and Epidemiology

1. The most common primary malignancy of the eye or eyes of children
2. Occurs in 1 in 18,000 to 30,000 births (estimated 350 cases/year) in the United States
3. Laterality
   a. Unilateral in two thirds of cases
   b. Bilateral in one third of cases
4. No racial, sexual, or involvement of right vs. left eye difference
5. Age at diagnosis depends on country of diagnosis:
   a. West: unilateral: 2 years old, bilateral: 1 year old
   b. Underdeveloped: 4 to 6 years old
6. Occurs in two forms: germinal and somatic
   a. Germinal: Has a germline mutation in the RB1 gene (located on the long arm of chromosome 13), which is present in one allele of all cells in the child. A subsequent genetic event (deletion, hemizygosity, recombination) affecting the same RB1 gene on the second allele initiates tumor development. A mean of 5 separate tumors arise synchronously or asynchronously in the retina of one or both eyes in germinal cases.
   b. Somatic: Occurs as a result of mutations in RB1 on

   both alleles in single retinal cells that give rise to solitary, unilateral tumors.
7. Genetics: In germinal form (50 per cent of cases) passed on as an autosomal dominant with >90 per cent penetrance (Fig. 147–1).
8. All retinoblastoma metastases occur within 5 years of intraocular diagnosis and initial treatment.

Pathophysiology

1. Tumor originates in the retina and grows initially within the retina. As it enlarges, it may grow beneath the retina, causing the retina to become elevated and detached with solid tumor underneath. It may also extend into the vitreous, causing tumor that may be continuous with the retinal tumor or may break separately into spheres of varying size (50 μ to 2 mm across) called vitreous seeds.
2. Retinal detachment and tumor growth may progressively impair vision, but the more dire concern is metastasis.
3. Retinoblastoma may extend out of the eye, where survival is at best 50 per cent. This tumor extends through the optic nerve and into the CSF or brain directly, via the deeper choroidal blood vessels into bone and distant organs or locally through the wall of the eye (sclera) and into the orbit, where systemic metastases occur almost simultaneously.
4. In advanced untreated cases, the retinoblastoma grows

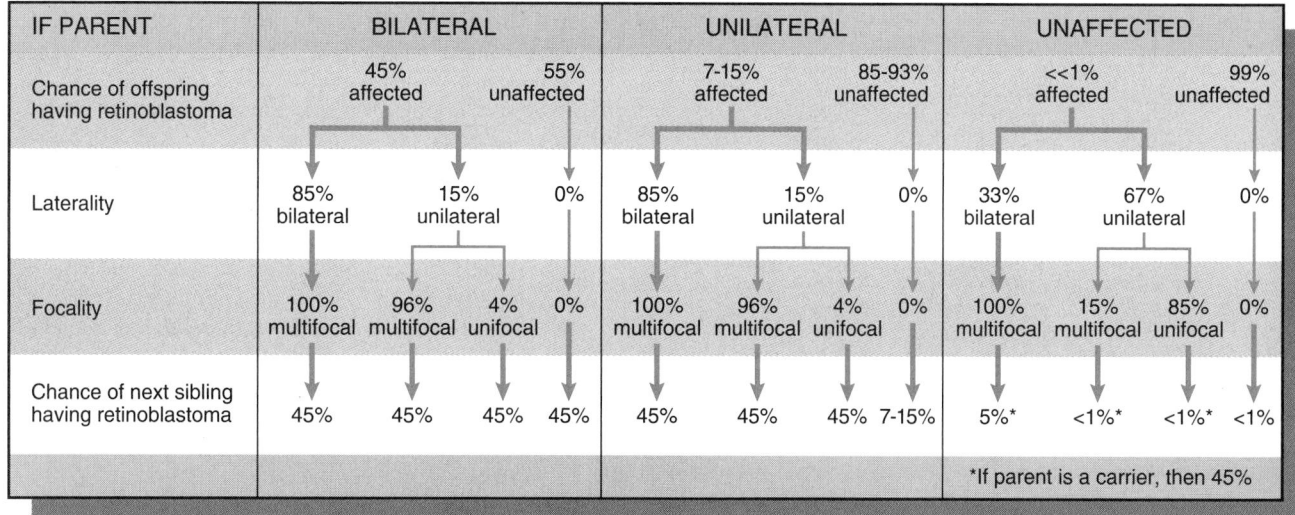

Figure 147–1 Genetic counseling for retinoblastoma.

through the wall of the eye and reaches the conjunctiva, where spread to regional nodes (preauricular, posterior auricular, and anterior cervical) occurs.

Clinical Findings

1. In Western countries, patients present with intraocular disease. In developing nations, patients present with extraocular disease.
2. The most common presentation with intraocular disease is leukocoria, also known as white pupillary reflex or "cat's eye reflex," seen in 60 per cent of cases (Table 147–1). Leukocoria is caused by intraocular tumor visible to the naked eye through the normally black pupil or because of a highly elevated retinal detachment caused by the tumor.
3. The second most common presentation is strabismus (20%), or crossed eyes, caused by tumor or detachment involving the macula. Although esotropia (eyes crossed in) is more common in all children, in retinoblastoma, exotropia (eyes crossed out) occurs as often as esotropia.
4. Other causes are inflammatory (mimicking orbital cellulitis or intraocular inflammation), glaucoma, nystagmus, and poor vision.
5. In cases in which there is a known family history, small tumors are identified on screening examinations under anesthesia.
6. In cases in which extraocular disease is found on presentation, patients exhibit orbital masses, seizures, failure to thrive, and masses of the scalp.

TABLE 147–1. PRESENTING FINDINGS IN RETINOBLASTOMA

Leukocoria	60%
Strabismus	20%
Inflammatory	5–10%
Ocular	
Orbital	
Heterochromia	5%
Anisocoria	<5%
Routine examination	<5%
Screening examination with family history	40%

7. The Reese-Ellsworth classification (not a staging system), is used most often to characterize intraocular disease (Table 147–2).
8. The Abramson classification is used to characterize extraocular disease (Table 147–3).

Key Clinical Findings

- White pupillary reflex
- Strabismus

Laboratory Findings/Radiologic Changes

1. X-ray: Skull x-rays can demonstrate intraocular calcification in >70 per cent of intraocular cases (no longer used).
2. CT scans: Useful to detect intraocular calcification, in-

TABLE 147–2. REESE-ELLSWORTH CLASSIFICATION OF RETINOBLASTOMA

GROUP I

a. Solitary tumor, <4 disc diameters in size, at or behind the equator
b. Multiple tumors, none >4 disc diameters in size, all at or behind the equator

GROUP II

a. Solitary tumor, 4 to 10 disc diameters in size, at or behind the equator
b. Multiple tumors, 4 to 10 disc diameters in size, behind the equator

GROUP III

a. Any lesion anterior to the equator
b. Solitary tumors >10 disc diameters behind the equator

GROUP IV

a. Multiple tumors, some >10 disc diameters
b. Any lesion extending anteriorly to the ora serrata

GROUP V

a. Massive tumors involving over half the retina
b. Vitreous seeding

TABLE 147–3. ABRAMSON CLASSIFICATION OF RETINOBLASTOMA

I. INTRAOCULAR DISEASE
    a. Retinal tumor(s)
    b. Extension into choroid
    c. Extension up to lamina cribrosa
    d. Extension into sclera

II. ORBITAL DISEASE
    a. Orbital tumor
        Suspicious (pathology of scattered episcleral cells)
        Proven (biopsy-proven orbital tumor)
    b. Local nodal involvement

III. OPTIC NERVE DISEASE
    a. Tumor beyond lamina but not up to cut section
    b. Tumor at cut section of optic nerve

IV. INTRACRANIAL METASTASIS
    a. Positive CSF only
    b. Mass CNS lesion

V. HEMATOGENOUS METASTASIS
    a. Positive marrow/bone lesions
    b. Other organ involvement

traocular masses, orbital tumors, pineal tumors, and second malignancies; poor at detecting optic nerve invasion.

3. MRI: Useful in differentiating proteinaceous subretinal fluid of Coats disease (hyperfluorescent on T1) from subretinal tumor of retinoblastoma (hypofluorescent on T1).

4. Ophthalmic ultrasound: Outpatient procedure that requires no anesthesia. A and B scans demonstrate intraocular mass and intraocular calcification and can be used to roughly measure tumor size as well as changes in size following treatment.

5. Aqueous analysis: Elevated levels of lactic dehydrogenase, phosphoglucoseisomerase, neuron-specific enolase, and uric acid have been demonstrated. It requires a needle aspiration and safety is unknown; rarely used.

6. Bone marrow biopsy/aspirate and spinal fluid: For detection of metastatic disease. Retinoblastoma cells are "sticky" and attach to the inside of collection tubes, so fluid for cell block should be directly dropped into fixative.

7. Intraocular biopsy: Rarely, if ever done. There is concern about possible spread of tumor through site.

Differential Diagnosis

Because a retinoblastoma diagnosis is made largely on the basis of examination with the indirect ophthalmoscope alone, consideration should be given to lesions that ophthalmoscopically simulate retinoblastoma. Eyes have been removed inappropriately as a result of incorrect diagnosis. Lesions are listed in the box below.

Differential Diagnosis of Retinoblastoma

With Total Retinal Detachment
- Coats disease
- Retinopathy of prematurity

Solitary or Multiple Retinal Tumors
- Astrocytic hamartoma
- *Toxocara canis* granuloma

Treatment

1. Goals of treatment are life, salvaging the eye, retaining vision, achieving acceptable cosmetic result, and minimizing the long-term side effects of therapy.

2. Treatment of intraocular and extraocular disease requires careful coordination of ophthalmic oncologist with pediatric oncologist and radiation oncologist.

3. Treatment of extraocular disease
Historically all children with extraocular disease died within 2 years of detection. Currently, 50 per cent survive following intensive treatment that is still evolving.

4. Orbital disease: Systemic chemotherapy combined with orbital radiation is used.

    a. Optic nerve disease: Treated when the pathologically reviewed cut section of the optic nerve is involved with tumor or if CSF is positive for tumor cells. Treatment includes socket radiotherapy and systemic chemotherapy.

    b. Optic nerve involvement that is not posterior to the lamina cribrosa is not treated. Treatment of optic nerve involvement beyond the lamina but not involving the cut section of the optic nerve is controversial.

    c. CNS disease: Managed with combinations of systemic chemotherapy and localized or diffuse CNS irradiation. Spinal axis radiation is no longer used.

    d. Hematogenous metastasis: Systemic chemotherapy, occasionally followed by a bone marrow transplant, has been used.

5. Intraocular disease

    a. Enucleation: Surgical removal of the eye. Quick, effective, minimal pain. Prosthesis fit 3 weeks after surgery.

    b. External beam radiation: Demonstrated effective in 1903. Patients treated without anesthesia utilizing fractionated doses of 200 to 250 cGy daily, five times a week for a total dose of 3500 to 4600 cGy. Well tolerated; when given lateral port irradiation, ocular side effects are rare. One or both eyes can be treated.

    c. Brachytherapy: Localized radioactive sources (cobalt, iodine, ruthenium), called plaques, can be surgically attached to the outside of the globe, allowing focal radiation to be delivered to the underlying retinal tumor. Plaque is left in place for 4 to 7 days and then removed in a second surgical procedure. Inpatient procedure that requires trained personnel, and two general anesthesias within a week. Effective for newly diagnosed tumors and tumors that have failed other treatments.

    d. Photocoagulation: Intense white light (xenon arc) or laser light (argon, diode) can be focused through the pupil to destroy small retinoblastomas by destroying the surrounding blood supply. Requires general anesthesia and experience.

    e. Cryotherapy: With a pencil-like probe, a rapid freeze is applied to the sclera underneath a retinoblastoma to rapidly cause intracellular ice crystallization and focally destroy the tumor(s). More than 90 per cent effective for small tumors (<3 mm). Requires general anesthesia and trained personnel.

f. Systemic chemotherapy: Causes a reduction in the volume of intraocular tumors and when combined with focal techniques can be used to destroy tumors.

6. Second malignancies

Retinoblastoma patients with the germinal mutation are at high risk for the development of second nonocular malignancies, apparently caused by the genetic defect. Since less than 10 per cent of retinoblastoma patients currently die with metastatic retinoblastoma and the majority of the survivors develop second malignancies (which are usually fatal), the main cause of death in these patients is the second malignancy and not retinoblastoma itself. The natural course of these malignancies is influenced by irradiation, as children who receive therapeutic radiation develop tumors at an earlier age, more commonly in the field of the radiation beam, and therefore have shortened life spans. However, even without radiation, the majority of germinally affected patients develop these malignancies. In the first 10 years of life, the most common malignancies are pinealoblastoma (trilateral retinoblastoma) and sarcomas in the head. In teenagers, the most common tumor is an osteogenic sarcoma of the extremity. In later life, sarcomas at any site, cutaneous melanomas, and malignancies (pathologically difficult to classify) are seen.

Key Treatment

- Enucleation
- Radiation
- Photocoagulation
- Cryotherapy
- Chemotherapy

Bibliography

Abramson DH: Treatment of retinoblastoma. *In* Blodi FC (ed): Retinoblastoma, New York, Churchill Livingstone, 1985, pp 3–39.

Abramson DH: The focal treatment of retinoblastoma with emphasis on xenon arc photocoagulation. Acta Ophthalmol (Suppl) 1989;194:3–63.

Abramson DH, Niksarli K, Ellsworth RM, Servodidio CA: Changing trends in the management of retinoblastoma: 1951–1965 vs. 1966–1980. J Pediatr Ophthalmol Strabismus 1994;31:32–37.

Eng C, Li FP, Abramson DH, et al: Mortality from second tumors among survivors of retinoblastoma. J Natl Cancer Inst 1993; 85:1102–1103;1121–1128.

Knudson AG: Mutation and cancer: statistical study of retinoblastoma. Proc Natl Acad Sci USA 1971;68:820–823.

148 Liver Tumors

Michael P. LaQuaglia

Epidemiology

1. The prevalence of primary malignant liver tumors in the United States is 1.4 cases per million children. The ratio of hepatoblastoma to hepatocellular carcinomas is variously reported to range from 1.3:1 to 6.5:1. However, in areas endemic for hepatitis B, the ratio may be reversed and as low as 0.2:1. Geographic clustering of cases of hepatoblastoma has not been reported. A male predominance is generally reported for both tumors, the male:female ratio ranging from 1.5 to 3.1:1 for hepatoblastoma and from 1.3 to 3.2:1 for hepatocellular carcinomas.

2. Hepatoblastoma has been reported to occur sporadically in adult life, but the tumor most commonly presents in the first 3 years of life. Congenital presentation and antenatal diagnosis have also been reported.

3. In contrast, hepatocellular carcinomas are rare in infancy. The Liver Cancer Study Group of Japan reported no cases in children aged 4 or younger in a series of 2286 patients.

Pathology

1. Hepatoblastoma usually presents as a single, pseudoencapsulated lesion, often reaching large proportions before becoming clinically apparent. The tumor grows in an expansive fashion such that the umbilical fissure is not generally breached. Thus, despite an incidence of bilobar disease of 30 to 40 per cent, a successful extended resection may still be possible. Multicentricity or massive diffuse disease within the liver occurs in less than 20 per cent, and cirrhosis of the surrounding liver is unusual.

2. In contrast, hepatocellular carcinomas usually lack a distinct capsule. It is common for the tumor to spread diffusely through the liver in as many as 70 per cent of patients, often with satellite nodules well separated from the main tumor mass. Bilobar involvement occurs in 50 to 70 per cent, and the umbilical fissure does not constitute a barrier to spread. As a result, hepatocellular carcinoma is usually unresectable. Finally, owing to the association of hepatocellular carcinomas with hepatitis B infection, cirrhosis may be present in the surrounding nonneoplastic liver.

3. The epithelial element of hepatoblastoma may display a range of differentiation from a frankly anaplastic form to

embryonal or fetal differentiation. Besides the epithelial element, hepatoblastoma may contain varying amounts of immature stromal tissue, constituting a "mixed" tumor. The pure fetal pattern is said to be favorable, and the presence of embryonal or undifferentiated histology is considered unfavorable.

4. Fibrolamellar hepatocellular carcinoma, which is characterized by broad fibrous septa that separate the cellular component into nodules, may be associated with a better prognosis. It is most commonly diagnosed in late childhood and adolescence. However, the survival difference may depend on the stage.

5. Metastatic spread at presentation in patients with hepatoblastoma occurs with an incidence of 10 to 20 per cent. The lungs are the metastatic site in 46 per cent, portal and periaortic nodes in 11 per cent, brain in 7 per cent, and peritoneum and diaphragm in 4 per cent each. The incidence of metastases is reportedly higher in patients with embryonal and anaplastic histology (80 and 100 per cent, respectively) as opposed to fetal differentiation (29 per cent).

6. Hepatocellular carcinoma presents as metastatic disease in 30 to 50 per cent. The lungs were involved in 48 per cent, lymph nodes in 37 per cent, intraperitoneal organs in 16 per cent, peritoneum in 15 per cent, adrenal in 11 per cent, bones in 10 per cent, brain in 2 per cent, and skin in 1 per cent. Tumor emboli were detected in the portal vein in 59.7 per cent and in the hepatic vein in 26.6 per cent. The higher incidence of lymphatic and intraabdominal spread in hepatocellular carcinomas is relevant to local resectability and recurrence. Nodal disease in the porta hepatis and periaortic region is not readily resectable, and recurrence is inevitable.

Clinical Findings

1. Children with hepatoblastoma usually present with an abdominal mass or diffuse abdominal swelling. Often the child is in good health, and the lesion is discovered by an observant parent or clinician on routine examination. Accompanying symptoms such as pain, irritability, minor gastrointestinal disturbances, fever, and pallor occur in smaller numbers of patients. Significant weight loss is unusual, although patients may fail to thrive.

2. In contrast, although children and adolescents with hepatocellular carcinomas frequently present with palpable abdominal masses, these are rarely incidental. Pain is a frequent accompaniment and may occur without an obvious mass. Constitutional disturbances such as anorexia, malaise, nausea and vomiting, and significant weight losses occur with greater frequency. Jaundice is an uncommon early feature of either disease. In most series of hepatoblastoma and hepatocellular carcinomas, small numbers of patients present acutely with tumor rupture. Hepatoblastoma may present as sexual precocity, although this is rare.

3. A mild anemia is common in both conditions. Pronounced thrombocytosis is most often evident in patients with hepatoblastoma but has also been reported in occasional patients with hepatocellular carcinomas. The platelet counts in patients with hepatoblastoma may reach 1 million cells/ml. The cause may be release of tumor-derived cytokines.

4. Nonspecific abnormalities are noted in liver function tests with both tumors. A high serum cholesterol value may be present in 50 to 60 per cent of cases, and there is some evidence to suggest that the elevation may correlate with a poorer prognosis.

5. A marker commonly detectable in significant levels is α-fetoprotein. Elevation, often extreme, occurs in 84 to 91 per cent of cases of hepatoblastoma. Slightly fewer patients with hepatocellular carcinomas have elevated levels, and the elevations are less marked. Although nonspecific for epithelial liver tumors, the marker is used extensively to monitor for disease reduction in patients undergoing nonoperative therapy and disease recurrence in treated patients. Some reports conclude that abnormal elevations in α-fetoprotein are more sensitive than radiology or surgical exploration at detecting recurrence.

6. A surgical resection is critical to the successful outcome, and the ideal radiologic study should be a predictor of diagnosis and resectability. Location, size, the relationship of the tumor to anatomic planes of resection and vascular anatomy, and the presence of metastatic disease are important radiologic parameters. Modalities used to investigate abdominal masses or diffuse abdominal enlargement in children include plain radiographs, ultrasonography, radionucleotide scanning, angiography, computed tomography (CT), and magnetic resonance imaging (MRI).

7. Plain films and liver-spleen scans usually indicate an abnormality but do not often contribute to diagnosis or assist in planning therapy. Angiography is indicated if embolization or infusion chemotherapy is contemplated; however, it is invasive, technically difficult to perform in children, and not universally available. An abdominal ultrasound examination, in view of low cost and ready accessibility, is probably the most useful screening investigation. This test can discriminate space-occupying lesions from diffuse hepatomegaly. Anatomic detail of the tumor margin is not usually sufficiently well delineated to assess resectability. Doppler ultrasonography is also used to evaluate patency of the inferior vena cava and hepatic veins. However, extreme compression of these vessels may prevent useful interpretation.

8. An abdominal CT scan is the investigation of choice, both for diagnostic discrimination and to assess operability. The chest should be included to identify pulmonary metastases. The typical appearance of hepatoblastoma is that of a solitary mass with lower attenuation values than normal liver. Dramatic contrast medium enhancement (as in benign vascular neoplasms), invasion of the portal vein, and lymph node involvement is unusual. Hepatocellular carcinomas have a similar appearance but are more likely to be multifocal, invade the portal vein, and metastasize to draining lymph nodes. Distinction between the two lesions cannot be definite because the pattern of disease may be atypical in either instance. The diagnostic ability of MRI is similar to that of a CT scan. The particular features of both hepatoblastoma and hepatocellular carcinomas on MRI are low signal intensity on T1-weighted images and high signal intensity on T2-weighted images. Appearance alone cannot distinguish the two lesions.

Key Clinical Findings

- Hepatic mass
- Abdominal pain

Staging

Currently, staging requires surgical exploration.

Clinicopathologic Staging System

- Stage I: Complete resection
- Stage II: Microscopic residual tumor
              Intrahepatic
              Extrahepatic
- Stage III: Gross residual tumor
              Primary lesion completely resected,
                  nodes positive, and/or tumor spill
              Primary lesion not completely resected
                  and/or nodes positive and/or tumor
                  spill
- Stage IV: Metastatic disease
              Primary lesion completely resected
              Primary lesion not completely resected

Treatment

1. Complete surgical resection remains the major objective of therapy for hepatoblastoma and hepatocellular carcinoma. At presentation, approximately 60 per cent of patients with hepatoblastoma have resectable tumors. A nonanatomic resection, wedging out the tumor with a satisfactory margin, may be feasible in the uncommon instance of a small peripheral or pedunculated lesion. More often, a major anatomic resection is required. It is possible to remove 85 per cent of hepatic substance with subsequent full and rapid hepatic regeneration even with the administration of postoperative chemotherapy.

2. After a successful complete surgical resection and without further treatment, long-term survival can be expected in approximately 60 per cent of patients with hepatoblastoma. Local relapses are unusual, and the most frequent cause of failure in the remaining 40 per cent is a systemic relapse. The overall cure rate with surgery alone is thus around 35 per cent. With the use of adjuvant chemotherapy, survival improves to the 70 per cent range. The most commonly used initial regimen includes cisplatin, vincristine, and 5-fluorouracil. Doxorubicin is also an active agent against hepatoblastoma.

3. Approximately 40 per cent of patients with hepatoblastoma are reported to have inoperable tumors at presentation. Over the past decade, it has become evident that preoperative therapy may render some of these patients resectable. Therefore, in cases judged unresectable the present practice is to administer chemotherapy and perform second-look surgery after a tumor response is documented radiographically.

4. The place of radiotherapy is not clearly defined. Hepatic toxicity has been described at doses to whole liver of greater than 25 Gy, but focal radiation up to 45 Gy can be administered with safety. There may be a place for radiation in a dose range of 25 to 45 Gy combined with chemotherapy in inoperable hepatoblastoma and patients with postresectional residual disease.

5. A definite place probably is emerging for liver transplantation, again in patients failing conventional therapy.

6. With improving management of the primary lesion, mortality is increasingly a result of metastatic relapses in the lungs. However, that this disease does respond to chemotherapy and complete resolution can occur with the current regimens. Should metastases show progression or relapse on therapy, a surgical resection is an option. Cure of pulmonary metastatic disease has not been accomplished with radiotherapy. Also, there are no reports of a cure in patients with hepatoblastoma with metastases to sites other than the lung or regional nodes.

7. Analogous to the case with hepatoblastoma, a complete surgical resection is a prerequisite for cure in hepatocellular carcinomas of childhood. Patients with unresectable tumors do not survive. Although patients undergoing resections survive longer than those that do not, the gain is small, owing to the high local and systemic relapse rate. Overall, the survival at 1 year is 40 per cent for resectable and 10 per cent for unresectable hepatocellular carcinomas.

8. Overall survival in the pediatric age group for hepatocellular carcinomas is rarely reported to exceed 20 per cent. Total hepatectomy with hepatic transplantation has not improved these results, with most patients undergoing disease recurrence and progression. This is especially true if vascular invasion is present at the time of transplant.

Key Treatment

- Surgical resection
- Chemotherapy
- Radiation therapy (metastases)

149 Langerhans Cell Histiocytosis

Stephan Ladisch

Definition

Langerhans cell histiocytosis (LCH) is characterized by the accumulation of Langerhans cells in lesions. LCH is definitively distinguished from other histiocytoses as well as other diseases by this specific pathologic finding. LCH was previously known as histiocytosis X, with the names eosinophilic granuloma, Hand-Schüller-Christian disease, and Letterer-Siwe disease applied to various forms of the disease.

Etiology

The etiology of LCH is not known. At present, controversy exists over whether LCH is reactive or neoplastic. Several features provide seemingly contradictory information on this point. These include spontaneous resolution of disease (especially single-system disease) and clonality of lesional LCH cells.

Pathophysiology

The clinically evident pathophysiology of LCH can broadly be divided into direct involvement with the disease (such as lytic lesions of the bone or involvement of the organs) and processes reflecting secondary consequences (such as tooth loss due to bone erosion).

1. Lytic lesions are believed to result from the release of cytokines by the mixed cell granuloma.
2. Internal organ involvement, although frequently not associated with infiltration by Birbeck granule-positive cells, is believed to occur by a similar mechanism.
3. Pathophysiology of secondary consequences: These permanent consequences are the result of permanent damage by primary disease. Examples include diabetes insipidus (permanent damage to the anterior pituitary), fractures (lytic bone lesions), and tooth loss (lytic bone lesions).

Clinical Findings

The clinical presentation of LCH is variable. It consists of the signs of active disease as well as the signs of the secondary "late" consequences of the disease.

1. *Local lesions.* This confined disease may include "punched out" lytic lesions of bones (especially flat bones), seborrheic rash, or lymph node enlargement.
2. *Systemic disease.* Internal organ involvement in LCH may involve the liver, lungs, hematopoietic system (bone marrow), and gastrointestinal tract, as well as the central nervous system. General findings include fever, failure to thrive, and irritability.
3. *Secondary clinical findings.* These may be the trigger to consider the diagnosis of LCH and include tooth loss, fractures, and diabetes insipidus.
4. *Late sequelae.* Of an as yet undefined relationship to the initial disease (i.e., are they primary or secondary), these include central nervous system involvement and hepatic cirrhosis.

It should be stressed that the diagnosis can be suspected by the clinical picture but can only be confirmed by pathologic evaluation.

Key Clinical Findings

- Rash
- Failure to thrive
- Diabetes insipidus

Pathology

The definitive diagnosis of LCH can only be established by pathologic examination. Several approaches may be used.

1. The classic approach to diagnosis is electron microscopy of lesional cells, demonstrating the presence of Birbeck granules in these lesional Langerhans cells.
2. Immunostaining, with CD1a antibody, revealing positivity of lesional Langerhans cells is also diagnostic. Morphology alone is inadequate to make the diagnosis.
3. Involvement of any additional organ system should be confirmed by biopsy of the involved tissue if possible.

> **NOTE**
>
> **Birbeck granule-positive Langerhans cells, detected by electron microscopy, are diagnostic.**

Laboratory Findings

Findings are related to the specific system involved. Because the systems involved may vary, the initial evaluation to detect abnormal organ function should be performed as listed in the following box. On findings indicating possible involvement of a specific organ system, a more extensive investigation is recommended.

Key Tests

- Complete blood cell count, differential, and platelet count
- Liver function tests (aspartate and alanine transaminases, alkaline phosphatase, bilirubin, total protein, and albumin)
- Coagulation studies (prothrombin time, partial thromboplastin time, fibrinogen)
- Chest radiograph, posteroanterior and lateral
- Skeletal radiographic survey
- Urine osmolality measurement after overnight water deprivation

Radiographic Changes

1. Bone lesions—"punched out" lytic lesions
2. Magnetic resonance imaging and computed tomographic investigation of the central nervous system—identifies pituitary abnormalities, mass lesions, and diffuse or patchy white or gray matter changes

Treatment

Current knowledge of treatment suggests tailoring the therapy to the extent of disease.

1. Single system disease
   a. Excisional biopsy
   b. Radiation therapy (500–800 rads)—restrict to bone lesions with risk of spontaneous fracture (e.g., vertebral lesion)
   c. Mild chemotherapy, topical or systemic (single agent)
2. Multisystem disease
   a. Single-agent chemotherapy (vinblastine and etoposide have been studied)
   b. Combination chemotherapy (includes vinblastine and etoposide)
3. Current experimental therapy
   a. Randomized treatment protocols for multisystem disease
   b. Immunosuppression and bone marrow transplantation for nonresponsive disease

Key Treatment

- Mild or no treatment for mild, single-system disease
- Early treatment with chemotherapy for multisystem disease

Bibliography

Broadbent V, Gadner H, Komp D, Ladisch S: Histiocytosis syndromes in children: II. Approach to the clinical and laboratory evaluation of children with Langerhans-cell histiocytosis. Med Pediatr Oncol 1989;17:492–495.

Gadner H, Heitger A, Grois N, et al: A treatment strategy for disseminated Langerhans cell histiocytosis. Med Pediatr Oncol 1994;23:72–80.

Histiocyte Society Writing Group: Histiocytosis syndromes in children. Lancet 1987;1:208–209.

Ladisch S, Gadner H: Treatment of LCH: Evolution and current approaches. Br J Cancer 1994;70(suppl XXIII):S41–46.

Ladisch S, Jaffe E: The Histiocytoses. *In* Pizzo P, Poplack D (eds): Principles and Practice of Pediatric Oncology, 3rd ed. Philadelphia, JB Lippincott, 1997, pp 615–631.

150 Symptoms of Gastroenterologic Disorders

Definition
Bleeding from the gastrointestinal (GI) tract.

Etiology
1. Gastrointestinal bleeding should be documented by specific chemical tests for blood applied to stool and/or gastric fluid.
   a. False positive guaiac-based tests on stool may occur in patients taking oral iron and those with recent ingestion of meat or certain vegetables.
   b. False negative guaiac-based tests occur when stool or gastric contents are acidic. Thus patients with GI bleeding taking vitamin C tablets may have a negative guaiac test of their stool.
2. The sources of true GI bleeding can be organized according to location (proximal [upper] or distal [lower] to the ligament of Treitz) and the age of the patient, as outlined in Table 150–1.
3. Infections of the gastrointestinal tract may be associated with GI bleeding. Among the pathogens are

TABLE 150–1.   CAUSES OF GI BLEEDING IN PEDIATRIC PATIENTS

UPPER GI TRACT

Esophageal lesions
  Esophagitis
  Varices
  Mallory-Weiss tears—especially in retching adolescents
Gastric lesions
  Gastritis
    Helicobacter infection—rarely seen in very young children
    Secondary to nonsteroidal antiinflammatory medications
  Ulcers
Duodenal lesions
  Ulcers
  Duodenitis
  Arteriovenous malformations

LOWER GI TRACT

Painless rectal bleeding, without diarrhea
  Newborn and infancy
    Perianal fissure secondary to hard stool or diaper rash
    Meckel diverticulum—usually males (2:1) <2 years of age
  Older children
    Anorectal trauma secondary to hard stools (constipation)
    Juvenile polyps (especially grade school children)
Bleeding associated with frequent loose, mucous stools often accompanied by abdominal pain
  Newborn and infancy
    Cow milk/soy protein allergy (especially in first 6 months)
    Necrotizing enterocolitis (especially in premature infants)
  Children
    Infectious enterocolitis
    Inflammatory bowel disease
    Henoch-Schönlein purpura—especially in children with involvement of skin, kidneys, and joints

a. Bacteria and their toxins, including *Salmonella, Shigella, Yersinia, Campylobacter,* hemorrhagic *Escherichia coli* (O157:H7), and *Clostridium difficile* toxin leading to pseudomembranous enterocolitis
   b. Viruses, including cytomegalovirus (CMV), herpes, and adenovirus (especially in immunocompromised children)
   c. Fungi, including *Candida*
   d. Parasites, including *Amoeba* and *Trichuris*
4. Congenital anomalies that may present with GI bleeding in children include duplications of the GI tract and vascular malformations.

Pathogenesis
Gastrointestinal bleeding usually results from inflammation and disruption of the mucosa with accompanying damage to vessels. The damage can be secondary to acid, infection, trauma, drugs, immune/allergic mediators, and ischemia.

Clinical Findings
1. Gastrointestinal hemorrhage can present as an acute event, occasionally with hypovolemic shock, as chronic bleeding with microcytic anemia, or sporadically with minimal functional consequences.
2. Hematochezia represents fresh blood that usually comes from the lower GI tract. However, brisk bleeding proximal to the ligament of Treitz can have a similar appearance as a result of rapid transit through the intestine. Aspiration of the gastric contents using a nasogastric (NG) tube is the first test to be performed to determine the location of the bleeding and the course of the diagnostic evaluation.
3. Melena describes maroon or tarry stools. A negative NG aspirate for blood suggests either obstruction at the pylorus (e.g., a duodenal bulb ulcer with edema preventing duodenogastric reflux) or a more distal small bowel source (vascular malformation, ulceration secondary to drugs, infection, Crohn disease, a Meckel diverticulum, or ileal duplication).
4. Hematemesis is blood generally from a site proximal to the ligament of Treitz mixed with emesis.
5. Children who present with hypovolemic shock should be taken from the emergency department to the pediatric intensive care unit for resuscitation and diagnostic tests. The history should include questions about any previous bleeding; gastrointestinal or liver problems in the child or family members; use of medications or drugs, including alcohol and NSAIDs; and whether the bleeding started as hematemesis, melena, or hematochezia.

Laboratory Assessment
1. For the child with hypovolemia secondary to GI bleeding, the immediate evaluation should include a complete

blood count with differential, reticulocytes and sedimentation rate, a coagulation profile, a chemistry profile, and a type and cross match.

2. After it is determined which part of the GI tract is bleeding (see Clinical Presentation) an evaluation for the etiology can be planned.

3. Identifying upper GI tract lesions can usually be done with endoscopy. If the bleeding has stopped, it may be difficult to find a small ulcer, and a repeat investigation during active rebleeding is warranted.

4. The most common cause of minor lower tract bleeding is constipation causing a rectal fissure.

5. If the child is of the appropriate age, has episodic pain, a sausage-shaped right-sided mass, and "currant jelly" stools, intussusception should be suspected and a barium enema performed by experienced personnel.

6. Substantial lower GI bleeding should be evaluated with colonoscopy to look for inflammation, a vascular malformation, or a polyp.

7. When colonoscopy fails to reveal the cause of suspected lower tract bleeding, radiographic investigations, including a radionuclide scan to search for a diverticulum or duplication and angiography (with brisk bleeding), should be considered. In rare instances, laparoscopy and/or exploratory laparotomy are indicated for persistent bleeding of unknown etiology.

8. In children, lower GI bleeding associated with diarrhea is usually secondary to infections. Stools should be sent for culture and parasites and, if appropriate, *C. difficile* toxin and subtypes of *E. coli* before endoscopic procedures are performed.

9. Hematochezia in the sick-appearing infant suggests volvulus secondary to malrotation, Hirschsprung enterocolitis, or necrotizing enterocolitis.

10. Hematochezia in an otherwise well infant without severe diaper rash or a fissure during the first 6 months of life suggests cow milk protein allergy. It is appropriate to change to a hypoallergenic (hydrolyzed protein) formula and observe for 10 days. If the infant is breast feeding, restricting the mother's diet (removing cow milk, eggs, soy, and wheat) may correct the problem.

Treatment

1. For the child in shock, infusions of isotonic saline and/or cross-matched packed red blood cells should be administered. Coagulopathy should be corrected with fresh frozen plasma for active bleeding or parenteral vitamin K. Somatostatin or vasopressin infusions may be useful in controlling persistent bleeding.

2. If bleeding esophageal varices are noted, the endoscopist may perform sclerotherapy to attempt to achieve hemostasis. When this is not possible, placement of a Sengstacken-Blakemore tube should be considered.

3. If endoscopy reveals a peptic ulcer with a visible vessel or active bleeding, injection of the ulcer or ablation of the vessel should be attempted. When this is unsuccessful, angiography with embolization of the bleeding vessel or surgical intervention is indicated, if life-threatening bleeding continues.

4. If an ulcer or inflammation in the upper GI tract is discovered that is not actively bleeding, the child should receive oral or intravenous H_2 blockers with the goal of raising the gastric pH above 4. After 24 hours with a stable hematocrit, the child can be fed. For the child with a stable hematocrit, epigastric tenderness, and occult blood in the stool, antacid therapy with close outpatient follow-up is appropriate. Antibiotics should be initiated if *Helicobacter pylori* is present.

5. Infectious causes of upper and lower GI bleeding in immunocompromised children may require antimicrobial therapy.

6. Bleeding from perianal trauma related to hard stools should be treated by softening the stools.

7. Polyps can be removed at the time of colonoscopy.

8. Inflammatory bowel disease is treated with antiinflammatory agents to allow the damaged mucosa to heal. If severe hemorrhage persists, colectomy should be considered.

9. Surgical intervention is required for Meckel diverticulum, duplications, intussusceptions that cannot be reduced by a barium enema, Hirschsprung enterocolitis not responding to intensive medical therapy, and necrotizing enterocolitis with impending or completed perforation.

 ## Bibliography

Berry R, Perrault J: Gastrointestinal bleeding. *In* Walker WA, Durie PR, Hamilton JR, et al (eds): Pediatric Gastrointestinal Disease, vol 1. Philadelphia, BC Decker, 1991, pp 111–127.

Hyams JS, Leichtner AM, Schwartz AN: Recent advances in diagnosis and treatment of gastrointestinal hemorrhage in infants and children. J Pediatr 1985;106:1–9.

Milov DE, Andres JM: Sorting out the causes of rectal bleeding. Contemp Pediatr 1988;5(10)80–104.

Olson AD, Hillemeier AC.: Gastrointestinal hemorrhage. *In* Wyllie R, Hyams JS (eds): Pediatric Gastrointestinal Disease. Philadelphia, WB Saunders, 1993, pp 251–270.

Definition

Gastroesophageal reflux (GER) refers to the flow of gastric contents retrograde into the esophagus. Gastroesophageal reflux disease (GERD) refers to the pathology that can occur from GER (e.g., pulmonary complications, apnea, failure to thrive).

Etiology

The etiology of GER is multifactorial, including dysmotility of the stomach and esophagus as well as abnormal functioning of the lower esophageal sphincter (LES).

Epidemiology

1. Gastroesophageal reflux events are an occasional occurrence in all newborn infants, but their frequency decreases with age.
2. High-risk groups and disorders associated with GERD include
   a. Premature infants
   b. Children with neuromuscular impairment
   c. Bronchopulmonary dysplasia
   d. Cystic fibrosis
   e. Esophageal atresia and tracheoesophageal (TE) fistula
   f. Obesity
   g. Hiatal hernia
   h. Children on chronic medications that may affect LES tone
   i. Children with nasogastric tubes or postgastrostomy tube placement
   j. Vigorous exercisers (especially runners).

Pathophysiology

1. LES abnormalities associated with GER include
   a. Transient relaxations—Most episodes of GER occur during brief, intermittent LES relaxations rather than as a result of persistently abnormal LES tone.
   b. Decreased basal tone that is often associated with esophagitis.
2. Abnormalities of perisphincteric factor
   a. Intraabdominal location of the LES
   b. Sphincteric action of the diaphragmatic hiatus
   c. Presence of a "mucosal rosette" at the gastroesophageal junction
   d. Presence of the gastroesophageal angle of His
   e. Phrenoesophageal ligament surrounding the esophagus.
3. Transient increases in intraabdominal pressure may account for significant numbers of reflux episodes (up to 54 per cent) in children.
4. Gastric emptying abnormalities are described in up to 40 per cent of adults with GERD.
5. Peristaltic abnormalities and delays in esophageal transit may occur with esophagitis or, more rarely, can be a primary abnormality.

Clinical Findings

The clinical presentation varies from infants to older children.

1. Infants
   a. Effortless regurgitation occurs during or right after a feeding and usually resolves between 6 and 18 months of age.
   b. Nonspecific irritability, rumination, and failure to thrive due to emesis or decreased intake is often seen.
   c. Respiratory symptoms may occur, including
      (1) Bronchospasm
      (2) Stridor
      (3) Apnea
      (4) Recurrent pneumonia.
   d. Neurobehavioral findings are characterized by twisting and extension of the neck (Sandifer syndrome).
   e. Anemia from GI bleeding (erosive esophagitis) can be seen.
2. Older children
   a. GER is usually not self-limited (>50 per cent require long-term medical or surgical management).
   b. Vomiting and abdominal pain are the most common symptoms followed by wheezing, regurgitation, dysphagia, heartburn, failure to thrive, chest pain, nocturnal cough, and nausea.
   c. Symptoms of esophagitis (chest pain, dysphagia, or odynophagia) tend to be more prominent than in infants.

Laboratory Findings

There are no consistent laboratory abnormalities noted in a child with uncomplicated GER.

Differential Diagnosis

The differential diagnosis of vomiting with abnormal laboratory findings include

1. Pyloric stenosis—hypochloremic metabolic alkalosis
2. Congenital adrenal hyperplasia— $\downarrow$ Na^+, $\uparrow$ K^+
3. Metabolic disease— $\uparrow$ ammonia, acidosis, or hypoglycemia
4. Eosinophilic gastroenteritis—peripheral eosinophilia
5. Renal disease— $\uparrow$ BUN, creatinine

Radiographic and Other Diagnostic Evaluation

1. Upper GI barium contrast x-rays are used to rule out anatomic abnormalities (hiatal hernia, malrotation, strictures, webs).
   a. There is a high incidence of false positive and false negative results in demonstrating GER on upper GI series; the presence of GER may also not correlate with GERD.
   b. Rarely, signs of GERD can be noted radiographically (e.g., erosive esophagitis, esophageal dysmo-

tility, severely delayed gastric emptying, GER event with aspiration).

2. Continual esophageal pH recording (pH probe) is the gold standard in quantifying frequency of *acid* reflux into the esophagus.

   a. The pH probe can be used to determine variations in acid reflux at different esophageal positions, associate temporal relationships between reflux and clinical symptoms (e.g., apnea), and measure effectiveness of surgical or pharmacologic therapy.

   b. A pH probe study cannot be used to determine volume of refluxed material, assess episodes of alkaline reflux, or detect postprandial reflux if the gastric acid becomes buffered by a meal.

3. Endoscopy with esophageal biopsy allows for detection of esophagitis. The absence of esophagitis does not imply that GER is not occurring.

4. Scintigraphy can allow detection of reflux or aspiration as evidenced by radioactivity in the esophagus or lungs; the rates of gastric emptying can also be determined.

   a. Advantages of scintigraphy include the possible documentation of aspiration as well as postprandial reflux.

   b. Disadvantages of scintigraphy include the technical difficulties (experienced personnel and so forth) and the need for the child to remain stationary for extended periods of time.

5. Esophageal manometry is useful in patients in whom esophageal dysmotility or LES dysfunction is suspected.

   a. GER can occur with normal, low, or high LES pressures, making interpretation difficult.

   b. Distal esophageal dysmotility may be seen in cases of existing esophagitis.

Treatment and Prevention

1. General recommendations

   a. Parents should provide small, frequent feedings and avoid overfeeding, prolonged attempts at feeding, bedtime feeding, and allowing the child to recline after eating.

   b. Thickened feedings by using 1 tbsp cereal/1 to 2 oz formula is often helpful.

   c. Upright positioning decreases reflux episodes. However, elevation of the head of the bed is not conclusively better than flat positioning.

   d. Parents are encouraged to avoid foods and medications that affect LES tone or increase gastric acidity (caffeine, fatty foods, chocolate, alcohol).

2. Pharmacologic therapy (most agents are not specifically approved for pediatric use)

   a. Prokinetic agents

      (1) Cisapride (0.2 mg/kg/dose qid 20–30 min a.c.)

         (a) Cisapride is a noncholinergic, nonantidopaminergic agent that enhances postganglionic acetylcholine release.

         (b) This medication does not cross the blood-brain barrier.

         (c) Cisapride enhances gastric emptying, increases LES tone, and enhances esophageal motility.

      (2) Metaclopramide (0.1 mg/kg/dose qid 20–30 min a.c.)

         (a) Metaclopramide is a dopamine antagonist.

         (b) Metaclopramide raises LES tone and enhances gastric emptying and esophageal peristalsis.

         (c) This medication crosses the blood-brain barrier and may cause extrapyramidal effects.

      (3) Bethanecol (0.1 mg/kg/dose qid, a.c.)

         (a) Bethanecol is a cholinergic agent.

         (b) Bethanecol increases LES pressure as well as esophageal peristaltic amplitude and duration.

         (c) This medication may exacerbate bronchospasm and has been associated with bradycardia and other cholinergic effects.

      (4) Domperidone

         (a) Domperidone is a peripheral dopamine antagonist.

         (b) Domperidone is not available for use in the United States.

   b. Agents that decrease gastric acidity

      (1) Histamine$_2$-receptor antagonists (ranitidine, cimetidine, famotidine, nizatidine)

         (a) These medications are indicated for acid-related complications (e.g., reflux esophagitis).

         (b) Treatment is for a minimum of 8 weeks.

      (2) Proton-pump inhibitors

         (a) These medications are more potent suppressors of gastric acid production and are indicated for refractory esophagitis.

         (b) Currently, omeprazole and lansoprazole are available as a sustained-release capsule.

         (c) These medications are not approved for chronic use owing to concerns about acid suppression, gastrin overproduction, and enterochromaffin cell stimulation.

3. Surgery

   a. Surgical procedures are designed to increase the high-pressure zone in the LES and to increase the length of the intraabdominal esophagus. Indications for surgical intervention include

      (1) Intractable reflux symptoms

      (2) Severe disease (e.g., strictures)

      (3) Life-threatening respiratory episodes.

   b. Children with neurologic impairment or peptic strictures are more likely to require surgical intervention.

   c. Nissen fundoplication is the most frequently performed procedure and consists of wrapping the gastric fundus around the gastroesophageal junction.

      (1) Reflux is reduced or eliminated in >90 per cent of cases.

(2) Short-term complications include herniation of the wrap through the hiatus and small bowel obstruction from adhesions.

(3) Long-term complications include dumping syndrome, gas bloat, and dysphagia.

Bibliography

Hillemeier AC: Reflux and esophagitis. *In* Walker WA, Durie PR, Hamilton JR, et al (eds): Pediatric Gastrointestinal Disease—Pathophysiology, Diagnosis, and Management, vol 1. Philadelphia, BC Decker, 1991, pp 417–422.

Orenstein SR: Gastroesophageal reflux. Curr Probl Pediatr 1991;21:193–241.

Orenstein SR: Gastroesophageal reflux. *In* Wyllie R, Hyams JS (eds): Pediatric Gastrointestinal Disease—Pathophysiology, Diagnosis, Management. Philadelphia, WB Saunders, 1993, pp 337–369.

Sondheimer JM: Gastroesophageal reflux: Update on pathogenesis and diagnosis. Pediatr Clin North Am 1988;35:103–116.

Treem WR, David PM, Hyams JS: Gastroesophageal reflux in the older child: Presentation, response to treatment and long-term follow-up. Clin Pediatr 1991;30:435–440.

| Symptom | Constipation, Encopresis, and Hirschsprung Disease | *Paul Harmatz* |

Definitions

1. *Constipation* may be defined in children quantitatively, as producing fewer than three stools per week; or qualitatively, as passage of either hard, large-diameter stools or pellet-like stools associated with pain and/or excessive straining.

2. *Encopresis* or *fecal soiling* is the passage of bowel movements in the underwear or other abnormal place after age 4 years.

Etiology and Epidemiology

1. Constipation in children is idiopathic or functional in 90 to 95 per cent; organic disease is found in the remainder. Idiopathic constipation is thought to be related to several possible causes, including slow colonic motility, psychologic factors, and/or a history of painful defecation.

2. Organic causes

   a. Neurologic—Disorders of the spinal cord, cerebral palsy, Hirschsprung disease, intestinal pseudo-obstruction, and neuronal intestinal dysplasia, types A and B

   b. Anal lesions—Fissures, stenosis, atresia, anterior displacement of the anus

   c. Endocrine and metabolic disorders—Hypothyroidism, hypercalcemia

   d. Medications that slow intestinal motility

   e. Hirschsprung disease, or congenital aganglionic megacolon, should be considered in any child with severe constipation, particularly with onset in the first year of life, and in those who respond poorly to medical therapy. The incidence is 1 in 5000 births, with males predominating 4:1. Presentation varies depending on the length of aganglionic segment and age of the child. This diagnosis should be considered in the newborn presenting with bilious vomiting and abdominal distention. In later infancy, the patient may have growth failure, abdominal distention, or life-threatening enterocolitis. Later in childhood, there is a pattern of infrequent stooling, abdominal distention, passage of thin stools with straining, and intermittent episodes of intestinal obstruction. A number of associated anomalies may occur with aganglionic megacolon. The conditions are heritable as autosomal recessive traits with location on chromosome 10.

3. Constipation and fecal soiling account for up to 3 per cent of outpatient pediatric visits or 10 to 25 per cent of visits to pediatric gastroenterologists. Chronic constipation can begin in the first year (25%), with the peak between 2 and 4 years. Males predominate. Encopresis is reported to affect 1 to 3 per cent of children in the 4- to 11-year age group, with males predominating.

Pathophysiology

1. A normal stool frequency on a low-fiber Western diet for 95 per cent of children (1 to 4 years old) ranges from three stools per day to one stool every other day. Mean stool weight is 25 g. Mean total transit time is 33 hours; the total transit time increases with age.

2. Stool weight is closely related to diet and fiber intake. Higher fiber intake produces a heavier stool and decreased transit time.

3. Normal defecation involves passage of a fecal bolus into the rectum, stimulating sensory receptors and conscious sensation of a bowel movement approaching. Transient contraction of the external anal sphincter and puborectalis sling occurs in conjunction with relaxation of the internal anal sphincter. This is followed by relaxation of the external anal sphincter and puborectalis sling, an increase in intraabdominal pressure, and passage of stool. Continence is primarily dependent on the puborectalis sling, with the external anal sphincter assisting in control of diarrheal stools.

4. Anorectal manometry has been used to define abnormalities in rectal function associated with chronic constipation. Incomplete internal sphincter relaxation, increased threshold volume to produce conscious awareness, and contraction of external anal sphincter when attempting to expel a stool mass (anismus) may be contributing to constipation. The presence of a *critical volume* response (that rectal volume distention necessary to produce relaxation of the internal anal sphincter) that is below the threshold volume has been described in encopresis.

5. Patterns of colonic transit and motility examined in adults by radiologic marker studies and manometry are abnormal in severe constipation. Similar studies have not been done in children.

6. A causal relationship between radiologic or manometric abnormalities and the development of constipation or encopresis have not been proved.

7. It is hypothesized that constipation develops in response to familial or constitutional makeup, diet, or external events such as a rectal fissure associated with pain, birth of a sibling, travel, illness, difficult toilet training, or difficult social adjustment. Significant psychologic problems have been demonstrated in only a small percentage of children, and these usually disappear when the constipation resolves. If left untreated, the constipation worsens, producing megarectum and the abnormalities described by manometric studies. Encopresis usually occurs in association with constipation and may represent leakage of liquid around a large fecal mass in the rectum.

Clinical Findings

1. Symptoms

    a. Stools that are passed with straining, grunting, pain; may also represent attempts to withhold stool.

    b. Abdominal pain is not seen in most patients.

    c. Decreased appetite is common.

    d. There is often a poor awareness of fecal soiling—either passage of stool or its presence in underwear.

    e. Encopresis can be associated with aggressive and angry behavior, refusal to cooperate, and poor school performance. It is rarely associated with enuresis or urinary tract infections.

2. Signs

    a. The abnormal stool consistency can vary and includes

    (1) Large-diameter stool often passed with blood on the outer surface, resulting in the "plugged toilet" sign

    (2) Small, hard, pellet-like stools

    (3) Liquid stool probably leaking around fecal obstruction, not to be confused with diarrhea

    (4) Soft stool passed after much straining and apparent discomfort, often seen in association with anteriorly displaced anus.

    b. Abdominal distention is seen only in severe cases of constipation and should raise suspicion of Hirschsprung disease.

    c. An abdominal mass can be mistaken for a tumor or pregnant uterus.

    d. The rectal examination may reveal

    (1) An anteriorly displaced anus (anus located in the anterior third of a line drawn from the coccyx and posterior edge of the scrotum or vulva)

    (2) A rectal fissure that may be seen only after carefully spreading the anal mucosa

    (3) A rectal canal that is normally 1 to 2 cm, with a small amount of stool in the ampulla. A long, tight canal suggests Hirschsprung disease, whereas a normal-length canal with large, hard stool mass in the ampulla suggests functional constipation. A rectal shelf may be present on the posterior margin and is associated with anterior displacement of the anus. It is important during the rectal examination to inquire about sensation and elicit a voluntary squeeze as a test of external sphincter mechanism and puborectalis sling.

    e. Other aspects of the physical examination—Observe for normal growth and development, since failure to thrive may be associated with Hirschsprung disease, and developmental delay may suggest cerebral palsy as a cause of constipation.

    f. Abnormal skin findings may suggest hypothyroidism.

    g. A "pit" in the lower back may suggest a meningomyelocele or spina bifida occulta.

    h. Neurologic abnormalities, including developmental delay, hypotonia, and abnormalities of lumbosacral nerve innovation, may demonstrate abnormal leg/foot strength/sensation, abnormal gait, and an absent anal wink.

Key Clinical Findings: Hirschsprung Disease

- Constipation—usually from birth
- Abdominal mass
- Long tight rectal canal with little or no stool

Laboratory Findings

Biochemical and hematologic tests are rarely helpful. A urinalysis should be obtained if a urinary tract infection is suspected.

Radiologic Findings

1. Abdominal films may demonstrate large amounts of stool to confirm the diagnosis of constipation or evaluate the effectiveness of therapy. They may also demonstrate an abnormality of the lower spine or bowel dilatation seen in pseudo-obstruction or neuronal intestinal dysplasia.

2. A barium enema should be performed unprepped as a single-contrast study. It is useful to examine for an obstruction, microcolon, zonal aganglionosis, and Hirschsprung disease with the diagnostic transition zone. A barium enema may miss total colonic aganglionosis because of an absent transition zone. This is rarely needed in "typical" functional constipation responding to medical therapy.

3. Evaluation of total gut transit time by radiopaque markers is rarely used in children because the physical examination usually demonstrates a diagnostic fecal mass and radiation exposure is undesirable.

Key Radiologic Findings: Hirschsprung Disease

- Abdominal film shows massive amount of stool
- Barium enema shows narrowed segment; transition zone

Anorectal Manometry

1. This procedure is performed on patients with a history or physical examination suggesting Hirschsprung disease or those who have severe constipation and have been poorly responsive to medical therapy. It is a very low risk procedure, with high sensitivity and specificity. False positive results are seen if the catheter shifts out of the sphincter region during balloon inflation. A better examination is obtained if it is delayed until initial bowel "clean-out" has been completed. The procedure can be done in neonates ≥39 weeks' gestation; however, chloral hydrate sedation may be needed in younger or uncooperative children to obtain an adequate examination.

2. Failure of the internal anal sphincter to relax or show decreased pressure with distention of a rectal balloon (rectosphincteric reflex) supports the diagnosis of Hirschsprung disease. An abnormal manometry result requires confirmation by rectal biopsy.

3. Incomplete or atypical relaxation of the internal anal sphincter suggests the possibility of hypoganglionosis (decreased ganglion cells in the intestine) or neuronal intestinal dysplasia.

Rectal Biopsy

1. Rectal biopsy provides the gold standard for diagnosis of Hirschsprung disease, hypoganglionosis, or neuronal intestinal dysplasia.

2. A diagnostic rectal biopsy can be obtained with a suction apparatus (Rubin tube) if sufficient submucosa is obtained (50 per cent of biopsy specimen). Small risks of bleeding and perforation are present. The biopsies are completed at 3 and 5 cm above the anal verge posteriorly to avoid the hypoganglionic segment of Aldrich (false positive results occur if biopsies are obtained in the hypoganglionic segment; false negative results occur if biopsies are above the area of aganglionosis). Acetylcholinesterase histochemical stain or other nerve trunk–specific stains may demonstrate thickened nerve bundles and nerve fibers traversing the lamina propria, to support the diagnosis of Hirschsprung disease.

Treatment

1. The treatment for Hirschsprung disease is corrective surgery, removing the aganglionic colon and pulling innervated colon through a "muscular" sleeve of rectum. The type of operation performed depends upon the length of aganglionic colon. These operations can be performed in two stages, with the creation of a diverting colostomy, or in a single stage.

2. Education—Constipation and encopresis

   a. Remove child and parental "blame and guilt" by explaining the high frequency of the problem and the general absence of intentional behavior or underlying psychologic problems in the child.

   b. Explain the mechanics of normal and abnormal defecation patterns.

   c. Discuss the concept of treatment as a long-term process to improve toileting behavior and alter diet, emphasizing the importance of fiber and the potential long-term use of laxatives. Emphasize that this is a long-term process—not a rapid cure in most cases.

3. Laxatives—Constipation and encopresis

   a. The amount, class, and combination of laxatives are matched to the age of the child, the severity of illness, and the risk of aspiration with underlying neurologic disease. Therapy is generally divided into an initiation phase and a maintenance phase.

   b. Initiation phase: This is designed to effectively disimpact the severely constipated child and prevent leakage of laxatives or stool softeners around a retained stool mass during maintenance-phase therapy. In children ≥1 year of age, this phase often involves starting a relatively large amount of mineral oil but, in addition, including a 2- to 3-day cycle of phosphate enemas, bisacodyl suppository, and bisacodyl tablets. Cycling these medications over the 3-day period helps prevent toxicity from multiple doses of a single medication, especially phosphate enemas.

   c. Maintenance phase: This involves use of a stool softener (mineral oil, lactulose, or Karo syrup), laxative (bisacodyl, Senokot, cisapride), high-fiber diet, multivitamin (especially if high doses of mineral oil are used), behavior modification, and frequent medical follow-up until the patient is responding well. It is appropriate to consider a trial of reduced medical support in 6 months to 1 year.

   d. Specific classes of medications used in treating the pediatric age groups:

      (1) Lubricants—Mineral oil is the prototypic agent of this class. Mineral oil acts to coat fecal contents, making them easier to pass. Use only in children >1 year of age to minimize risk of aspiration. For the same reason, this should not be used in children with neurologic disorders and risk of aspiration. Adverse effects are rare, but mineral oil may cause foreign body reaction in lymphoid tissue after absorption of small amounts from intestine, lipoid pneumonia after aspiration, or fat-soluble vitamin deficiencies. The approximate dose is 1 to 3 ml/kg in one to two divided doses. Mineral oil can be mixed with juice to administer. Supplement the patient with multivitamins. The child should be warned to avoid passing flatus outside the toilet or to wear a small pad in the underwear, as the mineral oil may pass and stain clothes or furniture. Mineral oil should not be administered with surfactants (sodium docusate), as absorption may increase.

      (2) Hyperosmotic laxatives act through osmotic properties to increase luminal pressure and stimulate peristalsis. Agents include glycerin suppository (3 g suppository), lactulose (10 g/15 ml, 1–2 ml/kg/day in two to three divided doses), and Karo syrup (5–30 ml/day mixed in formula). All are relatively safe and can be used in infants. Lactulose and Karo syrup may cause

diarrhea and fluid/electrolyte losses, and doses should be adjusted to produce soft stools two or three times a day. Recently the isotonic preparations GoLYTELY and NuLytely containing the nonabsorbable osmotic agent polyethylene glycol have been used safely for bowel cleansing before procedures or to relieve severe obstipation. These agents generally must be given by nasogastric tube. An adult dose of 1 L/hour for 4 hours can be scaled down to 10 to 20 ml/kg/hr for children, not to exceed the adult dose. Metoclopramide may be necessary if nausea or vomiting occurs.

(3) Bulk-forming agents—These agents include foods that are high in fiber as well as commercial fiber-containing products (e.g., Metamucil and Maltsupex). Dietary fibers are plant polysaccharides that are poorly digested in the small intestine but form gels and facilitate passage of stool by softening the stool and stimulating peristalsis. These agents are particularly safe, long-term therapies for constipation. They should be ingested with adequate fluids to prevent the rare complication of intestinal obstruction. Although fiber can bind minerals in the intestine, preventing absorption, the amount recommended is very unlikely to produce this side effect. Maltsupex liquid (16 g/tbsp) has been recommended in infants in doses of 7.5 ml to 30 ml/day to initiate therapy, with 5 to 10 ml/day for maintenance. Older children experience results from 7.5 ml to 30 ml/day.

(4) Saline laxatives—Magnesium, sulfate, phosphate, and citrate are the principal active agents in these laxatives. These ions are poorly absorbed and probably act as osmotic agents holding water in the intestine, softening stool, and stimulating peristalsis. The compounds can cause significant electrolyte abnormalities, especially Mg, in patients with renal failure or hypocalcemia, hypernatremia, and hyperphosphatemia in patients retaining phosphate enemas. They are generally used only in acute situations or as bowel preparations for procedures. A small dose of milk of magnesia (1–3 ml/kg/day) can be helpful in chronic constipation when other safer laxatives have been tried unsuccessfully.

(5) Emollient laxatives—These are surfactants that facilitate mixing of aqueous and fatty substances in stool to soften it. Docusate sodium (Colace) is the best known. These agents may promote the absorption of another laxative or mineral oil, producing toxicity. For this reason, they have not been used in management of chronic constipation.

(6) Stimulant laxatives—These agents include anthraquinone (sennosides) and diphenylmethane (bisacodyl) compounds. They probably act by decreasing fluid and electrolyte absorption in the intestine. Bisacodyl has been shown to stimulate the mucosal nerve plexus in the colon, producing increased contractions. It produces a bowel movement in 6 to 12 hours after oral administration and 15 minutes to 1 hour after rectal administration. We often use this agent for a limited period during the initiation phase of therapy to promote effective clean-out. It also may be helpful when used in rectal form (10 mg suppository, ½ to 1 suppository qod) to assist in the early phase of behavior modification to produce a successful bowel movement in the toilet early in the day to prevent later soiling or accidents. Side effects from these agents include cramping, fluid or electrolyte imbalances, melanosis coli, hepatoxicity, erythema multiforme, and, after years of use, "cathartic colon." For these reasons none of these agents is used for extended periods.

4. Behavior modification

a. It is extremely important to establish a plan for regular toileting and to encourage toileting early in the day to minimize the chance of soiling later. Toileting after meals will take advantage of the gastrocolic reflex.

b. Maintain a record of toileting behavior and successful bowel movements in the toilet with a "star chart." Place one star on the calendar for sitting on the toilet and two stars for having a bowel movement. Plan in advance a "special reward" if a certain number of stars are achieved by the next visit to the physician. Be sure to have the child bring the star chart to each appointment.

Do not reward child for not soiling—this may be reinforcing stool retention.

5. Biofeedback

a. This has been utilized in specialized centers to improve recognition of rectal distention and coordination of muscle function to allow defecation or to facilitate maintenance of continence.

b. The procedure involves a combination of rectal balloon manometry and skin surface electromyography.

c. Success in retraining patients with both surgical and functional disorders is reported to be ≥75 per cent.

Prevention

Anticipatory guidance by the physician is important in educating parents as follows:

1. An understanding of optimal feeding practices
2. An appreciation of normal and abnormal stool patterns
3. Early detection of problems with stooling and avoidance of pain associated with bowel movements
4. An ability to differentiate efforts by the child to pass stool from attempts to withhold stool
5. An understanding of the need to establish a regular toileting schedule (must encourage the child not to avoid the urge to use the toilet!)

6. An understanding of the need to increase fiber intake—fruits, breads, cereals, vegetables.

Prognosis

Generally 50 per cent of patients recover within 1 year and are off laxatives; 20 per cent require 1 to 2 years of laxatives; 30 per cent require prolonged treatment. Surgical correction of Hirschsprung disease is highly successful, with normal stooling patterns achieved in the majority of patients 1 year following surgery.

Bibliography

Berquist WE: Biofeedback therapy for anorectal disorders in children. Semin Pediatr Surg 1995;4:48–53.
Hatch TF: Encopresis and constipation in children. Pediatr Clin North Am 1988;35:257–280.
Loening-Baucke V: Chronic constipation in children. Gastroenterology 1993;105:1557–1564.
Loening-Baucke V: Constipation in children. Curr Opin Pediatr 1994;6:556–561.
Wrenn K: Fecal impaction. N Engl J Med 1989;321:658–662.

151 Achalasia

Toba Weinstein and *Jeremiah Levine*

Etiology and Epidemiology

1. Achalasia is an esophageal motility disorder characterized by absence of coordinated esophageal peristaltic wave upon swallowing, increased lower esophageal sphincter (LES) resting pressure, and incomplete relaxation of LES when swallowing.
2. *Achalasia* is Greek for failure to relax.
3. The etiology of achalasia is unknown.
4. The overall incidence of achalasia is 1:100,000.
5. Less than 5 per cent of cases occur in the pediatric population.
6. Familial achalasia is characterized by an autosomal recessive inheritance and is an extremely rare entity, with fewer than 35 reported cases.

Pathophysiology

1. Absent, decreased, or degenerated neurons in the Auerbach plexus of the esophagus are seen in achalasia.
2. The possibility that achalasia is an immunologic disorder is supported by several clinical findings, including
   a. "Triple–A" syndrome (alacrima, achalasia, adrenal insufficiency)
   b. Association between Sjögren syndrome and achalasia
   c. Association between glucocorticoid deficiency and achalasia.

Clinical Findings

1. The most common presenting symptom is dysphagia, which occurs in ≥90 per cent of patients.
   a. Patients experience pain with both solids and liquids and often have the sensation of food "sticking."
   b. Patients will often drink liquids after eating solids to wash food down.
2. Vomiting occurs in approximately 80 per cent of patients, with undigested food products often coming back up. Patients frequently awaken with vomitus on the pillow.

3. Chest pain occurs in approximately 50 per cent of patients.
   a. Impaired esophageal emptying often leads to a feeling of fullness.
   b. Esophagitis is often seen and is thought to be secondary to stasis of food and secretions.
4. Failure to thrive is commonly seen in children with achalasia and may be due to inadequate caloric intake secondary to fear of pain or emesis.
5. Respiratory complaints, including cough and recurrent pneumonia, occur in ≥25 per cent of patients. The cough in these patients is typically nocturnal and may represent aspiration of food and secretions that are pooled in the dilated esophagus.

Key Clinical Findings

- Dysphagia
- Pain on swallowing food and drink
- Undernutrition

Radiographic Changes

1. Chest x-ray findings useful in diagnosing achalasia include
   a. A widened mediastinum secondary to a dilated esophagus
   b. An air-fluid level in the posterior mediastinum
   c. Absent gastric air bubble
   d. Acute and chronic inflammatory lung changes.
2. A barium esophagram is often diagnostic. Findings include
   a. Esophageal dilatation
   b. Absence of normal esophageal peristalsis
   c. Failure of barium to empty from esophagus

d. A tapered narrowing of the esophagus at the cardioesophageal junction ("bird's beak" appearance)

e. Occasional esophageal ulcerations.

Diagnostic Findings

1. Esophageal manometry is the gold standard for diagnosing achalasia. Specific findings include

   a. Elevated resting LES pressure

   b. Impaired LES relaxation with swallowing

   c. Ineffective or absent esophageal peristalsis.

2. Esophagoscopy is frequently used to exclude other disorders, such as an esophageal stricture or a fixed obstructive lesion and to diagnose complications of achalasia, such as esophagitis or esophageal ulceration.

Treatment

1. Medications used in selected patients include calcium channel blockers and nitrates. These medications act to decrease LES pressure and are beneficial for short-term symptomatic relief until more definitive therapy is administered.

2. Pneumatic dilatation is the most effective nonsurgical treatment. Dilatation forcefully ruptures the muscle fibers of the LES. Unfortunately, only 25 per cent of children have significant improvement. In addition, there may be a lack of long-lasting relief. If repeat procedures are required within 1 year, surgical management is recommended.

3. Surgical intervention is the therapy of choice for achalasia in pediatric patients.

   a. Heller myotomy has a success rate of ≥85 per cent.

   b. Gastroesophageal reflux is a common occurrence following myotomy.

   c. An antireflux procedure is often performed in conjunction with the Heller myotomy.

Key Treatment

- Surgery (Heller myotomy)

Bibliography

Azizkhan RG, Tapper D, Eraklis A: Achalasia in childhood: A 20-year experience. J Pediatr Surg 1980;15:452–456.

Berquist WE, Byrne WJ, Ament ME, et al: Achalasia: Diagnosis, management, and clinical course in 16 children. Pediatrics 1983;71:798–805.

Bosher LP, Shaw A: Achalasia in siblings. Am J Dis Child 1981;135:709–710.

Maksimak M, Perlmutter DH, Winter HS: The use of nifedipine for the treatment of achalasia in children. J Pediatr Gastroenterol Nutr 1986;5:883–886.

Reynolds JC, Parkman HP: Achalasia. Gastroenterol Clin North Am 1989;18:223–255.

152 Pyloric Stenosis

Bradley Kessler and *Jeremiah Levine*

Definition

Pyloric stenosis (PS) is characterized by grossly thickened/hypertrophied circular muscle around the pylorus. This disorder is the most frequently diagnosed surgical disorder of the stomach and duodenum in infants and children. The thickened pylorus results in gastric outlet obstruction and leads to the clinical presentation of projectile vomiting and failure to thrive.

Etiology

The etiology is not clearly known.

1. The pathologic process progresses from birth in most infants.

2. Pyloric stenosis may be related to deranged nitric oxide synthesis or decreased nitric oxide synthase, poor neuronal innervation, and elevated prostaglandin levels.

Epidemiology

Infants and children at risk include

1. First-born children, with incidence in males four to six times more frequent than in females

2. Siblings and offspring of affected children, especially if the mother had been affected, and children from smaller family size and higher socioeconomic class.

3. The incidence is highest in Caucasians, particularly those of Northern European ancestry.

4. The sex ratio is more nearly 1:1 in blacks.

Pathophysiology

In PS, there is a gradual progression to high-grade obstruction of the pyloric channel by hypertrophic muscle.

Clinical Findings

1. Children with PS have nonbilious vomiting.

   a. The vomiting may or may not become projectile.

   b. The vomitus may be clear or brownish "coffee grounds" in color owing to gastritis in the later stages.

2. The onset of vomiting may occur as early as the first week of life or as late as 5 months of age. The average age at onset is 3 weeks.

3. The vomiting may lead to dehydration, weight loss, and failure to thrive.
4. The number of stools may decrease, or constipation may develop.
5. Associated anomalies may be present in 6 to 20 per cent of infants.

Key Clinical Findings

- Nonbilious vomiting
- Decrease in stool number
- Visible gastric peristalsis
- Olive-sized mass in midepigastric area

Diagnosis

The diagnosis of PS is best made by physical examination with palpation of a pyloric mass or tumor.

1. A palpable pyloric mass is pathognomonic for PS.
2. A palpable mass occurs in 80 per cent of cases.
3. The mass is most easily palpable with the infant quiet or sedated and the stomach empty or immediately after the infant has vomited.
4. The mass is small and movable, consistent with the size and shape of an olive.
5. The pyloric mass is generally located in the midepigastric area, although the position is variable.
6. Visible gastric peristalsis is often seen.

Laboratory Findings

1. The vomiting leads to a hypochloremic metabolic alkalosis.
2. Indirect hyperbilirubinemia occurs in 2 to 5 per cent of infants.
3. Occasional hypokalemia with paradoxical aciduria may be seen.

Key Laboratory Findings

- Hypochloremic metabolic alkalosis
- Rise in unconjugated bilirubin in serum (2–5%)

Radiographic Changes

1. Radiographic studies should be reserved for those infants suspected of having PS in whom a pyloric mass is not palpated.
2. An abdominal examination shows a dilated, air-filled stomach and a constricted pyloric channel. Small amounts of air distal to the stomach can often be seen. Ultrasound is the procedure of choice to confirm the diagnosis.
   a. Strict sonographic criteria include
      (1) muscle thickness ≥34 mm *or*
      (2) a pyloric length >16 mm *or both*.

b. In reported series, ultrasound has a specificity of 100 per cent and a sensitivity of 89 to 100 per cent.
3. Upper GI barium contrast x-rays are reserved for cases in which the clinical diagnosis is in question. These studies are best performed after aspiration of the stomach. Barium should be removed by nasogastric tube after completion of the study. Characteristic findings on upper GI series include
   a. Elongation of the pyloric channel, producing a "string sign"
   b. The "double tract sign" due to the folding of the compressed mucosa
   c. The "umbrella sign" due to a prepyloric bulge into the distal antrum
   d. Delayed gastric emptying.

Treatment

1. Correction of the dehydration and electrolyte/acid-base imbalance (potassium depletion, hypochloremic metabolic alkalosis) within the first 24 to 48 hours is essential.
   a. IV hydration, initially with 0.45 to 0.9 per cent saline in 5 per cent dextrose, 10 to 20 ml/kg, is most frequently used.
   b. Twenty to 40 mEq/L KCl is usually added following voiding.
2. With continued vomiting, a nasogastric tube should be placed for drainage.
3. A Ramstedt pyloromyotomy is the surgical procedure of choice and is curative.
4. Postoperative complications include
   a. Vomiting secondary to persistent localized edema and delayed gastric emptying
   b. Incomplete pyloromyotomy
   c. Abdominal wall dehiscence and wound infection
   d. Intestinal adhesions.

Key Treatment

- Surgery (pyloromyotomy)

 ## Bibliography

Alexander F: Pyloric stenosis and congenital anomalies of the stomach and duodenum. *In* Wyllie R, Hyams J (eds): Pediatric Gastrointestinal Disease. Philadelphia, WB Saunders, 1993, pp 414–418.

Benson CD: Pyloric stenosis. *In* Welch KJ, Randolph JG, Ravitch MM, et al (eds): Pediatric Surgery, vol 2. Chicago, Year Book Medical Publishers, 1986, pp 811–815.

Deluca SA: Hypertrophic pyloric stenosis. Am Fam Physician 1993;47:1771–1773.

Hernanz-Schulman M, Sells LL, Ambrosino MM, et al: Hypertrophic pyloric stenosis in the infant without a palpable olive: accuracy of sonographic diagnosis. Radiology 1994;193:771–776.

Macdessi J, Oates RK: Clinical diagnosis of pyloric stenosis: a declining art. Br Med J 1993;307:553–555.

153 *Helicobacter pylori*–Associated Peptic Ulcer Disease

Toba Weinstein and *Jeremiah Levine*

Etiology and Epidemiology

1. *Helicobacter pylori* is a bacterial organism that plays a significant role in the development and recurrence of peptic ulcer disease (PUD).

   a. *H. pylori* is a gram-negative spiral or curved rod with four to six unipolar sheathed flagella.

   b. *H. pylori* produces multiple extracellular enzymes, including urease (which is important in disease pathogenesis and diagnosis).

   c. *H. pylori* is located only in association with gastric epithelium.

2. Antritis seen in association with *H. pylori* represents a primary bacterial infection.

   a. Healthy human volunteers who ingested 10^9 CFU of organisms developed symptoms of abdominal discomfort and vomiting followed by documented antritis.

   b. Suppression or eradication of *H. pylori* infection leads to resolution of PUD.

   c. Children, who have a low prevalence rate of *H. pylori*, always have an associated pathogenic inflammatory response when organisms are isolated from gastric mucosa.

   d. Other etiologies typically associated with PUD (alcohol, drugs) are not common in the pediatric population.

3. Epidemiologic studies strongly support the role of *H. pylori* in PUD.

   a. There is an increasing prevalence of *H. pylori* with age.

      (1) There is a 10 to 20 per cent prevalence in children from industrialized countries vs. 80 to 100 per cent in developing countries.

      (2) It is rare for children <8 years of age from industrialized countries to be infected.

      (3) Greater than 50 per cent of adults ≥50 years in the United States test positive for *H. pylori*.

      (4) People from developing nations are infected almost a decade earlier than those in industrialized countries.

   b. Groups with an increased incidence of infection include

      (1) Patients from institutions of custodial care

      (2) Relatives of infected children

      (3) African Americans (prevalence rate is 40 per cent higher)

      (4) Hispanics (prevalence rate is 80 per cent higher).

   c. There is no relationship between *H. pylori* and gender.

   d. There is an inverse relationship between *H. pylori* prevalence and education and socioeconomic status.

   e. There is no increased association of *H. pylori* with nicotine, alcohol, or NSAIDs use.

4. Transmission of *H. pylori* is presumed to be person to person.

   a. A fecal-oral route of spread is possible.

   b. The organism has never been cultured from water sources, food, or pets.

Pathophysiology

1. *H. pylori*–induced inflammation represents a complex interaction of humoral factors, cell-mediated immunity, and inflammatory reaction within the gastric mucosa.

2. Virulence factors allow the organism to survive and thrive in the acid stomach environment. These include

   a. Motility factors, such as the spiral shape and flagella that allow the organism to travel through the stomach into the mucus layer.

   b. Specialized enzymes

      (1) Urease produces ammonia and bicarbonate from urea, neutralizing the acid environment.

      (2) Catalase helps resist opsonization and neutrophil destruction.

      (3) Proteases allow bacteria to penetrate the mucus layer and escape intraluminal acid.

   c. Adherence factors that allow organisms to attach to gastric mucosal cells.

Clinical Findings

1. The clinical presentation, duration, and location of abdominal pain do *not* distinguish between *H. pylori* positive and negative patients.

2. Epigastric pain with or without nausea is frequently seen.

3. Patients are usually older than 8 years without underlying medical conditions.

4. There is frequently a family history of PUD.

Key Clinical Findings

- Epigastric pain with or without nausea
- Above age 8 years

Diagnostic Findings

1. Currently available noninvasive studies do not determine the presence of active infection with *H. pylori*.

2. The definitive diagnosis of *H. pylori*–induced PUD is made by esophagogastroduodenoscopy and antral biopsy.

3. All children with *H. pylori* infection have antritis.

4. The most frequent endoscopic finding is antral nodularity.

   a. The antral nonulcerated mucosa has a cobblestone appearance consisting of nodules 2 to 4 mm in diameter.

   b. Nodularity occurs in 55 to 80 per cent of children with *H. pylori* antritis.

   c. Antral nodularity is thought to be an immunologic response to local infection more commonly seen in children, who have more reactive lymphoid tissue than adults.

Laboratory Findings

1. Culture initially was thought to be the gold standard for diagnosis but now is the least sensitive study available (approximately 80 per cent).

   a. *H. pylori* is a slow-growing organism (3 to 7 days).

   b. *H. pylori* must be grown on blood or chocolate agar in a microaerophilic environment ($T = 37°C$).

   c. Translucent colonies are oxidase, catalase, and urease positive.

2. Histology is important to assess the underlying inflammatory reaction.

   a. Comma-shaped organisms are identified within the mucus layer.

   b. Warthin-Starry stain precipitates silver on the organism, allowing it to be more easily recognized.

3. Biopsy with urease testing is the endoscopic test of choice to identify *H. pylori*.

   a. Antral biopsy specimens are placed into a urea-containing medium with pH-sensitive dye.

   b. The yield of this test is directly related to the number of organisms present.

4. Breath testing is noninvasive, quick, and easy to perform. A radiolabeled carbon dose of urea is ingested; if the organism is present, urease activity will result in the expiration of radiolabeled CO_2.

   a. The radiation exposure associated with the radioactive ^{14}C isotopes is unsatisfactory in the pediatric population.

   b. ^{13}C stable isotopes require the mass spectrometer for detection and quantification.

5. Serologic tests measure exposure to the organism.

   a. Enzyme linked immunosorbent assay (ELISA) is a sensitive and specific test for organism identification.

   b. ELISA is a useful technique for epidemiologic studies.

Treatment

1. Children with endoscopically documented *H. pylori*–associated PUD should receive antimicrobial therapy.

2. Standard ulcer therapeutic agents, including topical antacids and H_2 antagonists, heal duodenal ulcer disease, do not eradicate the organism, and do *not* prevent ulcer recurrence.

3. Monotherapy with bismuth subsalicylate (Pepto-Bismol)

   a. Suppresses *H. pylori* activity by disrupting the outer membrane and inhibiting enzyme production; has an antacid effect but rarely leads to eradication.

   b. Bismuth toxicity has not been reported with the pediatric dosing schedule used to treat *H. pylori*.

4. Combination therapy for 2 weeks using clarithromycin, metronidazole or amoxicillin, and a proton pump inhibitor has an overall eradication rate of 70 to 90 per cent. Compliance is the single most important factor predicting successful treatment outcome.

5. Triple therapy for 1 week using a proton pump inhibitor, metronidazole, and amoxicillin has an overall eradication rate of approximately 90 per cent.

   a. Efficacy of antibiotic therapy is affected by dose, duration of therapy, compliance, acquired resistance, and acid milieu.

   b. Metronidazole has potential side effects of dizziness, nausea, headache, and neuropathy.

   c. Antibiotic resistance is an increasing problem in underdeveloped countries but rarely poses difficulty in the United States. Resistance may develop when therapy is discontinued before a 10-day course has been completed.

Key Treatment

- Proton pump inhibitor
- Antibiotics

Bibliography

Drumm BD: Helicobacter pylori in the pediatric patient. Gastroenterol Clin North Am 1993;22:169–182.

Israel DM, Hassall E: Treatment and long-term follow-up of Helicobacter pylori–associated duodenal ulcer disease in children. J Pediatr 1993;123:53–58.

Judd RH: Helicobacter pylori, gastritis, and ulcers in pediatrics. Adv Pediatr 1992;39:283–306.

Prieto G, Polanco I, Larrauri J, et al: Helicobacter pylori infection in children: clinical, endoscopic, and histologic correlations. J Pediatr Gastroenterol Nutr 1992;14:420–425.

Sherman PM: Peptic ulcer disease in children. Diagnosis, treatment, and the implication of Helicobacter pylori. Gastroenterol Clin North Am 1994;23:707–725.

Key Laboratory Findings

- Serologic (ELISA)
- Culture of organism
- Histology of biopsy
- Urea breath test

154 Acute Diarrhea

John D. Snyder

Definition and Background

The definition of acute diarrhea can vary by culture and region, but most definitions include criteria related to increased frequency and altered form of stool. A good definition of a diarrheal stool is one that takes the shape of its container. Infectious causes of diarrhea are often categorized by the mechanisms of injury. These mechanistic categories include bacterial, viral, and parasitic organisms. This discussion concerns agents that cause disease in immunocompetent children.

Etiology

Many infectious agents can cause acute diarrhea in children; the most frequently recognized are listed in Table 154–1. Rotavirus, with seasonal prevalence in the winter months or rainy season, is the most common agent worldwide.

Epidemiology

Acute diarrhea continues to be one of the most important causes of morbidity and mortality in children. The impact is greatest in less developed countries, where an estimated 4 million children ≤5 years of age die each year from diarrhea. Even in North America, diarrhea causes 10 per cent of preventable child deaths. Most episodes are caused by enteric pathogens, which are usually transmitted by the fecal-oral route. Contaminated food or water is the most common vehicle.

TABLE 154–1. MECHANISMS OF DISEASE CAUSED BY ENTERIC PATHOGENS

INVASION

Campylobacter jejuni
Escherichia (E.) coli (enteroinvasive)
Salmonella enteritidis
Shigella
Yersinia enterocolitica
Vibrio (V.) enterocolitica

ENTEROTOXIN PRODUCTION

Vibrio cholerae non-01
E. coli (enterotoxigenic)
Aeromonas
Pleisiomanas shigelloides
Clostridium (C.) difficile
Yersinia enterocolitica
Shigella

CYTOXIN PRODUCTION

Shigella
E. coli (enterohemmorragic, enteropathogenic)
C. difficile

ADHERENCE

E. coli (enteropathogenic, enterohemorrhagic)
Rotavirus
Adenovirus

1. Risk factors for acquiring diarrhea include education level of the family, potability of water, quality of sanitation and hygiene practices, maturity of intestinal host defense system, use of breast feeding (protective), weaning practices, daycare attendance, travel to less developed countries, and exposure to animals.
2. Risk factors for dying from diarrhea include: infancy, low socieoeconomic status, and minority racial and regional status.

Pathophysiology

1. Injury. Injury to the intestine is caused by one or more of four mechanisms (see Table 154–1).
    a. Invasion
        (1) Attachment by pili, fimbriae, motility devices, chemotactic factors, and adhesions
        (2) Organism spread to contiguous cells, causing an inflammatory reaction.
    b. Enterotoxins
        (1) Inhibit Na and Cl absorption at the villous tip
        (2) Stimulate Cl and HCO_3 secretion in crypt cells.
    c. Cytotoxin
        (1) Shiga toxin of *Shigella* is the prototype.
        (2) These inhibit protein synthesis and elaborate inflammatory mediator substances.
    d. Adherence
        (1) Exact mechanism of injury is unknown.
        (2) Results in dissolution of microvilli, distortion of enterocytes, and round cell inflammation in the lamina propria.
2. Fluid and electrolyte losses. Regardless of the mechanism of intestinal injury, the major impact of acute diarrhea is caused by fluid and electrolyte losses. The mechanisms of these losses can be broadly categorized into those related to secretory losses and those related to osmotic effects.
    a. Secretory diarrhea. The prototype of secretory diarrhea is cholera, in which a toxin stimulates cyclic AMP production, resulting in increased losses of sodium, chloride, and water. These diarrheas produce large-volume watery stools that are relatively unrelated to the nature or volume of oral intake. The sodium content of secretory diarrheas is high, often ≥100 mmol/L.
    b. Osmotic diarrhea. These diarrheas occur when a poorly absorbed solute is present in the intestinal lumen and causes increased losses of electrolytes and water. The volume of diarrhea is usually less than for secretory diarrheas and usually decreases with fasting.

Clinical Findings

The great majority of diarrheal episodes share several common features, including fever, vomiting, and altered stools. However, a careful assessment is required to help determine the likely causative agent and, more important, to direct appropriate therapy.

1. Historical clues
   a. Associated illnesses. Meningitis, sepsis, pneumonia, otitis media, or urinary tract infection can cause similar symptoms.
   b. Risk factors. Travel to less developed countries, use of untreated water, exposure to animals, involvement in daycare, or recent use of antibiotics increases the risk of diarrhea.
   c. Dietary factors. Food allergies and excessive intake of fruit juice must be considered.
2. Physical examination
   a. Assessment of hydration status. Must include comparison of previous weights, if available; presence or absence of postural changes in heart rate or blood pressure; capillary refill time: skin elasticity; moisture of the mucous membranes; firmness of the orbits; presence of rapid, deep breathing (evidence of acidosis); and mental status.
   b. Evaluate for electrolyte disturbances.
      (1) Altered sensorium can be associated with hypernatremia.
      (2) Abnormal neuromuscular states can be caused by hypokalemia.
      (3) Cardiac arrhythmias can be caused by hyperkalemia (rare).

Key Clinical Findings

- History of liquid stools
- Dehydration

Laboratory Findings

The laboratory evaluation is rarely required in the immunocompetent child with acute diarrhea. However, laboratory evaluation should be considered in the following situations.

1. Serum electrolytes—Obtain when clinical signs and symptoms of severe dehydration or sodium or potassium abnormalities are present.
2. Wright or Gram stain of stool—Should be performed if a culture is considered. If the stain shows no red or white blood cells, the yield from a stool culture is very low. In most cases, knowing the nature of the infecting organism will not affect therapy.
3. Stool culture for enteric pathogens—Should be performed if bloody diarrhea is present.
4. Viral studies—Can be obtained to help define the epidemiology of a community outbreak.

Key Laboratory Findings

- Serum electrolytes
- Stool culture

Radiographic Changes

Radiographic studies are rarely required in the diagnosis and management of acute diarrhea. If studies are obtained during illness, the typical findings include air-fluid levels and thickened bowel wall.

Treatment

1. Oral therapy. The critical component of effective treatment for acute diarrhea is the replacement of fluid and electrolyte losses. This treatment can be done orally in the great majority of cases, with the important advantages of lower cost and easier administration than the alternative of intravenous therapy. Over the past 25 years of successful use, oral therapy has evolved to include two components: oral rehydration therapy (ORT) of fluid and electrolyte losses, and early appropriate feeding. Effective commercially available ORT solutions are included in Table 154–2. These solutions contain 45 to 90 mmol/L sodium and a sodium-to-glucose molar ratio approaching 1. Table 154–3 contains a list of fluids that are commonly given to children with diarrhea but that are not physiologically useful solutions for this purpose. The following therapeutic guidelines are based on the severity of illness.
   a. No dehydration. Children with no dehydration are less likely to drink the salty ORT solutions, but these children may require only appropriate feeding.
      (1) ORT (Pedialyte or similiar solution). If used, this will replace ongoing stool losses. Use 10 ml/kg for each stool.
      (2) Feeding. Use age-appropriate foods containing complex carbohydrates and easily digested sim-

TABLE 154–2. COMPOSITION OF ORAL REHYDRATION SOLUTIONS AVAILABLE IN THE UNITED STATES

ORAL REHYDRATION SOLUTIONS	CHO	Na	CHO:Na	K	BASE	OSMOLALITY
		Concentration in mmol/L				
Naturalyte, Unlimited Beverages	140	45	3.1	20	48	265
Pediatric Electrolyte, NutraMax Products	140	45	3.1	20	30	250
Pedialyte, Ross Laboratories	140	45	3.1	20	30	250
Infalyte, Mead Johnson	70	50	1.4	25	30	200
Rehydralyte, Ross Laboratories	140	75	1.9	30	30	310
WHO/UNICEF ORT	111	90	1.2	20	30	310

CHO, carbohydrate.

TABLE 154-3. COMPOSITION OF SOLUTIONS INAPPROPRIATELY USED TO TREAT CHILDREN WITH DIARRHEA

PRODUCT	CHO	Na	CHO:Na	K	BASE	OSMOLALITY
			Concentration in mmol/L			
Cola	700 F,G	2	350	0	13	750
Apple juice	690 F,G,S	3	230	32	0	730
Chicken broth	0	250	—	8	0	500
Sports drinks (e.g., Gatorade)	255 S,G	20	13	3	3	330

CHO, carbohydrate; F, fructose; G, glucose; S, sucrose.

ple proteins. These foods include rice, potato, wheat, cereals, chicken, yogurt, fruits, and vegetables. Regular formula or milk should be used, and breast feeding for infants is especially encouraged. Foods high in simple sugars and fats should be avoided.

b. Mild dehydration (<5% weight loss)

(1) ORT (WHO or Rehydralyte). Correct dehydration using 50 ml/kg in ≤ than 4 to 6 hours. Replace ongoing losses from stool and emesis with 10 ml/kg of Pedialyte or similar solution for each stool and emesis volume estimated in increments of 1/2 cup.

(2) Feeding. Once dehydration has been corrected, begin feeding as outlined above.

c. Moderate dehydration (5–9% acute weight loss)

(1) ORT similiar solution under supervision. Correct dehydration using 100 ml/kg in ≤4 to 6 hours. At the end of each hour of rehydration, continuing stool and emesis losses should be calculated and the volume added to the ORT to be given.

(2) Feeding. Once dehydration has been corrected, begin feeding as outlined above.

d. Severe dehydration (≥10% acute weight loss)

(1) ORT. This is a medical emergency that requires aggressive resuscitation of the shock or shock-like condition. A large-bore catheter or catheters should be used for the infusion of Ringer's lactate or isotonic sodium salt solution. Boluses of 20 to 40 ml/kg should be administered until signs of shock resolve. As the level of consciousness improves, oral therapy can be instituted (see Chapter 12).

(2) Feeding. When rehydration is complete, feeding is continued as outlined above.

2. Antidiarrheal agents (opiates, Lomotil). Although antidiarrheal agents are still widely used, their use is not recommended by the American Academy of Pediatrics, the World Health Organization, or the Centers for Disease Control, or by us. These drugs are dangerous for infants.

3. Antimicrobial agents. The great majority of episodes of diarrhea do not require treatment with antimicrobial agents. However, treatment is important in the following situations:

a. Cholera. This disease occurs rarely in North America and only near the Gulf of Mexico.

b. *Shigella* dysentery. *Shigella* infections without dysentery are almost always self-limited.

c. *Salmonella* infections in infants <1 year old. This age group is at particular risk for hematogenous spread of infection. In older patients the danger is usually self-limited. When invasive, antibiotic treatment is sometimes advisable.

d. *Clostridium difficile*

e. *Giardia*

f. Amebiasis.

 Key Treatment

• Correct dehydration
  Oral glucose
  Fluid and electrolyte replenishment for mild to moderate disorder
  IV solutions for severe disorder

• Early refeeding

• Antimicrobial (selective; rarely required)

Prevention

The single most important factor to reduce the impact of diarrhea is to raise the educational level of the family. Also of great importance are improving the quality and quantity of drinking and cooking water and raising the standards of sanitation and hygiene. To underscore the importance of these factors, the human cost of diarrhea in the United States at the turn of the twentieth century was similar to the current impact in less developed countries.

 Bibliography

AAP Committee on Nutrition: Use of oral fluid therapy and post-treatment feeding following enteritis in children in a developed country. Pediatrics 1985;75:358–361.

American Academy of Pediatrics Provisional Committee on Quality Improvement, Subcommittee on Acute Gastroenteritis: Practice parameter on acute diarrhea. Pediatrics 1996;97:424–434.

Cohen MB: Etiology and mechanisms of acute infectious diarrhea in infants in the United States. J Pediatr 1994;118:S34–S39.

Pickering LK: Therapy for acute infectious diarrhea in children. J Pediatr 1991;118:S118–S128.

155 Persistent Diarrhea

John D. Snyder

Definition

Most diarrheal episodes are self-limited and resolve in 3 to 5 days. No second peak of the incidence of episodes exists to define diarrheal illnesses that continue for longer periods. However, a definition, even if arbitrary, is needed to permit comparisons between studies. The current internationally accepted standard is episodes lasting ≥2 weeks with a change in stool frequency, consistency, and volume and often associated with adverse nutritional consequences. Many illnesses can be associated with persistent diarrhea (Table 155–1), but the majority of episodes are idiopathic.

Terminology

A variety of terms have been used to describe protracted episodes of diarrhea; they can be divided by the association with weight loss.

1. Weight loss—Chronic diarrhea, prolonged diarrhea, protracted diarrhea of infancy, persistent diarrhea
2. No weight loss present—Chronic nonspecific diarrhea, toddler's diarrhea. These disorders have no evidence of malabsorption or infection, occur in preschool children, and typically resolve by 3 to 4 years of age.

Epidemiology

Although accurate statistics are not available in the United States, the prevalence of idiopathic persistent diarrhea appears to be declining. In developed countries, a greater proportion of the cases are caused by conditions such as short bowel syndrome and inflammatory bowel disease; this is in contrast to developing countries, where the great majority of cases are idiopathic. Deaths from persistent diarrhea now account for the majority of the estimated 4 million childhood deaths from diarrhea in developing countries each year.

Pathophysiology (Idiopathic Form)

1. Since most episodes of persistent diarrhea are idio-

pathic, the causal mechanisms, by definition, are unknown. The pathogenesis is probably multifactorial and includes

  a. Variable mucosal injury, which may be caused by
    (1) Primary enteric infection
    (2) Small bowel overgrowth
    (3) Antigen sensitization
    (4) Other causes of inflammation.
  b. Altered immune response, especially cell-mediated immunity.
  c. A causal role for micronutrient deficiencies has not been clearly defined, but deficiencies are associated with both diarrhea and malnutrition. Currently, several studies are under way to evaluate micronutrient supplementation as a therapy.

2. Whatever the pathogenic mechanism, persistent diarrhea is closely linked to malnutrition, and therapy must include nutritional rehabilitation.

Clinical Findings

1. Since many disease states can be associated with persistent diarrhea (see Table 155–1), a thorough history must include questions about possible infections (including travel, exposures to animals); previous surgery; recurrent infections; family history, especially bowel disorders; and diet. Laxative abuse must always be considered in adolescents.

2. Special emphasis should be placed on a thorough dietary history, including
  a. A 3-day diet record
  b. Juice, fiber, and fat intake
  c. Evidence for intolerance to specific foods (especially dairy).

3. Cystic fibrosis and HIV infection must be considered.

4. The physical examination should be performed with the differential diagnosis list in mind and must include a careful evaluation of height, weight, and weight/height percentiles; adenopathy; surgical scars; clubbing; and rashes. The initial examination should also include a direct evaluation of the stool, which helps establish a common frame of reference for the family and medical team. Testing for occult blood should always be performed as a screening test for inflammation.

Laboratory Findings

1. The laboratory evaluation should be carried out in a stepwise fashion, which begins with less invasive, less expensive, and often less specific screening tests for malabsorption and chronic illness and progresses to more specific and often more invasive tests (Tables

TABLE 155–1. PERSISTENT DIARRHEA: DIFFERENTIAL DIAGNOSIS

Idiopathic	Short bowel
Postinfectious	Inflammatory bowel disease
Parasitic	Carbohydrate malabsorption
Medication-associated (antibiotics, laxatives)	Congenital
	Secondary
Small bowel overgrowth	Hepatobiliary tract disease
Celiac disease	Urinary (or other) infection
Food allergy	Pseudo-obstruction
Pancreatic insufficiency	Secretory (neuroendocrine tumors)
Cystic fibrosis	Immune deficiency
Shwachman-Diamond syndrome	Zinc deficiency
Congenital microvillus inclusion disease	

TABLE 155–2. INITIAL LABORATORY EVALUATION

NO WEIGHT LOSS	WEIGHT LOSS
Stools	**Stools**
Direct examination	Direct examination
Hematest	Hematest
Ova and parasites	Ova and parasites
	Sudan stain
	pH, reducing substances
	Gram stain
	? Bacterial culture
	Blood
	CBC
	Albumin
	? HIV test
	Other
	Sweat test
	Trial of increased balanced dietary intake
	Urine analysis, ? culture

155–2 to 155–4). The work-up for children with no weight loss is usually kept to a minimum.

2. First level of evaluation. If weight loss is present, stool should be tested for malabsorption.

   a. Carbohydrate—pH and reducing substances

   b. Fat—Sudan stain for neutral fats

   c. An important component of this initial evaluation is a clinical trial of increased caloric intake. If the child gains weight well on 25 to 30 per cent more calories, clinically significant malabsorption is unlikely. However, the caloric challenge may unmask malabsorption that was not clinically obvious on a low intake.

3. Second level of evaluation. If the diagnosis is not evident after the initial evaluation, additional laboratory tests are indicated (see Table 155–3). This evaluation focuses on possible nutrient deficiencies associated with chronic inflammation as well as diagnostic tests for celiac disease, food allergy (RAST or skin testing), and lactase deficiency (or other abnormalities of carbohydrate malabsorption), in addition to a 72-hour fecal fat collection.

TABLE 155–3. SECOND LEVEL OF EVALUATION

BLOOD

Ca, P, Mg, Zn, folate, Fe, vitamins B_{12}, A, D, E, K
IgA antibody screen for celiac disease
   Anti-endomysial antibody
   Antigliadin antibody
RAST for common food allergens (e.g., milk, soy, egg, nuts)

STOOL

72-hour fecal fat

OTHER TESTS

Breath hydrogen test
Endoscopy
   Duodenal biopsy (enzymes)
   Duodenal aspirate
X-rays
   ? UGI + SBFT

TABLE 155–4. THIRD LEVEL OF EVALUATION

Colonoscopy
CT scan
? Pancreatic stimulation test

4. Third level of evaluation. Duodenal intubation, pancreatic stimulation, and measurement of pancreatic enzymes has a high morbidity and is very infrequently performed.

Radiographic and Endoscopic Evaluation

1. The second and third levels of evaluation for persistent diarrhea often include radiographic and endoscopic tests.

2. Radiographic

   a. Upper GI + small bowel follow-through screens for anatomic abnormalities associated with entities such as small bowel overgrowth, inflammatory bowel disease, and pseudo-obstruction.

   b. CT scan is used primarily to evaluate for tumors, including neuroendocrine secreting tumors.

3. Endoscopic

   a. Upper GI endoscopy and biopsy are almost always performed when the child has evidence of weight loss or malabsorption. Although histologic evaluation (both light and electron microscopic) is often essential for diagnosis, it is a poor predictor for success with nutritional therapy.

   b. Colonoscopy is especially helpful in cases in which bloody diarrhea is present and when inflammatory bowel disease (IBD) is considered.

Treatment

1. If a cause for persistent diarrhea is found, the treatment is usually straightforward and can include specialized diets (e.g., celiac disease, lactose malabsorption), anti-inflammatory agents (e.g., IBD), or surgery (e.g., neuroendocrine tumors).

2. Idiopathic persistent diarrhea, the most common category of this disease, requires thoughtful and aggressive nutritional therapy.

   a. Enteral—If possible, enteral feedings should be used, as they aid intestinal repair and can shorten the duration of illness. Balanced diets of easily absorbed nutrients are most effective.

Key Treatment
• Treat specific etiology, if known
• Nutritional support

   b. Parenteral—In some cases, enteral feeds cannot be tolerated initially, and total parenteral nutrition (TPN) may be required. If possible, some enteral feeds should also be used to help reduce the morbidity of TPN and aid intestinal healing.

   c. Antimicrobial agents. The nonspecific use of antimicrobials has been shown to be of no benefit in cases of idiopathic persistent diarrhea.

Prevention

1. Idiopathic persistent diarrhea is most common in the poorest parts of the world, especially those with the lowest levels of family education. Diarrheal disease control efforts are of great importance, but raising the socioeconomic and educational status is a more critical goal, although difficult to accomplish.
2. Thoughtful and early nutritional interventions may play an important role in reducing the incidence of persistent diarrhea.

Bibliography

Black RE: Persistent diarrhea in children of developing countries. Pediatr Infect Dis J 1993;12:751–761.

Black RE: Persistent diarrhea in children of developing countries. Acta Paediatr 1992(Suppl 381);81:1–153.

Goldgar CM, Vanderhoof JA: Lack of correlation of small bowel biopsy and clinical course of patients with intractable diarrhea of infancy. Gastroenterology 1986;90:527–531.

Kleinman RE, Galeano NF, Ghishan F, et al: Nutritional management of chronic diarrhea and/or malabsorption. J Pediatr Gastroenterol Nutr 1989;9:407–415.

Lifshitz F, Ament ME, Kleinman RE, et al. Role of juice carbohydrate malabsorption in chronic nonspecific diarrhea in children. J Pediatr 1992;120:825–829.

156 Inflammatory Bowel Disease: Ulcerative Colitis and Crohn Disease

John D. Snyder

Definition

Inflammatory bowel disease (IBD) presents as one of two major forms: ulcerative colitis and Crohn disease, the latter also being known as regional enteritis and granulomatous colitis. These idiopathic inflammatory disorders follow a chronic course and often produce systemic symptoms (e.g., growth failure, anemia) as well as symptoms directly related to intestinal inflammation.

Etiology

The cause of inflammatory bowel disease remains unknown, although most experts believe that a number of factors may play a role. These factors include a genetic predisposition, possible infectious or other environmental triggers, and an altered immune response.

Epidemiology

The epidemiologic features of IBD are summarized in Table 156–1.

Pathophysiology

1. Fundamental Question—Current data cannot resolve the question of whether ulcerative colitis and Crohn disease are two manifestations of one disease or two diseases that overlap in pathogenesis and manifestations.
2. Current Hypotheses—The disease model currently in vogue is that people with a genetic predisposition have an unknown initiating event, which may be an infection or exposure to some food or environmental toxin. Inflammation is the result of a dysregulated immune response to the stimulus that may be caused by:
   a. Abnormal activation of the susceptible enteric mucosal immune system to induce excessive cytokine-mediated immune and nonspecific inflammatory cascades
   b. Failure to control (or downregulate) the inflammatory response.

Clinical Findings

1. Although there are many similar features of ulcerative colitis and Crohn disease, the two diseases can usually be distinguished using a combination of clinical signs and symptoms; selected laboratory, radiologic, and histologic findings; and the clinical course. In general, the clinical differences follow directly from the pathologic differences (see below).
2. *Clinical features*
3. *Historical clues*—Evaluation for other causes of bloody diarrhea is essential and requires questions about travel history, exposures (e.g., animals, contaminated water, infectious agents, and antibiotics), and possible food allergies. Additional important areas of questioning include assessment of altered growth, sexual development, family history of gastrointestinal disease, and chronic symptoms, including fevers, arthritis, stomatitis, and rash.

TABLE 156–1. EPIDEMIOLOGY OF IBD

	ULCERATIVE COLITIS	CROHN DISEASE
Age at onset	Peak in 20s and 30s	Same
Onset <20 yr	~20%	Same
Gender	M = F	Same
Ethnicity	Whites predominantly	Same
Genetics	Familial aggregations	Same
Prevalence	2/100,000	3.5/100,000
Frequency	Stable	Increasing

4. *Physical examination clues*—Areas to emphasize on physical examination include growth measurements, hydration and nutritional status, and evaluation for rashes, clubbing, and mucosal lesions. The abdominal examination should evaluate fullness, tenderness, hepatosplenomegaly, and possible masses or peritoneal signs. The examination must include the perianal area and rectum and testing the stool for the presence of blood.

5. *Differential diagnosis*—The diagnostic possibilities include infection by the invasive enteric pathogens, including *Salmonella, Shigella, Campylobacter, Yersinia, Escherichia coli* 0157:H7, *Aeromonas, Clostridium difficile*, and *Entamoeba histolytica*. Tuberculosis and HIV should also be considered. In addition, several diseases can mimic many of the enteric findings of IBD, including hemolytic-uremic syndrome, Henoch-Schönlein purpura, food allergy, and irritable bowel syndrome.

6. *Diagnosis*—The diagnosis is made using a combination of clinical, laboratory, radiologic, and histologic findings. One of the most important confirming factors is the clinical course of the disease. It may be very difficult initially to distinguish between infectious and noninfectious inflammation and between colonic involvement of Crohn disease and ulcerative colitis, so close follow-up is essential.

7. *Disease activity scoring system*—Most clinicians use some type of assessment scale to evaluate the activity of disease. These scales usually include criteria related to
   a. History: Stool frequency and nature, abdominal pain, general well-being
   b. Physical examination: Body weight, growth rate, abdominal mass, blood in stool, and extraintestinal manifestations (arthritis, aphthous ulcers, iritis, perianal disease, fever, rash)
   c. Laboratory: hematocrit, albumin.

Key Clinical Findings

Symptoms	Ulcerative Colitis	Crohn Disease
Pain	Common	Occasional
Vomiting	Rare	Occasional
Bloody diarrhea	Common	Occasional
Tenesmus	Common	Uncommon
Signs		
Weight loss	Occasional	Common
Growth faltering	Occasional	Common
Perianal disease	Occasional	Common
Abdominal mass	Rare	Common
Clubbing	Rare	Occasional

Laboratory Findings

1. Initial assessment—The laboratory evaluation includes collection of blood, urine, and stool specimens.

a. Blood: Complete blood count (CBC), erythrocyte sedimentation rate (ESR), electrolytes, albumin, alanine aminotransferase (ALT), bilirubin, alkaline phosphatase, gamma glutamyl transferase (GGT), and amylase. BUN and creatinine should be included if colitis is present. Tests for the presence of HIV should be considered.

b. Urine: Urinalysis should be performed, especially if colitis is present.

c. Stool: Cultures for *Campylobacter, Salmonella, Shigella, E. coli* 0157:H7, *Aeromonas*; *C. difficile* toxin titer; examination for *E. histolytica*.

2. With the exception of the HIV test and stool evaluations for pathogens, the remainder of the laboratory assessment provides only nonspecific information. None of the blood tests is diagnostic, but the levels of hemoglobin, albumin, and potassium are helpful indicators of severe disease.

Radiographic, Endoscopic, and Pathologic Evaluation

1. *Radiology*—The radiographic evaluation is not diagnostic for IBD but can be helpful in the assessment.
   a. Studies include
      (1) Abdominal flat plate
      (2) Upper GI barium contrast films with small bowel follow-through
      (3) Barium enema (less helpful; never during severe colitis)
      (4) Ultrasound to evaluate masses
      (5) Bone age to help evaluate growth failure.
   b. The upper GI x-ray with small bowel follow-through is the most frequently obtained test, as it evaluates the difficult-to-assess small intestine.
   c. Complications of IBD can be evaluated radiographically, including strictures; enteroenteric, enterovaginal, and enterocutaneous fistulas; and bone demineralization (secondary to treatment).

2. *Endoscopy*—Endoscopy greatly aids diagnosis by evaluating the nature and extent of disease, facilitating acquisition of histologic specimens, and monitoring response to therapy and progression of disease. The procedures most frequently done include

   a. Colonoscopy: Biopsies must always be obtained because there can be a poor correlation between visual and histologic findings.
   b. Flexible sigmoidoscopy: This is the procedure of choice, especially if severe colitis is present.
   c. Upper GI endoscopy: Essential to evaluate gastric and esophageal involvement, which occurs in 5 to 10 per cent of Crohn disease patients.

3. Pathology
   a. Acute infectious colitis can be difficult to distinguish from recent onset IBD on histologic grounds. Evidence for focal vs. continuous involvement is critical for differentiating Crohn disease and ulcerative colitis.
   b. Clinical signs and symptoms are used much more

than histologic criteria to assess response to treatment.

Treatment

Effective treatment for IBD invariably includes nutritional and medical therapy. Although ulcerative colitis and Crohn disease differ in many respects, the medical treatment is very similar. Surgery is rarely a first-line treatment but is curative for ulcerative colitis.

1. *Nutritional.* All IBD patients have increased caloric needs, which can be met in a variety of ways depending on disease severity.
   a. Elemental diets
      (1) Beyond nutritional support, they may also provide primary therapy for Crohn disease and are especially useful for mild to moderate disease.
      (2) They often require nasogastric administration.
   b. Parenteral nutrition (TPN) can be a primary therapy for Crohn disease. It is often required when fistulas are present and improves nutritional status in preparation for surgery.
2. *Medications.* Drug therapy for IBD focuses on two general types of antiinflammatory agents.
   a. General antiinflammatory agents
      (1) Steroids
         (a) Still the mainstay for severe disease; do not maintain a remission.
         (b) Every-other-day administration allows for growth.
         (c) Dosage: 2 mg/kg/day for flare.
         (d) Try to wean to alternate-day schedule to

decrease steroid side effects, especially growth.
      (2) 5-Aminosalicylates: Especially useful for colonic disease; can help maintain remission; several forms available.
         (a) Sulfasalazine: 5-ASA is the active component.
            (i) It remains the standard medication but has many side effects.
            (ii) Starting dose is 40 to 60 mg/kg/24hr; bid dosing often used to help with compliance.
         (b) 5-ASA derivatives have no therapeutic advantage over sulfasalazine but have fewer side effects.
            (i) Olsalazine: 5-ASA dimer; dose is 500 to 1000 mg/day in two doses.
            (ii) Asacol: 5-ASA, delayed release form; dose is 1200–2400 mg/day in three doses.
            (iii) Pentasa: 5-ASA sustained-release form; dose is 2000 to 4000 mg/day in four doses.
   b. Immunomodulators. This class of medications can modify the mucosal immune response and offers promise that more specific and effective therapy may be possible in the future.
      (1) Azathioprine: May act by reducing number of natural killer cells; can suppress bone marrow
         (a) Often requires 6 months to demonstrate effectiveness
         (b) Dose is 1 to 2 mg/kg/day.
      (2) 6-Mercaptopurine
         (a) Similar to azathioprine
         (b) Dose is 1 to 2 mg/kg/day.
      (3) Cyclosporin A: Suppresses cell-mediated immunity; interferes with interleukin-2 synthesis; may have a role in severe cases.
   c. Antimicrobials. Metronidazole is the only agent commonly used; it can be effective in treatment of perirectal disease.
3. *Surgery.* Although surgery is curative for ulcerative colitis, most patients, their families, and the medical team wish to avoid it, if possible, during the adolescent years. The goal of surgery for Crohn disease is to try to remove as little bowel as possible, because further surgery is likely to be needed in the future.
   a. Absolute indications. Several conditions require immediate surgery, including
      (1) Toxic megacolon
      (2) Perforation
      (3) Hemorrhage.
   b. Relative indications
      (1) No response to optimal medical management, which usually includes a 2-week trial of high-dose IV steroids and TPN.
      (2) The cumulative effect of disease on quality of life.

c. Outcome of surgery

  (1) Ulcerative colitis: Surgery is curative.

    (a) Total colectomy is always done.

    (b) The endorectal pull-through procedure has become popular because patients are potentially continent.

  (2) Crohn disease: Surgery is not curative.

    (a) Reoperation is very likely over a lifetime of disease.

    (b) Lesions requiring limited resection have the best outcome.

Key Treatment

- Nutritional support
  Enteral
  Parenteral
- 5-ASA compounds
- Steroids
- Surgery for indication

Outcome

1. Overall—The prospects for a normal life span are good, especially for ulcerative colitis.
2. Cancer
   a. Ulcerative colitis—The risk for intestinal cancer is substantially higher than for the general population, especially after the first 10 years of illness.
   b. Crohn disease—The risk is increased compared with that of the general population but is much smaller than for ulcerative colitis.

Bibliography

Hofley PM, Piccoli DA: Inflammatory bowel disease in children. Med Clin North Am 1994;78:1281–1302.

Kirchner BS: Ulcerative colitis and Crohn's disease in children: diagnosis and management. Gastroenterol Clin North Am 1995;24:866.

Kleinman RE, Balestreri WF, Heyman MD, et al: Nutritional support for pediatric patients with inflammatory bowel disease. J Pediatr Gastroenterol Nutr 1989;8:8–12.

Podolsky DK: Inflammatory bowel disease (Part I). N Engl J Med 1991;325: (Part I) 928–937; (Part II) 1008–1016.

Werlin SL, Grand RH: Severe colitis in children and adolescents: diagnosis, course and treatment. Gastroenterology 1977;73:828–832.

157 Allergic Gastroenteropathy Including Celiac Disease

Paul Harmatz

Definition

Allergic gastroenteropathy refers to adverse *immunologically mediated* gastrointestinal reactions related to ingestion of specific foods; it is also referred to as food hypersensitivity reactions. Food intolerance describes an abnormal response to an ingested food that is not immunologically mediated. These intolerances most commonly involve metabolic events, such as lactose intolerance, but may also include reactions to toxic contaminants or pharmacologic properties of the food.

Etiology

Allergic gastroenteropathy is an immunologically based reaction that occurs in the intestine or systemically following ingestion of a specific food substance.

Epidemiology

Surveys of general populations note that 25 to 30 per cent claim to have food allergies. In contrast, careful epidemiologic studies utilizing elimination and open or blinded challenges with the specific food substance in question demonstrate (probable) food allergy in only 2 to 3 per cent of the population.

Pathophysiology

1. Food allergy results from a poorly understood interaction of the food allergen, the intestine, and the immune system.
2. The molecular character of the antigen, including size, resistance to digestion, and glycosylation, is probably important but is poorly understood.
3. Most reactions occur in response to a limited number of foods, such as cow milk, egg, peanut, soy, fish, shellfish, and wheat. The composition of the list possibly relates to heavy exposure early in life as well as the intrinsic allergenicity of the food substance. For example, the high frequency of peanut allergy in the United States correlates with the high intake of peanut butter there in contrast to Europe; celiac disease is seen more frequently in Sweden than in Denmark and correlates with the higher gliadin content in infant formulas sold in Sweden. Foods such as cow milk are composed of many different proteins, each capable of generating an immune or allergic response.
4. Despite physiologic and immunologic barriers in the intestine, including digestion, mucus, an intact epithelial cell layer, and antibody-specific immunity, minute quantities of antigen penetrate the barrier. This occurs across both columnar epithelium overlying activated or differen-

tiated T and B cells and specialized antigen sampling epithelium known as M cells, overlying lymphoid aggregates of Peyer patches containing immature or quiescent elements of the immune system. After presentation of antigens or peptide fragments by specialized antigen-presenting cells (i.e., macrophage, B cells) to immature T and B cells, the activated immune cells migrate to the systemic circulation and then back to the intestine.

5. The normal immune system response is thought to provide an active defense against uptake of foreign antigens, intestinal toxins, and microorganisms but develops tolerance to the minute amounts of antigens that escape the barrier. It is the failure to develop tolerance or the loss of tolerance that may underlie food allergy.

6. The effector phase of gastrointestinal allergic reactions is divided into IgE-mediated and non–IgE mediated reactions, including immune complex and cell-mediated immune responses. Most recently, extensive pathologic studies have described a heavy infiltration of eosinophils in intestinal mucosa, especially the lamina propria, as a consistent feature of allergic colitis or enterocolitis in infants. Release of a variety of mediators, including platelet activating factor, may play a role in the tissue damage and bleeding seen in allergic intestinal disease. The immune mechanism mediating accumulation of eosinophils and release of mediators is not known.

7. Minute amounts of dietary antigen have been identified in maternal breast milk. Using elimination/challenge protocols, these antigens have been shown to induce allergic disease in the infant.

8. Celiac disease is a non–IgE mediated allergic gastroenteropathy involving a T cell–mediated reaction to gliadin protein that is found in wheat, rye, oats, and barley. In contrast to many other food allergies, celiac disease is a lifelong sensitization and pathologic response to wheat and cross-reacting antigens.

Clinical Findings

1. Symptoms
   a. IgE-mediated: Characterized by the onset of symptoms within minutes to 2 hours after ingesting food allergen. Symptoms may vary from the oral allergy syndrome involving pruritus and swelling of lips, tongue, palate, and throat to more generalized intestinal symptoms of nausea, vomiting, abdominal pain, and diarrhea. Although less common, reactions can be systemic to produce urticaria, respiratory symptoms, or anaphylaxis.
   b. Non–IgE mediated: The onset is most common in the first 3 months of life with recurrent vomiting, failure to thrive (FTT), diarrhea, or simply rectal bleeding. Celiac disease can show variable symptoms depending on age at presentation, including diarrhea, poor appetite, abdominal pain, constipation, and FTT. Hypoalbuminemia and anemia are commonly present.

2. Signs
   a. IgE-mediated: Urticaria, angioedema, wheezing, hypotension, tachycardia, vomiting, diarrhea within minutes to 2 hours of challenge with food allergen. Atopic dermatitis is thought to be an IgE-mediated

reaction but of late-phase type, with skin changes occurring 6 to 48 hours after the challenge.
   b. Non–IgE mediated: FTT, vomiting, diarrhea, rectal bleeding, and, rarely, peripheral edema, respiratory distress (pulmonary hemosiderosis—Heiner syndrome), and ascites.

Key Clinical Findings: Celiac Disease

- Undernutrition after introduction of cereal feeding
- Wasting, particularly in buttocks area
- Abdominal distention

Diagnosis

1. Elimination and challenge is the gold standard for diagnosis of food allergy in children. An elimination diet involves 7 to 14 days on a restricted diet, eliminating the suspected allergen, or placing the infant on a hypoallergenic formula (casein hydrolysate formula). Challenge can best be done by feeding the suspected allergen in a "blinded" fashion in liquid or capsule form to the fasting infant or child. If isolated cow milk protein is not available, one needs to challenge with lactose-free cow milk formula to eliminate lactose intolerance as a cause of intestinal symptoms. The initial dose should be small, with increases every 30 to 60 minutes. Medical personnel should be available and prepared to treat allergic reactions. The infant or child should be observed for symptoms over a 48-hour period. A positive reaction suggests at least the presence of food intolerance, but implicating immunologic mechanisms may require support from tissue biopsy, skin tests, or specific IgE assays. The diagnosis of celiac disease requires an abnormal intestinal biopsy, placing the patient on an elimination diet, confirmation of healing by biopsy, and rechallenge by oral feeding of a gliadin-containing food.

2. Skin tests, if indicated, should be done by an allergist skilled in applying and interpreting them. A positive skin test, unfortunately, has a poor predictive accuracy; that is, the individual has IgE sensitization to the allergen but does not demonstrate symptoms on oral challenge. A negative skin test is strong evidence against an IgE-mediated reaction to the ingested food.

3. Serum tests for specific IgE antibodies (RAST or ELISA) give essentially the same result as skin tests. These tests cost more than skin tests but are useful when the physician is not experienced in applying skin tests or if a severe skin reaction is possible.

4. Intestinal biopsy is very useful in supporting the diagnosis of intestinal allergy in infants by demonstrating infiltration of either eosinophils in rectal mucosa for allergic colitis or eosinophils, particularly in the gastric antrum, for allergic enterocolitis. Intestinal biopsy is essential to diagnose celiac disease and demonstrates severe villous atrophy, crypt hyperplasia, and a heavy infiltrate of mononuclear inflammatory cells.

5. Tests for specific serum antibodies have a very high sensitivity and specificity (>90%) in the diagnosis of celiac disease. These tests examine for a combination of

IgG and IgA antigliadin, IgA antiendomysial, and IGA antireticulin antibodies. It is important to examine for total serum IgA deficiency if IgG antigliadin antibodies are present but all IgA antibody screens for celiac disease return negative. Celiac antibody screens should be obtained over the course of a gliadin-containing diet; the decrease or disappearance of these antibodies can provide a marker for compliance during a gliadin-free diet.

6. Screening tests are often utilized for evaluation of food allergy, failure to thrive, anemia, rectal bleeding, malabsorption, protein-losing enteropathy, and vomiting. These tests include *CBC with differential* to examine for anemia or eosinophilia seen in food allergy; *erythrocyte sedimentation rate* to screen for inflammatory bowel disease (IBD); *serum urea nitrogen, transaminases, electrolytes, and bicarbonate* to examine for metabolic disease, renal function, or hepatitis as a cause of FTT or vomiting; *serum albumin*, which may be decreased in food allergy, IBD, cystic fibrosis, and protein-losing enteropathy; *fecal α1-antitrypsin* is elevated in patients with protein-losing enteropathy or severe intestinal mucosal inflammation; *urinalysis* to screen for protein loss in the urine; *stool guaiac tests* to confirm the presence of blood; *stool smear for white blood cells* to confirm an inflammatory process; *tests for infectious causes of rectal bleeding or diarrhea, including stool culture* for bacterial pathogens; *Clostridium difficile* toxin assay; *Giardia* antigen; *sweat chloride test* to evaluate for cystic fibrosis.

Radiologic Studies

1. Upper GI or barium enema contrast x-rays are rarely helpful for evaluation of intestinal food allergy.
2. Upper GI contrast x-rays may be indicated to evaluate for an anatomic abnormality when recurrent vomiting is present.

Treatment

1. Allergen elimination is the primary goal of therapy. Infants can be fed a casein hydrolysate formula. Rare infants will have poor resolution of symptoms and may be given an amino acid–containing formula (such as Neocate). Of infants who are allergic to cow milk, 15 to 35 per cent will also react to soy formula. Six to 12 months later, patients can be challenged in a controlled clinical setting prepared to manage anaphylactic reactions. Solid foods can be introduced at 4 to 6 months, adding one new food at a time and avoiding foods with high allergic potential, such as egg, peanut, fish, strawberry, citrus, chocolate, and soy. For breast-feeding infants, eliminate known major allergens from the mother's diet, including cow milk, soy products, and eggs. It is important for the mother to maintain an adequate nutrient intake, which may require a consultation with a dietitian. Breast-feeding infants with severe allergic symptoms should be placed on a casein hydrolysate formula. The mother can eliminate potential major allergens from her diet and continue to manually express breast milk to maintain flow. The infant can then be challenged with breast milk in 1 week if asymptomatic on the hydrolysate formula and eventually challenged with a cow milk formula in 6 to 12 months.
2. Elimination diets in older children are much more difficult unless only one or two foods are suspected as pri-

mary triggers for the allergic disease. A hypoallergenic diet can be tried, eliminating foods with high allergic potential, such as cow milk, eggs, peanuts, soy, fish, shellfish, and wheat, but care must be taken to ensure an adequate nutritional intake. If a good response is obtained on the elimination diet, the patient can be reintroduced to single foods, as "blinded" challenges if possible, until the allergen is identified.

3. When the diagnosis of celiac disease is confirmed, the patient must be placed on a diet free of wheat, barley, and rye for life. Oats may also have to be restricted.
4. Pharmacologic therapy is of very limited value in intestinal food allergy. Therapy for acute allergic or anaphylactic reactions involves the use of epinephrine, corticosteroids, antihistamines, bronchodilators, and standard supportive emergency medical care. Chronic drug therapy for gastrointestinal food allergy has not proved beneficial in controlled trials. A trial of disodium cromoglycate and/ or prednisone may be required for severe eosinophilic gastroenteropathy.

Key Treatment

- Elemental diet (infants)
- Elimination diet (children)

Prevention

1. Strict avoidance of food allergens such as cow milk, egg, and peanut–containing products during the third trimester of pregnancy and during lactation reduces the onset of allergic disease before the child is 2 years of age, but there are no differences in the prevalence of allergic disease by the age of 7 years.
2. It is unclear from present studies whether "prophylactic" feeding of casein hydrolysate formulas influences the prevalence of intestinal or systemic allergic disease in later childhood. The use of hypoallergenic formulas may delay or prevent gastrointestinal-specific symptoms in infancy, but there appears to be no effect by midchildhood.
3. Because of the severity of peanut allergy in children at risk for food allergy, peanuts or peanut butter feeding should be significantly delayed, possibly until 3 years of age.

Prognosis

1. Studies of reactivity to cow milk protein formulas in infants have shown that most reactions disappear by 3 years of age.
2. Reactions to the most common "allergenic" foods disappear gradually (25%/year) with avoidance.
3. Children are likely to outgrow allergic reactions to egg, milk, and soy but not peanuts, fish, and shellfish. Celiac disease is a lifelong condition. With the elimination of wheat, rye, barley, and oats, children thrive and lead normal lives.

Bibliography

Bock SA, Sampson HA: Food allergy in infancy. Pediatr Clin North Am 1994;41:1047–1067.

Host A: Cow's milk protein allergy and intolerance in infancy. Pediatr Allergy Immunol 1994;5(Suppl 5):5–36.

Littlewood JM: Coeliac disease in childhood. Baillieres Clin Gastroenterol 1995;9:295–327.

Moon A, Kleinman RE: Allergic gastroenteropathy in children. Ann Allergy Asthma Immunol 1995;74:5–12.

Sampson HA: Food allergies. Curr Opin Gastroenterol 1995; 11:548–552.

158 Acute Appendicitis

Paul Harmatz

Definition

Acute appendicitis consists of acute inflammation of the vermiform appendix.

Etiology and Epidemiology

1. Appendicitis results from luminal obstruction of the appendix by
   a. Lymphoid hyperplasia associated with mumps, infectious mononucleosis, CMV, HIV, *Salmonella*, *Shigella*, *Yersinia*, or *Campylobacter*
   b. Intestinal parasites, such as *Ascaris lumbricoides* or *Enterobius vermicularis*
   c. Foreign bodies, including chips of bone, metal, and wood
   d. A fecalith, which is a hard, often calcified, stool mass
   e. Tumors such as adenocarcinomas, carcinoids, metastatic lesions, or Kaposi sarcoma
2. A low-fiber diet and low water intake may be associated with an increased incidence of appendicitis.
3. Appendicitis may rarely result from granulomatous disease isolated to the appendix.
4. Various microorganisms have been suggested as etiologic agents: *Bacteroides fragilis, Escherichia coli, Campylobacter fetus, Streptococcus pneumoniae, Pasteurella multocida, Yersinia enterocolitica, and Schistosoma japonicum.*
5. The incidence of appendicitis in the United States has been decreasing. The overall incidence is 11 cases/10,000 population/year, and the incidence from ages 10 to 19 years is 23 cases/10,000/year. The incidence is equal among all social classes. There is a slight male predominance, and a familial incidence has been documented. The incidence of appendicitis is very low in preschool children; however, the incidence of perforation is highest in this age group.

Pathophysiology

1. Obstruction of the appendiceal orifice or lumen with continuing mucus production leads to increased luminal pressure and distention.
2. Distention results in stimulation of visceral afferent nerves that enter the spinal cord at T8–T10. This results in referred pain in dermatomes represented in the periumbilical area.
3. Increasing wall tension leads to lymphatic obstruction with edema, followed by reduced venous blood flow and ischemia.
4. Microorganisms trapped in the appendix invade the wall as inflammation spreads to the serosal surface.
5. When inflamed tissue comes into contact with the parietal peritoneum, pain is perceived in the right lower quadrant. An unusual location of the appendix (in a retrocecal or pelvic location) changes this pattern of pain sensation.
6. Gangrene occurs at the tip of the appendix and in the area of the fecalith after thrombosis of the appendiceal artery.
7. Gangrene leads to perforation with local peritonitis and abscess formation or generalized peritonitis.

Clinical Findings

1. Symptoms
   a. Pain is the most important feature. It is usually ≤3 days in duration unless perforation occurs.
      (1) Periumbilical pain occurs early, before serosal inflammation develops.
      (2) Pain may be colicky, representing spasm in the distended organ.
      (3) Pain shifts to the right lower quadrant as the parietal peritoneum becomes inflamed.
      (4) Unusual sites of pain include the following: for a retrocecal appendix, the flank; for pelvic appendix, pain referred to labium majoris or scrotum, testes, or penis.
      (5) Rare patients, with congenital anomalies of the intestine, can present with pain in any location.
   b. Vomiting occurs in 90 per cent of cases. It is usually not marked and follows the onset of pain.
   c. Small-volume, mucoid stools are occasionally seen when the appendix is in a retroileal or pelvic position.
   d. Dysuria and urinary frequency occur, especially with retrocecal or pelvic appendicitis.
2. Signs
   a. Patients tend to lie still, with the right hip flexed and a lumbar lordosis.
   b. Signs of dehydration may be present if vomiting or decreased fluid intake is a prominent feature.
   c. A normal temperature or a low-grade fever is common in the absence of perforation. With perforation

or peritonitis, the patient may have a very high or even a subnormal temperature.

d. Localized tenderness and guarding—particularly at McBurney point (junction of middle and lateral thirds of a line joining the umbilicus and the right anterior superior iliac spine)—are common.

e. The psoas sign (right hip flexed secondary to inflamed appendix causing right psoas muscle spasm) can be exacerbated by active flexion or extension of the hip.

f. The obturator sign (pain on internal rotation of the flexed hip) is present if the inflamed appendix rests on the obturator internus muscle.

g. A rectal examination contributes little in "clear-cut" cases. It may be helpful in pelvic appendicitis or abscess or in the evaluation of possible pelvic inflammatory disease.

Key Clinical Findings

- Anorexia
- Periumbilical pain
- Vomiting
- Afebrile or low-grade fever
- Localized pain later

Laboratory Findings

1. The diagnosis of acute appendicitis is established on the basis of history and physical examination.
2. A CBC is of very limited value. The white blood count is often mildly elevated.
3. A urinalysis can help differentiate pyelonephritis or passage of a renal stone from appendicitis. A limited number of RBCs or WBCs can be seen in the urine with an inflamed appendix lying near the ureter or bladder.

Key Laboratory Findings

- Elevated WBC (usually)
- Urinalysis to diagnose urinary tract infection or stone

Radiologic Findings

1. A chest x-ray may be helpful to differentiate pneumonia as a possible cause of unexplained abdominal pain.
2. Abdominal x-rays are rarely indicated in "clear-cut" appendicitis. A fecalith may be seen in 10 per cent of cases and is a strong indicator for surgery in questionable cases.
3. Filling of the appendix by barium during a barium enema is strong evidence against appendicitis, although not 100 per cent specific. In contrast, absence of appendiceal filling by barium because of edema of the cecum or a space-occupying lesion indenting the cecum supports the diagnosis of appendicitis.
4. Abdominal ultrasound has been particularly helpful as a noninvasive technique for evaluating abdominal pain in children. If the appendix can be seen, this is evidence in favor of appendicitis. This is a good screen for gynecologic or renal disease as causes of abdominal pain.

Treatment

1. The treatment of acute appendicitis without perforation includes
   a. Active observation to established the diagnosis
   b. Preoperative rehydration with Ringer's lactate solution and preoperative antibiotics (ampicillin, gentamicin, and clindamycin). Early appendectomy should be performed as soon as the patient's clinical condition permits.
   c. Antibiotics should be continued for two doses for a normal appendix and for 3 days with gangrenous appendicitis.
2. The treatment of acute appendicitis with perforation includes
   a. Fluid resuscitation
   b. Preoperative antibiotics with aerobic and anaerobic coverage
   c. Removal of the appendix and adherent omentum
   d. Culture of peritoneal fluid
   e. Peritoneal lavage with or without antibiotics
   f. Avoidance of peritoneal or wound drains, except for localized abscess
   g. Primary skin closure is still controversial.
   h. Antibiotic coverage for at least 5 days.
3. Infectious complications in the setting of a
   a. Normal appendix or simple acute appendicitis: 0 per cent
   b. A gangrenous and perforated appendix: 1.7 per cent.

Key Treatment

- Surgery
- Antibiotics—short course

Prevention

1. "Prevention" is rarely considered in appendicitis, but increasing dietary fiber or water may have a preventive effect.
2. The removal of a normal appendix during unrelated surgery is not indicated.

Bibliography

Hatch EI Jr: The acute abdomen in children. Pediatr Clin North Am 1985;32:1151–1165.

Neilson IR, Laberge J-M, Nguyen LT, et al: Appendicitis in children: Current therapeutic recommendations. J Pediatr Surg 1990;25:1113–1116.

Shandling B: Appendicitis. In Walker AW (ed): Pediatric Gastrointestinal Disease. Philadelphia, BC Decker, 1991, pp 754–757.

Silen ML, Tracy TF Jr: The right lower quadrant "revisited." Pediatr Clin North Am 1993;40:1201–1211.

Williams N, Kapila L: Acute appendicitis in the preschool child. Arch Dis Child 1991;66:1270–1272.

159 Biliary Atresia

Jay A. Hochman and *John C. Bucuvalas*

Definition

Biliary atresia results from progressive obliteration or absence of portions of the biliary system between the liver hilum and the duodenum with complete bile flow obstruction.

Etiology

Two theories, which are not mutually exclusive, have attempted to explain the clinical picture.

1. *Congenital Malformation.* The theory of ductal plate malformation indicts altered embryogenesis as leading to defective bile duct formation. This leads to the characteristic changes of atretic bile ducts with subsequent liver injury.
2. *Infantile Obstructive Cholangiopathy.* This theory proposes that biliary atresia, idiopathic neonatal hepatitis, and choledochal cyst are all secondary to an initiating insult (viral, immune-mediated) that leads to inflammation at various levels of the hepatobiliary tract.

Epidemiology

1. Incidence: ~1/12,000 live births.
2. Accounts for 30 to 40 per cent of cases of cholestasis in newborns, excluding parenteral nutrition–associated cholestasis.
3. Occurs more often in females than males (1.4:1.0). Familial cases are not well described.

Pathophysiology

1. Liver injury results from progressive sclerosing of the extrahepatic bile ducts. Epithelial injury, inflammation, and fibrosis cause complete obstruction of the biliary tree.

TABLE 159–1. DIAGNOSTIC EVALUATION OF INFANTS WITH CHOLESTASIS*

Clinical assessment: History, physical examination, stool color
Standard biochemical tests: Fractionated bilirubin and liver function tests
Emergent issues: Prothrombin time, urine-reducing substances; consider sepsis work-up (urine, blood, spinal fluid cultures) and serum glucose
Abdominal ultrasound
Specific tests of liver disease *as indicated:*
    α1-antitrypsin phenotype
    Thyroid function tests
    Metabolic screen (urine/serum amino acids, urine organic acids, urine for mass spectrometry to exclude defect in bile acid metabolism)
    Sweat chloride determination
    Viral serologies and cultures (e.g., CMV, syphilis)
Hepatobiliary scintigraphy
Liver biopsy
Exploratory laparotomy with an intraoperative cholangiogram

*An *individualized* evaluation is essential.

2. Two subsets of biliary atresia have been proposed based on clinical observation and presumed differences in pathophysiology.
   a. Congenital form (~35% of cases)—Biliary structures are absent. There is jaundice at birth and an association with congenital anomalies (e.g., polysplenia, malrotation, congenital heart disease).
   b. Perinatal form (~65% of cases)—Patients have a sclerosed biliary tree and the absence of associated anomalies.

Clinical Findings

1. Most infants with biliary atresia initially appear healthy. In the more common perinatal form, jaundice develops between 2 and 6 weeks of life. The diagnosis is often delayed because of overlap with unconjugated hyperbilirubinemia (Table 159–1).
2. The presentation is usually nonspecific with hepatomegaly, jaundice, acholic stools, and variable elevation of standard liver biochemical tests. If acholic stools are present, biliary obstruction must be excluded rapidly.
3. In patients with a delayed diagnosis ($\geq$6 months), the clinical picture is progressive jaundice, failure to thrive, splenomegaly, coagulopathy, ascites, and severe pruritus.

Key Clinical Finding

- Jaundice
- Hepatomegaly
- Acholic stools

Laboratory Findings and Liver Histology

1. Laboratory Findings (see Table 159–1)
   a. Cholestasis defined by direct hyperbilirubinemia
   b. Variable elevations of aminotransferases, alkaline phosphatase, and gamma glutamyl transferase
   c. Prolonged prothrombin time may reflect vitamin K malabsorption due to cholestasis. Breast-fed infants are at increased risk owing to decreased amounts of vitamin K in breast milk relative to standard infant formulas.

Key Laboratory Findings

- Bilirubin, unconjugated and conjugated
- Liver enzymes: AST, ALT, GGT
- Prothrombin time
- Histology on biopsy

2. Histology—Bile duct proliferation, bile duct plugging, and portal fibrosis with preservation of basic hepatic lobular architecture are found.

Radiographic Changes

1. Abdominal ultrasound—An atretic gallbladder, frequently not visualized, is suggestive but not diagnostic of biliary atresia. An ultrasound study is helpful to exclude choledochal cysts.
2. Hepatobiliary scintigraphy—Uses an iminoacetic analog to assess for patency of the biliary tract. Intestinal excretion of analog is absent. This test is most discriminating after 5 days of phenobarbital loading (5 mg/kg/day).
3. When biliary atresia cannot be excluded by liver biopsy, an intraoperative cholangiogram is necessary.

Treatment and Prevention

1. There is no current effective means of preventing biliary atresia.
2. Kasai portoenterostomy—Achieves biliary drainage in >60 per cent of infants before 2 months of age but in <20 per cent of infants beyond 3 months of age.
3. Liver transplantation—After portoenterostomy, the 10-year survival without transplantation is ~30 per cent. With sequential portoenterostomy and liver transplantation in those with progressive disease, the 5-year survival is ~80 per cent.
4. Medical management—Focuses on the prevention of postoperative complications as well as the sequelae of cholestasis.
   a. Cholangitis is the most frequent postoperative complication. Repeated episodes lead to progressive fibrosis and diminished bile flow. Treatment includes broad-spectrum antibiotics to treat infection due to enteric pathogens, a short course of corticosteroids to reduce inflammation, choleretic agents to stimulate bile flow (e.g., ursodeoxycholic acid), and reoperation in selected cases that are refractory to medical management.
   b. *Nutritional support.* Treatment with a calorically dense formula containing medium-chain trigylcerides and fat-soluble vitamins is indicated. Aggressive nutritional support improves outcome before and after transplantation.
   c. Pruritus is a frequent complication of cholestasis. Controlled studies have not identified an effective therapy.
   d. Complications of cirrhosis (see Chapter 161).

Key Treatment

- Kasai procedure
- Liver transplant

Bibliography

Arias IM (ed): The Liver: Biology and Pathobiology. New York, Raven Press, 1994.

Otte JB, et al: Sequential treatment of biliary atresia with Kasai portoenterostomy and liver transplantation: a review. Hepatology 1994;20:41S–48S.

Schweitzer P: Treatment of extrahepatic biliary atresia. Results and long term prognosis after hepatic portoenterostomy. Pediatr Surg Int 1986;1:30–36.

Suchy FJ (ed.): Liver Disease in Children. St. Louis, Mosby–Year Book, 1994.

160 Viral Hepatitis

Nada Yazigi and *John C. Bucuvalas*

Etiology

Cytomegalovirus, Epstein-Barr virus, herpes simplex virus, adenovirus, and enteroviruses can cause hepatitis, usually as part of a more generalized illness, and will not be discussed further in this chapter. The hepatotropic viruses, A, B, C, D, and E will be discussed (Table 160–1).

Epidemiology

In the United States, most cases of reported acute hepatitis occur in children and young adults. The risk for parenteral transmission and chronic hepatitis varies with the pathogen (see Table 160–1).

1. *Hepatitis A virus (HAV)*
   a. Most cases occur in children, adolescents, and young adults. Clinical severity increases with age.
   b. The risk of fulminant hepatitis is 10- to 20-fold increased in a person ≥50 years compared with those younger than 30 years.
   c. HAV is prevalent in low socioeconomic groups and where substandard hygiene prevails.
2. *Hepatitis B virus (HBV)*
   a. HBV is excreted in all body fluids except stools.
   b. Household contacts, sexual partners of infected patients, healthcare workers, intravenous drug users, dialysis patients, and hemophiliacs are at higher risk to acquire HBV.
   c. Perinatal transmission occurs more frequently if the mother has evidence of ongoing viral replication (Hb$_e$Ag +, high titers of HBV DNA or active infec-

TABLE 160-1. CHARACTERISTICS OF HEPATOTROPIC VIRUSES

	HAV	HBV	HCV	HDV	HEV	HGV
Nucleic acid type	RNA	DNA	RNA	RNA	RNA	RNA
Fecal-oral transmission	+++	−	−	−	+++	?
Parenteral transmission	+	+++	+++	+++	+	++
Risk of perinatal transmission	−	+++	+	?		?
Acute hepatitis	+++	+++	+	+++	+++	+
Risk for chronic hepatitis	−	++	+++	+++	−	++
Risk for fulminant liver failure	+	++	+/−	++	++	?
Mean incubation time (days)	28d	60d	60d	35d	42d	?
Risk for cirrhosis	−	++	+++	+++	−	++
Risk for hepatocellular carcinoma	−	++	++	++	−	?

tion in the third trimester). Chronic HBV infection occurs in 80 to 90 per cent of infected infants.

3. *Hepatitis C virus (HCV)*
   a. Infection is often anicteric and unrecognized. Household contacts of index cases, hemophiliacs, and dialysis patients are at higher risk for acquiring HCV.
   b. Progression to chronic hepatitis occurs in at least 70 per cent of patients with HCV.
   c. Protective immunity is not conferred by the presence of antibodies to HCV.
   d. Perinatal infection and sexual transmission occur, but the risk of transmission is less than for HBV.
4. *Hepatitis D (HDV)* is a defective virus that requires helper function of HBV to cause infection.
5. *Hepatitis E (HEV)* causes sporadic and epidemic hepatitis in developing countries.

Pathophysiology

Cellular injury from viral infections may be due to direct cytopathic effect, interference with cellular function, or damage from the host response. The hepatotropic viruses are usually not cytopathic. Cellular injury results from the interaction of virus-infected cells with the host immune response. When a brisk host immune response occurs, there is cellular damage and viral clearance. With evasion of immune response due to frequent mutations of the viral genome (HCV) or integration of the viral genome into the host genome (HBV), chronic infection results.

Clinical Findings

The onset of transaminase elevation is usually preceded by nonspecific influenza-like symptoms: headaches, fever, anorexia, vomiting, and right upper quadrant abdominal pain. Dark-colored urine and light clay-colored stool occur

in icteric hepatitis and may be seen in patients with anicteric hepatitis. Most pediatric cases are anicteric. Hepatosplenomegaly is usually present.

Key Clinical Findings

* Anorexia
* Headache and muscle aches
* Dark urine
* Jaundice

Laboratory and Radiographic Findings

1. Elevation of serum transaminases 5- to 100-fold with or without increased serum total and direct bilirubin.
2. A CBC and prothrombin time should be done to exclude bone marrow suppression and coagulopathy.
3. Serologic evaluation for hepatitis A, B, and C should be done as outlined in Table 160-2. Serology for HDV and HEV should be not be performed unless there is increased risk.
4. An abdominal ultrasound examination is indicated only to exclude biliary tract disease.

Key Laboratory Findings

* Marked by
  Elevated levels of AST and ALT
  Specific antigen/antibody titer

Treatment

1. *Acute hepatitis.* Treatment is primarily supportive. Follow-up evaluation should be performed to identify fulmi-

TABLE 160-2. SEROLOGIC FINDINGS OF HEPATITIS A, B, AND C

	Anti-HAV IgM	Anti-HAV IgG	HB$_s$Ag	Anti-Hbs	Anti-HB$_c$IgG	Anti-HCV
Acute HAV	+	−	−	−	−	−
Acute HBV	−	−	+	−	−	−
Chronic HBV	−	−	+	−	+	−
Resolved HAV	−	+	−	−	−	−
Resolved HBV	−	−	−	+	+/−	−
HCV	−	−	−	−	−	+

nant hepatic failure or development of chronic hepatitis and to demonstrate viral clearance. A patient with encephalopathy or coagulopathy that does not correct with administration of 5 mg vitamin K intramuscularly should be transferred to a center in which liver transplantation is performed.

2. *Chronic hepatitis.* In selected patients with chronic hepatitis due to HBV or HCV, treatment with α-interferon is effective, but relapse is frequent.

Key Treatment

- Supportive
- Vitamin K
- Alpha-interferon (chronic)

Prevention

1. General measures including hand washing, an ensured safe water and food supply, and sewage control will decrease spread of HAV. Universal precautions, screening of blood supply, and safe sexual practices will prevent spread of hepatotropic viruses, particularly HBV and HCV (Table 160–3).

2. Administration of pooled immunoglobulin prevents HAV infection before and after exposure. Administration of high-titer anti-HBs immunoglobulin prevents or attenuates HBV infection after exposure.

TABLE 160–3. PREVENTION AND TREATMENT OF VIRAL HEPATITIS

	HAV	HBV	HCV	HDV	HEV
Pooled IgG[1]	+	–	+/–	–	+/–
HBIG[2]	–	+	–	–	–
Vaccine available[3]	+	+	–	–	–
Universal precautions	+	+	+	+	+
α-Interferon	–	+	+ +	+	–
Follow-up evaluation	+	+	+	+	+

[1]0.02 ml/kg IM within 2 weeks of exposure to household members, those who have intimate contact with an index case, children and staff in daycare centers if a positive case is identified, and travelers to endemic areas.

[2]0.5 ml IM within 7 days of exposure or 12 hours with perinatal exposure if there is perinatal, accidental (needlestick), sexual, or household exposure.

[3]Universal HBV vaccination for infants is recommended by the Advisory Committee on Immunization Practices and the AAP Committee of Infectious Diseases.

3. Effective vaccines are available to prevent HAV and HBV. Administration of HBV vaccine is recommended for all children, but the HAV vaccine is currently recommended only for high-risk groups.

Bibliography

Schiff L, Schiff ER (eds): Diseases of the Liver. Philadelphia, JB Lippincott, 1993.

Suchy FJ (ed): Liver Disease in Children. St. Louis, Mosby–Year Book, 1994.

Zakim D, Boyer TD (eds): Hepatology. Philadelphia, WB Saunders, 1982.

161 End-Stage Liver Disease and Cirrhosis

L. Glen Lewis and *John C. Bucuvalas*

Definition

A chronic, diffuse process characterized by collagen deposition, fibrosis, and regenerative nodule formation.

Etiology

Cirrhosis represents the end stage of myriad hepatic insults (Table 161–1).

Epidemiology

Cirrhosis is uncommon in the pediatric population, and precise epidemiologic data are not available.

Pathophysiology

The response of the liver to ongoing cell injury is a cascade of cell death (necrosis), followed by scarring (fibrosis), and cellular regeneration (nodule formation).

1. Hepatocellular injury can result from a single insult or a combination of any number of insults, including viral infection, immune-mediated cytotoxicity, altered intermediary metabolism leading to accumulation of hepatotoxins, exposure to hepatotoxic drugs or environmental toxins, altered blood flow causing ischemia or outflow obstruction, and biliary obstruction.

2. Fibrogenesis is initiated by activated inflammatory cells or cytokines in the region of hepatocellular injury. As collagen deposition continues, dense connective tissue bands form that may further impair lobular blood flow, causing ischemia, and the cycle of injury and fibrosis continues.

3. Nodule formation ensues. To compensate for the reduction in the number of viable hepatocytes, regenerative nodules form as cells replicate within a restrictive connective tissue framework and cause further distortion of vascular structures.

Clinical Findings

1. *Compensated cirrhosis*: Cirrhosis may exist for a prolonged period with minimal clinical symptoms. Rou-

TABLE 161–1. DISEASES RESULTING IN CIRRHOSIS

METABOLIC DISORDERS

Alpha-1-antitrypsin deficiency
Cystic fibrosis
Fructosemia
Galactosemia
Gaucher disease
Glycogen storage disease, types III and IV
Hemochromatosis
Histiocytosis X
Native American childhood cirrhosis
Niemann-Pick disease
Tyrosinemia
Wilson disease
Wolman disease

INFECTIOUS DISEASES

Ascending cholangitis
Viral hepatitides
Cytomegalovirus
Chronic hepatitis B +/− delta
Chronic hepatitis C
Herpes simplex virus
Congenital rubella

INFLAMMATORY DISEASES

Autoimmune hepatitis
Primary sclerosing cholangitis

BILIARY MALFORMATIONS

Biliary atresia
Caroli disease
Choledochal cyst
Congenital hepatic fibrosis
Syndromic (Alagille) and nonsyndromic bile duct paucity

VASCULAR DISEASES

Budd-Chiari syndrome
Congestive heart failure
Veno-occlusive liver disease
Venocaval web

TOXIC DISORDERS

Toxins found in nature (mushrooms)
Organic solvents
Hepatotoxic drugs (methotrexate)

NUTRITIONAL DISORDERS

Hypervitaminosis A
Total parenteral alimentation
Malnutrition

IDIOPATHIC DISORDERS

Zellweger syndrome
Familial intrahepatic cholestasis (Byler syndrome)
Neonatal hepatitis

tine physical examination may reveal a firm liver and an enlarged spleen. Viral hepatitis, Wilson disease, autoimmune hepatitis, and anatomic abnormalities of the biliary tree should be immediately excluded, since specific therapy exists.

2. *Decompensated cirrhosis:* With ongoing fibrosis and progressive deterioration of hepatic function, the protean manifestations of end-stage liver disease and portal hypertension ensue.

   a. Portal hypertension

     (1) Portal hypertension causes formation of esophageal and gastric varices, which may rupture and bleed.

     (2) Hypersplenism due to portal hypertension causes anemia and thrombocytopenia.

     (3) Ascites results from increased portal venous pressure, decreased plasma oncotic pressure, and abnormal salt and water retention. Patients with ascites are at increased risk to develop spontaneous bacterial peritonitis.

   b. Failure to thrive and malnutrition result from inadequate caloric intake, malabsorption of fat and fat-soluble vitamins, and altered utilization of substrate.

Key Clinical Findings

- Anemia
- Thrombocytopenia
- Ascites
- Upper GI hemorrhage

   c. Coagulopathy may be due to vitamin K deficiency or decreased hepatic synthesis of clotting factors, including prothrombin and factors VII and IX.

   d. Hepatorenal syndrome (HRS) with progressive renal failure is seen in decompensated cirrhosis and is characterized by azotemia, decreased urine output, and decreased urine Na.

   e. Neurologic manifestations range from subtle cognitive and personality changes to hepatic encephalopathy and coma.

Laboratory Findings and Liver Histology

Evaluation of a patient with cirrhosis should be directed toward elucidating the underlying etiology by assessment of clinical, biochemical, and liver histologic findings.

1. Determination of serum α1-antitrypsin phenotype, sweat chloride, serology for hepatitis B and hepatitis C, serum ceruloplasmin concentration, and ANA should be performed.
2. *Biochemical findings.* Serum transaminases may be mildly or moderately elevated. Increased serum bilirubin, low serum albumin, and prolonged PT reflect poor hepatic function.
3. *Histology.* A liver biopsy can establish the presence of histologic criteria of cirrhosis and may yield information regarding the underlying etiology.

Key Laboratory Findings

- Serology for hepatitis B and C
- Liver tests
- Histology of liver biopsy
- Hepatic synthetic function: Albumin (PT/PT)

Radiographic Findings

1. An abdominal ultrasound study can elucidate the presence of ascites, gallstones, or cystic malformations.
2. MRI provides information regarding the degree of liver damage and presence of portal hypertension.

Treatment

1. Specific therapy should be instituted when applicable (e.g., penicillamine for Wilson disease).
2. Control of ascites can usually be achieved by sodium and water restriction plus diuretic therapy with a potassium-sparing diuretic and a loop diuretic. Refractory ascites warrants therapeutic paracentesis. When treating refractory ascites, care should be taken to avoid depletion of blood volume, which can cause hepatic ischemia and precipitate the hepatorenal syndrome.
3. Hepatic encephalopathy can be controlled by avoiding precipitating factors (dehydration, electrolyte disturbances, GI bleeding, infection); protein restriction (1 g/kg/day); and administration of neomycin ± lactulose. Serum ammonia levels and serial physical assessments are used to assess patient response.
4. Adequate calories and glucose should be administered to avoid hypoglycemia, since protein stores may be inadequate to provide precursors for gluconeogenesis.

5. Parenteral administration of vitamin K should correct prothrombin time within 12 hours if clotting dysfunction reflects vitamin deficiency rather than synthetic compromise.
6. Acute GI bleeding should be evaluated endoscopically. Bleeding esophageal varices can be managed by administration of octreotide and by sclerotherapy or band ligation.
7. Spontaneous bacterial peritonitis (SBP) must be considered in the febrile patient with cirrhosis. Cultures of blood and peritoneal fluid (10 ml peritoneal fluid directly inoculated into blood culture bottles at the bedside) should be obtained. Antibiotic coverage for *S. pneumon-*

Key Treatment

- Specific therapy if indicated (e.g., penicillamine)
- Careful monitoring
- Protein restriction
- Vitamin K
- Liver transplant

iae and gram-negative enteric pathogens should be started if SBP is suspected.
8. Orthotopic liver transplantation is often required for long-term survival in patients with end-stage liver disease.

Prevention

Removal of offending agents and initiation of specific therapy prior to irreversible hepatic fibrosis can prevent late complications. Siblings of patients with Wilson disease should be screened and identified before age 7 years to institute copper chelating therapy. Universal vaccination for hepatitis B will prevent cirrhosis from HBV.

Bibliography

Hardy SC, Kleinman RE: Cirrhosis and chronic liver failure: *In* Suchy FJ (ed): Liver Disease in Children. St. Louis, Mosby–Year Book, 1994, pp 214–248.
Hepatic cirrhosis. *In* Sherlock S, Dooley J (eds): Diseases of the Liver and Biliary System, 9th ed. Oxford, Blackwell Scientific, 1993, pp 357–369.
Thaler MM: Cirrhosis. *In* Walker WA, Durie PR, Hamilton JR, et al (eds): Pediatric Gastrointestinal Disease, vol 2. Philadelphia, BC Decker, 1991, pp 1096–1108.

162 Liver Failure

Simon Rabinowitz

Critical State

Definition

Liver failure is the reversible or irreversible cessation of many, and inevitably all, of the liver's vital functions. Failure occurring a few months or less after presentation is called acute or fulminant. Otherwise, liver failure occurs as a consequence of end-stage liver disease or cirrhosis. This chronic process is characterized by hepatic necrosis, regeneration, and fibrosis.

Etiology

1. Many acute or chronic insults can lead to liver failure. Acute factors that can cause severe, progressive hepatitis include infections, drugs and toxins, ischemia, and autoimmune processes.
2. The most common microbes that can lead to acute hepatitis and liver failure are viruses, including hepatitis A, B, C, D, E, and G and perhaps other non-A, non-B hepatotropic viruses. In newborns and immunocompromised children, Epstein-Barr virus, cytomegalovirus, adenovirus, herpes simplex, echovirus, and varicella can have a similar outcome. Although liver failure from hepatitis B is not uncommon in adults, hepatitis B rarely leads to

liver failure in young children who do not live in endemic areas.
3. There are a variety of medications as well as poisons that can severely damage the liver in some children. Drugs used in pediatrics that are potentially hepatotoxic include phenytoin, sulfonamides, propylthiouracil, valproic acid, oral contraceptives, NSAIDs, isoniazid, prolonged parenteral nutrition, and aspirin when it is used in a child at risk for Reye syndrome. Toxic substances that affect almost all children include carbon tetrachloride, *Amanita* mushrooms, organophosphates, and excessive amounts of acetaminophen.
4. Severe hepatic ischemia, as occurs in prolonged shock, can cause interruption of hepatic processes.
5. A form of autoimmune hepatitis, in which antibodies to smooth muscle are absent but liver-kidney microsomal antibodies are present, can be very virulent, with a rapid, irreversible course.
6. In children the most common cause of liver failure is complete obstruction of the extrahepatic bile duct system—biliary atresia. This is the result of a prenatal or perinatal insult that presents shortly after birth and can

Critical State *Continued*

sometimes be associated with other congenital anomalies. Other conditions that compromise bile excretion include Alagille syndrome, certain forms of nonsyndromic bile duct paucity, and sclerosing cholangitis. These can also progress to cirrhosis.

7. Metabolic conditions leading to cirrhosis that presents in childhood include tyrosinemia, cystic fibrosis, α1-antitrypsin deficiency, galactosemia, certain forms of glycogen storage disease, Wilson disease, and defects in mitochondrial, peroxisomal, and lysosomal function. Wilson disease can rarely present as a fulminant hepatitis, often accompanied by hemolytic anemia.

Pathogenesis

1. In many instances the mechanisms by which hepatic insults interfere with hepatic regeneration and lead to liver failure are unknown.
2. The hepatic microsomal P450 system is responsible for metabolizing many foreign substances, including pharmaceuticals, that are ingested. At times a toxic metabolite can be formed within the hepatocyte and overwhelms the liver's ability to excrete it. This type of toxicity usually involves the centrizonal regions of the organ, which contain the majority of the P450 enzymes.
3. Some infectious agents can directly cause apoptosis— individual cell death—throughout the hepatic lobule. Others alter hepatocytes and trigger an inflammatory response that causes most of the damage. Hepatitis B is an example of the latter.
4. Metabolic conditions and substantial disruption of bile flow often lead to an inappropriate accumulation of cytotoxins within hepatocytes that can interfere with cell function and result in widespread damage and necrosis.
5. Hepatic encephalopathy represents the neurologic sequela of liver failure. Accumulation of ammonia in the central nervous system plays a role in this process. Other contributors are aromatic amino acids, glycine, and gamma aminobutyric acid, which all function as false neurotransmitters; sulfhydryls; fatty acids; and certain medications. All these substances are usually removed from the circulation by the healthy liver. The more advanced the encephalopathy becomes, the higher the associated mortality rate.

Clinical Findings

1. The healthy liver performs several categories of functions that include synthesis of proteins (such as albumin, α1-antitrypsin, coagulation proteins, urea cycle enzymes, gluconeogenic enzymes); regulating intermediary metabolism (fatty acid synthesis and degradation, glycogen storage and breakdown); removal of potentially harmful compounds (drug and toxin metabolism, conversion of ammonia to urea); and secretion of bile and hydrophobic compounds.
2. Liver failure can present with an interruption of any of these activities, but in almost all instances there is univer-

sal compromise. As the process continues the morbidity becomes more marked and ultimately results in coma and possibly death. A liver that appears to be getting smaller on serial physical examinations suggests a poor prognosis.

3. The most common initial presentation is jaundice, accompanied by mental status changes. The typical progression is lethargy to excitability to stupor to coma. Hypoglycemia, which can also contribute to neurologic dysfunction, is reversible.
4. The cirrhotic child will often have failure to thrive, a protuberant abdomen, ascites, tortuous abdominal wall vasculature, hepatosplenomegaly, and clubbing.
5. Gastrointestinal bleeding, frequently related to coagulopathy or platelet dysfunction, is often the triggering event that leads the cirrhotic child into liver failure. Besides stress-related peptic ulcer and gastritis, esophageal varices may be the source of the bleeding.
6. Asterixis, a rhythmic tremor of the hands and wrists (best detected by placing a sheet of paper on the child's hands), and fetor hepaticus, a peculiar pungent odor, are two clinical clues suggesting hepatic encephalopathy. Asterixis may be hard to detect in young children.
7. Metabolic conditions as well as drug and toxin ingestions that affect organs besides the liver will present with multiorgan damage.
8. Reye syndrome presents in most children after a viral illness, often chickenpox or influenza, and aspirin ingestion. There will usually be a history of severe emesis followed by a rapid deterioration in mental status without noticeable jaundice.
9. Liver failure will occur 2 to 3 days after acetaminophen ingestion in children who do not receive *N*-acetylcysteine therapy.

Key Clinical Findings

- Jaundice
- Ascites
- Asterixis

Laboratory Assessment

1. The following biochemical values should be obtained in the child who is suspected of being in liver failure: serum ammonia, electrolytes (Na, K, Cl, Ca, P), glucose, SUN, creatinine, transaminases, total and direct bilirubin, CBC with differential, PT, PTT, and fibrinogen. In addition, a type and cross match should be sent. A chest x-ray, an electrocardiogram, and, if possible, an electroencephalogram are also very useful.
2. For the child without cirrhosis, blood and urine specimens to identify infections and drugs are also part of the initial evaluation. Marked prolongation of PT, very high biliru-

Critical State *Continued*

bin levels, and persistent hypoglycemia are poor prognostic indicators.

3. If there is a history of a drug or toxin ingestion, a serum and/or urine level of the suspected compound should be obtained. When there is no history of ingestion or hepatotoxic prescription drug use, appropriate serologic investigations to detect the infectious agents listed earlier should be obtained.

4. For the previously stable cirrhotic child who comes in with liver failure, gastrointestinal bleeding, increased intake of protein, or sepsis should be considered.

Key Laboratory Findings

- Liver tests
- Serum glucose
- Electrolytes

Treatment

1. The child in liver failure is critically ill and needs to be closely monitored in the intensive care unit by a number of subspecialists, including an intensivist, a gastroenterologist, and a neurosurgeon. Serial determinations of electrolytes, glucose, ammonia, hematocrit, liver size, and neurologic status are essential. Maintaining near-normal values of these measures is challenging but will minimize morbidity and give the liver a chance to begin functioning again.

2. The usual causes of mortality include bleeding, shock, respiratory failure, brain herniation related to cerebral edema, sepsis, and fluid and electrolyte disturbances compounded by renal failure. The comprehensive management plan must anticipate all these complications so that intervention can be initiated at the earliest possible stages.

3. A high concentration (10%) dextrose solution infused to meet basal fluid needs plus urine output can usually maintain a normal serum glucose. Renal function is often compromised in liver failure. This can be the result of prerenal azotemia, nephritis, or the hepatorenal syndrome. Therefore, fluid and electrolytes are often difficult to manage. Serial determinations can guide the salt composition of the intravenous fluids. Hyponatremia, hypernatremia, and hypocalcemia are frequently encountered and are all associated with increased morbidity.

4. Excessive ammonia can be reduced in the blood through the use of enteral lactulose or neomycin. Lactulose is a nondigestible disaccharide that is fermented by the colonic flora into small organic acids. The acidification traps the ammonia intraluminally and prevents absorption. Neomycin is an antibiotic that diminishes gut flora, thereby minimizing bacterial generation of ammonia. Both lead to diarrhea, which also contributes to ammonia

clearance. However, diarrhea can complicate fluid and electrolyte management.

5. Prophylaxis for gastrointestinal bleeding includes intravenous H_2 blockers to neutralize gastric acidity and minimize mucosal damage. Parenteral vitamin K should be the first step to correct a coagulopathy in the child who is not bleeding. If there is substantial bleeding, fresh frozen plasma along with packed red blood cells and sometimes platelets should be transfused. Care should be used to prevent fluid overload. Diuretics, which can precipitate hepatic encephalopathy, should be used judiciously.

6. For the child with progressive neurologic deterioration, management should include elective intubation followed by hyperventilation to achieve a P_{CO_2} of 25 mmHg. If this is not adequate, after correction of the coagulopathy an intracranial pressure monitor is placed. Increases in intracranial pressure can then be treated with infusions of mannitol or even induction of coma.

7. Benzodiazepines and sedatives are used sparingly, if at all. Drugs that are not metabolized by the liver should be used preferentially.

8. The goal of medical therapy is to provide support for the critically ill child while waiting for his or her own liver to recover. If at any time, even at presentation, it appears that this may not be possible, arrangements to transfer the child to a center that has expertise in pediatric liver transplantation should be initiated.

Key Treatment

- Close monitoring
- 10% Glucose infusion
- Lactulose
- Vitamin K
- Clotting factors

Bibliography

Hardy SC, Kleinman RE: Cirrhosis and chronic liver failure. *In* Suchy FJ (ed): Liver Disease in Children. St. Louis, Mosby–Year Book, 1994, pp 214–241.

Sherlock S: Acute (fulminant) hepatic failure. *In* Diseases of the Liver and Biliary System, 8th ed. Boston, Blackwell Scientific, 1989, pp 116–128.

Sherlock S: Chronic hepatitis. *In* Diseases of the Liver and Biliary System, 8th ed. Boston, Blackwell Scientific, 1989, pp 339–371.

Treem WR, Walker WA, Durie PR, et al: Hepatic failure. *In* Pediatric Gastrointestinal Disease: Pathophysiology, Diagnosis, and Management, vol 1. Philadelphia, BC Decker, 1991, pp 146–182.

Whitington PF: Fulminant hepatic failure in children. *In* Suchy FJ (ed): Liver Disease in Children. St. Louis, Mosby–Year Book, 1994, pp 180–205.

163 Toxic Megacolon

Simon Rabinowitz and *Rima Jibaly*

Critical State

Definition

Toxic megacolon is a medical and surgical emergency resulting from a severe episode of colitis that evolves into dilatation of the colon and three of the following: fever >38.6°C, tachycardia >120/min, leukocytosis >10,5000 cells/mm³, and anemia.

Etiology

1. In older children, toxic megalcolon is most commonly found in those with inflammatory bowel disease (IBD). The prevalence in ulcerative colitis is higher than in Crohn disease.
2. In younger children, Hirschsprung disease can present with a similar clinical picture, frequently referred to as enterocolitis. Enterocolitis and toxic megacolon may occur before or after surgical correction of Hirschsprung disease.
3. Severe infectious colitis or pseudomembranous colitis, caused by organisms such as cytomegalovirus, *Shigella*, and *Salmonella*, may progress to toxic megacolon.

Pathogenesis

1. Common pathway: Colonic stasis and compromise of mucosal integrity lead to overwhelming invasion of the systemic circulation by bacteria and bacterial products, with release of endogenous inflammatory mediators.
2. IBD
   a. Toxic megacolon occurs in the setting of severe mucosal or transmucosal inflammation.
   b. Ulcerations in the mucosa provide a point of entry into the systemic circulation for microbes and toxins. These agents lead to the release of cytokines, resulting in fever and leukocytosis and other signs of bacteremia and sepsis.
   c. Involvement of the myenteric or Auerbach plexus results in the loss of propulsive contractions of the colon.
   d. Other factors that can initiate the process include
      (1) Barium enema or insufflation of air during colonoscopy
      (2) Narcotic antidiarrheal or anticholinergic agents
      (3) Electrolyte imbalance, such as hypokalemia, hypocalcemia, or hypomagnesemia.
3. Hirschsprung disease
   a. Hirschsprung disease is thought to be caused by the failure of neural crest cells to migrate to the distal end of the gastrointestinal tract. The innervated colon then dilates as feces are ineffectively moved through the aganglionic segment.

b. The mucosal barrier may be markedly compromised by the dilatation, leading to enterocolitis.
c. These complications of Hirschsprung disease are more commonly associated with long-segment aganglionosis, Down syndrome, and delayed diagnosis.
d. *Clostridium difficile, Escherichia coli,* and rotavirus infections have been described as etiologic factors in a few cases.
e. Postoperatively, enterocolitis may occur if a stenosis develops at the anastomotic site. However, enterocolitis has also been described in patients who have normally functioning colostomies. In these situations it is presumed that some residual colonic dysmotility remains, leading to stasis in the ganglionic bowel.

Clinical Findings

1. The child with toxic megacolon appears septic with fever, tachycardia, and abdominal distention.
2. Physical examination of the abdomen reveals tympany and tenderness to palpation. These symptoms are most evident over the transverse colon with the patient in the supine position.
3. Typically, there are frequent bloody bowel movements with cramping abdominal pain relieved by the passage of stool.
4. As the process advances, hypotension and dehydration occur, and bowel movements decrease in frequency.
5. Shock and changes in mental status signal an advanced stage and failure of medical management. Patients should undergo laparotomy before reaching this stage.

Key Clinical Findings

- Toxic/septic appearance
- Bloody stools
- Dehydration, hypovolemic shock

Laboratory Assessment

1. Blood studies
   a. The child with toxic megacolon will have laboratory findings similar to those of other children with colitis. Initially, there will be a leukocytosis with a left shift. If the disease progresses, anemia will develop that may require transfusion.
   b. Electrolyte imbalances resulting from massive diar-

rhea include hypokalemia, hyponatremia, and hypomagnesemia. In addition, hypoproteinemia can occur.

c. The sedimentation rate is virtually always elevated. Improvement in the patient's clinical condition correlates with a decrease in the sedimentation rate.

2. Radiographic studies

a. IBD

(1) Plain abdominal x-rays show colonic dilatation that is usually most significant in the transverse colon, the most anterior part of the bowel. The colon loses its normal haustral pattern because of edema. There may be areas of intact mucosa adjacent to denuded or ulcerated mucosa that appear as nodules.

(2) Barium enema is contraindicated in this setting.

b. Hirschsprung disease

(1) Massive small and large bowel obstruction proximal to the aganglionic region is seen.

(2) If the predisposing condition (i.e., primary diagnosis) is uncertain and the patient is stable, a barium enema on the unprepared bowel may show a transition zone between the proximal dilated ganglionic colon and the distal aganglionic segment.

3. Pathology

a. Overview: Colonic biopsy is contraindicated in the presence of toxic megacolon. However, after resolution, a mucosal biopsy is part of the evaluation of the child with no known predisposing condition.

b. IBD

(1) Severe mucosal inflammation is seen with polymorphonuclear leukocyte infiltration, crypt abscesses, edema, and necrosis.

(2) The presence of noncaseating granulomas strongly supports a diagnosis of Crohn disease.

c. Hirschsprung disease

(1) Histology confirms the absence of ganglion cells in the submucosal and myenteric plexuses of the rectum and distal colon.

(2) Acetylcholine esterase activity is increased in the nerve fibers found in the muscularis mucosa and lamina propria of the aganglionic bowel compared with the innervated bowel.

Key Laboratory Findings

- Electrolyte disturbances

- Complete blood count and erythrocyte sedimentation rate

Treatment

1. The child must be hospitalized, often in an intensive care unit, and a surgical consultation should be obtained immediately. Failure of the patient to respond quickly to medical therapy usually leads to the need for a partial or full colectomy.

2. Vigorous IV hydration with electrolyte replacement, to prevent dehydration and shock, and broad-spectrum antibiotics, including anaerobic coverage, should be initiated.

3. Placement of a long intestinal tube for decompression and changing the patient's position in bed to redistribute gas and flatus can be helpful.

4. In distal Hirschsprung disease, frequent gentle rectal irrigations with warm saline solution can help with disimpaction of stool.

5. Close monitoring of vital signs and serial physical examinations are required.

6. Daily follow-up of the CBC, sedimentation rate, electrolytes including calcium and magnesium, and serum albumin along with plain radiographs of the abdomen is crucial to avoid complications and to evaluate the success of medical therapy. If the clinical situation is not improving, more frequent monitoring is required.

7. Packed red blood cells should be transfused if the hematocrit is falling.

8. Parenteral nutrition is indicated for the nutritionally debilitated patient.

9. Surgical intervention should be considered after a short course of medical therapy has failed, to prevent mortality. Children with evidence of perforation, or massive hemorrhage requiring transfusion of more than 6 to 8 units within 48 hours, should have immediate exploratory laparotomy and bowel resection.

Key Treatment

- IV hydration and electrolyte correction

- Decompression by intestinal tube

- Transfusion if indicated

- Surgery if no response to medical intervention

Bibliography

Carneiro PMR, Brereton RJ, Drake DP, et al: Enterocolitis in Hirschsprung's disease. Pediatr Surg Int 1992;7:356–360.

Jackson W, Grand R: Ulcerative colitis. *In* Walker WA, Durie PR, Hamilton JR, et al (eds): Pediatric Gastrointestinal Disease, vol 1. Philadelphia, BC Decker, 1991, pp 608–617.

Present D: Toxic megacolon. Gastrointest Emerg 1993;77:1129–1148.

Rescorla F, Morrison A, Englers D, et al: Hirschsprung's disease: Evaluation of mortality and long term function in 260 cases. Arch Surg 1992;127:934–940.

Rudolph C, Banroch L: Hirschsprung's disease. Pediatr Rev 1995;16:5–16.

164 Gastrointestinal Endoscopy

Simon Rabinowitz

Indications

1. Upper endoscopy
   a. The indications for upper intestinal tract endoscopy include the investigation and treatment of inflammation and/or upper gastrointestinal bleeding, diagnosis of the etiology of malabsorption, removal of foreign bodies, and placement of feeding tubes. Occasionally, endoscopy is required in the evaluation of emesis. The etiology of abdominal pain can often be determined by a careful history and physical examination. If the diagnosis is unclear and the pain persists, endoscopy may be warranted.
   b. Therapeutic endoscopic procedures should be restricted to centers with experienced endoscopists and support staff. Such procedures include esophageal dilatation for stenoses and achalasia, injection sclerotherapy, treatment of bleeding peptic ulcers (those with a prominent visible vessel), endoscopic retrograde cholangiopancreatography (ERCP), and placement of percutaneous gastrostomy and jejunostomy feeding tubes.

2. Colonoscopy
   a. The indications for colonoscopy include the investigation and treatment of lower gastrointestinal tract inflammation and/or bleeding, evaluation of persistent noninfectious diarrhea, and the diagnosis and treatment of colonic polyps. Irritable bowel syndrome (IBS) is commonly seen in children, and colonoscopy is not required for diagnosis or therapy.
   b. It is often difficult to decide whether a barium enema or a colonoscopy will be more useful in investigating a symptom or condition. In general, if there is a good possibility that a barium enema can provide the diagnosis and there is no need for therapeutic interventions, a barium enema should be obtained first, since it is safer and less expensive than colonoscopy.
   c. Proctoscopy can be useful to determine if there is an active proctitis. A normal rectum makes inflammatory colitis much less likely, although Crohn disease and certain bacterial infections can present with more proximal involvement only.

Contraindications

1. Endoscopy should be avoided, or performed with extreme care, if there is impending perforation or obstruction of the gastrointestinal tract.
2. The potential benefits of endoscopy in the sick child should be weighed against the possibility of perforation and infection. In many instances, children who require endoscopy may benefit from a period of stabilization and therapy prior to the procedure.
3. A child who has recently eaten is at risk for aspiration, and the procedure should be postponed until the stomach has emptied.
4. A child with a bleeding diathesis and coagulopathy should have the deficiency corrected prior to endoscopy. In children with AIDS, a bleeding time should be performed prior to endoscopy.
5. Endoscopy should never be attempted by an operator who is unfamiliar with sedating children or performing these procedures in children. In addition, there should be appropriate support personnel and monitoring devices available to assist during the procedure and handle any possible complications. If a child cannot be safely sedated or a procedure cannot be safely performed with intravenous sedation, general anesthesia is warranted.

Preparation

1. Upper endoscopy
   a. There should be nothing taken by mouth prior to the procedure for 4 to 6 hours for an infant and 8 hours for an older child.
   b. Children at risk for bacterial endocarditis or those who are immunosuppressed require antimicrobial prophylaxis. The administration of blood products may be necessary prior to endoscopy to correct hypovolemia or severe anemia.
   c. A chest x-ray should be taken immediately before an endoscopy is performed to remove a foreign body from the esophagus. Inert objects that pass spontaneously into the stomach almost always pass through the remainder of the gastrointestinal tract (and do not need to be removed).
   d. An oral sedative or anxiolytic medication may be helpful if given one hour prior to the examination.
   e. An intravenous line should be placed just before the procedure is performed. In addition, a device(s) to monitor heart rate, respiration rate, oxygen saturation, and blood pressure is positioned on the patient, and sedative medications are administered.
   f. There should be personnel experienced in pediatric cardiopulmonary resuscitation and a well-equipped crash cart in the room during the procedure.

2. Colonoscopy
   a. Children should be told that adequate colonic preparation permits the procedure to be completed more

Procedure *Continued*

quickly and avoids the possible need to repeat the examination.

b. For the cooperative child or the patient with a nasogastric tube, administration of an oral polyethylene glycol solution is the preferred method of bowel preparation. Alternatives include combinations of one or more of the following: phosphosoda, magnesium-containing cathartics, enemas and suppositories, and prolonged periods of clear fluid intake. Infants can be given oral rehydration solutions for half a day.

c. A colonoscopy requires intravenous sedation; proctoscopy or sigmoidoscopy may not.

d. The indications for antimicrobial prophylaxis and/ or blood product infusions are the same as those for upper endoscopy.

Equipment

1. A well-equipped endoscopy unit will have several upper and lower endoscopes of different sizes and equipment to clean and sterilize them. Ancillary endoscopy equipment includes cameras to photograph significant findings, forceps for grasping foreign objects and for biopsy of the mucosa, snares and probes to achieve hemostasis, needles for injection of sclerosants, snares to retrieve polyps and foreign bodies, and dilators to expand stenotic or strictured segments.

2. Monitoring device(s) should also be available to follow vital signs before and after the procedure. Medications to produce sedation, drugs to reverse opioids and benzodiazepines, and a cart with all the equipment and agents necessary for pediatric cardiopulmonary resuscitation, including oxygen, should be readily available. There should be easy access to surgeons who can deal with complications such as perforation, excessive bleeding, and pneumothorax.

Anesthesia/Analgesia

1. Many gastroenterologists employ conscious sedation to perform endoscopy in children. The most commonly used agents are intravenous meperidine or another opioid and midazolam or diazepam.

2. Anesthesiologists usually employ deeper sedation that is achieved with a variety of agents, including propofol, ketamine, fentanyl, inhaled anesthetic agents, and occasionally general anesthesia with endotracheal intubation.

Technique

1. Upper endoscopy

   a. The patient is placed in the left lateral position with the endoscopist facing the patient and all equipment appropriately arranged (Fig. *A*). The study is initiated by passing the lubricated endoscope into the posterior pharynx, which has been locally anesthetized. The endoscope is then gently moved down the esophagus and through the gastroesophageal junction into the stomach (Fig. *B*, p. 530).

   b. The stomach is then examined, and the endoscope is passed through the pylorus into the duodenal bulb. A standard examination ends with visualization of the ampulla of Vater; however, at times the distal duodenum is examined for causes of malabsorption. The jejunum can be examined by using an enteroscope or pediatric colonoscope.

   c. Biopsies are performed as the endoscope is being withdrawn. Once back in the stomach, the instrument is retroflexed so that the cardia and the entire fundic region of the stomach can be examined.

   d. Therapeutic manipulations are performed after the entire upper tract has been examined.

2. Colonoscopy

   a. The study is performed with the patient in the left lateral position. The endoscopist sits or stands behind the patient. The colonoscope, which is lubricated, is placed into the rectum and is advanced under direct visualization. Retroverting the scope is the best way to visualize the rectum (Fig. *C*, p. 530).

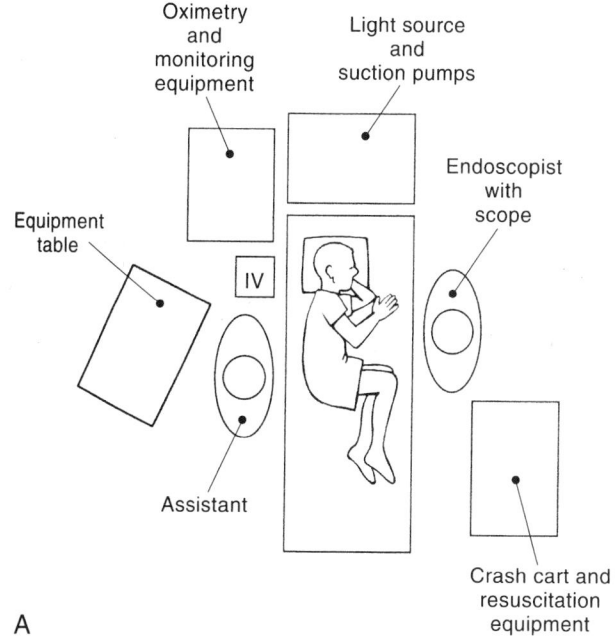

A

From Rakel RE: Saunders Manual of Medical Practice. Philadelphia, WB Saunders, 1996.

   b. During the course of the examination, the endoscopist must frequently partially withdraw the colono-

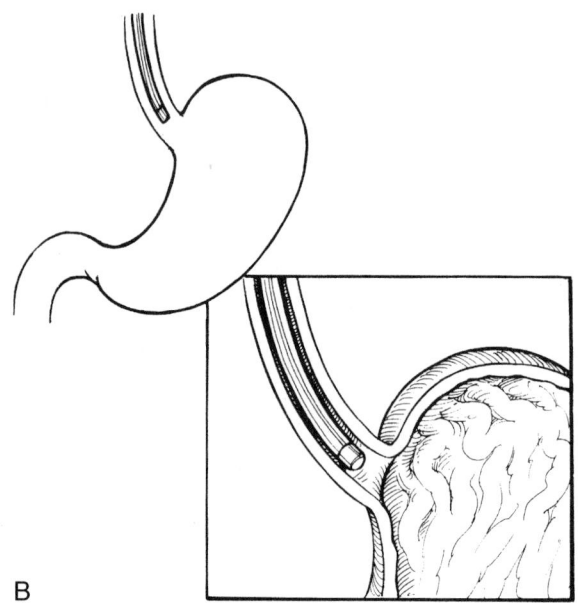

B

From Rakel RE: Saunders Manual of Medical Practice. Philadelphia, WB Saunders, 1996.

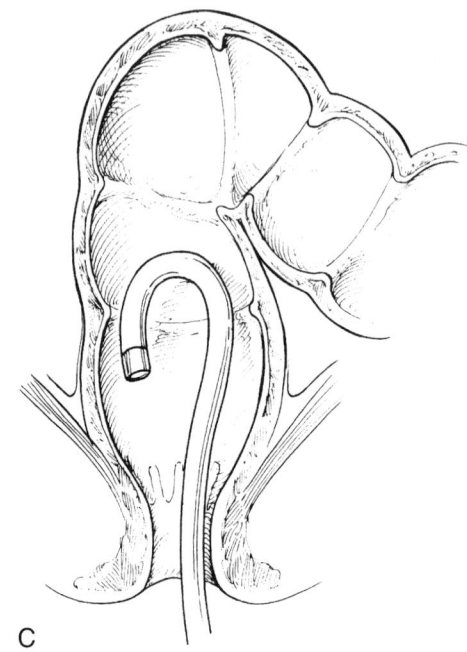

C

From Rakel RE: Saunders Manual of Medical Practice. Philadelphia, WB Saunders, 1996.

scope, apply gentle suction, and advance again while moving forward to the cecum.

c. The cecum is identified by anatomic landmarks such as the appendiceal orifice, the confluence of the teniae, and the ileocecal valve. Transillumination in the right lower quadrant and palpation of the tip of the instrument in that location are additional aids. At this point, intubation of the ileocecal valve to visualize and biopsy the terminal ileum can be performed.

d. Polypectomy, cauterization, and biopsies are performed during withdrawal of the colonoscope. However, if there is any doubt about relocating a lesion to be treated, therapy can be performed when the lesion is first encountered.

TABLE 164–1. COMPLICATIONS OF THERAPEUTIC ENDOSCOPY

PROCEDURE	COMPLICATION	EVALUATION AND THERAPY
Esophageal sclerotherapy	Bleeding	Repeat injections; possible placement of a Sengstaken-Blakemore tube
	Fever-bacteremia; mediastinitis	Blood cultures; upper GI contrast x-rays; surgical intervention if necessary
	Dysphagia	Upper GI contrast x-rays or repeat endoscopy; oral sucralfate
Esophageal dilatation	Fever	As above
	Dyspnea	CXR; repeat endoscopy; treatment of pneumothorax
Percutaneous gastrostomy tube	Bilious emesis	KUB; barium enema to examine for colon perforation
	Abdominal pain	KUB; CT scan to evaluate for perforation or liver injury
ERCP	Fever-bacteremia; cholangitis; pancreatitis	Blood culture; liver function tests; amylase, CT scan
Polypectomy (colon)	Hematochezia	Repeat colonoscopy to cauterize bleeding site
	Fever-sepsis; postpolypectomy syndrome; perforation	Blood cultures; KUB; antibiotics; observation; surgical intervention if necessary
	Bilious emesis	As for gastrostomy tubes

Follow-up

1. The child should have vital signs and oxygen saturation monitored until completely awake and responsive. Intravenous fluids should be continued until the patient can tolerate oral intake. Vigorous physical activities and operating potentially hazardous machines (including cars) by adolescents should be discouraged until the following day.
2. A mild sore throat is usually present for a day after upper endoscopy.
3. If antibiotic prophylaxis is indicated, the child will require an additional dose(s) after going home.
4. If there is any fever, the child should be evaluated for sepsis. If there is persistent hematemesis, melena, hematochezia, or signs of orthostatic changes, the child should be evaluated for gastrointestinal bleeding.
5. Therapeutic endoscopy is associated with more frequent and more serious complications. Common ones are listed in Table 164–1.

Bibliography

Ament ME, Vargas J: Fiberoptic upper intestinal endoscopy. *In* Walker WA, Durie PR, Hamilton JR, et al (eds): Pediatric Gastrointestinal Disease, vol II. Philadelphia, BC Decker, 1991, pp 1247–1257.

Bines JE, Winter HS: Lower endoscopy. *In* Walker WA, Durie PR, Hamilton JR, et al (eds): Pediatric Gastrointestinal Disease, vol II. Philadelphia, BC Decker, 1991, pp 1257–1272.

Caulfield M, Wyllie R, Sivak MV Jr, et al: Upper gastrointestinal tract endoscopy in the pediatric patient. J Pediatr 1989;115:339–345.

Gauderer MW, Ponsky JL, Izant RJ Jr: Gastrostomy without laparotomy: A percutaneous endoscopic technique. J Pediatr Surg 1980;15:872–875.

Lashner BA, Kane SV, Hanauer SB: Colon cancer surveillance in chronic ulcerative colitis: historical cohort study. Am J Gastroenterol 1990;85:1083–1087.

165 Symptoms of Cardiovascular Disorders

Ronald M. Lauer

Epidemiology

Congenital heart disease is the most common of all birth defects. It affects 5 to 8 infants per 1000 live births. Ventricular septal defect (VSD) is the most common lesion, followed by pulmonic stenosis, atrial septal defect (secundum), tetralogy of Fallot, complete transposition of the great vessels, coarctation of the aorta, and hypoplastic left heart syndrome. While other forms of heart disease occur in the pediatric age group, they are much less common in the United States.

Etiology

For the most part, the causes of congenital heart disease are unknown. However, subjects with Down, Marfan, Turner, Noonan-Ehmke, Williams, Holt-Oram, and trisomy 18 syndromes are often affected with heart malformations. Infants of diabetic mothers and mothers infected with the rubella virus also have cardiovascular malformations. Other forms of heart disease seen in pediatric patients include infectious pericarditis and myocarditis, rheumatic heart disease, Kawasaki syndrome, collagen vascular disease, endocrine disorders, and neoplastic diseases.

Manifestations of Heart Disease

When cardiac defects cause little hemodynamic change, there may be no symptoms.

1. Infants

The major features of congenital heart disease in the newborn are

    a. Cyanosis

    b. Respiratory symptoms

    c. Extreme tachycardia or bradycardia.

When the foregoing are present, they may indicate life-threatening situations that require urgent attention.

2. Children and adolescents

In older children, cyanosis, clubbing of the digits, and squatting to rest are indicative of right-to left-cardiac shunts; fatigue with exercise, tachycardia, dyspnea, orthopnea, nocturia, and pedal edema are signs of heart failure; and light-headedness, dizziness, syncope, and chest pain may indicate obstructive left heart disease or cardiac arrhythmias.

    a. Cyanosis

Cyanosis is a blue discoloration of the skin and mucous membranes caused by desaturated blood in the capillaries.

    (1) Central cyanosis is caused by either an intracardiac or an intrapulmonary right-to-left shunt. It becomes evident when there is 3 to 5 g of reduced hemoglobin in the arterial blood, and it depends upon the level of hemoglobin concentration. This type of cyanosis is always noted in lips and mucous membranes.

    (2) Peripheral cyanosis (acrocyanosis) is caused by a constriction of the arterioles in the skin allowing the blue color of the venous vessels to be readily seen. It does not affect the mucous membranes. This is often seen in the extremities of normal newborns, when children become cool, and in fair children. When the differentiation of central and peripheral cyanosis is required, oximetry can be used to assess oxygen saturation (normal = 93 to 95%).

    b. Tachypnea

In the newborn, tachypnea is rapid, shallow respirations that are persistent with rates exceeding 60 breaths per minute while asleep or resting. This sign may result from either cardiac or pulmonary disease. The normal respiratory rates for older infants, children, and adolescents are shown in Table 165–1.

    c. Dyspnea

    (1) In infants with heart failure or cyanotic heart disease, difficult breathing may be recognized by

        (a) Grunting respirations

        (b) Flaring of the alae nasae

        (c) Intercostal, supracostal, and infracostal retraction.

    (2) In older children and adolescents, dyspnea is subjective. It may be caused by

        (a) Metabolic acidosis

        (b) Structural lung and airway disease, e.g., cystic fibrosis

        (c) Congestive heart failure resulting in pulmonary edema

        (d) Hypoxia, e.g., right-to-left shunting as in tetralogy of Fallot

        (e) Severe anemia

        (f) Hyperventilation, e.g., hysteria, pain.

    d. Tachycardia

The normal heart rates for infants and children are shown in Table 165–2.

    (1) Resting tachycardia

        (a) Infants: 150 beats/minute

        (b) Children: >120 beats/minute

    (2) Causes of tachycardia

TABLE 165–1. NORMAL RESPIRATORY RATES

AGE	BREATHS/MINUTE
Birth to 6 weeks	35–60
6 to 12 weeks	40
2 to 6 years	30
6 to 10 years	25
>10 years	20

(a) Fever

(b) Anemia

(c) Anxiety

(d) Congestive heart failure

(e) Hypoxemia (cardiac, pulmonary)

(f) Paroxysmal supraventricular tachycardia (rates >200 beats/minute)

(g) Hyperthyroidism.

e. Bradycardia

(1) Resting bradycardia

(a) <3 years: 100 beats/minute

(b) 3–9 years: 60 beats/minute

(c) >9 years: <50 beats/minute

(2) Causes of bradycardia

(a) Sinus bradycardia (congenital, athletic training)

(b) Increased vagal tone (vasovagal faint)

(c) Atrioventricular (AV) block (infants of mother with lupus erythematosus)

(d) Sick sinus node syndrome

(e) Hypothyroidism

f. Fatigue

In infants, fatigue is recognized by tiring with feeding. A baby can normally take the required formula or breast feeding in 15 to 20 minutes without tiring. In older children and adolescents, fatigue is recognized by low endurance for daily activities and by the need for rest during play or usual activities.

g. Syncope

This may result from the following cardiac mechanisms:

(1) Cardiac standstill from vagal inhibition, e.g., orthostatic hypotension, psychogenic causes, pain

(2) Ventricular asystole, e.g., sudden onset of complete heart block (Stokes-Adams attack)

(3) Left heart obstructive disease, e.g., aortic valve and idiopathic hypertrophic subaortic stenosis (IHSS)

(4) Paroxysmal rhythm changes with rapid ventricular rates, e.g., atrial fibrillation, ventricular fibrillation

(5) Pericardial tamponade resulting in low cardiac output, e.g., pericarditis, hemopericardium

h. Chest pain

In children chest pain is usually not the result of cardiac disease. The major causes of chest pain are

(1) Noncardiac in origin

(a) Musculoskeletal discomfort, e.g., trauma, muscle strain, costochondritis

TABLE 165–2. NORMAL HEART RATES FOR INFANTS AND CHILDREN

AGE	RANGE (MEAN)
<1 day	93–154 (123)
1–2 days	91–159 (123)
3–6 days	91–166 (129)
1–3 weeks	107–182 (148)
1–2 months	121–179 (149)
3–5 months	106–186 (141)
6–11 months	109–169 (134)
1–2 years	89–151 (119)
3–4 years	73–137 (108)
5–7 years	65–133 (100)
8–11 years	62–130 (91)
12–15 years	60–119 (85)

(b) Pulmonary, e.g., pleuritic pain (pneumothorax, pleurisy), asthma, diaphragmatic irritation (subphrenic or hepatic abscess)

(c) Gastrointestinal discomfort, e.g., disorders of disorders of stomach, pancreas, and biliary tree

(d) Psychogenic causes, e.g., death in family, family member with angina (e.g., concern of parents, adolescent patients, or physicians)

(2) Cardiac in origin

(a) Pericardial disease, e.g., pericarditis, lymphomas, leukemia

(b) Left heart obstructive disease: aortic, subaortic, or supravalvular aortic stenoses

(c) Coronary artery disease, e.g., anomalies of coronary arteries, accelerated atherosclerosis (homozygous type II hyperlipidemia, homocystinemia), Kawasaki syndrome

(d) Syndromes resulting in aortic dissection, hypertrophic cardiomyopathies, or tumors, e.g., Marfan syndrome, familial idiopathic hypertrophic cardiomyopathy (IHSS), tuberous sclerosis (rhabdomyoma of heart)

(e) Tachyarrhythmias, e.g., paroxysmal supraventricular or ventricular tachycardias.

Bibliography

Davignon A, Rautaharju P, Boiselle E: Normal ECG standards for heart rate of infants and children. Pediatr Cardiol 1980; 1:123.

Ferencz C, Rubin JD, Loffredo CA, Magee CA: Epidemiology of congenital heart disease. The Baltimore-Washington Infant Study 1981–1989. *In* Perspectives in Pediatric Cardiology, vol 4. Mount Kisco, NY, Futura Publishing, 1993.

Illif A, Lee VA: Pulse rate, respiratory rate, and body temperature in children between two and eighteen years of age. Child Dev 1952;23:237.

166 Tetralogy of Fallot

David J. Driscoll

Definition

Tetralogy of Fallot consists of a subaortic ventricular septal defect (usually nonrestrictive), right ventricular outflow tract obstruction, an overriding aorta, and right ventricular hypertrophy (Fig. 166–1). Right ventricular tract obstruction produces relative obstruction to pulmonary blood flow. It can consist of infundibular stenosis (obstruction by right ventricular muscle bundles underneath the pulmonary valve), pulmonary valve or annular stenosis, and/or supravalvar pulmonary stenosis. Associated anomalies include multiple ventricular septal defects (approximately 4 per cent of cases) and anomalous origin of the left anterior descending coronary artery from the right sinus of Valsalva (approximately 4 per cent of cases). Some consider pulmonary artery atresia with ventricular septal defect to be a severe form of tetralogy of Fallot.

Etiology

The etiology is unknown. It has been hypothesized that tetralogy of Fallot results from abnormal septation of the conotruncus. Recently some cases (particularly with velocardiofacial syndrome) have been associated with a microdeletion of chromosome 22. Studies in animals suggest that tetralogy of Fallot may result from abnormal migration of ectodermal tissue.

Epidemiology

Tetralogy of Fallot constitutes 6 to 10 per cent of significant congenital heart defects.

Pathophysiology

1. The presence of right ventricular outflow tract obstruction and a nonrestrictive ventricular septal defect results in a relative decrease of pulmonary blood flow and a right-to-left intracardiac shunt through the ventricular septal defect. Hence most patients with tetralogy of Fallot manifest cyanosis, digital clubbing (Fig. 166–2), and polycythemia.

   Patients with lesser degrees of right ventricular outflow tract obstruction have lesser degrees of a right-to-left intracardiac shunt and may not manifest these signs (so-called pink tetralogy of Fallot). In general, with time the severity of right ventricular outflow tract obstruction increases, and the classic signs of cyanosis, digital clubbing, and polycythemia appear.

2. Patients can experience an abrupt decrease of pulmonary blood flow leading to acute hypoxemia, acidosis, seizures, and death. These so-called Tet spells, or hypercyanotic spells, represent a medical emergency and require prompt treatment.

Clinical Findings

1. Presentation

   a. Most patients manifest cyanosis in the newborn period.

   b. Infants who do not manifest cyanosis in the newborn period usually are identified by the presence of a cardiac murmur.

   c. Very rarely a patient may attract medical attention as a result of a Tet spell or hypercyanotic spell.

2. Physical findings for classic tetralogy of Fallot

   a. Cyanosis

   b. Digital clubbing

   c. Increased right ventricular impulse at the lower left sternal border

   d. Loud single second heart sound

   e. Crescendo/decrescendo holosystolic murmur best heard along the left sternal border radiating to the left upper sternal border and to the back

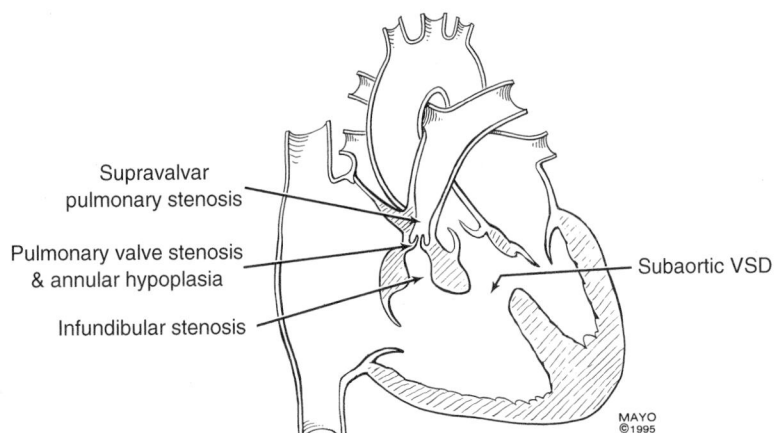

Supravalvar pulmonary stenosis

Pulmonary valve stenosis & annular hypoplasia

Infundibular stenosis

Subaortic VSD

MAYO ©1995

Figure 166–1. Diagrammatic representation of tetralogy of Fallot.

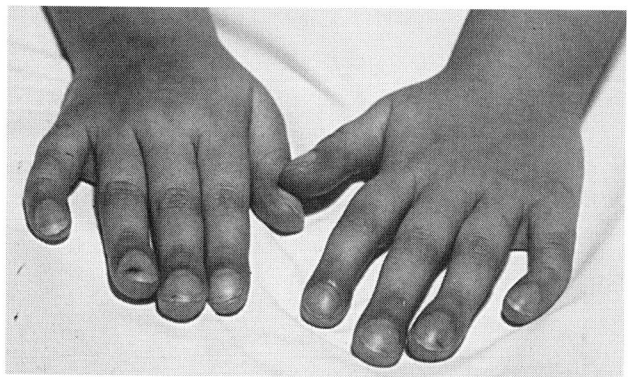

Figure 166–2. Marked digital clubbing in a young child.

3. Additional physical findings during a Tet spell or hypercyanotic spell
   a. Extreme cyanosis
   b. Hyperpnea
   c. Agitation
   d. Relative decrease in intensity of the systolic murmur

Key Clinical Findings

- Cyanosis
- Clubbing
- Holosystolic murmur

Laboratory Findings

1. Hematologic
   Usually there is polycythemia. Polycythemia may not be present if there is associated iron deficiency. The degree of polycythemia is inversely proportional to the volume of pulmonary blood flow.

2. Electrocardiography
   The electrocardiogram exhibits evidence of right ventricular hypertrophy. If, in addition to right ventricular hypertrophy, there is left axis deviation, one must suspect an associated endocardial cushion defect.

3. Echocardiography/Doppler
   The diagnosis can be confirmed by using echocardiography and Doppler. The right ventricular outflow tract obstruction and ventricular septal defect can be visualized. The pressure gradient across the right ventricular outflow tract obstruction can be estimated and the size of the main and proximal left and right pulmonary arteries ascertained. Using proper techniques, important abnormalities of the coronary arteries can be defined.

4. Cardiac catheterization and angiography
   Cardiac catheterization and angiography may be necessary for planning palliative or corrective surgical procedures. Since the advent of high-resolution echocardiographic and Doppler studies, the major use of cardiac catheterization and angiography is to define the size and distribution of the pulmonary arteries and the presence or absence of stenoses of the pulmonary arteries; coronary

artery abnormalities; and the presence of systemic to pulmonary artery collateral vessels.

Key Laboratory Findings

- Polycythemia
- ECG

Radiographic Changes

The heart size usually is normal. There may be a small or absent "main pulmonary artery segment" and an uptilted apex (because of right ventricular hypertrophy). The pulmonary vascular markings usually are decreased or normal.

Treatment

1. Management of infants with insufficient pulmonary blood flow
   Infants with severe right ventricular outflow tract obstruction may be dependent upon patency of the ductus arteriosus to provide sufficient pulmonary blood flow for adequate tissue oxygenation. Ductal closure in such an infant will result in significant hypoxemia and acidosis. Emergency treatment with prostaglandin E_1 is critical to maintain patency of the ductus arteriosus in these patients until a surgical procedure can be performed.

2. Systemic to pulmonary artery shunts
   Infants with unacceptable levels of hypoxemia will require creation of a systemic to pulmonary artery shunt to provide sufficient pulmonary blood flow. Although a variety of systemic to pulmonary artery connections have been described, most clinicians and surgeons prefer a tube graft connecting the subclavian to the pulmonary artery (so-called modified Blalock-Taussig shunt).

3. Definitive repair
   Definitive repair of tetralogy of Fallot consists of closure of the ventricular septal defect and relief of the right ventricular outflow tract obstruction. The technique to relieve right ventricular outflow tract obstruction is dictated by the type of obstruction. The techniques range from simple pulmonary valvotomy/valvectomy to subpulmonary infundibular resection and patch augmentation of a hypoplastic pulmonary annulus and, perhaps, areas of pulmonary artery hypoplasia and stenosis. The best age for the child to undergo definitive repair depends upon the individual anatomic features, particularly the size and distribution of the pulmonary artery tree.

4. Right ventricular outflow reconstruction with a conduit
   Infundibular resection may not be possible without damage to the left anterior descending coronary artery in patients who have anomalous origin of that vessel from the right sinus of Valsalva. For these patients it may be necessary to insert a valve containing conduit or homograft between the right ventricle and pulmonary artery to establish an unobstructed connection.

5. Pulmonary valve replacement
   Most patients who have had repair of tetralogy of Fallot have pulmonary insufficiency postoperatively. This is tolerated well by many patients for many years. However, some patients will develop progressive right ventric-

ular dilatation, failure, and tricuspid valve regurgitation. For these patients, placement of a competent valve in the pulmonary position may be necessary.

Key Treatment

- Prostaglandin E₁
- Surgery

Prevention

Currently there is no way to prevent the occurrence of tetralogy of Fallot. With improved understanding of the genetic basis of congenital heart defects, prevention may be possible in the future. Epidemiologic studies suggest that periconceptional maternal ingestion of folate may reduce the occurrence of conotruncal abnormalities such as tetralogy of Fallot.

Bibliography

Blackstone E, et al: Preoperative prediction from cineangiograms of postrepair right ventricular pressure in tetralogy of Fallot. J Thorac Cardiovasc Surg 1979; 79:542.

Garson A, Williams R, Reckless J: Long-term follow-up of patients with tetralogy of Fallot: Physical health and psychopathology. J Pediatr 1974; 85:429.

Kirklin J, et al: Surgical results and protocols in the spectrum of tetralogy of Fallot. Ann Surg 1983; 198:251.

Morgan B, Guntheroth W, Bloom R, Fyler D: A clinical profile of paroxysmal hyperpnea in cyanotic congenital heart disease. Circulation 1965; 31:66.

Stewart S, Alexon C, Manning J: Long-term palliation with the classic Blalock-Taussing shunt. J Thoracic Cardiovasc Surg 1988; 96:117.

167 Transposition of the Great Arteries

Stephen P. Sanders

Definition

Transposition of the great arteries (TGA) means literally that the great arteries are on the opposite side of the septum from normal. That is, the pulmonary artery arises from the left ventricle and the aorta from the right ventricle.

There are two basic types of transposition.

1. Common or complete transposition, in which the atria and ventricles are in solitus or usual position and only the great arteries are abnormally located and/or aligned, accounts for ≥90 per cent of transpositions.
2. Physiologically corrected transposition, in which the atria are normally situated but both the ventricles and the great arteries are abnormally positioned and/or connected, is rare (<10 per cent of transpositions).

This chapter will deal only with the first type, common or complete transposition of the great arteries.

Etiology

1. As is the case with most congenital heart defects, the etiology of transposition of the great arteries is unknown. Most cases are sporadic, with familial recurrences being extremely rare. No chromosomal abnormalities or syndromes are regularly associated with transposition.
2. Transposition of the great arteries appears to be due to abnormal development of the conus, the connecting segment between the ventricles and great arteries.
   a. During normal embryogenesis, conal muscle develops beneath the pulmonary artery, lifting it anteriorly and leftward and aligning it with the right ventricle. Involution of subaortic conus allows the aorta to remain posterior, aligned with the left ventricle and in fibrous continuity with the mitral valve.
   b. In common transposition of the great arteries, the converse occurs. The conal muscle beneath the aorta develops, lifting it anteriorly and rightward and aligning the aorta with the right ventricle while the pulmonary artery remains posterior and leftward, aligned with the left ventricle and in fibrous continuity with the mitral valve.

Epidemiology

Common transposition of the great arteries is the second most common congenital cardiac defect in the neonate, accounting for 5 to 7 per cent of all congenital heart defects. The occurrence rate is 0.22 to 0.44/1000 live births.

Pathophysiology

In common transposition of the great arteries, systemic venous blood is ejected into the aorta while pulmonary venous blood is ejected into the pulmonary artery. The two separate and parallel circulations would quickly lead to death from profound hypoxia and hypercarbia if there were no opportunity for mixing between them. Fortunately, most neonates with transposition of the great arteries also have a patent foramen ovale and persistent patency of the ductus arteriosus. These structures allow blood to pass back and forth between the pulmonary and systemic circulations, permitting gas exchange between the tissues and alveolar air.

1. Transposition with intact ventricular septum (65 per cent of common TGA)

The foramen ovale and ductus arteriosus are the only possible sites of mixing between the two circulations (Fig.

167–1A). As the pulmonary vascular resistance falls after birth, a shunt develops from aorta to pulmonary artery through the ductus arteriosus. The increased return to the left atrium raises the pressure above that in the right atrium and drives pulmonary venous blood across the septum into the systemic circulation. As the ductus closes, pulmonary blood flow decreases, reducing left atrial venous return. This, in turn, decreases mixing. After closure of the ductus, flow

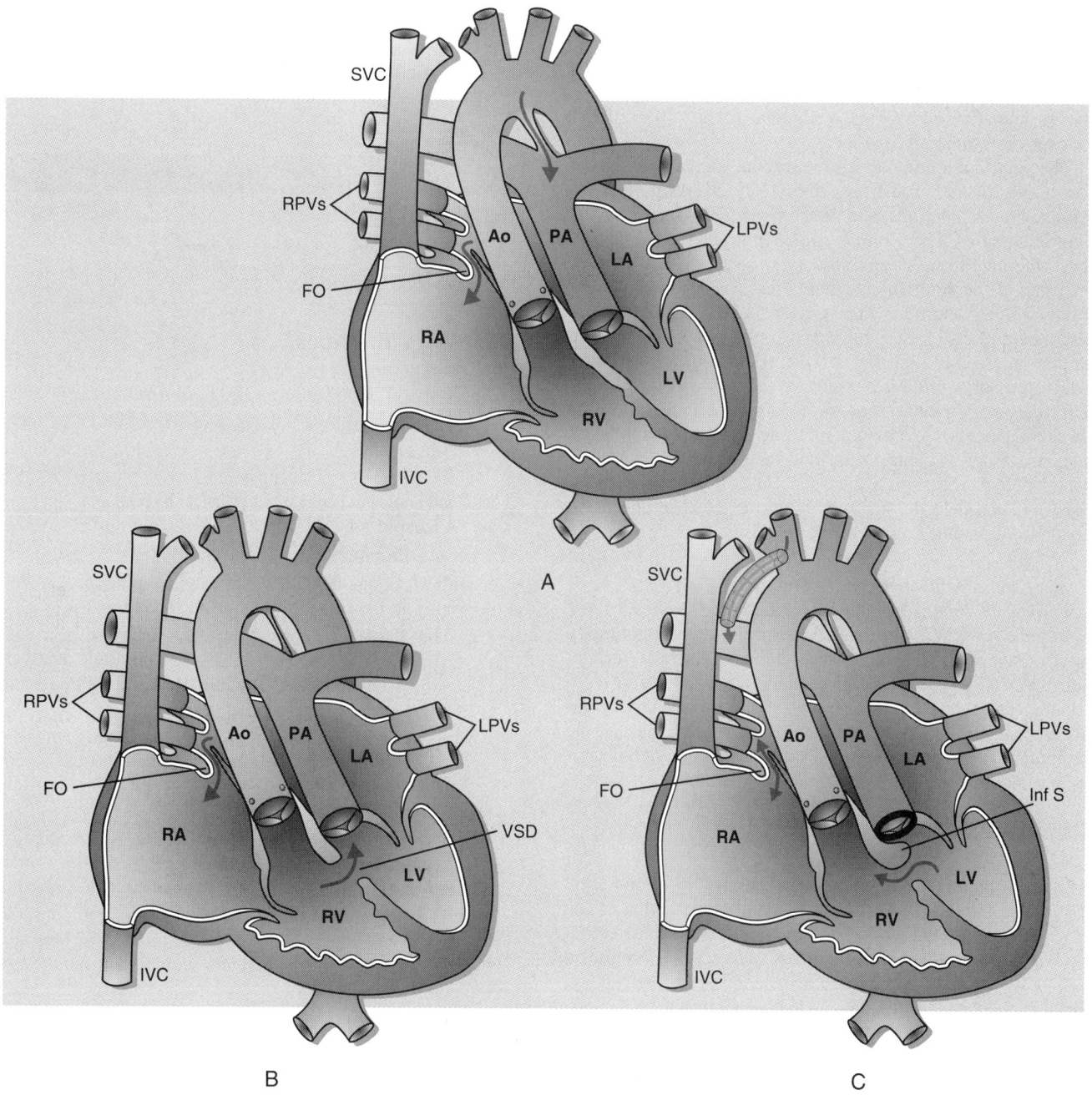

Figure 167–1. *A,* Transposition of the great arteries with intact ventricular septum. Note the flow from aorta (Ao) to pulmonary artery (PA) through the ductus arteriosus and from left atrium (LA) to right atrium (RA) through the foramen ovale (FO). *B,* Transposition with ventricular septal defect. Here the ventricular septal defect provides an additional site for mixing between the circulations. Flow across the defect is from right ventricle (RV) to the left ventricle (LV) and pulmonary artery (PA). Reciprocal flow is from left atrium (LA) to right atrium (RA) across the foramen ovale (FO). *C,* Transposition with ventricular septal defect and pulmonary stenosis. Here flow is from left ventricle (LV) to right ventricle (RV) and aorta (Ao) because of increased resistance to flow across the subpulmonary stenosis, due to posterior deviation of infundibular septum (Inf S). A modified Blalock-Taussig shunt (shunt) is shown as an additional source of pulmonary blood flow. Flow across the foramen ovale (FO) can be variable, but is usually from left atrium (LA) to right atrium (RA) if the shunt is large. IVC, Inferior vena cava; LPVs, left pulmonary veins; RPVs, right pulmonary veins; SVC, superior vena cava.

across the foramen ovale is bidirectional and equal in the two directions—from left to right during atrial diastole, and from right to left during atrial systole. Systemic arterial saturation is a function of the efficiency of mixing at atrial level. Left ventricular and pulmonary artery pressures fall as the ductus closes, usually to less than one-half systemic at a few days of life. Reduction in left ventricular pressure in the face of sustained systemic pressure in the right ventricle results in dynamic and eventually fixed left ventricular outflow obstruction.

2. Transposition with ventricular septal defect (30 to 35 per cent of common TGA)

The ventricular communication provides an additional site for mixing of the circulations (Fig. 167–1B). As pulmonary vascular resistance falls, shunting from right ventricle to left ventricle begins. The foramen ovale is the site for compensatory shunting from the pulmonary to systemic circulation. The size of the ventricular septal defect and the adequacy of atrial mixing determine the systemic arterial saturation. A large defect increases pulmonary blood flow and arterial saturation. In addition, the left ventricular and pulmonary artery pressures remain elevated, at or near systemic level. The risk for pulmonary vascular obstructive disease is high in such patients, developing in some by a few months of age. In some patients with transposition and ventricular septal defect, the right ventricular outflow tract is narrow, resulting in subaortic stenosis. Many of these infants have coarctation or interruption of the aortic arch.

3. Transposition with ventricular septal defect and pulmonary stenosis (10 per cent of common TGA)

Patients with this combination of defects have elevated resistance to flow from the left ventricle to the pulmonary artery owing to the pulmonary stenosis, which is usually subvalvar (Fig. 167–1C). There is shunting across the ventricular septal defect from left ventricle to right ventricle and aorta, and the pulmonary blood flow is reduced. If the pulmonary stenosis is severe, adequate systemic arterial saturation may be dependent on patency of the ductus arteriosus.

Clinical Findings

1. Presentation

   a. Cyanosis in the neonate is the most common sign. Hypoxia may be intense and life-threatening in the neonate with intact ventricular septum and restrictive foramen ovale or may be barely detectable in the infant with a large ventricular septal defect.

   b. Tachypnea without respiratory distress is characteristic.

   c. Infants with a large ventricular septal defect may develop congestive symptoms with tachypnea, respiratory distress, and poor feeding in the first weeks of life.

   d. Infants with aortic arch obstruction often develop gross heart failure, acidosis, and circulatory collapse when the ductus closes.

2. Physical examination

   a. Cyanosis is universal but may be variable in intensity depending on the pulmonary blood flow and adequacy of mixing.

   b. The second heart sound is loud and usually single.

   c. Infants with a ventricular septal defect usually develop a systolic murmur at a few days of age.

   d. Infants with pulmonary stenosis have a systolic ejection murmur along the left sternal border on the first day of life.

   e. Lower extremity pulses are diminished or absent in the presence of aortic arch obstruction.

   f. If heart failure develops, there may be tachypnea, retractions, pallor, hepatomegaly, and weak pulses generally.

Key Clinical Findings

- Cyanosis
- Tachypnea without respiratory distress
- Single loud second heart sound

Laboratory Findings

1. Electrocardiography

   a. Usually within normal limits in neonates

   b. Right ventricular hypertrophy is common in older infants.

   c. Diminished right ventricular forces or superior QRS axis suggest right ventricular hypoplasia or even tricuspid atresia.

2. Echocardiography

As with all congenital heart defects in the neonate, echocardiography is the primary diagnostic modality.

   a. The diagnosis is based on identification of the ventricles and great arteries by morphologic analysis and visualization of the abnormal ventriculoarterial alignments.

   b. Associated abnormalities are specifically investigated by imaging the atrial septum, ventricular septum, atrioventricular valves, ventricular outflow tracts, and great arteries.

   c. The coronary arteries should be imaged specifically, because of the importance of coronary artery anatomy to performance of the arterial switch operation.

   d. The Doppler examination shows important outflow tract obstruction and permits estimation of left ventricular pressure in patients with a ventricular septal defect.

3. Cardiac catheterization and angiography

   a. Diagnostic catheterization is rarely needed in the neonate. Unusual anatomic features or inability to obtain adequate echocardiographic images may prompt a cardiac catheterization.

   b. In the older infant, a cardiac catheterization may be useful after palliative procedures or to confirm that the left ventricle is capable of generating systemic pressure.

Key Laboratory Finding

- Electrocardiography

Radiographic Changes

1. In the neonate, the heart size and pulmonary vascular markings are usually normal. Within days to weeks, cardiac enlargement and increased pulmonary vascular markings are noted, especially in the presence of a ventricular septal defect.
2. Those infants with significant pulmonary stenosis usually have normal heart size and normal or even decreased pulmonary vascular markings.
3. A right aortic arch is present in about 10 per cent of infants with a ventricular septal defect.

Treatment

1. Palliation
   a. Medical therapy for the severely cyanotic neonate with transposition includes volume repletion, augmentation of inspired oxygen, and prostaglandin. The last-named treatment can cause left atrial hypertension and even pulmonary edema in the infant with a severely restrictive foramen ovale.
   b. Balloon septostomy is the standard first-line treatment for virtually all infants with transposition. The only instances in which this can be avoided safely are presence of a large atrial communication or immediate definitive surgical repair.
   c. Pulmonary artery banding is useful for selected neonates with multiple large ventricular septal defects

or in selected infants in whom the clinical condition is too poor to support definitive surgical repair (e.g. sepsis, CNS bleed).
   d. A systemic to pulmonary shunt (modified Blalock-Taussig shunt) is indicated in infants with severe pulmonary stenosis and unacceptably low oxygen saturation in anticipation of a Rastelli or REV operation.

2. Neonatal arterial switch operation (Fig. 167–2A)
   The arterial switch operation performed in the neonatal period, while the left ventricle is prepared to support the systemic circulation, is the surgical treatment of choice for virtually all infants with common transposition. Only those with severe subpulmonary stenosis due to posterior deviation of infundibular septum and annular hypoplasia are poor candidates.

3. Two-stage arterial switch operation
   A small number of infants with transposition, who would otherwise be candidates for a neonatal arterial switch operation, present for surgery after the left ventricle is no longer prepared to support systemic work. This may be due to neonatal illness, extreme prematurity, or simply late detection. The left ventricle can be prepared by banding the pulmonary artery and placing a systemic to pulmonary shunt to maintain pulmonary blood flow. Left ventricular mass accrual is complete after 7 to 10 days, when the arterial switch operation can be performed.

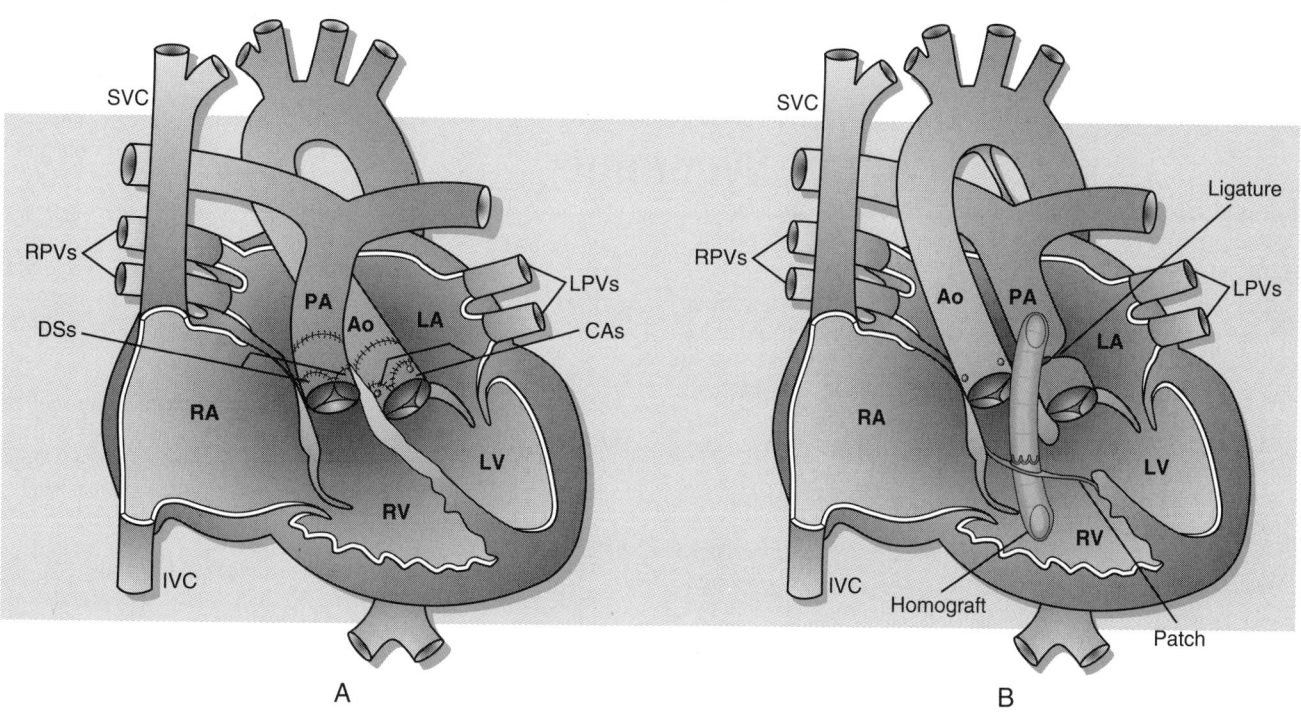

Figure 167–2. *A,* The arterial switch operation for transposition of the great arteries. Note that now the aorta (Ao) is connected with the left ventricle (LV) and the pulmonary artery (PA) with the right ventricle (RV). The great arteries have been transsected and then reconnected to the opposite root after the pulmonary artery (PA) was moved anteriorly. The coronary arteries (CAs) have been transferred from the anterior root to the posterior root (neo-aortic root) and the donor sites (DSs) in the anterior root filled with pericardial patches. *B,* The Rastelli operation for transposition, ventricular septal defect, and pulmonary stenosis. Note the patch directing flow from the left ventricle (LV) to the aorta (Ao) through the ventricular septal defect and the homograft connecting the right ventricle (RV) with the pulmonary artery (PA). The main pulmonary artery has been ligated (lig) proximal to the connection with the homograft.

An alternative approach to these infants is to perform the arterial switch operation primarily, using ECMO to support the circulation after surgery if needed.

4. Rastelli/REV operation (Fig. 167–2*B*)

These operations were designed for patients with transposition and significant pulmonary stenosis, in whom the left ventricular outflow tract is not usable. Here the left ventricle is baffled to the aorta through the ventricular septal defect, and the right ventricle is associated with the pulmonary artery directly or by means of a conduit or homograft.

5. Atrial switch operation (Mustard or Senning)

In the current era, there are few if any indications for an atrial switch operation in the treatment of common transposition, especially with ventricular septal defect.

Key Treatment

- Balloon septostomy
- Surgery

Prevention

1. There is no known prevention for this congenital heart defect.

2. The defect can be detected reliably by fetal echocardiography by 18 to 20 weeks of gestation. Elective termination of pregnancy can be carried out if desired. However, given the excellent results of surgery for this lesion, parents rarely choose this option, in our experience.

Bibliography

Boutin C, Jonas RA, Sanders SP, et al: Rapid two-stage arterial switch operation. Acquisition of left ventricular mass after pulmonary artery banding in infants with transposition of the great arteries. Circulation 1994;90:1304–1309.

Pasquini L, Sanders SP, Parness IA, et al: Conal anatomy in 119 patients with d-loop transposition of the great arteries and ventricular septal defect: an echocardiographic and pathologic study. J Am Coll Cardiol 1993;21:1712–1721.

Pasquini L, Sanders SP, Parness IA, et al: Coronary echocardiography in 406 patients with d-loop transposition of the great arteries. J Am Coll Cardiol 1994;24:763–768.

Vouhé PR, Tamisier D, Leca F, et al: Transposition of the great arteries, ventricular septal defect, and pulmonary outflow tract obstruction. Rastelli or Lecompte procedure? J Thorac Cardiovasc Surg 1992;103:428–436.

Wernovsky G, Hougen TJ, Walsh EP, et al: Midterm results after the arterial switch operation for transposition of the great arteries with intact ventricular septum: clinical, hemodynamic, echocardiographic, and electrophysiologic data. Circulation 1988; 77:1333–1344.

168 Hypoplastic Left Heart Syndrome

Paul M. Weinberg and *Meryl S. Cohen*

Definition

Hypoplastic left heart syndrome (HLHS) refers to a group of congenital heart defects that have in common an absolutely small left ventricle (LV) and normally aligned great arteries, i.e., pulmonary artery arising above morphologic right ventricle and aorta above morphologic LV. The following are the most common anatomic entities (Fig. 168–1).

1. Mitral atresia and aortic atresia with extreme hypoplasia or absence of an identifiable LV
2. Aortic atresia or stenosis with patent mitral valve. There is frequently endocardial fibroelastosis, probably secondary to intrauterine subendocardial ischemia.
3. Mitral stenosis and/or hypoplasia with aortic valve hypoplasia
4. Unbalanced common atrioventricular (AV) canal with hypoplasia of LV. These nearly always have a relatively large atrial septal defect (ASD) of the canal type (ostium primum ASD).

Etiology

1. Most cases occur sporadically. There is a preponderance of males. HLHS is the most severe form of left heart obstructive lesion and is seen in some cases of Turner syndrome.

2. Familial cases—Various reports cite risks of congenital heart disease in siblings as between 2 and 13 per cent (which is consistent with an autosomal recessive mode).

Epidemiology

HLHS is one of the most common cardiac anomalies, constituting 7 to 9 per cent of patients with significant congenital heart disease presenting in infancy. It accounts for 25 per cent of cardiac deaths in the first week of life.

Pathophysiology

1. *Ductal-dependent systemic circulation.* Because of the underdeveloped LV, there is inadequate antegrade flow to support the systemic circulation. Systemic output is augmented or completely supplied by the right heart via the ductus arteriosus. Postnatal survival prior to surgical intervention is dependent on persistence of ductal patency.

2. *Pulmonary overcirculation.* With systemic supply via the ductus, there is obligatory systemic level pulmonary artery pressure. As pulmonary vascular resistance falls postnatally, pulmonary blood flow increases correspondingly. Increased P_{O_2} from supplemental oxygen or decreased P_{CO_2} from hyperventilation exaggerates this phenomenon. In some cases pulmonary blood flow increases at the

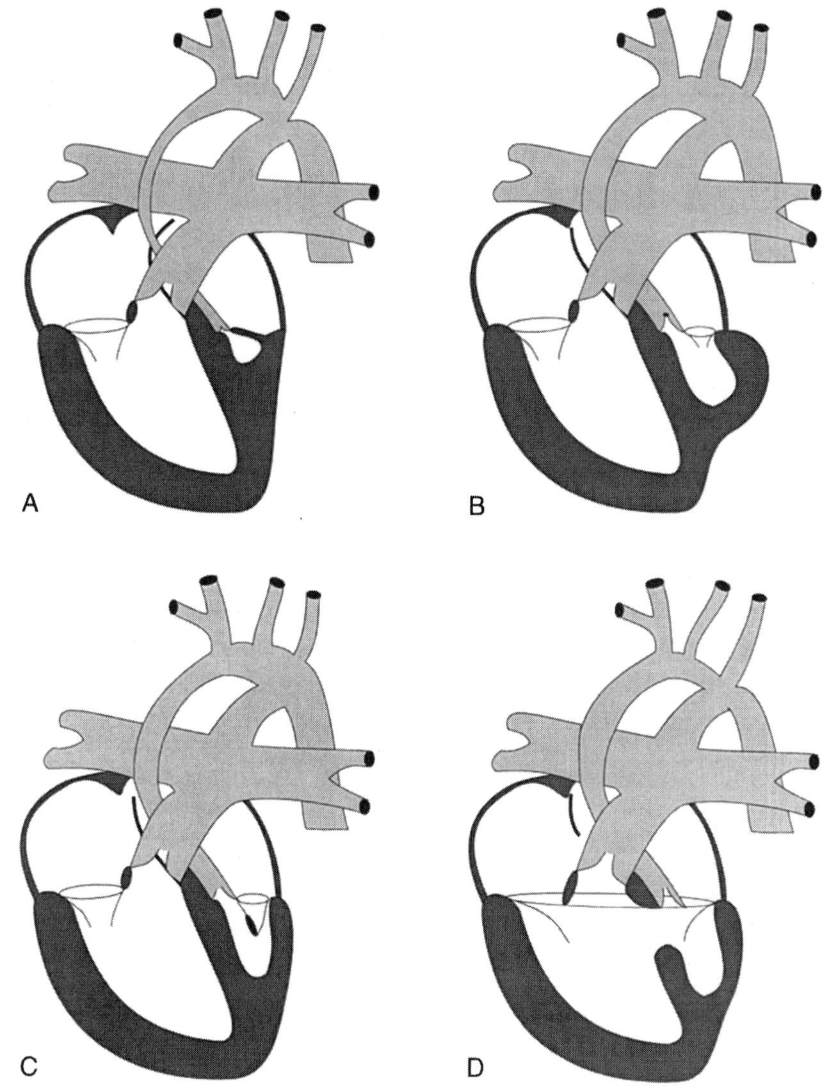

Figure 168–1 *A,* Mitral atresia and aortic atresia with extreme hypoplasia or absence of an identifiable LV. There is frequently a discrete coarctation of the aorta, and there may be a leftward deviation of the septum primum (flap valve of the foramen ovale). *B,* Aortic atresia or stenosis with patent mitral valve. There is frequently endocardial fibroelastosis probably secondary to intrauterine subendocardial ischemia. A congenitally small or absent foramen ovale may occur as a result of left atrial hypertension. *C,* Mitral stenosis and/or hypoplasia with aortic valve hypoplasia. *D,* Unbalanced common atrioventricular canal with hypoplasia of LV. These nearly always have a relatively large ostium primum atrial septal defect (ASD). Tubular hypoplasia of the aortic arch may occur.

expense of systemic blood flow, and systemic perfusion falls despite a widely patent ductus arteriosus.

3. *Pulmonary venous obstruction.* As already seen, systemic output in the unoperated state is dependent on ductal patency and maintenance of a balance between systemic and pulmonary blood flow. This balance is a reflection of total pulmonary resistance vs. systemic resistance. In HLHS, the combination of mitral valve hypoplasia or atresia with a functionally normal foramen ovale elevates pulmonary venous pressure and favorably influences the balance between systemic and pulmonary flow. With a large atrial septal defect this influence is lost, and pulmonary blood flow tends to be very high and difficult to control medically. Conversely, with severe pulmonary venous obstruction from a congenitally small or absent foramen, pulmonary blood flow is markedly limited, causing severe systemic desaturation due to the admixture of only a small proportion of pulmonary venous return with systemic venous flow.

Clinical Findings

1. There are four principal clinical scenarios, each with characteristic physical findings and age of presentation.

All have a single second heart sound regardless of age. Heart murmurs are variable and generally not diagnostic. There are no specific physical stigmata.

a. *Shock and multisystem organ failure.* Infants who present in shock and multisystem organ failure in the first week to 10 days of life should be thought to have a left-sided obstructive cardiac lesion until proven otherwise.

   (1) Appearance: Mottled and gray, with lethargy, irritability, and poor feeding just prior to circulatory collapse

   (2) Respiratory distress from a combination of metabolic acidosis and increased pulmonary blood flow

   (3) Acute renal failure and acute tubular necrosis, necrotizing enterocolitis sometimes requiring bowel resection, seizure or neurologic depression, coronary ischemia resulting in diminished right ventricular function, tricuspid regurgitation, and sometimes myocardial infarction

b. *Congestive heart failure.* Occasionally, the ductus arteriosus remains patent naturally in children with

HLHS, and the presenting symptoms are associated with congestive heart failure, usually between 2 and 6 weeks of age as pulmonary vascular resistance falls.

    (1) Appearance: Acyanotic despite systemic venous admixture to systemic output, because of the high proportion of pulmonary blood flow

    (2) Tachycardia, tachypnea, diaphoresis with feeding, and poor weight gain

    (3) Physical examination: Gallop rhythm, wheezing or rales, and hepatomegaly. Pulses usually mildly to moderately diminished but can be increased because of diastolic runoff into the ductus arteriosus.

  c. *Cyanosis in the newborn.* The dominant physical finding with pulmonary venous obstruction, due to either anomalous pulmonary venous connection with obstruction or a very restrictive (or sealed) foramen ovale. Cyanosis can also be seen when the pulmonary vascular resistance is unusually high in the newborn period.

  d. *Cyanosis in the older infant.* Rarely, a patient with a naturally patent ductus arteriosus does not develop frank heart failure but presents at 6 to 12 months of age with increased pulmonary vascular resistance from previous high pulmonary blood flow. Patients appear cyanotic because there is low pulmonary blood flow, but systemic perfusion is maintained.

2. Differential diagnosis

  a. Shock

    (1) Sepsis—Infants in septic shock can present with poor peripheral perfusion and decreased pulses but do not improve with prostaglandin therapy. Newborns presenting with shock in the first few days of life should be treated as if they have left heart obstruction until proven otherwise.

    (2) Other left-sided obstructive lesions can present similarly to HLHS, including critical coarctation of the aorta, interrupted aortic arch, and critical aortic stenosis. The initial medical treatment is virtually the same.

  b. Heart failure—Other acyanotic congenital heart disease, differentiated by echocardiography

  c. Cyanosis

    (1) Other cyanotic congenital heart disease, differentiated by echocardiography

    (2) Pulmonary disease; untreated HLHS tends to have low Pco_2.

Clinical course—HLHS is uniformly fatal in infancy or early childhood without surgical intervention.

Key Clinical Findings

- Shock (most common)
- Heart failure in early infancy (less common)
- Respiratory distress
- Single second heart sound
- Cyanosis (sometimes)

Laboratory Findings

1. Electrocardiography demonstrates right axis and right ventricular hypertrophy—occasionally indistinguishable from the normal right ventricular dominance of the newborn. Often, left ventricular forces are lower than normal.

2. Blood gases show metabolic acidosis when clinical presentation is due to ductal closure and shock. Despite this near-moribund condition, the Po_2 is likely to be relatively high, since what little systemic flow occurs is composed of a disproportionately large amount of pulmonary venous blood. With a widely patent ductus arteriosus, arterial Po_2 reflects the amount of pulmonary blood flow:

  a. Po_2 35 to 45, reflecting a good balance between pulmonary and systemic flow

  b. Po_2 >60, indicating high pulmonary blood flow likely to result in systemic hypoperfusion

  c. Po_2 <25, implying significant pulmonary venous obstruction.

3. Echocardiography is able to define the anatomy in almost all cases. Those findings relevant to management include the nature of the interatrial communication, right ventricular and tricuspid valve function, and identification of pulmonary venous connection.

4. Cardiac catheterization and angiocardiography have a limited role in the initial diagnosis of HLHS. Rarely, angiography may be necessary to define any anomalous pulmonary venous connection not well seen by echocardiography. Interventional catheterization may be indicated for creation of an atrial septal defect in a few cases of congenitally small or absent foramen ovale (with severe hypoxemia) for stabilization prior to surgery. Alternatively, such patients may be stabilized on ECMO or taken emergently to surgery.

Key Laboratory Findings

- Blood gases
- Electrolytes

Radiographic Findings

1. Pulmonary overcirculation—HLHS is one (and the most common) of just a few causes of marked cardiomegaly in the newborn, the others being Ebstein anomaly (distinguished by decreased pulmonary vascular markings and clinical cyanosis), cardiomyopathy, and congenital pericardial effusion (the latter two easily recognized by echocardiography). Pulmonary vascular markings are normal to increased.

2. Pulmonary venous obstruction is associated with a relatively small heart and hazy lung fields.

Treatment

1. Medical management

  a. Maintenance of ductal patency with intravenous prostaglandin E_1, 0.05 to 0.1 µg/kg/min

  b. Aggressive treatment of metabolic acidosis by volume infusion and sodium bicarbonate, since acidosis leads to increased systemic vascular resistance, and, in turn, to increased pulmonary blood flow.

c. Optimize balance between systemic and pulmonary blood flow. Ideally patients are managed

(1) In room air, since oxygen acts as a pulmonary vasodilator, decreasing pulmonary vascular resistance and potentially shifting blood flow into the pulmonary circulation. Occasionally oxygen may be used in the face of lung disease (pneumonia, hyaline membrane disease) if the P_{O_2} is below 25 to 30 in room air; in those few patients with pulmonary venous obstruction (small or no patent foramen ovale), O_2 will not have harmful effects, but prompt intervention (e.g., catheter septostomy or surgical septectomy) is required. Oxygen can be used in the preintervention management.

(2) Without mechanical ventilation; however, apnea from prostaglandins or marked hyperventilation secondary to torrential pulmonary blood flow may necessitate mechanical ventilation. Low P_{CO_2} (usually <35) and concomitant high P_{O_2} may be treated by either paralysis and hypoventilation or the addition of inspired CO_2. One aims for both P_{O_2} and CO_2 of 40 mmHg.

2. Surgical approaches

a. *Three-stage Norwood-Fontan.* Patients with HLHS have a functional single ventricle, i.e., one usable ventricle with one AV valve (the tricuspid) and one semilunar valve (the pulmonary). The systemic circulation is dependent on a patent ductus arteriosus.

(1) Newborn period—The Norwood operation consists of amalgamation of the proximal stump of the transected proximal pulmonary artery with the hypoplastic aorta, placement of a systemic-pulmonary shunt to the distal pulmonary artery to limit pulmonary blood flow, and atrial septectomy to facilitate egress of blood from the outlet-obstructed left atrium. This protects the pulmonary vasculature from systemic pressure while maintaining systemic output from the only ventricle, the right ventricle.

(2) Six months of age—Hemi-Fontan or bidirectional Glenn. The Fontan principle allows that the one usable ventricle support the systemic circulation while pulmonary circulation comes passively from a systemic vein to pulmonary artery connection. Because pulmonary resistance in the newborn is elevated, the Fontan principle is not applicable initially. However, by 6 months, pulmonary resistance has fallen

sufficiently to permit anastomosis of the superior vena cava alone to the pulmonary artery, thus decreasing the volume load on the ventricle while maintaining the balance of the cardiac output with some desaturated blood from the inferior vena cava.

(3) Eighteen months to 2 years of age—Fontan completion. Inclusion of inferior caval flow using a baffle passing through the right atrium or an extracardiac conduit.

b. *Heart transplantation*—An alternative to surgical reconstruction. It is mainly limited by organ availability. The patient can be maintained on PGE_1 pending transplantation. However, in patients with a large atrial septal communication, it may be difficult to manage pulmonary blood flow by manipulation of P_{CO_2} alone for long periods. Transplantation is also applicable for patients who, because of poor ventricular function, are not candidates for the Fontan procedure.

Key Treatment

- Prostaglandin E_1 infusion
- Correction of metabolic acidemia when perfusion is adequate
- Surgery

Prevention

There is no known prevention for HLHS. Because of familial recurrence in some cases, fetal echocardiography is appropriate with subsequent pregnancies. Since relative size differences between right and left ventricles in developing HLHS may be progressive, serial examinations may be necessary.

Bibliography

Abu-Harb M, Wyllie J, Hey E, et al: Presentation of obstructive left heart malformations in infancy. Arch Dis Child 1994;71:F179–F183.

Bailey LL, Nehlsen-Cannarella SL, Doroshow RW, et al: Cardiac allotransplantation in newborns as therapy for hypoplastic left heart syndrome. N Engl J Med 1986;315:949–951.

Farrell PE, Jr, Chang AC, Murdison KA, et al: Outcome and assessment after the modified Fontan procedure for hypoplastic left heart syndrome. Circulation 1992;85:116–122.

Norwood WI, Lang P, Castaneda AR, et al: Experience with operations for hypoplastic left heart syndrome. J Thorac Cardiovasc Surg 1981;82:511–519.

Norwood WI, Jr: Hypoplastic left heart syndrome. [Review.] Ann Thorac Surg 1991;52:688–695.

169 Pulmonary Atresia

Robert R. Wolfe

Definition

Pulmonary atresia with intact ventricular septum (PA-IVS) has an imperforate pulmonary valve with an obligatory atrial septal communication and a patent ductus arteriosus. The tricuspid annulus and right ventricle are variable in size, and right ventriculocoronary artery connections occur in 50 per cent of cases.

Etiology

The etiology is unknown. A fetal inflammatory process, such as a congenital rubella infection after cardiac septation is complete, has been suggested but is unproven.

Incidence

PA-IVS is an uncommon form of congenital heart disease (1–3%). However, it is a relatively common form of neonatal cyanotic congenital heart disease along with transposition of the great arteries, tricuspid atresia, and pulmonary atresia–stenosis with ventricular septal defect.

Pathophysiology

1. The atresia of the pulmonary valve and presence of an intact ventricular septum results in an obligatory right-to-left atrial level shunt, which may be either a stretched patent foramen ovale or a secundum atrial septal defect. The pulmonary blood supply is dependent on left-to-right flow via a patent ductus arteriosus. Unobstructed flow of blood in this manner results in moderate cyanosis and volume overload of the left ventricle. Progressive obstruction at either of these sites results in increasingly severe cyanosis and its sequelae. Interruption of flow at either of these sites results in death.

2. Two basic forms of PA-IVS occur, depending upon the presence or absence of tricuspid regurgitation.

   a. Those patients without tricuspid regurgitation have a small underdeveloped right ventricle and tricuspid annulus with suprasystemic right ventricle pressure. Right ventriculocoronary communications are common in this group and may result in right ventricle–coronary dependent physiology and obliterative coronary artery disease. The coronary arteries receive retrograde right ventricular flow during systole and antegrade flow during diastole. Therapeutic procedures that interfere with right ventricular flow or reduce right ventricular pressure may lead to myocardial ischemia and death. Spontaneous progression of obliterative coronary artery disease may have the same outcome.

   b. Those patients with tricuspid regurgitation tend to have larger, more developed right ventricles. The right atrium is large and may be massively dilated leading to dysrhythmias, hepatic congestion, and pulmonary compromise. Right ventriculocoronary artery communications do not tend to occur in these patients. A decrease in pulmonary blood flow and progressive cyanosis due to an inadequate ductus arteriosus commonly occurs.

Clinical Findings

1. Presentation

   a. Cyanosis with tachypnea but without dyspnea is usual in a term infant, appropriate for gestational age, for several hours after birth.

   b. Sudden onset of severe cyanosis and acidosis may indicate closure of the patent ductus arteriosus and require emergent therapy.

   c. Males and females are equally affected.

2. Physical findings

   a. Cyanosis

   b. Tachypnea without dyspnea

   c. May have hyperdynamic apical impulse

   d. Single first and second heart sounds

   e. Murmurs

      (1) Without tricuspid regurgitation—No murmur, or systolic-continuous murmur of patent ductus arteriosus at upper left sternal border

      (2) With tricuspid regurgitation—Long systolic murmur at the lower left sternal border with a diastolic rumble.

Key Clinical Findings

- Cyanosis
- Tachypnea without dyspnea
- Single first and second heart sounds

Laboratory Findings

1. Blood gases

   Room air hypoxemia-acidosis with little response to 100 per cent inspired oxygen

2. Electrocardiogram

   a. With small right ventricle (without tricuspid regurgitation)—Mild right atrial enlargement (peaked 3 mm P wave) somewhat leftward-posterior QRS forces ($+30$ to $+90$), decreased right ventricular–increased left ventricular forces ST-T changes of subendocardial ischemia

   b. With large right ventricle (with tricuspid regurgitation)—Striking right atrial enlargement (peaked 4 mm or greater P wave), QRS right axis deviation ($\geq^3 + 120$) right ventricular hypertrophy.

3. Chest x-ray

a. With small right ventricle (without tricuspid regurgitation)—Relatively normal heart size and shape; pulmonary arterial vascularity normal to decreased

b. With large right ventricle (with tricuspid regurgitation)—Giant right atrium with cardiac silhouette filling most of chest; difficult to assess pulmonary vascularity, as the heart covers most of the lung fields. (*Note:* Cerebral AV fistula and Ebstein malformation have comparable massive neonatal cardiomegaly.)

4. Echocardiography/Doppler

The diagnosis of pulmonary atresia with intact ventricular septum is routinely made with standard echo-Doppler techniques. The important determinations of small vs. large right ventricle, adequacy of the atrial septal communication, and patency of the ductus arteriosus are made.

A tiny antegrade jet of critical pulmonic stenosis may be lost in the retrograde flow of a patent ductus arteriosus. The anatomy of right ventriculocoronary artery communications and obliterative coronary artery disease can be made only with angiocardiographic techniques.

5. Cardiac catheterization and angiography

Cardiac catheterization is indicated to establish

a. Hemodynamics—The right ventricular pressure and adequacy of the interatrial communication

b. Definition of the right ventriculocoronary communication anatomy, done by selective angiocardiography of the right ventricle and coronary arteries.

c. Performance of interventional procedures

(1) Balloon atrial septostomy for a restrictive atrial communication

(2) Transcatheter balloon valvuloplasty after pulmonary plate perforation with laser or radio frequency–assisted wire.

Key Laboratory Findings

- Blood gases
- ECG

Treatment

1. Medical

When diagnosis of pulmonary atresia with intact ventricular septum is established in the newborn, intravenous prostaglandin E_1 infusion should be instituted (0.05–0.10 μg/kg/min) to maintain patency of the ductus arteriosus.

2. Interventional cardiac catheterization
3. Surgery

a. Small hypertensive right ventricle with inadequate coronary arteries (right ventricule–dependent or significant obstruction of two coronary arteries)

(1) Chronic PGE_1 infusion until systemic-pulmonary shunt

(2) List for cardiac transplantation

b. Small hypertensive right ventricle with adequate coronary arteries

(1) Without infundibulum

Perform systemic-pulmonary shunt as a bridge to a later Fontan procedure

(2) With infundibulum

With very small tricuspid annulus—Perform systemic-pulmonary shunt as a bridge to a later Fontan procedure.

With appropriate tricuspid annulus—Decompress the right ventricle with interventional catheter or surgical valvulotomy and slowly wean the PGE_1. If the patient is unacceptably hypoxemic and unstable, perform systemic-pulmonary shunt.

c. Large right ventricle with tricuspid regurgitation—Interventional catheter or surgical valvulotomy.

Key Treatment

- Balloon septostomy
- Prostaglandin E_1 infusion
- Surgery

Prevention

Currently there is no way to prevent pulmonary atresia with intact ventricular septum.

Bibliography

Freedom RM: Pulmonary atresia and intact ventricular septum. *In* Emmanouilides GC, Reimenschneider TA, Allen HD, Gutgesell HP (eds): Heart Disease in Infants, Children, and Adolescents. Baltimore, Williams & Wilkins, 1995, pp 962–982.

Hanley FL, et al: Outcomes in neonatal pulmonary atresia with intact ventricular septum. A multiinstitutional study. J Thorac Cardiovasc Surg 1993;105:406–427.

Riopel, DA: Pulmonary valve atresia with intact ventricular septum. *In* Garson A, Bricker, JT, McNamara DG (eds): The Science and Practice of Pediatric Cardiology. Philadelphia, Lea & Febiger, 1990, pp 1108–1117.

Rosenthal E, et al: Radiofrequency assisted balloon dilatation in patients with pulmonary atresia and intact ventricular septum. Br Heart J 1993;69:347–351.

170 Truncus Arteriosus

Paul Stanger

Definition

Truncus arteriosus is a cardiac anomaly characterized by (1) the biventricular origin of a single arterial root that gives rise to the coronary, brachiocephalic, and pulmonary arteries and (2) a single semilunar valve. In contrast, in pulmonary atresia or aortic atresia there are two arterial roots, one of which is hypoplastic and associated with an atretic semilunar valve.

Etiology

1. Chromosome 22 microdeletions may be found in association with a variety of congenital cardiac abnormalities, including truncus arteriosus. These microdeletions are found in virtually all patients with both truncus and DiGeorge syndrome and in most of those without DiGeorge syndrome. The remaining cases probably result from isolated mutations—that is, translocations, gene deletions, or other as yet undiscovered mechanisms that may involve the same chromosome.
2. Most patients with truncus have DiGeorge syndrome (thymic hypoplasia with cellular immune deficiency, hypoparathyroidism, cardiovascular malformations, and dysmorphism). The thymus, parathyroid glands, and aortic arches are derived from third and fourth pharyngeal pouch evaginations, the structures whose development are controlled by the neural crest. The mechanisms involved in neural crest control are unknown.

Epidemiology

Truncus arteriosus is rare, occurring once in 12,500 births and representing 1.4 per cent of congenital cardiac abnormalities. A high incidence (6%) has been found among stillbirths.

Anatomy

1. *Great arteries*—The most commonly used classification of truncus is based on the positions of the pulmonary artery origins (Collett and Edwards, 1949). Most cases of truncus arteriosus are actually "type 1 1/2" (i.e., a mixture of types 1 and 2).
   a. *Type 1*—A main pulmonary artery arises from the left aspect of the truncus and then divides into left and right branches.
   b. *Type 2*—Separate pulmonary arteries arise from the truncus posterolaterally.
   c. *Type 3*—Separate pulmonary arteries arise from the truncus laterally.
   d. *Type 4*—This category is no longer used, because it is not a true truncus but a pulmonary atresia with ventricular septal defect and absent central pulmonary arteries.
2. *Valves*—All patients with truncus have a single semilunar valve; however, leaflet number varies. Most common is three leaflets, followed by four and two. It is rare to see one, five, or six leaflets. Stenosis of the truncal leaflets is common and is usually mild, as is truncal insufficiency.
3. *Ventricular septal defects*—Usually large, the ventricular septal defect is straddled by the truncus so as to give it a biventricular origin. The defect is more anterior than the usual membranous defect, and this position is remote from the His bundle.
4. Additional vascular anomalies include coronary artery abnormalities (common), aortic arch interruption (infrequent), and absence of one pulmonary artery (rare).

Pathophysiology

1. The presence of large ventricular and aortopulmonary communications results in pulmonary hypertension and, once pulmonary vascular resistance declines, markedly increased pulmonary flow. In truncus, pulmonary vascular resistance declines during the first days, weeks, or sometimes months of life.
2. As pulmonary flow increases, there is associated left ventricular dilatation and congestive cardiac failure.

Clinical Findings

1. *Presentation*—Most patients with truncus arteriosus present with a prominent murmur and varying degrees of congestive heart failure during the first weeks of life.
   a. Patients with additional abnormalities, such as interrupted aortic arch or truncal regurgitation, present with marked failure within the first days.
   b. Ten per cent of truncus patients are asymptomatic during the first months, presumably because they do not show the usual decline in pulmonary vascular resistance.
2. Physical findings
   a. Failure to thrive is manifested primarily by poor weight gain; longitudinal growth and head growth are usually normal.
   b. Pallor and mild cyanosis are customary, with oxygen saturation percentages usually from the middle 80s to the low 90s. Lower saturations may reflect less pulmonary flow and higher pulmonary vascular resistance.
   c. Congestive cardiac failure
      (1) The earliest signs are those of catechol excess (i.e., pallor, diaphoresis, irritability, and tachycardia). The catechol excess is caused by impaired myocardial function, which stimulates release of endogenous catecholamines that in turn improve myocardial performance.
      (2) The passive congestion symptoms of failure occur when the heart can no longer perform adequately despite catechol stimulation.

(i) Left-sided failure is manifested by signs of pulmonary venous congestion, with tachypnea, hyperpnea, and rales.

(ii) Right-sided failure is manifested by systemic venous congestion, with hepatosplenomegaly but not peripheral edema.

d. The peripheral pulses are mildly to moderately accentuated, with a rapid rise and fall but not the full volume that is seen in association with a patent ductus arteriosus. Exceptions to the latter are patients with more than mild truncal incompetence.

e. Precordial activity is invariably increased, with hyperdynamic left and right ventricular impulses.

f. Auscultation

(1) The first heart sound is normal; the second is usually single but may reverberate and sound blurred or split, despite there being only one semilunar valve.

(2) A prominent systolic ejection click is heard in most patients.

(3) A harsh grade 2/6 to 4/6, diamond-shaped, pansystolic murmur is heard at the middle to lower left sternal border and transmits toward the right.

(4) A mitral mid-diastolic rumble reflects increased flow across that valve.

(5) Patients with truncal incompetence have a medium- to high-frequency decrescendo early diastolic murmur at the middle-left sternal border.

(6) Patients with truncal stenosis have a systolic ejection murmur at the base; the higher the frequency, the greater the degree of stenosis. Because stenosis is usually mild, the murmur is often of low to medium frequency.

Key Clinical Findings

- Prominent murmur
- Heart failure
- Mild cyanosis

Laboratory Findings

1. *Radiography*—Thoracic roentgenograms typically show the features of a large left-to-right shunt with prominent pulmonary vascularity and cardiomegaly with a left ventricular contour. A right aortic arch is found in 30 per cent of cases. Pulmonary complications may be evident as pneumonia, atelectasis, or aspiration. There is a relatively narrow mediastinal waist. Lack of thymic tissue suggests the possibility of DiGeorge syndrome.

2. *Electrocardiography*—There are no findings specific for truncus. The QRS axis is usually normal or rightward, with prominent inferior forces and, commonly, biventricular hypertrophy. In general, the strength of the left or right forces reflects the status of the pulmonary vascularity: the more pulmonary flow, the greater the leftward forces, and the higher the pulmonary vascular resistance, the greater the rightward forces.

3. *Echocardiography*—The diagnosis is readily made on echocardiography by the finding of a single artery overriding the ventricular septum and demonstration that the coronary arteries, pulmonary arteries, and brachiocephalic vessels all originate from this vessel. The common origin of the pulmonary arteries from this truncal root is best illustrated from the subcostal views, particularly in types 1 and 1 1/2. The large pulmonary flow resulting in aortic runoff is manifested by prominent descending aortic pulsations and Doppler detection of retrograde diastolic flow in the descending aorta.

4. *Cardiac catheterization and angiocardiography*—Invasive diagnostic testing is seldom necessary in the usual or typical case, because all of the features may be found with a good-quality echocardiogram. Catheterization may be necessary in patients with associated abnormalities that may influence the surgical approach (e.g., interrupted aortic arch, mitral regurgitation, multiple ventricular septal defects) and in patients in whom there are concerns about the status of the pulmonary vascular resistance.

5. *Pulse oximetry*—As there is common mixing of systemic and pulmonary venous returns, systemic saturation reflects pulmonary flow and inversely reflects pulmonary vascular resistance; that is, the higher the saturation, the higher the pulmonary flow and the lower the pulmonary vascular resistance. A saturation of less than 83 per cent may indicate a high pulmonary vascular resistance.

Key Laboratory Tests

- Echocardiography
- Pulse oximetry

Treatment

1. Without surgical repair, the natural history is bleak. Twenty per cent of patients die in the first month and 85 per cent in the first year; the survivors develop pulmonary vascular disease in the ensuing years. Palliative pulmonary artery banding alters this prognosis very little; however, early surgical repair can dramatically improve the likelihood of survival.

2. Surgical repair

a. Procedure

(1) Patch closure of the ventricular septal defect is performed so that the left ventricle empties entirely into the truncus.

(2) The pulmonary arteries are disconnected from the truncus, the stump is oversewn, and the disconnected pulmonary arteries are then connected to the right ventricle with the use of an aortic homograft. This completes the separation of pulmonary and systemic circuits, and the aortic homograft supplies a valve for the pulmonary circuit. Additional abnormalities such as atrial septal defects and mitral insufficiency are repaired at the same time.

(3) Truncal valve abnormalities may be dealt with at the initial surgery.

(i) A preoperative truncal valve systolic gradient overestimates the degree of stenosis, because both systemic flow and the markedly increased pulmonary flow pass through it. After repair, the valve carries only systemic flow, and the marked reduction in flow substantially decreases the gradient.

    (ii) Truncal incompetence that is mild is not repaired; however, marked incompetence is poorly tolerated in the postoperative period and therefore is dealt with surgically.

  (4) Aortic arch interruption must be repaired before the intracardiac repair is done. The repair involves ligation of the patent ductus arteriosus and an end-to-side anastomosis of the descending aorta to the aortic arch.

  b. The postoperative course may be protracted because of pulmonary hypertensive crises with bronchospasm and acute pulmonary vasoconstriction. Because the ventricular septal defect is remote from the induction system, atrioventricular block is rare.

3. Long-term follow-up

  a. Right-ventricle-to-pulmonary-artery graft durability

    (1) Currently, homografts are used in repairs because they deteriorate slower than porcine or bovine heterograft valves contained in Dacron prostheses.

    (2) Homografts require periodic replacement, particularly in childhood; some grafts may become insufficient, but eventually all become stenotic owing to a combination of static valve size in a growing child, fibrosis, and calcification.

    (3) Valve replacement necessitated by stenosis may be delayed by transcatheter balloon dilatation. If the largest valve possible is used initially, most patients will need to undergo valve replacement at least once in the first decade, with subsequent replacement as a teenager or adult. The longevity of homografts in adults is considerably greater (i.e., decades rather than multiple years).

  b. *Truncal (aortic) valve*—Truncal insufficiency or, less likely, truncal stenosis may necessitate truncal valve replacement. The annulus is large and, even at a young age, allows placement of a fairly large prosthetic or homograft valve.

4. *Other considerations*—All patients with truncus arteriosus should be evaluated for DiGeorge syndrome, because it may cause problems in several areas.

  a. Hypocalcemia, both preoperative and postoperative, may be associated with tremors, seizures, and impaired myocardial performance.

  b. Immunologic deficiency is related to lack of thymus and its influence on T cells. The degree of immunodeficiency varies and it is often transient, being limited to the first year.

  c. Transfusions should be with irradiated blood in order to prevent graft-versus-host reactions.

  d. Developmental problems are common.

Key Treatment

- Surgery

Bibliography

Butto F, Lucas RV Jr, Edwards JE: Persistent truncus arteriosus: Pathologic anatomy in 54 cases. Pediatr Cardiol 1986;7:95–101.

Collett RW, Edwards JE: Persistent truncus arteriosus: A classification according to anatomic types. Surg Clin North Am 1949;29:1245–1270.

Ebert PA, Turley K, Stanger P, et al: Surgical treatment of truncus arteriosus in the first 6 months of life. Ann Surg 1984;200:451–456.

Marcelletti C, McGoon DC, Mair DD: The natural history of truncus arteriosus. Circulation 1976;54:108–111.

Stanger P: Truncus arteriosus. *In* Moller JH, Neal WA (eds): Fetal, Neonatal and Infant Cardiac Disease. Norwalk, CT, Appleton-Century-Crofts, 1990, pp 587–602.

VanMierop LH, Kutsche LM: Cardiovascular anomalies in DiGeorge syndrome and importance of neural crest as a possible pathogenic factor. Am J Cardiol 1986;58:133–137.

171 Eisenmenger Syndrome

Marlene Rabinovitch

Definition

Usually a large ventricular septal defect with overriding of the aorta; a variety of congenital heart defects in which there is an initial left-to-right shunt, but over time, increasing elevation in pulmonary vascular resistance, ultimately resulting in reversal of the shunt and cyanosis.

Etiology

1. Natural history studies have shown that different congenital heart defects vary considerably in the rate of progressive elevation of pulmonary vascular resistance and in the potential for regression.

2. In ventricular septal defect (VSD) or patent ductus arteri-

osus (PDA), 15 per cent of infants will show progressive elevation in pulmonary vascular resistance in late infancy or early childhood. With atrial septal defects, however, this occurs extremely rarely in childhood, and the 20 per cent incidence is generally after the third decade of life.

3. With lesions such as atrioventricular septal defect commonly seen with Down syndrome or in transposition of the great arteries, particularly with associated VSD or PDA, there is a 40 per cent incidence of severe pulmonary hypertension within the first year of life; this is also true for patients with truncus arteriosus.

Pathophysiology

1. First, there is extension of muscle into peripheral normally nonmuscular arteries.
2. This is followed by medial hypertrophy of muscular arteries and reduced arterial concentration associated with increased pulmonary artery pressure and resistance, respectively.
3. There is also the concomitant development of neointimal formation. This is initiated by cellular changes that progress to occlusive fibroproliferative lesions and culminate in plexiform networks of obstructed and dilated vessels. The potential for reversibility of these changes is dictated by their severity.
4. Serum factors or endothelial factors that may gain access to the subendothelium when the barrier function of the endothelium is lost can induce release of a serine elastase from pulmonary vascular smooth muscle cells. This elastase can liberate biologically active smooth muscle cell mitogens, such as basic fibroblast growth factor, from extracellular matrix stores.
5. The resulting smooth muscle cell hyperplasia contributes to the hypertrophy of the arterial wall.
6. There is also induction of the matrix glycoprotein tenascin, which cooperatively interacts with growth factors, such as epidermal growth factor and basic fibroblast growth factor, in inducing the proliferative response in the vessel wall. In addition, elastin peptides may induce upregulation of fibronectin, important in switching the smooth muscle cells from a contractile to a migratory mode, necessary for neointimal formation.

Clinical Findings

1. Patients with Eisenmenger syndrome will show cyanosis, especially with exercise and, in fact, have progressively poor exercise tolerance.
2. They will have the sequelae of polycythemia (e.g., potential for abscess and stroke) and may be prone to hemoptysis owing to the rupture of numerous collateral vessels from bronchial arteries that develop in an effort to bypass obstructed pulmonary arteries.
3. Syncope may also occur in patients with Eisenmenger syndrome.
4. Progressive right heart failure is reflected in hepatomegaly and ascites.
5. The cardiovascular findings of Eisenmenger syndrome are related to the enlarged heart, particularly the right ventricle (right ventricular heave) and the loud and palpable second heart sound.

Key Clinical Findings

- Cyanosis with exercise
- Syncope
- Right-sided cardiac enlargement

Laboratory Findings

1. Progressive polycythemia is usually a manifestation of the deterioration in clinical status.
2. The ECG shows severe right ventricular hypertrophy with a strain pattern.
3. Pulsed Doppler echocardiography is useful in showing lack of restriction to flow across the defect (reflecting systemic levels of pulmonary artery pressure); this can be corroborated when there is a jet of tricuspid regurgitation.
4. In addition, the echocardiogram can be useful in assessing shunt reversal and progressive pulmonary regurgitation.

Key Laboratory Findings

- Polycythemia
- ECG
- Echocardiography

Cardiac Catheterization

Catheterization is often helpful in establishing whether a patient has true Eisenmenger syndrome or whether surgical interventional cardiologic correction of a defect is likely to result in a reduction in pulmonary vascular resistance.

1. In general, if the pulmonary vascular resistance is higher than 8 um^2 and does not fall to at least 6 um^2 with vasodilator stimuli, such as oxygen or nitric oxide, the patient is unlikely to show any benefit from surgical correction.
2. When the hemodynamic data are borderline or difficult to interpret, quantitative analysis of a pulmonary wedge angiogram may be useful. Correlation of biopsy with angiographic assessments indicate that the rate of taper of the pulmonary vascular lesion reflects the severity of the biopsy grade.
3. The more abrupt the taper, the more likely that there is distal vascular obstruction. The vessels may be so spindly owing to intimal formation that they appear striking in their lack of taper against a dark background. That is, gradual taper with dense background filling of peripheral vessels reflects reversible pulmonary vascular changes, whereas with absence of filling of small vessels, severe intimal formation and obstruction are likely.
4. In addition, it is helpful to count the circulation time from let-down of the balloon to the entry of contrast medium into the left atrium. If less than 0.5 seconds, a significant left-to-right shunt is likely.

Treatment

1. Symptomatic improvement can be accomplished by relief of the polycythemia through the use of plasma exchange transfusions.

2. Iron deficiency should also be aggressively treated to prevent thrombi.
3. Anticoagulation would appear to be beneficial in preventing thrombi and at least anecdotally has been shown to retard the progression of vascular disease in the Eisenmenger patient.
4. Oral contraceptives are contraindicated in the patient with Eisenmenger syndrome owing to the propensity to thromboses, and pregnancy carries a very high risk of mortality, particularly in the early postpartum period. Anesthesia presents an increased risk and should be weighed carefully against any potential benefit from an elective procedure.

Key Treatment

- Plasma exchange transfusion
- Iron supplementation
- Surgery

5. Heart-lung transplantation or single- or double-lung transplantation with correction of the congenital heart defect has proved to be a satisfactory option for some patients, particularly if mortality due to rejection and bronchiolitis obliterans and morbidity due to immunosuppressive therapy can be overcome.

Bibliography

Botney MD, Kaiser LR, Cooper JD, et al: Extracellular matrix gene expression in atherosclerotic hypertensive pulmonary artery. Am J Pathol 1992;140:357–364.

Houde C, Bohn DJ, Freedom RM, et al: Profile of paediatric patients with pulmonary hypertension judged by responsiveness to vasodilators. Br Heart J 1993;70:461–468.

Nihill MR: Clinical management of patients with pulmonary hypertension. *In* Emmanouilides GC, Riemenschneidier TA, Allen HD, Gutgesell HP (eds): Moss and Adams Heart Disease in Infants, Children, and Adolescents, 5th ed, vol II. Baltimore, Williams & Wilkins, 1994, pp 1695–1711.

Rabinovitch M: Pathophysiology of pulmonary hypertension. *In* Emmanouilides GC, Riemenschneidier TA, Allen HD, Gutgesell HP (eds): Moss and Adams Heart Disease in Infants, Children, and Adolescents, 5th ed, vol II. Baltimore, Williams & Wilkins, 1994, pp 1659–1695.

172 Single Ventricle

Tal Geva and *Stella Van Praagh*

Definition

The normal human heart is composed of three chambers at the ventricular level (between the atrioventricular [AV] valves and the semilunar valves): the left ventricular (LV) sinus, the right ventricular (RV) sinus, and the infundibulum. Single ventricle is said to be present when one of the two ventricular sinuses is absent. The infundibulum is always present and has been described by various terms such as infundibular outlet chamber, rudimentary or hypoplastic right ventricle, and rudimentary chamber. There are two anatomic types of single ventricle: single left ventricle (LV) (RV sinus is absent) and single right ventricle (RV) (LV sinus cannot be identified).

Etiology and Morphogenesis

The cause of single ventricle is unknown. It may be the end result of several morphogenetic mechanisms that are affected by genetic and hemodynamic abnormalities.

Epidemiology

Single ventricle, as defined above, accounts for approximately 1 per cent of congenital heart disease. Assuming approximately 4 million live births annually and given an estimated prevalence of congenital heart disease of 8 to 10 cases per 1000 live births, approximately 320 to 400 newborns are diagnosed each year in the United States with anatomic single ventricle. If patients with tricuspid atresia and other anatomic variants are included, the prevalence increases to approximately 1000 newborns per year.

Pathologic Anatomy

There are two types of single ventricle.

1. *Single LV*—Several anatomic types of single LV are recognized. Common to all is the absence of an RV sinus and the presence of an LV and an infundibulum.

   a. There is communication between the LV and the infundibulum, termed the bulboventricular foramen or ventricular septal defect (VSD). The different anatomic types of single LV vary according to the type of ventricular loop present and the types of AV and ventriculoarterial alignments.

   b. When two AV valves enter the LV (double-inlet LV), their different papillary muscle architectures reflect their identity. The tricuspid valve is typically closer to the septum (septophilic); it may have chordal attachments on the septum or to the inferior VSD margin, or both, and sometimes into the infundibulum (Fig. 172–1A). By contrast, the mitral valve attaches to the free wall papillary muscles (septophobic). If the two AV valves share the LV cavity, usually one, and rarely both, are abnormal. If only the mitral valve enters the LV (i.e., tricuspid atresia), it is typically structurally normal (see Fig. 172–1B). Other types of AV alignments in single LV include common inlet, when a common AV valve is present, and mitral atresia with a large LV (see Fig. 172–1C).

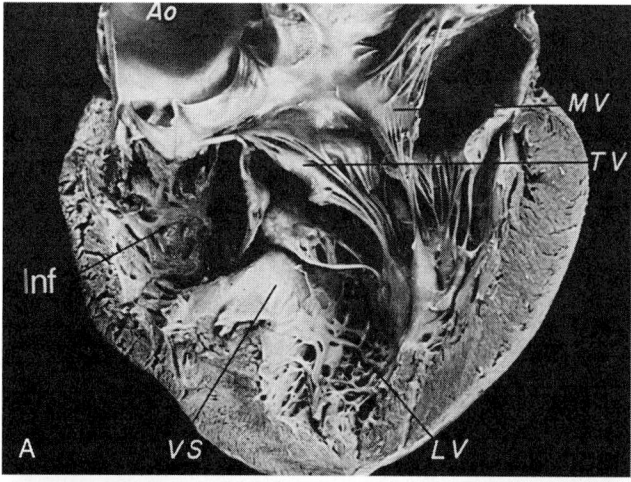

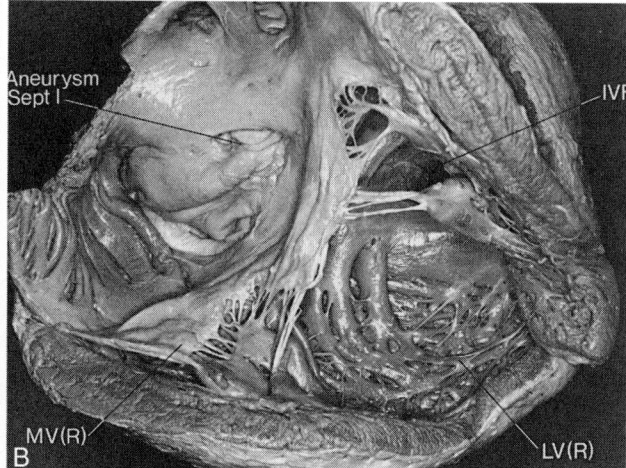

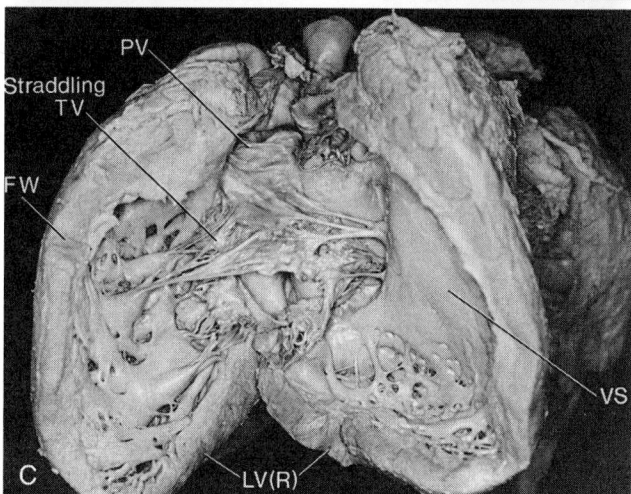

Figure 172–1 *A,* Double-inlet left ventricle (LV) with normally related great arteries and D-loop ventricles. The tricuspid valve (TV) has attachments on the LV and on the outflow infundibular chamber (Inf). The mitral valve (MV) attaches only on the free wall of the LV. Ao = aorta; VS = ventricular septum. *B,* The single LV of a 14-year-old boy with solitus atria and L-loop (inverted) ventricles. The atretic TV is left-sided. The normal right-sided mitral valve (MV(R)) is the only valve in this right-sided LV (LV(R)). Sept I = septum primum. *C,* The single LV of a 27-year-old man with solitus atria, L-loop (inverted) ventricles, and right-sided mitral atresia. This single LV(R) displays the characteristic left ventricular smooth septal surface. The left-sided TV straddles the ventricular septum (VS) and displays attachments on the free wall (FW) of the LV, the lower margin of the ventricular septal defect, and the infundibular outlet chamber. Compare the morphology of a tricuspid valve in the LV (*C*) with the morphology of a mitral valve in a single LV (Fig. 172–2*B*). This is one of the rare associations where the morphologic single LV contains a single valve which is the tricuspid. PV = pulmonary valve. (*A* from Van Praagh R, Plett JA, Van Praagh S: Single ventricle: Pathology, embryology, terminology and classification. Herz 1979; 4:113–150. *C* from Shinpo H, Van Praagh S, Parness I, et al: Mitral atresia with a large left ventricle and an undeveloped or absent right ventricular sinus. J Am Coll Cardiol 1992; 19:1561–1576.)

c. The types of ventriculoarterial connections include (1) normally related great arteries (Holmes heart), in which the aorta arises from the LV and the pulmonary artery from the infundibulum; (2) transposition of the great arteries, in which the pulmonary artery arises from the LV and the aorta from the infundibulum; and (3) double-outlet infundibulum, in which both aorta and pulmonary artery arise from the infundibulum. Pulmonary stenosis or atresia, aortic stenosis or atresia, and aortic arch anomalies (most commonly coarctation) may be associated with single LV.

2. *Single RV*—Single RV consists of the RV sinus and the infundibulum, both forming a common chamber. The septal band is present, indicating the location of a ventricular septum, but there is no macroscopically recognizable LV sinus on the other side of the septum. Several anatomic types of single RV are recognized.

   a. *Double-inlet RV*—Both AV valves open into the RV. The tricuspid valve attaches in the inlet (sinus) portion of the RV, and the mitral valve attaches in the outflow or infundibulum. Both valves exhibit attachments to the septal band.

   b. *Common-inlet single RV*—A single AV valve connects both atria with the RV. The morphology is often that of a tricuspid valve, but the presence of an ostium primum defect and the alignment of both atria with the single RV indicate that this is a common AV valve mimicking a tricuspid valve. This type of single RV usually occurs in association with visceral heterotaxy and asplenia. Associated malformations include anomalies of the systemic and pulmonary venous connections, absence or marked hypoplasia of the atrial septum, absence of the coronary sinus, and pulmonary outflow tract stenosis or atresia. In both types of single RV, both great arteries originate from the infundibulum, and the resulting ventriculoarterial alignment is that of double-outlet RV.

Pathophysiology

Single ventricle physiology is characterized by complete mixing of the systemic and pulmonary venous return flows. The proportion of the ventricular output distributed to the pulmonary or systemic vascular bed is determined by the relative resistance to flow in the two circuits.

  1. Resistance to pulmonary flow is determined by the following:

a. Degree of anatomic obstruction to pulmonary blood flow (subvalvar, valvar, or pulmonary arterial stenosis)

b. Pulmonary arteriolar resistance

c. Pulmonary venous and left atrial pressure.

2. Resistance to systemic flow is determined by the following:

a. Degree of anatomic obstruction to systemic output (subvalvar, valvar, or aortic arch obstruction or coarctation of the aorta)

b. Systemic arteriolar resistance.

Clinical Findings

The clinical presentation and course in patients with single ventricle depends on the hemodynamic profile.

1. Diminished pulmonary blood flow

a. Patients are cyanotic, and their arterial oxygen saturation is typically <75 per cent.

b. Patients do not manifest signs and symptoms of congestive heart failure.

c. Patients may have a systolic ejection murmur caused by turbulent flow across the obstructed pulmonary outflow tract.

d. Alternatively, patients may have a continuous murmur caused by a patent ductus arteriosus or aortopulmonary collaterals.

e. Clubbing of the nail beds develops later.

2. Increased pulmonary blood flow

a. Patients may be asymptomatic in the newborn and early neonatal periods.

b. Arterial oxygen saturation is typically >85 per cent, and cyanosis may not be evident.

c. Murmurs may not be heard initially.

d. During the first few weeks of life, as pulmonary vascular resistance decreases, pulmonary blood flow increases and signs and symptoms of congestive heart failure develop.

e. Heart murmurs may develop as a result of increased flow across the pulmonary outflow tract, systemic outflow tract obstruction, or AV valve regurgitation.

f. Diminished femoral pulses indicate the presence of aortic coarctation.

3. Balanced circulation

a. Patients exhibit mild to moderate cyanosis, with arterial oxygen saturation of 75 to 85 per cent.

b. A prominent systolic ejection murmur is present because of pulmonary outflow tract obstruction.

c. Patients do not manifest signs and symptoms of congestive heart failure.

4. *Closing duct*—Patients with a duct-dependent pulmonary circulation and a closing duct present with profound cyanosis and acidemia. Patients with a duct-dependent systemic circulation present with a clinical picture of shock, hypoperfusion, poor peripheral pulses, oliguria or anuria, and acidemia.

5. *Atypical clinical picture*—Although many patients with single ventricle can be fitted into one of the above categories, the progressive nature of certain anatomic and hemodynamic factors may alter the clinical picture in a given patient. Examples include development of AV valve regurgitation in a patient with decreased pulmonary blood flow, progressive narrowing of a bulboventricular foramen leading to severe subaortic stenosis, and development of pulmonary vascular obstructive disease.

Key Clinical Findings

- Findings vary with changing hemodynamics
- Patients may or may not be cyanotic

Laboratory Findings

1. *Hematology*—Most patients with single ventricle manifest varying degrees of polycythemia. Iron deficiency may be present and should be corrected. Howell-Jolly bodies can be seen in the red blood cells by peripheral blood smear in patients with heterotaxy syndrome and asplenia.

2. *Electrocardiography*—The electrocardiogram is typically abnormal, with evidence of left or right ventricular hypertrophy depending on the type of single ventricle present. If there is ventricular inversion (L-loop), the right chest leads show increased left ventricular forces. Around the chest precordial leads may be necessary in order to obtain the Q wave of septal depolarization. Since the advent of echocardiography, the electrocardiogram is seldom used for anatomic diagnosis of single ventricle. Rhythm abnormalities are encountered in increasing frequency with advancing age and surgical procedures.

Key Laboratory Findings

- Varying degree of polycythemia
- Electrocardiographic abnormalities

Diagnostic Imaging

1. Chest radiography is helpful in determining visceral situs and cardiac position. In patients with decreased pulmonary blood flow, the heart size may be normal or mildly increased and the pulmonary vascular markings are normal or decreased. In patients with pulmonary overcirculation, cardiomegaly and increased pulmonary vascular markings are present.

2. Echocardiography with Doppler ultrasound is the primary diagnostic modality. The initial management of most infants with single ventricle can be based on data obtained by echocardiography and Doppler ultrasound studies (Fig. 172–2). Transesophageal echocardiography is a useful diagnostic modality in older patients with inadequate acoustic windows and in patients who have undergone multiple operations.

3. Cardiac catheterization and angiography provide additional hemodynamic and anatomic information. Aortopulmonary collaterals, pulmonary vascular architecture, pressure, and resistance are best assessed by cardiac cath-

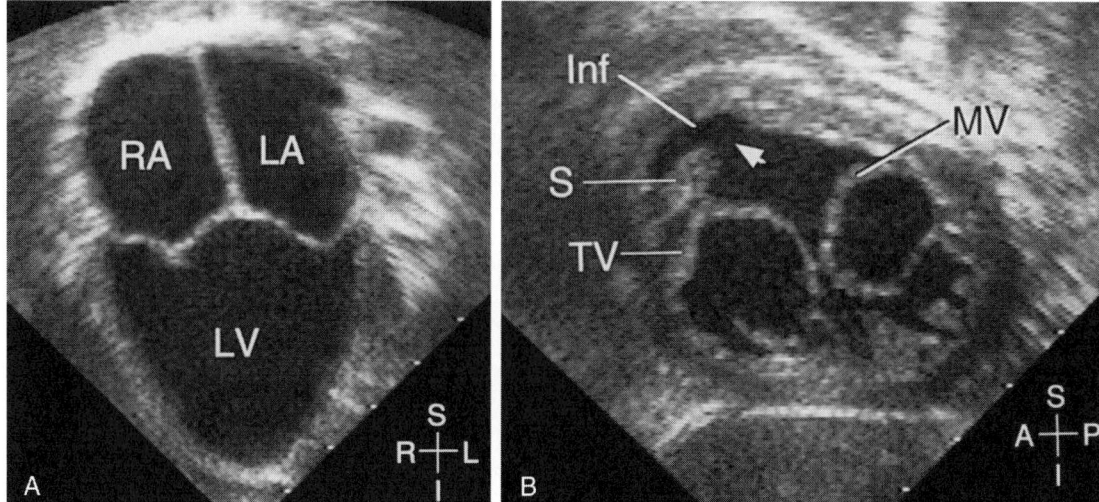

Figure 172–2 Two-dimensional echocardiogram in a 3-week-old infant with double-inlet left ventricle (LV) and transposition of the great arteries. *A,* Apical four-chamber view showing a large LV receives both the mitral and tricuspid valves. LA = left atrium; RA = right atrium. *B,* Subxiphoid short-axis view showing a cross-section of both atrioventricular valves opening into the large LV. The mitral valve (MV) has attachments only to the LV free wall, whereas the tricuspid valve (TV) has attachments both to the free wall and to the septum (S). A small infundibular outlet chamber (Inf) is seen on the anterosuperior aspect of the LV, with a bulboventricular foramen *(arrow)* communicating between the two chambers. (From Streeter GL: Developmental horizons in human embryos: Description of age groups XV, XVI, XVII, and XVIII. Contrib Endocrinol 1948; 32:133–203. © Carnegie Institution of Washington.)

eterization and angiography. In addition, transcatheter therapeutic interventions such as balloon and/or blade atrial septostomy, balloon dilatation of valvular or vascular stenosis, device closure of intracardiac shunts, and coil occlusion of excessive collaterals are used in conjunction with surgery to treat patients with single ventricle. Cardiac catheterization is recommended before a bidirectional Glenn operation or one of the modifications of the Fontan procedure is performed.

4. Magnetic resonance imaging is emerging as a very useful noninvasive diagnostic tool in patients with complex congenital heart disease.

Treatment

Although isolated case reports of individuals with single ventricle who survived beyond the third and fourth decades of life have been published, more than 90 per cent of surgically untreated patients die before their tenth birthday. These data form the rationale for the current treatment of patients with single ventricle.

1. Initial management of infants with single ventricle depends on the anatomic and hemodynamic profile of the patient.

   a. In patients whose pulmonary or systemic circulation depends on ductal patency, emergency administration of prostaglandin E intravenously can be lifesaving. Additional management is directed toward restoration of a normal acid-base balance, adequate ventilation and gas exchange, and myocardial pressor support if necessary.

   b. Patients with a well-balanced circulation may not need any intervention until symptoms develop or the hemodynamic profile changes.

   c. Patients with decreased pulmonary blood flow and prominent cyanosis in the first 2 to 4 months of life may require placement of a systemic-to-pulmonary-artery shunt to augment pulmonary blood flow.

   d. Patients with excessive pulmonary blood flow and unobstructed systemic arterial flow are at risk for development of elevated pulmonary vascular resistance, pulmonary vascular obstructive disease, changes in ventricular geometry, and ventricular dysfunction due to chronic volume overload. Banding of the main pulmonary artery decreases pulmonary blood flow and controls pulmonary arterial pressure. Banding is a short-term, palliative procedure used as a bridge for surgical procedures aimed at unloading the single ventricle and separating the systemic and pulmonary circulations (the bidirectional Glenn and modified Fontan operations; Fig. 172–3).

   e. Patients with excessive pulmonary blood flow and obstruction to systemic arterial flow require a procedure to decrease pulmonary blood flow and an additional procedure to relieve the systemic obstructive lesion. Several procedures are available for relief of aortic outflow tract obstruction, depending on the anatomy of the individual patient and on the preference and experience of the managing team:

      (1) Transection of the main pulmonary artery, anastomosis of the proximal main pulmonary artery to the ascending aorta (Damus-Kaye-Stansel procedure), and placement of modified Blalock-Taussig shunt

      (2) Enlargement of the bulboventricular foramen

      (3) Arterial switch operation.

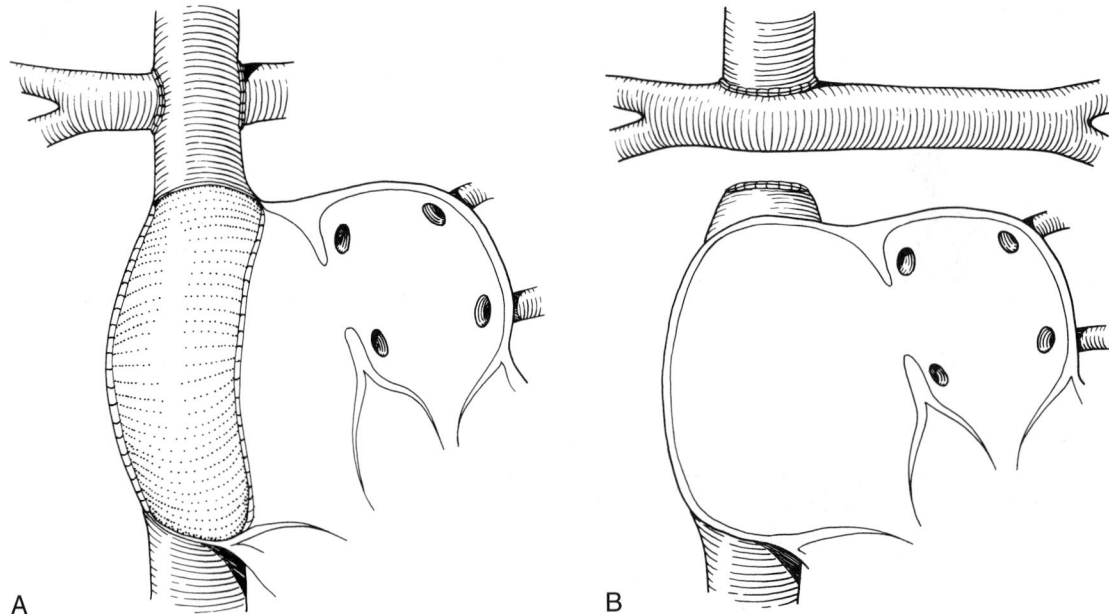

A   B

Figure 172–3 *A,* Modified Fontan operation with total cavopulmonary anastomosis. The inferior vena cava is connected to the superior vena cava by a lateral tunnel in the right atrium. A small fenestration (~4 mm in diameter) may be placed in the medial wall of the lateral tunnel to allow decompression of the systemic venous chamber (not shown). The Fontan operation achieves both unloading of the single ventricle and separation of the systemic and pulmonary circulations. *B,* Bidirectional Glenn procedure in which the superior vena cava is anastomosed to the right pulmonary artery so that the systemic venous return from the upper part of the body is diverted directly into the pulmonary circulation. The cardiac end of the superior vena cava may be oversewn or the right atrial–superior vena caval junction may be closed with a patch. The main pulmonary artery is usually divided, but in some cases it is allowed to remain patent. The aims of the bidirectional Glenn procedure are to decrease the volume load on the single ventricle and to serve as bridge toward completion of the Fontan operation.

2. The goals of current surgical therapy in patients with single ventricle are to separate the systemic and pulmonary circulations and to eliminate volume overload on the ventricle. These goals can be achieved by one of the modifications of the Fontan operation (see Fig. 172–3). The principal aim of the procedure is to divert the systemic venous return from the inferior and superior venae cavae to the pulmonary arteries, which separates the poorly oxygenated systemic venous return from the oxygenated pulmonary venous return.

3. Several preoperative risk factors are reported to be associated with a higher risk of mortality after a modified Fontan operation:

   a. High pulmonary artery pressure and pulmonary vascular resistance
   b. Pulmonary artery distortion
   c. More than mild AV valve regurgitation
   d. Systemic ventricular dysfunction
   e. Moderate or severe systemic ventricular hypertrophy
   f. Young age (the question of appropriate age for the modified Fontan procedure is still controversial)
   g. Pulmonary venous obstruction
   h. Certain anatomic subgroups such as heterotaxy syndrome and left AV valve atresia (mitral or tricuspid).

Key Treatment

• Corrective surgery

Prevention

Currently there is no available means of preventing single ventricle. Prenatal diagnosis is feasible by fetal echocardiography as early as 16 to 17 weeks' gestation.

Bibliography

Bevilacqua M, Sanders SP, Van Praagh S, et al: Double-inlet left ventricle: Echocardiographic anatomy with emphasis on the morphology of the atrioventricular valves and ventricular septal defect. J Am Coll Cardiol 1991;18:559–568.

Fisher DJ, Geva T, Feltes TF, et al: A protocol for the lifelong management of patients with a single functional ventricle. Tex Heart Inst J 1995;22:284–295.

Fyler DC: Single ventricle. *In* Fyler DC (ed): Nadas Pediatric Cardiology. Philadelphia, Hanley & Belfus, 1992, pp 649–657.

Shinpo H, Van Praagh S, Parness I, et al: Mitral atresia with a large left ventricle and an underdeveloped or absent right ventricular sinus: Clinical profile, anatomic data and surgical considerations. J Am Coll Cardiol 1992;19:1561–1576.

Van Praagh R, Plett JA, Van Praagh S: Single ventricle: Pathology, embryology, terminology and classification. Herz 1979;4:113–150.

173 Ventricular Septal Defects

Ronald M. Lauer

Definition

Ventricular septal defects are those that affect the septum in areas other than the atrioventricular septal area. Ventricular septal defects affect the perimembranous septum, the trabecular muscular septum, and the outlet septum. These are illustrated in Figure 173–1. Defects in the ventricular septum are associated with many other cardiac as well as extracardiac anomalies but, for the most part, occur as isolated defects.

Epidemiology

Defects in the ventricular septum are the most common of all congenital heart defects, occurring in about 1.8/1000 live births and constituting ≥20 per cent of all congenital heart disease. Various studies have shown that defects in the muscular septum make up 40 to 50 per cent and perimembranous defects 30 to 50 per cent of VSDs. Outlet VSDs are much less common in white subjects, composing 3 to 5 per cent, but in Japanese and Chinese they constitute about 30 per cent of VSDs. Outlet defects are often associated with aortic valve regurgitation.

Etiology

Although the etiology of ventricular septal defects is unknown, the condition is often found in association with a number of dysmorphic syndromes.

Pathophysiology

1. Size—The size of the defect is a major determinant of its severity. Very small defects cause no hemodynamic derangement. Large defects result in serious hemodynamic derangement with congestive heart failure, poor feeding, and poor growth and development. Because the size of the defect varies, the severity of symptoms and their time of onset also are variable.

2. Pulmonary vascular resistance—At birth the pulmonary vascular resistance is high and falls rapidly to near-adult levels by 2 to 3 months of age. As the pulmonary resistance falls the flow from the left to right ventricle increases. When the pulmonary resistance reaches its minimum, the flow across the defect reaches its maximum. Thus it is not unusual to see babies at birth who temporarily adjust well to the defect but develop signs of heart failure several weeks or months later.

In subjects who have been allowed to remain with a large defect beyond 2 years of age a number will develop occlusive pulmonary vascular disease, which results in an increasing level of pulmonary vascular resistance. When the pulmonary resistance exceeds the systemic resistance, the flow across the defect will flow right to left and the patient will become cyanotic. Once the pulmonary vascular resistance becomes severely elevated and is unresponsive to vasodilators (e.g., O_2, NO), the risk of surgical closure is prohibitive.

3. Spontaneous closure of ventricular septal defects—In muscular and perimembranous defects, spontaneous closure is frequent. In small defects evident on auscultation in the newborn, spontaneous closure occurs in about 60 per cent of cases. In large defects in which serious symptoms occur, closure occurs in only 10 to 12 per cent. Outlet defects of all sizes seldom undergo spontaneous closure; however, they can be partially occluded with a prolapsed aortic valve leaflet, which results in aortic valve regurgitation.

Clinical Findings

1. Presentation
   a. In the newborn period a systolic murmur may heard on routine physical examination.
   b. With large defects, when the pulmonary vascular resistance becomes minimum (2 to 3 months of age) the flow across the defect becomes maximal, and the signs of congestive heart failure occur: tachypnea, grunting respirations, tachycardia, and fatigue with feeding.

2. Physical findings on heart examination
   a. Small defects
      (1) The child appears normal.
      (2) The heart is quiet to palpation with neither a right or a left ventricular lift. No thrills are usually felt. A grade 1–3/6 systolic murmur may be heard at the lower left sternal margin. The second heart sound is normally split and accentuated.

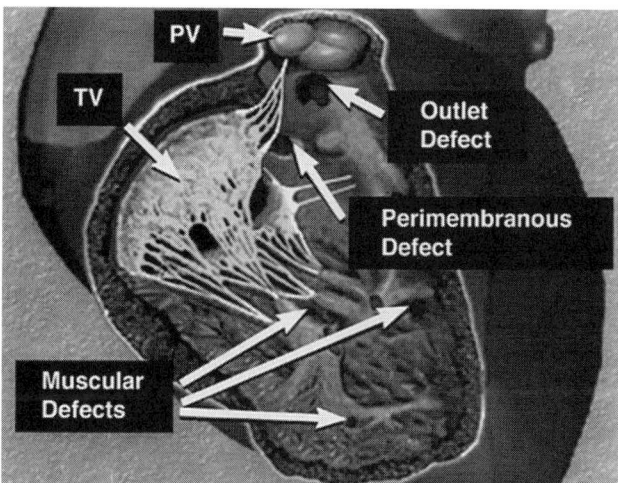

Figure 173–1 Ventricular septum viewed through the anterior surface of the right ventricle. A perimembranous defect is seen just below the tricuspid valve. Multiple defects in the trabecular muscular septum are shown. An outlet defect is demonstrated beneath the pulmonic valve. PV, Pulmonary valve; TV, tricuspid valve.

b. Large defects with low pulmonary vascular resistance
  (1) The infant appears ill, with poor weight gain.
  (2) Signs of congestive heart failure may be seen: tachypnea, tachycardia, grunting respirations, prolonged pulmonary expiration, pulmonary rales (a late manifestation), hepatomegaly, and periorbital and limb edema (a late manifestation).
  (3) The heart is overactive with either a left ventricular or a combined ventricular lift. A systolic thrill at the left sternal margin may be present. A grade 3–5 harsh pansystolic murmur is heard best at the lower left sternal margin. A mid-diastolic rumble is heard best at the apex of the heart with a bell of the stethoscope lightly applied.
c. Large defects with high pulmonary vascular resistance
  (1) Usually older children or young adults
  (2) Cyanosis
  (3) Digital clubbing
  (4) Poor exercise tolerance
  (5) The heart shows a right ventricular lift. The second heart sound is split, and the pulmonary component is accentuated. There are usually faint systolic murmurs to be heard at the lower left sternal margin. A decrescendo diastolic murmur of pulmonary valve insufficiency may be heard.

Key Laboratory Findings

• Echocardiography/Doppler

Laboratory Findings

1. Hematologic
Usually there are no abnormalities. If there is high pulmonary vascular resistance with a right-to-left shunt resulting in significant oxygen desaturation, polycythemia may occur.
2. Electrocardiographic—The ECG may be normal when there is a small defect. When the defects are moderate or large, left ventricular hypertrophy or combined ventricular hypertrophy may be seen. When there is high pulmonary vascular resistance, right ventricular hypertrophy alone may be seen. When there is left axis deviation, a defect in the atrioventricular canal should be suspected.
3. Echocardiography/Doppler
Defects in the ventricular septum may be directly visualized, and the flow across them may seen by color Doppler technique. From the velocities measured across the defect it is usually possible to estimate right ventricular and pulmonary artery systolic pressure if the cuff systolic pressure is known. When defects are very small, it sometimes is not possible to visualize the defects.
4. Radiographic findings
With small defects, the chest x-ray findings are normal.

With larger defects, the heart is enlarged and the pulmonary arteries are dilated. The intrapulmonary vascular markings are increased. When the pulmonary blood flow is extremely large, air trapping is seen.
5. Cardiac catheterization and angiocardiography
Necessary when
  a. The anatomic features cannot be defined by echocardiography.
  b. The pulmonary vascular resistance is elevated. Pulmonary vascular reactivity is tested with oxygen or nitric oxide. If it is possible to lower pulmonary resistance, it may be possible to consider surgical closure.

Treatment

1. Small defects—When defects are small with pulmonary to systemic flow ratios <2, surgical correction is not required because of the excellent prognosis. Only bacterial endocarditis precautions are required.
2. Moderate and large left-to-right shunts—When left-to-right shunts have pulmonary to systemic flow ratios ≥2, surgical correction is recommended.
  a. Less than 6 months—Because of the higher risk for surgery it is usually not performed unless congestive heart failure is intractable. If after decongestive measures an infant is unable to take in sufficient calories for growth or if weight gain is not sufficient, open heart surgical repair of the defect is indicated.
  b. Six to 24 months—If pulmonary hypertension or symptoms are present, surgery is indicated to prevent the development of hypertensive vascular disease, to relieve symptoms, and to allow normal growth.
  c. Greater than 24 months—If the pulmonary resistance is low and the pulmonary to systemic flow ratio is ≥2, surgical correction is recommended to prevent the development of hypertensive vascular disease. If the pulmonary to systemic flow ratio is ≤1.5 and the pulmonary resistance is extremely high, surgical correction is not indicated unless the pulmonary resistance can be shown to be reactive at the time of cardiac catheterization.

Key Treatment

• Small defects—spontaneous closure often occurs
• Bacterial endocarditis precautions
• Large defects—surgery

Bibliography

Gumbiner CH, Takao A: Ventricular septal defect. *In* Garson A Jr, Bricke JT, McNamara DG (eds): The Science and Practice of Pediatric Cardiology, vol II. Philadelphia, Lea & Febiger, 1990, pp 1002–1022.
Hoffman JIE, Rudolph AM: The natural history of ventricular septal defects in infancy. Am J Cardiol 1965;16:634–653.

Levy RJ, Rosenthal A, Miettinen OS, Nadas AS: Determinants of growth in patients with ventricular septal defect. Circulation 1978;57:793–797.

Pexieder T, Bloch D: EUROCAT Subproject on Epidemiology of Congenital Heart Disease: First analysis of the complete study.

In Clark EB, Markwald RR, Takao A (eds): Developmental Mechanisms of Heart Disease. Futura Publishing, Armonk, NY, 1995, pp 655–671.

Soto B, Becker AE, Moulaert AJ, et al: Classification of ventricular septal defects. Br Heart J 1980;43:332–343.

174 Atrial Septal Defects

Thomas D. Scholz

Nomenclature

Four types of atrial septal defects (ASDs) have been described—secundum, primum, sinus venosus, and coronary sinus.

Embryology

Septation of the atria occurs through development of the septum primum and septum secundum. In the fourth embryonic week, the septum primum grows inferiorly, gradually closing the ostium primum. As the ostium primum is closed by endocardial cushion tissue, openings develop in the midportion of the septum primum (ostium secundum). An infolding in the roof of the atrium develops into the septum secundum, which extends inferiorly and to the right of the septum primum. Septa are complete by 7 weeks of gestation.

Etiology

1. Secundum ASDs result from deficiency in the septum secundum or excessive resorption of the septum primum during formation of the ostium secundum.
2. Primum ASDs are due to insufficient extension of the endocardial cushions and often are associated with a cleft mitral valve.
3. Sinus venosus defects may reflect abnormal migration of the right pulmonary veins and are often associated with partial anomalous pulmonary venous return of the right pulmonary veins.
4. Coronary sinus ASDs are thought to result from failure of formation of the wall between the coronary sinus and the left atrium and are typically associated with a persistent left superior vena cava.

Epidemiology

1. Isolated secundum ASDs account for approximately 7 per cent of patients with congenital heart disease. The female:male ratio is approximately 2:1.
2. Virtually 100 per cent of ASDs ≤3 mm in diameter identified by echocardiography in infants ≤3 months of age will close spontaneously.
3. As many as 80 per cent of ASDs 5 to 8 mm in size will close by 18 months of age.
4. ASDs ≥8 mm in size rarely close spontaneously.
5. "Probe patent" ASDs are found in 25 to 30 per cent of adults; they represent failure of the septum secundum and fibrose to the septum primum postnatally. These lesions may allow paradoxical systemic emboli if right atrial pressure exceeds left atrial pressure, even transiently.
6. Most secundum ASDs are not familial. Familial ASDs have been described in association with the autosomal dominant Holt-Oram syndrome (upper limb anomalies, including absent or hypoplastic radii, and ECG findings of right bundle branch block or first-degree atrioventricular block).

Pathophysiology

1. The degree of shunting through an ASD is determined primarily by the relative compliance of the right and left ventricles (though small ASDs may restrict flow). At birth, the compliance of the right and left ventricles is comparable. Thus, little shunting through the ASD will occur. With increasing age, the right ventricular compliance decreases, resulting in increased left-to-right shunting through the ASD.
2. Pathophysiologic consequences are determined primarily by the degree of left-to-right shunting through the ASD. Defects with a pulmonary-to-systemic flow ratio (Qp:Qs) <1.5 to 2:1 typically do not have any significant sequelae and do not require operation. Recent findings of adults with paradoxical emboli (e.g., stroke) possibly due to transient right-to-left shunting through small ASDs may change this recommendation.
3. Systemic cyanosis due to significant right-to-left shunting can occur under two circumstances. In the presence of severe right ventricular outflow tract obstruction, the compliance of the right ventricle can increase sufficiently to cause right-to-left shunting through an ASD. With persistent left-to-right shunts of sufficient magnitude (typically a Qp:Qs >2:1), pulmonary vascular occlusive disease will develop in ≤10 per cent of patients. This results in increased right-sided pressures and right-to-left shunting. Pulmonary vascular occlusive disease due to an ASD appears to occur more commonly in women and typically after the age of 19 years.

Clinical Findings

1. History
   a. Failure to thrive due to an ASD is uncommon.
   b. Older children with large shunts may complain of increased fatigability.
2. Examination

a. Limb examination is particularly important in familial cases of ASD (looking for radial anomalies associated with Holt-Oram syndrome).

b. A hyperdynamic impulse of the right ventricle may be palpated at the lower left sternal border (an RV "heave").

c. An impulse over the left upper sternal border may be palpated in older patients with pulmonary vascular occlusive disease.

3. Auscultation

a. Wide fixed split S2 is found owing to delayed closure of the pulmonic valve, which does not vary with respiration. The second heart sound is best evaluated in the sitting or standing position.

b. A systolic ejection murmur is best heard at the upper left sternal border (second intercostal space) owing to increased flow across the pulmonic valve. If a thrill is felt in this location, associated pulmonic stenosis is generally present.

c. An early to mid-diastolic rumble is heard at the lower left sternal border owing to increased flow across the tricuspid valve. The diastolic murmur is typically heard in patients with a Qp:Qs >2:1.

Key Clinical Findings

- Systolic ejection murmur
- Early to mid-diastolic rumble
- Fixed split second sound

Laboratory Findings

1. Electrocardiogram

a. Most patients have normal sinus rhythm.

b. Sinus venosus defects are often associated with a leftward frontal P-wave axis ($<0°$).

c. Most have an RSR′ pattern in the right precordial leads (V1, V3R, and V4R) as a result of volume overload hypertrophy (R′ >5 mm is abnormal in infants, and >10 mm is abnormal in children).

2. Chest x-ray

a. In patients with small shunts (Qp:Qs <2:1), chest x-ray may be normal.

b. Cardiomegaly (cardiothoracic ratio >0.5) is found with larger shunts.

c. Increased pulmonary vascular markings are found with shunts >2:1.

d. The main pulmonary artery trunk can also be prominent.

e. Lateral views show an enlarged right ventricle filling the retrosternal space.

3. Echocardiogram

a. 2-D Echocardiography can identify most ASDs along with enlargement of the right atrium, right ventricle, and main pulmonary artery.

b. Color Doppler allows visualization of the left-to-right shunting of blood through the ASD.

c. Pulsed Doppler can be used to estimate the Qp:Qs ratio by integrating the time-velocity tracing of the pulmonary artery and aorta and multiplying by the respective valve areas and heart rate.

d. A rapid upstroke and descent of the pulmonary artery Doppler flow signal suggests pulmonary hypertension. Also, pulsed Doppler may be used to measure the peak velocity of a tricuspid insufficiency jet to estimate RV pressure using the formula

$$4 \times (\text{peak velocity})^2 + \text{estimated RA pressure}$$

e. Transesophageal echocardiography may help identify sinus venosus defects in older patients.

4. Cardiac catheterization

a. Cardiac catheterization is rarely needed for the preoperative evaluation of the patient with an ASD.

b. If pulmonary hypertension is suspected, a cardiac catheterization is needed.

c. Cardiac catheterization may also be needed to identify pulmonary venous return in patients with a sinus venosus ASD.

d. Cineangiography can demonstrate an ASD via an injection into the main pulmonary artery. Return of contrast agent to the right atrium and right ventricle will be seen as pulmonary venous return to the left atrium crosses the ASD.

Key Laboratory Findings

- Echocardiography

Treatment

1. Medical

a. Though uncommon, infants with congestive heart failure due to left-to-right shunting across an ASD should initially be treated medically. Furosemide (1 mg/kg/dose PO bid) and digoxin (5 μg/kg/dose PO bid) are the initial medications. Addition of potassium chloride (1 mEq/kg/dose PO bid) is usually necessary to prevent potassium depletion due to furosemide. Early ASD closure should be considered in these patients.

b. Subacute bacterial endocarditis (SBE) prophylaxis is not recommended for patients with an isolated ASD.

2. Closure of ASDs is recommended for lesions with a Qp:Qs >1.5 or 2:1 around the age of 3 to 5 years, prior to the child's entering school. Closure helps prevent the long-term sequelae of pulmonary vascular occlusive disease and atrial arrhythmias.

3. Paradoxical emboli through ASDs causing strokes in adult patients raises the question as to whether smaller ASDs should be closed. Until more is known about the number of adults with small ASDs and the frequency with which the small ASDs allow paradoxical embolization, routine surgical closure of hemodynamically insignificant ASDs cannot be advocated.

4. Surgical closure
   a. Cardiopulmonary bypass is required for closure of an ASD.
   b. Mortality due to surgery is generally ≤1 per cent.
   c. Morbidity from surgery includes postpericardiotomy syndrome and damage to the thoracic duct or phrenic nerve.
5. Catheter closure
   a. Transcatheter techniques for ASD closure continue to be evaluated to reduce the length of hospitalization needed and the risks associated with surgery.
   b. A double-umbrella device appears to have promise of widespread use, although the FDA has stopped clinical trials.

Key Treatment

- Small defects usually close spontaneously
- Large defects—surgery

Prognosis

Patients with surgical closure prior to 25 years of age have been shown to have a normal life expectancy.

Bibliography

Murphy JG, Gersh BJ, McGoon MD, et al: Long-term outcome after surgical repair of isolated atrial septal defect. Follow-up at 27 to 32 years. N Engl J Med 1990;323:1645–1650.

Porter CJ, Feldt RH, Edwards WD, et al: Atrial septal defects. *In* Emmanouilides GC, Riemenschneider TA, Allen HD, Gutgesell HP (eds): Heart Disease in Infants, Children, and Adolescents, 5th ed, vol 1. Baltimore, Williams & Wilkins, 1995, pp 687–703.

Radzik D, Davignon A, van Doesburg N, et al: Predictive factors for spontaneous closure of atrial septal defects diagnosed in the first 3 months of life. J Am Coll Cardiol 1992;22:851–853.

Vick GW III, Titus JL: Defects of the atrial septum including the atrioventricular canal. *In* Garson A Jr, Bricker JT, McNamara DG (eds): The Science and Practice of Pediatric Cardiology, vol II. Philadelphia, Lea & Febiger, 1990, pp 1023–1036.

175 Patent Ductus Arteriosus

Jill H. Morriss

Definition

The ductus arteriosus is the normal fetal blood vessel connecting the pulmonary artery to the descending aorta. In the mammalian embryo, the ductus is the channel through which blood is diverted away from the nonexpanded fetal lungs into the descending aorta and thence to the placenta to allow for respiratory gas exchange. The ductus arteriosus normally closes soon after birth. Failure of or delayed closure results in a patent ductus arteriosus (PDA).

Etiology

Complex interactions between mechanical, neural, hormonal, and chemical factors result in functional and usually complete postnatal ductal closure. In a subset of patients identified as having a PDA within the first 2 weeks after birth, true abnormalities in the morphology of the ductal wall are thought to explain the failure of ductal closure. The role of rubella infection in the increased incidence of PDA is known, and patients who live at high altitude are overrepresented in the distribution of PDA.

Epidemiology

PDA is reported to occur in 12 to 15 per cent of infants and children with significant congenital heart disease. In the preterm infant, the incidence of PDA is much higher than stated above and is directly related to weight and gestational age. For example, PDA is recognized in 60 per cent of infants with birth weights between 1000 and 1250 g who have an echocardiographic study within 2 weeks after birth.

Pathophysiology

1. The direction of flow across the patent ductus arteriosus is determined by well-known physical laws relating blood flow, pressures, and resistances in the connected systemic and pulmonary circulations.
2. When the ductus remains patent in patients with otherwise normal cardiac anatomy, the direction of flow is most commonly from the high-pressure aorta into the lower pressure pulmonary artery. The resulting left-to-right shunt causes pulmonary overcirculation, which varies in amount based on the anatomic size of the ductus as well as the pulmonary vascular (arteriolar) resistance.
3. When pulmonary vascular resistance exceeds systemic vascular resistance, flow across a PDA is reversed, with a right-to-left ductal shunt reflected in lower body desaturation.
4. Contrasted with the foregoing categories are those cases in which a PDA is but one feature of congenital heart disease.
5. Ductal-dependent lesions are those for which patency of the ductus makes an essential contribution to stability and survival. For example, a patient with pulmonary valve atresia requires a PDA for survival. Severe left heart obstruction with aortic valve atresia requires that systemic blood flow be provided from the pulmonary artery through the ductus that remains patent; the ascending aorta and coronaries as well as the distal aorta receive flow via the ductus arteriosus.

6. PDA in the preterm infant with lung disease is important to recognize because it complicates the course of respiratory distress syndrome. Persistent patency of the ductus and steal syndromes from runoff into the pulmonary circulation are implicated as contributing to the risks of renal underperfusion, poor myocardial function, necrotizing enterocolitis, and intracranial underperfusion and/or cerebral hemorrhage in the newborn infant.

Clinical Findings

1. Presentation

   a. Most patients beyond the newborn period are identified as having a PDA based on recognition of a heart murmur. The magnitude of the left-to-right shunt is the major determinant of whether cardiac signs and symptoms are present.

   b. Clinical recognition of a PDA in a premature infant is usually made when a murmur is present or when, during the course of recovery from lung disease, the oxygen requirement increases. Based on the likelihood that a PDA is present in a preterm infant and will complicate the course of a sick neonate, echocardiographic studies are used to determine the persistence of a ductus.

2. Physical findings for typical PDA with left-to-right shunt

   a. *Wide pulse pressure.* A wide pulse pressure on blood pressure measurement is caused more by the lower diastolic pressure (which results from runoff into the low-resistance pulmonary circuit) than by the small increase in LV systolic pressure, which is a function of the increased stroke volume that results from LV volume overload. The wide pulse pressure is reflected by bounding peripheral pulses.

   b. *Continuous murmur.* A distinctive to-and-fro or "machinery" murmur localized to the left infraclavicular area or the upper left sternal border is the hallmark of the physical examination in a patient with isolated PDA. The ability to hear splitting of the second heart sound should be sought as assurance that the pulmonary artery pressure and resistance are not elevated to systemic levels.

   c. *Apical diastolic murmur.* When pulmonary to systemic flow ratios approach or exceed 2:1, a mitral valve inflow murmur is expected and should be sought as an additional finding to predict a large left-to-right shunt through a PDA.

   d. Other less specific observations made during a careful physical examination include a displaced and hyperdynamic apical impulse, visible carotid pulsations, a suprasternal notch thrill, and muffled heart tones "buried" in the murmur.

Key Clinical Findings

- Continuous murmur

- Wide pulse pressure

- Hyperdynamic apical pulse

Laboratory Findings

1. Roentgenographic

The chest film may be normal, whereas the diagnosis of a more significant left-to-right shunt is supported when cardiomegaly and increased pulmonary vascular markings are present. A barium esophagogram, though rarely performed as part of a routine cardiac series, would show posterior displacement of the esophagus as a sign of left atrial enlargement. When a nasogastric tube is in place during chest x-ray, a similar displacement of the tube serves as indirect evidence of left atrial enlargement. In the AP film, dilation of both the aortic knob and the main pulmonary artery segment are offered as a differentiating observation supporting PDA rather than ventricular septal defect as the site of the left-to-right shunt.

2. Electrocardiography

If the electrocardiogram is not normal, there may be evidence for left-sided volume overload patterns, such as left atrial enlargement and increase in left ventricular voltage with deep q waves seen primarily in the lateral precordial leads. The rarity of "repolarization" abnormalities is mentioned, since this finding of ST-T wave changes in an ill neonate with an extremely large ductus can influence a decision for treatment of the ductus and may be reversible after successful ductal closure.

3. Echocardiography

Echocardiography is used to

   a. Confirm the presence of the ductus, to describe the direction of flow across the ductus, and to estimate the pressure gradient across the ductus.

   b. Assess the outcome of pharmacologic treatment to close the ductus with indomethacin or to maintain patency with prostaglandins.

4. Cardiac catheterization and angiography

The need for cathetization to make a diagnosis of PDA is rare, since echocardiography has been tested and found to be reliable when a PDA is the clinical diagnosis. Historically, the confident clinical diagnosis of a PDA precluded the need for catheterization even prior to the widespread use of echocardiography. In recent years, however, the therapeutic role of catheterization has been expanded to include treatment for PDA, resulting in scheduling patients with the diagnosis of isolated PDA for catheterization. Detailed angiographic descriptions of PDA anatomy have been published and are proving to be a very important factor in deciding on candidacy for success of therapeutic closure in the catheterization laboratory. Catheterizations have been reintroduced in evaluating all patients beyond the neonatal period in whom treatment for PDA is considered.

Key Laboratory Study

- Echocardiography

Treatment

1. Premature infant with large left-to-right shunt through PDA

   a. Fluid restriction

   b. Indomethacin, in a dose of 0.2 mg/kg IV q12 hours for three doses

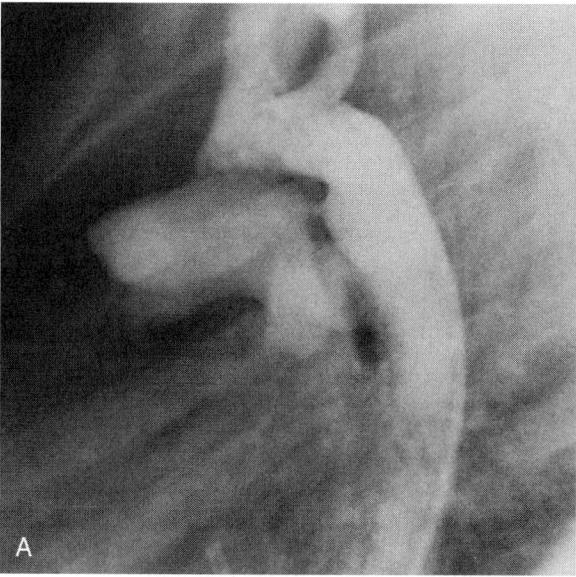
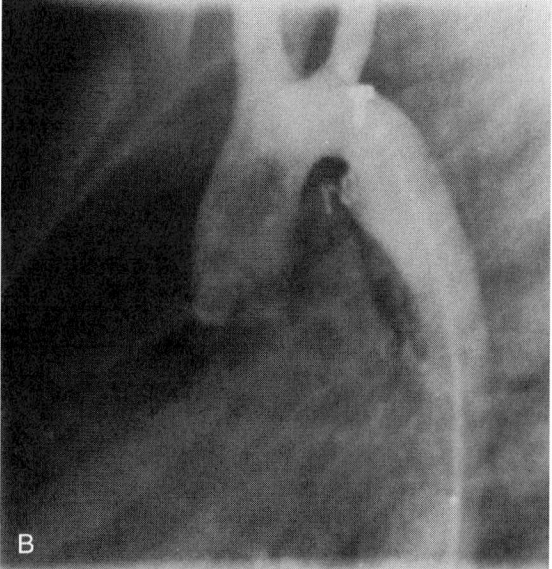

Figure 175–1 Lateral angiograms identifying PDA anatomy *(A)* and transcatheter successful coil placement *(B)* with obliteration of ductal left-to-right shunt.

c. Repeat indomethacin if treatment fails or ductus reopens.

d. Surgical ligation can be chosen when the ductus remains hemodynamically significant.

2. Full-term infants, children, and adolescents

a. PDA is often asymptomatic, and treatment is electively scheduled after 1 year of age.

b. Justification for treatment is based on the low operative risk for correction of this defect and the opinion that the surgical risk is lower than the risk of complications from the natural history of unoperated PDA, including bacterial endocarditis.

3. Methods of closure

a. Surgical ligation

b. Therapeutic catheterization with an "umbrella" device or coil procedure in the anatomically favorable smaller ductus (Fig. 175–1).

4. Endocarditis prophylaxis

Prophylaxis is used for PDA and continued for 6 months after repair of a ductus arteriosus but then discontinued if there is no residual shunt.

Key Treatment

• Surgical closure

• Coil or "umbrella" closure

Prevention

PDA is one of the few congenital lesions of the heart for which a reduction in frequency is possible. The immunization of women and children against rubella will affect the incidence of PDA as well as other sequelae of the teratogenic effects of this infection. The benefits of prenatal care will continue to improve the outlook for pregnant women and their offspring, including reducing the number of infants born preterm and at risk for problems such as PDA. The neonatal treatment of prematurely born infants with surfactant therapy and new management, including high-oscillation ventilators for lung disease, are decreasing the incidence and increasing the recognition of PDA in the early hospital course.

Bibliography

Clyman RI: Medical treatment of patent ductus arteriosus in premature infants. *In* Long WA (ed): Fetal and Neonatal Cardiology. Philadelphia, WB Saunders, 1990, pp 682–690.

Doyle TP, Hellenbrand WE: Percutaneous coil closure of the patent ductus arteriosus. ACC Curr J Rev 1994;3:47–49.

Kluckow M, Evans N: Early echocardiographic prediction of symptomatic patent ductus arteriosus in preterm infants undergoing mechanical ventilation. J Pediatr 1995;127:774–779.

Krichenko A, Benson LN, Burrows P, et al: Angiographic classification of the isolated, persistently patent ductus arteriosus and implications for percutaneous catheter occlusion. Am J Cardiol 1989;63:877–880.

Mullins CE: Patent ductus arteriosus. *In* Garson A, Bricker JT, McNamara DG (eds): The Science and Practice of Pediatric Cardiology. Malvern, PA, Lea & Febiger, 1990, pp 1055–1069.

176 Coarctation of the Aorta

Larry T. Mahoney

Definition

Coarctation of the aorta consists of a discrete narrowing in the proximal thoracic aorta, just opposite the insertion of the ductus arteriosus (juxtaductal); however, it may also consist of a long-segment stenosis, may be associated with tubular hypoplasia of the transverse arch, and may involve the abdominal aorta.

1. "Simple" coarctation

This describes a coarctation of the aorta occurring in isolation with or without the presence of a patent ductus arteriosus.

2. "Complex" coarctation

This describes the coexistence of important intracardiac anomalies, such as ventricular septal defect, aortic stenosis (valvular and subvalvular), atrioventricular septal defect, d-transposition of the great arteries, and atrial septal defects.

3. Other associated anomalies

A bicuspid aortic valve occurs in up to 85 per cent of patients with coarctation. Important vascular anomalies are associated with coarctation and include variations in the brachiocephalic artery anatomy, development of a collateral arterial circulation, and berry aneurysms of the circle of Willis.

Etiology

The underlying cause of the abnormal development of the embryologic left fourth and sixth aortic arches giving rise to coarctation is not well understood. Two concepts have been advanced, neither of which is entirely satisfactory. Coarctation may result from abnormal migration of ductus smooth muscle cells into the periductal aorta, with subsequent constriction and narrowing of the aortic lumen; or coarctation may develop as a result of hemodynamic disturbances that reduce the volume of blood flow through the fetal aortic arch and isthmus.

Epidemiology

Coarctation of the aorta is a common defect that occurs in approximately 6 to 8 per cent of patients with congenital heart disease; it is more common in males than in females. Its incidence is sporadic in most cases, but familial occurrences have been reported; it is present in approximately 35 per cent of females with the Turner XO syndrome. Simple and complex coarctation of the aorta occur with approximately equal frequency during infancy.

Pathophysiology

Hemodynamic disturbances

1. Hypertension

Depending on the severity of stenosis and extent of collateral circulation, which may decompress the ascending aorta, significant pressure differences across the coarctation may occur. The pressure gradient from ascending to descending aorta may exist throughout systole and diastole. Elevation of blood pressure in the distribution of the ascending aorta results in left ventricular myocardial hypertrophy. Left ventricular function is normal or increased (in the absence of congestive heart failure).

2. Congestive heart failure

If the coarctation is severe or develops rapidly, as in a neonate following closure of the ductus arteriosus, left ventricular dysfunction may result. The hemodynamic manifestations include diminished cardiac output, elevated left ventricular end-diastolic pressure and left atrial pressure, and pulmonary edema. The presence of associated intracardiac defects compounds the problem. Ventricular septal defects, patent ductus arteriosus, and mitral regurgitation increase left ventricular volume and preload. Left ventricular outflow obstruction, valvular or subvalvular, further increases left ventricular afterload. Congestive heart failure and pulmonary hypertension are common in infants presenting with complex coarctation.

Clinical Findings

1. Presentation

    a. Infant in congestive heart failure

Infants with complex coarctation often develop congestive heart failure, shock, and severe acidosis at approximately 7 to 14 days of life. Multiorgan failure, particularly renal failure and necrotizing enterocolitis, and subsequent death occur rapidly unless definitive medical and surgical intervention is provided immediately. Less commonly, an infant with simple coarctation may present with a more chronic picture of congestive heart failure manifested by dyspnea, poor feeding, and poor weight gain.

    b. Child with systemic hypertension and/or heart murmur

Coarctation of the aorta commonly presents later in childhood as systolic hypertension or as a heart murmur. Most patients are asymptomatic; physical findings are subtle, and delayed diagnosis is common. Referral is generally for evaluation of hypertension or an unexplained murmur, and the referring diagnosis of coarctation often is not made.

2. Physical findings

    a. The infant in congestive heart failure manifests with pallor, irritability, respiratory distress, tachycardia, tachypnea, diaphoresis, hepatomegaly, and peripheral edema.

    b. An older child generally is asymptomatic but may complain of claudication or frequent headaches.

    c. The hallmark physical finding in coarctation consists of differences in arterial pulses and blood pressures between the upper and lower extremities. Observations should be made in all four limbs. Arterial pulses distal to the coarctation are diminished in amplitude and delayed in timing when compared with proximal pulses. Systolic blood pressures in the lower extremities, normally equal to or higher than values in the upper extremities, are lower than systolic pressures measured in the arteries proximal to the coarctation.

d. A constant systolic ejection click at the apex and right upper sternal border signals the presence of a bicuspid aortic valve.

e. A systolic murmur, arising from the coarctation itself, is best heard at the upper left sternal border and left interscapular area posteriorly.

f. A continuous murmur, related to well-developed collateral blood vessels, may be heard across the precordium, laterally and in the back.

g. Other murmurs may be caused by associated defects.

Key Clinincal Findings

- Differential arterial pulses
- Upper extremities > lower extremities
- Murmurs
- Complex coarctation—heart failure

Laboratory Findings

1. Electrocardiography

An infant may have a normal electrocardiogram or may show right axis deviation and right ventricular hypertrophy. The presence of left ventricular hypertrophy suggests the presence of associated defects, such as aortic stenosis. The ECG in an older child may be normal or may show left ventricular hypertrophy related to long-standing pressure overload. Associated defects may also affect the ECG.

2. Echocardiography

Two-dimensional and Doppler echocardiography provide an accurate, noninvasive diagnosis of the coarctation anatomy and physiology. The discrete area of stenosis can be imaged, and Doppler echocardiography can estimate the pressure gradient from the high-flow velocity signal obtained across the stenosis. Associated intracardiac lesions can also be identified.

3. Diagnostic cardiac catheterization and angiography

Diagnostic cardiac catheterization and angiography are not required if noninvasive studies and physical findings are consistent with simple coarctation. If important questions arise regarding assessment of associated lesions, a diagnostic cardiac catheterization may be indicated.

Key Laboratory Findings

- Echocardiography

Radiographic Changes

The chest roentgenogram of an infant with coarctation in congestive heart failure is nonspecific. In an older child with simple coarctation, the heart size is normal or slightly increased. On the frontal film, a localized narrowing of the aorta ("3 sign") at the site of coarctation and poststenotic dilatation may be seen. A barium swallow will assist in localizing a discrete stenosis as evidenced by a "reverse 3 sign" or "E sign." Rib notching—erosion of the inferior

surfaces of the posterior ribs by dilated intercostal arteries—may be seen in up to 68 per cent of children, generally beyond the age of 5 years, and is presumptive evidence of a well-developed collateral circulation.

Treatment

1. Natural history

Untreated, coarctation of the aorta has a poor natural history. Excluding infants with critical coarctation and heart failure who have very high mortality rate if untreated, the mean age at death has been documented at 34 years; death was related to congestive heart failure, aortic rupture, bacterial endocarditis, and intracranial hemorrhage.

2. Medical management

Medical management of the infant in congestive heart failure consists of initially stabilizing the infant with inotropic support and diuretic therapy. The infant may benefit from an infusion of prostaglandin E_1 to promote ductal patency and improve perfusion to areas distal to the coarctation.

3. Surgical management

Surgical repair remains the conventional treatment for most children with coarctation of the aorta. A variety of surgical approaches have been developed and include resection and end-to-end anastomosis, prosthetic patch aortoplasty, subclavian flap aortoplasty, and bypass grafts between the ascending and descending aorta. The mortality approaches zero in the older child, rises to 10 to 15 per cent for infants with associated large ventricular septal defects, and is higher in the presence of more complex intracardiac defects. A residual mild gradient is not uncommon. The incidence of recurrence of coarctation is greatest if repairs are performed before age 3 years, and certainly if performed under 1 year of age. The timing of elective surgical repair generally is recommended for children between 3 and 5 years of age who do not have severe upper extremity hypertension.

4. Percutaneous balloon angioplasty

Percutaneous balloon angioplasty at the time of cardiac catheterization has gained wide acceptance for treatment of recurrent coarctation because the alternative approach of reoperation is more difficult and is associated with increased morbidity and mortality; however, it remains controversial for management of native coarctation, since surgery is associated with low risk and has a high success rate.

Key Treatment

- Control heart failure
- Surgery

Bibliography

Beekman RH: Coarctation of the aorta. In Emmanouilides GC, Riemenschneider TA, Allen HD, Gutgesell HP (eds): Heart Disease in Infants, Children, and Adolescents, 5th ed, vol II. Baltimore, Williams & Wilkins, 1995, pp 1111–1131.

Messmer BJ, Minale C, Muhler E, Bernuth GV: Surgical correction of coarctation in infancy: does surgical technique influence the results? Ann Thorac Surg 1991;52:594–603.

Rao PS, Hajjar HN, Mardini MK, et al: Balloon angioplasty for coarctation of the aorta: immediate and long-term results. Am Heart J 1984;115:657–664.

177 Atrioventricular Canal Defects

Robert H. Feldt

Definitions

Atrioventricular canal defects are a group of anomalies that share a defect in the atrioventricular septum and have similar abnormalities of the atrioventricular valves. Alternative terms include atrioventricular septal defect and endocardial cushion defect.

These defects are characterized by their anatomic features and include complete forms of atrioventricular canal defect and partial forms, such as ostium primum atrial septal defect, common atrium, and isolated cleft mitral valve.

Etiology

The etiology of these defects is not known, but a close association with Down syndrome suggests that chromosomal abnormalities may play a role in their development. The defect is the result of incomplete development of the four embryonic endocardial cushions.

Epidemiology

Atrioventricular canal defects occur in approximately 3 per cent of all cardiac defects found in live births. Echocardiographic experience has noted a higher prevalence in the fetus, suggesting that there is a significant loss of fetuses with these defects.

Pathophysiology

1. Partial forms of the defect usually are associated with a left-to-right shunt and a left atrioventricular valve regurgitation. Pulmonary hypertension is relatively uncommon.
2. Complete forms of the anomaly are invariably associated with large left-to-right shunting, atrioventricular valve regurgitation, and pulmonary hypertension. Progressive pulmonary vascular disease can be seen in the first year of life.

Clinical Findings

1. Presentation
   a. Ostium primum atrial septal defect, the most common partial form of this anomaly, frequently presents in childhood as a heart murmur. Symptoms vary from none to congestive heart failure depending on the size of the left-to-right shunt and degree of left atrioventricular valve regurgitation.
   b. Common atrium invariably presents in early childhood and can be associated with congestive heart failure. This defect should be considered when there are anomalies of cardiac or abdominal situs as well as splenic anomalies (polysplenia or asplenia).
   c. Isolated cleft of the mitral valve is the least common partial form of this defect; it presents as a heart murmur and often there are no associated symptoms.
   d. Complete atrioventricular canal is commonly associated with congestive heart failure in infancy, sig-

nificant cardiopulmonary symptoms, and growth failure. Down syndrome is more often associated with this anomaly than with partial forms of the defect.
2. Physical findings
   a. The first heart sound is usually normal, and the second heart sound may be widely split.
   b. A systolic crescendo-decrescendo murmur is often present at the upper left sternal border.
   c. A low-pitched diastolic murmur is commonly noted at the lower left sternal border or the cardiac apex, depending on the size of the left-to-right shunt and the degree of left atrioventricular valve regurgitation.
   d. A separate apical blowing holosystolic murmur is common.
   e. An accentuation of the pulmonary closure sound will be noted in the presence of pulmonary hypertension.
   f. Cyanosis will be noted in the presence of severe congestive heart failure or significant pulmonary vascular disease.

Key Clinical Findings

- Murmurs
- Split second heart sound

Laboratory Findings

1. There are no specific hematologic findings.
2. Chest roentgenographic findings include cardiomegaly and increased pulmonary vascular markings. There may be right atrial enlargement or prominence of the main pulmonary artery segment.
3. Electrocardiographic findings
   a. Normal sinus rhythm is usual. First-degree heart block is common. Right or left atrial enlargement is also seen.
   b. There is a marked shift in the frontal plane axis so that the AVF lead shows definite negative forces (Fig. 177–1). This axis shift is almost always present in patients with all forms of atrioventricular canal defects, as seen in Figure 177–2.
   c. Right and/or left ventricular hypertrophy is common.
4. Echocardiographic findings
   a. Size and extent of the defect are clearly seen on a four-chamber view (Fig. 177–3).
   b. Generalized chamber enlargement is common. Evidence of elevated pulmonary artery and right ven-

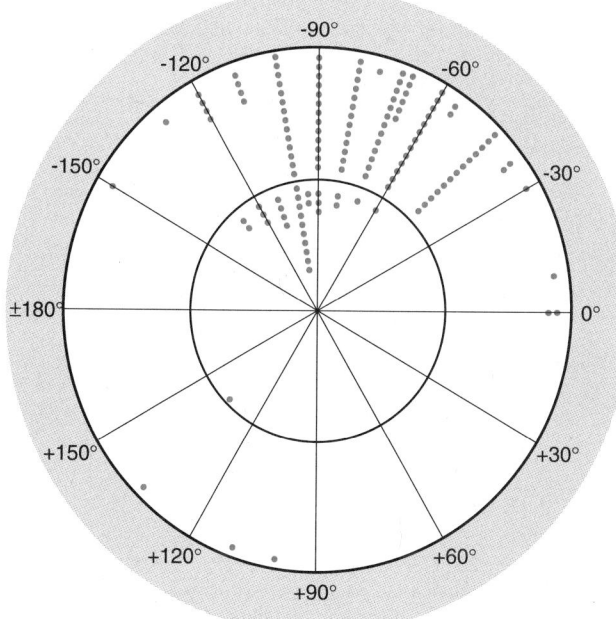

Figure 177–1 Conventional 12-lead electrocardiogram of a child with complete atrioventricular canal defect, showing the negative QRS wave in lead AVF denoting a marked shift in the mean frontal plane QRS axis. There is also clear evidence for right ventricular hypertrophy.

tricular hypertension is common in complete atrioventricular canal defects.

   c. Left-to-right shunting can be seen on color Doppler studies. Shunting may be noted from left ventricle to right atrium, which is common for these defects.

Mean QRS frontal plane axis

Inner circle—complete AV canal
Outer circle—partial AV canal

Figure 177–2 Diagram of mean frontal plane QRS axes seen in patients with atrioventricular canal defects, showing the strong predilection for marked superior axis deviation.

   d. Echocardiography may be all that is necessary to establish the diagnosis.

5. Cardiac catheterization findings

   a. Cardiac catheterization may be needed to exclude suspected associated defects or to assess degree of pulmonary vascular resistance.

   b. Because pulmonary vascular disease can occur early, cardiac catheterization should be done during the first 9 months of life, when complete forms of this defect are suspected.

Key Laboratory Findings

• ECG

• Echocardiography

Treatment

1. Patients with isolated cleft mitral valve may require operation if the regurgitation is significant and there are cardiac symptoms.

2. Patients with ostium primum atrial septal defect who have congestive heart failure and/or significant symptoms can have operative repair in infancy. Elective repair of this defect during childhood is recommended for those with significant left-to-right shunt regardless of symptoms.

3. Patients with complete atrioventricular canal defects often require management of their congestive heart failure and surgical correction. Operation is at less risk if the infant is at least 6 months of age and there are no major associated defects.

4. A small percentage of patients require left atrioventricular valve replacement at initial or subsequent operation. An

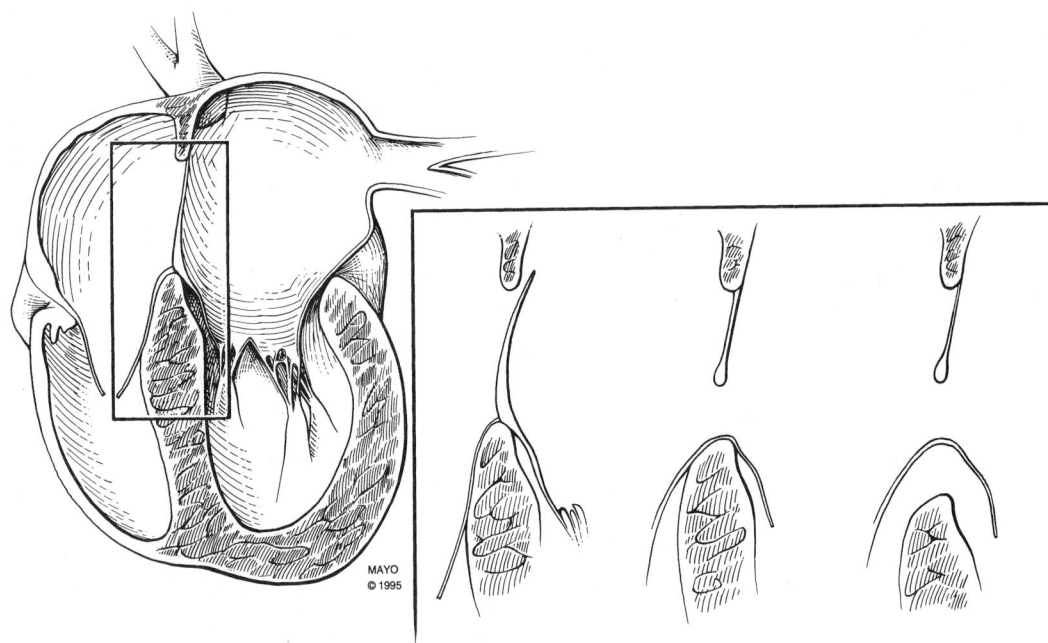

Figure 177–3 Diagrammatic drawings of the heart showing the four-chamber view noted on echocardiograms. Orientation of the normal heart is on the left; the three close-up views starting on the left show the normal anatomy, that of ostium primum atrial septal defect, and that seen with complete atrioventricular canal defects. (Courtesy of The Mayo Clinic, Rochester, MN.)

even smaller percentage will require pacemaker placement because of iatrogenic complete heart block.
5. All patients require antibiotic prophylaxis for dental or surgical procedures.
6. Periodic follow-up is necessary to detect later complications, such as progressive left atrioventricular valve regurgitation and left ventricular outflow obstruction.

Key Treatment

- Surgery
- Pacemaker (seldom)

Prevention

There are no known methods to prevent the occurrence of this anomaly.

Bibliography

Bender HW Jr, Hammam JW Jr, Hubbard SG, et al: Repair of atrioventricular canal malformation in the first year of life. J Thorac Cardiovasc Surg 1982;84:515–522.

Cook AC, Allan LD, Anderson RH, et al: Atrioventricular septal defect in fetal life: A clinicopathological correlation. Cardiol Young 1991;1:334–343.

Studer M, Blackstone EH, Kirklin JW, et al: Determinants of early and late results of repair of atrioventricular septal (canal) defects. J Thorac Cardiovasc Surg 1982;84:523–542.

Titus JL, Rastelli GC: Anatomic features of persistent common atrioventricular canal. *In* Feldt RH (ed): Atrioventricular Canal Defects. Philadelphia, WB Saunders, 1976, pp 13–35.

178 Aortic Stenosis

Jill H. Morriss

Definition

Aortic stenosis (AS) is the diagnosis made when there is obstruction to left ventricular outflow. Most commonly, the site of obstruction occurs at the aortic valve level, although obstruction above (supravalvular) or below (subvalvular) the valve also is recognized. Common to these dissimilar anatomic lesions is the increase in afterload that the left ventricle must overcome. Each site of obstruction has unique features related to recurrence risk, likelihood of progression, associated defects, congenital vs. acquired obstruction, and treatment, so that "aortic stenosis" is not a single diagnostic entity. This chapter deals with isolated valvular AS, as it is the level of obstruction most often encountered.

Etiology

1. Aortic valve obstruction can result from congenital or acquired valve disease. The bicuspid aortic valve, which reportedly occurs in 1 to 2 per cent of the population, is the substrate for much but not all of congenital AS recognized beyond the neonatal period.
2. Although the bicuspid aortic valve may not be importantly stenotic or even recognized in childhood, it serves as a site for "premature" acquired calcific aortic stenosis in adult years.
3. Obstruction of a normally formed trileaflet aortic valve can result from degenerative changes related to normal or accelerated aging (progeria) or rheumatic heart disease.

Epidemiology

1. Aortic stenosis, not further characterized as to type, constitutes approximately 5 to 8 per cent of congenital heart disease.
2. There is a strong male preponderance in all groups of patients with AS.
3. Bicuspid aortic valve is highly associated with coarctation of the aorta in up to 85 per cent of cases. The category of "left heart obstructive lesions," which includes AS, has a high recurrence risk (of up to 17%) in families.

Pathophysiology

1. The hemodynamic severity of AS is reflected by the left ventricular pressure and the gradient across the left ventricular outflow tract.
2. The gradient is influenced by the orifice size and the cardiac output, so that it is an oversimplification to relate the severity of AS to the gradient alone; the gradient is further affected if associated valve insufficiency is present.
3. Aortic stenosis produces resistance to left ventricular ejection, so that compensatory left ventricular hypertrophy is expected to occur.
4. Most children with AS have an elevation in measured LV end-diastolic pressure, which reflects the increased resistance to filling (decreased compliance) of the hypertrophied left ventricle.
5. Left atrial pressures are elevated when LV end-diastolic pressures are increased, and compensatory LA wall thickening can occur.
6. In spite of widely patent normal coronary arteries, the myocardial blood flow in children with AS may be inadequate owing to an imbalance between myocardial blood supply and demand.

Clinical Findings

1. Presentation
   a. Patients with AS are usually indexed by the recognition of a murmur in childhood. The gender ratio of AS in childhood approaches 4:1, with males predominating.
   b. In childhood, patients with AS maintain normal cardiac output, heart rate, and blood pressure even with severe obstruction.
   c. A newborn infant who has critical AS may have acute left ventricular failure and present in a shock-like state similar to the presentation of an infant with hypoplastic left heart syndrome or severe coarctation.
   d. Symptoms of fatigue, exercise intolerance with dyspnea, anginal chest pain, and dizzy spells and syncope are highly supportive of clinically severe AS.
   e. Syncope with exertion is an alarming symptom and is attributed to dysrhythmia resulting from the inability to increase cardiac output and coronary blood flow.
   f. Concern for sudden cardiac death in patients with aortic valve stenosis influences interpretation of symptoms, timing of therapies, and exercise restrictions.
2. Physical findings for aortic valve stenosis
   a. A systolic ejection murmur is heard beginning at the mid–left sternal border with radiation to and maximal intensity at the upper right sternal border (primary aortic area). The murmur may be accompanied by a palpable thrill at the upper right sternal border, in which case it is described as a grade 4/6 systolic ejection murmur.
   b. Often a thrill in the suprasternal notch and right carotid artery attests to a stenotic aortic valve as the origin of the murmur.
   c. The length and intensity of the murmur are helpful in interpreting the severity of AS, with long, harsh, louder murmurs more indicative of important obstruction.
   d. It is rare to have important valve obstruction without a murmur. The exception is found in the critically ill neonate with poor cardiac output and pulses, in whom no murmur may be audible until treatment for shock is effective.
   e. A systolic ejection click is a reliable finding in implicating the aortic valve as the site of the left ventricular outflow obstruction. A systolic click may be the only clinical clue to the presence of a nonstenotic bicuspid aortic valve.
   f. The second heart sound is usually normal, although the murmur may be long and encompass A_2; paradoxical splitting of S_2 is extremely rare but, if present, supports the clinical judgment that severe AS is present.

Key Clinical Findings

- Exercise intolerance
- Syncope
- Systolic ejection murmur

Laboratory Findings

1. Chest x-ray
   a. The chest film is usually normal in a patient with AS. LV wall thickness can be quite increased without producing radiographic evidence for cardiac enlargement (dilatation).

b. If congestive heart failure is present, particularly when it complicates the clinical course in an infant with severe AS, the cardiac silhouette can be massively enlarged.

c. Often the only radiographic clue to aortic valve disease is that the aortic shadow appears somewhat conspicuous as a result of poststenotic dilatation of the ascending aorta.

d. Aortic valve calcification is rarely seen with congenital or rheumatic AS in childhood.

2. Electrocardiogram

a. When left ventricular hypertrophy is seen on the ECG, it is supportive of the diagnosis of AS.

b. The ECG is very sensitive for "severe" AS if repolarization abnormalities are seen, primarily ST segment depression and/or T-wave inversion in the lateral precordial leads.

c. A normal ECG does not exclude the diagnosis of moderate or severe AS.

3. Echocardiography/Doppler

a. Echocardiography confirms the site of LV outflow obstruction and allows measurement of the valve annulus. Often, morphologic features of the valve are identifiable; when the valve is clearly seen, an opinion on whether it is a bicuspid valve may be rendered. The valve thickness and mobility may be inspected and may influence treatment decisions.

b. Valve area measurements can be made with some accuracy but are used less in judging severity than are measurements of LV wall thickness and Doppler quantitation of valve gradients.

c. Valve gradients are a reliable serial measurement to track severity of obstruction in patients when they are used as their own controls. Since the Doppler gradient is based on a "peak instantaneous gradient," it is corrected in many laboratories by multiplying that number by 0.8 to derive a "true" gradient closer to the peak-to-peak gradient that results from catheterization.

4. Cardiac catheterization and angiography

a. The measurement of the transvalvular gradient at catheterization has directed decisions for surgery for many years. The gradient can be obtained by a catheter "pullback" from the LV to the ascending aorta. Alternatively, one can place a catheter via a transseptal approach into the LV while measuring a simultaneous aortic pressure with a retrograde catheter.

b. Catheterization in a critically ill newborn is undertaken at increased risk; unless treatment is to be offered in the laboratory, this procedure is often bypassed preoperatively in an infant with symptomatic AS.

Key Laboratory Study

• Echocardiography

Treatment

1. Management of neonates with critical AS

Infants presenting with suspected severe LV outflow obstruction are stabilized by administration of prostaglandins to open the ductus arteriosus and allow for a ductal contribution to systemic blood flow. If severe AS is confirmed by echocardiography and the size of the aorta is not diminutive, aortic valvotomy should be performed on an emergency basis. The decision to offer surgical treatment with cardiopulmonary bypass and inspection of the valve vs. balloon valvuloplasty using interventional catheter therapies is based on experience and judgment at the treatment center.

2. Elective repair of asymptomatic AS

Criteria for aortic valvotomy are based on a catheterization gradient of 50 mmHg or more across the aortic valve. The therapy is often accomplished with balloon valvuloplasty in the catheterization laboratory.

3. Repair of symptomatic AS

If a patient with AS has symptoms attributed to the disease or if provocative treadmill testing is interpreted to show ischemic changes, aortic valvotomy is appropriately recommended. A single syncopal episode is sufficient justification for treatment in a patient with aortic valve stenosis if the cause of the event was not otherwise clearly explainable.

Key Treatment

• Prostaglandin infusion

• Surgery

Follow-up

1. All treatment of AS is palliative; expected future procedures are planned based on the rate of restenosis, the anatomy of the outflow obstruction, and the degree of valve regurgitation antecedent to or resulting from therapy.

2. Management in childhood is directed toward avoidance of prosthetic aortic valve replacement and resulting anticoagulation therapy.

3. Prophylaxis against bacterial endocarditis must be strictly observed when the diagnosis of bicuspid aortic valve or AS is made.

Bibliography

Latson LA: Aortic stenosis: Valvular, supravalvular, and fibromuscular subvalvular. *In* Garson A, Bricker JT, McNamara DG (eds): The Science and Practice of Pediatric Cardiology. Malvern, PA, Lea & Febiger, 1990, pp 1334–1352.

Nishimura RA, Pieroni DR, Bierman FZ, et al: Second natural history study of congenital heart defects. Aortic stenosis: Echocardiography. Circulation 1993;87(Suppl I):67–72.

Rao PS: Balloon valvuloplasty for aortic stenosis. *In* Rao PS (ed): Transcatheter Therapy in Pediatric Cardiology. New York, Wiley-Liss, 1993, pp 105–127.

Roberts WC: The congenitally bicuspid aortic valve: A study of 85 autopsy cases. Am J Cardiol 1970;26:72–83.

179 Pulmonary Stenosis

Thomas R. Lloyd

Definition

Pulmonary stenosis is mechanical obstruction to blood flow between the right ventricle and pulmonary arterioles. It is classified by site of obstruction, although mixed forms occur.

1. Subvalvar stenosis—Obstruction within the body of the right ventricle. Narrowing can be discrete or tubular and is occasionally associated with septal hypertrophy. Narrowing is more commonly due to anomalous muscle bundles (also called *double-chamber right ventricle*); it is observed as an isolated lesion or in association with ventricular septal defect and/or subaortic stenosis.
2. Valvar stenosis—Typical pulmonary valve stenosis is characterized by commissural fusion in a valve that has a normal or increased annulus size and mildly to moderately thickened valve leaflets. Pulmonary valve hypoplasia (significantly reduced annulus size) and dysplasia (severely thickened and stiff valve leaflets without significant commissural fusion) account for about 10 per cent of isolated pulmonary valve stenosis.
3. Supravalvar stenosis—Stenosis can occur in the main pulmonary artery, at the pulmonary artery bifurcation, in the central right or left pulmonary artery, at the branch points of the hilar pulmonary arteries, or in the intrapulmonary branches, where the process is often diffuse. Pulmonary artery branch stenosis in the newborn is usually physiologic, caused by the intrauterine diameter disparity between the large main pulmonary artery and the smaller right and left pulmonary artery branches. Ductal coarctation of the pulmonary artery can be seen at the site of ductal insertion (typically at the origin of the left pulmonary artery).

Etiology

1. The etiology of most cases of subvalvar and valvar pulmonary stenosis is unknown. Rarely, acquired subpulmonary stenosis is encountered as a consequence of myocardial tumors, most commonly in the setting of tuberous sclerosis, LEOPARD syndrome, neurofibromatosis, and other tumor syndromes. Typical pulmonary valve stenosis is occasionally familial (about 2%), but dysplastic pulmonary stenosis more commonly recurs in families and is found in about 50 per cent of patients with Noonan syndrome.
2. Peripheral pulmonary stenosis is often associated with intrauterine viral infection (particularly congenital rubella syndrome) or with congenital malformation syndromes such as Williams and Alagille syndromes. Acquired forms of pulmonary artery stenosis generally result from surgical procedures. Pulmonary artery branch stenosis is a benign, self-limited condition of the neonate presumed to be related to the small size of the right and/or left pulmonary artery branches; it is due to the relatively small amount of pulmonary blood flow in the fetal circulation.

Epidemiology

Pulmonary valve stenosis, isolated or in association with atrial septal defect, constitutes approximately 8 per cent of significant congenital heart disease. Some form of pulmonary stenosis accompanies approximately 30 per cent of significant congenital heart disease.

Pathophysiology

The pathophysiology of pulmonary stenosis depends on the severity of obstruction. With *mild* obstruction (right ventricular systolic pressure <50 to 60 mmHg or right ventricle to pulmonary artery systolic pressure gradient <40 to 50 mmHg), little alteration in ventricular function is seen at rest or with exercise, and symptoms are rare. With *moderate* obstruction (right ventricular pressure ≤ aortic pressure, gradient <70 mmHg), right ventricular function is adequate at rest, but stroke volume does not increase to the normal extent during exercise. Symptoms of chest pain on exertion or decreased exercise endurance can occur. The right ventricular hypertension results in hypertrophy of the right ventricle, including the infundibulum, which can result in progressive subpulmonary stenosis. With *severe* pulmonary stenosis (suprasystemic right ventricular pressure, gradient >70 mmHg), right ventricular function remains adequate at rest, but stroke volume response to exercise worsens and can even fall with increased heart rate. Greater limitations to exercise are observed, and subendocardial infarctions of the right ventricle, ventricular arrhythmias, and sudden death have been seen. *Critical* obstruction is present when right ventricular function is inadequate at rest, resulting in cyanosis, congestive heart failure, or syncope. Newborns with critical pulmonary stenosis may be dependent on a patent ductus arteriosus for adequate pulmonary blood flow.

Clinical Findings

1. Patients with mild pulmonary stenosis are asymptomatic as a rule and usually present with an asymptomatic murmur. Patients with mild, moderate, and severe pulmonary stenosis are generally robust (the exceptions generally being patients with the various syndromes). The typical murmur of pulmonary stenosis is a harsh ejection systolic murmur heard best along the upper part of the left sternal border. The murmur is shorter in duration and its peak intensity is earlier in systole than in more severe pulmonary stenosis. The murmur often radiates throughout the chest (especially when pulmonary artery stenosis is present) but tends to radiate particularly well to the left upper back. With subpulmonary stenosis, the murmur can be louder toward the mid–left sternal border. With mild valvar pulmonary stenosis, an early systolic ejection click (preceding the murmur) is usually heard along the left sternal border. The intensity of the click typically varies with respiration, being louder in expiration and softer in inspiration.

2. Patients with moderate pulmonary stenosis are usually asymptomatic, but some may have complaints of diminished exercise endurance or of precordial or epigastric pain with exertion. Right ventricular impulse is usually increased, and a precordial thrill is often present. The systolic murmur is louder and longer, and its peak intensity is later than with mild pulmonary stenosis. With moderate valvar pulmonary stenosis, the ejection click occurs earlier in systole than in cases of mild pulmonary stenosis, and aortic closure may be obscured by the murmur. In cases of pulmonary artery stenosis, the pulmonary component of S_2 may be very accentuated.

3. Patients with severe pulmonary stenosis are more likely to have complaints of exercise intolerance or chest pain. The murmur tends to be louder, of higher pitch, and longer yet, and it obscures the second heart sound. The click, if present, occurs early enough to be difficult to distinguish from the first heart sound.

4. In critical pulmonary stenosis, the murmur may be much less impressive because of the reduced volume of blood passing from the right ventricle to the pulmonary arteries. If an atrial septal defect is present, cyanosis will be the most prominent feature. When the atrial septum is intact, the clinical picture is that of low cardiac output with systemic venous congestion.

Key Clinical Findings

- Usually asymptomatic
- Ejection murmur

Laboratory Findings

1. Electrocardiography usually shows evidence of right ventricular hypertrophy in moderate and severe pulmonary stenosis; the ECG is usually normal in mild cases. Echocardiography establishes the diagnosis of pulmonary stenosis and associated lesions, and Doppler examinations can usually estimate right ventricular pressure and/or pulmonary stenosis gradient with considerable accuracy.

2. Cardiac catheterization is reserved for moderate, severe, or critical pulmonary stenosis. Right ventricular pressure and pulmonary stenosis gradients are measured directly; associated lesions are sought and quantified; and angiography definitively demonstrates pulmonary arterial anatomy as well as pulmonary annulus size and the nature of subpulmonary obstructions.

Key Laboratory Test

- Echocardiography

Radiographic Changes

Enlargement of the main pulmonary artery segment is frequently seen with typical valvar pulmonary stenosis. Cardiac size and pulmonary vascular markings are usually normal.

Treatment

1. Antibiotic prophylaxis against bacterial endocarditis is recommended for pulmonary stenosis regardless of severity, although the endocarditis risk is modest. No other treatment is necessary for mild pulmonary stenosis.

2. Percutaneous balloon pulmonary valvuloplasty is recommended for typical valvar pulmonary stenosis of at least moderate severity. Failure of a technically adequate balloon valvuloplasty procedure to immediately reduce pulmonary stenosis to the mild range suggests development of dynamic infundibular stenosis (which will subsequently resolve) or the presence of pulmonary valve dysplasia and/or hypoplasia. The risks of serious complications of this procedure are higher in neonates than in older patients; intervention should be postponed in newborns unless the stenosis is critical. Valvuloplasty may not be adequate treatment in neonates with hypoplasia of the right ventricle and tricuspid valve; infants with tricuspid valve annulus diameter ≤11 mm, pulmonary valve annulus <7 mm, or right ventricular volume ≤30 ml/m² are likely to require a systemic to pulmonary arterial shunt as well. Comparison of the results of balloon valvuloplasty to surgical valvotomy reveals a minor advantage in the reduction in pulmonary stenosis gradient with surgery, but it is at the expense of more pulmonary insufficiency and ventricular arrhythmias.

3. Endoluminal stenting of the pulmonary arteries can relieve pulmonary artery stenosis in the intraparenchymal pulmonary arteries as well as the mediastinal pulmonary arteries. While endoluminal stenting has permitted treatment of pulmonary arterial stenoses unsuitable for surgery, effective treatment is still lacking for severe, diffuse pulmonary artery stenosis.

4. Surgical valvotomy is effective for patients who require surgery for associated defects or in whom a technically adequate balloon valvuloplasty cannot be accomplished. Patients with pulmonary valve dysplasia or hypoplasia require pulmonary valve excision and/or annular augmentation. The pulmonary insufficiency produced by these procedures is usually better tolerated than severe pulmonary stenosis. Surgical angioplasty is suitable for pulmonary arterial stenoses within the mediastinum. Subvalvar pulmonary stenosis and double-chamber right ventricle require surgical relief.

Key Treament

- Balloon valvuloplasty
- Surgery

Prevention

Immunization against rubella prevents the congenital rubella syndrome, and genetic counseling should be offered to families suspected to have genetic disorders associated with pulmonary stenosis.

Bibliography

Beekman RH, Lloyd TR: Balloon valvuloplasty and stenting for congenital heart disease. *In* Topol EJ (ed): Textbook of Interventional Cardiology, 2nd ed. Philadelphia, WB Saunders, 1993, pp 1277–1297.

Fedderly RT, Lloyd TR, Mendelsohn AM, Beekman RH: Determinants of successful balloon valvotomy in infants with critical pulmonary stenosis or membranous pulmonary atresia with intact ventricular septum. J Am Coll Cardiol 1995;25:460–465.

Hayes CJ, Gersony WM, Driscoll DJ, et al: Second natural history study of congenital heart defects: results of treatment of patients with pulmonary valvar stenosis. Circulation 1993;87(Suppl I):28–37.

O'Connor BK, Beekman RH, Lindauer A, Rocchini A: Intermedi-ate-term outcome after pulmonary balloon valvuloplasty: comparison to a matched surgical control group. J Am Coll Cardiol 1992;20:169–173.

Rocchini AP, Emmanouilides GC: Pulmonary stenosis. In Emmanouilides GC, Riemenschneider TA, Allen HD, Gutgesell HP (eds): Moss and Adams Heart Disease in Infants, Children, and Adolescents Including the Fetus and Young Adult, 5th ed. Baltimore, Williams & Wilkins, 1995, pp 930–962.

180 Mitral Valve Prolapse

Kevin Mulhern

Definition

Mitral valve prolapse (MVP) is the displacement or billowing of one or both mitral valve leaflets into the atrium and beyond the normal position. Mitral regurgitation may or may not be present.

The standard for the diagnosis of MVP is physical examination, not echocardiography. Physical examination findings may vary from one visit to the next.

Etiology

1. Primary
   a. Primary mitral valve prolapse is usually inherited as an autosomal dominant trait with variable expression. Genetic studies have shown no linkage to major collagen genes. Isolated cases also occur.
   b. The valve leaflets are redundant. There is marked proliferation of the myxomatous connective tissue between the leaflet surfaces plus focal disruption of the ventricular surfaces of the leaflets. Other changes include fibrosis of the leaflet surfaces, thinning or elongation of chordae tendineae, ventricular friction lesions, and fibrin deposits on the atrial side of the annulus.
2. Secondary
   a. MVP may be secondary to a heritable connective tissue disorder. Examples include Marfan syndrome, Stickler syndrome, Ehlers-Danlos syndrome, cutis laxa, osteogenesis imperfecta, and the MASS (*Mi*tral valve, *A*orta, *S*keleton, *S*kin) phenotype. Myxomatous proliferation is present.
   b. MVP may also occur without myxomatous changes. Examples include rheumatic heart disease (secondary to postinflammatory changes), secundum atrial septal defect and anorexia nervosa (due to reduced left ventricular volume), and cardiomyopathies (hypertrophic and congestive).

Epidemiology

MVP has a prevalence of 3 to 8 per cent in the general population. Prevalence increases with age. Although inherited as an autosomal dominant trait, MVP is more common in females (2.7:1 in one community-based study of 813 children aged 9 to 14 years). Expression of the gene or genes for primary MVP seems to be affected by gender and age.

Pathophysiology

1. It should be emphasized to the parents and child that MVP is generally a benign condition. The prognosis for children and adolescents with isolated MVP is excellent. Complications are rare.
2. Significant mitral regurgitation (MR) due to MVP is rare in children and adolescents. MVP is, however, the most common cause of hemodynamically significant MR in adults.
3. Associated valve abnormalities are tricuspid valve prolapse (40%), pulmonic valve prolapse (10%), and aortic valve prolapse (2%).

Clinical Findings

1. Symptoms
   a. The vast majority of patients with MVP have no symptoms.
   b. Compared with control subjects, palpitations (due to ventricular premature beats or supraventricular tachyarrhythmias) are more common with MVP.
   c. There is no difference in the incidence of nonanginal chest pain, dyspnea, anxiety, or panic attacks when children and adults with MVP are compared with appropriate controls.
   d. Orthostatic syncope, possibly due to reduced blood volume, is more common with MVP.
2. Physical examination
   a. Body habitus
      (1) Thoracic bony abnormalities are more prevalent in patients with MVP. These include pectus excavatum, scoliosis, narrowed anteroposterior chest dimension, and straight back.
      (2) Children with MVP tend to be slender. Compared with children without MVP, height and arm span/height are not different.
   b. Cardiovascular examination
      (1) Systolic blood pressure is lower and orthostatic

hypotension more common in patients with MVP.

(2) Single or multiple midsystolic clicks are heard at the apex.

(3) A high-pitched crescendo late systolic murmur of mitral regurgitation is heard best at the apex.

Key Clinical Findings

- Majority asymptomatic
- Palpitations
- Orthostatic syncope
- Typical click and murmur

Laboratory Findings

1. Electrocardiogram
   The electrocardiogram (ECG) is usually normal, and there are no ECG changes characteristic of MVP.

2. Echocardiogram
   a. Echocardiography is useful for
   (1) Confirming the diagnosis of MVP, although 10 per cent of patients with auscultatory MVP will have nondiagnostic echocardiograms.
   (2) Quantifying the severity of MR and following its progression.
   (3) Identifying those at higher risk of complications (i.e., thick redundant leaflets, significant MR, a dilated left ventricle, or a dilated left atrium).

   b. M-mode echo criteria for MVP lack sensitivity and specificity. Two-dimensional echocardiography is recommended.

   c. Two-dimensional echocardiography criteria include
   (1) Posterior or superior systolic displacement of one or both mitral valve leaflets >2 mm in the parasternal long axis or apical long axis views, especially if the closure point is on the atrial side of the annulus.
   (2) Focal prolapse of the lateral scallop of the posterior leaflet in the apical four-chamber view or the medial scallop of the posterior leaflet in the apical two-chamber view.
   (3) The presence of thickened leaflets (5 mm during diastole) makes the diagnosis more certain.

Key Laboratory Test

- Echocardiography

Radiographic Changes

1. Chest x-ray
   The heart and lungs are usually radiographically normal unless significant MR (with left atrial and left ventricular dilatation) or left ventricular failure (with pulmonary venous congestion) is present. Thoracic bony abnormalities may be noted.

2. Angiogram

a. Although rarely necessary for the diagnosis of MVP and prone to inter- and intraobserver variability, left ventricular angiography can be used to confirm the presence of MVP.

b. Wall motion is usually normal, but abnormal contraction may be seen. This is usually indentation of the left ventricle at the base of a papillary muscle, probably due to traction on the papillary muscle. These wall motion abnormalities resolve after valve repair or replacement.

Treatment

1. Preventing complications and treating symptoms
   a. Infective endocarditis
   (1) The risk of infective endocarditis (IE) in patients with MVP is three- to eight-fold greater than in the general population. In a series of 136 patients over 15 years of age, the absolute risk of IE was 1 in 1400 per year if a systolic murmur was present and 1 in 56,000 per year without a systolic murmur.
   (2) Endocarditis prophylaxis is recommended for MVP with MR or for MVP without MR but with thickened or redundant leaflets.

   b. Mitral regurgitation and heart failure
   (1) Left ventricular failure may occur as a consequence of progressive MR. This is most common in men >50 years old and very uncommon in children and adolescents.

   c. Orthostatic symptoms
   These are treated best by liberalizing fluid and salt intake. Pharmacologic therapy with clonidine or fludrocortisone has been used.

   d. Palpitations
   Palpitations associated with sinus tachycardia, atrial or ventricular premature complexes, or brief episodes of atrial tachycardia may be alleviated by smoking cessation and by reducing caffeine and alcohol intake. Beta blockers may also be effective.

   e. Arrhythmias and sudden death
   (1) The true incidence of arrhythmias associated with MVP is unknown.
   (2) Sudden death in children and adolescents with isolated MVP is very rare. As of 1995, only four cases had been reported in patients <20 years old.
   (3) Predictors of increased risk of sudden death and life-threatening arrhythmias in adults with MVP include
   (a) Redundant mitral valve leaflets
   (b) Severe MR
   (c) Family history of sudden death
   (d) Prolonged QTc interval.
   (4) Asymptomatic children and adolescents with MVP, no mitral regurgitation, and no family history of sudden death associated with MVP may engage in all competitive sports.
   (5) Children and adolescents with MVP and symp-

toms (e.g., chest pain, palpitations, arrhythmias, near-syncope, or syncope), MR, or a family history of sudden death associated with MVP should be evaluated before participating in competitive athletics. This should include a resting ECG, an echocardiogram, a 24-hour ambulatory ECG (Holter monitor), and an exercise ECG. Cardiology evaluation is suggested.

f. Systemic emboli

(1) The risk of stroke in young adults with MVP is 1 in 6000 per year.

(2) Patients with MVP and documented but unexplained transient ischemic attacks (TIAs) should be treated with long-term low-dose aspirin therapy.

(3) Patients with MVP plus documented systemic embolism, chronic or paroxysmal atrial fibrillation, or recurrent TIAs despite aspirin therapy should be treated with long-term warfarin therapy.

Key Treatment

- Usually none
- Endocarditis prophylaxis
- Mitral valve replacement or repair

Follow-up

Unless significant MR is present already, follow-up every 2 to 3 years has been recommended. Echocardiography (to reassess MR) every 5 years has also been suggested.

Prevention

Primary mitral valve prolapse cannot be prevented. Preventive efforts are directed toward preventing complications of MVP.

Bibliography

Arfken CL, Lachman AS, McLaren MJ, et al: Mitral valve prolapse: associations with symptoms and anxiety. Pediatrics 1990;85:311–315.

Committee on Sports Medicine and Fitness, American Academy of Pediatrics: Mitral valve prolapse and athletic participation in children and adolescents. Pediatrics 1995;95:789–790.

Dajani AS, Bisno AL, Chung KL, et al: Prevention of bacterial endocarditis. Circulation 1991;83:1174–1178.

Devereux RB, Kramer-Fox R, Kligfield P: Mitral valve prolapse: causes, clinical manifestations, and management. Ann Intern Med 1989;111:305–317.

Maron BJ, Isner JM, McKenna WJ: Task force 3: Hypertrophic cardiomyopathy, myocarditis and other myopericardial diseases and mitral valve prolapse. 26th Bethesda Conference. Recommendations for determining eligibility for competition in athletes with cardiovascular abnormalities. J Am Coll Cardiol 1994;24:880–885.

181 Tachyarrhythmia

Dianne L. Atkins

Definition

1. Tachyarrhythmias and/or irregular rhythms are best defined by electrophysiologic mechanism rather than by absolute value of the heart rate. Normal heart rate is dependent on age, physical activity, and physical condition and can overlap with heart rates caused by abnormal supraventricular rhythms.

2. Heart rates ≥220 in the absence of fever warrant investigation

Supraventricular Tachycardiac Arrhythmias

Etiology and Epidemiology

1. Premature atrial contractions (PACs, atrial extrasystoles, and premature atrial beats) are common in infants and young children, occurring in 15 to 30 per cent. The prevalence is highest in infants and declines with age.

2. Supraventricular tachycardia (SVT, paroxysmal atrial tachycardia, PAT) is the most common tachyarrhythmia in the pediatric population. Infants <4 months represent about 40 per cent of patients presenting with their first episode of tachycardia. SVT encompasses several tachycardias with distinctly different mechanisms, therapies, and natural history.

a. Reentrant tachycardias are the most common, and although the clinical presentations are identical and ECG features are similar, they can be divided into two electrophysiologic types.

(1) Atrioventricular reciprocating tachycardia accounts for almost all reentrant tachycardia in infants ≤2 years.

(2) Atrioventricular node reciprocating tachycardia increases in frequency with age until adolescence, when it accounts for approximately 50 per cent of reentrant tachycardias.

b. Atrial ectopic tachycardias account for only 10 per cent of all tachycardias, and the incidence does not change with age.

Pathophysiology

1. Premature atrial contractions arise in atrial tissue and represent a benign abnormality of impulse generation.

2. Supraventricular tachycardia

   a. Reentrant tachycardias are caused by excitation around a fixed electrical obstruction. During normal conduction, excitation proceeds simultaneously down both pathways, which have different conduction velocities. Tachycardia occurs when antegrade excitation is blocked in one of the pathways but not the other. If the pathway with intact conduction conducts slowly enough, excitation can occur in the retrograde direction in the previously blocked pathway.

      (1) Atrioventricular reciprocating tachycardia (AVRT) is the classic example of this type. The AV node is the antegrade limb, and an accessory pathway forms the retrograde limb. The accessory pathway allows conduction between the atria and the ventricles via a pathway other than the AV node. Wolff-Parkinson-White syndrome is present if conduction proceeds from the atria to the ventricles during sinus rhythm (Fig. 181–1).

      (2) During atrioventricular nodal tachycardia (AVNRT), both limbs of the circuit are within the AV node.

   b. Atrial ectopic tachycardia is caused by an abnormality of impulse generation within the atria.

Clinical Findings

1. Premature atrial contractions rarely cause symptoms other than mild palpitations. If there are frequent "blocked PACs" (i.e., not conducted through the atrioventricular conduction system), it may imitate bradycardia.

2. Supraventricular tachycardia

   a. Infants present with symptoms of irritability, lethargy, poor feeding, congestive heart failure, and cardiovascular collapse. Additionally, the infant may be totally asymptomatic and the tachycardia detected coincidentally.

   b. Children frequently complain of a racing or pounding heartbeat. Older children may be able to indicate that the episode starts and stops suddenly. Patients may feel lightheaded or dizzy at the onset of an episode. They may also complain of fatigue, diaphoresis, or nausea. Occasionally, they complain of chest pain, but chest pain alone is rarely a symptom of SVT. Observers may notice neck pulsations or pallor. A frequent observation is the intensity of the cardiac movement in the chest. A minority of patients may experience more serious symptoms of syncope.

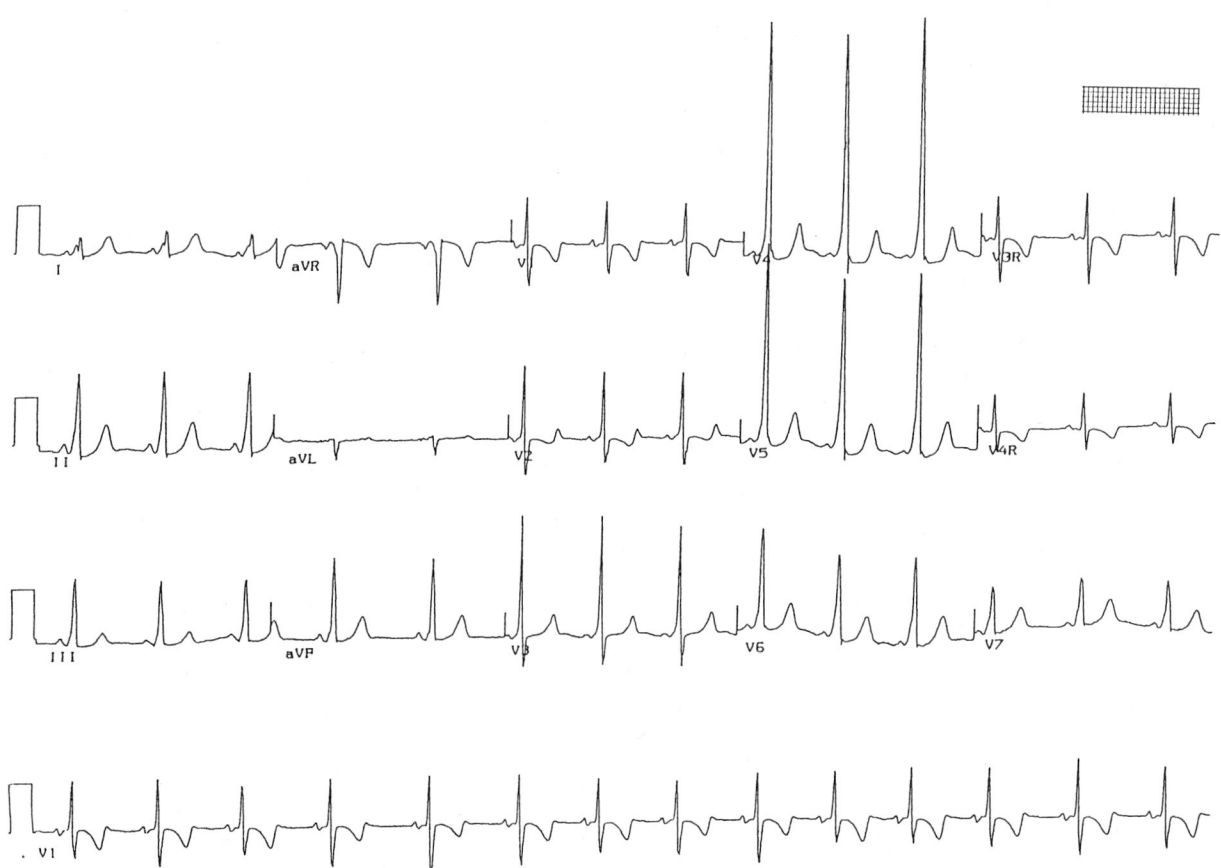

Figure 181–1 ECG illustrating Wolff-Parkinson-White syndrome. The PR interval is extremely short and the upstroke of the QRS complex is slurred, resulting in a wide QRS complex. Tracing was recorded at normal paper speed of 25 mm/sec.

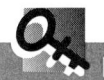

Key Clinical Findings: Supraventricular Tachycardia

• Tachycardia >200/min

Laboratory Findings

1. The ECG is the hallmark for diagnosing atrial arrhythmias.

   a. Premature atrial contractions can readily be diagnosed by an ECG. Typically, the morphology of the premature P wave will differ slightly from that of a sinus beat. The PR interval may be slightly shorter if the PAC arises low in the atrium. If the interval between the normal beat and the premature beat is very short, the PR interval may be lengthened. If the premature interval is very short (0.4 sec), the atrioventricular node or the His-Purkinje system may still be refractory from the previous beat; the premature P wave is not conducted to the ventricles, resulting in a pause. This does not indicate AV node disease.

   b. Supraventricular tachycardia—An ECG is essential to accurately make the diagnosis of SVT. Unless the patient has serious hemodynamic compromise, a 12-lead ECG should be obtained prior to any therapy.

      (1) Reentrant SVT is a regular tachycardia with rates of 220 to 300 beats/minute. The width of the QRS complex is almost always normal. P waves are generally apparent in leads II, III, and AVF as negative deflections close to the preceding QRS complex (Fig. 181–2).

      (2) Atrial ectopic tachycardias sometimes can be difficult to distinguish from normal sinus rhythm. Tachycardia rate is typically only moderately increased for age and may fluctuate over time. The tachycardia is frequently chronic or incessant. Examining the P waves in multiple leads will frequently demonstrate subtle abnormalities of the P wave compared with sinus rhythm. Second-degree heart block may occur with no interruption of the atrial rate.

2. Echocardiography is usually performed in all infants with their first episode of SVT to rule out associated congenital heart disease. Echocardiography is required in patients with atrial ectopic tachycardias, as there is frequently left ventricular dysfunction as a result of chronic tachycardia.

Key Laboratory Test: Supraventricular Tachycardia

• ECG

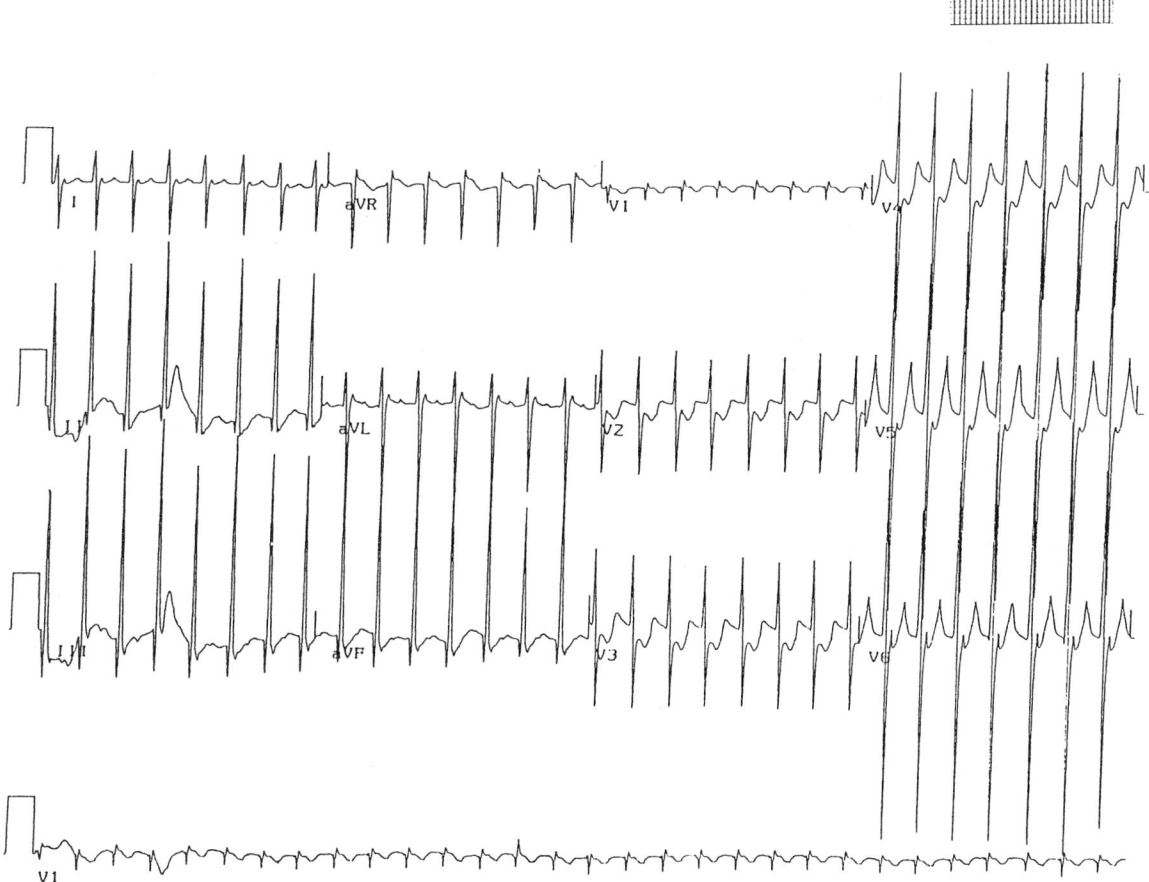

Figure 181–2 ECG of reentrant SVT. The ventricular rate is 235 and regular. The QRS complex is narrow. Inverted P waves are apparent just after the QRS complex and are negative in III, AVF, and the chest leads. Tracing was recorded at normal paper speed of 25 mm/sec.

Radiographic Changes

1. Premature atrial contractions rarely result in radiographic abnormalities.
2. In children with SVT, radiographic abnormalities are related to any underlying cardiac pathology. Infrequently, a child or infant will exhibit signs of congestive heart failure on the chest x-ray.

Treatment

1. Premature atrial contractions require no treatment unless there is significant bradycardia from nonconducted beats. Digoxin or propranolol is usually successful at preventing the PACs.
2. Supraventricular tachycardia
   a. Acute drug treatment
      (1) Maneuvers that heighten vagal tone to the AV node, such as the Valsalva maneuver, gagging, or ice to the face, often terminate an episode of reentrant SVT. Ocular pressure should never be used.
      (2) Intravenous administration of adenosine (50–250 µg/kg repeated two to three times) is a fast, effective, and safe medication.
      (3) Intravenous verapamil (0.1–0.2 mg/kg) is equally effective with a longer half-life. In infants ≤1 year of age, however, verapamil is associated with serious side effects of hypotension and bradycardia, and its use is avoided.
      (4) Digoxin requires several hours to be effective, limiting its usefulness for acute treatment. It is contraindicated in children with known Wolff-Parkinson-White syndrome.
      (5) Synchronized direct-current cardioversion is always an option, especially if the patient displays hemodynamic instability and/or transport is required for chronic therapy.
   b. Chronic treatment of reentrant SVT
      (1) Chronic drug treatment of SVT may be indicated if the episodes are frequent or do not convert without pharmacologic therapy. Therapy is usually directed at delaying conduction through one limb of the tachycardia circuit. Drugs that prolong conduction through the AV node include digoxin, β-adrenergic antagonists, and verapamil. Digoxin is contraindicated in children if Wolff-Parkinson-White syndrome is present, although its use in infants remains controversial. More aggressive medical therapy includes treatment with procainamide, flecainide, amiodarone, or sotalol. These drugs have significant toxicity, and radiofrequency ablation often supplants their use.
      (2) Infants usually require therapy for 4 to 12 months. Approximately 70 per cent will never have another episode of SVT. In the remaining 30 per cent there may be a prolonged symptom free interval.
      (3) Patients with life-threatening or disabling symptoms usually undergo radiofrequency ablation instead of chronic drug therapy.

   c. Atrial ectopic tachycardia—This arrhythmia can be particularly resistant to treatment. Drugs that suppress automaticity are the most effective and include quinidine, procainamide, flecainide, amiodarone, and sotalol. Agents that slow conduction through the AV node are effective at slowing the ventricular rate and include digoxin, verapamil, and β-adrenergic antagonists. Radiofrequency ablation holds great promise in controlling these tachycardias.

Key Treatment: Supraventricular Tachycardia

- Ice on face
- IV adenosine
- IV verapamil

Ventricular Arrhythmia

Etiology and Epidemiology

1. Premature ventricular contractions (PVCs, ventricular extrasystoles, premature ventricular beats) are common in healthy adolescents but are also observed in younger patients, including newborns.
2. Ventricular tachycardia in an otherwise normal heart is frequently seen in conjunction with PVCs. Couplets, triplets, and even long salvos can be observed and do not always indicate serious cardiac pathology. Accelerated ventricular arrhythmia is a benign form of ventricular tachycardia seen in infants and children.
3. Ventricular tachycardia occurs most commonly in patients with congenital heart disease, often as a late sequela to heart surgery. Those at highest risk include patients with tetralogy of Fallot, d-transposition of the great arteries, aortic stenosis, and anomalies of a coronary artery. Other causes include viral myocarditis, dilated cardiomyopathy, hypertrophic cardiomyopathy, congenital long QT syndrome, catecholamine infusion, cocaine, and psychotropic drugs (phenothiazines and tricyclic antidepressants).

Pathophysiology

1. PVCs arise from ventricular tissue and in the presence of a structurally normal heart appear to be benign.
2. Ventricular tachycardia in children rarely results from ischemic heart disease, the most common mechanism in adults. The electrophysiologic mechanisms include reentry (usually around an anatomic scar or electrically abnormal myocardium) or enhanced automaticity, seen most commonly in the presence of a myocardial tumor.

Clinical Findings

1. PVCs are detected because the patient complains of palpitations or an irregular heartbeat is detected during auscultation or ECG recordings.
2. Symptoms associated with ventricular tachycardia can be acute or chronic.
   a. Acute presentation with syncope and/or cardiac arrest
   b. Symptoms may be similar to SVT with sudden onset of racing heartbeat. Ability to terminate the

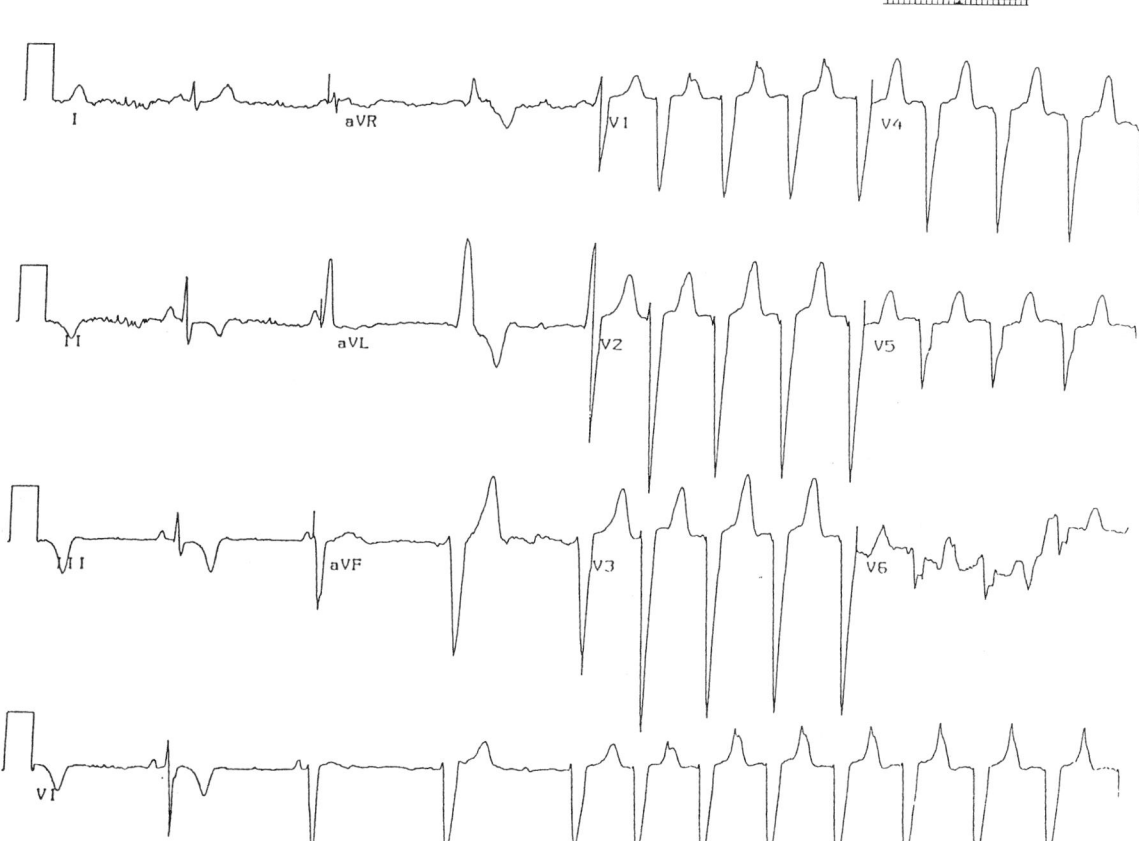

Figure 181–3 ECG of nonsustained ventricular tachycardia. QRS is wide, compared with normal QRS (second complex of tracing). AV dissociation is not apparent in this tracing. Tracing was recorded at normal paper speed of 25 mm/sec.

tachycardia with vagal maneuvers does not distinguish SVT from ventricular tachycardia.

c. Patients with slower tachycardia rates may complain of fatigue, lethargy, or symptoms consistent with congestive heart failure.

d. It is important to recognize that hemodynamic characteristics do not predict electrophysiologic mechanisms. Thus, a conscious patient with a wide-complex tachycardia is more likely to have ventricular tachycardia and should not be assumed to have SVT.

Key Clinical Findings: Ventricular Arrhythmia

• Palpitations

• Syncope

Laboratory Findings

1. PVCs can usually be diagnosed by a resting ECG or 24-hour ambulatory monitor. The premature beats occur early with respect to the basic rhythm, and the QRS complex is widened, with little similarity to the sinus

Key Laboratory Test: Ventricular Arrhythmia

• ECG

QRS. The T-wave polarity is usually opposite the major QRS deflection. A compensatory pause often follows a PVC, but its absence is not diagnostic of a PAC. Couplets and triplets are observed less commonly. Patients can have very frequent PVCs, numbering in the thousands per 24-hour period. A benign prognosis is supported by the criteria outlined in Table 181–1.

2. Characteristic ECG features of ventricular tachycardia are prolonged QRS complex and atrioventricular dissociation (P waves slower than the QRS rate). However, in young children, QRS width is age-dependent and may be less than the standard 0.12 sec in adults (Fig. 181–3). Compar-

TABLE 181–1.   CRITERIA FOR BENIGN PVCs

Absence of underlying heart disease
Uniform morphology
Suppression of PVCs by exercise
Constant coupling interval
Normal corrected QT interval

ison with a previous ECG in sinus rhythm is helpful in determining abnormalities of the QRS complex.

Radiographic Changes

1. Premature ventricular contractions rarely result in radiographic changes.
2. Radiographic findings of ventricular tachycardia are related to the presence of underlying heart disease.

Treatment

1. Premature ventricular contractions require no treatment. Indeed, the proarrhythmic effects of most antiarrhythmics are more threatening than the PVCs.
2. Lidocaine is the easiest and safest drug to administer for ventricular tachycardia if the patient is hemodynamically stable. The loading dose is 1 mg/kg IV push followed by an infusion of 30 to 50 µg/kg/hour. The infusion dose should be directed by measurement of serum blood levels (2–5 µg/ml). Synchronized direct-current cardioversion (2 joules/kg) is appropriate if the patient is hemodynamically unstable.
3. Chronic treatment usually requires long-term antiarrhythmic agents such as procainamide, β blockers, amiodarone, or sotalol. This therapy is directed by the results of electrophysiologic testing. New therapies such as radiofrequency ablation offer some promise.

Key Treatment: Ventricular Arrhythmia

• Lidocaine IV

Bibliography

Epstein ML: Disturbances of cardiac rhythm. *In* Gessner IH, Victorica BE (eds): Pediatric Cardiology: A Problem Oriented Approach. Philadelphia, WB Saunders, 1993, pp 167–182.

Jacobsen JR, Garson A Jr, Gillette PC, McNamara DG: Premature ventricular contractions in normal children. J Pediatr 1978;92:36–38.

Kugler JD, Danford DA, Deal BJ, et al: Radiofrequency catheter ablation for tachyarrhythmias in children and adolescents. N Engl J Med 1994;330:1481–1487.

Till JA, Shinebourne EA: Supraventricular tachycardia: diagnosis and current acute management. Arch Dis Child 1991;66:647–652.

Vetter VL: Postoperative arrhythmias after surgery for congenital heart defects. Cardiol Rev 1994;2:83–97.

182 Bradyarrhythmia

Dianne L. Atkins

Definition

1. Bradyarrhythmias are best defined by electrophysiologic mechanism rather than by absolute value of the heart rate. Normal heart rate is dependent on age, physical activity, and physical condition and can overlap with heart rates caused by abnormalities in impulse generation or conduction.
2. Rates ≤70 in infants and ≤50 in children warrant investigation.

Etiology and Epidemiology

1. Bradycardia in children is the result of abnormal impulse generation (sinus bradycardia, sick sinus syndrome) or abnormal impulse conduction (heart block).
2. Sinus bradycardia is a common sequela to corrective surgery for congenital heart disease, especially the atrial switch operation for d-transposition of the great arteries and the Fontan type operation for single ventricle. This is frequently referred to as sick sinus syndrome because of the associated atrial tachycardias. Sick sinus syndrome in children with normal cardiac anatomy is rare.
3. Congenital complete heart block is most commonly caused by maternal lupus erythematosus. Certain congenital malformations, especially ventricular inversion (l-transposition of the great arteries), are associated with complete atrioventricular (AV) block. Acquired AV block can be idiopathic or can result from open heart surgery, dilated cardiomyopathy, certain muscular dystrophies, myotonic dystrophy, and a variety of systemic infections including viral myocarditis bacterial endocarditis, Lyme disease, and Rocky Mountain spotted fever.

Pathogenesis

1. In patients with congenital heart disease, sick sinus syndrome is the result of alterations in intraatrial conduction following the atriotomy and atrial septum excision. Surgical disruption of the sinus node may also occur.
2. The pathogenesis of lupus-associated complete heart block is not completely understood but is known to be associated with placental transfer of circulating maternal antibodies to riboproteins termed anti-Ro and anti-La.

Clinical Findings

1. Sick sinus syndrome can be apparent immediately after surgery but more frequently appears 5 to 10 years later. Individuals may be asymptomatic or experience exercise intolerance and fatigue. The development of symptoms may be so insidious that patients do not recognize the changes. Other patients may have more acute symptoms with either syncope or sudden onset of congestive heart failure. Because sick sinus syndrome is frequently associated with atrial tachycardia, the patients may initially present with complaints of tachycardia.
2. Infants with congenital complete heart block are fre-

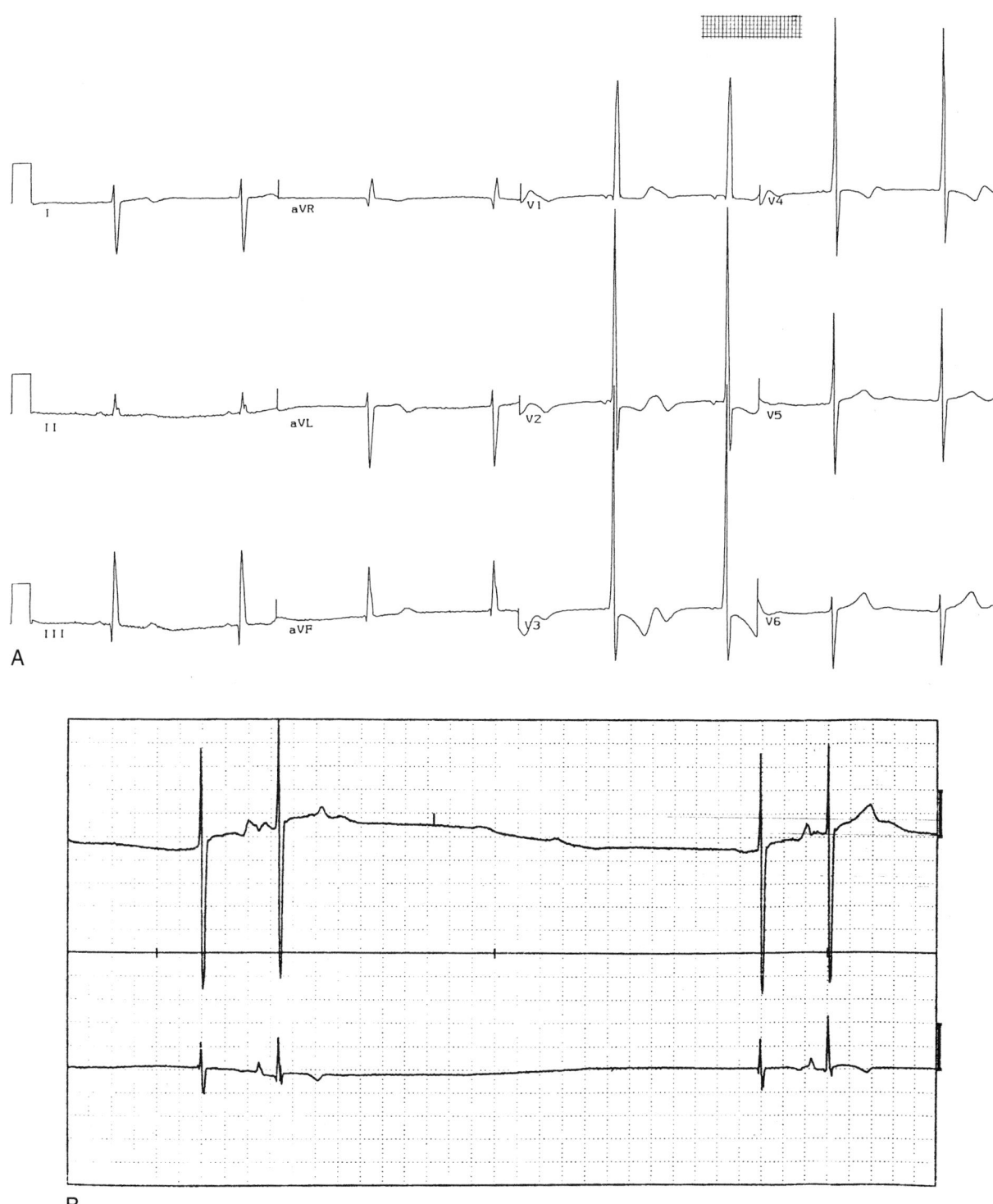

Figure 182–1 ECG and Holter tracing of patient with sinus node dysfunction. *A*, Heart rate is 50, and P waves have low amplitude. *B*, Holter tracing demonstrates extremely long (4.2 sec) pause.

quently diagnosed in utero because of low fetal heart rates. Symptoms are related to the ventricular rate. Infants with heart rates ≥55 are rarely symptomatic in infancy. In those with heart rates ≤55, symptoms include hydrops fetalis (an ominous finding in the fetus), congestive heart failure, and failure to thrive.

3. Patients who have acquired heart block may be asymptomatic or, more commonly, present with syncope or acute-onset congestive heart failure.

Key Clinical Findings
- Syncope
- Heart failure
- Fatigue

Laboratory Findings

1. The diagnosis of sinus node dysfunction is made by ECG and 24-hour ambulatory monitoring. Low resting heart rate, low mean heart rate, decreased heart rate variability, inappropriate heart rate response to exercise, and sinus pauses are observed singly or together (Fig. 182–1).

Key Laboratory Findings
- ECG

2. Complete heart block is characterized by total lack of conduction of the P waves to the ventricles (Fig. 182–2).

The atrial rate is faster than the ventricular rate. The QRS complex can be narrow if the site of block is above the His bundle, whereas block below the His bundle will have a prolonged QRS duration.

3. The mothers of infants with congenital complete heart block should be examined for clinical or serologic evidence of connective tissue disease.

Radiographic Findings

1. Radiographic findings are related to the presence of underlying heart disease. If congestive heart failure is present, cardiomegaly and suffused vascular markings may be observed.

Treatment

1. Treatment of sick sinus syndrome is directed at both the bradycardia and the tachycardia. Pacemaker therapy of symptomatic bradycardia is warranted. Antitachycardia pacing can be useful for patients with symptomatic bradycardia and tachycardia. Antiarrhythmic therapy may control the tachycardia but also may exacerbate the bradycardia. Prophylactic pacemaker implantation in asymptomatic patients remains controversial.

2. Acute treatment of heart block is directed at increasing the ventricular rate. Patients with acquired heart block may respond to intravenous isoproterenol, but infants with congenital complete heart block tend to have blunted responses to adrenergic agents. Atropine has very limited usefulness in congenital or acquired heart block. Temporary pacing may be indicated for unstable patients. Transcutaneous pacing is especially useful until temporary transvenous pacing can be accomplished.

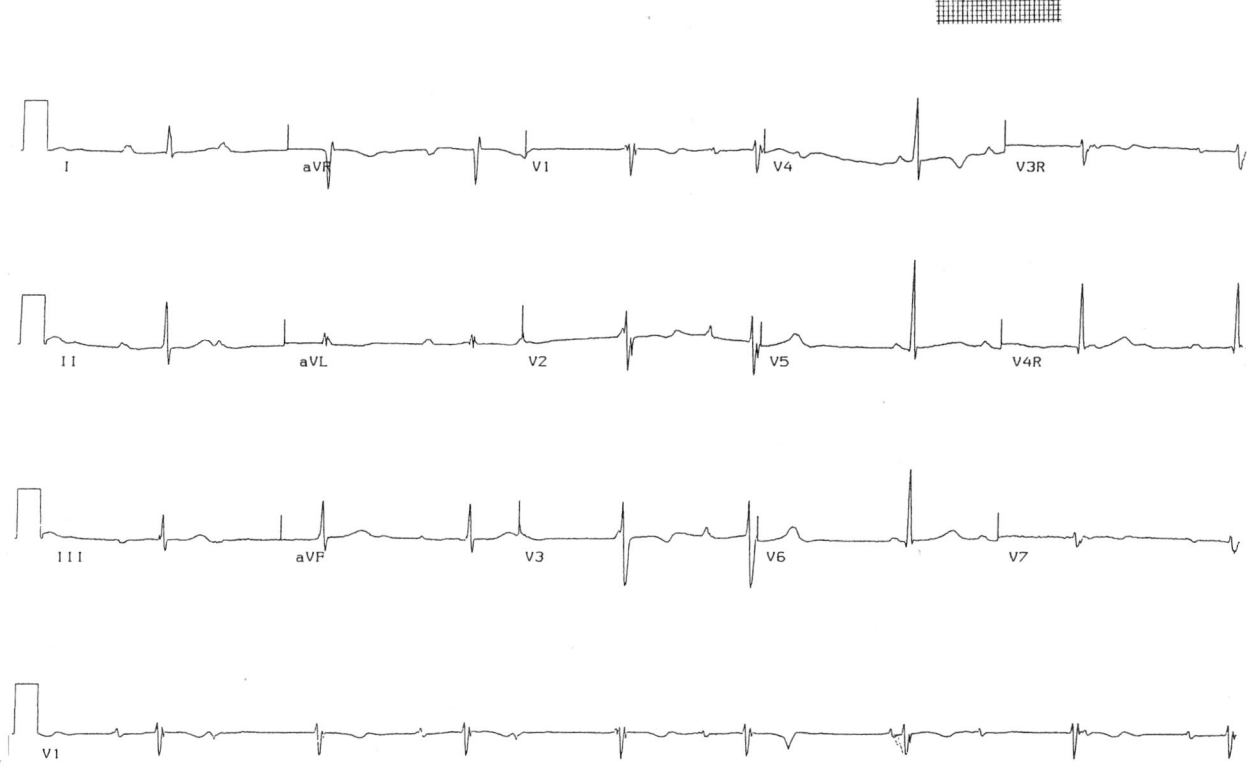

Figure 182–2 ECG of patient with complete heart block. P waves are apparent in leads II, AVR, and AVF and are faster (150 bpm) than the ventricular rate (80 bpm). QRS complex is narrow, indicating block above the His bundle.

3. Pacemaker implantation is the mainstay of therapy for complete heart block. Syncope, congestive heart failure, exercise intolerance, and block below the His bundle are definite indications for pacing. Pacing is possibly indicated for infants with heart rates ≤55, pauses two to three times the resting cycle length, and growth failure. Advances in pacemaker technology have dramatically increased the feasibility of this therapy for small infants and children.

Key Treatment–Heart Block

- Pacemaker
- Isoproterenol infusion (selected)

Bibliography

Dewey RC, Capeless MA, Levy AM: Use of ambulatory electrocardiographic monitoring to identify high-risk patients with congenital complete heart block. N Engl J Med 1987;316:835–839.

Flinn CJ, Wolff GS, Dick M II, et al: Cardiac rhythm after the Mustard operation for complete transposition of the great arteries. N Engl J Med 1984;310:1635–1638.

Kugler JD, Danford DA: Pacemakers in children: An update. Am Heart J 1989;117:665–679.

Vetter VL: Postoperative arrhythmias after surgery for congenital heart defects. Cardiol Rev 1994;2:83–97.

Waltuck J, Buyon JP: Autoantibody-associated congenital heart block: Outcome in mothers and children. Ann Intern Med 1994;120:544–551.

183 Myocarditis

Jeffrey A. Towbin

Definition

Myocarditis is a process characterized by inflammatory infiltrate of the myocardium with necrosis and/or degeneration of adjacent myocytes not typical of the ischemic damage associated with coronary artery disease.

Etiology

Most cases of myocarditis in the United States and western Europe result from viral infections. The most common viral causes include adenovirus and enterovirus (coxsackieviruses A and B, echovirus, poliovirus), particularly coxsackievirus B (Table 183–1). Other nonviral etiologies include infectious agents such as rickettsiae, bacteria, protozoa, and other parasites, fungi, and yeast (Table 183–2); various drugs, including antimicrobial medications; hypersensitivity or autoimmune disorders; toxic reactions to infectious agents (e.g., diphtheria); and other disorders such as Kawasaki disease, sarcoidosis, and scleroderma (see Table 183–2).

Epidemiology

Usually sporadic, viral myocarditis can also occur as an epidemic. Epidemics usually are seen in newborns, most

TABLE 183–1. CAUSES OF MYOCARDITIS

INFECTIOUS ETIOLOGIES	NONINFECTIOUS ETIOLOGIES
Viral	Collagen vascular
Rickettsial	Granulomatous disease
Bacterial	Pharmacologic agents
Mycobacterial	Physical agents (e.g., radiation)
Spirochetal	Chemicals
Fungal	Metabolic disorders
Parasitic	

TABLE 183–2. VIRAL CAUSES OF MYOCARDITIS

Enterovirus	Cytomegalovirus (CMV)	Rabies
Coxsackie A		Hepatitis
Coxsackie B	Herpesvirus	Rubella
Echovirus	Influenza	Rubeola
Poliovirus	Epstein-Barr virus (EBV)	Respiratory syncytial virus (RSV)
Adenovirus		
Parvovirus	Varicella	Human immunodeficiency virus (HIV)
	Mumps	

commonly in association with coxsackievirus B. Intrauterine myocarditis has also been seen during epidemics as well as sporadically. Postnatal spread of coxsackievirus is via the fecal/oral or airborne route. Other important viral causes, such as adenovirus and influenza A, are transmitted predominantly through the air. Although the disease can occur equally throughout the year, the etiology is probably season-dependent.

Pathophysiology

Viral infection results in interstitial inflammation or myocardial injury, leading to cardiac enlargement and an increase in the ventricular end-diastolic volume (Fig. 183–1). Normally, this increase in volume produces an increased force of contraction, improved ejection fraction, and improved cardiac output as demonstrated by the Starling mechanism. In the inflamed state, however, the myocardium is unable to respond to these stimuli, resulting in reduced cardiac output.

1. Interactions with the sympathetic nervous system may preserve systemic blood flow via vasoconstriction and elevated afterload. This sympathetic nervous system input results in tachycardia.
2. Congestive heart failure ensues, with disease progression.

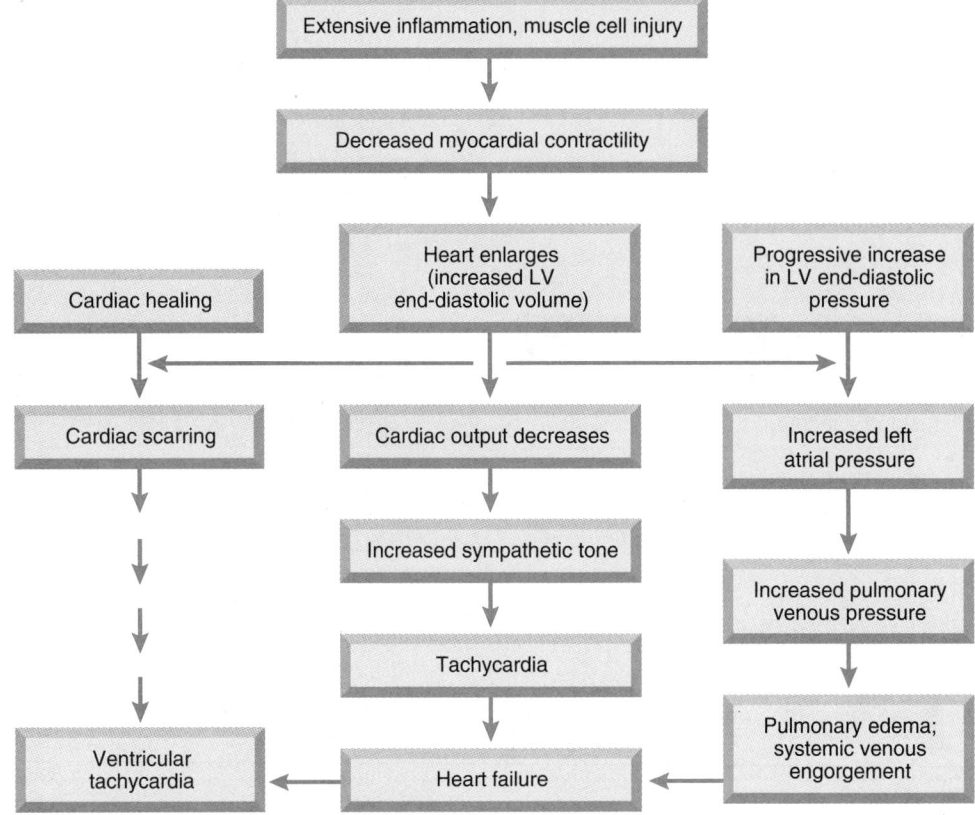

Figure 183–1 Pathophysiology of myocarditis.

The progressive increase in ventricular end-diastolic volume and pressure results in increased left atrial pressure, which is transmitted into the pulmonary venous system. This causes increasing hydrostatic forces, which overcome the colloid osmotic pressure that normally prevents transudation of fluid across the capillary membranes. This results in pulmonary edema.

3. Concomitantly, all cardiac chambers dilate, particularly the left ventricle. This dilatation, in addition to poor ventricular function, creates worsening pulmonary edema and worsening cardiac function. The ventricular dilatation also results in stretching of the mitral annulus and resultant mitral regurgitation, further increasing left atrial volume and pressure.

4. During the healing stages of myocarditis, fibroblasts replace normal myofibers and result in scar formation. Reduced elasticity and ventricular performance can lead to persistent heart failure. In addition, ventricular arrhythmias commonly accompany this fibrosis.

Clinical Findings

1. Differences in presentation are seen depending on the age of the child (e.g., newborn/infant vs. child or adolescent) (Fig. 183–2). Newborns or infants typically present with fever, irritability or listlessness, periodic episodes of pallor (which may precede the sudden onset of cardiorespiratory symptoms including tachypnea or respiratory distress), and diaphoresis. Poor appetite or vomiting is also seen frequently. Sudden death may occur. On physical examination, pallor and mild cyanosis are commonly noted. The skin is usually cool and mottled, consistent with poor perfusion due to decreased cardiac output. Respirations are usually rapid and labored; grunting may be prominent, but rales are uncommon. The cardiovascular examination is consistent with congestive heart failure and includes tachycardia, gallop rhythm, muffled heart sounds, and frequently an apical systolic murmur due to mitral regurgitation. The pulses are usually thready, and hepatomegaly is usually obvious.

2. Older children and adolescents commonly report a recent prior history of viral disease, generally 10 to 14 days earlier. Initial symptoms include lethargy, low-grade fever, and pallor; the child usually has decreased appetite

Newborn
- Sepsis
- Hypoxia
- Hypoglycemia
- Hypocalcemia

- Structural heart disease
- Idiopathic dilated cardiomyopathy
- Anomalous left coronary artery from the pulmonary artery
- Cerebral arteriovenous malformation

Child
- Idiopathic dilated cardiomyopathy
- Anomalous left coronary artery from the pulmonary artery
- Endocardial fibroelastosis
- Pericarditis

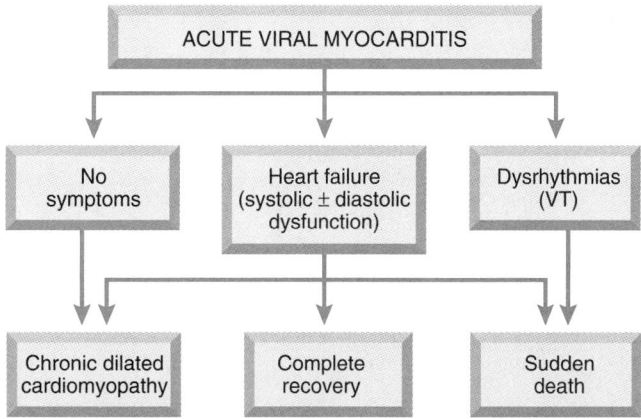

Figure 183–2 Clinical presentation of myocarditis.

and may complain of abdominal pain. Later in the course of the illness, respiratory symptoms become predominant; syncope or sudden death may occur. Physical examination findings are consistent with congestive heart failure, as described above.

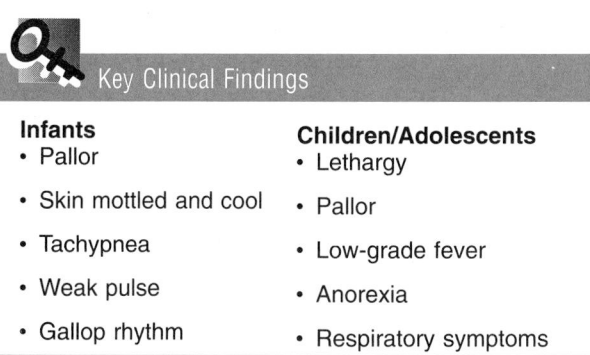

Key Clinical Findings

Infants	Children/Adolescents
• Pallor	• Lethargy
• Skin mottled and cool	• Pallor
• Tachypnea	• Low-grade fever
• Weak pulse	• Anorexia
• Gallop rhythm	• Respiratory symptoms

Diagnosis

The diagnosis of myocarditis is often difficult to establish but should be suspected in any infant or child who presents with unexplained congestive heart failure or ventricular tachycardia. Appropriate diagnostic studies include

1. Chest x-ray—Cardiomegaly with prominent pulmonary vascular markings consistent with congestive heart failure is notable.
2. Electrocardiogram—Sinus tachycardia with low-voltage QRS complexes (≤5 mm total amplitude in all limb leads) and low-voltage or inverted T waves are classically described. A pattern of myocardial infarction with wide Q waves (> 35 msec) and S-T segment changes may also be seen. Ventricular tachycardia or atrioventricular block occurs in some children.
3. Echocardiogram—A dilated and dysfunctional left ventricle consistent with a dilated cardiomyopathy is seen on two-dimensional and M-mode echocardiography. Pericardial effusion frequently occurs. Doppler and color-Doppler commonly demonstrate mitral regurgitation. Dilatation of other chambers may also be seen. Cardiac output calculations, if obtained, are typically reduced.
4. Endomyocardial biopsy—A cardiac catherization and endomyocardial biopsy may be performed to obtain cardiac output and intracardiac pressure measurements. Low car-

diac output is commonly seen along with elevated end-diastolic ventricular pressures. Endomyocardial biopsy is used to directly evaluate myocardium for evidence of inflammation histologically. Usually five tissue specimens are obtained for analysis, since the inflammatory infiltrate is usually patchy and scattered in the ventricular chamber. Evidence of significant mononuclear cell infiltrate is diagnostic of myocarditis, although this does not delineate etiology.

5. Viral studies—The diagnostic gold standard of the viral etiology is positive viral culture from the myocardium; this is rare, however. Other studies used to delineate the viral etiology include serologic studies in which a four-fold rise in antibody titer is required. Antibody studies commonly performed include type-specific neutralizing, hemagglutination-inhibiting, or complement-fixing antibody studies. However, these studies are nonspecific, since prior infection with the causative virus is commonplace. Molecular analysis using in situ hybridization has been used to identify coxsackievirus B sequences in myocardial samples. More recently, polymerase chain reaction (PCR) has been used to rapidly and specifically amplify viral sequences from cardiac tissue samples.

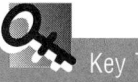

Key Treatment

• Supportive
• Digitalis for heart failure
• Diuretics
• ACE blockers

Differential Diagnosis

Any cause of acute circulatory failure may mimic myocarditis. The following box lists the differential diagnosis based on the age of the child.

Treatment

1. The therapy for myocarditis is supportive and nonspecific. In seriously ill patients, mechanical ventilation and intravenous inotropic support, including dobutamine, dopamine, and afterload-reducing agents (e.g., Nipride, amrinone, milrinone) are usually required. In addition,

intravenous diuretics are necessary. In stable patients, oral anticongestive medications are used; these include digoxin, diuretics, and afterload-reducing agents, particularly ACE inhibitors (e.g., captopril). In some children, anticoagulation is also necessary. Antiarrhythmic therapy may also be indicated in children with ventricular arrhythmias. If dilated cardiomyopathy results, cardiac transplantation may ultimately be required.

2. A variety of experimental therapies have been tried in association with the therapeutic agents outlined above. Steroids, immunosuppressive drugs (e.g., methotrexate, cyclosporin), and antiviral therapy such as interferon have been reported, with varying success. More recently, IV immunoglobulin has been used in a small number of patients, with good results.

Prognosis

1. Newborns are at significant risk of death resulting from acute myocarditis. In 30 to 50 per cent of these children, death ultimately occurs. In the remainder, approximately 30 per cent will recover, while 20 to 30 per cent will be left with a chronic dilated cardiomyopathy.

2. Children and adolescents generally have a less severe clinical course. However, a significant percentage die or are left with end-stage dilated cardiomyopathy.

Bibliography

Aretz HT, Billingham ME, Edwards WD, et al: Myocarditis: A histopathologic definition and classification. Am J Cardiovasc Pathol 1987;1:3–14.

Dec GW, Palacios IF, Fallon JT, et al: Active myocarditis in the spectrum of acute dilated cardiomyopathies: Clinical features, histologic correlates, and clinical outcome. N Engl J Med 1985;312:885–890.

Noren GR, Staley NA, Bandt CM, Kaplan EL: Occurrence of myocarditis in sudden death in children. J Forensic Sci 1977;22:118–196.

Towbin JA, Griffin LD, Martin AB, et al: Intrauterine adenoviral myocarditis presenting as nonimmune hydrops fetalis: Diagnosis by polymerase chain reaction. Pediatr Infect Dis J 1994;13:144–150.

184 Pericarditis

Jeffrey A. Towbin

Definition

Pericarditis is an inflammatory response of the pericardium, with or without an associated pericardial effusion.

Anatomy

The pericardium consists of a tough, fibrous outer coat with discrete attachments to the sternum, great vessels, diaphragm, and an inner membranous coat. These two loosely approximated layers are the visceral and parietal pericardium.

1. Visceral pericardium—Composed of a serosal membrane of mesothelial tissue that closely follows the contour of the heart and extends for a short distance beyond the atria and ventricles onto the great vessels.

2. Parietal pericardium—This outer layer consists of a fibrous coat that is lined by a serosal layer of cuboidal cells one layer thick. This fibrous structure contains layers of collagen interlaced with elastic fibers. The phrenic nerves are embedded in the parietal pericardium.

3. Pericardial cavity—Enclosed between the two serosal layers, this cavity usually contains a small amount of clear fluid (2 to 50 ml, depending on the size of the child), which is an ultrafiltrate of blood plasma.

Functions

1. Prevents overdistention of the heart
2. Protects the heart from infection and adhesions
3. Maintains the heart within a fixed geometric position within the chest

4. Regulates the interaction between the stroke volumes of the two ventricles.

Epidemiology

Pericardial disease of all etiologies reportedly occurs once in every 850 hospital admissions. There appears to be a predominance of cases in children ≤ 2 years of age. The sex distribution is approximately equal.

Etiology

1. Pericarditis is most commonly associated with infection; viral causes occur most frequently but are usually difficult to prove (Table 184–1). Nonviral infectious causes, such as bacterial, amebic, rickettsial, and fungal, are no longer common. In the past, particularly in the era prior to antibiotic therapy, purulent pericarditis was seen relatively frequently. Typical causes included pneumococcal, streptococcal, staphylococcal (especially *S. aureus*), *Haemophilus influenzae*, and tuberculous infections.

2. Noninfectious etiologies include trauma, hypersensitivity reactions to various drugs, and collagen vascular diseases such as lupus erythematosus. Kawasaki disease may also have associated pericarditis.

Pathology

1. Acute fibrinous or "dry" pericarditis is associated with acute fibrinous deposits that give rise to the characteristic "bread-and-butter" appearance of the pericardium. The fine deposits of fibrin are initially seen adjacent to the

TABLE 184–1. CAUSES OF PERICARDITIS

TRAUMA

Pericardiotomy
Indirect trauma to chest
Transseptal catherization
Pressure injection of contrast media
Perforation of right ventricle by indwelling catheter
Implantation of epicardial pacemaker
Blow to chest
Perforation of right ventricle with catheter for parenteral nutrition

VIRAL INFECTIONS

Coxsackie B5, B6
Echovirus
Adenovirus
Infectious mononucleosis
Influenza
Lymphogranuloma venereum
Chickenpox
Mycoplasma pneumoniae
AIDS

BACTERIAL INFECTIONS

Staphylococcus
Pneumococcus
Meningococcus
Streptococcus
Haemophilus influenzae
Psittacosis
Salmonella
Tuberculosis

AMEBIASIS

ECHINOCOCCUS CYSTS

FUNGUS INFECTIONS

Histoplasmosis, aspergillosis, blastomycosis, coccidioidomycosis

RICKETTSIA

RADIATION

AMYLOIDOSIS

KAWASAKI DISEASE

TUMORS

COLLAGEN VASCULAR DISEASE

Rheumatic fever
Lupus erythematosus
Rheumatoid arthritis
Vasculitis
Polyarteritis nodosa
Scleroderma
Dermatomyositis

ANTICOAGULANTS

Heparin
Warfarin

MYOCARDIAL INFARCTION

Post–myocardial infarction pericarditis (Dressler syndrome)

IDIOPATHIC THROMBOCYTOPENIC PURPURA

DRUGS

Procainamide
Cromolyn sodium
Hydralazine
Dantrolene
Methysergide

DISSECTING ANEURYSM

INFECTIVE ENDOCARDITIS WITH VALVE RING ABSCESS

THYMIC CYST

---

great vessels, thus causing the pericardial membrane to lose its smoothness and translucency.

2. The usual findings of inflammation, including numerous granulocytes (which may extend into the myocardium), are seen.
3. Pericardial fluid often accumulates in pericarditis, leading to pericardial effusion.

Pathophysiology

1. As pericardial fluid accumulates, intrapericardial pressure rises. The rate of rise is a function of the rapidity of accumulation as well as the compliance of the pericardium. In cases of slowly accumulating fluid, large volumes can be accommodated because the parietal pericardium can gradually expand. As the compliance of the pericardium reaches its maximum, however, further fluid accumulation results in an abrupt increase in intrapericardial pressure.
2. If pericardial fluid accumulation is rapid, marked elevation in intrapericardial pressure may occur with a much smaller volume of fluid.
3. The most significant hemodynamic effect of pericardial effusion is restriction to ventricular filling. Left ventricular and right ventricular diastolic pressures become equal to each other as well as to the pressure in both atria.
4. When restriction to ventricular filling becomes more pronounced, there is a fall in ventricular stroke volume and cardiac output. In an attempt to maintain cardiac output, tachycardia and peripheral vasoconstriction occur along with reduction of systemic arterial blood pressure and pulse pressure.
5. Cardiac tamponade occurs when these compensatory mechanisms fail to maintain adequate cardiac output. Cardiac tamponade means that there is compression of the heart by tense pericardial sac (usually full of fluid) that results in a decrease in venous return to the cardiac chambers and a decrease in cardiac output.

Clinical Findings

1. The classic signs and symptoms of pericarditis include the following:
   a. Precordial pain
   b. Pericardial friction rub
   c. Evidence of pericardial effusion
   d. Muffled heart sounds.
2. Chest pain is not a frequent symptom, especially in young children. The reported percentage of children complaining of chest pain is between 15 and 20 per cent.
3. The most common symptoms and signs of pericarditis are fever, tachypnea, and tachycardia in association with either cardiac enlargement or pericardial friction rub. The children are often lethargic and complain of loss of appetite and abdominal pain.

4. On physical examination, the following findings are common:

a. Muffled heart tones

b. Pericardial friction rub—High-frequency scratchy murmur that may be to-and-fro or triphasic but may not have any correlation with the cardiac cycle. The sound may be described as a "train-in-the-tunnel." The rub may be heard better with the patient leaning forward or kneeling, and it commonly increases in intensity with inspiration.

c. Ventricular apical impulse is commonly difficult to palpate.

d. Kussmaul sign—During inspiration, intrathoracic pressure falls and an increase in venous return to the vena cava occurs; owing to diastolic compression the tense pericardial sac limits the amount of blood that can enter the right atrium, and hence there is a paradoxical rise in jugular venous pressure during inspiration.

e. Pulsus paradoxus: During inspiration there is normally a small drop in systolic blood pressure and cardiac output due to an increase in pulmonary venous capacitance. This is exaggerated with pericardial tamponade, with ≥10 mmHg drop in blood pressure occurring with inspiration because of the restricted inflow into the cardiac chambers.

Key Clinical Findings

- Chest pain
- Friction rub
- Muffled heart sounds
- Pulsus paradoxus

Laboratory Test

The following studies may be helpful at arriving at the diagnosis of pericarditis:

1. Chest x-ray—Rapidly increasing cardiopericardial silhouette and cardiothoracic ratio without increasing pulmonary vascular markings is suggestive of pericarditis. The heart commonly has a globular shape.

2. Electrocardiogram (ECG)—Low-voltage QRS complexes are commonly seen in the presence of pericardial effusion. An injury pattern manifested by S-T segment deviation is common. Typically, pronounced S-T segment elevation occurs early in the disease along with PR segment depression. Subsequently the S-T segment has nearly returned to baseline, the T wave amplitude diminishes, and the PR segment continues to be depressed. Next the S-T segment returns completely to baseline, and T-wave inversion is seen. Over time, these changes resolve completely. Electrical alternans is seen in the presence of large pericardial effusions (i.e., alteration in electrical amplitude of the T wave and the QRS complex with each cardiac cycle).

3. Echocardiogram—Two-dimensional imaging demonstrates pericardial effusions in real time and may be measured on line. M-mode echocardiography is also sensitive in the detection of pericardial effusions.

4. Blood studies—The erythrocyte sedimentation rate is almost always elevated, and leukocytosis is common early in the course.

5. Cardiac catheterization—Not usually performed unless attempts at pericardiocentesis are to be made under fluoroscopy, or an attempt to differentiate constrictive pericarditis from restrictive cardiomyopathy is necessary.

6. Identification of etiology—Pericardial fluid obtained at pericardiocentesis can be studied under light microscopy for evidence of neoplastic cells or cultured for virus, bacteria, or fungus. Recently, molecular analysis of the fluid has been possible using the polymerase chain reaction (PCR) to identify specific nucleic acid sequences of the responsible infectious agent.

Key Laboratory Tests

- ECG
- Chest x-ray
- Echocardiography

Differential Diagnosis

1. Restrictive cardiomyopathy
2. Absence of the pericardium
3. Ebstein anomaly
4. Dilated cardiomyopathy
5. Myocarditis
6. Anomalous left coronary artery from the pulmonary artery
7. Glycogen storage disease
8. Cardiac tumors.

Treatment

1. Pericardiocentesis—In cases of pericardial effusion, tapping off most or all of the fluid may be lifesaving (in cases of tamponade) or may significantly alleviate symptoms. The fluid may also be used for diagnostic purposes.

2. Antiinflammatory agents—Aspirin therapy has been a mainstay for decades. More recently, nonsteroidal antiinflammatory agents (NSAIDs) have been used in cases in which aspirin is not indicated. Steroids may also be effective. In some cases, diuretic therapy may be useful.

3. Pericardial window/Pericardiectomy—This surgical method may be employed in cases of recurrent pericardial effusion. Here the parietal pericardium is resected (parietal pericardiectomy), allowing drainage of pericardial fluid to occur unimpeded. In cases of constrictive pericarditis, visceral pericardiectomy is necessary.

Key Treatment

- Pericardiocentesis
- Aspirin or NSAIDs
- Surgery (uncommon) for recurrent effusions

Prognosis

Viral pericarditis generally resolves spontaneously over a 3- to 4-week period. Large pericardial effusions and tamponade are rare. Acute purulent pericarditis has mortality rates in the 25 to 75 per cent range. Factors contributing to mortality include:

1. Delay in recognition
2. Presence of tamponade
3. Absence of early surgical drainage
4. The etiologic agent
5. The age of the patient.

Most children recover fully and return to normal activity.

 Bibliography

Pinsky WW, Friedman RA: Pericarditis. *In* Ganson A Jr, et al (eds): The Science and Practice of Pediatric Cardiology. Baltimore, Williams & Wilkins, 1990, pp 1590–1599.

Shabetai R: Diseases of the pericardium. *In* O'Rourke RA (ed): Hurst's The Heart, 8th ed. New York, McGraw-Hill, 1995, pp 1647–1674.

Spodick DH: Diseases of the pericardium. *In* Parmley WW, Chatterjee K (eds): Cardiology, vol 2. Philadelphia, JB Lippincott, 1988.

Strauss AW, Santa-Marie M, Goldring D: Constrictive pericarditis in children. Am J Dis Child 1975;129:822–826.

Tuna IC, Danielson GK: Surgical management of pericardial diseases. Cardiol Clin 1990;8:683–696.

185 Hypertension

Arno R. Hohn

Definition

Hypertension means high systemic blood pressure (BP). Systolic, diastolic, or both pressures are above established normal values. In the young, persistent BPs above the 95th percentile for age, per the revision of the 1987 Task Force Report pressure guidelines, are hypertensive. Rosner et al. (J Pediatr, 1993) added considerations of height.

Etiology

Hypertension is a sign, not a disease. Known causes (secondary hypertension) and unknown causes (primary hypertension) vary by age and are listed in Table 185–1.

1. The prevalence of primary hypertension increases with age. In older children most mild hypertension is primary.
2. Renal parenchymal diseases are the most common secondary cause of hypertension.
3. Genetics: A strong hereditary influence on BP exists.

Epidemiology

About 15 per cent of the United States adult population have hypertension, whereas only 1 or 2 per cent of young people have persistent hypertension.

1. Prevalence of hypertension is between 0.5 and 1.5 per cent of children.
2. Weight has a positive relationship with blood pressure. Over half of hypertensive young people are obese.
3. Age: BP increases in a nonlinear fashion through childhood.
4. Salt intake: For most individuals, little correlation exist between sodium intake and BP. However, there is a group of salt-sensitive individuals in whom sodium restriction appears beneficial. Black children from hypertensive families may be salt sensitive.
5. Other nutrient intake: A link between potassium intake and BP exists, but efforts to correlate calcium and other divalent cations as well as vitamins A, C, and E with BP have been equivocal.
6. Fat and fiber: Reduction in dietary intake of these substances together has been noted to reduce BP. Triglyceride levels are also correlated with pressure levels.
7. Stress: Both physical and mental stress evoke changes in BP.
8. Race: Although a factor in adults, race is not a factor in most children. Certain subgroups of black children had higher pressures than their white counterparts.

TABLE 185–1.   ESTIMATED AGE-RELATED HYPERTENSION CAUSES

AGE GROUP	NEONATE	INFANT	TODDLER	CHILD	ADOLESCENT	YOUNG ADULT
Condition	%	%	%	%	%	%
Congenital (incl. coarctation)	14	10	5	3	<1.0	<0.1
Renovascular (incl. thrombosis)	50	30	5	2	1	<0.4
Renal parenchymal disease	1	20	30	25	6	<4.0
Primary hypertension	15	30	50	65	91	95
Other	20*	10	10	5	2	1
	100	100	100	100	100	100

*Incl. central nervous system.

9. Tracking of (maintenance of rank order over time): Evidence that adult hypertension is predictable by childhood blood pressures is controversial, and correlation coefficients are generally low.

Pathophysiology

1. Blood pressure regulation is a complex interaction of neurohumoral mechanisms. When BP changes occur, baroreflexes, chemoreflexes, or CNS ischemic mechanisms are first called into play. Later, regulatory processes of the renin-angiotensin and kallikrein-kinin systems and the kidney blood volume mechanism act to control BP. Local vasoregulation of peripheral resistance is effected by autoregulatory mechanisms commonly mediated by nitric oxide.

2. A large number of disease processes, both known (secondary hypertension) and unknown (primary hypertension), result in hypertension.

3. Whatever the cause, the impact of hypertension is an end-organ effect. That is, serious hypertension results in central nervous system disorders from seizures to strokes, in renal disorders from increasing the severity of existing renal disease to renal shutdown, in cardiac disorders from heart failure to cardiomyopathy, and in eye disorders from impaired vision to blindness.

Clinical Findings

1. Three successive blood pressure determinations on different days show either high systolic and/or diastolic pressure. Most children with hypertension have pressures between the 95th and the 99th percentile. These people are generally symptom free and unaware of their pressure elevation.

2. If pressures are repeatedly above the 99th percentile in a symptomatic child, secondary hypertension is likely. Common symptoms and findings include

   a. Headache

   b. Chest pain or dyspnea

   c. Muscle weakness, abdominal masses, or bruits

   d. Obesity or edema

   e. Pallor, flushing attacks, or palpitation

   f. Polydipsia, polyuria, or weight loss

   g. Change in hair, body habitus, or menses

   h. Past history of renal, thyroid, or heart disease

   i. Skin striae/café-au-lait spots/neurofibromas

   j. Drug use

   k. Smoking history

   l. Family history of hypertension, myocardial infarction, diabetes, or strokes, and age of diagnosis

   m. Physical examination should include

      (1) Pulse and BP level in both arms and one lower extremity

      (2) Fundi for arteriolar narrowing

      (3) Cardiac/neurologic examination for stroke or cardiomegaly/failure

      (4) Body habitus (pattern of obesity, e.g., "buffalo hump")

   n. Clinical signs of secondary causes of hypertension are outlined in the Table 185–2.

TABLE 185–2. CLINICAL FINDINGS THAT MAY INDICATE THE PRESENCE OF HYPERTENSION IN THE INFANT OR CHILD

FINDING	SUSPECTED DISORDER
Abdominal masses or murmurs	Wilms tumor or neuroblastoma; renal artery stenosis
Weak distal pulses	Coarctation of the aorta
Heart murmur	Patent ductus arteriosus ± coarctation of aorta
Gonadal hypertrophy/dysgenesis	Adrenal hyperplasia; Turner syndrome
Salt loss/electrolyte imbalance	Adrenal disorders
Burns/large fractures	Secondary hypercalcemia from bone demineralization
Failure to thrive	Primary or secondary renal disorders
Neurofibromatosis	Renal artery stenosis
History of umbilical artery, catheterization	Renal artery thrombosis
Orbital tumor	Neuroblastoma
Steroid therapy	Cushing syndrome
Unexplained heart failure	Hypertensive cardiomyopathy
Unexplained seizures	Hypertensive encephalopathy

Key Clinical Findings

- Blood pressure >95 percentile
- Obesity (common)

Laboratory Findings

Without positive historical or examination findings, only a basic set of laboratory tests should be done, including

1. Sedimentation rate: may be elevated with secondary hypertension

2. Hematocrit/hemoglobin: elevated with hypertension

3. Urinalysis (with culture in females): abnormal with renal disorders

4. Blood chemistry panel (including BUN, creatinine, glucose) and electrolytes: If abnormal, may point to a renal or endocrine disorder.

5. Additional laboratory tests (if secondary hypertension suspected or if blood pressure remains elevated for over 6 months)

   (a) Echocardiogram (evaluate left ventricular wall thickness). LV wall thickness is thought to roughly correlate with time spent hypertensive. It is not seen in transient or "white-coat hypertension"

   (b) Chest x-ray: for cardiomegaly

   (c) Cholesterol and fasting triglyceride

   (d) Urine culture if not previously done

   (e) Uric acid (if elevated, a marker for hypertension in the young)

6. Tests for specific causes of hypertension should be ordered in conjunction with an expert in pediatric hypertension. Some of the tests include

   (a) Renal radiologic examinations such as CT and MR scans as well as radioisotope studies.

   (b) Hormonal studies such as urine catecholamine, plasma renin activity, serum aldosterone, and free plasma cortisol

Key Laboratory Findings

- Urinalysis and Hgb
- Serum electrolytes and urea, creatinine

Treatment

1. Medicines are definitely indicated for those who are
   a. symptomatic
   b. have dangerously high pressures, i.e., >12 mmHg over 99th percentile diastolic or >25 mmHg over 99th percentile systolic
   c. have evidence of end-organ damage.
   If in doubt and in the absence of symptoms, proteinuria, cardiomegaly, or echocardiographic evidence of left ventricular hypertrophy, it may be best to postpone drug treatment. Nonpharmacologic measures are used instead.
2. Drug therapy should be simple to adhere to in order to increase compliance in what may be a lifelong asymptomatic problem.
3. Explicit education should be given regarding hypertension and the reasons for therapy.
4. Age permitting, a young person should be responsible for taking his or her own medication.
5. Drug therapy is begun with a monodrug regimen that is superimposed on nonpharmacologic measures as initial treatment (Table 185–3). A calcium entry blocker (CEB) or angiotensin-converting enzyme (ACE) inhibitor or a diuretic or β blocker may be used.
   a. Begin with a low dose of the chosen initial drug. Many will begin with an ACE inhibitor. Titrate to a higher dose if necessary. If blood pressure control is still not achieved, proceed to:
   b. Add or substitute a small dose of a CEB inhibitor or diuretic or adrenergic inhibiting agent, whichever was not used in step a. Proceed to a full dose if necessary. If blood pressure control is still not achieved, proceed to:
   c. Add a third antihypertensive drug, usually a vasodilator or renin-angiotensin inhibitor, or preferably

TABLE 185–3. CLASSES OF HYPERTENSIVE MEDICATIONS

The most used specific drugs in each class are listed. References, such as the Pediatric Dosing Formulary (1995), provide dosages.

DIURETICS

Thiazide diuretics (hydrochlorothiazide—HydroDIURIL)

ADRENERGIC INHIBITORS

β-Adrenergic antagonists (atenolol—Tenormin)
Central adrenergic inhibitors (clonidine—Catapres)
α-Adrenergic receptor antagonists (prazosin—Minipress)

VASODILATORS

Vascular smooth muscle relaxing agents (hydralazine—Apresoline)
Slow-channel calcium-influx inhibitors (CEB) (nifedipine—Procardia)

ANGIOTENSIN-CONVERTING ENZYME (ACE) INHIBITOR

(enalapril maleate—Vasotec)

obtain consultation from an expert in hypertension in young people.
   d. Complications: Diuretics and β blockers have associated problems
      (1) For diuretics—hypokalemia, hypercholesterolemia, and hyperglycemia
      (2) For β blockers—elevated triglycerides and lowered HDL cholesterol.
      (3) ACE inhibitors and calcium blockers have the potential to control hypertension without these effects, although the long-term side effects and efficacy of the above drugs are not yet known.
   e. Once- or twice-a-day dosage is the preferred therapy. Long-acting or sustained-release medications are available.
6. Stepdown therapy or drug treatment withdrawal may be tried after an extended course of drug therapy with BP control.
7. Hypertensive emergencies (critical state)
   a. Definition: Signs of encephalopathy or heart failure with blood pressure 1.3 to 1.5 × the 95th percentile. Disastrous consequences may ensue unless efforts to lower the blood pressure are begun at once.
   b. Treatment
      (1) Hospitalize the patient and place a intravenous line.
      (2) If the patient is obtunded, begin intravenous sodium nitroprusside at a dose of 0.5 μ/kg, and titrate to slowly reduce the blood pressure toward the 99th percentile.
      (3) When the patient becomes responsive, change to oral medications.
      (4) If the patient needing help is conscious when first seen, give sublingual nifedipine 0.25 to 0.5 mg/kg every 30 minutes until a decrease in blood pressure is seen or a maximum dose of 1 mg/kg is reached.
      (5) Then begin maintenance therapy, or try other drugs.
      (6) The therapeutic goal in emergency cases is control of pressure while avoiding hypotension or too rapidly lowering the pressure.
      (7) When adequate pressure control is achieved, search for the cause of the hypertension, if not known.

Key Treatment

- Diuretic
- ACE inhibitor or β blocker
- Calcium entry blocker

Prevention

1. Prevention hinges on early detection of those at risk for later life hypertension. Risk factors include the following:
   a. Systolic blood pressure over the 90th percentile: doubles risk

b. Family history of two or more members with hypertension: increases risk two to four times.

c. Weight >20 per cent above the norm for height: Two thirds will be hypertensive.

d. Race: Blacks have over 10 per cent more hypertension in adulthood than other racial groups, i.e., 25 per cent will be found hypertensive in later life.

e. Dietary cations: Especially increased dietary sodium in salt-sensitive individuals and decreased potassium intake may lead to higher blood pressures.

f. Other risk factors include hyperlipidemia (or family history of), stress, smoking, alcohol/drug intake, preeclampsia and eclampsia, and diabetes mellitus.

2. Normotensive children and adolescents with one or more risk factors may benefit from nonpharmacologic antihypertension measures, especially

a. Those with consistently high normal blood pressure (above the 90th percentile)

b. Those with a trend of upward tracking pressures (above the 75th percentile) or pressures occasionally above the 95th percentile

c. Those who are obese, especially if parents are obese

d. Those with hyperlipidemia or a family history of the disorder, especially if with coronary artery disease or stroke

e. Those with diabetes mellitus

f. Those with two or more family members with treated hypertension, especially African Americans.

3. Nonpharmacologic measures include

a. Periodic blood pressure determinations

b. Dietary counseling for obesity

c. Avoidance of excess salt intake
Low-sodium, high-potassium foods are recommended as well as avoiding high-sodium, low-potassium foods.

d. Encouragement of regular physical exercise

e. Discontinuance of smoking and avoidance of alcohol excess, medications (save as directed by health care providers), and drugs

f. Other methods such as behavior modification, biofeedback, and hypnosis may be helpful.

Bibliography

Hohn AR: Guidebook for Pediatric Hypertension. Mount Kisco, NY, Futura Publishing, 1994, pp 209–278.

Joint National Committee (National High Blood Pressure Education Program): The fifth report of the Joint National Committee report on detection, evaluation and treatment of high blood pressure. Arch Intern Med 1993;153:154.

Lauer RM, Clarke WR: Childhood risk factors for high adult blood pressure: the Muscatine study. Pediatrics 1989;84:633.

Taketomo C (ed): Childrens Hospital of Los Angeles Pediatrics Dosing Handbook and Formulary. Hudson, OH: Lexi-Comp, 1995.

Update on the 1987 Task Force Report on High Blood Pressure in Children and Adolescents. Pediatrics 1996;98:649–658.

U.S. Task Force on Blood Pressure Control in Children—Report of the Second Task Force on Blood Pressure Control in Children—1987. Pediatrics 1987;79:1.

186 Kawasaki Syndrome

Masato Takahashi

Definition

Kawasaki syndrome (KS), also known as mucocutaneous lymph node syndrome (MCLS), may be diagnosed in a patient who fulfills five of the six diagnostic criteria and in whom other similar clinical conditions with known etiology have been ruled out with reasonable certainty. An exception to this definition is the patient with fewer than five clinical criteria who has been demonstrated to have typical coronary artery changes by echocardiography or angiography (see under *Clinical Findings*).

Etiology

Currently, the etiology of KS is unknown. Epidemiologic features such as a predilection for infants and young children, tendency for an increased incidence during winter and spring, and time-space clusters suggest a viral agent. Numerous etiologic theories have been proposed in the past, but none could be verified.

Epidemiology

1. Demographic factors

a. Median age of the patients is about 3 years. Children ≤5 years of age constitute 80 per cent of the patients.

b. The male to female ratio is approximately 1.6:1.

c. Attack rates in the United States is 9/100,000 children ≤5 years of age. Susceptibility varies along ethnic lines, Asian children being most susceptible, followed by blacks and Caucasians. Hispanic children have the same low level of susceptibility as Caucasians. The attack rate among Japanese children is 75 to 80/100,000 children.

d. Person-to-person transmission is rare.

2. Temporal and geographic factors

a. The incidence is higher during winter and spring.

b. The cases tend to cluster in time and place, but the number does not reach pandemic proportions.

c. Nationwide epidemics of KS were reported in Japan in 1979, 1982, and 1986, but no epidemics have been noted for the last 10 years. In the United States no nationwide active surveillance data are available. Although minor fluctuations in the incidence have occurred in some metropolitan areas, no clear-cut epidemics have occurred in the last several years.

Pathophysiology

1. Kawasaki syndrome is a systemic vasculitis with a self-limited clinical course. An unknown etiologic agent triggers a cell-mediated immune reaction, including activation of CD4 + T cells and B cells, spontaneous production of cytotoxic antibodies and immune complexes, and release of a multitude of cytokines. Some workers have proposed involvement of a superantigen that activates a cohort of T cells bearing Vβ receptors.

2. Eventually, inflammation becomes localized to medium-sized arteries, particularly the coronary arteries. The coronary arteries may become aneurysmal in about 20 per cent of untreated cases approximately 10 days from the onset of the acute symptoms.

3. When the aneurysms become large (≥8 mm in diameter, so-called giant aneurysms), there is increased risk of thrombotic occlusion due to stagnation of blood or of localized stenosis due to intimal proliferation at either end of the aneurysm, which may lead to myocardial infarction.

Clinical Findings

1. Since the etiology of this disease is unknown, the diagnosis is established when the patient has a fever for 5 days or longer and fulfills at least four of the following five principal clinical findings. A patient with fever and fewer than four principal symptoms may be diagnosed with atypical KS if there is evidence of coronary artery aneurysms by either echocardiography or angiography.

2. The patients frequently exhibit signs of acute pancarditis. These include tachycardia out of proportion to the degree of fever; transient cardiomegaly and pulmonary venous congestion on chest roentgenogram; ECG changes such as low-voltage R waves, flat T waves, and prolonged PR and QT intervals; and echocardiographic evidence of dilated left ventricle, reduced shortening fraction, mitral insufficiency, and pericardial effusion. Occasionally, patients may manifest a clinical picture of cardiogenic shock.

3. Patients ≤6 months of age offer a diagnostic challenge, as their clinical symptoms are often subtle and yet their fever is unrelenting. They frequently develop severe cardiovascular sequelae such as giant or multiple aneurysms, peripheral artery aneurysms (frequently in axillary and femoral arteries), and, rarely, gangrene of fingers and toes.

4. In addition to the principal symptoms described above, the patient may show involvement of the hepatobiliary system, such as hepatomegaly, jaundice, abnormal liver function tests, and hydropic gallbladder. The urogenital system may be involved with sterile pyuria and occasionally orchitis in boys. Anorexia and diarrhea are frequently present. Clinical findings of aseptic meningitis may be present, including mononuclear cells in the spinal fluid.

5. Arthritis involving interphalangeal joints, wrists, knees, and ankles is occasionally seen. Arthritis of the lower extremities may persist for several weeks, causing difficulty in walking.

6. Recurrence of KS may occur in 2 to 3 per cent of the patients who recover from the initial disease. Recurrent disease may produce new cardiac sequelae.

Key Clinical Findings

- Fever, 5 days or longer

- Changes in peripheral extremities
  Acute phase: Erythema and indurative edema of hands and feet
  Convalescent phase: Membranous desquamation of fingertips and toe tips

- Polymorphous exanthem, which may resemble measles, scarlet fever, or erythema multiforme, but is almost never bullous. Rash often starts in the inguinal area.

- Bilateral painless bulbar conjunctival injection without exudate

- Changes in lips and oral cavity: Erythema and cracking of lips, strawberry tongue, diffuse injection of oral and pharyngeal mucosa

- Acute nonpurulent cervical lymphadenopathy (≥1.5 cm in diameter), usually unilateral

Laboratory Findings

1. Blood studies show elevated white cell count with neutrophilia and increased band cells. Low-grade anemia, usually of normocytic and normochromic type, is common. Platelet count is normal or decreased in the first week but becomes elevated in the second week of illness. Acute phase reactants such as erythrocyte sedimentation rate, C-reactive protein, and α1-antitrypsin become elevated early in the acute phase and remain elevated several weeks after the patient becomes afebrile. The platelet count and acute phase reactants return to normal by the sixth to eighth week of illness.

2. Liver function tests such as transaminase and lactic dehydrogenase show mild to moderate elevation during the acute phase. High-dose aspirin therapy may accentuate transaminase levels. Bilirubin may be elevated in some patients.

3. A urinalysis may show positive albumin and leukocytes without bacteria.

4. For chest roentgenographic, ECG, and echocardiographic findings, see under *Clinical Findings*.

Key Laboratory Tests

- WBC

- Platelet count

- ESR

Differential Diagnosis

1. Viral or rickettsial diseases—Measles, Epstein-Barr infection, Rocky Mountain spotted fever
2. Bacterial infections—Scarlet fever, leptospirosis, *Yersinia* pseudotuberculosis
3. Other conditions—Stevens-Johnson syndrome, toxic shock syndrome, drug hypersensitivity reaction, juvenile rheumatoid arthritis, rheumatic fever, hypersensitivity to mercury.

Treatment

1. Acute phase
   a. Intravenous gamma globulin (IVGG) 2 g/kg body weight combined with high-dose aspirin (80 to 100 mg/kg per day in four divided doses)* should be given, preferably within the first 10 days of illness, for demonstrated effectiveness to shorten the duration of fever and reduce the prevalence of coronary artery abnormalities. Adverse effects of IVGG include chills, a high fever spike, pruritus, and, rarely, anaphylactoid shock. Minor adverse effects may be treated by slowing or temporarily stopping the infusion and giving Benadryl. Anaphylactoid shock must be treated promptly with respiratory and circulatory support.
   b. High-dose aspirin, if given, should be continued for several days after defervescence or up to the fourteenth day of illness, and then the dose should be reduced to 3 to 5 mg/kg/day for antiplatelet effect. Absorption of aspirin from the gastrointestinal tract is inefficient during the acute phase of the disease. But as the patient improves, so does the GI uptake of aspirin, such that one must be aware of the possibility of aspirin, toxicity in the second and third weeks of illness. Progressive elevation of transaminase is an indication for early dose reduction or discontinuation of aspirin. Although Reye syndrome is extremely rare, it has been reported in KS patients.
   c. General supportive measures include bed rest in semi-dark quiet surroundings, topical treatments for itching or tenderness caused by skin rash or desquamation, intravenous or oral fluid replacement, and cardiac monitoring as appropriate.
   d. For the treatment of persistent arthritis in the convalescent phase, around-the-clock dosing of a nonsteroidal antiinflammatory agent (NSAID) is often effective.
2. Chronic phase
   a. Although we do not have follow-up data of Kawasaki patients much beyond 10 years, the following empirical scheme of risk stratification has been proposed.
   b. *Risk level I:* No drug therapy is proposed beyond the first 6 to 8 weeks. At the moment there is no reason to impose any restriction on physical activities. It is not necessary to repeat echocardiography

---

*Since the introduction of IVGG treatment, no additional benefit has been demonstrated for a high-dose aspirin phase, though low dose is recommended and important (Ed.).

> ## Coronary Risk Stratification
> - Risk level I: No coronary artery changes at any stage of illness
> - Risk level II: Transient coronary artery ectasia with subsequent regression
> - Risk level III: Small to medium (<8 mm) solitary coronary artery aneurysm
> - Risk level IV: One or more giant coronary artery aneurysms or multiple medium to large aneurysms without thrombotic obstruction or stenosis
> - Risk level V: Thrombotic obstruction or significant stenosis of one or more coronary arteries

beyond the first year if the previous study clearly shows normal coronary artery anatomy. No coronary angiography is recommended.

c. *Risk level II:* No drug therapy is indicated beyond the point where the coronary artery lumens become normal by echocardiography or the first 6 to 8 weeks, whichever occurs later. No restriction on physical activity is necessary beyond the first 6 to 8 weeks during the first decade of life. The intimal thickening in the coronary arteries as the mechanism of regression of coronary artery ectasia may limit coronary vasodilatation, which normally occurs during strenuous exercise in teenagers and adults. Stress tests may be helpful in assessing the level of participation in competitive athletics. There has been an anecdotal report of sudden death following the use of albuterol inhaler for exercise-induced asthma in a KS patient with regressed coronary artery ectasia. More data need to be obtained on the interactions between coronary arteries with thickened intima, exercise, and β2-adrenergic agonists.

d. *Risk level III:* Aspirin, 3 to 5 mg/kg/day is recommended until the coronary abnormalities resolve. For patients in the first decade of life, no restriction beyond the first 6 to 8 weeks is necessary. For the patients in the second decade of life, physical activity should be guided by periodic stress testing. Very strenuous or contact sports are discouraged.

e. *Risk level IV:* These patients are at a particularly high risk for coronary artery thrombosis or stenosis and should receive warfarin with or without low-dose aspirin. To avoid bleeding complications, warfarin dosage should be regulated to achieve the target prothrombin time expressed as International Normalizing Ratio (INR) between 2.0 and 2.5. For patients in the first decade of life, no restriction beyond the initial 6 to 8 weeks is necessary in terms of intensity of physical efforts. Any situation that may precipitate a hard fall or high-impact collision must be avoided. For patients in the second decade, physical activity should be guided by periodic stress testing. Participation in strenuous or contact athletics is strongly discouraged. Noncontact recreational sports are encouraged, guided by periodic stress testing.

f. *Risk level V:* These patients should receive low-dose aspirin. In addition, if the patient has giant aneurysm(s), warfarin should be added to the regimen (see above for recommended doses). The level of physical activity should be guided by stress testing. Strenuous or contact athletics are strongly discouraged. Noncontact recreational sports are permitted as appropriate. Patients with evidence of myocardial ischemia should be evaluated for feasibility of coronary revascularization surgery.

g. Patients in the risk levels IV and V are at the greatest risk for myocardial infarction. The mortality rate of the first episode of myocardial infarction was 22 per cent, according to a survey by Kato, with progressive increase with the second or third attack. Symptoms of myocardial infarction in children include shock, chest pain, abdominal pain, vomiting, and inconsolable crying. Chest pain was reported infrequently in children ≤4 years of age. Approximately one third of the children were asymptomatic at the time of myocardial infarction. Myocardial infarctions have occurred frequently during rest or sleep and relatively infrequently during exercise. A pediatric cardiology consultation must be obtained immediately if myocardial infarction is suspected. Initiation of thrombolytic therapy within a few hours of the event may save the patient's life and may preserve the viability of the left ventricular myocardium.

h. Coronary artery bypass graft surgery is being done for KS patients in increasing numbers. Kitamura and others have shown that arterial grafts using the internal thoracic arteries have high patency rates, particularly in children ≥5 years, and have demonstrated the grafts' ability to grow in caliber and length. Patients with severe mitral valve insufficiency may require surgical repair or replacement of the valve. The patients who are left with severely depressed left ventricular function due to ischemic events may be considered for heart transplants. Thus far, at least 10 Kawasaki patients have undergone cardiac transplantation worldwide, with a success rate comparable to that of patients who have undergone transplantation for other forms of heart disease.

Key Treatment

- IVIG
- Aspirin, low dosage

Prevention

Currently no method is available for primary or secondary prevention.

 ### Bibliography

Dajani AS, Taubert KA, Gerber MA, et al: Diagnosis and therapy of Kawasaki disease in children. Circulation 1993;87:1776–1780.

Dajani AS, Taubert KA, Takahashi M, et al: Guidelines for long-term management of patients with Kawasaki disease. Circulation 1994;89:916–922.

Kato H, Ichinose E, Kawasaki T: Myocardial infarction in Kawasaki disease: clinical analysis in 195 cases. J Pediatr 1986;108:923–927.

Newburger JW, Takahashi M, Beiser AS, et al: Single intravenous infusion of gamma globulin as compared with four infusions in the treatment of acute Kawasaki syndrome. N Engl J Med 1991;324:1633–1639.

187 Marfan Syndrome

Kevin Mulhern

Definition

The Marfan syndrome is a heritable, multisystem connective tissue disorder with widely variable clinical expression. It typically involves the eyes, skeleton, and cardiovascular system.

Etiology

1. The Marfan syndrome is usually inherited as an autosomal dominant trait with variable expression, but there is a 15 per cent new mutation rate.
2. The underlying problem is a defective fibrillin gene. Fibrillin, a glycoprotein, is a major component of microfibrils. Microfibrils are components of the elastic fibers that are part of the extracellular matrix.

Epidemiology

1. The prevalence of the Marfan syndrome is 1 per 10,000.
2. The Marfan syndrome occurs in all races and ethnic groups.
3. Although infantile Marfan syndrome is sometimes seen, the diagnosis is usually made during adolescence or adulthood, when the manifestations of the disorder become more apparent.

Pathophysiology

1. The elastin-associated microfibrils affected by the fibrillin defect are present in the extracellular matrix of a number of tissues, including the aortic tunica media, the perichondrium, and the ciliary zonule. The most common cardio-

vascular manifestations of the Marfan syndrome are aortic dilation or aneurysms, aortic regurgitation due to aortic root dilatation, pulmonary artery dilatation or aneurysms, mitral annulus dilation, and mitral valve prolapse.

2. Aortic dilatation begins during infancy or childhood and usually progresses. Aortic dissection is most common during the fourth decade. It usually involves the ascending aorta but can occur at any level.

3. Cardiovascular complications continue to be the major cause of death. Life expectancy for adolescents and adults with the Marfan syndrome has improved significantly since the introduction of composite graft repair of the ascending aorta and routine use of β-adrenergic blockade. The mean age at death is now 41 ± 18 years, and the median cumulative probability of survival is 72 years. Survival is still adversely affected by a family history of the Marfan syndrome with severe cardiovascular involvement (i.e., nonischemic cardiovascular death, aortic dissection, aortic surgery, aortic valve and/or mitral valve replacement without coronary artery bypass surgery).

4. New mutations tend to result in more extensive genetic defects, a more defective fibrillin, and a more severe phenotype.

5. Infantile Marfan syndrome is a more severe form that presents during the first year of life. In infantile Marfan syndrome, fibrillin microfibrils are short, fragmented, and frayed even when compared with those seen in the classic Marfan syndrome. Only 30 per cent of these infants have a family history of the disorder. The mean age at diagnosis is 3.2 months and the mean age at death 16.3 months; death is usually due to congestive heart failure associated with mitral or tricuspid regurgitation.

Clinical Findings

Requirements for the diagnosis of the Marfan syndrome

1. If a first-degree relative has the Marfan syndrome, the patient must have at least two systems involved. The presence of at least one major manifestation is preferred but depends on the family's phenotype.

2. If the family history is negative or unknown, the skeleton and two other systems must be affected. At least one major manifestation must be present.

Key Clinical Findings: Marfan Syndrome

Major Manifestations
- Ectopia lentis, present in 60 per cent of patients

- Dilated ascending aorta

- Aortic dissection

- Dural ectasia (lumbosacral meningocele, dilated cisterna magna)

Minor Manifestations
- Skeleton
  Anterior chest deformity, especially asymmetric pectus excavatum/carinatum
  Dolichostenomelia (narrow body habitus) not due to scoliosis
  Arachnodactyly (long slender hands, fingers, feet, and toes)
  Spinal deformity

  Tall stature, especially compared with unaffected first-degree relatives
  High, narrow, arched palate and crowding of teeth
  Protrusio acetabuli, abnormal deepening of the acetabuli (hip sockets)
  Congenital flexion contractures or joint hypermobility

- Eyes
  Flat cornea
  Elongated globe
  Retinal detachment
  Myopia

- Heart and blood vessels
  Aortic regurgitation due to aortic root dilatation
  Mitral regurgitation due to mitral valve prolapse
  Calcified mitral annulus
  Mitral valve prolapse
  Abdominal aortic aneurysm
  Arrhythmia
  Endocarditis (usually involving the mitral valve)

- Lungs
  Spontaneous pneumothorax
  Apical bleb

- Central nervous system
  Most patients have normal intelligence
  Learning disability (verbal-performance discrepancy)
  Hyperactivity with or without attention deficit disorder

- Skin and other tissues
  Striae atrophicae not due to weight change
  Hernia (e.g., inguinal, umbilical, diaphragmatic, incisional)

Laboratory Findings

1. Molecular biology techniques

   a. There are no routine clinical laboratory tests specific for the diagnosis.

   b. There are investigational laboratory techniques.

      (1) Immunofluorescence studies of skin sections and cultured dermal fibroblasts show a decrease in immunostainable fibrillin.

      (2) The polymerase chain reaction (PCR) has been used to establish genetic linkage, raising the possibility of a molecular diagnostic test.

2. Echocardiogram

All patients suspected of having the Marfan syndrome should undergo echocardiography to assess aortic root size. Patients known to have the Marfan syndrome should undergo echocardiography to assess aortic root size and the presence and severity of aortic, mitral, or tricuspid valve regurgitation. Transesophageal echocardiography provides almost complete imaging of the thoracic aorta but is not recommended as a routine examination. The frequency of studies is determined by the stability of the disease.

Radiographic Changes

1. Chest x-ray should be used to examine the lung parenchyma for evidence of bullous disease. Heart size and contour may be affected by pectus deformities. Because the proximal aorta is often difficult to discern within the cardiac and mediastinal silhouette, the chest x-ray cannot be used to exclude aortic root dilatation.

2. CT can be used to follow aortic size but has been shown to be less sensitive and less specific than transesophageal echocardiography and MRI for the detection of dissection.

3. MRI is an accurate and comprehensive method of examining the entire aorta, its branches, and adjacent tissues.

Treatment

1. Follow-up

Annual follow-up by a multidisciplinary team, including a cardiologist, orthopedic surgeon, and ophthalmologist, is recommended for the stable patient. The patient with significant aortic root dilatation, increasing aortic root size, significant valve disease, or pregnancy must be seen more frequently.

2. Preventing complications

  a. Aortic dissection

    (1) Beta-adrenergic blockade

      (a) Beta-adrenergic blockade reduces the rate of rise of aortic blood pressure and slows the rate of aortic root dilatation and the development of aortic root complications. These benefits were demonstrated for adolescents and adults with mild or moderate aortic root dilatation. A separate study of children and adolescents with the Marfan syndrome showed that β blockade reduced the rate of aortic root dilatation.

      (b) Regardless of aortic root size, patients should be treated with a β blocker at the youngest age possible. The dose should be adjusted as tolerated to significantly blunt the heart rate response to exercise.

    (2) Composite graft repair

      (a) Replacement of the aortic valve and ascending aorta with a composite graft and reimplantation of the coronary arteries is indicated for

        (i) Aortic dissection

        (ii) Progressive aortic dilatation and aortic regurgitation.

      (b) Composite graft repair is indicated when an adult's aortic root diameter reaches 55 mm. There is no such cutoff for children who have fewer aortic complications.

      (c) Because of the significant risk of dissection remote from the original repair, annual MRI assessment of the thoracic aorta is recommended after composite graft repair. Variables predicting the need for a second operation include the presence of dissection at the time of the first operation, hypertension after the first operation, and a history of smoking.

    (3) Pregnancy

Pregnancy increases the risk of aortic dissection. The risk of aortic complications seems to be acceptably low if the aortic root diameter is <40 mm. Beta blockers should be continued during and after the pregnancy.

    (4) Infective endocarditis

Infective endocarditis prophylaxis is recommended for individuals with aortic or mitral regurgitation.

  b. Athletic competition

    (1) Athletes with the Marfan syndrome, no family history of premature sudden death, and no aortic root dilatation or mitral regurgitation may compete in low-static/low-dynamic sports (e.g., bowling, golf, riflery) and moderate-static/low-dynamic sports (e.g., archery). Aortic root dimension should be measured every 6 months.

    (2) Athletes with aortic root dilatation may compete only in low-static/low-dynamic sports.

    (3) The athlete with the Marfan syndrome should not participate in contact sports owing to the risk of lens dislocation, retinal detachment, skeletal injury, pneumothorax, and aortic dissection.

    (4) Weight lifting, other isometric exercise, and maximal exercise raise blood pressure and increase aortic wall stress and should be avoided.

    (5) Additional recommendations exist for the athlete with aortic or mitral regurgitation.

Key Treatment

- Beta-adrenergic blockade
- Composite graft repair

Prevention

The Marfan syndrome cannot be prevented. Preventive efforts are directed toward avoiding complications of the syndrome.

Bibliography

Beighton P, de Paepe A, Danks D, et al: International nosology of heritable disorders of connective tissue, Berlin, 1986. Am J Med Genet 1988;29:581–594.

Cheitlin MD, Douglas PS, Parmley WW: Task force 2: Acquired valvular heart disease. 26th Bethesda Conference. Recommendations for determining eligibility for competition in athletes with cardiovascular abnormalities. J Am Coll Cardiol 1994; 24:874–880.

Graham TP Jr, Bricker JT, James FW, Strong WB: Task force 1: Congenital heart disease. 26th Bethesda Conference. Recommendations for determining eligibility for competition in athletes with cardiovascular abnormalities. J Am Coll Cardiol 1994;24:867–873.

Morse RP, Rockenmacher S, Pyeritz RE, et al: Diagnosis and management of infantile Marfan syndrome. Pediatrics 1990; 86:888–895.

Salim MA, Alpert BS, Ward JC, Pyeritz RE: Effect of beta-adrenergic blockade on aortic root rate of dilation in the Marfan syndrome. Am J Cardiol 1994;74:629–633.

188 Rheumatic Fever

Edward L. Kaplan

Definition

Rheumatic fever is a nonsuppurative sequela to group A β-hemolytic streptococcal upper respiratory tract infection (URI). The disease classically occurs after a latent period of 10 to 20 days following streptococcal pharyngitis or tonsillitis. Although the etiology and pathogenesis are incompletely understood, it is generally agreed that manifestations of acute rheumatic fever result from an abnormal immune response to one or more group A streptococcal somatic antigens.

Etiology

1. The responsible organism is the group A *Streptococcus*. More than 80 different serologic types of group A streptococci have been described, but there is reason to believe that many more exist. At one time it was thought that all group A streptococci had the capacity to cause rheumatic fever. More recent data, largely based on epidemiologic observations, suggest that certain group A streptococcal serotypes are more likely to be responsible for the subsequent development of rheumatic fever.
2. The classic serotypes (based upon M protein classification) associated with rheumatic fever include serotypes 1, 3, 5, 6, 18, and 24. These are often referred to as rheumatogenic, although a molecular basis for this classification has not been defined.
3. Data are available to suggest that serotypes commonly involved with pyoderma (largely the "higher" serotypes, such as type 49) are not capable of causing rheumatic fever, even when they are recovered from the upper respiratory tract. These serotypes are frequently linked with pyoderma-associated nephritis.

Epidemiology

1. The epidemiology of acute rheumatic fever is identical to the epidemiology of group A streptococcal infections. Most common affected by group A streptococcal URI, and subsequently rheumatic fever, are children between the ages of 5 and 15 years. Although there are documented instances of rheumatic fever occurring in 3- and 4-year-olds, this is relatively rare.
2. Similarly, although initial and recurrent attacks of rheumatic fever affect older teenagers and adults, it is uncommon except in unique epidemiologic situations (e.g., military recruits).
3. Epidemics have been documented and usually are associated with introduction of specific serotypes into a community.
4. On the other hand, endemic cases are associated with multiple serotypes within a community.
5. Epidemiologic data indicate that rheumatic fever, in contrast to acute poststreptococcal glomerulonephritis, occurs only after URI.

Pathophysiology

The pathophysiology and pathogenetic mechanism(s) leading to the clinical manifestations of acute rheumatic fever remain incompletely defined (see below). Two major factors lead to the development of this nonsuppurative sequela to group A streptococcal URI.

1. Considerable study has been given to understanding the association of various somatic and extracellular antigens of this organism with their biologic significance. Studies have suggested that certain antigens of the group A *Streptococcus* (e.g., the cell membrane and certain epitopes of the M protein molecule) are closely related, if not identical, to several human tissues, such as myocardium and valvular glycoprotein. It has been proposed that because of this "antigenic mimicry" the human host reacts to the bacterial antigen(s), producing tissue damage; this causes several clinical manifestations. This proposed mechanism has been linked to damage to myocardium and heart valves and also has been associated with Sydenham chorea.
2. The other major consideration in examining the pathogenetic mechanism is the human host. Rheumatic fever does not occur in animals, and there is no animal model for studying the disease.
3. A genetic predisposition or susceptibility to develop acute rheumatic fever has been recognized for many years. Some families have multiple affected members. Similarly, certain ethnic groups tend to have a higher incidence of rheumatic fever and prevalence of rheumatic heart disease than others. The Maori population of New Zealand is a good example. There is no explanation for these epidemiologic observations.
4. Recent laboratory and epidemiologic studies have provided evidence that certain individuals have alloantigen markers on their B lymphocytes. Preliminary data suggest that the presence of these markers tends to correlate with susceptibility to rheumatic fever and rheumatic heart disease. Furthermore, not only are patients with rheumatic fever and rheumatic heart disease more likely than nonrheumatic controls to have the markers, but also a significant percentage of family members have similar findings. This provides convincing evidence for a genetic influence on susceptibility.
5. Whether this mechanism will ultimately explain genetic susceptibility to developing rheumatic fever remains a hypothesis. However, to be able to identify susceptible individuals is of obvious importance for implementing public health–administered rheumatic fever control programs. Identified individuals could be observed more closely for the presence of streptococcal infection. Perhaps, in the future, such individuals could be among the first to receive a streptococcal vaccine if one became available.

Clinical Findings

1. Major criteria

Clinically, rheumatic fever is a constellation of clinical

findings. In 1944, T. Duckett Jones first proposed criteria for diagnosing patients with this disease. In the absence of a specific diagnostic laboratory test for rheumatic fever, the Jones criteria remain the measure by which the diagnosis is made. There are five major criteria.

    a. Carditis is the most serious of the clinical manifestations of rheumatic fever because it is the only one that may lead to chronic sequelae. The incidence of carditis in patients with acute rheumatic fever varies but usually is reported in 40 to 60 per cent.

      (1) The carditis of rheumatic fever is a pancarditis involving pericardium, epicardium, myocardium, and endocardium.

      (2) Most frequently, the carditis of rheumatic fever is manifested by a new and previously undetected heart murmur, usually the murmur of mitral regurgitation. Occasionally, aortic valve regurgitation may occur in addition to mitral valve disease regurgitation. The diagnosis of rheumatic fever in patients who have only an isolated aortic valve murmur is doubtful.

      (3) Muffled heart tones, pericardial friction rubs, and tachycardia out of proportion to fever are other common cardiac findings. The carditis may be sufficiently severe to lead to cardiomegaly and congestive heart failure.

      (4) The addition of echocardiography to the physician's diagnostic armamentarium may ultimately prove not only to be clinically important but also to have pathogenetic importance. Recent series showing that approximately 20 per cent of individuals without murmurs have evidence of abnormal mitral valve function (mitral regurgitation) have led many to recommend routine echocardiography in patients suspected of having rheumatic fever. This new information explains the fact that many patients who do not have a murmur during the acute stage of rheumatic fever actually have clinically occult disease. These are patients who later are found to have rheumatic heart disease. It is also possible that most patients have valvular dysfunction at the time of the acute attack, whether or not it is clinically manifest.

      (5) Acute rheumatic carditis is more difficult to diagnose in individuals who have preexisting rheumatic heart disease. Differentiating congestive heart failure and recurrence of acute carditis in a patient with preexisting rheumatic valvular disease is clinically difficult. Careful examination of both clinical and laboratory findings is required. It should also be recalled, parenthetically, that infective endocarditis can present in this manner.

    b. The arthritis of acute rheumatic fever is a migratory polyarthritis. It most often affects large joints such as knees, ankles, wrists, and elbows but rarely affects small joints of the hands and feet. In most series, 50 to 70 per cent of patients will manifest this migratory polyarthritis.

      (1) The arthritis of rheumatic fever is exquisitely painful; patients seldom can tolerate even as much as sheets and blankets over an affected joint. The arthritis of rheumatic fever does not predispose to chronic arthritis.

      (2) Patients should *not* be given antiinflammatory therapy until the clinical manifestations of the arthritis of rheumatic fever are very clear. Antiinflammatory therapy, especially salicylates and corticosteroids, leads to rapid disappearance of the arthritis of rheumatic fever, literally within hours. For severe pain, codeine or similar analgesics are useful in allowing the arthritis to define itself while keeping the patient comfortable. This is important in making a correct diagnosis.

      (3) The arthritis of rheumatic fever can be confused with the so-called reactive arthritis associated with group A streptococcal infection. The latter tends to be less severe and rarely is migratory. The relationship between these two entities has not been fully explained, and there is confusion about the long-term management of the reactive arthritis. This is because some of these patients may later be found to have valvular heart disease.

      (4) When considering the Jones criteria, arthritis cannot be confused with arthralgia. The latter is subjective; the former is an objective finding.

    c. Erythema marginatum is a very characteristic rash, most prominent over the trunk. It is an unusual finding and occurs in <10 per cent of patients. It is an annular, nonpruritic rash that "moves" from site to site with time. Erythema marginatum is often incorrectly diagnosed because it is so uncommon that most physicians have never seen it. There is no therapy required for this manifestation.

    d. Subcutaneous nodules also are very rare, especially at the end of the twentieth century. These mobile, pea-sized, nontender nodules occur over the extensor surfaces of joints, most frequently in patients with long-standing chronic rheumatic heart disease. No therapy is required for this manifestation.

    e. The fifth major criterion for the diagnosis of rheumatic fever is Sydenham *chorea* (St. Vitus' dance). Of the five major manifestations of acute rheumatic fever, this one is unique. It differs from the other four in that the latent period following the group A streptococcal infection is usually much longer, sometimes several months.

      (1) The unusual choreoathetotic movements and the emotional lability noted in children with Sydenham chorea are very different from the other acute inflammatory changes in rheumatic fever.

      (2) Sydenham chorea has remained a pathogenetic enigma for many years, since the opportunity to obtain pathologic material in affected patients has been infrequent. Intriguing studies suggesting the presence of cross-reactive antibodies with human caudate nucleus may, in part, explain how this entity differs from other manifestations of rheumatic fever.

(3) Sydenham chorea may be either bilateral or unilateral. Its severity varies from very mild choreoathetotic movements to extreme incapacitation that requires prolonged (weeks) bed rest.

(4) As the streptococcal antibody titers in patients with Sydenham chorea may have decreased owing to the relatively long latent period since the preceding streptococcal infection, this diagnosis can be very difficult to substantiate. It has therefore become a diagnosis of exclusion, made in concert with the neurologist. The elimination of other causes of choreiform movements leaves one with a diagnosis of Sydenham chorea.

(5) Spontaneous recurrences of chorea have been noted at the time of pregnancy. Studies have also shown that approximately 40 per cent of individuals who develop Sydenham chorea may ultimately develop rheumatic valvular heart disease, even decades later. Therefore, careful cardiac examination is required for patients with chorea. Sydenham chorea can be effectively treated with haloperidol.

2. Minor criteria

The minor criteria included in the Jones criteria encompass less specific clinical and laboratory findings.

    a. Most important among these is arthralgia. When considering rheumatic fever and attempting to apply the Jones criteria, one cannot use both arthralgia and arthritis. The clinical difference between arthralgia and arthritis is remarkable. Frequently, if the physician is patient, what appears to be arthralgia will, in a day or so, prove to be frank migratory polyarthritis.

    b. The other minor criteria include fever but also laboratory findings such as elevated acute phase reactants and a prolonged P-R interval on the electrocardiogram.

    c. Finally, the "updated" 1992 revision of the Jones criteria indicates that evidence of a preceding group A streptococcal infection should be documented, either by throat culture (or rapid antigen test) or by streptococcal antibodies. Without evidence of a preceding infection, the diagnosis should be highly suspect.

Key Clinical Findings

- Carditis
- Arthritis
- Erythema marginatum
- Subcutaneous nodules
- Sydenham chorea

Laboratory Findings

There is no specific laboratory test to establish the diagnosis of rheumatic fever. It is not uncommon for physicians to misinterpret streptococcal antibody data as being pathogno-monic of rheumatic fever. These antibody tests are not an indication, per se, of rheumatic fever.

1. In patients suspected of having acute rheumatic fever or a recurrence of rheumatic fever, a throat culture should always be obtained. Even though throat cultures are positive at the time of presentation in less than half of patients, one or two throat cultures should be taken to attempt to confirm the presence of group A streptococci in the upper respiratory tract. Rapid antigen detection tests for group A streptococci are widely used. Although the presence of a positive rapid test is almost always indicative of the presence of group A streptococci, a negative rapid antigen detection test is *not* definitive and should be supplemented by a throat culture. The specificity of these rapid tests is much better than the sensitivity.

2. Streptococcal antibodies, such as antistreptolysin O and anti-DNase B, are valuable for confirming a previous group A streptococcal infection. The presence of a raised titer or, more significantly, the presence of a significant rise in titer during a 4- to 6-week period is indicative of a previous group A streptococcal infection.

Eighty per cent of individuals with rheumatic fever will have an elevated antistreptolysin O titer at presentation. If one performs two additional streptococcal antibody tests (e.g., anti-DNase B or antihyaluronidase), 95 per cent of patients with rheumatic fever will show serologic evidence of a previous group A streptococcal infection. Failure to demonstrate the presence of a previous streptococcal infection should make the clinician highly suspicious of a diagnosis of acute rheumatic fever.

3. The electrocardiographic findings in rheumatic fever, especially the presence of a prolonged P-R interval, are helpful in pointing toward carditis. However, this is a very nonspecific finding that can be due to many other causes. It is *not* pathognomonic of rheumatic fever.

4. The chest x-ray also is not specific. Its main use is to determine whether there is evidence of cardiomegaly and congestive heart failure.

5. Echocardiography is one of the more controversial issues in the laboratory diagnosis of acute rheumatic fever. Recent studies have suggested that individuals with carditis may not have murmurs indicative of carditis but that echocardiographic abnormalities may be demonstrated. Because of this, some have suggested that echocardiography should be performed in all patients suspected of having rheumatic fever. However, minimal mitral insufficiency does not necessarily confirm a diagnosis of rheumatic carditis. Long-term follow-up studies will be required to establish the true role of echocardiography in the acute phase of rheumatic fever as well as later in those individuals who have had an attack of the disease.

Key Laboratory Tests

- Throat culture for group A streptococci
- ASO titer
- ECG

Treatment

The treatment of patients with rheumatic fever has three purposes:

1. First is the treatment of the underlying group A streptococcal infection. *All* patients suspected of having rheumatic fever should be treated as if they have an acute group A streptococcal URI, whether or not group A streptococci are actually recovered from the upper respiratory tract. The drug of choice, according to the American Academy of Pediatrics, the American Heart Association, the World Health Organization, and the Infectious Diseases Society of America, is penicillin. Oral penicillin V for 10 days is recommended. Many choose to use intramuscular benzathine penicillin G because it will treat the acute group A streptococcal URI; it also allows one to begin secondary prophylaxis for prevention of recurrences. For those individuals who are allergic to penicillin, erythromycin is recommended. While there are many other antibiotics that can be used to treat group A streptococcal infections (e.g., cephalosporins and other macrolides), they appear to be no more cost-effective than the classically accepted form of therapy—penicillin.

2. A second group of medications for rheumatic fever are the antiinflammatory agents. For the carditis of rheumatic fever, none of the antiinflammatory agents has been documented to prevent development of rheumatic valvular heart disease. For those individuals who have carditis but do not have evidence of congestive heart failure, salicylates are given so that the serum salicylate level can be maintained between 15 and 20 mg/dl until the erythrocyte sedimentation rate returns to normal. There are no controlled studies with either nonsteroidal antiinflammatory drugs or acetaminophen in acute rheumatic fever.

3. In individuals with congestive heart failure, there is sufficient clinical information to strongly suggest that these patients improve with short courses of corticosteroid therapy. This is usually required only for 2 to 4 weeks. Once again, there is no convincing evidence from controlled studies that corticosteroid therapy reduces the incidence of rheumatic valvular heart disease.

4. Finally, for individuals with clinically evident congestive heart failure, anticongestive measures, such as inotropic agents and diuretics, frequently are required.

5. Bed rest is indicated until heart failure is controlled. Although in the past patients with rheumatic fever were kept in bed for months at a time, bed rest is generally not necessary in individuals who do not have congestive heart failure. Patients with arthritis will not wish to leave their bed, but they improve significantly upon initiation of salicylate therapy. Patients with Sydenham chorea are often kept in bed but primarily for the purposes of protecting them until the choreiform movements can be medically controlled.

Key Treatment

- Eradicate streptococci
- Antiinflammatory agents, salicylates
- Corticosteroids for heart failure
- Bed rest for those with heart failure

Prevention

1. The prevention of acute rheumatic fever is the treatment of group A β-hemolytic streptococcal URIs. Methods for treating these infections were discussed earlier.

2. Individuals who have had a previous attack of rheumatic fever require long-term secondary prophylaxis to prevent recurrent attacks of the disease. Data indicate that the most effective form of therapy is injection of intramuscular benzathine penicillin G given every 4 weeks. (It is more effective when administered every 3 weeks in patients at high risk for a recurrence.)

3. Oral penicillin or, in the case of the penicillin-allergic patient, oral sulfadiazine may also be given daily. Compliance tends to be a major impediment to successful oral secondary prophylaxis. For patients who cannot take sulfa drugs, erythromycin has been used.

4. The duration of secondary prophylaxis varies. Since the risk of recurrences is highest during the first 5 years after the attack, this is the most crucial time for secondary prophylaxis. Also to be taken into consideration are the age of the patient, the living conditions (crowding), and whether the patient has evidence of rheumatic valvular heart disease. Since recurrent attacks tend to be mimetic of the initial attack, patients with rheumatic heart disease generally require longer secondary prophylaxis, sometimes for life.

5. At the present time there is no vaccine available for prevention of β-hemolytic streptococcal URIs. Although there is considerable interest in the development of a group A streptococcal vaccine, current methods of treatment of streptococcal infections and prevention of these infections in individuals with preexisting rheumatic fever remain similar to techniques available for the past four or five decades.

189 Heart Failure

Fred S. Lamb

Critical State

Definition

Heart failure refers to the inability of cardiac output to meet the metabolic demands of the body.

Etiology

There are numerous potential causes of the clinical picture of congestive heart failure (CHF). Within the pediatric population, age of presentation is the most useful initial guide to determining cause. Causes of CHF by age are presented in Table 189–1.

Pathophysiology

Although the causes of ventricular dysfunction are diverse, the clinical manifestations of heart failure can all be accounted for by either inadequate cardiac output in the forward direction or increased systemic or pulmonary venous pressure upstream from the failing ventricle.

1. The heart employs three basic mechanisms to accommodate to increased demands. As these mechanisms are activated and then overwhelmed, the clinical entity of heart failure ensues.
   a. *Frank-Starling mechanism*—Increased preload produces ventricular dilatation, increased overlap of sarcomeric filaments, and increased force of contraction.
   b. Increased catecholamine release by cardiac adrenergic neurons and by the adrenal medulla augments cardiac contractility.
   c. Myocardial hypertrophy increases the mass of contractile tissue.
2. An inability of the myocardium to shorten adequately against a load results in incomplete emptying of the ventricle and diminished cardiac output. The resulting tissue underperfusion adversely affects the function of multiple organ systems and can account for many of the signs and symptoms of heart failure.
   a. Renal sodium and water retention
   b. Muscular weakness and diminished exercise tolerance
   c. Growth impairment
   d. Confusion, lethargy (late)
   e. Malabsorbtion, gastrointestinal dysfunction (late)
3. Impaired myocardial shortening also produces a cascade of compensatory events which acutely improve myocardial function but can also contribute to pathogenesis
   a. Increased ventricular end-diastolic volume and pressure (exacerbated by renal salt and water retention)
   b. Increased atrial volume and pressure
   c. Increased atrial and ventricular contractility (Frank-Starling mechanism)
      (1) Improvement in cardiac output (Fig. 189–1)
      (2) However, this improvement is at the expense of d and e (below).
   d. Increased volume and pressure in adjacent venous and capillary system
   e. Transudation of fluid and increased interstitial (lungs, liver, spleen, kidneys, intestine) or cavitary (pleural, pericardial, peritoneal, subcutaneous) fluid volume. There is partial compensation by increased lymphatic flow.

All of these secondary physiologic alterations can exacerbate end-organ dysfunction and contribute to symptomatology, particularly respiratory compromise resulting from pulmonary interstitial edema.

Clinical Findings

Symptoms depend on the age of the patient, the cause of the heart disease, the chamber or chambers involved, and the severity and time course of deterioration in ventricular function. Heart failure is a clinical diagnosis, and a wide

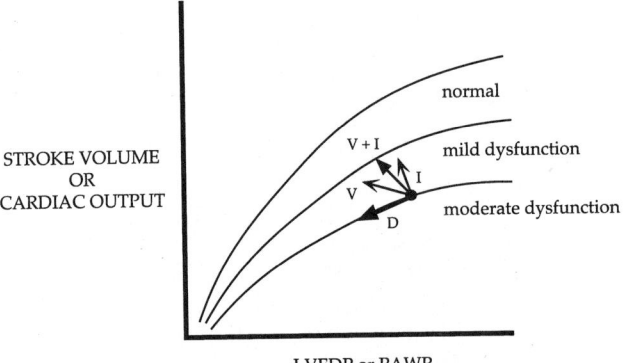

Figure 189–1 Function curves reflect a progression from normal to moderate myocardial dysfunction. Better function is associated with a larger increase in stroke volume per unit increase in left ventricular end-diastolic pressure (LVEDP). Inotropic agents (I), vasodilator drugs (V), or the combination of the two (V + I) shift the curve to a higher level of function. Diuretics (D) decrease LVEDP and thereby relieve symptoms without actually improving function. PAWP = pulmonary artery wedge pressure. (Chesebro JH, Burnett JC: Cardiac failure: Characteristics and clinical manifestations. *In* Brandenburg RO, Fuster V, Giuliani ER, McGoon DC [eds]: Cardiology, Fundamentals and Practice. Chicago, Year Book Medical Publishers, 1987, pp 645–665.)

TABLE 189–1. CAUSES OF CONGESTIVE HEART FAILURE BY AGE AT PRESENTATION

FIRST DAY OF LIFE

Structural—Tricuspid insufficiency, pulmonic insufficiency, large arteriovenous malformations (primarily liver or brain)
Rhythm—Supraventricular tachycardia, complete heart block (heart rate <50 bpm or associated structural disease)
Myocardial—Asphyxia/ischemia, sepsis, hypocalcemia, hypoglycemia, myocarditis
Hematologic—Anemia, hyperviscosity syndrome (hematocrit >65%)

FIRST WEEK OF LIFE

Structural—Left-sided obstruction (critical aortic stenosis [AS], coarctation, interrupted arch, hypoplastic left heart), critical pulmonic stenosis (PS), total anomalous pulmonary venous return (TAPVR)—obstructed type, patent ductus arteriosus (PDA, primarily in premature infants)
Myocardial/Rhythm—Same as for first day of life
Renal—Renal failure (volume overload), severe hypertension
Endocrine—Hyperthyroidism, adrenal insufficiency

FIRST 2 MONTHS OF LIFE

Structural—Aortic level shunts (PDA, truncus arteriosus, aorticopulmonary window), ventricular level shunts (ventricular septal defect, atrioventricular canal defect, single ventricle), atrial level shunts (atrial septal defects, TAPVR—unobstructed type), left-sided obstruction (as for first week of life), anomalous origin of the left coronary artery (from the pulmonary artery)
Myocardial—Congenital cardiomyopathy, endocardial fibroelastosis, myocarditis, Pompe disease
Pulmonary (chronic hypoxia, right-sided heart failure)—Bronchopulmonary dysplasia, upper airway obstruction, central hypoventilation
Renal/Endocrine—as for first week of life plus hypothyroidism

CHILDHOOD AND ADOLESCENCE

Acquired heart disease—Congenital syndromes (Marfan, Noonan, Hurler), endocarditis, rheumatic fever, Kawasaki disease, pulmonary hypertension—autoimmune (primary) or secondary to chronic lung disease
Unoperated congenital heart disease—Progressive valvar insufficiency, progressive valvar stenosis (AS > PS), rhythm disturbances (complete heart block, tachyarrhythmias), Eisenmenger syndrome
Postoperative congenital heart disease—Systemic ventricle overload (large palliative shunts, progressive valvar insufficiency, prosthetic valve deterioration, right ventricular failure after atrial switch operation), right ventricular failure (residual outflow obstruction, pulmonary conduit stenosis/insufficiency, post–right ventriculotomy, Fontan physiology)

Adapted from Artman M, Graham TP: Congestive heart failure in infancy: Recognition and management. Am Heart J 1982;103:1040–1055; and Artman M, Parrish MD, Graham TP: Congestive heart failure in childhood and adolescence: Recognition and management. Am Heart J 1983;105(3):471–480.

variety of factors contribute to the conclusion that a patient is in CHF.

1. Systemic manifestations
   a. *Growth failure*—Caused by limited caloric intake in the face of increased caloric requirements to achieve adequate growth. Infants in CHF may require as much as 150 to 170 kcal/kg/day to gain weight.
   b. *Exercise intolerance*—Lack of cardiac output response to increasing demand; frequently manifested as poor feeding or tachypnea with feeding in infants
   c. *Diaphoresis*—Caused by increased autonomic nervous system activation

2. Cardiac manifestations
   a. *Tachycardia*—Resting heart rate >150 bpm in infants, >100 bpm in children
   b. *Increased precordial activity*—Particularly in shunt lesions
   c. *Gallop rhythm*—Third heart sound may indicate rapid filling of a noncompliant ventricle but can be a normal finding, particularly in infancy.
   d. Altered perfusion
      (1) *Diminished pulses*—Extremities may be cool and mottled, with delayed capillary refill. However, pulses may actually be bounding in the presence of high-output failure (arteriovenous malformations, anemia) or lesions with large runoff (patent ductus arteriosus, aortic insufficiency).
      (2) *Pulsus paradoxicus*—Occurs in patients with a large left-right shunts (variation in ventricular filling and output due to respiratory changes in intrapulmonary pressures)
      (3) *Pulsus alternans*—Peak systolic pressure diminished with every other beat (usually a sign of severe ventricular dysfunction)

3. Respiratory manifestations
   a. *Tachypnea*—Principal manifestation of interstitial pulmonary edema; may be the earliest and most reliable symptom of left ventricular failure, particularly in infants
   b. *Wheezing/cough*—Often confused with bronchospasm; responds poorly to bronchodilators
   c. *Rales*—Infrequent in infants and young children; may reflect severe edema
   d. *Cyanosis*—May occur even with acyanotic heart disease as a result of severe pulmonary edema and/or profound tissue underperfusion (increased oxygen extraction)

4. Manifestations of systemic venous congestion
   a. *Hepatomegaly*—Degree of enlargement reflects elevated central venous pressure and increased blood volume and is proportional to the degree of right-sided heart failure (which may be secondary to left-sided heart failure). Tenderness may be noted with absence of a discrete edge, particularly in older children.
   b. *Jugular venous distention*—Difficult to assess in infants and small children
   c. *Peripheral edema*—Much less common in children than in adult population; may be manifested as facial edema.

Key Clinical Findings

- Tachycardia
- Gallop rhythm
- Tachypnea
- Pulmonary crackles
- Hepatomegaly
- Venous distention

Diagnostic Assessment

1. Chest radiographs should always be obtained. Typical findings in CHF include the following:

   a. *Cardiomegaly*—Cardiothoracic ratio >0.55 in infants, >0.5 in children older than 1 year of age. Absence of cardiomegaly should lead to questioning the diagnosis of CHF (exceptions are restrictive cardiomyopathy and obstructed total anomalous pulmonary venous return).

   b. Increased pulmonary vascular markings

   c. Hyperexpansion with flattening of the diaphragms

   d. *Pleural effusions*—Uncommon except with severe right-sided heart failure (frequently with tricuspid insufficiency) and in patients who have had the Fontan operation

   e. Pericardial effusion suggested by a "globular" cardiac silhouette.

2. Electrocardiography is useful for documentation of dysrhythmias. It may reveal underlying problems such as atrial enlargement or ventricular hypertrophy; however, it is rarely helpful in making the specific diagnosis of CHF.

3. Echocardiography is extremely helpful in delineating anatomic abnormalities and quantifying ventricular dysfunction (normal left ventricular shortening fraction, 28 to 42%). One must be cautious to consider factors such as hydration state (preload) and regurgitant volumes (overestimation of function with aortic or mitral insufficiency). Serial studies may be helpful to evaluate progression or therapeutic response but should be used as an adjunct to clinical evaluation.

4. Additional laboratory evaluations

   a. *Arterial blood gases*—Mild pulmonary interstitial edema with tachypnea may produce a respiratory alkalosis. Severe pulmonary edema and low output may cause a combined acidosis. The partial pressure of oxygen falls with right-to-left shunting or with progressive pulmonary edema.

   b. *Electrolytes*—Hyponatremia and hypochloremia, probably dilutional, may be found. Hyperkalemia may occur in severe CHF as a result of acidosis and reduced glomerular filtration rate. Hypocalcemia produces myocardial dysfunction (prolonged QT interval on electrocardiogram), and treatment with intravenous calcium may dramatically improve function.

   c. *Glucose*—Hypermetabolic infants can deplete hepatic glycogen stores.

   d. *Complete blood count*—Screen for anemia and polycythemia.

Treatment

Cardiac function (contractility) can be defined by the response of stroke volume, and therefore cardiac output, to changes in "filling pressure" (i.e., left ventricular end-diastolic pressure, LVEDP). This is often estimated clinically from the pulmonary artery wedge pressure. Therapy is focused at improving this relation and thereby maintaining adequate cardiac output at a lower filling pressure, which can significantly improve symptoms.

1. Inotropic agents increase the force of myocardial contraction, placing the relation between stroke volume and LVEDP along a higher function curve.

   a. Digoxin—first-line drug, safe and effective for outpatient therapy in children (Table 189–2)

   b. Sympathomimetic agents

   (1) Dopamine (activates dopaminergic, β_1 and α receptors).

   (a) Dose: 3 to 20 μg/kg/minute

   (b) Effects: inotropy, mild chronotropy, renal arterial dilatation (at low doses)

   (c) Potential problems: increasing afterload at high doses (α receptors)

TABLE 189–2. ORAL DOSING OF DIGOXIN

	DIGITALIZING DOSE (μg/kg)	MAINTENANCE (μg/kg/day)
Premature infant (<37 wk gestation)	20	5 (divided bid)
Full-term newborn infant	30	8–10 (divided bid)
Child <2 yr	40–50	10–12 (divided bid)
Child ≥2 yr	30–40	8–10 (qd or divided bid)
Maximum dose	1000 μg	250 μg total

Intravenous dosage is 75% of the oral dose. One half of the total digitalizing dose is given initially, then two 1/4 doses are given at 6- to 8-hr intervals. Maintenance therapy begins 12 hr after the digitalization is complete. Slow loading can be achieved over several days by simply beginning a maintenance dose. Therapeutic range is narrow, and care should be taken both to prescribe accurately (designating type of preparation, route of administration, and quantity both in micrograms and in milliliters of chosen preparation) and to be aware of toxicity. Levels are difficult to interpret and not routinely required in infants and children, who frequently achieve concentrations greater than 2.0 ng/ml, generally considered toxic in adults. Monitoring is best by electrocardiography (atrioventricular block, premature ventricular contractions). Nausea and vomiting may develop even at levels generally considered therapeutic in most patients. Hypokalemia (<3.5 mEq/L) may exacerbate toxicity.

(d) Indication: mild inotropy and increased renal blood flow desired.

(2) Dobutamine (activates primarily to β1-receptors).

   (a) Dose: 5 to 20 μg/kg/minute

   (b) Effects: inotropy, chronotropy, negligible afterload effects

   (c) Potential problems: questionable inotropy in neonates

   (d) Indication: relatively pure inotropic support.

(3) Isoproterenol (activates β_1 and β_2 receptors)

   (a) Dose: 0.1 to 5 μg/kg/minute

   (b) Effects: inotropy, strong chronotropy, vasodilation

   (c) Potential problems: tachycardia, dysrhythmias

   (d) Indication: primary bradycardia.

(4) A combination of low-dose dopamine (<5 μg/kg/minute) to augment renal blood flow and dobutamine for inotropy is frequently employed in all age groups.

c. Amrinone, milrirone

(1) Dosage: amrinone, 0.75 mg/kg load, then 5 to 10 μg/kg/minute; milrirone, 50 μg/kg load, then 0.375 to 0.75 μg/kg/min

(2) Inhibits cyclic adenosine monophosphate (cAMP) phosphodiesterase, thereby increasing cAMP levels

(3) Provides the advantage of inotropy and vasodilation (pulmonary and systemic)

(4) Acts in synergy with sympathomimetic agents (frequently dobutamine).

2. Diuretics reduce LVEDP by decreasing the circulating volume. This volume is expanded in CHF as the kidneys attempt to improve blood flow (through elevation of serum aldosterone, sodium retention). LVEDP is reduced with little change in contractility.

a. Loop diuretics inhibit sodium and chloride transport in the ascending loop of Henle. They induce a potent diuresis, which frequently produces potassium depletion requiring supplementation (1 to 2 mEq/kg/day) divided dosage.

(1) Furosemide (Lasix), 1 to 2 mg/kg per dose, IV, IM, PO, bid to qid

(2) Ethacrynic acid 1 mg/kg/dose, IV, may work in hospitalized patients who fail to respond to furosemide.

b. Thiazide diuretics inhibit transport of sodium and chloride in the distal convoluted tubule. They are generally less potent than the loop diuretics.

(1) Chlorothiazide, 10 to 15 mg/kg/dose, PO, bid

(2) Hydrochlorothiazide, 1 to 2 mg/kg/dose, PO, bid

c. Metolazone blocks sodium reabsorption in both the proximal and distal convoluted tubule. There is significant synergism between metolazone and furosemide, which together can produce a profound diuresis requiring close monitoring of electrolytes. Duration of diuresis may exceed 24 hours after a single dose (0.2 to 0.4 mg/kg per dose, PO, divided dosage daily). This drug is generally given intermittently or for a short period under supervised conditions.

d. Spironolactone is an aldosterone antagonist that produces a weak but potassium-sparing diuresis. In combination with thiazides or furosemide, it can prevent excessive potassium loss; potassium supplements should not be given to patients receiving spironolactone.

3. Vasodilators alter myocardial performance by changing both the resistance and the capacitance of the peripheral vasculature. Arteriolar dilatation reduces afterload and myocardial work, thereby increasing cardiac output. Venodilation increases the capacitance of the system and lowers filling pressures, which in turn reduces venous congestion. Initiation of vasodilator therapy requires close, in-hospital monitoring and can rapidly produce significant hypotension.

a. Oral agents useful for outpatient therapy

(1) Hydralazine, a relatively less potent agent, is primarily an arteriolar dilator. It can cause a lupus-like syndrome.

(2) Angiotensin-converting enzyme inhibitors produce mixed arteriolar and venous dilatation.

b. *Intravenous therapy for acute CHF*—Nitroprusside and nitroglycerin dilate both arteriolar and venous smooth muscle. Short half-life allows rapid titration of effect. Beware of potential for cyanide toxicity with prolonged use or high doses of nitroprusside.

Key Treatment

- Digoxin
- Sympathomimetic drugs (e.g., dopamine)
- Diuretics
- Vasodilators

Bibliography

Artman M, Graham TP: Congestive heart failure in infancy: Recognition and management. Am Heart J 1982;103:1040–1055.

Artman M, Parrish MD, Graham TP: Congestive heart failure in childhood and adolescence: Recognition and management. Am Heart J 1983;105(3):471–480.

Chesebro JH: Cardiac failure: Medical management. *In* Brandenburg RO, Fuster V, Giuliani ER, McGoon DC (eds): Cardiology,

Fundamentals and Practice. Chicago, Year Book Medical Publishers, 1987, pp 666–688.

Chesebro JH, Burnett JC: Cardiac failure: Characteristics and clinical manifestations. *In* Brandenburg RO, Fuster V, Giuliani ER, McGoon DC (eds): Cardiology, Fundamentals and Practice.

Chicago, Year Book Medical Publishers, 1987, pp 645–665.

Dreyer WJ: Congestive heart failure. *In* Garson A, Bricker TJ, McNamara DG (eds): The Science and Practice of Pediatric Cardiology, vol 3. Philadelphia, Lea & Febiger, 1990, pp 2007–2023.

190 Cardiogenic Shock/Hypertensive Crisis

James A. Royall

Critical State

Cardiogenic Shock

Definitions

1. Shock—Shock is an unstable pathophysiologic state with insufficient systemic delivery of oxygen to sustain vital organ function. Shock differs from heart failure in that shock represents an immediate threat to the patient's survival.
2. Cardiogenic shock—Shock is often organized into broad categories (hypovolemic, distributive, obstructive, dissociative, and cardiogenic). Cardiogenic shock is primarily due to inadequate myocardial function.

Etiology

Common causes of cardiogenic shock include global ischemia, sepsis, myocarditis, and postcardiac surgery myocardial dysfunction. Age-related causes are similar to congestive heart failure (see Chapter 189). Another cause is obstruction to ventricular filling (tension pneumothorax or pericardial tamponade). If adequate perfusion is not reestablished, all shock states eventually develop a significant cardiogenic component.

Pathophysiology

1. The initial abnormality results in inadequate cardiac function to support vital organ function.
2. Endogenous responses act as compensatory mechanisms attempting to maintain adequate perfusion to vital organs (brain and heart), often at the expense of perfusion to other organs (skin, gastrointestinal tract, kidneys).
   a. Increased sympathetic nervous system activity—increased heart rate, increased myocardial contractility, and vasoconstriction
   b. Activation of renin-angiotension system—vasoconstriction and increased renal sodium and water retention
   c. Increased antidiuretic hormone—increased water retention
   d. Accumulation of tissue metabolites—local vasodilation.

Clinical Findings

1. The clinical signs of cardiogenic shock are the result of the primary alteration, reduced perfusion, and the compensatory mechanisms (Table 190–1).
2. The "classic" presentation of cardiogenic shock is reduced cardiac output and poor tissue perfusion in the presence of an adequate intravascular volume.
   a. Hypotension and poor tissue perfusion are readily detectable by examination.
   b. Signs of high venous pressure hepatomegaly, and venous distention, may indicate intravascular volume overload or obstruction to right ventricular filling.
   c. The presence of rales on lung auscultation may reflect intravascular volume overload or obstruction to left ventricular filling.
   d. Invasive monitoring with a central venous catheter or pulmonary arterial catheter is frequently useful for evaluation of intravascular volume status as well as response to therapy.

Laboratory Findings

1. First priority is to evaluate for metabolic abnormalities that would inhibit cardiac function. Urgent laboratory studies include electrolytes, glucose, calcium, arterial blood gas, and hematocrit.
2. Other studies should include chest x-ray, ECG, complete blood count, phosphorus, magnesium, BUN and creatinine, liver function studies, and coagulation studies.
3. An echocardiogram will identify structural abnormalities of the heart, help quantify the degree of ventricular dys-

Critical State *Continued*

TABLE 190–1.   GENERAL CLINICAL SIGNS AS LOW CARDIAC OUTPUT PROGRESSES TO SEVERE CARDIOGENIC SHOCK

SIGNS	LOW CARDIAC OUTPUT	→	SEVERE CARDIOGENIC SHOCK
Heart rate	↑	↑ ↑	↑ ↑ ↑ or ↓
Blood pressure	Normal	↓	↓ ↓
Skin perfusion	Capillary refill >3 sec	Capillary refill >5 sec	Capillary refill >5 sec
		Cool extremities	Cold, mottled extremities
Respiration	Normal	↑	↑ ↑ or ↓
Urine output	Normal	↓	↓ ↓ Or anuria
Mental status	Normal	Agitated, lethargic	Obtunded, comatose
GI tract	Normal	↓ Motility	Ileus
Metabolic acidosis	None	↑	↑ ↑

function, and determine whether cardiomegaly is due to ventricular dilatation vs. a large pericardial effusion.

4. Other laboratory data, such as cultures, are needed based on the primary disease process.

Treatment

1. Stabilization and resuscitation are the first priority.

    a. Ensure an adequate airway, ventilation, and oxygenation. Use supplemental oxygen, and consider endotracheal intubation for severe shock, hypoxemia with a PaO_2 <60 mmHg (saturation <90%) on an FIO_2 of 0.50, hypoventilation with a $PaCO_2$ >50 mmHg, or when airway protective reflexes are poor.

    b. Correct any metabolic abnormalities detected.

    c. Except with clear signs of intravascular volume overload, volume expansion is given with 10 to 20 ml/kg of normal saline or 10 ml/kg of colloid solution. In children without a previous history of cardiac disease, hypovolemic and septic shock are more common than new-onset cardiogenic shock. Initial volume resuscitation should not be delayed pending the results of invasive monitoring or diagnostic studies.

    d. Secure intravenous access, usually with a central venous catheter, which will also aid in evaluation of intravascular volume.

    e. Begin infusion of an inotropic agent (Table 190–2). Dobutamine is often the first choice in the absence of significant hypotension. With significant hypotension, dopamine or the addition of norepinephrine may be used. Epinephrine is generally reserved for shock unresponsive to other inotropic agents. Isoproterenol is primarily used to treat bradycardia.

2. After initial stabilization, therapy is more precisely directed using invasive hemodynamic monitoring, often with a pulmonary arterial catheter. Vasodilators and diuretics are usually of benefit. Amrinone appears to have a favorable hemodynamic profile for cardiogenic shock but should be used with caution with significant renal dysfunction.

3. Further diagnostic studies are needed to evaluate for a

surgical heart lesion or for diseases that may be amenable to medical therapy.

4. Mechanical assist devices can be used to support cardiac function. Most pediatric patients are supported by extracorporeal membrane oxygenation (ECMO). These methods are temporary while awaiting improvement in cardiac function or as a bridge to transplantation.

Hypertensive Crisis

Definitions

Hypertensive crisis is not defined by a given blood pressure elevation but rather by the presence of end-organ dysfunction (usually neurologic or cardiac) in association with hypertension. Hypertensive crisis can be categorized as follows.

1. Malignant hypertension—Severe hypertension associated with grade IV Keith-Wagener retinopathy

2. Accelerated hypertension—Severe hypertension associated with grade III retinopathy

3. Hypertensive encephalopathy—Severe hypertension associated with central nervous system dysfunction

4. Malignant and accelerated hypertension are the result of chronic, poorly controlled hypertension and are uncommon in children.

Etiology

Severe hypertension in children is usually secondary to a variety of other disease processes. By far, the most common primary disease process involves the kidneys (see Chapters 218 and 232).

Pathophysiology

1. Hypertensive encephalopathy results from hyperperfusion to the brain when blood pressure exceeds the upper limits of cerebral autoregulation. Hyperperfusion causes cerebral edema, petechial hemorrhages, and microinfarctions.

    a. Encephalopathy is related to the preceding blood pressure status as well as the degree and rapidity of blood pressure elevation.

Critical State *Continued*

TABLE 190–2. COMMONLY USED VASOACTIVE DRUGS

DRUG	DOSE	COMMENT
Dobutamine	2–20 μg/kg/min	↑ Contractility with little effect on heart rate and SVR
Dopamine	2–20 μg/kg/min	Dose-dependent effects:
		Low dose— ↑ renal blood flow
		Mid-dose— ↑ contractility and ↑ heart rate
		High dose— ↑ SVR
Norepinephrine	0.05–1.0 μg/kg/min	↑ Contractility and ↑ SVR
Epinephrine	0.05–1.0 μg/kg/min	↑ Contractility, ↑ heart rate, and ↑ SVR
Isoproterenol	0.05–1.0 μg/kg/min	↑ Contractility, ↑ heart rate, and ↓ SVR
Amrinone	Loading dose: 0.75 mg/kg (over 2–3 min)	Phosphodiesterase inhibitor
	Infusion: 5–10 μg/kg/min	Half-life of 3–8 hr
		Renal excretion
		↑ Contractility and ↓ SVR
Nitroprusside	0.5–10 μg/kg/min	Direct vasodilator
		Rapid onset, easily titratable
Diazoxide	1–3 mg/kg/dose (max. 150 mg/dose)	Direct vasodilator
	May repeat in 5–15 min	Give by rapid IV push (over 10–30 sec)
		Delayed onset, less titratable (compared with nitroprusside)
Labetalol	0.5 mg/kg over 2 min	α- and β-adrenergic blockers
	May double dose and repeat q 10 min (max. 5 mg/kg)	Delayed onset, less titratable
Nifedipine	0.25 mg/kg sublingual q 4–6 hr	Calcium channel blocker
		Delayed onset, less titratable
Phentolamine	0.05–0.1 mg/kg/dose	α-Adrenergic blocker
	May repeat q 5 min	Used for catecholamine excess

SVR = Systemic vascular resistance.

b. With chronic hypertension, the upper limit of cerebral blood flow autoregulation is shifted such that a higher acute blood pressure elevation is required to exceed this limit.

2. Hypertension may cause congestive heart failure, especially in neonates and in those with preexisting cardiac dysfunction.

Clinical Findings

1. Early signs of hypertensive encephalopathy include headaches, nausea and vomiting, and visual disturbances. Later, altered mental status, focal neurologic abnormalities, and seizures may develop.

2. Hypertensive encephalopathy must be differentiated from other causes of hypertension and neurologic dysfunction, including increased intracranial pressure (head trauma or intracerebral mass), intracranial (intracerebral or subarachnoid) hemorrhage, uremic encephalopathy, primary seizure disorder, and CNS infection.

   a. Head trauma is usually evident from history and examination.

   b. Hypertensive encephalopathy tends to have a gradual onset over 24 to 48 hours with progressive symptoms. Intracerebral hemorrhage has a rapid onset.

   c. The neurologic signs of hypertensive encephalopathy usually resolve with control of blood pressure;

however, this will have little effect on other causes of neurologic dysfunction associated with hypertension.

Laboratory Findings

1. With hypertensive encephalopathy, therapy should not be delayed to await laboratory results. Initial studies may include

   a. Serum electrolytes, glucose, calcium, phosphorus, BUN and creatinine, and urinalysis will show evidence of renal dysfunction as well as immediate metabolic abnormalities that require correction.

   b. A chest x-ray is obtained to evaluate for heart size and pulmonary edema.

   c. If congestive heart failure is an immediate concern, an ECG and echocardiogram may be needed.

   d. If neurologic abnormalities persist after control of blood pressure, an emergency CT scan should be obtained.

2. Other studies are needed based on the suspected primary disease.

Treatment

1. With chronic hypertension in the absence of end-organ dysfunction, rapid reduction in blood pressure may result in inadequate cerebral blood flow. A reduction of approximately 25 per cent accomplished over sev-

eral hours can usually be achieved using oral medication.

2. With hypertensive encephalopathy a rapid and reliable reduction in blood pressure is needed. A 25 per cent reduction in mean arterial blood pressure or a reduction to about 100 mmHg diastolic pressure in the older child or adult is usually adequate. This is accomplished with intravenous or sublingual vasodilator therapy.

   a. Sodium nitroprusside—Often recommended as the initial agent owing to a rapid onset of action and short half-life that allows rapid and precise titration of blood pressure. It is generally for short-term use, and alternative therapy (usually oral) should be started as soon as possible.

   b. Diazoxide—Also recommended as an initial agent. Has a somewhat delayed onset of action (1–5 min) and is less titratable and more prolonged than nitroprusside.

   c. Labetalol—Increasingly used for pediatric hypertension. Although onset is somewhat delayed (1–5 min), there is usually a reliable, gradual reduction in blood pressure. One side effect is orthostatic hypotension (patients remain supine for 3 hours, then ambulate slowly).

   d. Sublingual nifedipine can be used for acute hypertension. It has a delayed onset (10–20 min) and relatively prolonged effect (2–4 hr).

   e. The α-adrenergic agonist phentolamine is primarily used for hypertension due to catecholamine excess (except pheochromocytoma).

3. Diuretics may be used after vasodilator therapy in the patient with clinical evidence of intravascular volume overload.

4. Control of blood pressure secondary to head injury is somewhat controversial. Some recommend that blood pressure be maintained at the upper limits of cerebral blood flow autoregulation (mean systemic arterial blood pressure of 115 to 120 mmHg in the adult).

 Bibliography

CARDIOGENIC SHOCK

Califf RM: Cardiogenic shock. New Engl J Med 1994;330:1724.
Pennington DG, Swartz MT: Circulatory support in infants and children. Ann Thorac Surg 1993;55:233.
Tobin JR, Wetzel RC: Cardiovascular physiology and shock. *In* Nichols DG, Cameron DE, Greeley WJ, et al (eds): Critical Heart Disease in Infants and Children. St. Louis, Mosby–Year Book, 1995, p 17.
Walker LK: Myocardial assist devices. *In* Nichols DG, Cameron DE, Greeley WJ, et al (eds): Critical Heart Disease in Infants and Children. St. Louis, Mosby–Year Book, 1995, p 531.

HYPERTENSIVE CRISIS

Kandt RS, Caoili AQ, Lorentz WB, Elster AD: Hypertensive encephalopathy in children: neuroimaging and treatment. J Child Neurol 1995;10:236.
Ruley EJ: Hypertensive emergencies in children. *In* Ayers SM, Grenvik A, Holbrook PR, Shoemaker WC (eds): Textbook of Critical Care, 3rd ed. Philadelphia, WB Saunders, 1995, p 529.
Tonnesen AS: Hemodynamic management of brain-injured patients. New Horizons 1995;3:499.

191 Cardiac Auscultation

L. George Veasy

Purpose

Cardiac auscultation is performed to establish an initial anatomic and hemodynamic diagnosis for direction of the work-up and planning of management.

Preparation

1. Establish rapport. Complete a thorough history.
2. The patient should be undressed. Cover only for warmth and modesty.
3. Observe for evidence of a syndrome, respiratory distress, and cyanosis or pallor.
4. Allow the toddler or young child to hold the stethoscope.
5. Warm the chest piece by holding it in your hand.
6. Crying must be avoided. Listen first, if indicated.
7. Room must be quiet.

Equipment

The chest piece of the stethoscope should have both a bell and a diaphragm, and the earpieces should fit snugly.

Sedation

Sedation for auscultation alone should be avoided. If the patient is sedated for other studies, complete auscultation at that time.

Precautions

Do not stress a patient with compromised cardiac reserve (congestive failure or hypoxemic episode).

Procedure *Continued*

Technique

1. *Systematic approach*—The first heart sound, second heart sound, systole, and diastole must be assessed over the entire precordium, from the apex to the upper right sternal edge, as well as the back and midaxillary areas. Each sound and murmur describes a discrete, identifiable hemodynamic event.

2. Heart sounds result from an abrupt cessation of movement of blood by heart valves or other cardiac structures.

   a. The first sound coincides with closure of the atrioventricular valves; the mitral valve closes slightly before the tricuspid valve.

   b. The second sound has two components: pulmonary closure (P_2) normally follows aortic closure (A_2). The normal splitting of the two components increases when inspiration augments venous return to the right ventricle (RV). Conversely, the splitting decreases or disappears with expiration.

   c. A third sound, common in children, occurs when the ventricles are suddenly distended from rapid filling in early mid-diastole.

   d. A fourth sound, rare in children, may occur when atrial contraction suddenly distends a noncompliant ventricle.

   e. Clicks are systolic sounds that occur when a stenotic semilunar valve or redundant atrioventricular valve tissue abruptly stops the flow of blood.

3. Murmurs occur when the vibratory activity produced by turbulent blood flow is transmitted to the chest wall. Murmurs are described by intensity, frequency, time course, and location (e.g., a grade 3, high-pitched, systolic regurgitant murmur at the apex).

   a. *Intensity (grade)*—A grade 1 murmur is barely audible. A grade 2 murmur is a soft murmur that can readily be heard. Grade 3 and 4 murmurs are loud murmurs, with grade 4 accompanied by a thrill. Grade 5 and 6 murmurs are very loud, with grade 5 audible with the edge of the stethoscope touching the chest.

   b. *Frequency (pitch)*—The larger the pressure gradient producing the turbulent flow, the higher the frequency of the murmur.

   c. *Location*—Structures of the heart transmitting the vibratory activity determine where the murmur is detected on the chest wall. For example, a murmur of a ventricular septal defect (VSD) is transmitted by the RV to the left sternal edge and mid-precordium, whereas the murmur of mitral regurgitation is transmitted by the left ventricle (LV) and is heard best at the apex.

   d. Time course

(1) Systolic murmurs

   (a) A systolic ejection (midsystolic, diamond-shaped) murmur is heard when blood being ejected from the heart becomes turbulent. It begins after the first heart sound, ends before the second, and is accentuated in mid-systole, at the time of maximum flow. The two most common systolic ejection murmurs are not associated with actual heart disease.

   (i) *Still's murmur*—Also termed a *vibratory murmur*, it is the most common murmur detected in childhood. It is heard best along the lower left sternal edge and diminishes or disappears with standing. Heart sounds are normal.

   (ii) *Flow murmur*—High cardiac output can cause systolic flow to become turbulent, producing a murmur. The murmur is heard best along the middle and upper left sternal edge and disappears after the cause of the high output (e.g., fever, anemia, thyrotoxicosis) is corrected.

   (iii) *Aortic stenosis (valvular)*—Because the jet from the stenotic aortic valve strikes the aorta, the murmur is heard best along the upper right sternal edge. The murmur varies in intensity from 2 to 6, depending on the gradient. The valve moves from a low position in diastole to a taut position in early systole, producing an ejection click at the apex; this clearly differentiates valvular obstruction from a fixed subvalvular obstruction.

   (iv) *Membranous subvalvular aortic stenosis*—This murmur can be differenti-

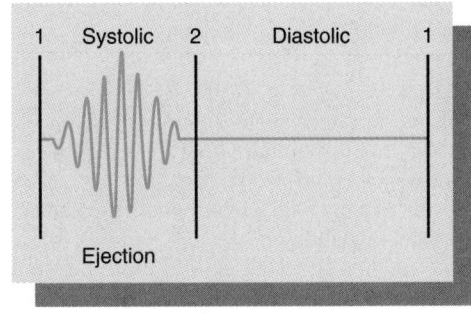

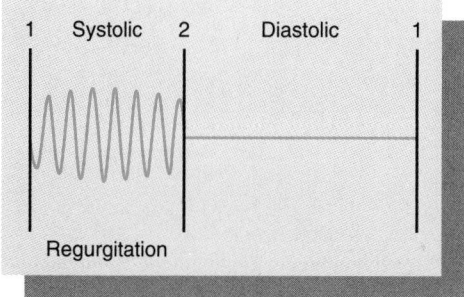

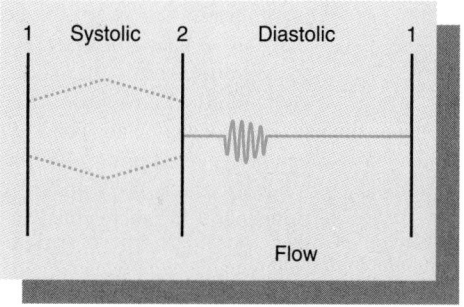

ated from valvular aortic stenosis because the obstruction is "fixed" and no ejection click precedes the murmur.

(v) *Valvular pulmonary stenosis*—Depending on the pressure gradient, this murmur can vary in intensity from 2 to 6. It is best heard along the upper left sternal edge. The ejection click preceding the murmur diminishes in intensity with inspiration, because increased RV volume decreases the excursion of the valve during systole. P_2 is soft and delayed.

(vi) *Infundibular pulmonary stenosis*—The absence of an ejection click distinguishes infundibular from valvular pulmonary stenosis.

(vii) *Atrial septal defect*—In this lesion, the outflow obstruction is "relative," owing to the increased RV volume. The murmur is not louder than grade 3. The increased volume prolongs RV emptying, delaying P_2. The increased RV volume persists even with expiration, and A_2 and P_2 remain "fixed" in their splitting. The increased flow across the tricuspid valve also causes a diastolic flow murmur (discussed later).

(b) Regurgitant (holosystolic, pansystolic) mur-

murs, which begin with the first heart sound and continue to the second, are caused by turbulent retrograde flow through atrioventricular valves or through an opening in the ventricular septum. Regurgitant murmurs are always pathologic.

(i) *VSD, small*—The jet coming from the high-pressure LV through the VSD strikes the RV wall, causing the murmur to be heard best along the lower left sternal edge. Unless the volume of the shunt is very small, the murmur is usually grade 3 or higher. With small shunts, LV and RV emptying may not be significantly altered, and P_2 and A_2 may be normal.

(ii) *VSD, moderate size*—This defect, while permitting a larger shunt, maintains a pressure gradient. The systolic murmur sounds like that of a small VSD, except that the larger volume usually produces a thrill. The LV empties early, and RV emptying is delayed. The second sound is split, and P_2 is accentuated. Diastolic flow murmur at the apex is also present (discussed later).

(iii) *Mitral regurgitation, rheumatic*—Because the pressure gradient between the LV and the left atrium is so large,

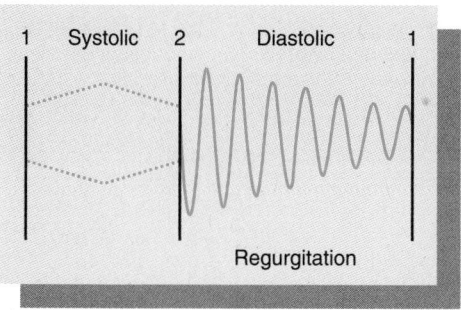

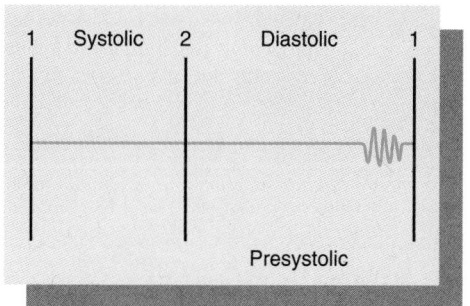

Procedure *Continued*

this murmur has a high frequency. The murmur is heard at the apex because the LV transmits the sound to the chest wall. The murmur is usually grade 3 or less, and when very soft it can be detected only if the patient is in a left decubitus position. If regurgitant flow increases sufficiently, a diastolic flow murmur will be detected in the apical area, and P_2 may be delayed and accentuated.

(iv) *Mitral valve prolapse (Barlow syndrome)*—In this myxomatous degenerative disorder, the mitral valve leaflets become redundant and, during LV systole, prolapse back into the left atrium, which allows separation of the opposing edges of the anterior and posterior leaflets. The redundant tissue causes cessation of blood motion, resulting in one or more clicks before regurgitant flow begins. Therefore, the murmur characteristically begins well after the first heart sound and the click or clicks.

(2) Diastolic murmurs

(a) Regurgitant (decrescendo) murmurs

(i) Aortic regurgitation may be either congenital or rheumatic. The murmur begins with aortic valve closure. The pressure gradient diminishes as arterial pressure drops in diastole. Therefore, the murmur is louder and has a higher frequency early in diastole and is softer and has a lower frequency in late diastole.

(ii) Pulmonary regurgitation is common after surgical repair of tetralogy of Fallot or pulmonary stenosis. The pressure gradient is less and produces a lower-pitched (lower-frequency) murmur.

(b) *Flow (ventricular filling, mid-diastolic) murmurs*—These murmurs occur at the time of most rapid ventricular filling and are caused by increased flow across the tricuspid valve (with an atrial septal defect) or across the mitral valve (VSD, mitral re-

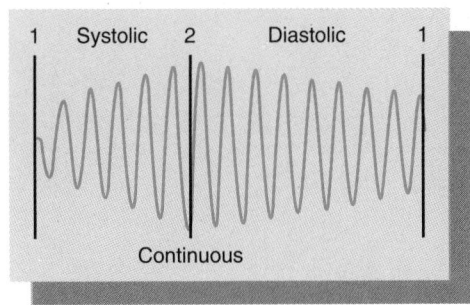

gurgitation). A systolic murmur is also present.

(c) Presystolic (atrial contraction) murmurs are rare in childhood and are detected only in cases of severe mitral (or tricuspid) stenosis.

(3) Continuous murmurs

(a) *Venous murmur*—This common murmur is known as a *benign venous hum*. It is accentuated in diastole and is heard along the upper right sternal edge. The murmur disappears when the patient sits up.

(b) *Arterial murmur*—The classic murmur of a patent ductus arteriosus is accentuated in systole and heard best along the upper left sternal edge.

Follow-up

If there is any doubt, echocardiography confirms the diagnosis. If the correct diagnosis was missed, the patient should be reexamined to learn why.

 Bibliography

Leatham A: Auscultation of the Heart and Phonocardiography. London, J & A Churchill, 1970.

Lehrer S: Understanding Pediatric Heart Sounds. Philadelphia, WB Saunders, 1992.

Park MK: Pediatric Cardiology for Practitioners: Physical Examination. Chicago, Year Book Medical Publishers, 1988, pp 17–33.

Shaver JA, Leonard JJ, Leon DF: Examination of the Heart: Part 4. Auscultation of the Heart. Dallas, American Heart Association, 1990.

Veasy LG: History and physical examination. *In* Emmanoulides GC, Reimenschneider TA, Allen HD, Gutgesell HP (eds): Heart Disease in Infants, Children and Adolescents, 5th ed. Baltimore, Williams & Wilkins, 1995, pp 131–146.

192 The Electrocardiogram: Preliminary Interpretation

D. Woodrow Benson, Jr.

Procedure

Indications

1. Initial evaluation of the patient with suspected cardiovascular disease and serial evaluation of the patient with known cardiovascular disease.
2. Evaluation of the patient with known or suspected disorders of rhythm and conduction, including patients with palpitations and syncope.
3. Evaluation of response to therapy with antiarrhythmic drugs or drugs with potential cardiac effects (e.g., tricyclic antidepressants).
4. There is little rationale for routine electrocardiography (ECG) screening of asymptomatic, ostensibly normal young patients (e.g., routine well-child examination) or for preoperative screening.

Patient Preparation

1. Artifact-free ECG recordings are essential.
2. Diagrams showing electrode placement are usually found on the ECG recording machine.
3. Cleaning the skin with alcohol and acetone is essential to lower the skin resistance.
4. Standard ECG recordings in active infants and toddlers may require two patient individuals and distracting toys.

Equipment

1. The standard ECG record consists of 12 "leads" recorded from nine body surface locations with the patient in the supine position.
2. The ideal recorder should display at least three leads simultaneously.
3. The standard configuration is sometimes modified to record additional right (V_3R or V_4R) or left (V_7) chest leads; this practice is based on opinion and personal choice.
4. Interpretation of rhythm disturbances is facilitated by viewing a rhythm strip with three simultaneously recorded leads.
5. Conventional recording speed is 25 mm/sec, and at full standardization an amplitude of 10 mm is equivalent to 1 mV.

ECG Interpretation

1. General considerations
   a. Examine the patient first; patient condition is relevant to ECG interpretation.
   b. If the chest is deformed (e.g., pectus excavatum, scoliosis) or the heart has an unusual location (e.g., dextrocardia, ectopic cordis), ECG interpretation may be limited.
   c. The zero-voltage baseline is the reference level for ECG amplitude measurements and is usually chosen in the TP or UP interval. At faster heart rates, use the PR segment, because the P wave may be superimposed on the previous TU wave. Baseline selection is relatively unimportant for large deflections, but it is critical for low-level potentials (e.g., ST segment).
   d. ECG features are age-dependent (Table 192–1); PR interval and ST-T wave are heart rate–dependent.
   e. To evaluate the ECG axis, represent leads I and aVF as ordinate (y-axis) and abscissa (x-axis), respectively, in a Cartesian system. The convention has been to designate lead I as 0° (left) to 180° (right) and lead aVF as 90° (inferior) to −90° (superior). An ECG segment or waveform of interest is evaluated with respect to the direction (positive or negative) and the average magnitude over the waveform interval. Since lead I and aVF are orthogonal, the direction and amplitude of the vector or electrical force can be estimated. With a small amount of practice, the idea can be extended to other limb leads (frontal plane) and precordial leads (horizontal plane).
   f. Use a systematic approach to ECG interpretation.
      (1) Evaluate ventricular depolarization first, because QRS waveforms are the largest potentials being evaluated, and other ECG features are interpreted from low-level potentials.
      (2) Determine that ventricular depolarization is normal before interpreting hypertrophy or the ST-T wave.
      (3) Determine heart rate and rhythm.
      (4) Determine interval measurements. Interval measurements are rarely the same in all leads; generally, the "worst" interval is reported. For example, the reported PR interval may be the shortest one measured in a patient with ventricular preexcitation or the longest one recorded in a patient with first-degree heart block.
      (5) Determine chamber enlargement or hypertrophy.
2. Evaluation of ventricular depolarization
   a. The duration of the QRS wave is brief and depends on the age of the patient. QRS duration may be prolonged by metabolic disturbances, right or left bundle branch block, ventricular preexcitation, or a ventricular pacemaker. The term *intraventricular conduction delay* is used when QRS prolongation cannot be categorized.

Procedure *Continued*

TABLE 192–1. SELECTED ECG MEASUREMENTS IN NORMAL PEDIATRIC PATIENTS

	0–3 DAYS	3–30 DAYS	1–6 MO	6–12 MO	1–3 YR	3–5 YR	5–8 YR	8–12 YR	12–16 YR
Heart rate (6pm)	90–160	90–180	105–185	110–170	90–150	70–140	65–135	60–130	60–120
PR (msec) lead II	80–160	70–140	70–160	70–160	80–150	80–160	90–160	90–170	90–180
QRS (msec) lead V_5	25–75	25–80	25–80	25–75	30–75	30–75	30–80	30–85	35–90
QRS axis (°)	60–195	65–185	10–120	10–100	10–100	10–105	10–135	10–120	10–130
QRS V_1 Q (mV)	0	0	0	0	0	0	0	0	0
R (mV)	0.5–2.6	0.3–2.3	0.3–2.0	0.2–2.0	0.2–1.8	0.1–1.8	0.1–1.5	0.1–1.2	0.1–1.0
S (mV)	0–2.3	0–1.5	0–1.5	0–1.8	0.1–2.1	0.2–2.1	0.3–2.4	0.3–2.5	0.3–2.2
QRS V_6 Q (mV)	0–0.2	0–0.3	0–0.25	0–0.3	0–0.3	0.02–0.35	0.02–0.45	0.01–0.3	0–0.3
R (mV)	0–1.1	0.1–1.3	0.5–2.2	0.5–2.3	0.6–2.3	0.8–2.5	0.8–2.6	0.9–2.5	0.7–2.4
S (mV)	0–1.0	0–1.0	0–1.0	0–0.8	0–0.6	0–0.5	0–0.4	0–0.4	0–0.4
TV_1 (mV)	−0.4–0.4	−0.5–−0.1	−0.6–0.1	−0.6–−0.1	−0.6–−0.1	−0.6–0	−0.5–0.2	−0.4–0.3	−0.4–0.3

Values reported as 2–98% (approximate).

Adapted from Davignon A, Rautaharju P, Barselle E, et al: Normal ECG standards for infants and children. Pediatr Cardiol 1979/80;1:123–134.

b. Severe hypertrophy can mimic conduction abnormality (bundle branch block).

c. The frontal-plane QRS axis is age-dependent.

   (1) Right axis deviation is present when the QRS axis is more positive than normal, and left axis deviation is present when the QRS axis is less positive than normal.

   (2) Right axis deviation is a criterion for right ventricular hypertrophy, but in pediatric patients left axis deviation is not a criterion for left ventricular hypertrophy.

   (3) The QRS axis is referred to as *superior* when it is between −60° and −100°. The axis is said to be *indeterminate* (neither left nor right) or northwest when it is between −100° and +210°.

   (4) Axis deviation may represent a conduction abnormality (see next section), but there is no known significance to isolated axis deviation in asymptomatic patients.

d. The concept of fascicular block (hemiblock) is useful but overly simplified. In pediatric patients, frontal-plane QRS axis deviation, the principal ECG feature of fascicular block, has other interpretations. For example, left axis deviation in patients with tricuspid atresia is thought to be caused by early right ventricular activation with relative delay in the left ventricle. In atrioventricular (AV) septal defect, left axis deviation is caused by early depolarization of the diaphragmatic surface of the left ventricle, a finding consistent with the known posterior and inferior displacement of the specialized conduction system.

e. Q waves are very common on the pediatric ECG, and a tendency to overdiagnose certain types of abnormalities has resulted. There are a few specific situations in which Q waves may be of clinical significance.

   (1) For the diagnosis of myocardial infarction, Q wave duration should be ≥40 msec; Q wave amplitude is lead-dependent but in all cases should exceed 0.4 mV. In patients with Kawasaki disease, the Q wave amplitude criterion (deep Q waves) alone is reported to be very specific for inferior myocardial infarction.

   (2) A QR pattern in lead V_1 signifies right ventricular hypertrophy, and Q waves in lead V_6 exceeding 0.4 mV indicate left ventricular hypertrophy. The latter condition also suggests inferior infarction.

   (3) If the QRS duration is prolonged, no specific significance can be attached to Q waves.

3. Evaluation of ventricular repolarization

   a. The sequence of ventricular depolarization is a major determinant of the ST-T wave.

   b. ST-T wave abnormalities (elevation or depression with respect to baseline) are nonspecific; they may be affected by electrolyte disturbances, myocardial infarction, drugs, neurologic abnormalities, myocarditis, and pericarditis.

   c. Analysis of the ST segment is sensitive to baseline selection; this is an important practical problem when the heart rate is increased (e.g., during exercise or fever). Normally, ST segments are between 0.1 and −0.05 mV. The term *early repolarization* is applied to the elevated ST segments seen as a normal variant in adolescents.

   d. The QT interval is both age- and heart rate–dependent. Correction for heart rate (Bazett formula) involves dividing the QT interval by the square root of the R-R interval, which yields the QTc (corrected QT) interval. The QT interval may be prolonged on a congenital basis or as the result of antiarrhythmic drugs or electrolyte imbalance. The significance of a prolonged QT interval in an asymptomatic child is unknown. It is generally agreed that a QTc of ≤440 msec is normal and a QTc of ≥480 msec is prolonged; however, there is disagreement as to the significance of intermediate values, especially in asymptomatic patients.

   e. U waves are common in young people after 8 years of age. Little is known of their source or significance. U waves are usually seen in midprecordial leads (V_2 to V_5), and they often overlap the T wave, resulting in TU fusion. This latter feature may complicate measurement of the QT interval. U-wave amplitude is heart rate–sensitive and is equal to about 10 per cent of the T wave amplitude (range, 4 to 28%).

4. Evaluation of rate and rhythm

   a. Heart rate is dependent on age, body temperature, autonomic nervous tone, and physical activity. For example, a resting heart rate of 150 bpm would be abnormally fast in a 14-year-old, but it may be a normal rate for an apprehensive toddler during ECG recording. Similarly, a resting heart rate of 50 bpm in a healthy adolescent would be normal, but the same heart rate in an infant would signify bradycardia.

   b. "Sinus" P waves should give an ECG pattern indicating atrial depolarization from top to bottom and right to left (positive in leads I and II). The term *normal sinus rhythm* is often used as a blanket statement for performance of the sinus node as well as the whole AV conduction system.

   c. Sinus arrhythmia results in an irregular rhythm; the phases of irregularity are synchronized with respiration.

5. Evaluation of AV conduction

   a. PR interval and QRS duration are age-dependent measures of AV conduction; the PR interval is heart rate–dependent also. Impaired AV conduction is described as first-, second-, or third-degree heart block; apparently abbreviated conduction, as seen in Wolff-Parkinson-White syndrome and glycogen storage disease, may be present.

   b. PR interval is determined by conduction from the sinus node to the onset of QRS. The PR interval may be prolonged or shortened, depending on delayed or enhanced conduction through the atrium (intraatrial conduction), through the low septal atrium to the bundle of His (AV node), and through the bundle of His to the Purkinje network. For example, first-degree heart block may occur in cases of atrial septal defect caused by prolonged intraatrial conduction associated with right atrial enlargement. The PR interval is usually short when ventricular preexcitation is present (e.g., Wolff-Parkinson-White syndrome). The most common cause of a short PR interval is a nonsinus atrial pacemaker.

6. Evaluation of hypertrophy and enlargement

Since the ECG does not the measure physical dimensions of the heart chambers, it is not surprising that the echocardiogram gives more accurate measures of chamber size. In spite of problems with sensitivity and specificity, the ECG is a relatively inexpensive and useful screening tool. Some leads are better than others for certain types of hypertrophy and enlargement (Table 192–2).

   a. Left ventricular hypertrophy tests derive from considerations of QRS amplitude and ST-T wave abnormalities (strain). Amplitude tests evaluate voltage increase, whereas strain tests measures a shift of the angle between the ST-T wave and the QRS axes. Amplitude tests use the R and S waves in leads V_1, V_2, V_5, and V_6, the ratio of R and S waves in lead V_1, and the Q wave amplitude in lead V_6. There has not been general agreement on defining what may be considered abnormal so far as the amplitude of Q, R, and S waves. The strain tests evaluate T-wave negativity in the lateral precordial leads and the angle ($>100°$) between the frontal-plane QRS and the T axis.

   b. Right ventricular hypertrophy criteria include an amplitude test for the S wave in left precordial leads (V_5, V_6), an amplitude test for the R wave in the

TABLE 192–2. VARIOUS TYPES OF HYPERTROPHY AND ENLARGEMENT

LEFT VENTRICULAR HYPERTROPHY
R V_6 >3.0 mV
S V_1 >2.7 mV
Q V_6 >0.4 mV

LEFT VENTRICULAR HYPERTROPHY WITH STRAIN
QRS-T angle $>100°$ and T negative in V_6, but not all precordial T waves negative

POSSIBLE LEFT VENTRICULAR HYPERTROPHY
R/S V_1 <0.5 mV with S >0.5 mV and age <3 yr
S V_2 >3.5 mV
R V_5 >4.0 mV
S V_1 + R V_6 >5.0 mV

RIGHT VENTRICULAR HYPERTROPHY
QR pattern in V_1 with S <0.5, Q >0.07 and R >0.1 mV
RV_1 >0.4 mV
RSR′ pattern in V_1 with R′ $>$R and R′ >0.7 mV for age >1 yr or 1.5 mV for age <1 yr
T >0.2 mV in V_1 and V_6 and age between 3 days and 8 yr

POSSIBLE RIGHT VENTRICULAR HYPERTROPHY
Right axis deviation
R/S V_1 >1 for age >5 yr or >2 for age 1 to 5 yr
R + S V_6 for age >9 mo or >1.1 mV for age <9 mo with R in V_5 <4.0 mV
Maximum R in chest leads <0.8 mV
R/S <1 in V_6

BIVENTRICULAR HYPERTROPHY
R >3 mV and S >3 mV in V_3 or V_4

RIGHT ATRIAL ENLARGEMENT
P >0.25 mV in any lead, usually II, V_1 or V_2

LEFT ATRIAL ENLARGEMENT
P < -0.1 mV, usually in V_1
P duration >100 msec

Procedure *Continued*

right precordial leads (V_1, V_2), an RSR′ pattern with R taller than R′ in lead V_1, a QR in lead V_1, and a positive T wave in lead V_1 after 48 hours of life. Right axis deviation also indicates right ventricular hypertrophy. Finally, evaluation of the R:S ratio in lead V_6 may be useful for detecting right ventricular hypertrophy, especially when lung disease is present. ECG interpretation of right ventricular hypertrophy in infants is difficult because infants normally have right ventricular hypertrophy.

c. Biventricular hypertrophy may be inferred when criteria for both left and right ventricular hypertrophy are met. An alternative criterion (the so-called Katz-Wachtel criterion) uses prominent midprecordial voltage to diagnose biventricular hypertrophy.

d. Several seeming paradoxes occur with regard to ECG criteria for ventricular hypertrophy. In conditions that result in hypertrophy because of pressure overload in the left ventricle (e.g., aortic stenosis), the ECG is often normal and left ventricular hypertrophy is not evident. On the other hand, volume overload of the left ventricle (e.g., aortic regurgitation) produces very large left precordial voltages. In the right ventricle, pressure overload (e.g., pulmonary stenosis) results in high voltage in the anterior chest leads, whereas volume overload (e.g., atrial septal defect) results in a particular QRS pattern in lead V_1 (RSR′).

e. Low voltage is said to be present when QRS amplitude is <0.5 mV in all limb leads and <1.0 mV in all precordial leads. It is a nonspecific finding that may be seen in a variety of conditions, including myocarditis, pericardial effusion, and generalized edema.

f. ECG features of right or left atrial enlargement differ because of asynchrony of atrial depolarization and the proximity of the right atrium to the anterior chest wall and the precordial leads. Effects of atrial enlargement may be manifest in the early (right) or late (left) portion of the P wave (see Table 192–2).

(1) Right atrial enlargement manifests as increased voltage in leads II, V_1, and V_2.

(2) Left atrial enlargement manifests as increased voltage in the terminal portion of the P wave or as prolonged P wave duration, usually in lead II or V_1.

(3) Biatrial enlargement may be diagnosed if criteria for both left and right atrial enlargement are present.

7. Recording errors

Lead reversals involving right and left arm or right and left leg are common errors. Leg lead reversal may have little effect on the ECG, but arm lead reversal has profound effect on the axes of both P and QRS. The ECG alterations resulting from right-left lead reversals may mimic those of ectopic atrial rhythm, left axis deviation (hemiblock), or myocardial infarction. Lead reversal should be suspected if two or more ECG recordings show drastic changes in the limb leads.

The Normal ECG

1. Developmental changes

a. The hallmark of the ECG changes in the normal infant and child are the age-related transitions of QRS morphology, QRS duration, and the pattern of the ST-T wave.

b. Developmental changes include a gradual decrease in heart rate and an increase in P-wave duration, PR interval, and QRS duration.

c. Compared with those of older children, QRS voltages are low during the first several months of life.

d. The mean QRS axis in the frontal plane moves from a rightward direction to the left.

e. Slight elevations of the ST segment, followed by decrease before the T wave, are common.

f. In the first days of life, the T wave is positive in lead V_1. T waves are negative in the right chest leads during childhood, and by adolescence qualitative ECG features of repolarization are similar to those of normal adults.

2. Preterm infant

a. Compared with that of a full-term infant, the ECG of the premature infant is notable for a shorter QRS duration, a shorter PR interval, a shorter QT interval, and a faster heart rate.

b. The ECG shows less right ventricular predominance at birth than that of the full-term infant.

c. ECG differences between full-term and preterm infants persist beyond the first year of life.

B ## Bibliography

Bailey JJ, Berson AS, Garson A Jr, et al: Recommendations for standardization of leads and of specifications for instruments in electrocardiography and vector cardiography: Report of the Committee on Electrocardiography and Cardiac Electrophysiology of the Council on Clinical Cardiology, American Heart Association. Circulation 1990;81:730–739.

Benson DW. The normal electrocardiogram. *In* Emmanoulides GC, Riemenschneider TA, Allen HD, Gutgesell HD (eds): Moss and Adams' Heart Disease in Infants, Children and Adolescents. Baltimore, Williams & Wilkins, 1994, pp 152–164.

Davignon A, Rautaharju P, Barselle E, et al: Normal ECG standards for infants and children. Pediatr Cardiol 1979/80;1:123–134.

Liebman J: Tables of normal standard. *In* Liebman J, Plonsey R, Gillette PC (eds): Pediatric Electrocardiography. Baltimore, Williams & Wilkins, 1982, pp 82–133.

193 Defibrillation

Dianne L. Atkins

Indications

1. Emergency treatment for life-threatening arrhythmias such as ventricular fibrillation and ventricular tachycardia
2. Urgent cardioversion for patients with symptomatic atrial and ventricular arrhythmias
3. Elective cardioversion for patients whose cardiac performance can be optimized with sinus rhythm.

Contraindications

1. Inadequate skill or training of the operator
2. Cardioversion of patients in established, hemodynamically stable atrial fibrillation without prior anticoagulation
3. Patients with chronic illness or poor prognosis who have indicated (or whose families have indicated) their desire that resuscitation not be performed.

Preparation

1. Patients requiring emergency defibrillation are unconscious and do not require anesthesia. Intubation and intravascular access are not necessary and should not delay defibrillation.
2. Anesthesia is essential for patients undergoing urgent or elective cardioversion. Endotracheal intubation may be appropriate. If general anesthesia is not used, then deep sedation with amnesia is required.

Equipment

1. A direct current defibrillator with the capacity to deliver synchronized cardioversion is required. For pediatric defibrillation, a broad range of energy doses must be available. Energy levels of 5, 10, 20, 40, 50, 70, and 100 J provide a reasonable range for patients weighing 3 to 50 kg.
2. Monitors and recorders are now standard accessories.
3. Pediatric electrodes (paddles) should be easily accessible. Units in which the adult electrodes clip over the pediatric electrodes are most convenient. Units that require the operator to unplug the adult electrodes and insert separate pediatric electrodes require additional storage space and risk loss of the pediatric electrodes. Self-adhesive, disposable pads are commercially available in adult and pediatric sizes. The transthoracic impedance and success rates appear to be equivalent to those of hand-held electrodes.
4. Electrode gel or cream is necessary to decrease the impedance of the electrode-skin interface. Many preparations are commercially available. Gels used for echocardiography are high-impedance gels and should not be used.

Technique (Table 193–1)

1. *Turn unit on*—Most defibrillators have two operating modes. One is for electrocardiographic (ECG) monitoring only and is frequently referred to as the *monitor mode*. In this mode, the unit will not charge or discharge a shock. The second mode ("ON") enables the unit to function as a defibrillator.
2. *ECG monitoring*—Cardiac rhythm should be monitored directly through the defibrillator, and all current defibrillator models provide the equipment for this. The most stable method is to use the standard ECG electrodes, which are connected to the defibrillator to display the rhythm on the monitor screen. Rhythm monitoring is then never interrupted by electrode positioning. Self-adhesive electrode pads provide similar convenience. The hand-held electrodes can be used to assess cardiac rhythm, but the ECG tracing is visible only when the electrodes are applied directly to the chest wall.
3. *Electrode paste*—Transthoracic impedance is very high if the electrodes are applied directly to the skin; therefore, it is necessary to use some type of conductive medium. Although commercially available pastes, creams, and gels have differing impedance scores, clinical differences have not been documented. Echocardiography gels should not be used. The paste should be applied directly to the electrodes and the paddles applied firmly to the chest wall. Self-adhesive pads contain the gel within the pad.
4. *Energy dose*—The optimal dose for defibrillation of children has never been tested experimentally, but 2 J/kg, as recommended by the American Heart Association, has

TABLE 193–1. PROCEDURE FOR TRANSTHORACIC DEFIBRILLATION

1. Turn defibrillator to ON, not monitor mode.
2. Evaluate rhythm with (in order of preference) electrode leads of the defibrillator, self-adhesive pads, or quick-look paddles.
3. Apply electrode paste (if not using self-adhesive pads).
4. Select energy level.
5. Turn synchronizer on, if necessary.
6. Position electrodes on chest with firm pressure.
7. Ensure that all personnel are clear of patient and bed.
8. Charge defibrillator.
9. Discharge defibrillator.
10. Reassess rhythm.
11. Repeat steps if rhythm not converted.

Procedure *Continued*

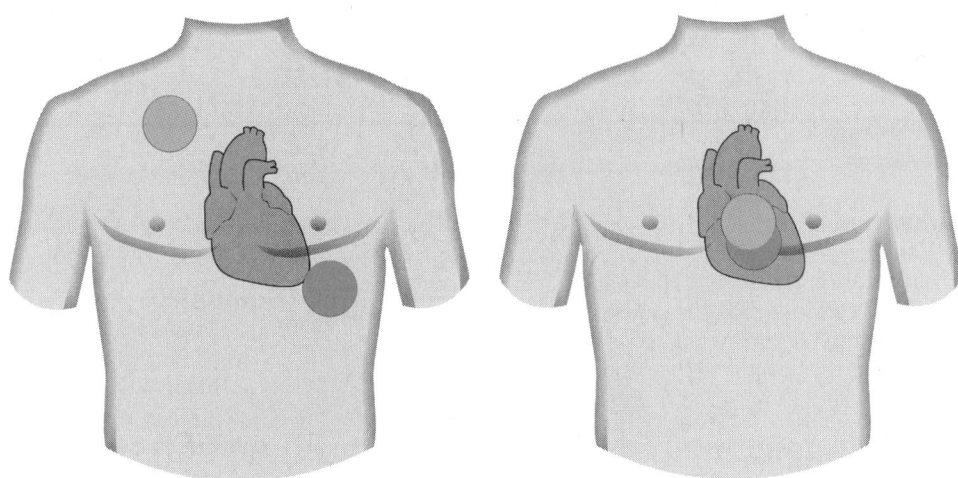

Figure 193–1 Proper placement of electrode paddles for pediatric defibrillation. *A,* Standard position of apex-anterior. The anterior electrode paddle is to right of sternum, and the apex electrode is placed under and beneath the left nipple. *B,* Anterior-posterior position. The anterior electrode paddle is directly over the heart, and the posterior electrode paddle is behind the heart.

stood the test of time. Organized rhythms such as supraventricular tachycardia and atrial flutter can be cardioverted with lower doses of 0.5 to 1.0 J/kg. If the shock is not successful the first time, the dose may be repeated or doubled. The dose of the third shock should be double that of the first.

5. *Synchronizer*—For all rhythms except ventricular fibrillation and pulseless ventricular tachycardia, the synchronizer switch should be on. The synchronizing circuitry ensures that the shock is delivered within a few milliseconds of the QRS complex, thus avoiding the "vulnerable" period of the cardiac cycle. Synchronization should be confirmed by seeing the marked QRS complex on the monitor.

6. *Electrode size and position*—The correct size of electrode should be chosen. Infants and children weighing 10 to 15 kg need the pediatric electrodes; adult electrodes should be used for larger children. Adequate current delivery through the heart depends on electrode position. If the electrodes are too close together or too far apart, the current passing through the heart may be inadequate to defibrillate. Standard positions include anterior-apex, anterior-posterior, and posterior-apex (Fig. 193–1). The anterior-apical position is the easiest and most frequently used. There is little evidence to suggest that one position is preferred. However, if a patient cannot be defibrillated or cardioverted in one position, an alternative position may be successful. Additionally, the presence of a right infraclavicular pacemaker pocket may preclude use of the anterior-apical position. The electrodes should be applied with firm pressure, to decrease transthoracic impedance. Many units have indicator lights to verify adequate pressure.

7. *Charging and discharging*—Charging of the defibrillator can be done from the machine or, preferably, from a charging button on one of the paddles. This allows the operator to be in total control of the charged electrodes. There is usually an audible indicator to signal that the capacitor is fully charged. Discharging the defibrillator, or delivering the shock, can be done only from the electrodes themselves. It is the responsibility of the operator to ensure that no one is touching the patient or the bed when the machine is discharged. Once the discharge buttons are pushed, there may be a perceptible delay before the shock is delivered. If the operator decides not to deliver the shock to the patient, the electrodes should be replaced into the machine and discharged there. It is not safe to discharge them into the air.

8. *Rhythm assessment*—As soon as the shock is delivered, the patient's rhythm should be assessed. There may be a short pause before normal sinus rhythm resumes. If there has been no conversion, the shock should be redelivered, at either the same energy dose or a doubled dose.

Complications

1. Rarely, a more malignant arrhythmia, such as ventricular fibrillation, may be induced, especially if the unit was not synchronized to the QRS complex. The treatment is immediate defibrillation.

2. Systemic thromboembolism can occur after cardioversion for chronic atrial fibrillation or, less likely, atrial flutter, if sufficient anticoagulation is not present.

3. The extent and severity of myocardial damage depends on excessive energy dose and number of shocks. Mitochondrial disruption, contraction band necrosis, and epicardial or subepicardial coagulation and necrosis have been observed in animal and human subjects. Arrhythmias and hemodynamic dysfunction are observed in patients who have been successfully resuscitated, but their relation to electric countershock is difficult to discern.

4. Erythema of the skin is frequently seen after defibrillation. Although commonly referred to as a burn, it is the result of hyperemia and not a true skin burn. No treatment is necessary.

Follow-up

Follow-up therapy depends on the clinical situation and the underlying cause of the arrhythmia. Patients with under-

Procedure *Continued*

lying cardiac disease may require anticoagulation or antiarrhythmic therapy.

Bibliography

Atkins DL: Pediatric defibrillation: Optimal techniques. *In* Tacker WA Jr (ed): Defibrillation of the heart: ICDs, AEDs, and Manual. St. Louis, Mosby–Year Book, 1994, pp 169–181.

Atkins DL, Kerber RE: Pediatric defibrillation: Current flow is improved by using "adult" paddle electrodes. Pediatrics 1994;94:90–93.

Emergency Cardiac Care Committee and Subcommittees, American Heart Association: Guidelines for cardiopulmonary resuscitation and emergency cardiac care, IV: Pediatric advanced life support. JAMA 1992;268:2262–2275.

Gutgesell HP, Tacker WA, Geddes LA, et al: Energy dose for ventricular defibrillation of children. Pediatrics 1976;58:898–901.

Mogayzel C, Quan L, Graves JR, et al: Out-of-hospital ventricular fibrillation in children and adolescents: Causes and outcome. Ann Emerg Med 1995;25:484–491.

194 Symptoms of Respiratory Disorders

| Symptom | **Chronic Cough** | *John C. Stevens* |

Definition

Respiratory tract symptoms, often with the major complaint of cough, account for half of all pediatric physician visits. Although cough lasting a week is not uncommon in children, one of 2 to 3 weeks' duration or frequent intermittent cough is of concern and often warrants evaluation and treatment of the underlying cause. In trying to establish the etiology of a child's cough it is best to consider those diagnoses most prevalent in the patient's age range.

Differential Diagnosis

Clinical Findings

1. History

    A well-taken history often provides valuable clues to the etiology of a chronic cough. Particularly important are the nature and timing of the cough.

    a. Nature of cough

    (1) Loose, rattling cough is indicative of excess sputum production

        (a) Purulent sputum may be secondary to cystic fibrosis, immune deficiency, immotile cilia syndrome, or chronic sinusitis.

        (b) Bloody sputum most often is indicative of nasopharyngeal irritation but may be secondary to a retained foreign body, cystic fibrosis, bronchiectasis, tuberculosis, or pulmonary hemosiderosis.

    (2) Nonproductive, dry, and brassy cough usually indicates tracheal irritation or upper airway secretions.

    (3) Throat-clearing, hacking cough is indicative of postnasal drip from rhinitis or sinusitis.

    (4) Cough accompanied by stereotyped movements may be indicative of a psychogenic cough.

    b. Timing of cough

    (1) Nighttime cough that is worse when lying flat may be from postnasal drip or asthma.

    (2) Prominent cough upon arising that is productive

Differential Diagnosis in Infancy

1. Congenital anomalies
    a. Cleft palate
    b. Laryngeal cleft
    c. H-type tracheoesophageal fistula
    d. Vascular ring
2. Infections
    a. Viral: respiratory syncytial virus, adenovirus, cytomegalovirus, influenza, parainfluenza
    b. Bacterial: pertussis, parapertussis
    c. *Chlamydia trachomatis*
    d. *Mycobacterium tuberculosis*
3. Cystic fibrosis
4. Asthma
5. Foreign body aspiration
6. Neurologic impairment with aspiration
7. Sinusitis

Differential Diagnosis in Toddler/Preschool Child

1. Foreign body aspiration
2. Infections
    a. Viral: respiratory syncytial virus, adenovirus, influenza, parainfluenza
    b. Bacterial: pertussis, parapertussis
    c. *Mycoplasma*
    d. *Mycobacterium tuberculosis*
3. Asthma
4. Cystic fibrosis
5. Passive smoking
6. Congenital anomalies
    a. Vascular ring
    b. H-type tracheoesophageal fistula
7. Immotile cilia syndrome
8. Immune deficiency

Differential Diagnosis in School-Age Child/Adolescent

1. Asthma
2. Postnasal drip/sinusitis
3. Infections
    a. *Mycoplasma*
    b. Viral
    c. *Mycobacterium tuberculosis*
4. Irritations
    a. Smoking
    b. Environmental pollution
5. Psychogenic cough
6. Cystic fibrosis
7. Immotile cilia syndrome
8. Immune deficiency

of sputum may be secondary to cystic fibrosis or other causes of bronchiectasis or sinusitis.

(3) Cough worse with feedings may be indicative of aspiration secondary to an incoordinated swallow, H-type tracheoesophageal fistula, or gastroesophageal reflux.

(4) Cough most pronounced when attention is drawn to it is indicative of psychogenic cough.

(5) Cough with a seasonal predilection may be indicative of allergy-induced bronchospasm or rhinitis. Cough in the winter may be secondary to viral infection or irritation from dry indoor air or bronchospasm induced by a cool mist vaporizer.

2. Physical

a. General assessment of growth is important, since underlying lung disease such as cystic fibrosis may be accompanied by failure to thrive.

b. Head and neck examination

(1) Atopy can be suggested by allergic shiners, a transverse nasal crease, baggy pale nasal mucosa, and an allergic gape.

(2) Hypertrophic lymphoid follicles (cobblestoning) of the posterior pharyngeal wall are indicative of chronic postnasal drainage from allergic rhinitis or chronic sinusitis.

c. Chest examination

(1) Increased anteroposterior diameter with hyperresonance to percussion is indicative of air trapping seen in diseases such as asthma and cystic fibrosis.

(2) Generalized coarse crackles are usually from bronchitis (infectious or noninfectious). These crackles change with coughing.

(3) Fine inspiratory crackles suggest pathology in the more distal airways.

(4) Decreased air entry is indicative of bronchial obstruction as seen with asthma or foreign body aspiration.

d. Distal clubbing should prompt an evaluation for suppurative lung disease such as cystic fibrosis or associated cardiac pathology.

Laboratory, Radiologic, and Function Tests

The diagnostic approach in evaluating a pediatric patient with chronic cough should be guided by the child's age.

1. Infancy

a. A chest roentgenogram is needed in all patients to evaluate for air trapping, e.g., seen in asthma and cystic fibrosis, and to detect any chronic infiltrative changes.

b. An upper GI study with barium swallow and airway fluoroscopy will enable evaluation for dysfunctional swallowing with aspiration. H-type tracheoesophageal fistula, vascular ring, tracheomalacia, gastroesophageal reflux, and other congenital anomalies.

c. Examination and culture of nasopharyngeal secretions will aid in diagnosing chlamydial, viral, and pertussis infections.

d. Infant pulmonary function testing can demonstrate upper or lower airway obstruction disease and detect bronchodilator response.

e. A sweat chloride determination should be performed to rule out cystic fibrosis.

2. Toddler/Preschool Age

a. Chest roentgenogram

b. Airway fluoroscopy and ventilation perfusion scan may be useful in detecting an aspirated foreign body.

c. Sinus roentgenogram or sinus CT scan to evaluate for sinusitis

d. Evidence of atopy can be detected with an absolute eosinophil count and an IgE.

e. As most children in this age range are uncooperative with pulmonary function tests, a therapeutic clinical trial of bronchodilation may be warranted in an effort to rule out asthma.

f. Sweat chloride determination.

3. School-Age Child/Adolescent

a. Chest roentgenogram

b. Pulmonary function testing with bronchodilator response, a methacholine challenge, or an exercise bronchial challenge can be used to detect underlying airway hyperreactivity.

c. Sinus roentgenogram/sinus CT scan

d. Sweat chloride determination.

Treatment

In general, it is most effective to direct therapy for chronic cough at the specific underlying etiology, such as treating reactive airway disease with bronchodilators, than to simply supply symptomatic treatment with cough-suppressive therapy. Therefore, considerable effort should be made to establish the actual cause of a chronic cough as outlined above. Symptomatic cough therapy may be useful, however, in a child with a tight nonproductive cough, not secondary to bronchospasm, and one that disrupts sleep or school.

1. Cough suppressants

a. Codeine is the most effective cough suppressant for children >5 years of age.

b. Dextromethorphan is the most effective non-narcotic antitussive.

2. Expectorants

a. Water is generally accepted as effective when given orally.

b. Guaifenesin, relatively free of side effects, is of questionable therapeutic value in the usual doses.

3. Local therapy, such as candies, local anesthetics, and lozenges, can be used to relieve cough arising from local irritation of the pharynx.

Definition

1. Wheezing is a high-pitched musical sound from the lungs. When expiratory pressure exceeds the pressure required for maximal flow through a large airway, the airway wall vibrates and produces the wheezing sound. Inflammation, mucosal edema, and bronchospasm all lead to airway obstruction and decreased flow. Increased expiratory effort fails to improve air flow through the obstructed airways, and the result is a wheeze.

2. In general, recurrent wheezing is a common symptom in children and is often a sign of serious chronic pulmonary disorder. Wheeze, which is an *expiratory* sound of the lower airways, must be distinguished from inspiratory sounds and sounds created by problems in the upper airways. For example, noisy breathing or snoring during sleep are often interpreted as wheezing by parents. In such cases, attention should be focused on possible disorders of the head and neck (e.g., enlarged adenoids, nasal polyposis, choanal narrowing, small chin). It is also important to establish whether the symptom is a result of multiple, acute, unrelated respiratory infections or of significant underlying lung disorder; the history, physical examination, and age of the child are important in making this determination. If expiratory wheeze is found, its likely cause varies with a child's age.

Differential Diagnosis

Infancy

1. Infections
   a. Viral
      (1) Respiratory syncytial virus (RSV)
      (2) Parainfluenza viruses
      (3) Adenoviruses
      (4) Influenza viruses
   b. Other infections
      (1) Tuberculosis
      (2) Histoplasmosis
      (3) Mycotic infections
2. Asthma/reactive airways disease
3. Aspiration
   a. Pharyngeal incoordination
   b. Gastroesophageal reflux
   c. Tracheoesophageal fistula
   d. Laryngotracheoesophageal cleft
4. Congenital malformations
   a. Tracheobronchial abnormalities
   b. Lung cyst
   c. Vascular rings
   d. Mediastinal lesions
5. Bronchopulmonary dysplasia
6. Cystic fibrosis
7. Human immunodeficiency virus (HIV) infection/ acquired immunodeficiency syndrome (AIDS)
8. Congenital heart disease with left-to-right shunt

Toddler/Preschool

1. Infection
   a. Viral
      (1) RSV
      (2) Adenoviruses
      (3) Parainfluenza and influenza viruses
   b. Other infections: tuberculosis, histoplasmosis, other mycotic infections; visceral larva migrans
2. Asthma/reactive airways disease
3. Foreign-body aspiration
4. Cystic fibrosis
5. HIV infection/AIDS
6. Tumor: leukemia, lymphoma
7. Congenital heart disease with left-to-right shunt
8. Pulmonary hemosiderosis
9. Aspiration, not foreign body

School-Age/Adolescence

1. Infection
   a. Viral: adenoviruses, influenza viruses
   b. Mycoplasma
   c. Other infections: mycobacterium tuberculosis, fungal infections
2. Asthma/reactive airways disease
3. Cystic fibrosis
4. Tumor: leukemia, lymphoma, lymphosarcoma
5. Kartagener syndrome
6. Hypersensitivity pneumonitis

Clinical Findings

1. History
   a. In general, the closer to birth symptoms first appear, the greater the chance that they are a manifestation of a congenital malformation or an inherited disorder.
   b. The presence of fever suggests acute infection and, if accompanied by grunting, often suggests a bacterial pneumonia.
   c. Sputum production varies with age in children, and toddlers and preschoolers cannot cough up their sputum. Clear secretions are observed in asthmatic children, whereas yellow-green sputum is more consistent with a bacterial process. Postnasal drainage from sinusitis can be confused with sputum production.
   d. Confirm whether environmental irritants trigger the wheezing. Time and place can be clues to environmental irritants as an underlying cause, whether the differential diagnosis is asthma or reactive airways disease. Irritants to consider include passive cigarette exposure, airborne allergens (animal dander, molds, cockroaches, antigen, pollen), wood burning stoves, unvented heaters, and pesticides. All of these can cause chronic airway irritation.
2. Physical examination

The physical examination can help confirm the presence of underlying chronic lung disorder.

   a. Assessment of growth gives a good overall indication of the child's recent health. Analysis of the growth curve helps determine whether nutrition and growth have been persistently abnormal or have changed in the recent past.

   b. Head and neck

     (1) Allergic shiners under the eyes, nasal mucosal swelling, or a crease across the bridge of the nose are commonly observed in children with allergic disorder.

     (2) Enlarged tonsils are seen in children with obstructive sleep apnea.

     (3) A deviated trachea may be shifted to the right or left if there is volume loss in one lung, severe unilateral gas trapping, or a space-occupying lesion.

   c. Increased anteroposterior diameter of the chest is consistent with severe obstructive lung disease.

   d. Clubbing of the extremities is uncommon in children, is rarely observed in asthmatics, and should trigger an extensive evaluation for chronic lung, heart, liver, or gastrointestinal disorders.

Diagnostic Tests

If a chronic respiratory disorder is suspected after the history and physical examination, a diagnostic assessment should proceed based on an age-dependent differential diagnosis.

1. Infancy

   a. A chest radiograph is required in all infants with recurrent wheezing to assess the presence and distribution of air trapping and to detect mediastinal or parenchymal mass or any chronic infiltrates (e.g., right upper lobe atelectasis in chronic aspiration).

   b. Culture and antigen detection (enzyme-linked immunosorbent assay or immunofluorescence assay) of nasopharyngeal secretions are needed for children suspected of having a respiratory tract viral infection (e.g., RSV, influenza virus, or adenovirus).

   c. Use a sweat chloride test to rule out cystic fibrosis.

   d. A barium esophagram often reveals mechanical or structural abnormalities leading to aspiration (e.g., tracheoesophageal fistula, oral motor dysfunction, vascular rings).

   e. Infant pulmonary function tests determine the presence of obstructive lung disorder and bronchodilator response.

   f. Quantitative immunoglobulins, complement (CH_{50} assay), and complete blood count with differential are needed for infants suspected of being immunodeficient.

   g. Order a tuberculin skin test, fungal titers, or HIV testing, if indicated.

2. Toddler/Preschool

   a. Chest radiograph to diagnose air trapping, mediastinal or parenchymal mass, or chronic infiltrates

   b. Airway fluoroscopy if a foreign body is suspected, followed by rigid bronchoscopy as needed for foreign body removal

   c. Sinus radiograph or modified computed tomography scan if sinusitis is suspected

   d. Absolute eosinophil count and an immunoglobulin E determination in children suspected of having allergen-induced wheezing

   e. Sweat chloride test to rule out cystic fibrosis

   f. Tuberculin skin test, fungal titers, or HIV testing, if indicated

3. School-Age/Adolescence

   a. Chest radiograph

   b. Absolute eosinophil count and an immunoglobulin E determination

   c. Pulmonary function testing with an inhaled bronchodilator. If initial testing is nondiagnostic, a methacholine challenge test to detect airway hyperreactivity may be indicated.

   d. Sweat test to rule out cystic fibrosis

   e. Sinus radiograph or modified sinus computed tomography scan

   f. Tuberculin skin test, fungal titers, or HIV testing

   g. Peripheral blood smear, lymph node biopsy, or bone marrow aspiration in a child with a mediastinal mass who is suspected of having a tumor.

Treatment

Once the diagnosis is established, appropriate therapy can be instituted; see the chapters on specific disorders.

Symptom **Stridor** *Howard Eigen*

Definition

Stridor is an abnormal noise associated with respiration, usually on inspiration.

Etiology

Stridor occurs when airflow is interrupted periodically during inspiration. The genesis of the noise usually is in the larynx, but it may come from the pharyngeal soft tissues as well. Unlike snoring, stridor may occur in a given child when the child is awake, during sleep, or both.

Epidemiology

Stridor is primarily a condition of the first year of life and is chronic or recurrent over weeks or months. Acute stridor occurring over hours or days is usually caused by an infection. Acute stridor from croup or epiglottitis can occur much later in life, well into school age.

Pathophysiology

As the child inspires, a negative pressure is established in the pleural space that is then transferred to the intrathoracic airways. In the chest this has an expansile effect on the airways, because the pressure in the pleural space is more negative than that in the airways, causing the airway walls to move outward. Above the thoracic inlet, the situation is reversed. The negative pressure inside the airway and the atmospheric pressure outside the airway cause a collapsing force on the airway structures, which move inward, toward the negative pressure narrowing the airway. When the airway is sufficiently narrow and the flow becomes turbulent, the noise of stridor is heard. Expiratory stridor is generated from airways within the thoracic cavity when the pressures are reversed and collapse or narrowing causes noise on exhalation.

Clinical Findings

1. Noise may be inspiratory or expiratory and is usually relatively high pitched.
2. The child may have subcostal, intercostal, or suprasternal retractions.
3. The infant with chronic stridor is usually without distress. The infant with acute stridor is usually distressed to a mild or severe degree.
4. In severe stridor, lack of normal weight gain may occur. This indicates high caloric expenditures secondary to increased work of breathing.
5. Careful physical examination reveals the phase of respiration in which the stridor takes place, and this gives a general location of the intermittent obstruction.
6. Associated signs (e.g., digital clubbing, failure to gain weight, cardiac murmur) may indicate a contributory secondary diagnosis.
7. The location and cause of the obstruction should be sought first. Fiberoptic laryngoscopy and bronchoscopy provide a definitive evaluation and are essential to rule out mass lesions narrowing the airway (extrinsic compression or space occupying lesion).

Causes of Stridor (Inspiratory and Expiratory)

Acute
Laryngotracheal bronchitis
Epiglottitis
Pharyngeal or retropharyngeal abscess
Chronic
Laryngomalacia
Laryngeal cyst, hemangioma
Subglottic stenosis
Laryngeal web
Laryngeal papillomatosis
Aspirated or swallowed foreign body
Vascular ring or sling

---

8. The physiologic consequences of the stridor are also important to determine. A sleep study (often in abbreviated form) determine whether the infant has oxygen desaturation during sleep, and, if so, what degree of oxygen therapy is required to correct it.

Laboratory or Respiratory Function Tests

Evaluations may include pH probe for gastroesophageal reflux, infant lung function testing, and echocardiogram for vascular anomalies and cardiac anatomy.

Treatment

Therapy is directed at relieving the initiating pathology. Correction of the obstruction usually necessitates surgery to remove obstructing lesions (e.g., laryngeal cysts, hemangiomas) or tonsils or, in the rare and most severe instances, tracheostomy. Oxygen should be used freely as indicated by oximetry during sleep. Parents should be reassured that the noise itself is benign if the pathophysiology is corrected.

Symptom **Hemoptysis**   *Harvey P. Bieler*

Definition

1. Hemoptysis is the coughing of blood from the lungs or airways as a result of pulmonary or bronchial hemorrhage.
2. Bleeding from the upper respiratory tract, or from the oropharynx, esophagus, or stomach, may be confused with true hemoptysis.
3. Hemoptysis is uncommon but can be a serious problem in children.
4. In developed countries, hemoptysis is associated almost solely with cystic fibrosis and less commonly with tuberculosis, bronchiectasis, or other infections in previously normal children.

Pathogenesis

1. Hemoptysis in children is related to the dynamic balance of forces that keep blood within pulmonary blood vessels and forces that lead to extravasation from pulmonary vessels into the airways:

   a. Physical integrity of the capillary walls and alveolar epithelium
   b. Hemostatic mechanisms in blood and vessel walls
   c. Pressure and flow in the pulmonary or bronchial circulation.
2. Pulmonary hemorrhage may occur from a discreet bleeding site, or it may occur as a result of diffuse bleeding, depending on the underlying disease process.
3. The severity of the hemoptysis does not necessarily correlate with the severity of the underlying problem.
4. Bleeding resulting only from a disorder in hemostasis can occur and may even be severe. Mild disorders in hemostasis can also lead to significant hemoptysis when coupled with a minor breakdown in vascular integrity or an increase in pulmonary blood flow.
5. There are many potential causes of hemoptysis, and they vary in incidence depending on patient age at presentation.

Etiology

1. Newborn (birth to 30 days)
   a. Congenital or acquired cardiopulmonary malformations
   b. Hemorrhagic disorders
   c. Sepsis (especially when associated with disseminated intravascular coagulopathy)
   d. Bacterial pneumonia
2. Infancy (1 to 12 months)
   a. Cardiopulmonary malformations (e.g., gastroenteric and bronchogenic cysts, arteriovenous malformations)
   b. Pneumonia
   c. Tumors
   d. Angiomas
   e. Pulmonary hemosiderosis/Heiner syndrome
3. Childhood (1 to 12 years)
   a. Retained foreign body
   b. Pulmonary hemosiderosis
   c. Immune/collagen vascular disorders (e.g., Goodpasture syndrome, Henoch-Schönlein purpura, allergic bronchopulmonary aspergillosis, systemic lupus erythematosus)
   d. Pneumonia
   e. Lung abscess
   f. Cardiopulmonary malformations (e.g., pulmonary sequestration, arteriovenous malformation, bronchogenic cyst)
   g. Hemangioma
   h. Pulmonary compression injury
4. Adolescence (12 + years)
   a. Cystic fibrosis
   b. Immune/collagen vascular disorders (including Wegener granulomatosis)
   c. Bronchiectasis
   d. Retained foreign body
   e. Lung abscess
   f. Hemangioma
   g. Pulmonary hypertension
   h. Tumors
   i. Congenital cardiac lesions (e.g., tetralogy of Fallot, pulmonary valve stenosis, mitral valve stenosis, Eisenmenger complex)
   j. Pulmonary compression injury
   k. Pulmonary embolism

Clinical Findings

1. History
   a. If the underlying disease process is known (e.g., cystic fibrosis), evaluation focused on localization of the bleeding site may be adequate.
   b. Dyspnea and cough are common complaints for patients with hemoptysis.
   c. Respiratory distress and circulatory stability may be helpful clinical indicators of the severity. However, the degree of distress may not correlate exactly with the severity of the hemoptysis, since the lung is capable of holding a relatively large volume of blood within the parenchyma.
   d. It may be difficult to elicit the specific time of bleeding or the cause of the hemorrhage.
   e. Detailed inquiry may be necessary to clarify whether the source of blood is the gastrointestinal tract (vomiting vs. coughing of blood), the oropharynx, or the sinuses instead of the lungs and airways.
   f. Relevant questions should elucidate any history of chest trauma, possibility of aspiration (foreign bodies, caustic agents), signs and symptoms of infection, or history of previous bleeding diathesis, as well as all medications taken (especially those containing aspirin, other nonsteroidal antiinflammatory agents, or other agents that may inhibit platelet function or lead to coagulopathies).
2. Physical examination

One may appreciate altered air exchange with crackles or wheezing over the lung areas involved. Blood loss may be large enough to cause pallor, tachycardia, or even hypotension.

Laboratory Findings

1. Assessment of oxygen saturation by pulse oximetry is important in evaluating the degree of pulmonary parenchymal involvement.
2. Complete blood cell count and differential is useful for ruling out thrombocytopenia, to consider infection as an underlying cause, and in evaluating for anemia. (Absence of anemia is not reassuring, because acute bleeding does not result in anemia).
3. Urinalysis and measurements of serum creatinine and blood urea nitrogen should be performed to look for signs of renal involvement.
4. Culture of expectorated material is appropriate in guiding any necessary antibiotic therapy.

Radiographic Findings

1. Chest radiographs (posteroanterior and lateral) are helpful in determining the extent of pulmonary infiltration and can be correlated with the results of physical examination.
   a. New infiltrates may be difficult to distinguish in a patient with severe chronic abnormalities.
   b. It may also be difficult to ascertain whether bleeding is the cause of a new infiltrate.
   c. Finally, large airway bleeding may produce more symptoms with less extensive radiographic changes.
2. Chest computed tomography may demonstrate bronchiectasis or underlying malformations that are inapparent on the plain chest film.
3. Angiograms may be useful to define the bleeding site and as a basis for therapeutic embolization.

Endoscopic Findings

Direct laryngoscopy and bronchoscopy may be useful to differentiate upper from lower respiratory tract bleeding, to define the source or sources of active bleeding, and to determine whether there is focal or diffuse involvement.

1. Use of a rigid bronchoscope in a patient with severe bleeding has been recommended, because its greater size offers better suctioning and airway control.
2. Flexible fiberoptic bronchoscopy, if tolerated, is recommended by some authors because it is better suited to evaluate the more distal airways.
3. In massive bleeding, bronchoscopy should be carried out initially for diagnostic localization and possibly as part of definitive treatment.

Treatment

Patients with intrapulmonary or airway bleeding may be critically ill, and attention must be given to airway patency and vital signs. Unnecessary manipulation must be avoided throughout the initial evaluation. Patients with massive intrapulmonary bleeding are more likely to succumb from asphyxiation than from exsanguination, so close attention to airway maintenance is paramount.

1. Prepare equipment for emergency intubation (large catheters with reliable suction source, supplemental oxygen, endotracheal tubes, and the means for ventilatory assistance).
2. Maintain circulation with the use of colloid or crystalloid, blood transfusions, and inotropic medications to avoid shock and renal insufficiency.
3. Maintain oxygenation.
4. Except in the terminal patient with cystic fibrosis or other destructive lung processes, the child with hemoptysis and respiratory failure should be intubated and supported with mechanical ventilation. Positive end-expiratory pressure may markedly improve gas exchange.
5. Postural drainage treatments should be withheld during acute hemoptysis.
6. In the patient with suppurative lung disease (i.e., cystic fibrosis or bronchiectasis), aggressive intravenous antibiotic therapy usually is necessary to limit an episode of hemoptysis.
7. Embolization of the bleeding vessel, as localized on bronchoscopy or arteriography or both, is usually the treatment of choice in severe hemoptysis.
8. Pulmonary resection may be required in massive bleeding, if the bleeding site can be positively located and embolization therapy has failed.

195 Pharyngitis and Tonsillitis

John Gaebler

Definitions

1. *Pharyngitis* is inflammation of the mucosa in the posterior nose, posterior mouth, and/or throat above the level of the larynx.
2. *Tonsillitis* is inflammation of lymphoid tissue between the glossopalatine and pharyngopalatine arches.
3. *Chronic nasopharyngitis* is inflammation of the mucosa in the nose and pharynx persisting longer than 3 weeks.

Etiology

1. Acute pharyngitis and acute tonsillitis are caused by Group A streptococci (GAS), adenoviruses, enteroviruses, Epstein-Barr virus (EBV), and herpes simplex virus type 1 (HSV-1). Pharyngitis episodes caused by *Mycoplasma pneumoniae* may become more severe with age. Infections with *Chlamydia pneumoniae* are less well defined and often are associated with lower tract symptoms. Less common causes are *Arcanobacterium haemolyticus*; streptococci groups B, C, and G; and *Neisseria gonorrhoeae*. Rarely, *Corynebacterium diphtheriae* may cause pharyngitis.
2. Chronic nasopharyngitis is caused by *Candida* species, *N. gonorrhoeae*, nasal foreign body, inhalant allergies, and illnesses in which host factors or therapeutic agents are a primary cause (e.g., neutropenia, immunodeficiencies).

Epidemiology

1. *Streptococcus pyogenes*—This GAS agent is most commonly found in children 5 to 11 years of age, with some increased incidence in the winter and early spring. Ten to 20 per cent of school children are asymptomatic carriers.
2. *Adenoviruses*—These viruses are estimated to cause 4 to 10 per cent of pharyngitis in children. They have accounted for 37 to 75 per cent of nonstreptococcal pharyngitis in military recruits in some studies. An increased incidence of illness has been observed in children younger than 5 years old in daycare or institutions for chronic care. Adenoviruses were cited as the most common cause of exudative pharyngitis in preschool children who were hospitalized.
3. *EBV*—In low socioeconomic groups or third world countries, 80 to 100 per cent of children are EBV antibody positive by 3 to 6 years of age. Most infections in upper and middle class communities and developed countries occur in persons 10 to 30 years old.
4. *Enteroviruses*—Children are the most susceptible cohort. In temperate climates, infections peak in late summer and fall.
5. *HSV-1*—There is no seasonal pattern. In lower socioeconomic groups, 40 to 60 per cent of children are antibody positive by age 5 years.
6. *A. haemolyticus*—Ninety per cent of recognized cases occur in persons between 10 and 30 years of age. The

bacterium has been isolated from 2 per cent of asymptomatic individuals in that age group. Its relative frequency is 5 to 13 per cent of that of GAS.

7. *N. gonorrhoeae*—Sexual abuse should strongly be considered if oral infection is proved in a prepubertal child beyond the newborn period.

Clinical Findings

1. GAS infections
    a. Given a febrile child with exudative pharyngitis, the probability of GAS varies with age. The most common cause of exudative pharyngitis in children younger than 3 years of age is adenoviruses. In the school-age group, GAS accounts for 15 to 50 per cent, viruses account for 38 per cent, and the cause cannot be determined in 30 to 35 percent of the episodes.
    b. *S. pyogenes (GAS)*—Symptoms are determined by the M protein of the organism and by the patient's age and immune status. The serotypes of organisms causing pyoderma are different from those causing pharyngitis. Infants younger than 6 months of age often have nasopharyngitis with mucopurulent discharge, irregular fever, and symptoms lasting about 1 week. Those 6 months to 3 years of age most often have a nasopharyngitis with enlarged, tender anterior cervical lymph nodes. Otitis media and sinusitis are frequent complications.
    c. Children 3 to 12 years of age have acute follicular or exudative tonsillitis. Anterior cervical adenopathy is usually present. The red, confluent, sandpapery rash of scarlet fever may be present. The onset is often abrupt, with fever, vomiting, headache, chills, malaise, and abdominal pain. Occasionally, palatal petechiae are present. Fever lasts 4 or 5 days in untreated cases. The presence of cough, rhinorrhea, or hoarseness make GAS an unlikely agent.
2. *Adenoviruses*—These viruses produce a wide range of signs and symptoms. Pharyngitis, croup, bronchitis, and pneumonia can be produced. Adenovirus pharyngitis is an acute illness with fever, sore throat, exudative tonsillitis, and cervical adenopathy. Malaise, headache, myalgias, chills, and cough are often associated, and rhinorrhea and abdominal pain may be present. The illness usually lasts 5 to 7 days.
3. *EBV*—Frequently there is a 3- to 5-day prodrome of malaise and fatigue before fever, sore throat, and adenopathy begin. The adenopathy is diffuse, not just anterior cervical. Splenomegaly is present in 50 per cent of cases. An erythematous, maculopapular rash is present on the arms, legs, and trunk in 5 per cent. Occasionally, frank jaundice, edema of the face and eyelids, or petechiae of the palate are present. Concurrent GAS infection has been reported in some cases. The duration of fever malaise and fatigue is more prolonged (>7 days) than in other common causes of pharyngitis.
4. Enteroviruses—Pharyngitis is common with infection by coxsackieviruses and echoviruses. An abrupt onset is common. Fever runs from 38.3 to 40°C. School-age children complain of headache and myalgia. Younger children have malaise and anorexia. Coryza, vomiting, and/or diarrhea may be present. The pharynx may be red or have a patchy exudate. Aseptic meningitis, pleurodynia, or an exanthem may be concurrent. The illness lasts 3 to 6 days.
5. *Hand-foot-and-mouth disease*—Ulcerative lesions (4 to 8 mm in diameter) of the tongue and anterior mouth are present. Vesicular lesions of the hands and feet are found, along with a papular red rash on the buttocks. The clinical expression of this disease is almost exclusively in young children. About 38 per cent of school children and only 11 per cent of adults have enough signs to recognize this viral infection as a specific entity.
6. *Herpangina*—Ulcerative lesions of the soft palate are associated with fever for 3 days.
7. *HSV-1*—This pharyngitis often evolves into a gingivostomatitis in preschool children. Fever, refusal to eat, and drooling are often present. Vesicular lesions on lips, gingiva, tongue, and palate develop. The gums become swollen and bleed with minor trauma. Fetor oris is present. Anterior cervical lymph nodes enlarge. Vesicular and/or ulcerative lesions may develop around the mouth and eyes. The inflammation peaks at 4 to 5 days and takes a similar period to resolve.
8. *A. haemolyticus*—This coryneform bacterium produces an acute pharyngitis often indistinguishable from that of GAS. In 30 to 67 per cent of cases, an exanthem begins on the extensor surfaces of the distal extremities and spreads centripetally. The rash may begin a few days after the onset of the sore throat. Desquamation after the rash is possible. Infected skin lesions, endocarditis, meningitis, and sepsis following mononucleosis have been reported with this organism. No postinfectious sequelae have been identified.
9. *Group C and G streptococci*—Clinical symptoms are similar to those with GAS. There is not a strong association with nonsuppurative sequelae, but two reports describe poststreptococcal glomerulonephritis associated with outbreaks of group C pharyngitis.
10. *N. gonorrhoeae*
    a. Only 25 per cent of those with positive cultures have symptomatic disease. Treatment of asymptomatic carriers is thought to be important to prevent disseminated disease.
    b. Culture of material from pharyngeal swabs on chocolate agar is appropriate in persons with multiple partners who engage in oral-genital sex and in cases of suspected sexual abuse.
11. *C. diphtheriae*—Infection may involve the nose, tonsils, pharynx, larynx, trachea, skin, or genitals. The onset is gradual. Nasal diphtheria begins with a serosanguineous discharge that becomes mucopurulent. A membrane then forms on the nasal septum. Tonsillar and pharyngeal diphtheria begin with anorexia, malaise, and low-grade fever; a membrane forms in 1 to 2 days. Variable cervical lymphadenopathy and edema of the neck are present. Myocarditis and neuritis may

develop. Respiratory and circulatory arrest may ensue. In mild cases, the membrane sloughs in 7 to 10 days.

Key Clinical Findings

- Pain in throat
- Dysphagia
- Tonsillar exudate
- Ulceration

Laboratory Findings

There is strong pressure on the physician to provide a rapid answer when a child presents with sore throat and fever. Rapid testing of throat swabs for streptococcal antigen is specific but not as sensitive as a standard throat culture. Office use of antigen detection kits is reasonable if followed by throat cultures for those with negative results.

1. *S. pyogenes* (GAS)
   a. Culture on complex media with sheep blood. Incubate aerobically for 48 hours without carbon dioxide supplementation. (A coverglass over the primary inoculation area enhances hemolysis, as do stabs into the media.) Antigen detection on β-hemolytic colonies may be performed to confirm the presence of GAS. Recovery of GAS does not differentiate those with infection from streptococcal carriers who have pharyngitis resulting from a viral infection; likewise, the number of colonies of GAS does not differentiate infection from carriage. Antigen detection on material from throat swabs is less sensitive (50 to 70%) but highly specific.
   b. Serologic proof of recent streptococcal infection is obtained 85 per cent of the time in patients with rheumatic fever by measurement of an antistreptolysin-O (ASO) titer. The titer is often >500 Todd units/ml. A value of less than 240 is considered normal in many laboratories. The antideoxyribonuclease B (anti-DNase B) and anti-A-CHO tests are used as adjuncts to the ASO titer in patients suspected of rheumatic fever or glomerulonephritis.
   c. The Streptozyme test uses erythrocytes coated with streptolysin-O, DNase B, streptokinase, hyaluronidase, and adenine dinucleotide nucleohydrase. It is considered less sensitive and not as well standardized as the ASO titer. Cultures are indicated for siblings and household contacts of children with rheumatic fever, glomerulonephritis, or streptococcal toxic shock syndrome. In these circumstances, antibiotics should be used even in cases of asymptomatic carriage. Posttreatment cultures are indicated only in symptomatic persons and those at high risk for recurrence of rheumatic fever.

2. *Adenoviruses*—Viral culture is appropriate in cases of severe disease and in immunocompromised hosts. These viruses are easily recovered from nasopharyngeal swabs or aspirates. Collection early in the course of disease and prompt transport of cold or frozen specimens enhance viral detection. Antigen panel tests are less specific than culture. Paired blood samples 2 to 4 weeks apart can establish the diagnosis serologically.

3. *EBV*—If a school-age patient has an exudative pharyngitis lasting longer than 5 days with an atypical lymphocytosis, a rapid slide test is sufficient. However, a 3- to 5-year-old with an exudative pharyngitis, diffuse lymphadenopathy, and negative throat culture for GAS needs an EBV antibody profile (measurement of antibodies to viral capsular antigen, immunoglobulins M and G, early antigen, and Epstein-Barr nuclear antigen). Viral isolation requires fetal B lymphocytes and is currently not practical. A positive result on the Paul-Bunnell antibody test is adequate in patients with compatible symptoms. Rapid qualitative test kits are 80 to 85 per cent sensitive. They have a false-positive rate of <10 per cent. The slide tests may have a false-negative rate of 50 to 75 per cent in children younger than 4 years of age.

4. *Enteroviruses*—Isolation of enteroviruses in tissue culture remains the gold standard. However, culture is seldom justified economically in normal patients with uncomplicated pharyngitis.

5. *HSV-1*—Viral culture usually is not justified. A rise in antibody titer is likely if it is a primary infection, but differentiation of HSV-1 from HSV-2 by antibody response is impossible.

6. *A. haemolyticus*—Blood agar is the preferred medium. Its colonies cause β hemolysis. Growth may not be visible for 48 to 72 hours. Additional biochemical tests are necessary to confirm the identity of the isolate. Distinguishing commensal coryneform organisms from disease-associated types is a major problem. Serologic tests for antibody are not available commercially.

7. *N. gonorrhoeae*—Selective media such as Thayer-Martin agar (chocolate agar supplemented with antibiotics) should be used for culture from the pharynx. The organism is extremely sensitive to drying and temperature changes. Direct inoculation on a warm culture plate with immediate incubation is preferred.

8. *C. diphtheriae*
   a. The laboratory should be notified if *C. diphtheriae* is suspected.
   b. Special medium is required. There are many coryneform organisms on a throat swab, and they are often not reported or identified. Colonies of *C. diphtheriae* are not distinctive on blood agar plates.

9. *Group C and G streptococci*—Large β-hemolytic colonies are formed on 5% sheep blood agar. Lancefield antisera are used. If the organism is nongroupable, biochemical tests can be used.

Key Laboratory Findings

- Rapid streptococcus test
- Throat culture
- Monospot test (selective)

Radiographic Changes

X-ray studies may be appropriate when associated sinusitis or abscess is suspected. A submental vertex view shows an ipsilateral fullness with a lateral pharyngeal abscess. An anteroposterior view of the neck demonstrates ipsilateral edema and obliteration of the pyriform sinus with a lateral pharyngeal abscess. A lateral radiograph of the neck can often demonstrate a posterior pharyngeal abscess. Computed tomographic scans, with their ability to define differences in tissue density, have made management of deep neck space infections more precise.

Treatment

1. *GAS*—Penicillin V 250 mg t.i.d. for 10 days or 500 mg b.i.d. for 10 days is the treatment of choice. Erythromycin estolate (20 to 40 mg/kg/day) or erythromycin ethylsuccinate (40 to 50 mg/kg/day) for 10 days is effective treatment; the maximal dose is 1 g/day. Tetracyclines and sulfonamides should not be used. When children have multiple recurrent episodes, 10-day regimen of clindamycin, amoxicillin-clavulanate, dicloxacillin, or penicillin, with rifampin given concurrently during the last 4 days, has been effective in eradicating the organism.
2. *Adenoviruses*—Supportive.
3. *EBV*—Steroids are useful if there is significant respiratory obstruction.
4. *Enteroviruses*—Supportive.
5. *HSV-1*—Acyclovir and vidarabine have been used primarily for potentially serious infections, such as occur in neonates and immunocompromised individuals. Primary gingivostomatitis in children has been treated with acyclovir, but data to prove efficacy are lacking.
6. *A. haemolyticus*—Erythromycin is the drug of choice. Penicillin susceptibility is variable.
7. *N. gonorrhoeae*—Ceftriaxone (125 mg IM) is given in a single dose for children weighing <45 kg.
8. *C. diphtheriae*—Antitoxin should be given on the basis of clinical diagnosis, because patients may deteriorate rapidly. Conjunctival or skin testing should be performed. Erythromycin is given orally or parenterally (40 to 50 mg/kg/day, maximum 2 g/day) or penicillin intramuscularly for 14 days.

Key Treatment: β-Hemolytic Streptococcus

• Penicillin × 7 to 10 days

9. *Group C or G streptococci*—Ampicillin or penicillin G is adequate for mild to moderate infections. Ampicillin and gentamicin may be required for optimal treatment in severe infections.

Prevention

1. *GAS*—Patients with a well-documented history of rheumatic fever or documented evidence of rheumatic heart disease should be placed on continuous prophylaxis, perhaps for life. The following three regimens are effective.
   a. Benzathine penicillin G (1,200,000 U IM) once every 3 or 4 weeks.
   b. Penicillin V, orally, 250 mg bid
   c. Sulfisoxazole, orally, 1 g once a day for patients weighing 27 kg or more, and 0.5 g once a day for patients weighing less than 27 kg.
2. *Adenoviruses*—Live enteric-coated vaccines have been used successfully in military personnel to reduce acute respiratory disease, but these vaccines are not available for civilian use.
3. *EBV*—Individuals with a recent history of EBV infection should not donate blood.
4. *Enteroviruses*—Attention should be paid to handwashing, especially after diaper changes.
5. *HSV-1*—Infected persons should avoid kissing or nuzzling, especially of young infants, until the lesions are healed.
6. *A. haemolyticus*—No control measures are known.
7. *N. gonorrhoeae*—Children and adolescents with sexual exposure to a patient known to have gonorrhea should be examined, cultured, and treated. Case reporting is required.
8. *C. diphtheriae*—Close contacts with a suspected case should be identified, cultured, given prophylaxis with penicillin or erythromycin, and kept under surveillance for 7 days. A booster dose of diphtheria toxoid should be given.

Bibliography

Cherry JD: Pharyngitis. *In* Feigin RD, Cherry JD (eds): Textbook of Pediatric Infectious Diseases, 3rd ed, vol 1. Philadelphia, WB Saunders, 1992, pp 159–166.

Committee on Infectious Diseases, American Academy of Pediatrics: 1994 Red Book. Elk Grove Village, American Academy of Pediatrics, 1994.

Moffet HL: Nose and throat syndromes. *In* Moffet HL: Pediatric Infectious Diseases, 3rd ed. Philadelphia, JB Lippincott, 1989, pp 13–44.

196 Croup

Michelle S. Howenstine

Definition

Croup (laryngotracheobronchitis) is a common viral illness in children that causes varying degrees of upper airway obstruction. The larynx is universally infected; the trachea and bronchi are usually involved to varying degrees.

Etiology

Parainfluenza type 1 is the most common causative agent. Other viral causes include parainfluenza types 2 and 3, influenza virus strains A and B, adenovirus, respiratory syncytial virus, and rhinovirus.

Epidemiology

Croup occurs almost exclusively in children younger than 5 years of age. The highest incidence is seen between 6 months and 2 years, and boys are affected more often than girls. There is wide regional variation in the rates of occurrence, with an average of 5 cases per 1000 children. The disease is more common in the late autumn and winter months.

Pathophysiology

The viral pathogens causing croup initially infect the upper airway; rhinorrhea and nasal congestion begin several days before lower airways symptoms. With progression of the infection to the lower airways, airway obstruction and hypoxemia ensue.

1. In croup, acute airway obstruction is related to anatomic and dynamic changes in the airway that follow attachment of the virus to the ciliated respiratory epithelium. The subglottic area and vocal cords become erythematous, edematous, and covered with exudate. The resulting airway obstruction is often progressive and is related to several physiologic factors:

   a. The size of the airway in a child is relatively small compared with that in the adult, and the infected subglottic cricoid cartilage area is the narrowest segment. Resistance to breathing is significantly increased as a result of the narrowing caused by swelling and exudate in the airway. Air flow is proportional to the fourth power of the radius of a tube.

   b. Dynamic obstruction of the airway occurs as the child forcibly breathes against the narrowed airway. As the infant generates increasingly negative intrathoracic pressure, the extrathoracic airway is dynamically narrowed during inspiration, resulting in additional airway compromise.

   c. The narrowed airway causes more turbulence of airflow, which produces vibration of the upper airway (stridor).

2. Hypoxemia occurs commonly with croup and is the result of ventilation and perfusion mismatch. Multiple factors contribute to this abnormality, including the following:

   a. Secretions in the small and large airways

   b. Bronchospasm resulting from airway inflammation

   c. Pulmonary edema secondary to airway obstruction and changes in intrapleural pressures

   d. Accumulation of interstitial fluid from vascular "leak" after infection.

3. Respiratory fatigue from increased work of breathing, impaired fluid intake, and hypoxemia occur.

Clinical Findings

The signs and symptoms of croup are variable and depend on the child's age, the extent of airway obstruction, the level of hydration, and the degree of fatigue. Symptoms usually worsen at night because of lower relative humidity and can progress over a 3- to 5-day period.

1. Early symptoms of infection include coryza (several days), with a gradual onset of hoarseness and cough which has a barking quality ("croupy" cough).

2. Inspiratory stridor occurs as the larynx becomes involved; uncommonly, wheezing may develop as the infection results in distal airway involvement.

3. Worsening airway obstruction is noted by the following signs:

   a. Stridor present at rest with prolongation of the inspiratory phase

   b. Increased retractions with progressively decreased breath sounds

   c. Restlessness and agitation indicative of air hunger; cyanosis is a late sign.

   d. Lethargy and decreases in levels of consciousness as the patient fatigues or develops respiratory failure.

4. The differential diagnosis includes foreign body aspiration, spasmodic croup, bacterial tracheitis and epiglottitis, and diphtheria.

   a. Spasmodic croup is a syndrome of unknown cause in which a previously well child awakens in the night with sudden stridor, hoarse voice, and a barking cough. Symptoms are usually self-limited and may recur. Mild viral infection and hyperreactivity of the airways are suggested causes. Vomiting or warm steam (e.g., a bathroom with a hot shower running) usually aborts the symptoms.

   b. Bacterial tracheitis is an uncommon disorder that is included in the differential diagnosis of severe croup. The patient develops progressive illness and stridor after a prodromal upper respiratory infection. Severe respiratory obstruction and distress are common. Typically, these children are older and appear more toxic than those with croup.

c. Epiglottitis presents with abrupt onset of fever, toxic appearance, stridor, muffled voice but not hoarseness, and progressive respiratory distress.

d. Laryngeal diphtheria (rare in United States) has a very gradual (several days) progression from hoarseness to complete obstruction.

Key Clinical Findings

- Inspiratory stridor
- Hoarseness
- Retractions

Laboratory Findings

There are no specific laboratory studies required for the diagnosis of acute croup.

1. A complete blood count may show mild to moderate leukocytosis; a very high leukocyte count may be indicative of bacterial infection (e.g., tracheitis, epiglottitis).

2. A viral culture or antigen study may disclose a specific virus. This information, however, does not alter management.

3. An arterial blood gas analysis may be helpful in determining impending respiratory failure; however, clinical evaluation is sufficient to identify patients who require intubation in most cases.

4. Obtaining a blood sample in a distressed infant may cause a great deal of agitation and worsen the airway obstruction and the respiratory distress. It is best to reserve laboratory evaluation for cases in which the diagnosis is unclear.

Radiographic Changes

Radiographs are not essential for the diagnosis of croup and do not correlate with the severity of the airway obstruction.

1. Anteroposterior views of the neck may show the "steeple sign" or narrowing of the upper trachea.

2. Overinflation of the hypopharynx may be present and is related to the increased inspiratory effort.

Treatment

Treatment for croup focuses on decreasing airway obstruction and providing supportive care.

1. Mild cases of croup can be managed in the outpatient setting with caregivers observing for worsening stridor, decreased fluid intake, or evidence of fatigue.

   a. The use of corticosteroids remains controversial in the treatment of croup and may not be necessary in the management of mild cases.

   b. Antibiotics are not indicated in the treatment of croup unless a secondary bacterial infection (e.g., otitis media) is identified.

   c. Warm or cool mist should be delivered by a humidi-fier or as steam from a shower and may help to thin secretions and soothe the inflamed pharynx.

2. Hospital admission is indicated for those children who develop worsening airway obstruction as evidenced by increasing stridor, retractions, cyanosis, agitation, and lethargy. Symptoms may worsen over 3 to 5 days. In-hospital management may include the following therapeutic measures:

   a. Close monitoring of disease progression, oxygenation, hydration, temperature, and effects of treatment is essential.

   b. Humidified oxygen corrects hypoxemia and soothes inflamed mucous membranes. A 30 per cent fraction of inspired oxygen is usually appropriate.

   c. Aerosolized epinephrine or racemic epinephrine (less expensive) causes mucosal vasoconstriction and increases air flow. The drug is effective but of short duration, with effects seen for 30 to 120 minutes.

      (1) Dosage of racemic epinephrine (2.25%) is 0.25 to 1.0 ml of solution aerosolized in 2 to 3 ml of 0.9 per cent NaCl.

      (2) Frequency is dictated by patient condition and ranges from every 1 to every 4 hours, depending on the patient's symptoms and response.

   d. Inhaled dexamethasone may limit severity and is probably beneficial.

   e. Inhalation of a helium-oxygen mixture (60:40 or 70:30) can improve air flow when upper airways are obstructed. This gas mixture is used in a monitored intensive care setting and may decrease the need for intubation.

   f. Children requiring very frequent treatment and those who become distressed between treatments should be considered for transfer to a facility in which intubation and ventilation of young children are routinely performed.

Key Treatment

- Aerosolized (racemic) ephinephrine
- Corticosteroids

Prevention

There are no specific measures to prevent croup. Consistent handwashing and secretion control can decrease transmission of respiratory viruses.

 ## Bibliography

Kilham H, Gellis J, Benjamin B: Severe upper airway obstruction. Pediatr Clin North Am 1987;34:1–14.

Kuusela AL, Vesikare T: A randomized double-blind placebo-controlled trial of dexamethasone and racemic epinephrine in the treatment of croup. Acta Paediatr Scand 1988;77:99–104.

Taussig LM, Castro O, Beaudiy PH, et al: Treatment of Laryngo-tracheobronchitis (croup). Am J Dis Child 1975;129:790–793.

197 Bronchitis

Fred Leickly

Definition

1. *Acute bronchitis* is a transient, febrile, inflammatory process involving the mucosa of the trachea and the major (medium- and large-sized) bronchi that results in excessive mucus production and cough.
2. *Chronic bronchitis* may not exist as a separate entity in children. The American Thoracic Society criteria for chronic bronchitis include a cough productive of sputum occurring for a majority of days during three consecutive months in two successive years. Most if not all children who have chronic inflammation of the airways (trachea, major bronchi) have a well-defined clinical disorder.

Etiology

1. The usual causes of acute bronchitis are viral and include the following: rhinovirus, respiratory syncytial virus (RSV), influenza virus, parainfluenza virus, adenovirus, coxsackievirus, measles (rubeola) virus, and paramyxovirus. Bacterial causes of acute bronchitis are rare except for pertussis, tuberculosis, diphtheria, and mycoplasmal infection. Secondary bacterial infections are a frequent concern. *Streptococcus pneumoniae*, *Haemophilus influenzae*, and *Staphylococcus aureus* are the suspected causative organisms. However, infection with these organisms usually remains unproven.
2. Chronic bronchitis is not a diagnosis by itself but a symptom of other disorders. The conditions that lead to chronic bronchitic inflammation include asthma, cystic fibrosis, immunodeficiencies, chronic aspiration, anatomic compression (blood vessels or lymph nodes), foreign bodies (intrathoracic or extrathoracic and esophageal), chronic infection (mycoplasmal infection, tuberculosis, or pertussis), and reactions to toxic inhalants (cigarette smoke and other air pollutants).

Epidemiology

1. *Acute bronchitis*—The peak occurrence of acute bronchitis is during the winter and early spring, known peak times for respiratory viruses. Acute bronchitis more commonly affects younger than older children, and boys more often than girls. The prevalence of bronchitis varies with age. Approximately 25 to 30 per cent of children younger than 7 years old, 6 to 8 per cent of those 7 to 12 years old, and 4 per cent of those 12 to 17 years old have acute bronchitis during a given year.
2. *Chronic bronchitis*—Given the lack of consensus on the definition of chronic bronchitis and the doubts regarding its existence in children, adequate epidemiologic data do not exist. However, responses to parental questionnaires in national health surveys indicate that there are approximately 2.5 million children with chronic bronchitis.

Pathophysiology

1. *Acute bronchitis*—There is minimal mortality associated with this disorder, and limited material is available for microscopic evaluation. In those few instances in which biopsy material is available, the pathologic findings are consistent with the nonspecific responses of the airway to a viral infection.
   a. Desquamation of the ciliated epithelial lining of the airways may cause decreased mucociliary clearance. Cough receptors are exposed, allowing for increased access, stimulation, and subsequent increased cough.
   b. Mucosal congestion is present.
   c. Increased mucus gland activity occurs.
   d. Cellular infiltration by polymorphonuclear cells within the airway wall and lumen is common and accounts for the mucopurulent character of the sputum.
2. *Chronic bronchitis*—This disorder is as poorly defined pathophysiologically as it is clinically. Pathologic findings in children said to have chronic bronchitis include an inflammatory cell infiltrate with polymorphonuclear cells and eosinophils, hypertrophy and hypersecretion of the airway submucosal glands, and increased mucus production. These findings occur in patients with asthma. In one series of patients labeled as having chronic bronchitis, almost all would have been diagnosed as having asthma based on pathologic findings.

Clinical Findings

1. Acute bronchitis
   a. Presentation
      (1) Clinical presentations are similar regardless of the etiologic agent; however, there are a few common patterns:
         (a) *RSV*—Infants; significant small airway obstruction component (bronchiolitis) with tachypnea and hyperinflation
         (b) *Influenza*—High fever, myalgia headache
         (c) *Measles*—Coryza, fever, rash
         (d) *Pertussis*—Barking, spasmodic cough; inspiratory whoop occurs in classic cases but need not be present.
         (e) *Tuberculosis*—Patient appears chronically ill.
      (2) The acute phase is usually an upper respiratory tract infection, rhinitis or nasopharyngitis, which may last for 3 to 5 days. Cough, the primary and sometimes the only symptom, reflects the involvement of the larynx, trachea, or bronchial tree. Initially, the cough is dry, brassy, harsh, or hacking.
      (3) The second phase occurs from the sixth to the twelfth day of illness. At this time, the lower

respiratory tract becomes more involved. The cough becomes loose, rattling, and productive of a thick, yellow mucopurulent sputum. The appearance of this sputum frequently leads to an erroneous diagnosis of a bacterial superinfection. During this phase, older children may complain of retrosternal chest pain; posttussive emesis is a frequent occurrence.

(4) The recovery phase occurs over the next week. The fever resolves and the cough decreases, but it may last an additional 7 to 14 days.

(5) Complications may occur if the lower respiratory tract symptoms extend beyond 2 weeks or if there is recurrence of fever. Segmental lung collapse is a consideration. Bacterial superinfection with *H. influenzae*, *S. pneumoniae*, or *S. aureus* is often suspected, although there are no studies to suggest that this happens. These organisms are *never* the primary cause of bronchitis in children, and their frequency as a secondary invader is undetermined.

b. The physical examination varies according to the stage of the disease.

(1) Upper respiratory tract symptoms predominate in the acute phase of the illness.

(2) As the condition progresses, there are lower respiratory tract signs and symptoms. Auscultation of the chest reveals coarse crackles, and wheezes.

(3) *Clinical course*—In most cases, the illness lasts for 2 weeks. There may be an extended recovery phase. This phase is notable for continued cough that may persist for another week.

2. Chronic bronchitis

a. Presentation

(1) The clinical evaluation of chronic bronchitis in children presupposes the presence of an excessive inflammatory response to an acute injury to the airway. There may also be continuous exposure to an agent or agents capable of eliciting an inflammatory response.

(2) Chronic bronchitis in children is usually a result of a known clinical condition.

b. The differential diagnosis of chronic bronchitis in children is extensive. Conditions to consider include asthma, cystic fibrosis, immune deficiency, gastroesophageal reflux, chronic infection (tuberculosis, *Mycoplasma* or *Bordetella* infection), chronic sinusitis, anatomic abnormalities (tracheoesophageal fistula, the immotile cilia syndrome), bronchiolitis, bronchopulmonary dysplasia, foreign body aspiration, toxin inhalation, irritant exposure, and psychogenic cough. The medical history, physical examination, and laboratory evaluation should establish one of these causes.

c. Each of these specific causes has its unique clinical course and prognosis.

Key Clinical Findings

- Cough
- Fever

Laboratory Findings

1. *Acute bronchitis*—This is usually a mild, self-limited disease. The diagnosis is clinical. Laboratory studies that may aid in the diagnosis include an evaluation of the sputum. Usually it appears purulent and many polymorphonuclear cells are present. The presence of these cells does *not* necessarily mean that there is a bacterial infection. Other studies for consideration include a complete blood count and differential, a nasal aspirate analysis for RSV, and a chest radiograph.

2. *Chronic bronchitis*—Specific studies suggested by the history and physical examination must be considered. Laboratory tests may include a chest radiograph, quantitative immunoglobulin analyses, pulmonary function tests (both before and after bronchodilator use), nasal smear, allergy tests, sputum evaluation, sweat chloride test, barium swallow, 24-hour pH probe, serology, tuberculin skin test, sinus radiograph inspiratory and expiratory films, bronchoscopy, esophagoscopy, and ciliary biopsy.

Key Laboratory Tests

- Sputum examination and culture

Radiographic Changes

1. *Acute bronchitis*—Chest radiographs vary from being normal to showing peribronchial thickening and hyperinflation. When the course is prolonged or there is recurrence of fever, the radiograph may reveal segmental collapse.

2. *Chronic bronchitis*—Here also the radiographic evaluation of the chest may be normal or may show peribronchial thickening. Atelectasis and hyperinflation are common. Special radiographic studies may reveal reflux, a fistula, or a foreign body.

Treatment

1. *Acute bronchitis*—This is generally a mild disorder that responds to supportive measures.

a. Supportive measures include rest, hydration, humidification of inspired air, avoidance of respiratory irritants (e.g., cigarette smoke), antipyretics, and bronchodilators for those with wheezing.

b. Contraindicated measures include the use of cough medicines. There are no data to support the efficacy of the mucolytic agents, and cough suppressants are contraindicated in children with productive cough. Antibiotics for acute bronchitis have no role unless the diagnosis is mycoplasmal infection, pertussis, or tuberculosis.

c. Antibiotics are considered if the time course is prolonged beyond 2 weeks or if there is recurrence of significant fever. Secondary bacterial infections with

Staphylococcus, Haemophilus, or *Streptococcus* are frequently suspected in older children and adolescents. Mycoplasma needs to be considered; it is treated with erythromycin. The other organisms mentioned respond to ampicillin, amoxicillin, penicillin, macrolides, trimethoprim-sulfamethoxazole, and cephalosporins.

2. *Chronic bronchitis*—Therapeutic choices depend on the specific cause of the chronic airway inflammation (usually asthma). Asthma and the other causes of chronic airway inflammation, such as cystic fibrosis, immune deficiency, and the chronic aspiration syndromes, all respond to disease-directed therapy. A few common treatment choices are avoidance of triggers, use of bronchodilators, inhaled antiinflammatory agents, and antibiotics for documented infection.

Key Treatment

- Supportive
- Antibiotics if 2-week persistence

Prevention

1. Prevention of acute bronchitis may be impossible. The disorder is frequent, usually mild, and self-limited. The agents of infection are usually viral, and the vectors are people.
2. Prevention in chronic bronchitis is disease specific. Because most cases of chronic bronchitis are caused by asthma, avoidance of known triggering events or factors helps prevent an exacerbation. Also, the use of antiinflammatory agents may prevent episodes of asthma.

Bibliography

Cohen GJ: Management of infections of the lower respiratory tract in children. Pediatr Infect Dis J 1987;6:317–323.

Daigle KL, Cloutier MM: Bronchitis. *In* Loughlin G, Eigen H (eds): Respiratory Disease in Children: Diagnosis and Management. Baltimore, Williams & Wilkins, 1994.

Klein RB, Huggins BW: Chronic bronchitis in children. Semin Resp Infect 1994;9:13–22.

Morgan WJ, Taussig LM: The chronic bronchitis complex in children. Pediatr Clin North Am 1984;31:851–864.

Phelan PD, Landau LI, Olinsky A: Respiratory Illness in Children. Oxford, Blackwell Scientific, 1990, chapter 4.

198 Bronchiolitis

Howard Eigen

Definition

Bronchiolitis is an acute viral infection of the respiratory tract that affects the small airways of the young infant. It accounts for significant morbidity and mortality, especially in those with underlying cardiac or pulmonary disease.

Etiology

1. The etiologic agent is respiratory syncytial virus (RSV), an RNA virus whose growth appears to be primarily in the respiratory tract epithelium. Other viruses, such as influenza virus, adenovirus, and parainfluenza virus, can produce similar clinical states.
2. Almost all children have been infected by RSV by the age of 3 years. The peak rate of hospitalization occurs at before 6 months of age.
3. Transmission occurs primarily by direct contact with infected secretions.
4. Viral shedding typically lasts 6 to 10 days. Attack rates among family members are 45 per cent, and transmission in daycare centers approaches 100 per cent among infants previously uninfected.

Pathogenesis

1. Bronchiolitis is an infection of the small bronchioles. The infection leads to sloughing of respiratory epithelium into the airway lumen and swelling of the lumen walls. In addition, the infectious irritation and inflammation may cause a bronchospastic component that results in wheezing.
2. Partial occlusion of the airways leads to decreased airflow and air trapping; some airways become completely occluded, resulting in small areas of atelectasis.
3. Severe disease tends to occur in children with preexisting pulmonary disease (e.g., bronchopulmonary dysplasia) or congenital heart disease, especially those with pulmonary hypertension.
4. Bronchiolitis is associated with increased immunoglobulin E in nasal and lower airway secretions. It appears that clinical bronchiolitis results not from a viral respiratory infection alone but from an immune response to the infection.

Clinical Findings

1. Clinical illness starts in phase 1 with rhinorrhea, cough, and fever and is indistinguishable from any other viral upper respiratory infection. Bronchiolitis then progresses to phase 2, in which tachypnea retractions and wheezing become apparent. Each phase takes 3 to 4 days for development.
2. *Additional signs and symptoms*—The presence and severity of fever is quite variable. Otitis media, conjunctivitis, and pharyngitis may also be present.
3. The second phase may intensify over 3 to 4 days. Hypoxemia is often present and commonly is more severe

than would be predicted by the overall state of the child. Respiratory rate is commonly >60 breaths per minute.

4. Dehydration may be part of the clinical picture because infants are unable to feed owing to respiratory distress and at the same time have increased water losses.

5. All infants who present to the medical office or emergency department with suspected bronchiolitis should be given supplemental oxygen and continuous pulse oximetry to ensure an oxygen saturation of 92 per cent or greater.

WARNING

All infants who present to the office or emergency room with suspected bronchiolitis should be given supplemental oxygen and continuous pulse oximetry to ensure an oxygen saturation of 92 per cent or greater.

 Key Clinical Findings

- Fever
- Cough
- Expiratory musical wheezing
- Retractions

Laboratory Findings

1. The first assessment should be oxygenation, measured by pulse oximetry. An oxygen saturation of <95 per cent has been identified as an indicator of severe disease and the need for hospitalization. In such children, an arterial blood gas measurement is strongly recommended so that acid-base balance and alveolar ventilation can be assessed.

2. Diagnosis of the etiologic agent (RSV) is done by performing either a nasal wash or a nasal swab. The sample of mucus and cells is sent to the laboratory for identification of RSV antigen by fluorescent staining or enzyme-linked immunosorbent assay (ELISA). Nasopharyngeal swabs are not as effective as nasal swabs for obtaining adequate cell specimens.

Radiographic Findings

A chest radiograph may be helpful but is not essential in the diagnosis and evaluation of bronchiolitis. Often there is multilobar infiltration or atelectasis.

Treatment

1. Treatment is essentially supportive, although some children may benefit from antiviral therapy.

2. Oxygen therapy is of primary importance. Infants who require hospitalization should be maintained in an oxygen saturation of at least 95 per cent. A humidified source of oxygen, not a form of mist, should be used in these children, because water particles may exacerbate the bronchospastic component of bronchiolitis.

3. Fluid support is essential in these children because they usually have a degree of dehydration. Feeding is often difficult if the respiratory rate remains above 60 breaths

per minute. Use of a nasogastric tube should avoided, because it increases the work of breathing in infants. If appropriate, an orogastric feeding tube may be placed to provide small feedings. In hospitalized children, an intravenous source of fluid and nutrition is best.

4. Hospitalized infants should be monitored with pulse oximetry to ensure appropriate oxygenation. In addition, those with more severe distress should have arterial blood gases monitored. In infants with a partial pressure of carbon dioxide from 40 to 50, transfer to a pediatric intensive care unit should be considered strongly. Infants who have a history of premature birth or who are younger than 6 weeks of age may be at risk for apnea, and a cardiac apnea monitor should be used.

5. The use of bronchodilators in bronchiolitis is problematic. One approach is to undertake a trial of bronchodilators (albuterol) and to continue them if a clinical response occurs. If no clinical response to bronchodilators is apparent, the mediation can be stopped and the condition treated supportively in other ways. Because of the edema and obstruction of the airway with debris, it is not surprising that bronchodilators are not effective in this disorder. Persistent use of bronchodilators despite a lack of clinical efficacy has been associated with more severe hypoxemia.

6. Although this is a disorder involving acute inflammation of the airways, corticosteroids have not been proven to be effective in improving the clinical outcome. It may be appropriate to use steroids in those infants who have severe wheezing or who require mechanical ventilation, although in neither case has this therapy been proved efficacious.

7. Antiviral therapy has been shown to be beneficial in certain subpopulations. Ribavarin reduces viral shedding and shortens the clinical course of the disease. It is probably most useful in children with underlying respiratory or cardiac disease. Although ribavirin does not reduce mortality in these populations, it does reduce morbidity. The 1996 recommendation of the American Academy of Pediatrics suggests that ribavirin be considered in those children with underlying cardiac or pulmonary disease, in premature infants, in infants younger than 6 weeks of age, and those who are immunosuppressed because of disease or therapy.

8. Respiratory failure and mechanical ventilation are very difficult to manage, and mechanical ventilation of infants with bronchiolitis should be performed only in centers with experienced pediatric intensive care unit staff.

 Key Treatment

- Oxygen
- Hydration

Prognosis

The long-term outcome for children with bronchiolitis is for recovery to full function. However, at least 50 per cent of these children experience wheezing during the first year. It is likely that infection with RSV uncovers a group of children with preexisting asthma who then go on to have full-blown asthma later in life.

199 Pneumonia

Robert P. Nelson, Jr., and *Michelle S. Howenstine*

Definition

Pneumonia is inflammation of the alveoli or interstitial spaces of the lung.

Etiology and Epidemiology

Pneumonia accounts for 10 to 15 per cent of pediatric respiratory illnesses.

1. The incidence varies by age (1% in older children to 4% in infants) and according to season (Table 199–1).
   a. *Neonate*—Infection usually is transmitted during gestation or labor but may also occur after exposure to caretakers in the hospital or home. Pneumonia during the first few days of life through approximately 6 weeks of age is caused by bacteria, viruses, or occasionally fungi. Viral infections are more common in winter.
   b. *Infant and preschool*—From 1 month to 5 years of age, viral pneumonias are more common than bacterial processes; there is a higher prevalence in fall and winter.
   c. *School-age and adolescence*—Most pneumonias are community acquired and occur year round, with occasional epidemics in the fall and winter. *Mycoplasma pneumoniae* is the predominant pathogen during outbreaks among groups such as classmates and military personnel.
2. Risk factors include poor socioeconomic status, large family size, passive smoke exposure, history of prematurity, previous hospitalization. Medical conditions contributing to an increased risk of pneumonia in children are listed in Table 199–2.

Pathophysiology

Pulmonary defenses include conditioning and filtering of inspired air in the upper airway, epiglottic prevention of aspiration, the cough reflex, mucociliary clearance, alveolar phagocytosis, and the immune system. Organisms breach these barriers and reach the lower respiratory tree following aspiration or inhalation of infectious material or occasionally by hematogenous dissemination.

1. Viral pneumonias are usually diffuse, involving airways initially and then alveoli.
   a. Viral organisms infect respiratory epithelial cells, causing ciliary dysfunction and sloughing of cells into the airways.
   b. A mononuclear cell inflammatory reaction develops in the submucosa and is accompanied by smooth muscle contraction and reduction of airway caliber.
   c. Viral spread into the alveoli, with the associated inflammatory response, leads to consolidation and subsequent ventilation-perfusion abnormalities resulting in hypoxemia.
   d. Airway hyperactivity is common and may persist long after resolution of the infection.
2. Bacterial organisms are aspirated, inhaled, or occasionally hematogenously acquired. Viral infection may also predispose to bacterial infection, in which case the disease is usually segmental or lobar in distribution; occasionally, it is diffuse.
   a. Bacterial invasion and immunologic response results in edema; proteinaceous fluid floods the alveoli.
   b. Red blood cell and polymorphonuclear cell infiltration follow (consolidation).
   c. Hypoxemia occurs secondary to ventilation-perfusion mismatch and shunting.

Clinical Findings

The clinical manifestations vary according to patient age, immune status, and specific pathogen.

1. Viral pneumonia
   a. There is a prodrome of low-grade fever and cough.
   b. Lower respiratory symptoms develop insidiously and include cough, tachypnea, and increased work of breathing (retractions, grunting).
   c. Wheezing often is present.
   d. Infants are particularly symptomatic and may expe-

TABLE 199–1.   CAUSES OF PNEUMONIA BY AGE

AGE GROUP	BACTERIAL	VIRAL	FUNGAL
Neonate	Group B *Streptococcus* *Escherichia coli* *Klebsiella pneumoniae*	Cytomegalovirus Respiratory viruses	*Pneumocystis carinii*
Infants and Preschool	*Haemophilus influenzae* *Streptococcus pneumoniae* *Staphylococcus aureus* *Moraxella catarrhalis*	Respiratory syncytial virus Adenovirus Parainfluenza 1, 2, 3 Influenza A and B Rhinovirus	
School-Age and Adolescence	*Mycoplasma pneumoniae* *Streptococcus pneumoniae*	Influenza A and B Adenovirus	

TABLE 199–2. CONDITIONS THAT INCREASE THE RISK OF PNEUMONIA IN CHILDREN

Congenital pulmonary abnormalities
Immunodeficiency diseases
Neurologic conditions
Sickle cell anemia
Congestive heart failure
Cystic fibrosis
Foreign body aspiration

rience poor fluid intake, dehydration, and respiratory fatigue.

e. Bacterial infections may complicate viral pneumonia, sinusitis, or otitis.

f. Late complications include persistent wheezing, bronchiectasis, and bronchiolitis obliterans.

2. Bacterial pneumonia (Table 199–3)

a. There is an abrupt onset, with high fever, toxic appearance, and increased respiratory rate.

b. Productive cough and chest pain may occur.

c. Nonspecific signs of headache, restlessness, gastrointestinal symptoms (nausea, vomiting, abdominal pain) are common.

d. Crackles may be heard. Decreased breath sounds and dullness to percussion may be localized to areas of consolidation or suggest pleural effusion.

e. May be complicated by dehydration and sepsis.

 Key Clinical Findings

• Fever
• Cough
• Tachypnea

Laboratory Findings

1. Nonspecific

a. *Complete blood count*—Leukocytosis with neutrophilia (bacterial) or lymphocytosis (viral). Eosinophilia is seen with *Chlamydia* or parasitic pneumonia. *B. pertussis* infection may result in very high leukocyte count with lymphocytosis.

b. Erythrocyte sedimentation rate may be elevated but is not specific.

c. Elevated cold agglutinins suggest *Mycoplasma* infection.

2. Specific—noninvasive

a. Blood cultures are highly specific, but there is only a 10 per cent positivity rate in bacterial pneumonias. Cultures should be obtained from all children suspected of having bacterial pneumonia.

b. Sputum culture and Gram stain require an adequate sample (<10 squamous cells, >25 neutrophils per high-power field). Presence of organisms on Gram stain suggests diagnosis.

c. *Bacterial antigen detection*—Concentrated urine studies are superior to serum analyses. Sensitivity is 20 to 45 per cent. Previous antibiotic therapy does not affect sensitivity. Tests are routinely available for group B *Streptococcus, Neisseria meningitidis, Streptococcus pneumoniae,* and *Haemophilus influenzae.*

d. Viral mycoplasma and chlamydia antigen tests are available and have varying sensitivities and specificities, depending on the specimen and the particular assay.

e. Nasopharyngeal viral cultures are useful, especially in infants.

3. Specific—invasive

a. Pleural fluids when present may be obtained for

TABLE 199–3. BACTERIAL PNEUMONIA

PATHOGEN	TYPICAL AGE	RISKS	SPECIAL CLINICAL CONCERNS
Staphylococcus aureus	Birth–3 mo	Immune deficiency; previous use of antibiotics; prior viral infection	Abrupt onset; rapid deterioration
Group B *Streptococcus*	Birth–3 mo	Maternal vaginal colonization; prolonged rupture of membranes; amnionitis; prematurity	Abrupt onset; rapid deterioration; predominantly neonatal
Chlamydia	3–12 wk	Maternal colonization	Usually mild; insidious onset; staccato cough; eosinophilia
Streptococcus pneumoniae	<2 yr most common; all age groups affected	African-American males; sickle cell diseases; asplenia	Abrupt onset blood-tinged sputum; pleural disease common
Haemophilus influenzae	<5 yr	Sickle cell anemia; humoral immunodeficiency; chemotherapy	Frequent extrapulmonary manifestations
Mycoplasma pneumoniae	School-age; all age groups affected	Groups (e.g., students, military recruits); sickle cell anemia	Systemic disease and neurologic complications
Bordetella pertussis	Infants (more severe)	Incomplete immunizations	Risk of hypoxia and airway obstruction
Mycobacterium tuberculosis*	All age groups	Exposure; immunodeficiency	Extrapulmonary disease more common in children

*For immunocompromised patients, see Chapter 110.

TABLE 199–4. ANTIMICROBIAL THERAPY FOR PNEUMONIA

POPULATION*	PATHOGEN	ANTIMICROBIAL
Infants (newborn–8 wk)	Group B *Streptococcus*	Broad-spectrum antibiotic (e.g., ampicillin, Claforan)
	Escherichia coli	
	Staphylococcus aureus	Nafcillin
	Respiratory syncytial virus	Ribivirin for severe cases
3 mo and older	*Haemophilus influenzae*	Cephalosporin or amoxicillin/clavulinate or erythromycin
Mild	*Streptococcus pneumoniae*	
	Mycoplasma pneumoniae	Clarithromycin
Moderate to severe	As for mild cases and/or	Cefuroxime or other second-generation cephalosporin,
	S. aureus	nafcillin, and gentamicin; consider vancomycin
	Klebsiella pneumoniae	
Aspiration risk	Anaerobes	Add clindamycin

*For immunocompromised patients, see Chapter 110.

diagnosis and/or therapy. High leukocyte count and elevated protein indicate infection. A Gram stain should be done. Cultures identify bacterial, fungal, viral, or tuberculous causes.

   b. Bronchoscopy and lung biopsy, although rarely necessary, are highly specific and sensitive.

Key Laboratory Findings

- Leukocytosis
- Blood culture
- Specific antigen tests

Radiographic Changes

1. Radiographic abnormalities or patterns may be suggestive of a specific pathogen or severity of illness but are often not diagnostic or predictive of disease severity.
2. Chest radiograph patterns
   a. *Interstitial*—Often nonspecific; both infectious and noninfectious causes possible; predominant pattern seen with viral pneumonia.
   b. *Perihilar*—Nonspecific; seen with viral infection and asthma.
   c. *Alveolar, localized or lobar*—Suggests bacterial pneumonia.
   d. *Pleural effusion, abscesses and pneumatocele*—Most often associated with bacterial pneumonias. Abscesses can be caused by anaerobic infections, and pneumatoceles are often seen with *Staphylococcus aureus* infections.
3. Computerized axial tomography
   Computed tomography scans of the chest are very sensitive but are not usually indicated for imaging of uncomplicated pneumonias. They may be helpful in the evaluation of pleural disorders, adenopathy, abscess cavities, or nodular infiltrates.

Treatment

Treatment plans for the patient with suspected viral or bacterial pneumonia vary depending on the patient's age, the severity of respiratory insufficiency, the suspected pathogen, and the capabilities of the caretaker.

1. Hospitalized patients usually have moderate to severe respiratory distress, apnea, oxygen requirements, systemic complications, poor intake or inability to tolerate oral medications, dehydration, or suspected organisms that require intravenous therapy.
   a. Supportive care includes the following:
      (1) Monitoring of cardiac and oxygen status
      (2) Supplemental humidified oxygen
      (3) Adequate hydration including intravenous fluids
      (4) Chest physiotherapy and bronchodilator therapy when indicated
      (5) Mechanical ventilation for respiratory failure
   b. Specific care includes antimicrobial therapy dictated by patient's age and underlying condition, the clinical circumstances and the specific pathogen (Table 199–4).
2. Follow-up evaluation for pneumonia includes reassessment at 2 to 3 weeks, or sooner if symptoms of fever or respiratory distress persists. Evaluation for extrapulmonary complications should be completed if recovery is delayed or systemic symptoms occur. A chest radiograph to document clearing of the infiltrate should be performed at 6 to 8 weeks.

Key Treatment

- Oxygen
- Appropriate antimicrobial therapy

Prevention

Consistent handwashing and secretion control are essential in the prevention of viral and bacterial pneumonias. The frequency of recurrent or persistent pneumonias may be reduced by alleviating specific risk factors such as aspiration. Prophylactic treatments include the following:

1. Viral
   a. Influenza vaccine can prevent influenza A infection.
   b. Amantadine or rimantadine hydrochloride can prevent progression of influenza A symptoms if initiated within 48 hours of infection.
   c. Respiratory syncytial virus (RSV) infections in

high-risk patients may be reduced by repeated pro-phylactic treatments with high-titered RSV-specific immune globulin.

d. Adenovirus vaccine is given to military recruits for protection against adenovirus types 4 and 7.

2. Bacterial

a. The pneumococcal vaccine is given to high-risk groups (e.g., sickle cell anemia patients) for preven-tion of specific serotype infections.

b. Serial immunizations for *B. pertussis* infection con-tribute to protection in childhood.

 Bibliography

Arguedas AG, Stutman HR, Marks MI: Bacterial pneumonias. *In* Kendig EL, Chernick V (eds): Disorders of the Respiratory Tract in Children, 5th ed. Philadelphia, WB Saunders, 1990, pp 371–380.

Campbell III PW, Stokes DC: Pneumonia. *In* Loughlin GM, Eigen H (eds): Respiratory Disease in Children: Diagnosis and Man-agement. Baltimore, Williams & Wilkins, 1994, pp 351–372.

Sabato AR, Martin AJ, Marmion BP, et al: *Mycoplasma pneumon-iae*: Acute illness, antibiotics, and subsequent pulmonary func-tion. Arch Dis Child 1984;59:1034–1037.

Stagno S, Brasfeld DM, Brown MB, et al: Infant pneumonitis associated with cytomegalovirus, *Chlamydia, Pneumocystis* and *Ureaplasma*: A prospective study: Pediatrics 1981;68:322–329.

200 Pleural Effusions

Harvey P. Bieler

Definition

1. Pleural effusion is an accumulation of excess fluid in the pleural space.

2. Under normal conditions, the pleural cavity is almost liquid free (containing only about 1 ml of liquid in the healthy individual) as a result of an equilibrium be-tween pleural fluid formation (filtration) and removal (absorption).

3. Excess liquid accumulates in the pleural cavity (effu-sion) when filtration exceeds removal as a result of ei-ther

a. Increased filtration associated with normal or im-paired absorption, or

b. Normal filtration associated with inadequate re-moval.

Classification

1. *Transudate* occurs when the mechanical forces of hy-drostatic and oncotic pressure are altered such that liquid filtration is favored over absorption. Pleural sur-faces are not directly involved by the underlying dis-ease process. Pleural fluid protein concentration is <3 g/100 ml.

2. *Exudate* results either from increased capillary perme-ability or from processes that impede lymphatic drain-age.

a. Pleural fluid protein concentration is >3 g/100 ml (or ratio of pleural fluid to serum protein is >0.5).

b. Pleural fluid lactic dehydrogenase (LDH) is >200 IU (or ratio of pleural fluid to serum LDH is >0.6).

3. *Chylothorax* refers to an accumulation of chyle in the pleural space that results from either obstruction of the thoracic duct or the left subclavian vein, congenital lymph fistula of undetermined cause, or traumatic rup-ture of lymphatic channels (e.g., after surgery). Chylo-thorax is the most common type of pleural effusion seen in the neonatal period.

a. The pleural fluid is sterile.

b. The predominant cells are lymphocytes.

c. Total fat content exceeds that of plasma (e.g., up to 660 mg/100 ml). Sudan stain is positive for fat globules.

d. Protein content usually ≥3 g/dl.

4. *Chyliform* occurs when the pleural fluid only looks like chyle (milky white and opalescent) but does not show fat globules (i.e., pseudochyle). The milky appearance represents the fatty degeneration of pus and endothe-lial cells.

5. *Hemothorax* occurs when blood is in the pleural cavity.

Pathogenesis

1. The extent of clinical compromise is determined by the severity and rapidity of pleural effusion develop-ment, the nature of the underlying disease process, and the status of cardiopulmonary function.

2. Various clinical disorders can create changes in vascu-lar filtration or absorption in the pleural capillaries and lymphatic flow through several mechanisms:

a. Damage to the basement membrane or endothelium.

b. Changes in local blood flow and capillary hydro-static pressure.

c. Increases in pleural fluid oncotic pressure as a result of protein loss from capillaries and accumulation of protein in the pleural cavity. Oncotic pressure determines how effectively fluid is reabsorbed.

d. Lymphatic drainage can be decreased as a result of mediastinal lymphadenopathy (e.g., lymphoma, fibrosis), thickening of parietal pleura (e.g., tubercu-losis), systemic venous hypertension, obstruction of the thoracic duct (e.g., chylothorax), or developmental hypoplasia of lymphatic channels (e.g., hereditary lymphedema).

Clinical Findings

1. Until pleural fluid accumulation is sufficient to cause cardiorespiratory symptoms (dyspnea and orthopnea are common), patients with pleural effusions may be asymptomatic.
2. Systemic symptoms are determined primarily by the underlying disease.
3. Though rare, malnutrition secondary to loss of chyle and shock from blood loss are additional clinical signs.
4. Chest findings on physical examination
   a. A pleural rub may be the only finding during the early phase.
   b. In older children with moderate effusion, decreased thoracic wall excursion, dullness to percussion, decreased breath sounds over the effusion site, and fullness of the intercostal spaces may be found. In infants and younger children, breath sounds often appear normal because of the small chest volume and easy transmission of breath sounds.
   c. The trachea and cardiac apex can be displaced away from the effusion.

Key Clinical Findings

- Dyspnea
- Pleural rub
- Percussion dullness
- Decreased breath sounds

Laboratory Findings

Evacuation of fluid by thoracentesis confirms the clinical and radiologic diagnosis of effusion.

1. The fluid specimen may be the only evidence on which to make or exclude the diagnosis of specific disease states.
2. The gross appearance of the fluid may be a clue to the cause of the effusion.
   a. Pale yellow fluid suggests a transudate.
   b. Chylous liquid is indicative of injury to the lymphatic channels. The characteristic milky appearance in congenital chylothorax is seen only after initiation of oral feedings with fat-containing formula.
   c. Bloody fluid indicates vascular erosion or damage to intercostal or chest wall vessels.
   d. A purulent specimen indicates bacterial infection of the pleura.
3. Pleural fluid should be sent to the laboratory for cytologic studies for malignant cells; biochemical determinations (pH, fat content, protein and LDH concentrations with their serum determinations); and immunologic and microbiologic studies (cultures and Gram staining). Generally, total counts of red blood cells and leukocytes are of little value.

Key Laboratory Tests

- Examine and culture pleural fluid

Radiographic Findings

1. With moderate effusions, the chest radiograph shows uniform water density and widened interspaces on the affected side, with displacement of the mediastinum toward the contralateral hemithorax.
2. A minimum of about 400 ml of liquid is required for visualization in upright radiographic views of the chest.
3. As little as 50 ml of fluid can be detected with proper exposure of lateral decubitus films taken with the patient lying on the affected side. A layering of liquid density in the dependent portion of the thoracic cavity is seen.

Treatment

Treatment is directed at specific management of the underlying cause and supportive relief of functional complaints caused by the instigating disease process, pleural involvement, and ongoing complications.

1. Supportive measures include bed rest for the acutely ill child, oral analgesics for pain, fluid management to replace increased losses from fever and tachypnea, and supplemental oxygen for hypoxemia or increased work of breathing.
2. Pleural effusions caused by infection require specific antimicrobial treatment. Chest tube drainage allows reexpansion of lung on the affected side. Antimicrobial therapy should be initiated if organisms are seen on Gram staining or the fluid is grossly purulent. Infection may be polymicrobial, so more than one antimicrobial drug may have to be given initially.
3. In thick loculated empyemas, prolonged thoracotomy drainage or (rarely) introduction of streptokinase into the pleural space may be needed to lyse adhesions. Open flap drainage, pleural decortication, and thoracoplasty now rarely need to be done.
4. Treatment of transudative, hemorrhagic, and chylous pleural effusions depends on the underlying disorder.
   a. Evacuation of a transudate after the initial diagnostic thoracentesis is indicated only for relief of dyspnea and other cardiorespiratory complaints caused by mediastinal displacement. Intercostal chest tube placement may be necessary if repeated thoracentesis procedures are required for recurrent symptoms.
   b. Diuretics may slow reaccumulation of transudate in some patients, but this treatment is rarely used in children.
   c. Hemothorax associated with shock requires immediate vascular volume expansion and direct surgical repair of bleeding vessels. Fibrinolytic enzymes instilled into the pleural cavity may help to remove blood clots.
   d. Chylothorax poses unique problems in management. Prompt and multiple thoracentesis procedures or chest tube placement may be necessary for life

threatening cardiorespiratory deterioration. Otherwise, initial therapy usually includes the following:

(1) Complete drainage of chyle by single thoracentesis

(2) Use of medium-chain triglycerides as the major source of dietary fat (in conjunction with avoidance of fatty meals containing long-chain fatty acids) significantly reduces lymph flow, because they are directly absorbed into the portal venous blood and contribute little to chylomicron formation.

(3) Replacement of nutrient losses

(4) Some cases of traumatic chylothorax require direct and immediate surgical intervention. Occasionally, in patients with rapidly reaccumulating chylothorax, a trial of fasting and parenteral hyperalimentation is indicated.

Key Treatment

- Specific antimicrobial
- Analgesia
- Open drainage (uncommon)

201 Pectus Excavatum

Frederick J. Rescorla

Definition

Pectus excavatum refers to an abnormality of the chest wall with posterior angulation of the sternum and lower costal cartilages toward the spine.

Etiology

The cause is unknown. Genetic factors probably exist, because one third of patients have a family history of chest wall deformity.

Epidemiology

1. Incidence in males is three times higher than in females.
2. The disorder is common in patients with Marfan syndrome and should be evaluated particularly in males with scoliosis. Perform eye examination for subluxation of lens and echocardiogram for dilatation of aortic root and aortic or mitral valve regurgitation.

Pathophysiology

1. Cardiopulmonary function before and after operation has been the subject of numerous clinical reports. The actual degree of impairment is difficult to determine and is probably related to the severity of the pectus excavatum, which is not specified in all reports. In addition, although several methods exist to measure and rate the severity of the defect, they are not universally used.
2. Cardiac function
   a. The response to upright exercise is below normal in some patients and improves with surgical repair in some.
   b. Several studies have identified an increase in cardiac stroke volume with surgical repair, and this may be the reason exercise tolerance improves after surgery.
3. Pulmonary function

   a. Mild decreases in total lung capacity and inspiratory vital capacity have been identified and correlated with the severity of the chest wall defect (measured as the degree of sternal depression).
   b. The effect of repair of pectus excavatum on pulmonary function has been controversial. Several studies failed to demonstrate significant improvement in pulmonary function tests with surgical correction of the pectus excavatum.
      (1) One study demonstrated a 10 per cent decrease in vital capacity at 2 months, with return to normal by 6 months and maintenance of baseline level at 42 months.
      (2) An increase in the restrictive defect has been identified with surgery, despite improvement in the anteroposterior diameter of the chest and improvement in symptoms.
      (3) The efficiency of breathing during maximal exercise has improved in some patients.

Clinical Findings

1. The chest wall defect consists of posterior angulation of the sternum and lower costal cartilages toward the spine.
2. The defect is noted by 1 year of age in 86 per cent of patients.
3. Symptoms often consist of chest wall discomfort and limited exercise tolerance for strenuous activities. Some school-age children and adolescents do not interact with peers (particularly in sports activities) due to appearance of defect.
4. Usually asymptomatic in infancy and childhood, with symptoms appearing in late childhood and in school-age children. Some patients remain asymptomatic.
5. Scoliosis is noted in 15 per cent of patients.

Key Clinical Findings

- Chest wall defect
- Scoliosis (15%)

Laboratory Findings

1. *Pulmonary function tests*—Perform with maximal exercise if possible.
2. *Echocardiography*—If heart murmur or physical features are consistent with Marfan syndrome.

Key Laboratory Tests

- Pulmonary function tests

Radiographic Findings

1. Chest radiographs demonstrate displacement of heart to the left on posteroanterior view, posterior angulation of sternum toward spine on lateral view.
2. Computed tomography (CT) scanning is used by some to rate severity of pectus. One scan is taken at the area of greatest sternal depression. The CT index is equal to the anterior vertebral body–sternal distance at the most depressed portion divided by the internal transverse distance of the thorax. The index is >3.25 in patients requiring surgery. Percent vital capacity is related to CT index and can provide some objective assessment of the relation between the restrictive disorder and severity of deformity.

Treatment

1. Indication for and timing of surgery
   a. Symptomatic pectus excavatum
   b. Severe defect with psychologic factors (i.e. child not interacting with peers due to appearance)
   c. Progression of defect documented by radiography (decreasing sternal–vertebral distance)
   d. Demonstrable defect in pulmonary function with exercise
   e. Most surgeons defer surgery until the patient is at least 4 years of age, and some prefer to wait until 8 to 12 years of age.
2. *Several* methods exist for repair; all involve the following:
   a. Elevation of muscle flaps
   b. Removal of the deformed cartilage with preservation of the perichondrial sheaths
   c. Sternal osteotomy and elevation with or without internal bar fixation. The bar is left in place for 6 months. Some use a "tripod fixation" technique involving the second and third costal cartilages to maintain sternal elevation.

d. In Marfan syndrome, the recurrence rate is high if an internal support bar is not used.

3. Complications
   a. Operative and early postoperative
      (1) *Pneumothorax*—Can treat with observation if small or with aspiration if large
      (2) *Pulmonary injury*—Extremely rare
      (3) *Bleeding*—Rarely significant, transfusions rarely if ever required
      (4) *Infection*—Rare
      (5) *Hematoma*—Rare; most surgeons place a drain to prevent this complication.
   b. Late postoperative
      (1) *Recurrence*—Major recurrence, 3 to 5 per cent
      (2) *Mild flattening of chest*—5 to 10 per cent
4. Results with surgery
   a. *Cardiorespiratory symptoms*—Almost all studies identify improvement in symptoms with surgery.
   b. *Psychologic and cosmetic issues*—Almost all patients report improvement with surgical correction and restoration of a normal anteroposterior diameter.
   c. Postoperative cardiopulmonary tests have not demonstrated consistent, reproducible improvement with surgical correction. Most studies demonstrate increase in stroke volume with surgical repair.
   d. Recent studies showed that repair of pectus excavatum increases exercise tolerance in teenage athletes, possibly through improved stroke volume.

Key Treatment

- Surgery—selection for symptomatic or (rarely) cosmetic reasons

Bibliography

Haller JA, Quigley PM, Loughlin GM, Marcus CL: Improvement in cardiorespiratory function after corrective surgery for pectus excavatum. J Pediatr Surg. In press.

Kaguraoka H, Ohnuki T, Itaoka T, et al: Degree of severity of pectus excavatum and pulmonary function in preoperative and postoperative periods. J Thorac Cardiovasc Surg 1992; 104:1483–1488.

Morshuis W, Folgering H, Barentsz J, et al: Pulmonary function before surgery for pectus excavatum and at long-term follow-up. Chest 1994;105:1646–1652.

Peterson RJ, Young WG, Godwin JD, et al: Noninvasive assessment of exercise cardiac function before and after pectus excavatum repair. J Thorac Cardiovasc Surg 1985;90:251–260.

Shamberger RC, Welch KJ: Cardiopulmonary function in pectus excavatum. Surg Gynecol Obstet 1988;166:383–391.

Shamberger RC, Welch KJ: Chest wall deformities. *In* Ashcraft KW, Holder TM (eds): Pediatric Surgery, 2nd ed. Philadelphia, WB Saunders, 1993, pp 146–162.

202 Pneumothorax

Frederick J. Rescorla

Etiology

1. Spontaneous pneumothorax

   a. *Primary (idiopathic)*—Usually occurs in tall, thin young men (male:female ratio, 6:1). Frequently caused by rupture of bleb or cyst near apex of lung.

   b. *Secondary*—Associated with chronic obstructive disorders such as cystic fibrosis, Langerhans cell histiocytosis, and bronchopulmonary dysplasia. Five to eight per cent of all patients with cystic fibrosis eventually develop a pneumothorax. Also seen with increased incidence in connective tissue disorders such as Marfan syndrome.

2. Traumatic pneumothorax—Most trauma in children results from blunt injury, commonly from motor vehicle crashes and collisions of motor vehicles with pedestrians or bicyclists. Penetrating trauma is rare; it is more common in urban areas and with older adolescents.

3. Iatrogenic pneumothorax—Associated with subclavian venous line placement, thoracentesis, mechanical ventilation, or cardiopulmonary resuscitation.

Pathophysiology

1. Spontaneous

   a. *Primary*—Apical alveoli are under greater distending pressures, leading to alveolar rupture with air collecting beneath visceral pleural to form blebs. Rupture of these blebs allows lung and visceral pleura to fall away from parietal pleura. The leak is frequently sealed by the time of presentation to a medical facility.

   b. *Secondary*—Effect of underlying condition; chronic obstructive pulmonary disease leads to rupture of alveoli and development of blebs.

2. Traumatic and iatrogenic—Alveolar and airway rupture from blunt or penetrating forces. Pneumothorax is associated with mechanical ventilation with high peak inspiratory airway pressures and high positive end-expiratory pressure (PEEP). Because of ongoing air leak, tension pneumothorax is possible in these cases.

3. Tension pneumothorax—Air continues to accumulate in pleural space and, as intrapleural pressure rises, the ipsilateral diaphragm flattens and the mediastinum shifts to the contralateral side. This compromises air exchange in the contralateral lung and impairs venous return by compression of the superior and inferior vena cavas.

4. Air released from alveoli may also move centrally to the mediastinum to form a pneumomediastinum. Air can dissect into the subcutaneous space (neck, chest, and abdomen), retroperitoneum, or pericardium.

Clinical Findings

1. Spontaneous pneumothorax

   a. *Symptoms*—Sudden onset of pleuritic chest pain and dyspnea. Pain gradually becomes dull. The degree of dyspnea generally depends on the size of pneumothorax, but it may be more severe with a smaller pneumothorax in patient with underlying lung disease (i.e., cystic fibrosis).

   b. *Physical examination*—Rapid, shallow breaths. Ipsilateral hyperinflation and decreased breath sounds. The examination may be normal in small pneumothorax.

2. Tension pneumothorax

   a. *Symptoms*—Dyspnea, cyanosis, tachycardia

   b. *Physical examination*—Jugular venous distension, hypotension, shift of trachea to contralateral side. Usually breath sounds are absent.

Key Clinical Findings

- Chest pain
- Dyspnea
- Unilateral hyperinflation
- Decreased breath sounds
- With tension, jugular venous distention

Laboratory Findings

Arterial hypoxemia, caused by ventilation-perfusion mismatch and shunting in collapsed lung.

Key Laboratory Finding

- Hypoxemia

Radiographic Changes

1. *Simple*—Absent lung markings in periphery of thoracic space. Difficult to estimate the amount of free air from chest radiograph. Volume of lung and hemithorax are proportional to the cube of the diameter.

2. *Tension*—Absent lung markings, flattening of diaphragm, shift of mediastinum to contralateral side. Heart may appear small.

3. *Blebs*—Visible in approximately 20 per cent of individuals on chest radiograph, usually apical. Computed tomography identifies blebs in 85 per cent of patients with proven blebs.

Treatment

1. Observation
   a. If site of pulmonary air leak is closed, absorption occurs at an average daily rate of 1.25 per cent; this can be increased to approximately 5 per cent with oxygen therapy.
   b. Indicated only for asymptomatic patients with small (<10 to 20%) pneumothorax. A period of observation is still required to make sure pneumothorax is not increasing.

2. Needle or catheter aspiration
   a. Aspiration is useful in some cases of initial spontaneous primary pneumothorax, since the leak is frequently closed at the time of presentation. Success reported in selected cases of traumatic pneumothorax.
   b. Catheter kits are available, or the physician can use 2-inch Angiocath. The needle is advanced into pleural space, the catheter passed through or over the needle, and air is evacuated with a syringe attached to a three-way stopcock. The catheter may be left in place for several hours to allow for reaccumulation of pleural air. If air reaccumulates, a one-way valve (e.g., Heimlich valve) may be used to allow air to escape. If evacuation is inadequate, suction can be applied to a Heimlich valve; if still inadequate, proceed to chest tube.
   c. Aspiration is successful in 50 to 70 per cent of cases, less successful with secondary spontaneous pneumothorax (30%).
   d. Needle aspiration is first-line emergency treatment for tension pneumothorax, followed by tube thoracostomy.

3. Tube thoracostomy
   a. Tube thoracostomy is indicated for severe symptoms, extensive air accumulation, tension pneumothorax, traumatic or iatrogenic pneumothorax, and patients with pneumothorax related to mechanical ventilation or underlying lung disease.
   b. Tube position is the second intercostal space in the midclavicular line or the fourth or fifth intercostal space in the midaxillary line.
   c. Technique
      (1) Local anesthesia and intravenous sedation are used for nonemergency cases.
      (2) Incision is made one interspace below the entry interspace. The subcutaneous tunnel decreases the chance of recurrent pneumothorax with tube removal. The interspace is entered on the superior border of rib to avoid the neurovascular bundle.
      (3) Tube size for infants is 12F; for preschool and school-age children, 16F; and for adolescents, 20 to 24F. Suction for infants is 10 cm H_2O; for preschool and school-age children, 15 cm H_2O; and for adolescents, 20 cm H_2O.
   d. After air leak stops, place to H_2O seal for 24 hours. If no reaccumulation, remove tube.
   e. Complications (rare) consist of postthoracostomy pulmonary edema caused by rapid reexpansion of lung.

4. Chemical or surgical pleurodesis (for persistent or recurrent pneumothorax)
   a. Guided by the recurrence rate, which is 23 to 50 per cent after initial spontaneous pneumothorax, 60 per cent after second episode, and 80 per cent after third episode.
   b. Indicated for air leak past 7 days, lung collapse, bilateral involvement, recurrent pneumothorax, or inability to tolerate a recurrent pneumothorax.
   c. May be performed chemically (through chest tube or with the use of thoracoscopy) or mechanically (by thoracoscopy or thoracotomy). Thoracoscopy with mechanical pleurodesis and apical parietal pleurectomy is preferred at the author's institution because of its safety and efficacy and because of the unknown long-term effects of chemical pleurodesis.
      (1) Chemical methods
         (a) Various agents (talc, tetracycline, silver nitrate, quinacrine and fibrin glue) are used.
         (b) Tetracycline is very effective but is no longer available in intravenous form. Minocycline is available and has been used for malignant effusions, but no data are available for treatment of pneumothorax. Quinacrine hydrochloride is no longer available. Silver nitrate 1 per cent solution (10 ml) can be used. Success with fibrin glue was reported in a neonate with a large air leak.
         (c) Talc may be administered in an aerosolized form at the time of thoracoscopy (5 g), or as a poudrage (5 g in 250 ml saline) through the chest tube. Although it is the most effective agent currently available, the long-term effects of talc are unknown. A mild restrictive defect and pleural thickening have been noted, and one case of pleural calcification with a significant reduction in lung function has been reported.
         (d) Chemical pleurodesis through the chest tube may be performed with the first episode; it is associated with a lower recurrence rate (2.5% with tetracycline) than is treatment with chest tube alone (20 to 50% recurrence). Lack of available agents limits use of this modality.
         (e) With chemical pleurodesis through a chest tube, material is placed into the pleural space, the tube is clamped, and the patient is placed in various positions to facilitate contact with the entire pleural surface. Advantage: less expensive. Disadvantages: May not coat all pleural surfaces, painful.
         (f) Advantages of chemical pleurodesis by thoracoscopy: more thorough covering of

pleural surfaces, less pain because patient is anesthetized. Disadvantage: cost.

    (g) The Cystic Fibrosis Foundation consensus conference report recommends no chemical pleurodesis unless the patient is gravely ill.

(2) Surgical intervention

    (a) Thoracotomy or thoracoscopy (preferred) allows evaluation of blebs. Blebs are excised and the pleural surface is mechanically abraded.

    (b) Many surgeons perform an apical parietal pleurectomy to increase the inflammatory response between the chest wall and the lung surface.

    (c) The recurrence rate after surgery is 0 to 10 per cent.

    (d) In view of the efficacy and safety of thoracoscopy, some authors advocate earlier intervention (>2 days with air leak).

Key Treatment

- Observation (mild cases)
- Needle or catheter aspiration
- Thoracostomy (severe cases)

Bibliography

Almind M, Lange P, Viskum K: Spontaneous pneumothorax: Comparison of simple drainage, talc pleurodesis, and tetracycline pleurodesis. Thorax 1989;44:627–630.

Lange P, Mortensen J, Groth S: Lung function 22–35 years after treatment of idiopathic spontaneous pneumothorax with talc poudrage or simple drainage. Thorax 1988;43:559–561.

Parry GW, Juniper ME, Dussek JE: Surgical intervention in spontaneous pneumothorax. Respir Med 1992;86:1–2. Editorial.

Schoenenberger RA, Haefeli WE, Weiss P, Ritz RF: Timing of invasive procedures in therapy for primary and secondary spontaneous pneumothorax. Arch Surg 1991;126:764–766.

Schramm CM: Pneumothorax and pneumomediastinum. In Burg FD, Ingelfinger JR, Wald ER, Polin RA (eds): Gellis and Kagan's Current Pediatric Therapy, 15th ed. Philadelphia, WB Saunders, 1996, pp 145–147.

203 Cystic Fibrosis

John C. Stevens

Definition

Cystic fibrosis (CF) is a multisystem, progressive disorder characterized by the production of thick, dehydrated mucus that causes premature death from respiratory failure in most affected persons.

Etiology

1. Autosomal recessive mode of inheritance.
2. The CF gene, found in a single locus on the long arm of chromosome 7, directs the production of the cystic fibrosis transmembrane conductance regulator (CFTR) protein.
3. More than 550 mutations have been found in individuals diagnosed with CF. The most common, ΔF508, is found in 70 per cent of cases.

Epidemiology

Affecting 1 in 3000 United States Caucasians, CF is the most common fatal genetic disorder. One in 28 Caucasians is a carrier of the CF gene. The incidence in the United States is 1 in 10,200 in Hispanics; 1 in 10,960 in Native Americans; 1 in 13,800 in blacks; and 1 in 62,600 in Asians.

Pathophysiology

1. CFTR acts as both a chloride channel and a regulator of chloride and sodium ion flux across the epithelial surfaces of exocrine glands.
2. In CF, a defective or absent CFTR protein leads to the production of very dehydrated exocrine secretions.
3. These highly viscous secretions cause luminal obstruction in the lungs and pancreas, resulting in the major manifestations of the disorder: chronic pneumonia, which leads to bronchiectasis, and pancreatic exocrine insufficiency, which causes malabsorption and failure to thrive.

Clinical Findings

1. Respiratory tract
    a. Abnormally thick bronchial secretions lead to chronic infection and inflammation of the respiratory tract, causing bronchiectasis, which eventuates in respiratory failure.
    b. Symptoms of respiratory tract disease (early to late) are chronic productive coughing, recurrent pneumonia, wheezing, dyspnea, hemoptysis, pneumothorax, cor pulmonale, and progressive respiratory failure.
2. Pancreatic digestive functions
    a. Insufficiency of exocrine pancreatic function, found in 85 to 90 per cent of patients with CF, causes malabsorption and failure to thrive.
    b. Symptoms of malabsorption are chronic diarrhea, abdominal bloating, ravenous appetite, fatty malodorous stools, rectal prolapse, and excessive flatulence.
3. Abnormalities in pancreatic endocrine function cause frank diabetes mellitus in approximately 15 per cent of

patients. This incidence increases as patients age and is seen in 35 per cent of those aged 25 years or older.

4. Other clinical conditions associated with CF

a. *Respiratory*—Chronic sinusitis, nasal polyps, pulmonary hypertension, cor pulmonale, allergic bronchopulmonary aspergillosis

b. *Gastrointestinal*—Meconium ileus, meconium plug syndrome, distal intestinal obstruction syndrome, gastrointestinal reflux, fibrosing colonopathy

c. *Hepatobiliary disease*—Prolonged neonatal jaundice, cholelithiasis, cirrhosis, portal hypertension

d. *Reproductive*—Male infertility (in 95%), reduced fertility in females, inguinal hernia

e. *Sweat abnormalities*—Dehydration with hypochloremic, hyponatremic metabolic alkalosis; heat stroke

f. *Skeletal abnormalities*—Arthritis, clubbing

g. *Hematologic*—Anemia secondary to vitamin E and/or iron deficiency, easy bruising secondary to vitamin K deficiency.

Key Clinical Findings

- Recurrent pneumonia
- Undernutrition
- Loose malodorous stools
- Rectal prolapse

Laboratory Findings

1. Diagnostic tests

a. The sweat chloride test (Gibson-Cooke method) is the only uniformly accepted diagnostic measure. Results should be accepted only if the test was performed by a highly experienced technician and at least 75 mg of sweat was collected. A sweat chloride concentration higher than 60 mmol/L is consistent with the diagnosis. A value lower than 40 mmol/L is normal. A value of 40 to 60 mmol/L is considered borderline, and the test should be repeated.

b. Genotype testing

(1) Several laboratories offer genotype testing for up to 62 of the most common CF mutations. This may be useful to confirm the diagnosis of CF in patients with equivocal sweat chloride results and those in whom an adequate sweat sample is not obtainable.

(2) Genetic screening for CF carriers is appropriate in families of a patient with CF[.] the probability of a positive carrier state with a negative screening panel is less than 1 per cent in this circumstance.

2. *Pulmonary function tests*—Serial pulmonary function testing is a very sensitive way of monitoring the pulmonary status of patients with CF. Early in the disease, patients may show mild signs of airway obstruction without overt clinical symptoms. As the disease progresses, decreases in pulmonary function may signal the need for more aggressive pulmonary treatment (e.g., hospitalization to initiate intravenous antibiotic therapy), even without new clinical symptoms. Pulmonary function tests are often used to document response to new or more aggressive therapy.

3. *Sputum culture*—Sputum cultures are needed to direct antibiotic coverage in the treatment of pulmonary exacerbation of the disease. The most common pathogens in CF are *Staphylococcus aureus, Haemophilus influenzae,* and *Pseudomonas aeruginosa.* The microbiology laboratory needs to be informed that the specimen is from a CF patient and should process the specimen in a manner that allows for isolation of the often slower growing *Burkolderia cepacia.*

4. *Yearly screening laboratories*—The following tests are performed once a year to screen for subtle change:

a. Liver function tests (aspartate aminotransferase, alanine aminotransferase, gamma-glutamyl transferase), prothrombin time, partial thromboplastin time

b. Urine analysis

c. Electrocardiogram if patient is >7 years old

d. Sputum culture

e. Complete blood count with differential

f. Glucose level

g. Vitamin E level

h. Oxygen saturation

i. PPD testing.

Key Laboratory Findings

- Sweat chloride elevation
- Genotype testing

Treatment

1. Treatment for CF is most successful when given at a cystic fibrosis center employing a multidisciplinary team of physicians, nurses, social workers, dietitians, respiratory and physical therapists, psychologists and/or psychiatrists, and genetic counselors.

2. Management of CF pulmonary disease includes a daily regimen of chest physiotherapy or breathing exercises. Patients are often treated with inhaled bronchodilators before chest physiotherapy to maximize secretion clearance.

3. Antibiotics are most often used to treat an acute exacerbation of the pulmonary disease, guided by the results of sputum cultures. Usually, the most common pathogens need to be covered (*P. aeruginosa* and *S. aureus*). With a significant pulmonary exacerbation, patients are often hospitalized for initiation of intravenous antibiotic therapy and frequent chest physiotherapy. After significant improvement in clinical status, the remainder of the typical 10- to 21-day intravenous course may be completed at home.

4. Corticosteroids can be used to treat airway inflammation and severe bronchospasm. Usually short-term use is indicated, but in selected cases in patients colonized with

Pseudomonas a more prolonged course with 1 mg/kg every other day may be warranted for 12 to 24 months, so long as there is close monitoring for side effects. Nonsteroidal antiinflammatory medications such as ibuprofen have also demonstrated some efficacy and may aid in slowing the progression of CF lung disease.

5. Mucus-thinning drugs such as *N*-acetylcysteine and deoxyribonuclease (DNase) may be useful. Acetylcysteine can cause bronchospasm and therefore should be used with caution. DNase, typically given once a day, can improve pulmonary function and may reduce the frequency of pulmonary exacerbations requiring intravenous antibiotic therapy.

6. Lung transplantation has become more successful in recent years, and CF patients with advanced lung disease should be counseled as to this option. Given the increasing demand with a stable donor pool, patients pursuing this option should be evaluated when their 1-second forced expiratory volume is stable at 30 to 40 per cent of the predicted value.

7. Pancreatic insufficiency is treated with pancreatic enzyme supplementation. Typically, patients require 500 to 2000 lipase units per kilogram per meal to achieve adequate nutrient absorption. Doses greater than 2500 lipase units/

kg should be avoided if possible to prevent the development of fibrosing colonopathy.

8. The use of antacids and H$_2$ blockers may improve the effectiveness of pancreatic enzyme supplements.

9. Many new therapies are under investigation, including gene transfer therapy for CF pulmonary disease. Dramatic improvement in the mean survival time of CF patients may be seen in the next 10 years, given these advances in therapy.

Key Treatment

- Chest physiotherapy
- Antibiotics
- Pancreatic enzyme enterally

Prevention

Given the autosomal recessive mode of inheritance and the ability to detect the carrier state, especially in a relative of a patient with CF, genetic counseling can be provided before conception. Genotype testing can also be performed in early pregnancy if the couple would want to pursue termination of pregnancy, given the diagnosis of CF.

204 Tuberculosis

Laura S. Inselman

Definition

Tuberculosis is an infectious, progressive disease of the lungs and other organs characterized by an acute and a chronic course.

Etiology

Tuberculosis is caused by the mycobacteria *Mycobacterium tuberculosis* and *Mycobacterium bovis*. These are acid-fast bacilli characterized by resistance to acid decoloration after staining with an aniline dye. *M. tuberculosis* occurs more frequently in the United States than does *M. bovis*.

Epidemiology

The highest mortality rates occur in children <4 years of age, during adolescence, and in the elderly population. An increased incidence of tuberculosis occurs

1. With the presence of human immunodeficiency virus (HIV) infection
2. With the presence of multidrug-resistant tuberculosis
3. In the homeless population
4. In the medically underserved population
5. With poverty
6. In poorly ventilated areas
7. In crowded living conditions

8. In the foreign-born population that comes from areas where the disease is endemic
9. In older individuals who were infected with tubercle bacilli when younger and now have active tuberculosis
10. Among individuals with certain human leukocyte antigen (HLA) phenotypes
11. Among individuals with the *Bcg* gene.

Pathophysiology

1. Means of infection
   a. Inhalation, which causes >95 per cent of cases of *M. tuberculosis* infections in the United States
   b. Ingestion of contaminated milk or meat, which usually involves *M. bovis* and is rare in the United States
   c. A wound, skin lesion, or mucous membrane lesion contaminated with tubercle bacilli
   d. Injection with a syringe containing tubercle bacilli
   e. Transplacental passage of tubercle bacilli or inhalation of infected amniotic fluid.

2. Pulmonary tuberculosis results from inhalation of aerosolized particles containing small numbers of tubercle bacilli that reach the alveoli. Most of these bacilli are

killed by pulmonary alveolar macrophages (PAMs). If the quantity and/or virulence of the inhaled bacilli is high, the bacilli can destroy the PAMs; form characteristic caseating tubercles composed of bloodborne macrophages, T lymphocytes, and Langerhans giant cells; spread to nearby hilar lymph nodes; disseminate through the lymphatics and the bloodstream; and infect other organs. Lymphohematogenous spread can result in miliary tuberculosis and in quiescent lesions that can activate in later years.

3. Most tuberculous lesions resolve and disappear in the immunocompetent host. However, caseation, liquefaction, necrosis, and calcification can occur. Liquefied caseum permits tubercle bacilli to multiply extracellularly and spread to other organs. An increased oxygen tension in cavities formed by release of liquefied caseum also promotes replication of bacilli. Clinical disease occurs when liquefied caseum is present.

4. Inhalation of tubercle bacilli and formation of the primary complex (see next section) occur during the 2- to 10-week incubation period. Cutaneous delayed-type hypersensitivity is present at the end of the incubation period, and the tuberculin skin test reaction is positive.

Clinical Findings

1. Tuberculous infection is characterized by a positive tuberculin skin test reaction and absence of clinical, laboratory, and radiographic evidence of disease. The risk of developing active tuberculosis after the onset of infection is highest during the first 2 years.

2. The primary complex is composed of the lung lesion, the draining regional lymphatic vessels, and the local lymph nodes. It can develop at any portal of entry (lung, skin, gastrointestinal tract). The complex usually heals by the end of the incubation period and is not visible radiographically. Then, the only indication that the child is infected with tubercle bacilli is a positive tuberculin skin test reaction.

3. If the primary complex enlarges instead of heals, pulmonary tuberculosis occurs. This consists of hilar, paratracheal, and/or mediastinal lymphadenopathy and may be accompanied by pneumonia. Caseation, cavity formation, and disseminated tuberculosis can develop subsequently.

4. The stages of pulmonary tuberculosis are as follows:
   a. *Primary pulmonary tuberculosis,* which is characterized by adenopathy with or without pneumonia
   b. *Progressive primary pulmonary tuberculosis,* which can cause pneumonia, tracheobronchitis, atelectasis, airway stenosis, air trapping, and bronchiectasis
   c. *Tuberculous pneumonia,* which results from hematogenous dissemination
   d. *Endobronchial tuberculosis,* which is caused by penetration of infected lymph nodes through an airway wall and spread of liquefied caseum into the airway lumen. Bronchopleural and bronchoesophageal fistulas and pneumothorax are complications.
   e. *Miliary tuberculosis,* which is caused by lymphohematogenous dissemination of tubercle bacilli throughout all organs, including the lung
   f. *Tuberculous pleural effusion* with or without empy-

ema. Scoliosis secondary to pleural adhesions, reduction of the involved hemithorax, and pneumothorax are complications.
   g. *Chronic pulmonary tuberculosis,* which is characterized by cavity formation, fibrosis, and calcification.

5. Children are more likely than adults to have lymphadenopathy, calcification, and disseminated disease.

> ### KEY POINT
>
> **Children are usually asymptomatic, even with chest x-ray findings suggestive of pulmonary tuberculosis.**

6. Tuberculosis can affect almost every organ in the body. Most cases of extrapulmonary tuberculosis are accompanied by pulmonary tuberculosis. Extrapulmonary tuberculosis can occur as
   a. Miliary tuberculosis
   b. Tuberculous meningitis
   c. Lymphatic disease—i.e., cervical adenopathy (scrofula)
   d. Tuberculosis of the bones and joints
   e. Disease of the gastrointestinal tract, skin, heart, eyes, ears, mastoid, peritoneum, genitourinary tract, and endocrine and exocrine glands.

Key Clinical Findings

- Positive tuberculin skin test
- Mediastinal adenopathy
- Pulmonary infiltrate
- Pleural effusion

Laboratory Findings

1. General diagnostic tests
   a. Complete blood cell count and serum aspartate aminotransaminase level are usually normal; leukocyte count is elevated with disseminated tuberculosis.
   b. Erythrocyte sedimentation rate is mildly elevated with pulmonary tuberculosis, markedly increased with disseminated tuberculosis.
   c. Urinalysis shows amicrobic pyuria with advanced renal tuberculosis.
   d. Cerebrospinal fluid (CSF) analysis in patients with tuberculous meningitis shows the presence of leukocytes (polymorphonuclear leukocytes initially, lymphocytes later), reduced glucose and elevated protein concentrations, normal chloride concentration initially (reduced later), and a turbid sediment on standing for 24 hours (secondary to the high protein level).
   e. Pleural fluid in patients with tuberculous pleural effusion is sanguinous or hemorrhagic, exudative, loculated or nonloculated, and has increased protein and lactic dehydrogenase levels, decreased glucose

levels, and increased leukocytes (polymorphonuclear leukocytes initially, T lymphocytes later).

2. Specific molecular tests (not readily available at present)

   a. Polymerase chain reaction (PCR) assay identifies the presence of the *M. tuberculosis* complex with the use of DNA probes in blood, CSF, sputum, gastric washings, urine, bronchoalveolar (BAL) fluid, pleural fluid, and abscesses. Results in children are variable with present methods.

   b. Restriction fragment-length polymorphism (RFLP) technique identifies the presence and spread of *M. tuberculosis* by gene mapping.

   c. Luciferase assay identifies the presence of drug-resistant *M. tuberculosis*.

   d. Immunologic testing to antigens and antibodies of *M. tuberculosis* is used to analyze the presence of such antigens as lipoarabinomannan (LAM), P32, purified protein derivative (PPD), A60, and 5 and to measure levels of intercellular adhesion molecule-1 (ICAM-1), interleukins-1 and -2, and adenosine deaminase.

3. Microbiology

   a. Ziehl-Neelsen, fluorescence, and Kinyoun acid-fast staining tests are performed on two to three consecutive first-morning gastric washings after an overnight fast and on first-morning urine collections. Sputum, BAL and pleural fluids, CSF, wound secretions, blood, abscesses, bone marrow, and liver biopsy material are other specimens used for stains. The staining tests are positive if tubercle bacilli are present.

   b. Culture of above specimens can be done on Löwenstein-Jensen medium (takes 6 to 8 weeks) or Bactec medium (takes 7 days).

   c. Drug sensitivity testing of the organism is performed if growth occurs.

4. Histology—Microscopic examination of biopsies of lymph nodes, lung, pleura, bone marrow, and liver is performed to look for granulomas, epithelioid cells, caseation, and necrosis.

Radiographic Findings

1. Chest radiography

   a. Posteroanterior and lateral views are used to detect adenopathy (hilar, paratracheal, mediastinal), a primary parenchymal focus, pneumonia, calcification, a cavity, miliary lesions, atelectasis, hyperaeration, mediastinal shift, pleural effusion, and pneumothorax.

   b. Oblique views are used to detect mediastinal lesions.

   c. Apical lordotic views are used to identify apical lesions.

   d. Lateral decubitus views are used to evaluate the presence of a loculated or nonloculated pleural effusion.

2. Ultrasonography of the chest is used to determine the presence of a pleural effusion.

3. Airway fluoroscopy differentiates hilar adenopathy from pulsatile blood flow through pulmonary blood vessels.

4. Computed tomography of the chest is used to identify pleural adhesions with a loculated pleural effusion and parenchymal and hilar lesions that are not observed on plain radiographs.

Tuberculin Skin Testing

1. The Mantoux tuberculin skin test is the only definitive test available to determine the presence of tuberculous infection in a child.

   a. *Application*—0.1 ml of 5 tuberculin units (TU) of PPD is injected intracutaneously on the volar surface of the forearm, with the subsequent formation of a wheal.

   b. *Interpretation*—Measure the amount of induration 48 to 72 hours after application. The interpretation depends on the size of induration, the risk of exposure to tuberculosis, and the age of the child (Table 204–1).

2. Induration of ≥15 mm of a Mantoux tuberculin skin test in a child who has received the bacillus Calmette-Guérin (BCG) immunization is interpreted as indicating active tuberculosis. Induration measuring 5 to 14 mm in a BCG-vaccinated child may also indicate the presence of active tuberculosis if high or moderate risk factors are present (see Table 204–1).

3. Multiple-puncture tests do not provide the standardization of PPD, are not diagnostic, vary in sensitivity and specificity, must be followed with a Mantoux tuberculin skin test unless vesiculation occurs, and, in general, are no longer used by most health care providers.

4. False reactions

   a. False-positive reactions result from incorrect application or interpretation and cross-reactivity with nontuberculous mycobacteria.

   b. False-negative reactions result from application during the incubation period; incorrect storage, application, or interpretation; and presence of anergy, viral infections, cellular immunodeficiency, or malnutrition.

TABLE 204–1. MANTOUX TUBERCULIN SKIN TEST REACTION AND RISK CATEGORY OF EXPOSURE TO ACTIVE TUBERCULOSIS

SIZE OF INDURATION	RISK CATEGORY
≥5 mm	High risk: children with clinical and/or x-ray evidence of tuberculosis, who are in recent close contact with someone who has active tuberculosis, or who have a cellular immunodeficiency (HIV infection, use of high-dose corticosteroids)
≥10 mm	Moderate risk: children who are younger than 4 years old; were born in a country where tuberculosis is endemic or whose parent comes from such a country; who live in prisons, institutions, or shelters; who use intravenous drugs; or who have malnutrition or a disease (malignancy, chronic renal failure, diabetes mellitus) that allows for tuberculosis to disseminate
≥15 mm	Low risk: children with none of the above risk factors

HIV, human immunodeficiency virus.

Treatment for Active Disease

1. General principles

   a. In general, three drugs are used for a total of 6 months, or two drugs are used for a total of 9 months. Four drugs are prescribed in drug-resistant disease and in certain forms of extrapulmonary tuberculosis. A daily or intermittent (twice weekly) regimen is administered (Tables 204–2 and 204–3).

   b. Corticosteroids are added for 2 to 3 months for the treatment of effusions (pleural, pericardial), meningitis, miliary tuberculosis, and endobronchial tuberculosis.

   c. Pyridoxine, 10 mg per 100 mg of INH per day, is added to prevent INH-induced peripheral neuropathy during periods of rapid growth, as in adolescence or pregnancy, or if pyridoxine deficiency is already present, as in malnutrition. Pyridoxine is also used with ethionamide to prevent peripheral neuropathy associated with this drug.

   d. Directly observed therapy (DOT), which employs a responsible individual who observes the ingestion of the drugs by the child, is preferable in the treatment of drug-resistant tuberculosis, in certain forms of extrapulmonary tuberculosis, and when HIV and *M. tuberculosis* infections coexist.

KEY POINT

Ideally, DOT should be available to treat all individuals with tuberculous infection or tuberculosis.

---

2. Alternative dosage schedules

   a. Drug-sensitive tuberculosis

      (1) *6-Month regimen*—Prescribe INH, RIF and pyrazinamide (PZA) daily for 2 months plus INH and RIF daily or 2 times per week for another 4 months

      (2) *9-Month regimen*—Prescribe INH and RIF daily for 9 months; *or* prescribe INH and RIF daily for 1 to 2 months plus INH and RIF 2 times per week for another 7 to 8 months

   b. Drug-resistant tuberculosis—Prescribe INH, RIF, PZA, and either streptomycin (SM) or ethambutol (EMB) for 2 months plus INH and RIF for another 10 to 16 months. Final selection of drugs depends on drug sensitivity testing results, if available, but usually includes INH and RIF. Four drugs are used empirically in areas where the INH resistance rate is ≥4 per cent. Second-line drugs are also available, although their use in children is limited and is accompanied by toxicity.

3. Specific treatment regimens

   a. Pulmonary tuberculosis—Use the 6- or 9-month drug regimen

   b. Extrapulmonary tuberculosis

      (1) *Miliary tuberculosis, tuberculous meningitis, bone and joint tuberculosis, renal tuberculosis*—Prescribe INH, RIF, PZA, and SM daily for 2 months plus INH and RIF daily or 2 times per week for an additional 10 months

      (2) *Other forms of extrapulmonary tuberculosis*—Use same drug regimen as for pulmonary tuberculosis.

   c. Coexistence of tuberculosis and HIV infection—

TABLE 204–2. ANTITUBERCULOSIS DRUG DOSAGES, ROUTES OF ADMINISTRATION, AND ACTIVITY

DRUG	DOSE Daily (mg/kg/day, [maximum/ day])	DOSE Intermittent (mg/kg/dose, [maximum/ dose])	ROUTE OF ADMINISTRATION	ACTIVITY
First-Line				
Isoniazid (INH)*	10–20 (300 mg)	20–40 (900 mg)	Oral, intramuscular, intrathecal	Bactericidal against intracellular and extracellular *M. tuberculosis*
Rifampin (RIF)*	10–20 (600 mg)	10–20 (600 mg)	Oral, intravenous	Bactericidal against intracellular and extracellular *M. tuberculosis*
Pyrazinamide (PZA)	15–30 (2 g)	50–70 (4 g)	Oral	Bactericidal against intracellular *M. tuberculosis* in an acid environment
Streptomycin (SM)	20–40 (1 g)	25–30 (1.5 g)	Intramuscular	Bactericidal and bacteriostatic against extracellular *M. tuberculosis* in a neutral or alkaline environment
Ethambutol (EMB)	15–25 (2.5 g)	50 (2.5 g)	Oral	Bacteriostatic against intracellular and extracellular *M. tuberculosis;* bactericidal at high doses
Prednisone (or equivalent)	1–2 (60 mg)	—	Oral	Antiinflammatory properties
Second-Line				
Para-aminosalicylic acid (PAS)	150 (12 g)	—	Oral	Bacteriostatic against extracellular *M. tuberculosis*
Kanamycin, capreomycin	15–30 (1 g)	—	Intramuscular	Bactericidal against extracellular *M. tuberculosis*
Ethionamide, cycloserine	15–20 (1 g)	—	Oral	Bacteriostatic against intracellular and extracellular *M. tuberculosis*

*When INH and RIF are used together, the dose of INH is 10 mg/kg/day and that of RIF is 15 mg/kg/day.

TABLE 204–3. SIDE EFFECTS AND INTERACTIONS OF ANTITUBERCULOSIS DRUGS

DRUG	SIDE EFFECTS	DRUG INTERACTIONS
Isoniazid (INH)	Hepatotoxicity, neurotoxicity, dermatitis, gastrointestinal irritation, hematologic toxicity, vasculitis, arthralgia, hypersensitivity, fever, urinary retention	Potentiates action of alcohol, phenytoin, barbiturates, carbamazepine, Antabuse; reduces ketoconazole activity. Overdose: metabolic acidosis, tachycardia, fever, hyperglycemia, photophobia, seizures, coma, mydriasis, urinary retention
Rifampin (RIF)	Red-orange color of urine, saliva, sweat, tears, stool, and sputum; hepatotoxicity (increased frequency when combined with INH); neurotoxicity; hematologic toxicity; dermatitis; hypersensitivity; gastrointestinal irritation; T-lymphocyte suppression; flu-like syndrome with high doses of intermittent therapy or after a drug-free interval	Reduces action of anticonvulsants, narcotics, anticoagulants, β blockers, theophylline, oral hypoglycemic agents, corticosteroids, oral contraceptives, digoxin, chloramphenicol, ketoconazole, cyclosporin; reduced action with ketoconazole; increased action with halothane and probenecid. Overdose: red-orange color of body fluids and skin; edema of face, larynx, eyes; hepatitis; pruritis; vomiting; lethargy; headache
Pyrazinamide (PZA)	Hyperuricemia, gout, hepatotoxicity, arthralgia, gastrointestinal irritation, fever, anorexia, malaise, dysuria, dermatitis	None known
Streptomycin (SM)	Dose-related auditory and vestibular toxicity of eighth cranial nerve, nephrotoxicity, hematologic toxicity, fever, dermatitis	Potentiates action of diuretics (chlorothiazide, ethacrynic acid, spironolactone, furosemide), neuromuscular blocking agents, antibiotics (other aminoglycosides, cephalosporins, colistin, cyclosporin); increased action with probenecid
Ethambutol (EMB)	Ophthalmologic toxicity, pruritus, dermatitis, hyperuricemia, malaise, neurotoxicity, gastrointestinal irritation	None known
Corticosteroids	Hypothalamic-pituitary-adrenal axis inhibition, growth inhibition, hypertension, obesity, osteoporosis, myopathy, electrolyte disturbance, peptic ulcer, cataract formation	Potentiate action of neuromuscular blocking agents; decrease action of calcium salts; reduced action with barbiturates, rifampin, phenytoin
Para-aminosalicylic acid (PAS)	Gastrointestinal irritation, thyroid disease, hematologic toxicity, fever, hypokalemia, hypoglycemia, dermatitis, hepatotoxicity, hypersensitivity, pericarditis, ophthalmologic toxicity	Potentiates action of digoxin, vitamin B_{12}, antituberculosis drugs (INH, RIF); reduced action with salicylates; increased action with probenecid
Kanamycin	Auditory and vestibular toxicity of eighth cranial nerve, nephrotoxicity, hematologic toxicity, neuromuscular blockade, respiratory inhibition	Same as for streptomycin
Capreomycin	Auditory and vestibular toxicity of eighth cranial nerve, nephrotoxicity, hepatotoxicity, hematologic toxicity, dermatitis, fever	Same as for streptomycin; potentiates action of antituberculosis drugs (INH, RIF, PZA, SM, EMB, PAS, cycloserine). Overdose: ototoxicity, nephrotoxicity, electrolyte imbalance, neuromuscular blockade, respiratory arrest
Ethionamide	Gastrointestinal irritation, central nervous system toxicity, peripheral neuropathy, ophthalmologic toxicity, hepatotoxicity, metallic taste, lethargy, orthostatic hypotension, stomatitis, hypersensitivity	Potentiates action of antituberculosis drugs (INH, RIF, PZA, EMB, PAS, cycloserine). Overdose: nephrotoxicity, central nervous system toxicity
Cycloserine	Central nervous system toxicity, dermatitis	Potentiates action of antituberculosis drugs (INH, RIF, PZA, EMB, PAS, ethionamide); increased action with alcohol. Overdose: nephrotoxicity, central nervous system toxicity

Prescribe INH, RIF, and PZA for 2 months plus INH and RIF for a minimum of an additional 7 months. SM or EMB may be included during the first 2 months. If improvement does not occur, treatment is extended for at least 12 months.

d. Perinatal tuberculosis—Prescribe INH, RIF, PZA, and SM daily for 2 months plus INH and RIF daily or 2 times per week for an additional 10 months.

e. Tuberculosis during pregnancy—Prescribe INH and RIF for 9 months in either the daily or the intermittent regimen for treatment of active tuberculosis. EMB can be included if drug resistance is suspected. SM and PZA are avoided because of teratogenicity. Treatment of *M. tuberculosis* with HIV is usually started during the second trimester. INH prophylaxis for an untreated recent tuberculin skin test conversion is often initiated after delivery.

Prevention

1. To prevent activity in a tuberculin-positive patient or in a person exposed and at increased risk:

   a. Chemotherapy

      (1) Indications for chemotherapy

         (a) Positive Mantoux tuberculin skin test reaction; absence of clinical, radiographic, and laboratory findings of tuberculosis; and no prior history of antituberculosis therapy

         (b) Recent conversion of a Mantoux tuberculin skin test reaction

         (c) Recent or close contact with someone with active tuberculosis, even if the child's Mantoux tuberculin skin test reaction is negative

         (d) HIV infection or increased risk for development of HIV infection

(e) Increased risk for development of widespread tuberculosis as a result of diabetes mellitus, malnutrition, immunosuppressive therapy, malignancy, or end-stage renal disease.

Antituberculosis Drugs

Isoniazid (INH)
Rifampin (RIF)
Pyrazinamide (PZA)
Streptomycin (SM)
Ethambutol (EMB)

---

(2) Drugs
   (a) For nonresistant *M. tuberculosis*: Isoniazid (INH), 10 mg/kg/day (maximum, 300 mg/day), daily for 9 months; *or* INH, 10 mg/kg/day (maximum, 300 mg/day), daily for 1 month followed by INH, 20 to 30 mg/kg per dose (maximum, 900 mg per dose), twice weekly for 8 months
   (b) For INH-resistant *M. tuberculosis*: INH, 10 mg/kg/day (maximum, 300 mg/day), daily plus rifampin (RIF), 10 mg/kg/day (maximum, 600 mg/day), daily for 9 months
   (c) For coexistent HIV infection: INH, 10 mg/kg/day (maximum 300 mg/day), daily for 12 months

2. Primary prevention
   a. Immunization
      (1) BCG vaccine is used for uninfected children who
         (a) Are living in a household with an adult with active pulmonary tuberculosis and in whom compliance with INH preventive therapy is not adequate
         (b) Are remaining exposed to adults with multidrug-resistant tuberculosis
         (c) Have asymptomatic HIV infection and are at increased risk of exposure to active tuberculosis.
      (2) The Mantoux tuberculin skin test reaction should be positive 6 to 8 weeks after immunization. If it is not, BCG is reapplied, and the tuberculin skin test is later repeated. A history of BCG vaccination should not prevent tuberculin skin testing if indicated.

KEY POINT

Mantoux tuberculin skin testing is not contraindicated with a history of BCG immunization.

---

(3) Side effects of immunization are
   (a) Local lymphadenitis and ulcer formation
   (b) Lupus vulgaris
   (c) Osteomyelitis
   (d) Fatal BCG infection in an immunodeficient child.
(4) Contraindications to vaccination are
   (a) Disruption of the skin, as with an infection or a burn
   (b) Immunodeficiency, either cellular or combined, or as a result of immunosuppression (e.g., corticosteroid therapy)
   (c) Symptomatic HIV infection.

b. An infant born to a mother with active tuberculosis is separated from her until the infant is protected and the mother is not infectious. Either of two methods is appropriate:
   (1) INH, 10 mg/kg/day, is prescribed for the infant for 3 months if the initial tuberculin skin test reaction, chest radiograph, and physical examination are normal.
      (a) If a repeat PPD test is negative after 3 months, INH can be discontinued provided the mother is receiving adequate therapy *and* is noninfectious. If both do not occur, INH is prescribed for a total of 9 months.
      (b) If a repeat PPD test is positive, the infant is evaluated and treated for tuberculous infection or tuberculosis (see specific treatment regimen for perinatal tuberculosis).
   (2) BCG immunization is administered with INH prophylaxis in cases of maternal noncompliance or maternal drug resistance or if it is anticipated that follow-up of the infant will be inadequate. INH is discontinued after conversion of the Mantoux tuberculin skin test.

c. Epidemiologic investigation of contacts—Contact identification is made through the local department of public health to detect and remove the source of active tuberculosis, treat the contact, and prevent further dissemination of tuberculosis in the community.

Bibliography

American Academy of Pediatrics: Tuberculosis. *In* Peter G (ed): 1997 Red Book: Report of the Committee on Infectious Diseases, 24th ed. Elk Grove Village, IL, American Academy of Pediatrics, 1997, pp 541–562.

Bass JB Jr, Farer LS, Hopewell PC, et al: Treatment of tuberculosis and tuberculosis infection in adults and children. Am J Respir Crit Care Med 1994;149:1359–1374.

Centers for Disease Control and Prevention: Initial therapy for tuberculosis in the era of multidrug resistance. Recommendations of the Advisory Council for the Elimination of Tuberculosis. MMWR Morb Mortal Wkly Rep 1993;42:1–8.

Inselman LS: Tuberculosis in children: An update. Pediatr Pulmonol 1996;21:101–120.

Smith MHD, Starke JR, Marquis JR: Tuberculosis and opportunistic mycobacterial infections. *In* Feigin RD, Cherry JD (eds): Textbook of Pediatric Infectious Diseases, 3rd ed. Philadelphia, WB Saunders, 1992, pp 1321–1362.

205 Sarcoidosis

Laura S. Inselman

Definition

Sarcoidosis is a chronic, multisystemic disease that is characterized clinically primarily by pulmonary manifestations, radiographically by stages of lung involvement, and histologically by non-necrotizing granulomas.

Etiology

The cause is unknown. Possible causes are

1. An immunologic response to an inhaled antigen
2. Host factors
3. Environmental factors, as observed with an increased incidence among persons living in rural areas
4. Genetic predisposition, as identified by an increased incidence in monozygotic twins
5. Infectious, as evidenced by detection of nontuberculous mycobacteria without cell walls in blood cultures of patients with sarcoidosis
6. The association of certain human leukocyte antigens (HLAs), resulting in increased incidence:
   a. HLA-B8 and acute sarcoidosis with arthritis and erythema nodosum
   b. HLA-B13 and chronic sarcoidosis
   c. HLA-B27 and sarcoidosis with uveitis
7. An autoimmune process, as suggested by the coexistence of sarcoidosis and systemic lupus erythematosus and of sarcoidosis and progressive systemic sclerosis.

Epidemiology

1. Sarcoidosis occurs endemically.
2. It occurs with increased frequency in rural areas of the United States, Japan, Ireland, and the Scandinavian countries. Most cases in the United States occur in the southeast, along the Gulf of Mexico, in the midwest, and in New England. The highest incidence nationally is in Virginia, with a rate of 500 cases per 100,000 population.
3. The incidence in the black population is 7 to 26 times that of the Caucasian population in the United States and South Africa. The incidence is high in Caucasians in Scandinavia and in the Asian population in Japan.
4. There is an equal sex predilection in children, but the disorder occurs slightly more frequently in adult women than in adult men.
5. Most pediatric cases occur during late childhood and adolescence (i.e., age 8 to 15 years). The overall incidence is highest in adults 20 to 50 years old.

Pathophysiology

1. Cellular and humoral immune systems are altered. Increased number and activity of lymphocytes and mononuclear phagocytes in target organs cause a characteristic tissue response consisting of the following:
   a. Non-necrotizing granulomas with centrally located multinucleated giant cells, macrophages, and epithelioid cells
   b. A peripheral layer of T and B lymphocytes, polymorphonuclear leukocytes, plasma cells, fibroblasts and collagen
   c. Deposits of immunoglobulin G (IgG) and the third component of complement.
2. The granulomas
   a. Are not specific for sarcoidosis
   b. May be present in any organ
   c. May be observed in many organs or as a sole infiltrating mass in one tissue
   d. Are characteristically present in clusters
   e. Occur most frequently in the lung
   f. Form in alveolar, bronchiolar, vascular, and lymphatic walls
   g. Can occur within the intima and media of blood vessels and cause vasculitis
   h. Can alter tissue architecture and function if large masses occur
   i. Resolve without scar formation in 80 per cent of cases but may persist either without fibrosis or with fibrosis and hyaline deposits.
3. CD4+ T lymphocytes and mononuclear phagocytes from the circulation selectively accumulate in the lung and other organs and secrete lymphokines, which promote granuloma formation, local immunoglobulin synthesis by B lymphocytes, collagen deposition, and fibrosis (Table 205–1).
4. Accumulation of these cells in tissues depletes them in the peripheral circulation, with a resultant elevated ratio of CD4+ to CD8+ lymphocytes in inflamed tissue and a diminished ratio in the peripheral blood. Peripheral polyclonal hypergammaglobulinemia occurs, and, as a result of nonspecific stimulation of tissue B lymphocytes, increased serum levels of antibodies to microorganisms and immune complexes are present. Tissue hypergammaglobulinemia also occurs, as evidenced in the lung by increased quantities of IgG, IgM, activated T and B lymphocytes, and the presence of immune complexes in bronchoalveolar lavage (BAL) fluid.
5. Interstitial pneumonitis, or alveolitis, is the initial lung lesion and results from CD4+ T lymphocyte accumulation in the pulmonary interstitium and alveoli. It can occur without clinical or radiographic findings. Airway obstruction can result from coalescence of granulomas. Increased alveolar-capillary membrane permeability, perhaps related to release of chemical mediators, can cause fluid and protein shifts in the lung.

TABLE 205–1. SOME CHEMICAL MEDIATORS SECRETED BY CELLS IN THE PATHOGENESIS OF SARCOIDOSIS

CELL	CHEMICAL MEDIATOR	FUNCTION
T lymphocyte	Angiotensin-converting enzyme–inducing factor	Stimulates formation of angiotensin-converting enzyme
	B-cell differentiation factor	Stimulates immunoglobulin secretion by nearby B lymphocytes
	B-cell growth factor	Stimulates immunoglobulin secretion by nearby B lymphocytes
	Gamma interferon	Stimulates macrophage differentiation, promotes granuloma formation
	Interleukin-2	Stimulates T lymphocyte replication
	Leukocyte inhibitory factor	Attracts circulating polymorphonuclear neutrophils to granulomas
	Macrophage inhibitory factor	Attracts and activates monocytes and macrophages to granulomas
	Migration inhibitory factor	Immobilizes and activates mononuclear phagocytes
	Monocyte chemotactic factor	Attracts and activates blood monocytes to granulomas
Mononuclear phagocyte	Alveolar-macrophage–derived growth factor	Interacts with fibronectin to promote fibroblast activity in the granuloma
	Colony-stimulating factor	Promotes monocyte and neutrophil synthesis in bone marrow
	Fibronectin	Attracts and promotes replication of fibroblasts and collagen formation in granulomas
	Interleukin-1	Activates T lymphocytes, promotes interleukin-2 receptor formation on T lymphocytes, induces muscle protein degradation, stimulates fibroblast growth, pyrogenic
	Oxygen free radicals	Inhibit antielastases, such as α_1 antitrypsin
	Plasminogen activator	Stimulates synthesis of plasmin and lipoxygenase pathway metabolites
	Prostaglandin E$_2$	Inhibits fibroblast replication
	Proteases (collagenase, elastase, acid hydrolase)	Injure and destroy tissue

Clinical Findings

1. *General*—Sarcoidosis is usually diagnosed in symptomatic children and in asymptomatic adults who have routine chest radiographs.
   a. It affects the lung, skin, lymph nodes, eyes, brain, myocardium, reticuloendothelial system, muscles, and joints.
   b. Symptoms are caused by local tissue compression, distortion, and penetration by sarcoid lesions.
   c. The disease has a different clinical picture in children younger than 5 years of age and in children aged 8 to 15 years.
   d. The disease usually involves at least two organ systems and is present for an average of 5 months before the diagnosis is made.
   e. The diagnosis is made by exclusion and is corroborated by the histologic presence of nonnecrotizing granulomas.
2. Children younger than 5 years of age
   a. Young children with sarcoidosis have a clinical triad of arthritis, uveitis, and dermatitis with an insidious onset and usually absence of intrathoracic involvement.
   b. Bone lesions may be asymptomatic; may be detected only radiographically initially; and are characterized by morning stiffness and pain, no limitation of motion, painless effusions, osteopenia, and radiographic lytic lesions. Large joints, wrists, fingers, knees, long bones, spine, and skull are affected, and fusiform swelling of the fingers is characteristic.
   c. Uveitis may be accompanied by keratoconjunctivitis; conjunctival painless, movable, yellow-brown granulomatous nodules; photophobia; papilledema; glaucoma; cataracts; optic neuritis and atrophy; retinitis; posterior synechiae; and blindness.

   d. The rash may precede the onset of arthritis, begins peripherally and then becomes diffuse, is maculopapular with erythema and scaling, may leave pitted scars, and has remissions and exacerbations.
3. Children aged 8 to 15 years
   a. The lungs, lymph nodes, skin, and eyes are affected and cause intrathoracic and extrathoracic disease. Initial symptoms are often anorexia, weight loss, lethargy, malaise, fatigue, fever, nausea, and headache.
   b. The lungs are almost always involved. The second most frequently affected organ is the lymphatic system.
   c. Pulmonary disease is characterized by a dry cough, dyspnea, chest pain or discomfort, tachypnea, diminished breath sounds, crackles, wheezes, rhonchi, and clubbing. Alveolitis develops, and fibrosis, a honeycomb lung, and cor pulmonale can ensue. Hemoptysis and thromboembolism may be present if secondary infection with *Aspergillus* occurs.
   d. Extrathoracic disease includes the following:
      (1) Hepatosplenomegaly and hepatitis secondary to granulomas
      (2) Peripheral lymphadenopathy, particularly submandibular, characterized by firm, nontender, mobile, large lymph nodes and usually generalized
      (3) Skin lesions (erythroderma, exfoliation, erythema nodosum, maculopapular lesions, papules, plaques, scars, keloids, subcutaneous granulomatous nodules, ulcerations)
      (4) Eye disease (uveitis, conjunctivitis, loss of visual acuity, photophobia, cataracts, glaucoma, lacrimal gland enlargement, proptosis)
      (5) Arthropathy (morning stiffness and pain, limited degree of motion)

(6) Salivary gland involvement (parotitis, enlargement)

(7) Uveoparotid fever syndrome (see box)

(8) Cardiac disease (conduction delay, arrhythmias, cardiomyopathy, pericardial effusion, myocarditis, cor pulmonale)

(9) Nervous system disease (seizures, aseptic meningitis, encephalitis, altered hypothalamic-pituitary axis, hydrocephalus, papilledema, space-occupying brain lesions, psychosis, facial nerve palsy, peripheral neuritis, polyneuropathy)

(10) Myopathy–skeletal

(11) Disorders of the endocrine glands (diabetes insipidus; thyroid, adrenal and pituitary disease)

(12) Bone disease (cysts of distal phalanges, metacarpals, and metatarsals)

(13) Renal disease (glomerulonephritis, nephrolithiasis, renal parenchymal granulomas, ureteral obstruction, urinary tract infections)

(14) Upper airway disease (sinusitis and rhinitis secondary to mucosal granulomas; nodules on nasal mucosa; nasal septal perforation; laryngitis; dysphagia and dyspnea resulting from edema of supraglottic and epiglottic areas, respectively).

Laboratory Findings

1. Biochemistry

   a. The elevation in the erythrocyte sedimentation rate (ESR) correlates with disease activity.

   b. Hypercalcemia occurs in <20 per cent of children with sarcoidosis. It results from abnormal extrarenal synthesis of calcitriol by activated pulmonary alveolar macrophages (PAMs), blood monocytes, and tissue granulomas, which causes increased intestinal absorption of calcium. Renal calculi and failure can develop.

   c. Hypercalciuria may be present with a normal serum calcium level. Urinary findings are usually mild and do not correlate with the severity of renal histology.

   d. Serum inorganic phosphorus and creatine kinase levels are normal.

Key Laboratory Findings: Biochemistry

Hematologic: eosinophilia*, increased ESR*, hemolytic anemia, leukopenia (<5000 cells/mm³),* thrombocytopenia

Hepatic: hyperproteinemia*, hypoalbuminemia, increased serum alkaline phosphatase level*, increased serum liver transaminase levels

Immunologic: polyclonal hyperglobulinemia*

Renal: increased blood urea nitrogen, hypercalcemia (serum calcium >11 mg/dl), hypercalciuria (>5 mg/kg of calcium per day), hyperuricemia, increased serum creatinine, decreased creatinine clearance rate, nephrolithiasis, granular casts, pyuria, proteinuria, hematuria

*Characteristic findings

   e. Serum levels of angiotensin-converting enzyme (ACE) are increased with active sarcoidosis and diminish with corticosteroid therapy.

   (1) ACE is a membrane-bound glycoprotein that converts circulating angiotensin I to active angiotensin II or inactive bradykinin. It is normally synthesized by pulmonary capillary endothelial cells, activated PAMs, and epithelial cells of the renal proximal tubules. Increased ACE production in sarcoidosis occurs in PAMs and epithelioid cells of granulomas in lymph nodes and skin. ACE is also recovered in BAL fluid in active sarcoidosis.

   (2) ACE levels may increase before clinical, radiographic, or physiologic evidence of disease. Elevated ACE levels do not correlate with pulmo-

---

Variants and Imitators of Sarcoidosis

- Löfgren syndrome: erythema nodosum, bilateral hilar adenopathy, acute iritis, arthropathy, and fever; caused by sarcoidosis, tuberculosis, and syphilis

- Lupus pernio: indurated, bluish discoloration of nose, cheeks, lips and ears; associated with bone cysts, peripheral adenopathy, ocular disease, and pulmonary fibrosis; causes disfiguring telangiectatic scars; a variant of acute sarcoidosis

- Mikulicz syndrome: ocular disease and bilateral swelling of lacrimal and salivary glands; caused by sarcoidosis, tuberculosis, and syphilis

- Sjögren syndrome: keratoconjunctivitis with or without parotid and lacrimal gland enlargement; mimics sarcoidosis

- Uveoparotid fever syndrome: uveitis, unilateral or bilateral parotid gland enlargement, facial nerve palsy, and fever; also known as Heerfordt syndrome; a variant of acute sarcoidosis

---

Key Clinical Findings: Lung Disease in Sarcoidosis

- Alveolitis
- Aspergillomas in lung cysts and bullae
- Atelectasis
- Bronchiectasis
- Chylothorax
- Hemoptysis
- Honeycomb lung
- Interstitial pneumonitis
- Nodules (solitary, multiple)
- Pleural effusion
- Pneumothorax (recurrent, tension)
- Pulmonary edema
- Pulmonary fibrosis
- Pulmonary hypertension
- Right middle lobe syndrome
- Stenosis (bronchus, trachea, subglottis)

nary function alterations but do parallel the extent of extrapulmonary lesions. Caution should be used in interpretation of levels (see box).

(3) Immunofluorescence staining of skin and lymph node lesions can identify ACE activity even when serum ACE levels are normal.

Serum ACE Levels

Baseline serum ACE levels are elevated in normal neonates and in children aged 4 to 13 years, compared with adults; they remain higher in boys than in girls before returning to adult levels at age 18 years. Premature infants have higher ACE levels than do full-term infants. The following diseases are associated with increased serum ACE levels:

- Diabetes mellitus
- Gaucher disease
- Histoplasmosis
- Hyperthyroidism
- Leprosy
- Primary biliary cirrhosis
- Sarcoidosis

---

f. Serum lysozyme levels are increased with active sarcoidosis and return to normal with disease inactivity and corticosteroid therapy. Lysozyme normally occurs in polymorphonuclear leukocytes and monocytes and is released by macrophages and epithelioid cells in active granulomas.

2. Immunology
   a. Skin test anergy results from cellular immune dysfunction. Lymphopenia, decreased T lymphocytes, a reduced CD4+/CD8+ ratio, and immune complexes are present in peripheral blood.
   b. BAL fluid in active sarcoidosis has elevated levels of T lymphocytes, PAMs, immunoglobulins, total hemolytic complement (CH50), histamine, and interleukins and an elevated CD4+/CD8+ ratio. The levels return to normal with inactive disease and corticosteroid therapy. The normal ratio of 9 PAMs/1 lymphocyte in BAL fluid is altered to 9 lymphocytes/1 PAM in sarcoidosis.

3. Elevated serum levels of ACE and lysozyme and elevated BAL markers are not specific for sarcoidosis, but their serial measurements are helpful in evaluating disease activity and therapeutic efficacy.

4. *Histology*—The diagnosis is suggested by the identification of non-necrotizing granulomas in tissue biopsy specimens, such as lung parenchyma, bronchi, skin, lymph nodes, scalene fat pad, conjunctiva, nasal mucosa, bone, bone marrow, liver, muscle, salivary glands, kidney, and testis. Granulomas are more likely to be identified before the development of fibrosis. An organ can appear functionally normal yet have diffuse granulomas. The use of fine-needle aspiration instead of an open surgical technique to obtain appropriate tissue for biopsy has been successful in children.

5. *Pulmonary function testing*—Decreased lung volumes with normal or slightly elevated airflow rates characterize the restrictive lung disease of sarcoidosis. Lung volumes, lung compliance, and diffusing capacity are reduced as a result of granulomas and fibrosis. Bronchial wall granulomas can also cause airflow limitation, reduced airflow rates, and an obstructive pattern. Nonuniform diminution in lung compliance results in ventilation-perfusion imbalance. Arterial hypoxemia occurs initially with exercise and later at rest. Serial pulmonary function measurements are useful in evaluating the course of the disease.

6. *Other testing*—Mediastinoscopy and transbronchial biopsy can help determine the cause of hilar adenopathy. The presence of a cardiac arrhythmia, conduction delay, or right and left ventricular hypertrophy may be detected by electrocardiography, whereas echocardiography can identify cardiac chamber enlargement and valvular dysfunction. An electroencephalogram can reveal the occurrence of abnormal electrical activity and seizures. A slit-lamp eye examination to determine the presence of eye disease, a renal scan to observe kidney function, and renal arteriography to detect renal microvasculature abnormalities should also be considered in the evaluation of sarcoidosis.

Radiographic Findings

1. *General*—The chest radiograph is abnormal in approximately 95 per cent of patients with sarcoidosis. Bilateral hilar adenopathy is the most common radiographic finding in children and adults and may occur with or without parenchymal abnormalities. Other radiographic changes include paratracheal and mediastinal adenopathy, a mass lesion that may cavitate, diffuse interstitial fibrosis, interstitial and alveolar edema causing "alveolar sarcoid," nodular lesions, atelectasis, a honeycomb pattern, and pleural and pericardial effusions. Oblique views of the chest and airway fluoroscopy in addition to anteroposterior and lateral chest films can help determine the presence of mediastinal adenopathy.

2. Radiographic changes are staged according to the extent of disease. The stages are helpful in identifying the severity and prognosis of pulmonary involvement.
   a. Stage I consists of bilateral hilar adenopathy, which is frequently accompanied by right paratracheal adenopathy. It occurs with acute, reversible disease and is often associated with reversible systemic signs and symptoms (e.g., acute iritis, erythema nodosum). Hilar adenopathy alone is the most common radiographic finding in adults.
   b. Stage II is characterized by bilateral hilar adenopathy and parenchymal disease consisting of interstitial infiltrates and/or nodules. This is the most common stage in children.
   c. Stage III consists of interstitial infiltrates without hilar adenopathy and is associated with interstitial fibrosis, bullae, cysts, a honeycomb lung, right ventricular hypertrophy, and pulmonary hypertension. It carries a poor prognosis.

3. A gallium scintiscan can identify pulmonary and extrapulmonary disease. Accumulation of radioactive-tagged gallium-67 isotope in pulmonary granulomatous

inflammatory lesions indicates activity of lymphocytes, PAMs, and polymorphonuclear leukocytes and can reveal the presence and extent of alveolitis. The scan is useful for evaluation of disease in stages II and III but is not specific for sarcoidosis. A negative scan may be helpful in determining that treatment is not needed.

4. Computed tomography scans of the chest, abdomen, and brain can help evaluate disease in these areas. Isolated anterior or posterior mediastinal, subcarinal, and abdominal lymphadenopathy can be detected. Magnetic resonance imaging can also identify brain lesions.

Treatment

1. Since sarcoidosis has an unknown cause, there is no specific therapy. Corticosteroids are used to suppress severe generalized manifestations, acute signs and symptoms, calcium alterations, and radiographic stages II and III disease. Therapy is used for
   a. Progressive lung disease, particularly with arterial hypoxemia
   b. Uveitis
   c. Myocardial disease
   d. Central nervous system involvement, particularly facial nerve palsy
   e. Renal disease with persistent hypercalcemia and hypercalciuria
   f. Arthritis
   g. Salivary and lacrimal gland lesions
   h. Hypersplenism
   i. Severe hepatic disease
   j. Disfiguring skin lesions.

2. Corticosteroid therapy usually causes transient improvement but may prevent progressive organ dysfunction. Disease of less than 2 years' duration responds better to steroids than does disease lasting longer. However, it is unclear whether corticosteroid therapy shortens the course of sarcoidosis.

3. Corticosteroids suppress alveolitis and granuloma formation. They may improve pulmonary symptoms, but they rarely alter the radiographic changes. They can alter pulmonary function, with resultant increases in the vital capacity, lung compliance, and diffusing capacity in radiographic stage II disease. Steroids normalize serum and urinary calcium levels, which remain normal years after discontinuation of the drug.

4. The dosage of corticosteroids is 1 to 2 mg/kg/day of prednisone (maximum, 60 mg/day), or 0.75 mg/kg/day of triamcinolone (maximum, 45 mg/day), in 3 to 4 divided doses. After clinical improvement appears, the steroid dose is tapered to a maintenance dose of 15 mg of prednisone on alternate days for a total of 6 months of therapy.

5. Ocular sarcoidosis is treated with 0.5 to 1 per cent corticosteroid ointment or drops in combination with systemic steroids. The addition of 1 per cent atropine ointment to maintain pupillary dilatation aids the treatment of uveitis.

6. Skin lesions may be treated with corticosteroid ointment as an adjunct to systemic steroids.

7. Colchicine has been used in children to treat arthritis, but other drugs, such as azathioprine, methotrexate, chloroquine, chlorambucil, oxyphenbutazone, and potassium para-aminobenzoate, which are given to adults, have had limited use in children.

Key Treatment

- Corticosteroids

Prognosis

1. Pediatric sarcoidosis usually is not progressive. It is usually a self-limiting disease with resolution of symptoms within 2 to 3 years without therapy. Radiographic stage I disease resolves without therapy.

2. Children have a better prognosis and lower morbidity and mortality than do adults. Mortality is approximately 5 per cent in children. Chronic sequelae occur in 10 to 20 per cent of children, with symptomatic patients having more complications.

3. A good prognosis with remission is associated with constitutional symptoms (malaise, fever, weight loss, erythema nodosum), acute iritis, arthralgias, and bilateral hilar adenopathy. A poor prognosis occurs with an insidious onset, pulmonary fibrosis, bone cysts, hypercalcemia, chronic iridocyclitis, and lupus pernio or skin plaques.

4. Radiographic findings determine the prognosis of the lung disease. Stage I has a good prognosis, even if granulomas and alveolitis are observed on histology. A poor prognosis occurs with radiographic parenchymal disease. Recurrences rarely are seen after resolution of pulmonary disease.

5. Changes in chest radiography, pulmonary function testing, and histologic findings do not correlate; that is, all three may not be abnormal simultaneously.

6. Exacerbations occur in 50 per cent of children, regardless of whether steroid therapy was used or spontaneous improvement occurred. Early diagnosis and treatment can prevent complications, including respiratory and renal failure and blindness.

Bibliography

Clark SK: Sarcoidosis in children. Pediatr Dermatol 1987;4:291–299.

DeRemee RA: Sarcoidosis. Mayo Clin Proc 1995;70:177–181.

Marcille R, McCarthy M, Barton JW, et al: Long-term outcome of pediatric sarcoidosis with emphasis on pulmonary status. Chest 1992;102:1444–1449.

Sharma OP: Pulmonary sarcoidosis and corticosteroids. Am Rev Respir Dis 1993;147:1598–1600.

Thomas PD, Hunninghake GW: Current concepts of the pathogenesis of sarcoidosis. Am Rev Respir Dis 1987;135:747–760.

206 Pulmonary Hemosiderosis

Howard Eigen

Definition

Pulmonary hemosiderosis is a rare condition or clinical syndrome consisting of ongoing pulmonary bleeding in which iron from red blood cells collects as hemosiderin in the lung parenchyma.

Etiology

Pulmonary hemosiderosis is a final common pathway for a number of disorders that result in bleeding from the lung. These disorders include Goodpasture syndrome, systemic lupus erythematosus, and so-called idiopathic pulmonary hemosiderosis. The ongoing bleeding results in sequestering of iron in the lung. Pulmonary hemosiderosis has been associated with milk allergy, under which circumstances it is called Heiner syndrome.

Epidemiology

This is an extremely rare condition in children, with approximately one case in 4 million children.

Clinical Findings

1. The child usually presents with recurrent episodes of respiratory distress, patchy infiltrates on chest radiograph, and iron deficiency anemia. Pulmonary symptoms may be mild, with only episodic tachypnea, cough, or wheeze and low-grade fever. The respiratory distress may be overshadowed by the anemia. New infiltrates seen on chest radiograph may clear in 1 to 2 weeks. It is unusual for children with pulmonary hemosiderosis to have hemoptysis or blood-stained sputum at diagnosis.
2. Diagnosis is made by the identification of hemosiderin-laden alveolar macrophages in the sputum or in material obtained from bronchoalveolar lavage (BAL) or open lung biopsy. Because young children do not produce sputum, the latter two procedures are often necessary. BAL is generally preferable to open lung biopsy because it is less invasive, but lung biopsy may become necessary to define the exact pulmonary pathology and to obtain tissue for immunofluorescence studies to allow the diagnosis of the underlying illness.
3. A key differential point is to assess the presence of other vascular disorders (e.g., glomerulonephritis, which would indicate the presence of Goodpasture syndrome) or of collagen vascular disease (e.g., rheumatoid arthritis, systemic lupus erythematosus, Wegener granulomatosis). This is particularly important because the nonpulmonary aspects of the syndrome may overshadow the pulmonary aspects as a cause for prolonged morbidity or even mortality.

Key Clinical Finding

• Alveolar macrophages containing hemosiderin in BAL fluid

Laboratory Findings

1. Anemia
2. Heme-positive stools
3. Indicators of underlying collagen vascular disease or the presence of milk precipitins may be helpful in the diagnostic evaluation.

Key Laboratory Findings

• Anemia

• Intermittent pulmonary infiltrates

Treatment

1. There is no single therapy for idiopathic pulmonary hemosiderosis. Many reports exist of treatment with systemic corticosteroids that can be used either chronically or to mitigate acute exacerbations. We generally use prednisone orally at a dose of 2 mg/kg of body weight up to 80 mg for acute exacerbations of bleeding. We use the same dose to treat the child who has an upper respiratory or lower respiratory viral infection in an attempt to preclude bleeding.
2. The repeated bleeding episodes lead to an accumulation of iron in the lung parenchyma, which in turn leads to progressive fibrosis. This can have a profound effect on lung function, and children typically do not live beyond the teenage years. More recently, we have had a patient who had a successful lung transplantation for idiopathic pulmonary hemosiderosis and has not had rebleeding in the transplanted lung.

Key Treatment

• Prednisone, 2 mg/kg/day, during bleeding episodes

207 Congenital Malformations

Harvey P. Bieler

A variety of bronchopulmonary malformations may occur as a result of disordered interactions among primordial lung components between 4 and 16 weeks of embryogenesis. Aside from pulmonary sequestration, most congenital bronchopulmonary malformations (e.g., bronchogenic cysts, congenital cystic adenomatoid malformations, congenital lobar emphysema) lead to presentation within the first year of life with moderate to severe (or even life-threatening) respiratory distress. When the diagnosis is made later in life, it is usually in patients who are asymptomatic or have only minimal respiratory complaints.

Bronchogenic Cysts

Pathogenesis
1. Congenital benign masses, which arise from abnormal fetal budding of a tracheobronchial segment
2. Usually located in the mediastinum or subcarinal area, but can "migrate" to extrapulmonary locations
3. Accounts for approximately 10 per cent of mediastinal masses in children
4. Can be unilocular or multilocular

Clinical Findings
1. Stridor is most common, but cough, dyspnea, or feeding intolerance may be seen.
2. Older children and adults are often asymptomatic, with the lesion being identified on a chest radiograph done for other reasons.
3. Malignant degeneration rarely occurs.

Key Clinical Finding: Bronchogenic Cyst
- Stridor

Radiographic Findings
1. Often discovered on routine radiograph; typically appears as a smooth, oval or round, homogeneous noncalcified density in close proximity to the major airways.
2. Computed tomography (CT) scanning may be helpful in defining exact cyst location and relevant anatomic details. Small cysts may be seen only on CT examination.

Treatment
1. Surgical excision usually is recommended in both children and adults.
2. Some experts have recommended close observation in asymptomatic patients with smaller cysts; others advocate early intervention out of concern that delaying surgery increases perioperative complications and the likelihood of infection.

Key Treatment: Bronchogenic Cyst
- Surgical excision

Pulmonary Sequestration

Pathogenesis
1. The sequestration consists of a mass of abnormal lung tissue that does not communicate with the tracheobronchial tree and is supplied by an anomalous systemic artery.
2. It can be intralobar (the more common variety) or extralobar (discussed in the next section).
3. In intralobar pulmonary sequestration, the abnormal lung tissue is located within healthy lung parenchyma and is contained within the visceral pleura, typically within a posterobasal segment.

Clinical Findings
1. This is a major unrecognized cause of recurrent pneumonia in children.
2. The common presenting complaint is either repeated or chronic localized pulmonary infections or an intrathoracic mass in an asymptomatic child.
3. Rarely, neonates and young children present in heart failure and pulmonary edema as a result of a large shunt from the aberrant artery through the sequestration into the pulmonary venous system.

Key Clinical Finding: Pulmonary Sequestration
- Recurrent pneumonia

Radiographic Findings
1. Delay in diagnosis may occur because of confusion on radiograph with pneumatocele, pneumonia, bronchiectasis, lung abscess, or neoplasm.
2. Routine radiography and CT scan are usually sufficient to make the diagnosis.
3. Selective arteriography may be needed to demonstrate the aberrant arterial supply from the abdominal or descending aorta.

Treatment
1. Lobectomy is often the treatment of choice for intralobar pulmonary sequestration.
2. Because reinfection is common in a poorly drained, sequestered segment, pulmonary resection in a quiescent phase is often the only reasonable treatment.

Key Treatment: Pulmonary Sequestration

- Surgery (lobectomy)

Extralobar Pulmonary Sequestration

1. Abnormal lung tissue has its own distinct pleural invest-
ment and maintains complete anatomic and physiologic
separation from the adjacent normal lung. Typically it
occurs below the lower lobe.
2. It often is associated with other anomalies, for example,
such foregut malformations as diaphragmatic hernia.
3. It often is asymptomatic and therefore may be underre-
ported.

Congenital Cystic Adenomatoid Malformation

Pathogenesis
1. Thought to be an overgrowth of terminal bronchiolar
structures
2. Occurs more commonly in the lower lobes
3. Classified into three types by the presence and size of the
cystic and adenomatoid components

Clinical Findings
1. Patients present with varying degrees of respiratory distress.
2. In the neonate, it is common to see tachypnea, retractions,
or cyanosis within hours of birth.
3. The older the infant, the less respiratory distress is present.
4. Only about 10 per cent of patients present after the
first year of life, often because of repeated respiratory
infections.
5. The diagnosis should be considered when a newborn
develops respiratory distress with decreased breath
sounds on one side.

**Key Clinical Finding: Congenital Cystic
Adenomatoid Malformation**

- Dyspnea

Radiographic Findings
1. Chest radiography typically demonstrates multiple cystic
structures in one hemithorax, with a shift of the mediastinum to the contralateral side.
2. Insertion of a nasogastric tube often aids in confirming
the mediastinal shift and the location of the stomach. The
stomach is located below the diaphragm, which distinguishes this lesion from congenital diaphragmatic hernia.

Treatment
Although some authors advocate observation in selected
cases, excision of the affected lobe or lobes is usually recommended.

**Key Treatment: Congenital Cystic Adenomatoid
Malformation**

- Surgical excision

Late complications of this malformation include the following:

1. Cardiorespiratory collapse as a result of pressure on surrounding structures by the expanding, affected lobe
2. Risk of pulmonary infection
3. A small but defined risk of malignant transformation of
these lesions in young adults

Congenital Lobar Emphysema

Pathogenesis
1. The precise nature of the lesion is not known, and the
cause is often unclear.
2. It is most common in the left upper lobe, occurring less
often in the right middle lobe.
3. Associated congenital anomalies of the heart and great
vessels can occur in as many as 15 per cent of cases.

Clinical Findings
1. Most patients are discovered by 6 months of age, but
asymptomatic school-age patients may be discovered
when chest radiographs are taken for other reasons.
2. During the neonatal period, those who are symptomatic
tend to have more severe, progressive disease, which
occasionally can cause acute and rapid deterioration resulting in respiratory failure and death. Dyspnea, tachypnea, cyanosis, and feeding intolerance are common.
3. Patients from 1 to 6 months of age tend to experience
mild respiratory symptoms.
4. Physical examination often reveals wheezing, crackles,
retractions, and cough. The involved hemithorax is often
more prominent and demonstrates little movement with
respiration. Anterior bowing of the sternum and herniation of the affected lobe across the midline may also be
seen. On the affected side, percussion reveals hyperresonance with diminished breath sounds.

**Key Clinical Findings: Congenital Lobar
Emphysema**

- Tachypnea
- Dyspnea

Radiographic Findings
1. In most cases, plain chest radiographs coupled with a
typical clinical presentation are sufficient for the diagnosis to be made.
2. Chest CT may be useful to identify any associated mediastinal mass or vascular anomaly.

Treatment
1. For patients with severe or life-threatening respiratory
distress and those who have had persistent or progressive

symptoms not responding to medical management, excision of the diseased lobe is recommended.
2. For asymptomatic patients and those with mild symptoms, conservative monitoring alone is favored. It has been shown that newborns with only mild symptoms at presentation may not necessarily benefit from surgery, because they can develop comparable improvements in pulmonary function over time without surgical resection.

Key Treatment: Congenital Lobar Emphysema

• Surgical excision for symptomatic patients

208 Foreign Body Aspiration

Michelle S. Howenstine

Definition

Foreign body aspiration is the accidental inhalation of foreign material into the airways or esophagus which may result in asphyxiation or severe lung damage.

Etiology and Epidemiology

1. Aspirated foreign bodies cause 500 deaths per year in the United States in children younger than 5 five years old. The highest incidence of aspiration occurs between 1 and 2 years of age. Children of this age group are at highest risk because of their limited mastication skills and the common practice of placing foreign objects in the mouth as part of their active exploration of the environment. Materials most often aspirated include the following:
   a. Small objects with smooth, round, or cylindrical shape (e.g., peanuts, grapes, beads, popcorn kernels)
   b. Hard or tough foods (e.g., carrots, frozen foods)
   c. Compressible foods that can fill the airway (e.g., hot dogs, skinned meats)
2. Older children also aspirate, but the items aspirated differ and can include any food items not properly chewed or nonfood items habitually chewed, such as grasses, pen tops, and small toy parts.

Pathophysiology

1. Following aspiration, the foreign body lodges in the trachea, major bronchus, or smaller airways, depending on the physical characteristics of the object and the physical size of the child.
2. The most common locations in the respiratory tract are the trachea or larynx (18%) and the main bronchi (70%).
3. Esophageal foreign bodies are common in younger children and can cause significant tracheal compression, stridor, or cough. Coins, safety pins, and small toys are among the more common items.
4. The initial insult is related to the degree of airway occlusion and injury (e.g., hypoxia, bleeding). Prolonged retention of the foreign object may result in atelectasis, inflammation, infection, and bronchiectasis.
5. Peanuts (which are not true nuts, but beans) contain arachidic acid, which is necrotizing and causes chemical pneumonia when aspirated into the bronchi. True nuts do not contain this substance.

Clinical Picture

1. The initial clinical presentation varies according to the size and shape of the foreign body and its location in the respiratory tract. The initial symptoms vary from sudden and severe respiratory distress secondary to an occluded upper airway to an annoying cough in a child with a small retained peripheral foreign body (Table 208–1).
2. In many cases, there is a variable period after aspiration in which there are no symptoms. Later, atelectasis, progressive inflammation, and infection may develop in segments distal to the obstruction. Signs and symptoms of chronic retention of the foreign body, which are present in approximately 30 per cent of aspiration events, include the following:
   a. Persistent cough or wheezing
   b. Shortness of breath with activity
   c. Fever
   d. Persistent infiltrate on chest radiograph

TABLE 208–1. SIGNS AND SYMPTOMS OF FOREIGN BODY ASPIRATION

LOCATION	SIGNS AND SYMPTOMS
Supraglottic region or larynx	Dyspnea Stridor Retractions Croupy cough Drooling
Trachea	Dyspnea Stridor or wheezing Retractions Cough
Bronchus	Asymmetry of chest movement Unilateral wheezing Cough
Small airway	Asymmetric breath sounds Wheezing Cough

e. Hemoptysis or sputum production

f. Asymmetric auscultated breath sounds or adventitial breath sounds

g. Constitutional symptoms, including weight loss, night sweats, and vomiting

Key Clinical Findings

- Cough
- Wheezing
- Asymmetric breath sounds

Laboratory Findings

1. There are no specific laboratory tests that are helpful in establishing the diagnosis of foreign body aspiration. An elevated erythrocyte sedimentation rate and/or leukocytosis may be indicative of infection in chronic cases.

2. Oxygen saturation should be measured in any patient with respiratory symptoms, and arterial blood gas monitoring is recommended for patients with severe respiratory distress.

Radiographic Changes

1. Radiographs are often helpful for diagnosis and localization of foreign bodies in the airways. Most foreign bodies are not radiopaque, and radiographic findings are related to the pattern and degree of airway obstruction. Standard chest radiographs are normal in 80 per cent of children with aspirated foreign bodies. Chest radiographs may show abnormalities in a third of cases in which an object is not localized at bronchoscopy (false positive).

2. Plain radiographs of the chest are initially obtained in the anteroposterior and lateral views. Obstructive hyperinflation is the most common finding in acute foreign body aspiration; atelectasis or infiltrate is found frequently in the case of chronically retained foreign bodies.

   a. Films obtained at the end of the inspiratory and expiratory cycles of respiration are helpful in cases of partial airway obstruction, in which the "ball-valve" effect may cause air trapping and incomplete deflation of the affected side during expiration.

   b. The end-inspiratory film may demonstrate incomplete expansion.

   c. Volume loss on atelectasis is seen with a chronically occluded airway.

   d. Right and left lateral decubitus films may demonstrate partial obstruction in a less cooperative patient; the dependent lung shows incomplete deflation.

3. Fluoroscopy may help locate a foreign body, especially in the uncooperative patient.

   a. Obstructive hyperinflation, mediastinal shift, and limited diaphragmatic excursion are demonstrated on the side of the partially occluded airway.

   b. Abnormalities also occur in patients with laryngeal or tracheal foreign bodies; these include paradoxical

mediastinal movement, with an increase in the size of the mediastinal structures on inspiration.

4. Pneumothorax, air extravasation, pleural effusion, and bronchiectatic changes occur infrequently.

Treatment

1. Attempts at manual removal of the foreign body should not be made unless the airway is totally occluded. In that case, basic airway resuscitation is initiated.

2. Rigid endoscopy with a ventilating bronchoscope is the procedure of choice when the diagnosis of a foreign body is suspected or established. A separate channel within the bronchoscope is used to insert foreign body forceps and remove the material. Rarely, a large tracheal foreign body is difficult to extract and may require simultaneous tracheotomy for airway maintenance and possibly as a route of foreign body removal. Sometimes a small peripheral object is removed with the assistance of a Fogarty catheter.

3. Thoracotomy with bronchotomy is necessary in the unusual case of extraction failure or persistent unexplained disease.

4. Flexible bronchoscopy is helpful in situations in which there is no definitive history of foreign body aspiration but there is evidence of chronic or recurrent localized pulmonary disease which suggests airway obstruction.

5. The use of chest physiotherapy or bronchodilators before removal of the foreign body is not indicated and may be dangerous in a patient suspected of having an aspirated foreign object because of the risk of dislodgement and movement into another airway. Chest physiotherapy may be beneficial after removal, especially if concurrent infection or inflammation is suspected.

6. Antibiotic use should be dictated by culture results. Vegetable matter is especially irritative to the lungs and may cause pneumonitis. Glucocorticosteroids may reduce edema related to instrumentation of the airway or effects of the retained material.

7. Complications of rigid bronchoscopy include fever, pneumothorax, retained foreign material, and bronchospasm or airway edema.

Key Treatment

- Rigid bronchoscopy

Prevention

1. Risks for foreign body aspiration include environmental and developmental factors. Suggestions for prevention include the following:

   a. Parents should avoid giving small round firm foods or foods that are cylindrical and easily compressible (e.g., peanuts, carrots, popcorn, hot dogs) to children younger than 4 years of age.

   b. Caretakers should check a child's environment for objects that are easily placed in the mouth and propelled into the airway. Children should be supervised during feedings and should not combine eating with playing or running.

2. Routine education regarding potential foreign body as-

piration and instructions on resuscitation of the child with airway obstruction should be included as part of well-child care.

Bibliography

Blazer S, Naveh Y, Friedman A: Foreign body in the airway: A review of 200 cases. Am J Dis Child 1980;134:68–71.

Hight EW, Philippart AI, Hertzler JH: The treatment of retained foreign body in the pediatric airway. J Pediatr Surg 1981; 16:694–671.

Svensson G: Foreign bodies in the tracheobronchial tree: Special reference to experience of 97 children. Int J Pediatr Otorhinolaryngol 1985;8:243–251.

Wagner MH: Foreign body aspiration. *In* Loughlin GM, Eigen H (eds): Respiratory Disease in Children: Diagnosis and Management. Baltimore, Williams & Wilkins, 1994, pp 343–350.

209 Status Asthmaticus

Fred Leickly

Critical State

Definition

Status asthmaticus is an acute, severe, and intractable episode of asthma that is refractory to bronchodilators and requires hospitalization for more intensive therapy.

Etiology

1. The agents responsible for status asthmaticus are the same as those that trigger less severe asthma. Included in this list are viral respiratory tract infections; allergens such as pollens, mold spores, house dust mites, cockroaches, and animal danders; and irritants such as cigarette smoke and cold air. Nonadherence to a previously prescribed asthma management plan is also a major contributor to refractory asthma events.
2. The medical history helps to establish the key features of the acute event. Inquire about the duration of the event, the presumed precipitating factors, and the rate of symptom progression. Also ask what therapy has been taken (dose and timing), in what ways this event resembles prior episodes, and about the time course of prior episodes.
3. Risk factors for status asthmaticus include frequent asthma attacks, recent hospitalization, intensive care unit (ICU) admissions, delay in seeking care, and recent use of high-dose steroids.

Pathogenesis

1. Key features include airway obstruction, inflammation, and hyperresponsiveness.
2. Release of mediators from inflammatory cells within the airway mucosa leads to bronchospasm, edema of the mucosal surface, and mucus plugging of the airways. Smooth muscle hypertrophy, hyperplasia, and spasm occur. The submucosal glands are also hypertrophic and produce excessive mucus.
3. Ventilation and perfusion become mismatched, leading to hypoxemia. As the obstruction progresses, the hypoxia worsens and hypercapnia occurs. Measures of airflow (1-second forced expiratory volume, peak flow level) decrease.
4. With increasing airway obstruction, air trapping occurs. Because the patient is breathing at higher lung volumes, work of breathing is increased. This increase in work of breathing requires the use of the accessory muscles of respiration. Fatigue and respiratory failure may occur.
5. Refractoriness to the bronchodilators may result from the edema of the mucosal surface and mucus plugging. The bronchial smooth muscle may become resistant to the actions of the bronchodilators because of acidosis or purported subsensitivity of the β receptors of the airway.

Clinical Findings

1. The usual presenting symptoms are dyspnea, shortness of breath, and wheezing.
2. The clinical signs that best reflect the severity of the situation are the use of the accessory muscles of respiration (i.e., the intercostal and sternocleidomastoid muscles) and the presence of pulsus paradoxus >20 to 40 mm Hg.
3. The physical examination may also show the following:
   a. *General*—agitation, restlessness, altered consciousness, fatigue, diaphoresis, cyanosis
   b. *Skin*—crackles consistent with subcutaneous air leak
   c. *Chest*—orthopnea, tachypnea, and cough. Infants may show grunting and flaring of the nose. The presence of a silent chest is an ominous sign (wheezing requires air movement).
4. Two additional vital signs are pulse oximetry and the peak flow. Hypoxia is present in status asthmaticus. Peak flows values are low, usually less than 25 per cent of the personal best or predicted value for age, sex, and height.

Critical State *Continued*

Key Clinical Findings

- Wheezing (unless very severe)
- Dyspnea
- Agitation
- Cyanosis
- Pulsus paradoxus

Laboratory Assessment

1. Oxygen level is assessed by arterial blood gas analysis or by pulse oximetry. If the oxygen saturation is less than 92 per cent, severe disease is present.

2. Carbon dioxide level is assessed by arterial blood gas analysis. Carbon dioxide levels of 40 mmHg or greater indicate severe asthma.

3. The arterial blood gas analysis provides objective evidence of the severity of the airway obstruction and may predict impending respiratory failure.

4. Peak flow levels, when they are determined, are valuable in assessing the response to the bronchodilators.

5. The chest radiograph may have utility when complicating factors are present. Examination of the chest with decreased breath sounds or localized wheezing and the suspicion of an air leak is an indication for a radiograph. Abnormal findings may include atelectasis, pneumonitis, pneumomediastinum, or pneumothorax.

6. Other laboratory studies include the following:
   a. *Serum electrolytes*—This determination forms the basis for decisions regarding the requirements for intravascular fluids. The use of β agonists may cause a decrease in the serum potassium levels.
   b. *Urinalysis*—This is done to assist in determining hydration status. Theophylline level is determined if appropriate.

Key Laboratory Tests

- Pulse oximetry
- Arterial blood gas analysis (oxygen, carbon dioxide)
- Peak flow level

Treatment

The objective of treatment is to improve the ventilation-perfusion mismatch, which in turn improves gas exchange and thereby decreases the work of breathing.

1. *Oxygen*—The first step in the treatment of status asthmaticus is the provision of oxygen. The goal is to keep the oxygen saturation higher than 95 per cent. Delivery of humidified oxygen is through a face mask, nasal cannula, or tent, depending on the child's age. The initial oxygen concentration delivered should be at least 40 per cent; the pulse oximeter is checked and the amount of oxygen changed accordingly.

2. Sympathomimetic agents, delivered by inhalation or by injection, help relieve bronchospasm. If nebulized therapy fails and there is minimal movement of air, injectable sympathomimetics should be tried before intubation or the use of intravenous sympathomimetics is considered.
   a. *Nebulized sympathomimetics*—Aerosols are given with appropriate oxygen. Note that aerosol treatments may initially increase the ventilation-perfusion mismatch and worsen the hypoxemia.
      (1) Albuterol (Proventil, Ventolin), 0.5 per cent (5 mg/ml), 0.02 ml/kg per dose (maximum, 1.0 ml) every 20 minutes times 3 or continuously at this level in an intensive care unit (ICU)
      (2) Terbutaline (Brethine), 1 mg/ml, 0.5 to 1.0 ml per dose (maximum, 1.0 ml) every 20 minutes times 3 or continuously at this level in an ICU
   b. Injectible sympathomimetics
      (1) Epinephrine, 1/1000, 0.01 ml/kg (maximum, 0.3 ml), SQ every 20 minutes times 3
      (2) Terbutaline (Brethine), 1 mg/ml, 0.01 ml/kg (maximum, 0.25 ml), SQ every 20 minutes times 3
   c. Intravenous sympathomimetics are given only in the ICU.
   d. After the first hour of sympathomimetic therapy, the frequency of subsequent use is a function of the response obtained. Gradually increase the interval between treatments to every 4 to 6 hours.

3. Corticosteroids may take 6 hours to begin to show their clinical effect. Because of this delay in the onset of action, corticosteroid administration should be started early in the treatment of status asthmaticus. Potential beneficial effects from the reversal of β-agonist insensitivity have been observed as early as 1 hour after their use. The optimal dose of the corticosteroids is unknown. Methylprednisolone may be given at 1 to 2 mg/kg as a loading dose followed by 1 mg/kg IV every 6 hours.

4. Theophylline continues to occupy a controversial position in the care of the asthmatic child. There is no evidence to support the contention that the addition of theophylline in a patient already on maximal doses of sympathomimetic agents causes additional bronchodilation. This is especially true during the first few hours of emergency treatment. When there is impending respiratory failure, add theophylline to avoid the need for more aggressive therapy.
   a. A dose of 1 mg/kg of aminophylline increases the blood level of theophylline by 2 μg/ml. The usual

Critical State *Continued*

loading dose is 6 mg/kg given intravenously over 20 to 30 minutes

b. Intravenous maintenance rates of theophylline are age dependent:

(1) Age 2 to 6 months–0.5 mg/kg/hour

(2) Age 9 to 16 months–0.8 mg/kg/hour

(3) Age 1 to 9 years–1.0 mg/kg/hour

(4) Age >9 years–0.8 mg/kg/hour.

c. For patients with congestive heart failure, cor pulmonale, or liver disease, give 0.3 mg/kg/hour of theophylline.

d. Keep the theophylline level between 5 to 15 μg/ml. Check the level of theophylline 1 to 2 hours after administration of the bolus. Reload as needed, but do not adjust the infusion rate until a steady state for theophylline has been reached (usually 4 to 5 half-lives) at about 12 to 18 hours.

5. Intubation is reserved for dire emergencies. If at all possible, this procedure should be done at a tertiary care facility.

6. Fluid status should be maintained normal—do not over hydrate. Maintain fluid and electrolyte status with 5 per cent dextrose in water or with 0.23 per cent or 40 mEq/L saline at 1500 ml/m²/day. Antidiuretic hormone secretion may occur and lead to water overload in patients with severe status asthmaticus. Serum electrolytes and urine specific gravity should be monitored.

7. Antibiotics are useful only when there is evidence of a bacterial infection.

8. Anticholinergic agents (e.g., atropine, ipratropium) are bronchodilators with a slower onset of action, compared with the β agonists. Their role in acute asthma is unclear.

9. Admission criteria

a. Peak flow <40 per cent of baseline (personal best or predicted value)

b. Pulsus paradoxus >15 mm Hg

c. Oxygen saturation <91 per cent

d. Occurrence of tachycardia, tachypnea, use of accessory muscles, or severe dyspnea

10. Hospital management

a. Respiratory status, oxygen saturation, and peak flow levels are monitored.

b. Treatment includes administration of oxygen, frequent nebulizations with albuterol (every 3 to 6 hours), methylprednisolone, and possibly theophylline.

11. ICU admission criteria—The above-mentioned issues plus the need for nebulized sympathomimetics more often than every 3 hours, increased O_2 requirements, the use of sympathomimetic agents by infusion, the presence of an arterial line, and the need to intubate the patient.

Key Treatment

- Oxygen

- Sympathomimetic drugs

- Assisted ventilation

Bibliography

DeNicola L, Monem G, Gayle M, Kisson N: Treatment of critical status asthmaticus in children. Pediatr Crit Care 1994; 41:1293–1324.

Murphy S, Kelly W: Management of acute asthma. Pediatrician 1991;18:287–300.

Provisional Committee on Quality Improvement: Practice parameters: The office management of acute exacerbations of asthma in children. Pediatrics 1994;93:119–126.

Rachelefsky G. Asthma update: New approaches and partnership. J Pediatr Health Care 1995;9:12–21.

Spector S, Nickles R (eds): Practice parameters for the diagnosis and treatment of asthma. J Allergy Clin Immunol 1995;96(Pt 2):707–870.

210 Epiglottitis

Michelle S. Howenstine

Critical State

Definition

Epiglottitis is an acute swelling of the glottic structures caused by bacterial infection. It is a true medical emergency and requires rapid, accurate diagnosis and treatment to avoid airway obstruction.

Etiology

Epiglottitis involves infection of the supraglottic structures, usually with *Haemophilus influenzae* type b (HIB). On rare occasions other pathogens are involved, including *Streptococcus pneumoniae*, *Staphylococcus aureus*, β-hemolytic streptococcus, and *H. influenzae* type a.

Epidemiology

Epiglottitis occurs throughout the year but is more common in the winter months. Eighty percent of infected children are younger than 5 years of age, with the peak incidence between 2 and 6 years of age. Since the institution of the HIB vaccine, the incidence appears to be declining, and epiglottitis currently accounts for only 1 to 10 of every 10,000 pediatric admissions. Older children may be affected by supraglottitis that is more indolent and is caused by group A streptococcus. There may be genetic and immunogenic factors which predispose individuals to invasive HIB disease.

Pathophysiology

A systemic blood infection with HIB precedes the seeding of the serosal surfaces of the supraglottic structures, with positive blood cultures obtained in 80 to 100 per cent of infected persons. Invasion of the organisms causes edema and swelling of the epiglottis, aryepiglottic folds, and arytenoids, which results in severe narrowing of the laryngeal airway. Purulent exudate is present, and abscess formation contributes to rapidly evolving airway obstruction.

Clinical Findings

1. The child with epiglottitis presents with an abrupt onset of fever, sore throat, and progressive respiratory distress. Typical signs and symptoms include the following:
   a. Minimal cough or other prodromal symptoms
   b. Sudden-onset high fever, toxic appearance, marked tachycardia, and often restless and irritable disposition
   c. Sore throat with a muffled voice and progressive noisy or stridulous breathing, with dysphagia and drooling occurring as the airway becomes compromised
   d. Absence of hoarseness, unless viral laryngitis also present.

2. Complete airway occlusion may occur without warning; therefore, minimal stimulation should be given to the child, and a physician skilled in intubation should attend the patient at all times. The child's level of consciousness may decrease as progressive respiratory obstruction and/or fatigue develops. The clinical presentation is variable in younger children, who may experience a more prominent upper respiratory prodrome, less fever, and a prominent croupy cough before supraglottic swelling occurs.

4. Extraepiglottic infections occur rarely and may cause meningitis, arthritis, tonsillitis, otitis media, and pneumonia.

5. Complications of epiglottitis are related primarily to sudden airway obstruction and include hypoxia and pulmonary edema.

6. The differential diagnosis includes laryngeal or tracheal foreign body, angioneurotic edema, severe viral croup, and bacterial tracheitis.

Key Clinical Findings

- Fever
- Stridor
- Dyspnea
- Irritability
- Muffled voice
- Drooling

Laboratory Findings

1. Phlebotomy should be postponed in a patient with suspected epiglottitis until an airway is secured and the child is sedated. The following diagnostic tests are then suggested:
   a. Complete blood count with differential
   b. Blood culture
   c. Culture of the epiglottis and aryepiglottic folds.

2. Evaluation of urine for bacterial antigens may be helpful, especially if the patient is taking antibiotics at the time of evaluation.

Key Laboratory Test

- Blood and epiglottis cultures

Radiographic Changes

1. Radiographs can be helpful in suspected epiglottitis, but they are not necessary to confirm the diagnosis. If transportation to the radiology department is required, a physician skilled in emergency intubation should accompany the patient at all times. The lateral radiograph has a high sensitivity for the detection of epiglottic abnormalities and may demonstrate replacement of the usual thin epiglottis with a swollen, thumblike appearance. The subglottic area should appear patent. Ballooning of the hypopharynx is indicative of significant supraglottic obstruction.
2. During the procedure, the patient should be kept upright to allow optimal positioning of the airway.

Treatment

1. Successful treatment of the child with airway obstruction from suspected or confirmed epiglottitis requires skilled personnel with a well organized and efficient plan to assess carefully the distressed patient and provide ready access to a secure artificial airway.
2. The patient should be closely observed at all times in an environment of minimal manipulation and stimulation.
   a. The upright sitting or prone position is recommended; often the child remains in the caretaker's lap. The supine position may cause abrupt airway closure.
   b. Direct visualization of the throat or epiglottis is not recommended because of the risk of precipitating complete airway obstruction.
   c. Phlebotomy or placement of intravenous catheters is not recommended until the airway is secured.
   d. Supplemental humidified oxygen can be given in a nonthreatening way (i.e., having a caretaker slowly advance the mask toward the patient's face).
3. Prompt plans for airway placement should be initiated with patient arrival. Observation of the patient without intubation is associated with increased mortality and is not recommended. The artificial airway should be placed in the operating room by an anesthesiologist skilled in the care of young children, accompanied by a surgeon who is prepared to perform a tracheostomy if necessary.
   a. Initially the child is taken to the operating room accompanied by the caretaker and is anesthetized with anesthetic gases. Intravenous access is simultaneously secured.

b. Oral intubation with a stylet is accomplished, followed by elective nasal intubation.
   c. Cultures and blood tests are then obtained.
   d. Antibiotics are then started. Recommended drugs are cefuroxime, 75 mg/kg/day, maximum 1.5 g/dose every 8 hrs; or cefotaxime, 150 mg/kg/day divided every 8 hrs, maximum 12 g/day, for 7 to 10 days. Oral antibiotics can usually be given after 7 days of intravenous therapy.
4. The intubated patient with epiglottitis is transferred to the intensive care unit for further treatment.
   a. Mechanical ventilation usually is not necessary, and the patient may be placed in an humidified tent. Sedation and restraints are used to minimize the risk of spontaneous extubation.
   b. The duration of intubation is usually 36 to 48 hours, with termination determined by clinical response (i.e., decreased fever, toxicity, and lower endotracheal tube leak pressure) or by direct visualization of the epiglottis with a laryngoscope.
5. In the event of complete airway obstruction before a secure artificial airway is obtained, mask-bag ventilation can be initiated before emergency placement of the airway.

Key Treatment

- Tracheal intubation or tracheostomy
- Antibiotics

Prevention

1. Prevention of HIB disease may be accomplished by the administration of the HIB conjugate vaccine.
2. Rifampin prophylaxis (10 to 20 mg/kg/day; maximum dose, 600 mg) should be given to all household members and possibly to daycare contacts if at least one contact is younger than 4 years old.

Bibliography

Butt W, Shann F, Walker C, et al: Acute epiglottitis: A differential approach to management. Crit Care Med 1988;16:43–47.

Mauro RD, Poole SR, Lockhart CH: Differentiation of epiglottitis from laryngotracheitis in the child with stridor. Am J Dis Child 1988;142:679–682.

Schloss MD, Gold JA, Rosales JK, Baxter JD: Acute epiglottitis: Current management. Laryngoscope 1983;93:489–493.

Sivan Y, Newth C: *In* Loughlin GM, Eigen H (eds): Respiratory Disease in Children: Diagnosis and Management. Baltimore, Williams & Wilkins, 1994, pp 315–334.

211 Respiratory Failure

Howard Eigen

Definition

Respiratory failure refers to any life-threatening respiratory distress.

Etiology

Causes are multiple. The most common causes are acute bronchospasm from various conditions; aspiration, especially in a child with an underlying respiratory or cardiac disorder; and upper airway obstruction, either from an infectious agent (e.g., croup, epiglottis) or from aspiration of a foreign object.

Clinical Findings

1. These depend on the cause. In general, children with acute wheezing episodes present with both expiratory and inspiratory distress; are moderately to severely hypoxemic but lucid; and are using the accessory muscles of inspiration as well as those of expiration.
2. In children with upper airway obstruction or aspiration, generally, there is a picture of inspiratory distress, with the neck muscles being used in a rather dramatic fashion along with flaring of the ala nasi and intercostal and suprasternal retractions. Hypoxemia and hypercapnia, and even total cardiovascular collapse, can be manifestations of acute upper airway obstruction. An especially difficult group is children with neuromuscular disorders, in whom the typical signs of distress are obscured by the weak musculature. Such children may be in severe respiratory failure but not show the typical signs of accessory muscle use or retractions.
3. Massive aspiration is rarely a cause of critical respiratory disease in children who were previously neurologically intact. In those with developmental delay, aspiration should be considered if the symptoms are primarily those of respiratory obstruction.

Key Clinical Finding

• Inspiratory and/or expiratory distress

Laboratory Findings

1. Immediate evaluation of oxygenation should be made, using a pulse oximeter.
2. It is typical to place the child in at least 40 per cent oxygen before oximetry measurements are made, and arterial blood gas analysis should be obtained to assess the partial pressure of carbon dioxide (PCO_2) and the pH.
3. In addition, electrolytes (sodium, potassium, chloride, bicarbonate) should be measured.
4. Acute heart failure can manifest as acute respiratory distress. If the history warrants, an echocardiogram may be of benefit.

Key Laboratory Tests

• Arterial blood gases
• Pulse oximetry

Treatment

1. Goal: Maintenance of the partial pressure of oxygen at >60 mmHg or the oxygen saturation at >90 per cent
   a. In a patient who is acutely wheezing, administration of albuterol, 0.5 to 1.0 ml, acutely is the first treatment. This should be administered with sufficient oxygen to maintain the arterial oxygen saturation (SaO_2) at >90 per cent. Repeated bronchodilator treatments while monitoring heart rate are indicated until the distress lessens. Repeated doses of β_2 agonists can increase oxygen requirements and so continuous monitoring of SaO_2 is imperative.
   b. If acute airway obstruction from croup or epiglottis is the suspected diagnosis, increasing the airflow past the obstruction is critical (see Chapters 196 and 210). This can be achieved by
      (1) Racemic or nonracemic epinephrine aerosols
      (2) Helium-oxygen breathing mixture
      (3) Intubation by a skilled practitioner. In general, it is better to assist breathing with other measures if a physician completely familiar and skilled in the intubation of critically ill children is unavailable. Mask and bag ventilation may be sufficient to gain the time needed for the appropriate persons to attend the child.
   c. Clearing the airway of any foreign material is imperative. This may require intubation with a orotracheal tube. Children with foreign bodies in the pharynx, trachea, or main stem bronchus may be in extreme distress and require immediate intubation. In the case of upper airway obstruction, intubation should immediately improve the patient's status. If this is not the case, the diagnosis should be rethought and the success of the procedure reevaluated.
2. Goal: Restoration of acid-base balance
   a. After assessment by arterial blood gas analysis, pH should be corrected either by ventilation of the child

to a normal P_{CO_2} or by correction of the pH with bicarbonate.

b. Fluid resuscitation also may be necessary. It is often difficult to assess fluid status under these circumstances. If there is any suspicion that the child is hypovolemic or hypotensive, a fluid bolus should be given. The typical dose is 10 ml/kg of body weight given over 15 to 30 minutes. Isotonic sodium salt solution (e.g., Ringer's solution, 0.9% saline) are the fluids most likely to be available quickly.

3. Stabilization and preparation for transport

a. Once the acute respiratory crisis is under control, a stable, large-bore intravenous catheter should be placed and fluid resuscitation and appropriate medications for sedation given.

b. A chest radiograph to assess the position of the endotracheal tube and the presence of pulmonary disease is then appropriate. In the acute phase of this evaluation, a chest radiograph is usually not helpful, and therapy should not be delayed in order to obtain a radiograph.

c. Patients who have had an acute respiratory emergency should be transferred to a pediatric intensive care unit for further care and evaluation.

d. *Pitfalls*—In the author's experience, the greatest pitfall is underestimation of respiratory distress and failure to take sufficiently aggressive action. The second is the overuse of diagnostic tests rather than dealing with the immediate and acute problem of respiratory failure. Third is allowing practitioners who are not familiar with children to perform excessive or inappropriate procedures as part of the evaluation and stabilization.

Key Treatment

- Oxygen
- Secure patent airway
- Antiwheezing medication if appropriate

---

212 Adult Respiratory Distress Syndrome

Peter W. Hiatt

Definition

Adult respiratory distress syndrome (ARDS) is a clinical syndrome of acute respiratory failure from either local or systemic disease that leads to injury of the alveolar capillary membrane, endothelial cells, and alveolar cells, resulting in pulmonary edema.

Etiology

1. Sepsis
2. Direct injury
   a. Aspiration
      (1) Near-drowning (fresh or salt water)
      (2) Gastric fluid (especially if pH <2.5)
      (3) Hydrocarbons
   b. Pulmonary infections
   c. Inhalation (smoke, oxygen toxicity, nitrogen dioxide, chlorine, sodium dioxide, ammonia, phosgene)
   d. Pulmonary contusion
   e. Emboli (air, fat)
   f. Radiation pneumonitis
3. Secondary injury
   a. Shock
   b. Trauma (multiple trauma, fractures, burns, head trauma)
   c. Increased intracranial pressure
   d. Blood disorders (diffuse intravascular coagulation, massive blood transfusion)
   e. Drug overdoses (heroin, methadone, barbiturates, salicylates, propoxyphene)
   f. Paraquat ingestion
   g. Metabolic disorders (diabetic ketoacidosis, uremia, pancreatitis)
   h. Complications of surgery or treatment (cardiopulmonary bypass, hemodialysis, cardioversion)

Pathogenesis

1. The exact mechanism is unknown, but it appears to involve the host's defense mechanism and response to

injury or infection. Tissue damage may be the result of activation of complement, neutrophils, macrophages, platelets, or tumor necrosis factor.

2. Capillary permeability is increased after tissue injury, resulting in accumulation of protein-rich material in the interstitium and alveoli (pulmonary edema).

3. Pulmonary edema leads to decreased lung compliance, reduction in functional residual capacity, and ventilation-perfusion mismatch, as reflected in an increased shunt fraction.

4. The pathologic changes in the lung are divided into three stages:

   a. *Early exudative phase*—12 to 48 hours after onset, increased fluid in the alveoli and interstitium

   b. *Cellular proliferative phase*—3 to 10 days after onset, proliferation of type II cuboidal epithelial cells (surfactant-producing) as the lung tries to repair itself

   c. *Fibrotic proliferative phase*—7 to 10 days after onset, decreased cellularity, organized alveolar fluid, fibrosis of the lung parenchyma.

Clinical Findings

Pediatric cases of ARDS have a reported age range of 2 months to 17 years and account for 8.5 to 10.4 cases per 100 pediatric intensive care unit admissions. Onset of clinical features can be acute or gradual, depending on the cause. The most generally agreed-upon criteria for ARDS are

1. Severe hypoxemia, decreased lung compliance, and increased severity of shunt

2. Diffuse patchy infiltrates on chest radiograph

3. Exclusion of heart disease and left ventricular dysfunction (pulmonary artery occlusion pressure <18 mmHg).

Typical Physical Findings of ARDS

- Tachypnea
- Tachycardia
- Retractions
- Hypoxemia
- Quiet chest with few crackles

Laboratory Findings

There is no laboratory test specific for ARDS; it is diagnosed through a constellation of signs and symptoms. Laboratory values reflect the underlying disease process and concomitant problems (see next section).

Treatment

The goals are to treat the underlying, precipitating condition; to minimize barotrauma and oxygen toxicity to the lung; and to treat any secondary problems. Mortality has remained at roughly 40 to 70 per cent over the past 20 years.

1. Intubation

2. Use mechanical ventilation if the fraction of inspired oxygen (FIO_2) is >0.6.

   a. Use positive end-expiratory pressure (PEEP) to increase functional residual capacity, decrease ventilation-perfusion mismatch, and improve compliance.

   b. Limit peak inspiratory pressure to 50 cm H_2O, if possible, to reduce barotrauma.

   c. Reduce supplemental oxygen until the FIO_2 is ≤0.6, if possible, to limit oxygen toxicity to the lung

3. Stabilize blood pressure with colloid or crystalloid (20 ml/kg IV)

4. After blood pressure is stable:

   a. Restrict fluids to decrease lung water.

   b. Maintain fluid balance; this may require diuretics (e.g., furosemide, 1 ml/kg IV).

   c. Give positive inotropic support as necessary.

      (1) Dopamine (5 to 20 μg/kg/minute IV)

      (2) Dobutamine (2 to 10 μg/kg/minute IV)

5. For patients unresponsive to conventional mechanical ventilation, consider investigational ventilation methods such as pressure-limited ventilation with increased inspiration/expiration ratio (I:E), high-frequency oscillation, liquid ventilation, or extracorporeal membrane oxygenation (ECMO).

6. Treat secondary infections aggressively; the gastrointestinal tract is thought to be the source of many of the infectious agents frequently isolated: *Klebsiella*, *Pseudomonas*, *Escherica coli*, *Candida albicans*, and *Staphylococcus epidermidis*.

7. Treat concomitant problems caused by inflammatory cell activation:

   a. Renal impairment (50% of patients)

   b. Central nervous system abnormalities (30% of patients)

   c. Hepatic failure (uncommon, but check for mild elevations of transaminases, increased clotting times, and elevated bilirubin).

Key Treatment

- Intubation
- PEEP
- Oxygen

Prognosis

Children who survive ARDS eventually have normal chest radiographs; their pulmonary function improves, with a mild reduction in forced vital capacity. The level of support required during the acute phase of ARDS generally correlates with the severity of long-term physiologic abnormalities.

Critical State *Continued*

 Bibliography

Arnold JH, Hanson JH, Toro-Figuero LO, et al: Prospective, randomized comparison of high-frequency oscillatory ventilation and conventional mechanical ventilation in pediatric respiratory failure. Crit Care Med 1994;22:1530–1539.

Hickling, KG, Walsh J, Henderson S, Jackson R: Low mortality rate in adult respiratory distress syndrome using low-volume, pressure-limited ventilation with permissive hypercapnia: A prospective study. Crit Care Med 1994;22:1568–1578.

Moler FW, Custer JR, Bartlett RH, et al: Extracorporeal life support for severe pediatric respiratory failure: An updated experience 1991–1993. J Pediatr 1994;124:875–880.

Paulson TE, Spear RM, Peterson BM: New concepts in the treatment of children with acute respiratory distress syndrome. J Pediatr 1995;127:163–175.

Sarnaik AP, Lieh-Lai M: Adult respiratory distress syndrome in children. Pediatr Clin North Am 1994;41:337–363.

213 Pulmonary Function Testing

Gary A. Mueller

Procedure

Physiology

1. The purpose of pulmonary function tests is to provide objective and reproducible measurements of lung function. They can be used as a diagnostic tool and as a means of monitoring the response to therapy. The commonly tested parameters are lung volumes, flow, and airway reactivity.

2. *Volume testing (plethysmography)*—Total lung capacity and its components

   a. Maximal inhalation achieves total lung capacity (TLC).

   b. A maximal expiratory maneuver results in a measurement of residual volume (RV) remaining in the lungs.

   c. Vital capacity (VC) is the difference between TLC and RV; it is generated by a maximal inspiration followed by a maximal expiration.

   d. The lung volume at the end of a passive expiration is the functional residual capacity (FRC).

   e. *Tidal breathing* is active inspiration followed by passive expiration back to FRC.

3. *Flow testing (spirometry)*—When the VC is generated with as much forced effort as possible, a forced vital capacity (FVC) is obtained.

   a. Plotting of maximal flows within the VC range against the volumes at which they were generated produces a *flow-volume curve*. Some of the useful measures by this method are:

      (1) FVC

      (2) Peak expiratory flow rate

      (3) The volume forcibly exhaled in the first second (FEV_1)

      (4) The average of flows between 25 and 75 per cent of the FVC ($FEF_{25-75\%}$)

      (5) The ratio of FEV_1 to FVC.

   b. After approximately 20 per cent of VC has been exhaled, flows are independent of effort so long as a reasonable effort is made. Additional muscular effort cannot increase flows in this portion of the flow-volume curve. Peak flow is part of the effort-dependent portion, FEV_1 partially lies in both portions, and $FEF_{25-75\%}$ is effort independent.

4. *Airway reactivity testing*—A variety of methods that measure lung function parameters before and after introduction of a challenge agent. Airway hyperreactivity (e.g., asthma) is present when a lung function test changes more than what would be expected for a normal person. Commonly used agents are bronchodilators, methacholine, and histamine, in addition to exercise.

Indications

1. The primary objective is to determine the presence and quantify the amount of suspected or known respiratory disease. Physiologic classifications are as follows:

   a. Obstructive

   b. Restrictive

   c. Mixed

   d. Normal

2. The ability to perform adequate FVC maneuver. With an experienced technician, spirometry can be performed reliably by most children 5 to 6 years old or older. Lung volumes by body plethysmography may be more difficult for the younger ages.

Procedure *Continued*

3. To evaluate treatment efficacy or withdrawal of therapy; this could include, for example, use of bronchodilators, steroids, antibiotics, or surgery

4. Preoperative evaluation.

Equipment

1. Items commonly used
   a. Spirometry measures volumes and flows in the VC range, the common types being volume displacement of a bell over water, dry wedge, bellows, or pneumotachometer. Pneumotachometers are common for office use, given their compact size, ease of use, and ease of upkeep.
   b. Body plethysmograph is used for measuring FRC. When it is combined with spirometry, TLC and all of its subcomponents can be measured.
   c. Peak flow meter
      (1) Standard range (0 to 800 L/minute, for children >8 years old)
      (2) Low range (0 to 400 L/minute, for children 5 to 8 years old)

2. General requirements
   a. Low inertia, making the equipment responsive to smaller volumes and low flows
   b. Reproducibility, because longitudinal assessments are made; a small deviation in accuracy (± 3 to 5%) can be accepted for reproducible serial measurements
   c. Graphic display of the flow-volume loop
   d. Computerized equipment, set up with pediatric normalization.

Technique/Performance

Strict adherence to appropriate technique in performing pulmonary function tests is necessary to provide reproducible, accurate results

1. Testing area
   a. Free of distractions
   b. Friendly environment (safe, "no-pain" zone)

2. Patient preparation
   a. The youngest testable patient able to cooperate and produce good effort is usually 5 to 6 years of age.
   b. Make use of the child's eagerness or curiosity; young children are especially willing to attempt to please the technician or parent.
   c. Reward a positive attitude verbally and perhaps by small "treasures" (e.g., colorful stickers).
   d. Keep the thorax erect.
   e. Keep the head in neutral position.
   f. The use of soft nose clips is preferred, if they do not frighten the child.
   g. A formal period (15 minutes) of instruction and practice, including technician demonstration, can enhance performance by 10 per cent, compared with a brief, informal instruction period. Instruction and practice are particularly helpful for first-time testers and for the youngest patients. Providing such training when the child is relatively well can enhance cooperation later on, when the child is ill.

3. Testing procedure for spirometry—A great amount of coaching may be needed to obtain an adequate effort. Young children have difficulty with the concept of blowing out with maximum effort, particularly until all air is exhaled. This requires 3 to 5 seconds usually.
   a. Technician demonstration
   b. Frequent, positive comments
   c. Mouthpiece between the teeth, making a seal with the lips
   d. A few tidal breaths are made, followed by inspiration to TLC and forcible, complete exhalation to RV.
   e. Effort may vary widely with each attempt. Three FVC measurements within 5 per cent of each other confirm reproducibility. The best of these is reported.
   f. A graphic tracing of the flow-volume curve assists with sorting out cough artifacts, premature termination, and delayed onset.
   g. Measurements are corrected for barometric pressure and body temperature (BTPS), according to the American Thoracic Society standards.

Testing Types

Different testing modalities are available, depending on the specific clinical question to be answered. For example, the question of airflow obstruction consistent with asthma is answered by spirometry. Restrictive lung disease is evaluated by plethysmography and spirometry.

1. *Spirometry*—Expiration begins at TLC and ends at RV, taking less than 3 seconds in normal persons, or as long as 6 to 8 seconds in persons with obstructive disorders.

2. *Plethysmography*
   a. TLC, FRC, and RV are commonly evaluated. The other volumes and capacities are needed for the pulmonary function laboratory to measure these items but are less helpful for interpretations.
   b. It is useful in determining whether restrictive lung disease is present when spirometry results are unclear.

3. *Peak expiratory flow rate (PEFR)*—Commonly re-

ferred to as "peak flow," this is the greatest flow obtained on forced expiration after complete inspiration to TLC.

a. It is useful in the management of some obstructive lung disorders, most notably, asthma.

(1) PEFR correlates well with FEV_1.

(2) It is not a substitute for spirometry, which is more sensitive.

(3) Routine home use is particularly helpful to parent and physician.

b. Benefits are that the test is simple to use, inexpensive, and portable.

c. Disadvantages are the large standard deviation and effort dependence of this test. This reduces usefulness of an isolated, single measurement, but serial assessments are very useful.

d. Regular peak flow monitoring is emphasized in the National Heart, Lung and Blood Institute's 1997 guidelines as a home measurement in asthma and for use in the office, emergency room, and hospital.

e. Testing procedure requires a short, sharp puff into the peak flow meter.

(1) Record highest of three attempts.

(2) Measure at the same time each morning and evening.

f. Testing involves detecting changes from baseline (usually 12% or more) or increases in circadian variation. A 20 per cent difference between morning and evening values indicates that asthma is not under complete control.

g. A "traffic light" system of three color-coded PEFR zones has been adapted for asthma management. This helps simplify decision making at home for the parent and provides physicians with helpful information if called.

(1) The zones are based on the patient's personal best values when well.

(2) Green zone (80 to 100% of personal best) indicates no need for change from current therapy in the asymptomatic patient.

(3) Yellow zone (50 to 80% of personal best) indicates a significant deterioration, and an acute exacerbation may be present, even with a normal physical examination. Physician examination, an increase in maintenance therapy, or a temporary increase in therapy may be needed. A return to the green zone and resolution of any signs or symptoms is the goal.

(4) Red zone (less than 50% of personal best) indicates an emergency. An inhaled bronchodilator should be administered immediately, and physician attention is needed for those with distress and those who do not stabilize in the yellow zone. Physician advice should be sought as soon as possible.

(5) The ranges (zones) presented are suggested guidelines only. The specific range should be tailored for each patient (e.g., an upward shift in children known to deteriorate quickly or severely).

4. *Airway reactivity*—Children suspected of having asthma and those with a history of lung injury in infancy (e.g., bronchiolitis, aspiration, prematurity, prolonged mechanical ventilation) may have increased bronchial reactivity. If the child shows an obstructive pattern on baseline testing, a bronchodilator test is helpful.

a. With bronchodilator testing, a dose of inhaled medication is given and spirometry is performed both before and 15 minutes after dosing.

(1) A high dose is recommended to reduce the possibility of missing a response for lack of sufficient dose. The author uses three full breaths of nebulized albuterol, 5 mg/ml.

(2) An increase of 1 standard deviation (usually 10% of baseline) in a measurement is considered to be a significant positive bronchodilator response (Table 213–1).

b. Bronchial provocation challenge is useful for children in whom bronchospastic, obstructive lung disease (e.g., asthma) is suspected despite normal spirometry and a negative bronchodilator response. Such testing may be necessary instead of placing a child on empiric therapy. It is also helpful for children who are not responding to conventional therapy and who may need more aggressive management after the diagnosis is confirmed.

(1) Commonly used provocations are inhaled methacholine, inhaled histamine, and standardized exercise.

(2) Provocation testing should not be performed until well after resolution of any upper or lower respiratory infection.

TABLE 213–1. NORMAL RANGE AND CHANGES OF SPIROMETRY

TEST	NORMAL RANGE (% OF PREDICTED VALUE)	SIGNIFICANT RESPONSE TO BRONCHODILATOR (% IMPROVEMENT OVER BASELINE)*
FVC	>80	+10
FEV_1	>80	+10
$FEF_{25–75\%}$	>70	+25
PEFR	>80	+12
FEV_1/FVC ratio	>80	N/A

*These values may be different in some laboratories or clinical states.

(3) It must be performed in specialized centers with a staff capable of handling severe, acute bronchospasm and complications of acute airway obstruction.

(4) Nonstandardized challenges, such as jumping in place, climbing flights of steps, and running in the hallway, are to be avoided, because false-negative results are more likely to occur and the tests are not reproducible.

5. *Infant pulmonary function testing*—Noninvasive methods of measuring volumes and flows in infants are available at specialized pediatric centers. The inability to provide voluntary maneuvers (e.g., FVC) is compensated by more sophisticated technology.

   a. A partial expiratory flow-volume curve can be produced by the rapid thoracoabdominal compression technique.

      (1) Requirements generally are an infant weighing less than 15 kg, and perhaps mild sedation.

      (2) FRC is used as a reference point, and the maximal exhaled flow at FRC (V_{max} FRC) is reported. Interpretation of obstruction is possible from this test, as is response to inhaled bronchodilator.

   b. Volumes

      (1) Gas dilution techniques (helium, nitrogen washout) and, more recently, plethysmography can be used to measure FRC.

      (2) This may be useful in children with cystic fibrosis or some unusual conditions involving air trapping.

Interpretation

Pulmonary function tests do not provide a specific diagnosis but serve to place a disorder into a physiologic category (Table 213–2). Interpretation of these tests relies on comparing the results with a previously established reference standard or population (see Table 213–1).

1. Reference populations

   a. Test results are expressed as a percentage of predicted value for age, weight, height, sex, and race.

   b. Most normal children are within 2 standard deviations from the mean.

   c. It is important to know the reference population used.

(1) Pediatric normal standards should be included in computer software.

(2) Sex and race are as important as age and height.

(3) Percentages for adolescents should not be calculated using adult standards.

2. The physiologic categories are normal, obstructive, restrictive, and mixed.

   a. Obstructive lung disease

      (1) Examples are asthma and cystic fibrosis.

      (2) Expiratory flows are reduced relative to lung volume (FEV_1/FVC <80%).

      (3) Gas trapping is indicated by an elevated residual volume (RV/TLC >30%).

      (4) FRC and TLC also may be elevated.

      (5) As obstructive disease becomes more severe, FVC decreases as RV increases.

      (6) It is important to note that peak flow can be normal despite measurable obstruction as indicated by spirometry.

   b. Restrictive lung disease

      (1) Examples are interstitial fibrosis, neuromuscular disorders, and scoliosis.

      (2) Expiratory flows are normal relative to *reduced* lung volume (FEV_1/FVC usually >90%).

      (3) TLC, FVC, and RV are reduced.

   c. Mixed patterns

      (1) Mixed patterns have qualities of both obstructive and restrictive lung disease.

      (2) Spirometry often is enough to classify a disorder physiologically. However, plethysmography is needed to reliably sort out mixed disease states (e.g., severe emphysema).

3. *Longitudinal testing*—The results of a child's tests are compared with those of previous tests.

   a. Removes the limitation of a reference population and compares the child with his or her own baseline.

   b. "Personal best" values should be established at a time when the patient is as well and asymptomatic as possible.

   c. Concept of relative change

      (1) A change of more than 1 standard deviation is significant (see Table 213–1).

      (2) A high-normal test value may decrease by 1 standard deviation between testings (indicating a significant change) but still be within the "normal range" of the reference population.

      (3) Conversely, a child with low-normal function may fall below the "normal range" on a subsequent test and yet be disease free.

TABLE 213–2.   PHYSIOLOGIC PATTERNS OF SPIROMETRY

TEST	OBSTRUCTION	RESTRICTION
FVC	Normal or decreased	Decreased
FEV_1	Decreased	Normal or decreased
FEV_1/FVC	Decreased	Increased
$FEF_{25-75\%}$	Decreased	Not predictive

Procedure *Continued*

Bibliography

Eigen H: Lung function testing. *In* Loughlin GM, Eigen H (eds): Respiratory Disease in Children: Diagnosis and Management. Baltimore, Williams & Wilkins, 1994, pp 77–85.
Lemen RJ: Pulmonary function testing in the office, clinic, and home. *In* Chernick J (ed): Disorders of the Respiratory Tract in Children, 5th ed. Philadelphia, WB Saunders, 1990, pp 147–154.
Mueller GA, Eigen H: Pulmonary function testing in pediatric practice. Pediatr Rev 1994;15:403–411.
Mueller GA, Eigen H: Pediatric pulmonary function testing in asthma. Pediatr Clin North Am 1992;39:1243–1258.
Pfaff JK, Morgan WJ: Pulmonary function in infants and children. Pediatr Clin North Am 1994;41:401–423.

214 Blood Gas Analysis

Howard Eigen

Procedure

Sampling of arterial blood gases is an important way to assess patients with respiratory disorders. The three primary measures to monitor are oxygenation, ventilation, and acid-base balance. Oxygenation can be assessed by measuring the arterial partial pressure of oxygen (PaO_2), or per cent saturation (SaO_2) can be measured directly using pulse oximetry. Partial pressure of carbon dioxide ($PaCO_2$) in arterial blood is a good reflection of total alveolar ventilation. Acid-base balance is assessed by the pH measurement from an arterial blood sample.

1. In considering oxygenation, the first thing to determine is the distinction between the PaO_2, the per cent oxygen saturation, and the oxygen content.

   a. These distinctions are important in understanding and interpreting these measurements. PaO_2 reflects the physical partial pressure of oxygen in the sample. This would be the same in a given sample whether or not hemoglobin were present.

   b. The per cent saturation is determined by comparing the amount of oxygenated hemoglobin with the total hemoglobin.

   c. The oxygen content, although difficult to measure directly, is perhaps the most important factor because it indicates how much oxygen (in milliliters) is actually contained in an aliquot of blood—usually expressed as the amount in 100 ml of blood. Although anemia has very little effect on the PaO_2 and the per cent saturation, it has a significant effect on oxygen content (Table 214–1).

2. When we assess the PaO_2, which is the commonly measured blood gas, we need to understand why the normal PaO_2 is what it is (approximately 95 mmHg) and what factors influence it. Doing this helps us evaluate the cause of a low PaO_2 in a given patient. The key here is really to determine whether the hypoxemia is a result of ventilation-perfusion mismatch or of hypoventilation. It is rare that a patient is not breathing sufficient oxygen, but this can happen when a patient is at high altitude.

   a. In order to assess oxygenation, we calculate the alveolar-arterial difference for oxygen ($A-aDO_2$). The calculation is relatively simple. We can assume the barometric pressure and therefore know the partial pressure of inspired oxygen (PIO_2): $PIO_2 = P_B \times \%$ inspired O_2.

   b. We can calculate PAO_2 from the arterial blood gas measurements using the modified alveolar gas equation, $PAO_2 = PO_2 - PCO_2/R(.8)$, which can be modified to $PAO_2 = PIO_2 - 1.2 \times PCO_2$. This simplifies the calculation so it can be done without pencil and paper.

$$PAO_2 = PIO_2 - (PCO_2 \div R)$$

TABLE 214–1. EFFECTS OF PARTIAL PRESSURE OF OXYGEN AND ANEMIA ON OXYGEN CONTENT OF ARTERIAL BLOOD

PO_2 (mmHg)	HGB (g)	O_2 (ml/100 ml BLOOD)	DIFFERENCE
Effect of PO_2			
70	15	18.82	
100	15	19.48	0.66 ml
100	15	19.48	
600	15	20.10	0.62 ml
Effect of Anemia			
100	15	19.48	
100	10	13.05	6.43 ml

R = respiratory quotient assumed to be 0.8 *or*

$$PAO_2 = PIO_2 - (1.2 \times PCO_2)$$

c. The alveolar-arterial difference, then, is the difference between the calculated PAO_2 and the PaO_2 obtained from the arterial blood sample.

d. An increase in $A-aDO_2$ (above 15 mmHg) indicates intrinsic pulmonary disease or an anatomic shunt. In most cases, an anatomic shunt can be dismissed on clinical grounds, and a ventilation-perfusion abnormality is found to be the cause of an increase in the $A-aDO_2$.

3. The analysis of the PCO_2 is used to assess total alveolar minute ventilation.

   a. There is often confusion between total alveolar minute ventilation and respiratory rate. These two are not synonymous, and the rate may be very high while alveolar ventilation remains low.

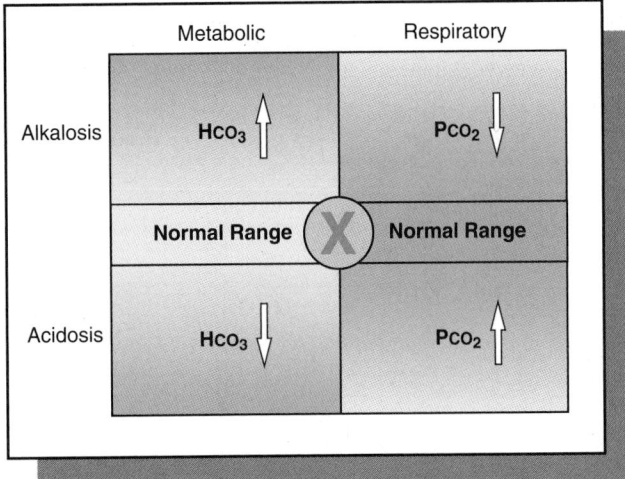

b. The ultimate example of this is panting, in which the respiratory rate is extremely high but, because the tidal volume is very small, only the dead space is ventilated and alveolar ventilation is essentially zero.

c. Under most circumstances, an elevation of PCO_2 10 mmHg above what is expected for that clinical condition or patient indicates impending respiratory failure and should be dealt with rapidly.

d. For example, a patient with chronic carbon dioxide retention who progresses from 60 to 70 mmHg PCO_2 during an acute illness requires immediate attention. The same can be said for a patient undergoing an acute episode of asthma whose PCO_2 rises from 35 to 45 mmHg. Although the absolute values are considerably different, the elevation indicates failure to maintain sufficient alveolar ventilation.

4. In assessing pH, we evaluate the metabolic state of the patient and what compensation has taken place.

   a. As a metabolic or respiratory derangement progresses, compensation takes place over hours to days and moves the patient from one of the rectangular areas toward a normal state.

   b. If a patient starts out with a respiratory acidosis (lower right hand box), compensation occurs in a diagonal fashion toward a metabolic alkalosis; therefore, the patient stabilizes with an elevated PCO_2 and an elevated bicarbonate but with a pH that is below 7.40. Analysis tells us that an elevated PCO_2 (respiratory acidosis) was the initiating condition and that compensation occurred by elevation of the serum bicarbonate. An acute respiratory acidosis results in an elevated PCO_2 but a normal bicarbonate; therefore, there is an uncompensated acidosis, and the pH falls dramatically. Any one of the four conditions in the figure can be the initiating condition, with compensation taking place in a diagonal fashion through the normal range.

215 Thoracentesis

Howard Eigen

Thoracentesis can be used either diagnostically to ascertain the nature of pleural fluid or therapeutically to remove pleural fluid that has accumulated in the chest and is causing respiratory compromise. Localization of pleural fluid is best done from an anteroposterior chest radiograph with the patient in the upright position. Once the site of fluid has been determined, it is helpful to obtain a decubitus radiograph to confirm that the fluid is free flowing.

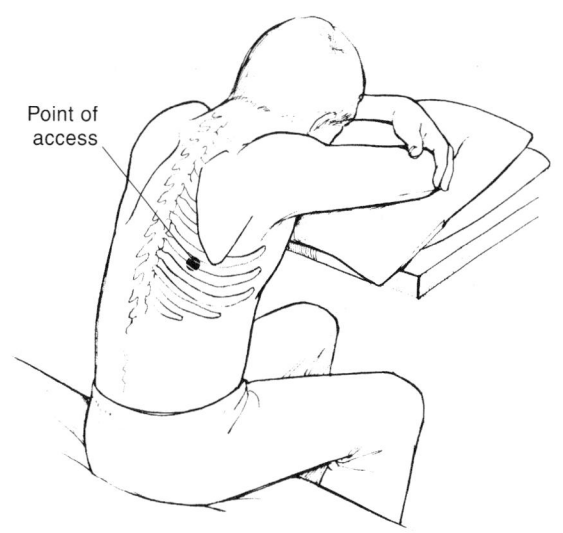

Point of access

Preparation

1. The procedure itself is performed with the child in a sitting position; an infant can be held in a sitting position by the nurse. Older children are seated and asked to lean forward over a pillow. The pillow can be placed either on the back of a chair with the child sitting facing the back of the chair or on a bedside stand with the child seated at the edge of the treatment table. Monitoring is routinely done by pulse oximetry, and one person is assigned to monitor vital signs and patient status and to coach the child during the procedure. A sterile field is prepared in the usual manner, and universal precautions are taken.

2. Sedation is not usually necessary, but chloral hydrate or a low-dose midazolam can be used. Analgesia is obtained by local infiltration using lidocaine (Xylocaine).

Equipment

The equipment is a large-bore (usually 12-gauge) angiocatheter attached to three-way stopcock and syringe. The syringe can be either 5 ml or 10 ml, depending on the hand size of the person performing the procedure.

Technique

1. The syringe is arranged so that the stopcock is held in the palm of the gloved hand and the thumb is placed 2 to 3 cm from the tip of the needle, acting as a "stop" when the needle enters the pleural space. With this method, there is virtually no likelihood that the needle will be placed into the pleural space farther than is desired by the operator, even if the child should move suddenly. After infiltration with analgesic, the needle is placed in the midaxillary line posteriorly with the tip of the needle aimed at the middle of the rib just below the inner space that the operator wishes to enter (see figure). The needle is advanced until its tip touches the rib. The needle and the skin are then pulled upward so that the needle passes just over the top of the rib into the interspace and through into the pleural space. This technique ensures that the needle will pass through the interspace at its lowest point, thereby avoiding the neurovascular bundle that runs on the inferior margin of each rib. In addition, it creates a Z-track, which minimizes leakage.

2. As the needle is passed into the pleural space, negative pressure is applied by keeping traction on the syringe plunger. Once fluid appears, the needle and its catheter are advanced slightly, and then the catheter is passed into the pleural space while the needle is held in place. Only a small portion of the needle actually enters the pleural space, but a sufficient amount to allow the catheter to reach into the pleural space and drop downward into the fluid. As the needle is withdrawn from the catheter, the left thumb is placed over the catheter to prevent air from leaking into the pleural space. The stopcock and syringe are reattached and the fluid is aspirated.

3. If this is a diagnostic thoracentesis, then the fluid is aspirated to obtain specimens for chemistry, cytology, and culture. Usually, a specimen of between 15 and 30 ml is sufficient for all tests necessary (see below).

Follow-up

1. Cover the area with a sterile dressing of appropriate size; a Band-Aid is usually sufficient. A chest radiograph

Tips for Success

- Ensure that the needle is placed perpendicular to the plane of the child's back rather than parallel to the child's seating surface. In this way, the needle enters the pleural space cleanly, and the opportunity to run the catheter up under the skin is minimized.
- If fluid stops flowing, have the child lean back slightly or even markedly, with the nurse supporting the child in this position. This is unlikely to cause pain, because only the soft catheter is in the pleural space. The fluid level is raised relative to the catheter, and more fluid can be withdrawn.
- At the end of the procedure, rub hard over the site of the needle puncture to break up the Z-track and prevent further leakage.

should be obtained after the procedure to document the reduction of fluid and that no free air is present. If free air is present, another film 2 to 3 hours later is appropriate. Continue monitoring oxygen saturations if signs of an air leak are detected.

2. *Chemistry*—Specimens are sent for analyses including protein, lipids, and glucose. Lactate dehydrogenase (LDH) is a good marker of malignancy but usually is not helpful in children, because the likelihood of doing a thoracentesis for an unknown malignancy is very small.
3. *Cytology*—Specimens are sent for complete cell count and differential and, if a malignancy is considered, a cell block is sent as well. Gram staining of the fluid is also done in an attempt to identify a bacterial cause for the pleural effusion.
4. *Culture*—Specimens are sent for culture of bacteria, both aerobes and anaerobes, and mycobacteria. Under some circumstances, a viral culture may be warranted, but this is unusual.
5. The most helpful diagnostic information to come back quickly from a thoracentesis is whether the pleural fluid represents a transudate (typically associated with low protein and few cells) or an exudate (typically associated with high protein and large numbers of leukocytes).
6. A discussion of pleural effusion appears in Chapter 200.

216 Pulmonary Health Care

Jean Homrighausen Zander

When discharge with supportive technology is being considered for the child with lung disease, thorough assessment of the child and family is indicated.

Patient Selection

1. The child's medical condition must be stable, according to predetermined criteria (see box for example).

Discharge Criteria

- Disease process stable on reasonable care plan
- Stable blood gases
- Stable oxygen requirements or ventilator settings
- Stable growth
- Established nutrition and medication schedules

From Loughlin GM, Eigen H (eds): *Respiratory Disease in Children: Diagnosis and Management.* Baltimore: Williams & Wilkins, 1994.

2. The constellation of resources available to the family must be assessed:
   a. The caretaker (or caretakers)
      (1) Who will be the primary caretaker?
      (2) What are the physical, emotional, educational resources, and needs of this person?
      (3) Is there another person available for respite?
      (4) What other social supports can be called on?
   b. *The physical environment*—The specifics of the home and physical environment are often best assessed by a nurse or respiratory therapist affiliated with a home care agency. Elements to consider include the following:
      (1) Room size and arrangements
      (2) Adequacy of utilities (phone, electricity, wiring, water, heat, air conditioning)
      (3) Proximity of home community to emergency, primary, and tertiary care

Procedure *Continued*

(4) Availability of *pediatric* services such as occupational therapy, physical therapy, and ST.

c. *Financial resources*—Reimbursement for pediatric respiratory home care varies widely dependent on the third-party payor. Many payors have developed case management programs, administered by a medical doctor, registered nurse, or registered social worker, to assist the discharging institution in comprehensive planning. However, sensitivity to and knowledge about children's needs vary.

d. *Psychosocial issues*—The child and family should undergo thorough assessment by a professional trained in the needs of chronically ill children. Anticipatory guidance with regard to potential stressors should be provided on an ongoing basis. Some elements to consider in counseling families are the following:

(1) The burden on the primary caretaker and the shortage of respite care

(2) Lack of family privacy secondary to the presence of home care nurses

(3) Social isolation secondary to care commitments

(4) Feelings of isolation and abandonment after leaving the acute care setting.

Home Oxygen Therapy

1. *Patient assessment*—Pulse oximetry is used to assess the adequacy of oxygenation at rest, with activity, with feeding, and during sleep. The need for home oxygen therapy is thereby established and then adjusted as needed for each level of activity. Families should be taught to assess for the following criteria:

a. Increased respiratory rate and effort (nasal flaring, retractions, forced respiration, head bobbing)

b. Poor feeding

c. Diaphoresis

Factors to Consider in Selecting Home Oxygen Therapy Systems

- Convenience for intended use
- Weight of system
- Ease of refill
- Low-flow capacity
- Need for backup
- Home environment
- Local supply and service
- Economics and reimbursement

From Loughlin GM, Eigen H (eds): Respiratory Disease in Children: Diagnosis and Management. Baltimore: Williams & Wilkins, 1994.

TABLE 216–1. ADVANTAGES AND DISADVANTAGES OF OXYGEN SOURCES

OXYGEN SYSTEM	ADVANTAGES	DISADVANTAGES
Compressed gas (tanks)	Long shelf-life Easily available	Heavy Need refills High pressure (2000 PSI) Low volume for size when compared with liquid system
Liquid oxygen	Low pressure (20 PSI) Portable Easy home refilling	Evaporation Potential for frostbite during refilling Technical problems such as ice
Oxygen concentrators/ enrichers	Simple, easy to use Mobile	Heavy Not portable Need power source

From Lund CH (ed): Bronchopulmonary dysplasia: Strategies for total parent care. Petaluma, CA, Neonatal Network, 1990.

d. Pallor

e. Additional criteria in older children:

(1) Daytime sleepiness

(2) Morning headaches

(3) Decreased attention span

(4) Diminished school performance.

2. *Implementation*—A variety of factors (see box) must be considered in selecting home oxygen therapy systems. The advantages and disadvantages of various oxygen systems are noted in Table 216–1.

Home Tracheostomy Care

Before hospital discharge, the parents and other home care providers must demonstrate specific skills:

1. Parents are able to state the reason for their child's tracheostomy.

a. The variety of indications for tracheostomy in children necessitates specific explanations for each child.

b. Thorough explanation contributes to understanding of long-term prognosis, management, and health care needs.

2. Parents are able to explain the basic anatomy of the trachea and its relation to the tube and to the vocal cords and the esophagus.

3. Parents are able to state the elements of respiratory assessment and the signs of illness.

4. Parents are able to state the actions to be taken in the event of tube obstruction, accidental decannulation, and bleeding.

Procedure *Continued*

Signs of Increased Respiratory Distress or Illness

- Fever
- Change in amount, color, consistency, or odor of secretions
- Hemoptysis
- Change in respiratory rate or rhythms (including retractions, nasal flaring)
- Diaphoresis
- Color change (pallor, cyanosis; cyanosis is a late, inconsistent sign)
- Restlessness

Adapted from the Home Care Teaching Program, James Whitcomb Riley Hospital for Children. From Loughlin GM, Eigen H (eds): Respiratory Disease in Children: Diagnosis and Management. Baltimore: Williams & Wilkins, 1994.

WARNING

Tube obstruction is the most common cause of severe respiratory distress in a child with a tracheostomy and must be treated as an emergency.

 a. Equipment for emergency tracheostomy tube changes must *always* be available; a "travel kit" should be assembled for use away from home.

 b. Supplies for changing a tracheostomy tube
   (1) Clean tube with tracheostomy strings in place
   (2) Tube that is one size smaller with tracheostomy strings in place
   (3) Scissors
   (4) Obturator
   (5) Water-soluble lubricant
   (6) Suction equipment
   (7) Small roll for shoulders.

IMPORTANT

The above supplies are to be kept with child at all times.

 c. The child must never be left alone with a caretaker who is unable to perform an emergency tracheostomy tube change. This includes at school, on the school bus, and during after-school activities.

5. Parents are able to demonstrate cardiopulmonary resuscitation.
6. Parents are able to name the type of tracheostomy tube, the parts of the tube, and the purpose of each part. They are able to perform proper inflation and deflation of cuff (if applicable).
7. Parents understand the importance of humidification, the method of oxygen delivery, and the care of the equipment.
8. Parents are able to assess the need for suctioning, demonstrate suction technique, state the indications and the technique for normal saline lavage, and demonstrate cleaning of the inner cannula and the suction equipment.
   a. The family should be cautioned to avoid too frequent suctioning, which can result in mucosal irritation and increased secretions.
   b. Clean suction technique, as opposed to sterile technique, is used in the home.
9. Parents are able to demonstrate correct technique for changing the tracheostomy tube.

Changing the Tracheostomy Tube

- Assemble supplies
- Place obturator in new tube; check cuff integrity; check tube integrity
- Suction child's tracheostomy tube
- Position neck in slight extension, using small roll under shoulders
- Deflate cuff (if present) in old tube
- Cut strings
- Remove tube in upward and outward arc
- Insert new tube in inward, downward arc
- Immediately remove obturator
- Reposition head in neutral position by removing shoulder roll
- Tie strings in triple knot with one finger space between neck and strip
- Inflate cuff if necessary or according to instructions
- Lock inner cannula in place

From Loughlin GM, Eigen H (eds): Respiratory Disease in Children: Diagnosis and Management. Baltimore: Williams & Wilkins, 1994.

10. Parents know the principles and techniques of skin care and general safety, including feeding.
   a. Tube may be secured with the use of twill tape encircling the neck and tied with a triple knot. Alternatively, commercially available Velcro ties may also be used, to minimize skin irritation. Care must be taken to avoid detachment of the Velcro by a curious young child.
   b. Stomahesive (peristomal protection material) can

Procedure *Continued*

Home Care Skills for a Child with a Tracheostomy

Before the child is discharged, the parents must demonstrate the following skills:
1. Explain basic anatomy of trachea and relation to adjoining structures.
2. State reason for tracheostomy.
3. State elements of respiratory assessment and signs of illness.
4. State actions to be taken in the event of tube obstruction, accidental decannulation, and/or bleeding.
5. Demonstrate cardiopulmonary resuscitation.
6. Name type of tracheostomy tube, parts of tube, and purpose of each part; demonstrate proper use of tube cuff if applicable.
7. State importance of humidification, method of oxygen delivery, and care of equipment.
8. Assess need for suctioning, demonstrate suction technique using catheter, state indications and technique for normal saline lavage, and demonstrate methods for cleaning inner cannula and suction equipment.
9. Demonstrate correct technique for changing tracheostomy tube.
10. State principles and techniques for skin care and general safety, including feeding.
11. State importance of verbal stimulation and know the communication/speech therapy home plan for child.
12. State plans regarding decannulation timetable.

From Loughlin GM, Eigen H (eds): Respiratory Disease in Children: Diagnosis and Management. Baltimore: Williams & Wilkins, 1994.

be applied to the neck to provide a cushion between skin and strings.
  c. Meticulous attention must be paid to keeping the skin clean and dry. An infant's short, fat neck is

especially vulnerable to irritation and skin breakdown.
  d. The routine use of powders and creams is not recommended. Occasional short-term application of hydrocortisone cream may be helpful; prolonged use results in thinning of the tissues and increases the risk of ulceration.
  e. A child with a tracheostomy tube must *never* be left alone near *any* standing water, including pools, toilets, and buckets.
  f. Clothing and bedding should be carefully selected to avoid obstruction of the tube. A loosely draped bandanna provides protection on a windy, dusty, or cold day.
  g. When the child with a small-diameter tracheostomy tube is sleeping, or when the child is not being directly observed by an adult, cardiac/apnea monitoring is necessary.
  h. Feeding should take place when suctioning is performed. The child should always be positioned so as to avoid aspiration.
11. Parents know the importance of verbal stimulation of their child and know the communication/speech therapy home plan for child.
12. Parents know the plans regarding the decannulation timetable.

Bibliography

Eigen H, Zander JE: Home mechanical ventilation of pediatric patients. Am Rev Respir Dis 1990;141:258–259.

Frates RC, Splaingard ML, Smith ED, et al: Outcome of home mechanical ventilation in children. J Pediatr 1989;106:850–856.

Splaingard MC, Frates RC, Harrison GM, et al: Home negative-pressure ventilation: Twenty years experience. Chest 1983; 84:376–382.

Splaingard ML, Frates RC, Jefferson LS, et al: Home-regulated pressure ventilation: Report of 20 years experience in patient with neuromuscular disease. Arch Phys Rehab Mech 1985; 6:239–242.

Zander JH: Comprehensive home care. *In* Loughlin GM, Eigen H (eds): Respiratory Disease in Children: Diagnosis and Management. Baltimore: Williams & Wilkins, 1994.

217 Symptoms of Renal Disorders

Symptom **The Urinary Tract**   *Stanley Hellerstein*

Symptoms that should direct the physician's attention to a possible disorder of the urinary tract are often defined by the child's age.

1. Neonatal period
   a. *Oligohydramnios*—Suggests an obstructive lesion such as posterior urethral valves or prune-belly syndrome
   b. *Polyhydramnios*—Suggests congenital nephrotic syndrome or neonatal Bartter syndrome (hyperprostaglandin E_2 syndrome)
   c. *Oliguria, anuria, rising serum urea nitrogen and creatinine*—Hypovolemia (prerenal azotemia) or renal damage from intrauterine obstruction, acute tubular necrosis or cortical necrosis from any cause (e.g., anoxia, sepsis, hypovolemia)
   d. *Hypertension*—Often secondary to umbilical artery catheterization resulting in clot formation and renal arterial emboli; autosomal recessive polycystic kidney disease.

2. Infancy and childhood
   a. *Unexplained febrile illness*—Urinary tract infection, especially in the infant
   b. *Voiding symptoms (new-onset urgency, frequency, hesitancy, dysuria, dribbling, or incontinence), foul-smelling urine*—Cystitis
   c. *Fever and systemic symptoms with abdominal, flank or costovertebral angle pain*—Acute pyelonephritis
   d. *Isolated nocturnal enuresis*—Usually no underlying urinary tract disorder
   e. *Voiding dysfunction (persistence of any of the following: urgency, frequency, day and/or nighttime urinary incontinence, dysuria, posturing to avoid incontinence, "bladder spasms")*—Urinary tract infection (UTI), hypercalciuria, unstable bladder of childhood, neurogenic urinary bladder
   f. *Edema*—Nephrotic syndrome, glomerulonephritis
   g. *Painless hematuria*—Urolithiasis, immunoglobulin A nephropathy, hereditary nephropathy (Alport syndrome, thin basement membrane disease [TBMD]), ureteropelvic junction obstruction, urethral obstruction ("penis grabbing" may be a symptom of urethral obstruction)
   h. *Painless hematuria with proteinuria*—Acute glomerulonephritis, nephrotic syndrome, immunoglobulin A nephropathy, hereditary nephropathy
   i. *Hematuria with dysuria (with or without fever and with or without flank pain)*—Rule out urolithiasis, hypercalciuria, ureteropelvic junction obstruction, urethral obstruction, urinary tract infection.
   j. *Hypertension*—Reflux nephropathy, renal artery stenosis, chronic renal failure
   k. *Growth failure, rickets, metabolic acidosis, metabolic alkalosis, hypokalemia, hyperkalemia, polyuria*—Renal tubular disorders (Fanconi syndrome, renal tubular acidosis, Bartter syndrome, nephrogenic diabetes insipidus)
   l. *Chronic fatigue, anemia, hypertension, elevated serum urea nitrogen (SUN) and creatinine*—Chronic renal failure
   m. *Oliguria/anuria, anemia, elevated SUN and creatinine*—Hemolytic uremic syndrome.

Symptom **Neonatal Urinary Tract Dilation**   *J. Patrick Murphy*

Etiology and Epidemiology

The dilated urinary tract in the neonatal period is usually detected as a result of a routine sonography during pregnancy. There are many possible causes of this dilation:

1. *Partial obstruction involving the ureter* is the most common reason for dilation. It is usually unilateral (95%).
   a. Proximal ureteral stenosis at the ureteropelvic junction (UPJ) is the most common site (1 in 1500 births). The degree of stenosis is variable.
   b. Distal ureteral stenosis is less common (1 in 5000 births) and likewise occurs in variable degrees. It may occur at the ureterovesical junction (UVJ), or it may be secondary to an ectopic ureter with or without a ureterocele.
   c. Stenosis elsewhere in the ureter and in the intrarenal collecting system does occur but is extremely rare.

2. *Bladder outlet obstruction* causes dilation or hypertrophy of the bladder and bilateral upper urinary tract dilation.
   a. Posterior urethral valves represent the most common type of outlet obstruction (1 in 5000 male births).

b. True congenital urethral stenosis and anterior urethral valves (diverticulum) also occur but are extremely rare (1 in 40,000 births).

c. Infants with neurogenic bladder associated with spina bifida defects may occasionally present in the neonatal period with dilation of the upper urinary tract.

3. *Prune-belly or Eagle-Barrett syndrome* is manifest by urinary tract dilation, cryptorchidism, and laxity of the abdominal wall musculature. It is rare (1 in 40,000 to 50,000 births) and may occur with only partial manifestation of the syndrome.

4. High-grade *vesicoureteric reflux (VUR)* is another cause of neonatal urinary tract dilation.

Pathophysiology

1. The degree and probably the duration of intrauterine obstruction generally determines the severity of dilation of the collecting system and the extent of kidney damage.

   a. Obstruction at the UPJ can be intrinsic or extrinsic.

      (1) Intrinsic obstruction is related to muscular wall abnormalities in the ureter with alterations of muscle fiber orientation and fibrosis leading to poor peristalsis across the UPJ.

      (2) Extrinsic obstruction is usually caused by aberrant renal vessels and/or fibrous bands that result in a high insertion of the ureter on the renal pelvis.

   b. Distal ureteral obstruction

      (1) Distal ureteral obstruction caused by stenosis at the UVJ is secondary to a decreased muscularity and increased collagen deposition in the ureteral segment, which results in an adynamic segment.

      (2) Obstruction secondary to ureteral ectopia almost always occurs in a duplex ureter and usually involves the upper pole ureter.

2. Bladder outlet obstruction is most commonly caused by posterior urethral valves. The valves usually are seen as leaflets that extend distally from the verumontanum and attach to the anterior urethral wall, partially obstructing antegrade flow of the urine like sails (type I valves). Dilation of the upper tracts is caused by high-pressure changes in the bladder that lead to bladder wall thickening and ureteral dilation secondary to obstruction and/or VUR.

3. The cause of prune-belly syndrome is unknown. Theories suggest transient obstruction of the urinary tract, mesodermal arrest during early development, or persistence of the yolk sac after abdominal wall closure.

Clinical Findings

1. Ureteral obstruction is now usually detected by prenatal ultrasound. However, the more classic signs and symptoms include abdominal mass, hematuria, urinary infection, pain, failure to thrive, and hypertension. On occasion, a dilated system may be detected incidentally during imaging evaluation for another problem.

2. Bladder outlet obstruction may cause the previously mentioned signs and symptoms. A palpably distended bladder

is commonly present. In the severe forms of posterior urethral valves, the features related to oligohydramnios (Potter syndrome) include pulmonary hypoplasia, intrauterine growth deficiency, limb compression anomalies, and flattened facial features. The infant may present with urinary ascites secondary to intraabdominal leakage of urine.

3. *Multicystic dysplastic kidney (MDK)* is second only to hydronephrosis as the most common cause of a palpable abdominal mass in the neonate. It appears to develop from a very early and complete obstruction of the ureter before differentiation of the metanephros, producing the dysplastic kidney. It is characterized by a severely dysplastic parenchyma with multiple noncommunicating cysts of various sizes and ureteral atresia. Obstruction of the contralateral kidney may be present in as many as 20 per cent of the cases, and contralateral VUR is seen as often as 25 per cent of the time.

4. Children with prune-belly syndrome present with the triad of lax abdominal wall, dilated urinary tract, and bilateral cryptorchidism. Cardiovascular anomalies occur about 10 per cent of the time, and with severe bilateral obstruction there may be all of the features associated with intrauterine oligohydramnios (see discussion of bladder outlet obstruction).

Imaging Evaluation

1. Ultrasound is the primary screening examination for urinary tract dilation. It also detects many abnormalities of the kidneys, such as MDK, a significantly hypoplastic or scarred kidney, and an absent kidney. Absent kidney could reflect an ectopic kidney and requires nuclear renography or computed tomography scanning for diagnosis.

2. Voiding cystourethrography (VCUG) is the primary study for evaluating the urethra and bladder.

3. Nuclear renography is the primary study for determination of comparative function of the two kidneys and drainage from the upper tract.

   a. Diuretic renography with furosemide used to augment washout is helpful in determining significant obstruction.

      (1) Obstruction is suggested if longer than 15 to 20 minutes is required for drainage of half the radiotracer activity from the renal pelvis.

      (2) Diuretic renography in the newborn is unreliable because of the blunted response of the immature kidney to the diuretic.

   b. The uptake of tracer should be similar for the two kidneys. Tracer uptake of less than 35 to 40 per cent on one side suggests a significant decrease in renal function on that side.

4. Intravenous pyelography is used less commonly now than in the past. It is a good anatomic study, but it is not as sensitive physiologically in determining obstruction as diuretic renography.

Laboratory Tests

1. Urinalysis and urine culture are used to diagnose urinary tract infection.

2. Serum chemical analyses—Urea nitrogen and creatinine

concentrations are useful to evaluate the status of kidney function.

Treatment

1. In most infants with dilated upper urinary tracts, the disorder is discovered prenatally. All of these infants should have a repeat ultrasound during the first few days of life.

   a. If the ultrasound results are normal, it should be repeated within 1 to 3 months. The decreased urinary output that occurs early in the newborn period may account for lack of dilatation even though an obstructive lesion is present.

   b. If the ultrasound study shows unilateral dilation or a unilateral MDK, a normal second kidney, and a normal collecting system and the infant's clinical status is satisfactory, further imaging of the urinary tract may be delayed for 4 to 6 weeks. The infant should be placed on a low dose of antibiotic to prevent a UTI until nuclear renography and a VCUG are obtained.

2. Unilateral UPJ or distal ureteral obstruction

   a. If the nuclear renography scan shows function (>35 to 40%) and good drainage, most surgeons would observe and repeat ultrasound and/or nuclear renography in 3 to 4 months.

   b. If function is good (>35 to 40%) and drainage is poor, some surgeons would intervene surgically but others would observe and repeat the ultrasound and nuclear renography studies as above.

3. Posterior urethral valves are initially managed by catheter or percutaneous suprapubic drainage of the urinary bladder, followed by endoscopic fulguration, usually within the first few days of life.

4. Prune-belly syndrome requires individualized treatment of each patient because of the broad spectrum of the disorder.

   a. Some clinicians advocate early urinary tract reconstruction to eliminate VUR and stasis, to reduce the risk of infection, and to prevent deterioration of renal function.

   b. Other clinicians advocate a nonoperative approach and the use of urinary antibiotic prophylaxis, unless persistent infection or deterioration of function occurs.

   c. Treatment of the cryptorchidism associated with this syndrome follows the approach used for any other child with undescended testes.

5. Treatment of MDK is somewhat controversial. Both surgical removal and observation have advocates.

   a. The argument for removal centers on the potential for malignant degeneration. This risk is low, and it is estimated that between 2500 and 8000 MDKs would need to be removed to prevent one malignancy.

   b. The National Multicystic Kidney Registry has registered more than 245 MDKs to date. Long-term follow up of these kidneys through the registry should give more guidance as to the optimal treatment of MDK. Until then, most clinicians suggest observation with ultrasound every 6 months until age 1 year, then yearly thereafter until puberty. Growth of the kidney, change in echogenicity, infection, hypertension, or hematuria may be indications to intervene surgically.

Prevention

Fetal intervention is a potential way to prevent some of the manifestations of urinary tract obstruction. Indications for fetal intervention are few and are restricted those patients with signs of significant renal insufficiency in utero.

Bibliography

Elder JS, Duckett JW: Perinatal urology. *In* Gillenwater JY, Grayhack JT, Howards SS, et al (eds): Adult and Pediatric Urology, 2nd ed, vol 2. St. Louis, Mosby–Year Book, 1991, pp 1711–1810.

Kaplan GW, Scherz HC: Infravesical obstruction. *In* Kelalis PP, King LR, Belman AB (eds): Clinical Pediatric Urology, 3rd ed, vol 2. Philadelphia, WB Saunders, 1992, pp 821–864.

Koff SA, Campbell KD: Nonoperative management of unilateral neonatal hydronephrosis: Natural history of poorly functioning kidneys. J Urol 1994;152:593–595.

Peters CA: Urinary tract obstruction in children. J Urol 1995;154:1874–1884.

Prune-belly syndrome. *In* Rowe MI, O'Neill JA, Grosfeld JL, et al: Essentials of Pediatric Surgery. St. Louis, Mosby–Year Book, 1995, pp 760–766.

| Symptom | **Urinary Tract Infection and Vesicoureteric Reflux** | *Stanley Hellerstein* |

Definitions

1. *Urinary tract infection (UTI)*—Growth of bacteria at a site within the urinary tract that is normally sterile—that is, within the urinary bladder, the ureter, the renal pelves, or the kidneys.

   a. *Significant bacteriuria*—The presence and multiplication of bacteria in bladder urine (Table 217–1). Bacterial colony counts are used to differentiate bacteria proliferating within the urinary tract from bacteria acquired during collection of the urine specimen.

   b. *Symptomatic bacteriuria*—Significant bacteriuria in a child with symptoms of cystitis or acute pyelonephritis.

> ### WARNING
>
> **The infant, usually younger than 2 years of age, with acute pyelonephritis may present with fever and significant bacteriuria in the absence of localizing signs of infection.**

TABLE 217–1. INTERPRETATION OF QUANTITATIVE URINARY CULTURES

METHOD OF COLLECTION	QUANTITATIVE CULTURE: UTI PRESENT
Suprapubic aspiration	Growth of urinary pathogens in any number (the exception is up to 2–3 × 10³ CFU/ml of coagulase-negative staphylococci)
Catheterization	Febrile infants or children usually have ≥50 × 10³ CFU/ml of a single urinary pathogen, but infection may be present with counts from 10 × 10³ to 50 × 10³ CFU/ml
Midstream clean-void	Symptomatic patients usually have ≥10⁵ CFU/ml of a single urinary tract pathogen; however, if there is urinary frequency a UTI may be present with much lower colony counts.
Midstream clean-void	Asymptomatic patients: at least two specimens on different days with ≥10⁵ CFU/ml of the same organism.

CFU/ml = colony forming units per milliliter.

Adapted from Hellerstein S: Urinary tract infections. Old and new concepts. Pediatr Clin North Am 1995;42:1433–1457.

c. *Asymptomatic bacteriuria*—Significant bacteria in a patient free of clinical symptoms of a UTI. Pyuria is present. It usually is detected in a child monitored because of tract infections and/or vesicoureteric reflux (VUR). Screening of the urine of healthy children for bacteriuria is not recommended.

d. *Bacterial colonization*—Significant bacteriuria in the asymptomatic patient. Pyuria is not present. It is a transient event that does not proceed to a symptomatic UTI and that clears spontaneously.

2. *Vesicoureteric reflux*—The retrograde flow of urine from the urinary bladder into the ureter and, in some instances, into the pelvicalyceal system.

Epidemiology

UTI is the most frequently encountered disorder of the urinary tract. Approximately 3 per cent of girls and 1 per cent of boys have a UTI by age 11 years. The prevalence of UTI is approximately 5 per cent in infants with fever in the absence of localizing signs of infection.

1. The prevalence of UTI in uncircumcised males is 10 to 20 times higher than in circumcised males.
2. Male infants have a much higher incidence of UTI than do female infants during the first 2 months of life, but the incidence is about equal between 2 and 6 months, and thereafter the prevalence in girls far exceeds that in boys.
3. VUR is found in about 20 per cent of girls after a first UTI and in 40 to 45 per cent of those with recurrent UTIs.

Etiology

1. Most UTIs are caused by bacteria that normally inhabit the colon.
2. Viruses have been implicated in some cases of hemorrhagic cystitis. *Candida* species may cause UTI in patients with altered normal barriers to infection, particularly if they have had frequent exposure to broad-spectrum antibiotics.

Pathophysiology

1. UTIs during the first 2 months of life may be hematogenous or ascending in origin, but thereafter a UTI is almost always the result of ascent of bacteria from the perineal area through the urethra and into the bladder.
2. Infection of the urinary bladder (cystitis) that occurs in the absence of neurogenic or anatomic abnormalities of the bladder or voiding dysfunction may be the result of defective local immune mechanisms.
3. Acute pyelonephritis may develop secondary to cystitis in children with VUR and intrarenal reflux (i.e., reflux through the orifices of collecting tubules deep into the renal parenchyma).
4. Acute pyelonephritis occurs in the absence of VUR in two thirds of the cases. Uropathogenic *Escherichia coli*, P-fimbriated *E. coli*, may be responsible for some of these infections.
5. VUR in the unobstructed urinary tract is thought to be the result of immaturity of the vesicoureteral junction or of abnormal insertion (implantation) of the ureter in the bladder.

Clinical Findings

1. *Cystitis*—Usually easily recognized at all ages beyond infancy. Little or no fever is present, and there is an altered voiding pattern with any or all of the following: urgency, frequency, hesitancy, dysuria, dribbling and/or urinary incontinence, bladder spasms.

> **WARNING**
>
> **Infants and children with hypercalciuria and those with voiding dysfunction may present with symptoms identical to those of bacterial cystitis.**

2. *Acute pyelonephritis*—Systemic symptoms with fever, at times vomiting, abdominal pain, and/or back pain. Kidney or costovertebral angle tenderness may be present. The symptoms of cystitis may or may not be present. The young infant may present with fever in the absence of localized signs of infection.

 Key Clinical Findings: Pyelonephritis

- Fever
- Abdominal pain
- Costovertebral angle tenderness

Diagnosis

1. Significant bacteriuria must be present to diagnose a UTI, whether the clinical presentation is cystitis or acute pyelonephritis (see Table 217–1).
2. Localization of the site of infection as cystitis or pyelonephritis is usually made on clinical grounds. In doubtful cases, the diagnosis of acute pyelonephritis may be confirmed with the use of cortical scintigraphy (dimercaptosuccinic acid or glucoheptonate renal scan). A blood culture should be obtained in the febrile infant with a

UTI and in the older child with high fever and systemic symptoms.

> ### WARNING
>
> **Although the presence of a UTI may be suggested by findings on urinalysis (positive nitrite test or pyuria), the diagnosis depends on documentation of significant bacteriuria. Treatment for a UTI should not be instituted until a properly collected specimen of urine has been obtained for culture.**

Imaging Evaluation

1. A urinary tract ultrasound study (if not done in the past) should be obtained in the infant, young child, or adolescent with a clinical diagnosis of acute pyelonephritis (documented by culture) to detect structural abnormalities. A contrast voiding cystourethrogram (VCUG) should be done to evaluate the urethra and detect VUR.

2. The child from about 1 to 5 years of age who has had one or two episodes of cystitis should have a urinary tract ultrasound and bladder imaging. Bladder imaging may be obtained as soon as bacteriuria and pyuria have cleared and the voiding pattern is the same as when uninfected.

   a. A contrast VCUG should be obtained in all boys and in girls with voiding dysfunction when uninfected.

   b. A nuclear cystogram should be obtained in girls who have a normal voiding pattern when not infected.

3. Children older than 5 years should, at the physician's discretion, have imaging evaluation of the urinary tract after one or several episodes of cystitis. A urinary tract ultrasound should be obtained in all except the pubescent girl who has become sexually active. (If a pubescent girl has three episodes of cystitis within 1 year an ultrasound should be obtained.) If the urinary tract ultrasound is normal, bladder imaging may be omitted in children with a normal voiding pattern who are 5 years of age or older.

Treatment

1. Acute pyelonephritis

   a. *Complicated patient*—The seriously ill, dehydrated, or toxic-appearing child, the child unable to hold down oral medication and fluids, and the child in whom compliance is doubtful should be hospitalized and receive fluids and antibiotic therapy by the parenteral route.

   (1) Ceftriaxone, 75 mg/kg divided every 12 to 24 hours IV or IM, in children beyond the neonatal period who are not allergic to cephalosporins. Cefotaxime, 150 mg/kg per day divided every 6 to 8 hours IV or IM in the neonate.

   (2) For those allergic to cephalosporins, use gentamicin, 5 to 7.5 mg/kg per day divided every 8 hours IV or IM.

(3) If cocci are identified in the urinary sediment or no organisms are seen, initial therapy should include ampicillin plus a third-generation cephalosporin.

   b. *Uncomplicated patient*—The child, usually older than 2 months of age, who is not seriously ill or significantly dehydrated, who can take oral fluids and medication, and in whom compliance is expected may be managed as an outpatient.

   (1) Ceftriaxone 50 mg/kg IM or IV (if allergic to a cephalosporin, give gentamicin, 2.5 mg/kg IM or IV). After 8 to 12 hours, give one of the oral antibacterial agents for treatment of a UTI.

Key Treatment: Oral Antimicrobial Therapy for UTIs

Antibacterial Agent	Daily Dosage and Intervals
Sulfisoxazole	120–150 mg/kg, divided q 4–6 hr
Trimethoprim-sulfamethoxazole (TMP-SMX)	6–12 mg/kg TMP, 30–60 mg/kg SMX, divided q 12 hr
Amoxicillin*	20–40 mg/kg, divided q 8 hr
Cephalexin (Keflex)	25–50 mg/kg, divided q 6 hr
Cefixime (Suprax)	8 mg/kg, divided q 12 hr
Cefpodoxime (Vantin)	10 mg/kg, divided q 12 hr
Loracarbef (Lorabid)	15–30 mg/kg, divided q 12 hr
Nitrofurantoin†	5–7 mg/kg, divided q 6 hr

*In some communities many strains of *Escherichia coli* are resistant to amoxicillin.

†Indicated for treatment of clinical cystitis (lower UTI) but not for acute pyelonephritis because of limited tissue distribution.

From Hellerstein S: Urinary tract infections. Old and new concepts. Pediatr Clin North Am 1995;42:1433–1457.

   (2) The physician should be contacted if the child is unable to tolerate oral fluids or the oral antibiotic or if clinical symptoms increase. A child doing poorly and a child with a positive blood culture should be hospitalized for intravenous therapy.

   c. *All children with acute pyelonephritis*—The results of bacterial sensitivity studies should be used to modify treatment if warranted. The hospitalized child who is improved clinically should be placed on oral medication after being afebrile for 24 hours. Most children are ready for discharge 48 to 72 hours after admission. Oral medication at therapeutic doses should be given for about 10 days, followed by treatment to prevent reinfection (Table 217–2).

   (1) Preventive (suppressive or prophylactic) antibacterial treatment may be discontinued in children without VUR if there is no recurrence of infection after 6 months. The urine should be checked for infection if there are symptoms of a UTI or an unexplained illness. Children with VUR should be kept on the preventive dose of antibiotic with ongoing monitoring and should be scheduled for follow-up bladder imaging

TABLE 217–2. ANTIMICROBIAL THERAPY: PREVENTION OF RECURRENT UTIs

DRUG*	DOSAGE
Nitrofurantoin†	1–2 mg/kg/day
Trimethoprim-sulfamethoxazole (TMP-SMX)†	1–2 mg/kg TMP, 5–10 mg/kg SMX per day
Trimethoprim	1–2 mg/kg/day

*These may be given as a single daily dose, usually at bedtime in the older child.
†Nitrofurantoin and sulfa drugs should not be used in infants younger than 2 months of age. Reduced doses of an oral first-generation cephalosporin, such as cephalexin at 10 mg/kg/day, may be used for antibacterial prophylaxis until 2 months of age. At times, because of drug intolerance or allergy, it may be necessary to use amoxicillin or an oral cephalosporin to prevent recurrent UTIs.
Adapted from Hellerstein S: Urinary tract infections. Old and new concepts. Pediatr Clin North Am 1995;42:1433–1457.

after 1 year. A breakthrough UTI is an indication for consideration of surgical reimplantation of the refluxing ureter.

(2) Urologic consultation should be sought for patients with obstructive lesions or dilating VUR (grade IV or greater VUR by the International Reflux Study Committee criteria).

(3) Children with renal scarring, a solitary kidney, or a unilateral small or atrophic kidney and those with hypertension, elevated serum creatinine levels, or other evidence of abnormal kidney function should be evaluated by a pediatric nephrologist.

2. Cystitis

a. Therapeutic doses of antibacterial agents for oral treatment of a UTI should be used. Children who do not show a good clinical response within 2 to 3 days should have a repeat urinalysis and culture.

b. A follow-up urinary culture should be obtained after 5 to 7 days of treatment.

c. Symptomatic relief from urinary frequency and dysuria is often afforded by sitz baths in warm water for 20 to 30 minutes three to four times a day. Systemic analgesia with acetaminophen or bladder analgesia with phenazopyridine hydrochloride (Pyridium) is occasionally needed. The latter should not be used for a period longer than 48 hours because of the risks of methemoglobinemia, hemolytic anemia, and other toxic reactions.

Bibliography

Haycock GB: A practical approach to evaluating urinary tract infection in children. Pediatr Nephrol 1991;5:401–402.
Hellerstein S: Urinary tract infections: Old and new concepts. Pediatr Clin North Am 1995;42:1433–1457.
Jodal U, Winberg J: Management of children with unobstructed urinary tract infection. Pediatr Nephrol 1987;1:647–656.
Nash MA, Seigle RL: Urinary tract infections in infants and children. Adv Pediatr Infect Dis 1996;11:403–448.
Winberg J, Anderson HJ, Bergström T, et al: Epidemiology of symptomatic urinary tract infection in childhood. Acta Paediatr Scand 1974;S252:3–19.

Symptom | **Isolated Hematuria**

Douglas L. Blowey

Definition

1. The isolated finding of blood in the urine of an asymptomatic child occurs frequently but rarely signifies the presence of serious renal disease. Hematuria may be macroscopic (i.e., gross) or microscopic; it may be persistent, recurrent, or transient. The diagnosis of hematuria should be confirmed by a microscopic examination of the urinary sediment, because red urine and a positive urine dipstick test for blood may reflect the presence in the urine of pigments, dyes, hemoglobin, or myoglobin.

2. Microscopic hematuria is defined as the presence of five or more red blood cells per high-power field on a fresh, centrifuged urine sample. This should be confirmed by at least two sequential urine samples.

Etiology

The causes of isolated hematuria are numerous and are best categorized by the presumed site of bleeding.

1. Glomerular

a. Glomerulonephritis (likely to be associated with other symptoms of renal disease)

(1) Immunoglobulin A (IgA) nephropathy (Berger disease)

(2) Acute postinfectious glomerulonephritis

b. Primary glomerulopathy

(1) Hereditary nephritis (e.g., Alport syndrome)

(2) Thin glomerular basement membrane disease

2. Nonglomerular

a. Infectious

b. Metabolic (e.g., hypercalciuria)

c. Toxic (e.g., drugs)

d. Tumors (e.g., Wilms tumor)

e. Polycystic kidney disease

3. Postrenal

a. Obstruction

b. Nephrolithiasis

c. Inflammation (e.g., cystitis)

d. Trauma

4. Nonrenal

a. Bleeding diathesis

b. Factitious

Epidemiology

The prevalence of persistent microscopic hematuria in school-age children is 0.5 to 2 per cent.

Clinical Findings

1. Symptoms related to renal disease (e.g., fatigue, anorexia, poor growth, anemia, hypertension, and oliguria or poly-

uria) should be sought in any child presenting with hematuria. A complete history and physical examination, including an accurate measurement of the child's blood pressure, is required. The family history should be scrutinized for hematuria, urolithiasis, kidney disease, renal failure, and hearing impairment.
2. The urine should be examined for protein and the urinary sediment for leukocytes, cellular casts, and crystals.

IgA Nephropathy (Berger Disease)

Epidemiology
1. IgA nephropathy is a very common glomerular disorder, detected in up to one third of persons biopsied for persistent microscopic hematuria.
2. There is a 2:1 male predominance.
3. IgA nephropathy is uncommon in blacks.

Pathophysiology
The diagnosis is based on kidney biopsy showing a predominance of IgA deposits, primarily in the mesangium. The pathogenesis of the glomerular injury that results in hematuria is unknown.

Clinical Findings
1. Recurrent episodes of painless macroscopic hematuria constitute the prevailing manifestation of IgA nephropathy. The episodes of macroscopic hematuria are often precipitated by a nonspecific viral infection. Unlike the 7- to 10-day latent period observed in acute postinfectious glomerulonephritis, the macroscopic hematuria linked to IgA nephropathy occurs at the same time or very shortly after an infection. The duration of macroscopic hematuria is usually less than 72 hours.
2. Microscopic hematuria, with or without proteinuria, is also a frequent presentation. This pattern may persist between episodes of macroscopic hematuria.
3. Rarely, the nephrotic syndrome or renal failure is the presenting manifestation of IgA nephropathy.

Outcome
Ten to 30 per cent of patients with IgA nephropathy manifest a slow progressive loss of renal function. The remainder have stable renal function despite the continued presence of hematuria. No therapy has proved to be beneficial in halting the progressive loss of renal function.

Sickle Cell Nephropathy

Epidemiology
1. Up to one third of American blacks presenting with macroscopic hematuria have sickle cell disease.
2. Episodes of macroscopic hematuria occur in people with either sickle cell disease or sickle cell trait.

Pathophysiology
1. Sickling of the red blood cells in the renal medulla appears to play a causative role. Red blood cell sickling, even in persons who are heterozygous for the sickle cell mutation, occurs in the medulla owing to the low oxygen tension, hypertonic milieu, and low pH.
2. The bleeding is usually unilateral, most often from the left kidney.

Clinical Findings
The hematuria may be gross or microscopic. Gross hematuria is often recurrent.

Treatment
1. Treatment of the episodic macroscopic hematuria entails correction of the factors that promote sickling. Usual management consists of hydration and treatment of infection.
2. More specific therapies have been recommended for significant recalcitrant macroscopic hematuria, although none can be considered a treatment of choice. These include ϵ-aminocaproic acid, modified exchange transfusion, thiazide diuretics, renal embolization, and even unilateral nephrectomy.

Hereditary Nephritis

Hereditary nephritis is a term used to describe a heterogenous group of inherited renal diseases including Alport syndrome and familial recurrent hematuria (benign recurrent hematuria).

Alport Syndrome
Epidemiology
1. Alport syndrome accounts for 3 per cent of all children with chronic renal failure and 1.5 per cent of children on dialysis.
2. The syndrome is classically inherited as an X-linked trait; however, patterns of autosomal recessive and autosomal dominant inheritance have been reported.
3. Males are typically more severely affected, but in some kindreds females are severely affected.

Pathogenesis
An inherited defect in type IV collagen results in both renal and extrarenal abnormalities. Electron microscopy of a kidney biopsy specimen shows the characteristic ultrastructural findings of multilamination of the glomerular basement membrane with attenuation and periodic disruption.

Clinical Findings
1. The most common manifestation is microscopic hematuria. Episodes of macroscopic hematuria can occur during infectious episodes or periods of stress.
2. Since many children with Alport syndrome have a normal urinary sediment until the second decade of life, a normal urinalysis in a young child with a family history of Alport syndrome does not confirm the absence of that disorder.
3. Extrarenal manifestations
   a. Hearing loss is present in 40 per cent of individuals with Alport syndrome.
   b. Ocular abnormalities are exhibited in 30 per cent.

Treatment and Prognosis
1. Those with isolated hematuria and no evidence of deterioration in renal function (usually the females) require only ongoing monitoring and support. Genetic counseling is imperative.
2. Those with progressive renal deterioration should be referred to a pediatric nephrologist for ongoing care, because progression to end-stage kidney disease is inevitable.

Familial Recurrent Hematuria

1. Inherited as an autosomal dominant trait.
2. Clinical picture similar to Alport syndrome but lacking the extrarenal manifestations of hearing loss and ocular abnormalities.
3. In some patients, ultrastructural evaluation of kidney reveals thinning of the basement membrane, hence the eponym "thin basement membrane disease." The multi-lamination of the glomerular basement membrane seen in Alport syndrome is absent.
4. The long-term outcome is believed to be benign.

Bibliography

Boineau FG, Lewy JE: Evaluation of hematuria in children and adolescents. Pediatr Rev 1989;11:101–108.
Galla JH: IgA nephropathy. Kidney Int 1995;47:377–387.

Symptom	**Isolated Asymptomatic Proteinuria**	*Ari M. Simckes*

Definition

1. *Proteinuria*—Greater than normal urinary excretion of protein (UEP) with otherwise normal urinary findings. The history and physical examination are normal, as are laboratory studies except for the presence of proteinuria. Proteinuria may be diagnosed based on qualitative, semiquantitative, or quantitative criteria.

    a. *Qualitative*

       (1) $\geq 1+$ protein (30 mg/dl) on dipstick of dilute urine (specific gravity ≤ 1.015) on two out of three random specimens

       (2) $\geq 2+$ protein (100 mg/dl) on dipstick of concentrated urine (specific gravity ≥ 1.015) on two out of three random specimens.

    b. *Semiquantitative*—Urine protein:creatinine ratio (mg/dl) >0.2 in a daytime random urine specimen

    c. *Quantitative*—UEP ≥ 4 mg/m^2/hour in a timed (12 or 24 hours) urine collection.

2. *Microalbuminuria*—Urinary albumin excretion rate of 20 to 200 μg/min or (30 to 300 mg/24 hours). This level of proteinuria is not detected by routine urine dipsticks.

3. *Orthostatic (postural) proteinuria (OP)*—Greater than normal UEP that occurs only while the child is upright. A normal amount of protein is excreted in recumbent position. Protein excretion is usually less than 1 to 1.5 g/24 hours in this condition.

Epidemiology

1. Isolated asymptomatic proteinuria is often a transient phenomenon. It is common during childhood and is generally of little significance. The prevalence of asymptomatic proteinuria detected on a routine urinalysis is high in school-age children (about 5%), increases with age, and peaks during adolescence. Since children may have intermittent proteinuria, the more often a urinalysis is performed on a child, the greater the likelihood of detecting proteinuria.

2. Persistent proteinuria is rare during childhood. When protein is detected by qualitative or semiquantitative methods on multiple samples including first morning voids, an underlying renal disorder must be suspected.

3. OP is common in teenagers, accounting for 75 per cent of cases of isolated proteinuria in this age group. Therefore, ruling out OP is the first step in the evaluation of a teenager with proteinuria. OP is usually a transient phenomenon with a benign prognosis. However, it may be persistent in 2 to 5 per cent of teenagers and young adults. As long as proteinuria is the only abnormal finding, no impairment in renal function is to be expected (even in patients with persistent OP).

4. Microalbuminuria, in addition to being a prognostic indicator for progressive renal damage in those with diabetes, is present in up to 40 per cent of nondiabetic untreated hypertensive adults.

Pathogenesis

1. *Glomerular proteinuria*—Increased glomerular filtration of plasma proteins occurs because of increased intraglomerular hydrostatic pressure and/or damaged, leaky glomerular capillary walls, which occur in most glomerular diseases. Albumin is the most abundant urinary protein in this setting. OP is a form of glomerular proteinuria, yet the pathogenesis is unclear. Probably, subtle alterations of the filtration system within the glomerulus result in proteinuria concurrent with the hemodynamic changes that occur during upright posture.

2. *Overflow proteinuria*—Excessive plasma concentration of a normal or abnormal protein may result in filtration of proteins which overwhelm the renal tubule reabsorptive capacity. Although uncommonly associated with asymptomatic proteinuria, causes include:

    a. Dysproteinemias (immunoglobulin light chains)

    b. Acute proliferative diseases

    c. Muscle injury (myoglobinuria).

3. *Tubular proteinuria*—Renal tubule dysfunction may result in decreased reabsorption of filtered proteins. This occurs in many situations, including congenital tubular disorders (e.g., Fanconi syndrome, Lowe syndrome) and toxic injury (e.g., tubular-interstitial nephritis, cadmium poisoning). Increased excretion of low-molecular-weight proteins is present without elevated plasma levels. Excessive tubular secretion of proteins into the urine is a rare cause of proteinuria.

4. *Microalbuminuria*—This occurs in both diabetic and nondiabetic individuals when the glomerular filtration of albumin exceeds reabsorption by the proximal tubule.

Clinical Findings

Isolated proteinuria, being asymptomatic, is usually detected on a routine urinalysis (e.g., physical examination for school or sports) and often leads to apprehension for the patient, family, and physician. It should be documented by semiquantitative or quantitative tests to avoid an unnecessary and costly laboratory work-up. The urinalysis should be otherwise normal, and the physical examination (including blood pressure) should be normal. If appropriate, pregnancy should be ruled out. The pattern of the proteinuria should be determined.

1. *Transient or intermittent proteinuria*—This phenomenon may occur in many situations and does not require work-up if the urine has cleared of protein 1 to 2 weeks after the particular stress has resolved. Conditions associated with transient proteinuria include the following:
   a. Fever
   b. Infections (not only of the urinary tract)
   c. Congestive heart failure
   d. Seizures
   e. Strenuous exercise
   f. Psychological and/or physiologic stress.

2. *Persistent proteinuria*—Proteinuria that persists long after initial detection and is not orthostatic. Children with persistent proteinuria that is not orthostatic require further evaluation.

3. *Orthostatic proteinuria*—This may be either persistent or transient.

Laboratory Findings

1. Except for the elevated UEP, other laboratory findings are normal (e.g., blood chemical analyses, spun urine sediment, urine culture) in those with isolated proteinuria.

2. The pattern of the proteinuria may be determined (e.g., persistent, transient, orthostatic) with the use of urine dipsticks. If the first morning samples are negative for protein and those obtained during the day are positive, OP should be suspected. A confirmatory test for OP is to quantify protein excretion in a "split" 24-hour collection. The amount of protein excreted during the day (about 12 hours) is compared with that excreted while recumbent (overnight urine collection, 8 to 10 hours). The child's bladder must be emptied before she or he goes to bed,

and this urine must be discarded and not included in the overnight collection.

3. Excretion of >3 g of protein in 24 hours usually indicates glomerular proteinuria. Those with persistent proteinuria with >1 g of protein in 24 hours should have measurements of total serum protein, serum albumin, cholesterol, urea nitrogen, creatinine, and liver function. In selected cases, C3, C4, antinuclear antibodies, hepatitis screen, rapid plasma reagin, and human immunodeficiency virus testing should be considered.

4. Determining the type or types of proteins excreted (e.g., albumin, β_2 microglobulin, immunoglobulin light chains) and the source of the proteinuria (e.g., glomerular, tubular, overflow) may be required if the source of the urinary protein is not clear from the preceding studies. This may be accomplished by electrophoretic analysis of urinary proteins.

5. Renal biopsy is not indicated in those with isolated proteinuria, if it is transient and/or orthostatic. Renal biopsy may be required for the diagnostic evaluation of children with persistent proteinuria.

Imaging Studies

Imaging studies are not indicated in those with isolated asymptomatic proteinuria.

Treatment

Unless there is an underlying disorder such as diabetes mellitus or a glomerular disease such as "minimal change disease," membranous nephropathy, or membranoproliferative glomerulonephritis associated with isolated proteinuria, no specific therapy is required.

 Bibliography

Ettenger R: The evaluation of the child with proteinuria. Pediatr Ann 1994;23:9:486–494.

Glassock RJ, Cohen AH, Adler SG: Primary glomerular diseases. *In* Brenner BM (ed): The Kidney, 5th ed., vol 2. Philadelphia, WB Saunders, 1995, pp 1422–1423.

Larson TS: Evaluation of proteinuria: Mayo Clin Proc 1994; 69:1154–1158.

Vehaskari VM, Robson AM: Proteinuria. *In* Edelmann CM (ed): Pediatric Kidney Disease, 2nd ed., vol 1. Boston, Little, Brown, 1992, pp 531–551.

218 Acute Glomerulonephritis

Douglas L. Blowey

Definition

Varied degrees of hematuria, proteinuria, hypertension, and, at times, impaired renal function constitute the main clinical features of acute glomerulonephritis. The fundamental pathologic feature, glomerular inflammation, originates from a heterogeneous group of causes. In children, most

cases appear to be acute postinfectious glomerulonephritis (APGN). The remaining causes are principally categorized as primary or secondary glomerulonephritis.

1. *Primary glomerulonephritis* denotes a disorder in which the original and predominant structure involved is the glomerulus of the kidney. The extrarenal mani-

festations (e.g., hypertension, edema) are presumed to spring from the functional impairment of the kidney.

   a. Mesangiocapillary glomerulonephritis (MPGN, types I and II)

   b. Mesangial proliferative glomerulonephritis

   c. Immunoglobulin A (IgA) nephropathy (Berger disease)

2. *Secondary glomerulonephritis* designates a collection of systemic diseases with renal involvement. The extrarenal findings are usually manifestations of the systemic process.

   a. Systemic lupus erythematosus (SLE)

   b. Henoch-Schönlein purpura

   c. Primary vasculitis (e.g., Wegener granulomatosis, polyarteritis nodosa)

   d. Goodpasture syndrome

   e. Drug hypersensitivity reactions

Acute Postinfectious Glomerulonephritis

Epidemiology

1. The incidence of APGN is difficult to estimate due to the substantial rate of subclinical cases. Most cases of APGN occur during the early school-age years (e.g., 5 to 10 years of age), with a slight male predominance.

2. Group A, β-hemolytic streptococcus is the most common agent associated with APGN. Typically, cases of APGN related to streptococcal pharyngeal infections occur during the winter to spring months, whereas those resulting from streptococcal skin infections occur during the summer months. Several different strains of Group A, β-hemolytic streptococci have been associated with APGN (e.g., M-type 12 and 49); however, only a small percentage of individuals infected with a nephritogenic strain develop glomerulonephritis.

3. APGN is associated with an expansive list of bacterial, viral, fungal, parasitic, and rickettsial agents.

Pathophysiology

1. The glomerular damage associated with APGN appears to be mediated, in part, by immune complexes. The varied clinical expression of the disorder suggests that many host and pathogen factors play a modifying role.

2. Immunofluorescence and electron microscopic studies have established the presence of immune complex deposits on the subepithelial side of the glomerular basement membrane. These granular deposits are predominately composed of IgG and the complement component C3.

3. The pathogenesis of the immune deposits in the kidney is poorly understood. The subepithelial immune deposits may result from the glomerular trapping of circulating immune complexes, in situ immune complex formation involving planted antigens, or in situ immune complex formation resulting from the exposure of native glomerular antigens.

4. A sequence of cellular and immunologic events is triggered by the immune deposits and ultimately brings about an alteration in glomerular structure and function. Modulators believed to be involved in the complex sequence of events include monocytes, polymorphonuclear neutro-

phils, complement components, platelets, and coagulation factors. Of these, monocytes appear to play the pivotal role in the cascade of glomerular events leading to damage. In addition to the influx of inflammatory cells into the glomeruli, there is mesangial and endothelial cell proliferation.

Clinical Findings

1. The clinical hallmark of streptococcus-associated APGN is the presence of a latent period between the clinical manifestations of the infection (e.g., pharyngitis) and the abrupt onset of glomerulonephritis. The typical latent period is 7 to 10 days, but it may be longer with streptococcal skin infections. An accurate estimation of the duration of the latent period is of considerable importance, because uncharacteristic latent periods (e.g., <5 days, or >14 days) may suggest an alternate diagnosis.

   a. Clinical evidence of acute glomerulonephritis coincident with or shortly following an acute infection (i.e., <5 days) is suggestive of IgA nephropathy or an exacerbation of a preexisting glomerular process.

   b. A prolonged interval between an acute infection and the onset of glomerulonephritis (i.e., >14 days) should spur the consideration of other primary or secondary causes.

2. The clinical features of APGN are macroscopic or microscopic hematuria, edema, reduced urine output, and hypertension. Many children have an almost subclinical presentation, with only scant hematuria and few other findings.

   a. Macroscopic (gross) hematuria, often described as cola-colored urine, is a common symptom bringing the child to the attention of a physician. Children with clinically evident APGN have microscopic hematuria, and 50 per cent have episodes of macroscopic hematuria. In most instances, the urinary abnormalities resolve within 6 months, but microscopic hematuria may persist for 1 year or longer.

   b. Hypertension may be severe and a significant source of morbidity. Uncontrolled hypertension can result in hypertensive encephalopathy and/or congestive heart failure. Hypertension is usually transient and resolves within 2 weeks.

   c. Edema results from fluid retention or, in the rare circumstance of massive proteinuria, from hypoalbuminemia. In most instances, periorbital edema and some generalized puffiness along with weight gain is noted, but dependent edema is usually absent.

Key Clinical Findings

- Preceding pharyngitis or pyoderma

- Periorbital edema

- Reduced urine output

- Hypertension

d. Varied degrees of decreased urine output are frequently encountered, although anuria is uncommon. Diuresis commonly occurs within 5 to 7 days.

e. A rapidly progressive impairment of renal function and the nephrotic syndrome are rare clinical presentations of APGN.

Laboratory Findings

1. The key elements in the diagnostic laboratory investigation of APGN are

   a. Documentation of depressed serum complement (C3)

   b. Documentation of a prior streptococcal infection

   c. An abnormal urinary sediment.

2. During the acute phase of APGN, C3 is depressed.

   a. The depression is short-lived and returns to normal by 8 weeks in 94 per cent of cases. Persistent hypocomplementemia increases the likelihood of another cause of the hypocomplementemic glomerulonephritis (e.g., SLE, MPGN).

   b. In the situation of persistent hypocomplementemia, a renal biopsy should be strongly considered.

   c. Owing to the brief nature of the complement depression, a normal serum complement in a child evaluated later in the course of the illness does not exclude the possibility of APGN.

3. Antibody titers to streptococcal antigens are used to provide evidence of a preceding streptococcal infection.

   a. A rise in the antistreptolysin O (ASO) titer occurs in 70 to 80 per cent of individuals after a streptococcal pharyngeal infection. The rise in the ASO titer is frequently absent after a streptococcal skin infection.

   b. In cases in which the ASO titer is inconclusive, antideoxyribonuclease B titers may be more sensitive.

Key Laboratory Findings

- Gross hematuria (cola-colored urine)
- Proteinuria
- Red cell casts in urine
- Depressed serum complement C3
- Rise in antistreptolysin O titer

4. Examination of the urine demonstrates varied degrees of proteinuria and hematuria. Red blood cell casts are frequently observed when a fresh, centrifuged urine sample is examined. Leukocytes are also common.

5. Chest radiography usually shows an enlarged heart and often increased vascular markings from hypovolemia.

Treatment

1. The clinical course of APGN is not altered by therapeutic maneuvers. Because the great majority of children with APGN recover completely, therapy is supportive and directed toward prevention of complications.

2. Hypertension, a major source of morbidity in APGN, should be aggressively treated. The oral administration of short-acting calcium channel blockers (e.g., nifedipine) is often used for the acute lowering of moderately elevated blood pressure. Intravenous medications (e.g., labetalol, diazoxide, hydralazine, nitroprusside) should be considered for children with severe hypertension. Milder hypertension can be treated with oral medications such as diuretics or calcium channel blockers.

3. Fluid and sodium intake should be closely monitored to prevent further fluid retention. In cases in which edema is evident, the diuretic furosemide may be of some benefit.

WARNING

In the acute presentation, if the disorder is not recognized, pulmonary edema with fatal outcome may occur (treatment: phlebotomy).

Key Treatments

- Control intake of water and salt if oliguria is present
- Treat mild hypertension, if present, with oral medication
- Treat severe hypertension with intravenous medication
- Phlebotomy for pulmonary edema

Outcome

1. Most children with APGN recover from the episode of acute glomerulonephritis. During the acute phase, morbidity and mortality are related to sepsis and hypertension.

2. The children who have massive proteinuria, prolonged hypertension, or a preceding infection that is not caused by group A, β-hemolytic streptococci are at increased risk for permanent kidney damage.

B | Bibliography

Dodge WF, Spargo BH, Travis LB, et al: Poststreptococcal glomerulonephritis: A prospective study in children. N Engl J Med 1972;286:273–278.

Makker SP: Glomerular diseases. *In* Kher KK, Makker SP (eds): Clinical Pediatric Nephrology. New York, McGraw-Hill, 1992, p 175.

Rodríquez-Iturbe B: Epidemic poststreptococcal glomerulonephritis. Kidney Int 1984;25:129–136.

219 Nephrotic Syndrome

Ari M. Simckes

Definition

Nephrotic syndrome (NS) is characterized by heavy proteinuria resulting in hypoalbuminemia, edema, and hyperlipidemia. NS unrelated to a systemic disease is called *primary NS* and accounts for about 90 per cent of childhood cases. NS associated with a systemic disorder, infection, drug, or toxin is called *secondary NS*.

1. Primary nephrotic syndrome

   a. *Congenital nephrotic syndrome (CNS)*—The patient usually presents at birth or within the first 3 months. The classic example is the Finnish-type NS, but CNS may also result from a congenital infection (e.g., syphilis). Children with infantile NS present between 3 to 12 months of age; causes include diffuse mesangial sclerosis and other glomerular diseases.

   b. *Mimimal change nephrotic syndrome (MCNS)* is the most common primary nephrotic syndrome of childhood. It is also called "nil" disease, lipoid nephrosis, and idiopathic primary NS. MCNS is usually steroid responsive.

   c. *Focal segmental glomerulosclerosis,* a form of *primary* NS of childhood, is usually steroid nonresponsive; other forms of NS, such as membranous nephropathy and membranoproliferative glomerulonephritis (GN), may or may not be steroid responsive.

2. Secondary nephrotic syndrome

   a. *Associated with infections* such as bacterial, viral, protozoal, and helminthic infections. Numerous infections have been associated with NS. The NS can occur concurrent with or after the infection (i.e., postinfectious GN).

   b. *Associated with a systemic disorder* such as connective tissue disorders, lupus erythematosus, Henoch-Schönlein purpura, and immunoglobulin A nephropathy (Berger disease). Numerous other medical conditions (e.g., infections, neoplasms) have been associated with NS.

   c. *Associated with allergens* such as bee stings, snake bites, immunizations, food allergies, and poison oak.

   d. *Associated with medications or toxins* such as nonsteroidal antiinflammatory drugs, penicillamine, lithium, heroin, gold, trimethadione, and mercury.

Etiology and Epidemiology

1. The most common form of NS during childhood is MCNS, a descriptive term based on essentially normal light microscopy histologic findings. However, virtually all of the primary and secondary glomerulopathies can provoke the biochemical features that constitute the NS.

2. Age at presentation is clinically important, because the probability that a patient with NS has a steroid-responsive glomerular disease (mainly MCNS) is age related. Steroid responsiveness is infrequent during the first year, but is present in some 95 per cent of children aged 1 to 3 years; responsiveness declines to 15 per cent in persons older than 35 years of age. NS occurs at an annual rate of approximately 2 per 100,000 children younger than 16 years old, with a cumulative prevalence of 16 per 100,000. The majority of these children (about 80%) have MCNS, with the highest incidence in those between 2 to 6 years of age.

3. The cause of MCNS remains unclear and is probably heterogeneous. Many observations implicate involvement of immune-mediated processes, particularly dysregulation of T-cell function.

Pathophysiology

The biochemical and clinical features of the NS are primarily caused by abnormal permeability of the glomerular basement membrane (GBM) resulting in proteinuria.

1. Proteinuria

   a. The specific abnormalities causing the altered GBM permeability vary depending on the cause of the NS. In MCNS, there is increased clearance of negatively charged proteins (e.g., albumin) due to loss of the charge-selective barrier normally provided by anionic constituents of the GBM (e.g., heparan sulfate, proteoglycans).

   b. MCNS is characterized by selective proteinuria, meaning that albumin is the main protein found in the urine.

   c. Secondary NS, such as immune-mediated glomerular injury, results in nonselective proteinuria caused by damage to the GBM and alterations in transglomerular pore size and/or number. Because of these alterations in the size-selective barrier, high-molecular-weight proteins in addition to albumin can be found in the urine.

2. Hypoalbuminemia

   a. Hypoalbuminemia results from an inability of protein synthesis by the liver to balance protein catabolism and the increased urinary protein losses (primarily by the renal tubules).

> **WARNING**
>
> **As a result of the alterations of coagulation factors and hyperaggregation of platelets, patients with NS are in a hypercoagulable state and at increased risk for thromboembolic events.**

   b. Normal or elevated rates of albumin synthesis occur in patients with NS.

c. Serum proteins other than albumin may be increased or decreased, with resultant effects on immune responses, the coagulation cascade, and the fibrinolytic system.

3. Hyperlipidemia

a. Serum cholesterol concentration is inversely related to the serum albumin level. Triglycerides and lipoproteins (e.g., low-density lipoproteins, very-low-density lipoproteins) may be increased in the NS.

b. The cause of the elevation in lipid levels is believed to be increased synthesis, stimulated by the decreased oncotic pressure resulting from the hypoproteinemia, and decreased breakdown of lipoproteins, caused by inhibition of lipoprotein lipase activity.

4. Edema is the cardinal clinical feature of NS. It occurs in dependent areas, particularly in lax tissues, when the serum albumin falls below 2.4 g/dl. Two theories have been proposed to explain the formation of edema in the NS.

a. Classic theory

(1) Hypoproteinemia secondary to urinary losses leads to decreased intravascular oncotic pressure, moving water and solute to the interstitial space.

(2) Secondary to the decreased intravascular volume, physiologic mechanisms (e.g., renin-angiotensin-aldosterone system, antidiuretic hormone) enhance distal renal tubular sodium and water reabsorption.

b. Intrarenal theory—Sodium retention seems to be unrelated to the serum renin and aldosterone levels. This suggests that the factor causing edema is increased renal tubular sodium reabsorption. An unknown stimulus may affect intrarenal hemodynamics, resulting in increased sodium and water reabsorption.

Features of the Nephrotic Syndrome

- Proteinuria
- Edema
- Hypoproteinemia and/or hypoalbuminemia
- Hyperlipidemia
- Lipiduria

Clinical Findings

The presentation of the child with NS is quite uniform, despite the myriad causes. History of a recent prodromal infection (e.g., upper respiratory tract infection) is often elicited, and decreased urine output is often present.

1. *Edema*—The parents frequently note swelling, initially around the eyes, which is worse in the morning. This is often mistaken for an allergic reaction. Later, facial, abdominal, sacral, labial, scrotal, and pitting pretibial edema usually become apparent.

2. *Gastrointestinal system*—Loss of appetite, diarrhea, edema of the intestinal wall, ascites, and abdominal pain are common as a consequence of the hypoproteinemia. Ab-

dominal pain, particularly in the right upper quadrant, may occur secondary to hepatomegaly caused by liver edema and increased albumin synthesis.

WARNING

Evaluation of abdominal pain in these children is important since they are at risk for peritonitis (usually pneumococcal) because of the presence of ascitic fluid and decreased resistance to infection. Immunodeficiency occurs secondary to the NS as well as from iatrogenic immunosuppression. Some pediatric nephrologists recommend treatment with a prophylactic antibiotic (penicillin) and administration of vaccinations (pneumococcal).

---

3. *Respiratory system*—Respiratory difficulty may occur because of abdominal distention (ascites), pleural effusions, and pneumonia.

Key Clinical Findings

- Periorbital edema
- Dependent edema
- Ascites

Laboratory Findings

1. Urine

a. By definition, patients during the onset or with a relapse of the NS have heavy proteinuria, defined as >40 mg/m²/hour.

b. Heavy proteinuria is usually present with a protein:creatinine ratio of ≥2.0 in a random urine specimen.

c. The urine is often concentrated in response to intravascular depletion.

d. Approximately 20 per cent of children with MCNS have trace hematuria at presentation.

e. Moderate and persistent hematuria or cellular casts suggest focal segmental glomerulosclerosis or a secondary form of NS.

2. Blood

a. Hypoproteinemia and hypoalbuminemia (usually <2.5 g/dl).

b. Hyponatremia is common and may be secondary to water retention or to a pseudohyponatremia caused by hyperlipidemia.

c. Hypocalcemia is often caused by hypoalbuminemia. The ionized serum calcium is usually normal.

d. Serum urea nitrogen (BUN or SUN) and serum creatinine are usually normal but may be mildly elevated as a result of hypovolemia.

e. The hemoglobin and hematocrit may be raised secondary to plasma volume contraction, and the platelet count is often elevated.

f. Serum cholesterol, triglycerides, very-low-density

lipoprotein, and low-density lipoprotein are usually increased.

 g. Serum complements C3 and C4 are normal or elevated in primary MCNS. When complement levels are decreased, membranoproliferative GN, postinfectious GN, and lupus nephritis should be considered.

3. Renal biopsy is indicated if the history and laboratory features suggest a disorder other than MCNS or if the child does not respond to the initial or subsequent courses of steroids or is steroid dependent. Hypocomplementemia, macroscopic hematuria, age >10 years or <1 year (especially <6 months) are often indications for biopsy, because the histologic findings may aid with diagnostic and therapeutic decisions.

Key Laboratory Findings

- Marked proteinuria
- Hypoalbuminemia
- Increased serum cholesterol

Radiographic Changes

 The child with the NS does not routinely require radiologic studies.

Treatment

1. General management does not alter the natural history of the disorder but does counteract the risks of complications and makes the patient more comfortable. Children with CNS, most of those with secondary NS, and those with renal failure require special management and should be referred to a pediatric nephrologist.

 a. *Diet*—Children with MCNS should have a diet appropriate to their age. Fluids, protein, and salt usually do not need to be restricted.

 b. Diuretics

  (1) Proper use of diuretics (e.g., furosemide, spironolactone, thiazides, metolazone), often in combinations, may effectively minimize symptomatic edema and ascites.

  (2) Monitoring should be performed to screen for complications from diuretic treatment (e.g., hypokalemia, hyperuricemia, hyperglycemia).

  (3) Infusion of concentrated serum albumin (0.5 to 1 g/kg), followed by a loop diuretic, is very effective treatment of edema and is indicated when there is profound edema, respiratory and gastrointestinal symptoms, and skin breakdown. Patients receiving albumin must be closely monitored for complications such as hypertension, pulmonary edema, and cardiac decompensation.

 c. *Activity*—Physical activity need not be limited.

2. Steroid therapy is recommended for children with a clinical presentation suggestive of MCNS, since most will respond.

 a. PPD skin testing with positive controls is recommended before initiation of steroid treatment.

 b. The initial prednisone dose is 2 mg/kg/day or 60 mg/m²/day, divided 3 times per day for 4 to 6 weeks. Although proteinuria usually resolves after 2 weeks, some patients respond more slowly. If the proteinuria resolves, the prednisone dose is decreased to approximately 1.3 mg/kg or 40 mg/m², given as a single morning dose every other day for 4 to 6 weeks, and subsequently tapered and discontinued.

 c. Relapse of the NS is treated by a shorter course of high-dose prednisone, until the urine is dipstick negative for protein for three consecutive days; the dose then is lowered to the alternate-day schedule for 1 month, then tapered.

 d. Those children in whom the proteinuria continues despite compliance with corticosteroid treatment, those who relapse on discontinuation or tapering of the steroids, those who relapse frequently (e.g., twice in 6 months), and those with signs of steroid toxicity (e.g., growth retardation, profound cushingoid appearance, hyperglycemia, cataracts) should be referred to a pediatric nephrologist.

Key Treatment

- Corticosteroid to suppress immune inflammatory process
- Albumin infusion with furosemide for symptomatic edema

Bibliography

Anderson S, Garcia DL, Brenner BM: Renal and systemic manifestations of glomerular disease. *In* Brenner BM, Rector FC (eds): The Kidney, 4th ed. Philadelphia, WB Saunders, 1991, pp 1831–1870.

Barratt TM, Clark G: Minimal change nephrotic syndrome and focal segmental glomerulosclerosis. *In* Holliday MA, Barratt TM, Avner ED (eds): Pediatric Nephrology, 3rd ed. Baltimore, Williams & Wilkins, 1994, pp 767–787.

Holmberg C, Laine J, Ronnholm K, et al: Congenital nephrotic syndrome. Kidney Int 1996;49:53:S51–S56.

Nash MA, Edelmann CM, Bernstein J, Barnett HL: The nephrotic syndrome and minimal change nephrotic syndrome, diffuse mesangial hypercellularity, and focal glomerular sclerosis. *In* Edelmann CM (ed): Pediatric Kidney Disease, 2nd ed. Boston, Little, Brown, 1992, pp 1247–1290.

Warshaw BL: Nephrotic syndrome in children. Pediatr Ann 1994;23:9:495–504.

220 Renal Tubular Acidosis

Uri S. Alon

Definition

Renal tubular acidosis (RTA) is defined by the presence of alkaline urine in a patient with hyperchloremic metabolic acidosis who has a normal anion gap and normal or near-normal glomerular function. Depending on the site of the nephron affected, three types of RTA (proximal, distal, and type IV) are recognized (Table 220–1).

Pathophysiology

1. The basic disorder in proximal RTA is a reduction in the capacity of the proximal tubule to reabsorb the filtered bicarbonate. As a result, the tubular threshold for bicarbonate declines, and with it the serum bicarbonate concentration. Because the distal tubular activity remains intact, the kidney adequately continues to secrete H$^+$ ions and, therefore, the serum bicarbonate concentration of patients with proximal RTA remains close to or equal to the "reset" tubular threshold, without further progression of the systemic acidosis. Correction of the acidosis with alkali administration and elevation of serum bicarbonate concentration gives rise to massive bicarbonaturia, which at normal serum bicarbonate concentration exceeds 15 per cent of the filtered load. When the serum bicarbonate concentration is below the tubular threshold, the urine pH falls to less than 6.0. Although proximal RTA can be an isolated disorder, it is often associated with more wide-spread tubular dysfunctions, including phosphaturia, aminoaciduria, and glucosuria (i.e., Fanconi syndrome).

2. The basic disorder in distal RTA is the inability of the distal renal tubular cells to secrete H$^+$ ions. As a result of this tubular defect, the patient's urine pH remains alkaline (>6.0), and net acid excretion is reduced even during extreme systemic metabolic acidosis. The continuous failure of the renal tubule to secrete H$^+$ ions leads to retention of H$^+$ and to progressive acidosis. Patients with distal RTA usually have more profound acidemia than those with proximal RTA. With normalization of serum bicarbonate concentrations with alkali therapy, losses of bicarbonate in the urine vary with age: in children and adults it is less than 3 per cent; in infants it may reach 15 per cent, because of the greater role of bicarbonate reabsorption in the distal tubule during infancy. The degree of bicarbonaturia decreases progressively with advancing age.

3. A true situation of mixed distal and proximal RTA is observed in the rare syndrome of carbonic anhydrase II deficiency (see below).

4. RTA type IV is associated with low circulating aldosterone concentrations or partial or complete end-organ resistance to the mineralocorticoid. RTA type IV can be divided into five subtypes, as shown in Table 220–2.

Clinical Findings

Infants with both distal and proximal RTA present with failure to thrive, vomiting, polyuria, dehydration, and acidotic breathing. Short stature is characteristic of untreated older children. Hypokalemic paralysis has been described, although this is an infrequent symptom of RTA in early life. Children with Fanconi syndrome may have rachitic bone deformities, and older patients with distal RTA may have urolithiasis. Patients with RTA type IV diagnosed during infancy usually have some degree of failure to thrive.

Key Clinical Findings

- Failure to grow
- Polyuria
- Vomiting

TABLE 220–1. CLINICAL AND LABORATORY FINDINGS OF RENAL TUBULAR ACIDOSIS (RTA) IN CHILDHOOD

FINDING	PROXIMAL RTA	DISTAL RTA	TYPE IV RTA
Growth failure	+	+	+
Serum potassium	N to ↓	N to ↓	↑
Urine pH during profound acidosis	<6.0	>6.0	<6.0
Net acid excretion during profound acidosis	N	↓	↓
Potassium excretion	↑	↑	↓
Calcium excretion	N to ↑	↑	N (?)
Citrate excretion	N	↓	N
Bicarbonate excretion (%) at normal serum bicarbonate	>15	<5*	<15
(Urine-blood) Pco$_2$	N	↓	(?)
Glucosuria, aminoaciduria, and hyperphosphaturia	+	—	—
Nephrocalcinosis	—	+	—
Rickets	+	—**	—
Daily alkali treatment (mEq/kg body weight)	2–15	1–4*	1–3
Requirement for potassium with treatment	↑	—	—

+, commonly exists; —, absent; N, normal; ↑, increased; ↓, decreased; *, higher in infants; **, rarely seen.
Modified from Alon U, Chan JCM: Inherited forms of renal tubular acidosis. *In* Fernandes J, Sandubray J-M, Tada K (eds): Inborn Metabolic Diseases: Diagnosis and Treatment. Berlin, Springer-Verlag, 1990, with permission.

TABLE 220–2. SUBTYPES OF RENAL TUBULAR ACIDOSIS TYPE IV

	CLINICAL AND LABORATORY FINDINGS				
MECHANISM AND DESIGNATION	**Plasma Renin Activity**	**Serum Aldosterone**	**Blood Volume**	**Blood Pressure**	**Salt Wasting**
Aldosterone deficiency without intrinsic renal disease					
(1) Primary mineralocorticoid deficiency (Addison disease, congenital adrenal hyperplasia, hypoaldosteronism)	↑	↓	N to ↓	N to ↓	+
Aldosterone deficiency with chronic hyporeninemia					
(2) Primary hyporeninemia secondary hypoaldosteronism (diabetes mellitus, pyelonephritis, interstitial nephritis)	↓	↓	N to ↑	N to ↓	—
(3) Adolescent hyperkalemic syndrome (chloride shunt syndrome)	↓	↓	↑	↑	—
Reduced tubular responsiveness to aldosterone					
(4) Pseudohypoaldosteronism	↑ ↑	↑ ↑	↓	↓	+
(5) "Early childhood" type IV RTA	N	N	N	N	—

+ = present; — = absent; N = normal; ↑ = increased; ↑ ↑ = markedly increased; ↓ = decreased.

Laboratory Findings

Laboratory work-up in all patients with RTA shows metabolic acidosis with hyperchloremia and a normal serum anion gap. In infants and young children, the best indicator of the magnitude of acidosis is serum bicarbonate concentration, because blood pH and partial pressure of carbon dioxide change rapidly in the crying infant, whereas changes in serum bicarbonate concentration occur much more slowly. In most instances, urine pH is inappropriately high relative to serum bicarbonate concentration. In children with mild acidosis, it may be necessary to stress the acidification capacity of the renal tubule by an acidification test that uses arginine hydrochloride. In patients with distal RTA, the urine pH remains elevated and net acid excretion remains reduced despite the lowered serum bicarbonate concentration (see Table 220–1). Following the acid load, patients with type IV RTA are able to lower urinary pH, but net acid excretion remains inappropriately low.

Key Laboratory Findings

- Metabolic acidosis
- Inappropriately high urine pH

Diagnosis

1. The diagnosis of the various types of RTA is also based on the degree of urinary bicarbonate loss, expressed as fractional excretion of bicarbonate (FEHCO₃). This is calculated from the simultaneous determination of serum and urine bicarbonate (HCO3) and creatinine (Cr) concentrations: $FEHCO_3\% = U_{HCO3}/U_{Cr} \times S_{Cr}/S_{HCO3} \times 100$. After normalization of serum bicarbonate concentration, either orally or by intravenous infusion, patients with distal RTA and type IV RTA have an FEHCO₃ of less than 15 per cent, whereas patients with proximal RTA show massive bicarbonaturia, with FEHCO₃ exceeding 15 per cent (see Table 220–1). A simple method of differentiating proximal from distal RTA is the measurement of carbon dioxide tension in alkaline urine. In pa-

tients with an intact distal H^+ ion secretion mechanism, urine carbon dioxide tension in alkaline urine (pH >7.4) exceeds plasma carbon dioxide tension by 20 mmHg. Ultrasonography of the kidneys should be done to identify nephrocalcinosis, as well as a skeletal survey to search for rickets.

2. A syndrome with features characterized by renal tubular acidosis, osteopetrosis, and cerebral calcifications resulting from deficiency of carbonic anhydrase II isoenzyme has been described.

3. In contrast to other types of RTA, patients with type IV RTA are hyperkalemic, and their urinary potassium excretion is reduced, with a fractional excretion of potassium of <15 per cent. Ultrasonographic evaluation in many of those with RTA type IV subtype 5 (see Table 220–2) may disclose unilateral or bilateral obstructive uropathy. In other cases, there may be evidence of previous vascular injury to one or both kidneys, and in still others ultrasound may be normal, indicating an idiopathic case (related to delayed maturation of aldosterone receptors in tubules).

Treatment

1. *Proximal RTA*—Give 5 to 15 mEq/kg of base per 24 hours, provided with half the cations as sodium and half as potassium. (See Chapter 221 for management of RTA in Fanconi syndrome.)

2. *Distal RTA*—In infants and young children, give the sum of daily urine bicarbonate excretion plus 2 mEq/kg to buffer the daily endogenous acid production. Total daily dose may reach up to 15 mEq/kg. With the gradual disappearance of bicarbonaturia and reduction in endogenous acid production, eventually only 0.8 to 1.0 mEq/kg/24 hours of alkali is required in later childhood.

3. *Type IV RTA*—Treatment depends on the primary cause of the tubular acidosis.

   a. In aldosterone deficiency, treatment with mineralocorticoids, such as fludrocortisone (Florinef Acetate), corrects the acidosis and hyperkalemia as well as the salt wasting. In subtype 2, mineralocorticoids may cause hypertension, and a diuretic may be needed. Subtype 3 is best treated by thiazide diuretics.

Key Treatment

- Daily base administration

---

b. Pseudohypoaldosteronism requires large quantities of sodium chloride and sodium bicarbonate.

c. Subtype 5 requires only low-dose sodium bicarbonate until alleviation of the obstruction or until spontaneous remission in idiopathic cases.

Bibliography

Alon U, Chan JCM: Inherited forms of renal tubular acidosis. In Ferdandes J, Saudubray J-M, Tada K (eds): Inborn Metabolic Diseases: Diagnosis and Treatment. Berlin, Springer-Verlag, 1990, pp 585–595.
Hanna JD, Scheinman JI, Chan JCM: The kidney in acid-base balance. Pediatr Clin North Am 1995;42:1365–1395.

---

221 Fanconi Syndrome

Uri S. Alon

Definition

Fanconi syndrome is characterized by generalized proximal tubular dysfunction manifested by phosphaturia, generalized aminoaciduria, glucosuria, and bicarbonaturia. Less common features include uricosuria and increased renal clearance of sodium, potassium, and calcium, as well as rickets and osteomalacia. The syndrome can be inherited in association with several genetic disorders or acquired through a variety of insults to the proximal tubule (Table 221–1). The most common genetic cause for Fanconi syndrome in childhood is cystinosis.

TABLE 221–1. CAUSES OF FANCONI SYNDROME

INHERITED CAUSES	ACQUIRED CAUSES
Idiopathic	Heavy metals
Known genetic disorders	Cadmium
Cystinosis	Uranium
Glycogen storage disease type I	Mercury
Hereditary fructose intolerance	Lead
Galactosemia	Drugs and toxins
Tyrosinemia	Outdated tetracycline
Wilson disease	Aminoglycosides
Oculocerebrorenal (Lowe) syndrome	Valproate
Methylmalonic acidemia	Cisplatin
Metachromatic leukodystrophy	6-Mercaptopurine
Pyruvate carboxylase deficiency	Ifosfamide
Cytochrome *c* oxidase deficiency	Methyl-3-chromone
Kearns-Sayre syndrome	Lysol
	Paraquat
	Streptozocin
	Toluene
	Glue
	Kidney diseases
	Nephrotic syndrome
	Medullary cystic disease
	Interstitial nephritis
	Amyloidosis
	Malignancy

Pathophysiology and Clinical Findings

The losses of glucose, amino acids, and uric acid in Fanconi syndrome have no clinical implications. It is the losses of phosphate, bicarbonate, water, and electrolytes and the inappropriate production of calcitriol that result in clinical manifestations. Children with Fanconi syndrome present with failure to thrive, fatigue, polydipsia, and polyuria. Typically, these children have nocturia and need to drink several times during the night. In infants, the clinical picture also includes anorexia, vomiting, dehydration, constipation, and unexplained intermittent fever. Muscle weakness caused by severe hypokalemia is more commonly seen in adults than in children. The age at which the patient presents with the syndrome can provide a clue to its cause (see Table 221-1). Appearance during the first weeks of life is typical for some metabolic disorders (e.g., galactosemia, fructosemia). Cystinosis usually appears during the second half of the first year of life, the tubulopathy of Lowe syndrome in early childhood, and acquired causes in late childhood and adulthood.

Key Clinical Findings

- Growth impairment
- Polyuria
- Fatigue
- Rickets (some patients)

Laboratory Findings

1. Proximal renal tubular acidosis (see Chapter 220)
2. *Urine*—glucosuria, tubular proteinuria, hyposthenuria (see Chapter 241).
3. *Blood chemical analysis*—In the early phases of the disease, serum creatinine concentration is normal. Serum

sodium, potassium, and uric acid concentrations may be low. Serum bicarbonate is low, and chloride is elevated (hyperchloremic metabolic acidosis). Serum phosphate is low, with calcium and parathyroid hormone concentrations usually within the normal range. Serum calcitriol concentrations are low in absolute terms or relative to the degree of hypophosphatemia. Serum glucose and protein concentrations are normal, whereas that of carnitine can be low.

4. *Imaging studies*—Renal ultrasound and intravenous pyelogram results are usually normal. Radiologic survey of the skeleton shows rickets and osteopenia in children and osteomalacia in adults.

Key Laboratory Findings

- Metabolic acidosis
- Glycosuria
- Aminoaciduria
- Phosphaturia

Treatment

1. *Elimination of the cause*—In both inherited and acquired types of Fanconi syndrome, the ideal treatment is removal of the offending metabolite or toxin, which in most instances results in reversal of the tubulopathy. The damage to the kidney commonly seen in children undergoing anticancer treatment with cisplatin or ifosfamide is reversible to some extent after each course of therapy; however, with repeated courses of chemotherapy there is progressive damage to the kidney.

> **WARNING**
>
> **Treatment with sodium bicarbonate or sodium citrate results in marked urinary bicarbonate excretion, which promotes potassium excretion and causes hypokalemia. For this reason, at least half of the alkali should be provided as a potassium salt.**

2. *Proximal renal tubular acidosis*—Treatment of the acidosis consists of large quantities of alkali, 5 to 15 mmol/kg/day, divided into four to six doses per day.

Hypokalemia also can be treated by the use of potassium-sparing diuretics. In some patients, the acidosis cannot be corrected despite treatment with alkali. In such patients, proximal tubule bicarbonate reabsorption can be improved by contracting the intravascular fluid compartment with thiazide diuretics and/or dietary restriction of salt and water.

3. *Mineral metabolism*—Treatment of hypophosphatemia and metabolic bone disease consists of administration of oral phosphate and active vitamin D metabolites. Some patients may require supplementation with calcium and magnesium.

4. *Polyuria and electrolyte losses*—Treatment of the polyuria consists of adjusting the fluid intake to the urinary losses. This is important, especially in infants with febrile disorders, to prevent dehydration. Older children should have free access to fluids at all times. Some patients may require supplementation with sodium and potassium. Losses of water, sodium, and potassium can be significantly decreased by the use of prostaglandin synthetase inhibitors. This maneuver improves the patient's quality of life and makes medical management less difficult. However, the latter medication should not be used in patients with decreased glomerular filtration rate.

Key Treatments

- Remove cause when possible
- Base administration for RTA

Bibliography

Bergeron M, Gougoux A, Vinay P: The renal Fanconi syndrome. *In* Scriver CR, Beaudet AL, Sly WS, Valle D (eds): The Metabolic and Molecular Bases of Inherited Disease, 7th ed. New York, McGraw-Hill, 1995, pp 3691–3704.

Foreman JW: Fanconi syndrome and cystinosis. *In* Holliday MA, Barrat TM, Avner LD (eds): Pediatric Nephrology, 3rd ed. Baltimore, Williams & Wilkins, 1994, pp 537–557.

Wilson DM, Alon U: Renal hypophosphatemia. *In* Alon U, Chan JCM (eds): Phosphate in Pediatric Health and Disease. Boca Raton, FL, CRC Press, 1993, pp 159–192.

222 Bartter Syndrome

Uri S. Alon

Definition

Bartter syndrome is characterized by chronic hypokalemic hypochloremic metabolic alkalosis caused by an intrinsic renal tubular defect.

Pathophysiology

The exact mechanism and location of the tubular defect causing the disorder are unknown. However, based on some experimental data and the fact that the syndrome mimics the effects of loop diuretics, the most common hypothesis is that of defective chloride reabsorption in the ascending limb of the loop of Henle. This results in increased delivery of chloride and sodium to the distal tubule, where sodium is exchanged for potassium. The loss of fluids and electrolytes results in increased secretion of renin, aldosterone, and renal prostaglandins, which further enhances urinary potassium losses. The fact that patients are normotensive despite elevated circulatory levels of angiotonin II is mainly related to the presence of hypovolemia and elevated prostaglandin concentrations.

Clinical Findings

The syndrome can be seen in all age groups but is more common in the young. In a few familial cases it has been diagnosed prenatally. Infants with the disorder exhibit reduced appetite, failure to thrive, hypoventilation, polyuria, dehydration, and possibly developmental delay. On rare occasions, tetany caused by alkalosis and hypomagnesemia may be seen. In the adult, the symptoms are mainly those of hypokalemic muscular weakness. Both children and adults are normotensive or hypotensive.

Key Clinical Findings

- Failure to thrive
- Vomiting
- Dehydration

Laboratory Findings

Characteristically, at presentation patients have hypochloremia, hypokalemia, normal to low serum sodium concentrations, and elevated bicarbonate concentrations. Plasma renin activity and serum aldosterone concentration are elevated. Serum creatinine and creatinine clearance are normal. Some patients have hypomagnesemia. The urine is dilute, and even after administration of antidiuretic hormone the patients are unable to concentrate their urine. Urine potassium and chloride excretion rates are enhanced. Patients may have hypocalciuria, normocalciuria, or hypercalciuria with increased excretion of urinary prostaglandins. A few patients have been described who were found to have nephrocalcinosis on ultrasound imaging.

Key Laboratory Findings

- Metabolic alkalosis
- Hypokalemia
- Increased plasma renin
- Increased serum aldosterone

Pathology

In the early stages of Bartter syndrome, kidney histology may show hyperplasia of the juxtaglomerular apparatus, consistent with the chronic hyperreninemia. In later stages and especially in untreated patients, interstitial nephritis with gradual progression to chronic renal failure may develop.

Differential Diagnosis

1. Metabolic alkalosis is relatively uncommon in childhood cases and most commonly originates from losses of gastrointestinal fluids, as in pyloric stenosis (Table 222–1). Salt loss from the skin, as in cystic fibrosis, should also be considered. The best diagnostic test in the work-up of

TABLE 222–1. DIAGNOSIS OF METABOLIC ALKALOSIS

URINARY CHLORIDE <10 mEq/L

Low chloride intake
Gastric losses (e.g., vomiting, gastric drainage)
Intestinal losses (e.g., colonic adenoma, laxative abuse, congenital chloride diarrhea)
Diuretic therapy and abuse (prolonged)
Cystic fibrosis

URINARY CHLORIDE >20 mEq/L

With Normal Blood Pressure

Bartter syndrome
Gitelman syndrome
Diuretic therapy and abuse (recent)

With Hypertension

High renin, high aldosterone
   Renal artery stenosis
   Renin secreting tumors
Low renin, high aldosterone
   Cushing syndrome
   Primary aldosteronism (adenoma or hyperplasia)
Low renin, low aldosterone
   Congenital adrenal hyperplasia (11β-hydroxylase deficiency)
   Exogenous mineralocorticoids
   Liddle syndrome
   Excessive licorice intake

UNCLASSIFIED

Hypoparathyroidism
Alkali administration
Glucose ingestion after starvation
Massive blood transfusion
Recovery from organic acidosis
Milk-alkali syndrome

metabolic alkalosis is urine chloride excretion. It is low in cases of extrarenal losses of the electrolyte and elevated when the alkalosis is caused by renal chloride losses. The determination of blood pressure, plasma renin activity, and serum aldosterone concentration further assist in establishing the cause of metabolic alkalosis (see Table 222–1).

2. Gitelman syndrome is also characterized by hypokalemic, hypochloremic metabolic alkalosis. However, patients with Gitelman syndrome are usually older and tend to have a milder disease (but a greater tendency for tetany). Their laboratory data are characterized by the presence of hypomagnesemia and hypocalciuria.

Treatment

Treatment of Bartter syndrome requires large quantities of potassium chloride, up to 10 mEq/kg/24 hours, often combined with a potassium-sparing diuretic like spironolactone or amiloride. Additional therapy includes a prostaglandin synthetase inhibitor such as indomethacin. This may not be very helpful in patients with Gitelman syndrome, who may require magnesium supplementation. In some cases of Bartter syndrome, the use of captopril or another angiotensin-converting enzyme inhibitor may be effective in diminishing urinary potassium losses, but it may also cause hypotension.

Key Treatment

- Potassium chloride daily
- Indomethacin

Prognosis

Early diagnosis and treatment may improve growth and physical development and perhaps also intellectual development. On the other hand, inappropriate treatment, resulting in long-standing hypokalemia, leads to progressive renal failure.

Bibliography

Bettinelli A, Bianchetti MG, Girardin E, et al: Use of calcium excretion values to distinguish two forms of primary renal tubular hypokalemic alkalosis: Bartter and Gitelman syndromes. J Pediatr 1992;120:38–43.

Hanna JD, Scheinman JI, Chan JCM: The kidney in acid-base balance. Pediatr Clin North Am 1995;42:1365–1395.

Stein JH: The pathogenic spectrum of Bartter's syndrome. Kidney Int 1985;28:85–93.

223 Hemolytic Uremic Syndrome

Richard A. Kaplan

Definition

1. Hemolytic uremic syndrome (HUS) is defined by the clinical triad of microangiopathic hemolytic anemia, thrombocytopenia, and acute renal failure.
2. HUS is one of the most common causes of acute renal failure in infants and children.
3. HUS may be classified into typical HUS, known as diarrhea-associated HUS or D(+) HUS, and atypical HUS, known as non–diarrhea-associated HUS or D(−) HUS.
4. D(+) HUS is much more common in children than is D(−) HUS.

Epidemiology

1. HUS occurs throughout the world. There are endemic regions in Argentina, California, Holland, and South Africa.
2. In the United States, the prevalence of HUS ranges from 0.3 to 10 cases per 100,000 children.
3. The age of onset may be any time from the neonatal period through adulthood, but most cases of D(+) HUS occur between in children aged 6 months to 4 years.
4. The incidence is similar in males and females.
5. Caucasians are affected more often than African-Americans.
6. In North America, the peak incidence of D(+) HUS is from June through September.

Etiology

1. In North America, D(+) HUS is most often associated with gastrointestinal infection with verotoxin-producing *Escherichia coli* (VTEC). There are more than 100 VTEC serotypes, of which *E. coli* O157:H7 is by far the most important.
2. D(+) HUS is also associated with infection by *Shigella dysenteriae*, type 1, particularly in the Indian subcontinent.
3. VTEC is present in the intestinal tracts of about 1 per cent of healthy cattle. Beef may be contaminated during slaughter. The bacteria are transported to the inside of the meat in the process of producing ground beef. The bacteria survive on the inside of undercooked ground beef hamburgers.
4. VTEC infection may also occur from drinking unpasteurized milk or unpastuerized apple cider.
5. VTEC is also transmitted from person to person by the fecal-oral route.
6. D(−) HUS may be familial (autosomal dominant and autosomal recessive forms).
7. D(−) HUS is associated with infection by neuraminidase-producing Streptococcus pneumoniae, oral contraceptives, cyclosporine, vincristine, cisplatin, quinine, radiation therapy, pregnancy, and organ transplantation.

Pathophysiology

1. D(+) HUS
   a. Colitis
      (1) VTEC adheres to colonic epithelial cells. Verotoxins, which are structurally similar to toxins produced by *S. dysenteriae* and are known as Shiga-like toxins, may contribute to colonic epithelium.
      (2) Verotoxins, *E. coli*-derived lipopolysaccharide (LPS), and other mediators of inflammation enter the circulation through damaged colonic epithelium.
   b. Endothelial cell injury
      (1) Verotoxin injures endothelial cells in glomerular capillaries and other capillaries.
      (2) LPS activates neutrophils, which results in release of elastase and other catabolic enzymes, which in turn mediate endothelial cell detachment from the underlying glomerular basement membrane.
      (3) LPS stimulates production of tumor necrosis factor and interleukin-1, which also contribute to endothelial cell injury.
   c. The damaged endothelium is a site for localized intravascular coagulopathy.
      (1) Intact endothelial cells are negatively charged and produce prostacyclin (PGI_2).
      (2) The injured endothelial cells swell, become detached from the underlying basement membrane, lose their negative charge, and do not produce PGI_2.
      (3) The exposed basement membrane is a site for deposition of fibrin and activation of platelets.
      (4) The activated platelets release thromboxane (TXA_2), which is a promoter of platelet aggregation and is a vasoconstrictor.
      (5) The balance between PGI_2 and TXA_2 is altered in favor of TXA_2.
      (6) The coagulation balance is altered in favor of platelet aggregation, microthrombus formation, and vasoconstriction. Glomerular capillary lumens become narrowed or obstructed, reducing the glomerular filtration rate and producing renal insufficiency. Platelets are rapidly added to the microthrombi, producing a consumptive thrombocytopenia. Erythrocytes passing through the thrombus-filled capillary are sheared, producing the fragmented red blood cells characteristic of microangiopathic hemolytic anemia.

2. D(−) HUS
Some patients with autosomal dominant HUS have decreased production of PGI_2 by endothelial cells. Neuraminidase, produced by certain strains of *S. pneumoniae*, removes *N*-acetylneuraminic acid from the cell membranes of endothelial cells, erythrocytes, and platelets, exposing the Thomsen-Friedenreich antigen, against which there is immunoglobulin M antibody present in most human plasma. There is subsequent endothelial cell damage, erythrocyte agglutination, hemolysis, and platelet consumption.

Clinical Findings

1. *Gastrointestinal tract*—Infection by VTEC produces abdominal cramping and diarrhea 1 to 8 (usually 3 to 4) days after exposure. Diarrhea may be bloody by the third day of the illness. Nausea and vomiting are present in one half of the cases, but fever is low grade or absent. The child may appear to have an acute surgical abdomen.

2. *Hematopoietic system*—Three days to 2 weeks (usually 4 to 6 days) after the onset of diarrhea, the child suddenly develops pallor, restlessness, irritability, and drowsiness. Hemolysis may produce rapid decreases in the hematocrit. Hemolysis may continue for 2 weeks. The severity of the anemia does not correlate with the severity of the renal failure. Thrombocytopenia is present; however, other than hemorrhagic diarrhea, significant clinical bleeding is relatively rare.

3. *Renal*—Acute renal failure is usually accompanied by oliguria or anuria. Hypertension may be present, secondary to fluid overload or caused by renin release.

4. Central nervous system (CNS)
   a. Mild CNS findings include irritability, drowsiness, and tremor.
   b. Major neurologic complications, including seizures, coma, decerebrate rigidity, and hemiparesis, occur in 20 to 50 per cent of patients. Severe CNS involvement is more common in D(−) HUS.
   c. CNS abnormalities may be caused by hyponatremia, hypocalcemia, uremia, or hypertension. Intravascular coagulopathy in the cerebral vasculature, with resultant cerebral thrombosis, infarction or hemorrhage, may also cause severe CNS abnormalities.

Key Clinical Findings

- Diarrhea
- Abdominal pain
- Nausea and vomiting
- Pallor

Laboratory Findings

1. *Blood findings related to acute renal insufficiency*—Elevated blood urea nitrogen, serum creatinine, and serum uric acid; hyperkalemia, hyperphosphatemia, hyponatremia, hypocalcemia, and metabolic acidosis.
2. *Urine*—The urine may be scant and show little proteinuria, or there may be proteinuria and hematuria.
3. *Blood*—A Coombs-negative microangiopathic hemolytic anemia, with schistocytes, helmet cells, and burr cells on peripheral blood smear; reticulocytosis; elevated serum lactate dehydrogenase; and serum bilirubin. Thrombocytopenia with normal prothrombin time and partial thromboplastin time.
4. *Other blood abnormalities*—Elevated liver enzymes if hepatic involvement has occurred; elevated serum amylase, lipase, and sometimes glucose if pancreatic involvement has occurred.

Key Laboratory Findings

- Elevated serum urea and creatinine
- Hemolytic anemia
- Schistocytes, burr cells

Imaging Studies

Ultrasonography demonstrates increased kidney size, hyperechogenicity, and poor corticomedullary differentiation. These are nonspecific findings of medical-renal disease.

Pathology

Renal biopsy, which is rarely needed for the diagnosis, may show glomerular findings of thickening of the capillary walls and narrowing of the capillary lumens. Early in the course, erythrocytes and fibrin are seen in the narrowed lumens, and a granular, eosinophilic periodic acid-Schiff–positive material is seen in the subendothelial space produced by endothelial detachment from the basement membrane.

Treatment

1. *HUS without acute renal failure*—Correction of fluid deficits with close monitoring of intake and output. Packed red blood cells if the hemolytic anemia results in impaired circulation. Platelet transfusions are rarely needed. Close monitoring of the blood pressure and serum electrolytes, urea nitrogen, and creatinine.
2. *HUS with acute renal failure*—Prompt referral to a pediatric dialysis unit. Decrease in mortality from HUS is associated with the early institution of dialysis. Dialysis should be started for any child with 12 or more hours of oliguria, hyponatremia, hyperkalemia, severe uremia, severe fluid overload, pulmonary edema, or persistent hypertension.

Key Treatment

- Transfusion, if needed
- Dialysis

Prognosis

1. The availability of dialysis has resulted in a decrease in the mortality rate from D(+) HUS to 4 to 8 per cent. CNS complications are the most frequent cause of death. Mortality from D(−) HUS remains as high as 25 per cent.
2. Most survivors of D(+) HUS have normal serum creatinine levels; however, 5 to 10 per cent of survivors have end-stage renal failure and as many as one fourth of the remaining patients have decreased GFR when measured by inulin clearance or iothalamate clearance.
3. CNS deficits may persist in 2 to 15 per cent of patients.
4. Insulin-dependent diabetes mellitus is a rare sequela. Rarely, bowel infarction, perforation, intussusception, rectal prolapse, or toxic megacolon occurs. The liver may be enlarged and tender. Pancreatic involvement may be manifested as ongoing abdominal pain, pancreatitis, or glucose intolerance.

Prevention

1. Most cases of D(+) HUS in North America may be prevented by avoiding exposure to VTEC.
   a. Ground beef should be cooked until the core temperature of the meat reaches at least 160°F.
   b. Unpasteurized milk and apple cider should not be consumed.
2. Stool culture samples from patients with bloody diarrhea should be screened for *E. coli* O157:H7.
3. Public health authorities should be notified of *E. coli* O157:H7 isolates.
4. Children with VTEC should be excluded from daycare centers until two consecutive stool cultures are negative for VTEC.
5. Proper handwashing should occur after bathroom use and diapering.

Bibliography

Boyce TG, Swerdlow DL, Griffin PM: *Escherichia coli* O157:H7 and the hemolytic-uremic syndrome. N Engl J Med 1995;333:364–368.

Brandt JR, Fouser LS, Watkins SL, et al: *Escherichia coli* O157:H7-associated hemolytic-uremic syndrome after ingestion of contaminated hamburgers. J Pediatr 1994;125:519–515.

Siegler RL: Spectrum of extrarenal involvement in postdiarrheal hemolytic-uremic syndrome. J Pediatr 1994;125:511–514.

224 Polycystic Kidney Disease in Childhood

Douglas L. Blowey

Definitions

The finding of multiple renal cysts is a common occurrence in many genetic and nongenetic disorders. The term *polycystic kidney disease (PKD)* is, by convention, limited to the description of two inherited disorders: autosomal recessive polycystic kidney disease (ARPKD) and autosomal dominant polycystic kidney disease (ADPKD). Although most persons with ADPKD are recognized clinically in the fourth or fifth decade of life, the historic label of "adult-onset PKD" is clearly misleading, because ADPKD may be symptomatic in children and neonates. The distinction between ARPKD and ADPKD in childhood is often difficult because of their similar clinical and radiologic findings. Correct identification of the disorder is important for prognosis and genetic counseling. In addition to a physical examination and renal ultrasound of the affected child, a proper evaluation includes an in-depth family history and renal ultrasound studies of both parents. The recent advances in identification of the genes associated with PKD will provide invaluable assistance in this diagnostic dilemma.

Autosomal Recessive Polycystic Kidney Disease

Etiology

The chromosomal defect associated with ARPKD has been mapped to the short arm of chromosome 6. The precise genes and gene products responsible for the manifestations of ARPKD remain to be identified. The incidence appears to be on the order of 1 to 2 per 10,000 births.

Clinical Findings

1. The most common clinical finding in ARPKD is an abdominal mass caused by the massive enlargement of the kidneys. The kidneys are often so large that they impair respiratory function and nutritional intake. Many infants die shortly after birth from pulmonary hypoplasia associated with oligohydramnios (Potter's oligohydramnios sequence). Of those surviving the neonatal period, most show an increase in renal function over the first year of life, consistent with normal renal maturation. Renal function may remain stable for many years. Approximately one third of children with ARPKD will progress to end-stage renal disease by 7 years of age.

2. A wide spectrum of clinical manifestations is noted in ARPKD. In the most common form, designated *infantile PKD*, the renal abnormalities predominate in the clinical picture. In contrast, liver manifestations predominate in those children diagnosed during adolescence. The latter condition has often been called congenital hepatic fibrosis with renal tubular ectasia, but in fact it is a form of ARPKD.

3. Hypertension is common and occurs even in the absence of renal insufficiency. A defect in urinary concentrating ability may predispose children with ARPKD to dehydration during periods of limited intake. Portal hypertension with esophageal varices, evolving from the liver abnormalities, may become apparent later in life.

Key Clinical Findings: ARPKD

• Abdominal mass

• Hypertension

Pathology

1. The renal cysts in ARPKD are located in the collecting ducts and are lined by hyperplastic epithelium. The cysts are often limited to diffuse microscopic dilation; however, macroscopic cysts may be present. Renal dysplasia is not a feature of ARPKD, and the presence of dysplastic elements suggests an alternative diagnosis.

2. Variable degrees of biliary dysgenesis and hepatic fibrosis are invariably present on liver biopsy. Macroscopic liver cysts are rare.

Radiologic Findings

1. Ultrasound is the imaging study of choice. In ARPKD, the kidneys may be massively enlarged, with increased echogenicity of the entire parenchyma. Discrete cysts may or may not be present. Although not pathognomonic for PKD, this pattern of renal abnormalities can be seen on prenatal ultrasound. The ultrasound appearance of the liver in neonates frequently shows little or no increase in echogenicity. In contrast, older children may have enlarged echogenic livers with or without visible cysts.

2. The evaluation of any child suspected of having PKD should include a renal ultrasound of both parents, because the presence of kidney cysts in either parent is strongly supportive of the diagnosis of ADPKD. In young parents (<30 years of age), CT may be more sensitive than ultrasound in detecting cysts.

Treatment

1. Currently, there is no therapy available to reverse or retard the pathologic changes in ARPKD. Therapy is supportive. Children who progress to end-stage renal disease are candidates for dialysis and transplantation.

2. Hypertension is common and should be treated aggressively. Adequate nutritional intake is often hampered by the massive kidney enlargement, and nasogastric feedings may be required to ensure intake of sufficient calories for growth and development.

Key Treatment: ARPKD

- Antihypertensive drugs

Prevention

Genetic counseling for the family is extremely important when a child is diagnosed with ARPKD. The disorder is inherited as an autosomal recessive trait, so the risk of having an affected child with each subsequent pregnancy is 25 per cent.

Autosomal Dominant Polycystic Kidney Disease

Etiology

At least three separate chromosomal defects have been associated with ADPKD. The most common abnormality (ADPKD1) is located on the short arm of chromosome 16.

Clinical Findings

1. The presentation of ADPKD in the neonate can be similar to that of ARPKD, with enlarged and hyperechoic kidneys evident on prenatal ultrasound. Potter's oligohydramnios sequence may be present.
2. The clinical findings in children that may lead to the diagnosis of ADPKD include abdominal masses caused by the markedly enlarged kidneys, abdominal and flank pain, hypertension, and hematuria. Occasionally, ADPKD is diagnosed in an asymptomatic child when a family history of ADPKD prompts a screening ultrasound. Similarly, asymptomatic parents may be diagnosed with ADPKD when they are screened during the evaluation of a child with suspected PKD.
3. The extrarenal manifestations associated with ADPKD (e.g., rupture of a berry aneurysm, liver cysts, renal stones) are rarely seen during childhood.

Key Clinical Finding: ADPKD

- Abdominal mass

Radiologic Findings

1. ADPKD is best diagnosed with ultrasound. Cysts may or may not be present. In contrast to the requirement of three or more renal cysts in an adult, a single renal cyst in a child at risk (i.e., parent with ADPKD) is sufficient to make the diagnosis of ADPKD in the child.
2. Ultrasound is sufficient to screen the parents in most cases. Renal cysts are present in 80 per cent of persons with ADPKD by the age of 20 years and in almost all by 30 years of age.

Pathology

1. The renal cysts in ADPKD arise from any segment of the nephron and are lined by hyperplastic epithelium. As with ARPKD, renal dysplasia is not a feature of ADPKD, and its finding should suggest an alternative diagnosis.
2. Hepatic involvement, consisting of clusters of dilated ductuli, is infrequent compared with hepatic involvement in children with ARPKD. The findings in ADPKD are distinct from the appearance of congenital hepatic fibrosis in ARPKD.

Treatment

There is no therapy to prevent cyst development, so therapy is aimed at minimizing the complications. Hypertension is one factor that can affect progression and should be addressed. Urinary tract infections require antibiotic therapy. Pain, presumably caused by cyst enlargement, is usually managed with rest and analgesics. Children who progress to end-stage renal disease are candidates for dialysis and transplantation.

Key Treatment: ADPKD

- Supportive
- Antihypertensives when needed

Prevention

Genetic counseling should be provided to the parents and the child with ADPKD. If one of the parents has ADPKD, there is a 50 per cent risk of having an affected child with each pregnancy.

Bibliography

Cole BR, Conley SB, Stapleton FB: Polycystic kidney disease in the first year of life. J Pediatr 1987;111:693–699.

Fick GM, Duley IT, Johnson AM, et al: The spectrum of autosomal dominant polycystic kidney disease in children. J Am Soc Nephrol 1994;4:1654–1660.

Fick GM, Johnson AM, Strain JD, et al: Characteristics of very early onset autosomal dominant polycystic kidney disease. J Am Soc Nephrol 1993;3:1863–1870.

Guay-Woodford LM, Muecher G, Hopkins SD, et al: The severe perinatal form of autosomal recessive polycystic kidney disease maps to chromosome 6p21.1–p12: Implications for genetic counseling. Am J Hum Genet 1995;56:1101–1107.

Kaplan BS, Kaplan P, Rosenberg HK, et al: Polycystic kidney disease in childhood. J Pediatr 1989;115:867–879.

225 Voiding Disorders

Stanley Hellerstein

Definition

Voiding dysfunction is a broad term indicating a voiding pattern that is abnormal for a child's age. For example, nocturnal enuresis is not normal for a 10-year-old, whereas urinary urgency is expected in infants from 18 to 36 months of age who are in the transitional phase of acquiring daytime urine control.

Etiology

Voiding dysfunction in pediatric patients may be a consequence of an anatomic (usually obstructive), neurogenic, or functional disorder. Isolated nocturnal enuresis appears to reflect delay in acquisition of a usual developmental milestone. Presumably, this reflects a maturational process, one that is often genetically linked.

Functional Voiding Disorders

Functional voiding disorders are encountered in children with no anatomic or neurogenic lesion. They are also referred to as the unstable bladder of childhood, instability of the detrusor muscle, or persistence of an infantile bladder. The clinical manifestations are variable.

Small-Capacity Hypertonic Bladder

Symptoms

Symptoms include frequency, urgency, urge incontinence, staccato voiding, nocturia and/or enuresis, and dysuria. Recurrent urinary tract infections (UTIs) are common.

Pathophysiology

Urodynamic studies demonstrate a small-capacity bladder for age, with increased detrusor pressure (net intravesical pressure) during filling and marked urgency at capacity. Emptying is often incomplete despite high detrusor pressure.

Imaging

Voiding cystourethrography (VCUG) may show a relatively small bladder with varying degrees of trabeculation. Spasm of the sphincter during voiding may cause a narrowing of the distal urethra with dilatation of the posterior urethra, giving a "spinning top" deformity. Ultrasound usually shows a normal upper tract but a thickened bladder wall.

Treatment

An effective bladder retraining program is needed to help the child relax during voiding and completely empty the bladder. Repeated infections should be controlled with suppressive antibacterial therapy. Anticholinergic and antispasmodic agents such as oxybutynin, propantheline, or hyoscyamine are useful to help reduce intravesical pressure.

Key Treatment: Small-Capacity Hypertonic Bladder

- Bladder retraining program

Detrusor Hyperreflexia

Symptoms

Long-standing symptoms of daytime urinary frequency, urgency, urge incontinence, posturing (including squatting), and at times nocturia or nocturnal enuresis may be present. Bladder spasms may be rare or frequent, and recurrent UTIs may occur.

Pathophysiology

Uninhibited contractions of the detrusor muscle during bladder filling may cause urgency, or may not be recognized, or may be abolished by voluntary contraction of the external sphincter. Various postures, including squatting with the heel of one foot pressed against the urethra, are employed to occlude the urethra and avoid incontinence during an uninhibited detrusor contraction. During the initial phase of an uninhibited contraction, reflex relaxation of the sphincter may cause a sense of urgency or urge incontinence with scant, if any, rise in detrusor pressure.

Imaging

Imaging evaluation usually shows no abnormality other than a mildly trabeculated or thick-walled bladder. Bladder capacity may be slightly reduced, but bladder emptying is complete at capacity.

Treatment

These children usually benefit from a voiding retraining program and anticholinergic therapy, usually with oxybutynin. If recurrent UTIs are a problem, suppressive and antibacterial therapy should be employed.

Key Treatment: Detrusor Hyperreflexia

- Bladder retraining program
- Oxybutynin

The Infrequent Voider (Lazy Bladder Syndrome)

Symptoms

Lazy bladder syndrome is characterized by infrequent voiding with urgency, posturing, and/or daytime incontinence only after a prolonged period without voiding. It occurs predominately in girls, who commonly do not void during an entire day at school. Frequent UTIs, chronic constipation, and, at times, encopresis may be present.

Pathophysiology

A large-capacity, highly compliant bladder with normal relaxation of the bladder outlet during voiding but incomplete bladder emptying is common.

Imaging

VCUG reveals a very large bladder capacity, often with incomplete emptying. Ultrasound may show mild bladder wall thickness, but trabeculation is usually mild or absent.

Treatment

Treatment consists of a voiding-retraining program that focuses on techniques to achieve complete bladder emptying, a relatively rigid daytime voiding schedule with bladder emptying every 2 to 3 hours, and control of constipation. A cholinergic agent, bethanechol hydrochloride, is often helpful in stimulating voiding. Suppressive antibacterial therapy is indicated if recurrent UTIs are a problem.

Key Treatment: Infrequent Voider

- Rigid voiding schedule

Psychologic Non-neuropathic Bladder (Hinman Syndrome, Non-neurogenic or Occult Neurogenic Bladder)

Symptoms

Urgency and/or stress incontinence, infrequent voluntary voiding, straining to void with an intermittent urine stream, recurrent UTIs, and chronic constipation, often with fecal soiling, are the symptoms. The condition mimics neurogenic bladder disorders.

Pathophysiology

The sphincter may periodically contract during filling. Uninhibited detrusor contractions may occur during voiding. This incoordination of detrusor contraction with sphincter activity causes outflow obstruction with high voiding pressures and incomplete emptying.

Imaging

Radiographic examination of the kidneys, ureter, and bladder usually shows an excess of fecal material in the colon. The VCUG often shows a large-capacity, severely trabeculated bladder with severe vesicoureteric reflux. Upper tract imaging may show hydroureteronephrosis with or without renal parenchymal scarring.

Treatment

Management is directed toward improving bladder and bowel emptying, preventing infection, and alleviating psychosocial pressures that may be aggravating the voiding dysfunction. A timed voiding schedule is given; anticholinergic agents are used to control bladder stability and, at times, an α-adrenergic blockade is given to block contraction of the bladder outlet. In some instances, intermittent catheterization may be needed to accomplish bladder emptying.

Key Treatment: Psychologic Non-neuropathic Bladder

- Timed voiding schedule

Isolated Nocturnal Enuresis

The persistence of nighttime bedwetting beyond the age at which nocturnal continence is expected is the most common voiding disorder in children. Nocturnal enuresis usually is not diagnosed until 5 years of age, when the prevalence of nighttime wetting is 15 to 20 per cent. Subsequently, about 15 per cent of children with nocturnal enuresis achieve nighttime continence each year, without any intervention.

Symptoms

Children with isolated nocturnal enuresis have a normal daytime voiding pattern. The urinalysis is normal, as is the urine flow rate and the renal concentration ability. The children may soak their beds almost nightly or do so irregularly, at times with dry nights all summer and recurrence of wetting in the fall and winter. It is common for them not to waken on bed wetting.

Imaging

None is warranted.

Treatment

The goal is to help the child cope with his or her problem and, hopefully, to accomplish nighttime urinary continence. Nighttime urinary control is a result of development of the ability to suppress detrusor contractions while asleep, just as unconscious inhibition of the voiding reflex occurs while awake. The exact neurologic mechanisms involved in either voluntary or unconscious control of micturition are not known. The most successful and well accepted treatment measures combine a behavioral approach to help increase the child's perception of bladder fullness with the use of a moisture alarm. Medication with agents such as imipramine, oxybutynin, or desmopressin are usually of limited value and may have untoward side effects or be dangerous to have in the home (imipramine). Demopressin or oxybutynin, if successful in achieving dry nights, may also be useful for nights out or periods at camp, although they do not contribute to the development of the child's ability to suppress detrusor contractions while asleep.

Key Treatment: Isolated Nocturnal Enuresis

- Moisture alarm
- Behavior training

Bibliography

Bauer SB: Neuropathology of the lower urinary tract. *In* Kelalis PP, King LR, Belman AB (eds): Clinical Pediatric Urology, 3rd ed, vol I. Philadelphia, WB Saunders, 1992, pp 399–440.

Fernandes E, Vernier R, Gonzalez R: The unstable bladder in children. J Pediatr 1991;118:831–837.

Hellerstein S, Stern L, Alon U, et al: Voiding dysfunction in pediatric patients: A clinical approach to diagnosis and management. Children's Hospital Quarterly 1990;2:213–225.

Rushton HG: Wetting and functional voiding disorders. Urol Clin North Am 1995;22:75–93.

226 Hypercalciuria and Urinary Tract Stone Disease

Uri S. Alon

Hypercalciuria

Definition

Hypercalciuria is defined as urine calcium excretion exceeding the upper limit of normal of 4.0 mg/kg/24 hours. In children 5 years and older, it can also be defined as a ratio of urine calcium to creatinine >0.20. In younger children, the upper limit of normal is higher: 0.80 up to age 7 months, 0.60 between ages 7 to 18 months, and 0.4 between ages 1.5 and 5 years. Whereas these values are valid for the Caucasian population, they may not be applicable for the African-American population, which in general has lower urinary calcium excretion rates.

Etiology

All causes of hypercalcemia can cause also hypercalciuria. Nevertheless, most hypercalciuric children do not have hypercalcemia (Table 226–1). In most children the hypercalciuria is idiopathic. For research purposes, the latter is often divided into absorptive and renal hypercalciuria, but this subtyping does not affect the current clinical approach to the patient. There is evidence that urine calcium excretion is affected by several dietary factors, such as protein and sodium (which increase urinary calcium excretion) and potassium (which decreases the mineral excretion). In some cases, hypercalciuria may be familial because of either genetic or environmental factors.

Clinical Findings

Hypercalciuria may be asymptomatic or associated with a wide spectrum of symptoms and signs. These manifestations include gross hematuria, microscopic hematuria, high urinary frequency with dysuria, nocturnal enuresis, urinary incontinence, abdominal pain, and urinary tract infections. All of these may be related to the presence of calcium crystals in the urinary tract, which may or may not be detected on urinalysis. In its most serious form, hypercalciuria can result in formation of urolithiasis with its associated morbidity.

Key Clinical Findings: Hypercalciuria

- Urinary frequency
- Nocturnal enuresis

Diagnosis

See Table 226–2.

Treatment

1. *High fluid intake*—At least 1.5 times time maintenance. The child and family should be taught to look at the urine and make sure that it looks "like water."
2. *Dietary changes*—Reduced intake of protein and salt to the recommended dietary allowance, increase in potassium-rich food. In most cases, calcium restriction is not indicated because it may lead to a negative calcium balance.
3. Pharmacologic treatment
   a. Thiazide diuretics, which decrease urinary calcium excretion and increase the deposition of the mineral in the skeleton
   b. Potassium citrate, which decreases calcium crystallization in the urine by forming soluble calcium citrate complexes
   c. In extremely stubborn cases, cellulose phosphate, which binds calcium in the gut can be used. However, as with dietary calcium restriction, its use can result in a negative calcium balance.

TABLE 226–1. CAUSES OF HYPERCALCIURIA

Hypercalcemia of any cause	
Endocrinopathies:	Hyperparathyroidism, hyperthyroidism, corticosteroids excess
Renal diseases:	Renal tubular acidosis (distal and proximal), medullary sponge kidney, Bartter syndrome, hypophosphatemic rickets with hypercalciuria, familial hypomagnesemia with hypercalciuria and nephrocalcinosis, hyperprostaglandin E syndrome, nonacidotic proximal tubulopathy with hypercalciuria
Extrarenal diseases:	Malignancy, sarcoidosis, insulin-dependent diabetes mellitus, juvenile rheumatoid arthritis, Wilson disease
Physical factors:	Immobilization, physical exercise
Drugs:	Vitamin D, furosemide, acetazolamide, corticosteroids
Nutritional factors:	High protein, sodium, and carbohydrate intake; low phosphate and potassium intake
Idiopathic:	Absorptive, renal

TABLE 226–2. NORMAL VALUES FOR URINE CHEMICAL COMPOSITION

TIMED URINE COLLECTION

Calcium <4 mg/kg/24 hr
Oxalate <30 mg/m^2/24 hr
Uric acid <815 mg/1.73 m^2/24 hr
Cystine <75 mg/g creatinine
Citrate >180 mg/g creatinine

RANDOM URINE SPECIMEN

Calcium <7 mo, <0.86; 7–18 mo, <0.60; 19 mo to 5 yr, <0.42; older children, <0.22 (mg/mg creatinine)
Oxalate 0–6 mo, ≤360; 7–24 mo, ≤174; 2–4.9 yr, ≤101; 5 yr, ≤82; 9 yr, ≤69; 12 yr, ≤50; 14 yr, ≤56; 16 yr, ≤40 (mmol/mol creatinine)
Uric acid <0.57 mg/dl GFR (urine uric acid × serum creatinine/ urine creatinine [in mg/dl])

4. Treatment of the primary disorder or adjustment of the dose of medication causing the hypercalciuria (see Table 226–1).

Key Treatment: Hypercalciuria

- High-fluid intake
- Moderate salt and protein restriction
- Increased dietary potassium

Urinary Tract Stone Disease

Etiology

1. Increase in urine stone formation promoters
   a. *Hypercalciuria*—Usually results in formation of calcium oxalate stones and, less commonly, especially in the face of very alkaline urine, in calcium phosphate stones.
   b. *Hyperoxaluria*—Either genetic or enteric. Patients with genetic hyperoxaluria frequently develop multiple stones. Infants may develop nephrocalcinosis with rapid deterioration in kidney function and deposition of oxalate in multiple organs—a condition named *oxalosis*. Enteric hyperoxaluria is secondary to fat malabsorption. The fatty acids chelate intestinal calcium to form soaps. Because there is less calcium available to bind intestinal oxalic acids, they are absorbed and excreted in the urine.
   c. *Sturvite stones*—Recurrent infections with urea-splitting organisms like *Proteus* lead to alkaline urine rich in ammonium and trivalent phosphate ions, which can result in formation of staghorn stones composed of magnesium ammonium phosphate and carbonate apatite. The tendency to form these and all other types of stones is higher in the face of anatomic abnormalities causing urinary stagnation.
   d. *Uric acid stones*—Can result from hyperuricosuria and/or low urine pH. A rare X-linked recessive disorder, Lesch-Nyhan syndrome, is characterized by hyperuricosuria and recurrent formation of uric acid stones. Uric acid stones can develop also in patients with malignancies because of the high turnover of purines, or in patients treated with some pancreatic enzymes.
   e. *Cystine stones*—Cystinuria (not to be confused with cystinosis) is an autosomal recessive disorder in which urine cystine excretion in homozygotes exceeds 250 mg/g creatinine. The stones are radiopaque, but not as clearly so as calcium stones. Urinalysis in these patients often discloses the typical hexagonal cystine crystal. Screening for the disorder can be done by the nitroprusside test.
2. Decrease in urine stone formation inhibitors
   a. *Citrate*—Decrease in urinary citrate is characteristically seen in patients with distal renal tubular acidosis. Hypocitraturia can some times be observed in patients with chronic diarrhea. In other patients it may idiopathic.
   b. The influence of magnesium and possibly several urine proteins is currently under research.

Clinical Findings

The most common manifestations include pain, hematuria, and urinary tract infection. Other manifestations include urinary frequency, dysuria, sterile pyuria, and, rarely, anuria caused by obstructive uropathy. Urolithiasis may also be an incidental finding during imaging studies of the abdomen and urinary tract.

Key Clinical Findings: Urinary Tract Stone Disease

- Pain
- Hematuria
- Frequency
- Dysuria

Laboratory and Radiographic Findings

1. *Radiologic evaluation*—Plain abdominal radiographs detect only radiopaque stones containing calcium or cystine. Ultrasonography or intravenous pyelography detects all kinds of stones, as well as the presence of anatomic abnormalities in the system and obstruction. Intravenous pyelography may have a therapeutic effect by way of osmotic diuresis, which may result in passage of the stone.
2. Whenever possible during acute attacks, patients' urines should be strained to catch the stone. Stones passed spontaneously or removed surgically should be analyzed for their chemical composition.
3. All children with stones in the urinary tract should undergo metabolic evaluation:
   a. *Blood analysis*—Creatinine, electrolytes, calcium, phosphorus, alkaline phosphate, uric acid. If abnormalities in calcium metabolism are suspected, intact parathyroid hormone, vitamin D metabolites, and the tubular threshold for phosphorus should also be determined.
   b. Urinalysis (including urine pH) and urine culture
   c. A 24-hour urine collection (or, if that is not feasible, a random specimen) is analyzed for calcium, oxalate, urate, cystine, citrate, and creatinine (see Table 226–2).

Treatment

1. *Stone removal*—Stones causing pain, obstruction, or recurrent infections should be removed from the urinary tract. If the stone is small enough, hydration combined with analgesia and smooth muscle relaxants can result in stone mobilization and elimination. In other cases, surgical intervention or extracorporeal shock wave lithotripsy is indicated. On the other hand, asymptomatic stones of the appropriate size may pass spontaneously, at times painlessly.
2. *Medical treatment*—The medical treatment does not dissolve existing stones but rather is aimed at abolishing growth of existing stones and protecting against forma-

tion of new ones. The cornerstone of nonpharmacologic treatment is high fluid intake. Specific treatments for the various metabolic abnormalities are shown in the box that follows. Follow-up of patients with kidney stones should include periodic radiographic evaluation of the urinary tract and chemical analysis of the urine.

Key Treatment: Drug Treatment in Urolithiasis

- Idiopathic hypercalciuria
  Calcium-sparing diuretics
Chlorothiazide	20–30 mg/kg/day, divided b.i.d.
Amiloride	0.2–0.4 mg/kg/day, divided b.i.d.
Potassium citrate	1–2 mEq/kg/day, divided b.i.d., t.i.d.
Cellulose phosphate	10–15 g/1.73 m²/day, with meals t.i.d.

- Hyperuricosuria
Allopurinol	10 mg/kg/day, divided t.i.d., q.i.d.
Potassium citrate	1–2 mEq/kg/day, to keep urine pH 6.0–6.5

- Primary hyperoxaluria
Pyridoxine	25–250 mg/day (titrated dose)

Potassium citrate	1–2 mEq/kg/day, divided b.i.d., t.i.d.
Magnesium hydroxide	5–10 mEq/1.73 m²/day, divided t.i.d.
Neutral orthophosphate	30–40 mg/kg/day, divided t.i.d.
Chlorothiazide	20–30 mg/kg/day, divided b.i.d.

- Enteric hyperoxaluria
Potassium citrate	1–2 mEq/kg/day, divided b.i.d., t.i.d.
Magnesium hydroxide	5–10 mEq/1.73 m²/day, divided t.i.d.
Calcium citrate	1 g/1.73 m²/day, divided b.i.d., t.i.d.
Cholestyramine	240 mg/kg/day, divided t.i.d.

- Cystinuria
Penicillamine	30 mg/kg/day, divided q.i.d.
Potassium citrate	1–2 mEq/kg/day, divided b.i.d., t.i.d.

Bibliography

Polinsky MS, Kaiser BA, Baluarte HJ, Gruskin AB: Renal stones and hypercalciuria. Adv Pediatr 1993;40:353–384.

Stapleton FB, Kroovand RL: Stones in childhood. *In* Coe FL, Favus MJ, Pak CYC, et al (eds): Kidney Stones: Medical and Surgical Management. Philadelphia, Lippincott-Raven Publishers, 1996, pp 1065–1080.

227 Cryptorchidism

J. Patrick Murphy

Definition

Cryptorchidism means "hidden testis," but it has come to be defined as failure of normal descent of the testes into the scrotum.

Etiology and Epidemiology

1. Normal testicular descent occurs in two stages. Abdominal descent occurs by the third month of gestation, and the testes remain at the internal inguinal ring until the seventh month, when inguinal descent occurs. Although the exact mechanism of testicular descent remains undefined, it is generally accepted that the descent of the testes to the scrotum is hormonally mediated. Maldescent occurs secondary to some abnormality of this hormonal mediation relating to the hypothalamic-pituitary-gonadal axis.

2. The incidence of cryptorchidism in full-term infants is 3.4 to 5.8 per cent. By 1 year of age, the incidence becomes 0.8 to 1.8 per cent. Spontaneous descent can still occur up to the end of the first year of life but is rare after that. The incidence in premature infants is 17 to 100 per cent, depending on the degree of prematurity.

Pathophysiology

1. Cryptorchidism is probably a variant of hypogonadotropic hypogonadism. In the normal male, a gonadotropin surge occurs at about 3 months of life which stimulates a testosterone response, triggering the formation of spermatogonia. These spermatogonia become the pool of cells that will be the source of sperm throughout the life of the testes. In the cryptorchid testis, this gonadotropin surge is diminished or absent, leading to diminished germ cell maturation. This process involves both testes, even in unilateral cryptorchidism. Histologic studies of biopsy specimens confirm the bilateral involvement. These studies explain the abnormalities of spermatogenesis in treated and untreated men with both unilateral and bilateral undescended testis.

2. There is also an observed decrease in the ratio of Leydig cells to tubules in cryptorchidism, and a blunted testosterone response may be seen after stimulation with human

chorionic gonadotropin (hCG). However, there is usually adequate hormonal function for normal male development at puberty unless significant bilateral testicular atrophy is present.

3. The various factors that affect germ cell development in cryptorchidism probably account for the increased incidence of malignancies seen in undescended testes. Dysgenesis of the germ cells secondary to failed maturation may be the mechanism of formation of the germ cell malignancies in adults with a history of cryptorchidism. The risk of malignancy in the cryptorchid testes is about 50 per 100,000 per year, which is about 20 to 25 times greater than in scrotal testes.

Clinical Findings

1. Cryptorchid testes may be either *palpable* or *nonpalpable*. Careful physical examination is the cornerstone to diagnosis. The testes in young patients can be difficult to locate because of their small size and active cremasteric response. A relaxed patient and warmed examiner's hands lead to a more productive examination. Placing the patient in a cross-legged sitting position may make testes easy to see or palpate. The use of a milking action toward the scrotum often delivers a difficult-to-locate gonad. Palpable testes can be classified as retractile, ectopic or true undescended.

   a. *Retractile testes* can be brought to the scrotum without any tension on the spermatic vessels and will remain in the scrotum unless the cremasteric reflex is stimulated. These are not truly undescended testes, and no treatment is required. However, some severely retractile testes can become undescended as the patient grows. This phenomenon of secondary testicular ascent is rare but does occur, and therefore these patients should be examined periodically.

   b. *Ectopic testes* are descended through the external ring but become positioned in a location outside the scrotum. They may be positioned in the superficial inguinal pouch, pubic area, femoral area, or perineum. This form of maldescent is related to abnormal gubernacular attachment.

   c. *True undescended testes* can be in the abdomen, in the inguinal canal, or at the scrotal inlet. To be palpable, they must be in the inguinal canal or below. However, true undescended testes cannot be brought to the scrotum without significant tension on the spermatic vessels, which immediately leads to retraction out of the scrotum when the gonad is released.

2. The nonpalpable testis may be intraabdominal or absent. Careful physical examination by an experienced examiner is necessary to be certain the testicle is not palpable.

   a. The unilateral nonpalpable testis is absent in as many as 47 per cent of cases. However, bilateral nonpalpable testes represent anorchia only 5 per cent of the time. The contralateral testes often shows significant hypertrophy in the child with unilaterally absent testis. The cause of the absent testis is usually a prenatal vascular accident.

   b. The intraabdominal testis is usually near the internal inguinal ring but may be located as high as the ipsilateral kidney.

Key Clinical Findings

- No palpable testes, or
- Palpable ectopic testes

Laboratory Findings

Laboratory studies usually are not necessary in patients with straightforward unilateral cryptorchidism.

1. Karyotyping is indicated in bilateral cryptorchidism, especially with bilateral nonpalpable testes. Measurement of follicle-stimulating hormone, luteinizing hormone, and testosterone before and after administration of hCG in children with bilateral nonpalpable testes may predict the presence or absence of the testes.

2. Histologic evaluation of the testes is indicated any time that testicular tissue is removed, because of the increased risk of malignancy in cryptorchid testes.

Key Laboratory Tests

- Karyotyping (selective)
- Follicle-stimulating hormone and luteinizing hormone

Imaging Evaluation

Imaging studies are occasionally used in the evaluation of nonpalpable testes. Ultrasonography, computed tomography scanning, magnetic resonance imaging, and venography have been used. However, since these studies do not change the management of the child, imaging evaluation should be deferred until the patient is examined by the person who will ultimately be responsible for management of this problem.

Treatment

1. *Hormonal therapy*—hCG and gonadotropin-releasing hormone (GnRH) are the two forms of hormonal therapy for cryptorchidism.

   a. hCG is given intramuscularly over a 3- to 4-week period in a series of injections weekly or twice weekly, not to exceed a total of 10,000 IU.

   (1) The success reported for use of hCG to promote testicular descent is quite variable (20 to 50%). This probably relates to the fact that most studies do not adequately differentiate between undescended and retractile testes. The retractile testes respond very well to hormone therapy. In addition, the response is better in the older age groups.

   (2) Subsequent return of the testes to a suprascrotal position after initial descent may occur 20 to 50 per cent of the time after hCG therapy. However, even if this occurs or there is failure of descent, subsequent surgical treatment may be somewhat easier.

   (3) hCG therapy is not indicated in patients with

clinically noticeable hernias, previous inguinal surgery, or ectopic testes.

b. GnRH is given intranasally. It has been used extensively in Europe but is not approved at this time for use in the United States. It has a response rate for testicular descent similar to that of hCG (20 to 50%). However, combination therapy with the two hormones may be more successful. GnRH treatment in the younger infants (6 to 12 months) has been shown to enhance germ cell maturation in the cryptorchid testes. Whether this translates into improved fertility in the cryptorchid male is yet to be seen. However, treatment with GnRH may have benefits even in nonresponders who require subsequent surgical treatment.

2. Surgical therapy varies depending on whether the testis is palpable or nonpalpable.

a. The palpable nondescended testis can almost always be brought to the scrotum with a standard orchiopexy through an inguinal incision.

b. The nonpalpable testis presents a more complex surgical problem.

(1) If any tissue is palpable in the inguinal or scrotal area to suggest cord structures or a patent processus vaginalis, the initial surgical approach would be inguinal. If no spermatic vessels are found, then it is imperative that an intraabdominal approach be used to rule out an intraabdominal testicle. Laparoscopy has become popular recently in this approach, but some surgeons prefer a counterincision above the inguinal canal, through either the same or a different skin incision, to allow direct visualization of the peritoneal cavity.

(2) If no tissue is initially palpable in the inguinal canal or scrotum, then an intraabdominal approach would be considered first, either laparoscopically or by open technique. If a testicle is found in the abdomen, it may be brought to the scrotum by one of several techniques. If it is

very abnormal in appearance or size, removal may be warranted. In postpubertal males, nondescended testes have little chance for spermatogenesis, and most surgeons would recommend these testes be removed.

OPTIMAL TREATMENT

The *optimal recommended treatment* in the United States at this time for the palpable undescended testis is orchiopexy at 1 year of age.

---

3. The logic for use of orchiopexy instead of hormonal therapy is that hCG is minimally effective in this age group and GnRH is not available, so there may be benefit to fertility in bringing the testicle to the scrotum early in life. If intranasal GnRH becomes approved for use in this country, then early hormonal therapy may replace initial orchiopexy if subsequent studies show a benefit in fertility with hormonal therapy.

Prevention

To date, no known intervention can prevent cryptorchidism. However, early treatment may have some benefit in preventing the fertility problems associated with cryptorchidism.

 Bibliography

Hadziselimovic F: Cryptorchidism. *In* Gillenwater JY, Grayhack JT, Howards SS, et al (eds): Adult and Pediatric Urology, 2nd ed, vol 2. St. Louis, Mosby–Year Book, 1991, pp 2217–2228.

Kogan SJ: Treatment of cryptorchidism: An additional viewpoint. *In* Gillenwater JY, Grayhack JT, Howards SS, et al (eds): Adult and Pediatric Urology, 2nd ed, vol 2. St. Louis, Mosby–Year Book, 1991, pp 2229–2244.

Rozanski MD, Bloom DA: The undescended testis. Urol Clin North Am 1995;22:107–118.

Spencer JR: Mechanisms of testicular descent. Dialogues in Pediatric Urology 1992;15:1–8.

Zaontz MR: Orchiopexy revisited. Dialogues in Pediatric Urology 1990;13:1–8.

---

228 Trauma to the Urinary Tract

J. Patrick Murphy

Etiology and Epidemiology

1. Trauma is the leading cause of death in children. Blunt trauma accounts for 90 per cent of the injuries in children. However, penetrating trauma has increased dramatically in the last decade. Urinary tract injuries account for 3 to 5 per cent of pediatric trauma.

2. *Renal trauma* is more common in children than adults and accounts for the majority of injuries to the urinary tract (50 to 60%).

3. *Ureteral injuries* are not common in children and account for only 4 per cent of all urinary tract trauma.

4. *Bladder injuries* occur more commonly in children than adults because the bladder is more of an abdominal organ in children; 95 per cent of bladder injuries are caused by blunt trauma.

5. *Urethral injuries* can be divided into posterior and anterior injuries and are much less common in females than males.

Pathophysiology

1. Renal trauma occurs more frequently in children than adults. The kidneys are less well protected by the chest wall. Gerota fascia and perirenal fat are poorly developed, and the child's kidney is more mobile and at greater risk for injuries to the vascular pedicle and ureteropelvic junction (UPJ) in deceleration accidents.

2. Ureteral injuries are usually the result of blunt trauma.
   a. The shearing forces that occur with deceleration accidents usually cause the proximal injuries.
   b. Pelvic fractures and crush injuries usually cause the distal injuries at the ureterovesical junction (UVJ).
   c. Penetrating trauma causes injury to all portions of the ureter.

3. Bladder injuries can occur from several mechanisms in blunt trauma.
   a. Blowout injuries from compression of a full bladder can occur with seat belt trauma or crush trauma and are often intraperitoneal injuries.
   b. Penetration by bone fragments in pelvic fractures more often are extraperitoneal injuries.
   c. Shearing forces from pelvic crush trauma can also injure the bladder neck.
   d. Spinal trauma may disrupt the normal voiding function of the bladder.

4. Urethral injuries occur at various sites related to the mechanism of trauma.
   a. Posterior injuries are almost always a result of severe pelvic trauma and pelvic fractures.
   b. Anterior injuries occur most commonly from straddle accidents, which crush the bulbar urethra against the pubic bone.
      (1) Pendulous urethral trauma can occur with toilet seat injuries.
      (2) Distal urethral and meatal injuries can occur with circumcision accidents.

Clinical Findings

1. Renal trauma may result in nonspecific physical findings, including flank or upper abdominal tenderness, ecchymosis, mass, nausea and vomiting, or shock. Hematuria is more specific for urinary tract injury and should lead to a radiologic evaluation of the urinary tract.

2. Ureteral injuries may be difficult to detect, and a high index of suspicion is necessary to avoid missing the injury.
   a. Hematuria and/or obstructive symptoms which would suggest ureteral trauma may be absent or masked by other abdominal injuries.
   b. Delayed leaks or strictures may occur from both blunt and penetrating injuries that may not be suspected initially.

3. Bladder trauma may also be masked by symptoms of other lower abdominal or pelvic trauma. Hematuria may suggest bladder injury with associated pelvic trauma, but hematuria may not be present. Any major pelvic crush injury or pelvic fracture requires evaluation radiologically to rule out bladder injury.

4. Urethral injuries may have more specific physical findings.
   a. Blood at the meatus and/or inability to void
   b. Perineal, scrotal, or penile ecchymosis and swelling
   c. Rectal examination suggesting bogginess anteriorly or a high-riding prostate

Key Clinical Findings

- Flank tenderness
- Abdominal mass

Laboratory Findings

Except for the hematuria seen on urinalysis, laboratory studies are not specific for urinary tract trauma.

Key Laboratory Finding

- Hematuria

Imaging Evaluation

1. Historically, the intravenous pyelogram was the study of choice for evaluation of renal and ureteral trauma. The computed tomography (CT) scan is now the choice because it is much more sensitive and anatomically specific in identifying urinary tract trauma.

2. Ultrasound is used in some situations of less severe trauma.
   a. Evaluation of microscopic hematuria in minor trauma to screen for congenital anomalies of kidney
   b. To follow injuries of kidney originally evaluated by CT.

3. Nuclear renography and/or arteriography may be used in selected cases of suspected renal vascular injury.

4. Contrast cystography is used to specifically rule out bladder rupture and to differentiate between intraperitoneal and extraperitoneal rupture. Multiple radiographic views must be taken with the bladder filled and emptied to avoid missing subtle extravasation.

5. Retrograde and voiding contrast urethrography studies evaluate potential urethral disruption.

WARNING

Any suspected urethral injury should be evaluated by retrograde urethrography before a catheter is passed per urethra.

Treatment

1. Treatment of renal injuries depends on the severity of injury. The goal is preservation of functioning renal tissue.
   a. Most renal injuries can be managed nonoperatively.
      (1) Bed rest is indicated until gross hematuria has resolved.

(2) Activity should be restricted for 2 to 3 months and until microscopic hematuria has resolved.

(3) Follow-up imaging is done by ultrasound or CT depending on the injury severity.

(4) Long-term follow-up should be at least 1 year, with blood pressure, urinalysis, and imaging as indicated for all significant renal injuries.

b. Indications for operative intervention include the following:

(1) Exsanguinating or persistent bleeding

(2) Persistent urinary extravasation

(3) Renal vascular pedicle injury

(4) Significantly large segments of devitalized renal tissue

(5) Infection of perinephric blood or urine collection

(6) Urinary obstruction.

2. Ureteral injuries usually require operative intervention.

3. Treatment of *bladder rupture* depends on whether it is intraperitoneal or extraperitoneal.

a. Extraperitoneal perforation can often be treated with transurethral catheter drainage for 1 to 2 weeks without open surgical repair.

(1) Injuries caused by penetrating bone fragments should be treated surgically.

(2) Male infants may be better treated by suprapubic catheter drainage to avoid risk of urethral trauma from long-term urethral catheter use.

b. Intraperitoneal rupture usually requires open surgi-

cal repair and suprapubic or urethral catheter drainage.

c. All penetrating injuries should be treated surgically because of the likelihood of injury to adjacent structures.

4. Urethral disruptions should generally be treated with initial suprapubic diversion and delayed repair.

Key Treatment

- Rest
- Surgery (selective)

Prevention

Prevention of urinary tract trauma involves all of the measures that help to prevent pediatric trauma.

Bibliography

McAleer TM, Kaplan GW: Pediatric genitourinary trauma. Urol Clin North Am 1995;22:177–188.

Murphy JP: Genitourinary trauma. *In* Ashcraft KW (ed): Pediatric Urology. Philadelphia, WB Saunders, 1990, pp 437–447.

Noe HN, Jerkins GR: Genitourinary trauma. *In* Kelalis PP, King LR, Belman AB (eds): Clinical Pediatric Urology, 3rd ed, vol 2. Philadelphia, WB Saunders, 1992, pp 1353–1378.

Peclet M, Murphy JP: Abdominal and urinary tract trauma. *In* Ashcraft KW, Holder TM (eds): Pediatric Surgery, 2nd ed. Philadelphia, WB Saunders, 1993, pp 133–145.

Reitelman C: Pediatric renal trauma. Dial Pediatr Urol 1992;15:1–8.

229 Acute Renal Failure

Uri S. Alon

Critical State

Definition

Acute renal failure (ARF) indicates abrupt decrease in glomerular filtration rate (GFR). Although ARF is often associated with reduction in urine output, the real hallmark of ARF is increase in serum creatinine concentration as an indicator of decreased GFR.

Etiology

1. Acute renal failure is divided into three types: prerenal, renal (parenchymal), and postrenal.

a. Prerenal failure is caused by decreased perfusion of the kidneys; most commonly this type of renal failure is seen in cases of dehydration, shock, and

postcardiac surgery. It is often reversible with restoration of adequate renal perfusion.

b. Parenchymal renal failure is due to direct insult to the kidney tissue, to the glomeruli, the tubules, or both. Postrenal ARF is less commonly seen in children, but this entity, which is easily diagnosed by renal ultrasound, needs to be ruled out in all unexplained cases of ARF.

2. Whereas most cases of ARF are associated with oliguria/anuria, some patients may have a nonoliguric condition. This latter type is considered to have a better prognosis than oliguric ARF and is usually easier to manage. Nonoliguric ARF is typically seen in associa-

tion with nephrotoxic drugs, such as aminoglycosides and some antineoplastic agents, that damage mainly the renal tubule.

Differential Diagnosis

1. The most common problem is to differentiate prerenal failure from parenchymal failure due to acute tubular necrosis (ATN). Besides clinical and laboratory evidence of dehydration or "ineffective" arterial blood pressure, which support the diagnosis of prerenal failure, urine and blood tests in the latter condition will demonstrate intact tubular function. This is manifested by urine specific gravity >1.015, osmolality >500 mOsm/kg H_2O, a urine–to–plasma urea ratio >5, urine Na concentration >20 mEq/L, and disproportionate increase in BUN relative to serum creatinine concentration (>10:1). The most reliable index of tubular integrity is fractional sodium excretion

$$\frac{\text{urine Na}}{\text{urine creatinine}} \times \frac{\text{serum creatinine}}{\text{serum Na}} \times 100$$

which in prerenal failure is <1 per cent in mature infants and children and <2.5 per cent in premature infants. This calculation is made using random urine and blood specimens obtained simultaneously before any diuretics are given.

2. Although the aforementioned tests will help differentiate between ATN and prerenal failure, a similar pattern may be seen in prerenal failure and parenchymal renal failure due to glomerular diseases, such as acute post-streptococcal glomerulonephritis. This is because in glomerular disorders the tubular functions may remain intact. However, contrary to the situation in ATN and prerenal failure, in which urinalysis is basically normal or shows only minimal findings, patients with glomerulonephritis have urinary findings such as hematuria, proteinuria, and cellular casts. It is essential to do a careful urinalysis in all patients with ARF.

Management

1. In cases with sufficient clinical and laboratory evidence to suspect prerenal failure, a fluid challenge is indicated with an isotonic solution, 20 ml/kg. This often is done by using normal saline or plasma, but a solution that contains bicarbonate may have a physiologic advantage (1/2 isotonic NaCl in 5 per cent glucose to which 25 to 40 mEq/L of 1 M $NaHCO_3$ is added). It is important not to add potassium until renal failure has been ruled out. If the child still seems dehydrated, a second fluid challenge can be given. The fluid challenge should be accompanied by close monitoring of vital signs, including blood pressure and auscultation of the lungs, urine output, and serum chemistries. Overzealous fluid treatment should be avoided owing to risks of overhydration in the patient with renal failure.

2. If urine output is still inadequate despite adequate fluid replenishment, a trial of intravenous furosemide is indicated. The trial dose is 1 mg/kg, but in patients with renal failure, up to 5 mg/kg/dose may be required to achieve the diuretic response. Furosemide can also be given by constant infusion in a dose of 0.1 to 0.4 mg/kg/hour.

3. In patients with established acute parenchymal renal failure, the treatment is basically symptomatic/supportive.

   a. Total fluids given should not exceed insensible water loss plus urine output and other losses (i.e., gastric drainage) and should be adjusted every 6 to 12 hours. Fluid administration should be kept to the minimum in those with systemic fluid overload manifested by hypertension, heart failure, and/or pulmonary edema.

   b. *Electrolyte abnormalities.* These usually include hyponatremia and hyperkalemia. The former is best treated by fluid restriction and enhancement of urine output. In children with acute symptomatic hyponatremia, careful infusion of NaCl 3 per cent solution (512 mEq/L) 5 ml/kg over 2 to 3 hours can alleviate the symptoms. High concentration of serum potassium (>6.5 mEq/L) can cause cardiotoxicity first evident by peaked T waves on the electrocardiogram. Higher potassium levels can cause ventricular fibrillation and cardiac standstill. Urgent treatment is necessary when serum K >7.0 mEq/L or changes are seen on the electrocardiogram.

   c. *Metabolic acidosis.* Mild acidosis carries no risk, and serum bicarbonate concentrations of 15 mEq/L and higher do not require correction unless associated with hyperkalemia. Treatment of acidosis is usually done by $NaHCO_3$, but one should be aware of the additional sodium given with this therapy. It is also important to know that ARF is often associated with hypocalcemia and that metabolic acidosis has a protective effect against hypocalcemic tetany.

   d. Hypocalcemia, hyperphosphatemia, and hyperuricemia are usually of lesser importance in acute renal failure; however, in patients with impaired heart function, correction of hypocalcemia by IV or oral calcium supplementation is indicated. The latter mode of administration may also assist in lowering serum phosphorus concentration. Treatment of hyperuricemia with allopurinol is indicated when it is regarded as the cause of ARF, as in acute tumor lysis syndrome.

   e. *Nutrition.* It is important to provide adequate nutrition to the child with ARF. This should include the RDA for calories but may require protein, potassium, and phosphate restriction if the child is not on dialysis. In hypercatabolic conditions the nutrition should be upgraded to hyperalimentation. One should remember that enteral feeding is always superior to parenteral nutrition; however, the latter is often used in patients who cannot be fed enterally.

Critical State *Continued*

Key Treatment: Hyperkalemia

Cardiac Protection
Calcium gluconate 10%, 0.5 to 1.0 ml/kg body weight injected intravenously and slowly over 5 to 10 minutes, with continuous monitoring of heart rate.

Shift of Potassium into the Intracellular Compartment
Sodium bicarbonate, 1 to 2 mEq/kg body weight intravenously over 10 to 20 minutes, provided that salt and water overload is not a problem.
Glucose, 1 g/kg body weight, and insulin, 1 U/every 4 g of glucose, intravenously over 20 to 30 minutes.
Stimulants of β₂-adrenergic receptors such as salbutamol, intravenously or by inhalation.

Elimination of Excess Potassium
Cation exchange resin, sodium polystyrene sulfonate, 1 g/kg body weight, administered orally or rectally in 20 to 30% sorbitol or 10% glucose, 1 g resin/4 ml.
Dialysis, peritoneal or hemodialysis

f. Indications for acute dialysis include uremic syndromes, prolonged oligoanuria, systemic fluid overload, uncontrolled hypertension, and inability to medically control hyperkalemia, acidosis, and other severe electrolyte and mineral abnormalities. In addition, dialysis may be required to remove circulating drugs and toxins. This is also the case in patients with severe hypercatabolic states in which administration of higher amounts of fluids and protein are desired. In children with the hemolytic uremic syndrome, dialysis is often instituted earlier relative to other conditions that cause ARF.

g. The mode of dialysis most commonly used in children is peritoneal dialysis, as the catheter can be placed at the bedside, and an effective dialysis can be given with practically no machine used and with few trained personnel. However, whenever acute dialysis is indicated, all efforts should be made to transfer the child to a medical center in which appropriate equipment and highly trained personnel are available.

4. *Postrenal failure.* Alleviation of the obstruction or urinary diversion is the only definitive measure to reverse the ARF, but supportive treatment as outlined above may be temporarily required.

Bibliography

Brady HR, Brenner BM, Liberthal W: Acute renal failure. *In* Brenner BM (ed): The Kidney, 5th ed. Philadelphia, WB Saunders, 1994, pp 1200–1252.

Brenner BM, Stein JH: Acute renal failure. Contemp Issues Nephrol 1980;6:1–107.

Urizar RE, Largent JA, Gilboa N: Pediatric Nephrology. New York, Medical Examination Publishing, 1983, pp 398–440.

230 Chronic Renal Failure

Richard A. Kaplan

Critical State

Definition and Epidemiology

Chronic renal failure (CRF) is defined as a persistent (>3 months) and irreversible decrease in the glomerular filtration rate. This is clinically identified by an increase in the serum creatinine, above 1.5 mg/dl in children younger than 2 years of age and above 2.0 mg/dl in children older than 2 years of age. *Uremia* refers to the accumulation of nitrogen-containing waste products that occurs in renal failure. The incidence of CRF ranges from 4 to 20 new cases per 1 million population younger than 15 years of age.

Etiology

The causes of CRF in children differs dramatically from those in adults, which are predominately diabetic nephropathy and hypertensive nephropathy.

1. Chronic pyelonephritis is the result of scarring of the kidneys after one or more episodes of acute pyelonephritis. Typically, renal scarring occurs after episodes of acute pyelonephritis in the first 5 years of life, although the consequences of these infections may take years to appreciate. Chronic pyelonephritis occurs almost exclusively in children with urinary tract obstruction and those with severe vesicoureteral reflux. Chronic pyelonephritis is the most common cause of CRF in children.

2. Glomerulonephritis, examples of which are focal segmental glomerular sclerosis (FSGS) and membranoproliferative glomerulonephritis (MPGN), is a common cause of CRF in school-age and adolescent children.

3. Hereditary disorders of the kidney include polycystic

kidney disease, hereditary nephritis (Alport syndrome), oxalosis, cystinosis, and nephronophthisis.
4. Hypoplastic kidneys are congenitally small kidneys; dysplastic kidneys are congenitally malformed kidneys.
5. Hemolytic uremic syndrome is one of the most common causes of acute renal failure in children; however, only a small minority of affected children develop CRF.
6. Bilateral Wilms tumor and bilateral renal vein thrombosis are rare causes of CRF in children.

Pathophysiology

The pathophysiology of CRF is related to alterations in mineral and electrolyte excretion, decreased synthesis of erythropoietin and 1,25-dihydroxyvitamin D_3 (calcitriol), and the physiologic changes that occur as a result of uremia (the uremic environment).

1. Renal osteodystrophy is a bone disorder related to CRF.
   a. The primary causes of renal osteodystrophy are a decrease in renal excretion of phosphate, which results in hyperphosphatemia, and decreased renal production of the active form of vitamin D, calcitriol, from the less active precursor, 25-hydroxyvitamin D_3.
   b. Hyperphosphatemia and low levels of calcitriol produce hypocalcemia.
   c. Hypocalcemia and low levels of calcitriol promote secondary hyperparathyroidism, which results in excessive reabsorption of bone (osteitis fibrosa).
   d. Hypocalcemia and low levels of calcitriol result in defective mineralization of the bones (rickets in the growing child and osteomalacia in adults).
2. Growth failure of CRF is the result of renal osteodystrophy, metabolic acidosis, decreased efficacy of growth hormone and insulin-like growth factors in the uremic environment, and poor nutrition caused by decreased appetite and vomiting.
3. Anemia of CRF is a result of the decreased synthesis of erythropoietin by the kidney and decreased efficacy in the uremic environment.

Clinical Findings

1. Decreased appetite and vomiting are usual in CRF.
2. Renal osteodystrophy is characterized by skeletal pain, particularly in the extremities and lower back. Bones may fracture easily and heal slowly and poorly.
3. Anemia of CRF may result in decreased activity level, exercise tolerance, and appetite.
4. Easy bruising is a result of platelet dysfunction in the uremic environment.
5. Itching may be the result of uremia or of secondary hyperparathyroidism.
6. There is a delay in sexual maturation in both males and females with CRF.
7. Hypertension is a common feature of CRF, particularly CRF secondary to glomerulonephritis or to chronic pyelonephritis.

Key Clinical Findings

- Anorexia
- Vomiting
- Skeletal pain
- Hypertension

Laboratory Findings

1. Elevations in serum creatinine, blood urea nitrogen, and serum uric acid are present in CRF by definition.
2. Alterations in mineral metabolism include an elevation in serum phosphate, a decrease in serum calcium, an elevation in serum alkaline phosphatase (bone fraction), a decrease in calcitriol, and an increase in parathyroid hormone levels. Transient elevations in serum phosphate may be present when only 50 per cent of glomerular filtration rate has been irreversibly lost.
3. Metabolic acidosis results from the inability of the kidney to excrete acid.
4. Hyperkalemia is usually a late finding, occurring after more than 90 per cent of total glomerular filtration rate has been irreversibly lost.
5. Normochromic, normocytic anemia may occur after 60 per cent of total glomerular filtration rate has been irreversibly lost.
6. The platelet count is typically normal; however, the platelets function poorly in the uremic environment, often resulting in prolonged bleeding times.

Key Laboratory Findings

- Azotemia
- Hyperuremia
- Metabolic acidosis
- Anemia

Radiographic Changes

1. Radiologic findings in the kidney depend on the cause of the CRF.
   a. Renal ultrasound may show small kidneys with abnormal architecture, hydronephrosis if obstructive uropathy or reflux nephropathy is the cause, polycystic kidneys, or a damaged solitary kidney.
   b. Intravenous pyelography may be an unsatisfactory imaging modality because of poor uptake of contrast material.
   c. Cortical imaging renal scans (dimercaptosuccinic acid, glucoheptonate) demonstrate small kidneys in chronic glomerulonephritis and renal hypoplasia, with poor uptake of the tracer. Diffuse renal scarring

is present if chronic pyelonephritis was the cause of CRF.

2. Renal osteodystrophy

   a. Osteitis fibrosa is characterized by resorption of bone, particularly in the calvaria and distal clavicles. Severe disease may result in cyst formation in the distal femur, proximal tibia, and distal radius.

   b. Osteomalacia and rickets are characterized by generalized decreased mineralization of the bones, cupping of the distal ulna and radius, widening of the metaphyses of the long bones, and fraying of the distal ends of the long bones.

   c. Osteosclerosis is the result of replacement of lamellar osteoid by woven osteoid. Since woven osteoid has inferior mechanical stability, a larger amount of woven bone is deposited to replace the amount of lamellar bone that was resorbed. Osteosclerosis is most noticeable in the vertebrae (rugger jersey spine).

Treatment

1. *Metabolic acidosis*—Dietary supplementation with bicarbonate or citrate (Bicitra, Polycitra, Polycitra-K).
2. *Hyperkalemia*—Foods high in potassium content, such as bananas, fruit juices, and tomatoes, should be avoided or consumed in moderate quantities. Severe hyperkalemia may be treated with a potassium-binding resin (sodium polystyrene sulfonate), but persistent hyperkalemia may be an indication for end-stage management with dialysis or kidney transplantation.
3. *Renal osteodystrophy*—Supplementation with Vitamin D_3 metabolites, calcitriol, or enantiomers of this compound (dihydrotachysterol). Hyperphosphatemia and hypocalcemia are treated with phosphate-binding, calcium-containing antacids (calcium carbonate, calcium acetate). Phosphate is ubiquitous in food, and since dairy products are particularly high in phosphate these should be consumed in limited quantities or avoided. Infants require low-phosphate formulas.
4. *Growth failure*—Treatment with recombinant human growth hormone.

5. *Anemia*—Treatment with recombinant human erythropoietin.
6. *Hypertension*—Avoid fluid overload and treat with appropriate antihypertensive agents.

Key Treatments

- Correct acidosis
- Reduce potassium intake
- Vitamin D metabolites

Prevention

1. Prompt recognition of acute glomerulonephritis and referral to a center familiar with the diagnosis and treatment of childhood glomerulonephritis may decrease the incidence of CRF secondary to glomerulonephritis. However, there are types of glomerulonephritis resistant to all known therapeutic modalities.
2. Prompt identification and treatment of infants and children with urinary tract obstruction (anatomic or neurogenic) and those with severe vesicoureteral reflux is also important. Significant renal damage may have occurred in utero.
3. Prompt antibiotic treatment of any episode of acute pyelonephritis is believed to decrease the risk of renal scarring. Early identification of the child with vesicoureteral reflux or obstruction is fostered by obtaining a renal ultrasound and cystogram in any child with a urinary tract infection during the first 5 years of life.

Bibliography

Deleau J, Andre JL, Briancon S, Musse JP: Chronic renal failure in children: An epidemiological survey in Lorraine (France) 1975–1990. Pediatr Nephrol 1994;8:472–476.

Eschbach JW, Kelly MR, Haley R, et al: Treatment of the anemia of progressive renal failure with recombinant human erythropoietin. N Engl J Med 1989;321:158–163.

Fine RN, Attie KM, Kuntze J, et al: Recombinant human growth hormone in infants and young children with chronic renal insufficiency. Pediatr Nephrol 1995;9:451–457.

Harmon WE: Treatment of children with chronic renal failure. Kidney Int 1995;47:951–961.

231 End-Stage Renal Disease

Douglas L. Blowey

Critical State

Definition

A diagnosis of end-stage renal disease (ESRD) indicates that the child requires some form of renal replacement therapy (i.e., dialysis or transplantation) in order to maintain an acceptable quality of life. A reduction of the glomerular filtration rate (GFR) to less than 10 per cent of normal is frequently used as a definition of ESRD, although in clinical practice the decision as to when renal replacement therapy should begin is based on the severity of symptoms and laboratory findings in the individual child, regardless of the GFR.

Etiology

Obstructive congenital anomalies, hereditary disorders and glomerulonephritis cause the majority of cases of ESRD in children.

Epidemiology

1. The incidence of ESRD in children is 2 to 10 new cases per 1 million child population per year. The incidence of ESRD in children increases with age.
2. Children (aged 0 to 19 years) account for 2 per cent of the total ESRD population.

Pathophysiology

1. Decreased GFR and impaired tubular function result in disturbances in the essential functions of the kidney, such as the maintenance of normal body water and solute concentration, excretion of metabolic products (e.g., H^+ ions, urea), and excretion of exogenous substrates (e.g., drugs).
2. The kidney is metabolically active in the biotransformation and production of systemically active hormones (e.g., vitamin D, erythropoietin).
3. The symptoms associated with ESRD, or "uremia," result from the accumulation of water and metabolic products and the impaired production of hormones. Some of the manifestations of ESRD are bone disease, poor growth, anemia, and hypertension.

Treatment

1. Regardless of the therapy prescribed, a child with ESRD requires an inordinate amount of care, not only from the ESRD team, but also from the family. A team approach led by the pediatric nephrologist but involving the family, primary care physician, ESRD nurse (dialysis or transplantation), social worker, and nutritionist is usually needed to bring about a successful outcome.
2. The goal for all pediatric patients with ESRD is to have a well-functioning renal allograft.
   a. Forty to 50 per cent of children beginning ESRD therapy receive a transplant during the first year.
   b. In situations in which transplantation is impossible or must be delayed, dialysis is employed.
      (1) Peritoneal dialysis is the most common form of dialysis therapy used in children, especially in the younger age group. This is usually done at home.
      (2) In some instances, hemodialysis is the modality used, because of infections of the peritoneal membrane or other complications. Hemodialysis is usually done in an outpatient dialysis unit.
3. Other aspects of ESRD management that require experience and expertise for management are the following:
   a. Erythropoietin therapy for anemia
   b. Growth hormone therapy for growth failure
   c. Nutritional management
   d. Immunosuppressive therapy after kidney transplantation

Key Treatment

- Dialysis (peritoneal dialysis, hemodialysis)
- Kidney transplantation

Outcome After Pediatric Kidney Transplantation

1. The 2- and 10-year survival rates for children (>4 years) after kidney transplantation are 95 and 80 per cent, respectively. The youngest age group (0 to 4 years) experiences the lowest 2-year survival rate (85 per cent).
2. The estimated rate of renal graft survival (i.e., a graft that is working) for a live, related-donor kidney is 84.6 per cent at 2 years and 74.7 per cent at 5 years. The comparable estimates for cadaver kidneys are 76.4 per cent and 70.7 per cent.

Bibliography

Avner ED, Chavers B, Sullivan EK, Tejani A: Renal transplantation and chronic dialysis in children and adolescents: The 1993 annual report of the North American Pediatric Renal Transplant Cooperative Study. Pediatr Nephrol 1995;9:61–73.

United States Renal Data System 1995 Annual Data Report: Pediatric End-Stage Renal Disease. Am J Kidney Dis 1995;26(Suppl 2):S112–S128.

232 Hypertensive Crisis

Uri S. Alon

Critical State

Hypertensive emergencies can develop in children already known to be hypertensive (e.g., those with end-stage renal disease) or as part of the presenting picture of a new disease (e.g., acute postinfectious glomerulonephritis). Emergency intervention is indicated when the level of blood pressure can become a threat to life or the function of vital organs. Generally this occurs with symptoms when the systolic pressure is >160 mmHg and diastolic >100 mmHg, but these values may vary with age.

Etiology

All causes of secondary hypertension (i.e., nonessential hypertension) in childhood can result in hypertensive crisis. Most commonly, it is seen in children with acute and chronic glomerulonephritis, hemolytic uremic syndrome, chronic pyelonephritis, or renovascular hypertension, or in association with treatment with corticosteroids.

Symptoms

1. Headache, irritability
2. Nausea and vomiting
3. Visual disturbances
4. Seizures
5. Coma
6. Congestive heart failure
7. Asymptomatic

Signs

1. *Retinopathy*–May not be seen in the first hours of newly developed acute hypertension
2. Left-sided congestive heart failure
3. Edema
4. Oliguria and/or hematuria

Treatment

1. The goal is to quickly lower the blood pressure from its dangerously high level, which can be damaging especially to the brain and heart. This does not necessarily mean rapid normalization of blood pressure. On the contrary, too rapid correction, especially in patients with long-standing hypertension, may result in hypoperfusion of essential organs. Therefore, the optimal approach is one of gradual reduction of blood pressure, depending on its values, symptoms, and chronicity.
2. In patients who have encephalopathic symptoms, who are uncooperative, or who are vomiting, intravenous therapy is indicated. The use of calcium channel blockers like nifedipine has the advantage of causing less cerebral ischemia because of their property to increase cerebral blood flow, and therefore they can be used even in patients with early encephalopathic symptoms. After successful treatment of hypertensive encephalology, some children may suffer from cortical blindness, which usually resolves within a few days.

Key Treatment: Drugs for Treatment of Hypertensive Crisis

Drug	Dose	Comments
Oral		
Nifedipine	0.25–0.5 mg/kg	Drug of choice
Minoxidil	0.25 mg/kg	—
Intravenous		
Labetalol	0.25–0.5 mg/kg	Drug of choice
	1.0–3.0 mg/kg/hr	Drug of choice
Sodium nitroprusside	0.5–8.0 μg/kg/min	Drug of choice. Needs to be carefully titrated and supervised. Thiocyanate blood level must be measured after 48 hr.
Hydralazine	0.15–0.3 mg/kg	Can also be given intramuscularly.
Diazoxide	2.0–5.0 mg/kg	Use the lower dose especially when combined with other antihypertensives.
Furosemide	1.0 mg/kg	For use in hypervolemia. Can be increased up to 5.0 mg/kg in renal failure.

Bibliography

Houtman PN, Dillon MJ: Medical management of hypertension in childhood. Child Nephrol Urol 1992;12:154–161.

Ingelfinger JR: Pediatric Hypertension. Philadelphia, WB Saunders, 1982, pp 218–228.

233 Bladder Catheterization

Ari M. Simckes

Indications

1. To obtain an uncontaminated specimen of urine for diagnostic purposes, for example, to assess the presence of a urinary tract infection (UTI). Quantitative bacterial culture of a catheterized urine sample may be used to determine the presence or absence of a UTI (see Table 217–1).

2. To differentiate urinary retention from lack of urine formation, as in the infant who has not voided by 36 to 48 hours of age.

3. To measure accurately urine output. An indwelling catheter may be required to evaluate and manage the oliguric patient.

4. As a diagnostic procedure
   a. Radiologic bladder imaging
   b. Urodynamics
   c. Measurement of postvoid residual urine
   d. To determine whether a menstruating female has hematuria.

> **WARNING**
>
> **Urethral trauma, including a burn injury, is a contraindication to bladder catheterization.**

Preparation

1. Explain the need for the procedure to the patient, if appropriate, and to the caretakers. Unless the patient is in a life-threatening situation, time should be spent to describe the diagnostic and therapeutic benefits of the procedure and the potential risks.

2. Confirm that support personnel are aware of what is expected of them.

3. Have available all necessary equipment, with backup items such as smaller-size catheters and extra sterile gloves. If a Foley-type catheter is to be used, the balloon should be inflated to check for patency.

Equipment

1. Urethral catheter of the appropriate size and type. Use a Foley catheter with an inflatable distal balloon if the catheter is to remain in place. A sterile feeding tube may suffice when a urine specimen is needed in an infant, although it is difficult to secure in the bladder. A 10F catheter is appropriate for most children. Smaller catheters (5 or 8F) are used for newborns and larger catheters (12 to 14F) for teenagers.

2. A supply of sterile 2×2 or 4×4 gauze pads, cotton-tipped applicators, gloves (latex-free for myelodysplasia patients), and tape.

3. Sterile lubricant. Lidocaine (Xylocaine) HCl 2% gel functions as both a lubricant and an anesthetic.

4. Skin-cleaning agent, such as povidone-iodine solution.

5. Sterile syringe and liquid (e.g., normal saline) for a Foley-type indwelling catheter.

6. Sterile container for the urine specimen. Tubing and graduated container if the catheter is to be used for monitoring urine output.

Anesthesia

When catheterization is performed on a conscious, sensate patient, anxiolytic agents, sedatives, and analgesics are rarely required. A lubricant with topical anesthetic additives (e.g., Xylocaine HCl 2% gel) may be useful for the child undergoing a radiologic investigation.

Technique

1. After all the equipment is prepared, the patient is restrained as necessary. The catheter should be well lubricated with sterile gel to minimize local trauma. Sterile towels or drapes may be used to maintain a sterile field.
   a. In the case of an infant who must be restrained, holding the knees in a frog-leg position often allows for good visualization. The urethral meatus and surrounding region are gently cleansed at least three times with an agent such as povidone-iodine solution. The solution should be allowed to air dry, both for proper antisepsis and because contamination of the internal channel of the catheter may result in a false-negative culture and erroneous measurements in the urinalysis (e.g., false elevation of urine protein).
   b. To avoid fecal contamination, clean females in an anterior to posterior direction. The foreskin should be retracted gently in the uncircumcised male.

2. *Females*—The labia must be carefully spread to visualize the external urethral meatus. The well lubricated catheter is advanced through the urethra (approximately 2 to 3 cm) into the bladder (see part A of figure).

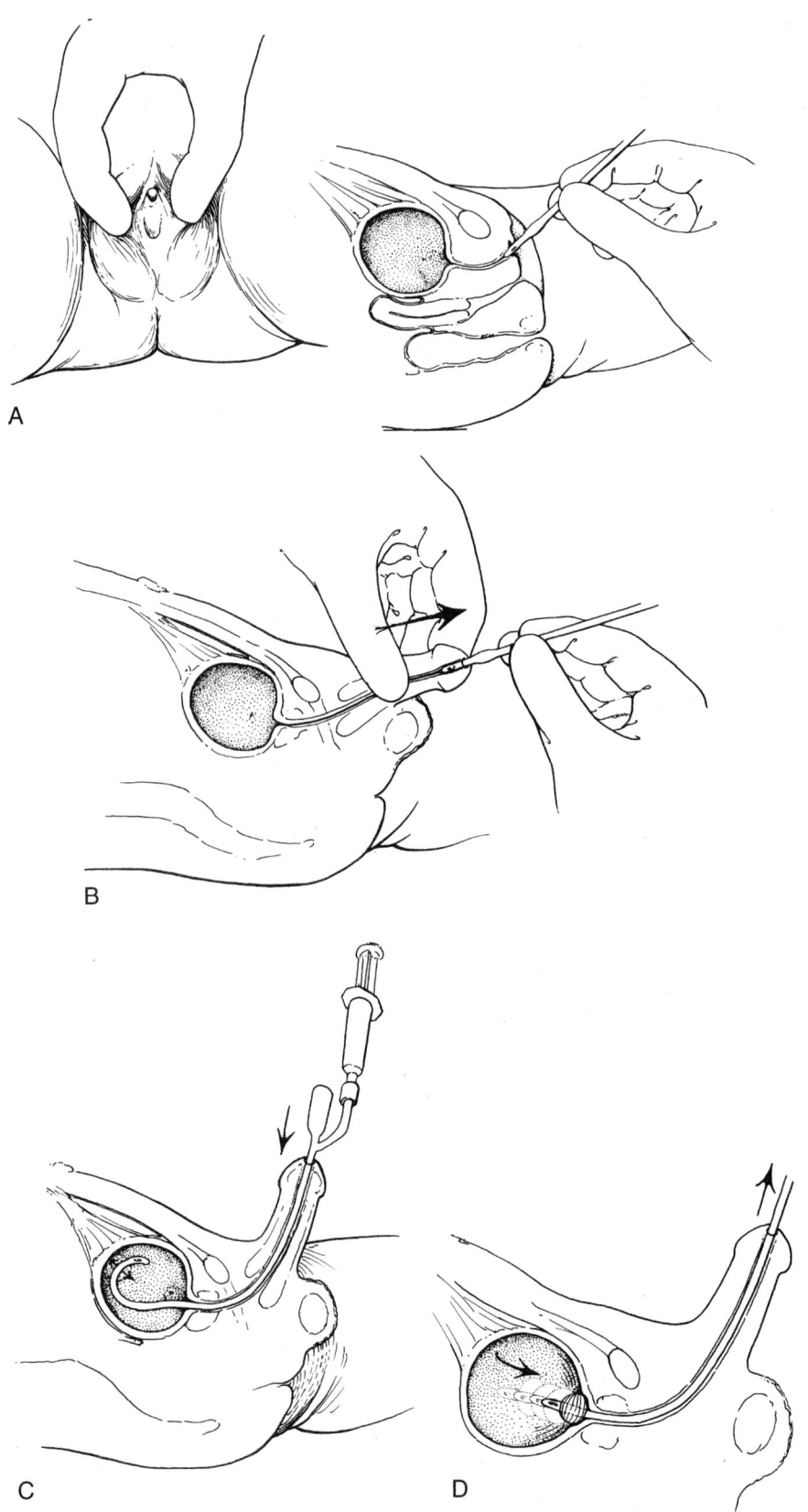

A

B

C

D

Procedure *Continued*

3. *Males*—The penis is grasped gently and extended in a caudal direction to straighten the urethra. The catheter is slowly advanced through the urethra (see part B of figure). Mild resistance often is met when the catheter reaches the external sphincter. Passage of the catheter tip from the proximal urethra into the bladder may be aided by holding the penis in a vertical position. If much resistance is encountered, excess force should not be applied, although constant gentle pressure may result in sphincter relaxation and success. However, a fresh start with a smaller-size catheter may be necessary.

> **WARNING**
>
> **Catheterization should not be performed without visualization of the external urethral meatus because of the risks of complications such as trauma, vaginal catheterization, and iatrogenic infection.**

4. *Balloon catheters*—The balloon must be inserted into the bladder before inflation. After the balloon is inflated, the catheter is withdrawn until resistance is appreciated, indicating that the balloon is resting at the trigone of the bladder (see parts C and D of figure). The catheter should be secured by taping it to the patient's thigh, leaving slack to prevent trauma in case the catheter is accidentally pulled. A retention catheter should be connected to the appropriate tubing with a closed system collection bag. Be sure to deflate the balloon before removal of a retention catheter.

> **WARNING**
>
> **The incidence of an iatrogenic UTI is high with indwelling bladder catheters. Urinalyses and cultures should be obtained as clinically appropriate, and the catheter should be removed as soon as its presence is no longer needed.**

 Bibliography

Illustrated techniques of pediatric procedures. *In* Fleisher G, Ludwig S (eds): Textbook of Pediatric Emergency Medicine, 2nd ed. Baltimore, Williams & Wilkins, 1988, p 1307.

Rowe PC: Pediatric procedure. *In* Oski FA (ed): Principles and Practice of Pediatrics, 2nd ed. Philadelphia, JB Lippincott, 1994.

234 Suprapubic Aspiration (Bladder Tap)

Ari M. Simckes

Procedure

Indications

1. This method of urine collection is the gold standard for determining the presence or absence of a urinary tract infection, because it is least likely to contain contaminating bacteria. Suprapubic catheterization is less likely than urethral catheterization to introduce contaminants into the urinary tract. The procedure is not now widely used but is most applicable in children less than 2 years of age in whom the distended urinary bladder is situated in the abdomen. Suprapubic aspiration is specifically indicated to obtain urine for culture in infant girls with moderate to marked vaginitis and urethritis and in the presence of phimosis/balanoposthitis in boys.

2. The procedure is used for drainage of the bladder in the presence of urinary retention secondary to urethral or bladder outlet obstruction. Transient acute urinary retention is uncommon in children but may occur because of postoperative pain or, rarely, because of lower urinary tract infection.

Contraindications

Suprapubic aspiration of the urinary bladder should not be done in the presence of infection of the skin of the lower abdominal wall or when urinary tract anomalies make it difficult to locate the distended urinary bladder.

Preparation and Equipment

1. Explain the need for the procedure to the caretaker or caretakers and, if appropriate, to the child.
2. Wait at least 30 to 60 minutes after the child voids, so the bladder is not likely to be empty.
3. Confirm that those assisting know their responsibilities, including the appropriate method for restraining the child.

Procedure *Continued*

4. Have available all of the necessary equipment and supplies, including backup items. These include 3-ml or 5-ml sterile syringes for infants and 10-ml syringes for older children, 21- or 23-gauge 1.5-inch needles, antiseptic solution (povidone-iodine), gauze pads, and an adhesive bandage.
5. A sterile urine collection bag is placed over the genitalia before suprapubic catheterization, or a well coordinated assistant may have a sterile cup available, since children often void because of the stimulation of the bladder.
6. If placement of an indwelling suprapubic catheter is indicated, a urology or surgery consultation should be obtained.

Anesthesia

Generally, no anesthesia is used for this procedure. However, if time allows, a local topical anesthetic agent may be used. Sedation may be appropriate, depending on the circumstances.

Precautions

Suprapubic bladder aspiration, performed correctly, is a safe procedure in young children and allows for precision in the diagnosis of a urinary tract infection. A distended bladder is a necessity for this procedure to be both productive and safe. Complications of this procedure include the following:

1. Hematuria, usually microscopic (not uncommon and usually benign)
2. Aspiration of the bowel (usually without adverse effects)
3. Intraabdominal bleeding (exceedingly rare)
4. Abdominal wall infection.

Technique

1. The infant should be restrained and secured in a frog-leg position. It may be helpful to have an assistant occlude the patient's urethra to prevent urination during the preparations and during the procedure itself. This may be accomplished by gentle penile pressure in the male and by anterior rectal pressure in females. (Sterile urine cups should be available to collect a *midstream* specimen, or a sterile urine collection bag should be placed over the genitalia.)
2. The site chosen for the puncture should be in the midline, 0.5 to 1.5 cm cephalad to the superior aspect of the pubic symphysis. Usually there is a horizontal skin crease which aids in locating the puncture site. The lower abdomen is then cleaned at least three times using an antiseptic solution such as povidone-iodine. The skin should be allowed to air dry and then may be wiped with 70% alcohol.
3. Use a 1.5-inch, 21- or 23-gauge needle attached to a 3-, 5-, or 10-ml syringe.

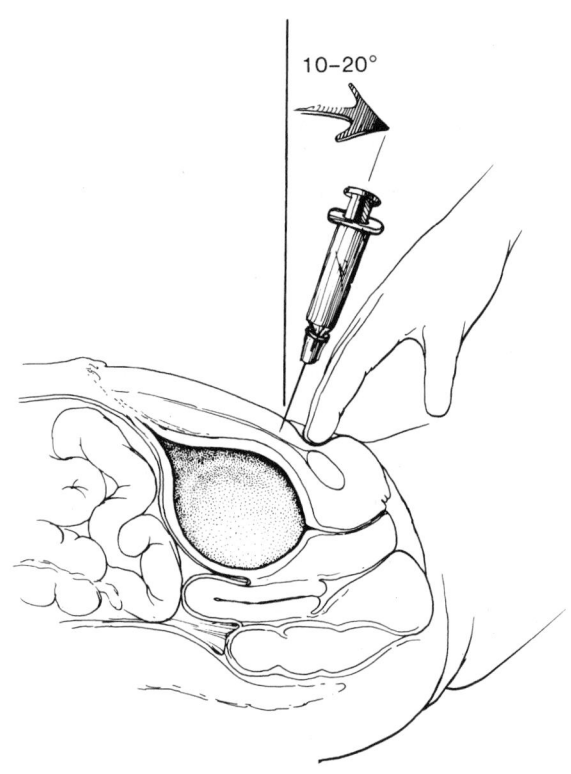

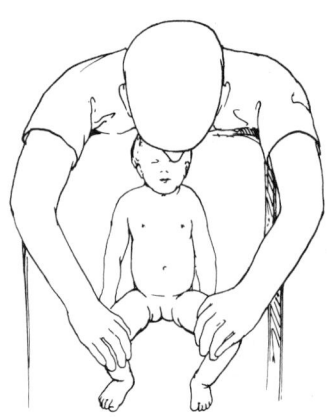

a. Puncture the skin and bladder perpendicular to the abdominal wall (see figure).
b. After entering the skin, apply gentle suction to the syringe as the needle is advanced into the bladder to a depth no greater than 2.5 cm. If no urine is obtained, the needle may be retracted while maintaining negative pressure within the syringe.

Procedure *Continued*

c. Without removing the needle from the skin, additional attempts may be made by piercing the bladder at a slightly more caudal or cephalad angle (maximum angle, 20 degrees).

4. If urine is not obtained after three attempts, urethral catheterization may be performed (if not contraindicated), or the bladder aspiration may be reattempted after waiting 1 to 2 hours, allowing the bladder to fill.

5. After removal of the needle, gentle pressure is applied with a sterile gauze pad on the puncture site and an adhesive bandage is applied. The aspirated urine should be injected into the appropriate containers and processed immediately.

Follow-up

Although the incidence of complications is very low if suprapubic aspiration is performed correctly, the puncture site should be monitored for evidence of abdominal wall or skin infection and the development of a urinary tract infection should be investigated if symptoms or signs occur. Abdominal pain and/or heme-positive stools suggest the possibility that the bowel was punctured.

Bibliography

Illustrated techniques of pediatric procedures. *In* Fleisher G, Ludwig S (eds): Textbook of Pediatric Emergency Medicine, 2nd ed. Baltimore, Williams & Wilkins, 1988, p 1309.

Nyamekye I, MacKinnon AE: A simple technique for temporary suprapubic catheterization. Br J Hosp Med 1992;47:284–285.

Rowe PC. Pediatric procedure. *In* Oski FA (ed): Principles and Practice of Pediatrics, 2nd ed. Philadelphia, JB Lippincott, 1994.

235 Urinalysis

Uri S. Alon

Procedure

Urinalysis is part of the "physical examination" of the kidney and urinary system. Urinalysis includes the assessment of the physical characteristics of the urine, the dipstick evaluation, and the microscopic examination of the urine sediment.

1. Observation of the urine specimen
   a. *Color*—An abnormal urine color can result from the clearance from the blood of colored substances (e.g., drugs, foodstuffs) or because of systemic or kidney disorders. Bright red urine and at times the presence of blood clots in the urine indicate bleeding in the lower urinary tract. The urine in patients with glomerular disease usually has a smoky, brown color.
   b. Clarity, foam, and odor
      (1) The urine is usually clear. A cloudy urine is usually the result of the presence of amorphous phosphates in alkaline urine, which disappear with the addition of acid. Amorphous urates cause white or pink cloudiness, which disappears on heating. Leukocytes in the urine can result in an appearance similar to that of amorphous phosphates.
      (2) Protein and bilirubin alter the surface tension, and their presence can produce foam.

   (3) An unusual odor of urine may result from ingested substances (e.g., some antibiotics), the breakdown of urea into ammonia by urea-splitting bacteria, the foul odor of some gram-negative bacteria, the presence of acetone or diacetic acids, or the presence of various unusual metabolites in the urine. Examples are the "maple syrup" odor in maple syrup disease, "mousy" odor in phenylketonuria, "sweaty feet" odor in isovalericacidemia, and "fishy" odor in hypermethioninemia.

2. Specific gravity*
   The specific gravity (SG) of the urine may be used to evaluate the capacity of the kidneys to save or to excrete water. Disturbances in kidney functions and in the secretion of antidiuretic hormone and aldosterone are reflected by the kidneys' inability to modify urine concentration according to the metabolic needs of the body. SG is also important for interpretation of other findings in the urine. The presence

---

*The dipstick paper measures a surrogate for osmolality, not SG, although it is calibrated as SG. When SG and osmolality do not correlate, as in albuminuria and glycosuria, the true SG is sometimes much higher, though the osmolality surrogate gives a better index of tubular function.

Procedure *Continued*

of a trace of protein in highly concentrated urine (SG >1.025) is less significant than the same magnitude of proteinuria (by dipstick) in very dilute urine.

3. Dipstick examination of the urine
Evaluation of the urine of a patient not suspected of having kidney disease or urinary tract infection can in fact be done solely by the use of the dipstick, in the so-called routine urinalysis; the microscopic examination of the urinary sediment may be omitted if the dipstick test is negative. It should be noted, however, that the sensitivity of the nitrite test is too low to be used for evaluation of children with urinary tract infection.

a. *Glucose*—The dipstick uses the glucose oxidase reaction and therefore is specific for the presence of glucose. False-negative results with the glucose oxidase test can occur in association with the presence of ascorbic acid and ketones in the urine. To interpret the significance of the presence of glucose in the urine, it is necessary to simultaneously measure blood glucose concentration. Glucosuria in the face of normal blood glucose concentration is caused by inadequate glucose reabsorption in the proximal tubule.

b. *Protein*—The dipstick test for protein is specific for albumin, providing a semiquantitative estimation. Highly alkaline urine (pH 7.5 to 8.0) and several interfering substances such as phenazopyridines, radiocontrast agents, tolmetin, sulfonamides, and high concentrations of penicillin or cephalosporins can give false-positive results for albumin. Taking into account that normally up to 100 mg of protein per square meter are excreted daily, the presence of trace protein in nondilute urine (SG >1.015) can be regarded as a normal finding. A rough estimation of protein excretion can be obtained by analysis of the protein and creatinine concentrations in a "spot" urine and employment of the following equation:
24-hour urine protein (gm/m^2) = 0.63 × urine protein (mg/dl) ÷ urine creatinine (mg/dl).

c. *Ketone bodies*—The conventional dipstick test for ketone bodies detects acetone and acetoacetic acid. The finding of ketone bodies in the urine without glucose is common in children after several hours of starvation.

d. *pH*—Normal urine pH ranges between 4.5 and 8.0. Higher urine pH may result from the presence of bacteria that degrade urea to ammonia, which in turn combines with hydrogen to form ammonium. Urine pH below 4.5 or above 8.0 may indicate contamination of the collection utensil. Urine pH should be determined on a freshly voided specimen as quickly as possible.

e. *Hemoglobin, myoglobin, and red blood cells*—A positive dipstick test for blood with absence of red blood cells in the microscopic examination indicates the presence of free hemoglobin or myoglobin. Free hemoglobin can be present in the urine because of lysis of red blood cells in highly alkaline or very dilute urine, especially when the urine stands for a long time before testing, or it may be the result of hemoglobinemia due to hemolysis. Hemoglobinuria and myoglobinuria may be differentiated by the plasma color: it is pink-red or brownish in hemoglobinuria but stays normal in color in myoglobinuria.

f. *Nitrite*—The nitrite test is an indirect method for detection of bacteria in the urine. Common uropathogens such as *Escherichia coli*, Enterobacteriaceae, *Klebsiella*, and *Proteus* species contain enzymes that reduce the nitrate in the urine to nitrite. In order for quantitatively significant amounts of nitrite to be formed, the reaction must take place in the bladder over at least 4 hours.

WARNING

Although a positive nitrite test indicates the presence of bacteria, a negative test does not rule out the presence of bacteria in the urine.

---

g. *Leukocytes (leukocyte esterase)*—The main advantage of the leukocyte esterase test is that, whereas leukocytes in a urine specimen can disintegrate and disappear quite rapidly, leukocyte esterase persists; so the dipstick result remains positive.

4. Microscopic examination of the urine
The microscopic examination of the urine should be performed on a fresh urine specimen. The usual procedure is to centrifuge 5 to 10 ml of urine at 2000 to 3000 rpm for 3 to 5 minutes. Discard all but about 0.25 ml of supernatant fluid, and resuspend the sediment in the residual supernatant fluid. The sediment is placed on a clean slide and covered with a coverslip for microscopic examination. The urine is scanned under low power (about 200×) for abnormalities, and then the formed elements are examined and counted under high-power magnification (×400 to 450). The use of the phase contrast microscope enables better identification of the various elements and eliminates the need for special staining.

Bibliography

Abitol C, Zilleruelo G, Freundlich M, Strauss J: Quantitation of proteinuria with urinary protein/creatinine ratios and random testing with dipsticks in nephrotic children. J Pediatr 1990; 116:243–247.

Alon U, Hellerstein S, Warady BA: Assessment and interpretation of urinalysis and routine kidney function tests. Children's Hospital Quarterly 1990;2:317–325.

Houser M: Assessment of proteinuria using random urine samples. J Pediatr 1984;104:845–848.

Klinenberg JR, Bluestone R, Schlosstein L, et al: Urate deposition disease: How is it regulated and how can it be modified? Ann Intern Med 1973;78:99–111.

236 Tests of Kidney Function

Stanley Hellerstein

Procedure

Effective kidney function maintains the normal volume and composition of body fluids through glomerular ultrafiltration of plasma and modification of the ultrafiltrate by tubular reabsorption and secretion.

1. *Glomerular filtration rate (GFR)*—Estimation of GFR is the most important measure of kidney function in clinical practice, because an adequate volume of glomerular filtrate is essential for the kidney to carry out the function of regulation of water and solute balance. Urea and creatinine are commonly used to estimate GFR in a clinical setting.

    a. *Serum or blood urea nitrogen concentration (SUN or BUN)**—Estimation of urea concentration in serum or blood is usually done by measurement of urea nitrogen concentration. SUN and BUN are similar in evaluation of renal function, recognizing that BUN is about 14 per cent less than SUN. Most of the urea produced in the body is excreted by the kidneys.

    (1) Although most of the urea produced in the body is excreted by the kidneys, SUN or BUN is not reliable for estimation of GFR because the concentration of urea in body fluids is determined by both renal and nonrenal factors. For example, urea clearance by the kidney depends not only on the quantity of functioning renal tissue but also on urine flow, which is a function of water and electrolyte balance. Another factor that affects the concentration of urea in body fluids is protein intake. Increased protein intake (or blood in the gastrointestinal tract) increases urea levels, and decreased protein intake decreases SUN.

    (2) SUN and BUN are very useful as markers for the toxic metabolites that cause the uremic syndrome, although urea itself is not toxic. In general, nephrologists intervene to keep the BUN or SUN below 100 mg/dl to avoid uremic symptoms.

    b. *Creatinine clearance (Ccr) and serum creatinine concentration ([Cr]s)* are used almost universally to estimate GFR in clinical practice (Table 236–1).

    (1) *Ccr*—Although Ccr is often viewed as a good measure of GFR, this is the case only with normal levels of GFR. Creatinine is not only filtered at the glomerulus but also secreted by the renal tubules, so Ccr is greater than GFR by a quantity reflecting tubular secretion of creatinine. The more severe the renal failure, the

TABLE 236–1. SERUM CREATININE CONCENTRATIONS AT VARIOUS AGES

AGE	HEIGHT (cm)	TRUE SERUM CREATININE (mg/dl)	
		Mean	Range (± 2SD)
Cord blood	—	0.75	0.51–0.99
0–2 wk	50	0.50	0.34–0.66
2–26 wk	60	0.39	0.23–0.55
26 wk–1 yr	70	0.32	0.18–0.46
2 yr	87	0.32	0.20–0.44
4 yr	101	0.37	0.25–0.49
6 yr	114	0.43	0.27–0.59
8 yr	126	0.48	0.31–0.65
10 yr	137	0.52	0.34–0.70
12 yr	147	0.59	0.41–0.78
Adult male	174	0.97	0.72–1.22
Adult female	163	0.77	0.53–1.01

Modified from Chantler C, Barratt TM: Laboratory evaluation. *In* Holliday MA, Barratt TM, Vermer RL (eds): Pediatric Nephrology, 2nd ed. Baltimore: Williams & Wilkins, 1987, pp 286–287. Published with permission.

---

*Virtually all determinations of urea are performed on serum samples. Laboratories nonetheless refer to the determination by the term *BUN* for historical reasons only.

Procedure *Continued*

lower the GFR, the higher the [Cr]s, and the greater the tubular secretion of creatinine. With GFR <40 ml/min/1.73 m², the Ccr averages 1.5 times more than the true value for GFR as measured by inulin clearance.

(2) *Ccr*—Another problem related to the use of Ccr to estimate GFR is that of collection of reliable timed-urine samples. The coefficient of variation for Ccr in a routine clinical setting is as high as 27 per cent. However, Ccr is commonly used for estimation of GFR because it is more convenient, less costly, and less invasive than more accurate methods. The normal range for Ccr in a clinical setting is from 80 to 150 ml/min/1.73 m². If the Ccr is below 80 ml/min/1.73 m², GFR should be estimated using a more accurate method.

(3) *Serum creatinine ([Cr]s)*—Creatinine, a metabolic end product, is formed from nonenzymatic degradation of creatine in muscle. This occurs at an essentially constant rate, so the entry of creatinine into serum is proportional to muscle mass. Creatinine is also added to body fluids by ingestion of meat, fish, or fowl, which contain preformed creatinine and creatinine precursors. Creatinine is not metabolized and is excreted exclusively by the kidneys. In the fasting state, with a fixed rate of entry of creatinine into body fluids (proportional to muscle mass), [Cr]s depends on renal excretion and serves as an index of GFR.

  (i) *[Cr]s*—This is the most widely used parameter for evaluation of kidney function in clinical medicine, mainly because of convenience and low cost. The laboratory methods used to measure [Cr]s are such that the physician should know the range of normal [Cr]s levels as determined by the local laboratory.

  (ii) *[Cr]s*—The variation of [Cr]s with muscle

mass as well as GFR results in a normal range of values based on age (see Table 236–1). The [Cr]s levels shown in the table are a good guide to the values to be expected at various ages in persons of essentially normal body morphology (i.e., no decrease in muscle mass, as occurs with myelodysplasia or wasting diseases, nor excessive muscle mass, as in some weight lifters and others).

2. *Renal tubular function*—Serum electrolyte concentrations and acid-base status are useful for detecting abnormalities in renal tubular function in the absence of extrarenal losses of water and solute, metabolic disorders such as diabetes mellitus, and pulmonary disorders altering carbon dioxide excretion.

  a. *Hypernatremia and hyperchloremia*—Diabetes insipidus

  b. *Hyperchloremic metabolic acidosis with a normal anion gap*—Renal tubular acidosis (RTA)

  (1) *Normokalemic or hypokalemic*—Proximal RTA and distal RTA, except type IV

  (2) *Hyperkalemic*—Type IV distal RTA

  c. *Hypophosphatemia*—Nutritional rickets, vitamin D–dependent rickets, familial hypophosphatemia

  d. *Hyperchloremic metabolic acidosis with a normal anion gap, hypokalemia, and hypophosphatemia*—Fanconi syndrome

  e. *Hypokalemic, hypochloremic metabolic alkalosis*—Bartter syndrome, renal artery stenosis.

B **Bibliography**

Chantler C, Barratt TM: Laboratory evaluation. *In* Holliday MA, Barratt TM, Vermer RL (eds): Pediatric Nephrology, 2nd ed. Baltimore, Williams & Wilkins, 1987, pp 286–287.

Kasiske BL, Keane WF: Laboratory assessment of renal disease: Clearance, urinalysis and renal biopsy. *In* Brenner BM (ed): The Kidney, 5th ed, vol 2. Philadelphia, WB Saunders, 1996, pp 1140–1143.

237 Symptoms of Growth Disorders

Definition

Idiopathic short stature (ISS) is defined as the presence of significant growth failure in childhood without a definable etiology. Short stature is considered significant if a child is below the 3rd percentile for age (-2 standard deviations [SD]) when compared with appropriate normal standards *and* consistently has a growth rate less than the 25th percentile for age.

Etiology

ISS is by definition a diagnosis of exclusion. Thus, these are children with significant growth failure who do *not* have any evidence of systemic disease, malnutrition, or hypothyroidism. In addition, the presence of classic growth hormone deficiency must be carefully sought for and excluded.

Epidemiology

Although it might be thought that as many as 3 per cent of the childhood population might be candidates for the designation of ISS, in practice the number is much smaller than this because most short children do not have a consistently low growth rate. Thus, accurate longitudinal growth measurements over at least 12 months are an absolute necessity before a short child is designated as having ISS.

Pathophysiology

1. The control of growth depends on a complex interaction of many factors including genetic, nutritional, and humoral. The genetic heritage of a child is extremely important in determining the growth rate and growth potential. The mid-parental height provides a convenient estimate of the genetic potential for growth. Nutrition plays a crucial role in growth, and without adequate nutrition the genetic and humoral factors that control growth are ineffective. The humoral factors include thyroid hormones, gonadal hormones, and the growth hormone/insulin-like growth factor (GH/IGF) axis.
2. The presence of an adequate level of thyroid hormones is an absolute prerequisite for growth, and is demonstrated by the almost total failure of linear growth in patients with severe untreated congenital or acquired hypothyroidism.
3. Gonadal steroids are important mainly at the time of puberty, and play only a minimal role in the control of growth between birth and the onset of sexual development.
4. The GH/IGF axis plays an extremely important role in the control of growth beyond infancy. The GH/IGF axis includes not only GH but also the entire mechanism of GH secretion and action. Thus in addition to obvious undersecretion of GH, subtle defects in the neural control of GH releasing hormone (GHRH) and somatostatin, the signal transduction of the GH receptor, IGF-1 secretion

and action can all play a role in the etiology of significant growth failure in childhood.

Clinical Findings

1. The patient with ISS has:
   a. Significant short stature, with a height less than the 3rd percentile for age.
   b. A consistently low rate of growth, usually less than the 25th percentile for age.
   c. *No* evidence for malnutrition, significant systemic disease, or hypothyroidism.
   d. Normal GH peak levels after standard provocative testing by the generally accepted criteria of >10 ng/ml.
2. With the exception of the normal GH peak values, these patients may be clinically indistinguishable from patients with GH deficiency.
3. No features of the history or physical examination are reliably useful in predicting which patient with growth failure will be found to have ISS.
4. On the other hand, the history and physical examination can be very useful in leading to the positive diagnosis of specific disease leading to growth failure.
   a. It is important to examine the patient carefully for signs of malnutrition, systemic disease, and hypothyroidism.
   b. A birth history is important, because there is an association between an infant inappropriately small for fetal age and certain syndromes of short stature, and because of the link between problems in the perinatal period and idiopathic hypopituitarism.
   c. Clues to the existence of genetic diseases such as Turner syndrome and chondrodystrophies should be carefully sought. In addition to a careful measurement of length or standing height, every child with short stature should have a sitting height or an upper/lower segment ratio determined, should have a measurement of the span, and should be examined for asymmetry.

Laboratory Findings

1. Laboratory investigation should be conducted in patients with severe growth failure to detect any underlying systemic disease. These tests include serum analyses for CO_2, blood urea nitrogen (BUN) or creatine as a determination of renal acidification and function, an erythrocyte sedimentation rate (ESR) to screen for inflammatory diseases, and others as clinically indicated.
2. Hypothyroidism can present clinically as growth failure without other obvious clinical signs or symptoms.

Therefore, it is important to chemically assess thyroid function in every child with significant growth failure. This includes thyroid-stimulating hormone (TSH), T_4, and/or free T_4 levels.

3. Turner syndrome is a relatively common cause of short stature, and many of these patients do not have any clear manifestations of the Turner phenotype other than growth failure. Therefore, *any* girl with unexplained significant short stature should have her chromosomal karyotype determined. Chromosomes should also be determined in children with growth failure and major or minor anomalies, irrespective of gender.

4. Assessment of the function of the GH/IGF axis is a crucial part of the work-up of any case of significant short stature not due to malnutrition, systemic disease, hypothyroidism, or genetic disorder.

a. The measurement of IGF-1 and insulin-like growth factor binding protein (IGFBP)-3 has proven to be a useful screen for abnormalities of the GH/IGF axis. Almost all children with classic growth hormone deficiency have low (< -1 SD for age) levels of IGF-1 and IGFBP-3. Patients with ISS may also have low levels of IGF-1 and IGFBP-3, although on the average not as low as those found in classic growth hormone deficiency.

b. Measurement of GH binding protein and basal GH may be useful when GH insensitivity syndrome (GHIS) is suspected.

c. GH provocative testing (or determination of GH endogenous secretion) is often necessary to differentiate between the diagnoses of ISS and classic GH deficiency.

d. At this time, a peak GH level of <10 ng/ml on two or more provocative tests of GH release is considered diagnostic of GH deficiency, and peak levels above that are consistent with the diagnosis of ISS. The variability in GH assays and GH response to stimulation makes this cut-off level of GH less definitive than might be thought.

Radiographic Changes

1. The determination of bone age can be a useful adjunct test. The bone age of children with ISS is frequently significantly delayed. In addition, the bone age can be used to predict the final height of children with significant short stature.

2. In patients in whom classic GH deficiency is strongly suspected, magnetic resonance imaging (MRI) may be useful to detect abnormalities of the pituitary gland or hypothalamus consistent with the diagnosis, or tumors of the central nervous system (CNS) leading to GH deficiency. MRI studies of the head are not necessary in ISS.

Treatment

1. ISS is by definition a diagnosis of exclusion, and no definitive therapy has become generally accepted. Some experts believe that many cases of ISS may have subtle defects in the GH/IGF axis, even though they do not fulfill the classic criteria for GH deficiency or GHIS.

2. A variety of studies have been conducted on the use of GH therapy for patients with ISS. Most studies have found a short-term increase in growth rates with GH treatment. However, the long-term results have been variable.

3. A collaborative U.S. study of 121 patients with ISS treated for up to 9 years with GH found an increase in expected adult height of 8.8 cm (95 per cent confidence limits 5.0 to 12.7) for boys and 7.4 cm (95 per cent confidence limits 3.7 to 11.1) for girls when compared with untreated historical control ISS patients. However, the mean final height of these patients was still 0.8 SD less than their expected target heights. Other reports of final height results have been less optimistic. The use of GH treatment for ISS is not yet generally accepted.

Prevention

There does not appear to be any way to prevent ISS.

Bibliography

Hintz RL: Disorders of growth. *In* Lee P, Sanfilipo J (eds): Pediatric and Adolescent Gynecology. Philadelphia, WB Saunders, 1993, pp 34–43.

Hintz RL, Attie KM, Johanson AJ, et al: Near final height in GH-treated short children without classical GH deficiency. Pediatr Res 1995;37:A530.

Hopwood NJ, Hintz RL, Gertner JM, et al: Growth response of non-growth hormone deficient children with marked short stature during three years of growth hormone therapy. J Pediatr 1993;123:215–22.

Loche S, Cambiaso P, Setzu S, et al: Final height after growth hormone therapy in non-growth hormone deficient children with short stature. J Pediatr 1994;125:196–200.

Rosenfeld, RG, Albertsson-Wikland K, Cassorla F, et al: Diagnostic controversy: The diagnosis of childhood growth hormone deficiency revisited. J Clin Endocrinol Metab 1995;80:1532–1540.

Zadik Z, Chalew S, Zung A, et al: Effect of long-term growth hormone therapy of bone age and pubertal maturation in boys with and without classic growth hormone deficiency. J Pediatr 1994;126:189–95.

Symptom **Tall Stature**

Jennifer Bell

Definition

Height more than 3 standard deviations above the mean height for age and sex.

Etiology

Tall stature is usually due to either familial tall stature or to a constitutional pattern of rapid growth and early puberty with resultant adult size in the normal range. These two benign variations of normal growth must be distinguished from pathologic conditions in which tall stature is just one of many signs and symptoms of disease.

Differential Diagnosis

1. Physiologic causes

a. Familial tall stature

(1) Definition: Tall stature in an otherwise physically normal child, with family history of adults more than 3 SD above the mean.

(2) Clinical picture

(a) Size normal at birth with tall stature established usually in first 18 months of life. Growth curve follows a normal pattern, above but paralleling the normal growth curves, without increasing deviation from the mean.

(b) Onset of puberty at normal age. Predicted adult height 3 SD or more above mean adult heights.

(3) Laboratory tests

(a) Bone age normal for chronological age.

(b) Random serum GH level <10 ng/ml; IGF-1 normal; serum GH suppresses to <5 ng/ml after glucose load.

b. Constitutional acceleration of growth and development

(1) Definition: Tall stature in an otherwise physically normal child, with a family history of adults of normal stature and early puberty.

(2) Clinical picture

(a) Size normal at birth with increased linear growth from early childhood. Growth curve, as in familial tall stature, follows a normal pattern above but paralleling normal growth curve.

(b) Onset of puberty at younger range of normal. Growth ceases early. Adult stature normal.

(3) Laboratory tests

(a) Bone age advanced for chronological age.

(b) Growth hormone parameters normal [see 1. a. (3) (b)].

(4) Childhood *exogenous obesity* is often associated with an identical pattern of increased linear growth and advanced skeletal maturation. Puberty is early and adult height normal.

2. Pathologic conditions associated with tall stature

a. Endocrine disorders

(1) Pituitary gigantism

(a) A rare condition caused by the autonomous secretion of excessive growth hormone by a pituitary adenoma or because of hyperplasia of GH-producing cells of the pituitary gland.

(b) Growth pattern is one of rapidly accelerated growth with increasing deviation from mean heights for child's age and sex. The occurrence is very rare before second decade. Acromegaloid features are present even in childhood, for example, frontal bossing, broad hands and feet with thickened heel pads, coarse trabeculations of distal phalangeal bones on x-ray.

(c) Random serum GH elevated (>10 ng/ml) and not suppressible below 5 ng/ml with oral glucose load. IGF-1 consistently elevated. Neuroradiologic imaging demonstrates pituitary enlargement and/or adenoma.

(2) Precocious puberty

(a) Definition: The occurrence of sexual development at an inappropriately early age (younger than 8 years old in girls, 10 years old in boys). The etiology, pathogenesis, diagnosis and treatment of precocious puberty are discussed elsewhere.

(b) Linear growth accelerated (pubertal growth spurt) in conjunction with appearance of secondary sexual characteristics. Heights deviate upward from mean.

(c) Bone age (BA) is advanced beyond 2 SD. BA advances more rapidly than the child grows and there is a net loss of growth potential. Predicted adult height is thus limited despite tall stature in childhood.

(d) With successful treatment of the precocious puberty, the child's growth rate normalizes and the rate of epiphyseal maturation approaches normal, allowing more time for growth to occur.

(3) Thyrotoxicosis: In addition to the usual signs and symptoms of excess thyroid hormone, childhood thyrotoxicosis results in a characteristic disturbance of the growth pattern:

(a) Linear growth is accelerated abnormally with increasing deviation of the growth curve upward, crossing percentiles.

(b) There is an equivalent advancement in bone age. Since linear growth and bone age advance at a similar pace, there is neither a gain nor a loss in growth potential. Predicted adult height is not affected.

(c) With successful treatment of the thyroid overactivity, the rate of growth and of bone maturation normalizes.

b. Genetic syndromes associated with tall stature

(1) Marfan syndrome

(a) A hereditable disorder of connective tissue, of autosomal dominant inheritance, believed due to an abnormal elastin structure in many tissues. Recent evidence confirms an abnormality in the fibrillin gene on chromosome 15q21.1.

(b) Affected children are of normal size at birth but tall stature and skeletal disproportion become more manifest with time. In full-blown syndrome the child is remarkably tall and thin with elongated limbs, fingers, and toes (arachnodactyly). Joints are lax. There are ocular abnormalities, typically ectopia lentis and severe myopia. Important cardiovascular abnormalities include prolapse and regurgitation of cardiac valves (especially mitral), and progressive aortic root dilatation, with early death due to aortic rupture or dissection.

(2) Homocysteinuria: Affected children have a marfanoid habitus but also progressive mental impairment. This is due to a biochemical defect in methionine metabolism.

(3) Congenital lipodystrophy: Overgrowth has been described but is a minor aspect of this disorder, which is characterized by severe insulin resistance, acanthosis nigricans, almost total loss of subcutaneous fat, hyperlipidemia, and fatty liver.

(4) Genetic syndromes are associated with prenatal and/or postnatal overgrowth. Associated physical findings are diagnostic:

(a) Soto syndrome (cerebral gigantism): Large birth size with excessively rapid growth in first 2–4 years. Thereafter, growth rate decelerates to normal with growth curve paralleling the 97th percentile. Characteristic facies with large cranium, frontal bossing, hypertelorism, antimongoloid slants, high arched palate, prominent jaw. Neuroradiologic studies show large ventricles without increased pressure.

(b) Beckwith-Wiedemann syndrome: Fetal and neonatal gigantism associated with omphalocele, hemihypertrophy, macroglossia, and neonatal hypoglycemia. Abnormalities in chromosome 11p15, possibly in the gene for the fetal growth factor, IGF-II. Affected children and adults are ≥ 90th percentile in height.

(c) Weaver's syndrome: Pre- and postnatal overgrowth with lengths > 97th percentile, but, in contrast to Soto syndrome, growth parallels the curve without abnormal acceleration. Face is round in infancy with large head, broad forehead, small recessed chin, and large ears. Finger pads are prominent.

Treatment

1. Girls

   a. Interventional therapy is usually sought by families of children, most often girls, with familial tall stature or constitutional acceleration of growth and development. Since in the latter condition growth is self-limited, establishing the diagnosis with a bone age x-ray and estimation of a predicted adult height within normal range is sufficient. In the former condition, however, the family and child may consider the predicted adult height excessive and wish it to be curtailed if possible for cosmetic reasons.

   b. There is a medical rationale for attempting to curtail the overgrowth associated with Marfan's syndrome and thus curtail the severe scoliosis that may develop in that condition with the adolescent growth spurt.

   c. In general, endocrinologists will consider treatment if a girl has a predicted adult height of 183 cm (6′) or greater. Since intervention carries potential risks, the family and in particular the child must be thoroughly counseled about the potential risks of therapy and the limitations of what can realistically be achieved.

   d. Predicting adult heights is difficult and estimates are at best accurate to within only about ± 5 cm (2″).

   e. The standard method of treatment is the use of supraphysiologic doses of estrogen, three to four times adult replacement doses, continued until the child's epiphyses are on the point of fusion, usually at a bone age of 15–16. The effect of this therapy is believed secondary to an associated decrease in IGF-1 levels, and an estrogen-dependent increase in the rate of epiphyseal maturation. The average length of treatment is about 2 years. Menarche occurs within 2–3 months of the start of therapy, at which point a progestational agent is administered for 10 to 12 days each month to mimic the menstrual cycle and allow renewal of the uterine endometrium.

   f. Adult height is reduced by an average 2–3″, although as much as 4–5″ reduction has been reported with initiation of therapy before puberty.

   g. Short-term side effects are surprisingly few: occasional nausea and vomiting at onset of therapy; pigmentation of the areolae and significant weight gain, both reversing when therapy is discontinued. There is a low incidence of ovarian cysts. Headaches and hypertension severe enough to require discontinuation of therapy are rare, as is thromboembolism.

   h. Long-term side effects: although there is real concern about a potential disruption of the hypothalamic-pituitary-ovarian axis as a consequence of estrogen suppression, menses are established usually within 2 months after discontinuing therapy, although occasionally amenorrhea has been reported for as long as 13 months. There is no evidence of infertility, and in those births reported in the literature the offspring have been normal. The question of whether, with increasing age, treated women will have an increased incidence of breast or uterine cancer is as yet unanswered.

2. Boys

   a. The treatment of boys for tall stature has not been reported in the United States. In the European literature, treatment is generally considered for height predictions above 195 cm (6′5″).

   b. The usual treatment is with long-acting testosterone esters in a dose of 500 mg intramuscularly every 2 to 3 weeks, a dose about four to five times the adult daily testosterone production rate.

   c. Adult height is reduced on average about 2″. Earlier therapy is more effective.

   d. Side effects: During therapy a decrease in testicular volume is seen that may take as long as 5.9 years to restore. A similar period of time has been reported before normalization of sperm counts.

Bibliography

Blizzard RM, Johanson A: Disorders of growth. *In* Kappy MS, Blizzard RM, Migeon, CJ (eds): Wilkins Diagnosis and Treatment of Endocrine Diseases in Childhood and Adolescence, 4th ed. Springfield, IL, Charles C Thomas, 1994, pp 424–429.

Conte FA, Grumbach MM: Estrogen use in children and adolescents: A survey. Pediatrics 1978;62:1091–1097.

Crawford JD: Treatment of tall girls with estrogen. Pediatrics 1978;62:1189–1195.

Kaplan SA: Growth and growth hormone: *In* Kaplan, SA (ed): Clinical Pediatric Endocrinology, 2nd ed. Philadelphia, WB Saunders, 1990, pp 54–57.

Zachmann M: Testosterone treatment of excessively tall boys. J Pediatr 1976;88:116–123.

238 Constitutional Short Stature

Philippe Bareille and *Richard Stanhope*

Definition

1. Height below 2 standard deviation scores (SDS)* below the mean for age without any underlying pathologic organic cause. Two SDS is the arbitrary cutoff usually used. One should notably exclude: chromosomal abnormalities, celiac disease, skeletal dysplasia, malnutrition, psychosocial deprivation, and intrauterine growth retardation. Classical endocrine assessment, if performed, should not show any hormonal abnormalities with normal growth hormone response to provocative tests.

2. This term, however, remains unclear in the literature and is also termed *idiopathic short stature* or *normal variant short stature*.

3. Encompasses two entities: *constitutional growth delay*, which may progress to constitutional delay of growth and puberty (CDGP), also termed constitutional delay of growth and development, and *familial short stature* (FSS).

   a. CDGP

      (1) Bone age is retarded by 2 or more years.

      (2) Predicted final height (based on bone age) close to target height† (based on parental height).

      (3) Will progress to delayed puberty.

      (4) Midparental height is within the normal range.

      (5) Usually a family history of growth delay.

   b. FSS

      (1) Height SDS for chronological age close to target height SDS.

      (2) Bone age is not delayed.

      (3) Puberty starts at a normal age.

      (4) Midparental height is below 2 SDS.

   Nevertheless, these two diagnoses can frequently merge into one another; notably many children with familial short stature may also have constitutional delay.

Natural History

1. Normal size and weight at birth or, in FSS, slightly below the average.

2. Gradual fall in height SDS during infancy and early childhood.

3. Between approximately age 2 years and early adolescence linear growth lies below 2 SDS but typically does not display any further decrease.

4. In CDGP, growth velocity decelerates in early adolescence due to delayed puberty. At puberty there may be incomplete catch-up with a reduced amplitude of the growth spurt.

5. In FSS, puberty and its growth acceleration occur at a normal age and these individuals grow along the same percentile.

Clinical Findings

1. Children affected by constitutional short stature are small but healthy.

2. The main consequence is psychologic distress, but this is difficult to demonstrate in controlled, prospective studies.

3. Classically, in constitutional short stature, growth velocity is normal and predicted final height is appropriate for parents' heights. However:

   a. Some children grow at a subnormal rate, and despite this fact, are considered as constitutionally short. This growth deceleration may impair final height outcome and may be confused with growth hormone (GH) insufficiency.

   b. Infancy and early childhood are characterized by relatively reduced growth velocity.

   c. In CDGP, at the normal time for puberty, growth velocity is decelerating because the pubertal growth spurt is delayed.

---

*SDS = Observed height minus average height at the subject's age/standard deviation of the average.

†Target height = Midparental height minus 6 cm in girls and plus 6 cm in boys.

Key Clinical Findings

- Short, well proportioned, and healthy

Family History

When parents are very short (below 3 SDS) one should suspect an underlying cause responsible for their stature and refer them to an adult endocrinologist.

Two disorders are notably to be excluded:

1. Isolated growth hormone deficiency. Classic associated features: Osteoporosis, overweight, early aging of the skin.
2. Skeletal dysplasia: Disproportionate between upper and lower segments and radiologic evidence of abnormal bone structure.

Pathogenesis

1. Children with constitutional short stature should be regarded as normal.
2. However, attempts have long been made to explain their short stature especially in those with subnormal growth velocity and who are thought unlikely to reach their genetic potential. The reasons responsible for their growth failure are probably multiple and have not been fully elucidated. Three main causes have been proposed:

    a. Inadequate spontaneous secretion of endogenous growth hormone.*

There may be an abnormal pattern of 24-hour GH secretion with diminished total release despite normal response to provocative tests. This disorder has been labeled *neurosecretory dysfunction* and may be causally related to CDGP. However, one should underline that there is significant overlap between the lower range of subjects with normal stature and values reported even in GH deficiency so that it is not very easy to attribute poor growth in an individual to a low 24-hour GH secretion. Study results have been contradictory and have not been able to clearly establish a correlation between 24-hour GH secretion and auxologic parameters. On the other hand, other studies have shown that the best predictors for the short-term response to GH of children with normal response to pharmacologic tests are the pretreatment growth velocity and the integrated 24 hour GH concentration. This may buttress the positive correlation found by some authors between 24-hour GH secretion and growth rate.

    b. Abnormal GH structure has also been suspected.

    c. Abnormal GH receptor (or postreceptor defect) is another putative cause of inadequate growth. Apart from the extreme situation of complete hormone insensitivity (Laron syndrome), partial GH resistance has been surmised in some children with constitutional short stature, subnormal growth rate, and relative increment in the ratio of GH concentration to insulin-like growth factor (IGF)-1 concentration. Their low serum growth hormone binding protein (GHBP) levels may arouse the suspicion of a defect in the extracellular domain of the GH receptor.*

Treatment

1. *Growth hormone* is currently the main possible growth-promoting therapy. GH treatment has been considered in children with CSS since an unlimited supply has become available due to DNA recombinant technology. *This should concern only a small percentage of children with CSS.* Hitherto, trials have reported short-term growth enhancement in most children with CSS treated with GH. This initial beneficial effect may be sustained several years but whether this treatment improves final stature is still unknown. Preliminary data indicate that these children do not exceed their genetic target height at the standard dosage. This is partly caused by excessive bone age advancement due to accelerated pubertal development. No characteristics appear to be able to predict reliably the short- and long-term response. The decision of GH treatment ought to be left to the pediatric endocrinologist and should be part of a controlled trial.
2. *Alternative therapies* (see Chapter 243, on CDGP)

Key Points

- The diagnosis of CSS is made after exclusion of other causes of short stature.
- Growth velocity is an essential parameter to be monitored carefully. Subnormal growth velocity should point to the suspicion of an alternate diagnosis and requires investigation.
- Reassurance is all that is usually required. Treatment should be considered only when the diagnosis is uncertain.

Bibliography

Costin G, Kaufman FR, Brasell JA: Growth hormone secretory dynamics in subjects with normal stature. J Pediatr 1989; 115:537–544.

Goddard AD, Covello R, Luoh SM, et al: Mutations of the growth hormone receptor in children with idiopathic short stature. N Engl J Med 1995;333:1093–1098.

Hindmarsh P, Smith PJ, Brook CGD, Matthews DR. The relation-

---

*There would be a wide *spectrum of GH secretion* extending from the severe deficiency, which is defined by failure to secrete GH in response to standard provocative stimuli, to the normal state. In the middle a group of subjects in spite of a normal response to pharmacologic tests do not produce sufficient quantities of GH under physiologic conditions as assessed by a reduced 24-hour spontaneous secretion (in terms of pulse frequency, amplitude, and integrated concentration) of GH.

*Human growth hormone receptor (GHR) has been purified, cloned, and expressed (Nature 1987;330:537–543). In man, the GHBP corresponds to the extracellular domain of the GHR and is produced by proteolytic cleavage. Measurements of serum concentrations of GHBP provide a faithful indicator of extracellular GHR function and/or structure. Thus, in Laron syndrome when mutations are in the extracellular domain of GHR (which has hitherto been the vast majority of cases), GHBP is very low or undetectable.

ship between height velocity and growth hormone secretion in short prepubertal children. Clin Endocrinol 1987;27:581–591.

Wider indications for treatment with biosynthetic human growth hormone in children. Clin Endocrinol 1991;34:417–427.

Loche S, Cambiaso P, Setzu S, et al. Final height after growth

hormone therapy in non growth hormone deficient children with short stature. J Pediatr 1994;125:196–200.

Moore KC, Donaldson DL, Ideus PL, et al. Clinical diagnoses of children with extremely short stature and their response to growth hormone. J Pediatr 1993;122:687–692.

239 Familial Short Stature

Philippe Bareille, Finella Craig, and *Richard Stanhope*

Definition

Familial short stature is a term used to define short children who:

1. Are small for the average population (below 2 SDS).
2. Are of appropriate stature for their parents' height.
3. Are growing at a normal rate (linear growth velocity > 10th percentile).
4. Have bone age that is not delayed.
5. Are healthy without any known disease.
6. Have not been subject to intrauterine growth retardation.

Nevertheless, the defined limits are unclear and only very few children fulfill all these criteria. One should stress that many children with familial short stature also have delayed bone age. Thereby, familial short stature and constitutional delay of growth are often interwoven.

Pathophysiology

(see also Chapter 238 on constitutional short stature)

1. This condition is probably just a variant of normality. However, environmental factors may also play a role.
2. Progress in molecular biology may shed light on the mechanisms controlling growth in the future. New insights have already been gained over the recent years pointing to the suspicion of genetic defects responsible for short stature of some children hitherto considered as affected by idiopathic short stature. Preliminary data for example indicate that some of these children have partial insensitivity to growth hormone (GH) due to mutations in the GH receptor gene. However we believe that suspicion of an underlying molecular defect should only be aroused for very short children (height < 3 SDS), for those with subnormal growth velocity, or for those with very short parents.

Clinical Findings

1. Normal size at birth (usually below the average but within the normal range).
2. Gradual growth deceleration between 3 months and 2 years of age.
3. Subsequently normal growth rate for size until attainment of final stature.
4. Puberty usually occurs at a normal age.

5. In practice the real picture is often not as typical as mentioned above because familial short stature is unlikely to represent a homogeneous group. Notably many of these children have also associated a certain degree of constitutional delay in growth and development. Some of these children, despite normal investigations, may present with subnormal growth velocity and not reach their target height. The diagnosis of familial short stature should therefore be reconsidered with time.
6. One in three normal short children at age 7 years becomes a short adult (below 5th percentile).

Laboratory Investigation

1. When the clinical picture is typical, no investigations are required (these may only fuel anxiety).
2. When should one consider investigating a child who is healthy with apparent familial short stature?
   a. Subnormal growth velocity.
   b. Very short parents ought to be investigated to exclude familial GH deficiency, GH resistance, insulin-like growth factor (IGF)-1 resistance as well as skeletal dysplasias and other causes of inherited short stature.

Treatment

1. Once the diagnosis has been established, these children should be considered as normal and thereby no treatment should be proposed.
2. Since the advent of unlimited availability of growth hormone, growth hormone treatment has been attempted in children with familial short stature. Such treatment regimens have used pharmacologic doses of growth hormone of 30–40 IU/m^2/week (0.3 mg/kg/week) as a daily subcutaneous injection. Despite the observation of short-term enhancement of growth, no data so far have documented significant increase of final height above target height. It is still unclear whether growth hormone treatment is a panacea for children with familial short stature.
3. Arresting and delaying puberty by using a GnRH analogue (which may be combined with growth hormone treatment) has not proved to increase final height. Delaying puberty therapeutically may have its own psychologic sequelae greater than those associated with short stature.

Key Points

- Height SD score below 2 SDS.
- Height SD score close to target height SD score.
- Normal growth velocity.
- Bone age typically not retarded.
- Frequent overlap with constitutional delay of growth.
- No treatment has been proven to increase final stature.

Bibliography

Greco L, Power C, Peckham C: Adult outcome of normal children who are short or underweight at 7 years. Br Med J 1995; 310:697–700.

Guidelines for the use of growth hormone in children with short stature. A report by the Drug and Therapeutics Committee of the Lawson Wilkins Pediatric Endocrine Society. J Pediatr 1995;127:857–867.

Laron Z: Short stature due to genetic defects affecting growth hormone activity. N Engl J Med 1996;334:463–465.

Lifshitz F, Cervantes CD: Short stature. *In* Lifshitz F (ed): Pediatric Endocrinology, 3rd ed. New York, Marcel Dekker, 1996, pp 1–19.

240 Growth Hormone Resistance Syndromes

Ron G. Rosenfeld

Definition

Growth hormone resistance syndromes are a clinical phenotype resulting from generalized resistance (insensitivity) to growth hormone (GH) action.

Etiology

Classification of GH resistance syndromes:

1. Primary GH resistance syndromes (Laron syndrome; hereditary/congenital defects)
   a. GH receptor deficiency. Heterozygosity for some mutations of the GH receptor may present as milder cases of GH resistance.
   b. Abnormalities of GH signal transduction
   c. Primary defects of synthesis of insulin-like growth factor (IGF)-1
2. Secondary GH resistance (acquired conditions; sometimes transient)
   a. Circulating antibodies to GH that inhibit GH action
   b. Antibodies to the GH receptor
   c. GH resistance caused by malnutrition
   d. GH resistance caused by liver disease
   e. Other conditions

Laron syndrome represents the primary hereditary form of GH resistance. It results from abnormalities of the gene for the GH receptor, involving either gene deletions or point mutations of portions of the gene encoding the extracellular, transmembrane, or intracellular domains of the GH receptor. The disorder is transmitted in an autosomal recessive manner.

Epidemiology

Approximately 200 cases of Laron syndrome have been reported to date. Although initial cases involved Oriental Jews from Israel and the Middle East, patients have now been identified throughout the world. The largest single concentration of patients has been identified in southern Ecuador. Marked genetic heterogeneity has been reported, with multiple gene deletions and mutations described.

Pathophysiology

1. The GH receptor belongs to a family of transmembrane receptors, including those for prolactin, interleukins, erythropoietin, granulocyte-macrophage colony-stimulating factor, and interferon. After binding a molecule of GH to its extracellular domain, the GH receptor dimerizes and then initiates a still poorly defined signal transduction pathway.
2. Under normal conditions, the extracellular domain of the GH receptor is proteolytically cleaved and circulates as a GH binding protein (GHBP), providing a ready means for assaying the cellular GH receptor.
3. Virtually all abnormalities of the GH receptor discovered to date have involved the ability of the GH receptor to bind GH. Such abnormalities are, typically, reflected in low serum GHBP concentrations. One mutation of the extracellular domain of the receptor has been described that, while not affecting the binding of GH, prevents normal dimerization of the GH receptor. A pedigree has also been identified where a mutation in a portion of the gene encoding the transmembrane domain results in loss of this domain and truncation of the receptor. In these two situations, circulating GHBP concentrations have been normal, or even elevated.

Clinical Findings

1. Although patients have near-normal birth weight and length, postnatal growth failure is profound and is usually evident in the first months of life. Body segments and arm span are normal for skeletal age.
2. Puberty may be delayed 3 to 7 years but is otherwise normal, with apparently normal fertility.
3. The forehead is prominent, with a hypoplastic nasal

bridge and shallow orbits. Hair is sparse before age 7 years. Scleras are blue. Dentition is delayed.

4. Hypoglycemia may occur in infancy. Muscular hypoplasia and hypotonia are frequent during infancy, with delayed gross motor milestones. Intelligence is normal, unless there are intellectual consequences of hypoglycemia. Voices are high-pitched, reflecting laryngeal hypoplasia.

Key Clinical Findings

- Profound postnatal growth failure
- Immature facies
- Prominent forehead; flattened nasal bridge

Laboratory Findings

1. Serum GH concentrations (both basal and stimulated) are generally markedly elevated in children but may be normal in adults.
2. Serum concentrations of the GH-dependent proteins IGF-1, IGF binding protein (IGFBP)-3, and the acid-labile subunit (ALS) of IGFBP-3 are markedly reduced.
3. No or minimal rise in serum IGF-1 or IGFBP-3 is observed following GH administration.
4. Serum concentrations of GHBP are, typically, reduced, but they may be normal or even elevated when mutations affect receptor dimerization or are in portions of the gene encoding the transmembrane or intracellular domains of the GH receptor.
5. Fasting serum glucose concentrations may be reduced.

Key Laboratory Findings

- Elevated basal and stimulated serum GH concentrations
- Low IGF-1, IGFBP-3, ALS

Radiographic Changes

1. Skeletal maturation (bone age) is, generally, markedly delayed.
2. Abnormal craniofacial proportions and delayed closure of the fontanelles are evident radiologically.

Treatment

1. Therapy with GH is ineffective, although it may be possible that in some cases with "mild" defects of the GH receptor, high doses of GH might overcome the resistant state.
2. Treatment with IGF-1, at a dose of 80–120 μg/kg twice daily, has proven effective in stimulating short-term growth. Therapy may be limited, however, by the failure of IGF-1 treatment to stimulate a rise in serum IGFBP-3 concentrations, resulting in persistently abnormal IGF-1 pharmacokinetics.
3. It is not yet clear whether IGF-1 therapy will be able to lead to sustained normalization of growth velocity and attainment of normal adult height.

Key Treatment

- IGF-1 gives short-term growth, with ultimate effect uncertain.

Prevention

Laron syndrome is transmitted as an autosomal recessive trait, and genetic counseling should be available to known carriers of this disorder. In genetically homogeneous areas (such as southern Ecuador), prenatal diagnosis may be possible.

Bibliography

Laron Z, Pertzelan A, Mannheimer S: Genetic pituitary dwarfism with high serum concentration of growth hormone. A new inborn error of metabolism? Isr J Med Sci 1966;2:152–155.

Rosenfeld RG, Rosenbloom AL, Guevara-Aguirre J: Growth hormone (GH) insensitivity due to primary GH receptor deficiency. Endocr Rev 1994;15:369–390.

Guevara-Aguirre J, Vasconez O, Martinez V, et al: A randomized, double-blind, placebo-controlled trial on safety and efficacy of recombinant human insulin-like growth factor-I in children with growth hormone receptor deficiency. J Clin Endocrinol Metab 1995;80:1393–1398.

Wilson KF, Fielder PJ, Guevara-Aguirre J, et al: Long-term effects of insulin-like growth factor (IGF)-I treatment on serum IGFs and IGF binding proteins in adolescent patients with growth hormone receptor deficiency. Clin Endocrinol 1995;42:399–407.

241 Diabetes Insipidus

Joseph A. Majzoub

Etiology

1. Central (hypothalamic, neurogenic, or vasopressin-sensitive) diabetes insipidus
   a. Disorders of vasopressin gene structure
   b. Surgical or accidental trauma to vasopressin neurons
   c. Congenital anatomic hypothalamic or pituitary defects
   d. Neoplastic, infiltrative, autoimmune, and infectious diseases affecting vasopressin neurons or fiber tracts
   e. No apparent etiology in approximately 10 per cent of children with central diabetes insipidus
   f. Boys and girls are equally affected
2. Nephrogenic diabetes insipidus
   a. X-linked mutations in the renal (V2) vasopressin receptor, found almost exclusively in males
   b. Drugs such as lithium chloride or demeclocycline
   c. Autosomal recessive mutations in the renal water channel, aquaporin-2
   d. Pharmacologic causes of nephrogenic diabetes insipidus are more common but less severe than genetic forms of the disease.

Pathophysiology

1. Central diabetes insipidus
   a. Diabetes insipidus due to vasopressin deficiency is known as central diabetes insipidus.[5]
   b. Infiltrative lesions such as histiocytosis, granulomatous meningitis, and leukemia must destroy over 90 per cent of vasopressin neurons in the hypothalamic paraventricular and supraoptic nuclei to cause diabetes insipidus. Lymphocytic hypophysitis, affecting both anterior and posterior pituitary function, may cause diabetes insipidus.
   c. Germinomas, because of their location, may as very small tumors cause the disease, several years before they are detectable by magnetic resonance imaging (MRI).
   d. Head trauma can cause diabetes insipidus by disruption of the hypothalamo–posterior pituitary axonal tracts.
   e. A familial form of autosomal dominant central diabetes insipidus has recently been described,[3] with several different families having unique point mutations in the gene that encodes the vasopressin precursor. Patients are born with normal vasopressin function and develop full diabetes insipidus by the middle of the first decade of life.
   f. Vasopressin deficiency is also found in Wolfram's, or DIDMOAD syndrome, consisting of *d*iabetes *i*nsipidus, *d*iabetes *m*ellitus, *o*ptic *a*trophy, and *d*eafness. The gene for this syndrome complex has been localized to human chromosome 4p by polymorphic linkage analysis.
   g. The most common cause of central diabetes insipidus is the neurosurgical destruction of vasopressin neurons following pituitary-hypothalamic surgery.
      (1) Lesions closer to the hypothalamus will cause greater permanent loss of vasopressin secretion.
      (2) "Triple phase" response (Fig. 241–1): following surgery, an initial phase of transient diabetes insipidus is seen, lasting 1/2 to 2 days, and possibly due to edema in the area interfering with normal vasopressin secretion. If significant vasopressin cell destruction has occurred, this is often followed by a second phase of the syndrome of inappropriate vasopressin (antidiuretic hormone) release (SIADH), which may last up to 10 days, and is due to the unregulated release of vasopressin by dying neurons. A third phase of permanent diabetes insipidus may follow if more than 90 per cent of vasopressin cells were destroyed. Usually, a marked degree of SIADH in the second phase portends significant permanent diabetes insipidus in the final phase of this response.
2. Nephrogenic diabetes insipidus
   a. Diabetes insipidus due to the inability of the kidney to respond normally to vasopressin is known as nephrogenic diabetes insipidus.[1]
   b. Congenital, X-linked nephrogenic diabetes insipidus is caused by mutations in the V2 vasopressin receptor. Over 16 mutations have been identified.
   c. Mutations in the renal water channel, aquaporin-2, lead to autosomal recessive nephrogenic diabetes insipidus.
   d. Nephrogenic diabetes insipidus may be caused by drugs such as lithium and demeclocycline, as well as by hypercalcemia and hypokalemia, all of which are thought to interfere with vasopressin-stimulated cyclic adenosine monophosphate (AMP) generation or action.[2]
   e. Osmotic diuresis due to glycosuria in diabetes mellitus, or to sodium excretion with diuretic therapy, will interfere with renal water conservation.
   f. Primary polydypsia can result in secondary nephrogenic diabetes insipidus because the chronic excretion of a dilute urine lowers the osmolality of the hypertonic renal interstitium, thus decreasing renal concentrating ability.

Clinical Findings

1. Pathologic polyuria or polydipsia, exceeding 1.5 L/m² must be documented.

Figure 241–1 Diabetes insipidus following neurosurgery. Vasopressin neurons terminate at different levels of the posterior pituitary. Depending on the level of neurosurgical damage, different numbers of vasopressin neurons will be permanently damaged. The three phases of the "triple phase" response to neural damage are noted within the box.

Hypothalamus

Posterior Pituitary

Anterior Pituitary

Phase	Condition	Cause	Duration
1st	DI	Edema	0.5-2d
2nd	SIADH	Necrosis	1-10d
3rd	DI	Cell Loss	Permanent

2. One should determine whether there is a psychosocial reason for either polyuria or polydipsia. Has either polyuria or polydipsia interfered with normal activities? Is nocturia or enuresis present? If so, does the patient also drink following nocturnal awakening? Does the history (including longitudinal growth data) or physical examination suggest other deficient or excessive endocrine secretion? Does the history or physical examination suggest an intracranial neoplasm?

3. Patients with central diabetes insipidus often crave very cold beverages.

4. In the inpatient, postneurosurgical setting, central diabetes insipidus is likely if hyperosmolality (serum osmolality over 300 mOsm/kg) is associated with urine osmolality lower than serum osmolality. One must beware of intraoperative fluid expansion with subsequent hypo-osmolar polyuria masquerading as diabetes insipidus.

5. Nephrogenic diabetes insipidus must be suspected when polyuria and polydipsia are present in patients treated with lithium chloride, or in infant males with a family history of the disease. Such males often present during the first few months of life with failure to gain weight adequately.

Key Clinical Findings

- Polyuria
- Polydipsia
- Dehydration

Laboratory Findings

1. In the outpatient setting, the following should be obtained in a patient suspected of having diabetes insipidus: serum osmolality; levels of sodium, potassium, glucose, calcium, and blood urea nitrogen (BUN); and urinalysis, including measurement of urine osmolality, specific gravity, and glucose concentration.

2. Serum osmolality greater than 300 mOsm/kg, with urine osmolality less than 300 mOsm/kg, makes the diagnosis of diabetes insipidus likely. If serum osmolality is less than 270 mOsm/kg, or urine osmolality is greater than 600 mOsm/kg, or if the intake/output report clearly discloses less than 1 L/m²/24 hours, the diagnosis of diabetes insipidus is unlikely.

3. If upon initial screening, the patient has a serum osmolality less than 300 mOsm/kg, but the intake/output record at home suggests significant polyuria and polydipsia that cannot be attributed to primary polydipsia (i.e., the serum osmolality is greater than 270 mOsm/kg), the patient should undergo a water deprivation test to establish a diagnosis of diabetes insipidus and to differentiate central from nephrogenic causes.

4. After a maximally tolerated fast (based upon the outpatient history), the patient is admitted to the outpatient testing center in the early morning of a day when an 8- to 10-hour test can be carried out, and is deprived of water. The physical signs and biochemical parameters shown in the accompanying protocol are measured.

   a. If at any time during the test, the urine osmolality exceeds 1000 mOsm/kg, or 600 mOsm/kg and is stable over 1 hour, the patient does not have diabetes insipidus.

   b. If at any time the serum osmolality exceeds 300 mOsm/kg and the urine osmolality is less than 600 mOsm/kg, the patient has diabetes insipidus.

   c. If the serum osmolality is less than 300 mOsm/kg and the urine osmolality is less than 600 mOsm/kg, the test should be continued unless vital signs disclose hypovolemia. A common error is to stop a test too soon, based on the amount of body weight lost, before either urine osmolality has plateaued above 600 mOsm/kg or a serum osmolality above 300 mOsm/kg has been achieved.

d. If the diagnosis of diabetes insipidus is made, aqueous vasopressin (Pitressin), 1 U/m², should be given subcutaneously. If the patient has central diabetes insipidus, urine volume should fall and osmolality should at least double during the next hour, compared with the value prior to vasopressin therapy. If the patient fails to concentrate urine during water deprivation, and there is less than a twofold rise in urine osmolality following Pitressin administration, the patient probably has nephrogenic diabetes insipidus.

Key Laboratory Findings

- Low osmolality and specific gravity of urine
- Hypernatremia, hyperchloremia

Radiographic Findings

1. Central diabetes insipidus due to loss of hypothalamic vasopressin neurons or interruption of their tracts by infiltrative lesions such as histiocytosis, or large tumors such as craniopharyngiomas, is usually evident in MRI of the hypothalamic-pituitary region. However, as noted, MRI may not detect small germinomas for several years following the onset of symptomatic diabetes insipidus. For this reason, children with presumed idiopathic central diabetes insipidus should have an annual MRI examination.

2. In both central and nephrogenic diabetes insipidus, the MRI demonstrates loss of the normal T1-weighted "bright spot" in the region of the posterior pituitary following administration of gadolinium, due to loss of vasopressin/neurophysin in this region. This loss is due to inadequate delivery of vasopressin to the posterior pituitary in central disease, and to excessive release from the gland in nephrogenic disease.

3. Patients with nephrogenic disease often display dilated renal calyces, ureters, and bladder, reflecting the large volume of urine flow in these patients due to the difficult long-term management of nephrogenic diabetes insipidus.

Treatment

1. Central diabetes insipidus

   a. In the outpatient setting, treatment should begin with either oral or intranasal DDAVP (desmopressin).

      (1) Oral DDAVP, 25 μg, should be started at bedtime, increasing the dose to the lowest amount which gives an antidiuretic effect (usually 100 to 200 μg). Oral DDAVP may require 30 to 60 minutes before the onset of action. If the dose is effective, but has too short a duration, a second, morning dose should be added. Patients should escape from the antidiuretic effect for at least 1 hour before the next dose, to ensure that any excessive water will be excreted. Otherwise, water intoxication may occur.

      (2) As an alternative to oral administration, intrana-

sal DDAVP, 0.025 ml (2.5 μg), may be started at bedtime, increasing the dose to the lowest amount that gives an antidiuretic effect, and adding a morning dose as necessary. DDAVP is also available as a fixed-dose nasal spray in the same concentration (10 μg/0.1 ml), with each spray delivering 10 μg (0.1 ml).

      (3) Lysine vasopressin (Diapid) nasal spray (50 units/ml) may be used if a duration less than that of DDAVP is desired. One spray delivers 2 units (.04 ml), with a duration of action between 2 and 8 hours.

   b. In infants, management of diabetes insipidus should be initially attempted with fluid replacement alone, because nutrition is largely provided in a liquid form, in which case the obligate large oral fluid intake coupled with DDAVP therapy may cause hyponatremia.[4] If an infant cannot be managed without vasopressin replacement therapy, Diapid is recommended because of its shorter duration of action.

   c. Inpatient postneurosurgical setting

      (1) Patients may be managed with fluids alone, avoiding the use of vasopressin therapy and the attendant risk of hyponatremia. This method consists of matching input and output hourly, with input ranging between 1 to 3 L/m²/day. These limits are derived assuming an obligate daily solute excretion of approximately 500 mOsm/m², normal renal function, and extrarenal water loss of 500 ml/m². The initial liter of fluid is given as 5% dextrose/ normal saline, and the remainder as 5% dextrose in water.

      (2) Alternatively, a patient can be initially managed on intravenous aqueous vasopressin (Pitressin), 1.5 mU/kg/hr, with fluids restricted to 1 L/m²/ 24 hour. Note well that fluid administration in excess of this amount while receiving continuous vasopressin therapy will lead to fluid overload and hyponatremia.

Treatment: Central Diabetes Insipidus

- DDAVP, oral or intranasal spray

---

2. Nephrogenic diabetes insipidus

   a. The treatment of acquired nephrogenic diabetes insipidus focuses on elimination, if possible, of the underlying disorder, such as offending drugs, hypercalcemia, hypokalemia, or ureteral obstruction.[2] Congenital nephrogenic diabetes insipidus is often difficult to treat. The main goals should be to ensure the intake of adequate calories for growth and to avoid severe dehydration. Foods with the highest ratio of caloric content to osmotic load should be

Key Treatment: Nephrogenic Diabetes Insipidus

- Thiazide and amiloride diuretics

ingested, to maximize growth and minimize the urine volume required to excrete urine solute. However, even with the early institution of therapy, growth and mental retardation are not uncommon.

b. Thiazide diuretics in combination with amiloride or indomethacin are the most useful pharmacologic agents in the treatment of nephrogenic diabetes insipidus. The combination of thiazide and amiloride diuretics is the most commonly used regimen for the treatment of congenital, X-linked nephrogenic diabetes insipidus, because amiloride counteracts thiazide-induced hypokalemia, avoids the nephrotoxicity associated with indomethacin therapy, and is well tolerated, even in infants.

Bibliography

1. Bichet DG: The posterior pituitary. *In* Melmed S (ed): The Pituitary. Cambridge: Blackwell Scientific, 1995, pp 277–306.
2. Knoers N, Monnens LA: Nephrogenic diabetes insipidus: Clinical symptoms, pathogenesis, genetics and treatment. Pediatr Nephrol 1992;6:476–482.
3. Miller WL: Molecular genetics of familial central diabetes insipidus. J Clin Endocrinol Metab 1993;77:592–595.
4. Muglia LJ, Majzoub JA: Diabetes insipidus. *In* Burg FD, Ingelfinger J, Wald E (eds): Gellis and Kagan's Current Pediatric Therapy 14. Philadelphia, WB Saunders, 1993, pp 318–319.
5. Muglia LJ, Majzoub JA: Disorders of the posterior pituitary. *In* Sperling M (ed): Pediatric Endocrinology. Philadelphia, WB Saunders, 1996, pp 195–227.

242 Onset of Puberty

Joan DiMartino-Nardi

Normal Puberty

Onset
1. Girls: 8 to 13 years (mean 10.5 years)
2. Boys: 9 to 14 years (mean 11.5 years)

Physical Examination
Pubertal changes have been staged according to Marshall and Tanner (Table 242–1).[2, 3] Zachmann and Prader have introduced a set of elliptical models of known volume to assess testicular development.

1. Girls
   a. Earliest changes: Breast budding and increased diameter of areola
   b. Duration of breast development: 4 years
   c. Menarche: Mean age is 12 6/12 to 12 9/12 years
   d. Breast and pubic hair development may show discordance.
2. Boys
   a. Earliest change: Testicular volume ≥ 3 ml
   b. Genital development spans 3 to 5 years.
   c. Pubic hair development spans 4 years.
   d. Adult hair distribution occurs approximately at 20 years.
   e. Breast development (gynecomastia) occurs in 60 per cent of boys during puberty.

Hormonal Changes
1. Gonadarche: activation of hypothalamic/pituitary/gonadal axis (H/P/G). The pulsatile release of gonadotropin releasing hormone (GnRH) from the hypothalamus results in an increase in the amplitude and frequency of follicle

TABLE 242–1. STAGES OF MALE AND FEMALE GENITAL AND PUBIC HAIR DEVELOPMENT ACCORDING TO MARSHALL AND TANNER (T I–V)

TANNER STAGE	MALE GENITALS	MALE AND FEMALE PUBIC HAIR	FEMALE BREASTS
I	Preadolescent	Preadolescent	Preadolescent
II	Testes 2.7 cm or 4 ml in volume; scrotum—some reddening; scrotum and testes begin to enlarge	Sparse, slightly pigmented, straight or slightly curled at base of penis or along labia	Breast bud; elevation of breast and papilla as small mound; enlargement of areolar diameter
III	Penis—growth begins, some increase in width; testes and scrotum continue to enlarge	Darker, coarser, curlier and spreads sparsely over junction of the pubis	Enlargement of breast and areola with no separation of their contours
IV	Penis increases in length and width; scrotal skin darkens	Adult in type but area covered is smaller than most adults; no spread to medial thighs	Projection of areola and papilla to form a secondary mound above the level of the breast
V	Genitalia are adult in size and shape	Adult in quantity and type; spread to medial thighs	Mature, projection of papilla only, resulting from recession of the areola to the general contour of the breast

stimulating hormone (FSH) and luteinizing hormone (LH) release from the pituitary gland. LH and FSH stimulate release of sex steroids from gonads as well as stimulate folliculogenesis, maturation of seminiferous tubules, and maturation of oocytes and spermatocytes. The presence of gonadarche can be confirmed with the GnRH test. In the presence of gonadarche, a bolus dose of GnRH causes an increase of LH and FSH levels.

2. Adrenarche: Activation of hypothalamic/pituitary/adrenal axis (H/P/A) causes a rise of adrenal androgen production from the zona reticularis of adrenal gland.

Growth

1. Peak height velocity—Girls: 9 cm/yr, Tanner stage 3–4; Boys: 10.3 cm/yr, Tanner stage 4–5.
2. Growth spurt is due to combined effect of growth hormone and gonadal steroids (especially estradiol).
3. Gonadal steroids cause maturation of epiphyseal growth plate and advancement of bone age.
4. Estrogen is important for accumulation of calcium in bones and an increase in bone mineral density.

Precocious Puberty

Appearance of pubertal changes:

1. Girls < 8 yrs.
2. Boys < 9 yrs.

Differential Diagnosis

1. True precocious puberty
   a. Activation of H/P/G axis
   b. Etiology
      (1) Idiopathic true precocious puberty
      (2) Central nervous system (CNS) lesion: for example, septo-optic dysplasia, tumor, cyst, abscess, head trauma, hamartoma, neurofibromatosis
2. Pseudo-precocious puberty
   a. Primary production of sex steroids from gonads or adrenal glands without activation of H/P/G axis
   b. Etiology
      (1) Exogenous sex steroids or gonadotropins, ovarian tumors (granulosa cell, granulosa theca cell, mixed germ cell, cystadenoma, gonadoblastoma, lipoid tumor), ovarian cyst, feminizing adrenal tumor, McCune-Albright syndrome, chronic primary hypothyroidism.
      (2) Familial testotoxicosis: Autosomal dominant mutation in LH receptor resulting in a constitutionally activated LH receptor and autonomous production of testosterone. Boys can have secondary activation of H/P/G axis and true puberty as well.
3. Combined precocious puberty
   a. Long-standing pseudo-precocious puberty causing activation of H/P/G axis with secondary true precocious puberty
   b. Etiology: congenital adrenal hyperplasia, McCune-Albright syndrome, familial testotoxicosis
4. Contrasexual pubertal development

   a. Virilization of girls, feminization of boys
   b. Etiology: congenital adrenal hyperplasia, adrenal and ovarian neoplasms

Evaluation

1. Direct measurement of sex steroids
2. GnRH test: GnRH—(100 μg is administered with FSH and LH measured 0, 20, 40, 60 minutes after administration of bolus GnRH
3. Magnetic resonance imaging (MRI) of pituitary with gadolinium (performed with true precocious puberty) to rule out CNS pathology
4. Adrenal computed tomography (CT), or gonadal ultrasound (performed with pseudo-precocious puberty)
5. Bone age
6. Height prediction

Risks of Precocious Puberty

1. Psychosocial and behavioral changes
2. Early pregnancy
3. Short adult stature: 10–30 per cent of girls with true precocious puberty are less than 60″

Treatment

1. True precocious puberty
   a. Goal of therapy is to halt pubertal progression in order to avoid psychosocial problems and to improve adult height. The Bayley-Pinneau method of height prediction can be used to identify those patients at risk for short stature who would be eligible for therapy. In slowly progressive forms of precocious puberty no therapy may be indicated.
   b. GnRH analogs cause reversible suppression of LH and FSH and a decline in sex steroids within 1 month of initiation. GnRH testing is used periodically to confirm H/P/G suppression. GnRH analogs are not indicated for gonadotropin-independent precocious puberty.
   c. Clinically, one sees a regression of breast development in girls, and a decrease in testicular size in boys after several months of therapy. When treatment is discontinued, FSH, LH, and sex steroids levels increase, menses occur in 65 per cent of patients within 2 years after discontinuation of GnRH analog therapy. Fertility after GnRH analog therapy has not been assessed.
   d. Data regarding final height in treated children are begining to emerge.
2. Pseudo-precocious puberty
   a. Tumors—surgery and chemotherapy
   b. Testotoxicosis—testolactone, spironolactone
   c. McCune-Albright—provera, testolactone
   d. Congenital adrenal hyperplasia—glucocorticoids and mineralocorticoids

Key Treament: Precocious Puberty

- Gonadotropin releasing hormone analogs (GnRHa)

Delayed Puberty

Definitions
1. Delayed puberty—lack of pubertal changes
   a. Boys > 14 years
   b. Girls > 13 years
2. Amenorrhea—absence of menses
   a. Primary amenorrhea: female with secondary sexual characteristics who has *never* menstruated by age 16.5 yrs *or* lack of secondary sexual characteristics and absence of menarche by age 13 years
   b. Secondary amenorrhea: loss of menses for 6 months or longer

Etiology
1. Hypothalamic (FSH and LH low)
   a. Constitutional delay—most common
   b. Chronic disease
   c. Hypothalamic dysfunction
   d. Congenital malformation
   e. Space-occupying lesion (craniopharyngioma, tumor)
   f. Infiltrative lesion
   g. Infectious lesion
   h. Inflammatory disease
   i. Postirradiation
   j. Posttraumatic
   k. Postsurgical
   l. Drugs: lysergic acid diethylamide (LSD), marijuana, tricyclic antidepressant
   m. Specific disorders
      (1) Kallman syndrome—GnRH deficiency and anosmia
      (2) Adrenal hypoplasia and hypogonadism
      (3) Prader-Willi syndrome
      (4) Isolated gonadotropin deficiency
      (5) Eating disorder
      (6) Excess exercise
      (7) Stress
      (8) Laurence-Moon-Biedl syndrome
2. Pituitary (FSH and LH low)
   a. Postinfectious
   b. Postinflammatory
   c. Posttraumatic
   d. Postirradiation
   e. Congenital malformations
   f. Space-occupying lesions (craniopharyngioma, adenoma, prolactinoma)
   g. Hypothyroidism
3. Gonadal (FSH and LH elevated)
   a. Ovarian failure
      (1) Destructive process: autoimmune disease, space-occupying lesion, postirradiation, post-chemotherapy, postsurgical, galactosemia, infection
      (2) Genetic conditions: Turner syndrome, pure XX gonadal dysgenesis, XY gonadal dysgenesis, multiple X chromosomes, aneuploidy (trisomy 21, 18, 13)
      (3) LH receptor insensitivity
      (4) Ataxia-telangiectasia
      (5) 17-hydroxylase deficiency; 17,20-desmolase deficiency
   b. Testicular failure
      (1) Generalized systemic illness (cystic fibrosis, autoimmune, hemochromatosis)
      (2) Destructive lesions (post chemotherapy, post surgery, posttraumatic, post torsion, post orchitis)
      (3) Anorchia: "Vanishing testes" syndrome
      (4) Genetic syndromes: Klinefelter syndrome (47,XXY), XX males, Noonan syndrome, ataxia-telangiectasia, prune-belly syndrome, myotonic dystrophy
      (5) Drugs—estrogen, marijuana, ketoconazole
   c. Breast development and primary amenorrhea
      (1) Absence of uterus
         (a) Congenital absence of uterus (Rokitansky-Kuster-Hauser syndrome). Defect can range from uterine agenesis with a blind-ending vagina to complete absence of uterus and vagina. Occurs in 1/4,000 to 1/5,000 female births.
         (b) Complete androgen insensitivity (testicular feminization = 46,XY): Testes produce normal levels of testosterone but, due to androgen insensitivity, there is a lack of male differentiation of external and internal genitalia. Patients have normal external genitalia, but lack uterus, fallopian tubes and upper 1/3 of vagina. Gonadectomy should be performed to prevent formation of gonadoblastoma.
      (2) Uterus present
         (a) Outflow tract obstruction
            1. Imperforate hymen
            2. Transverse vaginal septum
            3. Cervical agenesis
         (b) Polycystic ovary syndrome (PCO)
            1. Common cause of 1° and 2° amenorrhea in adolescents
            2. Originally characterized by amenorrhea, hirsutism, and obesity
            3. PCO represents a spectrum of disorders resulting in chronic anovulation.
   d. Evaluation
      (1) FSH, LH
      (2) Sex steroids (T, E2)
      (3) T$_4$, TSH
      (4) Prolactin
      (5) MRI of pituitary with gadolinium (for hypothalamic and pituitary lesions)

(6) Karyotype for gonadal failure

e. Treatment

  (1) Females

    (a) Idiopathic—no therapy or low-dose oral estrogen (Premarin 0.3–0.625 mg PO daily for 6 months)

    (b) Organic failure—cyclic estrogen/progesterone replacement therapy

    (c) Fertility—human chorionic gonadotropin (hCG), pulsatile GnRH (need intact ovaries)

  (2) Males

    (a) Idiopathic—no therapy or systemic testosterone (depot testosterone 50 mg IM every 4 weeks for 3–6 months)

    (b) Organic failure

      1. Depot testosterone: initially 50 mg IM monthly with a progressive increase of testosterone to adult doses of 200–300 mg IM every 2–4 weeks; or transdermal testosterone patch on scrotum

  2. Fertility—hCG, pulsatile GnRH therapy (need intact testes)

  3. Testicular prosthesis for anorchia

Key Treatment: Delayed Puberty

- Organic failure
  Females: cyclic estrogen/progesterone
  Males: depot testosterone

Bibliography

1. Bar A, Linder B, Sobel EH, et al: Bayley-Pinneau Method of height prediction in girls with central precocious puberty: Correlation with adult height. J Pediatr 1995;126:955–958.
2. Marshall WA, Tanner JM: Variations in pattern of pubertal changes in girls. Arch Dis Child 1969;44:291–303.
3. Marshall WA, Tanner JM: Variations in pattern of pubertal changes in boys. Arch Dis Child 1970;45:13–23.

243 Symptoms of Abnormal Puberty

Assunta Albanese and *Richard Stanhope*

Symptom | **Constitutional Delay of Growth and Puberty (CDGP)**

Definition

1. Primary delayed onset of puberty occurring in children with retarded linear growth, short stature for chronological age, and delayed bone age maturation, which should allow a final height within the normal range.
2. The absence of secondary sexual characteristics at 2.0 standard deviations (SD) from the mean chronological age value for the onset of pubertal development (13.4 years in girls and 13.8 in boys) is defined as delayed puberty.

Etiology

The commonest cause for delayed puberty is CDGP, which represents the most frequent growth disorder seen by pediatric endocrinologists. The cause is unknown.

Epidemiology

1. The incidence is higher in boys than in girls, even though by definition it should occur with equal frequency in both sexes. This may be partially explained by social reasons, or by the physiologic later onset of pubertal growth spurt within puberty in boys.
2. Precocious sexual maturation is more frequent among girls. This may be due to a sex difference in the pituitary response to GnRH, with the girls having an increased sensitivity.

3. A familial pattern can be found in many cases.
4. The cause of CDGP remains unclear.

Pathophysiology

1. In CDGP endocrine investigations fail to show any endocrine pathology. Sex and gonadotropin hormone concentrations are appropriate to the pubertal stage and growth hormone (GH) and insulin-like growth factor (IGF)-1 levels correlate to the reduced height velocity. Adrenal androgens, sex hormones, and gonadotropin values are generally low for chronological age but normal for bone age. Gonadotropin response to a bolus intravenous GnRH injection will be indistinguishable from that obtained in normal prepubertal or pubertal children before and during puberty, respectively. Nocturnal pulsatile gonadotropin secretion will be the initial endocrine event of puberty as in normal pubertal development. Normal progression into puberty will then occur, with conservation of the normal harmony between growth and puberty.
2. Biochemical assessment of GH secretion in this condition may be misleading, especially in boys. The physiologic decrease in GH secretion seen in late prepuberty and early puberty, when growth decelerates, is amplified in delayed puberty, making this condition difficult to distinguish from true GH deficiency/insufficiency. However, in delayed puberty, a transient increase in GH secretion can

be induced by priming with sex steroids prior to the test in both sexes. Low values of IGF-1 are also found reflecting the state of "GH insufficiency." During the spontaneous growth spurt both GH secretion and IGF-1 levels increase, reaching values similar to those seen during the pubertal growth spurt of normal children.

Clinical Findings

1. The typical patient with this condition is an otherwise healthy boy who is referred to a pediatric endocrinologist because of his short stature. Occasionally the lack of signs of puberty is the primary reason for referral.
2. The onset of growth delay usually precedes that of delayed puberty. Growth deceleration can commence to become manifest at around 3 to 4 years of life.
3. On school entry these children are among the smallest in their peer group and overall they tend to grow parallel below the 10th percentile of normal distance chart until puberty.
4. A progressive retardation in bone maturation runs parallel with slow growth, and skeletal maturation may be delayed greater than 2 years. At the time of normal puberty, while the peer group is having a pubertal growth acceleration, the growth velocity of these patients is extremely reduced, with a nadir that may be

below 3 cm per year. A deviation from the normal percentiles then becomes more apparent.
5. The pubertal growth spurt is usually delayed by 2 to 4 years and the total period of growth may come to its end only at the age of 20 or more years.
6. Figure 243–1 illustrates the pattern of growth in a boy with CDGP. The onset of puberty occurred at the age of 13.8 years but the pubertal growth spurt was delayed until the age of 16 yrs.
7. Sometimes growth delay becomes manifest only during late prepuberty and delayed bone maturation is a sequela of the retarded puberty, the so-called condition *constitutional delay of puberty and growth*.
8. When the pubertal growth spurt occurs in patients with CDGP, its duration, peak height velocity, and consequently the total pubertal height gain are reduced. However, the 2 to 3 years of extra growth gained in late prepuberty should counterbalance the reduced pubertal growth spurt so that final height should not be compromised.
9. Nevertheless, data on final height from nontreated boys with CDGP have shown that genetic potential may not be fully achieved, with an adult final height being below the mean adult height of the normal population by an average of 2 inches. In addition, data on segmental body

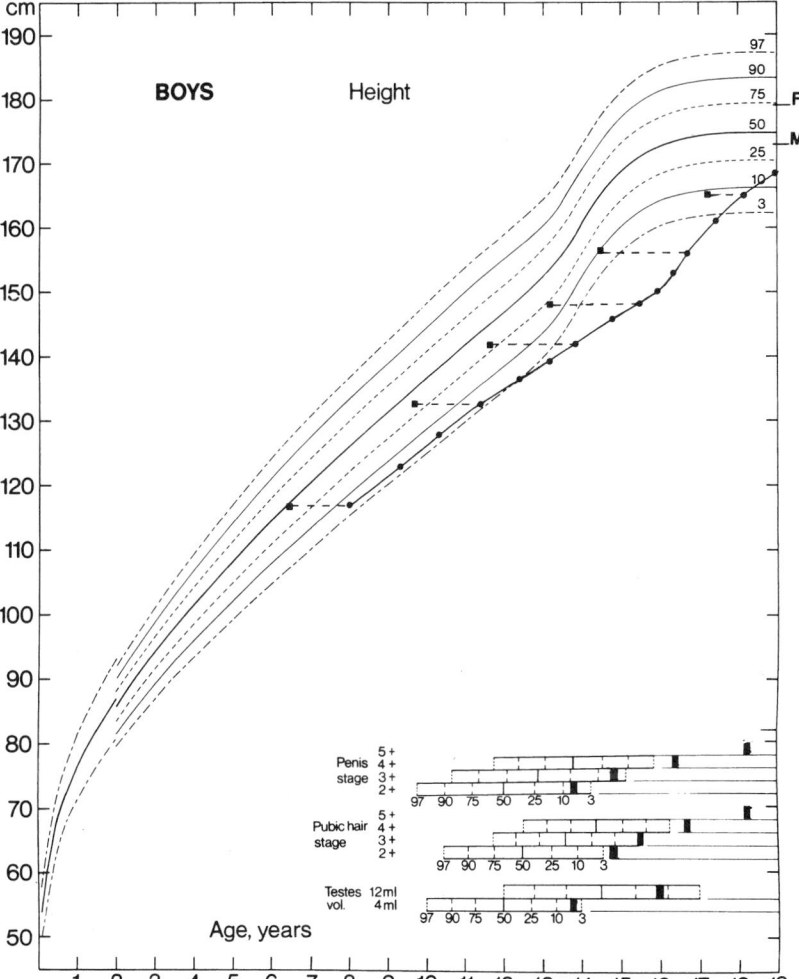

Figure 243–1 Growth data from a boy with CDGP. Bone age is shown by the solid squares. Parental centiles are indicated on the right hand border. The onset of puberty occurred at the age of 13.8 years but the pubertal growth spurt was delayed until the age of 16 years.

proportion at final height have also suggested that a moderate degree of spinal growth impairment may also occur.

10. During normal pubertal development a dramatic increase in bone mineral density and mineral content is observed from 11 to 14 years in girls and from 13 to 17 years in boys. Osteopenia has been reported in adult men who had untreated delayed onset of pubertal development. These data suggest that delayed onset of pubertal maturation may alter normal bone accretion, predisposing to later osteoporosis.

Key Clinical Findings

- Growth parallel to the 10th percentile on a "distance chart" during childhood

- Progressive growth deceleration in late prepuberty

- Absence of early features of sexual maturation

- Shorter upper than lower segment

Differential Diagnosis and Laboratory Findings

1. The diagnosis of CDGP is usually made on clinical grounds and confirmed retrospectively by normal progress through puberty. An accurate history, physical examination, anthropometric measurements and bone age assessment should already be highly suggestive of CDGP, without recourse to biochemical investigations.

2. It is important to identify if the growth delay is secondary to systemic chronic disease, such as asthma or inflammatory bowel disease, or to prolonged corticosteroid treatment.

3. Turner syndrome should be excluded with a karyotype in each girl presenting with short stature and/or delayed puberty. Dysmorphic features should be looked for as they may be suggestive of genetic conditions that are associated with short stature and delayed puberty, that is, Noonan syndrome and Prader-Willi syndrome.

4. An x-ray of hand and wrist should be taken to document the degree of delay in bone maturation and to predict final height.

5. The "consonance" between the pattern of acquisition of secondary sexual characteristics and occurrence of the growth spurt should be ascertained because loss of this consonance points to an abnormality.

6. The absence of secondary sexual characteristics at 14 years in girls and 14.5 in boys requires endocrine investigations because CDGP becomes less likely.

7. There is usually a relatively short upper to lower segment ratio. Indeed the opposite finding usually indicates a skeletal dysplasia (i.e., hypochondroplasia).

8. The most difficult differential diagnosis is between CDGP and isolated hypogonadotropic hypogonadism (IHH), which is a much less common disorder. Auxology may be helpful because patients with IHH present with delayed puberty but have normal stature. The hypogonadism in Kallmann syndrome (autosomal dominant disorders with variable penetrance, more prevalent in boys) is associated with undescended testes, anosmia, color blindness, and midline defects, which may help in the diagnosis. Endocrine investigations do not consistently differentiate CDGP from IHH. A common practical approach is to induce puberty and confirm the diagnosis of IHH at a later stage after the completion of sexual development or to observe an increase in testicular volume despite exogenous testosterone administration.

9. In case of hypogonadism secondary to gonadal failure, such as post pelvic irradiation or Klinefelter syndrome, measurement of basal gonadotropin levels (follicle stimulating hormone [FSH] and luteinizing hormone [LH]) can be diagnostic because high levels will be found after the age of 8 to 10 years.

10. If acquired GH deficiency is suspected, an intracranial space occupying lesion should be excluded by neuroradiologic imaging. In order to exclude GH deficiency, pharmacologic tests of GH secretion can be carried out, but the patients, both boys and girls, should be primed with sex steroids prior to the test.

Key Points in the History

- Presenting problem

- Who is more concerned

- Previous growth measurements if available

- Past chronic illnesses

- Medication, past or current, by any route

- Bullying or peer pressure

- Family history of delayed sexual maturation

- Social problems

Treatment

1. Some adolescents with CDGP can be extremely distressed by the short stature and/or lack of sexual development. Once made, the diagnosis of CDGP should be carefully explained to both patients and parents and reassurance on almost "normal" final height outcome for genetic potential given.

2. However, a significant number of patients, especially boys, remain distressed. Deficit in emotional development, poor self-image, lack of independence, and antisocial behavior can develop and their consequences can also persist in adult life. Distressed patients, particularly boys, may need specialist psychological help as well as pharmacologic intervention to improve their psychological well-being.

3. If pharmacologic intervention is sought, testosterone preparations or weakly anabolic steroids are the most suitable agents to treat boys with CDGP. Testosterone can be used orally or by depot intramuscular preparations. Oxandrolone is an anabolic steroid that can be safely used in low dose. At these doses the latter mainly induces a growth spurt, compared to testosterone, which induces more marked virilization. For this reason it is more suitable for treating growth delay in younger boys. The induced growth acceleration is usually sustained when

the treatment is interrupted at the attainment of 4-ml testicular volume. No short- or long-term significant side effects or deterioration of final height attainment have been reported when sex/anabolic steroids are used at the dose regimens indicated in the Treatment box.

4. In girls low doses of ethinylestradiol can be administered for 3 to 6 months or until spontaneous sexual maturation has exceeded that produced by treatment. As with the observation of increased testicular volume in boys, in girls an increase in ovarian volume and follicular activity on ultrasound ovarian imaging despite exogenous ethinyl-estradiol administration point to spontaneous puberty.

5. Both human chorionic gonadotropin (hCG) and pulsatile GnRH can be used to induce puberty in children with CDGP but do not have any advantages over sex steroid administration. HCG requires frequent injections. It can be used only in boys because it may cause ovarian hyper-stimulation syndrome in girls. Subcutaneous pulsatile GnRH treatment can mimic the exact sequence of normal pubertal maturation in boys and girls but it requires a pulsatile subcutaneous injection using a portable mini-pump and is expensive and complicated.

6. Biosynthetic human growth hormone has also been used to treat growth delay in boys with CDGP. It improves short-term growth rate in CDGP but it is less effective than that induced by oxandrolone. Final height is not significantly improved.

Treatment in CDGP

Boys
- Depot testosterone (enanthate): 50 mg/month, IM, for 3–6 months*
- Oral testosterone (undecanoate) 40 mg/day, for 3–6 months*
- Oral oxandrolone, 1.25–2.5 mg/day, for 3–6 months*

Girls
- Ethinylestradiol, 1–2 μg/day for 3–6 months or until spontaneous sexual maturation has occurred

*Or until a 4-ml testicular volume has been attained.

Bibliography

Albanese A, Stanhope R: Predictive factors in the determination of final height in boys with constitutional delay of growth and puberty. J Pediatr 1995;126:545–550.

Eastman CJ, Lazarus L, Stuart MC, et al: The effect of puberty on growth hormone secretion in boys with short stature and delayed adolescence. Aust N Z J Med 1971;1:154–159.

Prader A: Delayed adolescence. Clin Endocrinol Metab 1975;4:143–155.

Stanhope R, Albanese A, Shalet S: Delayed puberty. Many good arguments to treat. BMJ 1992;305:790.

Wilson DM, Kei J, Hintz RL, et al: Effects of testosterone therapy for pubertal delay. Am J Dis Child 1988;142:96–99.

Symptom Premature Thelarche   *Paul Hofman* and *Ora Hirsch Pescovitz*

Definition

Premature thelarche is the isolated onset of breast development in girls younger than 8 years of age without other signs of sexual maturation. Although generally considered a benign, self-limited condition, it must be distinguished from other progressive disorders that cause premature sexual development.

Epidemiology

The actual incidence of premature thelarche is unknown, although it is common. It occurs in two peaks, one in the first 2 years of life and the other, at 6 to 8 years of age.

Etiology

1. Premature thelarche is the consequence of increased estrogen bioactivity at the level of breast tissue in girls prior to the time of expected breast maturation. The breasts, being exquisitely sensitive to estrogen exposure, may show some degree of enlargement, while other estrogen-sensitive tissues generally remain unaffected. Serum estradiol levels are usually not elevated. It has been proposed that the increased estrogen sensitivity is, in part, due to the ratio of plasma androgens to estrogens. Sex hormone binding globulin (SHBG), a plasma protein that binds testosterone and estrogen, is influenced by sex steroids, with estrogens increasing and androgens decreasing plasma levels. In some girls with premature thelarche, the SHBG level is elevated, suggesting an imbalance in the ratio of estrogen to androgen. The increased estrogen bioactivity seen in premature thelarche may, in some instances, be secondary to an abnormality in this ratio.

2. Occasionally premature thelarche is secondary to a transient increase in serum estrogen, either due to increased endogenous secretion (e.g., a follicular cyst) or exogenous ingestion or application. Breast development has been observed following ingestion of estrogen-primed meat (especially chicken) and oral contraceptives, as well as the application of estrogen containing creams (which generally have excellent skin and mucosal absorption). Estrogens are also found in a variety of herbal medications and occasionally in sources such as some hair care products.

3. Widespread contamination of estrogen-containing compounds has led to epidemics of premature thelarche. Puerto Rican girls, for instance, had a dramatic increase in reported episodes of premature thelarche over a 7-year period from 1979 to 1986. This was ultimately traced to contamination of meat (especially chicken), milk, eggs and other dairy products with Zearalanol and diethylstilbestrol (DES), estrogenic compounds sold over the counter for agricultural purposes.

4. Estrogen is synthesized from androgen precursors by the enzyme aromatase. Either an increased availability of androgens or increased aromatase activity can result in elevated plasma estrogen levels and contribute to breast

development. The main source of androgens prior to puberty is the adrenal cortex. Aromatase is present in many tissues other than the ovary, especially fat. Obesity is a well-recognized cause of increased extra-ovarian estrogen production.

5. The breast tissue commonly identified in infants shortly after birth is the result of maternal and placental estrogens (predominantly estriol), and is not considered premature thelarche.

Pathophysiology

1. The majority of girls with premature thelarche are thought to have incomplete inhibition of the hypothalamic-pituitary-ovarian axis. This axis is fully activated and pubertal at birth. Over the following 3 to 12 months, cortical neural pathways mature and inhibit the amplitude of hypothalamic gonadotropin releasing hormone (GnRH) pulses, suppressing follicle stimulating hormone (FSH) and luteinizing hormone (LH) release. Normally the hypothalamic-pituitary-ovarian axis remains relatively inactive until release from this inhibition occurs with the onset of puberty.

2. In some girls there is incomplete inhibition of the hypothalamic-pituitary-ovarian axis in infancy, leading to either persistence of neonatal breast tissue or increasing breast tissue during the second year of life.

3. Activation of the hypothalamic-pituitary axis in premature thelarche is usually characterized by a predominant increase in secretion of FSH. FSH, in turn, induces follicular growth and estrogen synthesis and release. In the absence of LH release, follicular development is not sustained.

4. The profile of hypothalamic-pituitary axis activation observed in premature thelarche differs from that seen in central precocious puberty and normal puberty, where LH pulsatile secretion predominates.

Clinical Findings

1. Patients generally present with the gradual onset of breast development over several months. There is often associated breast tenderness.

2. As with normal pubertal breast development, premature thelarche can be characterized by either unilateral or asymmetric breast enlargement. It is rare for the breasts to be more advanced than Tanner stage III.

3. No other signs of either estrogen exposure or ensuing puberty should be present. In particular, there should be no increase in growth velocity, no pubic/axillary hair, no adult body odor, and no acne. It is not uncommon to note some estrogenization of the vaginal mucosa on physical examination.

4. By definition, premature thelarche is a benign condition that does not progress. In some cases, breast regression occurs over time.

5. Both gonadotropin-dependent and gonadotropin-independent precocious puberty can mimic premature thelarche. In contrast to premature thelarche, they may result in progressive secondary sexual development, growth velocity acceleration, accelerated bone age maturation, and diminished final height. Although it is important to differentiate between premature thelarche and other forms of precocious puberty, this is not always easy or clear-cut.

Premature thelarche may evolve into more progressive forms of precocious puberty. Although most studies suggest that this evolution is uncommon, 14 per cent of girls in one series went on to develop progressive gonadotropin-dependent precocious puberty.

6. A spectrum appears to exist, ranging from premature thelarche at one extreme, to gonadotropin-dependent precocious puberty at the other. This continuum is reflected in reports of exaggerated and atypical premature thelarche variants, with patients having features intermediate between those of premature thelarche and gonadotropin-dependent precocious puberty.

7. No currently known predictive factors can identify those patients who will progress from premature thelarche to gonadotropin-dependent precocious puberty. It is therefore essential that these children be followed regularly to ensure pubertal progression is not occurring.

Key Clinical Features

- Isolated breast development, either unilateral or bilateral
- Absence of other secondary sexual characteristics
- Normal linear growth
- Normal skeletal maturation

Laboratory and Radiologic Findings

1. Measurements of basal FSH, LH, and estradiol are generally not helpful in the investigation of simple premature thelarche.

2. In uncomplicated cases of premature thelarche, the only investigation required is a bone age. If this is age-appropriate or delayed for chronological age, no further investigations are required, although the patient should be followed carefully for evidence of progressive feminization (see below).

3. An advanced bone age or progressive thelarche requires consultation with a pediatric endocrinologist and further investigation to exclude progressive forms of precocious puberty. Additional tests that may prove useful in this evaluation include a GnRH stimulation test and a pelvic ultrasound.

Differential Diagnosis

1. Bilateral breast development
   Increased estrogen bioactivity and/or ovarian estrogen secretion

- Premature thelarche
- Precocious puberty

   Exogenous estrogen

- Ingestion of estrogen- or androgen-contaminated food
- Medication (oral contraceptives and postmenopausal preparations)
- Topical creams/ointments
- Insecticides, pesticides (DDT, polychlorinated ketone, methoxychlor)

   Increase in extraglandular aromatase

Obesity

Medication side effects (e.g., cimetidine)

2. Unilateral breast enlargement

The differential diagnosis includes that for bilateral breast enlargement plus the following:

Papilloma
Cyst
Hematoma
Mastitis
Lipoma
Lymphangioma
Fibrosis
Fat necrosis
Hemangioma
Metastatic tumor (rare)
Breast cancer (very rare)

A breast bud is usually easily recognized by the experienced examiner, even when unilateral. Hence, a biopsy should be unnecessary in most circumstances and should generally be avoided because it may lead to iatrogenic unilateral amastia.

Treatment

1. If the initial bone age is within 2 standard deviations of the patient's chronological age, the patient should be followed regularly every 3 to 6 months, with accurate growth data and physical examination evaluated at each visit. The patient's height, weight, and growth velocity should be plotted on growth charts. As long as the growth velocity remains age appropriate and the physical examination shows no progression, continued long-term observation is sufficient.

2. Consultation with a pediatric endocrinologist is warranted if any of the following is present:

   a. Progressive secondary sexual development

   b. Increasing growth velocity

   c. Accelerated bone age maturation.

Bibliography

Mills JL, Stolley PD, Davies J, Moshang T Jr: Premature thelarche: Natural history and etiologic investigation. Am J Dis Child 1981;135:743–745.

Pasquino AM, Pucarelli I, Passeri F, et al: Progression of premature thelarche to central precocious puberty. J Pediatr 1995;126:11–14.

Pescovitz OH, Hench KD, Barnes KM, et al: Premature thelarche and central precocious puberty: The relationship between clinical presentation and the gonadotropin response to luteinizing hormone–releasing hormone. J Clin Endocrinol Metab 1988;67:474–479.

Rosenfield RL: Normal and almost normal precocious variations in pubertal development premature pubarche and premature thelarche revisited. Horm Res 1994;41(Suppl 2):7–13.

Symptom **Gynecomastia**

Paul H. Saenger

Definition

Gynecomastia occurs in up to 75 per cent of boys to some degree usually during the first stages of puberty. Gynecomastia may be unilateral or bilateral and occurs most frequently in mid- to later stages of puberty. Gynecomastia lasts generally at least 2 years. In few instances the breast tissue is compatible to that in Tanner stage 3 or 4 female breast development. It is in those instances where spontaneous regression is less likely and surgical intervention may be appropriate, particularly when the breast is pendulous and hypertrophy is a significant somatic problem adversely affecting the teenager's self-image.

Etiology

The etiology of gynecomastia is unclear. A high estrogen-to-androgen ratio, elevated prolactin concentrations, and increased sensitivity to normally circulating low estrogen levels have been proposed. Late-onset 17-ketosteroid reductase deficiency producing greater conversion of androgens, particularly Δ^4-androstenedione, to estrogen has also been proposed but has not been confirmed in larger series.

1. Galactorrhea, as seen in prolactin hypersecretion, does not usually go along with gynecomastia. Prepubertal male gynecomastia is rare.

2. Gynecomastia also occurs in pathologic conditions, such as:

   a. Testicular tumors

   b. Inadvertent chronic estrogen ingestion

   c. Retroareolar fibromas or lipomas such as in neurofibromatosis

   d. Klinefelter syndrome

   e. Anorchia or acquired testicular failure

   f. Biosynthetic defects in testosterone production

      (1) 3β-hydroxysteroid dehydrogenase deficiency

      (2) 17-ketosteroid reductase deficiency

      (3) 17,20-desmolase deficiency

      (4) 17-hydroxylase deficiency

   g. Testicular failure, secondary to mumps or trauma

   h. Increased substrate for aromatase activity leading to excessive androgens

      (1) Thyrotoxicosis, starvation, cirrhosis

      (2) Congenital adrenal hyperplasia

   i. Drugs affecting androgen or estrogen production or metabolism associated with gynecomastia

      (1) Spironolactone, coumadin, ketoconazole, human chorionic gonadotropin (hCG)

      (2) Antidepressants, marijuana, heroin, isoniazid

      (3) Methyldopa, digitalis, phenothiazines

Treatment

1. In routine transient pubertal gynecomastia sympathic reassurance and psychosocial support should be the only therapy necessary. Encourage weight loss and physical activity to increase pectoralis muscle develop-

ment. Advise teenagers to wear a tee shirt during gym to reduce public embarrassment.

2. In severe or prolonged cases with no apparent remission for more than 2 years and when pubertal development is nearly completed, other interventions may be considered.

   a. *Medical* therapy has been proposed involving clomiphene citrate, danazol, tamoxifen (blocking estrogen receptors), or dihydrotestosterone heptanoate. Drug therapy using the modalities outlined above has generally been carried out in uncontrolled studies. Tamoxifen, particularly, is furthermore not approved for routine use in the United States. Testosterone should *not* be considered as a therapeutic agent because it usually aggravates the gynecomastia and leads to increased breast tenderness.

   b. *Surgical* removal has been a realistic alternative particularly since newer techniques using liposuction, which avoids extensive surgery, have been perfected. In this technique, after a circumareolar incision, glandular and adipose tissues are removed. This leaves relatively little scarring. However, it can only be recommended in the hands of a skilled surgeon. It should also not be done in early stages of gynecomastia because after insufficient surgical removal of tissue, regrowth may occur as puberty progresses.

Bibliography

Carlson SE: Gynecomastia. N Engl J Med 1980;1303:795–799.

Eberle AJ, Sparrow JT, Keenan BS: Treatment of persistent pubertal gynecomastia with dihydrotestosterone heptanoate. J Pediatr 1986;109:144.

Nuttall FQ: Gynecomastia is a physical finding in normal men. J Clin Endocrinol Metab 1979;48:338–340.

| Symptom | **Premature Adrenarche** | *Paul H. Saenger* |

Premature adrenarche or pubarche is commonly defined as the appearance of pubic hair before 8 years in girls and 9 years in boys. Premature adrenarche generally occurs between the ages of 2 and 8 years and is seen much more frequently in girls than in boys at a ratio of almost 10 to 1. Increased frequency of premature adrenarche has been reported in children with abnormal central nervous system function.

Etiology

1. The cause of adrenal oversecretion in premature adrenarche is currently unclear. Various theories have been advanced. Oversecretion of a purported central androgen stimulating hormone, perhaps part of the pro-opiomelanocortin molecule, perhaps in concert with adrenocorticotropic hormone (ACTH), may be the cause of adrenarche. Confirmatory data, however, are lacking. Other theories postulate that the development of the zona reticularis, the innermost layer of the adrenal gland and the site of the production of adrenal androgens, is accelerated in premature adrenarche. Furthermore, at the advent of physiologic adrenarche the 17,20-desmolase enzyme is increased and the 3β-hydroxysteroid dehydrogenase (3β-HSD) enzyme shows decreased efficiency in the zona reticularis, leading to rises in dehydroepiandrosterone (DHEA) with early appearance of pubic hair through peripheral conversion to more potent androgens. Thus changes in human adrenal microsomal enzyme activity also contribute to the initiation of adrenarche. These enzymatic activity changes appear to be responsible for the increase in adrenal androgen secretion in premature adrenarche, where this process is initiated prematurely.

2. Enzymatic defects of steroidogenesis, such as 21-hydroxylase, 11β-hydroxylase, and 3β-hydroxysteroid dehydrogenase deficiency, both in their classic and nonclassic forms of congenital and late-onset adrenal hyperplasia, may be rare causes of premature adrenarche, although the exact frequency is still not well defined.

Pathophysiology

The physiologic basis of premature adrenarche is a mild to moderate oversecretion of adrenal androgens. Chiefly, DHEA, Δ^4-androstenedione, and testosterone are elevated to levels commonly seen in Tanner stage II of puberty. Published normal levels of these hormones in boys and girls in the various stages of puberty should be utilized when evaluating hormonal determinations. 17-Hydroxyprogesterone is also occasionally elevated to a level seen in Tanner stage II of puberty. It is, however, generally less than 100 ng/dl and thus the likelihood of late onset adrenal hyperplasia (21-OHase deficiency) becomes remote (see Chapters 257 and 258).

Clinical Findings

1. The appearance of pubic hair is mostly limited to the labia majora in girls or at the base of the scrotum in boys and thus may easily elude detection on casual examination.

2. Clinical presentation may also include axillary hair and adult apocrine secretion in the axilla. Growth velocity may be increased, that is, the height may be above the 50th percentile, and a mild advancement in bone age (i.e., 1–2 years) is often present. The bone age advancement is, however, closely correlated with the height age of the child. It is important to recognize that testicular volume and breast size remain at the prepubertal level in typical premature adrenarche.

Differential Diagnosis

1. In those patients in whom testicular, breast, or clitoral enlargement is present, the possibility of precocious puberty or of a virilizing adrenal or gonadal tumor has to be ruled out.

2. Late-onset adrenal hyperplasia (21-OHase deficiency, 3β-OL-dehydrogenase deficiency) may also present as premature adrenarche and the correct diagnosis is readily established by hormone determinations (see below).

3. Cushing syndrome may rarely present with cortisol and androgen excess simulating premature adrenarche. Generally, however, in cortisol excess the growth velocity is impaired and assessment of glucocorticoid levels will quickly show loss of diurnal function and/or elevated levels of serum and urinary glucocorticoids. (See Chapter 260.)

Diagnosis

1. Diagnostic tests for premature adrenarche are serum levels of DHEA, 17-hydroxyprogesterone, Δ^4-androstenedione, and cortisol in the baseline state.
2. If basal 17-hydroxyprogesterone is above 100 ng/dl, at any time of the day an ACTH stimulation test to unmask any adrenal steroid enzyme deficiency should be performed.
3. An ACTH stimulation test should also be carried out in those forms where systemic androgen effects are present such as atypical or exaggerated adrenarche characterized by cystic acne, signs of virilization, clitoral hypertrophy, increased muscle mass, and bone age advancement of more than 2 years over chronological age.

Treatment and Natural History

1. Premature adrenarche itself requires only sympathetic reassurance.
2. The natural history of children with premature adrenarche is generally benign.
3. Although the slightly advanced bone age leads sometimes to earlier onset of puberty, final height is generally within the normal range.

Careful follow-up into the adolescent and adult stages, however, suggests that functional ovarian hyperandrogenism and polycystic ovarian syndrome may be much more common sequelae of premature adrenarche in girls than previously thought. Therefore, in addition to the clinical follow-up in premature adrenarche, repeated measurements of plasma androgens are necessary until the patient has entered the normal course of puberty in order to corroborate the initial diagnosis. There is evidence for nascent forms of insulin resistance in premature adrenarche. Acanthosis nigricans on the neck and in the axilla that is associated with insulin resistance may also frequently be seen in premature adrenarche.

Bibliography

Ibanez L, Potau N, Virdis R, et al: Postpubertal outcome in girls diagnosed of premature pubarche during childhood: Increased frequency of functional ovarian hyperandrogenism. J Clin Endocrinol Metab 1993;76:1599–1603.

Lashansky G, Saenger P, DiMartino-Nardi J, et al: Normative data for the steroidogenic response of mineralocorticoids and their precursors to adrenocorticotropin in a healthy pediatric population. J Clin Endocrinol Metab 1992;75:1491–1496.

Lashansky G, Saenger P, Fishman K, et al: Normative data for adrenal steroidogenesis in a healthy pediatric population: Age and sex-related changes after ACTH stimulation. J Clin Endocrinol Metab 1991;73:674–686.

Oppenheimer E, Linder B, DiMartino-Nardi J: Decreased insulin sensitivity in prepubertal girls with premature adrenarche and acanthosis nigricans. J Clin Endocrinol Metab 1995;80:614–618.

Saenger P, Reiter E: Editorial: Premature adrenarche: A normal variant of puberty. J Clin Endocrinol Metab 1992;74:236–238.

Symptom **Brief Guide to Work-up of the Child with Short Stature** *Paul H. Saenger*

1. Growth is a sensitive indicator of a child's state of health, nutrition, and genetic background. Short stature is usually defined as a height less than the 3rd percentile for the reference range, that is, 2.0 SD scores (SDS) below the population mean. In some instances the 5th percentile (−1.8 SDS) is used. Disease-specific cross-sectional standards for a variety of growth disorders such as Noonan, Russell-Silver, Turner, Down, and skeletal dysplasias are available. Ethnic standards should be also utilized whenever possible because, for example, mean final height of the Japanese male is 8 cm less than mean final height of the World Health Organization (WHO) reference range.

2. Fortunately in most instances individuals who present to the pediatrician and to the pediatric endocrinologist with concerns about their growth do have variants of normal growth: familial short stature (FSS) or constitutional delay of growth and development (CDGD), and, therefore, sympathetic reassurance is all that is necessary.

3. Work-up of the child with short stature should take into account
   a. Growth velocity
   b. Height of the parents and siblings
   c. Advent of puberty and pubertal tempo of parents
   d. Age of menarche in the mother
   e. Height of grandparents on mother's and father's side

4. Longitudinal records allow calculation of growth velocity and will give early clues as to the presence of a pathologic process. Assessment of an individual's growth velocity should be made at intervals of at least 6 months, preferably 1 year. In children over 3 to 4 years the standing height is recommended and use of an appropriate instrument, such as the Harpenden stadiometer, is strongly recommended. In children under 3 years of age, recumbent heights should be recorded also with a reliable instrument. Repeat measurements should be accurate to within 0.2 cm. Measurements of sitting height and lower segment of the body (from the pubic symphysis to the ground) are important in assessing body proportions.

5. In addition to longitudinal records of height, weight, and head circumference, an assessment of the biologic age can be made by determining the dental age and the bone age (left hand and wrist). Interpretation of the bone age uses most commonly the standards of Greulich and Pyle. This will allow a calculation of predicted adult height in children older than 6 years.

6. There are clinical situations for which the population cross-sectional definition of short stature may be at variance with the circumstances of an individual's family. An individual may be on the 10th percentile, but may still be abnormally short if the parents are very tall. To determine this, the midparental height (MPH), also known as the target height, should be calculated, with the 10th to the 90th percentile range being determined using the following formula:

a. MPH if male:

$$\frac{(\text{father's height} + \text{mother's height} + 13)}{2} \pm 7.5 \text{ (all in cm)}$$

b. MPH if female:

$$\frac{(\text{father's height} - 13 + \text{mother's height})}{2} \pm 6 \text{ (all in cm)}$$

c. If the individual falls outside of this range, a reason should be sought.

7. Parent-specific standards may also be helpful to assess a child's height in relation to the height of the parents. Note that this can be done only during a period of relatively stable growth, that is, between 3 and 9 years of age.

Diagnostic Tests

1. Laboratory screening tests that should be carried out in every child being evaluated for short stature should include the following:

   a. Complete blood count (CBC) and sedimentation rate

   b. Urinalysis: check for reducing substances and determination of specific gravity and pH

   c. Urine microscopy

   d. Blood chemistries including electrolytes, calcium, phosphorus, CO_2, blood urea nitrogen (BUN), creatinine, alkaline phosphatase, serum glutamic-oxaloacetic transaminase (SGOT) and serum glutamic-pyruvate transaminase (SGPT), bilirubin, total protein, albumin, globulin, T_4, thyroid stimulating hormone (TSH). Care should be taken that T_4 is interpreted according to age-specific standards (see Chapters 253 and 254).

   e. Bone age, skeletal survey

   f. In short girls, chromosomes should always be determined, rather than just follicle stimulating hormone (FSH) and luteinizing hormone (LH), which may not be diagnostic in a young child. Phenotypic features of Turner syndrome may not be present in all cases.

2. The nature of the growth problem can be best assessed by looking at longitudinal growth records. Birth size and perinatal events are important, as is the family history focusing on stature, puberty, and other heritable diseases. Other systemic illness (e.g., asthma, congenital heart disease) may affect growth. Nutritional review with at least a 3-day review of dietary intake and appropriate calculation of daily caloric intake is an integral part of the evaluation.

3. As a screening test for growth hormone deficiency, exercise to stimulate release of growth hormone (i.e., 20 minutes of vigorous exercise and growth hormone determination immediately after the exercise), combined with measurements of insulin-like growth factor (IGF)-1 and other growth factors such as IGF binding proteins, particularly IGFBP-3, is generally sufficient.

4. If a clear cause for growth retardation and short stature has been identified (e.g., Turner syndrome, chronic renal failure), testing for growth hormone deficiency is generally superfluous. Additional measures other than laboratory tests for growth hormone measurements either in screening tests or in definitive tests are determinations of components of the growth hormone (GH)-IGF axis.

   a. In patients with unequivocal growth hormone deficiency, IGF-1 and IGFBP-3 are invariably reduced.

   b. Age-appropriate standards have to be utilized for proper interpretation of test results.

   c. For patients with mild abnormalities of GH secretion, serum concentrations of IGF-1 and IGFBP-3 provide a meaningful measure of functional GH secretion and possibly assess GH secretory status more effectively rather than the pharmacologic provocative testing.

5. For growth hormone testing using pharmacologic criteria, employ stimulation tests with the following secretagogues:

   a. Clonidine: 100 μg PO

   b. Glucagon: 0.1 mg/kg up to 5 mg IM

   c. L-DOPA:
      (1) 125 mg for body weight up to 15 kg
      (2) 250 mg for weight up to 35 kg
      (3) 500 mg for weight above 35 kg

   d. Propranolol: 40 mg PO

   e. Insulin: 0.1 U/kg Regular insulin IV

   f. Arginine: 0.5 g/kg up to 20 g IV over 20 minutes.

6. Blood samples are to be obtained at 0, 30, 60, 90, and 120 minutes. During the glucagon and insulin test the cortisol response can be measured at 60 and 90 minutes. Generally, test results for growth hormone above 10 ng/ml are considered normal, whereas test results between 5 and 10 may document partial growth hormone deficiency. If a severe defect of GH secretion has been documented, appropriate imaging studies of the pituitary and the hypothalamus should always be done to rule out any space-occupying lesions.

7. In summary, the work-up of the child with short stature should therefore take into account not only laboratory data but also auxologic criteria, that is, the careful and accurate documentation of height velocity over time and the correct plotting of height on appropriate growth curves.

8. In the absence of other evidence suggesting hypothalamic/pituitary dysfunction (e.g., hypoglycemia, microphallus, cryptorchidism, and intracranial tumors), a child who is growing normally typically does not require evaluation of growth hormone secretion. On the other hand, if a child has central nervous system disease, a history of an intracranial tumor, or a history of past cranial irradiation, growth hormone deficiency

should definitely be ruled out whenever growth velocity slows down to a velocity less than the 50th percentile of normal even though the height might still be within the normal range on the growth curve.

9. It cannot be stressed enough that only a combined approach in the evaluation of the child stature using both auxologic and biochemical criteria can be expected to define hormonal deficiency states adequately and identify those children who need hormonal therapy early.

Symptom **Ambiguous Genitalia** *Paul H. Saenger*

Definition

Sexual ambiguity in a neonate is a medical emergency, challenging the physician to arrive expediently (within a week or two) at a rational sex assignment.

Etiology

1. Four major diagnostic categories cause confusion regarding sex assignment in the newborn.
   a. Female pseudohermaphroditism: 46XX
   b. Male pseudohermaphroditism: 46XY
   c. True hermaphroditism: 46/XX or mosaicism
   d. Mixed gonadal dysgenesis: 45X/46XY.
2. The external genitalia are rarely distinctive enough to allow a diagnosis of a particular disorder or to distinguish clearly between male (46XY) pseudohermaphroditism (MPH) and female (46XX) pseudohermaphroditism (FPH). The most common forms of FPH are virilizing forms of congenital adrenal hypoplasia (CAH). In MPH the diagnosis is not found in 50 per cent of cases. The phenotype in MPH may be indistinguishable from that seen in FPH.
3. This potential source of grave error in diagnosis and management emphasizes the need for biochemical characterization of the enzymatic defect in each patient with genital ambiguity. The parents need counseling about the nature of the baby's abnormality and guidance as to how to deal with their friends and relatives. Once the sex of rearing has been decided, treatment can be organized. Genetic counseling will need to be deferred until a specific diagnosis is available. This may not be possible in every instance.

Clinical Findings

1. Reproductive organs
   a. Palpable gonadal structures almost always contain testicular tissue. An abdominal CT or an abdominal sonograph will demonstrate the presence or absence of müllerian derivatives, particularly the presence or absence of a uterus. Presence of a uterus is strong evidence against MPH. A uterus is present in females with CAH, females virilized by transplacental androgens, patients with mixed gonadal dysgenesis, and most patients with true hermaphroditism. A uterus is absent, of course, in all forms of MPH, such as androgen insensitivity syndrome (complete or incomplete), 5α-reductase deficiency, enzymatic blocks in testosterone biosynthesis, and primary intrauterine gonadotropin deficiency.
   b. Inguinal or intraabdominal gonads can best be located by MRI. Ultrasound studies may give unsatis-

factory results. A voiding cystourethrogram will yield important information about the vaginal vault and anatomy of the urethra.

2. In the evaluation, look carefully for systemic features
   a. Features of Turner syndrome (e.g., webbed neck, edema of the hands and feet), suggestive of mixed gonadal dysgenesis
   b. Skin pigmentation in infants with CAH. Always watch for systemic illness in infants with ambiguous genitalia, such as electrolyte imbalance (salt wasting and vomiting) and hypoglycemia.
   c. The development of hypoglycemia after birth suggests adrenal deficiency.
   d. Signs and symptoms of mineralocorticoid deficiency can occur, generally within the first few days of life but mostly 1 to 2 weeks after birth.

Laboratory Findings

Diagnostic studies in intersex patients should include

1. Electrolytes
2. Endocrine studies
   a. Congenital adrenal hyperplasia profiles (17-OH progesterone, DHEA, DHEAS, androstenedione, testosterone, cortisol)
   b. Androgen and estrogen levels
   c. ACTH stimulation test (250 mg ACTH IM)
   d. Gonadal stimulation (with HCG 5000 U × 3 IM) (measure testosterone and dihydrotestosterone).
   e. Cytogenetics (FISH fluorescent in situ hybridization) (SRY sex-determining region on the Y chromosome) probes for Y-chromosome fragments.
   f. Gonadotropins (mostly after the second week of life)
3. Consultation with
   a. Urologic surgery (depending on degree of malformation)
   b. Social work (re management plans concerning decisions of sex assignment).

Radiologic Findings

1. Voiding cystourethrogram (VCU).
2. Pelvic ultrasound, renal ultrasound.

Management Decisions

1. Initial laboratory results, particularly electrolytes and 17-hydroxyprogesterone, are generally available within 24 to 48 hours. Other studies may take longer. At any time during the work-up the physician must bear in mind that

the neonate may be at risk for adrenal crisis, and forms of CAH with impaired glucocorticoid and mineralocorticoid production have to be discovered early on.

2. Elevated 17-hydroxyprogesterone measurements in serum are diagnostic for CAH caused by 21-hydroxylase deficiency (for therapy, see Chapters 257 and 258). Particularly careful attention must be paid to potential electrolyte imbalance in patients with salt-losing forms of adrenal hyperplasia.

3. While the chromosome analysis will be very important in determining whether the patient has MPH or FPH and is clearly of importance in the sex of assignment, it should be remembered that a low level of mosaicism may be missed in an initial study. In addition to karyotypic analysis, consider special techniques to probe for Y-chromosome fragments.

4. In some instances, final analysis has to await the results of stimulation tests, particularly HCG stimulation tests evaluating the rise in serum testosterone and ACTH stimulation tests to unmask any adrenal steroid enzyme deficiency. In male newborns a physiologic rise in serum testosterone from day 30 to 100 of life aids in the detection of Leydig cells and the assessment of this function.

5. The task of deciding the gender of patients with MPH should be addressed tactfully by experts. The serum androgen response to HCG stimulation and effects of systemic testosterone on penis size (50 mg IM q 4 weeks for not more than 3 to 4 months) may help in arriving at a final decision, although these measures may delay sex assignment slightly.

6. In some instances, surgical exploration through either laparoscopic procedures or external gonadal biopsy is necessary. Patients should not be discharged until sex assignment and naming have been carried out. Therefore, an orchestrated approach under the leadership of an endocrinologist is necessary in the work-up of infants with ambiguous genitalia.

7. A very common cause of confusion in the neonatal period is the distinction between clitoromegaly and excessive estrogen effect on prepuce and the labia minora in the normal female. A redundant prepuce is often mistaken for clitoromegaly, prompting unnecessary evaluations. Hypertrophy of the vaginal mucosa or even prolapse is a common cause for referral. All these findings are benign and resolve spontaneously.

8. The distinction between a microphallus and a small penis can also present as a possible source of ambiguity. Standards for stretched normal penile length are 3.5 cm ± 2.5 cm. Infants with micropenis may be at risk for low glucose and cortisol levels secondary to hypopituitarism (Table 243–1).

Specific Intersex Disorders

1. Mixed gonadal dysgenesis, true hermaphroditism
   Variants of mixed gonadal dysgenesis (45X/46XY), true hermaphroditism (80 per cent of these are 46XX) present with palpable external gonads and ambiguous genitalia of varying degree. The suspicion is particularly high when hormonal studies in these patients for adrenal hyperplasia are negative. Very often the HCG stimulation gives a positive response, i.e., a generous rise in testosterone due to presence of Leydig cells in cryptic, testicular material.

2. Incomplete virilization of the male
   a. This presentation is commonly described as hypospadias, with varying degrees of severity (first degree: coronal; second degree: shaft; third degree: base of shaft and perineal) with a bifid scrotum. The penis may be small and frequently presents with a chordee, which gives the penile shaft a bent, shortened appearance. The cause may be an androgen synthesis defect or may be due to fetal gonadotropin deficiency.

   b. In patients with 5α-reductase deficiency or partial androgen insensitivity, the lack of virilization at birth is severe, and testes generally are undescended. The diagnosis in these categories is made with measurements of testosterone and DHT, before and after HCG stimulation. In complete androgen insensitivity the testes are intraabdominal, external genitalia are normally feminized, and no ambiguity exists.

   c. In congenital anorchia or vanishing testes syndrome there are no gonads at all at birth. The diagnosis is made after endocrine testing, when an absent testosterone response to HCG is noted. One has to postulate, of course, that the testes must have been present and functioning in utero during early development to orchestrate normal male phenotypic differentiation.

3. In 47XY Klinefelter syndrome and 46XX males the external genitalia are normal male.

4. Denys-Drash syndrome—This condition consists of the association of XY karyotype in a phenotypic female with renal disease and/or Wilms tumor. Phenotypic variability is present, and sometimes genital ambiguity is found. An infant with any XY ambiguity without an obvious etiology could therefore be at risk for renal disease and/or Wilms tumor and should be followed carefully. The molecular basis for this disorder, an alteration of the tumor suppressor WT1 (the Wilms tumor gene), has recently been described.

5. Micropenis
   When the gonads are symmetrically descended in the scrotum and the penis is very small (use penile length standards) but the urethra is normally placed at the tip of the penis, congenital hypopituitarism has to be ruled out. The patient should be carefully monitored for hypoglycemia. Thyroid function should be assessed as well as growth hormone levels together with insulin and cortisol, specifically during a hypoglycemic episode. Note that these patients will not be identified during the neonatal thyroid screening programs using TSH. Micropenis is also seen in many syndromes, such as

   a. Pallister Hall syndrome

   b. Septo-optic dysplasia

   c. CHARGE syndrome

   d. Robinow syndrome

   e. Fetal face syndrome

TABLE 243–1. AMBIGUOUS GENITALIA: STEPS IN ESTABLISHING THE DIAGNOSIS IN AN INFANT OF UNCERTAIN SEX

CLINICAL FEATURE	21-HYDROXYLASE DEFICIENCY	GONADAL DYSGENESIS WITH Y CHROMOSOMES	TRUE HERMAPHRODITISM	PARTIAL ANDROGEN INSENSITIVITY	BLOCK IN TESTOSTERONE BIOSYNTHESIS
Palpable gonad(s)	−	+	+/−	+	+
Uterus present*	+	+	Usually	−	−
Increased skin pigmentation	+	−	−	−	−/+
Sick baby	+/−	−	−	−	−/+
Dysmorphic appearance	−	+/−	−	−	−
CLINICAL DIAGNOSIS					
Investigation					
Serum 17OHP	↑	Normal	Normal	Normal	Normal
Electrolytes	Abnormal	Normal	Normal	Normal	Possibly abnormal
Karyotype	46,XX	45,X/46,XY or other pattern	46,XX	46,XY	46,XY
Testosterone response to hCG	Not indicated	Definite response	Normal or blunted	Good response (both T and DHT)	Blunted or absent
Gonadal biopsy	Not indicated	Dysgenetic gonad, +/− tumor	Ovatestes	Normal testes (+/−) Leydig cell hyperplasia)	Normal testis
Other	−	−	−	Genital skin fibroblast culture for AR assay	Measure testosterone precursors after ACTH and hCG

As determined by US examination or rectal palpation.
AR, androgen receptor; DHT, dihydrotestosterone; 17-OHP, 17-hydroxyprogesterone; T, testosterone.

Therapeutic Planning

1. Sex assignment in infants with MPH should be guided by the anatomy of the external and internal genitalia, the degree of masculinization, the possibility that development at puberty will conform to the assigned sex, and the capacity for normal future sexual activity.
2. If the full-term neonate stretched penile length is <1.5 cm, a female sex assignment should be consistent, particularly if there is no growth response or no good testosterone response after HCG.
3. A newborn with female pseudohermaphroditism, even if severely virilized, should always be assigned the female sex before gonadectomy.
4. Gonadectomy prior to puberty is always recommended in 46XY patients reared as girls (complete testicular feminization). Sex steroid therapy concordant with the sex of rearing at the age of puberty is necessary.
5. If reconstructive surgery of the external genitalia is necessary, it should be initiated before the age of 3 years, before gender awareness is embedded too firmly. A parallel between the process of gender identity formation and the acquisition of language has been suggested. Certainly, by the age of 5 years, children grasp linguistic principles. Analogously, at this same age the primary identification with sex is irrevocably part of self-image.
6. With even the most sophisticated diagnostic techniques available, the pathogenesis of MPH remains obscure in many patients. Recalling the complex schedule of genital differentiation in the human, it becomes clear that even only transient disturbances in any of the processes involved may alter the male phenotype. With available techniques, testosterone synthesis and metabolism as well as androgen binding can be assessed, and the ability to respond to exogenous or endogenous androgens at puberty can be tested.

Bibliography

Almaguer MC, Saenger P, Linder BL: Phallic growth after hCG: A clinical index of androgen responsiveness. Clin Pediatr 1993; 32:329–333.

Saenger P: Physiology of sexual determination and differentiation. In Brook CGD (ed): Clinical Paediatric Endocrinology, 3rd ed. London, Blackwell Scientific Publishing, 1995, pp 41–52.

Saenger P: Abnormal sexual differentiation. J Pediatr 1984; 104:1–17.

Sinclair AH: New genes for boys. Am J Hum Genet 1995; 57:998–1001.

Warne GL, Hughes IA: The clinical management of ambiguous genitalia. In Brook CGD (ed): Clinical Paediatric Endocrinology, 3rd ed. London, Blackwell Scientific Publishing, 1995, pp 53–68.

244 Hypogonadotropic Hypogonadism

Peter Lee

Definition

Hypogonadotropic hypogonadism (HH) is the state of gonadal deficiency secondary to the lack of sufficient gonadotropin stimulation (failure of the hypothalamic-pituitary unit). This may occur as isolated deficiency of luteinizing hormone (LH) and folllicle stimulating hormone (FSH) secretion or concomitant with other pituitary hormone deficiencies including growth hormone, thyroid stimulating hormone (TSH) and adrenocorticotropic hormone (ACTH) deficiency. This deficiency may result from defects in the hypothalamus (gonadotropin releasing hormone [GnRH] deficiency) or the pituitary (inability to secrete adequate LH and FSH when appropriately stimulated).

Etiology

1. *Kallmann syndrome* is hypogonadotropic hypogonadism due to GnRH deficiency associated with anosmia.
2. *Idiopathic hypogonadotropic hypogonadism* (IHH) refers to patients with this disorder without central nervous system (CNS) abnormalities or anosmia.
3. Multiple hormonal deficiencies including gonadotropin deficiency may be congenital, idiopathic, or secondary to CNS lesions. The hypogonadotropic defect may be at the level of the hypothalamus, the pituitary or both. Lesions may be a consequence of craniopharyngiomas, germinomas, head injury, surgery, or irradiation.
4. Gonadotropin deficiency may be congenital (associated with Kallmann, Prader-Willi, or Laurence-Moon-Biedl syndromes and idiopathic panhypopituitarism) or acquired (secondary to craniopharyngioma or other tumors, empty sella syndrome or infiltrative disorders such as histiocytosis, sarcoidosis, or hemochromatosis).

Pathophysiology

1. Hypogonadotropism presenting at pubertal age must be differentiated from the delayed onset of puberty (prolongation of the physiologic hypogonadotropic state of childhood).

   a. This differentiation cannot be made during pubertal years with certainty until adequate time has passed while the patient is otherwise healthy for potential gonadotropin secretion to become manifest. Since secretion is normally minimal after infancy during childhood years until pubertal secretion is established, assessment of gonadotropin secretion dynamics is not conclusive during these years.

b. This diagnosis may be made during infancy only if gonadotropin levels are clearly subnormal for age, since active secretion of GnRH, LH, and FSH normally approximates early pubertal levels during the first 6 months of life. Such evaluation is appropriate in a patient with a family history of Kallmann syndrome, with a micropenis or cryptorchidism, or evidence of panhypopituitarism (hypoglycemia suggestive of ACTH and growth hormone deficiency and TSH deficiency).

2. Kallmann syndrome results from the failure of migration of GnRH neurons from the olfactory placode to the hypothalamus (arcuate nucleus) and is associated with anosmia. This syndrome may be associated with midfacial developmental abnormalities (cleft lip and palate, agenesis of maxillary incisors, nasal malformations), defects or deletion of genes adjacent to the KAL gene on the X chromosome (X-linked ichthyosis, short stature, chondrodysplasia punctata, and ocular albinism) as well as other defects (renal agenesis or aplasia, absent vas deferens, mirror movements, sensory neural hearing loss, mental retardation).

3. Partial gonadotropin deficiency may be manifested by some but not complete pubertal development. Partial defects may result in LH deficiency with apparently normal FSH secretion, this profile likely being a reflection of partial GnRH secretion.

    a. An example of this deficiency may be the *fertile eunuch syndrome*, males with normal FSH levels, and low LH and testosterone levels. Males have incomplete virilization, have eunuchoid proportions, and have testicular growth with no Leydig cells but spermatogenesis.

    b. Isolated FSH deficiency has been reported among females with primary amenorrhea, lack of pubertal development, and small ovaries containing numerous primordial follicles.

Clinical Findings

1. Gonadotropin deficiency usually presents with lack of pubertal development at an appropriate age. Patients with gonadotropin deficiency without other hormonal deficiencies are normal height for age throughout childhood and when presenting with lack of pubertal development.

2. Since gonadotropin deficiency may be partial, patients may present with inadequate progression of pubertal development, which began at an appropriate age.

3. Among females, partial HH may present with lack of menarche or irregular menses in women with moderate breast development. Normally, menses can be expected within 3.5 years of the onset of breast development. If menarche is delayed more than 5 years beyond the onset of puberty, subsequent fertility may be decreased and the etiology may be hypogonadotropism or other abnormalities.

4. Males with partial HH have some decrease in testicular volume and decreased spermatogenesis and may have gynecomastia. Puberty may be prolonged, with failure to attain full pubertal development (Tanner stage V with adult-sized testes) within a period of 4 to 5 years from the onset.

5. If hypogonadotropism is suspected, the sense of smell should be tested because of the association with the Kallmann syndrome.

6. Midline facial defects (including cleft palate and solitary maxillary incisor) may occur in association with hypogonadotropism.

7. When puberty has been delayed, retarded closure of epiphyseal growth zones of long bones is common. Such bones are disproportionally long resulting in an upper:lower ratio less than normal and increased arm span.

8. Social, environmental, endocrine, nutritional, and psychologic disruptions apparent by medical history may be associated with delay of or diminution of gonadotropin secretion; presentation is similar to permanent gonadotropin deficiency. Diagnoses may include exercise-related and psychogenic amenorrhea, and anorexia nervosa.

9. Syndromes (Table 244–1): In addition to Kallmann syndrome, the following syndromes commonly include hypogonadotropic hypogonadism:

    a. Laurence-Moon-Bardet-Biedl syndrome includes mental retardation, retinal abnormalities, polydactyly, and hypogonadism that may be hypogonadotropic.

    b. Prader-Willi syndrome features may include neonatal hypotonia, obesity, short stature, mental retardation, cryptorchidism, and hypogonadotropic hypogonadism.

Key Clinical Findings

- Lack of pubertal development
- Anosmia (Kallmann)
- Mental retardation, polydactyly (Laurence-Moon-Biedl)
- Obesity, mental retardation, hypotonia (Prader-Willi)

TABLE 244–1. CONDITIONS INVOLVING HYPOTHALAMIC OR PITUITARY DEFECTS

Autoimmune disease	Syndromes
Craniopharyngioma	Biemond
Fertile eunuch syndrome	Blepharophimosis
Granulomatous disease	Borgeson-Forssman-Lehman
Hemosiderosis, thalassemia	CHARGE
Holoprosencephaly	Laurence-Moon-Biedl
Central maxillary incisor	Leopard (multiple lentigenes)
Cleft lip/palate	Lowe
Septo-optic dysplasia	Martsoff
Idiopathic hypopituitarism	Prader-Willi
Irradiation	Rothmund-Thompson
Isolated FSH deficiency	Rud
Isolated gonadotropin deficiency	Tumors
(IHH)	ACTH-secreting
Kallmann syndrome	Astrocytoma
Laron dwarfism	Craniopharyngioma
Prolactinomas	Germinoma
Sickle cell disease	Growth hormone–secreting
Surgical resection	Optic glioma

ACTH, adrenocorticotropic hormone; CHARGE, coloboma of the eye, heart anomaly, choanal atresia, retardation, and genital and ear anomalies; FSH, follicle stimulating hormone; IHH, idiopathic hypogonadotropic hypogonadism.

Laboratory Testing

1. During infancy and after pubertal age, patients with hypogonadotropism have low baseline gonadotropin and sex steroid levels. Levels however may not be discernibly lower than normal prepubertal levels. Hence, the diagnosis based upon baseline levels alone should not be made unless the patient is otherwise disease free and until adequate time has passed to preclude pubertal delay. Since numerous assays are available for gonadotropins, care must be taken to be sure that normal ranges are specifically for the assay being used.
2. There *may* be subnormal responses of LH and FSH to GnRH, although these must be compared with normal responses of pubertal individuals of the same sex. Usually this response is not different from the normal response during childhood. This test does not consistently differentiate pubertal delay from permanent states of HH. Subnormal responses may be present among growth hormone deficiency. Among males, a diminished response of testosterone to hCG stimulation (<200 ng/dl) is characteristic of HH.
3. The laboratory confirmation of hypogonadotropism is the persistence of low or low-normal gonadotropin levels with concomitant low steroid levels (testosterone in males and estradiol in females) in a patient who has lack of progression of pubertal development without exogenous steroid therapy.

Key Laboratory Findings

- Persistent low gonadotropin levels

Radiologic Findings

1. Magnetic resonance imaging (MRI) assessment of the pituitary-hypothalamic region is indicated in patients being investigated for hypogonadotropism.
2. MRI findings among patients with Kallmann syndrome (not an obligatory part of a diagnostic assessment) include findings of hypoplasia of the rhinencephalon, absence or aplasia of the olfactory bulbs, and rudimentary or absent olfactory sulci.

Treatment

1. Replacement therapy routinely involves sex steroids at dosages appropriate for the age and sex of the patient. This therapy stimulates pubertal development and maintains appropriate adult male or female characteristics.
   a. Female patients should be begun on estrogen therapy with eventual addition of progesterone given in a cyclic fashion. Estrogen may be oral or transdermal; while some patients are treated with daily estrogen, most still receive cyclic medication. Oral preparations can be begun at the lowest available dosage (e.g., conjugated estrogens 0.3 mg daily or ethinyl estradiol 0.02 mg) and gradually increased

as required to attain full pubertal development. Transdermal estrogen can be begun by using only one patch a week rather than the twice-weekly regimen that is used for full replacement.
   (1) Maintenance dosages should be at the lowest level that provides for adult sexual status and regular menses.
   (2) Progesterone (e.g., medroxyprogesterone, 5 or 10 mg) should be given from 10 to 14 days each month. Combination estrogen-progesterone regimens can be used.
   (3) Initiation of therapy among patients with growth hormone deficiency or panhypopituitarism should be begun only after careful consideration of height and growth potential.
   b. Male patients receive testosterone beginning at pubertal age (12.5 to 14 years) unless delayed because of other growth disorders.
   (1) Testosterone can be given by injection or transdermally. There is limited experience with the initiation of pubertal development using the transdermal patch. To restrict the dosage, the patch may be worn only at night. Depot testosterone is commonly begun at 50 mg every 4 weeks in the prepubertal boy, the dosage being gradually increased over subsequent years to the full replacement dosage of 200 mg every 2 weeks or 300 mg every 3 weeks.
   (2) Testosterone therapy does not have a detrimental effect upon testicular potential to subsequently respond to gonadotropin therapy. Androgen therapy results in full male physical development, except testicular growth, and potential for sexual function.
2. To attempt fertility, gonadotropin injections or pulsatile GnRH infusion may be used. While such therapy could potentially also stimulate the gonad to secrete appropriate sex steroids, it is generally reserved for stimulation of germ cell maturation because of the expense and cumbersome nature of this regimen.

Key Treatment

- Sex steroids

Bibliography

Grumbach MM, Styne DM: Puberty: Ontogeny, neuroendocrinology, physiology, and disorders. *In* Wilson JD, Foster DW (eds): Williams Textbook of Endocrinology, 8th ed, Chapter 22. Philadelphia, WB Saunders, 1992, pp 1139–1221.

Lee PA, O'Dea L St L: Primary and secondary testicular insufficiency. Pediatr Clin North Am 1990;37:1359–1387.

Whitcomb RW, Crowley WF Jr: Male hypogonadotropic hypogonadism. Endocrinol Metab Clin North Am 1993;22:125–143.

Yen SS: Female hypogonadotropic hypogonadism. Endocrinol Metab Clin North Am 1993;22:29–58.

245 Premature Ovarian Failure

Susan Davis

Definition

Premature ovarian failure (POF) is cessation of normal reproductive ovarian function accompanied by elevated serum gonadotropin levels in a woman <40 years of age.

Epidemiology

This condition is present in 1 per cent of women, with the annual incidence rate in North American females aged 15 to 29 years being 10/100,000 person years.

Etiology

The majority of cases of POF are of unknown etiology (karyotypically normally spontaneous POF). The other recognized causes are listed in Table 245–1.

1. Of the chromosomal anomalies causing POF, Turner syndrome (45X) and 47 XXY are the most common. Abnormalities of the short arm of the X chromosome (Xp) generally do not affect ovarian function, whereas deletions or translocations of the Xq region do. Recent studies indicate that there is a gene (POF1) localized to either Xq21.3-q27 or within Xq26.1-q27 that is responsible for premature ovarian failure.

2. The link between POF and other autoimmune diseases (Table 245–2) is well established. Circulating autoantibodies to ovarian tissue are detected in only some patients, indicating that such antibodies are present only during a limited phase of the disease process. POF occurs in 10 to 20 per cent of women with Addison disease. The autoimmune response to both adrenal and gonadal antigens is believed to involve antibodies to the adrenal-specific 21-hydroxylase enzyme, the 17α-hydroxylase enzyme (adrenal and gonadal), and P450 side-chain cleavage enzyme.

3. The iatrogenic antigonadal effects of chemotherapy and radiotherapy vary according to the dose and agent administered. Younger patients are more resistant to the oophorotoxicity, possibly because of the presence of a greater number of immature ovarian follicles. Following cancer therapy, ovarian failure may be relatively immediate or may follow a more insidious course. The effect may also be transient with unpredictable spontaneous recovery occurring after months to years.

4. The resistant ovary syndrome is characterized by elevated FSH in the presence of ovarian follicles. Whether this condition is due to an autoimmune-induced defect of the FSH-receptor protein, deficient or absent follicular gonadotropin receptors, or a defect in postreceptor signaling is not known. This syndrome is rare, and fertility in affected women is low.

Clinical Findings

1. The age of presentation of POF depends on the timing and rapidity of follicular atresia. Patients with chromosomal defects usually present with primary amenorrhea, although individuals with mosaicism may have some functional gonadal tissue giving rise to varying degrees of sexual development and a brief history of menstruation culminating in secondary amenorrhea.

2. Primary amenorrhea is not associated with symptoms of estrogen deficiency, as exposure to postpubertal levels of estrogen and subsequent withdrawal appears to be necessary for the development of symptoms. The most common estrogen deficiency symptoms experienced include hot flashes, night sweats, fatigue, and mood changes including emotional liability, irritability, and depression.

3. Specific questioning should target symptoms of thyroid disease and adrenal insufficiency as well as a family history of POF.

4. A complete examination should include assessment of pubertal development, signs of underlying pathology including stigmata of Turner syndrome, short stature and other dysmorphic features of gonadal dysgenesis, and clinical features of thyroid and adrenal autoimmune disease.

 Key Clinical Finding

• Primary amenorrhea

5. When judged appropriate, a gynecologic pelvic examination should be performed; however, an ultrasound examination is usually more informative.

TABLE 245–1. CAUSES OF PREMATURE OVARIAN FAILURE

Chromosomal anomalies
Autoimmune
Metabolic (galactosemia, hemochromatosis)
Familial
Infectious (mumps)
Iatrogenic (chemotherapy, radiotherapy)
Resistant ovary syndrome
Karyotypically normal spontaneous premature ovarian failure

TABLE 245–2. AUTOIMMUNE DISEASES ASSOCIATED WITH PREMATURE OVARIAN FAILURE

Autoimmune thyroid disease
Adrenal insufficiency
Vitiligo
Myasthenia gravis
Systemic lupus erythematosus
Hypoparathyroidism
Autoimmune hemolytic anemia
Candidiasis
Idiopathic thrombocytopenic purpura
Diabetes mellitus

6. In the majority of cases, physical examination will be normal.

Laboratory Findings

1. FSH is consistently elevated in the clinical setting of amenorrhea. FSH should be measured on at least three occasions separated by about 1 month.
2. Chromosomal analysis is mandatory in all women under the age of 30 years, since the presence of a Y chromosome is associated with a substantial risk for the development of a gonadal cell germ tumor. Only 30 per cent of women with a Y chromosome manifest virilization.
3. An ovarian ultrasonographic assessment should be obtained to assess ovarian morphology and demonstrate any follicular activity.
4. Ovarian biopsy cannot be recommended.

Key Laboratory Findings

- FSH, LH, serum estradiol, measured on minimum of three occasions separated by 3 to 4 weeks
- Chromosomal evaluation
- Autoantibody screen
  Tissue-specific autoantibodies: thyroid, adrenal, ovarian, gastric parietal cell, ANF
- TSH, free T_4
- AM serum cortisol

Treatment

1. Patients with POF need to understand the nature and prognosis of their condition, since these women require long-term hormone replacement therapy (HRT), and patient compliance is dependent on the individual's understanding the ultimate health sequelae without estrogen replacement (Table 245–3).

TABLE 245–3.   TREATMENT OF PREMATURE OVARIAN FAILURE

Provision of appropriate patient information and counseling
Hormone replacement therapy
Genetic counseling as indicated
Assisted pregnancy by oocyte donation

Recommended Daily Maintenance Doses of Natural Estrogens

Conjugated equine estrogen (CEE) 1.25 mg
Estradiol valerate 3–4 mg
Piperazine estrone sulfate 2–5 mg
Transdermal estradiol 75–100 µg

2. Bilateral gonadectomy must be performed in all patients with a Y chromosome, as they are at significant risk for development of a gonadal cell tumor. Most of these malignant tumors occur before the age of 20 years and are virtually unknown after 30 years.
3. Estrogen replacement will relieve estrogen deficiency symptoms, restore and enhance sexuality, a facet so often neglected, and protect against the long-term risks of prolonged estrogen deficiency, namely osteoporosis and cardiovascular disease.

Key Treatment

- Provision of appropriate patient information and counseling
- Bilateral gonadectomy if Y chromosome present
- Hormone replacement therapy
- Genetic counseling as indicated
- Assisted pregnancy by oocyte donation

Bibliography

Baber R, Abdalla H, Studd J: The premature menopause. Prog Obstet Gynaecol 1991;9:209–226.

Davis SR, McCloud P, Strauss BJG, Burger HG: Testosterone enhances oestradiol's effects on postmenopausal bone density and sexuality. Maturitas 1995;21:227–236.

Eden JA: Menopause before 40—Premature but not always permanent. Aust NZ J Obstet Gynaecol 1993;33:201–203.

Khastgir G, Abdalla H, Studd JWW: The case against ovarian biopsy for the diagnosis of premature menopause. Br J Obstet Gynaecol 1994;101:96–98.

Volpé R: Autoimmune endocrinopathies: Aspects of pathogenesis and the role of immune assays in investigation and management. Clin Chem 1994;40:2132–2145.

246 Hirsutism and Hyperandrogenism in Adolescent Girls

Robert L. Rosenfield

Relation of Hirsutism, Acne, and Alopecia to Androgens

1. Role of androgens in pilosebaceous unit (PSU) development
   a. Androgens are a prerequisite for the development of PSUs in specific areas.
      (1) Sebaceous glands: normally most sensitive to androgen.
      (2) Sexual hairs: intermediate sensitivity to androgen, varying with location.
      (3) Scalp hair balding (in the genetically predisposed): least sensitive to androgen.
   b. Other factors are involved.
      (1) Sexual hair: growth hormone (GH) augments response to androgen.
      (2) Sebaceous gland: retinoids inhibit; catechols and GH stimulate.
2. Hyperandrogenism and PSU disorders
   a. PSU disorders (hirsutism, acne vulgaris, and pattern alopecia) begin at puberty as androgen levels rise.
      (1) Hirsutism is defined as excessive male-pattern hair growth in a woman.
      (2) Hirsutism must be differentiated from hypertrichosis, the situation in which intermediate vellus hair follicles predominate on "nonsexual" areas of the body. Hypertrichosis is not caused by sex hormone imbalance but appears with heredity, glucocorticoid excess, starvation, and certain medications.
   b. Acne, hirsutism, and alopecia are variably expressed manifestations of androgen excess. Severity of these signs is variable for a given degree of androgen excess.
      (1) Some females develop hirsutism or acne at normal levels of androgen (true idiopathic hirsutism or acne).
      (2) Some females have no skin manifestations of excess androgen (cryptic hyperandrogenemia).
      (3) Androgenetic alopecia may be the only skin manifestation of androgen excess.
   c. Hyperandrogenism is found in half of women with mild hirsutism and the vast majority of those with moderately severe hirsutism.
   d. Inflammatory acne that is unusual in its age of onset, severity, or persistence suggests hyperandrogenism. Think of androgens before prescribing Accutane!

Androgen Physiology

1. Biosynthesis of steroid hormones (Fig. 246–1)
2. Androgen production
   a. Production = secretion + peripheral conversion from secreted precursors.
   b. The ovaries and the adrenal glands normally contribute about equally to testosterone production in females.
      (1) Half of testosterone arises from direct secretion.
      (2) Remainder of testosterone arises from peripheral conversion of secreted precursors, primarily the 17-ketosteroids (17-KSs) androstenedione and dehydroepiandrosterone (DHEA). This occurs mainly in liver, skin, and adipose tissue.
3. Androgen secretion. As by-products of cortisol and estradiol secretion, androgen levels in females are not directly under negative feedback control by adrenocorticotropin (ACTH) or luteinizing hormone (LH).
   a. Adrenal androgens
      (1) *Adrenarche* is "the puberty of the adrenal gland" during which the adrenal cortex develops the ability to secrete 17-KSs in response to ACTH.
         (a) Although young children secrete cortisol as

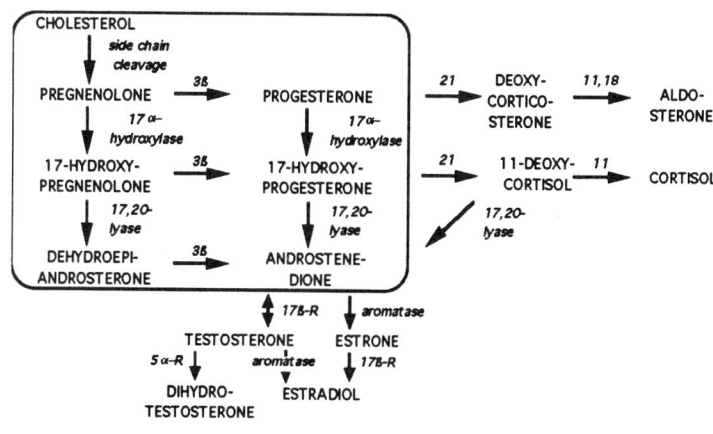

Figure 246–1 Outline of the major steroid biosynthetic pathways. The core pathway is outlined: The adrenal cortices utilize the pathways to the right; the gonads and certain peripheral tissues utilize the pathways below. The 17-ketosteroids are formed by cytochrome P450c17α, an enzyme with both 17-hydroxylase and 17,20-lyase activities. The steroidogenic enzymes are italicized: $3\beta = \Delta^5$-isomerase-3β-hydroxysteroid dehydrogenase; $17\beta = 17\beta$-reductase; 5α-$R = 5\alpha$-reductase; $21 = 21$-hydroxylase; $11,18 = 11\beta$-hydroxylase/aldosterone synthase. (Modified and reproduced with permission from Rosenfield RL, Lucky AW: Acne, hirsutism, and alopecia in adolescent girls. Endocrinol Metab Clin North Am 1993;22:507.)

well as adults, they form hardly any 17-KSs.

    (b) Adrenarche results from a change in the pattern of adrenal secretory response to ACTH.

    (c) DHEA-sulfate (DHEAS) becomes the predominant androgen secreted by the adrenal gland.

  (2) Adrenarche begins in mid-childhood and is not complete until adulthood.

  (3) The cause of adrenarche is unclear.

    (a) Adrenarche is not directly related to true puberty (*gonadarche*).

    (b) Adrenarche seems related to the development of the zona reticularis.

    (c) An adrenarche factor has been postulated that either controls the growth and differentiation of the zona reticularis, which possesses sulfokinase activity, or regulates steroidogenic enzymes, particularly by increasing the 17,20-lyase activity of P450c17α.

b. Ovarian androgens (Fig. 246–2)

  (1) Ovarian secretion of androgen increases during puberty.

    (a) LH stimulates thecal cells to secrete androgens.

    (b) Follicle-stimulating hormone (FSH) stimulates granulosa cell aromatase to form estradiol from androgen.

    (c) Insulin and insulin-like growth factors (IGFs) augment this secretion.

  (2) Androgens are a necessary evil in the ovary.

    (a) On one hand, they are obligate intermediates in estradiol biosynthesis.

    (b) On the other hand, in excess they hinder emergence of a dominant follicle.

  (3) Ovarian androgen secretion appears to be coordinated with estrogen formation by intraovarian mechanisms.

    (a) LH secretion is not efficiently regulated by sex steroids.

    (b) Androgen excess normally seems to be prevented by a down-regulation process whereby excessive LH stimulation leads to desensitization of the intraovarian responses to LH. A number of hormones and growth factors modulate theca cell responsiveness (see Fig. 246–2).

4. Plasma testosterone. This is the most important circulating androgen because of its relative potency directly at the target organ level and its plasma concentration.

  a. About 1 to 3 per cent of the total plasma testosterone is free and bioavailable.

  b. Sex hormone binding globulin (SHBG) is the major determinant of the distribution of testosterone to the plasma albumin and free fractions.

    (1) SHBG is increased by estrogens and hyperthyroidism.

    (2) SHBG is decreased by androgens and insulin.

  c. Because SHBG is typically low in hyperandrogenic and obese women, the plasma *free* testosterone concentration is more often elevated in women with hirsutism or acne than is the plasma *total* testosterone concentration.

5. Androgen action. The biologic activity of testosterone on target tissues is effected mainly by its conversion to dihydrotestosterone (DHT).

  a. 5α-reductase performs this conversion in both androgen target tissues and liver.

  b. PSU 5α-reductase is localized mainly to sebocytes and the dermal papilla of hair follicles.

  c. Androgens cause the prepubertal vellus follicles of target PSUs to either form a large terminal hair (sexual hair) or to develop instead a large sebaceous portion (sebaceous gland). Balding mainly results from terminal hairs of the scalp gradually miniaturizing to form adult vellus follicles in genetically prone individuals.

Causes of Hyperandrogenism

Androgen excess arises from abnormal ovarian or adrenal sources in most cases. It occasionally appears to be due to abnormalities in the peripheral formation of androgen, such as may occur in obesity or perhaps on a genetic basis.

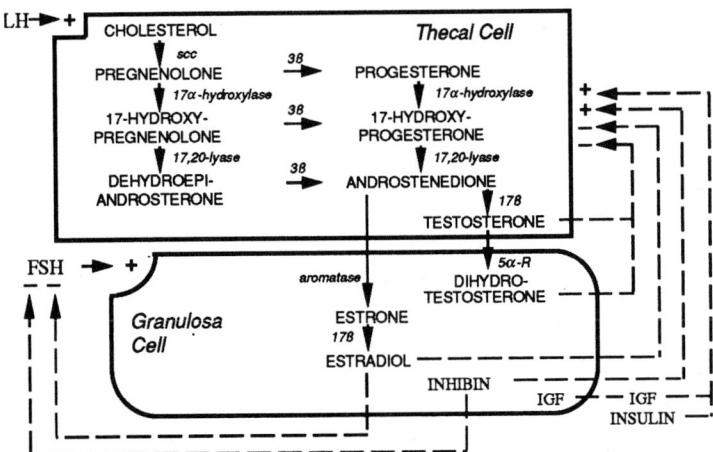

Figure 246–2 Organization and regulation of ovarian androgen and estrogen biosynthesis depicted according to the two-cell, two-gonadotropin model. LH stimulates androgen formation within theca-interstitial-stromal (thecal) cells via the steroidogenic pathway common to the gonads and adrenal glands. FSH regulates estradiol biosynthesis from androgen by granulosa cells. Long-loop negative feedback of estradiol and inhibin on gonadotropin secretion does not suppress LH at physiologic levels of estradiol. Androgen formation in response to LH appears to be modulated by intraovarian feedback at multiple levels, including 17-hydroxylase and 17,20-lyase. Androgen and estradiol inhibit (minus signs) and inhibin, insulin, and insulin-like growth factors (IGF) stimulate (plus signs) enzyme activities. Other peptides probably also modulate the steroidogenic response to LH. For abbreviations, see legend to Figure 246–1. (Reproduced with permission from Ehrmann DE, Rosenfield RL, Barnes RB: Polycystic ovary syndrome as functional ovarian hyperandrogenism. Endocr Rev 1995;16:322–353.)

TABLE 246-1. CAUSES OF HYPERANDROGENISM

1. Functional gonadal hyperandrogenism
   a. Polycystic ovary syndrome/functional ovarian hyperandrogenism
   b. Adrenal rests
   c. Hermaphroditism
   d. Chorionic gonadotropin–related
2. Functional adrenal hyperandrogenism
   a. Idiopathic
   b. Congenital adrenal hyperplasia
   c. Cushing disease
   d. Prolactin or growth hormone excess
   e. Abnormal cortisol action or metabolism
3. Peripheral androgen overproduction
   a. Obesity
   b. Other
4. Tumoral hyperandrogenism

Functional abnormalities are much more common than virilizing tumors (Table 246–1).

1. Functional ovarian hyperandrogenism
   a. Clinical picture. Polycystic ovary syndrome (PCOS) is the most common cause of hyperandrogenemia presenting in the perimenarcheal period. Symptoms typically begin during puberty. The classic (Stein-Leventhal) form is characterized clinically by amenorrhea, hirsutism, and obesity and test-wise by hyperandrogenemia, polycystic ovaries, and elevation of serum LH or the ratio of LH to FSH. Insulin resistance is frequent, and its manifestation as acanthosis nigricans may be prominent. Not all patients have all the symptoms or signs. Functional ovarian hyperandrogenism (FOH) due to a PCOS-type of ovarian dysfunction is found equally often with and without polycystic ovaries or gonadotropin abnormalities. Those not meeting the classic laboratory criteria are often mistakenly considered to have "idiopathic hirsutism."
   b. Etiology. The theories that abound are not mutually exclusive.
      (1) Hypothesis of PCOS as "hyperpuberty," due to an overshoot in the pubertal increase in LH levels and in pubertal insulin resistance.
      (2) Hypothesis of congenital disorders of pituitary-ovarian function first manifest at puberty.
         (a) Type A insulin resistance always is accompanied by PCOS.
         (b) Family and identical twin clusterings occasionally occur.
         (c) Congenital virilization (e.g., classic congenital adrenal hyperplasia) programs the neuroendocrine system to secrete excessive LH at puberty.
         (d) Onset after idiopathic true sexual precocity suggests tonic LH excess.
      (3) Complex trait hypothesis: PCOS/FOH results from a combination of two or more gene defects:
         (a) A polycystic ovary/premature male pattern baldness gene inherited as an autosomal dominant trait.

(b) A genetic predisposition to non–insulin-dependent diabetes mellitus.
   (c) A steroidogenic enzyme polymorphism.
   (d) As yet unidentified factors.
c. Pathophysiology of PCOS/FOH.
   (1) The central abnormality in PCOS/FOH seems to be intraovarian androgen excess. The excess androgen secretion results in the pilosebaceous manifestations. The disproportionately high intraovarian androgen concentration accounts for the premature commitment of follicles to atretic degeneration, the abnormal ovarian architecture, and anovulation.
   (2) Causes of PCOS/FOH.
      (a) Processes which interfere with follicular maturation are theoretical causes.
      (b) Extraovarian androgen excess (as in poorly controlled congenital adrenal hyperplasia).
      (c) Ovarian steroidogenic blocks (such as 3β-hydroxysteroid dehydrogenase, 17β-ketosteroid reductase, or aromatase deficiency).
      (d) Congenital severe (type A) insulin resistance.
      (e) Abnormal regulation (dysregulation) of ovarian androgen secretion.
   (3) Dysregulation of ovarian androgen secretion accounts for over 80 per cent of cases.
      (a) Characterized by hyperresponsiveness to LH of the entire steroidogenic cascade involved in thecal androgen secretion, most prominently of 17-hydroxyprogesterone as a manifestation of apparent P450c17 overactivity, and a tendency to hyperestrogenism.
      (b) Results from escape from the down-regulational processes that normally coordinate ovarian androgen and estrogen secretion (see Fig. 246–2).
   (4) Hyperinsulinemia is a prime candidate as the cause of the dysregulation. As a group, FOH patients are hyperinsulinemic, in association with a peculiar state of insulin resistance in which the ovaries and adipocytes function as if responding to the hyperinsulinemic state in spite of the resistance to the effects of insulin on skeletal glucose metabolism.
2. Functional adrenal hyperandrogenism (FAH)
   a. Clinical picture. Hyperandrogenism without menstrual abnormality suggests FAH.
   b. Etiology
      (1) Five to 10 per cent of adolescent FAH is secondary to mild (nonclassic) 21-hydroxylase deficiency congenital adrenal hyperplasia. Hyperprolactinemia, acromegaly, Cushing syndrome, and glucocorticoid resistance states are rare causes.
      (2) Idiopathic (primary) form: DHEA hyperresponses to ACTH are characteristic, occurring in 80 per cent of cases.

(a) Nonclassic 3β-hydroxysteroid dehydrogenase deficiency was commonly assumed to be the cause. However, deficiency of this enzyme is rarely proven by ovarian function testing or molecular genetic analysis.

(b) The pattern of 17-KS hyperresponsiveness to ACTH has suggested an exaggeration of adrenarche or dysregulation of adrenal steroidogenesis.

b. Pathophysiology. DHEA hyperresponsiveness to ACTH is accompanied in half the cases by androstenedione hyperresponsiveness. Dysregulation of adrenal steroidogenesis seems more likely than exaggerated adrenarche because:

(1) DHEAS is usually not elevated.

(2) Subtle cortisol hyperresponsiveness to ACTH often exists.

(3) Minor abnormalities of the pattern of cortisol metabolism are found.

(4) Evidence of increased adrenal P450c17 activity exists. This suggests that the intraglandular modulation of androgen secretion has gone awry in the adrenal just as in the ovary. According to this theory, dysregulation of androgen secretion takes place in the ovary alone (isolated PCOS or FOH), in the adrenal alone (isolated "exaggerated adrenarche"), or in both together.

3. Peripheral overproduction of androgen

a. Obesity can cause hyperandrogenemia and anovulation, mimicking PCOS. Testosterone formation from androstenedione is increased and SHBG is suppressed. Consequently, testosterone production is increased and the plasma free testosterone may be high. Estrone formation from androstenedione is increased. Insulin resistance occurs.

b. Idiopathic hyperandrogenemia. Ten per cent of women have hyperandrogenemia in which adrenal and ovarian function testing reveal no clear adrenal or ovarian source for the androgen excess. These cases may arise from increased peripheral conversion of inactive steroid precursors to active androgens.

4. Tumoral hyperandrogenism

a. Ovarian tumors. The most common virilizing ovarian tumor is arrhenoblastoma.

b. Adrenal virilizing tumors occur with increased frequency in multiple neoplasia syndromes and may be congenital and mimic classic congenital adrenal hyperplasia (CAH). They are sometimes associated with Cushing syndrome. If there is hypercortisolism, the growth spurt of androgen excess is blunted.

c. Clinical and laboratory findings

(1) Virilization may be suggested by key historical or physical features, such as rapid onset, voice change, clitoromegaly, genital ambiguity, cushingoid changes, or abdominal or pelvic masses.

(2) Very high testosterone levels (>200 ng/dl) should lead to consideration of tumor.

(3) Typically, ovarian virilizing tumors are characterized by a disproportionate elevation of plasma androstenedione relative to testosterone; mild elevation of urinary 17-KS secretion characteristically results.

(4) Very high DHEAS levels (>800 μg/dl) should lead to consideration of adrenal carcinoma as the cause.

(5) Some degree of ACTH dependency or gonadotropin dependency may be found in either ovarian or adrenal virilizing tumors.

Laboratory Findings

1. The first step in diagnosis is to document excessive plasma androgen levels. If the plasma concentrations of free testosterone and DHEAS are normal, virilizing states are ruled out.

2. Elevation of serum LH or the LH/FSH ratio has about 80 per cent specificity and 45 per cent sensitivity for the diagnosis of FOH.

3. Ultrasound examination of the abdomen: A polycystic or enlarged ovary has about 85 per cent specificity and 50 per cent sensitivity for the diagnosis of FOH.

4. Prolactin level in serum; measure because hyperandrogenism may be the only manifestation of excess prolactin.

5. The dexamethasone androgen-suppression test (Fig. 246–3) has about 95 per cent specificity and 85 per cent specificity for the diagnosis of FOH. Thus, it detects cases of FOH that lack the classic criteria for PCOS. In addition, it is a useful adjunct when the other tests are positive in that it rules out CAH and Cushing syndrome.

a. In our laboratory, dexamethasone suppressibility of androgens is considered normal in a postmenarcheal female if the free plasma testosterone is below 8 pg/ml and 17-hydroxyprogesterone below 50 ng/dl. Plasma DHEAS should fall to below the normal control range and cortisol to below 2 μg/dl as indices of normal adrenocortical suppression.

6. Normal suppression of androgens and cortisol usually indicate idiopathic FAH, but CAH must be ruled out. A 17-hydroxyprogesterone level over 1500 ng/dl 60 min after a standard dose of ACTH indicates 21-hydroxylase deficiency.

Key Laboratory Findings

- High plasma androgen levels
- High LH level
- Enlarged ovary (ultrasound)

Treatment

1. Weight reduction is indicated in obese hyperandrogenemic patients. This is sometimes successful in reversing hyperandrogenemia and menstrual disorders.

2. Endocrinologic treatment of hirsutism, acne, or alopecia is indicated if standard cosmetic or dermatologic

Figure 246–3 Algorithm for the differential diagnosis of hyperandrogenemia using a low-dose dexamethasone suppression test. After 4 days (longer in patients who are very obese or have relatively high DHEAS levels) of dexamethasone, subnormal suppression of plasma free testosterone points toward FOH/PCOS (if both DHEAS and cortisol suppress normally), tumor (if only cortisol suppresses normally), or Cushing syndrome (if cortisol does not suppress normally). Normal suppression of hyperandrogenemia is indication for ACTH testing. CAH = congenital adrenal hyperplasia; GH = growth hormone. (Modified with permission from Rosenfield RL, Lucky AW: Acne, hirsutism, and alopecia in adolescent girls. Endocrinol Metab Clin North Am 1993;22:507–532.)

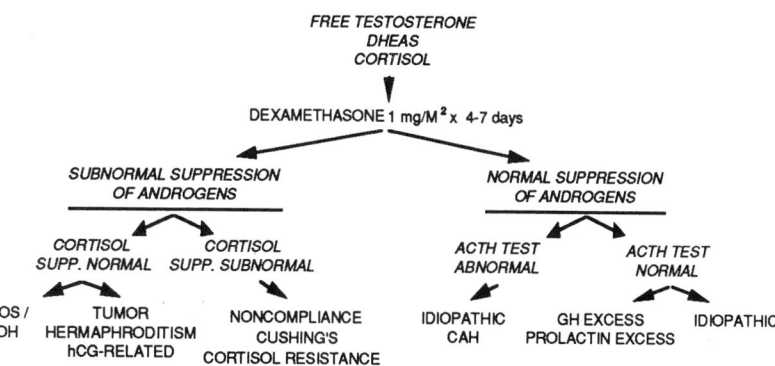

measures short of electrolysis, Accutane, or Rogaine are inadequate. Therapy is directed at interrupting androgen secretion or action. The maximal effect of pharmacologic agents on hirsutism takes 9 to 12 months due to the long growth cycles of sexual hair follicles, but acne should respond to effective treatment within two months.

a. Combination estrogen-progestin therapy will lower free testosterone levels in FOH by reducing serum gonadotropin levels, increasing SHBG levels, and modestly lowering DHEAS levels. This treatment arrests progression of hirsutism in FOH, but it will not to lead to substantial improvement. A new generation of oral contraceptives containing nonandrogenic progestins is now available, for example, norgestimate in Ortho-Cyclen.

b. Glucocorticoids are indicated to suppress androgens in patients whose major source of androgen is adrenal, particularly in CAH. They are occasionally beneficial in PCOS, but should not be used for more than 6 months if menses remain abnormal. The sequelae of glucocorticoid therapy can typically be minimized by using a modest bedtime dose (about 5 to 7.5 mg prednisone) to reduce adrenal androgen secretion selectively without causing adrenal atrophy. Significant glucocorticoid deficiency can be excluded by a rapid ACTH (cosyntropin) test performed 2 to 3 months after initiation of therapy.

c. Antiandrogens are required for reversal of hirsutism. Spironolactone has been shown to be effective and is probably the most potent and safe antiandrogen available in the United States. In doses of 50 to 100 mg bid, it is usually well tolerated; fatigue and hyperkalemia at higher doses may limit its usefulness. It is potentially teratogenic to fetal male genital development and may cause menstrual disturbance; therefore it should be prescribed with an oral contraceptive.

3. Progestin therapy alone is the method of choice for treating menstrual irregularity that is not associated with hirsutism or acne, particularly in adolescence. A full replacement dose of Provera (medroxyprogesterone acetate) is 10 mg at bedtime for 10 days a month. However, lower dosage for a shorter period in alternate months may be best in adolescents.

4. Infertility is a major cause for concern in PCOS cases, but it is not invariable. During adolescence, contraceptive regimens may be indicated. These patients can be reassured that they will probably ultimately be able to bear children with endocrinologic help. Ovulation can usually be induced with clomiphene, glucocorticoid, FSH, or pulsatile gonadotropin releasing hormone (GnRH) therapy under the care of an experienced reproductive endocrinologist. Ovarian surgery by laser cautery or wedge resection is a last resort, used only when pregnancy cannot be achieved by medical management.

Key Treatment

- Weight reduction
- Birth control pills
- Glucocorticoids
- Antiandrogens

Bibliography

Ehrmann DA, Rosenfield RL, Barnes RB: Polycystic ovary syndrome as functional ovarian hyperandrogenism due to dysregulation of androgen secretion. Endocr Rev 1995;16:322–353.

Ehrmann DA, Rosenfield RL, Barnes RB, et al: Detection of functional ovarian hyperandrogenism in women with androgen excess. N Engl J Med 1992;327:157–162.

Franks S: Polycystic ovary syndrome. N Engl J Med 1995;333:853–861.

Rosenfield RL, Deplewski D: Role of androgens in the developmental biology of the pilosebaceous unit. Am J Med 1995;98(Suppl 1A):80S–88S.

Rosenfield RL, Lucky AW: Acne, hirsutism, and alopecia in adolescent girls. Endocrinol Metab Clin North Am 1993;22:507–532.

247 Turner Syndrome

Barbara Lippe

Definition

Turner syndrome (TS) is the clinical manifestation, in a phenotypic female, of the consequences of complete or partial X chromosome monosomy.

Etiology

No obvious predisposing factors account for the X chromosome monosomy (45,X) or X chromosome mosaicism (45,X/46,XX). Structural deletions or rearrangements of the X such as the iso X duplication of the long arm (q), 46,X, i(Xq), with absence of the short arm (p), may be increased with advanced paternal age. More than 99 per cent of monosomic conceptuses do not reach term, ending in early or midtrimester fetal loss. Although this situation occurs more frequently in young mothers, affected liveborns do not. Molecular studies show the maternal X retained in 2/3 and the paternal in 1/3, approximating a frequency from random loss of either a maternal X or a paternal X or Y at meiosis or following fertilization. No obvious imprinting from maternal or paternal X is apparent.

Epidemiology

Its incidence is estimated to be 1 in 2000 live female births. This high frequency translates into a population, in the United States, of about 50,000 affected infants, children, and adult women.

Pathophysiology

1. X chromosome genes: Clinical and molecular investigators have attempted to map the findings in TS to specific areas on the X, but most "Turner genes" have yet to be identified.

   a. Short stature: Almost all patients have significant short stature. While the "stature gene" is probably on the pseudoautosomal region of Xp, another mechanism that impairs the growth of cells also pertains, and may be related, to the disruption that occurs whenever mitosis takes place with unequal chromosome pairing.

   b. Ovarian failure: The ovary develops normal architecture and a normal number of primordial follicles during the first trimester. What then occurs is accelerated follicular loss or atresia (much like in menopause) so by birth many, but not all, affected infants have few or no follicles. Several genes may be responsible for follicular integrity on both Xp and Xq. However, the process of accelerated atresia is multifactorial since some monosomic, 45,X individuals maintain function and are fertile.

   c. Other features: The search for other genes, including the cause of the lymphatic abnormalities, is under way. From the clinical perspective, however, it is currently impossible to predict phenotype from genotype except that the intrauterine edema, webbed neck phenotype (and coarctation of the aorta) are found almost exclusively in 45,X individuals and rarely in 46,X, i(Xq) girls.

2. Developmental mechanisms

   a. Lymphedema phenotype: When maldevelopment of the lymphatic channels occurs in the fetus the physical consequences are obvious.

      (1) Fetal nuchal hygroma in the first trimester distorts the head and neck and may cause hemodynamic abnormalities. If the fetus survives, the result may be:

         (a) Loose skin and then scarring "webbing" of the neck or pterygium colli

         (b) Deformities of the ears, the low hairline, and the flattened shieldlike appearance of the chest

         (c) Coarctation of the aorta

      (2) If the fetal edema is more generalized the result may be:

         (a) Swollen hands and feet at birth

         (b) Distortion of the nail bed and upturned or absent nails

   b. Skeletal disturbances:

      (1) Specific bones may be abnormal: Short metacarpals, small cervical vertebrae (making the neck short), distorted trochlear head of the ulna causing the increased carrying angle (cubitus valgus).

      (2) Generalized bone growth is more impaired along the longitudinal body axis so that the patients have a short square appearance.

      (3) Linear growth can be described in 4 phases but the pathophysiologic mechanisms in each phase are unknown.

         (a) In utero: mean birth length is -1 SD.

         (b) Infancy: growth rate is usually normal.

         (c) Childhood: velocity decreases so that height becomes progressively shorter.

         (d) Adolescence: the normal pubertal growth spurt is almost always absent (even in those girls who show signs of puberty).

   c. Other phenotypic and clinical abnormalities: Save for the relationship of coarctation of the aorta to intrauterine lymphedema, the pathophysiology of other organ system and clinical features of TS are unknown. However, many appear to be related to a disordered mesenchyme as manifested by:

      (1) Aortic dilation and risk of aortic rupture

      (2) Bicuspid aortic valve

      (3) Renal and renovascular abnormalities

(4) Mesenteric vascular abnormalities and potential for hemorrhage

Clinical Findings (Table 247–1)

1. Short stature: The most consistent clinical finding in girls and women with TS. Growth and velocity curves have been developed, and growth is very consistent along these curves from the age of 3 or 4 years. The mean adult height for U.S. women with TS is 143 cm and an individual's final height can be projected from the growth channel (on the TS chart) that is followed in childhood.
2. Pubertal absence: Premature ovarian failure occurs in 80 to 90 per cent. In those that begin puberty, about half stop at Tanner III breasts and half progress and go on to have menses.
3. Webbed neck: Present in only 20 to 30 per cent. These children are often recognized at birth (or earlier with fetal ultrasonography). Thus, relying on the presence of this feature during the evaluation of a short girl will not be helpful since all the "obvious" TS children will already have been identified.
4. Typical facial features: When present, a small jaw, short neck, high arched palate, low hairline, rotated or protruding ears, and occasional strabismus give some girls a recognizable facial appearance.
5. Skeletal features: In addition to short stature, square appearance, short metacarpals, and increased carrying angle, a bayonet (Madelung) deformity may develop at the wrist, the medial tibial and femoral condyles of the

TABLE 247–1. TURNER SYNDROME

COMMON CLINICAL FEATURES	INCIDENCE (%)
DISORDERED SKELETAL GROWTH	
Short stature	100
Abnormal upper/lower segment	97
Characteristic face—small jaw ± high arched palate	60
Cubitus valgus	47
Genu valgum	40
Short metacarpals	37
Scoliosis	12.5
CONSEQUENCES OF LYMPHATIC OBSTRUCTION	
Low hairline	42
Webbed neck/loose skin at neck	25
Edema of the hands and feet	22
Severe nail dysplasia	13
Coarctation of the aorta	<20
Rotated ears	common
GERM CELL—CHROMOSOMAL DEFECTS	
Complete gonadal failure	80–90
Infertility	>95
Gonadoblastoma	<5
METABOLIC, ENDOCRINE, AND OTHER FEATURES	
Otitis media	75
Hashimoto thyroiditis	35
Cardiovascular abnormalities	50
Renal abnormalities	39
Multiple pigmented nevi	26
Strabismus	17.5
Ptosis	11

knees may be protuberant, the metatarsals may be short, and the incidence of scoliosis may be increased.

6. Dermatologic features: Multiple pigmented nevi that increase in size with age or when growth hormone or estrogen are administered. However, malignant degeneration has not been reported. Vitiligo and psoriasis are reported to be increased, as is autoimmune alopecia areata.
7. Cardiovascular abnormalities: While coarctation of the aorta is classically described as the most common cardiac abnormality, its incidence is less than 20 per cent and lower than that of bicuspid aortic valve (up to 50 per cent). Coupled with the tendency toward dilation of the aortic root and aortic aneurysm or rupture, cardiovascular disorders are the single source of identifiable mortality that has been reported.
8. Renal abnormalities: Developmental abnormalities in location (horseshoe, pelvic, or absent kidney) as well as in structure (double collecting system, retrocaval ureter) or vascular supply (multiple vessels, aberrant vessels causing obstruction) are all increased but their contribution to morbidity is small.
9. Ear, nose, and throat abnormalities: Recurrent otitis media is the single most common source of illness. This is due to anatomic distortion, not immunologic dysfunction. Cholesteatomas and mastoiditis are common so that aggressive treatment of ear infections is recommended. However, adenoidectomy is not recommended because the high arched palate and small lower face cause a change in voice resonance that the adenoids buffer. In addition to conductive middle ear disease there is also a high incidence of gradually progressive sensory neural hearing loss.
10. Hashimoto thyroiditis: May reach 50 per cent as girls age (frequency also increased in their mothers and sisters). Thyroid failure requiring exogenous thyroxin is, therefore, common and repeated screening with thyroid-stimulating hormone (TSH, thyrotropin) determinations should be part of the long-term care of these girls and women.
11. Intestinal phlebectasia: Gastrointestinal (GI) bleeding due to abnormal vascular development in the bowel has been reported in increased frequency and should be considered if unknown bleeding occurs.
12. Psychosocial development: Intelligence is generally normal with the exception of those with a small ring X chromosome where the X inactivation site is believed lost. However, as a group TS women have areas of specific cognitive dysfunction, characterized by difficulties in spatiotemporal processing, perceptual stability, and visual-motor coordination.

Laboratory Findings

1. Chromosomal karyotype: The common karyotypes and approximate frequencies are:
   a. 45,X (50 per cent); 46,X, i(Xq) alone or with another cell line (16 per cent); 45,X/46,XX (12 per cent)
   b. Y chromosome: A Y chromosome is found in approximately 5 per cent of phenotypic females with features of TS, as 45,X/46,XY, 46,XX/46,XY or other mosaicisms, or as an identifiable peri-cen-

tromeric fragment or marker. These convey an increased risk for a gonadoblastoma. Thus, prophylactic gonadectomy in childhood is usually recommended. Not recommended, at this time, is a molecular search for Y DNA (when a Y or marker is not seen on karyotype) since the gonadoblastoma risk gene(s) have not yet been identified or mapped, and gonadoblastoma has not been reported in patients in whom only Y DNA but not a Y fragment was detected. Hysterectomy is not recommended since donor ovum transplantations have resulted in pregnancy in TS women and that option should be left available.

2. Gonadotropins: Since the hypothalamic-pituitary axis responds to the failed ovary (in infancy and again at the expected time of puberty, but not during childhood) by increasing follicle-stimulating hormone (FSH) and luteinizing hormone (LH), measurements of these hormones at these times can indicate the functional status of the ovary.

3. Thyroid function studies: Since Hashimoto thyroiditis is frequent, antithyroid antibodies may be positive and, if thyroid failure is incipient, the TSH may be elevated. Hyperthyroidism may also occur and is said to be more frequent in girls with the 46,X, i(Xq) karyotype.

4. Oral glucose tolerance: Insulin resistance may be present and exaggerated by obesity, progesterone, or androgen. Type II diabetes may develop in middle age; Type I diabetes is not increased.

Key Laboratory Findings

- Karyotype
- Thyroid function tests

Radiographic Changes

1. Skeleton: Bones may have an osteoporotic radiologic appearance that is secondary to disordered trabecular organization (not true osteoporosis). If a left hand and wrist radiograph is taken for bone age (in a short girl before the diagnosis of TS is made), the presence of short metacarpals or osteoporotic "fish net" carpals may suggest the diagnosis. Bone age should not be used for height prediction because there are no accurate prediction methods for TS. Spine films may be needed if scoliosis is suspected. Protuberant medial tibial and femoral condyles sometimes cause knee pain.

2. Cardiac: Ultrasonography to evaluate the aortic valve and root. In the absence of risk factors for aortic dilation (hypertension, repaired coarctation), ultrasonography should probably be repeated at 5-year intervals.

3. Renal: Ultrasonography can be used, initially, to evaluate for congenital renal abnormalities. In the absence of serious malformations or occurrence of urinary tract infection, ultrasonography need not be repeated.

4. Pelvic ultrasonography: To evaluate size of ovaries if ovarian function is suspected. May be used to determine presence of an adnexal mass if gonadoblastoma is suspected. However, relying on this for following the girl

with a Y in her karyotype (rather than prophylactic gonadectomy) is not recommended.

Treatment

1. Hormone replacement therapies
   a. Estrogen/progesterone replacement therapy:
      (1) Timing: Start treatment for feminization (not growth promotion) at an age-appropriate time if height at that time is approaching an acceptable goal, since epiphyseal closure will result rapidly (1 to 2 years) without a concomitant growth spurt and height gains following estrogen will be modest.
      (2) Recommended dosage: Initial dose of 0.3 mg Premarin (or synthetic equivalent) to begin breast development, followed in 3 to 6 months by 0.625 mg for 3 to 6 months, followed by an adult replacement dose of 0.9 to 1.25 mg or equivalent. At this time, institute cyclic therapy with added progesterone.
      (3) Regimens: If menses are desired (they usually are by adolescent females) one can add 10 mg of medroxyprogesterone acetate (Provera) for 12 days of the cycle (example: days 11 to 23) with an "off week" for both drugs. Another way is to use a "low dose" oral contraceptive, recognizing that the current preparations may be higher than needed for replacement therapy. If menses are not desired, one can use Provera continuously, at a dose of 2.5 mg/day in conjunction with the estrogen, without any "off" weeks. Breakthrough bleeding may occur initially, but eventually endometrial atrophy will be sufficient to avoid menses.
   b. Thyroid replacement therapy: If hypothyroidism develops, oral thyroxin replacement therapy should be initiated in a dose sufficient to suppress TSH to normal (but not undetectable) range, and therapy should be considered lifelong.

2. Syndrome-specific adjunctive therapy
   Growth promotion therapy:
   a. Growth hormone (GH) therapy: Data now show that while TS individuals are not generally GH deficient (and should not be tested for GH deficiency unless their growth velocity is abnormal for a TS individual), long-term treatment with GH will accelerate growth and increase final height. Following 6 or more years of therapy and in the absence of spontaneous puberty or early estrogen treatment, height may be increased by a mean of 8 to 10 cm. The dose of GH employed, 0.375 mg/kg week, given divided in 6 to 7 daily injections, requires a long-term commitment to a program which should not be taken lightly.
   b. Anabolic hormone therapy with or without GH: Low-dose anabolic steroids (oxandrolone or fluoxymesterone) have been used to promote growth acceleration in TS for several decades. However, data fail to show a significant effect on final height. When used in conjunction with GH, height acceleration is slightly increased over GH alone and there

may be a 1 to 2 cm increase in final height over GH alone. When employed alone or with GH the dose is 0.05 to 0.0625 mg/kg/day.

Key Treatment

• Estrogen/progesterone replacement

Prevention

Chorionic villus sampling or amniocentesis may detect aneuploidy that is present only in the membranes and may overdiagnose an X chromosomal disorder. In addition, the lack of risk factors, the heterogeneity of the syndrome and the absence of mental retardation makes "prevention" unlikely. Fetal ultrasonography can be reassuring if hygroma is not present, since most physical stigmata will then be absent. Early detection and treatment of the common medical problems will prevent much of the associated morbidity. Attention to early school performance with intervention strategies in areas where difficulties are detected help with learning. Early treatment of growth failure (see previously) will prevent the consequences of marked differences in stature between patient and peers and may help socialization. Taller stature at the time of expected puberty permits early introduction of estrogen for feminization.

Bibliography

Lippe BM: Turner syndrome. *In* Sperling M (ed): Clinical Pediatric Endocrinology and Metabolism, 3rd ed. Philadelphia, WB Saunders, 1996, pp 387–421.

Rosenfeld RG, Frane J, Attie KM, et al: Six-year results of a randomized, prospective trial of human growth hormone and oxandrolone in Turner syndrome. J Pediatr 1992;121:49–55.

Rosenfeld RG, Tesch L-G, Rodriguez-Rigau LJ, et al: Recommendations for diagnosis, treatment, and management of individuals with Turner syndrome. The Endocrinologist 1994;4:351–358.

Stratakis CA, Rennert OM: Turner syndrome: Molecular and cytogenetic, dysmorphology, endocrine, and other clinical manifestations and their management. The Endocrinologist 1994;4:442–453.

248 Micropenis (Hypogenitalism)

Peter Lee

Definition

1. A micropenis is an anatomically normal penis which is abnormally small. Size is determined by stretched length; a micropenis being more than 2.5 SD below mean length for stage of development. For the newborn male, a micropenis is a penis less than 1.9 cm stretched or erect length (Table 248–1). Normal length of the newborn male depends upon gestational stage. A micropenis has a meatus at the tip of the glans without hypospadias.

2. While *micropenis* is a descriptive term, its meaning is clearly apparent, carrying a stigma in a society too much preoccupied with genital size. Perhaps a diagnostic term such as *hypogenitalism* would be more appropriate.

3. A micropenis must be differentiated from a "buried penis," a penis containing adequate corpora that is largely held beneath the surface of the surrounding skin because of inadequate skin along the shaft. This rare problem may be congenital or secondary to too vigorous trimming of the skin on the penis during circumcision.

4. Penile agenesis is the absence of the organ, rather than a small, normally formed structure.

TABLE 248–1. STRETCHED PENIS LENGTH (CM) AMONG MALES

AGE	MEAN + SD	− 2.5 SD
Birth		
30 weeks' gestation	2.7 ± 0.5	1.5
34 weeks' gestation	3.0 ± 0.4	2.0
Term	3.5 ± 0.4	2.5
0–5 months	3.8 ± 0.8	1.8
6–11 months	4.1 ± 0.8	2.1
1–3 years	4.8 ± 0.8	2.8
3–5 years	5.5 ± 1.0	3.0
5–7 years	6.0 ± 0.9	3.8
7–9 years	6.3 ± 1.0	3.8
9–11 years	6.3 ± 1.0	3.8
Adult*		
20–25 years	13.3 ± 1.6	9.3
17–60 years	15.7 ± 1.9	11.0
18–63 years	16.7 ± 1.9	12.0

SD = standard deviation.
*Composite from literature.

Etiology

A micropenis results from inadequate androgen effect during the last half of gestational life during which marked penile growth occurs. Inadequate androgen (testosterone) effect may result from:

1. Deficient testosterone secretion by testicular Leydig cells (primary testicular failure, Leydig cell dysgenesis/agenesis).

2. Deficient gonadotropin (luteinizing hormone [LH]) stimulation of Leydig cell testosterone production (hypogonadotropism/hypothalamic-pituitary deficiency/dysfunction). Gonadotropin deficiency may be accompanied by

other anterior pituitary trophic hormone deficiencies including growth hormone, thyroid-stimulating hormone (TSH, thyrotropin), and adrenocorticotropic hormone (ACTH).

3. Defect in androgen action; androgen receptor or postreceptor defects (partial androgen insensitivity syndrome).

4. Idiopathic; unexplained in patient with normal hypothalamic-pituitary-testicular axis and normal androgen receptor–mediated actions. Micropenis may occur in association with multiple congenital anomalies, including some syndromes, without apparent etiology other than evidence of significant in utero insult (Table 248–2).

5. Etiologic classification as partial androgen insensitivity is extremely rare, with primary hypogonadism and hypogonadotropism being minority categories. Most patients are considered idiopathic, some of these representing the low extreme of normal biologic variation.

Pathophysiology

1. While normal differentiation of the primordial genital structures into a normally formed penis requires adequate testosterone during the first trimester of fetal life, growth to a normal size requires adequate levels during the third trimester. The former can occur in the absence of a functioning hypothalamic-pituitary-testis unit. However, inadequate growth appears to be a result of deficient testosterone stimulation because of inadequate LH stimulation, insufficient testosterone synthesis, or decreased androgen action during the last half of fetal life.

2. Insufficient androgen or androgen action during the first trimester results in hypospadias, which may be accompanied by inadequate penis size. However, since diagnostic and therapeutic considerations are different, a small, incompletely differentiated penis is properly termed a microphallus, not a micropenis. The etiology of microphallus includes many additional conditions that present with genital ambiguity, such as enzyme deficiencies of steroid synthesis and gonadal and chromosomal defects such as mixed gonadal dysgenesis. It may occur in association with cryptorchidism.

3. Postnatal penile growth normally occurs as a result of

testosterone stimulation related to the increased activity of the hypothalamic-pituitary axis during the neonatal period. This, in addition to androgen stimulation in late gestation, may be lacking with micropenis. After the penile growth of early childhood up to age 4 or 5 years, there is minimal further growth until the onset of puberty. Therefore, the penis of a prepubertal boy of 10 or 11 years is relatively smaller in proportion to the rest of his body than at 5 years of age.

Clinical Findings

1. Accurate measurement verifies the diagnosis:

   a. Care must be made to carefully measure the length of the penis dorsally, depressing the suprapubic subcutaneous tissue and measuring to the tip of the glans. The glans should be gripped and pulled taut enough to cause discomfort but not pain. The dorsal surface of the penis should be pulled firmly against a rigid ruler for measurement. If the penis is uncircumcised, the foreskin should be retracted if possible.

   b. Stretched penile length should correlate with, but may underestimate, erect length. Since a spontaneous erection commonly occurs during examination of an infant, when this occurs, the measured dorsal length should be used.

   c. Reproducible measurements occur only after consistent technique involving actual stretching. The greatest length measurable is the most accurate and the best approximation of erect length (see Table 248–1).

2. A micropenis may not be associated with any other clinical findings, although findings including small testes, hypoplastic scrotum, midline facial defects, and anosmia may provide clues concerning etiology; the latter two suggest gonadotropin deficiency.

3. The two most frequent ages of referrals concerning inadequate penis size are:

   a. Neonatal and infancy (gestational age must be considered).

   b. Just prior to puberty. Since there is little penile growth after age 5 years until the onset of puberty, adequacy of penis size may be questioned at this age, especially among large, heavy boys with abundant peripubertal fat.

4. A newborn male with a micropenis and hypoglycemia should be evaluated for congenital panhypopituitarism. These findings suggest gonadotropin, ACTH, and growth hormone deficiency.

5. When a micropenis is diagnosed, penis size should be reassessed after androgen stimulation to verify androgen responsiveness.

TABLE 248–2. MICROPENIS-ASSOCIATED SYNDROMES BY DIAGNOSTIC CATEGORY

PRIMARY HYPOGONADISM	IDIOPATHIC
Klinefelter and multiple X syndromes	Carpenter
Laurence-Moon-Biedl	CHARGE
Robinow syndrome	Cornelia de Lange
HYPOGONADOTROPISM	Down
	Fanconi pancytopenia
Anencephaly	Hallerman-Streiff
Growth hormone deficiency	Long-arm 18 deletion
Kallmann	Noonan
Laron	Smith-Lemli-Opitz
Laurence-Moon-Biedl	Triploidy
Prader-Willi	Williams
Rud	
Septo-optic dysplasia	

CHARGE = coloboma of the eye, heart anomaly, choanal atresia, retardation, genital and ear anomalies.

Key Clinical Findings

• Very small penis

Laboratory Findings

1. Hormone levels during infancy and after the onset of puberty may lead to etiologic classification. Unstimulated levels during childhood are generally not helpful.

2. The basis of the etiologic classification during infancy is the profile of LH, follicle-stimulating hormone (FSH), and testosterone.

   a. Primary hypogonadism: high LH and FSH; low T. Among patients with Leydig cell deficiency, circulating levels of LH and FSH are elevated and testosterone (T) levels are low, diagnostic of primary testicular failure (primary hypogonadism).

   b. Hypogonadotropic hypogonadism: low LH, FSH, and T. With gonadotropin deficiency (hypothalamic-pituitary dysfunction or hypogonadotropic hypogonadism), LH, FSH, and T values are all low.

   c. Partial androgen insensitivity: high LH, FSH, and T. Defects of androgen action (partial androgen insufficiency) are reflected in androgen unresponsiveness. This is the only clinical situation in which LH, FSH, and T are all elevated. This profile in a newborn is diagnostic of androgen insensitivity.

   d. Idiopathic: normal LH, FSH, and T for age. These hormone levels are normal for age among the idiopathic group.

3. Human chorionic gonadotropin (hCG) stimulation testing followed within 24 hours with a measurement of the testosterone levels may be useful to document testicular function (ability of Leydig cells to respond to gonadotropin stimulation). hCG can be given daily or every other day. A reasonable regimen for infancy is 1000 units daily for 5 days. Dosage should not exceed 3000 units/M² per injection. While it has been suggested that a response above 200 ng/dl is normal, the basis for this was established upon a small number of subjects and should be further studied. A response into the adult range (> 285 ng/dl) is more confirming. hCG stimulation testing is not necessary and superfluous in the patient who already has elevated LH levels.

4. Binding of androgen receptor and mutations of the androgen receptor gene may not be helpful in ruling out partial androgen insensitivity.

5. A karyotype is not indicated in an otherwise normally developed boy with normal hormonal levels for age. It should be done if elevated gonadotropins, small testes, or other evidence suggest Klinefelter syndrome or to determine if other stigmata are associated with known syndromes with chromosomal abnormalities.

Key Laboratory Tests

- Gonadotropin and testosterone levels during infancy or after puberty

Treatment

1. The initial treatment of a male with a micropenis is also a diagnostic test. A trial with testosterone is used to verify androgen responsiveness with penile growth while stimulating growth to a more appropriate size for age. While verifying that the etiology is not androgen insensitivity, this demonstrates to parents as well as health professionals that the penis is capable of response to androgen. Generally 25 mg of depot testosterone will cause a dramatic response. The patient should be reexamined 2 to 4 weeks after the first injection to document growth.

2. Gender reassignment should be reserved for the exceptional situation in which partial androgen insensitivity has been diagnosed (in infancy, elevated LH, FSH, and T levels, lack of penile growth after exogenous testosterone with variable results of androgen binding studies) or in which there is no discernible erectile tissue. Reassignment in any other situation in which a normally formed but small penis is present with a fully formed scrotum containing bilateral testes is an extreme resolution for this situation. It should be undertaken only after extensive evaluation of all physical, physiologic, and psychologic factors involving the parents, and then only with the parents' unwavering endorsement. A team involving the parents; an endocrinologist; urologist; and psychologist, psychiatrist, or social worker should thoroughly evaluate and discuss the entire situation including the child's potential for fertility, sexual function, and adequate endogenous hormone secretion. If female assignment becomes an option, the extent and outcome of such surgical construction and hormone replacement therapy must be considered.

3. The child with a small penis should be seen at intervals throughout childhood to assess physical development including penile growth and psychosexual outlook. The penis may decrease in size during long intervals after androgen stimulation during childhood years. If the penis is below the size range for age, or if the child has developed excessive concern about the size of his penis, androgen (testosterone cypionate or enanthate 25 mg IM) can be given at carefully spaced intervals to stimulate growth. Although such injection can be given several months in succession, it is generally satisfactory to give only one injection and repeat only if response has not been reasonable. Such single injections can be repeated on 3 or 4 occasions throughout the childhood years without untoward skeletal age or physical effects. If numerous injections are given in succession or totally, there is a risk of accelerating growth rate, skeletal age, and early pubertal changes. There is no evidence that stimulated penile growth during childhood resulting in greater penile size for age ultimately results in a larger penis after puberty.

Key Treatment

- Testosterone

Prevention

1. Since micropenis is a congenital problem, there are no specific preventive measures. There is increased risk among kindred with Kallmann syndrome or androgen insensitivity.

2. Appropriate, timely counseling may be indicated to prevent negative psychosocial and psychosexual sequelae of hypogenitalism. Because human society has placed such an emphasis upon male genital size, counseling of parents and age-appropriate counseling of the patient should help form the perception that penis size is not a rational basis for body image, self-esteem, and a healthy sexual adjustment.

Bibliography

Lee PA: Micropenis. *In* Forest MG (ed): Androgens in Childhood. Pediatr Adolesc Endocrinol, Vol 19. Basel, Karger, pp 149–154.

Migeon CJ, Berkovitz GD, Brown TR: Sexual differentiation and ambiguity. *In* Kappy MS, Blizzard RM, Migeon CJ (eds): The Diagnosis and Treatment of Endocrine Disorders in Childhood and Adolescence, 4th ed, Chapter 12. Springfield, Charles C Thomas, pp 659–662.

249 Undescended Testes

Edward O. Reiter and *Paul H. Saenger*

Definition

This term describes any testis occupying an extrascrotal position. Cryptorchidism occurs at a frequency of 0.8 per cent, thus being the most common disorder of male sexual differentiation. The two most important sequelae are infertility and testicular neoplasia.

Etiology

1. The cause is abnormalities in the bihormonal regulation of testicular descent, which includes müllerian inhibitory substance and testicular androgens. The importance of androgens in this process is demonstrated by the association of cryptorchidism with multiple syndromes of diminished androgen action (ambiguous genitalia).
2. Anatomic and mechanical abnormalities, especially of the processus vaginalis and epididymis, may cause incomplete testicular descent.
3. Possible immunogenetic mechanisms may operate because of overrepresentation of certain HLA types in patients with cryptorchidism.

Epidemiology

Approximately 3 to 4 per cent of infant boys have undescended testes at birth, the number being as high as 30 per cent in preterm infants. This figure falls to 1.8 per cent by 1 month of life and the adult frequency of 0.8 per cent by the middle of the first year. In approximately 10 per cent of patients, both testes are undescended; the testes are not palpable (see below) in 20 per cent; unilateral absence of testes occurs in 4 per cent, with anorchia in less than 1 per cent.

Clinical Findings

1. Cryptorchid testes are classified as being palpable or nonpalpable. Palpable undescended testes may be retractile, ectopic, or placed within the inguinal canal. Impalpable testes may be in the inguinal canal, in the abdomen, or totally absent.
2. Retractile testes are not truly undescended but ones that withdraw into a position above the scrotum because of a hyperactive cremasteric reflex. They may be manoeuv-

ered at maturation, and fertility of retractile testes is normal.
3. Ectopic testes, which account for about 20 per cent of cryptorchid gonads, have descended into areas outside the usual inguinal scrotal pathway.
4. Careful family history and physical examination. Inherited syndromes must be sought. Examination with the child seated in a cross-legged position permits gentle manual examination as the cremasteric reflex is inhibited.

Key Clinical Findings

- Nonpalpable or ectopic testes

Laboratory Findings

1. Necessary in cases of bilateral cryptorchidism with impalpable testes.
2. Extremely high levels of LH and FSH strongly suggest an absence of steroid-producing and germinal gonadal tissue. In patients with indeterminate levels of gonadotropins, an HCG test is performed (1500 U IM × 3 days for children <2 years; a post-HCG measurement of serum testosterone is obtained within 24 hours after the last HCG injection: if testicular tissue is present, serum testosterone should rise to >100 ng/dl).
3. Imaging techniques, such as ultrasonography and magnetic resonance imaging, though increasingly used, have not been shown to have high enough sensitivity. Ultimately, laparoscopy and operative exploration are needed to seek the impalpable testis.

Sequelae of Undescended Testes

1. *Infertility*—The number of spermatogonia in undescended testes begins to decline early in the second year of life. Bilateral intraabdominal testes beyond the midchildhood years is associated with marked oligospermia and, almost assuredly, infertility.
2. *Risk of neoplasia*—There is an increased risk of cancer in cryptorchid testes, especially if left in place for >6 years. The frequency of testicular cancer is 3- to 10-fold

greater in individuals with a history of cryptorchidism. Twenty per cent of tumors in unilateral cryptorchidism, however, are in the normally descended testis.

Management

1. The primary aim is to improve potential fertility and to diminish the risk of subsequent development of gonadal neoplasms. A secondary goal is a beneficial effect on psychosexual development.
2. Operative treatment is indicated for the truly cryptorchid testis, palpable or nonpalpable; such intervention is not recommended for retractile testes that can be mobilized into the scrotum and remain there without tension.
3. Surgical treatment
   a. Should be undertaken early in the second year of life, because the chance of spontaneous descent is low after the first 12 months. Furthermore, diminished spermatogenesis is documented during the second year of life. The fact that operative intervention before age 2 years improves spermatogenesis or fertility, however, has not been unequivocally documented.
   b. Correction of undescended testes does not clearly diminish the incidence of testicular carcinoma. Nonetheless, a scrotal testis permits self-examination and the ease of obtaining testicular biopsy.
   c. *Operative intervention*—In the young patients, surgical treatment should be provided early in the second year of life; in the hands of experienced pediatric surgeons or urologists, it is successful in 90 per cent of all cases and in >95 per cent of cases with palpable testes. In almost all cases, day-stay surgery is the accepted manner of care. Operative care is more difficult in patients with impalpable intraabdominal testes, with as many as 10 per cent of cases associated with complications such as vascular injury, testicular atrophy, or, most commonly, retraction. Secondary ascent of testes after surgical intervention is sometimes seen.
4. *Hormonal treatment*
   a. As surgical treatment does carry a small, but definite

morbidity, hormonal attempts at inducing testicular descent have been attempted. HCG or GnRH administration have both been tried, with varying degrees of success. Wide discrepancies in apparent efficacy are probably due to inclusion in different studies of patients who have retractile testes that descend readily following hormonal administration. Impalpable testes generally are not benefited by hormonal treatment. Treatment failures are frequent, and retraction will occur in half of the testes that have descended. Thus, at best, there may be 5 to 10 per cent success in truly undescended testes.
   b. In older prepubertal boys with cryptorchidism, HCG administration may be useful in palpable testes. In postpubertal individuals, hormonal therapy is inappropriate, and surgical care is necessary. Orchiectomy is the appropriate therapy in older boys in whom the testes cannot be fully brought into the scrotum, as the risk of not being able to appropriately screen for neoplasm is a serious concern.
5. Testicular biopsy is not recommended as a routine measure during orchidopexy in prepubertal boys. In pubertal boys or adults, bilateral testicular biopsy should be undertaken as carcinoma in situ can be detected. Continued careful self-examination is also recommended postoperatively, especially in those individuals who have had surgery after 6 years of age.

Key Treatment

- Surgery

Bibliography

Cilento BG, Najjar SS, Atala A: Cryptorchidism and testicular torsion. 1993;40:1133–1149.

Lee PA: Fertility in cryptorchidism: Does treatment make a difference? Endocrinol Metab Clin North Am 1993;244:479–490.

Saenger P, Reiter EO: Management of cryptorchidism. Trends Endocrinol Metab 1992;3:249–253.

250 Hypospadias

Stanley J. Kogan

Definition

Hypospadias is derived from the Greek *hypo*, meaning "under" and *spadon*, meaning "opening" or "rent." The combination of these indicates a congenital abnormality of the penis where the urethral opening is located on the ventral surface of the shaft short of its normal terminal position,

and the glans fails to fuse ventrally, forming a flattened open surface.

Etiology

1. In most cases, hypospadias cannot be attributed to a specific identifiable inciting factor and is considered to

be *multifactorial* in origin. Prematurity reportedly occurs in hypospadiacs four times as frequently as in controls. No differences in maternal age, number of previous pregnancies or stillborn fetuses, twinning, Rh incompatibility, or blood types were noted in one study. Of interest though, fathers of index patients had a higher incidence of testicular abnormalities (postpubertal unilateral cryptorchidism, varicocele, testis atrophy). Delayed maternal age at menarche has been reported.

2. The most attractive etiologic theories relate to endocrine abnormalities occuring during formation of the penis. Since the penis undergoes completion of morphogenesis by the end of the first trimester and this process is androgen-dependent, any endocrinologic abnormalities (endogenous or exogenous) occurring during this time could result in hypospadias formation. Administration of progestins to animals during the first trimester can cause experimental hypospadias, and it has also been incriminated in human hypospadias, such as when given for pregnancy stabilization in cases of threatened abortion.

3. Whereas some of these theories are based on speculation rather than fact, observation indicates that there is a clear-cut genetic aspect associated with hypospadias. Hypospadias has also been reported in three successive generations, suggesting that familial isolated hypospadias can be inherited as a sex-linked autosomal dominant (or Y-linked) gene, and hypospadias is also associated with some syndromes of mendelian inheritance.

Epidemiology

Hypospadias is a common urologic condition, cited in various series as occurring in between 0.2 and 8.2 per 1000 (i.e., 1 in 125 male births). True geographic differences in frequency may exist. In the United States, hypospadias occurs less commonly in blacks.

Pathophysiology

1. Hypospadias appears to result from decreased androgenization during a critical period of embryogenesis, that is, during the first trimester when penile morphogenesis is occurring.

2. Normally, endogenous testosterone is converted locally (by 5α-reductase) in genital tissues to dihydrotestosterone, the locally active hormone that first is involved with proper penile formation and later with growth.

3. Some abnormalities identified include poor testosterone production after hCG stimulation, diminished androgen receptor levels in genital tissues, and defective conversion of testosterone to dihydrotestosterone.

4. An increased frequency (14% of hypospadiac boys) of finding a prostatic utricle or vagina masculinis, an outpouching of the posterior urethra encountered in some boys with androgen insufficiency or intersexuality, also substantiates defective androgenization as an important component of the pathophysiology of this condition.

Clinical Findings

Hypospadias is usually diagnosed at the initial birth examination of the genitalia. Rarely, it may come to attention only at the time of circumcision when the megameatus variety is exposed as the foreskin is removed.

1. Classification
   a. Hypospadias is best classified according to the loca-
   tion of the urethral meatus (i.e., glanular and coronal; distal, mid or proximal penile; penoscrotal, scrotal, perineal) and the degree of chordee that is present (mild, moderate, or severe).
   b. Distal hypospadias accounts for about three quarters of all cases, with midpenile and more proximal locations each accounting for 10 to 15 per cent each.

2. Physical findings. The diagnosis is made by evaluating three key components:
   a. The location of the urethral meatus.
   b. Degree of bend to the penile shaft.
   c. Presence of an incomplete ventral foreskin.
   d. The hypospadiac urethral meatus may be identified anywhere along the ventral shaft.
   e. Varying degrees of chordee (bend) may be present. The ventral foreskin is usually absent, and the ventral skin may be thinned and deficient. Hypospadias may exist without chordee (i.e., straight penile shaft), and chordee may exist without hypospadias (penis is bent with urethral opening at the normal terminal position on the glans). A deficient foreskin ventrally with a straight penile shaft is a clue that a subtle hypospadias may be present.

3. Associated genitourinary anomalies. Both genital and urinary abnormalities occur with increased frequency in hypospadiac boys.
   a. Meatal stenosis occurs more commonly, especially in the more distal glanular cases.
   b. Penile torsion also is a common occurrence in boys with both hypospadias and those with isolated chordee. Varying degrees of penoscrotal transposition occur in association with the more severe forms of hypospadias.
   c. Inguinal hernias and cryptorchid testes are significantly more common.
   d. A slight but significant increase (about 4% incidence) in significant upper urinary tract abnormalities occurs in boys with hypospadias. Vesicoureteral reflux occurs in about 10 per cent and should be investigated with a voiding cystourethrogram if a febrile urinary tract infection occurs.

4. Associated syndromes. Hypospadias is an accompanying feature of many pediatric syndromes with both normal and abnormal chromosomes. Additionally, when cryptorchidism or absent testes are associated with hypospadias, even if mild, intersexuality must be suspected. The frequency of intersex in this context has been recorded as between 28 and 64 per cent in three series. "Boys" with impalpable gonads and varying degrees of hypospadias actually may be 46xx females with adrenogenital syndrome.

Key Clinical Findings

- Displaced urethral meatus
- Chordee

Laboratory Findings

No specific laboratory investigations are indicated for boys with *isolated* hypospadias.

Treatment

1. American Academy of Pediatrics recommendations concerning the timing of genital surgery in children have been refined in light of more recent studies. Current recommendations are that the best time for hypospadias surgery is between 6 and 12 months, and that the child be cared for at a facility with experienced pediatric anesthesia, nursing, and urologic personnel.

2. Initially, circumcision must be avoided since the foreskin tissue is utilized in all but the most minor repairs. Initial neonatal consultation by an experienced pediatric urologist should occur, if not before hospital discharge, at least within the first few weeks of life. Parents benefit by clarifying potential misconceptions about causation and treatment, as well as by having a specific treatment program outlined. Outpatient reassessment at 6 months of age is done, at which time surgical repair is planned. Optimally, surgical repair should be done between 6 and 12 months of age, before ambulation occurs, since postoperative management is facilitated at this earlier age.

3. The goals of hypospadias treatment, therefore, are to restore normal penile function and appearance and to preclude development of these psychological problems.

4. Hypospadias treatment has undergone very significant changes in the last decade. Refinements in pediatric anesthesia and surgical techniques now allow for all but the most complex hypospadias currently to be repaired on an ambulatory basis, that is, with the patient discharged home the same day as surgery.

5. The principles of hypospadias repair are to correct the chordee, then to extend the urethra and to reconstruct the glans.

6. Complications of hypospadias surgery are usually minor and infrequent.

   a. Persisting chordee occasionally occurs despite apparent adequate initial complete correction.

   b. Stenosis of the newly created meatus may require minor revision. Strictures of the neourethra are uncommon but can be troublesome, requiring dilatation, incision, or reoperation.

   c. Urethral fistulas ("leaks") are the most common problem, and if persistent, require repair several months later.

Key Treatment

- Surgery, 6 to 12 months of age

See also Chapter 227.

Bibliography

Kass EJ, Kogan SJ, Manley C, Wacksman JA: Timing of elective surgery on the genitalia of male children with particular reference to the risks, benefits and psychological effects of surgery and anesthesia. Action Committee Report, Urology Section, American Academy of Pediatrics. Pediatrics 1996;97:590–594.

Khuri FJ, Hardy BE, Churchill BM: Urologic anomalies associated with hypospadias. Urol Clin North Am 1981;8:565–571.

Sweet RA, Schrott HG, Kurland R, et al: Study of the incidence of hypospadias in Rochester, Minnesota, 1940–1970 and a case controlled comparison of possible etiologic factors. Mayo Clin Proc 1974;49:52–58.

251 Hypopituitarism

Joseph M. Gertner

Definition

1. The term *hypopituitarism* refers to a reduced capacity of the pituitary gland to carry out its hormonal functions. Since the posterior pituitary is distinct anatomically and physiologically from the anterior pituitary, this review will be restricted to coverage of diminished anterior pituitary function. Because of the frequency and striking symptomatology of growth hormone deficiency in childhood, pediatric endocrinologists sometimes consider *hypopituitarism* to be synonymous with *growth hormone deficiency*. Although a broader view will be taken here of childhood anterior pituitary failure, the emphasis will be on disordered function of the growth hormone secretory axis.

2. Because of the rapid developments in our understanding of genetic disorders of hormone production and the critical importance of genetic diseases in the pediatric age group, these conditions will receive some emphasis. Well-characterized genetic diseases are cross-referenced in the text with their MIM numbers, referring to their classification in *Online Mendelian Inheritance in Man*.

3. The anterior pituitary gland (or adenohypophysis) is derived embryologically from the oropharyngeal ectodermal evagination called Rathke's pouch. The cells of the developing adenohypophysis differentiate into the functional hormone-secreting cells of the anterior pituitary by the seventh to tenth week of fetal development, showing the distinctive staining properties that separate the various

cell types. The principal hormones, their biochemical characteristics, their releasing hormones, and the cell types from which they are derived are listed in Table 251–1.

4. A major part of the control of the release of the above hormones is exerted through the action of small peptide hormones secreted by the hypothalamus. In general, these are "releasing hormones," transported to the anterior pituitary by a specialized vascular system, the hypothalamic-pituitary portal system (HPPS), which permits releasing hormone concentrations in contact with pituicytes to be much higher than those prevailing in other parts of the body. In addition to the stimulatory releasing hormones, the peptide hormone somatostatin is secreted into the HPPS. At the pituitary, it tonically inhibits growth hormone release, but its role in the control of secretion of other anterior pituitary hormones is less clear. Prolactin release is tonically inhibited by a hypothalamic factor or factors referred to as prolactin inhibiting factor (PIF).

5. The hypothalamic cells producing releasing hormones receive neural impulses from other regions of the brain. The output of releasing hormones is modulated by short feedback loops dependent on the pituitary hormones released by their action, and long feedback loops dependent on the products of hormone/target cell interaction.

Anatomic Classification of Hypopituitarism

1. Disordered hypothalamic stimulation

   a. Higher cerebral dysfunction. Physical or psychologic stress can lead to a reduction in hypothalamic releasing hormone output. Examples include:

      (1) Stress-induced amenorrhea
      (2) So-called psychosocial dwarfism
      (3) "Sick-euthyroid" syndrome

   b. The assumption is that these conditions involve reduced production of luteinizing hormone releasing hormone (LHRH), growth hormone releasing hormone (GHRH), and thyrotropin releasing hormone (TRH), respectively, but the evidence for this is not conclusive.

   c. Disorders of releasing hormone release and transport. Disordered secretion of releasing hormones may arise as a consequence of inborn or acquired disease of the hypothalamic areas in which they are secreted.

      (1) Genetic

         (a) Mutated releasing hormone gene (mouse corticotropin releasing hormone [CRH]

"knockout"—no human examples recognized)

         (b) Kallmann syndrome (hypogonadotropic hypogonadism [LHRH deficiency])—defective neuronal migration (MIM 308700)

         (c) Congenital adrenal hypoplasia with hypogonadotropic hypogonadism [LHRH deficiency](mutations in the DAX1 gene; MIM 300200)

         (d) Septo-optic dysplasia [GHRH deficiency](may also have diabetes insipidus)

      (2) Destructive. The most common situation in which failure to secrete hypothalamic releasing hormones leads to anterior pituitary failure is the disruption of hypothalamic tissues by disease. Section of the pituitary stalk that bears the HPPS disrupts anterior pituitary function. This type of physical damage may occur in the tumors mentioned below or as a result of trauma. Hyperprolactinemia generally accompanies functional section of the pituitary stalk. Disruption of the pituitary stalk can cause diabetes insipidus. Destructive processes can include the following:

         (a) Tumors

            (1) Craniopharyngiomas
            (2) Optic gliomas
            (3) Astrocytomas
            (4) Choriocarcinomas

         (b) Trauma

         (c) Granulomatous

            (1) Histiocytosis
            (2) Tuberculosis
            (3) Disordered releasing hormone transport to the pituitary

2. Primary pituitary disorders

   a. Structural developmental disorders
      Maldevelopment of the anterior pituitary is sometimes seen on imaging studies in case of hypopituitarism. Causes may be:

      (1) "empty sella" syndrome (little is known about how this arises)

      (2) PIT1 mutations (autosomal recessive GH, thyroid-stimulating hormone [TSH, thyrotropin], and prolactin deficiency; MIM 173110)

   b. Functional disorders

TABLE 251–1. HORMONES SECRETED BY THE ANTERIOR PITUITARY GLAND

SECRETED HORMONE	BIOCHEMICAL CHARACTERIZATION	RELEASING HORMONE	SECRETING CELL TYPE
Adrenocorticotropic (ACTH)	Small monomer (MW 4,500)	Corticotropin releasing (CRH)	Chromophobe
Thyroid stimulating (TSH)	Heavily glycosylated heterodimer	Thyrotropin releasing (TRH)	Basophil
Luteinizing (LH)	Heavily glycosylated heterodimer	LH releasing (LHRH)	Basophil
Follicle stimulating (FSH)	Heavily glycosylated heterodimer	LH releasing (LHRH)	Basophil
Growth (GH)	Large monomer (MW 21,800)	Growth hormone releasing (GHRH)	Acidophil
Prolactin (Prl)	Large monomer (MW 22.500)	None recognized	Acidophil

MW = molecular weight.

(1) Genetic

    (a) Defective releasing hormone receptor (e.g., GHRHR defect MIM 139191)

    (b) Isolated adrenocorticotropic hormone (ACTH) deficiency (very rare). ACTH is one of the peptides encoded by the gene pro-opiomelanocortin (POMC), which also controls the synthesis of beta-endorphin, melanocyte-stimulating hormone, and other active peptides. Once again, isolated ACTH deficiency has (rarely) been described, but involvement of the POMC gene has never been proven.

    (c) Recessively inherited growth hormone deficiency (MIM 262400)

    (d) Dominantly inherited growth hormone deficiency (MIM 173100)

    (e) Bioinactive growth hormone

(2) Metabolic

The release of pituitary hormones is subject to a variety of chemical controls, which include negative feedback by the secretions of each pituitary hormone target tissue. Thus, TSH secretion is inhibited by tri-iodothyronine, LH by estradiol, and ACTH by cortisol. Insulin-like growth factor 1 (IGHF-1) inhibits growth hormone secretion. Other metabolites and fuels may influence pituitary hormone production, most notably free fatty acids that inhibit growth hormone secretion.

3. Childhood anterior pituitary failure.

The clinical signs of pituitary hormone deficiency are conveniently divided between deficiency of growth hormone, which acts directly on peripheral tissues, and deficiency of the other hormones, which act by stimulating their target endocrine organs. The symptoms of the latter are very similar to the symptoms of failure of the target organs. However, target organ failure leads to high levels of the stimulating anterior pituitary hormone while, of course, hypopituitarism does not. Anterior pituitary hormone deficiency and target organ failure are contrasted in Table 251–2.

a. Growth hormone deficiency and panhypopituitarism.

The definition of growth hormone deficiency is a vexed topic with physiologic, pathologic, and economic implications. It should be realized that the secretory capacity for growth hormone represents a continuum, and that the level below such capacity called deficient is arbitrary. For most of what follows I will be using the definition currently accepted in the United States: failure to reach a peak growth hormone concentration of 10 ng/ml in two successive provocative tests.

With this definition, the search for a precise underlying cause will often be elusive. The economic implications are obvious, with insurance approval for treatment of "deficient" but not "nondeficient" short children.

(1) Clinical findings

    (a) Hypoglycemia (infancy—usually with panhypopituitarism involving other pituitary hormone deficiencies including hypothyroidism [TSH deficiency] and, in males, microphallus [LH/FSH deficiency]). Measurement of serum growth hormone concentration during a hypoglycemic episode should be part of the evaluation of infantile hypoglycemia.

    (b) Progressive growth failure. Growth hormone deficiency is compatible with normal birth weight and reasonable growth in the first few months of life. Growth hormone–deficient children are usually overweight for their stature. The evolution of both these aspects of the growth hormone deficient phenotype is shown in Figure 251–1.

    (c) Accompanying other diseases (e.g., signs of brain tumor)

(2) Evaluation

    (a) Determine whether the short stature is clinically significant; if not, do not perform laboratory investigation.

    (b) Screen out systemic nonendocrine causes.

TABLE 251–2. ANTERIOR PITUITARY HORMONE DEFICIENCY VERSUS TARGET ORGAN FAILURE

PITUITARY HORMONE	TARGET ORGAN	MAJOR SYMPTOMS OF CONGENITAL DEFICIENCY	MAJOR SYMPTOMS OF ACQUIRED DEFICIENCY	DIFFERS FROM TARGET ORGAN FAILURE BY
LH and FSH (male)	Testicular Leydig and tubular cells	Micropenis	Hypogonadism, delayed adolescence, infertility	Congenital form: genitalia unambiguously male
LH and FSH (female)	Ovarian stroma and follicles	None	Amenorrhea, infertility	
ACTH	Adrenal cortex zona fasciculata	Hypoglycemia, hypotension, hyponatremia	Fatigue, hypoglycemia, hypotension, hyponatremia	Normal sodium conservation (mineralocorticoid function) No excess pigmentation
TSH	Thyroid	Mental retardation, jaundice, physical signs of hypothyroidism	Growth failure, other physical signs of hypothyroidism	

ACTH = adrenocorticotropic hormone; FSH = follicle-stimulating hormone; LH = luteinizing hormone; TSH = thyroid-stimulating hormone, thyrotropin.

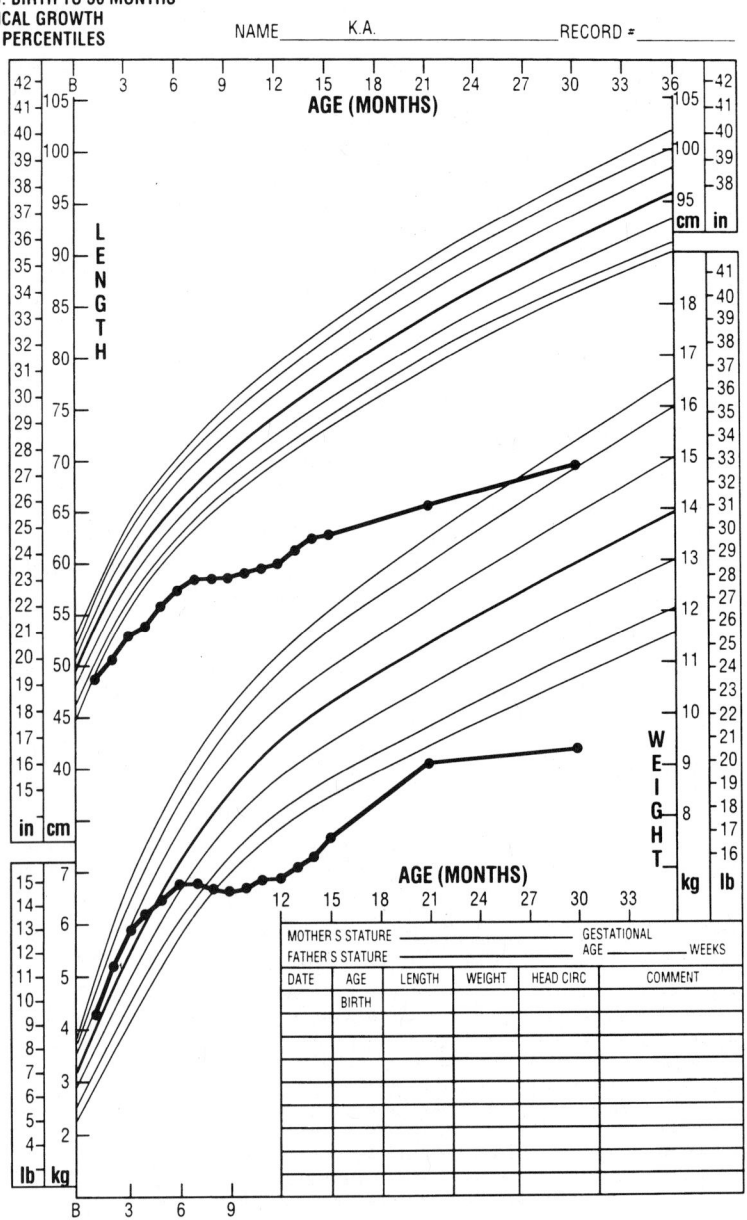

GIRLS: BIRTH TO 36 MONTHS
PHYSICAL GROWTH
NCHS PERCENTILES

NAME_____K.A._____ RECORD #_____

Figure 251–1 Growth curve from 1 to 30 months of an infant girl with isolated growth hormone deficiency. Note that length and weight are mildly affected at first. As the child grows older, linear growth is more severely affected than weight gain.

(c) Where shortness is significant, and without readily determined nonendocrine cause, two standard provocative tests for growth hormone release together with measurement of serum IGF-1 and IGF-BP3 are performed. Where both provocative tests fail to elevate serum growth hormone above 10 ng/ml, growth hormone deficiency is diagnosed, and, after appropriate investigation as to the cause, replacement therapy is commenced. Growth hormone therapy for children considered not to be growth hormone deficient is not approved by the FDA and is regarded as experimental.

(d) Ancillary measures to diagnose growth hormone deficiency are widely used, particularly the measurements of the growth hormone–dependent peptides, insulin-like growth factor 1 (IGF-1) and the IGF binding protein 3 (IGFBP-3). These concentrations vary with age, and low age-adjusted values may be supportive of a diagnosis of growth hormone deficiency. The diagnosis of deficiency, however, should not be based solely on low IGF-1 or IGFBP-3 levels, nor do values in the normal range necessarily exclude such deficiency.

b. Deficiencies other than growth hormone.
TSH and ACTH deficiency give rise to end-organ failure and to hypothyroidism and pure glucocorticoid deficiency, respectively. Similarly, gonadotropin deficiency leads to hypogonadism, generally not manifest until the usual age of puberty. In most respects, therapies of these conditions are similar to

TABLE 251–3.   ADVERSE EFFECTS RECORDED OR SUSPECTED IN THE TREATMENT OF CHILDREN WITH GH

TYPE OF EFFECT	SUBCATEGORY	COMMENT
Exaggeration of desired effect	Statural	Controlled by prescriber
	Cosmetic	No evidence of facial disproportion
Metabolic	Insulin resistance	Rarely gives rise to hyperglycemia
	Sodium retention	
Mitogenic	Brain tumor recurrence	Unlikely that GH increases incidence
	Leukemia	May be increased incidence in susceptible individuals
	Other tumors	May be increased incidence of melanotic skin tumors
Psychological/social	"Medicalization"	
	Frustration with attainment	
	Financial issues	
Miscellaneous	Benign intercranial hypertension	May be associated with sodium and water retention
	Slipped femoral capital epiphysis	Little evidence that incidence increases in GH therapy

those for corresponding end-organ failure and are dealt with in the corresponding chapters of this volume.

Treatment of Growth Hormone Deficiency

1. Hypoglycemia

   Often other pituitary hormone deficiencies contribute to the problem. These must be corrected as appropriate, using the corresponding hormone(s), most commonly hydrocortisone. Growth hormone is given in the same doses as those used for growth failure (0.02–0.05 mg/kg/day) but a divided dose regimen (two injections daily) may be used.

2. Growth failure

   a. Dosage for treatment with growth hormone.

      The dose-response curve for growth hormone is rather flat, particularly for the most deficient children who respond well to smaller doses. The recommended dose is 0.03–0.04 mg/kg/day. Studies continue as to the optimal dose, and as to whether pubertal children should receive higher doses to mimic the increase in endogenous growth hormone secretion seen in healthy pubertal children.

   b. Mode of administration.

      Subcutaneous injection of recombinant growth hormone is effective and free from local side effects. This route is now used almost exclusively.

   c. Duration of therapy.

      Patients with demonstrable growth hormone deficiency should be treated until growth is almost at an end (because of epiphyseal fusion) or until patient and family are content with the height attained. The issue of whether growth hormone replacement should continue into adult life is currently the focus of intense investigation.

   e. Adverse effects associated with GH therapy (Table 251–3)

      (1) The issue of safety of biosynthetic growth hormone therapy has been intensely studied since the 1988 report of growth hormone–treated patients in Japan developing acute leukemia at a rate exceeding the expected. Intensive follow-up of patients treated with growth hormone has led to the conclusion that the incidence of leukemia is indeed higher than in the untreated population. However many children with growth hormone deficiency have "risk factors," such as a history of malignancy or irradiation, which may predispose them to leukemia. Even growth hormone deficiency per se may be such a predisposing factor. When this is taken into account, the current consensus is that growth hormone therapy is not leukemogenic, particularly in children without prior history of malignancy or exposure to ionizing radiation.

      (2) The issue of treating non–growth hormone–deficient children with growth hormone remains controversial. Some contend that growth hormone should be reserved for those with demonstrable insufficiency. Others maintain that since growth hormone can induce short-term increases in growth velocity, possibly leading to increased adult stature, it should be available also to children with severe short stature from other causes.

Key Treatment

- Growth hormone
- Hydrocortisone

Bibliography

Fradkin JE, Mills JL, Schonberger LB, et al: Risk of leukemia after treatment with pituitary growth hormone. JAMA 1993; 270:2829–2832.

Hopwood NJ, Hintz RL, Gertner JM, et al: Growth response of children with non-growth-hormone deficiency and marked short stature during three years of growth hormone therapy. J Pediatr 1993;123:215–222.

Laron Z: Prismatic cases: Laron syndrome (primary growth hormone resistance) from patient to laboratory to patient. J Clin Endocrinol Metab 1995;80:1526–1531.

Online Mendelian Inheritance in Man, OMIM (TM), Baltimore and Bethesda, MD. Center for Medical Genetics, Johns Hopkins University and National Center for Biotechnology Information, National Library of Medicine, 1996. World Wide Web URL: http://www3.ncbi.nlm.nih.gov/omim/

Rotnem D, Cohen DJ, Hintz RL, Genel M: Psychological sequelae of relative "treatment failure" for children receiving human growth hormone replacement. J Am Acad Child Psych 1979; 18:505–520.

252 Maternal Antibody–Induced Neonatal Thyroid Dysfunction

Rosalind Brown

Etiology and Epidemiology

1. Transient neonatal thyroid dysfunction is an unusual complication of maternal autoimmune thyroid disease, a generic term that includes both Graves disease and chronic lymphocytic thyroiditis. It occurs due to the transplacental passage of maternal IgG.

2. Although Graves disease is characterized clinically by thyroid stimulation whereas thyroid destruction predominates in chronic lymphocytic thyroiditis, significant overlap may exist in some mothers. In the neonate either hyperthyroidism or hypothyroidism may occur.

3. Of the antibodies known to affect the thyroid, only those directed at the thyrotropin (TSH) receptor are of importance to the fetus. Antibodies to thyroglobulin and the thyroid peroxidase (TPO) enzyme, although of use clinically as markers of underlying autoimmune thyroid disease, do not cause fetal or neonatal thyroid dysfunction.

4. IgG is the only class of antibody that can be transmitted to the fetus. Transplacental passage of IgG becomes significant after 16 weeks' gestation, increasing until term. Therefore, babies do not usually become symptomatic until the second, or more frequently, the third trimester.

5. TSH receptor antibodies may be stimulatory or inhibitory.
   a. Transient, antibody-induced, neonatal *hyper*thyroidism is more common.
      (1) It occurs in approximately 2 per cent of mothers with Graves disease or 1 in 25,000 newborn infants.
      (2) It is the most common cause of neonatal hyperthyroidism.
   b. Transient, antibody-induced, neonatal *hypo*thyroidism is much less frequent.
      (1) It occurs in only 1 in 220,000 neonates.
      (2) It accounts for 2 per cent of babies with hypothyroidism detected by neonatal screening programs in North America, and approximately 20 per cent of transient cases.

6. In view of the aforementioned features, neonatal *hyper*thyroidism should be considered in infants whose mothers have the following risk factors (Table 252–1):
   a. potent TSH receptor antibody secretion in the third trimester (a time when most patients experience a significant modulation in antibody titer)
   b. high dose requirement for antithyroid medication during pregnancy
   c. history of previous affected offspring, and/or
   d. previous thyroid ablation either as a result of disease or therapy for their hyperthyroidism

TABLE 252–1. SITUATIONS THAT SHOULD PROMPT CONSIDERATION OF NEONATAL HYPERTHYROIDISM

1. Unexplained tachycardia, goiter, or stare in neonate.
2. Mother had persistently high TSH receptor antibody titer in pregnancy.
3. Mother required persistently high dosage for antithyroid medication.
4. Mother has undergone thyroid ablation.
5. Previous sibling was affected.

TSH = thyroid-stimulating hormone, thyrotropin.

7. Similarly, blocking antibody–induced neonatal *hypo*thyroidism should be suspected in any hypothyroid baby whose mother:
   a. has autoimmune thyroid disease,
   b. has had thyroid ablation, and/or
   c. has had previous affected offspring (Table 252–2)

Pathophysiology

1. The TSH receptor belongs to subgroup 2 of the G-protein coupled receptor superfamily and is located on chromosome 14 in humans. Like other members of this family, the receptor consists of a large extracellular domain, a transmembrane domain that traverses the membrane seven times, and a short intracytoplasmic tail.

2. Pituitary TSH, the physiologic thyroid regulator, binds to the extracellular domain of its receptor at multiple discrete segments recognized in a three-dimensional conformation. In some way this results in stimulation of second messenger (primarily adenyl cyclase), thyroid hormonogenesis and growth. Like TSH itself, TSH receptor antibodies bind to the extracellular domain, but stimulatory and blocking varieties appear to bind at different sites.

3. Stimulatory antibodies mimic the effect of TSH, leading to thyroid stimulation and growth. As a consequence of the hyperthyroxinemia, pituitary TSH secretion is suppressed. Blocking antibodies, on the other hand, inhibit the effects of both TSH and stimulatory antibodies. This action of blocking antibodies prevents the formation of goiter and, in hypothyroid individuals, worsens the hypothyroidism.

Clinical Findings

1. Rarely hyperthyroidism may develop in utero and is suspected by the presence of fetal tachycardia (heart rate

TABLE 252–2. SITUATIONS THAT SHOULD PROMPT CONSIDERATION OF BLOCKING ANTIBODY–INDUCED NEONATAL HYPOTHYROIDISM

1. Previous sibling was affected.
2. Mother has autoimmune thyroid disease.
3. Thyroid gland is present on ultrasound study.

> 160/min). More frequently, hyperthyroidism develops at the end of the first week of postnatal life when maternally administered antithyroid medication but not antibody has been cleared from the neonatal circulation.

2. Sometimes, an affected fetus comes to attention because of the detection of a goiter on ultrasound. This may be due not only to maternally transmitted TSH receptor antibodies but to maternal antithyroid medication to which the fetus is particularly sensitive. Fetal thyroid function is dependent on the balance of these various influences.

3. Severe fetal hyperthyroidism is associated with fetal loss, intrauterine growth retardation, craniosynostosis, and poor developmental outcome. Therefore, early recognition and treatment is necessary.

4. Analogous to athyreotic babies on the other hand, fetal hypothyroidism is well tolerated. Therefore, identification and treatment of affected infants soon after birth is sufficient to ensure a normal outcome.

5. Neonatal hyperthyroidism is characterized by tachycardia, irritability, poor weight gain, and prominent eyes. Goiter, when present, may be related to maternal antithyroid drug treatment as well as to the neonatal Graves disease itself. Thrombocytopenia, hepatosplenomegaly, jaundice, and hypoprothrombinemia have also been reported. Rarely, arrhythmias and cardiac failure may develop and may cause death, particularly if treatment is delayed or inadequate. There is a significant mortality rate.

Key Clinical Findings

- Tachycardia
- Poor weight gain
- Exophthalmos
- Goiter

6. Babies with neonatal hypothyroidism secondary to blocking antibody are frequently asymptomatic at birth and the diagnosis of hypothyroidism is made by routine newborn screening. When present, signs and symptoms are indistinguishable from babies with the more frequent thyroid agenesis/dysgenesis. However unlike the latter, a sporadic disease, blocking antibody–induced congenital hypothyroidism is transient and there is a high risk of future affected children due to the tendency of these antibodies to persist in the maternal circulation for many years. Therefore it is important to distinguish the two (Table 252–3).

7. The duration of maternal antibody–induced neonatal thyroid dysfunction is usually 2 or 3 months, but both shorter and longer courses may occur.

Laboratory Findings

1. Neonatal Graves disease
   a. Thyroid function tests are similar to those in patients with hyperthyroidism, whatever the etiology:
   (1) The serum concentration of thyroid hormones (both T_4 and T_3) is elevated when compared with normal values for this age group. (Note that values for T_4 are higher and T_3 lower in the newborn period than at other ages.)
   (2) Pituitary TSH is suppressed.
   b. Skeletal maturation is normal or advanced.
   c. Potent TSH receptor antibody activity can be documented in serum (see below) and distinguishes neonatal Graves disease from nonimmune forms of neonatal hyperthyroidism (e.g., activating mutations of the TSH receptor).

2. In transient, blocking antibody–induced neonatal *hypo*-thyroidism, laboratory findings may be difficult to distinguish from other forms of neonatal hypothyroidism, particularly thyroid dysgenesis (see Table 252–3).
   a. Serum concentration of thyroxin (both total and free) is normal or diminished. The combination of a normal T_4 and an elevated TSH is sometimes called "compensated" hypothyroidism.
   b. TSH is elevated.
   c. Skeletal maturation is normal or delayed.
   d. If the TSH receptor blocking antibodies are sufficiently potent, inhibition of TSH-induced radioactive iodine uptake may result in failure to visualize thyroid tissue on thyroid scan and a misdiagnosis of thyroid agenesis.
   e. Unlike thyroid agenesis, however, a normally placed thyroid gland can usually be demonstrated by ultrasound examination and may also be appreciated clinically.
   f. Diagnosis is confirmed by demonstration of a high titer of TSH receptor antibodies.

3. Two types of assays for TSH receptor antibodies can be used to verify an immune etiology for the thyroid dysfunction.
   a. Radioreceptor assay
   (1) Measures the ability of antibodies to compete for binding of radiolabeled TSH to thyroid membranes; therefore, detects both stimulatory and blocking antibodies
   (2) Usual names: TSH receptor antibodies (TRAbs), or TSH binding inhibitory immunoglobulins (TBII)
   b. Bioassay
   (1) Assesses biologic effect directly by measuring

TABLE 252–3. BLOCKING ANTIBODY–INDUCED NEONATAL HYPOTHYROIDISM AND THYROID DYSGENESIS: COMPARISON OF THEIR CLINICAL FEATURES

FEATURE	THYROID DYSGENESIS	BLOCKING ANTIBODY
Severity of hypothyroidism	+ to + + + +	+ to + + + +
Palpable thyroid	No	No
^{125}I-uptake	None to low	None to normal
Clinical course	Permanent	Transient
Familial risk	No	Yes
TPO antibodies	Variable	Variable
TSH receptor antibodies	Absent	Present

TPO = thyroid peroxidase; TSH = thyroid-stimulating hormone, thyrotropin.

stimulation of adenyl cyclase or inhibition of TSH-induced stimulation of adenyl cyclase.

(2) Usual names

(a) Stimulatory antibodies—thyroid-stimulating antibodies (TSAbs), thyroid-stimulating immunoglobulins (TSI)

(b) Blocking antibodies—thyroid-stimulating blocking antibodies (TSBAbs), thyroid-stimulating blocking immunoglobulins (TSI-block).

Key Laboratory Findings

- Elevated T_3 and T_4
- Low TSH
- Advanced bone age

Treatment

1. Treatment of neonatal *hyper*thyroidism is expectant.

   a. Propylthiouracil (5 to 10 mg/kg/day given tid) is used initially.

   b. Because the maximum effect may be delayed for several days, a strong iodine solution (Lugol's solution or SSKI, 1 drop every 8 hours) is usually added to block acutely the release of thyroid hormone.

   c. Therapy with both propylthiouracil and iodine should be adjusted subsequently depending on the response.

   d. Propranolol (2 mg/kg/day given bid or tid) is added if sympathetic overstimulation is severe, particularly in the presence of marked tachycardia.

   e. If cardiac failure develops, treatment with digoxin should be initiated and propranolol discontinued.

f. In unusually severe cases, prednisone (2 mg/kg/day) may be added to inhibit acutely thyroid hormone secretion.

g. Recently sodium ipodate (0.5 gm every 3 days) has been used successfully in the treatment of a baby with neonatal hyperthyroidism. Because of its simplicity and rapidity of onset, it offers promise in the treatment of transient neonatal hyperthyroidism.

2. Treatment of blocking antibody–induced neonatal *hypo*thyroidism is identical to that for neonatal hypothyroidism in general and should be initiated as soon as possible after birth in order to prevent mental retardation.

   a. L-Thyroxine, 10 to 15 μg/kg, is used initially. The dosage is adjusted subsequently depending on the results of repeat T_4, TSH, and TSH receptor antibody measurements.

   b. If the initial TSH is < 40 mU/L, treatment can be delayed for 2 weeks in expectation that thyroid function will normalize.

Key Treatment

- Propylthiouracil
- Propranolol

Bibliography

Brown RS: Autoimmune thyroid disease in pregnant women and their offspring. Endocr Pract 1996;2:53–61.

Fisher DA: Neonatal thyroid disease in the offspring of women with autoimmune thyroid disease. Thyroid Today 1986;9:1–7.

LaFranchi S, Dussault JH, Fisher DA, et al: American Academy of Pediatrics American Thyroid Association Newborn screening for congenital hypothyroidism: recommended guidelines. Pediatrics 1993;91:1203–1209.

253 Congenital Hypothyroidism

Robert M. Ehrlich

Etiology

Athyrosis, thyroid dysgenesis (ectopic or lingual thyroids), and presumed enzyme defects are the three commonest causes of congenital hypothyroidism (CH). Athyrosis and thyroid dysgenesis are sporadic. Presumed enzyme defects are genetic and may recur in the same family. In some cases there is the transplacental passage of a substance that interferes with thyroid hormone synthesis. This causes transient hypothyroidism that is indistinguishable from an enzyme defect.

Epidemiology

Neonatal screening has provided extensive data. Screening programs for detecting CH use capillary blood spotted onto filter paper. The filter paper is then sent to a laboratory for assay for either thyroid-stimulating hormone (TSH) or thyroxin (T_4).

1. The incidence of CH is 1:4000 to 1:5000 live births.

2. Most screening programs report TSH values over 20 mU/L as a positive test. TSH values over 40 mU/L are strongly suggestive of CH. If thyroxin (T_4) is used, the lowest 10 per cent of T_4 values in each assay have a TSH performed. If TSH is used as the primary screening hormone, early discharge will increase the number of false-positive tests because the sample may be taken during the neonatal TSH surge which occurs during the first 48 hours after birth. To minimize recalls, samples

taken in the first 24 hours should be over 30 mU/L and over 25 on the second day of life before they are considered abnormal. In some children the TSH rise may not be evident at birth. This has been noted particularly in premature babies and those with Down syndrome. In these clinical situations a second sample should be taken within the first 4 to 6 weeks after birth.

Pathophysiology

1. Thyroid hormones appear in the thyroid gland by the end of the first trimester. Thyrotropin (TSH) is present in the pituitary at 10 to 12 weeks. In the first trimester the fetus is dependent on placental transfer of maternal thyroid hormones. The hypothalamus begins to regulate circulating hormone levels in the second trimester. Thyroid hormone levels are low until the last few weeks of gestation when they begin to approach postnatal levels. At birth there is a surge of TSH that lasts 24 to 72 hours. Thyroid hormone levels then rise and remain relatively high throughout the first 6 to 12 months of life.
2. Fetal growth and development are independent of thyroid hormone, although subtle abnormalities such as a delayed bone age may be present in severe hypothyroidism.

Clinical Findings

1. Children with CH usually have very few clinical signs in the newborn period unless there is severe intrauterine hypothyroidism. Prolonged jaundice, a large anterior fontanelle, a big tongue, or a hoarse cry is present in a minority of patients.
2. Symptoms and signs of thyroid hormone deficiency develop after birth if the child is untreated. Some children with CH do not have abnormal hormone levels at birth and may present later with symptoms and signs of classical cretinism (failure to grow and develop neurologically, coarse features, puffy eyes, big tongue and hoarse cry, etc.).
3. If there is clinical suspicion repeat thyroid function tests are indicated even if screening test was reported as normal.

Key Clinical Findings

- Prolonged neonatal jaundice
- Coarse features
- Hoarse cry, deep voice
- Large tongue
- Infantile upper/lower segment ratio

Management of a Positive Screening Test in the Newborn Period

There are a number of scenarios depending on the TSH level.

1. Values over 40 mU/L at any age strongly suggest CH. The minimum follow-up is a serum TSH and T_4 or free T_4 (FT_4). A thyroid scan with ^{99}Tc will give the anatomic diagnosis and is useful in counseling parents about future pregnancies. A radiograph of the knee will help establish the severity of the hypothyroidism. An absent lower femoral epiphysis usually indicates severe CH and correlates with poorer intellectual outcome.
2. Screening values of TSH between 20 and 40 mU/L require only a serum sample since most of these children do not have CH. If the repeat TSH is lower than the screening value but over 10 mU/L, further samples are necessary every 1 to 2 weeks until the TSH is < 10 mU/L. If the follow-up value is the same or higher than the screening value a full work up is recommended. If the TSH remains elevated beyond 4 to 6 weeks, treatment with thyroxin is recommended even if the T_4 is normal. At 3 years of age the thyroxin could be discontinued in these children and the TSH followed to see if it rises. In the vast majority of cases it does not.
3. The thyroid scan may fail to show uptake in a recognizable gland, suggesting athyrosis. It may show uptake at the base of the tongue, indicating a lingual thyroid. A normally placed gland with normal or increased uptake of the radionuclide is either an enzyme defect or due to the transplacental passage of a substance that interferes with thyroid hormone synthesis. The value of an ultrasound examination of the neck is questionable because it usually fails to detect a lingual thyroid and sometimes a thyroid gland may be reported when nothing is seen on thyroid scan. This may be due to the technique or may be suggestive of a iodine trapping defect.

Key Laboratory Findings

- Low thyroxin
- High TSH

Treatment

1. Once the diagnosis is made, treatment with L-thyroxin 10 to 15 μg/kg body weight should be started. This will rapidly raise the FT_4 level to normal and suppress the TSH. Repeat serum values should be obtained within 2 to 3 weeks. At this time the T_4 is usually > 120 nmol/L (> 10 μg/dl) and the TSH is lower or even normal. If the T_4 is not above 120 nmol/L (10 μg/dl), the dose of thyroxin should be increased by 12.5 μg and the tests repeated at 3 months of age. The TSH is usually normal by this age. If not increases of 12.5 to 25 μg/day of thyroxin should be made until the TSH is normal unless symptoms or signs of excess thyroxin are detected.
2. Repeat TSH and T_4 should be obtained at 3, 6, 9, 12, 18, and 24 months and every 6 to 12 months thereafter. Some may wish to follow children more frequently but thyroid function tests should only be repeated 6 to 8 weeks after a change in thyroxin dose. Should the TSH rise significantly above reference values, increases of 12.5 to 25 μg/day should be instituted.
3. Thyroxin values may be relatively high in the first year of life but unless the TSH is suppressed or there are symptoms and signs suggestive of excess thyroid hormone, the thyroxin dose need not be reduced.

Key Treatment

• Thyroxin

Outcome

1. Most children who are started on treatment within the first 14 to 21 days and have a normal IQs. Some children who are diagnosed late or who have more severe CH as evidenced by a T₄ < 43 nmol/L (3.5 μg/dl) may have some subtle cognitive defects.
2. Physical growth is normal as is the bone mass.
3. Since the intellectual outcome of children detected on neonatal screening and treated from an early age is excellent, routine tests of cognitive function should be limited to those children who were diagnosed later than 1 month, whose initial T₄ was < 43 nmol/L (3.5 μg/dl), or who are having school difficulties.

Special Problems

1. Premature infants pose special problems since their T₄ levels are normally low and their TSH values may be slightly elevated. Recently Adams and colleagues have produced reference ranges for FT₄ and TSH in premature infants aged 25 to 36 weeks. These are compared with the values for infants born after 36 weeks (Table 253–1).
2. Children who are placed on a soy-based formula may require more thyroxin since soy interferes with thyroxin's absorption from the gastrointestinal tract.
3. Some children with a normal gland on radionuclide scan and who stay on the same dose of thyroxin for 3 years can safely be taken off thyroxin to see if they are permanently hypothyroid. If repeat TSH values 3 and 6 weeks later rise above reference ranges, thyroxin should be restarted. If the TSH has not risen, repeat tests after another 3 to 6 weeks should be performed. Any rise above reference values is an indication to restart thyroxin.
4. Some children are very sensitive to thyroxin and may manifest irritability, tachycardia, and poor sleeping pat-

terns. If their T₄ values are high or their TSH values are suppressed, the dose of thyroxin dose should be reduced.
5. False-negative screening values occur due to transcription errors or a delayed rise in TSH. If T₄ is used, 25 per cent of children with lingual thyroids who have normal T₄ values will be missed. They may present at an older age with symptoms and signs of hypothyroidism as the residual thyroid tissue at the base of the tongue decompensates. Thyroxin-binding globulin deficiency will give low T₄ values but the TSH and FT₄ are normal. If TSH is used secondary and tertiary hypothyroidism will be missed, but the incidence of these conditions is very low.

TABLE 253–1. REFERENCE RANGES FOR SERUM FREE T₄ AND THYROTROPIN IN PREMATURE INFANTS DURING THE FIRST WEEK OF LIFE

AGE GROUPS	GESTATIONAL AGE (WK)	FREE T₄ (pmol/L= [ng/dl])	THYROTROPIN (mU/L)
Premature infants	25–27	7.7–28.3 (0.6–2.2)	0.2–30.3
	28–30	7.7–43.8 (0.6–3.4)	0.2–20.6
	31–33	12.9–48.9 (1.0–3.8)	0.7–27.9
	34–36	15.4–56.6 (1.2–4.4)	1.2–21.6
Combined premature infants	25–30	6.4–42.5 (0.5–3.3)	
	31–36	16.7–60.5 (1.3–4.7)	
	25–36		0.5–29
Term infants	37–42	25.7–68.2 (2.0–5.3)	1.0–39

From Adams LM, Emery JR, Clark SJ, et al: Reference range for newer thyroid function tests in premature infants. J Pediatr 1995;126:122–127.

Bibliography

Fisher DA: Management of congenital hypothyroidism. J Clin Endocrinol Metab 1991;72:523–529.

Fisher DA, Klein AH: Thyroid development and disorders of thyroid function in the newborn. N Engl J Med 1981;304:702–712.

Gruters A: Congenital hypothyroidism. Pediatr Ann 1992; 21(1):15–18.

LaFranchi S: Congenital hypothyroidism: A newborn success story? The Endocrinologist 1994;4(6):477–486.

Rovet JF, Ehrlich RM, Sorbara D: Intellectual outcome in children with fetal hypothyroidism. J Pediatr 1987;110:700–704.

254 Acquired Hypothyroidism

Robert M. Ehrlich

Definition

Hypothyroidism, defined as decreased levels of thyroid hormones in the blood, can occur at any age, but is unusual under 2 years of age. Clinical symptoms may be subtle unless a goiter is present.

Etiology

The commonest cause of acquired hypothyroidism in childhood is chronic lymphocytic thyroiditis (CLT, Hashimoto thyroiditis). Chronic lymphocytic thyroiditis is an auto-

immune disease of the thyroid gland. Other causes are extremely rare and include goitrogens, iodine deficiency, late presentation of enzyme defects and thyroid gland dysgenesis that was missed at birth, cystinosis, thyrotropin deficiency, and thyroid hormone resistence.

Epidemiology

Hypothyroidism and goiter were common in iodine-deficient areas such as the Great Lakes. When iodine was added to salt, goiter due to iodine deficiency disappeared. Hypothyroidism affects females three times more commonly than males. There is often a family history of thyroid disease or some other autoimmune condition such as insulin-dependent diabetes. Family studies show that about 30 per cent of nonaffected members may have circulating antithyroid antibodies, without clinical or laboratory evidence of disease.

Pathophysiology

Children who develop autoimmune thyroiditis are considered to have a genetic susceptibility. Tissue types HLA-DR4, DR5 and HLA DQW-7 are particularly prone to develop CLT. Some enviromental trigger occurs that allows T lymphocytes directed against thyroid antigens to proliferate in the thyroid gland. These infiltrating lymphocytes damage the thyroid by a variety of mechanisms including cytotoxic killer cells, antibody-mediated cytotoxicity, and cytokines.

Clinical Findings

1. The course is quite variable. Children may present with a goiter without symptoms or signs of thyroid dysfunction. Occasionally the thyroid gland may be slightly tender. Short stature, poor growth, constipation, fatigue, deteriorating school performance, and cold intolerance may occur. The children have a dull facial expression, pale cool skin, puffy eyes, and delayed relaxation of their deep tendon reflexes. Very rarely the children with Hashimoto thyroiditis may present with symptoms and signs of hyperthyroidism if the destruction of the gland is particularly acute.
2. The thyroid gland is usually enlarged, feels quite firm and pebbly, like a cobblestone road. In some cases the thyroid is atrophic and not palpable.
3. CLT may be associated with other autoimmune conditions, most commonly insulin-dependent diabetes mellitus and Addison disease. Children with Down, Turner, Klinefelter, or Noonan syndrome have a higher incidence of autoimmune thyroid disease and should have periodic thyroid-stimulating hormone (TSH, thyrotropin) determinations. Children with cystinosis may deposit cystine crystals in their thyroid gland and develop hypothyroidism.

Key Clinical Findings

- Poor growth
- Cold intolerance
- Constipation
- Deteriorating school performance
- Enlarged thyroid

4. Unusual presentations of acquired hypothyroidism: Sexual precocity with breast development and vaginal bleeding may occur in prepubertal girls, while big testes may be noted in boys. This is usually part of severe hypothyroidism. The mechanism appears to be a cross-reactivity of TSH with the follicle-stimulating hormone receptor on the ovary and the seminferous tubules. Galactorrhea with elevated prolactin levels has also been reported. Some children with hypothyroidism may complain of "rheumatic like" symptoms—stiff muscles and joints. Treatment with thyroid hormone causes the signs of sexual precocity to regress and the rheumatic symptoms to disappear. All children who develop slipped femoral capital epiphysis, particularly if it is bilateral, should have thyroid function tests.

Diagnostic Tests

Hypothyroidism can be *primary* due to disease of the thyroid gland such as CLT, *secondary* due to pituitary disease such as a pituitary tumor, or *tertiary* due to hypothalamic dysfunction.

1. Thyroid function tests should be obtained in any child who is being investigated for short stature or poor growth even if no obvious symptoms or signs are present.
2. Modern thyroid function tests, especially the availability of sensitive thyrotropin (TSH) assays, make resin uptakes or estimates of thyroxin indices unnecessary.
3. Initially only a TSH and a thyroxin (T_4), or a free thyroxin (FT_4) should be obtained. If the TSH is elevated the child has primary hypothyroidism. If the TSH is normal and the T_4 or FT_4 is low, the hypothyroidism is secondary or tertiary. An elevated TSH with a normal FT_4 is called subclinical or compensated hypothyroidism.
4. Antimicrosomal antibodies (antithyroid peroxidase) are most commonly elevated in CLT. Antithyroglobulin antibodies do not help in making a diagnosis and are unnecessary.
5. Thyroid ultrasound or radionuclide scans are not necessary unless there is suspicion of nodular thyroid disease.
6. If short stature is the presenting problem, a bone age determination will help with the ultimate height prognosis.
7. If secondary or tertiary hypothyroidism is indicated from the thyroid function tests, further tests of pituitary function as well as a magnetic resonance imaging study of the head are necessary. Occasionally imaging techniques may show an enlarged sella turcica. This is due to hypertrophy of thyrotrophs with long-standing hypothyroidism and resolves with treatment.

Treatment

1. For overt hypothyroidism, a TSH > 10 mU/L and a low FT_4, L-thyroxin 2 to 4 mg/kg/day orally is indicated.
2. If the FT_4 is normal but the TSH elevated > 10 mU/L (compensated hypothyroidism), thyroxin is also indicated; otherwise the thyroid gland may enlarge.
3. Slight elevations in TSH up to 10 mU/L with a normal FT_4 do not require immediate treatment. Repeated TSH determinations should be performed every 6 months. Treatment is indicated if the TSH is rising above 10 mU/L or the gland appears to be growing in size.

Key Treatment

- Thyroxin

4. Thyroxin treatment of a euthyroid goiter has not been shown to reduce the size of the thyroid gland or prevent the development of hypothyroidism. Children with a goi-

ter and normal thyroid function tests should be followed clinically and have thyroid function tests repeated at regular intervals.

Follow-up

1. Thyroid function tests should be repeated every 6 to 8 weeks to adjust the dose of thyroxin until both the FT_4 and the TSH are within the normal range. Dosage changes should be 12.5 to 25 μg/day. If the TSH becomes suppressed, the dose of thyroxin should be reduced by a similar amount. Once the TSH and FT_4 are normal, repeat studies should be perfomed every 6 to 12 months until growth ceases and then yearly thereafter.
2. About 20 to 30 per cent of children with CLT may revert to a euthyroid status. Once the child has stopped growing it may be worthwhile to discontinue therapy for 6 to 8 weeks and see if the TSH rises. If it does, lifelong replacement therapy is indicated. If the TSH remains normal, periodic checks should be performed every 6 to 12 months.
3. Some children who have severe hypothyroidism may develop pseudotumor cerebri (headache, vomiting, papilledema) if started on too large a dose of thyroxine too quickly. They should be started on a subtherapeutic dose; that is, 1/4 of the recommended dose initially. The dose should be increased every 2 weeks with increments of 12.5 μg/day up to the full therapeutic dose. Should a persistent headache develop and pseudotumor cerebri be diagnosed, the dose should be reduced and increased more gradually.

4. Most children show catch-up growth when started on replacement therapy. Some children do not, and their bone ages faster than their height accelerates. They may go into puberty and end up significantly shorter than their height potential would predict. If the child does not show catch-up growth on follow-up visits, the bone age is accelerating faster than the child's height, and there are signs of puberty, a trial with a gonadotropic releasing hormone agonist should be considered.
5. Some children as they become euthyroid become more distractable and may show deteriorating school performance. Thyroid function tests should be checked to make sure they are not being overtreated. This phase is usually self limited.

Bibliography

Dussault JH: Primary pediatric hypothyroidism and endemic cretinism. *In* Bardin CW (ed): Current Therapy in Endocrinology and Metabolism, 4th ed. Philadelphia, BC Decker, 1991, pp 82–84.

Fischer DA: The thyroid gland. *In* Brook CGD (ed): Clinical Pediatric Endocrinology, 2nd ed. Oxford, Blackwell Scientific Publications, 1990, pp 321–325.

Foley TP, Malvaux P, Blizzard, RM: The thyroid gland. *In* Kappy MS, Blizzard RM, Migeon CJ (eds): Wilkins' The Diagnosis and Treatment of Endocrine Disorders in Childhood and Adolescence, 4th ed. Springfield, CC Thomas, 1994, pp 487–492.

La Franchi S. Thyroiditis and acquired hypothyroidism. Pediatr Ann 1992;21:1.

Rivkes SA, Bode HH, Crawford JD: Long term growth in juvenile acquired hypothyroidism. N Engl J Med 1988;318:599–602.

255 Hyperthyroidism

Robert M. Ehrlich

Definition

Hyperthyroidism is the excessive synthesis and secretion of thyroid hormone by the thyroid gland. *Thyrotoxicosis* is the clinical picture that results when the tissues respond to excessive thyroid hormone. In practice the terms are used interchangeably. In the pediatric age group over 90 per cent of the cases of thyrotoxicosis are due to Graves disease. The remainder are secondary to thyroiditis, a toxic nodule, or exogenous thyroid hormone.

Graves Disease

Etiology and Pathogenesis

1. Graves disease is a genetically determined organ-specific defect in suppressor T-cell function. Enviromental trigger factors (stress, infection) impair suppressor T-cell function allowing T-helper cells to produce cytokines that induce B cells to produce a thyroid-stimulating hormone (TSH, thyrotropin) receptor stimulating antibody (TSAb).

HLA-DR expression occurs on thyrocytes. The thyrocytes become antigen presenting cells for thyroid hormone, which further stimulates the T-helper cells to produce cytokines and antibody. A vicious cycle is created. The clinical manifestations of Graves disease are hyperthyroidism, ophthalmopathy, and pretibial myxedema.

2. The TSAb (also known as long-acting thyroid stimulator [LATS], or thyroid-stimulating immunoglobulin [TSI], depending on how it is assayed) causes unregulated stimulation of the thyrocyte, resulting in thyroid cell growth and excess secretion of thyroid hormones. Excess secretion of thyroxin (T_4) and triiodothyronine (T_3) accounts for the thyrotoxicosis. The cause of the ophthalmopathy and dermopathy is not completely understood.

Clinical Findings

1. The disease is rare in infancy but is more common in early adolescence. It is six times more common in females than males.

2. The onset is insidious, with symptoms being present for many weeks or even months before they are recognized. There may be a trigger factor such as a car accident or a death in the family. Deteriorating school performance, emotional lability, nervousness, weight loss with an increased appetite, heat intolerance, sleep disturbance, palpitations, and the recognition of an enlarged thyroid gland are common. There is usually a tachycardia, a wide pulse pressure, and a tremor of the hands. A mid-systolic click suggests the presence of mitral valve prolapse, which occurs more frequently in children with Graves disease. Proximal muscle weakness may also be present. The thyroid gland is usually diffusely enlarged. The eyes may be prominent. Lid retraction and lid lag are common. Exophthalmos may be unilateral or bilateral. Severe exophthalmos with muscle paresis is rare in children.

Key Clinical Findings

- Emotional lability
- Tachycardia
- Enlarged thyroid
- Weight loss
- Increased appetite
- Wide pulse pressure
- Tremor
- Exophthalmos

Laboratory Findings and Diagnosis

1. A clinical diagnosis of Graves disease is made if there is thyrotoxicosis plus exophthalmos and pretibial myxedema. In practice, if there are signs of thyroid hormone excess plus prominent eyes, the diagnosis is almost certainly Graves disease. Pretibial myxedema is rare in children.

2. If the symptoms are severe the diagnosis is easily confirmed with simple laboratory tests. The serum thyrotropin (TSH) is suppressed and the free T_4 (FT_4) and triiodothyronine (T_3) are elevated, confirming the diagnosis. With the availability of the sensitive TSH assays and a FT_4, a T_3 may not be necessary. In an obvious case, measuring the TSAb and a radioactive iodine uptake are not necessary for the diagnosis. An ultrasound is indicated only if the gland is irregular or nodular.

Key Laboratory Findings

- Elevated T_3 and T_4
- Decreased TSH

3. With the availability of the sensitive TSH assays, a condition of subclinical hyperthyroidism—normal FT_4 and suppressed TSH with few or no symptoms—has been recognized. This usually occurs in older persons who may have an arrythmia. Subclinical hyperthyroidism has also been observed in children but requires no further tests or treatment unless symptoms develop.

4. In difficult cases measuring the TSAb and performing T_3 suppression tests and thyrotropin releasing hormone stimulation tests may be helpful in making the diagnosis.

Differential Diagnosis

1. Thyrotoxic symptoms can occur with anxiety, subacute thyroiditis, the thyrotoxic phase of Hashimoto thyroiditis, by a toxic nodule, or an exogenous source of thyroid hormone. The history and physical examination usually can differentiate the various causes. In anxiety, thyroid hormone and TSH levels should be normal. The thyroid gland may be tender in subacute thyroiditis. If subacute thyroiditis is suspected a radioiodine uptake is helpful because the inflammatory process in the gland will inhibit uptake of the radionuclide even though the FT_4 is increased and the TSH suppressed. In Graves disease the radioiodine uptake is increased. A toxic nodule should be palpable and show a circumscribed area of increased radionuclide uptake with little or none in the surrounding gland.

2. The thyrotoxic phase of Hashimoto thyroiditis may be indistinguishable from Graves disease (they are both autoimmune thyroid diseases). The thyroid gland is often firm and rubbery in consistency. The TSAb is usually negative, the course milder, the response to treatment with antithyroid drugs is rapid. A very high level of thyroid antimicrosomal (antiperoxidase) antibodies is suggestive. Since the treatment is the same for both conditions differentiation may not be necessary.

Treatment

1. Symptomatic
   a. Children tolerate excess thyroid hormone levels better than adults. Beta blockers may be helpful to control tachycardia and tremor until other forms of therapy become effective. In newborns the dose of propranolol is 2 mg/kg/day, while in older children it is 10 mg/kg/day.

2. Antithyroid drugs
   a. Thiourea drugs block the synthesis thyroid hormone. They are effective in reducing thyroid hormone levels but do not affect the underlying disease process. They are effective orally but take 6 to 12 weeks for their full effect. Propylthiouracil 10 mg/kg/day or methimazole 0.5–1.0 mg/kg/day is equally effective. Propylthiouracil must be given every 6 to 8 hours while methimazole is effective every 12 or 24 hours. The bid dosage with methimazole has advantages in children where compliance may be an issue. If there is no improvement in symptoms or thyroid function tests in 6 to 8 weeks the dose should be increased and compliance monitored. As thyroid function tests return to normal the dose of the thiourea drugs should be adjusted to maintain the T_4 in the normal range. The TSH will likely remain suppressed even if the T_4 is normal or low. Alternatively if the T_4 falls to low values thyroxin could be added and the dose of antithyroid drugs maintained.

b. Treatment should be continued for 18 to 24 months. About 40 to 50 per cent of children will remit in that period of time. Those children who remit on therapy usually respond quickly to antithyroid medication. They are easily maintained euthyroid and have glands that become smaller during therapy. If the thyroid gland remains large the child will likely relapse when the drugs are discontinued.

c. Side effects of these drugs occur in about 1 per cent of children. They are usually mild and disappear on withdrawal of the drugs. A rash, usually urticarial and itchy, but sometimes mimicking viral exanthems, is the commonest. Stopping the drug and switching from one thiourea drug to the other may be associated with the rash disappearing.

   (1) The thiourea drugs may affect the liver. Liver enzymes should be measured initially and followed regularly while on antithyroid treatment. They may be elevated before therapy and then return to normal. Should the aspartate aminotransferase (AST) rise above 100 units/L the drugs should be discontinued and other forms of treatment considered. Thiourea-induced hepatitis has been reported.

   (2) Asymptomatic intermittent fluctuations of the white blood count may occur throughout the course of Graves disease. Thiourea drugs may suppress the bone marrow and cause a fall in the white blood cell count, platelets, and red cells. If the white cell count falls to less than 1000×10^9/L, mouth ulcers and fever occur. Patients should be warned to report such symptoms and discontinue the drug. Because of the spontaneous fluctuation of the white blood cells, repeated white blood cell counts are not helpful.

   (3) Arthritis with a lupus-like syndrome has also been reported in children with Graves disease treated with thiourea drugs.

3. Thyroidectomy, usually total is still preferred by some patients. The children should be made euthyroid by thiourea drugs and given Lugol's iodine for 10 days prior to surgery. Recurrent laryngeal nerve damage and hypoparathyroidism, usually transient but occasionally permanent, may occur. Surgery is becoming less common and therefore if this is the desired therapy, a surgeon with experience in thyroid surgery should be selected.

4. An ablative dose of radioactive iodine ^{131}I is the preferred treatment in adults and children who have completed their pubertal growth. There is no increased incidence of malignancy in patients or abnormalities in their offspring. Children should be made euthyroid with antithyroid drugs before using radioactive iodine unless the hyperthyroidism is mild. A dose of 5 to 15 mC is usually effective. Younger children who relapse after the initial course of antithyroid therapy may be carried through puberty with drugs and then given radioactive iodine. Most children can be rendered hypothyroid with one dose but a few need a second or a third dose.

5. The eye disease associated with Graves disease requires no treatment and usually improves as the hyperthyroidism improves. Even severe exophthalmos with muscle paresis recovers over a period of time. Radiation to the orbit or glucocorticoid therapy is usually not required.

Key Treatment

- Propranolol
- Antithyroid drugs
- Surgery for some
- Radioactive iodine postpuberty

Euthyroid Graves Disease

Some children present with unilateral or bilateral exophthalmos, without clinical evidence of hyperthyroidism. Thyroid function tests are normal. Orbital computed tomography or magnetic resonance imaging studies show the characteristic muscle thickening associated with Graves ophthalmopathy without any other lesion to account for the proptosis. In the past T_3 suppression tests and/or TRH stimulation tests were performed to determine the state of the hypothalamic-pituitary-thyroid axis. With the advent of the sensitive TSH assays these tests are unnecessary. The FT_4 is normal and the TSH is usually suppressed or normal. Thyroid antimicrosomal (antiperoxidase) antibodies are often positive. Some children may go on to develop thyrotoxicosis, others may become hypothyroid, while most remain euthyroid. Most children show a regression of the eye findings over a 2-year period. Unless there is evidence of thyrotoxicosis or hypothyroidism develops, no treatment is indicated.

Neonatal Graves Disease

The TSAb is transferred across the placenta during pregnancy and may cause fetal and neonatal hyperthyroidism. Women are often treated with low doses of propylthiouracil (PTU) in the last trimester in attempt to control fetal hyperthyroidism. At birth the baby may show few if any signs of hyperthyroidism, especially if the mother has been on PTU. Thyroid function tests may not be very abnormal at birth. If the neonate is affected, symptoms of extreme restlessness, diarrhea, failure to gain weight, and prominent eyes occur within the first 7 to 10 days. Occasionally children go into heart failure and may die unexpectedly. Signs include tachycardia, proptosed eyes, periorbital edema, lid retraction, staring eyes, cardiomegaly, hepatomegaly, and splenomegaly. A goiter may be present.

Mild disease without failure to gain weight may be managed without medication. The antibody has a half-life of 3 weeks and most symptoms are gone by 6 to 8 weeks. In more severe cases, propylthiouracil, Lugol's iodine, and β blockers may be required. Thyroid function tests should be performed weekly and medication adjusted to control symptoms and promote weight gain without overtreating and causing hypothyroidism at a time of vulnerable brain development. The prognosis with adequate treatment is usually good but some children may have developmental delay and develop craniosynostosis.

Bibliography

Bahn RS, Heufelder AE: Pathogenesis of Grave ophthalmopathy. N Engl J Med 1993;329:1468–1475.

Fischer DA: Grave's disease in children. *In* Bardin CW (ed): Current Therapy in Endocrinology and Metabolism, 4th ed. Philadelphia, BC Decker, 1991, pp 64–68.

Foley TP: Thyrotoxicosis in childhood. Pediatr Ann 1992;21:43–49.

Foley TP, Malvaux P, Blizzard RM: The thyroid gland. *In* Kappy MS, Blizzard RM, Migeon CJ (eds): Wilkins' The Diagnosis and Treatment of Endocrine Disorders in Childhood and Adolescence, 4th ed. Springfield, CC Thomas, 1994, pp 493–503.

Volpe R: Autoimmunity causing thyroid dysfunction. Endocrinol Metab Clin North Am 1991;20:565–587.

256 Thyroid Cancer

Donald Zimmerman

Definitions

Thyroid cancer comprises malignant proliferation of thyroid cells arising in the thyroid follicle (papillary, follicular, and anaplastic cancers) and of thyroid cells arising in parafollicular areas (medullary cancer). Normally functioning thyroid follicular cells—and many cancers arising from them—produce thyroxine, triiodothyronine, and thyroglobulin. Similarly, normally functioning parafollicular cells—and many cancers arising from them—produce calcitonin and a number of other peptides.

1. Genetics
   a. Medullary thyroid cancer. The most prominent example of a thyroid cancer arising from genetic predisposition is medullary carcinoma. The vast majority of childhood cases of medullary thyroid carcinoma arise in the setting of multiple endocrine neoplasia type 2 (MEN 2). This condition is transmitted with an autosomal dominant pattern of inheritance, is characterized by age-related penetrance, and includes medullary thyroid carcinoma and pheochromocytoma (both tumors tending to be multicentric and to arise bilaterally). Families with MEN 2a develop a third endocrinopathy, parathyroid hyperplasia. Families with MEN 2b develop ganglioneuromatosis which includes ganglioneuromas of the gastrointestinal tract (from the lips and tongue to the colon) and of the eyelids. In addition, individuals affected with MEN 2b have overgrowth of corneal nerves, subtle sensorimotor neuropathy (which may produce hypotonia in the newborn), and marfanoid habitus. Medullary thyroid carcinoma may also be inherited in an autosomal dominant fashion without the other neoplasms of MEN 2.
   b. Papillary thyroid cancer. Papillary carcinoma is only occasionally transmitted in families. One condition associated with familial papillary thyroid carcinoma is Gardner syndrome. This syndrome is transmitted with an autosomal dominant pattern of inheritance and consists of adenomatous colonic polyps appearing in childhood or adolescence; multiple osteo-

mas, epidermoid cysts, and cutaneous or subcutaneous fibromas; retinal pigmentation; dermoid tumors; gastric and small bowel adenomas and carcinomas; pancreatobiliary adenomas; hepatoblastomas; and dental anomalies. The papillary carcinoma associated with Gardner syndrome has several histologic features that are only rarely found in isolated papillary carcinoma.

2. Environmental factors
   a. The most well-documented environmental factor contributing to thyroid cancer is exposure to ionizing radiation. The frequency of radiation-induced thyroid carcinogenesis is proportional to radiation doses between .10 Gy and 10 Gy. Radiation exposure is particularly carcinogenic in thyroids of individuals exposed in the first 5 years of life; this thyroid carcinogenic effect is generally evident until approximately 20 years of age. Excess relative risk for thyroid carcinoma is greatest 15 years after radiation exposure but is still present 40 years following exposure to ionizing radiation.
   b. Other environmental influences may affect thyroid cancer. Iodine deficiency is associated with predominance of follicular and undifferentiated thyroid cancer, while iodine sufficiency and iodine excess are associated with a predominance of papillary thyroid carcinoma. A number of volcanic areas in the Pacific basin and elsewhere have high incidences of thyroid cancer.

Epidemiology

1. Occult carcinomas. Occult carcinomas of the thyroid are less than 1.5 cm in diameter and are unsuspected clinically. These small tumors are almost always papillary rather than follicular or medullary cancers. The prevalence of these "subclinical" tumors in adults older than 40 years is twice the prevalence in younger adults. The prevalence in children appears to be less than that in young adults and to be particularly low in children 10 years of age or younger.
2. Clinically evident childhood thyroid cancers are rare,

occurring with an incidence of approximately 0.5 to 5 cases/million population/year. These tumors comprise less than 1 per cent of childhood cancers and less than 10 per cent of thyroid cancers in all age groups. Between 62 and 72 per cent of children with thyroid cancer are girls.

3. Papillary thyroid carcinoma predominates, comprising 76 per cent of childhood thyroid cancers. Medullary thyroid cancer comprises 20 per cent, while follicular carcinoma of the thyroid accounts for 4 per cent of childhood thyroid cancers. Anaplastic cancers have been reported in very few children.

4. Sex predominance. The predominance of females among patients with thyroid cancer between the ages of 10 and 40 years suggests a possible role for estrogen in thyroid carcinogenesis. This possibility is made particularly plausible by the observation that estrogen receptors are present in normal and neoplastic thyroid follicular cells. Females develop autoimmune disease—including autoimmune thyroid disease—more frequently than do males.

5. Noncancerous thyroid disease. Patients with thyroid adenomas and generalized thyromegaly have been shown to have high incidence of thyroid cancer in a number of studies. However, other studies contradict these observations. Data also conflict concerning possible predisposition to thyroid cancer in patients with autoimmune thyroid disease.

Pathogenesis

1. Oncogenes and tumor suppressor genes. Most solitary thyroid adenomas and carcinomas comprise single clones of cells arising from a single mutated cell. Mutations appear in genes involved in regulating cell growth—especially in genes involved in cellular response to growth factors (proto-oncogenes) and in genes coding for tumor-suppressing proteins. In addition, thyroid tumors may overexpress nonmutated growth factors and their receptors. The precise manner in which oncogenes and tumor suppressor genes produce thyroid cancers is still uncertain. The mechanisms responsible for transition from C-cell hyperplasia to medullary carcinoma are not clearly understood. One of the RET oncogenes seen in papillary thyroid cancer has been induced in cultured thyrocytes following radiation exposure.

2. RET proto-oncogene

   a. Structure and function of RET. One of the most important and well-studied proto-oncogenes in thyroid carcinogenesis is RET. The gene product of RET is a transmembrane protein with tyrosine kinase activity. While the structure of RET is similar to structures of a number of receptors for growth factors, the growth factor or other ligand that binds to RET—thereby stimulating its tyrosine kinase—is presently unknown. It is expressed in early development in tissues derived from the neural crest; the possibility that RET may play a developmental role in such tissues is suggested by the observation that RET mutations cause abnormalities such as Hirschsprung disease.

   b. RET mutations in medullary thyroid cancer. Germline RET mutations have been detected in families with MEN 2 and with familial medullary thyroid carcinoma. Families with MEN 2a and familial medullary carcinoma frequently have mutations in the cysteine-rich region of the RET molecule, a region between the extracellular and transmembrane domains. Families with MEN 2b most commonly have a mutation in the intracellular tyrosine kinase portion of the molecule.

   c. RET mutations in papillary thyroid cancer. In patients with RET-associated papillary thyroid cancer, the mutations are somatic rather than germ-line. Three chromosomal rearrangements involving the RET region of chromosome 10 have been described. Two of the mutations involve rearrangements within chromosome 10, while a third comprises a translocation from chromosome 17 to chromosome 10. In two of the mutations, an activating genetic sequence is fused with a portion of the RET gene immediately preceding the tyrosine kinase domain. The precise structure of the third mutation is under study.

3. TRK mutations in papillary thyroid cancer. Like RET, TRK is a proto-oncogene that encodes a growth factor receptor (in this instance, the receptor for nerve growth factor); it is also mutated via a chromosomal inversion (chromosome 1 in this instance) in some cases of papillary thyroid carcinoma.

4. Ras and Gsp mutations in various thyroid tumors. Two transducing molecules in the signaling cascade, Ras and Gsp, convey signals from activated receptors (via binding of guanosine triphosphate [GTP]) to downstream elements. These proto-onocogenes are mutated in a number of papillary, follicular, and undifferentiated thyroid cancers as well as in some adenomas.

5. Overexpression of nonmutated proto-oncogenes. A number of other proto-oncogenes are overexpressed, but not mutated, in some thyroid cancers. These include the growth factor receptors c-erb B2/neu and c-erb B (receptor for epidermal growth factor) as well as the transcription factors C-myc and N-myc.

6. Thyroid suppressor genes in various thyroid cancers. Tumor suppressor genes may be mutated in some thyroid tumors. Many undifferentiated thyroid cancers have mutations in the tumor suppressor gene p53. Another tumor suppressor gene, RB (the retinoblastoma gene), is mutated in several kinds of thyroid tumors.

Clinical Findings

1. Papillary thyroid carcinoma. Papillary thyroid carcinoma usually presents with a neck mass. Approximately 75 per cent of patients have palpable thyroid nodules, and at least 35 per cent have palpably enlarged cervical lymph nodes. Hoarseness, dyspnea, cough, and hemoptysis are distinctly unusual. Occasionally, thyroid nodules and/or cervical lymphadenopathy are detected during evaluation for thyrotoxicosis or for hypothyroidism.

2. Follicular thyroid carcinoma. The clinical presentation of patients with follicular thyroid cancer is similar to that of patients with papillary carcinoma. Some observers, but not all, have reported a lower incidence of palpable cervical lymphadenopathy in patients with follicular cancer than in those with papillary cancer.

3. Medullary thyroid carcinoma. The majority of children with medullary thyroid carcinoma are diagnosed as a result of family screening. Probands in affected families may present with neck mass, with flushing and/or diarrhea due to hormonal secretion from medullary thyroid carcinoma, with symptoms due to pheochromocytoma (hypertensive symptoms associated with tremor and palpitations), or with symptoms and signs of the mucosal neuroma phenotype found in MEN 2b. The mucosal neuroma phenotype is often most easily recognizable in older children and in adults; affected individuals have thickened lips with a degree of lip nodularity associated with nodules of the eyelids and tongue and a marfanoid habitus. Infants with MEN 2b may present with diarrhea and/or obstipation in addition to hypotonia.

Key Clinical Findings

- Neck mass
- Cervical lymphadenopathy (35%)

Laboratory and Radiographic Findings

1. Evaluation of thyroid nodules

    a. Fine needle aspiration is the most sensitive and specific test to evaluate the possibility of thyroid cancer in thyroid nodules. Nodules associated with a cytologic diagnosis of malignancy or suspected malignancy require surgical biopsy. Those that are cytologically nondiagnostic require repeat fine needle aspiration or surgical removal.

    b. Young children may not tolerate fine needle aspiration without administration of general anesthesia. The pathology of thyroid nodules in such patients can be determined with open surgical biopsy. Some clinicians prefer open biopsy of all thyroid nodules in children, since removal of such lesions obviates the need for prolonged medical follow-up if a definitive diagnosis of benign neoplasm is made.

    c. Ultrasound examination of the neck is particularly useful in evaluation of nodules that are partially cystic. Fine needle aspiration of a solid portion of the mass under ultrasound may facilitate obtaining adequately cellular samples.

    d. Radionuclide scans (e.g., with ^{131}I or ^{123}I) are sometimes employed in diagnosis in order to ascertain the probability of cancer in lesions found to be "follicular neoplasms" on examination of fine needle aspiration specimens. Nodules with decreased uptake are associated with a higher probability of malignancy.

    e. Serum levels of thyroxin, thyroid stimulating hormone, and calcitonin may be helpful.

    f. Chest x-ray may demonstrate pulmonary metastases in patients with nodules shown to be malignant or suspicious.

2. Evaluation of cervical lymphadenopathy

    a. If cervical lymphadenopathy is associated with a palpable thyroid nodule, fine needle aspiration of the thyroid nodule may be diagnostic.

    b. Open surgical lymph node biopsy is more certain to provide a diagnosis in evaluation of isolated cervical lymph node enlargement than is fine needle aspiration of a lymph node.

3. Evaluation of members of families with medullary thyroid carcinoma

    a. Probands with medullary thyroid carcinoma should undergo molecular genetic testing for germ-line mutation of the RET proto-oncogene.

    b. If an RET mutation is detected, first-degree relatives should be studied for the presence of the mutation.

    c. If medullary carcinoma in an RET-mutation–free proband is bilateral or if the medullary carcinoma in such a proband is associated with other MEN 2 neoplasms, first-degree relatives should be studied with calcitonin stimulation tests using infusions of pentagastrin and/or calcium. Individuals with hypercalcitoninemia should be treated as having medullary thyroid cancer.

4. Other studies in patients found to have medullary thyroid carcinoma

    a. All patients with medullary thyroid carcinoma should be examined for pheochromocytoma with adrenal imaging (either computed tomography [CT] or magnetic resonance imaging [MRI]) and with determination of urinary metanephrines.

    b. Patients with positive or suspicious adrenal imaging studies but negative metanephrine determinations should be studied to determine urinary levels of free fractionated catecholamines.

    c. Serum levels of calcium and phosphorus should be determined in patients with medullary thyroid carcinoma. Patients with hypercalcemia should undergo studies of parathyroid hormone levels.

Key Laboratory Test

- Needle aspiration and histology

Treatment

1. Papillary and follicular thyroid cancer

    a. Thyroidectomy. Patients with these tumors should undergo bilateral total or near-total thyroidectomy. Less complete thyroidectomy predisposes to increased frequency of local neck recurrence in patients with papillary thyroid cancer. In both papillary and follicular thyroid cancer, total or near-total thyroidectomy increases the sensitivity of postoperative ^{131}I scans and permits use of serum thyroglobulin (Tg) measurement to detect cancer persistence or recurrence. Neck nodes in the central compartment should be removed. Palpably enlarged lymph nodes should be removed employing modified radical neck dissection.

    b. Postoperative ^{131}I ablation of remaining normal thyroid tissue. ^{131}I ablation has been observed to reduce tumor recurrence by some investigators but not by others. Such treatment may be particularly useful in patients with large or high-grade tumors. ^{131}I treatment should be postponed until thyroid stimulating hormone (TSH) levels rise above 35 mIU/L. At present, patients are treated with triiodothyronine (approximately 75 μg/1.73 m²/day) for 4 weeks and then withdrawn from treatment for 2 weeks. After 2 weeks without thyroid hormone replacement, ¹³¹I scan and uptake should be performed and therapeutic ¹³¹I administered. In the near future, injection of recombinant h-TSH will be used, and patients will be able to remain on thyroid hormone replacement for ¹³¹I studies and treatment. ¹³¹I doses of 29.9 mCi to 100 mCi may be used for treatment.

c. ¹³¹I treatment of persistent tumor

    (1) Patients with postoperative ¹³¹I uptake should be aggressively treated with ¹³¹I if thyroid tumor invading neck structures (such as the recurrent laryngeal nerve or trachea) was knowingly left in the neck at the time of surgery or if distant metastases are detected. Generally, ¹³¹I doses vary from 100 mCi to 300 mCi.

    (2) The need to treat patients with thyroglobulin levels remaining above the athyreotic range in the absence of ¹³¹I uptake or other evidence of residual tumor (e.g., findings on neck ultrasonography, chest x-ray, and/or CT) remains controversial.

    (3) Patients should be restudied and retreated at 6- to 12-month intervals until ¹³¹I total body scans show no evidence of persistent or recurrent thyroid carcinoma.

d. Surgical treatment of persistent tumor. Patients with postoperative ¹³¹I uptake, determined by neck palpation and/or neck ultrasonography to result from cancer metastases to cervical lymph nodes, should be treated surgically.

e. L-thyroxine (L-T₄) treatment

    (1) If ¹³¹I treatment is employed, L-thyroxine treatment should be initiated 5 to 7 days later. If ¹³¹I treatment is not required, then L-thyroxine should be given immediately postoperatively.

    (2) The L-thyroxine dose should be adjusted to achieve circulating TSH levels partially suppressed to 0.1 mIU/L to 0.4 mIU/L in patients with tumors less than 1 cm in diameter and with no metastases. Patients with larger tumors and those with metastases or with local invasion should receive enough L-T₄ to suppress TSH below the limit of detectability of a high-sensitivity TSH assay.

f. Follow-up care

    (1) Once ¹³¹I scans and thyroglobulin levels have normalized, then patients should be reexamined with physical examination, chest x-ray, neck ultrasound, and serum thyroglobulin levels at yearly intervals. ¹³¹I scans should be performed at approximately 5-year intervals.

    (2) There is general agreement that serum Tg levels should be measured while patients are not taking L-T₄ replacement, since Tg may remain sup-

pressed despite the presence of metastases in patients who continue to take L-T₄.

2. Medullary thyroid cancer

a. Total thyroidectomy is required because of the high frequency of bilaterality and multicentricity of this tumor. Lymph nodes in the central compartment and palpably enlarged nodes should be removed.

b. Thyroid hormone replacement should be given in physiologic doses to achieve TSH levels within the normal range.

c. Postoperatively, serum calcitonin levels (calcium and/or pentagastrin infusion) should be measured; if basal levels are normal, calcitonin should be measured after infusion of pentagastrin and/or calcium.

d. Persistent hypercalcitoninemia should prompt clinical and ultrasonographic examination of the neck. Patients with enlarged lymph nodes should undergo surgical re-exploration of the neck. If enlarged cervical lymph nodes are not detected in patients with persistent hypercalcitoninemia, CT of the chest and MRI of the abdomen (especially of the liver) should be performed. If these studies are negative, octreotide scanning may be helpful in localizing medullary carcinoma metastases. Normal imaging studies can be followed with selective venous sampling done in conjunction with dynamic calcitonin testing.

e. Normalization of circulating calcitonin should be followed by yearly provocative calcitonin studies.

f. Patients with familial medullary carcinoma found to be associated with germ-line RET mutations and patients with bilateral medullary cancer or with other MEN 2 neoplasms should be followed with yearly metanephrine determination and with CT or with MRI of the adrenals to search for pheochromocytoma. Such patients should be followed for hypercalcemia and hypophosphatemia. If these mineral abnormalities appear, parathyroid hormone levels should be obtained.

Key Treatment

- Thyroidectomy

Prevention

1. Medullary thyroid carcinoma. First-degree relatives of probands with medullary thyroid carcinoma should be studied by approximately 1 year of age as outlined in the "Laboratory and Radiographic Findings" section. Those with demonstrable RET mutations should undergo dynamic calcitonin testing (with calcium and/or pentagastrin infusion) and testing for presence of pheochromocytoma; subsequently, patients should be treated with total thyroidectomy. First-degree relatives of patients who are RET-mutation negative but who have bilateral medullary thyroid carcinoma and/or other MEN 2 neoplasms should undergo yearly dynamic calcitonin testing. Those with elevated stimulated levels of calcitonin should be treated with total thyroidectomy.

2. Patients with known Gardner syndrome should have

yearly physical examination including careful thyroid examination. Thyroid nodules should be investigated as described in the "Laboratory and Radiographic Findings" section.

Bibliography

Duh Q-Y, Grossman RF: Thyroid growth factors, signal transduction pathways, and oncogenes. Surg Clin North Am 1995; 75:421–437.

Gharib H, Zimmerman D, Goellner JR, et al: Fine-needle aspiration biopsy: Use in diagnosis and management of pediatric thyroid diseases. Endocrine Practice 1995;1:9–13.

Ledger GA, Khosla S, Lindor NM, et al: Genetic testing in the diagnosis and management of multiple endocrine neoplasia type II (review). Ann Intern Med 1995;122:118–124.

Ron E, Lubin JH, Shore RE, et al: Thyroid cancer after exposure to external radiation: A pooled analysis of seven studies. Radiation Research 1995;141:259–277.

257 21-Hydroxylase Deficiency

Walter L. Miller

Congenital adrenal hyperplasia (CAH) is a group of disorders of adrenal steroid biosynthesis. In most cases cortisol secretion is diminished, leading to increased adrenocorticotropic hormone (ACTH) secretion and consequent growth (hyperplasia) of the adrenals. These disorders are genetically complex, as some disrupt only adrenal steroidogenesis while others disrupt both adrenal and gonadal steroidogenesis. They are also complex clinically, as there are signs and symptoms due to both the underproduction of adrenal steroids and the overproduction of hormonally active precursors. Understanding of the various disorders of steroidogenesis is facilitated by understanding the pathways of steroidogenesis (Fig. 257–1).

Etiology

1. The first step in the biosynthesis of all steroid hormones is the conversion of cholesterol to pregnenolone by a single mitochondrial cytochrome P450 enzyme termed P450scc (where scc denotes cholesterol side-chain cleavage). The same P450scc enzyme is responsible for the initiation of adrenal mineralocorticoid, glucocorticoid, and sex steroid synthesis, as well as for the synthesis of gonadal steroids and some placental and brain steroids as well.

2. Pregnenolone may be converted to progesterone, the first biologically active steroid in the pathway by 3β–hydroxysteroid dehydrogenase (3βHSD), a short-chain dehydrogenase enzyme distantly related to two other steroidogenic enzymes, 11βHSD and 17βHSD, and to alcohol dehydrogenase. Human beings have multiple 3βHSD genes and express at least two distinct forms of this enzyme. The type II enzyme is expressed in the adrenals and gonads; the type I enzyme is expressed in the placenta and in peripheral, extraglandular tissues, where it may modify steroids secreted by the adrenals and gonads.

3. Both pregnenolone and progesterone may then be acted on by the microsomal enzyme P450c17, which catalyzes both 17α-hydroxylase and 17,20-lyase activities. P450c17 is absent in the adrenal zona glomerulosa so that the progesterone is then eventually converted to the mineralocorticoid, aldosterone. In the adrenal zona fasciculata, the 17α-hydroxylase activity of P450c17 predominates, favoring synthesis of cortisol. In the adult adrenal zona reticularis (and in the gonads) the 17,20-lyase activity of P450c17 is also manifested, resulting in the cleavage of C-21 steroids to C-19 sex steroids.

4. Both progesterone and 17α-hydroxyprogesterone (17OHP) are then hydroxylated at carbon 21 by the adrenal 21-hydroxylase, P450c21, to yield 11-deoxycorticosterone (DOC) and 11-deoxycortisol, respectively. Although there are two P450c21 genes, one is nonfunctional, so that there is only one adrenal P450c21, which 21-hydroxylates the precursors to both mineralocorticoids and glucocorticoids. However other, as-yet unidentified enzymes can catalyze the 21-hydroxylation of steroid hormones, both in peripheral, extraglandular tissues and possibly also in the adrenal cortex itself.

5. Finally, DOC and 11-deoxycortisol are converted to aldosterone and cortisol by two distinct isozymes of P450c11 termed P450c11AS (aldosterone synthase) and P450c11β (11β-hydroxylase); these are discussed in greater detail in the next chapter.

Genetics

1. The genes for all of these enzymes have been cloned (Table 257–1) and genetic disorders identified and characterized in each of them. However, disorders of P450c21 account for about 95 per cent of patients with CAH, with severe forms occurring in about 1 in 12,000 persons and mild forms occurring in 1 in 100 to 1 in 1000 persons, depending on the population. This chapter deals only with 21-hydroxylase deficiency; the other disorders are considered in Chapter 258.

2. The gene for P450c21 (sometimes termed CYP21), plus the gene for the fourth component of serum complement (C4) and a gene for an extracellular matrix protein termed tenascin-X, are duplicated in tandem in an array (C4A, 21A, XA, C4B, 21B, XB) lying in the midst of the human

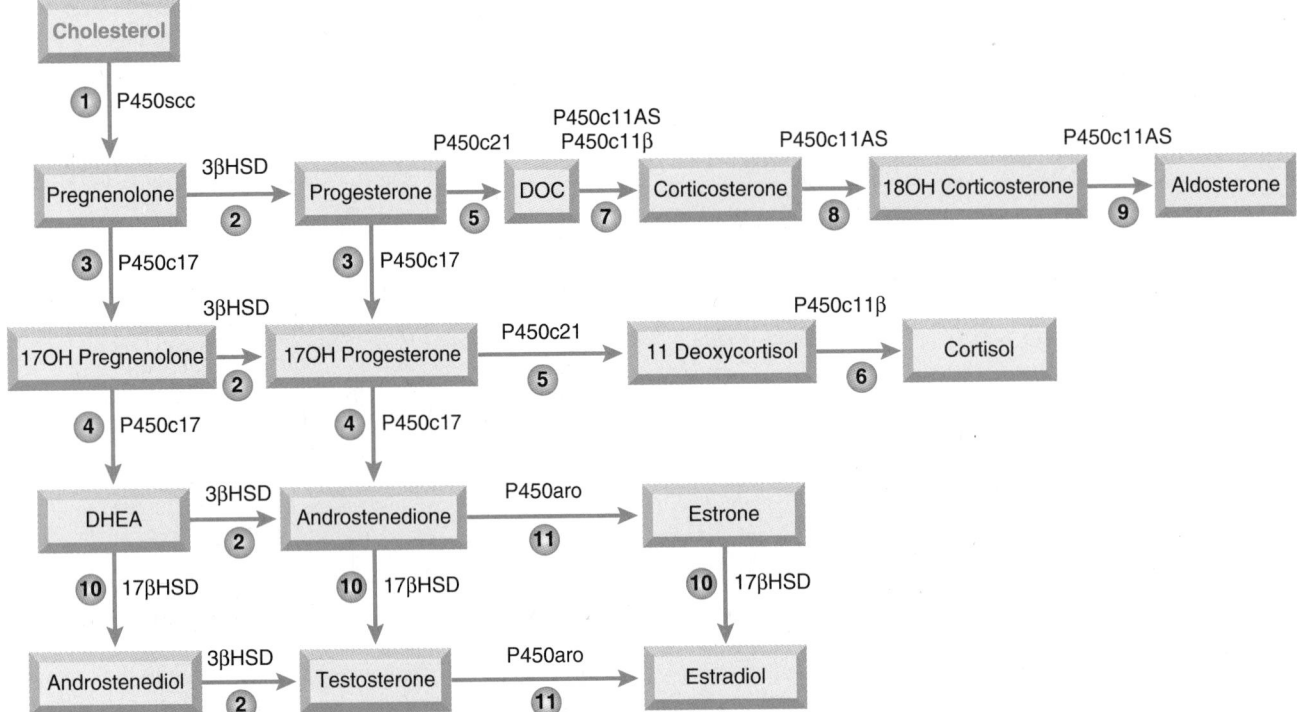

Figure 257–1 Principal pathways of human adrenal steroid hormone synthesis. Other quantitatively and physiologically minor steroids are also produced. The chemical identities of the enzymes are shown by each reaction. Reaction 1: Mitochondrial cytochrome P450scc mediates 20α-hydroxylation, 22-hydroxylation, and scission of the C20-22 carbon bond, to convert cholesterol to pregnenolone. Reaction 2: 3β-HSD mediates 3β-hydroxysteroid dehydrogenase and isomerase activities. Reaction 3: In the adrenal fasciculata and reticularis, P450c17 catalyzes the 17α-hydroxylation of pregnenolone to 17OH-pregnenolone and of progesterone to 17OH-progesterone. Reaction 4: The 17,20-lyase activity of P450c17 converts 17OH-pregnenolone to DHEA, but very little 17OH-progesterone is converted to Δ⁴ androstenedione. Reaction 5: P450c21 catalyzes the 21-hydroxylation of both progesterone and 17OH-progesterone. Reaction 6: P450c11β converts 11-deoxycortisol to cortisol. Reactions 7, 8, and 9: In the adrenal zona glomerulosa, DOC is converted to corticosterone and then to 18OH-corticosterone and finally to aldosterone by P450c11AS. DOC may also be converted to corticosterone by P450c11β in the zona fasciculata. Reactions 10 and 11 are found principally in the testes and ovaries. Reaction 10: Several isozymes of 17β-HSD mediate both 17-ketosteroid reductase and 17β-hydroxysteroid dehydrogenase activities, converting DHEA to androstenediol, androstenedione to testosterone, and estrone to estradiol. Reaction 11: Testosterone is converted to estradiol by P450aro (aromatase).

leukocyte antigen (HLA) locus on chromosome 6p21.3. Both C4 genes encode active complement protein, but the 21A and XA genes do not appear to encode proteins. Thus the B locus is the area of interest—the P450c21B gene encodes all P450c21B protein and the XB gene encodes an important extracellular matrix protein and an intracellular adrenal protein of unknown function.

3. The cellular differences among individuals are maintained by a highly diverse array of cell surface (HLA) antigens. This HLA diversity is due to a very high rate of genetic recombinations and gene duplications in the HLA locus, including the P450c21 genes. This leads to the unique genetics of CAH. Each person carries two P450c21B alleles, one inherited from each parent. Because there are many different defects in 21B genes, most patients are compound heterozygotes, having a different genetic lesion on each 21B gene inherited from each parent. Thus the common conception that a patient with CAH is homozygous for a defective 21B gene is not strictly true. The patient is homozygously affected due to compound

heterozygosity, having inherited a different mutation in each P450c21B allele.

4. Random gene deletions, insertions, and point mutations, which cause virtually all other genetic disorders, are extremely rare in CAH. About 15 per cent of severely affected 21B genes have unusual gene deletions that extend from various locations in the 21A gene to the precisely corresponding base in the 21B gene, resulting in a perfectly spliced 21A/B hybrid. These hybrids retain the 8 base pair (bp) deletion in exon 3 of 21A so that the hybrid cannot produce the P450c21 enzyme. The remaining 85 per cent of severely affected alleles, and all alleles causing mild (nonclassic) CAH, are due to gene conversions. About 10 per cent of alleles causing severe disease have large "macroconversions" that change all of the 21B gene sequence into a 21A sequence, so that the chromosome has two 21A genes and no functional 21B gene. The remaining 75 per cent of severely affected alleles have microconversions. These look like ordinary point mutations, but in fact they represent a small region

TABLE 257–1. GENES ENCODING STEROIDOGENIC ENZYMES

ENZYME	NO. OF GENES	CHROMOSOMAL LOCATION
P450scc	1	15q23 → q24
P450c11	2	8q13 → q22
P450c17	1	10q24 → q25
P450c21	2	6p 21.3
P450aro	1	15q21.1
3β-HSD	2	1p11 → p13
17β-HSD—type 1	2	17q21
17β-HSD—type 2	?	16q24
17β-HSD—type 3	1	9q22
17β-HSD—type 4	?	?
Adrenodoxin	1	11q22
	2 pseudogenes	20cen → 13.1
Adrenodoxin Reductase	1	17q24-q25
P450 Reductase	?1	7p15 → q35
5α-Reductase—type 1	1	5p15
	1 pseudogene	Xq24 → qter
5α-Reductase—type 2	1	2p23
11β-HSD—type 1	1	1
11β-HSD—type 2	1	16q22

HSD, hydroxysteroid dehydrogenase.

of the 21B gene that is changed to the sequence of the defective 21A gene. This is unique in human genetics, but it simplifies understanding of the defective alleles causing CAH. There is only a small array of defects in the 21A gene, which dictate the changes that can be found in the 21A gene; by contrast there is an endless variety of defects causing other genetic diseases such as the hemoglobinopathies. Table 257–2 summarizes the mutations causing CAH. Because all persons have two 21B alleles, the severity of the disease in a compound heterozygote is determined by the activity of the less severely affected of the two alleles. Thus the clinical phenotypes listed in the table are those seen if the defect either is truly homozygous or is a compound heterozygote with a severely affected allele. More than one phenotype

TABLE 257–2. MUTATIONS CAUSING 21-HYDROXYLASE DEFICIENCY

MUTATION	LOCATION	ASSOCIATED PHENOTYPES	ACTIVITY
Pro 30 → Leu	Exon 1	NC/SV	30–60%
A → G	Intron 2	SV/SW	minimal
8 bp deletion	Exon 3	SW	0
Ile 172 → Asn	Exon 4	SV	3–7%
Ile 236 → Asp			
Val 237 → Glu	Exon 6	SW	0
Met 239 → Lys			
Val 281 → Leu	Exon 7	NC	18 ± 9%
Gly 292 → Ser	Exon 7	SW	
T insertion @ 306	Exon 7	SW	0
Gly 318 → Stop	Exon 8	SW	0
Arg 339 → His	Exon 8	NC	20–50%
Arg 356 → Trp	Exon 8	SV/SW	2%
Pro 453 → Ser	Exon 10	NC	20–50%
GG → C @ 484	Exon 10	SW	0
Gene deletion	Exons 1–10	SW	0
Macro conversion	Exons 1–10	SW	0

SW, salt-wasting; SV, simple virilizing; NC, nonclassic.

is listed with some of the mutations, due to variations in diagnostic criteria and in extra-adrenal 21-hydroxylation. The base change in intron 2 results in more than one RNA splicing variant. Variations in the phenotypic presentation of a single homozygous lesion are found in most genetic disorders, reflecting the fact that multiple genes contribute to a clinical trait.

Pathophysiology

1. Glucocorticoids are not needed for normal fetal development, and the metabolism of salt and water is handled by the placenta. Thus fetuses affected with 21-hydroxylase deficiency do well until birth. Thereafter, the pathophysiology of the various clinical forms of CAH can be considered variations on the theme of the severe, salt-wasting form. In the mineralocorticoid pathway, the inability to convert progesterone to DOC results in aldosterone deficiency. In the absence of aldosterone, the kidney cannot retain sodium normally, and serum sodium concentrations fall to the low 100s. The kidney also inappropriately retains K^+ and H^+, resulting in hyperkalemia, acidosis, hypotension, shock, cardiovascular collapse, and death. Once diagnosed and treated, such children may continue to be highly resistant to mineralocorticoid therapy, presenting a clinical picture similar to type IV renal tubular acidosis. This "salt-losing crisis" only develops after birth, usually during the second week of life.

2. In the zona fasciculata, inability to convert 17OHP to 11-deoxycortisol results in cortisol deficiency. This impairs carbohydrate metabolism and other processes, such as the action of catecholamines as pressor agents. Prenatal cortisol deficiency does not harm the fetus directly, but it appears to stimulate ACTH secretion, causing the adrenal hyperplasia. More importantly, the prenatal stimulation of the affected fetal adrenal by ACTH leads to overproduction of precursor steroids. The overproduction of 17OHP is useful in prenatal and newborn diagnosis, but the associated overproduction of steroids in C-19 pathway (dehydroepiandrosterone [DHEA] → androstenedione → testosterone) can virilize a female fetus severely. In the male fetus, the testes produce high concentrations of testosterone in early to midgestation, which cause the differentiation of the external male genitalia; in the male fetus with 21-hydroxylase deficiency, the additional adrenal androstenedione and testosterone have no clinically discernible effect. In the female fetus, the ovaries produce no steroids at all; in the female fetus with 21-hydroxylase deficiency, the adrenal testosterone causes varying degrees of virilization of the external genitalia. This can range from mild clitoromegaly, with or without posterior fusion of the labioscrotal folds, to complete labioscrotal fusion including a urethra traversing the enlarged clitoris. At birth, these female infants, who retain normal internal female organs, may have "ambiguous" genitalia or may be sufficiently virilized so that they appear to be male, resulting in errors of sex assignment at birth.

Clinical Forms of 21-Hydroxylase Deficiency

CAH is generally categorized into three clinical forms: salt-wasting, simple virilizing, and nonclassic, which includes the groups sometimes termed late-onset and cryptic.

These are not different diseases, but instead represent points on a continuous spectrum of disease severity.

1. *Salt-wasting* CAH generally refers to patients who manifest hyponatremia, hyperkalemia, and acidosis during a hypovolemic "salt-wasting crisis," which is usually seen in the second week of life, but not in the newborn period. If unrecognized and untreated, such patients will die. The salt-wasting crisis is due to diminished aldosterone and cortisol synthesis; affected females also have severe genital virilization due to conversion of steroidal precursors upstream from 21-hydroxylase to androgens. The combination of adrenal salt loss and genital virilization leads to the term *adrenogenital syndrome* for this disease. Affected females are diagnosed more frequently than affected males because the associated genital virilization usually brings these patients to medical attention. The most sensitive clinical index of prenatal exposure to androgens is posterior fusion of the labia. There is a poor correlation with the degree of genital virilization and the degree of salt loss: Some infants with minimal virilization may be severe salt-losers and some severely virilized females may be non–salt-losers. Thus the diagnosis of salt loss can only be made by seeing a fall in serum sodium and a rise in serum potassium, usually between 5 and 10 days of age.

2. *Simple virilizing* CAH refers to severely virilized patients without clinical signs of salt-wasting. The females are generally diagnosed as newborns, but the males, having normal genitalia, escape diagnosis until 3 to 7 years of age, when they present as rapidly growing masculinized boys with pubic hair, phallic enlargement, increased muscle mass, and advanced bone age. These boys can often be distinguished from boys with true central precocious puberty by the physical examination, as testicular size remains prepubertal in CAH but increases in central precocious puberty. Simple virilizing patients do, in fact, have a defect in mineralocorticoid synthesis, usually evidenced by an elevation in the plasma renin activity (PRA). Patients with simple virilizing CAH have severe disorders of P450c21, but they still retain at least 2 per cent of their 21-hydroxylase activity. This is insufficient to make the large amounts of cortisol normally produced by the adrenal, but it suffices to produce nearly normal amounts of aldosterone, whose circulating concentrations are only 0.1 to 1.0 per cent of those of cortisol.

3. *Nonclassic* patients may come to clinical attention as adolescent or adult females with virilism, acne, and menstrual irregularity, or they may have no manifestations at all.

Diagnosis

1. The diagnosis of CAH should be the first consideration in any newborn infant with genital ambiguity. However, since the genitalia of affected newborn boys are normal, and salt-wasting does not become apparent until after discharge from the newborn nursery, affected males are at great risk. Unfortunately, the diagnosis of salt-wasting CAH is rarely considered in male infants presenting to an emergency room with hyponatremia, hyperkalemia, acidosis, and dehydration; the associated vomiting and diarrhea lead to diagnoses of viral syndromes, gastroenteritis, and pyloric stenosis, so that many of these babies die. Thus the diagnosis must be considered in any infant with hyponatremia as well as in infants with ambiguous genitalia, in any rapidly growing virilized boy, and in any adolescent or adult female with hirsutism, virilism, or menstrual irregularity.

2. The initial evaluation of any child with genital ambiguity includes a karyotype and a basal elevation of the adrenal and gonadal sex steroids (Table 257–3). The most useful diagnostic procedure is an intravenous ACTH test. This benign test should be done as soon as possible, but after 24 hr of age, as 17OHP and many other steroids are elevated during the first 24 hr, clouding the diagnosis. Blood is obtained at 0 and 60 min and assayed for pregnenolone, 17OH-pregnenolone, DHEA, testosterone, 11-deoxycortisol, cortisol, and, most importantly, 17OHP. 17OHP will be elevated in the basal state (> 2000 ng/dl) and will hyper-respond to ACTH in well-characterized patterns. Measurement of all of the above steroids is needed to distinguish 21-hydroxylase deficiency from other forms of CAH and other disorders causing genital ambiguity. If the patient is already receiving physiologic glucocorticoid replacement, it is not necessary to discontinue therapy to do the ACTH test: the 17OHP response will still be diagnostic. Because enzymes other than P450c21 can 21-hydroxylate some steroids, both in the adrenal and peripherally, the measurement of low but detectable levels of 21-hydroxylated steroids does not necessarily mean a "partial block" in steroidogenesis.

3. In the newborn, other crucial tests include a bimanual rectal exam to palpate the estrogenized cervix of the newborn female, and pelvic ultrasonography. With rare exceptions, an ultrasonographically detectable uterus will indicate a 46,XX female, but the absence of a sonographically detectable uterus is uninformative, as a retroflexed uterus may be missed fairly easily. Parents should be counseled to delay naming the child for 4 to 5 days until diagnosis and the genetic sex are unambiguously established by the ACTH test and the karyotype, and they should be told that a virilized female will be able to have normal adult sexual function irrespective of the newborn genital appearance, once proper corrective surgery is completed. The diagnosis in older children requires an ACTH test, bone age, karyotype, and measurement of plasma renin activity (PRA). The diagnosis of nonclassic CAH in adolescents and adults is based entirely on the results of the ACTH test.

Treatment

1. The infant with newly diagnosed CAH will typically be hyponatremic, hyperkalemic, acidotic, hypovolemic, and hypotensive. Acute treatment consists of replacing the fluid volume with saline solutions and administering intravenous hydrocortisone. Resuscitation of patients in shock with pressor agents requires the permissive effect of glucocorticoids on catecholamine action. Initial glucocorticoid doses should be high, both to deal with acute stress and to suppress the hyperstimulated adrenal. Initial doses of 25 mg hydrocortisone, given stat and then as 6 mg IV every 6 hr, work well but should be reduced to maintenance levels within a week. This also suffices for much of the mineralocorticoid requirement during the

TABLE 257–3.   MEAN SEX STEROID CONCENTRATIONS*

	PROG	17OHP	DHEA	DHEA-S	Δ⁴-A	E₁	E₂	T M	T F	DHT M	DHT F
Cord blood	36000	1900	600	235	90	1500	810	30	25	6	6
Prematures	350	250	800	400	200			120	10	30	4
Term newborns		35	570	160	150			200	40	25	10
Infants	30	30	110	30	20			190	<10	40	<3
Children 1–6 yr			30	10	25	<1.5	<1.5	5		<3	
6–8 yr			90	20	25	<1.5	<1.5	5		<3	
8–10 yr			160	50	25	<1.5	<1.5	5		<3	
Males											
Pubertal stage I	20	40	160	35	25	1.1	0.8	5		<3	
II	20	50	300	95	45	1.6	1.1	40		8	
III	25	60	390	120	70	2.1	1.6	190		20	
IV	35	80	400	200	80	3.3	2.2	370		35	
V	40	100	500	230	100	3.2	2.1	550		45	
Adult	35	100	450	270	115	3.0	2.0	620		50	
Females											
Pubertal stage I	20	30	160	50	25	1.3	0.8		5		<3
II	30	50	330	70	65	2.1	1.6		20		8
III	40	70	390	90	120	3.0	2.5		25		10
IV	290	90	430	120	130	3.6	4.7		25		10
V	160	110	540	150	160	6.1	11.0		30		10
Adult											
Follicular	30	45	450	150	165	6.0	5.0		30		10
Luteal	750	165	450	150	165	11.0	13.0		30		10

*All values except DHEA-S are in ng/100 mL of plasma; DHEA-S is in µg/100 mL.
PROG, progesterone; 17OHP, 17 hydroxyprogesterone; DHEA, dehydroepiandrosterone; DHEA-S, DHEA sulfate; Δ⁴-A, androstenedione; E₁, estrone; E₂, estradiol; T, testosterone; DHT, dihydrotestosterone; M, male; F, female.
Data adapted from Endocrine Sciences, Tarzana, CA.

acute resuscitation, as cortisol (hydrocortisone) has substantial mineralocorticoid action (Table 257–4). The only mineralocorticoid preparation currently available in the United States is fludrocortisone (Florinef), administered orally. This should be given in doses of 0.1 to 0.3 mg daily as soon as possible. These doses are larger than the adult replacement doses, as newborns are normally highly resistant to mineralocorticoids and normally have very high aldosterone levels. In addition, about 1 g/day of NaCl as an oral supplement will be needed in most infants.

2. The basic principles in the long-term management of CAH are to replace the steroids that the adrenal fails to make and to suppress the overproduction of androgens. In practice this is an extremely difficult balancing act. Treatment with low doses of glucocorticoids will lead to incomplete suppression of adrenal androgens, causing disproportionate acceleration in the bone age, and ultimate short stature; however, treatment with generous doses of glucocorticoids will also lead to poor growth as minimally supraphysiologic glucocorticoid regimens can suppress normal growth. Recent studies indicate that the physiologic secretory rate of cortisol is 7 to 8 mg/m²/day, much less than the widely used 12.5 mg/m²/day figure. While this provides a good guide in the treatment of Addison disease (see Chapter 259), it will rarely provide adequate suppression of adrenal androgen secretion in CAH. Because there are substantial variations in individual gastrointestinal absorption rates and metabolism, therapy must be individualized for each patient. It is crucial to follow bone age, height, and height velocity as well as steroid values in treating CAH, as growth and bone maturation indicate the long-term results of therapy. Growth and bone age may progress normally in patients receiving doses of glucocorticoids that only partially suppress 17OHP; thus no single variable can be followed to indicate the success of therapy.

3. The clinical pharmacology of the glucocorticoid used for replacement therapy is also crucial. Cortisone acetate and hydrocortisone are preferred because they are relatively weak glucocorticoids, making it is easier to make small incremental changes in doses as the child grows. They also have significant mineralocorticoid effects. Many pediatric endocrinologists treat newborns with intramuscular cortisone acetate once every 3 days for the first year of life. This eliminates variability due to swallowing and

absorption, and it ensures the infant has retained the dose during illnesses and vomiting. Difficulties arise with powerful oral synthetic glucocorticoids such as prednisone or dexamethasone. The generally available tables of glucocorticoid dosage "equivalents" are based on their anti-inflammatory effects; however, the anti-inflammatory and growth-suppressant effects of various glucocorticoids are not equivalent. The more potent steroids with longer biologic half-lives have a disproportionately greater growth suppressant effect and lack mineralocorticoid activity (see Table 257–4). "Stress doses" of glucocorticoids are usually given during illness because cortisol secretory rates normally rise in response to trauma, surgery, or severe illness. Patients with CAH cannot mount such a stress response, and hence they need coverage with "stress doses" of steroids. Modern surgical and anesthesiologic techniques have reduced surgical stress. Appropriate doses are three times physiologic during surgery and for 2 to 3 days afterwards. It is not usually necessary to triple a child's physiologic replacement regimen during routine colds, upper respiratory infection, or otitis media or following immunizations, unless the patient is febrile.

4. As glucocorticoids can suppress growth, even at doses that generate no "cushingoid" features, a goal of therapy is to use as little glucocorticoid as possible. ACTH can be suppressed with somewhat lower glucocorticoid doses if other stimuli to ACTH, such as hypovolemia, are eliminated. All patients with CAH, even those with the non–salt-losing form, have a defect in aldosterone synthesis and hence tend to have a mild degree of salt loss leading to chronic compensated hypovolemia. Thus mineralocorticoid replacement should be used to suppress the PRA irrespective of whether there is a history of salt-losing episodes. The use of fludrocortisone in doses of 0.05 to 0.10 mg/day in children with non–salt-losing CAH will ensure suppression of the PRA, removing the hypovolemic drive to ACTH. The same principle applies to salt-losers, although maintenance doses of fludrocortisone are usually 0.10 to 0.15 mg/day.

5. Overdosage can result from the misinterpretation of laboratory data. The adequacy of steroidal replacement is generally assessed by measuring the suppression of adrenal steroidogenesis. However, because some 21-hydroxylation is catalyzed by enzymes other than P450c21, adequate steroidal therapy may not completely suppress all

TABLE 257–4. RELATIVE POTENCY OF VARIOUS STEROIDS

STEROID	ANTIINFLAMMATORY GLUCOCORTICOID EFFECT	GROWTH-RETARDING GLUCOCORTICOID EFFECT	SALT-RETAINING MINERALOCORTICOID EFFECT
Cortisol (hydrocortisone)	1.0	1.0	1.0
Cortisone acetate (oral)	0.8	0.8	0.8
Cortisone acetate (IM)	0.8	1.3	0.8
Prednisone	3.5–4.0	5	0.8
Prednisolone	4		0.8
Methylprednisolone	5	7.5	0.5
Betamethasone	25–30		0
Triamcinolone	5		0
Dexamethasone	30	80	0
Fludrocortisone	15		200

plasma 21-hydroxylated steroids. Similarly, familiarity with the normal developmental pattern of adrenal androgen secretion is essential in the management of the older child. About 2 years before the onset of puberty (i.e., before the initial activation of the hypothalamic-pituitary-gonadal axis), children undergo adrenarche. This is a normal increase in the secretion of adrenal androgens that is not associated with changes in glucocorticoid or mineralocorticoid secretion, and it is independent of gonadotropins and puberty. All of the plasma steroids that are normally assessed in the management of CAH, including DHEA, 17OHP, Δ^4-androstenedione, and testosterone, increase in normal children undergoing adrenarche. Unrecognized adrenarche may be mistaken for poor control of CAH, leading to unnecessary increases in glucocorticoid doses and compromised growth.

6. In addition to hormonal, medical, and surgical management, the treatment of CAH requires careful, repeated, long-term counseling of the family. Many families will be concerned about the psychosexual development of virilized females. The degree to which the human brain is sexually dimorphic, in addition to the roles of androgens in brain development, remains controversial. Recent studies show that adult females with CAH have a more negative body image, have less sexual activity, and have less interest in sexual activity. They tend to marry with a lower frequency, have fewer children when they do marry, and have a higher incidence of lesbianism than the general population. However, the relative contributions of fetal adrenal androgens versus the contributions of parental uncertainty about the sex assignment, and of the possible psychologic trauma of genital surgery have not been distinguished. Thus the diagnosis and management of severe forms of CAH is precarious and complex and should be undertaken only by experienced pediatric endocrinologists.

Key Treatment

- Restore fluid volume and sodium chloride
- Hydrocortisone
- Fludrocortisone

Prenatal Diagnosis and Treatment

1. Prenatal diagnosis of CAH can be done hormonally, by HLA linkage, or by molecular genetic techniques when a pregnancy is known to be at risk because of a previously affected child. Amniotic fluid concentrations of 17OHP, androstenedione, and 21-deoxycortisol are fairly reliable for the diagnosis of severe salt-losing CAH, but they may not be elevated above the broad range of normal in simple

virilizing CAH and hence should not be relied on for prenatal diagnosis. HLA typing of fetal amniocytes can be useful only if the HLA types of both parents and of the previously affected child are known, but it is technically difficult and may not always be informative. Thus hormonal and HLA diagnostics are being replaced by molecular genetic diagnostics.

2. The principal indication for prenatal diagnosis is to permit parents to make informed decisions about the pregnancy. However, early prenatal diagnosis is sometimes sought because of the possibility of prenatal treatment. Several groups have administered dexamethasone to pregnant women carrying fetuses at risk for CAH. The rationale is that early administration of a glucocorticoid that traverses the placenta will suppress the fetal hypothalamic-pituitary-adrenal axis so that excess adrenal androgens are not produced, thus substantially ameliorating the virilization of the fetal genitalia. Clinical experience indicates that such treatment is most effective when started very early, at 4 to 5 weeks of gestation. However, it is not clear that the hypothalamic-pituitary-adrenal axis is functioning at this time; furthermore, some fetal adrenal steroidogenesis appears to be independent of ACTH. Hence the mode of action of early prenatal administration of dexamethasone has not been established. It is not possible to obtain DNA by chorionic villus biopsy until about 10 weeks, and time must also be allowed for analysis of the samples. Thus substantial time elapses between instituting therapy and obtaining the subsequent molecular diagnosis. Of the initially treated pregnancies, only one in four will be affected with CAH, and, of those affected, only the females will be helped by the treatment; thus seven of eight fetuses will be treated unnecessarily. Thus prenatal treatment has generated both excitement and controversy. At the present time, prenatal treatment of CAH remains experimental and can be done only with the approval of appropriate human experimentation committees and with informed parental consent, all done in the context of prospective academic research studies.

Bibliography

Miller WL, Tyrrell JB: The adrenal cortex. *In* Felig P, Baxter JD, Frohman L (eds): Endocrinology and Metabolism, 3rd ed. New York, McGraw Hill, 1995, pp 555–717.

Morel Y, Miller WL: Clinical and molecular genetics of congenital adrenal hyperplasia due to 21-hydroxylase deficiency. Adv Hum Genet 1991;20:1–68.

New MI, White PC, Speiser PW, et al: Congenital adrenal hyperplasia. *In* Emery AEH, Rimoin DL (eds): Principles and Practice of Medical Genetics, 2nd ed. Edinburgh, UK, Churchill Livingstone, 1990, pp 1559–1591.

Seckl JR, Miller WL: How safe is long-term prenatal glucocorticoid treatment? JAMA 1997;277:1077–1079.

258 Other Congenital Adrenal Hyperplasias

Walter L. Miller

Definition and Biochemistry

1. Mineralocorticoids are adrenal steroids that exert crucial roles in salt and water metabolism and in the regulation of blood pressure. In considering salt and water metabolism, one should remember that mineralocorticoids act by promoting the retention of salt by the kidney, while the retention of water is stimulated by vasopressin (antidiuretic hormone) produced by the posterior pituitary. Adrenal steroids are synthesized from cholesterol according to the pathway shown in Chapter 257. The adrenal cortex is divided anatomically and functionally into three zones. The outermost, the zona glomerulosa, is the principal site of mineralocorticoid synthesis, the inner zones, the fasciculata and reticularis, are the principal sites of glucocorticoid and adrenal androgen synthesis. The enzymology and cell biology of the zona glomerulosa is distinct in three respects. First, its cells have receptors for angiotensin II (AII), whereas the cells of the other adrenal zones have few AII receptors. Second, glomerulosa cells fail to express the enzyme P450c17, which is required for glucocorticoid and sex steroid synthesis. Third, glomerulosa cells uniquely express the aldosterone synthase enzyme, P450c11AS.

2. The biosynthesis of mineralocorticoids from pregnenolone requires the sequential action of only three enzymes: 3β-hydroxysteroid dehydrogenase (3βHSD), P450c21, and P450c11AS. Only the type II 3βHSD is involved in the adrenal and gonadal production of progesterone; the type I enzyme is expressed only in extraglandular tissues. Progesterone in the zona glomerulosa is then hydroxylated at carbon 21 by the adrenal 21-hydroxylase, P450c21 to yield 11-deoxycorticosterone (DOC). DOC itself is a potent mineralocorticoid, and overproduction of DOC, such as in 11β-hydroxylase (P450c11β) deficiency, can cause salt retention and hypertension. DOC is then converted to aldosterone, a more potent mineralocorticoid, in three steps, all catalyzed by a single mitochondrial enzyme, P450c11AS.

Physiology

1. The two principal regulators of mineralocorticoid biosynthesis and secretion are the renin/angiotensin system and potassium ion; adrenocorticotropic hormone (ACTH) and sodium ion play minor roles.

    a. Renin is a serine protease secreted by the juxtaglomerular cells of the kidney in response to decreased blood pressure and/or intravascular volume. Renin cleaves off the first 10 amino acids of angiotensinogen, a blood-borne glycoprotein produced by the liver to produce biologically inactive angiotensin I. Converting enzyme, found in the lung, then cleaves off two carboxy-terminal amino acids from angiotensin I to form the active octapeptide, angiotensin II (AII). Inhibition of converting enzyme with agents such as captopril is useful in the treatment of hypertension. AII rapidly stimulates arteriolar vasoconstriction, thus increasing blood pressure, and stimulates the biosynthesis of aldosterone. AII binds to cell surface receptors linked to the protein kinase C/Ca^{++} second messenger pathway; by contrast, ACTH activates the cAMP/protein kinase A pathway.

    b. Potassium ion exerts similar effects on the zona glomerulosa by depolarizing the cell membrane, which results in the uptake of extracellular Ca^{++}. Thus AII and K$^+$ activate the same intracellular second messenger pathway at different levels, but exert fundamentally different actions from ACTH.

2. The human mineralocorticoid and glucocorticoid receptors are closely related members of the superfamily of nuclear zinc-finger transcription factors. This family includes ligand-dependent receptors, such as those for thyroid and steroid hormones, vitamin D, and retinoic acid. There is 57 per cent amino acid sequence identity in the ligand binding domains of the mineralocorticoid and glucocorticoid receptors, leading to substantial overlap in their binding activities. These binding activities are so similar that these receptors are frequently referred to as type I and type II glucocorticoid receptors, respectively. When the steroid-binding activities of these receptors were measured either in vitro or in transfected cell systems, the results initially appeared to be inconsistent with physiology. Cortisol, prednisolone, DOC, and aldosterone all bind well to both the glucocorticoid and mineralocorticoid receptors, but cortisone and prednisone do not bind to either type of receptor. Thus only the chemically reduced form of the steroids is active; their oxidized forms (cortisone, prednisone), which are frequently used as drugs, are inactive. Furthermore, both glucocorticoid and mineralocorticoid steroid hormones can bind to both the glucocorticoid and mineralocorticoid receptors, yet mineralocorticoids clearly exert distinct actions. These two apparent paradoxes are explained by the actions of 11β-hydroxysteroid dehydrogenase (11βHSD).

3. 11βHSD is a microsomal enzyme that interconverts the active steroids cortisol and corticosterone to their inactive metabolites, cortisone and 11-dehydrocorticosterone, respectively. There are at least two 11βHSD enzymes.

    a. Type I, 11βHSD, encoded by a gene on chromosome 1, catalyzes both the oxidase (cortisol → cortisone) and reductase (cortisone → cortisol) reactions using either NADP or NADPH as a co-factor and has a high Km (1μM) so that only abundant steroids will be metabolized. The type I enzyme is expressed predominantly in glucocorticoid target tissues such as liver, testis, lung, and proximal convoluted tubule and favors activation of cortisone to cortisol, and of prednisone to prednisolone.

b. The type II enzyme is crucial in regulating mineralocorticoid action. Type II 11βHSD, encoded by a gene on chromosome 16q22, is only 14 per cent identical to the type I enzyme. This enzyme catalyzes only the oxidase reaction (cortisol to cortisone) uses NAD as a co-factor and has a low Km (10–100nM). Thus the type II 11βHSD inactivates cortisol in mineralocorticoid target tissues, "defending" the mineralocorticoid receptor from being overwhelmed by the much higher concentrations of glucocorticoids. When there is congenital absence of type II 11βHSD (the syndrome of apparent mineralocorticoid excess) or when the enzyme's activity is inhibited by licorice or carbenoxolone, the protective mechanism fails and cortisol gains inappropriate access to mineralocorticoid receptors, resulting in hypertension and hypokalemia. Type II 11βHSD is abundantly expressed in mineralocorticoid target tissues such as kidney and colon, and is also expressed in pancreas, placenta, prostate, and gonads. The type II enzyme is dose-dependently inhibited by its end product (11-dehydrocorticosterone) while the type I enzyme is not.

Salt-Wasting Disorders of Mineralocorticoid Synthesis

The findings in the various forms of CAH are summarized in Table 258–1.

1. Congenital lipoid adrenal hyperplasia (lipoid CAH)

   a. Lipoid CAH is the most severe form of CAH. Affected individuals can synthesize no steroid hormones, and hence are all phenotypic females with a severe salt-losing syndrome that is fatal if not treated early. While it has been thought that the disorder was due to mutations in the cholesterol side-chain cleavage enzyme (P450scc), this has been ruled out by molecular genetic analysis. Because P450scc is needed for the placental production of progesterone, and placental progesterone is required for the maintenance of the second and third trimesters of pregnancy, it is likely that mutations of P450scc would be lethal prenatally.

   b. The molecular lesion in lipoid CAH was recently found in the steroidogenic acute regulatory protein (StAR),which promotes the flow of cholesterol into mitochondria, so that it can be converted to pregnenolone by P450scc. Infants with lipoid CAH are normal at birth, consistent with the notion that glucocorticoids are not essential for fetal development.

   c. The testes of genetic 46,XY males with lipoid CAH cannot produce testosterone but continue to produce müllerian inhibitory factor (a glycoprotein). Thus, affected males have normal female external genitalia with a blind vaginal pouch but lack a uterus, fallopian tubes, and cervix. Affected 46,XX females have normal female external genitalia.

   d. Lipoid CAH usually becomes clinically apparent in the second week of life with symptoms of glucocorticoid and mineralocorticoid insufficiency, including poor feeding, lethargy, diarrhea, vomiting, hypotension, dehydration, hyponatremia, hyperkalemia, and acidosis, that is, the same symptoms seen in salt-losing 21-hydroxylase deficiency or any other congenital absence of mineralocorticoid biosynthesis. Early treatment with appropriate replacement doses of glucocorticoids and fludrocortisone (as described in Chapter 257) is effective. Genetic males with this disorder should be reared as females and undergo orchiectomy in early childhood. Lipoid CAH is distinguished from congenital absence of the adrenals by finding massively enlarged adrenals on an abdominal CT or MRI.

   f. Lipoid CAH is rare in most populations but is the second most common form in individuals of Japanese ancestry, most of whom carry the Q258X mutation; Palestinians are also commonly affected. As with many "rare" diseases, the apparent incidence increases once the disorder becomes recognized, its basis is determined, and treatment is successful.

2. 3β-Hydroxysteroid dehydrogenase (3βHSD) deficiency

   a. 3βHSD deficiency is a rare autosomal recessive disorder of the type II 3βHSD gene, which is expressed in the adrenals and gonads. More than 24 lesions in the type II gene have been reported causing the classic form of 3βHSD. The type I gene is expressed in the placenta and in peripheral tissues such as the skin and mammary gland, whereas the type II gene is expressed in the adrenals and gonads. The type I gene is required for the synthesis of placental progesterone, which is needed to maintain pregnancy. Mutations in this gene are probably incompatible with fetal survival, and have not been found in any patient. In its classic form, 3βHSD deficiency impairs cortisol, aldosterone, and testosterone synthesis and usually causes ambiguous genitalia in newborn males.

   b. 3βHSD is a membrane-bound short-chain dehydrogenase that catalyzes 3β-hydroxysteroid dehydrogenation and isomerization of the double bond from the B ring (Δ5-steroids) to the A ring (Δ4 steroids) in both adrenal and gonads. Thus the plasma concentrations of pregnenolone, 17-hydroxypregnenolone, DHEA, and DHEA sulfate are elevated in affected patients. Plasma levels of 17OHP may be also increased as a result of the action of type I 3βHSD in the liver and skin, which will still convert 17-hydroxypregnenolone to 17-hydroxypregnenolone even when the type II enzyme is disordered in the adrenals and gonads. Such high levels of 17OHP may lead to an incorrect diagnosis of 21-hydroxylase deficiency. Thus, in all cases of suspected CAH, it is important to examine a complete panel of adrenal steroids, both before and after ACTH stimulation. In 3βHSD deficiency, the plasma 17-hydroxypregnenolone/17-hydroxyprogesterone ratio will remain strikingly elevated, permitting the diagnosis to be made. The excretion of urinary 17-ketosteroids is also increased due to the overproduction of DHEA and its sulfate.

TABLE 258–1. CLINICAL AND LABORATORY FINDINGS IN THE VARIOUS FORMS OF CONGENITAL ADRENAL HYPERPLASIA

ENZYME DEFICIENCY	PRESENTATION	LABORATORY FINDINGS	THERAPEUTIC MEASURES
Lipoid CAH (StAR)	Salt-wasting crisis Male pseudohermaphroditism	Low/absent levels of all steroid hormones, with decreased/absent response to ACTH Decreased/absent response to hCG in male pseudohermaphroditism ↑ ACTH ↑ PRA	Glucocorticoid and mineralocorticoid replacement Salt supplementation Estrogen replacement at age ≥12 years Gonadectomy of male pseudohermaphrodite
3βHSD	*Classic form:* Salt-wasting crisis Male and female pseudohermaphroditism *Nonclassic form:* Premature adrenarche, menstrual irregularity, hirsutism, acne, infertility	↑ Δ^5 steroids before and after ACTH ↑ Δ^5/Δ^4 ratio of serum steroids Suppression of elevated adrenal steroids after glucocorticoid administration ↑ ACTH ↑ PRA	Glucocorticoid and mineralocorticoid replacement Salt supplementation Surgical correction of genitalia Sex hormone replacement as necessary
P450c21	*Classic form:* Salt-wasting crisis Female pseudohermaphroditism Pre- and postnatal virilization *Nonclassic form:* Premature adrenarche, menstrual irregularity, hirsuitism, acne, infertility	↑ 17OHP before and after ACTH ↑ Serum androgens and urine 17KS Suppression of elevated adrenal steroids after glucocorticoid R_x ↑ ACTH ↑ PRA	Glucocorticoid and mineralocorticoid replacement Salt supplementation Surgical repair of female pseudohermaphroditism
P450c11β	*Classic form:* Female pseudohermaphroditism Postnatal virilization in males and females *Nonclassic form:* Premature adrenarche, menstrual irregularity, hirsuitism, acne, infertility	↑ 11-deoxycortisol and DOC before and after ACTH ↑ Serum androgens and urine 17KS Suppression of elevated steroids after glucocorticoid administration ↑ ACTH ↓ PRA Hypokalemia	Glucocorticoid administration Surgical repair of female pseudohermaphroditism
P450c11AS (CMOI & II)	Failure to thrive Weakness Salt loss	Hyponatremia, hyperkalemia ↑ Corticosterone ↑ PRA ↓ Aldosterone CMOI: ↓ 18OH corticosterone CMOII: ↑ 18OH corticosterone	Mineralocorticoid replacement Salt supplementation
P450c17	Male pseudohermaphroditism Sexual infantilism Hypertension	↑ DOC, 18-OHDOC, corticosterone, 18-hydroxycorticosterone Low 17α-hydroxylated steroids and poor response to ACTH Poor response to hCG in male pseudohermaphroditism Suppression of elevated adrenal steroids after glucocorticoid administration ↓ PRA ↑ ACTH Hypokalemia	Glucocorticoid administration Surgical correction of genitalia and sex steroid replacement in male pseudohermaphroditism consonant with sex of rearing Estrogen replacement in female at ≥12 years Testosterone replacement if reared as male (rare)

ACTH = adrenocorticotropic hormone; CAH = congenital adrenal hyperplasia; CMO = corticosterone methyl oxidase; DOC = deoxycorticosterone; hCG = human chorionic gonadotropin; 3βHSD = 3β-hydroxysteroid dehydrogenase; 17-OHP = 17α-hydroxyprogesterone; PRA = plasma renin activity; StAR = steroidogenic acute regulatory protein.

c. In its severe, classic form, 3βHSD deficiency presents with the typical signs of glucocorticoid and mineralocorticoid deficiency discussed above, and will be fatal if not diagnosed and treated with appropriate glucocorticoid and mineralocorticoid replacement. An unusual feature of 3βHSD deficiency is that both affected females and males may have ambiguous genitalia. Severely affected 46,XX genetic females will produce large amounts of DHEA, which may undergo peripheral conversion by 3βHSD type I to produce androstenedione and small amounts of testosterone, partially virilizing the genitalia. Severely affected males cannot produce adequate testicular testosterone in utero to undergo normal male sexual development, but again, the peripheral conversion of DHEA to androstenedione and testosterone will result in partial masculinization. This emphasizes why a karyotype is a crucial part of the evaluation of genital ambiguity, and should be obtained as soon as the infant is seen. Hirsutism associated with mildly elevated ratios of Δ^5 to steroids has been described in women and adolescent girls, and has been thought to be due to a mild, "nonclassic" form of 3βHSD deficiency. However, no mutations have been reported in either the type I or type II 3βHSD genes in these individuals, suggesting that the traditional hormonal diagnostic criteria do not truly identify a disorder of 3βHSD.

Key Treatment: Lipoid CAH and 3β-Hydroxysteroid Dehydrogenase Deficiency

- Glucocorticoids
- Fludrocortisone
- Sodium chloride

3. **21-Hydroxylase deficiency.** Steroid 21-hydroxylase deficiency comprises about 95 per cent of all cases of CAH and has an overall incidence of about 1 in 12,000 persons. About two thirds of patients have salt loss, making it the most common congenital salt-losing disease. This disorder is discussed in Chapter 257.

4. **Corticosterone methyloxidase (CMO) deficiencies.** The term *CMO deficiency* is somewhat archaic, as it derives from a time when the enzymes needed for mineralocorticoid synthesis had not yet been identified as discrete molecular entities, yet the CMO classification remains useful. Two different syndromes are generally recognized:

   a. CMO I deficiency refers to patients who have salt-wasting associated with high serum concentrations of corticosterone but low concentrations of 18OH-corticosterone and aldosterone.

   b. CMO II deficiency is similar except that 18OH corticosterone concentrations are high.

   c. In both cases, aldosterone deficiency leads to hyponatremia, hyperkalemia, and metabolic acidosis. These disorders are milder and present later in infancy than the salt-wasting forms of CAH associated with cortisol deficiency, because the continued production of cortisol in the CMO deficiencies provides some mineralocorticoid activity. The clinical severity of the CMO deficiencies varies inversely with the age: Infants and newborns tend to be severely affected while older children and adults may have normal serum electrolytes, even without treatment. Similarly, the plasma renin activity (PRA) is markedly elevated in very young patients, but may be normal in adults. In both forms of CMO deficiency, aldosterone synthesis is impaired while the adrenal zona glomerulosa continues to produce corticosterone and deoxycorticosterone in response to the renin-angiotensin system. The age-dependent clinical severity of the CMO deficiencies correlates with the age-dependent sensitivity to mineralocorticoids.

   d. Normal infants are mineralocorticoid resistant and have high concentrations of aldosterone, which fall drastically in later life (Table 258–2). Thus untreated affected individuals who survive infancy (due to high-salt diets or increased DOC secretion) may appear to outgrow their disease, and become normal adults. Thus treatment in the newborn consists of fludrocortisone (usually 0.10 to 0.15 mg PO daily) and supplemental NaCl (0.5 to 1.0 g daily), but these doses may need to be reduced as the child gets older. Therefore it is important to monitor blood pressure and PRA every 6 to 12 months. Because plasma 18OH corticosterone is low in CMO I and high in CMO II deficiency, but aldosterone is low in both disorders, the ratio of 18OH corticosterone to aldosterone is the usual differential diagnostic hallmark. However, this is not always reliable in CMO I deficiency; the ratio of corticosterone to 18-hydroxycorticosterone should also be increased in CMO I deficiency, and decreased in CMO II deficiency, corresponding to the absence or presence of 18-hydroxylase activity, respectively.

   e. Recent studies have examined the CYP11B2 gene encoding P450c11AS in the CMO deficiencies. Mutations causing CMO I deficiency include a deletion of five nucleotides, and the mutation R384P, which still resulted in low levels of 18-hydroxycorticosterone. The type II deficiency is common among Jews of Iranian origin, in whom the affected individuals are homozygous for two different point mutations, R181W and V386A. Family members homozygous for only one of these mutations were phenotypically and clinically normal: Both mutations were required to produce disease. An unrelated patient with a typical clinical and hormonal picture of CMO II deficiency was a complex compound heterozygote, where the father's allele contributed T318M and V386A while mother's allele contributed R181W and the deletion/frame-shift mutation ΔC372. Both of these mutants were inactive in vitro so that the predicted clinical phenotype would have been CMO I than CMO II deficiency; the basis of the elevated 18OH corticosterone in this patient is unknown. Other patients with the clinical and hormonal findings of CMO II deficiency have no mutations of P450c11AS at all. These findings suggest that other enzymes may be involved in the synthesis of other mineralocorticoids.

Key Treatment: Corticosterone Methyloxidase Deficiencies

- Fludrocortisone
- Supplemental NaCl

Hypertensive Genetic Disorders of Mineralocorticoid Synthesis

1. 11β-Hydroxylase deficiency
   a. Steroid 11β-hydroxylase deficiency is the second

TABLE 258–2. NORMAL AGE-RELATED MINERALOCORTICOID VALUES (μg/dL)

	CORTISOL	DOC	CORTICOSTERONE	18-OH CORTICOSTERONE	ALDOSTERONE	PLASMA RENIN ACTIVITY*
Cord blood	13	180	650		85	1800
Prematures	6.5			200	100	8000
Newborns	5		230	350	95	2100
Infants	9	20	545	80	30	1200
Children (8 AM)						
1–2 yr	4–20			65	28	535
2–10 yr	10–20	10		45	10→30†	300
10–15 yr	10–20			25	5→20†	120
Adults (8 AM)	10–20	7	425	20	7→13†	199→145†
(4 AM)	5–10		130			

*In ng/dL/hr.
†Two values separated by an arrow indicate those in supine and upright posture.
DOC = deoxycorticosterone.

most common cause of CAH, but still comprises less than 5 per cent of patients with CAH. However, a large number of cases has been reported among Jews of Moroccan descent, among whom the incidence is 1/5000 to 1/7000. 11β-Hydroxylase deficiency is caused by mutations in the CYP11B1 gene that encodes P450c11β, thus disrupting the conversion of 11-deoxycortisol to cortisol. As a consequence of deficient cortisol production, the pituitary secretes large amounts of ACTH, stimulating adrenal steroidogenesis. Thus affected patients characteristically have very high serum concentrations of 11-deoxycortisol, which is the diagnostic hallmark of the disorder. The ACTH-driven adrenal hyperactivity will lead to accumulation of steroidal precursors that are converted to androgens. Just as in 21-hydroxylase deficiency, this leads to virilization of female fetuses in utero, but causes no anatomic changes in males.

b. The unique aspect of 11β-hydroxylase deficiency is that the patients also produce excess DOC, principally in the ACTH-responsive cells of the adrenal zona fasciculata. As DOC is an effective mineralocorticoid, the excess DOC can cause retention of salt and water and consequent hypertension. This ACTH-driven overproduction of DOC also suppresses the renin-angiotensin system and the secretion of aldosterone so that the patients have mineralocorticoid-based hypertension in the absence of the principal mineralocorticoid, aldosterone. Although 11β-hydroxylase deficiency is often termed the *hypertensive form of CAH*, the hypertension may not develop for several years, and affected newborns may actually present with a paradoxical salt-losing episode. This is probably due to the mineralocorticoid resistance typical of newborns and the lower potency of DOC as a mineralocorticoid.

c. Numerous mutations in P450c11β that cause 11β-hydroxylase deficiency have been described. The high incidence in Jews from Morocco is due to the mutation R448H, and at least 10 other mutations have been identified in other populations.

Key Treatment: 11β-Hydroxylase Deficiency

- Glucocorticoid replacement

2. 17α-Hydroxylase deficiency. Deficient 17α-hydroxylase activity is a rare form of CAH, caused by defects in cytochrome P450c17, the single enzyme that has 17α-hydroxylase and 17,20-lyase activities. More than 125 cases of 17α-hydroxylase deficiency and 14 other cases of apparently isolated 17,20-lyase deficiency have been reported. The molecular lesions in the P450c17 gene on chromosome 10q24 → 25 causing 17-hydroxylase deficiency have now studied in about two dozen patients, identifying at least 17 different mutations. 17-Hydroxylase deficiency is characterized by absent sex steroid synthesis and by impaired production of cortisol and compensatory hypersecretion of ACTH, which stimulates the synthesis of large amounts of DOC, 18-hydroxy-DOC, corticosterone, and 18-hydroxycorticosterone. Although these patients cannot make cortisol, the elevated concentrations of ACTH stimulate the overproduction of corticosterone in the zona fasciculata. As corticosterone is a fairly good glucocorticoid, patients with 17α-hydroxylase deficiency rarely have signs of glucocorticoid deficiency. While the steroidogenic pathway might suggest that these patients will overproduce aldosterone, most do not. ACTH also stimulates the overproduction of DOC in the zona fasciculata, resulting in sodium retention and hypertension, but also suppressing aldosterone secretion from the zona glomerulosa. Absence of 17α-hydroxylase and 17,20-lyase activities also prohibits the production of adrenal and gonadal sex steroids. As a result, genetic 46,XY males may have completely female external genitalia or may have incomplete development (male pseudohermaphroditism). Affected 46,XX females are phenotypically normal but fail to undergo adrenarche and puberty. The classic presentation is that of a teenage female who has no breast development and no pubic or axillary hair (sexual infantilism) and hypertension. The diagnosis is made by finding low or absent 17-hydroxylated C21 and C19

plasma steroids and low urinary 17OHCS and 17KS, which respond poorly to stimulation with ACTH. Serum levels of DOC, corticosterone, and 18OH-corticosterone will be elevated, will hyper-respond to ACTH, and will suppress with glucocorticoid treatment. Heterozygous parents and siblings may have slight increases in plasma DOC, corticosterone, 18-hydroxy DOC and 18-hydroxycorticosterone and exaggerated responses of 17-deoxysteroids to ACTH stimulation, but the ratio of urinary metabolites of C21,17-deoxysteroids to C21,17 hydroxysteroids is the most accurate means of heterozyote detection.

Key Treatment: 17α-Hydroxylase Deficiency

- Glucocorticoids

3. Syndrome of apparent mineralocorticoid excess (AME). This rare disorder presents with the symptoms of mineralocorticoid excess, including hypertension, salt retention, hypokalemia, and suppressed plasma renin activity, but no mineralocorticoid excess is found, as plasma aldosterone and DOC are low. This disorder is due to mutations in the type 2 (renal) 11βHSD enzyme that is normally responsible for "defending" the mineralocorticoid receptor. In the absence of type 2 11βHSD, cortisol cannot be inactivated to cortisone and hence acts as a potent mineralocorticoid. The clinical diagnosis is confirmed by examining urinary steroids by mass spectrometry, showing a high ratio of metabolites of cortisol to those of cortisone. Treatment is symptomatic, emphasizing spironolactone, diuretics, and captopril.

Key Treatment: Syndrome of Apparent Mineralocorticoid Excess

- Diuretics

4. Glucocorticoid-suppressible hypertension. This rare disease causes hypertension with low or normal serum potassium and low plasma renin. It is caused by a genetic recombination between the adjacent genes for P450c11β and P450c11AS. This creates a hybrid c11β/c11AS gene. The hybrid, which contains the P450c11β regulatory sequences, is expressed in the zona fasciculata in response to ACTH, but the coding region is primarily that of P450c11AS. Thus an enzyme with aldosterone synthase activity is inappropriately overproduced in response to ACTH. This results in hyperaldosteronism, salt retention, hypertension, and suppressed PRA. The expression of this pathologic hybrid gene can be suppressed by suppressing pituitary ACTH with glucocorticoids such as dexamethasone.

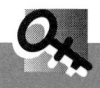

Key Treatment: Glucocorticoid-suppressible Hypertension

- Glucocorticoids

Bibliography

Bose HS, Sugawara T, Strauss JF III, Miller WL: The pathophysiology and genetics of congenital lipoid adrenal hyperplasia. N Engl J Med 1996;335:1870–1878.

Fardella CE, Miller WL: Molecular biology of mineralocorticoid metabolism. Annu Rev Nutr 1996;16:443–470.

Simard J, Sanchez R, Durocher F, et al: Structure-function relationships and molecular genetics of the 3β-hydroxysteroid dehydrogenase gene family. J Steroid Biochem Mol Biol 1995;55:489–505.

White PC, Mune T, Agarwal AK: 11β-hydroxysteroid dehydrogenase and the syndrome of apparent mineralocorticoid excess. Endocr Rev 1997;18:135–156.

Yanase T, Simpson ER, Waterman MR: 17α-hydroxylase/17,20 lyase deficiency: From clinical investigation to molecular definition. Endocr Rev 1991;12:91–108.

259 Addison Disease

Walter L. Miller

Definition

Addison disease is a term that refers to primary adrenal insufficiency (as opposed to secondary to adrenocorticotropic hormone [ACTH] deficiency) due to causes other than congenital adrenal hyperplasia.

Etiology

1. When Thomas Addison described the clinical symptoms of adrenal insufficiency in 1849, "Addison disease" was almost always due to tuberculosis of the adrenal.

2. However in current usage, over 80 per cent of all patients and an even higher percentage of children with Addison disease have autoimmune adrenalitis. The various causes of Addison disease are shown in Table 259–1.

Epidemiology

Autoimmune adrenalitis is most commonly seen in adults 25 to 45 years old, about 70 per cent of whom are women. The incidence in adults is about 1 in 25,000. The incidence in children in unknown, but apparently the disease is much

TABLE 259-1. ETIOLOGIES OF ADDISON DISEASE

PRIMARY ADRENAL INSUFFICIENCY (ADDISON DISEASE)

Autoimmune adrenalitis
Autoimmune polyglandular syndromes, types 1 and 2
Metabolic causes
   Adrenoleukodystrophy/adrenomyeloneuropathy
   Wollman disease/cholesterol ester storage disease
   Unresponsiveness to ACTH
Infectious causes
   Tuberculosis, fungal infections
   Sepsis
   AIDS
Other causes
   Congenital adrenal hypoplasia
   Sarcoidosis
   Amyloidosis
   Abdominal irradiation

SECONDARY ADRENAL INSUFFICIENCY

Withdrawal of glucocorticoid therapy
Hypopituitarism
Pituitary hypothalamic tumors
Irradiation of the hypothalamus

ACTH = adrenocorticotropic hormone; AIDS = acquired immunodeficiency syndrome.

rarer; in children under the age of 5, boys constitute about 75 per cent of patients.

Pathophysiology

1. Chronic adrenal insufficiency is typically seen when more than 90 per cent of adrenal function is lost. It usually presents a clinical picture of poor weight gain or weight loss, weakness, fatigue, anorexia, hypotension, hyponatremia, hypochloremia, hyperkalemia, frequent illnesses, nausea, and vague gastrointestinal complaints. The symptoms listed in the box that follows this section include those of chronic deficiency of both glucocorticoids and mineralocorticoids. The signs of glucocorticoid deficiency (weakness, fatigue, weight loss, hypoglycemia, anorexia) predominate early in the course of autoimmune adrenalitis, whereas signs of mineralocorticoid deficiency (hyponatremia, hyperkalemia, acidosis, tachycardia, hypotension, low voltage on ECG, small heart on chest x-ray) tend to be seen later. However, mineralocorticoid deficiency can also be the presenting picture. Thus, an initial clinical presentation in which one category of adrenal steroids is uninvolved does not mean it will be spared in the long run.

2. The symptoms in the box that follows this section can been seen in other primary or secondary causes of chronic adrenal insufficiency. In primary chronic adrenal insufficiency, low plasma cortisol concentrations stimulate the synthesis of pro-opiomelanocortin (POMC), which is cleaved to yield increased amounts of both ACTH and melanocyte-stimulating hormone (MSH). The increased production of MSH results in hyperpigmentation, most prominently of the skin exposed to sun and in flexor surfaces such as knees, elbows, and knuckles, and also the mucous membranes. The clinical diagnosis is confirmed by low cortisol and high ACTH levels and confirmed by a minimal response of cortisol to a 60-minute intravenous ACTH test. Other findings include the ap-

pearance of a small heart on chest x-ray, anemia, azotemia, eosinophilia, lymphocytosis, and hypoglycemia.

3. The diagnosis of an autoimmune mechanism causing chronic adrenal insufficiency is based largely on the finding of circulating anti-adrenal antibodies. Recent studies show that the steroidogenic enzymes P450c17 and P450c21 are major adrenal autoantigens. Autopsy studies show lymphocytic infiltration of the adrenal cortex. Autoimmune dysfunction of other endocrine tissues is frequently associated with autoimmune adrenalitis, consistent with the steroidogenic enzymes being among the major autoantigens. Approximately half of adult patients with lymphocytic adrenalitis also have autoimmune disease of other endocrine systems and high titers of antibodies specific to the affected tissues.

Key Clinical Signs and Symptoms of Adrenal Insufficiency

Features of Chronic Insufficiency (Addison Disease)

Decreased pubic and axillary hair

Diarrhea

Hyperpigmentation

Low-voltage electrocardiogram

Small heart on x-ray

Weight loss

Features Shared by Acute and Chronic Insufficiency

Anorexia

Apathy and confusion

Dehydration

Weakness and fatigue

Hyperkalemia

Hypoglycemia

Hyponatremia

Hypovolemia, hypotension, and tachycardia

Nausea and vomiting

Postural hypotension

Salt craving

Features of Acute Insufficiency (Adrenal Crisis)

Abdominal pain

Fever

Autoimmune Polyglandular Syndromes

1. The term *Schmidt syndrome* refers to the fairly common association of thyroiditis and/or diabetes mellitus with autoimmune adrenal insufficiency. This disease triad, which is seen mainly in adults, is sometimes termed *type 2 autoimmune polyglandular syndrome* and is linked to human leukocyte antigen (HLA)-DR3 and HLA-DR4. In older children and adults, primary ovarian failure but not

primary testicular failure is seen in about one quarter of patients with primary lymphocytic autoimmune adrenalitis (Table 259–2).

2. Hypoparathyroidism, pernicious anemia and chronic mucocutaneous infection with *Candida albicans* (moniliasis) are often seen together without associated adrenalitis in girls. When adrenalitis is also present, boys and girls are affected equally. This associated group of disorders, often termed the *type 1 autoimmune polyglandular syndrome,* is more common in children than adults. It may also include atrophic gastritis, hypergonadotropic hypogonadism, chronic active hepatitis, alopecia, and vitiligo. Unlike type 2 autoimmune polyglandular syndrome, there is no specific HLA association with this disorder.

3. Metabolic disorders also cause chronic primary adrenal insufficiency, including adrenoleukodystrophy (Schilder disease), primary xanthomatosis (Wollman disease), cholesterol ester storage disease, and hereditary unresponsiveness to ACTH.

Metabolic Causes of Addison Disease

1. *Adrenoleukodystrophy* is caused by mutations in one of two genes. An X-linked form seen only in males is caused by mutations in the gene for a specific, very long chain fatty acid acyl-CoA synthase. A severe infantile autosomal recessive form also occurs. Both forms of the diseases are characterized by accumulation of very long chain (22 to 26 carbon) fatty acids in tissues, permitting diagnosis of carriers and affected fetuses as well as individual patients. Symptoms usually first develop in midchildhood. A milder allelic variant of X-linked adrenoleukodystrophy, termed *adrenomyeloneuropathy,* presents in early adulthood. The leukodystrophy of the central nervous system causes behavioral changes, poor school performance, dysarthria, and poor memory, and eventually progresses to severe dementia. Symptoms of adrenal insufficiency usually appear after the central nervous system (CNS) symptoms, but in adrenomyeloneuropathy adrenal insufficiency is present in childhood and adolescence, followed by signs of neurologic disease 10 to 15 years later. The incidence of these disorders is unknown, but it is a fairly common cause of Addison disease in males.

2. *Wollman disease* and *cholesterol ester storage disease* are two rare allelic disorders of the cholesterol esterase that mobilizes cholesterol esters from adrenal lipid droplets.

TABLE 259–2. AUTOIMMUNE POLYGLANDULAR SYNDROMES

	TYPE 1 (%)	TYPE 2 (SCHMIDT SYNDROME) (%)
Adrenal insufficiency	60	100
Thyroiditis	10	70
IDDM	—	50
Gonadal failure	40	10–40
Hypoparathyroidism	90	—
Moniliasis	70–80	—
Malabsorption syndrome	25	—
Alopecia (in adults)	20	—
Pernicious anemia	15	—

IDDM = insulin dependent diabetes mellitus.

Consequently, free cholesterol is not available to P450scc, resulting in adrenal insufficiency. The steroidogenic defect is less severe than in congenital lipoid adrenal hyperplasia, and patients may survive for several months after birth. However, the disorders affect cells throughout the body, as all cells must store and utilize cholesterol; hence, the disorders are relentless and fatal with vomiting, steatorrhea, failure to thrive, hepatosplenomegaly, and adrenal calcification. The diagnosis is made by bone marrow aspiration yielding foam cells containing large lysosomal vaccules engorged with cholesterol esters, and is confirmed by finding absent cholesterol esterase activity in fibroblasts, leukocytes, or marrow cells.

3. *Hereditary unresponsiveness to ACTH* is a very rare disorder that can present as an acute adrenal crisis precipitated by an intercurrent illness in an infant, but more commonly presents with the signs and symptoms of chronic adrenal insufficiency in childhood. Unlike patients with autoimmune adrenalitis or other forms of destruction of adrenal tissue, patients with hereditary unresponsiveness to ACTH do not have mineralocorticoid deficiency, because aldosterone production by the zona glomerulosa is regulated principally by angiotensin II. The clinical picture includes failure to thrive, lethargy, pallor, hyperpigmentation, development delay, and hypoglycemia, often associated with seizures, but serum electrolytes are normal, and dehydration is only seen associated with intercurrent illness. Both autosomal recessive and sex-linked forms have been reported, suggesting that the clinical syndrome is due to more than one type of molecular lesion including those of the ACTH receptor as well as the various postreceptor proteins involved in generation of cyclic adenosine monophosphate (cAMP) as an intracellular second messenger.

Acute Versus Chronic Primary Adrenal Insufficiency

1. Acute adrenal insufficiency (adrenal crisis) occurs most commonly in the child with undiagnosed chronic adrenal insufficiency who is subjected to an additional severe stress such as major illness, trauma, or surgery. The major presenting symptoms are abdominal pain, fever, hypoglycemia with seizures, weakness, apathy, nausea, vomiting, anorexia, hyponatremia, hypochloremia, acidemia, hyperkalemia, hypotension, shock, cardiovascular collapse, and death. Treatment consists of fluid and electrolyte resuscitation, ample doses of glucocorticoids, chronic glucocorticoid and mineralocorticoid replacement, and treatment of the precipitating illness.

Key Treatment

- Fluid and electrolyte replacement (NaCl)
- Glucocorticoids
- Mineralocorticoid

2. Acute adrenal crisis commonly presents in the second week of life, as in infants with the salt-losing forms of congenital adrenal hyperplasia. A similar presentation in infancy is seen with *congenital adrenal hypoplasia.* There

are autosomal and X-linked forms of adrenal hypoplasia. The X-linked form is due to mutations in a gene called DAX-1, and is associated with glycerol kinase deficiency and Duchenne muscular dystrophy, which are encoded on adjacent genes. The basis of the autosomal recessive form remains unknown. The diagnosis is suggested by the absence of plasma or urinary steroids with no response to ACTH. Congenital lipoid adrenal hyperplasia presents precisely the same clinical picture; the differential diagnosis is made radiologically by the grossly enlarged adrenals that are characteristic of lipoid CAH. In both diseases the absence of fetal adrenal synthesis of dehydroepiandrosterone (DHEA) results in very low maternal estriol concentrations. These two causes of low maternal estriol are readily distinguished from a more common cause, anencephaly, by ultrasonographic examination of the fetus.

3. *Infectious adrenalitis* is seen in about 3 per cent of patients with extrapulmonary tuberculosis, and can also be seen rarely in fungal infections. Adrenal failure is also common among patients dying of acquired immunodeficiency syndrome (AIDS), and may occasionally be an early presenting symptom. Although human immunodeficiency virus (HIV) can directly infect adrenal cells, it appears that the Addison disease of AIDS is more commonly due to secondary infections or AIDS-related tumors.

4. *Massive adrenal hemorrhage* with shock due to blood loss can occur in large infants following a traumatic delivery, or due to a coagulation defect. A flank mass is usually palpable and can be distinguished from renal vein thrombosis by the presence of microscopic rather than gross hematuria. The diagnosis is confirmed by intravenous pyelography, ultrasonography, or magnetic resonance imaging (MRI). Massive adrenal hemorrhage is more commonly associated with sepsis, especially due to meningococcemia (Waterhouse-Friderichsen syndrome), but may also be seen in sepsis due to other gram-positive organisms.

Secondary Adrenal Insufficiency and Glucocorticoid Withdrawal

1. Chronic adrenal insufficiency may result from insufficient tropic stimulation of the adrenal or tissue insensitivity to adrenal steroids. Insufficient tropic stimulation of the adrenal is usually due to idiopathic hypopituitarism, to CNS tumors that damage the cells that produce corticotropin-releasing factor (CRF) and/or POMC, or to chronic suppression of these cells by long-term glucocorticoid therapy. Idiopathic hypopituitarism and CNS tumors associated with hypopituitarism are discussed elsewhere. However, it is important to note that some hypopituitary patients with thyroid-stimulating hormone (TSH) deficiency and hypothyroidism may have normal cortisol levels and still be ACTH deficient. The hypothydroidism slows the metabolism and clearance of cortisol, thus sometimes maintaining normal cortisol levels when ACTH is low. Treatment of the hypothyroidism can then return cortisol metabolism to normal, dropping the cortisol concentrations and unmasking adrenal insufficiency.

2. Long-term glucocorticoid therapy can suppress the synthesis and storage of ACTH in the pituitary, the synthesis and storage of CRF in the hypothalamus, and the number of receptors for CRF in the pituitary. Therefore, recovery of the hypothalamic-pituitary axis from long-term glucocorticoid therapy requires the recovery of multiple components, which may require considerable time. Patients successfully withdrawn from glucocorticoid therapy or successfully treated for Cushing disease may exhibit a fairly rapid normalization of plasma cortisol values while continuing to have diminished adrenal reserve for 6 to 12 months.

3. The speed at which glucocorticoid therapy can be withdrawn depends on the dose and length of duration of the therapy, and individual factors. Therapy of less than a week's duration can be discontinued abruptly. Very long term therapy requires a long period of tapering the dose. Symptoms of steroid withdrawal, including anorexia, malaise, headache, nausea, fever, and lethargy, can be seen, even when the reduced doses remain "supraphysiologic," because long-term, high-dose glucocorticoid treatment will diminish glucocorticoid receptor number and sensitivity ("down-regulation"). Withdrawal from alternate-day therapy is easier than from daily therapy. A tapering protocol should reduce the weekly dose by 25 per cent of the previous week's dose, that is, if the initial dose is 100 per cent, weekly reductions would be to 75, 56, 42, 31.5, 24, 18, 13.5 per cent, and so forth (rounded off for a conveniently administered format), but not 100, 75, 50, 25, 0, which is very likely to precipitate an adrenal crisis. Following successful withdrawal, patients who have been on high-dose glucocorticoids may still have diminished adrenal reserve, and should receive glucocorticoid "coverage" of two to three times their physiologic requirement during times of surgery or febrile illnesses, for at least 6 and up to 12 months following glucocorticoid withdrawal.

Bibliography

Kasperlik-Zaluska AA, Migdalski B, Czarnocka B, et al: Association of Addison disease with autoimmune disorders—a long-term observation of 180 patients. Postgrad Med J 1991;67:984.

Miller WL, Tyrrell JB: The adrenal cortex. *In* Felig F, Baxter JD, L Frohman L (eds): Endocrinology and Metabolism, 3rd ed. New York, McGraw Hill, 1995, pp 555–717.

Muir A, Maclaren NK: Autoimmune diseases of the adrenal glands, parathyroid glands, gonads, and hypothalamic-pituitary axis. Endocrinol Metab Clin North Am 1991;20:619.

Rao RH, Vagnucci AH: The clinical profile and management of bilateral massive adrenal hemaorrhage. Adv Endocrinol Metab 1992;3:213.

Sadeghi-Nejad A, Senior B: Adrenomyeloneuropathy presenting as Addison disease in childhood. N Engl J Med 1990;322:13.

260 Cushing Syndrome and Cushing Disease*

Constantine A. Stratakis and
George P. Chrousos

Definition

Cushing syndrome (CS) results from prolonged exposure of tissues to excess glucocorticoids. It affects most tissues and is characterized by growth deceleration or complete arrest, gonadal and thyroid dysfunction, progressive adiposity, dermopathy (atrophy, violaceous striae, ecchymoses, hirsutism), myopathy, hypertension, insulin resistance, hyperlipidemia, and osteoporosis.

Etiology

1. *Endogenous* CS results from increased secretion of cortisol by the adrenal cortex.
   a. Due to adrenocorticotropin (ACTH) hypersecretion (ACTH-dependent CS) or caused by autonomous hyperfunction of the adrenocortical cells (ACTH-independent CS).
   b. *Cushing disease.* The ACTH-dependent form of endogenous CS, caused by an ACTH-secreting, benign corticotroph tumor of the anterior pituitary gland.
2. *Exogenous CS* results from chronic administration of glucocorticoids (for treatment of neoplastic, autoimmune, and other diseases) or ACTH (for the treatment of certain seizure disorders).

Epidemiology

1. The overall incidence of spontaneous Cushing syndrome is approximately 2 to 4 new cases per million of population per year, with a female to male preponderance. Approximately 10 per cent of these cases occur in children and adolescents.
   a. ACTH-dependent Cushing syndrome accounts for about 85 per cent of endogenous cases in children older than 7 years through adulthood (Table 260–1).

*All material in this chapter is in the public domain, with the exception of any borrowed figures or tables.

TABLE 260–1. CLASSIFICATION OF ENDOGENOUS CUSHING SYNDROME AND RATE OF OCCURRENCE IN CHILDREN OLDER THAN 7 YEARS

CLASSIFICATION	PER CENT
ACTH-dependent	85
Pituitary (Cushing disease) (includes MEN-I)	80
Ectopic ACTH (includes MEN-I)	20
Ectopic CRH	Rare
ACTH-independent	15
Adrenal adenoma (includes MEN-I)	30
Adrenal carcinoma	70
Primary pigmented adrenocortical disease (PPNAD)	0.5–1
McCune-Albright syndrome	Rare
"Transitional States"	Rare

ACTH = adrenocorticotropic hormone; CRH = corticotropin-releasing hormone; MEN = multiple endocrine neoplasia.

b. Cushing disease is responsible for 80 per cent of cases. The remaining are caused by ectopic ACTH or, very rarely, ectopic corticotropin-releasing hormone (CRH) secretion.
   c. ACTH-independent Cushing syndrome accounts for the remainder. Adrenal causes (benign adenomas and primary pigmented nodular adrenocortical disease [PPNAD]) are the most frequent in the age group under 7 years.
   d. With the increasing use of glucocorticoids for a wide range of nonendocrine diseases, the exogenous, iatrogenic CS has become increasingly frequent, and its prevalence far exceeds that of the endogenous forms.

Pathophysiology

1. Hormonosynthesis
   a. Cholesterol is utilized by the adrenal cortex as the precursor for the synthesis of cortisol, aldosterone, and adrenal androgens. Although the adrenals retain the ability to synthesize cholesterol de novo, in normal situations they obtain cholesterol from the circulation via the low-density lipoprotein (LDL) receptor and store it inside cytoplasmic lipid droplets in the form of cholesterol esters. Activation of a cytoplasmic cholesterol ester hydrolase causes the entry of cholesterol into the mitochondria with the assistance of a carrier protein (steroidogenic acute regulatory protein [StAR]). There it is converted to pregnenolone, which, in turn, is converted by a series of reactions to cortisol in the *zona fasciculata*, to aldosterone in the *zona glomerularis*, and to Δ4-androstenedione, dehydroepiandrostenedione (DHEA), its sulfate (DHEA-S), and other androgens in the *zona reticularis*.
2. Physiologic regulation of secretion
   a. The main stimulus for release of cortisol from the adrenal cortex is ACTH, produced by the corticotrophs of the anterior pituitary, which, in turn, are under the regulatory influence of hypothalamic CRH and vasopressin. The ambient plasma free cortisol levels regulate ACTH secretion in a negative feedback fashion. Normally, less than 10 per cent of plasma cortisol is in the free form, with the majority being bound to cortisol-binding globulin (or "transcortin"). Most plasma assays measure total plasma cortisol concentrations. In contrast to cortisol, aldosterone release is controlled mostly by the renin-angiotensin system and the concentration of K^+ and Na^+ ions, and to a much lesser extent by ACTH.
   b. In the physiologic state, ACTH and cortisol have a circadian pattern of secretion that is established early in infancy and is in accordance with other

human circadian biologic activities. The peak of ACTH and cortisol secretion occurs in the morning (between 7:00 and 8:00 AM), and their nadir, in the late evening hours (around midnight). Reversal of this rhythm is observed in people who work night shifts or are involved in strenuous activities in the evening.

3. Pathologic actions of adrenal hormones

a. Glucocorticoids have profound catabolic activities: They inhibit growth and reproduction, promote proteinolysis, and suppress the immune and inflammatory reaction. These effects are behind some of the cardinal clinical manifestations of CS: delayed growth and bone maturation, hypogonadism, dermopathy, loss of muscular tissue, and frequent fungal or saprophytic infections.

b. The mineralocorticoid receptor recognizes and responds to cortisol. An enzyme (11β-dehydrogenase) inactivates cortisol as a mineralocortioid (or glucocorticoid), by converting it to cortisone in tissues that are primarily aldosterone-responsive. The activity of this enzyme is overcome in CS by the excessive amounts of circulating cortisol. The latter, along with several steroid precursors with mineralocorticoid activity, may cause the hypertension and hypokalemic alkalosis often seen in the severe forms of the syndrome.

c. Adrenal androgens Δ4-androstenedione, DHEA, and DHEA-S) are capable of causing significant virilization, when hypersecreted in CS.

Clinical Findings

1. Table 260–2 summarizes the clinical features of CS in children and adolescents.

a. One of the earliest and commonest signs, in almost all patients, is obesity, which is generalized or truncal, and is characterized by facial rounding (moon facies) and plethora.

b. Growth retardation or complete arrest are present in all but 10 per cent of the children.

c. Other clinical manifestations include sleep disturbances, muscle weakness and fatigue, hirsutism, and typical purple skin striae.

d. Hypertension, carbohydrate intolerance or diabetes, amenorrhea, advancement or arrest of pubertal development, easy bruising or spontaneous fractures of ribs and vertebrae may be encountered.

2. The clinical presentation can point to the cause of CS in children and adolescents.

a. Rapidly progressing, very severe Cushing syndrome points toward an adrenal neoplasm, or, although rare in children, the ectopic ACTH syndrome. Patients with adrenocortical carcinomas may be asymptomatic, or may present with abdominal pain or fullness, symptoms and signs of Cushing syndrome (30%), virilization (20%), combined symptoms of Cushing syndrome and virilization (30%), feminization (10%), or hyperaldosteronism (5–10%).

TABLE 260–2. CLINICAL PRESENTATION OF CS IN PEDIATRIC PATIENTS

SYMPTOMS/SIGNS	FREQUENCY (PER CENT)
Weight gain	90
Growth retardation	83
Menstrual irregularities	81
Hirsutism	81
Obesity (body mass index > 85th percentile)	73
Violaceous skin striae	63
Acne	52
Hypertension	51
Fatigue—weakness	45
Precocious puberty	41
Bruising	27
Mental changes	18
"Delayed" bone age	14
Hyperpigmentation	13
Muscle weakness	13
Acanthosis nigricans	10
Accelerated bone age	10
Sleep disturbances	7
Pubertal delay	7
Hypercalcemia	6
Alkalosis	6
Hypokalemia	2
Slipped femoral capital epiphysis	2

Modified from Magiakou MA, Mastorakos G, Oldfield EH, et al: Cushing's syndrome in children and adolescents: presentation, diagnosis and therapy. N Engl J Med 1994;331:629–636.

b. CS is periodic or intermittent in a significant percentage (10%) of children and adolescents.

Key Clinical Findings

- Obesity
- Short stature
- Hirsutism
- Violaceous

Laboratory Findings

1. The first step in diagnosing non-iatrogenic CS is the biochemical documentation of endogenous hypercortisolism, which can usually be accomplished by outpatient tests.

a. *Measurement of 24-hour urinary free cortisol excretion* (UFC), corrected for body surface area, and/or the determination of 24-hour urinary 17-hydroxy-corticosteroid (17OHCS) excretion (corrected per gram of excreted creatinine). UFC excretion is an excellent first-line test for documentation of CS. Assuming correct collection, there are very few false-negative results.

b. *Single-dose dexamethasone suppression test.* The overnight 1-mg (in young children 15 μg/kg body weight) dexamethasone suppression test is a useful screening procedure for hypercortisolism. It is simple and has a low incidence of false normal suppression (less than 3%). The same test, however, has a high incidence of false-positive results (approximately 20 to 30%). A plasma cortisol level greater than 5 µg/dl suggests endogenous hypercortisolism, and needs to be followed by a 24-hr urine collection for determination of UFC or 17OHCS levels.

2. Cushing syndrome is generally excluded if the tests mentioned above are normal, although one should keep in mind that periodic and intermittent cortisol hypersecretion, which may occur in patients with Cushing syndrome of any etiology, may confuse the picture.

3. Once the diagnosis of CS has been established, the differential diagnosis is investigated by dynamic testing of the function of the hypothalamic-pituitary-adrenal (HPA) axis and by imaging studies. It is essential that dynamic endocrine testing is performed while the patient is hypercortisolemic, and that, in order to avoid mistakes, this state should always be documented at the time of testing. All adrenal blocking agents should be discontinued for at least 6 weeks prior to testing. The major tests in the differential diagnosis of Cushing syndrome and their interpretation are:

a. *Liddle dexamethasone suppression test.* The standard high-dose, low-dose dexamethasone suppression test is a reliable procedure for differentiating Cushing disease from the ectopic ACTH syndrome. (see Bibliography)

b. *Overnight 8-mg dexamethasone suppression test* (see Bibliography)

c. *Corticotropin-releasing hormone stimulation (CRH) test.* The ovine (o) CRH test is of equal to or greater value than the standard dexamethasone suppression test in differentiating between Cushing disease and ectopic ACTH secretion.

d. Petrosal-sinus sampling with CRH test.

Key Laboratory Test

- 24-hr urine excretion of free cortisol

Radiographic Findings

Imaging techniques can help clarify the etiology of hypercortisolism. These include computed tomographic (CT) scanning and magnetic resonance imaging (MRI) of the pituitary gland, and CT scan, MRI, and ultrasound imaging of the adrenal glands. CT and MRI scans of the chest and abdomen are also employed, when tumors secreting ectopic ACTH are suspected.

Treatment

1. Cushing disease
   a. *Transsphenoidal surgery (TSS).* TSS is the treatment of choice for most cases of CS caused by pituitary microadenomas.
      (1) Most frequently, successful TSS leads to cure of hypercortisolism with no need for permanent glucocorticoid replacement. Approximately 5 per cent of patients suffer recurrences.
      (2) Complications include transient or permanent, partial or complete anterior pituitary insufficiency, including in order of frequency, hypothyroidism, growth hormone (GH) deficiency, hypogonadism, and adrenal insufficiency.
   b. *Pituitary x-radiation with or without mitotane.* This is an alternative treatment, which may be used after failure of TSS, in the presence of cavernous sinus wall invasion by the tumor, or in patients judged unsuitable for surgery.

Key Treatment: Cushing Disease

- Transsphenoidal surgery
- Radiation

2. Ectopic ACTH-dependent CS
   a. The treatment of choice for ectopic ACTH secretion is surgical and directed toward complete excision of the tumor, if the latter is resectable and its location known.

Key Treatment: Ectopic ACTH-Dependent CS

- Surgical removal of tumor

3. Primary adrenal disease
   a. The therapeutic approach to ACTH-independent Cushing syndrome is also surgical. Unilateral or bilateral adrenalectomy is the recommended therapy, depending on whether one or both adrenals are affected.

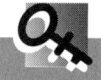

Key Treatment: Primary Adrenal Disease

- Adrenalectomy

Bibliography

Chrousos GP, Schulte HM, Oldfield EH, et al: The corticotropin-releasing factor stimulation test: an aid in the evaluation of patients with Cushing syndrome. N Engl J Med 1984;310:622–626.

Magiakou MA, Mastorakos G, Oldfield EH, et al: Cushing's syndrome in children and adolescents: presentation, diagnosis and therapy. N Engl J Med 1994;331:629–636.

Oldfield EH, Doppman JL, Nieman LK, et al: Petrosal sinus sampling with and without corticotropin-releasing hormone for the differential diagnosis of Cushing's syndrome. N Engl J Med 1991;325:897–905.

Tsigos C, Chrousos GP: Differential diagnosis and management of Cushing's syndrome. Annu Rev Med 1996;47:443–461.

261 Hypoparathyroidism

Morri E. Markowitz

Etiology

1. Hypoparathyroidism (HypoP) occurs when insufficient amounts of parathyroid hormone (PTH)–producing tissue are present. This may be due to
   a. Primary failure of embryologic development occurring as an isolated defect or as part of a larger genetically based syndrome (velocardiofacial/DiGeorge syndrome).
   b. Secondary destruction of the glands, as occurs in certain autoimmune disorders, after removal of the glands or damage to them during neck surgery, or with infiltration of the glands in iron-overload states (e.g., thalassemia).
   c. In the newborn period as a consequence of in utero exposure to maternal hypercalcemia.
2. Functional HypoP can also occur in the presence of electrolyte abnormalities, such as hypomagnesemia, hypermagnesemia, and hypernatremia.

Epidemiology

HypoP from any etiology is uncommon. Of the approximately 20,000 annual pediatric hospital discharges from the Bronx affiliates of the Albert Einstein College of Medicine, fewer than a half dozen cases carry this diagnosis.

Pathophysiology

1. PTH is produced from a preprohormone and is secreted in response to a reduction in extracellular calcium.
2. After release, PTH is transported to target tissues in bone and kidney (and other organs). Osteoblast receptors in bone respond to PTH with increased activity marked by elevated alkaline phosphatase levels in serum. The osteoblast activation is also coupled to increased osteoclast activity. The latter results in bone resorption with release of bone mineral into the circulation. The descendent of the osteoblast, the osteocyte, probably also responds to PTH, leading to a more immediate increase of bone mineral release into blood and a rise in blood calcium levels.
3. In the kidney, PTH stimulates the activity of the $1,\alpha$-hydroxylase vitamin D enzyme involved in the hydroxylation of vitamin D to 1,25-dihydroxyvitamin D. The latter is fully activated hormonal vitamin D.

Clinical Findings

1. *Symptoms*—The symptoms of PTH deficiency are primarily attributable to hypocalcemia. These are neuromuscular-induced cramps and twitches. When sustained cramps in the hands and feet occur, this is termed tetany (carpopedal spasm). Classically, the fingers are extended with ulnar deviation. If the contractions are rhythmic they are indistinguishable from other motor seizures, with the exception that initially there may be no postictal phase. Contraction in the larynx can produce cyanosis if complete occlusion occurs or stridor if there is partial closure. A typical presentation to the pediatrician is of the infant who turns dusky in the mother's arms but appears to be breathing since chest wall motion continues. A few seconds later, normal color returns as well as audible sounds. This may occur several times before medical help is sought. In older children, hypoplasia of dental enamel may be apparent.
2. *Signs*—The signs of hypocalcemia relate to the increased excitability of motor nerves. Tapping the facial nerve and observing a contraction of the perioral musculature is termed a positive Chvostek sign. Inflating a blood pressure cuff applied to the arm to right above systolic for 3 to 5 minutes and inducing a tetany response of the hand is termed a positive Trousseau sign. In general, tapping on any motor nerve, such as the peroneal, should result in an abnormal contraction of the target muscle.
3. *Associated findings*—These will depend on whether the HypoP is an isolated disorder. Midline facial defects and heart murmurs may be present as part of the congenital syndrome described above. A surgical scar on the neck would lead one to suspect postsurgical HypoP. Other signs and symptoms such as polyuria, polydipsia, constipation, weight gain, postural hypotension, and moniliasis indicate evidence of other endocrine organ failure resulting in concomitant diabetes mellitus, hypothyroidism, hypoadrenalism, or autoimmune disease.

Key Clinical Findings

- Cramps and twitches of hands and feet
- Carpopedal spasm
- Chvostek sign
- Trousseau sign
- Peroneal sign

Laboratory Findings

Low or inadequately elevated PTH levels for the degree of hypocalcemia define HypoP. Since PTH is a phosphaturic agent, serum phosphate levels are elevated in its absence in patients who are eating normally. Alkaline phosphatase levels are in the normal range. One,25-dihydroxyvitamin D levels are low. The QTc interval on an ECG is prolonged (>.45 in infants).

Key Laboratory Findings

- Hypocalcemia
- Hyperphosphatemia
- Low PTH

Radiographic Findings

No findings specific to HypoP are present. However, examination of a chest x-ray in young infants will help in the determination of associated absence of the thymus or cardiovascular anomalies.

Treatment

1. Correction of hypocalcemia-related events consists of the intravenous administration of calcium salts. Initially, a 10 per cent solution of calcium gluconate, 0.5 ml/kg, up to 10 ml, given over 10 to 15 minutes is usually sufficient to stop spasms or seizures. A repeat bolus can immediately be given if it is not. This should be followed by a continuous intravenous infusion of the same salt at a rate of 500 mg/kg administered over 24 hours for neonates and 200 mg/kg/24 hours for infants and children. Calcium- and carbonate-containing salts are incompatible in the same IV solution, since the calcium carbonate will precipitate. Continuous ECG monitoring is mandatory during calcium infusions; bradyarrhythmias may occur if the infusion rate is too great.

2. PTH is theoretically available for administration but would need to be given parenterally, since it is a peptide. The accepted alternative is to employ the next hormone in calcium regulation, vitamin D. One,25-dihydroxyvitamin D at a dose of 20 to 40 ng/kg/day will supply physiologic requirements and is the vitamin D metabolite of choice. Since the mechanism of action of this hormone is to increase intestinal calcium absorption, ingestion of at least the RDA for calcium is also required. By adjusting 1,25-dihydroxyvitamin D dosage every 2 to 3 days, blood calcium levels can be titrated to the near-normocalcemia level.

3. Since PTH decreases urinary calcium excretion, its absence results in a greater fractional excretion of filtered calcium. This necessitates careful monitoring of urinary calcium excretion in order to prevent the development of nephrocalcinosis or renal stones. For older infants and children, a urinary calcium divided by urinary creatinine

<0.25 (mg Ca/mg creatinine) is generally considered safe. In some instances, blood calcium levels will need to be maintained slightly below the normal range in order to prevent hypercalciuria.

4. As ancillary treatment, phosphate intake should be restricted until calcium levels are brought under control and serum phosphate levels are under 10 mg/dl.

Key Treatment

- Initial
  Continuous infusion of calcium salt
- Long-term
  Calcitriol
  Supplementary dietary calcium

Prevention

The genetic etiology of the velocardiofacial/DiGeorge syndrome will allow for prenatal diagnosis and counseling. Serial determination of calcium levels will identify those children at risk for developing clinically relevant HypoP. Iron-overload syndromes associated with chronic transfusions may be avoided by the use of iron-chelating agents such as desferrioxamine. Incidental damage during thyroid surgery is much more rare, since surgeons now take care to identify the parathyroid glands and avoid intraoperative trauma to them or their vascular supply. HypoP secondary to the removal of hyperplastic or adenomatous parathyroid glands can be ameliorated by the autotransplantation of a portion of a gland in the forearm.

Bibliography

Favus MJ (ed): Primer on the Metabolic Bone Diseases and Disorders of Mineral Metabolism, 2nd ed. New York, Raven Press, 1993.

Harrison HH, Harrison HC: Disorders of Calcium and Phosphate Metabolism in Childhood and Adolescence. Philadelphia, WB Saunders, 1979.

 # 262 Pseudohypoparathyroidism

Morri E. Markowitz

Definition

Hypocalcemia in the presence of appropriately elevated serum parathyroid hormone (PTH) levels signifies failure of hormone activity. If the vitamin D pathway is intact, this failure to respond to PTH is termed pseudohypoparathyroidism (PHP). PHP is therefore a disorder of end-organ unresponsiveness. There are several variants.

Etiology

PHP occurs when there is either a PTH receptor or a postreceptor problem. Failure to recognize the PTH signal

can be due to a genetic disorder inherited as an autosomal dominant. In these types of PHP, other endocrine disorders related to a common peptide receptor abnormality may occur. A G protein abnormality defines the disorder.

In some cases, a postreceptor defect is postulated, since cAMP production may be uncoupled from other PTH-mediated events, such as phosphaturia.

Epidemiology

Little is known of the prevalence of these disorders.

Pathophysiology

PTH receptors are located on the cell surface and share the characteristics of peptide receptors in general: One of three components of the receptor complex extends from the cell surface and binds PTH. This causes activation of the second intracellular component, a protein called G_s that binds GTP. This in turn stimulates the third component, an adenylate cyclase, leading to cAMP production. Abnormalities of any portion of these components will result in the failure of endogenously produced or exogenously administered PTH to stimulate intracellular cAMP production, the second messenger. In the kidney, this will be marked by the absence of phosphaturia, increased urinary cAMP excretion, or 1,25-dihydroxyvitamin D production. In bone, mineral release will not occur at a rate sufficient to maintain blood calcium levels.

Clinical Findings

Patients can present with the same hypocalcemia-related symptoms and signs as noted for HypoP patients. In one variant of PHP, associated findings of short stature, round face, obesity, shortened metacarpals, decreased cognitive abilities, and intracerebral calcifications of the basal ganglia are found.

Key Clinical Findings

- Carpopedal spasm
- Chvostek sign
- Trousseau sign

Laboratory Findings

Low serum calcium, high phosphate, and high PTH characterize PHP. In a minority of patients a high alkaline phosphatase is also present, possibly signifying a dissociation of renal and bone responsiveness to PTH. If exogenous PTH is administered, the measurement of urinary cAMP and phosphate will differentiate subcategories of PHP.

Key Laboratory Findings

- Hypocalcemia
- High PTH
- Hyperphosphatemia

Radiographic Findings

Calcification of the basal ganglia may be present. Shortened metacarpals will be evident in the appropriate PHP variant.

Treatment

See Chapter 261.

As with hypoparathyroidism, bypass of the PTH-related defect by the administration of vitamin D metabolites will restore normocalcemia. Associated findings will not be addressed by this measure and will require individualized attention.

Key Treatment

- Calcitriol

---

263 McCune-Albright Syndrome

Cornelis Van Dop

Definition

1. This disorder was first described in the 1930s as a hormonal overactivity syndrome with clinical presentation that varies widely from patient to patient. The disease was originally defined by the triad of café-au-lait skin pigmentation, sexual precocity, and polyostotic fibrous dysplasia.
2. Other clinical problems include: hyperthyroidism, hyperadrenalism, growth hormone excess, and hypophosphatemia (Table 263–1).
3. The extreme heterogeneity of clinical findings and the often described segmental pattern of café-au-lait skin hyperpigmentation led Happle to postulate that the disease results from postzygotic mutations that occur following initiation of fetal development and consequent variable involvement of tissues among these patients.

Affected tissues do in fact have specific activating mutations of G_s that are identical to G_s mutations previously found in somatotrophs of some patients with acromegaly. The postzygotic activating mutation in the α-subunit of G_s inhibits its GTPase activity by replacing an arginine residue on the α-subunit of G_s. The postzygotic nature of the activating G_s mutation means that no two patients with the disorder will have involvement of the same cells and tissues.

Polyostotic Fibrous Dysplasia

1. Histologically these lesions simulate focal hyperparathyroidism. Although skeletal surveys were long used to detect these lesions, a bone scan is now generally used owing to its greater sensitivity.

TABLE 263–1. CLINICAL PROBLEMS DESCRIBED IN McCUNE-ALBRIGHT SYNDROME

ORGAN	CLINICAL PROBLEM
Skeleton	Polyostotic fibrous dysplasia
Skin	Café-au-lait skin pigmentation
Gonads	Gonadotropin-independent precocious puberty
Thyroid gland	Multinodular colloid goiter, hyperthyroidism
Adrenal gland	Nodular adrenocortical hyperplasia, hypercortisolism
Kidney	Hypophosphatemia
Somatotropes	Growth hormone excess
Heart	Arrhythmia (?)
Liver	Focal nodular hyperplasia, cholestasis

Thymic hyperplasia, gastrointestinal polyps, splenic enlargement, and islet cell hyperplasia have been described in some patients with McCune-Albright syndrome, but the presence of activating G_s mutation in these abnormalities has not been demonstrated.

2. The fibrous dysplastic lesions can involve any bone, with disfigurement and fracture of the bone resulting from growth and expansion of the fibrous dysplasia.
3. Most skeletal problems due to polyostotic fibrous dysplasia develop during childhood. Most reviews indicate that the lesions remain quiescent during adulthood. However, exacerbations of polyostotic fibrous dysplasia with resulting skeletal fractures or optic nerve compression have been described during pregnancy.
4. The only effective therapy for these lesions is surgical resection with bone grafting. Radiation therapy, used to control the lesions prior to 1950, was associated with subsequent development of sarcomas within the lesions.

Key Treatment

- Surgical resection and bone grafting

Café-au-lait Skin Hyperpigmentation

These lesions, which often follow dermatomal patterns, are presumed due to activating G_s mutations in melanocytes, which cause increased production of melanin, as the receptor for melanocyte-stimulating hormone is coupled to G_s.

Gonadotropin-Independent Precocious Puberty

1. Most cases of precocious puberty in McCune-Albright syndrome have been reported in females. The few reports in males suggest that normal spermatogenesis occurs in adulthood. Pubertal development may first become appar-

ent at any time during childhood. Before bone age advances to normal pubertal age these children have a prepubertal (absent) gonadotropin response during a gonadotropin-releasing hormone stimulation test, and girls usually have multiple ovarian cysts on ultrasound examination.
2. Treatment is directed to preventing gonadal steroidogenesis. Ketoconazole or a combination of antiandrogen (e.g., flutamide or fludrocortisone) and aromatase inhibitor (e.g., testolactone) have been used successfully.

Other Endocrinopathies

1. Hyperthyroidism with multinodular goiter and homogeneous hypertrophy of the thyroid gland have been described. Successful long-term treatment of the hyperthyroidism in McCune-Albright syndrome requires ablative therapy. Partial thyroidectomies have been reported to be unsuccessful owing to recurrence of hyperthyroidism in several patients.
2. Growth hormone excess has been described in several infants caused by eosinophilic adenomas of the pituitary gland.
3. Multinodular adrenal hyperplasia causing Cushing syndrome occurs rarely and has been successfully treated with adrenalectomy.
4. Hypophosphatemia occurs in some children with the disorder. Oral phosphate supplementation is appropriate therapy, with addition of calcitriol necessary in some cases.

Inheritance

Transmission of McCune-Albright syndrome from parent to child has not been confirmed, although two reports suggest that possibility. One report described a mother with skin pigmentation, possible sexual precocity, and polyostotic fibrous dysplasia who had a daughter with multiple cystic bone lesions but without endocrine abnormalities. A second report described a mother and daughter who both had hyperparathyroidism and cystic bone lesions, without skin pigmentation or endocrinologic abnormalities. Others have questioned whether these two families had McCune-Albright syndrome.

 ### Bibliography

Danon M, Crawford JC: The McCune-Albright syndrome. Ergeb Inn Med Kinderheilkd 1987;55:82–115.

Happle R: The McCune-Albright syndrome: A lethal gene surviving by mosaicism. Clin Genet 1986;29:321–324.

Weinstein LS, Shenker A, Gejman PV, et al: Activating mutations of the stimulatory G protein in the McCune-Albright syndrome. N Engl J Med 1991;325:1688–1695.

264 Hyperparathyroidism

Morri E. Markowitz

Definition
Overproduction and secretion of PTH resulting in hypercalcemia.

Etiology
A parathyroid gland may lose appropriate responsiveness to extracellular calcium levels when adenomatous changes occur. Multiple glands can become hyperplastic. Either of these situations may occur as part of a more general endocrinopathy inherited as an autosomal dominant, the MEA syndromes (multiple endocrine adenomatoses), in which multiple endocrine glands are overactive.

Epidemiology
All causes of hyperparathyroidism are rare in the pediatric age groups in contrast to the much higher prevalence in older adults.

Pathophysiology
Excessive PTH secretion results in overabsorption of ingested calcium and release of calcium from bone stores.

Clinical Findings
Multiple organs are affected by high calcium levels.
1. GI—Abdominal pain, anorexia, vomiting, constipation
2. GU—Stone-related pain, hematuria, isosthenuria
3. CNS—Change in behavior, headache, stupor, coma
4. CV—Hypertension
5. Eye—Nonpurulent conjunctivitis, band keratopathy

Laboratory Findings
The hallmark biochemical constellation is high serum calcium, low phosphate, elevated alkaline phosphatase, and elevated PTH. Of these, only the high calcium and PTH levels are required for diagnosis. Urinary phosphate and calcium may be elevated; the urinary calcium is not as high as occurs in nonhyperparathyroid hypercalcemic conditions.

Further evaluation could include studies to localize enlarged glands: sonography, CT scan, radionuclide scans. Currently, the method of choice is the sestamibi scan.

Key Laboratory Findings
- Hypercalcemia
- Hypophosphatemia
- Elevated PTH

Radiographic Findings
Subperiosteal resorption, especially of the distal phalanges and bone cysts, is seen on plain film. Radionuclide scans may identify enlarged glands and also localize ectopic tissue.

Treatment
Treatment is dependent on age at diagnosis. In mild neonatal hyperparathyroidism, the disease sometimes becomes quiescent after the first few months of life. If hypercalciuria is not present and normal growth continues, observation and follow-up may be sufficient. In all other circumstances, surgical intervention is warranted to remove the overactive tissue. In cases of hyperplasia of the glands, all the glands are removed. A half-gland may be implanted in the forearm. This is usually sufficient to maintain normocalcemia after transplant recovery. If hyperparathyroidism should recur, surgical excision of the gland in the forearm is easier to perform and offers a better cosmetic outcome than repeat neck explorations.

Key Treatment
- Surgery

265 Neonatal Hypocalcemia

Morri E. Markowitz

Hypocalcemia occurring in newborns can be divided into early (first 3 to 5 days) and late (after 5 to 7 days) onset. Associated with early-onset hypocalcemia are prematurity, sepsis, and maternal hypercalcemia, hypomagnesemia, diabetes, or vitamin D deficiency. Late-onset hypocalcemia may be caused by hypoparathyroidism (HypoP) that is either transient or permanent.

A difficulty arises in defining the normal calcium level range in premature infants. A total calcium level <1.63 mmol/L (6.5 mg/dl) or ionized calcium <0.75 mmol/L

(<3.0 mg/dl) is generally accepted. Higher cut-offs are proposed by others. However, these values are considerably below the normal range of healthy term infants, in whom the lower limit in many laboratories is 8.5 and 4.0 mg/dl, respectively. They appear to be based on the normal distribution of values from babies in the NICU rather than on calcium-related physiologic events.

Pathophysiology

1. Immaturity of the parathyroid glands, inadequacy of vitamin D stores or vitamin D activity, or secondary events such as hypomagnesemia have all been invoked as contributors to neonatal hypocalcemia.
2. PTH deficiency may be due to immaturity or absence of the glands. In the former, hypocalcemia is of late onset and responds to reduction in the amount of phosphate in the formula. Presumably, less calcium bound to phosphate decreases stress on immature parathyroid glands. Absence or hypoplasia of the glands is associated with a congenital embryopathy syndrome—cardiovelofacial syndrome, which overlaps with DiGeorge syndrome. In the latter syndrome, HypoP may be lifelong, whereas in the former, hypocalcemia is usually limited to the first year of life; occasionally it recurs in the teenage years. Both syndromes have a 22-p deletion.

Clinical Findings

As in hypocalcemia occurring in children, seizures, stridor, and tetany can occur in newborns. But, in addition, more nonspecific features, such as apneic episodes, poor feeding, and vomiting, may be seen.

Key Clinical Findings

- Tetany
- Seizures
- Apnea

Laboratory Findings

Associated findings in serum may be hyperphosphatemia with levels >10 mg/dl, normal alkaline phosphatase, low or high magnesium concentrations, low PTH, 25-OH vitamin D, or 1,25-dihydroxyvitamin D levels.

Key Laboratory Findings

- Hypocalcemia
- Hyperphosphatemia

Radiographic Findings

Absence of a thymic shadow or abnormal cardiac silhouette on x-ray should increase the suspicion of a congenital embryopathy.

Treatment

1. Acute treatment is the same as outlined in Chapter 261 with the exception that maintenance drip levels begin at 500 mg/kg/day of calcium gluconate (or about 50 mg/kg/day of elemental calcium) as a continuous infusion. Repeated boluses of calcium may result in hyper- and hypocalcemic swings, since calcium is rapidly cleared from plasma. Titration from the starting dose is performed in order to maintain blood calcium levels at the lower end of the normal range.
2. More definitive treatment depends on the underlying diagnosis.
   a. In early-onset hypocalcemia, correction of the underlying abnormality, e.g., sepsis, results in its resolution. Calcium support for 3 to 5 days is usually sufficient for infants of diabetic mothers.
   b. Transient HypoP due to phosphate overload requires little more than dietary manipulation of mineral intake to achieve a calcium-to-phosphate formula ratio of 4:1. This should be maintained for 6 to 12 weeks.
   c. Replacement use of 1,25-dihydroxyvitamin D is appropriate for babies with more profound HypoP. Since the medication comes inside a sealed gelatin capsule that is unsuitable for direct administration to an infant, the liquid form of the drug, originally developed for intravenous use, is an effective substitute at a dose of 20 to 40 ng/kg/day with a minimum of 0.1 μg/day.

Key Treatment: Tetany of the Newborn

- Feeding ratio of Ca/PO$_4$ = 4:1

Prevention

Elimination of symptomatic hypocalcemia can be achieved by monitoring high-risk babies with serial calcium levels during the first 3 to 5 days after birth.

266 Hypoglycemia

Barbara Linder

Definition

Hypoglycemia is defined as a blood glucose lower than 40 mg/dl. The concentration of glucose in serum or plasma is 12 to 15 per cent higher than simultaneous measurements in whole blood that are obtained by fingerstick. Samples for glucose measurement are best obtained in a gray-top tube, which contains sodium fluoride to inhibit red cell glycolysis.

Etiology

The causes of hypoglycemia can be divided into two general categories:

1. Overutilization due to excessive tissue uptake of glucose. This occurs secondary to hyperinsulinism.
2. Underproduction due to deficient precursor conversion to glucose. This can occur because of:
   a. Limitations of substrate (glycogen, protein, fat)
   b. Enzymatic defects related to glycogenolysis or gluconeogenesis. An expanded list of enzymatic deficiencies is shown in Table 266–1.
   c. Hormonal deficiencies (particularly growth hormone or cortisol)

Etiology of Hypoglycemia

- Excess utilization of glucose
- Deficient glucose production

Epidemiology

1. Certain neonates are at high risk for *transient* hypoglycemia.
   a. In the infant of a diabetic mother, hyperinsulinism occurs because of chronic exposure to maternal hyperglycemia. Hypoglycemia usually presents at a few hours of life and resolves by 3 to 7 days of age. Other causes of transient neonatal hyperinsulinism are listed in Table 266–1.
   b. Premature, small for gestational age (SGA), and stressed neonates (e.g., asphyxia, sepsis) become hypoglycemic primarily because of diminished glycogen stores.
2. Beyond the neonatal period, hypoglycemia usually results from a significant disease process.
   a. Hyperinsulinism can present at any time during infancy. The more severe forms present in the neonatal period.
   b. Hypoglycemia secondary to deficient glucose production typically presents beyond the neonatal period, when the infant stretches out the feeding interval or begins to sleep through the night.
   c. Most causes of hypoglycemia are sporadic; how-

TABLE 266–1. CAUSES OF HYPOGLYCEMIA

I. Neonatal (usually transient)
  A. Hyperinsulinism
    1. Infant of a diabetic mother
    2. Infant with erythroblastosis fetalis
    3. Umbilical artery catheter malposition
    4. Abrupt cessation of TPN
  B. Deficient glucose production
    1. SGA infants
    2. Premature infants
    3. Fetal distress (e.g., asphyxia, sepsis)
    4. Maternal drugs (e.g., beta blockers)
II. Infancy/Childhood
  A. Hyperinsulinism
    1. Islet cell dysmaturation
    2. Beckwith-Wiedemann syndrome
    3. Islet cell adenoma
    4. Factitious (ingestion of oral hypoglycemic agents or injection of insulin)
  B. Deficient glucose production
    1. Enzyme deficiencies
      a. Glycogen synthetase
      b. Glycogen storage diseases
        1) Glucose-6-phosphatase
        2) Debrancher
        3) Phosphorylase
      c. Defects in gluconeogenesis
        1) Fructose-1,6-diphosphatase
        2) Pyruvate carboxylase
        3) Phosphoenol pyruvate carboxykinase
      d. Precursors for gluconeogenesis
        1) Galactosemia
        2) Hereditary fructose intolerance
        3) Defects in fatty acid oxidation
        4) Defects in amino acid metabolism
    2. Deficiencies of counterregulatory hormones
      a. Growth hormone
      b. Cortisol
    3. Substrate limitations—ketotic hypoglycemia
    4. Hepatic poisons
      a. Salicylates
      b. Alcohol
      c. Beta blocker overdose
      d. Jamaica vomiting sickness
      e. Reye syndrome
      f. Other causes of liver failure

SGA = small for gestational age; TPN = total parenteral nutrition.

ever, enzymatic deficiencies are usually inherited in an autosomal recessive pattern. Hyperinsulinism can be familial.

To maintain a normal blood glucose requires:

- Adequate substrate (glycogen, lipid, muscle)
- Functional enzymes for utilizing substrate
- A normal endocrine system for regulating substrate utilization

---

Pathophysiology

Glucose Homeostasis

1. Blood glucose levels reflect the balance between glucose production and glucose utilization.

2. Ingested glucose is used to meet tissue energy demands. Any excess glucose is stored, primarily as liver glycogen.

3. The brain accounts for most of the glucose utilization during a fast. Basal glucose requirements decrease with age, reflecting lower brain to body mass ratios.

4. During fasting, glycogenolysis initially supplies glucose to meet energy requirements.

5. As glycogen stores are exhausted, gluconeogenesis (i.e., the synthesis of glucose from other metabolites) contributes to glucose supplies. Substrates for gluconeogenesis include:

    a. Glycerol derived from the breakdown of lipids. A by-product of lipolysis is the production of ketones, which can be used by some tissues as an alternative fuel when glucose supplies are limited.

    b. Amino acids (e.g., alanine) and lactate derived from protein (i.e., muscle).

6. The metabolic pathways involved in glucose homeostasis (glycogenolysis, lipolysis, proteolysis, gluconeogenesis) are hormonally regulated. Insulin is an anabolic hormone that promotes substrate deposition, whereas the counterregulatory hormones (growth hormone, cortisol, glucagon, epinephrine) stimulate substrate mobilization and utilization. Thus, the maintenance of a normal blood glucose reflects the interplay between the glucose-lowering actions of insulin and the actions of the counterregulatory hormones to raise blood glucose.

Differential Diagnosis

1. The most common cause of hypoglycemia in infancy is hyperinsulinism.

    a. Hypoglycemia occurs not only because of increased glucose utilization; excess insulin also inhibits glycogenolysis and gluconeogenesis, thereby impairing the body's defense against hypoglycemia.

    b. Hyperinsulinism in infancy is not an anatomic defect but is thought to be a maturational or functional defect in the islet cell "glucostat." Pancreatic pathology may include nesidioblastosis (a normal histologic variant in infancy), β cell hypertrophy or hyperplasia, or normal histology.

    c. In older children (> 1 year), hyperinsulinism may be secondary to an adenoma.

2. The most common cause of hypoglycemia in older children is so-called "ketotic" or idiopathic hypoglycemia.

    a. The peak incidence occurs between 18 months and 3 years of age, with spontaneous resolution before puberty.

    b. These children are thin for age and develop hypoglycemia during caloric restriction (e.g., because of an intercurrent illness or a prolonged fast), presumably because of limited substrate (especially muscle) to fuel gluconeogenesis.

Clinical Findings

1. General features of hypoglycemia:

    a. Neonates present with nonspecific symptoms that often suggest sepsis—lethargy, poor feeding, apnea, irritability, hypotonia, cyanosis. Seizures may occur.

    b. Older children first develop epinephrine-mediated symptoms (sweating, shaking, pallor, tachycardia, hunger), followed by neuroglycopenic symptoms (headache, irritability, mental clouding, loss of consciousness, and seizures).

2. Differential diagnosis: Many entities causing hypoglycemia have unique clinical features that are helpful in establishing the diagnosis.

    a. Hyperinsulinism: Like infants of diabetic mothers, many newborns with islet cell dysmaturation are large for gestational age. Hypoglycemia is severe and the child requires excessive amounts of glucose to maintain a normal blood glucose.

    b. Enzymatic defects: Many children with enzymatic defects have hepatomegaly. There may be a family history of infant deaths. The temporal relationship of the hypoglycemia to the meal may be helpful. Defects in glycogenolysis present after a short (6–8 hour) fast, whereas defects in fatty acid oxidation present after prolonged (12–24 hours) fasting. Children with fatty acid oxidation defects may have myopathies.

    c. Hormonal deficiencies: Children with panhypopituitarism may have midline facial defects. Males may have a small phallus. Hyperpigmentation, vomiting, and electrolyte abnormalities may be clues to primary adrenal insufficiency.

Key Clinical Findings

↑ **Epinephrine**	**Neuroglycopenia**
Sweating	Headache
Tachycardia	Irritability
Shaking	Confusion
Pallor	Coma
Hunger	Seizures

Laboratory Findings

1. Initial studies

    a. To determine the etiology of the hypoglycemia, it is crucial that a blood specimen be drawn for glucose and other determinations at the time of hypoglycemia, before therapy is initiated.

    b. If blood is not obtained at the time of presentation, a fast under medical supervision is usually necessary.

    c. The initial blood sample should be sent for glucose, insulin, cortisol, growth hormone, and ketones. If possible, additional serum should be frozen for later use. A more extensive initial laboratory evaluation may be warranted based on the physical examination (e.g., liver function tests, free fatty acids and lactate in the presence of hepatomegaly).

    d. A urine sample (obtained at the time of hypoglycemia) should be analyzed for the presence of ketones and reducing substances. The absence of ketosis is highly suggestive of hyperinsulinism or a defect in fatty acid oxidation. If a fatty acid oxidation defect is suspected, urine should be obtained for organic acid analysis.

  e. There are transient defects in glycogenolysis and gluconeogenesis, caused by a variety of hepatic toxins (see Table 266–1). These should obviously be considered before embarking on expensive laboratory investigations.

2. Differential diagnosis

  a. During hypoglycemia, insulin levels should be suppressed. Measurable insulin levels and hypoketonemia are highly suggestive of hyperinsulinism.

  b. During hypoglycemia, elevated levels of growth hormone (>10 ng/ml) and cortisol (>15 μg/dl) should be present. Lower levels are indicative of a hormone deficiency.

  c. Lactic acidosis is generally indicative of an enzymatic defect and will require further laboratory evaluation. Definitive diagnosis may require a liver biopsy.

  d. Children with so-called ketotic hypoglycemia will have a completely normal laboratory evaluation at the time of hypoglycemia. This is the most common cause of hypoglycemia in older children (1–5 years) but is a diagnosis of exclusion.

Key Initial Laboratory Evaluation

Blood	Urine
Glucose (gray top)	Ketones
Growth hormone	Reducing substances
Cortisol	
Insulin	
Frozen serum	

Treatment

1. A symptomatic child with hypoglycemia should be given 0.2 g/kg of glucose intravenously. High dextrose containing solutions (25% or 50%) should be avoided because they provoke hyperinsulinemia. Serum glucose should be maintained by an infusion of 10 per cent dextrose. Neonates generally require 6 to 8 mg/kg/min, and older children 3–5 mg/kg/min to maintain a serum glucose above 50 mg/dl. A prolonged requirement for higher infusion rates (>12 mg/kg/min) is highly suggestive of hyperinsulinism.

2. Glucagon (0.03 mg/kg) given intramuscularly or subcutaneously in a symptomatic child with no intravenous access will effectively raise the blood glucose acutely, if glycogen stores are present. Glucagon should not be given in the presence of hepatomegaly, as it will worsen the metabolic acidosis seen with gluconeogenic defects. Glucagon administration must be followed by a maintenance intravenous glucose infusion.

3. Definitive therapy is determined by the etiology of hypoglycemia, but in extreme situations pharmacologic doses of glucocorticoid (e.g., Solu-Cortef 100 mg/m², intravenously) will usually raise the blood glucose.

4. In infants with hyperinsulinism, medical therapy with diazoxide (10–20 mg/kg PO TID) is usually effective in maintaining euglycemia. If diazoxide is ineffective, a long-acting somatostatin analog may be tried. If medical therapy is ineffective, the infant should have a near-total pancreatectomy. Older children with an adenoma will require surgery.

5. Patients with hormonal deficiencies are easily treated with hormone replacement.

6. Patients with enzymatic defects require specific dietary modifications.

7. Patients with "ketotic" hypoglycemia need only to avoid prolonged fasting.

Key Treatment of Hypoglycemia

- Intravenous glucose—2 cc/kg of D10W followed by maintenance infusion

- Nonspecific therapy if hypoglycemia persists:
  Glucagon (0.03 mg/kg IM, SC, or IV)
  Solu-Cortef (100 mg/m² IV)

- Specific therapy based on etiology

See also Chapter 67.

Bibliography

Geffner ME: Hypoglycemia. *In* Kaplan SA (ed): Clinical Pediatric Endocrinology. Philadelphia, WB Saunders, 1990, pp 165–179.

Hale DE, Bennett ME: Fatty acid oxidation disorders: a new class of metabolic diseases. J Pediatr 1992;121:1–10.

Senior B, Sadeghi-Nejad A: The glycogenoses and other inherited disorders of carbohydrate metabolism. Clin Perinatol 1976; 3:79–98.

Thornton, PS, Sumner AE, Ruchelli ED, et al: Familial and sporadic hyperinsulinism: histopathologic findings and segregation analysis support a single autosomal recessive disorder. J Pediatr 1991;119:721–724.

267 Diabetes Mellitus

Cecilia C. Capriles and *Lynne L. Levitsky*

Etiology

1. Diabetes mellitus results from an insufficiency of insulin release or action.
   a. Children and adolescents with type 1 diabetes need insulin to control hyperglycemia and prevent spontaneous ketosis.
   b. Type 2 diabetes, commonly seen in adults, is a genetically heterogeneous disorder of insufficient insulin release and insulin resistance.
   c. Maturity-onset diabetes in youth (MODY) is usually an autosomal dominant form of type 2 diabetes.
2. In type 1 diabetes, environmental factors trigger autoimmune destruction of the pancreatic beta cells. Beta cell destruction leads eventually to absolute insulinopenia. Exposure to certain viruses (coxsackievirus has been epidemiologically associated) and other toxins (cow milk exposure is a debated risk factor) has been associated with the development of type 1 diabetes.
3. Susceptibility to type 1 diabetes is inherited.
   a. Over 10 different genetic loci associated with risk of type 1 diabetes have been identified.
   b. The human leukocyte antigen (HLA) class II DQ locus on chromosome 6 is most important.
      (1) Specific alleles are associated with high risk or are protective for diabetes.
      (2) Class II HLA molecules bind short peptide antigens and present them to T cells. Presentation of certain islet-related antigens might determine susceptibility to diabetes. Protective HLA alleles may compete for antigen binding but not activate a T-cell response.

Epidemiology

1. In the United States, the incidence is 12 to 14 per 100,000 per year and the prevalence is 1 in 600 among late adolescents. The incidence is higher in Caucasians than in other genetically defined groups.
2. The peak incidence of type 1 diabetes is during puberty, there is no sex predominance, and there is a seasonal variation with peaks of onset in the fall and winter months.
3. The lifetime risk of developing diabetes if a close relative has diabetes varies from 30 to 50 per cent for an identical twin, to 1 per cent for a sibling without HLA identity.

Pathophysiology

1. Prodrome
   a. Serum antibodies directed against insulin (IAA), the islet cell (ICA), and other antigens such as glutamic acid decarboxylase (GAD$_{65}$) can be detected up to 10 years before the development of the classic symptoms of diabetes.

   b. A decline in first phase insulin secretion during an intravenous glucose tolerance test, indicating progression of autoimmune beta cell destruction, precedes the development of overt diabetes.
2. Overt diabetes: The loss of 80 to 90 per cent of pancreatic beta cell function produces insulinopenia, leading to hyperglycemia and indequate intracellular substrate transport or metabolism for tissue function. Without insulin replacement therapy, ketoacidosis and death is inevitable.
3. Chronic diabetes: Hyperglycemia and insulin deficiency lead to microvascular, renal, and retinal disease and sensory, motor, and autonomic nerve damage as a result of:
   a. Altered metabolic pathways including activated production of sugar alcohols, altered myo-inositol metabolism, and increased production of advanced glycosylation end products.
   b. Increased levels of growth hormone and other counterregulatory hormones, and increased production of local growth and angiogenic factors.
   c. Changed microvascular dynamics leading to intraorgan hypertension and hypoxia.

Clinical Findings

1. Presentation: The classic presenting symptoms of diabetes are polyuria, polyphagia, polydipsia, weight loss, and lethargy. Onset may be acute, precipitated by the stress of an acute illness, or more chronic and insidious over weeks or even months.
2. The remission phase: Within a few weeks of starting insulin therapy, approximately two thirds of children enter a remission ("honeymoon") period during which endogenous insulin production increases. Remission can last weeks to months.
3. Complete insulin deficiency: When there is no endogenous insulin secretion, glycemic control with subcutaneous insulin becomes more difficult and glycemic excursions more profound. Instability of glycemic control is a hallmark of type 1 diabetes. Hypoglycemia (blood glucose less than 60 mg/dl) is a frequent acute complication.

Key Clinical Findings

- Polyuria
- Polyphagia
- Polydipsia
- Weight loss
- Lethargy
- Genital moniliasis

4. Chronic complications of diabetes in childhood and adolescence result from poor glycemic control. Complications include short stature with delayed maturation, limited joint mobility commonly affecting the interphalangeal joints, and adolescent microvasculopathy, neuropathy, and microalbuminuria.

Laboratory Findings

1. Blood glucose: A formal glucose tolerance test is rarely necessary for diagnosis. Classic symptoms and one random blood glucose greater than 200 mg/dl, confirmed on a subsequent day, or a fasting blood glucose greater than 126 mg/dl on two occasions is sufficient.

2. ICA, IAA, and GAD$_{65}$
   a. If the patient is ketosis-free at diagnosis, presence of anti-islet or anti-insulin antibodies confirms the diagnosis in 90 per cent of individuals with type 1 diabetes.
   b. Stress hyperglycemia (a transient increase in blood glucose during acute stress) may be differentiated from new onset diabetes by its short duration (1–5 hr) without insulin treatment, glucose levels that are usually not higher than 300 mg/dl, and absence of IAA and ICA. This is not, in general, associated with later type 1 diabetes.

3. Urine/blood ketones (acetoacetate, acetone, beta-hydroxybutyrate): Increased ketogenesis results from insulinopenia. The presence of ketonuria/ketonemia generally confirms that diabetes is type 1 diabetes. Acetone and acetoacetate, but not betahydroxybutyrate, are measured by usual "dipstick" ketone reagents.

4. Serum electrolytes, pH, phosphate, calcium
   a. Hyponatremia may result from dilution of the extracellular space by the hyperglycemia occupying "osmotic space."
   b. Metabolic acidosis is seen if diabetes is decompensated.
   c. Re-equilibration of blood glucose may lead to low potassium or phosphate.

5. Serum creatinine and serum ureal nitrogen (SUN)
   a. May be elevated because of dehydration.
   b. Creatinine may be factitiously elevated because of cross-reaction with acetoacetate in the most commonly used laboratory method.

6. Triglycerides and cholesterol are elevated with insulin deficiency. Hypertriglyceridemia may factitiously lower serum sodium.

7. Glycohemoglobin is formed when glucose is bound nonenzymatically to free amino groups of the hemoglobin molecule. Per cent glycohemoglobin correlates with the mean blood glucose over the life span of the red cell (reflects glycemic control over the preceding 8–16 weeks).
   a. There is no universally accepted reference value for glycohemoglobin.
   b. Hemoglobin A$_{1c}$ is hemoglobin glycated only at the amino terminal of the beta chain of hemoglobin A.
   c. If a hemoglobinopathy is present, measurement of all glycation sites of all hemoglobins (total glyco-

hemoglobin by affinity chromatography) is necessary.

Key Laboratory Findings
• Glycosuria
• Random blood glucose >200 mg/dl
• Fasting blood glucose >126 mg/dl

Treatment

1. Goals
   a. To avoid episodes of severe hypoglycemia: Recurrent hypoglycemia is a particular risk in children less than 5 years old and has been associated with learning disabilities and neurologic deficits.
   b. To prevent chronic complications by achieving near-normal blood glucose: Duration of hyperglycemia is the most important risk factor for chronic complications of type 1 diabetes. Establishing appropriate behaviors for maintenance of glycemic control in early childhood facilitates maintenance of these behaviors during the pubertal years.

2. Management of newly diagnosed type 1 diabetes
   a. Hospitalization is not always required.
      (1) Those with moderate hyperglycemia without acidemia, who are clinically stable and can take fluids orally, can be managed as outpatients if the family has adequate emotional, intellectual, and economic resources, and there is a readily available diabetes management team.
      (2) Children with ketoacidemia or with presenting blood glucose of 800 mg/dl or greater will require at least a short hospitalization.
   b. Education: The family should not be overwhelmed with information initially. Diabetes education should be a slow and continuing process. Printed educational material should be used to facilitate long-term mastery.
      (1) The family and the patient must understand the basic pathophysiology of diabetes and the importance of adequate metabolic control to avoid acute and chronic complications.
      (2) They must learn basic skills for survival including insulin administration, blood glucose monitoring, recognition and treatment of hypoglycemia, hyperglycemia, and ketoacidosis, adjusting insulin and diet for growth, exercise, and sick days.
   c. Insulin preparations: In general, use recombinant human insulins. Relatively impure beef and pork insulin is more antigenic than either recombinant human insulin or purified pork insulin. Time of onset and peak of insulin is influenced by injection site (more rapid in abdomen, slower in thigh). Differences in the onset and duration of insulins from different sources may influence therapeutic outcome (Table 267–1).
   d. Initiation of insulin therapy

TABLE 267-1. ACTION OF SUBCUTANEOUSLY
ADMINISTERED INSULINS

INSULIN	ONSET (HR)	PEAK (HR)	DURATION (HR)
Lispro*	0.25	1	2–3
Regular			
Human	0.5–1	2–3	3–6
Pork	0.5–2	2–4	4–6
NPH/Lente			
Human	2–4	4–8	10–16
Pork	2–4	6–10	16–20
Ultralente†			
Human	2–4	8–16	18–20

*Lispro is a semisynthetic insulin with an amino acid substitution that speeds its availability when given SC.
†Onset, peak, and duration of human Ultralente are particularly unpredictable.

(1) Early and adequate insulin therapy seems to postpone complete loss of insulin secretion.

(2) The use of oral beta cell stimulatory hypoglycemic drugs is contraindicated because stimulation of residual beta cell function early in the course of type 1 diabetes might lead to more rapid loss of insulin-release capacity.

(3) The usual insulin requirement for newly diagnosed type 1 diabetes is 0.5 to 1 U/kg per day. However, requirements may be lower in children less than 5 years old diagnosed before development of ketoacidosis (0.2–0.5 U/kg per day) and higher in adolescents recovering from ketoacidosis (1–1.2 U/kg per day).

  (a) Begin with 0.5 U/kg per day (0.3 U/kg per day in children younger than 5 years without ketoacidemia at presentation) in a bid regimen.

  (b) Give 2/3 of daily dose in the morning, before breakfast, and 1/3 before dinner.

  (c) Give 2/3 of morning insulin as intermediate-acting (NPH or Lente) and 1/3 as Regular insulin. Split the predinner insulin dose equally between regular and intermediate-acting insulin.

  (d) Adjust insulin based upon results of qid blood glucose monitoring before meals and bedtime snack.

  (e) Give 0.1 U/kg of Regular insulin before meals or 0.05 U/kg at bedtime for blood glucose greater than 300 mg/dl.

  (f) If insulin regimen is being developed in a newly diagnosed outpatient, the patient or guardian should call a designated member of the diabetes team to make insulin adjustments.

3. Long-term management of type 1 diabetes

  a. Insulin dose: The usual replacement dose of insulin is 0.7 to 1 U/kg SC per day. Adolescents or obese children may be more insulin resistant and require up to 1.3 U/kg per day. Approximately two thirds of children enter a remission phase within a few weeks of starting insulin therapy and need less than 0.5 U/kg per day to achieve metabolic control.

  b. Modes of administration: The amount, proportion, and timing of each insulin type will depend upon the individual meal plan and activity level. Initially, the bid intermediate and Regular insulin regimen is usually sufficient, but other regimens often prove more effective with time:

  (1) The tid regimen is useful if predinner intermediate insulin sufficient to control morning blood glucose induces nocturnal hypoglycemia:

    (a) Intermediate and Regular insulin mixed pre-breakfast.

    (b) Regular insulin (sometimes intermediate is given as well) before dinner and intermediate insulin at (parental) bedtime.

  (2) Regular and human Ultralente:

    (a) Human Ultralente and Regular insulin at dinner can sometimes supplement the standard bid regimen in those families for whom tid is not acceptable.

    (b) Ultralente and Regular insulin before breakfast and dinner can be useful in infants and young children with irregular eating patterns.

    (c) Some late adolescents may wish to use Ultralente insulin given bid as basal insulin, with regular given before each meal.

    (d) Mixing Ultralente and Regular insulin in the same syringe will change the pharmacokinetics of both insulins and should be avoided.

  (3) Lispro insulin is more rapid-acting than Regular and its effect more short-lived. It may be given immediately with meals and may be useful as a replacement for Regular insulin or as a supplemental short-acting insulin.

  c. Adjustment of insulin dose: Blood glucoses reflect the adequacy of the insulin most active at the time of glucose determination.

  (1) Regular or Lispro insulin can be adjusted at each dose based upon preceding blood glucose (BG) and nutritional or activity plans according to a predetermined algorithm. Example: A fixed dose of insulin is chosen for blood glucose within the target range (70–130 mg/dl). The dose is decreased by 10 to 20 per cent for BG less than 70, and increased 10 to 20 per cent for each 100 to 150 mg/dl increment over 130.

  (2) Intermediate/long-acting insulin can be adjusted by 10 to 20 per cent every 2 to 3 days based upon persistent blood glucose patterns.

  (3) Regular or Lispro insulin can be administered as a supplement before lunch (0.1 U/kg) or at bedtime (0.05 U/kg) for blood glucose over 300 mg/dl.

  (4) Blood glucose testing at 1 to 3 AM will clarify whether predinner intermediate- or long-acting insulin is causing nocturnal hypoglycemia.

d. Blood glucose monitoring:

(1) Frequent blood glucose determinations allow more accurate adjustment of insulin dose, enhance patient education, and can identify emergency situations.

(2) Ideally, self–blood glucose monitoring (SBGM) should be performed at least four times a day (before meals and at bedtime).

(3) We recommend at minimum twice daily monitoring, before breakfast and dinner insulin administration. Tests before lunch and at bedtime twice a week (once during school days and once on weekends) and at 2 to 3 AM once or twice a month offer supplementary information for insulin adjustment.

(4) Additional testing is recommended to cope with illness, exercise, and other intercurrent events.

e. Urine testing: Urine glucose testing has limited utility because it correlates poorly with blood glucose. Urine testing for ketones is always recommended when blood glucose is greater than 250 mg/dl or during illness.

f. Nutritional management: See Chapter 268.

4. Special situations

a. Exercise increases muscle glucose uptake and may cause hypoglycemia. With poor control, exercise may worsen hyperglycemia and ketosis.

(1) Delay exercise for blood glucose greater than 250 mg/dl with ketonuria.

(2) For planned exercise, decrease the insulin dose peaking at that time by 10 to 20 per cent. If total daily activity will increase, decrease total daily insulin by 10 to 20 per cent. Give insulin in a site that will not be stimulated by exercise (e.g., in arm for bicycling). Increase the bedtime snack to avoid erratic postexercise hypoglycemia.

(3) For unplanned exercise, increase carbohydrate intake (see Chapter 268).

b. Intercurrent illness is usually associated with insulin resistance. Management is directed toward avoiding hypoglycemia or ketoacidosis and treatment of the underlying illness. Telephone management is often sufficient.

(1) Monitor blood glucose and urine ketones every 2 to 4 hr.

(2) Adjust insulin dose:

(a) For decreased oral intake and/or vomiting, not associated with ketonuria, reduce basal insulin dose by 30 to 50 per cent and supplement with regular insulin as necessary.

(b) Give 10 per cent of total insulin dose as Regular insulin every 4 to 6 hr for glucose greater than 250 mg/dl. Give 20 per cent of insulin dose as Regular insulin every 4 to 6 hr for glucose greater than 250 mg/dl and moderate or large ketones.

(3) Maintain hydration, carbohydrate, and electrolyte intake by offering frequent, small amounts of fluids. If blood glucose is greater than 180, these should be sugar-free electrolyte-containing broths alternating with diet drinks. If blood glucose is less than 180, sugar-containing drinks should be used.

(4) Evaluate and treat in a medical facility if condition worsens or oral intake is not tolerated.

c. Perioperative management

(1) For elective surgery, schedule first in the morning if possible and give 50 per cent of intermediate insulin SC in AM with 5 per cent dextrose–containing intravenous fluids. Monitor blood glucose every 2 hr.

(2) Blood glucose should be maintained between 150 and 200 mg/dl to protect against hypoglycemia and avoid ketoacidosis associated with surgical stress.

(3) For blood glucose greater than 200 mg/dl, supplement with regular insulin 0.05 to 0.1 U/kg SC every 4 hr until oral intake is reinstituted.

(4) For nonelective procedures, or, alternatively, for prolonged elective surgery, infuse 5 per cent dextrose–containing fluid and give intravenous Regular insulin (0.03–0.05 U/kg per hour) as a separate infusion. Monitor blood glucose hourly, and adjust insulin infusion rate to maintain stable blood glucose.

d. Inappropriate insulin dose

(1) Missed insulin dose: Supplement with regular insulin at discovery and before meals until next normal insulin dose.

(2) Inadvertent overinsulinization: Give frequent carbohydrate feeds and test blood glucose every 2 hr. Receipt of more than three times the total daily insulin may require availability of intravenous glucose.

5. Other approaches to insulin therapy

a. Insulin pump therapy provides a patient-controlled subcutaneous insulin infusion and has proved useful in highly motivated adults but has not been a successful long-term alternative for children and adolescents.

b. Pancreatic or islet transplantation requires immunosuppression and is not yet considered an alternative therapy for young people with type 1 diabetes.

6. Treatment of complications of diabetes associated with insulin therapy

a. Hypoglycemia: Frequency increases following intensification of insulin treatment. Predisposing factors include insulin errors, erratic insulin absorption, inappropriate timing of meals and insulin administration, increased actvity level, and, in older patients, concomitant use of alcohol or drugs.

(1) Presentation

(a) Mild to moderate symptoms result from autonomic responses and include tremor, weakness, and hunger. Parents may notice pallor and behavior changes. Moderate neuroglycopenic symptoms include headaches and decreased alertness.

(b) Severe neuroglycopenic symptoms include

decreased mentation, loss of consciousness, and seizures.

(2) Treatment

(a) Mild to moderate: 10 to 15 g of simple carbohydrate (2 to 3 glucose tablets, 4 to 6 small hard candies, 4 to 5 oz juice or soft drink) are usually sufficient to raise the blood glucose in 15 min. If a meal is not anticipated within 1 hr, a complex carbohydrate and fat/protein-containing snack is recommended. Overtreatment will lead to hyperglycemia and should be avoided by checking blood glucose after 30 min and assessing the need for additional carbohydrate.

(b) Severe: If the child is uncooperative, but still capable of swallowing, a semisolid gel or sugar paste (tube cake frosting, or other preparation) may be administered. This cannot be absorbed through the buccal mucosa and must be swallowed. For seizures or coma, 0.5 to 1 mg glucagon should be administered subcutaneously and can be repeated in 15 min. This often causes nausea or vomiting 45 to 60 min after administration. Therefore, when the child is awake and arousable (15–20 min), oral carbohydrate should be immediately administered to maintain blood glucose for the next several hours.

b. Chronic complications of insulin therapy:

(1) Lipoatrophy: Local loss of fat in subcutaneous depots is a result of immune responses to impure animal insulin preparations and can be treated by injection of human insulin at atrophic sites.

(2) Lipohypertrophy: Fat hypertrophy at injection sites secondary to stimulation of adipogenesis by high local levels of insulin may lead to erratic absorption and metabolic control and should be avoided by adequate site rotation.

(3) Obesity: Excess weight gain from overinsulinization during intensification of treatment should be avoided by appropriate nutritional counseling.

7. Other associations with type 1 diabetes

a. Chronic lymphocytic thyroiditis and other autoimmune disorders that are more common in type 1 diabetes should be identified and treated appropriately.

b. Peptic ulcer disease may be more common in young people with type 1 diabetes. Symptoms respond well to H_2-receptor antagonists.

8. Prevention and treatment of complications of diabetes associated with chronic hyperglycemia

a. Improvement in glycemic control reduces the risk of developing retinopathy, nephropathy, and neuropathy, and slows the progression of these complications.

b. Adjunctive approaches to management

Management and Monitoring of Type 1 Diabetes Mellitus

- **Clinical evaluation** every 2–3 months

  Evaluate diabetes control by history and review of meter and recorded glucose values. Monitor for growth, puberty, blood pressure, injection sites, thyroid, joint elasticity, funduscopy, and peripheral neuropathy. Adjust management as necessary.

- **Nutrition consultation** twice a year
- **Diabetes education** review at least yearly
- **Other referrals:** Ophthalmologic examination yearly beginning at puberty
- **Psychosocial support** as required
- **Laboratory studies**

---

(1) Retinopathy: 60 per cent of patients postpuberty manifest retinopathy within 5 to 10 years. Yearly ophthalmology visits after puberty will facilitate identification and appropriate early laser therapy of clinically significant retinopathy.

(2) Nephropathy: Microalbuminuria is a marker for early nephropathy. Treatment of microalbuminuria with angiotensin-converting enzyme (ACE) inhibitors decreases progression to end-stage renal disease even in normotensive patients, but *ACE inhibitors are fetal teratogens.*

(3) Neuropathy: The symptoms of painful sensory neuropathy may respond to treatment with tricyclic antidepressants, anticonvulsants (phenytoin and carbamazepine), or local capsaicin. Some gastrointestinal symptoms of autonomic

---

Routine Laboratory Studies

- *Glycohemoglobin* every 2–3 months

  We choose these goals for average blood glucose in childhood type 1 diabetes as assessed by glycohemoglobin:

  5 yr or younger: Mean blood glucose of 250 mg/dl or less, in order to avoid hypoglycemic damage to the developing central nervous system.

  School-age children: Mean blood glucose of 180 mg/dl or less.

  Older children and adolescents: Mean blood glucose of 150 mg/dl or less to decrease the risk of chronic complications.

- *Lipid profile* yearly
- *Thyroid-stimulating hormone (TSH), antithyroid antibodies* yearly in children over age 10 yr or earlier based on history and physical examination
- *Serum creatinine* yearly in adolescents
- *Microalbumin and creatinine* in 12 hr overnight urine yearly in adolescents

neuropathy (gastroparesis diagnosed by slow gastric emptying of a solid food bolus) may respond to prokinetic agents (metoclopramide or cisapride) or motilin agonists such as erythromycin.

(4) Hyperlipidemia is usually secondary to poor glycemic control, but may be an independent risk factor for diabetes complications and should be treated by appropriate nutritional or, if severe, drug therapies.

(5) Hypertension increases the risk of progression of retinopathy and nephropathy. Treatment with ACE inhibitors will inhibit this progression.

(6) Smoking is a risk factor for retinopathy, nephropathy, and macrovascular disease. Smoking cessation and prevention should be pursued in parents of young children with type 1 diabetes and in adolescents.

Prevention

1. There is no presently acceptable prevention.
2. Immunosuppressants (cyclosporine, cyclophosphamide)

have prolonged the remission phase in a few studies but are still investigational tools.

3. Several prospective trials are underway to determine if individuals at high risk for the development of diabetes can be protected by early treatment with insulin or other agents.

Bibliography

American Diabetes Association: Report of the Expert Committee on the diagnosis and classification of diabetes mellitus. Diabetes Care 1997;20:1183–1197.

American Diabetes Association: Standard of medical care for patients with diabetes mellitus (position statement). Diabetes Care 1996;19(Suppl 1):S8–S15.

Atkinson MA, Maclaren NK: The pathogenesis of insulin-dependent diabetes mellitus. N Engl J Med 1994;331:1428–1436.

Hirsch IB: Implementation of intensive diabetes therapy for IDDM. Diabetes Rev 1995;3:288–307.

Raboudi N, Levitsky LL: Insulin-dependent diabetes mellitus. *In* Burg FD, Ingelfinger JR, Wald ER, Polin RA (eds): Current Pediatric Therapy, 15th ed. Philadelphia, WB Saunders, 1996, pp 348–357.

268 Dietary Management of Childhood Diabetes Mellitus

Fenella Greig

1. Dietary management of insulin dependent diabetes mellitus (type 1) is a major component of the treatment together with insulin used in the quest for acceptable glycemic control. The aims of dietary management for diabetic children include the following:

   - Provide adequate nutrition for normal growth.
   - Carbohydrates divided in meals and snacks to balance with insulin action and reduce the risk of severe or recurrent hypoglycemia or hyperglycemia.
   - Reduce long-term complications of type 1 diabetes associated with chronic hyperglycemia, dyslipidemia, or obesity.
   - Nutritional education to enable practical and effective home management.

2. Recommendations for dietary management are presented in publications of the American Diabetes Association (ADA) and the American Dietetic Association, but may require adaptation for the special needs of young and growing children. The latest ADA recommendations call for more individualized meal planning reflecting the patient's lifestyle. New food labels offer additional practical help listing the carbohydrate and sugar content of packaged food.

3. Management by a team approach is part of the current standard of diabetes care for children. The dietitian should be an integral part of the diabetes team to

allow recommendations from the dietitian, the doctor and diabetes nurse educator to be coordinated with the family. A thorough initial assessment of the diabetic child's nutritional needs includes assessment of growth and weight for height plotted on a standard growth curve, level of activity, food preferences, and appetite. At diagnosis several sessions with the dietitian will set the foundation for the necessary skills and practical goals so the family can plan appropriate meals and snacks. The dietitian's role is ongoing, with visits recommended at least every 6 months, to adapt the meal plan for a child's changing needs and food preferences.

4. For infants and preschool children a calculation of 1000 kilocalories plus 100 kilocalories per year of life can be used. For school-aged children calculation is based on 65 kilocalories/kg of ideal body weight. During the pubertal growth spurt a transient increase in caloric needs is followed by reduced need to about 35 kilocalories/kg as growth is completed. At each stage, energy needs can vary widely, and the child's activity level will play a large part in determining caloric needs to maintain appropriate body weight.

5. The percentages of calories from fat, protein, and carbohydrate recommended for the diabetic meal plan differ from the average American diet, with a decrease of fat, protein, and simple sugar and an increase of complex carbohydrates.

a. Fat should provide no more than 30 per cent of total calories with up to one third of this as saturated fat.

b. A protein intake of 10–20 per cent of total calories is recommended for adults but needs adjustment for children.

Recommended protein intake for infants is:
- 2.0–2.2 g/kg
- A gradual decrease in childhood to 1.2–1.5 g/kg
- A further decrease to 0.8–1.0 g/kg as growth in height is completed.

c. Carbohydrates should contribute the remaining 50 to 65 per cent of the total calories, with the majority provided by complex carbohydrates.

6. Distribution of carbohydrates

a. Distribution of carbohydrates between meals and snacks is used to minimize extremes of hypoglycemia or hyperglycemia. Consistency in the amount of carbohydrate for each meal or snack allows the effect of food on blood glucose to be balanced with the actions of each dose of insulin.

Distribution of carbohydrates could be:

- breakfast 20%
- midmorning snack 10%
- lunch 20%
- midafternoon snack 10%
- dinner 30%
- bedtime snack 10%

b. Individualized meal planning, adjusting the amount or timing to fit a child's preferred schedule, could modify this schedule, for example: to omit the morning snack if school lunch is early, or provide two afternoon snacks if there is a long period with sports between lunch and dinner. While some might prefer to have bigger meals and no snacks, a better strategy for carbohydrate/insulin dynamics is to divide the carbohydrate load into smaller amounts. In school the timing and amount of food should cover the peak action of insulin or vigorous activity.

7. The approach to the dietary management for diabetes has varied widely from unrestricted intake except for avoidance of foods rich in simple sugars ("concentrated sweets") to a system where all food was measured. Effective nutritional management was found to be an important component of the ability to maintain improved diabetes control during a long-term study—the Diabetes Control and Complications Trial (DCCT). This prospective, randomized study, involving 1441 patients over 5 to 9 years, demonstrated long-term benefits of improved diabetes control as measured by a lowered level of glycosylated hemoglobin A_{1c}. The outcome of intensified therapy, compared with conventional but less precise insulin and diet therapy, was clearly superior in reducing the progression or onset of diabetic complications. While such intensive therapy and lowered blood glucose attained in the DCCT are not readily achieved or yet recommended in younger children, any degree of improvement in diabetes control was beneficial in the reduction of complications. Certain diet behaviors in the DCCT, including overall adherence to the meal plan, a consistent snack at bedtime, and the ability of the patient to adjust food or insulin in response to blood glucose excursions, were associated with improved control.

8. Various strategies provide a structured basis for meal plans, and enable consistency with flexible food choice. The Exchange Lists for Meal Planning, published by the ADA, lists foods in each of six groups (starch, fruit, vegetable, milk, meat, and fat). The portion size contains relatively consistent amounts of carbohydrate, fat, and protein within each group. Another version, Carbohydrate Counting, considers only the main sources of carbohydrate (starch, fruit, starchy vegetables and milk), which have the major effect on blood glucose. Carbohydrate Counting was found to be readily understood and to provide greater choice and precision in estimating carbohydrate intake, but might need additional guidelines for fat and protein intake in growing children.

9. The labels, Nutrition Facts, on all processed food have greatly enhanced the ability to judge the effect of a particular food on blood glucose by the total carbohydrate and sugar content. The use of "sugar" is defined as the sum of all the mono- and disaccharides, both naturally occurring and added. This should remove a source of much confusion when a product declared "sugar free" reflected only the sucrose content.

10. While the main focus is on carbohydrate because of the rapid effect on blood glucose, dietary fat requires attention because of the increased risk for cardiovascular disease in diabetes. For children less than 2 years of age dietary fat should not be restricted. For older children the guidelines from the pediatric panel of the National Cholesterol Education Program should be followed. If weight gain is excessive for height, limitation of fat intake becomes more important. If total cholesterol is elevated, diabetes management overall as well as dietary intake should be reevaluated. Poor diabetes control is the predominant cause of hyperlipidemia in type 1 diabetes.

11. Protein consumption by Americans generally exceeds the recommended dietary allowance (RDA) levels. Increased protein load may increase the risk of diabetic nephropathy. While this is rarely seen before puberty, pediatricians should be aware that 30 per cent of patients with type 1 diabetes have some signs of nephropathy 15 years after diagnosis. Decrease in dietary protein may be advised at the very earliest signs of nephropathy with rise in microalbuminuria.

12. Sweet food is preferred by most American children. The long-standing limitation of sucrose in the IDDM meal plan is questioned by recent studies that do not show an adverse effect on short-term glycemic control. The inclusion of sucrose, within the planned carbohydrates in the meal, would extend food choices, but the issue is not yet clear since only one study evaluated the effect of moderate amounts of sucrose

in the diets of children with type 1 diabetes. The nutritive sweeteners, fructose and other sugars, and sorbitol and other sugar alcohols, offer little glycemic and no caloric advantage over sucrose. The use of nonnutritive sweeteners, aspartame, saccharine and asulfame K increase the range of food choices, with amounts likely to be used on a daily basis by children falling well within the safety limits, and their use is supported by the ADA.

13. A small but increasing number of pediatric diabetic patients will have non–insulin-dependent diabetes (type 2 diabetes). They are usually significantly obese adolescents with a strong family history of obesity and diabetes in adults. Modified caloric intake and the decrease in insulin resistance with weight reduction may decrease or eliminate the need for insulin or oral hypoglycemic treatment. Increased exercise plus a diet with moderate calorie restriction, 500 to 1000 kilocalories below usual food intake, may be adequate to produce gradual weight loss.

14. The diabetic child and family need advice and support

from various members of the diabetes team to develop problem-solving abilities with which to close the gap between desires and recommendations about food. These needs are not met by a sheet of instructions and minimal explanation. Advocacy for adequate dietary management is needed for diabetic children in the managed care setting. A potential problem is a patient's disordered eating pattern, including manipulation of weight control by omitting insulin, which may lead to bulimia or anorexia.

Bibliography

The DCCT Research Group: Anderson EJ, Richardson M, Castle G, et al: Nutrition interventions for intensive therapy in the Diabetes Control and Complications Trial. J Am Diet Assoc 1993;93:768–772.

Franz MJ, Horton ES, Bantle JP, et al: Nutrition principles for the management of diabetes and related complications (technical review). Diabetes Care 1994;17:490–518.

Diabetes mellitus. *In* Kleinman RE (ed): Pediatric Nutrition Handbook, 4th ed. American Academy of Pediatrics, 1997, Elk Grove Village, IL.

269 Diabetic Ketoacidemia

Irma Fiordalisi and *Glenn D. Harris*

Critical State

Definition

Diabetic ketoacidosis/ketoacidemia (DKA) is a life-threatening catabolic state that occurs primarily in patients with insulin-dependent diabetes mellitus. DKA is triggered by insulin deficiency and characterized by hyperglycemia, water and electrolyte loss, metabolic acidosis/acidemia with ketonemia, ketonuria, glycosuria, and, frequently, subclinical brain swelling. "Acidosis" is defined as a decrease in measured total carbon dioxide (tCO_2) with respiratory compensation sufficient to preserve a normal blood pH. Once respiratory compensation is no longer sufficient, a decrease in arterial blood pH occurs, hence the term *acidemia*. The abbreviation DKA applies regardless of the degree of acid-base disturbance (Table 269–1).

Pathophysiology

1. Insulin deficiency causes failure to deliver an adequate supply of glucose into cells (particularly muscle and adipose tissue) resulting in cellular starvation, a stress that triggers lipolysis, proteolysis, glycogenolysis, and gluconeogenesis through the release of counterregulatory hormones (glucagon, epinephrine, norepinephrine, cortisol, and growth hormone). Insulin is required in the portal

circulation (albeit in low concentrations) to inhibit the hepatic acyl carnitine cycle. In the absence of insulin, this cycle is not inhibited, resulting in ketone body formation. A cycle of decreasing blood pH and increasing insulin resistance ultimately leads to death if untreated (Fig. 269–1).

2. In most cells of the body, the hypertonic state of DKA promotes intracellular dehydration with initial preservation of intravascular volume. Brain cells, however, adapt to hypertonicity by an increase in intracellular osmotically active solute (i.e., osmoprotection). These osmoprotective molecules help preserve brain cell volume despite systemic dehydration. Rapid decreases in osmolality, as

TABLE 269–1. MILD, MODERATE, AND SEVERE DKA

DKA	tCO_2 (mEq/L)	ARTERIAL BLOOD pH
Mild	15–19	Usually normal (acidosis)
Moderate	10–14	Decreased (acidemia)
Severe	<10	Decreased (acidemia)

DKA = diabetic ketoacidosis/ketoacidemia; tCO_2 = total carbon dioxide.

Critical State *Continued*

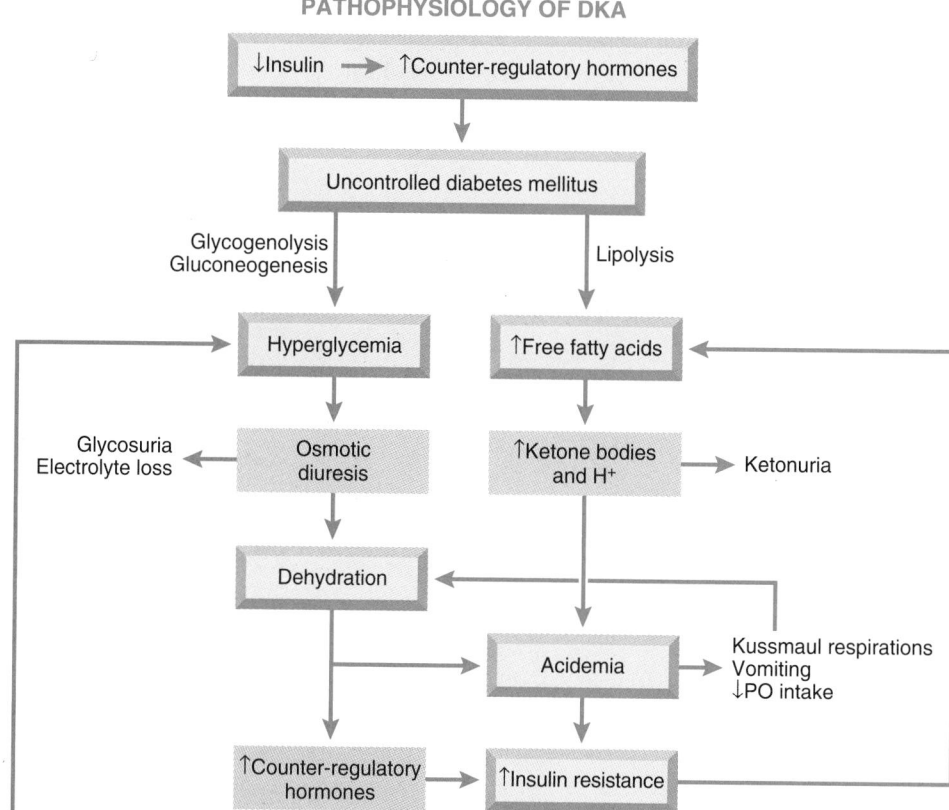

PATHOPHYSIOLOGY OF DKA

Figure 269–1 Pathophysiology of diabetic ketoacidemia.

would occur with excess free water administration, can precipitate brain swelling by initial rapid movement of water but not electrolyte across the tight junctions of brain capillary endothelium into the osmotically adapted brain. Asymptomatic brain swelling occurs commonly, even prior to treatment, in pediatric patients with DKA. Although its etiology is incompletely understood, it is clear that the therapeutic strategy should restore and maintain euvolemia and avoid hypervolemia and rapid decreases in osmolality, both of which would exacerbate brain swelling and potentially lead to increased intracranial pressure (ICP) and brain herniation.

Clinical Findings

1. Many physiologic stresses (such as infection) can lead to increased insulin resistance with subsequent need for additional insulin. While such stresses commonly lead to hyperglycemia, it is unusual for DKA to occur unless insulin doses are grossly inadequate or omitted altogether. Efforts to identify problems with insulin administration should be made in each case.
2. Note that in DKA, hyperglycemia may be only modest (blood glucose <300 mg/dl).

Clinical Findings

- Polyuria, polydipsia
- Dehydration
- Weight loss
- Abdominal pain
- Vomiting
- Hyperventilation/Kussmaul breathing
- Mental status changes
- "Fruity" odor of ketones on the breath

Treatment

Treatment of DKA is a dynamic process that requires frequent and vigilant reassessment of the neurologic status, vital signs, circulation, and laboratory data, so that adjustments in therapy can be made hourly based on individual patient needs. Such care is generally best provided in an intermediate unit or intensive care setting. Maintenance of a flowsheet for physical examination and biochemical data is

Critical State *Continued*

important. The patient's weight should be measured prior to treatment whenever possible. If the patient is obese, ideal body weight (i.e., the mean weight for height) should be used for water and electrolyte calculations; the actual weight is used for calculating the dose of insulin.

Key Laboratory Findings

Always Present
- Hyperglycemia, glycosuria
- Ketonemia, ketonuria
- Metabolic acidosis/acidemia
- Hypocarbia (compensatory)

Sometimes Present
- Apparent hyponatremia
- Hypernatremia
- Hyper- or hypokalemia
- Hypophosphatemia
- Increased serum amylase (primarily salivary in origin)
- Increased serum urea nitrogen
- Increased serum creatinine

Emergency Phase

- In the first minutes, assess:
  Airway
  Breathing
  Circulation
- Obtain venous access
- Obtain blood for:
  Electrolytes, glucose
  Urea nitrogen (SUN), creatinine
  Arterial blood gases (ABG)

1. Airway
   a. Ensure airway patency and adequacy of ventilation.
2. Breathing
   a. Give supplemental oxygen until shock, if present, is corrected.
3. Circulation
   a. If peripheral pulses, capillary refill time, blood pressure, and skin temperature are normal and urine is being produced, shock is *not* present and rapid emergency volume resuscitation is not indicated. Such a patient should receive 5 ml/kg IV of an isotonic saline solution (lactated Ringer's solution or 0.9% NaCl) over 1 hr while awaiting laboratory results.

b. If poor peripheral perfusion is present, with or without hypotension, shock *is* present, and emergency volume resuscitation is indicated. Give aliquots of 10 ml/kg of an isotonic saline solution rapidly until blood pressure is normal, peripheral pulses are easily palpable, and capillary refill time and skin temperature begin to improve. Volumes greater than 30 ml/kg are infrequently necessary to restore circulation in patients with DKA. The need for additional volume resuscitation may indicate an etiology other than hypovolemia as the cause of shock (e.g., septic shock, pancreatitis).

4. Insulin
   a. Begin human Regular insulin by continuous IV infusion by the end of the first hour of treatment. The usual starting dose is 0.1 U/kg/hr based on *actual* body weight. If continuous IV infusion is not practical, the same dose may be given intramuscularly (0.1 U/kg IM hourly) until IV access is secured. The expected effect would be an increase in blood pH of approximately 0.03 pH units *per hour* along with improvement in the base deficit. If this effect is not achieved, insulin should be progressively increased by 50 to 100 per cent until an appropriate rate of improvement in blood pH and correction in base deficit occur.
   b. Insulin infusion
      (1) Use a separate IV access site whenever possible.
      (2) Mix 1 U human Regular insulin per ml 0.9% NaCl.
      (3) Flush the IV tubing with 50 ml of solution to saturate potential binding sites prior to beginning infusion.
      (4) Serum glucose concentration should be measured hourly during continuous IV insulin infusion. Rapid bedside techniques for glucose determination facilitate the prompt institution of necessary changes in therapy. Serum glucose should drop approximately 50 to 100 mg/dl per hr.

5. Rehydration (Fig. 269–2)
   a. Guidelines for estimating the volume of deficit in DKA are presented in Table 269–2.
   b. Electrolyte content of rehydration solutions
      (1) Sodium: The extracellular deficit of sodium is calculated based on the estimated volume of deficit, with half the sodium salt deficit to be given in the first 12 hours and the remainder planned to be given over the next 36 hours. In addition to the deficit fraction of sodium, 20 to 40 mEq/L of sodium is needed to replace ongoing sodium losses during the osmotic diuresis that accompanies the early portion of therapy. This results in a rehydration solution during the

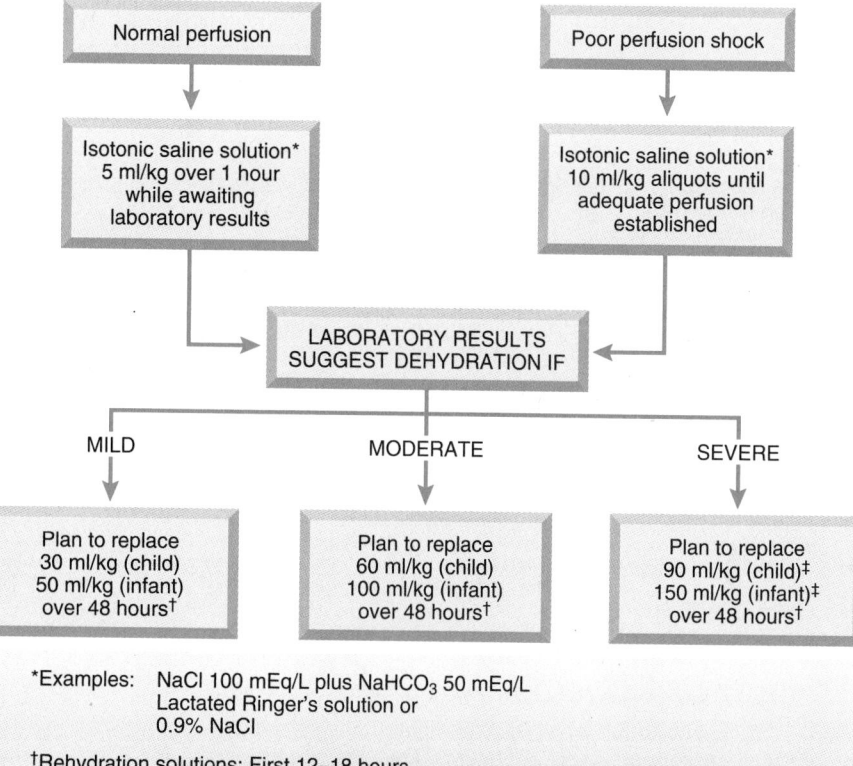

REHYDRATION IN THE NORMALLY NOURISHED INFANT OR CHILD WITH DKA

Figure 269–2 Rehydration in the normally nourished infant or child with diabetic ketoacidemia.

first 12 to 18 hours containing Na$^+$ 125 mEq/L for patients over 2 years of age and Na$^+$ 100 mEq/L for infants. Thereafter, the concentration of sodium is reduced to 75 mEq/L for patients over 2 years and 50 mEq/L for infants.

(2) Potassium: Total body potassium depletion is common in DKA, though initial serum concentrations of K$^+$ are often increased due to acidemia. Provided urine is being produced and there is no ECG evidence of hyperkalemia, K$^+$ 40 mEq/L (half as acetate and half as phosphate) is added to the rehydration solution.

c. Urine output should *not* be replaced milliliter for milliliter as a separate ongoing loss. The focus of therapy should be to effect progressive improvement in the clinical hydration status and biochemical disturbances that accompany dehydration.

d. Maintenance fluid should be given in addition to deficit volume replacement. Maintenance requirements are increased by 25 to 35 per cent during hyperventilation (PaCO_2 < 30 torr).

e. Undernourished children 2 years or older follow more closely a "50–100–150 ml/kg" volume of deficit for mild, moderate, and severe dehydration, respectively.

f. Oral fluids should not be permitted until DKA is largely resolved. Small volumes of ice chips may be given if requested. If oral intake begins prior to complete correction, volumes taken orally plus IV should equal the desired fluid intake.

6. Monitoring the rehydration process and the correction of DKA (Table 269–3)

a. The goals of therapy are to correct shock rapidly, complete the remainder of the rehydration gradually,

Critical State *Continued*

TABLE 269–2. GUIDELINES FOR ESTIMATING THE VOLUME OF DEFICIT (DEGREE OF DEHYDRATION) IN DKA

GUIDELINE MEASURES	DEGREE OF DEHYDRATION		
	Mild	Moderate	Severe
Volume of deficit (ml/kg)*			
>2 yr old	30	60	90
≤2 yr old	50	100	150
Clinical measures			
Peripheral perfusion			
Palpation of peripheral pulses† (pulse volume)	Normal	Normal to decreased	Decreased to absent
Capillary refill time (sec)‡	<2	≤2 to 3	≥3
Skin temperature (tactile)	Normal	Normal to cool	Cool
Heart rate	Normal to mildly increased	Moderately increased	Moderately to severely increased
Blood pressure	Normal	Normal to mildly increased	Decreased to moderately increased
Biochemical measures in serum urea nitrogen (mg/dl)	Normal to mildly increased; e.g., <20	Mildly increased; e.g., 20–25	Moderately to severely increased; e.g., 30
Corrected Na⁺ (mEq/L)	Usually normal	Usually normal	Normal to increased
Glucose (mg/dl)	Mildly increased; e.g., 400	Moderately increased; e.g., 600	Severely increased; e.g., 800

*Use actual weight for normally nourished patients; for obese patients, use ideal body weight.
†Hypothermia and severe ketonemia may mimic signs of poor peripheral perfusion.
‡Capillary refill time is modified by the hypertonic state. Capillary refill time between 2 and 3 seconds suggests moderate to severe dehydration.
Modified from Harris GD, Fiordalisi I, Harris WL, et al: Minimizing the risk of brain herniation during treatment of diabetic ketoacidemia: a retrospective and prospective study. J Pediatr 1990;117:28.

and correct the base deficit. Once shock is reversed, the plan should be replacement of the remaining deficit volume over 48 hours. This approach to rehydration permits a gradual decrease in effective osmolality (E_{osm}). E_{osm} in mOsm/kg H_2O is calculated as follows:

$$2[Na^+] \text{ in mEq/L} + \frac{[\text{glucose in mg/dl}]}{18}$$

or glucose in mmol/L.

b. A gradual decrease in E_{osm} is best accomplished by a treatment resulting in a simultaneous increase in the measured concentration of sodium in serum as that of glucose declines. This approach avoids rapid lowering of E_{osm}, a potential effect of excess free water administration that can lead to brain swelling or its exacerbation. The following should be monitored throughout treatment:

(1) Mental status: This should be monitored at least hourly until DKA is corrected. Mental status should improve during treatment (if abnormal initially). Increasing lethargy, obtundation, disorientation, or headache that begins during treatment warrant emergent evaluation for raised ICP. Hypertension with bradycardia, focal neurologic findings, and papilledema are late signs of increased ICP. If increased ICP is suspected, treatment with mannitol (0.5 to 1.0 g/kg IV of a 20% or 25% solution) should be given immediately. Radiologic studies (head computed tomography [CT]) should not delay administration of mannitol. Assisted ventilation with a bag-valve-mask device followed by tracheal intubation may be required to maintain adequate hyperventilation. Intravenous fluids may need to be decreased or even withheld temporarily if indicated. Administra-

TABLE 269–3. MONITORING OF REHYDRATION

Clinical	
Neurologic examination	Hourly
Cardiac and respiratory	Continuously
Peripheral perfusion	Continuously until shock is corrected and peripheral perfusion is stable, then every 2–4 hr
Fluid balance	Hourly initially, then every 4 hr
Indwelling arterial catheters	For blood pressure monitoring and blood sampling in severely dehydrated and/or acidemic patients or in patients with abnormal mental status
Laboratory	
Glucose	Hourly as long as insulin is given IV
Blood gases	Every 1–2 hr until blood pH approximates 7.30
Electrolytes, SUN	Every 2 hr until appropriate trends are established, then every 4 hr
Phosphorus	If clinically indicated

SUN = serum urea nitrogen.

Critical State *Continued*

tion of insulin in appropriate dose should be continued.

(2) Vital signs and peripheral perfusion: Tachycardia and tachypnea should progressively improve toward normal. Subnormal body temperature is common in severe ketoacidemia and should normalize as the base deficit resolves. Once hypotension is corrected with emergency phase fluids, the blood pressure should remain normal. Peripheral perfusion should normalize early in treatment and remain normal throughout the treatment period.

(3) Glucose: With appropriate fluid and insulin therapy, the serum concentration of glucose should decrease by approximately 50 to 100 mg/dl per hour. Add glucose to the electrolyte-containing rehydration solution when the serum glucose concentration approximates 300 mg/dl; dextrose 5%, 10%, or occasionally 12.5% added to the electrolyte-containing rehydration solution may be required. If significant hyperglycemia is corrected but acidemia is unresolved, the addition of glucose (not the decrease or discontinuation of insulin) is required. Glucose should be maintained in the approximate range of 150 to 200 mg/dl during the remainder of the IV treatment.

(4) Insulin: The primary goal of insulin therapy is to terminate ketogenesis, correct the base deficit, and, secondarily, to correct hyperglycemia. The dose of insulin (usually 0.1 U/kg per hour by continuous IV infusion) is determined by its efficacy in improving the base deficit. An effective dose of insulin should increase the arterial blood pH by approximately 0.03 pH units per hour. If circulation is adequate and this effect is not achieved with the usual dose, the dose of insulin should be increased by 50 to 100 per cent until an appropriate rate of improvement in blood pH and base deficit are achieved. Correction of the measured tCO_2 initially lags behind improvement in blood pH and base deficit. If hyperglycemia resolves before the acid base disturbance is repaired, it is important to *supply additional glucose* (7.5% or 10% dextrose) to provide sufficient substrate for an effective dose of insulin.

(5) Trends in the concentration of sodium: In the presence of hyperglycemia, the measured concentration of sodium in serum is decreased because of the dilutional effect of water that moves from the intra- to extracellular compartment to resolve the osmotic gradient. With treatment, the reverse effect occurs; the serum sodium concentration should increase by approximately 1.6 mEq/L per 100 mg/dl decrease in serum glucose concentration. The corrected sodium concentration (Na^+_c) should remain approximately unchanged with each paired determination of sodium and glucose in serum during treatment. If the measured sodium concentration exceeded the expected increase, the patient should be evaluated for an increase in free water requirement (i.e., an increase in the rate of fluid administration). If the measured sodium concentration falls or fails to rise as glucose declines, this is biochemical evidence of excessive free water administration and should prompt evaluation for a decrease in the administration of free water (i.e., a decrease in the rate of fluid administration).

(6) Potassium: As the base deficit is corrected, serum potassium concentrations decrease, making it important to consider the acid-base status when the need for additional potassium supplementation (in addition to K^+ 40 mEq/L in the rehydration solution) is assessed. Generally, additional K^+ 0.25 to 0.50 mEq/kg IV infused over 1 hr suffices to avoid serum potassium concentrations less than 3.5 mEq/L. If hypokalemia persists despite additional supplementation, coexisting magnesium depletion should be considered. When total body magnesium depletion occurs, serum concentrations of magnesium may be normal or low, and renal tubular reabsorption of potassium is impaired. Once magnesium depletion is corrected, hypokalemia is more easily managed. Oral potassium supplementation may be appropriate for a few days after DKA is resolved to replenish total body stores.

(7) Serum urea nitrogen: If initially increased, this should decrease progressively with rehydration. Failure of this to occur suggests underestimation of the volume of deficit or, rarely, renal insufficiency.

(8) Fluid balance: Ensure that urine is being produced. Patients with a depressed mental status should have a catheter placed in the bladder. It is not unusual for "volume in" to be equal to or even less than the volume of urine produced for the first several hours. Provided the patient's peripheral perfusion is normal, vital signs are trending toward normal, and SUN is decreasing, this discrepancy will resolve as the osmotic diuresis abates.

(9) Hypernatremia: Approximately 5 to 10 per cent of patients with DKA have an Na^+_c of 150 mEq/L or greater. Such patients tend to be severely dehydrated and severely hyper-

Critical State *Continued*

tonic. The initial approach to these patients is identical to that for others with DKA. As the serum concentration of glucose declines by 100 mg/dl, the measured concentration of sodium should increase by 1 to 2 mEq/L. Once the glucose concentration is sufficiently lowered such that further decreases in its concentration will not impact greatly on E_{osm}, hypernatremia should be corrected. Since hypernatremia itself is associated with hyperglycemia, serum concentrations of glucose in the 300 to 400 mg/dl range often persist until hypernatremia is resolved. Therefore, once glucose concentrations approach these values, correction of hypernatremia should proceed by decreasing the concentration of sodium in the rehydration solution by 25 to 50 mEq/L to achieve a gradual decrease in Na_c^+ of approximately 1 mEq/L every 2 hr (or 10–15 mEq/L decrease over 24 hr). Other markers for efficacy of rehydration (physical examination, SUN) should be followed throughout this process.

(10) Duration of IV therapy

(a) Insulin: Once the measured tCO_2 is greater than 17 mEq/L, the patient may be given subcutaneous insulin. We have generally continued insulin IV until such time as would be appropriate to begin a long-acting and Regular insulin (e.g., early morning or late afternoon). Subcutaneous insulin is usually given 10 to 30 minutes prior to meals, depending on the type of insulin. Insulin IV should be continued for approximately 2 hr *after* the subcutaneous dose is given. This will control hyperglycemia until the subcutaneous depot of insulin becomes fully effective.

(b) Fluids

1. Even though deficit volume replacement is planned over 48 hours, the majority of patients appear fully rehydrated within 12 to 24 hours. By the time subcutaneous insulin is given, patients are generally able to eat and drink, and IV rehydration fluids should

be discontinued, permitting thirst to guide the remainder of rehydration.

2. Patients presenting with DKA and hypernatremia ($Na_c^+ \geq 150$ mEq/L) often require controlled IV rehydration for somewhat longer periods, since hypernatremia should be corrected *after* hyperglycemia is resolved to the extent possible.

Complications

- Increased intracranial pressure
- Dysrhythmias/cardiac dysfunction
  - hypo- or hyperkalemia
  - hypomagnesemia
  - hypophosphatemia (< 1.0 mg/dl)
- Thromboses/pulmonary embolus
- Pancreatitis
- Renal insufficiency
- Pulmonary edema

Prevention

Education of the patient and family is the key to early recognition of suboptimal control of diabetes and prevention of progression to DKA. Physician recognition of new-onset disease and access to a skilled professional team when hyperglycemia and ketonuria occur can prevent DKA or at least minimize its severity through early intervention.

Bibliography

Finberg L, Kravath RE, Hellerstein S (eds): Water and Electrolytes in Pediatrics: Physiology, Pathology and Treatment, 2nd ed. Philadelphia, WB Saunders, 1993.

Hardy PC, Bartlett JM, Usala A-L: Toward a more physiologic state: the use of human Ultralente and the "Run and Shoot" plan. Tool Chest 1992;8:481–485.

Harris GD, Fiordalisi I: Physiologic management of diabetic ketoacidemia: a 5-year prospective pediatric experience in 231 episodes. Arch Pediatr Adolesc Med 1994;148:1046–1052.

Harris GD, Fiordalisi I, Harris WL, et al: Minimizing the risk of brain herniation during treatment of diabetic ketoacidemia: a retrospective and prospective study. J Pediatr 1990;117:22–31.

Harris GD, Fiordalisi I, Yu C: Maintaining normal intracranial pressure in a rabbit model during treatment of severe diabetic ketoacidemia. Life Sci 1996;59:1695–1702.

270 Steroid Withdrawal

Barbara Linder

Procedure

Etiology

Chronic (>10 days) glucocorticoid use results in suppression of the hypothalamic-pituitary-adrenal (HPA) axis. The glucocorticoid dose must be slowly tapered to avoid adrenal insufficiency.

Epidemiology

Because of potent anti-inflammatory effects, glucocorticoids are widely used for a variety of pediatric diseases. The following list is not meant to be exhaustive.

1. Parenteral/oral glucorticoids are widely used for acute exacerbations of asthma. Inhaled steroids have now become a mainstay in the chronic treatment of asthma.
2. Malignancies—including leukemia and lymphoma
3. Rheumatologic diseases—including juvenile rheumatoid arthritis (JRA), systemic lupus erythematosus (SLE)
4. Inflammatory bowel disease
5. Nephrotic syndrome
6. Posttransplantation
7. Bronchopulmonary dysplasia

Pathophysiology

1. Glucocorticoids exert negative feedback inhibition on the hypothalamic-pituitary unit, resulting in decreased adrenocorticotropic hormone (ACTH) secretion.
2. Diminished ACTH secretion results in atrophy of the adrenal gland.
3. Following steroid withdrawal, the time course of adrenal gland recovery is dependent on:
   a. Dose: In general, supraphysiologic doses of steroid are required to suppress the HPA axis. As normal cortisol production rates are in the range of 10 mg/day (6.8 ± 1.9 mg/m²/day), most therapeutic regimens for inflammatory diseases exceed physiologic production.
   b. Duration of therapy: Even several doses of glucocorticoid probably result in some HPA axis suppression; however, recovery is also rapid following short courses of steroids. Although definitive evidence is lacking, the consensus is that significant axis suppression occurs when treatment lasts longer than 2 weeks.
   c. Administration schedule: Since peak cortisol production occurs early in the morning (6–8 AM), nighttime dosing causes maximal axis suppression. Alternate-day dosing using a steroid with an intermediate biological half-life (e.g., prednisone) allows for significant HPA axis recovery on the "off" day.
   d. Steroid preparation: Table 270–1 shows the charac-

TABLE 270–1.   COMMONLY USED GLUCOCORTOIDS

NAME	BIOLOGIC HALF-LIFE (hr)	ANTI-INFLAMMATORY POTENCY	APPROXIMATE EQUIVALENT DOSE (mg)
Hydrocortisone	8–12	1	20
Prednisone	12–36	4	5
Methylprednisolone	12–36	5	4
Dexamethasone	36–54	30	0.5

teristics of some commonly used glucocorticoid preparations. It is important to note that dosage equivalency is based on immunosuppressive potency. Although equivalent doses provide the same immunosuppressive action, those preparations with the longest half-life (e.g., dexamethasone) are associated with the greatest degree of axis suppression. Long-acting steroids also cause the greatest degree of growth suppression and should, therefore, be avoided in children.

4. During a glucocorticoid taper, the initial goal will be a reduction in dose from pharmacologic to physiologic levels. The rate of this initial taper is usually dictated by any exacerbation of the underlying disease.
5. Once physiologic replacement doses have been reached, the tempo of the taper depends on the rapidity at which HPA axis function is recovered. It can take up to 1 year for full axis recovery when suppression is long-standing.
6. Adrenal recovery generally lags behind that of the pituitary.

Clinical Findings

1. Patients who have been on chronic pharmacologic doses of glucocorticoid may appear "cushingoid," with typical plethora, moon facies, increased supraclavicular fat pads, and weight gain.
2. Symptoms of adrenal insufficiency include weakness, anorexia, fatigue, depression and hypotension.
3. The "steroid withdrawal" syndrome, manifest by severe symptoms of adrenal insufficiency, along with arthralgia, myalgia, fever and dermatologic disturbances, may occur even when the glucocorticoid dose is in the physiologic range and may limit the rate of the taper. It is often not clear whether symptoms reflect a relative glucocorticoid deficiency or a flare of the underlying disease for which steroids are being used.

Laboratory Findings

1. A normal morning (8–9 AM) cortisol level is 6 to 20 μg/dl. In a patient who has been receiving chronic steroids,

an AM cortisol greater than 10 μg/dl generally indicates adequate basal adrenal function. It does *not* imply adequate adrenal reserve during stress (e.g., serious infections, surgery).

2. After weaning a patient off steroids, a normal response to ACTH (0.25 mg cosyntropin IM or IV) generally indicates complete HPA axis recovery. A normal response to ACTH consists of a plasma cortisol value greater than 20 μg/dl (drawn at 0 minutes or at 60 minutes following ACTH administration).

Treatment

1. Patients treated with high-dose steroids for less than 5 days can generally have their medication abruptly stopped.

2. Patients who have received pharmacologic doses of glucocorticoids for more than 1 week but less than 1 month can generally undergo a rapid taper (decreasing the dose by 30% each day) until the dose is equivalent to half the physiologic secretion rate of cortisol (5–8 mg/m^2/day). The steroid can then be stopped.

   a. Usually, the actual oral dose prescribed is somewhat higher than the physiologic secretion rate because of incomplete gut absorption. Thus, physiologic replacement for a child who has a surface area of 1 m^2 might be 10 mg/day of hydrocortisone.

   b. Practically, the taper percentage will be dictated by the actual tablet size. For example, prednisone doses can be altered by 5- or 2.5-mg decrements.

3. Treatment for longer than 1 month results in significant HPA axis suppression. Recovery may take 6 to 12 months and patients, therefore, require a gradual taper of medication.

4. There is not a single correct protocol for weaning patients off of pharmacologic doses of steroids. The following represents a suggested approach that must be modified for the individual patient.

5. The initial step involves tapering the amount of glucocorticoid administered from pharmacologic doses to physiologic doses. This may be done as rapidly as possible without precipitating an exacerbation of the underlying disease. A reduction of the dose by 25 per cent each week usually works well.

6. If the underlying disease flares during the taper, the dose should be increased and the taper done more gradually. An alternative approach would be to increase the dose until remission is achieved and then convert to alternate-day prednisone dosing (i.e., give twice the dose every other day). This usually provides adequate immunosuppression because of the relatively long biologic half-life of prednisone, but it allows for HPA axis recovery on the "off" days.

7. Once physiologic replacement doses (5–8 mg/m^2/day of cortisol or its equivalent) have been reached, the patient is switched to a single morning dose of a short-acting glucocorticoid (e.g., hydrocortisone) to allow HPA axis recovery, especially during the early morning hours when there is normally peak activity.

8. A morning plasma cortisol should then be measured monthly, before that morning's hydrocortisone dose is taken. Once the morning cortisol is greater than 10 μg/dl, the hydrocortisone can be stopped.

9. Throughout the weaning period, glucocorticoid coverage must be provided during surgery or significant medical illness.

   a. For most medical illnesses, two to three times physiologic replacement should be adequate. If the patient is already on pharmacologic doses, no increase is necessary.

   b. For surgical procedures, intravenous hydrocortisone (100 mg/m^2/day, given q 6 h) is administered. One dose should be given the night before surgery and one dose given just prior to surgery. Following surgery, the dose can be weaned as rapidly as the patient's condition permits.

   c. While waiting for complete HPA axis recovery, the patient should wear a medical alert bracelet and have an emergency injectable hydrocortisone kit at home.

10. Once daily glucocorticoid administration has stopped, the patient should undergo ACTH testing. When the adrenal response to ACTH stimulation is normal, HPA axis recovery can be assumed to be complete and the patient no longer requires glucocorticoid coverage during stress.

11. If ACTH testing is not possible and the patient is experiencing a significant illness, it is safest to assume that HPA axis suppression may last for 1 year and to cover the patient with stress dose glucorticosteroids.

Protocol for Steroid Withdrawal

- Taper from pharmacologic to physiologic doses (5–8 mg/m^2/day hydrocortisone or its equivalent).
- Provide physiologic replacement with a single morning dose of hydrocortisone.
- Measure morning cortisol levels monthly. Stop hydrocortisone when cortisol is greater than 10 μg/dl.
- Provide glucocorticoid coverage during illness until a normal ACTH stimulation test is obtained.

 Bibliography

Byyny RL: Withdrawal from glucocorticoid therapy. N Engl J Med 1976;295:30–32.

Linder BL, Esteban N, Yergey A, et al: Cortisol production rate in childhood and adolescence. J Pediatr 1990;117:892–896.

Soyka LF: Alternate-day corticosteroid therapy. Adv Pediatr 1972;A:47–70.

271 Symptoms of Neurologic Disorders

Symptom | **Neurologic Symptoms**   *Gerald S. Golden*

Convulsions

Definition

Repetitive jerking movements of the limbs, often associated with an alteration in the state of consciousness. The movements may be symmetric or asymmetric, or can involve just one limb. There may also be twitching of the muscles around the mouth and eyes. These events are the result of abnormal paroxysmal activity in the brain.

Causes of Seizures

Trauma
Toxins
Central nervous system infections
Metabolic disorders
Congenital abnormalities of the central nervous
   system

Tics

Definition

Rapid, repetitive, highly stereotyped movements. There may be some abililty to inhibit tics voluntarily, but this is limited and is often followed by an increase in tic activity. The face and upper extremities are most commonly involved.

Causes of Tics

Simple tics
Chronic motor and vocal tic disorder (Tourette
   syndrome)

Weakness

Definition

Muscle strength less than would be expected for the individual's age, general stature, and usual level of activity. Weakness may be associated with muscle atrophy and with either hypotonia and decreased reflexes or hypertonia and increased reflexes.

Causes of Weakness

Upper Motor Neuron Disorders
Brain abnormalities
Spinal cord compression or injury

Lower Motor Neuron Disorders
Anterior horn cell degeneration or disease
Disorders of spinal nerve roots or peripheral nerves
Abnormalities of the Myoneural Junction
Muscle Disease
Muscular dystrophy
Acquired

Diplopia

Definition

Double vision. The images are most commonly side-by-side but may be separated vertically, or one image may be rotated compared to the other image. The type of diplopia depends on the specific extraocular muscles involved.

Causes of Diplopia

Increased intracranial pressure
Head trauma
Orbital or ocular trauma
Infection or tumor of the orbit
Disorders of the myoneural junction

Diminished Vision

Definition

Diminished vision, in a broad sense, can refer to loss of visual acuity (central vision) or a defect in peripheral vision. Decrease in central vision can be monocular or may involve both eyes. Loss of peripheral vision can be symmetric or asymmetric, monocular or binocular and, if binocular, homonymous or bitemporal.

Causes of Diminished Vision

Diminished Central Vision
Retinal (macular) degeneration
Central scotomas secondary to optic neuritis
Central scotomas secondary to papilledema
Unilateral Visual Field Defect
Lesion involving one optic nerve
Bitemporal Hemianopsia
Compression of optic chiasm
Homonymous Hemianopsia
Lesion of optic tracts or optic radiations
Lesion of occipital lobe

Ataxia

Definition

Incoordination during attempts at directed voluntary movement. Any patient can show a mixture of three types of symptoms:

1. Limb ataxia is marked by an intention tremor that increases as the target is reached and there is a tendency to overshoot the target. There is often failure to check the movement of a restrained limb when it is suddenly released.
2. Truncal ataxia is manifested by swaying of the trunk and head (titubation) when the patient is upright.
3. Gait ataxia presents as a staggering, "drunken" gait. The person is unable to walk a line with one foot placed directly in front of the other.

Causes of Ataxia

Limb Ataxia
Tumor of the cerebellar hemispheres
Head trauma
Truncal and Gait Ataxia
Tumor of the midline cerebellum
Hydrocephalus
All Types of Ataxia
Toxins and sedative drugs
Neurodegenerative disorders

Headache

Definition

Headache is used to refer to pain in the head or face. It can be described by its mode of onset, location, characteristics, and intensity.

Causes of Headache

Headache Syndromes
Migraine

Muscle contraction headaches
Cluster headaches
Headaches Secondary to Medical Conditions
Hypertension
Febrile illness
Intracranial Processes
Increased intracranial pressure
Expanding mass lesion
Infection
Intracranial hemorrhage
Paracranial Structures
Sinuses
Eye and orbits
Ears and mastoids
Teeth
Trigeminal (fifth cranial) nerve

Brain Death

Definition

Brain death, or irreversible coma, is a state of permanent unconsciousness and inability to maintain independent respiratory function. A number of diagnostic criteria have been agreed upon, although they may not be applicable to infants.

Criteria for the Diagnosis of Brain Death

Unresponsiveness to all environmental stimuli
Absence of brainstem function
No evidence of spontaneous respirations
Isoelectric electroencephalogram
No evidence of significant hypothermia
No evidence of the ingestion of depressant drugs

B | Bibliography

Golden GS: The neurologic history. *In* Golden GS (ed): Textbook of Pediatric Neurology. New York, Plenum, 1987, pp 13–21.
Swaiman KF: General aspects of the neurologic history. *In* Swaiman KF (ed): Pediatric Neurology: Principles and Practice, 2nd ed. St Louis, CV Mosby, 1994, pp 3–17.

Symptom | **The Floppy Infant** | *Gerald S. Golden*

Definition

An infant with decreased muscle tone and decreased spontaneous movements, with or without depression of consciousness.

Etiology

Decreased muscle tone in an infant can result from systemic illness, metabolic imbalance, or dysfunction of the nervous system. Neurologic disorders can be defined by the level of the nervous system involved.

1. Abnormalities of the central nervous system result most commonly from developmental abnormalities but may, in some instances, be secondary to perinatal asphyxia. Premature infants, especially very low birth weight infants, have a high incidence of periventricular hemorrhage and leukomalacia.
2. Spinal cord damage is rare, but may result from complications of breech delivery.
3. The clinical abnormalities of infantile spinal muscular atrophy (Werdnig-Hoffmann disease) are the result of progressive loss of anterior horn cells.
4. Disorders of peripheral nerves are rare except for traumatic lesions of the upper brachial plexus (Erb palsy) or lower brachial plexus (Klumpke paralysis) resulting from a stretch injury sustained during a complicated delivery.

5. Disorders involving the neuromuscular junction in infants are rare.
6. Congenital myopathies are also quite uncommon.

Epidemiology

The most common cause of the floppy infant is an abnormality of the central nervous system. Incidence and prevalence rates cannot be easily derived because of confounding issues such as the incidence of preterm birth in the population, the level and quality of prenatal and obstetric care, and access to specialized medical care including clinical genetics.

Pathophysiology

1. A structural or functional abnormality any place in the pathway from the cerebral cortex to the muscles can cause loss of muscle tone, weakness, and decreased voluntary movements.
2. Abnormalities of the brain are associated with hypotonia in the infant, but spasticity generally develops between 3 months and 1 year of age. Some children will remain hypotonic. Spinal cord injury follows a similar pattern, although maintenance of hypotonia is more common.

Clinical Findings

1. Features suggesting central nervous system involvement in an infant, in addition to the hypotonia, are a depressed level of consciousness and seizures.
2. Diagnostic clues of a spinal cord lesion are preservation of arm movement, especially shoulder movement, with absent leg movement, and failure to react to painful stimuli below the level of the lesion. Consciousness is preserved unless there is also significant cerebral trauma.
3. Infantile spinal muscular atrophy presents with severe hypotonia, muscle wasting, absent reflexes and intact sensation, and a normal state of consciousness and social responsivity. Fasciculations of the tongue are easily visualized.
4. Erb palsy is manifested by weakness of shoulder elevation, elbow flexion, supination of the forearm, and dorsiflexion of the wrist, giving the so-called "waiter's tip" position. If the C-4 nerve root is involved, there may be paralysis of the diaphragm on the affected side. Sensory deficits may be present, but are difficult to demonstrate. Klumpke paralysis presents with weakness of the intrinsic muscles of the hand, wrist and finger flexors, and wrist extensors. Horner syndrome may also be present on the affected side. These lesions are almost always unilateral.
5. Congenital myasthenia gravis is extremely rare. It presents as a severely floppy infant with swallowing difficulty and respiratory insufficiency. Infants of myasthenic mothers may have a transient myasthenic syndrome that responds to treatment with anticholinesterase drugs. The onset of hypotonia and constipation with unimpaired consciousness in an older infant suggests infantile botulism.
6. Congenital myopathies present with a clinical picture resembling infantile spinal muscular atrophy but reflexes are generally preserved and fasciculations of the tongue should not be present.

Laboratory Findings

1. Neurophysiologic studies such as nerve conduction velocities, somatosensory evoked potentials, and electromyography may be useful and help differentiate infantile spinal muscular atrophy, brachial plexus lesions, disorders affecting the neuromuscular junction, and congenital myopathies.
2. Muscle biopsy can provide diagnostic information in infantile spinal muscular atrophy and congenital myopathies.

Radiographic Changes

Magnetic resonance imaging (MRI) studies are the most sensitive tool for defining abnormalities, both congenital and acquired, of the brain and spinal cord. Abnormalities of brain structure may be at the cellular level, however, and it is not uncommon to have a normal MRI in the infant with severe involvement of the central nervous system.

Treatment

1. The only disorders in this group for which specific treatment is available are those involving the neuromuscular junction. Treatment of congenital myasthenia gravis, along with treatment of the infant born to a myasthenic mother until the condition resolves, utilizes the same anticholinergic drugs as are used for treating adults. These infants, as well as those with infantile botulism, also require careful attention to respiratory function and swallowing.
2. The other conditions are not amenable to any primary treatment. Attempts to maximize eventual function and independence depend on the appropriate use of the rehabilitation based specialties.

Prevention

1. Appropriate prenatal care, prevention of prematurity, and quality obstetric care can reduce the incidence of brain and spinal cord trauma. Good obstetric management can also reduce the incidence of brachial plexus lesions.
2. Genetic counseling is appropriate for families of children with infantile spinal muscular atrophy, congenital myopathies, and congenital myasthenia gravis.
3. Mothers with myasthenia gravis should be made aware of the risk of a transient neonatal myasthenic syndrome in their infants.

 Bibliography

Dubowitz V: The Floppy Infant. Philadelphia, JB Lippincott, 1980.
Gay CT, Bodensteiner J: The floppy infant: recent advances in the understanding of disorders affecting the neuromuscular junction. Neurol Clin 1990;8:715–725.

Definition

Abnormal electrical discharges of the brain which result in simultaneous changes in the child's behavior. These changes range from subtle, manifested merely by a brief change in the general level of activity, to more obvious, such as multifocal or generalized clonic movements.

Etiology

1. Neonatal seizures are most commonly the result of abnormalities of the brain caused by events during labor and delivery or as a complication of prematurity. Conditions which are seen frequently include intracranial hemorrhages, especially periventricular and intraventricular hemorrhages in premature infants, and hypoxic-ischemic encephalopathy.
2. Neonatal meningitis is commonly associated with seizures. Prenatal intracranial infections, such as toxoplasmosis or cytomegalovirus infections, can cause seizures beginning at any age.
3. Developmental abnormalities of the brain such as micropolygyria and more severe anatomic defects may be associated with seizures with an onset at any age.
4. A number of metabolic disorders can also produce seizures. The most common are hypoglycemia and hypocalcemia. Disorders of electrolytes, amino acids, organic acids, and ammonia metabolism are less common but frequently associated with seizures.

Epidemiology

1. The frequency of neonatal seizures is difficult to determine because of the multiple causes and difficulty making a diagnosis with more subtle seizure types. Reports of incidence range from 0.15 per cent to 1.4 per cent of neonates.
2. Among the children at increased risk would be:
   a. infants born following a complicated labor or delivery
   b. premature infants
   c. infants of diabetic mothers
   d. infants with a family history of a metabolic disorder associated with seizures

Pathophysiology

Seizures are the end result of any one of a series of events leading to excessive neuronal discharge. The chain of events can be triggered by abnormalities of the neurons themselves, abnormalities of neuronal organization, or changes in the biochemical milieu of the central nervous system.

Clinical Findings

1. There is a broad range of clinical manifestations of seizures in the neonate. Subtle seizures may not be easy to recognize. These may consist of a sudden cessation of movement that may be associated with a brief apneic spell. Abnormal spontaneous eye movements, sucking or cessation of sucking, and peculiar movements of the limbs are common.
2. Sudden jerking or clonic movements may be focal or multifocal, involving different portions of the body in sequence. Generalized tonic seizures are less common, except in the premature infant with intraventricular hemorrhage.

Laboratory Findings

1. Laboratory evaluation is most useful to confirm a diagnosis that is suspected clinically. If there is no obvious cause for the seizures, serum glucose and calcium determinations are appropriate.
2. A detailed evaluation for metabolic disorders should not be carried out routinely. Certain clinical features suggest that such an evaluation would be appropriate:
   a. a family history of neonatal seizures or a family history of a metabolic disorder.
   b. the presence of unexplained acidosis or hyperammonemia
3. Electroencephalography can assist in confirming the diagnosis of seizures, especially subtle seizures. This evaluation will also help classify the type of seizures and may give some clues to the etiology of the seizures.
4. Ultrasound examination of the brain is useful for demonstrating major congenital malformations and intracranial hemorrhage.
5. Lumbar puncture is essential if an intracranial infection is being considered.

Radiographic Changes

Computerized tomography of the head can demonstrate congenital malformations, intracranial hemorrhage, and calcification suggestive of an intrauterine infection. This technique can also demonstrate cerebral edema, both generalized resulting from perinatal asphyxia and focal resulting from intracranial trauma. MRI scans have a higher sensitivity for demonstrating structural abnormalities.

Treatment

1. The primary aspect of treatment should be directed towards the underlying problem if one can be determined. As with any medical emergency, meticulous attention should be paid to maintenance of ventilation, heart rate, and circulation.
2. Phenobarbital in appropriate doses is the primary antiepileptic drug. Doses as high as 20 mg/kg intravenously have been recommended. Respirations should be monitored closely. Incremental doses can be given if required to achieve a blood level of at 20 µg/ml.
3. If seizures continue following maximum doses of phenobarbital, phenytoin or other anticonvulsants may be necessary.

Prevention

The majority of neonatal seizures are not preventable. Reduction in the rate of prematurity will decrease the number of infants with intraventricular hemorrhage and seizures. Close attention during labor and delivery can reduce the incidence of perinatal asphyxia and perinatal trauma.

Bibliography

Aicardi J: Epilepsy in Children, 2nd ed. New York, Raven Press, 1994, pp 217–243.

Mizrahi EM: Electroencephalographic/polygraphic/video-monitoring in childhood epilepsy. J Pediatr 1984;105:1–9.
Painter MJ: Neonatal seizures. Int Pediatr 1988;3:97–103.

Symptom Seizures

Michael H. Kohrman

Definition
Abnormal electrical discharges of the brain that result in simultaneous changes in the child's behavior.

1. Seizures are classified as:
   a. Partial: focal symptoms (motor movement, sensory symptoms) without impairment of consciousness
   b. Partial complex: focal symptoms with impairment of consciousness
   c. Generalized seizures involving the entire brain
      (1) Tonic-clonic (stiffening and jerking)
      (2) Tonic (stiffening)
      (3) Clonic (jerking)
      (4) Myoclonic (lightning-like jerks)
      (5) Absence (short staring spells)
2. In children 50 per cent of seizures are generalized and 50 per cent partial.

Etiology
Seizures are also classified by etiology:

1. Genetic: Twenty-five per cent of seizures in children are of genetic etiology. Such syndromes include juvenile myoclonic epilepsy, absence epilepsy, benign rolandic epilepsy, fifth day fits.
2. Symptomatic: Fifty per cent of seizures are symptomatic: electrolyte imbalance, hypoglycemia, hypocalcemia, head trauma, infection, metabolic abnormality of protein, sugar, or lipids.
3. Idiopathic: No clear etiology determined.

Epidemiology
It is estimated that 10 per cent of the population will experience at least one seizure during their life time. Epilepsy is defined as repeated seizures. Peak incidences of seizures are in the neonatal period, between 5 and 10 years (absence and benign rolandic epilepsy), and adolescence (partial complex epilepsy).

Pathophysiology
Seizures are an orderly, abnormal electrical discharge from the brain. Clinical seizures follow anatomic pathways and localization within the nervous system (jacksonian march).

Clinical Findings
1. Neonatal seizures: Often multifocal symptoms, rarely generalized. Apnea is a rare symptom
2. Partial seizures: Focal motor or sensory symptoms most common. Autonomic manifestations may occur. No clouding of consciousness.
3. Partial complex seizures: Clouding of consciousness greater than 30 sec duration; postictal lethargy common. Focal onset on electroencephalogram (EEG).
4. Generalized seizures: Tonic-clonic activity with incontinence, cyanosis, respiratory depression, postictal lethargy.
5. Absence seizures: Short duration, 5 to 15 sec. No postictal lethargy. Generalized EEG abnormality (3/sec spike and wave pattern).
6. Myoclonic seizures and infantile spasms: Quick, lightning-like jerks. Infantile spasms occur in infancy, often in clusters, with jack-knife flexion of the trunk or extensor spasms.
7. Simple febrile seizures: Generalized seizures associated with temperature greater than 38.5 degrees, less than 20 minutes duration, nonfocal examination pre- and postictus. Risk of epilepsy small. Work-up should be aimed at the source of the fever. Lumbar puncture is recommended for infants less than 1 year of age or if there is any question of meningeal signs.
8. Status epilepticus is defined as a single seizure lasting longer than 20 minutes or repeated seizures without regaining consciousness and lasting longer than 20 minutes. Status epilepticus is a life-threatening emergency and must be treated promptly (see Chapter 289).

Laboratory Findings
1. Metabolic abnormalities (Table 271–1).
2. Electroencephalogram is the primary diagnostic test for identification of seizures.
3. Lumbar puncture is indicated for any seizure associated with fever for all children less than 1 year of age. In addition it may be useful in the diagnosis of neurodegenerative diseases, demonstrating elevated cerebrospinal fluid (CSF) protein.

Radiographic Changes
Neuroimaging should be performed if there are focal neurologic findings, focal seizures, or focal EEG. Computed tomography (CT) is preferred for demonstrating acute hemorrhage or intracranial calcification. Magnetic resonance im-

TABLE 271–1. METABOLIC ABNORMALITIES PRODUCING SEIZURES

Electrolytes: Na, Ca, Mg
Hypo- or hyperglycemia
Aminoacidopathies
Urea cycle abnormalities
Organic acidurias
Mitochondrial disorders
Peroxisomal disorders
Lysosomal enzyme disorders
Pyridoxine deficiency

TABLE 271–2. COMMONLY USED ANTICONVULSANTS

DRUG	DOSAGE	THERAPEUTIC LEVEL	HALF-LIFE
Phenobarbital	5 mg/kg/day divided bid infants and young children; 1–2 mg/kg/day divided bid in older children and adults	15–40 μg/ml	48–96 hr
Carbamazepine	10 mg/kg/day divided bid up to 50 mg/kg/day or 1600 mg in adults in higher dosages tid or qid	5–12 μg/ml	8–12 hr
Phenytoin	5–7 mg/kg/day divided bid; in infants tid or qid	15–20 μg/ml	24 hr
Valproic acid	10 mg/kg/day divided bid (liquid tid) increased in 10-mg/kg increments up to 50 mg/kg/day	50–100 μg/ml	8–12 hr
Ethosuximide	15–40 mg/kg/bid	50–100 μg/ml	30 hr

aging provides a more detailed image, especially if a neurodevelopmental anomaly or temporal lobe pathology is suspected.

Treatment

1. When to treat: The risk of a second seizure is estimated between 23 and 75 per cent, depending on the population studied. Most pediatric neurologists delay treatment until the second seizure unless the first episode was status epilepticus. All patients with status epilepticus should be treated.

2. Outcome: Overall, 70 per cent of epilepsy is permanently resolved with therapy. If seizures are controlled and EEG is normal for 1 year, 60 per cent of patients remain seizure free. If treatment is continued for 2 years, 80 per cent of patients remain seizure free.

3. Anticonvulsant therapy: The goal of anticonvulsant therapy is seizure control with minimal side effects.

   a. Drugs. Table 271–2 lists recommended dosages.

      (1) Phenobarbital: Good drug for partial and generalized seizures especially in infancy. IM, IV, and PO routes available. Causes behavioral side effects in 50 per cent of patients.

      (2) Carbamazepine: For partial or generalized seizures in children older than age 2. Neutropenia or rash can be a problem. Aplastic anemia reported in adults. Can only be given orally. Behavioral side effects in 50 per cent of patients. Auto-induction of drug elimination pathways a problem.

      (3) Valproic acid: First line for generalized seizures in children above 10 years of age. Good drug for myoclonic and absence seizures. Liver failure occurs in 1:500 children younger than age 2, 1:10,000 age 2 to 10, and less than 1:40,000 greater than age 10. Thrombocytopenia also a problem. Only PO route is available for maintenance.

      (4) Phenytoin: Equally effective as carbamazepine for partial and generalized seizures. Available for oral and intravenous administration. Poor absorption in infants and young children limits efficacy. Coarsening of facial features a problem in children. Therapeutic dose is close to toxic dose under 5 years of age.

      (5) Ethosuximide: Effective only for absence seizures. Gastrointestinal upset a problem.

      (6) Benzodiazepines: Diazepam or lorazepam for management of status epilepticus. Clonazepam for myoclonic seizures. Clorazepate for partial seizures. Tolerance to their anticonvulsant effects develops quickly.

   b. Surgery: Indicated for refractory seizure disorders, primarily seizures of temporal lobe origin with single focal area of onset.

   c. Diet: Ketogenic diet is effective but limited by the high fat content and poor palatability. Ketone bodies have anticonvulsant properties. Long-term effects of the diet are unknown.

Prevention

The most effective prevention strategy is directed toward the causes of symptomatic seizures, including the prevention of head trauma, central nervous system infection, and metabolic disturbances associated with acute and chronic illnesses.

Bibliography

Aicardi J: Epilepsy in Children. New York, Raven Press, 1986.
Engel J: Seizures and Epilepsy. Philadelphia, FA Davis Co, 1989.
Holmes GL: Diagnosis and Management of Seizures in Children. Philadelphia, WB Saunders, 1987.

Symptom | Movement Disorders

Gerald Erenberg

Definition

1. Movement disorders include those abnormalities of motor control not due to muscle weakness or sensory loss.

2. Types of abnormal involuntary movements include chorea, dystonia, ataxia, tics, athetosis, myoclonus, tremor, and ballismus.

Etiology

Movement disorders may be caused by genetic abnormalities, central nervous system (CNS) infections, metabolic disorders, CNS injury, neurotransmitter disturbances, reactions to toxins or drugs, and neurodegenerative disorders. Many occur with no known cause.

Epidemiology

Movement disorders are less frequent in children than in adults. Tics are the most common form seen in childhood and are estimated to occur in 1 of every 2000 persons.

Pathophysiology

The pathophysiology is different for each movement disorder and in most cases is unknown. Anatomic or functional changes in the basal ganglia, cerebellum, and other subcortical structures are probably involved in most movement disorders.

Ataxias

Clinical Findings

1. Disturbances in motor coordination and balance usually due to abnormalities of cerebellar function.
2. May be caused by many different etiologies.
   a. Acute ataxia
      (1) Acute cerebellitis
      (2) Metabolic (e.g., hypoglycemia)
      (3) Infections (e.g., meningitis)
      (4) Toxins or drugs
      (5) Hydrocephalus
      (6) Posterior fossa tumors
      (7) Labyrinthitis
      (8) Trauma
      (9) Demyelinating diseases
   b. Intermittent ataxia
      (1) Benign paroxysmal vertigo
      (2) Basilar migraine
      (3) Following seizures
      (4) Metabolic (e.g., aminoacidurias)
   c. Chronic ataxia
      (1) Degenerative (e.g., Friedreich ataxia)
      (2) Metabolic (e.g., Wilson disease)
      (3) Acquired (e.g., hypothyroidism)
      (4) Fixed (e.g., cerebral palsy)
3. Findings on examination
   a. Nystagmus
   b. Gait disturbance
   c. Dysmetria of limb movements
   d. Hypotonia
   e. Impaired rebound
   f. Dysdiadochokinesia

Laboratory Findings

Consider the following:

1. MRI of head
2. Blood chemistries, blood ammonia, serum copper and ceruloplasmin, complete blood count (CBC), toxicology screen
3. Metabolic studies for amino acid and organic acid abnormalities
4. Metabolic studies for vitamin and biotinidase deficiencies
5. Cerebrospinal fluid analysis

Treatment

1. Varies with etiology.
2. Some require no treatment because of self-limited nature.
3. Possible surgical interventions include tumor removal and ventricular shunting.
4. Metabolic treatments include special diets and vitamin supplementation.

Dystonia

1. Characterized by sustained or spasmodic simultaneous contractions of agonist and antagonist muscles leading to abnormal postures of the trunk or extremities. Tremors and myoclonus may also be present.
2. May be a symptom of an underlying disease or may be a specific disease entity (primary or idiopathic torsion dystonia).
3. May be classified according to age at onset, etiology, and anatomic distribution.
   a. Age of onset
      (1) Infantile (less than 2 yr)
      (2) Childhood (2 to 12 yr)
      (3) Juvenile (13 to 20 yr)
      (4) Adult (older than 20 yr)
   b. Etiology
      (1) Generally thought to be due to basal ganglia dysfunction
      (2) Sporadic
      (3) Inherited
      (4) Secondary
         (a) Acute reaction to medication, especially phenothiazines
         (b) Late reaction to medication, especially phenothiazines (tardive dystonia)
         (c) Metabolic (e.g., Wilson disease)
         (d) Neurodegenerative (e.g., Hallervorden-Spatz disease)
         (e) Toxic (e.g., carbon monoxide)
         (f) Immediate or late reaction to brain injury or hypoxia, including after open heart surgery
         (g) Brain tumor
         (h) Encephalitis
         (i) Hysteria
   c. Distribution
      (1) Focal
      (2) Segmental
      (3) Multifocal
      (4) Unilateral
      (5) Generalized

Epidemiology

The prevalence of generalized dystonia has been estimated to be 3.4 per 100,000 persons. For focal dystonia, the prevalence has been estimated at 29.5 per 100,000.

Laboratory Findings

Consider the following:

1. MRI of head
2. Serum copper and ceruloplasmin; slit lamp examination for Kayser-Fleischer rings.
3. Cerebrospinal fluid analysis

Treatment

1. Removal of toxins
2. Medication
   a. High-dose anticholinergic agents
   b. Levodopa for dopa responsive dystonia
   c. Muscle relaxants (e.g., baclofen).
   d. Anticonvulsants (e.g., carbamazepine)
   e. Benzodiazepines
   f. Dopamine antagonists (e.g., haloperidol)
   g. Dopamine depleting agents (e.g., reserpine)
3. Thalamotomy
4. Botulinum toxin injections

Chorea

Characterized by abrupt, brief, nonrhythmic, random, isolated muscle movements that result in uncoordinated jerks of the face, trunk, or extremities.

Etiology

1. Perinatal asphyxia or hyperbilirubinemia
2. Post–cardiopulmonary bypass
3. Reaction to medication (e.g., phenytoin)
4. Metabolic (e.g., Lesch-Nyhan syndrome; hepatic encephalopathy)
5. Neurodegenerative (e.g., Huntington disease)
6. Toxic (e.g., heavy metal poisoning)
7. Encephalitis
8. Postinfectious (e.g., Sydenham chorea)

Laboratory Findings

Consider the following:

1. MRI of head
2. Blood smear for acanthocytes
3. Serum calcium, uric acid, electrolytes, chemistry panel, copper, ceruloplasmin
4. Sedimentation rate, antinuclear antibodies, thyroid function
5. Throat culture, electrocardiogram, anti-streptolysin titers

Treatment

1. Removal of toxins
2. Medication for symptomatic relief
   a. Antibiotics if due to streptococcal illness
   b. Haloperidol
   c. Valproic acid

Tics and Tourette Syndrome

1. Characterized by sudden, rapid, recurrent, purposeless, nonrhythmic, stereotyped motor movements or vocalizations. There is often an irresistible need to perform the action, and some degree of voluntary control in suppressing the action is often present.

2. The frequency and intensity of tics are increased by mental or physical stress. Alternatively, some persons manifest more tics when they are relaxed, such as quietly watching television. Tics are reduced and may disappear during sleep.

Etiology

Tics and Tourette syndrome (TS) are thought to be due to abnormalities of neurotransmitters, especially dopamine and especially in the area of the basal ganglia. Tics are often genetic in origin. TS is an autosomal dominant disorder with variable penetrance and sex-specific expression.

Epidemiology

Tics are the most common movement disorder in childhood and have been experienced by up to 24 per cent of children. TS occurs in approximately 3 of every 10,000 persons, with a male to female ratio of 4:1. Although reported in all races and and ethnic groups, TS is uncommon in African Americans.

Classification

1. Tics begin in childhood, most commonly between the ages of 5 to 10 years. Tics are classified by type and complexity.
   a. Simple motor tics include eye blinking, grimacing, head turning, and shoulder shrugging.
   b. Complex motor tics include jumping, squatting, thrusting out an arm, or ritualistic movements such as smelling an object or touching one's own or another person's body.
   c. Simple vocal tics include sniffing, throat clearing, grunting, and coughing.
   d. Complex vocal tics include:
      (1) Echolalia (repeating another's sounds or words)
      (2) Palilalia (repeating one's own sounds or words)
      (3) Coprolalia (the involuntary use of obscene language)
2. Tic syndromes are also classified by number of tics and duration:
   a. Transient simple motor or vocal tic (a single tic that does not last longer than 12 months)
   b. Chronic simple motor or vocal tic (a single tic that lasts more than 12 months)
   c. Chronic motor or vocal tics (a changing pattern of motor *or* vocal tics that lasts for more than 12 months)
   d. Chronic motor and vocal tics (a changing pattern of motor *and* vocal tics that lasts for more than 12 months). This form is known as Tourette syndrome.

Clinical Findings

In addition to tics, persons with TS often have associated, comorbid behavior and learning problems.

1. Attention-deficit/hyperactivity disorder (ADHD)
2. Obsessive-compulsive traits and disorder
3. Increased incidences of anxiety, depression, and mood swings
4. Learning disabilities

Laboratory Findings

Laboratory tests are normal, including MRI scan, electroencephalogram (EEG), and metabolic studies. Tests to consider include serum copper and ceruloplasmin to rule out Wilson disease as well as electrocardiogram and anti-streptolysin titers to rule out Sydenham chorea.

Treatment

Treatment includes:

1. Education of child, parents, siblings, and teachers
2. Counseling if needed to help adapt and cope
3. Medication
   a. Not necessary unless symptoms are creating emotional or social consequences.
   b. When used, the medication chosen should be specific for the exact symptoms targeted for treatment.
   c. Anti-tic medications include haloperidol, pimozide, risperidone, clonidine, and clonazepam.
   d. ADHD medications include clonidine, tricyclic antidepressants, and psychostimulants. Medications such as methylphenidate may increase tics in approximately one third of children.
   e. Obsessive-compulsive medications include clomipramine and selective serotonin reuptake inhibitors such as fluoxetine.

Bibliography

ATAXIAS

Connolly AM, Dodson WE, Prensky AL, Rust RS: Course and outcome of acute cerebellar ataxia. Ann Neurol 1994;35:673–679.

Harding AE: Clinical features and classification of inherited ataxias: *In* Harding AE, Duefel T (eds): Advances in Neurology, vol 61. New York, Raven Press, 1993, pp 1–10.

DYSTONIA

Fahn S: High dosage anticholinergic therapy in dystonia. Neurology 1983;33:1255–1261.

Greene P, Kang U, Fahn S, et al: Double-blind placebo-controlled trial of botulinum toxin injections for the treatment of spasmodic torticollis. Neurology 1990;40:1213–1218.

Nygaard TG, Marsden CD, Fahn S: Dopa-responsive dystonia: long-term treatment response and prognosis. Neurology 1991;41:174–181.

Saint Hilaire M-H, Burke RE, Bressman SB, et al: Delayed-onset dystonia due to perinatal or early childhood asphyxia. Neurology 1991;41:216–222.

CHOREA

Byers RK, Dodge PA: Huntington's chorea in children. Neurology 1967;17:587–596.

Nausieda PA, Grossman BJ, Koller WC, et al: Sydenham chorea. An update. Neurology 1980;30:331–334.

Robinson RO, Samuels M, Pohl KRE: Choreic syndrome after cardiac surgery. Arch Dis Child 1988;63:1466–1469.

Wheeler PG, Weaver DD, Dobyns WB: Benign hereditary chorea. Pediatr Neurol 1993;9:337–340.

TICS AND TOURETTE SYNDROME

Cohen DJ, Bruun RD, Leckman JF (eds): Tourette's Syndrome and Tic Disorders. New York, John Wiley and Sons, 1988.

Erenberg G, Cruse RP, Rothner AD: Tourette syndrome: An analysis of 200 pediatric and adolescent cases. Cleve Clin Q 1986;53:127–131.

Erenberg G: Gilles de la Tourette Syndrome. *In* Rakel RE (ed): Conn's Current Therapy 1995. Philadelphia, WB Saunders, 1995, pp 823–828.

Symptom | **Migraine Syndromes**

Gerald Erenberg

Definition

Migraine has been defined as a familial disorder characterized by recurrent attacks of headache widely variable in intensity, frequency, and duration. They are commonly associated with anorexia, nausea, and vomiting.

Etiology

The etiology of migraine is not certain. Many patients have a family history of migraine and other headache disorders.

Epidemiology

Migraine headaches are relatively common among children. By the age of 15 years, 5 per cent of adolescents will have experienced a migraine attack. Attacks begin before 20 years of age in 50 per cent of all individuals who will ever develop migraine. There is an equal sex incidence prior to puberty, but in adolescence, migraine occurs more frequently in females.

Pathophysiology

The pathophysiology of migraine has still not been fully determined. The classic theory has been that migraine has to do with paroxysmal attacks of vasoconstriction and vaso-dilation involving cerebral blood flow. Others have postulated that this is a primary neuronal event. The role of neurotransmitters remains unclear.

Clinical Findings

1. Criteria include paroxysmal headaches separated by pain-free intervals. Other criteria include at least three of the following six symptoms:
   a. Abdominal pain, nausea, or vomiting with the headache
   b. Unilateral pain
   c. Throbbing pulsatile pain
   d. Complete relief after a brief period of rest
   e. An aura, either visual, sensory, or motor
   f. Positive family history of migraine headaches

2. Migraine headaches in children may be bilateral. There is a high incidence of associated sleep disturbances such as nightmares, sleepwalking, and bed-wetting. There is also a high incidence of motion sickness, but there is little evidence to support the concept of a migraine personality.

3. Episodes may be precipitated by trigger phenomena,

which include anxiety, fatigue, stress, exercise, excitement, travel, menses, illness, and certain medications such as birth control pills. There may be dietary triggers, including chocolate, nitrites, and monosodium glutamate.

4. The classification of migraine syndromes in children includes classic migraine, common migraine, complicated migraine, and migraine variants.

   a. Classic migraine occurs less frequently than does common migraine. Classic migraine is preceded by a visual or somatosensory aura, including the possibility of distortion of body image. The aura usually lasts less than 20 minutes, and the subsequent headache is frequently frontal, temporal, or orbital.

   b. Common migraine occurs without a preceding aura. Instead, children often demonstrate personality changes followed by headache and associated symptoms. Both forms of migraine often lead the children to seek a quiet and darkened room where they attempt to sleep.

   c. Complicated migraine is the association of transient neurologic disturbances and headaches. The neurologic deficits are presumed to be due to intracranial vasoconstriction with resultant ischemia and edema. The vast majority of patients will recover completely.

     (1) Ophthalmoplegic migraine includes the presence of a partial or complete 3rd nerve palsy in association with orbital pain. The 3rd nerve dysfunction leads to strabismus, ptosis, diplopia, and mydriasis. The ophthalmoplegia often persists for much longer than the headache and may go on for days to weeks.

     (2) Hemiplegic migraine is associated with a hemiparesis and headache, and the hemiparesis is typically contralateral to the side of the headache. The side of the hemiparesis may alternate from one attack to the other.

     (3) Basilar artery migraine involves the infratentorial blood flow and leads to symptoms and signs referable to the brainstem and cerebellum. The headaches tends to be occipital in location, and the neurologic symptoms are of short duration.

     (4) Acute confusional migraine occurs most commonly in teenagers and includes confusion, agitation, and altered sensorium. This diagnosis is impossible to make in a patient who has not previously had a migraine attack, and alternative causes for an acute encephalopathy must be investigated.

   d. Migraine variants

     (1) Benign paroxysmal vertigo occurs in preschool age children and consists of sudden and brief episodes where the child appears frightened and is unable to maintain equilibrium. Consciousness is maintained, but nystagmus may be observed.

     (2) Paroxysmal torticollis consists of recurrent episodes of head tilt associated with headache and vomiting. The episodes may last for days.

     (3) Cyclic vomiting may occur with or without headache and consists of episodes of pernicious vomiting that may lead to dehydration.

     (4) Migraine sine hemicrania refers to patients who have the visual aura that occurs in classic migraine, but these patients do not actually have headaches.

     (5) Abdominal migraine is a rare occurrence. It occurs in patients with the gastrointestinal symptoms of pain, nausea, and vomiting but with little or no headache. They must be differentiated from complex partial seizures, where the aura consists of abdominal discomfort.

Laboratory Findings

Although the diagnosis is clinical, based on history and normal physical and neurologic examinations, a number of laboratory tests can be considered.

1. Electroencephalogram
2. Sedimentation rate
3. Evaluation for gastrointestinal disorder

Radiographic Changes

There are no radiographic abnormalities. In some patients the following examinations might be justified based on unusual features of the history or abnormal findings on examination.

1. Computed tomography or MRI scan of head
2. CT scan of sinuses

Treatment

1. Attempts at preventing migraine attacks focus on those events that may serve as trigger factors for individual patients. These include a diet that eliminates specific foods that may precipitate headaches, sufficient sleep, and stabilization and avoidance of stressful situations.

2. Nonpharmacologic treatment can include the use of biofeedback and relaxation techniques. These techniques focus on decrease of muscle tension as well as elevation of skin temperature.

3. Acute pharmacologic treatment

   a. Analgesics

   b. Antiemetics

   c. Sedatives

   d. Vasoconstrictors include compounds given early in the course to abort the headache. These include ergotamine preparations, isometheptene mucate, D.H.E. 45 given parenterally, and sumatriptan given parenterally or orally.

4. Chronic pharmacologic therapy is given daily to help prevent recurrent attacks.

   a. Cyproheptadine

   b. Propranolol

   c. Amitriptyline

   d. Calcium-channel blockers

   e. Antiepileptics

Bibliography

Rothner AD: A practical approach to headaches in adolescents. Pediatr Ann 1991;20:200–205.

Shinnar S, D'Souza BJ: The diagnosis and management of headaches in children. Pediatr Clin North Am 1982;29:79–94.

Silberstein SD, Lipton RB: Overview of diagnosis and treatment of migraine. Neurology 1994;44(Suppl 7):S6–S16.

Symptom | **Sleep Disorders** | *Gerald Erenberg*

Definition

1. Any condition that disrupts the developmentally normal pattern or duration of sleep. Sleep disorders also include certain abnormal events that occur during sleep.

2. Sleep is not a single uniform state but is made up of REM (rapid eye movement) sleep and NREM (non–rapid eye movement) sleep. Dreaming occurs during REM sleep, often with good recall. During this phase of sleep, there is loss of motor tone as well as irregular breathing and heart rhythm. REM sleep makes up 20 to 25 per cent of nighttime sleep in most normal persons. Newborn infants, however, spend as much as 50 per cent in REM sleep. During NREM sleep, the imagery of dreaming is more thought-like but with limited recall. The physiologic changes such as hypotonia and autonomic irregularity do not occur.

3. The number of hours per day spent in sleep varies at different ages. A newborn may sleep for 16 or 17 hours a day. This gradually decreases with age so that a 1-year-old spends approximately 13 hours in sleep. This is down to 11 hours at age 5 years and 8.5 hours at age 16 years. The sleep of younger children has a greater proportion of deep sleep with fewer wakings than does that of older children or adults. The newborn infant's awake and asleep periods are spread out evenly over the entire 24-hour span. Starting at approximately 3 months, the infant begins to spend most of his sleep time at night, and daytime sleep is reduced to two naps a day. The morning nap is usually given up some time between 6 and 18 months of age, while naps in the afternoon continue until three to five years of age.

Etiology

Sleep disorders may be due to a variety of altered biologic and emotional states.

Epidemiology

Sleep problems in children of all ages are very common, affecting 25 to 40 per cent of infants and preschool children and approximately 20 per cent of adolescents. Significant deviations from normal sleep patterns can lead to fatigue, irritability, and interference with the normal sense of emotional and physical well-being. There is often a corresponding disruption in family relationships because parents often become sleep-deprived as well.

Pathophysiology

Variations in sleep stages and problems during transitions between sleep stages appear to be related to sleep problems.

Clinical Findings

1. Altered sleep phase. Infants and children may have normal sleep quality but at the wrong time. A careful history of daytime activities, naps and night sleep is essential to successful management.

   a. A sleep phase delay occurs when children go to bed late at night and wake up late in the morning. This often leads to bedtime struggles since the children are being put to sleep at a time that they are not tired. Phase delays are treated by gradually waking the child up earlier each day by a small amount of time.

   b. Sleep phase advance. This occurs when the child goes to sleep early in the evening but awakens very early in the morning. This problem is often associated with prolonged morning naps. By shortening or eliminating these morning naps gradually, the time of going to sleep can be delayed.

   c. Irregular sleep-wake schedules. This is a more serious situation where individuals experience prolonged periods without sleep. This may go on for up to 36 hours and be followed by 12 hours of sleep. The sleep and wake times vary considerably day by day. This is usually due to a complete breakdown in a child's social life and has serious consequences. This type of pattern requires intensive therapy, including setting up of rigid schedules for activity, mealtimes, and sleep.

2. Parasomnias are events that occur sporadically in sleep.

   a. Nightmares occur during REM sleep. The child is awakened by a frightening dream and can remember the details for a short period after awakening.

   b. Night terrors (pavor nocturnus) occur in NREM sleep. In this situation, the child suddenly sits up in bed, screams, and appears to be focused on a distant object. There are autonomic reactions, including rapid breathing, sweating, tachycardia, and apparent anxiety. The child is inconsolable and difficult to arouse for 10 minutes or longer. When finally awakened, the child is amnesic for the event.

   c. Sleepwalking and sleeptalking are associated with the transition from deeper to lighter stages of sleep. The child is not aware during these times and the motor movements or speech patterns are not of the usual type seen while awake. Sleepwalkers may need to be protected to avoid their encountering dangerous situations.

   d. Sleep myoclonus is a benign event and is characterized by brief arrhythmic movements that can be focal or generalized. Children more commonly experience myoclonus in the distal portions of their extremities while adolescents and adults experience a single proximal myoclonus.

e. Nocturnal enuresis is quite common and declines in frequency as children grow older. At age 12 years, however, approximately 3 per cent of children are still experiencing bed-wetting. Bed-wetting is thought to occur during the transition from stage 3 or 4 sleep to the first REM period. Medical problems such as diabetes, nocturnal epilepsy, or kidney or bladder problems need to be excluded.

f. Bruxism is tooth grinding that occurs during sleep. This is common but the cause is unknown. Protective mouth guards are only occasionally necessary for control of this phenomenon.

g. Obstructive sleep apnea is characterized by cessation in airflow at the nose and mouth during sleep. It may be caused by obstruction in the air passages due to enlarged tonsils and adenoids, nasal deformity, birth defects, or an enlarged tongue. Snoring is almost universal in these children. Cor pulmonale is often present.

h. Central sleep apnea occurs without obstruction to the flow of air and is especially common in premature infants. The sudden infant death syndrome is believed to be a form of central apnea. Central apneas are seen more frequently in children with neurologic diseases, defects in the chemical regulation of breathing, heart failure, and muscle diseases. Other conditions that may present as sleep apnea include seizure disorders and gastroesophageal reflux.

3. Narcolepsy is a condition characterized by attacks of irresistible sleepiness that may occur in unusual situations such as eating or driving. Other symptoms include cataplexy, where there is a sudden loss of tone often precipitated by laughter or strong emotions. Hypnagogic hallucinations consist of vivid visual or auditory images occurring at the onset of sleep. Sleep paralysis is the sudden awareness while falling asleep that the person cannot cry out or move.

Laboratory Findings

1. Laboratory testing will often include time spent in the sleep laboratory. In that setting, the child can have a polysomnogram with or without a simultaneous recording of the electroencephalogram.
2. The multiple sleep latency test can also be performed in the sleep laboratory and measures the amount of time taken to fall asleep and the sleep stage reached during the nap.
3. If reflux is being considered, a pH monitor can also be simultaneously performed.

Treatment

1. Sleep phase disorders and sleep-associated behaviors
   a. Dealing with the problems associated with sleep phases and sleep-associated behaviors begins by the keeping of an exact sleep-wake diary. This should note the timing of when the child sleeps and awakens as well as the timing of meals and other play activities.
   b. Many phase disturbances can be dealt with by gradually altering the time of going to sleep and changing the timing and duration of daytime naps. Once achieved, the schedule must be maintained with a high degree of consistency.
   c. Bedtime rituals and methods of placing the child into the crib need to be investigated. The consistent sleeping in the parents' bed is not recommended nor is the use of hypnotics.

2. Parasomnias
   a. The parasomnias are treated according to the type being experienced. Nightmares, sleep myoclonus, and bruxism rarely require treatment. Night terrors, sleepwalking, and sleeptalking can be treated, if necessary, with benzodiazepines taken at bedtime.
   b. Nocturnal enuresis can be treated with an alarm system, imipramine, or intranasal DDAVP. Sleep apnea is often a health- or life-threatening situation. Obstructive apnea is treated by removal of the obstruction, such as an adenoidectomy.
   c. Sleep apnea may require the use of continuous positive airway pressure and/or the use of devices that keep the tongue pulled forward.

Prevention

Establishing and adhering to a reasonable nighttime schedule is helpful in preventing at least some of the disorders of sleep.

Bibliography

Guilleminault C: Sleep and Its Disorders in Children. New York, Raven Press, 1987.

Kotagal S, Hartse KM, Walsh JK: Characteristics of narcolepsy in preteen-aged children. Pediatrics 1990;85:205–209.

Report of the Therapeutics and Technology Assessment Subcommittee of the American Academy of Neurology: Assessment: techniques associated with the diagnosis and management of sleep disorders. Neurology 1992;42:269–275.

Symptom **Learning Disabilities**   *Gerald S. Golden*

Definition

A significant difficulty in the ability to learn one or more academic skills at the expected rate, not primarily due to mental retardation, sensory impairment, emotional disturbance, social disturbance, or inadequate instruction.

Etiology

1. Learning disabilities are a result of abnormalities in the structure or function of the brain. These abnormalities can be congenital or acquired; head trauma and intracranial infections are the most common causes of acquired learning disabilities.
2. There is a family history of similar learning disabilities in some cases. This is most apparent in reading disability (dyslexia).

Epidemiology

The prevalence in public schools is approximately 5 per cent.

Pathophysiology

1. A specific pathophysiology has not been defined. Autopsy studies have shown areas of disorganized cerebrum that appear to have a congenital basis. Functional studies of the central nervous system such as cortical evoked potentials and positron emission tomography are beginning to define abnormalities in specific brain regions.
2. Acquired lesions can disrupt specific cognitive functions that interfere with the acquisition of specific academic skills. Closed head trauma, often associated with damage to the temporal lobes, produces memory deficits, which makes learning in many areas difficult.

Clinical Findings

1. The presenting problem is the inability to learn basic academic material at the expected age and grade level. The difficulty is usually in specific areas, such as reading, although other related skills, such as writing, may also be affected. There also may be problems with mathematical concepts or mathematical operations.
2. Evaluation demonstrates that the areas of weakness, as measured by standardized academic achievement tests, are significantly impaired as compared with overall ability as measured by an individually administered IQ test.
3. Additional psychoeducational testing should show abnor-

malities in one or more of the fundamental processes underlying the area in which learning is inadequate.
4. Evaluation should exclude other causal factors such as mental retardation, hearing or visual defect, social or psychological factors, and inadequate teaching.
5. There is an increased incidence of attention-deficit/hyperactivity disorder in children with learning disabilities.

Laboratory Findings

There are no useful routine laboratory studies. Electroencephalography, cortical or brainstem evoked potentials, and computer assisted brain mapping have no diagnostic role but can be considered to be research tools.

Radiographic Changes

There are no radiographic changes.

Treatment

Special education techniques can take two basic forms.

1. Remedial education uses a number of educational strategies to improve skills in the areas of academic deficit.
2. Compensatory techniques allow the acquisition of information but work around the deficit. Examples would be tape-recorded books for the student with a severe reading disability, a computer for the child with difficulty writing, and a calculator for the student who has problems with mathematical operations.

Prevention

1. There are no known prevention strategies for the majority of learning disabilities.
2. Strategies to prevent central nervous system infections and head trauma in children will reduce the number of acquired problems with learning.

 Bibliography

American Psychiatric Association: Diagnostic and Statistical Manual of Mental Disorders, 4th ed. Washington DC, American Psychiatric Association, 1994, pp 46–53.

Shaw SF, Cullen JP, McGuire JM, Brinckerhoff LC: Operationalizing a definition of learning disabilities. J Learning Disab 1995;28:586–597.

Shaywitz BA, Pletcher JM, Shaywitz SE: Defining and classifying learning disabilities and attention-deficit/hyperactivity disorder. J Child Neurol 1995;10(Suppl 1):S50–S57.

Symptom **Attention-Deficit/Hyperactivity Disorder**   *Gerald S. Golden*

Definition

A persistent pattern of inattention or hyperactivity that is greater than would be expected of others at the same developmental level.

Etiology

Evidence suggests that there is a biologic basis for attention-deficit/hyperactivity disorder (ADHD) as there is an

increased incidence of this condition and a number of psychiatric disorders in the same families. These include mood disorders, anxiety disorders, and substance abuse.

Epidemiology

1. The male to female ratio is between 5:1 and 10:1 in different studies.
2. Prevalence in school-age children is 3 to 5 per cent.

Higher prevalence rates in some studies may be a result of inadequate diagnostic criteria.

3. This clinical syndrome may develop following head trauma or other events that can diffusely damage the central nervous system.

Pathophysiology

No specific pathophysiology has been defined. Neurochemical studies and electrophysiologic studies suggest that specific underlying functional abnormalities may be present.

Clinical Findings

1. An operational definition, as defined in the Diagnostic and Statistical Manual of Mental Disorders (4th ed), requires symptoms of attention deficit and/or hyperactivity-impulsivity. Behavioral descriptions of these symptoms are listed, including the minimum number that must be present, and there are a number of checklists for parents and teachers that assist in defining these symptoms.

2. Some of the symptoms must have been present before age 7 years.

3. If symptoms are apparent in only one setting, such as school, home, or during play with peers, another diagnosis should be considered. A child may be able to suppress behavior for a period of time, and it is not unusual for the child to appear well behaved in the physician's office.

4. Symptoms must be severe enough to cause difficulty for the child, other children, and adults who have contact with the child.

Laboratory Findings

There are no useful routine laboratory findings. A number of computer-administered tests that attempt to quantitate inattention and impulsivity have been developed, but these should not be used to replace the clinical diagnostic criteria.

Radiographic Changes

There are no radiographic changes.

Treatment

1. The initial approach to management should focus on behavioral techniques. Useful strategies include defining expectations and setting limits, rewarding socially appropriate behavior, structuring the environment to avoid unnecessary distractions, dividing tasks into small segments that can be finished within the limits of the child's attention span, and allowing breaks during which the child can release excess energy.

2. Symptoms may be severe enough to warrant a trial of pharmacotherapy. The most commonly used drug is methylphenidate. The daily dose, and timing of doses, must be individualized for the child. In general, 0.3 mg/kg to 1.0 mg/kg twice a day is sufficient. Serious side effects are unusual, but poor appetite and decreased linear growth with high doses have been reported. There is a growth rebound during drug holidays or when the medication is discontinued. Insomnia may be a problem if a dose is given too close to bedtime.

3. If the response to methylphenidate is inadequate, or there are reasons to try other medications, dextroamphetamine, pemoline, clonidine, and tricyclic antidepressants may be useful.

Prevention

There are no generally useful prevention strategies. The number of acquired cases can be reduced by prevention of head trauma and other conditions that can damage the central nervous system.

Bibliography

American Psychiatric Association: Diagnostic and Statistical Manual of Mental Disorders, 4th ed. Washington DC, American Psychiatric Association, 1994, pp 78–85.

Cantwell DP, Baker LB: Differential diagnosis of hyperactivity. J Dev Behav Pediatr 1987;8:159–165.

Safer DJ, Krager JM: A survey of medication treatment for hyperactive/inattentive students. JAMA 1988;260:2256–2258.

Satterfield JM, Satterfield BT, Cantwell DP: Three-year multimodality treatment study of 100 hyperactive boys. J Pediatr 1981;98:650–655.

Symptom **Microcephaly**   *Gerald S. Golden*

Definition

Any condition in which the head circumference is more than 2 standard deviations below the mean for the child's age.

Etiology

There are two types of microcephaly.

1. Primary microcephaly refers to a brain that is smaller than normal but otherwise has normal structure. This condition may be genetic or sporadic.

2. Secondary microcephaly results from any external factor that impairs the growth of an otherwise normal brain.

Epidemiology

Based on the criterion of a head circumference more than 2 standard deviations below the age-specific mean, 2.5 per cent of the population will be defined as microcephalic. The

---

Causes of Microcephaly

Infection
Anoxia
Trauma
Drugs
Metabolic disorders
Genetic disorders and syndromes

---

specific diagnoses of individuals within this group depend on the prevalence of various etiologic factors in the population.

Pathophysiology

The pathophysiology resulting in primary microcephaly is unknown, although there is a genetic basis in some families.

In secondary microcephaly there is destruction of brain tissue and disruption of the programmed processes of brain growth.

Clinical Findings

1. The occipitofrontal circumference is more than 2 standard deviations below the age-specific mean. Except in premature infants, this should be viewed as an independent measurement, and not compared with the weight and height percentiles. The acceptable range of brain growth is more restricted than the normal ranges of height and weight.
2. There may be associated abnormalities found in children with secondary microcephaly. These are characteristic of the underlying condition.
3. Abnormalities on neurologic examination, especially spasticity, are common in secondary microcephaly.
4. Mental retardation is associated with microcephaly in a high percentage of cases. At the definitional borderline, head circumference 2 standard deviations below the mean, 10 to 15 per cent of children will have a normal IQ. These are usually children with no other evidence of congenital anomalies. At 3 standard deviations below the mean for head circumference, virtually no children have normal intelligence.

Laboratory Findings

There are no specific laboratory abnormalities except in those children who have a chromosomal or metabolic cause for their microcephaly.

Radiographic Changes

Neuroimaging studies can define the underlying structural abnormalities in secondary microcephaly. These findings may provide a clue to the underlying diagnosis.

Treatment

Treatment should be directed at any underlying medical problems. If seizures are present, they should be treated appropriately. Special education is needed for children with mental retardation. Children with spasticity or other motor problems should be referred for physical and occupational therapy.

Prevention

There are no specific methods of prevention other than those directed toward the conditions producing secondary microcephaly. There is a genetic component in some cases of primary microcephaly, and so genetic counseling about the risk of affected children in subsequent pregnancies is appropriate. Ultrasound of the fetus may detect severe microcephaly.

Bibliography

DeMeyer W: Microcephaly, micrencephaly, megalocephaly, and megalencephaly. *In* Swaiman KF (ed): Pediatric Neurology, Principles and Practice. St Louis, CV Mosby, 1994, pp 205–218.
Dolk H: The predictive value of microcephaly during the first year of life for mental retardation at seven years. Dev Med Child Neurol 1991;33:974–983.

Symptom **Hydrocephalus**

Gerald S. Golden

Definition

A condition in which excessive amounts of cerebrospinal fluid collect in the ventricles and cause ventricular enlargement.

Etiology

There are a number of causes of hydrocephalus, but they can be categorized into two groups.

1. Hydrocephalus may be due to a congenital malformation of brain that interferes with the normal flow of spinal fluid. This group includes:
   a. Aqueductal stenosis in which the aqueduct of Sylvius is not patent or inadequate in capacity.
   b. The Arnold-Chiari malformation, in which the brainstem is elongated and kinked and the cerebellar tonsils are herniated through the foramen magnum. This blocks the flow of cerebrospinal fluid. This malformation often accompanies neural tube defects.
   c. The Dandy-Walker malformation, in which the outlet foramina of the fourth ventricle (foramen of Magendie and foramen of Luschka) are not patent.
2. Hydrocephalus may also be acquired. Common causes are:
   a. Tumors that can block the spinal fluid pathways at any point.

   b. Meningitis that may block the aqueduct, subarachnoid spaces, or site of absorption of spinal fluid.

Epidemiology

An overall incidence is difficult to determine because of the multiplicity of possible causes.

Pathophysiology

1. Three primary mechanisms can produce hydrocephalus.
   a. Blockage of cerebrospinal fluid flow. As noted above, this can be either congenital or acquired.
   b. Failure of absorption of cerebrospinal fluid. The block is at the arachnoid villi.
   c. Overproduction of cerebrospinal fluid. This is uncommon, but may be seen with choroid plexus papillomas.
2. Based on the specific mechanism, a clinical distinction is often made between communicating hydrocephalus, in which there is no block within the ventricular system, and noncommunicating hydrocephalus, in which the block is within the ventricular system.
3. Increased pressure within the ventricular system compresses the brain and the ventricles enlarge. In the young child, before the cranial sutures fuse, head cir-

cumference increases more rapidly than normal and the head may enlarge considerably.

4. Mechanisms such as transependymal absorption may allow the increased intraventricular pressure to become compensated, and a steady state can be reached. In most cases, however, ventricular enlargement continues unless there is medical or surgical intervention.

Clinical Findings

1. Acute hydrocephalus presents with dramatic symptoms. These include:
   a. Marked behavioral changes with irritability and lethargy
   b. Severe headache
   c. Vomiting
   d. A bulging fontanelle and increasing head circumference in infants
   e. The neurologic examination is usually normal initially, but neurologic signs may appear
      (1) VI nerve (abducens) palsy with in-turning of one or both eyes
      (2) Spasticity of the legs
      (3) Opisthotonus
      (4) Papilledema can develop rapidly in the older child
2. Chronic hydrocephalus is more insidious in its manifestations.
   a. Mild personality change and lethargy
   b. Chronic headaches
   c. Gradually increasing head circumference, especially in infants and young children
   d. VI nerve palsies may occur
   e. Chronic papilledema

Laboratory Findings

There are no specific laboratory findings, except those relating to the underlying etiology. Ultrasonography is a useful tool for determining and following ventricular size in infants.

Radiographic Changes

Neuroimaging studies will define the degree of hydrocephalus and demonstrate the presence of any anatomic or pathologic causes, such as brain tumors, for the hydrocephalus.

Treatment

1. Some cases of hydrocephalus arrest spontaneously and need no intervention.
2. In cases in which the imbalance between cerebrospinal fluid production and absorption is marginal, drugs that decrease cerebrospinal fluid production may allow the condition to stabilize. Acetazolamide is most commonly used, although this may cause metabolic acidosis.
3. It may be possible to surgically remove the block to cerebrospinal fluid flow in cases of noncommunicating hydrocephalus.
4. The majority of children with progressive hydrocephalus will require placement of a shunt. This is a tube with a one-way valve. The proximal end is inserted into the ventricles and the distal end can be placed in the abdominal or pleural cavities or into the circulation via the jugular vein and superior vena cava. A major problem with shunts in infants is the need to revise them as the child grows. Serious complications are common and include blockage of the shunt, shunt infections, and thromboembolism or immune complex shunt nephritis with shunts placed in the vascular system.

Prevention

Prevention of some of the causes of acquired hydrocephalus is the only effective strategy.

Bibliography

Fletcher JM, Brookshire BL, Landry SH, et al: Behavioral adjustment of children with hydrocephalus: relationships with etiology, neurological, and family status. J Pediatr Psychol 1955;20:109–125.

McLone DG, Partington MD: Arrest and compensation of hydrocephalus. Neurosurg Clin North Am 1993;4:621–624.

O'Brien MS, Harris ME: Long-term results in the treatment of hydrocephalus. Neurosurg Clin North Am 1993;4:625–632.

Shiminski-Maher T, Disabato J: Current trends in the diagnosis and management of hydrocephalus in children. J Pediatr Nurs 1994;9:74–82.

272 Craniosynostosis

Gerald S. Golden

Definition

A condition characterized by premature fusion of the cranial sutures, leading to growth abnormalities of the skull and abnormal head shape.

Etiology

No etiology has been defined for most cases. Familial clustering of craniosynostosis has been reported in up to 10 per cent of cases.

Epidemiology

Some form of craniosynostosis occurs in approximately 1 in 200 live births.

Pathophysiology

1. No specific mechanism has been defined.
2. Skull growth occurs perpendicular to the suture lines. Premature closure of the sagittal suture, for example, would prevent growth in the coronal dimension, and a long thin head (scaphocephaly) would result.

Clinical Findings

1. The shape of the head is a function of which suture closes prematurely (Table 272–1).
2. Craniosynostosis may be an isolated problem or may occur as part of a number of syndromes. In these cases, there is usually involvement of multiple sutures. Multiple congenital anomalies are also present in these conditions (e.g., Apert syndrome, Crouzon disease).
3. Neurologic complications of isolated craniosynostosis are rare.
   a. Papilledema and optic atrophy are sometimes associated with severe coronal synostosis.
   b. Multiple suture closures can produce increased intracranial pressure.

Laboratory Findings

No specific laboratory examinations are useful.

Radiographic Changes

Radiographs and computed tomography (CT) scans of the skull provide diagnostic information. The earliest sign is increased bone density alongside the suture. Fusion then occurs.

Treatment

1. Unless there is compromise of the optic nerve or increased intracranial pressure, treatment is strictly cosmetic.

TABLE 272–1. CRANIOSYNOSTOSIS

SUTURE CLOSED	CONDITION	HEAD SHAPE
Sagittal	Scaphocephaly	Long, thin
Coronal	Brachycephaly	Broad; short AP dimension
Lambdoid or single coronal	Plagiocephaly	Trapezoidal
Metopic	Trigonencephaly	Keel-shaped forehead

AP = anteroposterior.

2. Linear craniectomy, removing the fused suture, is the standard surgical approach. More radical surgery is needed in cases in which there is closure of multiple sutures or facial malformations.
3. Surgery is most effective if done in the first 6 months.

Key Treatment

- Surgery
  Relief of intracranial pressure (uncommon)
  Cosmetic

Prevention

There are no known preventive strategies for primary craniosynostosis. Families should be made aware of the risk of recurrence in subsequent children. Genetic counseling is appropriate for families of children with a syndrome that includes craniosynostosis.

Bibliography

Becker LE, Hinton DR: Pathogenesis of craniosynostosis. Pediatr Neurosurg 1995;22:104–107.
Marion RW: Craniosynostosis. Pediatr Rev 1995;16:115–116.

273 Neural Tube Defects

Gerald S. Golden

Definition

A group of congenital malformations arising from abnormalities in the growth and development of the embryonic neural tube and characterized by abnormal structure of the brain or spinal cord, often associated with abnormalities of the overlying dura, bone, muscle, and skin.

Etiology

1. The etiology in most cases is not known. There may be a genetic component as the recurrence risk is increased in families of affected children.
2. Possible teratogenic agents include maternal hyperthermia, valproic acid, and gestational diabetes mellitus.
3. There is now evidence that a relative deficiency of folic acid may be an etiologic factor in humans. Vitamin A deficiency or excess has been shown to be teratogenic in experimental animals.

Epidemiology

Current incidence figures are difficult to determine. There has been a continuous decline from the commonly reported incidence of 1 per 600 live births for all forms of neural tube defects, largely as a result of prenatal diagnosis and termination of affected pregnancies.

Pathophysiology

1. The most commonly accepted theory is that failure of closure of the anterior or posterior neuropores of the embryonic neural tube occurs, and the overlying defects are the result of abnormal induction.
2. An alternate hypothesis is that the roof of the fourth ventricle remains impermeable to cerebrospinal fluid, causing intrauterine hydrocephalus, which produces rupture of the neural tube.

Clinical Findings

1. Spina bifida occulta involves only the vertebral arches and is not associated with neurologic deficits. A clinical clue is the presence of overlying cutaneous abnormalities including a sinus tract or an abnormal tuft of hair, or a subcutaneous lipoma.
2. Meningocele refers to a sac of meninges protruding through a defect in the vertebral arches or skull. It may or may not be skin covered. There are no neurologic deficits associated with lumbar meningoceles. Cranial meningoceles are frequently associated with anomalies of the underlying brain.
3. Meningomyelocele involves not only the meninges but the spinal cord and the overlying bone, muscle, and skin. The majority are in the lumbar and lumbosacral regions, but the defects may be present at any level of the neuraxis. Cranial lesions are referred to as encephaloceles. Neurologic deficits are always present, their severity relating to the level of the lesion and the extent of the disruption of the spinal cord and nerve roots.
   a. The lesion on the back is usually obvious. It may be completely skin covered but, more commonly, meninges are visible. A leak of cerebrospinal fluid is common.
   b. Flaccid weakness of the legs, usually severe, is universally present. Weakness may be asymmetric, and there may be sparing of some muscles.
   c. Sensory deficits in areas below the lesion are also present, but may be spotty. The anesthetic areas are susceptible to inadvertent trauma and the development of decubitus ulcers.
   d. Sphincter involvement is usually severe with a flaccid bladder, urinary retention, and overflow incontinence.
   e. Orthopedic deformities of the feet result from abnormal uterine positioning secondary to the weakness. Subluxation of the hips frequently occurs because of muscle weakness.
   f. Hydrocephalus is present in the majority of children. The risk of clinically significant hydrocephalus increases as lesions involve higher levels of the neuraxis.
4. Encephalocele is characterized by a cranial defect through which a dural or meningeal sac containing brain tissue protrudes. These lesions are most frequent in the occipital and frontal regions. Associated problems in the majority of cases include hydrocephalus, mental retardation, and motor abnormalities.

5. Anencephaly refers to absence of the cerebral hemispheres and overlying meninges, skull, and scalp. Many of these children are stillborn. Those children alive at birth demonstrate intact brainstem reflexes and primitive responses to noxious stimuli, but will die within a few days.

Key Clinical Finding

- Protruding sac of meninges through defect in vertebral arches, less commonly the skull

Laboratory Findings

1. These lesions, except for some cases of spina bifida occulta, are obvious at birth and no laboratory confirmation is required.
2. Cranial ultrasonography is an effective way to evaluate the presence and progression of hydrocephalus in the infant.
3. Children with myelomeningocele need frequent monitoring of the status of their urinary tract, including regular ultrasonography of the kidneys and bladder and urine cultures when clinically indicated.

Key Laboratory Test

- Monitor for urinary tract infection (UTI)

Radiographic Changes

1. Radiographs of the spine will provide details of bony involvement at site of the lesion and allow evaluation of the kyphoscoliosis that may also be present.
2. Neuroimaging, including computed tomography scans and magnetic resonance imaging, are important for monitoring the presence or progression of hydrocephalus and for defining the extent of neural involvement before surgical closure of the overlying defects.
3. Periodic assessment of the urinary tract is usually required to demonstrate the extent of ureteral reflux and the efficiency of bladder emptying.
4. Radiographs of the legs and hips are necessary for planning orthopedic procedures, if they are indicated.

Treatment

1. Surgical repair to cover the defect is urgent. This will help prevent the development of meningitis, and there is some evidence that early surgery prevents the deterioration of function that is commonly seen.
2. Treatment of hydrocephalus is required if ventricular enlargement is progressive.
3. Scheduled intermittent clean catheterization of the bladder is the most effective method of prevention of urinary reflux and repeated urinary tract infections.
4. Orthopedic status should be monitored. Treatment of foot deformities, dislocated hips, and kyphoscoliosis is important to prevent progression, improve functional status, prevent pain, or facilitate nursing care.

Key Treatment

- Surgery
  Cover defect
  Shunt to relieve hydrocephalus
  Correct orthopedic defects

Prevention

1. The major tool for prevention is prenatal detection and termination of the pregnancy. Families that have had a child with a neural tube defect should be counseled that there is an increased risk in subsequent pregnancies. Prenatal detection of neural tube defects is practical and can provide parents with important information.

   a. Maternal serum α-fetoprotein levels are an effective screening tool, although the false-negative rate may be as high as 20 per cent.

   b. Amniotic fluid α-fetoprotein levels are elevated in all cases except when the lesion is completely skin covered.

   c. Fetal ultrasonography is effective in detecting these lesions.

2. Administration of folic acid 0.4 mg/day to women before conception and during the first trimester of pregnancy appears to be able to reduce the incidence of neural tube defects.

Bibliography

Byrd SE, Radkowski MA: The radiological evaluation of the child with a myelomeningocele. J Nat Med Assoc 1991;83:608–614.

Hernandez RD, Hurwitz RS, Foote JE, et al: Nonsurgical management of threatened upper urinary tracts and incontinence in children with myelomeningocele. J Urol 1994;152:1582–1585.

McLone DG: Continuing concepts in the management of spina bifida. Pediatr Neurosurg 1992;18:254–256.

Rieder MJ: Prevention of neural tube defects with periconceptual folic acid. Clin Perinatol 1994;21:483–503.

Steinberg A: Meningomyelocele in the neonate: medical and ethical considerations. J Perinatol 1991;11:51–56.

274 Agenesis of the Corpus Callosum

Gerald S. Golden

Definition

Congenital absence of all or part of the large commissure of fibers between the cerebral hemispheres.

Etiology

This condition may exist as an isolated anomaly or as part of a syndrome of other neural or nonneural malformations.

1. In those cases not associated with a defined syndrome, no specific etiologic agents have been recognized. An X-linked or autosomal dominant pattern of inheritance has been found in some families.
2. Aicardi syndrome is an X-linked dominant condition that, as it is only found in females, is probably lethal in males. The major features are agenesis of the corpus callosum, infantile spasms, and mental retardation.

Epidemiology

Isolated agenesis of the corpus callosum is rare and is often not diagnosed unless the child has a neuroimaging study for some reason. Its overall prevalence relates to the frequency of conditions that have callosal abnormalities as one of their features.

Pathophysiology

The fiber tracts of the corpus callosum develop predominantly from late in the first trimester of pregnancy until the middle of the second trimester. The teratogenic influences must occur during this period. Myelination of these fibers is primarily postnatal. The area normally occupied by the corpus callosum is encroached upon by an enlarged third ventricle and is filled with cerebrospinal fluid. The lateral ventricles are laterally placed and elongated, giving a "bat-wing" appearance on coronal section. Other cerebral malformations such as areas of polymicrogyria are commonly present.

Clinical Findings

1. Some children are neurologically normal, although neuropsychologic testing may show subtle cognitive deficits.
2. Children who have associated cerebral anomalies may have multiple handicaps including mental retardation and spastic quadriplegia (cerebral palsy).
3. The abnormalities in Aicardi syndrome have been described above.

Key Clinical Findings

- Cognitive delay or deficit
- May have associated neural defects
- Seizures

Laboratory Findings

No specific laboratory findings are present. An electroencephalogram is indicated if the child has seizures.

Radiographic Changes

Magnetic resonance imaging of the brain documents the lesion and associated cerebral malformations. The unusual shape of the ventricles is best demonstrated in the coronal plane.

Treatment

There is no specific treatment other than therapy for seizures, physical therapy for children with motor deficits, and special education for those with cognitive abnormalities such as mental retardation.

Key Treatment

- Manage seizures, if any
- Physical therapy as needed

Prevention

Genetic counseling should be offered to those families in which there is a clear pattern of inheritance, and especially to families of children with Aicardi syndrome.

Bibliography

Bodensteiner J, Schaefer GB, Breeding L, Cowan L: Hypoplasia of the corpus callosum: a study of 445 consecutive MRI scans. J Child Neurol 1994;9:47–49.

Menezes AV, MacGregor DL, Buncic JR: Aicardi syndrome: natural history and possible predictors of severity. Pediatr Neurol 1994;11:313–318.

275 Neurodegenerative Disorders

Shanti Thirumalai and *Sakkubai Naidu*

Definition

1. A neurodegenerative disorder causes progressive loss of function of the central nervous system (CNS) and should be suspected if:

   a. A child sustains loss of previously acquired developmental milestones or

   b. The rate of acquisition of new skills declines or

   c. There appears to be a stagnation in development.

   d. Conditions b and c are often difficult to differentiate from static encephalopathies, where development proceeds at a slow but constant rate.

2. Most clinicians classify degenerative diseases of the nervous system into those that primarily affect the gray matter or neurons and those that affect the white matter or myelin (Table 275–1). Initial symptoms and signs provide the best guidelines, and these may not be separable in later stages.

3. Pathologic processes that can mimic neurodegeneration include hydrocephalus, hypothyroidism, mass lesions, structural abnormalities, chromosomal defects, poorly controlled seizures, environmental deprivation, subdural hematoma, and congenital and chronic infections, including human immunodeficiency virus (HIV). These conditions must be ruled out by appropriate tests before searching for a metabolic basis.

Etiology

1. Most neurodegenerative diseases have a biochemical basis.

2. It is important to make a specific diagnosis because specific treatments such as dietary manipulation, use of cofactors, enzyme replacement, and bone marrow transplantation are available in some conditions. Furthermore, genetic counseling, prenatal diagnosis and carrier testing are possible for many diseases.

Epidemiology

These are unusual conditions, the incidence depending on the specific disorder.

Pathophysiology

1. Most of these disorders are characterized by progressive damage to cerebral cortex, white matter, or both.

2. The specific pathophysiology is related to each individual condition.

Clinical Findings

1. History

   a. Exclude antenatal and perinatal factors contributing to brain injury.

   b. The age of onset and the rate of progression of neurodegeneration should be ascertained.

   c. The presence or absence of the following features should be elicited: seizures, exaggerated startle, visual and hearing loss, irritability, speech abnormality, loss of skills, spasticity, movement disorders

TABLE 275–1. DIFFERENTIATION OF GRAY AND WHITE MATTER DISEASES

TIME	GRAY MATTER	WHITE MATTER
Early	Dementia	Spasticity
	Seizures	Babinski signs
	Retinal pigmentary change	Optic nerve atrophy
	Ataxia	Ataxia
Later	Spasticity	Dementia
	Babinski signs	Seizures

TABLE 275–2. NEURODEGENERATIVE DISORDERS WITH MICROCEPHALY

Congenital infections including human immunodeficiency virus (HIV)
Chromosomal abnormalities
Miller Dieker syndrome
Rett syndrome
Cornelia de Lange syndrome
Smith-Lemli-Opitz (SLOP) syndrome

including dystonia, involuntary movements, tremor, gait difficulty, ataxia, and school problems.

   d. Family history with attention to consanguinity, the mode of inheritance, and phenotypic variations noting causes of death in various family members.

2. Physical examination

   a. Anthropometry with serial head circumference measurements to identify microcephaly (Table 275–2), megalencephaly (Table 275–3), and rate of deceleration or acceleration of head growth and general growth parameters is essential and valuable.

   b. Skin examination is important to identify neurocutaneous disorders and examination with a Wood's lamp in fair-skinned children to visualize ash-leaf–like lesions in tuberous sclerosis.

   c. Abnormal kinky hair is seen in Menkes disease, and children with biotinidase deficiency may have alopecia.

   d. A careful search for dysmorphic features may reveal coarse facies, epicanthal folds, abnormal slant of eyes, ear pits, high arched palate, and bony abnormalities (Table 275–4).

   e. Abdominal examination for organomegaly (Table 275–5) is very helpful because of systemic storage in some neurodegenerative disorders.

   f. Eye examination including sclera, cornea, lens and fundus for anomalies (Table 275–6) is important.

3. Neurologic examination

   a. A thorough neurologic examination to evaluate cognitive function; cranial nerves; motor system including tone, strength, and involuntary movements (see Table 275–7); response to noxious stimuli; reflexes; and coordination provides direction.

Menkes Kinky Hair Disease

Definition

A hereditary disease of newborn males resulting from decreased copper absorption and inadequate function of a number of copper-containing enzymes.

TABLE 275–3. NEURODEGENERATIVE DISORDERS WITH MEGALENCEPHALY

Familial megalencephaly	GM_2 gangliosidosis
Soto disease	Glutaricaciduria type I
Mucopolysaccharidosis	Alexander disease
GM_1 gangliosidosis	Canavan disease

TABLE 275–4. NEURODEGENERATIVE DISORDERS WITH DYSMORPHISM

Mucopolysaccharidosis
Sialiduria
Peroxisome biogenesis defects: Zellweger syndrome, neonatal adrenoleukodystrophy (NALD), rhizomelic chondrodystrophica punctata
I-cell disease
GM_1 gangliosidosis
Mucolipidosis
Smith-Lemli-Opitz syndrome
William syndrome
Hypothyroidism
Oligosaccharidosis (fucosidosis, mannosidosis)

Etiology

Inheritance is X-linked recessive. The gene for Menkes disease has been localized to Xq13.2–13.3.

Epidemiology

The disease is rare and appears to occur in all ethnic groups.

Pathophysiology

1. The primary biochemical problem relates to copper metabolism, with decreased absorption from the gut and low serum copper and copper containing enzymes including ceruloplasmin.
2. Other copper-dependent enzymes including cytochrome oxidase c (mitochondrial), superoxide dismutase, dopamine hydroxylase, tyrosinase, lysyl oxidase, and monamine oxidase are deficient, resulting in energy failure, infections, abnormal structure of skin and blood vessels, and neurotransmitter imbalances.
3. Pathologic findings include disruption of the intima of tortuous blood vessels, neuronal depletion in the cortex and cerebellum and demyelination of deep white matter.

Clinical Findings

1. There are abnormal pale kinky hair, chubby rosy cheeks, hypothermia, severe seizures, hypotonia, feeding difficulties, and optic atrophy.
2. The course is one of progressive neurologic deterioration and early death.

Key Clinical Findings: Menkes Kinky Hair Disease

- Hypotonia
- Kinky hair
- Hypothermia
- Seizures
- Optic atrophy

Laboratory Findings

Diagnosis is made by microscopic examination of the hair to show fractures of the shaft of the hair follicles and by confirming low levels of copper and ceruloplasmin in blood.

Radiographic Changes

1. Flaring of the ribs and metaphyseal abnormalities in the long bones are present.

TABLE 275–5. NEURODEGENERATIVE DISORDERS WITH VISCEROMEGALY

Galactosemia
Gaucher disease II and III
Sandhoff disease
Niemann-Pick disease
Peroxisomal biogenesis defects: Zellweger syndrome, neonatal adrenoleukodystrophy (NALD)
Glycogen storage disease
Wilson disease
Mucopolysaccharidosis, oligosaccharidosis, mucolipidosis
GM_1 gangliosidosis

2. Neuroimaging studies demonstrate progressive loss of cerebral tissue.

Treatment

Treatment with copper-histidine injections to give 50 to 150 µg of elemental copper/kg/day normalizes copper and ceruloplasmin levels. The nervous system continues to deteriorate despite this therapy.

Key Treatment: Menkes Kinky Hair Disease

• Copper-histidine injections—minimal effectiveness

Prevention

1. Prenatal diagnosis is now possible by measuring radiolabeled ^{64}Cu uptake in amniocytes.
2. Cultured chorionic villi are often contaminated by mater-

TABLE 275–6. NEURODEGENERATIVE DISORDERS WITH OCULAR ABNORMALITIES

DISORDER	OCULAR ABNORMALITY
Sclera	Ataxia telangiectasia
Kayser-Fleischer rings	Wilson disease
Corneal clouding	Mucopolysaccharidosis
	Lowe syndrome
Cataracts	Galactosemia
	Zellweger syndrome/rhizomelic chondrodysplasia punctata
	Fabry disease
	Cerebrotendinous xanthomatosis
	Lowe syndrome
	Marinesco Sjögren syndrome
	Cockayne syndrome
Retinal pigmentary change	Mitochondrial cytopathy
	Zellweger syndrome/infantile Refsum disease
	Adult Refsum disease
	Abetalipoproteinemia
	Hallervorden-Spatz disease
Optic atrophy	Leber hereditary atrophy
	Leukodystrophies (some)
	Infantile neuroaxonal dystrophy
Macular degeneration	Neuronal ceroid lipofuscinosis (NCL)
Cherry-red spots	GM_1 gangliosidosis
	Tay-Sachs disease
	Sandhoff disease
	Gaucher disease
	Mucolipidosis type 1
	Niemann-Pick disease
	Multiple sulphatase deficiency

TABLE 275–7. DISORDERS CAUSING DYSTONIA, CHOREA, OR RIGIDITY

DISEASE	TEST	INHERITANCE
Wilson disease	Serum ceruloplasmin, urine copper ↑	AR
Lesch-Nyhan syndrome	Hypoxanthine guanine Phosphoribosyl Transferase ↓	XR
Niemann-Pick disease type C	Filipin staining positive, cholesterol esterification ↓	AR
Hallervorden-Spatz disease	↑ iron deposition in basal ganglia by MRI	AR
Glutaricaciduria type I	Urine glutaric and 3-hydroxy glutaric acids ↑	AR
Huntington disease	DNA for increased CAG triplet repeats	AD
Cerebrotendinous xanthomatosis	Cholestanol	AR

AD = autosomal dominant; AR = autosomal recessive; MRI = magnetic resonance imaging; XR = X-linked recessive.

nal deciduum and therefore this is not a satisfactory prenatal diagnostic approach.

Wilson Disease

Definition

This is a multisystem disease caused by copper deposition in tissues including the liver, renal tubules, the eye, and the brain.

Etiology

1. The gene for Wilson disease has been localized to chromosome 13q.
2. The disease is inherited in an autosomal recessive manner with marked phenotypic variability: for example, liver cell failure in one child and chorea alone in a sibling.

Epidemiology

The condition is uncommon and occurs in all ethnic groups.

Pathophysiology

1. Patients have high metallothionine levels and increased copper absorption from the gut.
2. Ceruloplasmin, a copper-containing enzyme, is deficient but its precise role in the disease has not been defined.
3. Copper appears to be stored first in the liver before the CNS is involved. Therefore, clinical manifestations of CNS involvement do not often occur until about 5 years of age.
4. Pathologic features include atrophy of the basal ganglia, notably the putamen, cerebellum, and frontal lobes.
5. In the liver, cirrhosis and chronic active hepatitis are seen.

Clinical Findings

1. Clinical features include liver disease in children with onset under 5 years of age, and dystonia in children presenting between 5 and 10 years of age.

2. In older children, CNS involvement may present as tremor, chorea, dystonia, ataxia, psychosis or dementia. Seizures are uncommon.

3. Examination of the eyes shows Kayser-Fleischer rings on slit lamp examination in 95 per cent of patients with CNS involvement. Rarely seen are sunflower cataracts.

4. Hypersplenism, hemolytic anemia, renal tubular acidosis, renal rickets, and growth failure are present in some cases.

Key Clinical Findings: Wilson Disease

- Dystonia
- Tremor
- Ataxia
- Kayser-Fleischer rings

Laboratory Findings

1. Low serum ceruloplasmin levels with elevated serum copper levels and increased urinary excretion of copper are diagnostic.

2. Magnetic resonance imaging (MRI) shows generalized atrophy and decreased signal of the lentiform nucleus.

Treatment

1. Wilson disease is a CNS condition that is reversible with early treatment and therefore is an important diagnostic consideration whenever indicated.

2. Treatment includes restricting dietary copper by curtailing shellfish, nuts, and liver.

3. Urinary excretion of copper is enhanced by penicillamine, a chelating agent whose side effects include neutropenia and proteinuria.

4. Zinc has been used in patients who do not tolerate penicillamine. It decreases copper absorption by competing with copper for metallothionine binding, while continued renal excretion helps achieve a negative balance.

Key Treatment: Wilson Disease

- Curtail intake of shellfish, nuts, and liver
- Penicillamine
- Zinc

Prevention

The only preventive strategy is genetic counseling.

Metachromatic Leukodystrophy

Definition

A group of related inherited disorders of myelin metabolism affecting the CNS and the peripheral nerves.

Etiology

The disease is transmitted in an autosomal recessive manner. The gene is situated on chromosome 22q13.

Epidemiology

The disorders in this group are uncommon.

Pathophysiology

There is an abnormal accumulation of sulfatides in the brain, as a result of deficiency of the enzymes catabolizing these substances.

Clinical Findings

1. Late infantile form

    a. This form presents between 1 and 2 years of life with gait difficulty. Death occurs in the first decade.

    b. There is hypotonia initially and in a few months, there is motor regression with loss of cognitive skills and speech deterioration.

    c. Nystagmus and optic nerve atrophy occur.

    d. Muscle tone progressively increases; ataxia and head titubation set in. As the disease progresses, quadriplegia and inability to swallow become problematic. This state can last for years.

2. Juvenile form

    a. Juvenile metachromatic leukodystrophy (MLD) has its onset between 4 and 12 years, presenting usually as poor school performance and behavioral difficulties.

    b. Gait disturbances and incontinence occur, with slurring of speech, increased tone and abnormal posture. Within a year, most patients are unable to walk, and have trouble with swallowing and speech. Muscle tone increases, tonic spasms occur, and seizures may be noted.

    c. Most patients do not live beyond their teen years.

3. An adult-onset form presenting in the third or fourth decade with primarily psychiatric problems, dementia, some gait difficulty and incontinence is recognized.

Key Clinical Findings: Metachromatic Leukodystrophy

- Hypotonia
- Ataxia
- Dementia

Laboratory Findings

1. Leukocyte enzyme studies show reduced activity of arylsulfatase A, due to deficiency of the enzyme. Urinary sulfatide excretion is increased.

2. Nerve conduction studies are decreased, reflecting peripheral nerve involvement. Brainstem auditory evoked responses (BAER), visual evoked potentials (VEP), and somatosensory evoked potentials (SSEP) may be abnormal. Electroencephalography (EEG) may show diffuse slowing and epileptiform discharges.

3. Cerebrospinal fluid protein is increased.

4. Peripheral nerve biopsy shows metachromatic granules for which the disease is named.

5. Some patients may have increased sulfatide excretion in the urine with normal levels of arylsulfatase A. These

patients may have deficiency of activator protein, which can be diagnosed by sulfatide incorporation studies in skin fibroblasts.

6. Normal individuals and asymptomatic relatives of patients with MLD may have decreased arylsulfatase A activity. This would be due to a pseudodeficient state as the low level of the enzyme may be adequate to prevent disease. This can be ascertained by sulfatide loading studies in cultured fibroblasts and more recently by molecular studies to identify characteristic mutations on the pseudodeficiency allele, which occurs with a frequency of 7 to 15 per cent in the general population.

**Key Laboratory Findings:
Metachromatic Leukodystrophy**

- Reduction of arylsulfatase A in leukocytes
- Increased cerebrospinal fluid (CSF) protein
- Metachromatic granules in peripheral nerve biopsy

Radiographic Changes

MRI scan shows abnormal signal in the white matter on T2 weighted images affecting the deep and subcortical white matter.

Treatment

1. General supportive measures include attention to nutrition, prevention of aspiration, and treatment of seizures and infections.
2. Results of bone marrow transplantation have been encouraging in the late onset forms, especially when performed early in the course of the disease.

Key Treatment: Metachromatic Leukodystrophy

- Supportive
- Bone marrow transplant?

Prevention

Prenatal diagnosis with amniotic fluid cells or chorionic villus sampling is possible.

Krabbe Disease

Definition

Also known as globoid-cell leukodystrophy, this is an autosomal recessive condition with abnormal myelin metabolism affecting both the central and peripheral nervous systems.

Etiology

This is a genetic condition with the abnormality on chromosome 14q21–31.

Epidemiology

This is an uncommon condition found in all population groups.

Pathophysiology

1. The biochemical defect is the deficiency of a lysosomal enzyme, galactocerebroside-beta-galactosidase.
2. Multinucleate globoid cells derived from macrophages are seen in the white matter, enabling a morphologic diagnosis. Severe myelin loss and astrocytic gliosis are also present.

Clinical Findings

1. The infantile form is a rapidly progressive disease with onset between 3 and 6 months; death occurs within 2 years.
   a. Early symptoms are irritability, stiffness, fever, and hypersensitivity to stimuli. Seizures may occur. Feeding difficulties and vomiting are common.
   b. Hypertonicity, optic atrophy, hyporeflexia with extensor plantar responses, and motor and mental deterioration then develop. In late stages, the infant is decerebrate and blind.
   c. Peripheral neuropathy is common and CSF protein is elevated.
2. The late infantile form is similar, with onset between 6 months and 3 years and death within 3 years of onset.
3. The juvenile-onset form presents between 3 and 10 years of age with hemiparesis, ataxia, loss of vision, and dementia. CSF protein may not be elevated and there may be no involvement of the peripheral nerve. The illness can last 5 or more years before death.
4. In the adult-onset form, CSF protein is normal and peripheral neuropathy has not been described. Dementia, loss of vision, and pyramidal tract signs are common.

Key Clinical Findings: Krabbe Disease

- Irritability
- Seizures
- Hypertonicity
- Optic atrophy
- Decerebrate and blind (late)

Laboratory Findings

1. The diagnosis is made on leukocyte or cultured fibroblast assays of galactosylceramidase.
2. Brain and peripheral nerve biopsies show periodic acid–Schiff (PAS)–positive inclusions in multinucleate globoid cells that are derived from the monocyte-macrophage system.
3. VEP, BAER, and nerve conduction velocity studies may be abnormal.

Key Laboratory Findings: Krabbe Disease

- Deficiency of galactosylceramidase in leukocytes or cultured fibroblasts
- Increased CSF protein

Radiographic Changes

MRI shows diffuse cerebral atrophy with abnormal white matter beginning often in the parieto-occipital regions.

Treatment

1. Supportive treatment with attention to nutrition, and symptomatic management of seizures is important.
2. Bone marrow transplantation has not been successful in the more rapidly progressive infantile form of the disease.

Key Treatment: Krabbe Disease

- Correct hypotonia

Prevention

Prenatal diagnosis using cultured amniocytes or chorionic villus sampling to detect the biochemical defect is possible.

Adrenoleukodystrophy

Definition

This is an X-linked disease causing demyelination in boys.

Etiology

The genetic defect has been localized to Xq28.

Epidemiology

As the disorder is X-linked, the majority of affected individuals are male. A small percentage of carrier females may show some manifestations of the disorder later in life.

Pathophysiology

The biochemical defect is the deficient activation of very long chain fatty acids (VLCFAs) to their CoA derivatives. The VLCFAs accumulate in plasma and in tissues including the brain, testes, and the adrenal glands.

Clinical Findings

1. The classic form affects boys aged 5 to 10 years.
   a. Initial symptoms are poor school performance and personality change.
   b. Neurologic symptoms include ataxia, spasticity, loss of vision and hearing. Seizures may occur in some patients. The disease progresses with dementia, ultimately leading to a vegetative state and death.
   c. Adrenal failure is present in all boys with the childhood-onset form of the disease but is not universal in the adult-onset form.

Key Clinical Findings: Adrenoleukodystropy

- Personality change
- Ataxia
- Spasticity
- Adrenal failure

2. Some adults with the same genetic background present with only spinal cord, adrenal gland, and peripheral nerve involvement in the third and fourth decades of life.
3. Heterozygotes or female carriers present late with mild spinal cord and peripheral nerve disease but rarely have adrenal involvement.

Laboratory Findings

Plasma and skin fibroblasts show increased levels of VLCFA.

Key Laboratory Finding: Adrenoleukodystrophy

- Increased levels of very long chain fatty acids

Radiologic Changes

MRI of the head shows high signal intensity on T2 weighted scans. Parieto-occipital regions of the white matter are initially involved in 85 per cent while the other 15 per cent may present initially with frontal white matter abnormalities.

Treatment

1. In addition to supportive measures, treatment includes the use of corticosteroids to treat adrenal insufficiency.
2. Patients who are presymptomatic may benefit from diet enriched with erucic acid and oleic acid, which help normalize plasma VLCFA levels. It is not certain if this therapeutic intervention alters the clinical course of the disease.
3. Bone marrow transplantation has been shown to be effective in the cerebral form of the disease if performed early.

Key Treatment: Adrenoleukodystrophy

- Corticosteroid replacement
- Bone marrow transplantation (early)

Prevention

Prenatal diagnosis is possible. There are increased VLCFA levels in amniocytes and chorionic villus samples.

Alexander Disease

Definition

This is a degenerative disorder of the white matter of the central nervous system related to astrocyte dysfunction.

Etiology

The etiology is unknown.

Epidemiology

The condition is extremely rare.

Pathophysiology

No enzymatic or biochemical defects have been defined. The disease is sporadic although a few familial cases have been reported.

Clinical Findings

1. Infantile, juvenile, and adult-onset forms have been described.
2. Prominent features are progressive megalencephaly, psychomotor retardation, optic atrophy, spasticity, and seizures leading to rapid death.
3. Bulbar or pseudobulbar palsy is seen in patients with the juvenile form.
4. Mentation may be intact in some patients with later onset.

Key Clinical Findings: Alexander Disease

- Megalencephaly
- Spasticity
- Seizures
- Bulbar palsy

Laboratory Findings

The definitive test is a brain biopsy in which cytoplasmic eosinophilic Rosenthal fibers derived from glial elements are seen.

Key Laboratory Finding: Alexander Disease

- Brain biopsy histology

Radiographic Changes

MRI shows abnormal white matter signal in T2 weighted images particularly in the frontal regions, with cystic changes in the later stages.

Treatment

No specific treatment exists for Alexander disease. Supportive therapies include attention to nutrition and control of seizures and infections.

Key Treatment: Alexander Disease

- Supportive only

Prevention

The condition is sporadic, so no preventive techniques are available.

Canavan Disease

Definition

This is a degenerative disease of the CNS associated with spongy change in the brain.

Etiology

The disease is inherited by autosomal recessive transmission. The gene has been identified on chromosome 17p13.

Epidemiology

The condition is more common in Ashkenazi Jews.

Pathophysiology

The biochemical abnormality is the deficiency of aspartoacylase, which leads to increased levels of N-acetylaspartic acid.

Clinical Findings

1. In the infantile form, onset occurs in the first few months with megalencephaly, hypotonia, and developmental arrest. Increasing spasticity, extensor posturing, blindness, and autonomic failure set in, and death usually occurs by age 3 to 4 years.
2. The juvenile form occurs after age 5 years and is characterized mainly by progressive ataxia with dementia, tremor, and spasticity. Visual symptoms relate to optic atrophy.

Key Clinical Findings: Canavan Disease

- Megalencephaly
- Hypotonia—early
- Spasticity
- Blindness

Laboratory Findings

Increased amounts of *N*-acetylaspartic acid in the urine and deficient activity of aspartoacylase in cultured skin fibroblasts offer a biochemical diagnosis.

Key Laboratory Finding: Canavan Disease

- Increased N-acetylaspartic acid in urine

Radiographic Changes

MRI shows white matter involvement on T2 weighted scans.

Treatment

At present, treatment is mainly supportive with attention to nutrition and control of seizures.

Key Treatment: Canavan Disease

- Supportive

Prevention

There are no preventive measures at this time.

Niemann-Pick Disease

Definition

Progressive degenerative disorders associated with lipid-laden foam cells derived from the monocyte macrophage system. It is now clear that Niemann-Pick types A and B are biochemically distinct from type C.

Etiology

These are all autosomal recessive disorders. Niemann-Pick disease type A and B occur with a high frequency in Ashkenazi Jewish individuals. The gene has been identified on chromosome 11p15. Niemann-Pick type C is a panethnic disease.

Epidemiology

There are a number of subtypes of Niemann-Pick disease. The epidemiologic characteristics depend on the specific type of disorder.

Pathophysiology

1. Niemann-Pick disease types A and B are lysosomal storage diseases that result from deficient activity of sphingomyelinase.
2. Niemann-Pick type C is caused by an error in cellular trafficking of exogenous cholesterol and is associated with the accumulation of unesterified cholesterol in lysosomes with normal sphingomyelinase activity.

Clinical Findings

1. Niemann-Pick type A
   a. Typically, the infant with Niemann-Pick type A disease is born after normal gestation and labor, and has neonatal jaundice that may be prolonged. Progressive hepatosplenomegaly becomes evident.
   b. Early neurologic signs include hypotonia, generalized weakness, and feeding difficulties.
   c. Aspiration pneumonias and failure to thrive are common in the first 6 months. This is followed by regression of motor and mental milestones, progressive hypotonia, and diminished deep tendon reflexes.
   d. Spasticity and rigidity are obvious in the late stages. Seizures are rare.
   e. Although macular degeneration with cherry red spots occurs in 50 per cent, vision is not necessarily impaired.
2. Patients with Niemann-Pick type B have adequate activity of sphingomyelinase to prevent neurologic symptoms but do have involvement of the liver, spleen, and lung.
3. Niemann-Pick type C
   a. Transient neonatal jaundice is often the first symptom of the disease.
   b. Early childhood may be unremarkable, although behavior problems are seen on entering kindergarten.
   c. Dementia is insidious, and ataxia, dystonia, and drooling are common motor problems. Gradually, the child becomes nonambulatory, and psychosis may set in at the time of puberty. Death is due to inanition and aspiration pneumonia.
   d. Seizures may be generalized or partial and may occur at any stage. Cataplexy may be a feature.
   e. Head thrusting or eye blinking on attempted vertical gaze is pathognomonic. Difficulty with vertical gaze is most evident when attempting to climb stairs. Vertical supranuclear gaze palsy is the neurologic hallmark of this disease.
   f. Some patients have visceromegaly.

Key Clinical Findings: Niemann-Pick Disease

- Hepatosplenomegaly
- Hypotonia
- Later spasticity
- Aspiration pneumonias

Laboratory Findings

1. Niemann-Pick types A and B are diagnosed by deficient activity of sphingomyelinase in peripheral leukocytes or cultured skin fibroblasts. In addition, bone marrow aspiration shows foam cells that support the diagnosis.
2. The diagnosis of Niemann-Pick type C can be established by filipin staining in cultured skin fibroblasts. This method demonstrates nonesterified cholesterol stored in lysosomes and abnormal cholesterol esterification intracellularly. Sphingomyelinase levels are normal or secondarily reduced.

Key Laboratory Finding: Niemann-Pick Disease

- Reduced activity of sphingomyelinase in cultured fibroblasts

Radiologic Changes

Neuroimaging may show a nonspecific picture of degeneration of the central nervous system.

Treatment

1. No specific treatment is available for types A and B. Bone marrow transplantation has not been useful. Enzyme replacement is under investigation.
2. For type C, supportive treatment and attention to swallowing and nutrition with involvement of physical and occupational therapists is the mainstay of management. Control of seizures with anticonvulsant medications, treatment of cataplexy with tricyclic antidepressants and of dystonia with anticholinergics are important symptomatic measures. Cholesterol-lowering agents and a low-cholesterol diet are under investigation.

Key Treatment: Niemann-Pick Disease

- Supportive
- Enzyme replacement—experimental

Prevention

Prenatal diagnosis and carrier detection are possible with the identification of specific mutations. It is also possible to measure sphingomyelinase activity in cultured amniocytes and chorionic villi.

Neuronal Ceroid Lipofuscinoses

Definition

This is a group of neurodegenerative disorders characterized by abnormal accumulation of autofluorescent waxy pigment in neurons and other tissues including lymphocytes, skin, conjunctiva and rectal ganglion cells, which leads to distension of the cytoplasm of the cells.

Etiology

The disorders in this group are genetic. Gene mapping has been successful in localizing the genetic defect for the infantile form to chromosome 1p32, the late infantile variant form to chromosome 13q21 and the juvenile form to 16p12. The genes for the late infantile form and the adult form have not been mapped. The disease is transmitted in an autosomal recessive manner.

Epidemiology

It is difficult to obtain epidemiologic data, as the classification of this group of disorders changes with advances in understanding the underlying pathophysiology of the conditions.

Pathophysiology

1. The cause of the disease is undetermined, but the evidence so far points to an inborn error of metabolism, with disturbances in protein transport and degradation leading to neuronal membrane instability.
2. The lysosomes of these cells contain membrane-bound osmiophilic bodies that may be curvilinear, granular, or have a fingerprint profile. The ultrastructural appearance has not been useful in classifying the subtypes of the disease.

Clinical Findings

1. The condition may present in the neonatal period, in infancy, in later childhood (juvenile form), or in adult life and may have an acute, subacute, or chronic course.
2. Males and females are equally affected.
3. The symptoms are visual, mental, and motor deterioration with ataxia and involuntary movements.
4. Seizures occur early in the infantile forms and later in the course of the disease in the juvenile and adult onset forms.
5. Eye examination reveals macular degeneration and retinal pigmentary changes in all but the adult form of the disease.

Key Clinical Findings:
Neuronal Ceroid Lipofuscinoses

- Ataxia
- Involuntary movements
- Seizures
- Macular degeneration

Laboratory Findings

1. Ultrastructural examination of the skin, conjunctiva, lymphocytes, or rectal mucosa demonstrates the inclusions.
2. EEG is abnormal, VEP is increased in amplitude in the late infantile form, and electroretinography (ERG) is flat in all but the adult-onset forms.

Key Laboratory Finding:
Neuronal Ceroid Lipofuscinoses

- Ultrastructural demonstration of lysosomal inclusions in skin or lymphocytes

Radiographic Changes

Neuroimaging shows nonspecific findings of cerebral degeneration.

Treatment

Treatment is limited to control of seizures and management of the visual impairment.

Key Treatment: Neuronal Ceroid Lipofuscinoses

- Supportive

Prevention

Genetic counseling is limited to statement of risk for autosomal recessive mode of inheritance in all forms and, in addition, a possible autosomal dominant mode in the adult forms. The identification of genes in some forms of the disease will help in carrier detection and prenatal diagnosis.

GM₁ Gangliosidosis

Definition

A neurodegenerative disorder characterized by accumulation of GM_1 ganglioside in the cells of the brain and visceral organs. It is inherited by autosomal recessive transmission.

Etiology

The gene is on 3p14.

Epidemiology

No detailed epidemiologic information is available.

Pathophysiology

The biochemical defect is the deficient activity of β-galactosidase.

Clinical Findings

1. In the infantile form the babies present at birth with organomegaly, coarse facies, and bony abnormalities resembling the Hurler phenotype.
   a. There is failure to thrive with feeding difficulties and hypotonia associated with motor and mental retardation from birth. Hyperreflexia and flexion contractures are present.
   b. Seizures become prominent in the second 6 months.
   c. A cherry red spot in the macula may be seen in half the patients. Hyperacusis is present.
   d. Most children die by 2 years of age, following respiratory infection.
2. Juvenile and adult forms are recognized. These patients have a slower course and present mainly with dystonia,

rigidity, and gait and speech disturbances, and less prominent dysmorphism.

Key Clinical Findings: GM₁ Gangliosidosis

- Failure to thrive
- Seizures
- Hyperacusis
- Cherry red spot in macula (50%)

Laboratory Findings

Leukocytes and cultured skin fibroblast levels of β-galactosidase levels are decreased.

Key Laboratory Finding: GM₁ Gangliosidosis

- Decreased beta-galactosidase levels in cultured fibroblasts

Radiographic Changes

Bony abnormalities indistinguishable from those in Hurler syndrome are present.

Treatment

Symptomatic treatment of seizures and dystonia and supportive care including prevention of aspiration and attention to nutrition are important.

Key Treatment: GM₁ Gangliosidosis

- Supportive

Prevention

Prenatal diagnosis can be made on cultured amniocytes.

GM₂ Gangliosidosis

Definition

The GM₂ gangliosidoses are neurodegenerative diseases caused by excessive intralysosomal accumulation of GM₂ gangliosides particularly in neurons.

Etiology

These are autosomal recessive genetic disorders. The genetic defects are on chromosome 15 for HEX A, and on chromosome 5 for HEX B and GM₂ activator.

Epidemiology

The diseases are common in the Ashkenazi Jewish population.

Pathophysiology

The biochemical defect may lie in the deficient activity of hexosaminidases A and B (Sandhoff disease), hexosaminidase A alone (Tay-Sachs disease), or absence of an activator protein GM_{2A}.

Clinical Findings

1. In the infantile acute-onset type, affected infants are usually normal at birth. Mild motor weakness begins at 3 to 5 months of age. At that time an exaggerated startle response to sound may be observed.
   a. Developmental delay is evident by 6 to 10 months of age. Vision begins to deteriorate and cherry red spots are seen in the macula.
   b. Seizures develop around 12 months of life. Macrocephaly is secondary to ganglioside accumulation.
   c. Decerebrate posturing, swallowing difficulties, and seizures lead to a vegetative state, and death is due to aspiration pneumonia.
2. In Sandhoff disease, hepatosplenomegaly and skeletal abnormalities with storage cells in the bone marrow and oligosacchariduria occur.
3. Subacute and chronic variants of the disease have been described with dementia, ataxia, seizures, dystonia, psychosis, motor neuron disease, and loss of vision without macular cherry red spots.

Key Clinical Findings: GM₂ Gangliosidosis

- Motor weakness
- Seizures
- Macrocephaly
- Cherry red spot in macula

Laboratory Findings

There are two approaches to the diagnosis: enzymatic and molecular. The activity of the lysosomal enzymes hexosaminidase A and B and the activator protein can be quantitated using leukocytes, cultured skin fibroblasts, or amniocytes. The molecular approach is used to define specific mutations in individual families.

Key Laboratory Finding: GM₂ Gangliosidosis

- Reduced hexosaminidase A and B in cultured fibroblasts

Radiographic Changes

MRI initially shows changes in the cerebral white matter and basal ganglia. Severe brain atrophy is seen in later stages.

Treatment

At present, supportive care, attention to nutrition, treatment of infections, and control of seizures and psychosis are the basis of therapy. Specific treatments are unavailable.

Key Treatment: GM₂ Gangliosidosis

- Supportive

Prevention

The enzymatic and molecular methods are combined to identify carriers in high-risk groups and for prenatal diagnosis.

Gaucher Disease

Definition

A lysosomal glycolipid storage disorder characterized by accumulation of glucocerebroside.

Etiology

The gene for this enzymes lies on chromosome 1q21–31.

Epidemiology

The disease is most common in the Ashkenazi Jewish population.

Pathophysiology

The biochemical defect is the deficiency of glucocerebrosidase.

Clinical Findings

1. Type 1, which is the most common, is distinguished from the other types by the lack of CNS involvement. Symptoms are due to liver and spleen enlargement with functional hypersplenism and bone marrow infiltration by storage cells leading to bone infarctions and fractures.
2. Types 2 and 3 are also known as acute and subacute neuronopathic types, respectively.
   a. Early- and late-onset varieties of type 2 are recognized but the clinical course is similar. The degree of visceral involvement varies. Oculomotor abnormalities with strabismus or apraxia of gaze are initial symptoms. Cherry red spots may be seen. Hypertonia, especially of the neck muscles, rigidity, bulbar signs, seizures, ataxia, and choreoathetosis may occur.
   b. Type 3 disease has a later onset and is less severe than type 2 in terms of neurologic involvement.

Key Clinical Findings: Gaucher Disease

- Hepatosplenomegaly
- Visceral defects, types 2 and 3

Laboratory Findings

1. Leukocyte and cultured skin fibroblasts are used for enzymatic diagnosis. However, enzyme-based diagnosis is not useful in differentiating neuronopathic from nonneuronopathic types.
2. DNA analysis has been used to identify specific mutations.
3. Bone marrow aspiration can demonstrate lipid-engorged cells derived from the monocyte-macrophage system.

Key Laboratory Findings: Gaucher Disease

- Bone marrow shows lipid-engorged cells
- Enzyme analysis in cultured cells

Radiographic Changes

Thinning of long bones may be present.

Treatment

1. Supportive care and general measures include management of bone crises, treatment of infections, splenectomy for hypersplenism, orthopedic treatment with joint replacement, and surveillance for pathologic fractures.
2. Enzyme replacement with intravenous β-glucosidase has been successful in type 1 disease with regression in visceromegaly and decrease in bone pain. The enzyme does not cross the blood-brain barrier.
3. Bone marrow transplantation is associated with 10 to 30 per cent mortality but is followed by a cure when successful in type 1 disease. The role of transplantation in type 3 disease is being studied.
4. Gene therapy using the patient's own hemopoietic cells with a retroviral vector to correct the genetic defect is under investigation.

Key Treatment: Gaucher Disease

- Enzyme replacement for type 1
- Bone marrow transplantation
- Gene therapy? (experimental)

Prevention

Prenatal diagnosis can be carried out.

276 Subacute Sclerosing Panencephalitis

Shanti Thirumalai and *Sakkubai Naidu*

Definition

Subacute sclerosing panencephalitis is a progressive inflammatory disease causing degeneration of both gray and white matter of the entire brain.

Etiology

It is considered to be a chronic infection with the measles virus. Most patients report measles infection in the past. The virus has been isolated from the brains of the patients, and antibody to the virus has been identified in the cerebrospinal fluid.

Epidemiology

The disease is now rarely seen in Western countries following successful immunization against measles, but occasional cases are recognized.

Pathophysiology

Following measles infection during a vulnerable period, infancy, an incompletely effective antibody response occurs. Under these circumstances only part of the measles proteins are destroyed, and the virus finds refuge in the central nervous system (CNS), where it accesses neurons and glia. Here it continues to grow intracellularly and spreads from cell to cell.

Clinical Findings

1. The most common age of presentation is 5 to 15 years, with a range of 6 months to 32 years. Both sexes are equally affected. The disease is stereotyped, with four stages of variable duration.
   a. Stage 1: Onset is often insidious. School failure, personality and behavior changes are usual presenting symptoms.
   b. Stage 2: The diagnosis is usually made at this stage when myoclonus and major motor seizures occur. Involuntary movements reflecting basal ganglia involvement are now seen.
   c. Stage 3: Dementia worsens considerably, with tremor and spasticity becoming evident, indicating destructive changes in the gray and white matter.
   d. Stage 4: The patient is bedridden and vegetative with severe dementia and mutism. Death usually occurs at this stage and may be related to autonomic nervous system failure.
2. Differential diagnosis includes ceroid lipofuscinosis, Tay-Sachs disease, Sandhoff disease, and other conditions that present with dementia and seizures.
3. Progressive rubella panencephalitis following congenital rubella or natural rubella in early life manifests with dementia and cerebellar degeneration and has a slower course. Rubella antibody studies in serum and cerebrospinal fluid are elevated. Retinal abnormalities seen in this disorder are an important differentiating feature.

Key Clinical Findings

- School failure
- Behavioral changes
- Myoclonus
- Seizures

Laboratory Findings

1. Cerebrospinal fluid (CSF) analysis shows elevation of protein, especially of the globulin fraction. Plasmacytosis may be present. Antibody to all major subunits of the measles virion except the M protein is diagnostic.
2. Electroencephalography (EEG) may be normal or reveal mild slowing early in the disease. Classic periodic bursts of high-voltage sharp and slow waves may be seen in stage 2. In stages 3 and 4 the EEG shows disorganization with high-amplitude random arrhythmic slowing. The amplitude decreases with progression of the disease.

Key Laboratory Findings

- CSF
  Elevated protein
  Antibodies to measles virus

Radiographic Changes

1. Computed tomography (CT) scan is useful in the later stages of the disease, reflecting tissue destruction.
2. Magnetic resonance imaging (MRI) demonstrates severe atrophy of the gray matter with compensatory increase in ventricular size.

Treatment

1. Specific treatment is unavailable to date, as no drug has been shown to reverse the disease process. Isoprinosine (Inosiplex) has been tried, alone in a dose of 100 mg/kg/day, and in combination with alpha-interferon given intrathecally or by intraventricular injection. There have been reports of increased survival and decreased disability following treatment.
2. General supportive measures include treatment of seizures, for which clonazepam and valproic acid may be useful. Attention to nutrition, prevention of bedsores, and prevention of aspiration pneumonia are helpful.

Key Treatment

- Supportive

Prevention

Universal immunization against measles will decrease or eliminate the incidence of this disease.

277 Rett Syndrome

Shanti Thirumalai and *Sakkubai Naidu*

Definition

A disorder, primarily involving girls, characterized by a period of normal development followed by loss of developmental skills and associated with characteristic stereotyped hand movements.

Etiology

Although most cases are sporadic, the disease is considered to have a genetic basis because of the involvement of females predominantly, the occurrence of a few familial cases, and concordance in monozygotic twins, with discordance in dizygotic twins.

Epidemiology

Rett syndrome (RS) primarily affects female infants. This disease has been reported worldwide.

Pathophysiology

The underlying pathophysiologic mechanisms are unknown.

Clinical Findings

Diagnosis is based on clinical grounds alone. Birth and antenatal history are normal. Girls with the syndrome go through four stages, not all of which are mandatory.

1. Stage 1. Perinatal to 18 months.
   a. At birth, the patients appear normal and have a normal head circumference. In retrospect there may be a history of colic or poor feeding with irritability in early infancy.
   b. Deceleration of head growth begins between the second and fourth month of life resulting in acquired microcephaly. This insidiously progressive failure of brain growth is often missed by pediatricians as the head circumference is often not measured during well baby visits after 4 months.
   c. There is decreased interest in the environment. Hypotonia may be severe.
   d. The differential diagnosis at this age may include benign infantile hypotonia, cerebral palsy, or Prader-Willi syndrome.
2. Stage 2. Age 1 to 3 years.
   a. Loss of expressive language, developmental regression, loss of hand use, abnormal hand movements, seizures, irritability, and insomnia.
   b. At this stage they may be thought to have hearing loss, autism, childhood psychosis, epileptic encephalopathy, neuronal ceroid lipofuscinosis, or other neurodegenerative disease.
3. Stage 3. Age 2 to 10 years.
   a. Girls with RS at this age appear to be severely mentally retarded, with seizures in a third of the cases, and persistent stereotyped hand movements, typically wringing. A stiff-legged wide-based gait develops in most patients, while others may never walk. A prominent finding is tremulousness. Growth retardation occurs.
   b. Respiratory irregularities are common with hyperventilation, breath-holding, and cyanosis in some cases.
   c. The child at this age may be misdiagnosed with Angelman syndrome, spinocerebellar degeneration, or ataxic cerebral palsy.
4. Stage 4. After age 10 years.
   a. Progressive scoliosis, distal muscle wasting, and trophic disturbances of the extremities are noted. Some patients with decreasing mobility become wheelchair-bound.
   b. Seizures and respiratory abnormalities ameliorate. Social interaction improves, and there may be small gains in hand use.

Key Clinical Findings

- Mostly girls
- Infancy
  Failure of head growth
  Irritability
- Toddler
  Hypotonia
  Regression of language and cerebration
- Child
  Mental retardation
  Seizures
- Stereotypic hand movements

Laboratory Findings

No specific findings are present.

Radiographic Changes

Magnetic resonance imaging (MRI) studies show a decrease in brain volume, and slight increase in the size of the ventricles.

Treatment

1. Specific treatment is not available.
2. RS patients have increased caloric requirements for the excessive energy requirements from abnormal movements.
3. Physical, occupational, and speech therapies may be useful. Simple communication devices can be used by some children despite limited hand use.
4. Treatment of seizures is effective using standard anticonvulsants.
5. Sleep and behavioral disturbances are often difficult to manage.

6. Constipation can be severe and requires the use of large amounts of mineral oil, stool softeners, and a high-fiber diet.
7. Orthopedic intervention for contractures and scoliosis is essential. Children should be encouraged to ambulate.
8. Most patients survive to adulthood. There is an increased risk of sudden death in sleep in the first two decades of life that is unexplained.

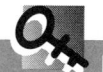

Key Treatment

• Supportive

Prevention

No preventive strategies are available.

278 Spinal Cord Disorders with Late Onset

Gerald S. Golden

Definition

A group of congenital malformations of the spinal cord or spinal canal that do not present clinically until after infancy.

1. In diastematomyelia the lower thoracic or lumbar spinal cord is split by a septum of mesoderm that may become calcified. There are usually vertebral abnormalities in the same region.
2. Syringomyelia is a cavity within the spinal cord that progressively enlarges. It may extend into the medulla.
3. The tethered cord syndrome results from fixation of the sacral end of the spinal cord, which prevents normal cephalic migration with longitudinal growth of the spine.

Etiology

The etiology of these disorders is not clear. One theory proposes that diastematomyelia and syringomyelia result from intrauterine hydrocephalus; diastematomyelia is caused when the lower end of the cord ruptures. Tethered cord syndrome can be primary or can be secondary to fixation of the cord resulting from any form of myelodysplasia.

Epidemiology

These are uncommon conditions. Except for the genetic and environmental factors that increase the risk of myelodysplasia, no specific risk factors are known.

Pathophysiology

1. Splitting of the spinal cord during early development can interfere with sensory tracts that cross at that level, producing sensory deficits below the level of the lesion. Abnormal development of anterior horn cells and the corticospinal tracts can cause weakness. As the child grows, the septum fixing the cord in place can also produce a tethered cord syndrome.
2. Syringomyelia also disrupts crossing fibers at the level of the lesion and interferes with the function of descending long tracts. Clinical manifestations progress as the cavity expands.
3. A tethered cord has its effect when longitudinal growth of the spine occurs. Progressive traction on the spinal cord can affect both motor and sensory function.

Clinical Findings

1. The child with diastematomyelia may have no clinical abnormalities at birth, but talipes equinovarus is sometimes present. Symptoms are progressive, especially during periods of rapid growth.
   a. Weakness of the legs with muscle atrophy is the most common presenting complaint. This is most pronounced distally. Deep tendon reflexes are decreased or absent.
   b. Areas of anesthesia below the level of the lesion are common.
   c. An atonic bladder may develop as symptoms progress.
   d. Some children have cutaneous abnormalities, such as areas of hypertrichosis or angiomas, on the back in the region of the lesion.
2. Syringomyelia is also a progressive disorder, with clinical onset usually delayed until the late adolescent or early adult years. Most patients have a rather typical clinical picture.
   a. Weakness with atrophy and fasciculations of muscles in the hands occur early. Other muscle groups in the upper extremities then become involved. Findings are typically symmetric.
   b. Loss of sensation in a "shawl" distribution is typical. Trophic ulcers may develop on the fingers.
   c. Spasticity of the lower extremities occurs as the lesion progresses. This may be accompanied by a neurogenic bladder.
3. Symptoms of a tethered cord are similar to those of diastematomyelia. Weakness is more prominent than sensory abnormalities.

Key Clinical Findings

• Weakness and atrophy of legs

• Atonic bladder

Laboratory Findings

1. No routine laboratory abnormalities are useful in diagnosis.
2. Electromyography, nerve conduction studies, and sensory evoked potentials are helpful in determining the level and extent of neurologic dysfunction.
3. Urodynamic studies are indicated if there is evidence of bladder dysfunction.

Key Laboratory Test

- Electromyography for determining level

Radiographic Changes

1. Magnetic resonance imaging (MRI) of the spine is the most useful diagnostic modality in these disorders.
   a. The septum in diastematomyelia is easily visualized. If it is calcified, it can also be seen on standard radiographs of the spine.
   b. Spinal MRI is a very sensitive tool for demonstrating the cavity in syringomyelia. The ability to obtain longitudinal views allows the extent of the cavity to be determined.
   c. The major finding in tethered cord syndrome is that the caudal end of the cord has not migrated upwards to its expected level. An underlying abnormality, such as an intradural lipoma, may also be seen.
2. Voiding cystourethography may be part of the evaluation of the child with a neurogenic bladder.

Treatment

1. Surgical removal of the septum in diastematomyelia may prevent further progression of symptoms, but will not correct abnormalities that are already present.
2. Although opening and draining the intramedullary cyst in syringomyelia is intuitively obvious, symptoms continue to progress in many patients.
3. Attempts to surgically free the caudal portion of the spinal cord in the tethered cord syndrome also are not always effective in preventing progression of symptoms.

Key Treatment

- Surgery—some relief; may halt progression

Prevention

There are no useful preventive strategies in the absence of known causative agents.

Bibliography

Farley FA, Song KM, Birch JG, Browne R: Syringomyelia and scoliosis in children. J Pediatr Orthoped 1995;15:187–192.

Miller A, Guille JT, Bowen JR: Evaluation and treatment of diastematomyelia. J Bone Joint Surg 1993;75:1308–1317.

Satar N, Bauer SB, Shefner J, et al: The effects of delayed diagnosis and treatment in patients with occult spinal dysraphism. J Urol 1995;154:754–758.

279 Cerebral Palsy

Barry Russman

Definition

Cerebral palsy (CP) is characterized by aberrant control of movement or posture of a patient, appearing early in life (secondary to a central nervous system lesion, damage, or dysfunction), and not the result of a recognized progressive or degenerative brain disease.

Etiology

1. Etiology is generally difficult to determine. Most often only risk factors can be identified; the majority of children born with known risk factors, however, will not develop CP. More than half the children with CP in the National Collaborative Perinatal Project (NCPP) population were born at term. Of these children, 85 per cent were appropriate for gestational age and 15 per cent were small for gestational age.
2. Although only 10 per cent of the children with CP weighed less than 1500 grams at birth, the risk of developing CP in this group was found to be extremely high (90 per 1000). This compared with 3 per 1000 children who were born appropriate for gestational age and weighed more than 2500 grams.
3. Twelve per cent developed CP as a result of a postnatal event.

Epidemiology

Three per 1000 of those who participated in the NCPP had CP; 32 per cent had diplegia; 29 per cent had hemiplegia; 24 per cent quadriplegia; and 14 per cent had either dyskinesia or ataxia.

Pathophysiology

1. In some instances, it is possible to establish a specific etiology of CP, namely genetic syndromes, congenital malformations, and in utero or perinatal central nervous system infections.
2. Identified risk factors include the following:
   a. Prenatal events
      (1) Maternal mental retardation, epilepsy, and hy-

perthyroidism prior to the pregnancy are associated with the development of CP in the child.

(2) Problems during pregnancy identified as risk factors associated with CP include severe toxemia and incompetent cervix, when associated with premature birth. Third trimester bleeding, but not first or second trimester bleeding, is also a risk factor.

(3) Kidney and bladder infections, radiation exposure, and hyperemesis gravidarum are not associated with increased risk of CP. Level of maternal education, marital status, parity, paternal age, pregnancy spacing, smoking history, intercourse frequency, history of maternal diabetes, and the length of time to become pregnant are not risk factors.

b. Perinatal events

(1) Risk factors identified during the labor and delivery include vaginal bleeding at the time of admission and placental complications such as abruption, premature rupture of the membranes, chorionitis, and breech presentation.

(2) Many of these risk factors are significant only if a baby weighed less than 2500 grams at birth. In addition, some of the risk factors, such as oxytocin augmentation, cord prolapse, or breech delivery, were relevant only if they were associated with low Apgar scores.

c. Perinatal asphyxia. Freeman and Nelson suggest that four questions must be answered in the affirmative if perinatal asphyxia is thought to be the cause of CP:

(1) Was there evidence of marked and prolonged intrapartum asphyxia?

(2) Did the newborn exhibit signs of moderate or severe hypoxic-ischemic encephalopathy?

(3) Is the neurologic condition one that intrapartum asphyxia could explain?

(4) Has the clinical evaluation been extensive enough to exclude other conditions?

d. Risk factors and type of CP

(1) Children with spastic diplegia were almost universally appropriate for gestational age; 55 per cent were born preterm.

(2) The dyskinetic syndromes are most likely to occur with perinatal risk factors such as asphyxia and hyperbilirubinemia.

Clinical Findings

1. The child must have an obvious motor deficit for the diagnosis of CP to be considered. The chief complaint usually is that the child is not reaching motor milestones at the normal time. The history must establish that the child is not losing function, providing assurance that the patient does not have a progressive disease.

2. Physical and neurologic examinations

a. CP is easily diagnosed in a child who is not developing motor skills, whose muscle tone is generally increased, and who is not regressing. However, a common diagnostic problem is presented by the child who is not developing normally and who has normal or decreased muscle tone.

b. Persistent primitive reflexes, or the lack of development of the protective reflexes at the expected time, are important findings on the neurologic examination, suggesting corticospinal tract impairment.

(1) Moro reflex should be unobtainable after 6 months of age.

(2) The asymmetric tonic neck response should never be obligatory when the patient is placed in the appropriate position; that is, the infant should "break" the tonic neck posture spontaneously after 15 to 30 seconds, and it should be unobtainable after 6 months of age.

(3) The side protective reflexes should be evident after 5 months of age.

(4) The parachute reflex is typically obtained after 10 months of age.

(5) A child should not cross the midline when reaching for an object until after 1 year of age and should not show clear hand preference on examination until 18 to 24 months of age. The development of handedness prior to this time suggests a hemiplegia or a brachial plexus injury.

3. Common health problems

a. Drooling may be responsible for severe skin irritation, but of greater significance is its unpleasant cosmetic effect.

b. Poor nutrition also may be a major problem.

c. Bladder dysfunction is more frequent than in the uninvolved population. Surveillance should lead to recognition of problems of practical importance to the patient and family.

d. Constipation is a problem that must be monitored by the physician. Presumably, this problem occurs as a result of the patient's inability to control the abdominal muscles that provide the propulsion for the stool. Symptomatic treatment must be provided.

Key Clinical Findings

- Motor deficit
- Usually normal intelligence

Laboratory Findings

Laboratory tests are not necessary to confirm the diagnosis. However, they can occasionally be helpful to establish an etiology and suggest a prognosis.

Radiographic Changes

1. Computed tomography (CT) scans of the head are frequently abnormal, the most common finding being cortical atrophy. A correlation between the severity of the anatomic abnormality as determined by CT scan and the extent of the motor disability, cognitive deficits, and the presence of epilepsy has been demonstrated.

2. Ultrasonography can be utilized in infants whose anterior fontanelle is still open. Periventricular cysts, which are

usually preceded by echodense lesions, when larger than 3 mm, are predictive of future CP.

Treatment

1. Evaluate the associated problems: Epilepsy, mental retardation, learning disabilities, vision difficulties, strabismus, dysarthria, and hearing loss occur with higher frequency in the CP population compared with control groups.

   a. A number of methods have been used to reduce drooling.

      (1) Anticholinergic medication, in addition to the unpleasant side effects, has not been effective.

      (2) Surgical intervention, including reposition of the salivary ducts and dividing the chorda tympani, has sometimes been effective.

      (3) Behavior modification programs to help the individual control drooling have been effective.

   b. Either tube feeding or gastrostomy feeding resulted in a significant increase in weight gain and, in some patients, a significant increase in height.

2. Treatment protocol for spastic CP

   a. Avoid surgery to improve ambulation until after the gait has matured. A program of physical therapy should be started early in conjunction with a good home maintenance program. Various modalities that alter muscle tone may be attempted, including medication, selective posterior rhizotomy, and botulinum toxin.

   b. When the gait is mature, usually sometime between the age of 6 and 10, perform gait analysis. Utilize these data in conjunction with the clinical examination to determine an appropriate course of treatment. This is usually some combination of surgery and orthotics.

   c. If surgery is elected, try to avoid staging. Lengthen and/or transfer all muscles necessary to obtain balance during the course of a single surgical procedure.

   d. Following surgery, minimize casting and remobilize the patient rapidly. Maintain an active physical therapy program as long as the gait is improving, usually at about 12 months. Prevent recurrence of contractures throughout the remaining years of growth with appropriate night splinting and a good home maintenance program designed to adequately stretch tight musculature.

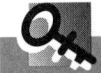

Key Treatment

- Individualized to nature and extent of disability

Prevention

1. Low birth weight babies account for the greatest number of patients with CP. In a review of intraventricular hemorrhage and the use of phenobarbital to prevent this phenomenon, Kuban and associates[2] noted that the incidence of CP in those mothers who were toxemic and had received magnesium sulfate was less than that of a comparable group.

2. Nelson found that only 7.1 per cent of preterm mothers receiving magnesium sulfate gave birth to babies who developed CP as opposed to 30 per cent who did not receive magnesium sulfate.

Bibliography

1. Freeman JM, Nelson KB: Intrapartum asphyxia and CP. Pediatrics 1988;82:240–249.
2. Kuban KCK, Leviton A, Pagano M, et al: Maternal toxemia is associated with reduced incidence of germinal matrix hemorrhage in premature babies. J Child Neurol 1992;7:70–75.
3. Nelson KB, Ellenberg JH. Antecedents of CP. Univariate analysis of risks. Am J Dis Child 1985;139:1031–1038.
4. Nelson KB, Ellenberg JH. Epidemiology of CP. Adv Neurol 1978;19:421–435.
5. Nelson KB, Grether JK. Can magnesium sulfate reduce the risk of CP in very low birthweight infants? Pediatrics 1995; 95(2):263–269.

280 Neurofibromatosis

Gerald S. Golden

Definition

A heritable multisystem disorder with characteristic skin lesions, bony abnormalities, and specific types of tumors. Neurofibromatosis-1 (NF-1, von Recklinghausen disease) manifests this typical picture. Abnormalities in neurofibromatosis-2 (NF-2) are generally restricted to the eighth cranial nerve.

Etiology

NF-1 is inherited as an autosomal dominant condition, with the abnormal gene locus on chromosome 17. NF-2 is also an autosomal dominant trait, with the mutation at a locus on chromosome 22.

Epidemiology

The incidence of NF-1 is 1 in 3000. Approximately one half of cases represent new mutations. The prevalence of NF-2 is 1 in 50,000.

Pathophysiology

1. The primary abnormality is in migration of neural crest cells during embryonic development, although the mecha-

nism linking the gene mutation to this abnormality has not been defined.

2. Abnormal growth of Schwann cells or the peripheral nerves, cranial nerves, and nerve roots produces tumors involving the peripheral and autonomic nervous systems. Tumors located on nerve roots can cause spinal cord compression. Plexiform neuromas typically involve the orbit, but can be located in other regions.

3. There is also an increased incidence of tumors of the central nervous system and nonneural tumors such as Wilms tumor and hematologic malignancies. The pathophysiology of these tumors is not clear, as the neoplasms do not have a Schwann cell origin.

Clinical Findings

1. NF-1 is characterized by:
   a. Six or more café-au-lait spots, greater than 5 mm in diameter in children and greater than 15 mm in diameter in adults
   b. Freckling in the axillary and inguinal areas
   c. A plexiform neuroma or two or more neurofibromas
   d. Other features including:
      (1) Optic glioma
      (2) Iris hamartomas (Lisch nodules)
      (3) Sphenoid dysplasia or other bony abnormalities
   e. A family history of NF-1
2. NF-2 is characterized by:
   a. Bilateral tumors of the eighth cranial nerve
   b. A family history of NF-2
3. The incidence of mental retardation is increased over that in the general population. Approximately one half of the patients with neurofibromatosis have learning disabilities.
4. Hypertension may result from renal artery stenosis.

Key Clinical Findings

- Café-au-lait spots
- Axillary and inguinal freckling
- Neurofibromas and plexiform neuromas
- Optic gliomas
- Iris hamartomas (Lisch nodules)
- Bone lesions
- Family history

Laboratory Findings

There are no specific laboratory abnormalities.

Radiographic Changes

1. Magnetic resonance imaging (MRI) is the most important technique for demonstrating tumors impinging on or arising from the spinal cord, brain tumors, optic gliomas, and acoustic nerve schwannomas.
2. Radiographs of the skull may demonstrate a number of developmental abnormalities of bone such as an abnormal or absent sphenoid wing, enlarged cranial nerve foramina, and a J-shaped sella turcica.
3. Spine radiographs may demonstrate enlargement of intervertebral foramina and more obvious changes such as anterior meningocele.
4. Long bones may have areas of decreased density or fractures and pseudoarthroses.
5. Renal vascular studies may demonstrate renal artery stenosis in the patient with hypertension.

Treatment

1. Treatment of neurofibromas of the peripheral nervous system is rarely required.
2. Acoustic nerve schwannomas should be removed surgically. Early diagnosis and microsurgical techniques often allow sparing of hearing and facial nerve function on the affected side.
3. The approach to treatment of optic gliomas is controversial. Growth may be slow with little or no progressive loss of function. The appropriate use of surgery or radiation therapy, and the timing of these procedures, is not clear.
4. Spinal nerve root tumors compressing the spinal cord can be removed surgically. Many patients have multiple nerve root involvement, however, and surgery is restricted to those lesions that clearly impinge on the spinal cord and produce a functional deficit.
5. Other brain tumors are treated appropriately, based on their histology and location.
6. Plastic surgery may be useful for patients with plexiform neuromas of the face or orbit. The roof of the orbit may be absent, causing a pulsating enophthalmos. The orbital abnormality can be surgically repaired.
7. Surgical repair of the renal artery, if stenosis is present, can relieve hypertension in some patients.

Key Treatment

- Usually none
- Removal of acoustic neuroma
- Plastic surgery for functional and cosmetic reasons
- Renal artery repair if indicated

Prevention

The only prevention tool currently available is genetic counseling. Both NF-1 and NF-2 are autosomal dominant traits, although approximately one half of cases of NF-1 appear to result from a new mutation.

Bibliography

Hoffman KJ, Harris EL, Bryan RN, Denckla MBL: Neurofibromatosis type 1: the cognitive phenotype. J Pediatr 1994;124:S1–S8.

Martuza RL, Eldridge R: Neurofibromatosis 2 (bilateral acoustic neurofibromatosis). N Engl J Med 1988;318:684–688.

National Institutes of Health Consensus Development Conference: Neurofibromatosis conference statement. Arch Neurol 1988;45:575–578.

281 Tuberous Sclerosis

Gerald S. Golden

Definition

A hereditary disorder characterized by the triad of a seizure disorder, mental retardation, and angiofibromas (adenoma sebaceum) of the face.

Etiology

Transmission is as an autosomal dominant condition, but linkage studies have failed to consistently implicate a specific locus. A broad range of clinical manifestations may be seen in a single affected family.

Epidemiology

This is a rare disorder, with an incidence of 1 in 10,000.

Pathophysiology

1. The mechanistic link between the abnormal gene and the clinical manifestations has not been determined.
2. Abnormalities in brain structure include abnormal neurons and glia, abnormal organization of some areas of cerebral cortex, and areas of demyelination. These changes correlate with the seizure disorder and mental retardation.
3. Tuberous sclerosis may involve many other organ systems. No single pathophysiologic mechanism has been defined.

Clinical Findings

1. The most common initial presentation is with seizures, most commonly infantile spasms, in infancy. After the first year of life a changing seizure pattern is common, and the Lennox-Gastaut syndrome, with a mixed seizure pattern that is difficult to control with medication, is a frequent outcome.
2. A number of characteristic skin lesions may be present:
   a. Hypopigmented areas, often with an "ash-leaf" shape, are the most common lesion present at birth and in the preschool years.
   b. Angiofibromas (adenoma sebaceum) appear during the preschool years. These are reddish acneiform papules in a butterfly distribution on the face. They do not have the comedones that are part of acne.
   c. Less common skin lesions include the leathery shagreen patch in the lumbar region and subungual and periungual fibromas.
3. The majority of patients have mental retardation which can vary widely in severity. Virtually every patient with a seizure disorder also is mentally retarded.
4. Other organs are involved in a minority of patients. These include
   a. Cardiac rhabdomyomas
   b. Renal angiomyolipomas or renal cysts
   c. Pulmonary cysts
   d. Retinal tumors

Key Clinical Findings

- Seizure disorder, especially infantile spasms or Lennox-Gastaut syndrome
- Mental retardation
- Skin lesions, especially hypopigmented macules and facial angiofibromas
- Tumors of heart or kidneys

Laboratory Findings

1. Electroencephalography (EEG) assists in making a specific diagnosis of the epileptic syndrome in patients with seizures. The patterns consistent with infantile spasms or Lennox-Gastaut syndrome are most common.
2. Ultrasonography will help define cardiac or renal tumors if they are present.

Key Laboratory Findings

- EEG often shows Lennox-Gastaut
- Ultrasonography of chest and kidneys

Radiographic Changes

1. Characteristic features on neuroimaging studies provide important diagnostic information. MRI and CT studies are complementary; MRI is a more sensitive tool, but CT is better at delineating areas of calcification which are commonly present. The most typical findings are
   a. Calcified and noncalcified subependymal nodules
   b. Areas of abnormal myelination in the white matter; these areas sometimes calcify.
2. MRI and CT scans are useful in the diagnosis of cardiac and renal tumors.
3. Pulmonary cysts can be seen on radiographs of the chest.
4. A number of bony abnormalities have been reported, and can be demonstrated by appropriate X-ray studies. These include cystic and sclerotic areas in the ribs, hands, and feet.

Treatment

1. The most difficult aspect of management is treatment of the seizure disorder, which often does not improve with the use of the major antiepileptic drugs. (See section on Seizure Disorders.)
2. The child with mental retardation should receive the full spectrum of educational services appropriate for the level of function.
3. Cosmetic surgery should be considered for the patient

with disfiguring facial angiofibromas, especially if the individual has a relatively high level of cognitive function and independence.

4. The patient with renal abnormalities should be monitored regularly for the development of hypertension or progressive impairment of renal function. If these complications occur, appropriate treatment can be instituted.

Key Treatment

- Control seizures

Prevention

The only tool for prevention is genetic counseling. Because of the wide spectrum of severity of the findings, if neither parent appears to be clinically affected they should still be evaluated fully before counseling is provided. Appropriate studies include inspection of the skin for characteristic lesions, fundoscopic examination, and a CT scan or MRI of the brain. Electroencephalography is not useful if there is no history of a seizure disorder or other findings raising the suspicion of tuberous sclerosis. If there is hypertension or impairment of renal function, renal ultrasonography should be obtained. Cardiac ultrasonography is appropriate if there is a history of a cardiac arrhythmia.

Bibliography

Fitzpatrick TB: History and significance of white macules, earliest visual sign of tuberous sclerosis. Ann NY Acad Sci 1991; 615:26–35.

Gomez MR, Kuntz NL, Westmoreland BF: Tuberous sclerosis, early onset of seizures, and mental subnormality: Study of discordant homozygous twins. Neurology 1982;32:604–611.

Roach ES, Kerr J, Mendelsohn D, et al: Detection of tuberous sclerosis in parents by magnetic resonance imaging. Neurology 1991;41:262–265.

Roach ES, Smith M, Huttenlocher P, et al: Diagnostic criteria—tuberous sclerosis. J Child Neurol 1992;7:221–224.

282 Sturge-Weber Syndrome

Gerald S. Golden

Definition

A syndrome defined by a facial angioma (port-wine stain), hemiparesis, and seizures. Mental retardation is present in approximately one half of patients.

Etiology

The etiology of the underlying vascular and cerebral abnormalities is not well understood. The condition appears to be sporadic, rather than inherited.

Epidemiology

The incidence has been stated to be 1 in 50,000, but mild forms of the condition are probably more common but unrecognized clinically.

Pathophysiology

1. Abnormal vasculature is present in the leptomeninges of the affected area. Abnormal blood vessels are also present in brain underlying these areas, and there is calcification in cerebral cortex. The pathophysiologic chain of events leading to these changes is unknown.

2. The facial angioma invariably involves the area innervated by the first division of the trigeminal nerve; there may also be involvement of the second and third divisions of this nerve. This distribution may be unrelated to the morphogenesis of the nerve, however, but may be a result of abnormalities in the development of the other structures in the facial region.

Clinical Findings

1. The facial angioma (port-wine stain) is present at birth. In addition to cutaneous involvement, the angioma may be found on the buccal mucosa, tongue, palate, and pharynx. Not every child with a facial angioma has Sturge-Weber syndrome.

2. Hemiparesis contralateral to the side involved by the angioma is the most common neurologic abnormality. Hemianopsia may also be present. Poor growth of the affected limbs is common. Bilateral involvement can occur.

3. Seizures of all types can occur, although simple and complex partial seizures are most common.

4. Glaucoma is common if the eye is involved by the angioma.

Key Clinical Findings

- Facial port-wine stain
- Contralateral hemiparesis
- Seizure disorder
- Glaucoma

Laboratory Findings

1. Electroencephalography may assist in defining the specific epileptic syndrome.

2. Intraocular pressure of both eyes should be monitored regularly.

Radiographic Changes

1. Skull radiographs reveal a characteristic "railroad track" pattern of parallel linear calcifications outlining cerebral convolutions.
2. Neuroimaging studies such as MRI and CT scans provide more discrete definition of the calcifications and demonstrate underlying brain abnormalities.
3. Cerebral angiography may provide important information if surgical treatment of the seizures is planned.

Treatment

1. The primary treatment problem is management of the seizures. If treatment with antiepileptic drugs does not provide adequate control, surgical removal of the affected areas of brain may be useful.
2. The hemiparesis should be treated with the same approaches used for any child with a congenital motor deficit.
3. If glaucoma is present, referral for specialized treatment is appropriate.
4. The psychosocial stigma of the facial angioma can be minimized by laser treatment of the angioma or properly used make-up.

Key Treatment

- Control seizures

Prevention

Sturge-Weber syndrome is not genetic and no predisposing factors have been defined, so there are no useful preventive strategies.

Bibliography

Bebin EM, Gomez MR: Prognosis of Sturge-Weber syndrome: comparison of unihemispheric and bihemispheric involvement. J Child Neurol 1988;3:181–184.

Sperner J, Schmauser I, Bittner R, et al: MR-imaging findings in children with Sturge-Weber syndrome. Neuropediatrics 1990; 21:146–152.

Tallman B, Tan OT, Morelli JG, et al. Location of port-wine stains and the likelihood of ophthalmic and/or central nervous system complications. Pediatrics 1991;87:323–327.

283 Von Hippel–Lindau Disease

Gerald S. Golden

Definition

A condition characterized by hemangioblastomas of the retina and cerebellum. Commonly associated abnormalities include angiomas of the spinal cord and cystic tumors of other organs.

Etiology

The condition is transmitted as an autosomal dominant trait.

Epidemiology

The condition is rare. The incidence is difficult to determine as many patients have a partial syndrome or are never recognized clinically.

Pathophysiology

The pathophysiologic mechanisms have not been defined.

Clinical Findings

1. Vascular retinal tumors are the most characteristic manifestation.
2. Hemangioblastomas of the cerebellum present as would any progressive cerebellar mass lesions. Some of these patients have polycythemia, which resolves when the cerebellar tumor is removed.
3. Other lesions include cysts of internal organs, especially the pancreas, liver, and epididymis; renal tumors; and pheochromocytomas.

Key Clinical Finding

- Vascular retinal tumors

Laboratory Findings

1. Polycythemia is present in some patients with cerebellar hemangioblastomas.
2. Studies of catecholamines and catecholamine metabolites are appropriate if pheochromocytoma is suspected.

Key Laboratory Findings

- Polycythemia
- Catecholamine studies for pheochromocytoma

Radiographic Changes

Magnetic resonance imaging (MRI) studies of the brain will demonstrate the cerebellar tumor, if present.

Treatment

1. Total removal of the cerebellar tumor is curative.
2. Vascular tumors of the retina can be treated with laser coagulation.

Key Treatment

• Surgery for cerebellar tumor
• Laser coagulation for retina

Prevention

Genetic counseling for families of affected individuals is appropriate.

Bibliography

Choyke PL, Glenn GM, Partonas NJ, et al: Von Hippel-Lindau disease: genetic, clinical, and imaging features. Radiology 1995;194:629–642.

Karsdorp N, Elderson A, Wittebol-Post D, et al: Von Hippel-Lindau disease: new strategies in early detection and treatment. Am J Med 1994;97:158–168.

284 Cerebrovascular Disorders

David L. Coulter

Definition

A stroke is a disorder causing a structural or functional abnormality resulting from transient or permanent decrease of blood flow to an area of the central nervous system.

Etiology

See Table 284–1.

Epidemiology

The incidence and prevalence of stroke reflects the etiologic disorders in the population at risk.

Pathogenesis

1. Stroke is an abrupt alteration in neurologic function caused by one of two mechanisms:
   a. Interrupted blood supply to a part of the brain resulting in ischemic tissue injury and infarction.
   b. Brain hemorrhage resulting in disruption of tissue integrity, mass effect with ischemic compression of brain, or secondary vasospasm.
2. Neuronal injury and death is likely due to disturbances in calcium metabolism, increased excitatory amino acid activity, and/or generation of toxic free radicals.

Clinical Findings

1. The patient presents with an abrupt onset of focal neurologic signs, which may persist for a variable period of time.
   a. If the neurologic examination becomes normal within 24 hours, the episode may have been a transient ischemic attack (TIA). Neuroimaging shows no permanent brain damage after a TIA.
   b. If the neurologic signs persist for more than 24 hours, or if neuroimaging shows evidence of permanent brain damage, the episode can be considered to be a stroke.
2. Abrupt loss of consciousness with focal neurologic signs is more likely to be a hemorrhage than an ischemic infarction.

Key Clinical Finding

• Abrupt onset of focal neurologic deficits

Laboratory Findings

Specific laboratory studies should be obtained based on the history, examination, and neuroimaging studies; most likely etiologies are given in Table 284–1. The diagnostic work-up should be guided by the specific differential diagnosis in each case and thus will be different in each case.

Radiographic Changes

1. Neuroimaging (CT or MRI) is indicated if the clinical presentation suggests a TIA or stroke.
2. CT with contrast enhancement is helpful for detecting vascular malformations and other etiologies.
3. Magnetic resonance arteriography (MRA) and magnetic resonance venography (MRV) are additional procedures that can be done easily in conjunction with MRI and can confirm the existence of vascular defects or anomalies.
4. Invasive arteriography has greater risk than CT or MRI but may be indicated in selected cases.

Treatment

1. General supportive measures include attention to systemic factors such as ventilation, circulation, nutrition, and fluid management.
2. Treatment of increased intracranial pressure may be indicated (see chapter on Increased Intracranial Pressure).
3. If a specific etiology is present (such as sickle cell disease or hypertension), specific treatment for that etiology may be indicated.
4. Experimental "neuroprotective" treatment strategies to

TABLE 284–1. CAUSES OF STROKE IN CHILDREN

CATEGORY	EXAMPLE	CATEGORY	EXAMPLE
Congenital heart disease	Atrial septal defect	Inborn metabolic errors	Mitochondrial disorders
	Ventricular septal defect		Homocystinuria
	Mitral valve prolapse		Propionic aciduria
	Mitral stenosis		Methylmalonic aciduria
	Coarctation of the aorta		Isovaleric acidemia
	Patent ductus arteriosus	Hematologic disorders	Hemoglobinopathies
Acquired heart disease	Cardiac rhabdomyoma		Coagulation defects
	Atrial myxoma		Polycythemia
	Bacterial endocarditis		Thrombocytosis
	Myocarditis		Leukemia
	Rheumatic heart disease		Anticardiolipin antibody
	Arrhythmia		Antithrombin III antibody
	Prosthetic heart valve		Antiphospholipid antibody
Systemic vascular disease	Familial hypercholesterolemia		Protein C deficiency
	Progeria		Protein S deficiency
	Diabetes mellitus	Vascular anomalies	Arteriovenous malformation
	Hypertension		Cerebral aneurysm
	Hypernatremic dehydration		Sturge-Weber syndrome
Vasculitis	Systemic lupus erythematosus		Fibromuscular dysplasia
	Polyarteritis nodosa	Traumatic disorders	Traumatic brain injury
	Kawasaki disease		Vascular injury (oral trauma)
	Takayasu disease		Arterial dissection syndrome
	Cerebral angiitis		Fat or air embolism
	Dermatomyositis	Medical complications	Arterial catheterization
	Inflammatory bowel disease		Open heart surgery
	Meningoencephalitis		Cranial irradiation
	Substance abuse (e.g., cocaine)		Status epilepticus
	Acquired immunodeficiency syndrome (AIDS)	Idiopathic	Acute infantile hemiplegia
Other vasculopathies	Fabry disease		Other
	Moya-Moya syndrome		
	Neurofibromatosis (NF-1)		
	Alternating hemiplegia		
	Vasospasm (from subarachnoid hemorrhage)		
	Hemiplegic migraine		

counteract calcium-mediated injury, excitotoxic injury, or free radical toxicity may become available in the future.

Key Treatment

• Supportive

• Management of underlying disorder

Prevention

Preventative strategies are based on minimizing the potential etiologic factors.

Bibliography

Aicardi J: Cerebrovascular disorders. *In* Aicardi J (ed): Diseases of the Nervous System in Childhood. New York, Cambridge University Press, 1992, pp 850–908.

Golden GS: Cerebrovascular disease. *In* Swaiman KF (ed): Pediatric Neurology: Principles and Practice. St Louis, CV Mosby, 1989, pp 603–617.

Hund E, Grau A, Hacke W: Neurocritical care for acute ischemic stroke. Neurol Clin 1995;13:511–527.

Roach ES, Riela AR: Pediatric Cerebrovascular Disorders, 2nd ed. New York, Futura, 1995.

Solomon GE: Acute therapy of childhood stroke. *In* Pellock JM, Myer EC (eds): Neurologic Emergencies in Infancy and Childhood, 2nd ed. Boston, Butterworth-Heinemann, 1993, pp 179–207.

285 Muscular Dystrophies

Barry Russman

Duchenne Muscular Dystrophy

Definition

1. The muscular dystrophies are a group of degenerative genetic disorders that have similar histologic appearances. They are classified by the age of onset, clinical picture, and course of the disease. The identification of the gene defect associated with each of the dystrophies will allow the diagnosis to be made more easily, provide insight into the pathophysiology of the disease, and hopefully lead to definitive treatments (Table 285–1).
2. Duchenne muscular dystrophy (DMD) is the most common form presenting in childhood.
3. Becker muscular dystrophy (BMD) is an allelic form of DMD, and is characterized by later onset and slower progression of symptoms.

Etiology

The gene defect is located at the p21 location on the X chromosome.

Epidemiology

The incidence of DMD is one per 3000 live male births. BMD occurs in 3 to 6 per 100,000 live male births. This figure will change as more patients with onset of weakness after age 5 years receive diagnoses with the DNA deletion test and the application of dystrophin analysis of muscle tissue. Heretofore, many of these patients have been placed in the limb-girdle muscular dystrophy category.

Pathophysiology

The majority of the molecular deletions are single or multiple exon deletions. Most of the boys have an absence of dystrophin as determined by immunoelectrophoresis of Western blot analysis of the muscle tissue corresponding to an out-of-frame exon or multiple exon deletion so that there is a disruption of normal dystrophin translation. How this lack of dystrophin is associated with muscle deterioration is unknown.

Clinical Findings

1. Early motor development is usually normal or minimally delayed. At age 3 to 4 years, the child will demonstrate difficulty in climbing stairs and will begin to "fall frequently."
2. The examination shows weakness primarily in the hip area as manifested by the need to use the Gower maneuver to rise from the floor to the standing position. When placed in a prone position, the child rolls on to his stomach, gets up on his hands and knees and then hands and feet, and "walks up" his legs with his arms to enable him to bring his trunk erect.
3. Typically, the patients lose ability to walk between ages 10 and 12 years, and life expectancy is approximately 20 years, give or take 2 to 3 years. Eighty per cent will

die from respiratory failure and about 20 per cent from cardiac failure.
4. In BMD the weakness typically starts in the latter part of the first decade of life. The patients are ambulatory until about age 20 years and life expectancy is about age 35.

Key Clinical Findings:
Duchenne Muscular Dystrophy

- Frequent falls
- Cannot climb stairs
- "Walks up" legs

Laboratory Findings

1. The creatine kinase (CK) level is elevated to at least 10 to 20 times above normal, even at birth. If the CK is only 1 to 2 times above normal, it is highly unlikely that DMD is responsible for the motor deficit.
2. The electromyogram (EMG), which is not required for diagnosis, will show myopathic potentials.
3. The muscle biopsy shows a variation in muscle fiber size, internal nuclei in approximately 20 per cent of the muscle fibers, necrosis, and an abnormal amount of connective tissue.
4. DNA deletion studies should be performed and will be abnormal in 70 per cent.
5. Dystrophin analysis of muscle tissue is mandatory as a way of differentiating DMD from BMD.

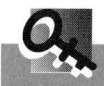

Key Laboratory Finding:
Duchenne Muscular Dystrophy

- Elevated CK

Treatment

1. A specific cure is not yet available.
2. Supportive treatment including the use of adaptive equipment is extremely helpful.
3. Orthopedic intervention to correct the scoliosis that commonly occurs in about 75 per cent between ages 12 and 15 is recommended in order to maintain an upright posture and in order to avoid future sitting problems when the patient becomes 18 or 19. It is doubtful whether scoliosis surgery will prevent pulmonary deficits.
4. The use of prednisone is recommended to delay the onset of loss of ambulation for up to 2 to 3 years.
5. Nighttime ventilation with bi-positive airway pressure is helpful for those patients who have early morning headache or "fatigue" (presumably from hypoxemia and hypercarbia).

TABLE 285–1. MUSCULAR DYSTROPHIES

DIAGNOSIS	INHERITANCE	TYPICAL AGE OF ONSET	DIAGNOSIS	PROGNOSIS	ASSOCIATED PROBLEMS
Congenital muscular dystrophy	Recessive; rarely dominant; occasionally sporadic	Birth	Clinical picture; Muscle BX; MRI of head	20% static 80% progressive	Seizures, retinitis
Duchenne muscular dystrophy	X-linked recessive	3–4 yr	DNA deletion; analysis of muscle for dystrophin	Life expectancy = 20 yr	50% have LD, gastrointestinal problems
Becker muscular dystrophy	X-linked recessive	5–10 yr	DNA deletion; analysis of muscle for dystrophin	Life expectancy = 35 yr	None
Limb-girdle muscular dystrophy	Recessive; rarely dominant	8–12 yr	Clinical picture; muscle BX	Variable	None
Facioscapulohumeral muscular dystrophy	Dominant	8–12 yr (neonatal form exists)	Linkage analysis; clinical picture; muscle BX	Variable	Hearing loss, visual impairment
Myotonic muscular dystrophy	Dominant	>20 yr (neonatal form exists)	Trinucleotide repeats	Variable	GI problems, cataracts, endocrinopathies, dementia

BX = biopsy; GI = gastrointestinal; LD = learning disability; MRI = magnetic resonance imaging.

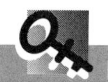

Key Treatment: Duchenne Muscular Dystrophy

• Supportive

Prevention

If a deletion is found in the mother, biopsy of the chorionic villus can determine if a male fetus, at about the seventh week of gestational age, also has a deletion of the dystrophin gene.

Limb-Girdle Muscular Dystrophy (LGMD)

Definition

This entity consists of different types of muscular dystrophies that have not heretofore been given a genetic identity but phenotypically are similar. The typical textbook description describes the onset of the disease in a male or female in the second decade of life.

Etiology

Recently, two loci have been identified for the recessive form of LGMD, LGMD2A, mapped to 15q and LGMD2B mapped to 2p. The link between the genetic abnormality and the clinical syndrome is unknown.

Epidemiology

No specific etiologic factors are known.

Pathophysiology

The muscle biopsy is similar to that of DMD and BMD. Specific aspects of the pathophysiology are unknown.

Clinical Findings

Initially, the patient develops muscle weakness of the proximal muscles of the lower extremities. Ambulation continues until the fourth or fifth decade of life. The hands will stay strong almost indefinitely.

Key Clinical Finding:
Limb-Girdle Muscular Dystrophy

• Muscle weakness of lower extremities

Laboratory Findings

1. The EMG shows myopathic changes, and the muscle biopsy shows dystrophic changes similar to the biopsy of patients with DMD.
2. The CK may be four to five times above normal.
3. Dystrophin is normally distributed in the muscle tissue.

Key Laboratory Findings:
Limb-Girdle Muscular Dystrophy

• EMG shows myopathy

• Elevated CK

Radiographic Changes

No specific findings occur.

Treatment

No specific treatments are available. Use of orthotics, manual wheelchairs, and power chairs are recommended according to the problems and needs of the patients.

Key Treatment: Limb-Girdle Muscular Dystrophy

• Supportive

Prevention

There are no known preventive strategies. As the genetic issues become clarified, carrier detection and prenatal screening may become available.

Facioscapulohumeral (FSH) Muscular Dystrophy (Landouzy-Dejerine Dystrophy)

Etiology

This is an autosomal dominant disorder. The disease is linked to chromosome 4q35.

Epidemiology

The incidence is 1 per 20,000.

Pathophysiology

The pathology is similar to that of the other muscular dystrophies. There are several phenotypic and presumably genotypic forms of the disease that have yet to be delineated. Only linkage studies have been available to date.

Clinical Findings

1. The range of severity of impairment is extremely variable in any one family. The clinical picture ranges from minimal facial weakness to weakness of the scapula and peroneal muscles without facial involvement. Muscle weakness starting in the face and scapular area, proceeding to involve the lower extremity muscles, the proximal muscles of the upper extremities, and finally the hands is the classic clinical progression of FSH.
2. There is a neonatal form that is associated with a high incidence of hearing loss.
3. The "typical" form starts in the second or third decade of life and is slowly progressive; affected individuals have a normal life span. Death may occur as early as the fourth decade from cardiac or respiratory failure.
4. Retinal vascular abnormalities have bee described in over 20 per cent of the cases.

Key Clinical Findings:
Facioscapulohumeral Muscular Dystrophy

• Muscle weakness

• Hearing loss (neonatal form)

• Retinal vascular changes (20%)

Laboratory Findings

1. The EMG and muscle biopsy findings are similar to those of other muscular dystrophies.
2. Linkage but not deletion studies are available.
3. Dystrophin is normally found in the muscle biopsy.

> **Key Laboratory Finding:**
> **Facioscapulohumeral Muscular Dystrophy**
>
> • EMG changes

Radiographic Changes

No specific findings are present.

Treatment

As with LGMD, there is no specific treatment. Orthoses and aid for mobility should be used when appropriate.

> **Key Treatment:**
> **Facioscapulohumeral Muscular Dystrophy**
>
> • Supportive

Prevention

No preventive strategies are available.

Congenital Muscular Dystrophy (CMD)

Definition

1. This is a group of neuromuscular disorders characterized by autosomal recessive inheritance, early onset, "floppiness," generalized muscle weakness, joint contracture, nonprogressive or slowly progressive disease with normal or near normal intelligence.
2. These disorders are classified into three distinct entities, based upon clinical evaluation.
   a. Classical CMD with normal or slightly reduced intellectual capability
   b. Fukumara type with cerebral abnormalities including polymicrogyria and heterotopias
   c. Muscle-eye brain disease including lissencephaly and cerebellar abnormalities. The latter might be a milder form of the Walker-Warburg syndrome.

Etiology

They are all most probably autosomal recessive, although dominant forms have been described.

Epidemiology

These are uncommon conditions, and no epidemiolgic data are available.

Pathophysiology

The muscle biopsy results are abnormal, showing changes similar to those described under DMD. Dystrophin is present in the muscle tissue of most CMD patients, although there are rare reports of CMD with missing dystrophin.

Clinical Findings

The patient presents with floppiness and joint contracture. Facial diplegia is present at birth. The arms are usually more involved than the legs. The patients with the "pure" form will improve, although some may deteriorate. Currently, there are no specific prognostic signs.

> **Key Clinical Findings:**
> **Congenital Muscular Dystrophy**
>
> • "Floppiness"
>
> • Joint contracture
>
> • Facial diplegia

Laboratory Findings

1. The CK may be normal or elevated to five times normal.
2. The electromyogram demonstrates myopathic potentials.

> **Key Laboratory Findings:**
> **Congenital Muscular Dystrophy**
>
> • CK normal to five times normal
>
> • EMG abnormalities

Radiographic Changes

The computed tomography (CT) or magnetic resonance imaging (MRI) scans may show abnormal myelin, polymicrogyria, heterotopias, lissencephaly, and/or cerebellar abnormalities. Classification and prognosis depends on the findings.

Treatment

As with the other dystrophies, treatment is symptomatic. Severe floppiness at birth including swallowing, sucking, and breathing difficulties may necessitate the use of gastrostomy and tracheostomy. The patient may develop strength and swallowing abilities during the toddler years, allowing the removable of the gastrostomy and tracheostomy.

> **Key Treatment:**
> **Congenital Muscular Dystrophy**
>
> • Supportive

Prevention

No preventive strategies are available

Myotonic Muscular Dystrophy

Definition

1. Myotonic muscular dystrophy (MMD) is an autosomal dominant, multisystem disorder, manifested by myotonia, muscle weakness, cataracts, endocrinopathies, cardiac disease, gastrointestinal disturbances (especially diarrhea), and dementia.
2. Myotonia is defined as increased relaxation time of mus-

cles following a contracture. The contracture can either be elicited or can occur volitionally.

Etiology

The gene for MMD is located on the long arm of the 19th chromosome.

Epidemiology

The incidence is 5 in 100,000.

Pathophysiology

1. The muscle biopsy does not show as much connective tissue and necrosis as the other muscular dystrophies.
2. Five to 27 copies of the cytosine-thiamine-guanine triplet are normally found. The number of repeats of this triplet is correlated with the severity of the disease. Sixty to 200 repeats are correlated with mild disease; more than 1000 repeats are correlated with the severe neonatal form of MMD.

Clinical Findings

1. The severe form presents in the neonatal period and typically occurs in infants born to mothers who have the disease. These children are extremely floppy and may demonstrate lack of respiratory effort and inability to swallow.
   a. If the child can survive the newborn period, improvement will occur. Some children will not walk until age 5.
   b. These children are commonly mentally retarded.
2. The more benign form of the disease typically starts in the second decade of life with the complaint of inability to let go of objects, that is, the complaint that is correlated with the sign of myotonia. Patients will have minimal weakness of the muscles.
   a. The presence of cataracts must be evaluated.
   b. Heart disease includes arrhythmias or mitral valve prolapse.
   c. Gastrointestinal abnormalities consist of difficulties in swallowing or diarrhea.

Key Clinical Findings: Myotonic Muscular Dystrophy

- Floppy infant
- Delayed walking
- Mental retardation (usually)
- Cataracts
- Cardiac disease

Laboratory Findings

1. The EMG shows evidence of increased relaxation time, and a "dive bomber" noise is heard during the needle EMG examination.
2. A muscle biopsy is unnecessary.

Key Laboratory Finding: Myotonic Muscular Dystrophy

- EMG shows increased relaxation time

Radiographic Changes

There are no useful radiographic changes.

Treatment

Phenytoin (Dilantin) has successfully been used to decrease the amount of myotonia if this significantly hampers the performance of the patient (unusual).

Key Treatment: Myotonic Muscular Dystrophy

- Phenytoin helpful

Prevention

Identification of excessive trinucleotide repeats in the fetus can identify a person who will have a severe form of the disease.

Bibliography

DUCHENNE MUSCULAR DYSTROPHY

Brooke MH, Fenichel GM, Griggs RC, et al: Duchenne muscular dystrophy: patterns of clinical picture progression and effects of supportive therapy. Neurology 1989;39:475–481.

Hoffman EP, Fishbeck KH, Brown RH, et al: Characterization of dystrophin in muscle-biopsy specimens from patients with Duchenne's or Becker's muscular dystrophy. N Engl J Med l988;318;1363–1368.

Griggs RC, Moxley RT, Mendell JR, et al: Duchenne dystrophy: randomized, controlled trial of prednisone (18 months) and azothioprine (12 months). Neurology 1993;43:512–527.

LIMB-GIRDLE MUSCULAR DYSTROPHY

Chiannilkulchar N, Pasturand P, Richard I, et al: A primary expression map of chromosome 15q 15 region containing recessive form of Limb-Girdle muscular dystrophy (LGMD2A) gene. Hum Molec Genet 1995;4:717–725.

FACIOSCAPULOHUMERAL MUSCULAR DYSTROPHY

Brouwer OF, Padberg GW, Wijmenja C, Franks RR: Facioscapularhumeral muscular dystrophy in early childhood. Muscle Nerve 1995;Suppl 2:s67–s72.

CONGENITAL MUSCULAR DYSTROPHY

Fenichel GM: Congenital muscular dystrophies. Neurol Clin 1988;6:519.

Leyten QH, ter Laak HJ, Gabreels FJM, et al: Congenital muscular dystrophy. A study on the variability of morphological changes and dystrophin distribution in muscle biopsies. Acta Neuropathol 1993;86:386–392.

Leyton QH, Gabreels FJM, Renier WO, et al: White matter abnormalities in congenital muscular dystrophy. J Neurol Sci 1995;129:162–169.

MYOTONIC MUSCULAR DYSTROPHY

Harley HG, Brook JD, Rundle SA, et al: Expansion of an unstable DNA region and phenotypic variation in myotonic dystrophy. Nature 1992;355:545.

286 Spinal Muscular Atrophy

Barry Russman

Definition

Spinal muscular atrophy (SMA) is a disorder of progressive muscle weakness that begins during the first 5 years of life, resulting in death at an inconstant age, and characterized pathologically by anterior horn cell loss. The disorder is classified by age of onset and maximum function achieved (MFA). The prognosis for life expectancy is more closely related to MFA than to age of onset (Table 286–1).

Etiology

The gene locus for acute and chronic spinal muscular atrophy was mapped to the long arm of chromosome 5 in 1990 using linkage studies. The specific gene was described in 1995 and was given the name of survival motor neuron gene. This gene is missing in the severe as well as the more benign forms of this disease. It is obvious that this story is incomplete.

Epidemiology

The incidence is 4 per 100,000 live births, suggesting a carrier frequency of 1 in 80 to 10 in 100,000.

Pathophysiology

The pathophysiology of this disorder will remain unknown until the gene product has been identified.

Clinical Findings

1. SMA type I (Werdnig-Hoffman disease): The disease onset is usually at birth or during the first few months of life; the patients never sit independently, and life expectancy is less than 2 years of age.

   a. Sucking and swallowing difficulties as well as abdominal breathing in the perinatal period or during the first few months of life are the presenting symptoms.

   b. Muscle weakness is symmetric, sparing ocular movement and the diaphragm. The heart is normal; a peculiar tremor of the electrocardiographic baseline has been attributed to fasciculation of limb and chest wall muscles. Facial weakness is minimal or absent. Fasciculation of the tongue is seen in most but not all patients.

Key Clinical Findings: SMA I

- Sucking and swallowing problems
- Abdominal breathing
- Muscle weakness
- Fasciculation of tongue

2. The onset of SMA II (chronic or juvenile SMA) is usually after 6 months of age.

   a. Consultation is sought when the child does not sit independently by age 9 to 12 months or is not standing by age 1 year.

   b. Finger trembling and flaccidity in a child who is alert and cognitively normal suggests the diagnosis. Sensation is intact in all patients with SMA II.

   c. Approximately 70 per cent lack all tendon reflexes.

   d. These patients may gain motor milestones slowly.

Key Clinical Findings: SMA II

- Motor delay
- Finger trembling
- Lack of tendon reflexes (70%)

3. SMA III patients (Kugelberg-Welander disease) develop walking skills but may fall frequently or have trouble walking up and down stairs at age 2 to 3 years.

   a. Examination shows proximal limb weakness; the legs are more severely affected than the arms.

   b. As with SMA I and II, absent tendon reflexes and a normal sensory examination complete the clinical picture.

TABLE 286–1. SPINAL MUSCULAR ATROPHIES

VARIABLE	SMA I	SMA II	SMA III
Age of onset	Birth to 6 months	6–18 months	>18 mo
Maximum function achieved	Never sits without support	Sits independently	Walks independently
Genetics	SMN gene deleted—autosomal recessive	SMN gene deleted—autosomal recessive	SMN gene deleted—autosomal recessive
Other features	Fasciculation of tongue in 65%; no sensory loss	Tremor of fingers; no sensory loss	Tremor of fingers; no sensory loss; fasciculations rarely observed
Course	50% die by age 7 mo; 80% die by age 1 yr	Life expectancy into the teens; atelectasis is a major problem	Normal life expectancy; loss of ambulation by age 12–40 yr

Key Clinical Findings: SMA III

- Frequent falls
- Proximal limb weakness
- Absent tendon reflexes

Laboratory Findings

1. Blood chemistry values should be unrevealing, but serum CK activity may be 1–2 times normal. If it is more than 10 times normal another diagnosis, such as one of the muscular dystrophies or polymyositis, should be considered.
2. Electromyography reveals regular spontaneous motor unit activity, a unique feature in SMA. Fasciculations are uncommon in SMA I, but they are common findings in SMA II and III. Nerve conduction velocities and sensory conduction times are normal, ruling out motor neuropathies.
3. Muscle biopsy reveals group atrophy of type 1 and type 2 muscle fibers as opposed to the normal checkerboard pattern. Rare angulated and large type 1 fibers are scattered throughout. Glycogen and lipid deposits are not seen, eliminating glycogen and lipid storage diseases from the differential diagnosis.

Radiographic Changes

No specific diagnostic changes are present.

Treatment

1. The management of children with spinal muscular atrophy starts with diagnosis and assignment into one of the three categories. Life expectancy can thus be estimated.
2. The management of SMA I involves monitoring for respiratory infection. Early discussion with family about "do not resuscitate" orders is helpful.
3. The life expectancy of patients with SMA II is not known accurately. Anecdotal information suggests that patients live into adolescence and early 20s. Ventilatory support has been recommended and been used successfully. Forced vital capacity decreases in all SMA patients and the eventuality of respiratory support should be discussed before it is needed so that management options can be considered. Forced vital capacity should be monitored as part of routine care.
4. The development of deformities in patients with SMA II and III necessitates a team approach for their care. SMA I patients rarely require orthopedic intervention because they do not live long enough to develop spinal deformity. However, scoliosis is a major problem in most SMA II patients and in half of SMA III patients.

Key Treatment

- Supportive

Prevention

Localization of the major gene for the spinal muscular atrophies has led to prenatal detection using the chorionic villus or amniotic fluid cells.

Bibliography

Iannaccone ST, Browne RH, DCN/SMA group, et al: A prospective study of spinal muscular atrophy before age six years. Pediatr Neurol 1993;9:187–193

Melki J, Abdelhak S, Burlet P, et al: Prenatal prediction of Werdnig-Hoffmann disease using linked polymorphic DNA probes. J Med Genet 1992;29:171–174

Russman BS, Fredericks EJ: Use of the ECG in the diagnosis of childhood spinal muscular atrophy. Arch Neurol 1979;36:317–318

Thieme A, Mitulla B, Friedemann S, Spiegler AWJ: Epidemiological data on Werdnig-Hoffmann disease in Germany (West-Thuringen). Human Genet 1993;91:295–297

Zerres K, Rudnik-Schoneborn S: Natural history in proximal spinal muscular atrophy. Clinical picture analysis of 445 patients and suggestions for a modification of existing classifications. Arch Neurol 1995;52:518–523.

287 Head Trauma

David L. Coulter

Definition

1. Head trauma is an injury to the skull or brain severe enough to produce an abnormality of structure or function.
2. Minor head injuries are generally reversible and full recovery is the rule. On the other hand, severe head injuries induce permanent changes that will forever alter the functioning of the child and family. The concept that rehabilitation following severe head injury begins on the day of the injury and continues indefinitely guides the acute and long-term management of children with severe head injuries and their families.

Epidemiology

1. Head injury is the most common cause of death in children and accounts for 6,000 to 12,000 deaths per year in the United States. For the most part, this is entirely preventable.
2. Head injury can be classified on the basis of severity.

a. Mild head injury: Initial and subsequent Glasgow Coma Scale (GCS) (Table 287–1) scores of 13 to 15, with no or brief (less than 30 minutes) loss of consciousness, no focal neurologic deficit, no intracranial hematoma, and no depressed skull fracture (although linear skull fracture may be present)

b. Moderate head injury: Initial or subsequent GCS scores of 9 to 12, with variable loss of consciousness, focal neurologic deficit, intracranial hematoma, or depressed skull fracture

c. Severe head injury: Initial or subsequent GCS scores of 8 or less with prolonged loss of consciousness, often with focal neurologic deficit, intracranial hematoma, or depressed skull fracture

Pathophysiology

1. The force of a blow to the head may be concentrated locally or spread diffusely. Both mechanisms may be present in severe head injuries.

   a. The consequences of localized trauma include skull fracture (which may be linear, comminuted, or depressed), hemorrhage at the site of the injury (which may be epidural, subdural, or intraparenchymal), and focal brain injury (which may consist of edema, contusion, laceration or necrosis). If there is no diffuse injury, consciousness may be relatively intact even though the child has focal neurologic signs.

   b. The consequences of diffuse trauma include contrecoup effects and diffuse axonal injury.

      (1) Contrecoup effects reflect the movement of the brain within the skull, with secondary injury on the side of the brain opposite from the site of the initial trauma.

      (2) Diffuse axonal injury reflects generalized disruption of tissue integrity, particularly in the cerebral white matter. Diffuse injury may cause prolonged impairment of consciousness even in the absence of focal neurologic signs.

2. Focal brainstem injuries, particularly hemorrhages in the midbrain and pons, result in cranial nerve abnormalities and prolonged unconsciousness. The severity

TABLE 287–1. GLASGOW COMA SCALE

CATEGORY	BEST RESPONSE	SCORE*
Eye opening (E)	Spontaneous	4
	To speech (command)	3
	To pain	2
	None	1
Motor (M)	Obeys (command)	6
	Localizes	5
	Withdraws	4
	Abnormal flexion	3
	Extensor response	2
	None	1
Verbal (V)	Oriented	5
	Confused conversation	4
	Inappropriate words	3
	Incomprehensible sounds	2
	None	1

*Total score (E + M + V): Maximum 15; Minimum 3.

of neurologic dysfunction is typically much greater than one would expect from the extent of brain injury and reflects the critical location of the relatively small area of damage.

Clinical Findings

1. Assessment of the head-injured child begins in the field at the scene of the injury and continues in the ambulance and in the emergency room.

   a. Initial considerations emphasize assessment of the airway, breathing, and cardiac function. Because of the possibility of critical neck injury as well, the neck must be stabilized until this possibility is excluded, usually by x-ray.

   b. Trained professionals should estimate the GCS score on arrival at the scene, again on arrival in the emergency room, and periodically thereafter.

   c. Complete physical examination is necessary to look for evidence of injuries to other organs. Inspection of the body should be conducted to look for bruises and lacerations. Battle sign (ecchymosis behind the ear), blood in the middle ear, or cerebrospinal fluid (CSF) rhinorrhea suggests the presence of a basilar skull fracture.

   d. Neurologic examination should be performed to look for signs of focal dysfunction such as hemiparesis, reflex asymmetry, or Babinski sign, or cranial nerve abnormalities such as a gaze palsy or pupillary asymmetry. The GCS score is not a substitute for a neurologic examination, since it may fail to detect significant focal findings.

2. Seizure activity should be noted and described carefully, looking particularly for evidence of focal seizure activity. Seizures occurring within the first few minutes after the injury, "impact" seizures, should be differentiated from seizures that occur subsequently, "early" seizures.

Key Clinical Findings

- Variable findings; look for
  Battle sign
  CSF rhinorrhea
  Level of consciousness (coma, severe)

Laboratory Findings

1. Electroencephalography (EEG) is rarely useful in the emergency assessment of a head-injured patient. It may be useful later to help decide whether or not to continue anticonvulsant drug treatment, although this is unproven.

2. Other laboratory studies may be indicated by the nature, extent, and severity of the child's other injuries.

Radiographic Changes

1. Neuroimaging (computed tomography [CT] or magnetic resonance imaging [MRI]) is indicated in children with moderate and severe head injuries. Contrast studies are usually not necessary in the initial study. CT with "bone window" settings will detect most skull fractures. MRI is better than CT for detecting tissue damage.

2. Skull x-rays are rarely useful in children with mild head injuries. Children with severe head injuries are best managed at facilities that have neuroimaging available.

Treatment

1. Children with mild head injuries often do not need to be admitted to the hospital. Parents can be educated about what to look for at home and instructed about what findings warrant a return to the emergency room.

2. Children with skull fractures or transient neurologic findings whose level of consciousness is normal in the emergency room may be admitted for overnight observation. A child with altered consciousness requires frequent, careful observation and should be admitted to an intensive care unit.

   a. Observation or "neuro checks" include assessment of the child's vital signs, arousability, the size and reactivity of the pupils to light, and the extent and symmetry of motor responses.

   b. Neuro checks are performed every 15 to 30 minutes until the child is alert, then every 1 to 2 hours for 12 hours and every 2 to 4 hours thereafter.

   c. Neurologic deterioration may reflect the development of cerebral edema or an expanding epidural or subdural hemorrhage. Repeat neuroimaging is indicated.

3. Intracranial pressure monitoring is indicated in children with persistent unconsciousness (see Chapter 291). Neurosurgical consultation, if not already obtained, is usually warranted in this situation.

4. Anticonvulsant drug treatment is indicated if the child has a skull fracture, intracranial hematoma, or GCS score of 10 or less on admission. Phenytoin is preferred.

   a. If the child does not have any seizures, phenytoin may be discontinued after 7 to 10 days because no convincing evidence exists that further treatment is helpful.

   b. If the child has had seizures or if the child is felt to have a significant risk of seizures, EEG may be useful. The presence of epileptiform discharges in the EEG supports continuation of anticonvulsant treatment.

5. Families can be referred to the National Head Injury Foundation (1-800-444-NHIF) for more information and support.

Key Treatment

- Varies with severity

Prevention

Prevention is part of all pediatric primary care and includes parent support to prevent inflicted injury (abuse), education and training of parents and children to avoid household and pedestrian accidents, and the requirement that all children wear bicycle helmets.

Bibliography

Jennett B, Teasdale G: Management of Head Injury. Philadelphia, FA Davis, 1981.

Kraus JF, Fife D, Conroy C: Pediatric brain injuries: The nature, clinical course and early outcomes in a defined United States population. Pediatrics 1987;79:501–507.

Levin HS, Eisenberg HM, Benton AL (eds): Mild Head Injury. New York, Oxford University Press, 1989.

Rosman NP. Acute brain injury. *In* Swaiman KF (ed): Pediatric Neurology: Principles and Practice. St Louis, CV Mosby, 1989, pp 715–734.

Temkin NR, Dikmen SS, Wilensky AJ, et al: A randomized, double-blind study of phenytoin for the prevention of post-traumatic seizures. N Engl J Med 1990;323:497–502.

288 Brain Tumors

Patricia K. Duffner and *Michael E. Cohen*

Definition

Brain tumors comprise a group of neoplasms arising from immature or mature cell lines of the tissues making up the central nervous system (CNS).

Etiology

Although the cause of most brain tumors in children is not known, certain conditions and exposures predispose the patient to their development.

1. Neurocutaneous syndromes: Several neurocutaneous syndromes, that is, neurofibromatosis, tuberous sclerosis, von Hippel–Lindau, linear nevus sebaceous, and the multiple basal cell nevus syndrome are associated with an increased risk of brain tumors.

2. Radiation exposure

   a. Low-dose cranial irradiation for tinea capitis has been associated with a significantly increased risk of developing tumors of the brain.

   b. Moderate-dose cranial irradiation administered to children with leukemia and lymphoma as part of CNS prophylaxis has been associated with the development of meningiomas and astrocytomas.

   c. High-dose cranial irradiation for children with brain

tumors has been associated with second primary brain tumors.

Epidemiology

1. The incidence of brain tumors in children less than 15 years of age is approximately 2.5 to 3/100,000.
2. Brain tumors occur in all age groups although there is a peak in the 5 to 9 year interval.
3. The ratio of males to females is 1.1:1.
4. Gliomas represent the most common histology.
5. The most common location is the posterior fossa.
6. PNET (primitive neuroectodermal tumors)/medulloblastomas are the most common malignant brain tumors in children.

Pathophysiology

1. Astrocytomas represent 40 to 60 per cent of brain tumors in children. They are graded in increasing degrees of malignancy as astrocytoma, anaplastic astrocytoma, and glioblastoma multiforme.
2. Medulloblastomas and primitive neuroectodermal tumors are largely undifferentiated and are typical of "small blue cell" tumors.
3. Ependymomas are classified as ependymomas and malignant ependymomas.

Clinical Findings

1. The signs and symptoms of a child with a brain tumor vary with the location of the tumor, that is, supratentorial, midline, or infratentorial. Signs and symptoms can either be localizing or nonlocalizing.
2. Symptoms: Nonlocalizing
   a. Headaches are common in children in general and do not usually reflect structural intracranial disease. Certain warning symptoms should suggest the presence of a serious problem.
      (1) Headaches that wake the child from sleep.
      (2) Headaches that occur upon wakening.
      (3) Persistently focal headaches.
      (4) Headaches that increase with coughing, sneezing, or straining.
      (5) Headaches associated with vomiting.
   b. Vomiting
      (1) Vomiting may reflect increased intracranial pressure or direct invasion of the floor of the 4th ventricle.
      (2) Vomiting associated with increased intracranial pressure is not typically projectile.
      (3) Vomiting is unusual with nonneoplastic hydrocephalus.
   c. Behavior change
      (1) Personality change is a very sensitive indicator of structural CNS disease.
      (2) Apathy, listlessness, and sleep problems may occur with tumors in any location.
      (3) Declining school performance, although most common with supratentorial tumors, may occur with tumors in the midline and posterior fossa.
      (4) Anorexia and/or obesity are associated with midline tumors.

3. Signs: Nonlocalizing
   a. Nonlocalizing signs generally reflect increased intracranial pressure.
   b. Sixth nerve (abducens) palsy occurs because the long free intracranial course of the 6th nerve makes it extremely susceptible to compression against bony prominences. The child with a sixth nerve palsy will complain of diplopia on horizontal gaze.
   c. Papilledema is a nonspecific sign of increased intracranial pressure. The blind spot may increase despite normal visual acuity.
   d. Increasing head circumference may occur. The absolute size of the child's head is less important than the rate of growth. In a young child with a brain tumor the sutures will separate in order to accommodate an expanding intracranial mass, leading to an inappropriately rapid rate of head growth.

4. Localizing signs and symptoms: Supratentorial location
   a. Partial seizures with or without secondary generalization may reflect a cerebral mass lesion. Although most partial seizures in children are not due to structural disease, children with a long history of seizures should be reevaluated if they develop a personality change or change in school performance, a change in the frequency or type of seizure, a change in neurologic exam, or a slow wave focus on electroencephalography (EEG). The incidence of seizures in children with hemispheric tumors ranges from 30 to 60 per cent.
   b. Focal motor and/or sensory signs, hemiparesis, or hemisensory loss may reflect the site of involvement of hemispheric lesions. In children less than 18 to 24 months of age, the development of hand preference is suggestive of an abnormality of the ipsilateral hemisphere leading to decreased use of the contralateral hand.
   c. Visual field abnormalities suggest involvement of the optic pathways in the cerebral hemispheres.

5. Localizing signs and symptoms: Posterior fossa location
   a. Children with posterior fossa tumors, because of obstruction of cerebrospinal fluid pathways, typically develop increased intracranial pressure early in their course. Nonlocalizing signs and symptoms such as headache, vomiting, diplopia, and papilledema are common.
   b. Signs that tumor involves the cerebellar hemispheres are appendicular ataxia, hypotonia, and pendular reflexes.
   c. Patients whose tumors involve the vermis (midline of the cerebellum) typically have gait and/or truncal ataxia.
   d. Children whose tumors involve the brainstem typically have ipsilateral cranial nerve abnormalities, contralateral pyramidal tract signs, and ipsilateral cerebellar signs.

6. Localizing signs and symptoms: Midline location
   a. If the tumor involves the optic nerves, ipsilateral visual loss or proptosis may occur.

b. Patients whose tumor involves the optic chiasm may develop nystagmus. Bilateral field cuts suggest involvement of the optic chiasm.

c. Tumors that involve the hypothalamic pituitary axis may be associated with endocrinopathies (e.g., increased or decreased appetite, precocious or delayed puberty, and diabetes insipidus). Tumors in the pineal region may be associated with Parinaud syndrome (i.e., failure of upper gaze and abnormalities of convergence and accommodation). Boys, more commonly than girls, may develop precocious puberty.

Key Clinical Findings

- Ataxia
- Vomiting
- Behavior changes
- Seizures
- Endocrinopathies (midline tumors)

Laboratory Findings

1. EEG offers the ability to identify structural disease as demonstrated by a slow wave focus. The major role of EEG is to identify paroxysmal discharges, suggesting a seizure disorder. Although EEG is not an important part of the evaluation of the child with a brain tumor, a change in EEG pattern in a long-term epileptic child may suggest the presence of a previously undetected neoplasm that is undergoing transformation to a more malignant state. In these children, focal seizure discharges may be associated with a slow wave focus.

2. Visual evoked responses provide a physiologic assessment of the optic pathway. When combined with a radiographic image of the optic nerves on computed tomography (CT) or magnetic resonance imaging (MRI) scan, both an anatomic and a physiologic evaluation of the optic nerves can be made.

3. Cerebrospinal fluid (CSF) cytology should be assessed in those tumors that seed the CSF.

4. Bone scans and bone marrow aspirations are performed as part of the metastatic work-up of children with medulloblastomas and primitive neuroectodermal tumors.

5. Endocrine studies including evaluation for diabetes insipidus are important with tumors of the hypothalamus, pituitary, and optic chiasm.

Key Laboratory Test

- CSF cytology

Radiographic Findings

1. CT scans provide the ability to rapidly diagnose most brain tumors and permit visualization of edema, calcification, and hemorrhage. They are least accurate in the posterior fossa and parasellar regions. MRI scans have largely replaced CT scans as they are more accurate, allow superior anatomic definition, and provide multiple planes of imaging without exposure to ionizing radiation.

2. Magnetic resonance angiography (MRA) offers the potential for noninvasive examination of the cerebral blood vessels. At this time the technique is not so accurate as traditional angiography.

3. Carotid angiography is much less frequently used than previously, but it is still necessary in highly vascular tumors to assess their blood supply prior to surgery.

4. Myelography or MRI of the spine should be performed in all children whose tumors have a tendency to seed the CSF pathways. Thus, children with medulloblastomas, ependymomas, primitive neuroectodermal tumors, pineal region tumors (including germinomas), and choroid plexus carcinomas should have baseline studies as well as routine surveillance testing.

Treatment

1. Surgery is the primary treatment approach for children with brain tumors. When possible, a gross total resection should be performed. With the advent of microsurgical techniques, surgery can now be performed in virtually all regions of the brain. Only in patients with diffuse brainstem gliomas is obtaining tissue not considered mandatory prior to definitive treatment.

2. For those children not cured by surgery alone, radiation is the postoperative treatment of choice except in the very young. The volume of radiation, that is, whether the radiation port remains localized to the tumor bed or involves whole brain with or without the entire neuraxis, depends on the tumor's tendency to seed the CSF. If leptomeningeal dissemination is identified, full neuraxis radiation is warranted.

3. Chemotherapy is increasingly being used both at the time of tumor recurrence and at initial diagnosis in children with certain tumors. Medulloblastomas and germinomas, in particular, are chemotherapy sensitive. Chemotherapy is now the primary postoperative treatment for children with brain tumors who are less than 3 years of age, as it is believed to be less neurotoxic than radiation.

4. Postoperative observation is recommended for those children with potentially indolent tumors in whom the natural history of the tumor may not be known. Thus, children with hemispheric supratentorial astrocytomas that have been totally resected may be followed until recurrence rather than immediately committing them to radiation and/or chemotherapy.

5. Observation alone with close follow-up is currently recommended in some children with visual pathway tumors, particularly those who have neurofibromatosis, no evidence of increased intracranial pressure, and adequate vision. Only when there is evidence of progressive disease is further treatment recommended.

6. Prognosis varies with tumor type, extent of surgical resection, presence or absence of metastases, and the age of patient.

a. Children with medulloblastoma who are older than 3 years of age, who have had a gross total resection, and who have no metastases may have a 60 to 70 per cent 5-year survival.

b. Children with cystic cerebellar astrocytomas who have had a gross total resection have a greater than 90 per cent chance of surviving 5 years.

c. Children with ependymomas have approximately a 30 to 40 per cent survival, but better survivals are seen in children older than 3 years who have had a gross total resection and have no metastases. In these children, progression-free survivals may approach 50 per cent.

d. The worst survival rates occur in children with diffuse brainstem gliomas, in whom survival rates are less than 20 per cent.

e. Children with low-grade hemispheric supratentorial astrocytomas have survival rates approaching 70 per cent.

f. Survival rates of infants with brain tumors are significantly worse than in any other age group, except in the case of high-grade gliomas, where in small series survival rates have approached 50 per cent.

7. Long-term complications of CNS therapy

a. Dementia

(1) Cranial radiation is associated with the development of dementia and learning disabilities. Risk factors for treatment-induced dementia are young age, large volume radiation (whole brain), high-dose radiation, vasculopathy and leukoencephalopathy, and supratentorial location of tumor.

(2) Radiation-induced dementia is progressive over time.

(3) Prospective neuropsychologic testing should be performed routinely in children with brain tumors. Special education classes and resource rooms may improve their level of functioning.

b. Endocrinopathy

(1) Growth hormone deficiency

(a) The most common radiation-induced endocrinopathy is growth hormone deficiency, occurring in approximately 80 per cent of children irradiated for brain tumors.

(b) Growth failure relates to growth hormone deficiency, vertebral shortening (secondary to spinal radiation), hypothyroidism, and precocious puberty.

(c) Growth hormone replacement therapy can improve longitudinal growth but is not as effective as in children who have idiopathic growth hormone deficiency.

(2) Hypothyroidism

(a) Thirty per cent of children who receive spinal radiation develop primary hypothyroidism because the thyroid gland is included within the port to the cervical spine.

(b) Treatment with chemotherapy in conjunction with spinal radiation increases the risk of primary hypothyroidism to 60 per cent.

(c) Compensated hypothyroidism, with normal T4 but elevated TSH, may occur following spinal radiation with or without chemotherapy. Although patients are clinically euthyroid, they require thyroid treatment to prevent the development of thyroid carcinoma.

(3) Gonadal dysfunction

(a) Spinal radiation may be associated with scatter to the ovaries, leading to ovarian dysfunction.

(b) Chemotherapy adversely affects gonadal function. In particular, cyclophosphamide is damaging to the Leydig cells.

(4) Oncogenesis

(a) Second tumors may develop as a result of radiation (see under Epidemiology). Chemotherapeutic agents, particularly the alkylating agents, may induce leukemia and lymphoma in children treated for brain tumors.

(b) Spinal radiation, as part of neuraxis radiation, may induce thyroid carcinoma.

Key Treatment

- Surgery
- Radiation
- Chemotherapy

Prevention

The only prevention strategies available are limiting a child's exposure to ionizing radiation and genetic counseling in families with neurocutaneous syndromes. (See also Chapter 142.)

Bibliography

Bloom HJG, Glees J, Bell J: The treatment and long-term prognosis of children with intracranial tumors: A study of 610 cases. 1950–1981. Int J Radiat Oncol Biol Phys 1990;18:723–745.

Burger PC, Fuller GN: Pathology. Trends and pitfalls in histologic diagnosis, immunopathology, and application of oncogene research. Neurol Clin 1991;9:249–271.

Cohen ME, Duffner PK: Brain Tumors in Children. Principles of Diagnosis and Treatment, 2nd ed. New York, Raven Press, 1994.

Mulhern RK, Crisco JJ, Kun LE: Neuropsychological sequelae of childhood brain tumors: A review. J Clin Child Psychol 1983;12:66–73.

Shalet SM, Clayton PE, Price DA: Growth and pituitary function in children treated for brain tumors or acute lymphoblastic leukemia. Horm Res 1988;30:53–61.

289 Status Epilepticus

Michael H. Kohrman

Critical State

Definition

1. Status epilepticus is a single seizure lasting longer than 20 minutes or repeated seizures without regaining consciousness lasting longer than 20 minutes.
2. Status epilepticus may be convulsive (active tonic or clonic movements) or nonconvulsive (partial seizures or impairment of consciousness).

Etiology

Causes of status epilepticus are multiple. They include hyper- or hypoglycemia, electrolyte imbalance (hyponatremia, hypocalcemia, hypomagnesemia), trauma (concussion; contusion; subdural, epidural or parenchymal hemorrhage), infection (meningitis or abscess), tumor (primary or metastatic), poor compliance with antiepileptic drugs, and difficult-to-control epilepsy.

Epidemiology

Status epilepticus occurs 60,000 to 250,000 times per year in the United States. The majority of cases occur in children under 5 years of age.

Pathophysiology

1. Prolonged seizures may cause injury to the brain. The primary mechanism of injury is the result of an inadequate delivery of metabolic substrates (glucose and oxygen) caused by the increased metabolic demand of tonic and clonic movements, hypopnea associated with the tonic phase of seizures, and resulting hypoglycemia and lactic acidosis.
2. Brain injury also may result from excitatory neurotransmitters (glycine and glutamate).
3. Some regions of the brain are very susceptible to this type of injury, especially the hippocampus.

Clinical Findings

1. Children presenting in convulsive status epilepticus display active tonic-clonic seizure activity. They are usually cyanotic and may have vomited. They often have fever as the result of the underlying cause of the seizure or as a result of constant muscle activity. They are acidotic as a result of hypoxia and the resultant lactic acidosis from muscle activity. There may be signs of overt trauma or other focal neurologic signs. There may be cardiac arrhythmias, hyper- or hypotension, or complete cardiac arrest.
2. Nonconvulsive status epilepticus may present as a stuporous state with waxing and waning of level of responsiveness.

Key Clinical Finding

- Seizure lasting more than 20 minutes

Laboratory Findings

1. Obtain blood glucose, electrolytes, Ca^{2+}, Mg^{2+}, complete blood count with differential, arterial blood gas analysis, toxic screen, and anticonvulsant levels.
2. An electroencephalogram will assist in confirming the diagnosis of nonconvulsive status epilepticus and if there is a suspicion that there is a conversion reaction rather than seizures.
3. If the patient is febrile, a lumbar puncture is highly recommended.

Key Laboratory Tests

- Serum glucose, calcium, magnesium
- Arterial blood gases
- Toxic screen

Radiographic Changes

Once seizures are controlled, a computed tomography (CT) scan should be obtained to look for intracranial pathology; especially if there is any history of head trauma, intracranial bleeding must be excluded.

Treatment

1. Stabilization of the patient comes first.
   a. Establish a secure airway.
   b. Confirm that breathing is adequate and deliver low-flow oxygen.
   c. Confirm that cardiac status is stable or initiate cardiopulmonary resuscitation (CPR).
   d. Establish intravenous access.
   e. Administer 50% glucose in water 1 mg/kg IV and pyridoxine 100 to 200 mg in infants less than 18 months old.
2. Obtain history: Special attention should be given to confirm a history of previous seizures and anticonvulsants or other medications being taken. A family history of seizures should be assessed. Compliance with the use of anticonvulsants should be determined. The possibility of recent head trauma should also be ascer-

Critical State *Continued*

tained, as should a history of metabolic disease, toxic ingestion, recent illness, or other chronic illnesses.

3. Control of seizures: During the entire time that seizures continue, the patient's airway must be maintained. Intubation should be considered if any signs of respiratory depression are observed or gag reflex is impaired.

   a. Lorazepam 0.05 mg/kg IV up to 2 mg or diazepam 0.2–0.3 mg/kg up to 10 mg/kg IV. Watch for respiratory depression. May be repeated one time if seizures persist. These drugs need to be followed by another long-acting anticonvulsant, usually phenytoin.

   b. Phenytoin (or fosphenytoin in phenytoin equivalents) 15 mg/kg IV, up to 1200 mg in normal saline administered at a rate no greater than 1/20 total dose/minute. Should follow the dose of benzodiazepine within 10 to 15 minutes. Cardiac arrhythmias can be a problem. Phenytoin precipitates in glucose. If seizures persist after the loading dose is complete, then give phenobarbital.

   c. Phenobarbital is given in 5 mg/kg increments, no more than 120 mg per dose by slow IV push every 5 minutes until seizures stop or a total dose of 20 mg/kg is reached. Maximum total dosage is 400 mg. Obtain stat drug levels after both medicines have been pushed to determine if loading doses of phenytoin and phenobarbital are adequate. Phenobarbital can be given as the primary anticonvulsant, prior to benzodiazepines. However barbiturates and benzodiazepines have synergistic effects on respiratory depression.

   d. If seizures are not controlled by now, the patient should be intubated. After the above medications have been given, a neurology consultation should be obtained for assistance in anticonvulsant management and to assess the patient.

   e. Other drugs that may be utilized include lidocaine or a diazepam drip. Pentobarbital should be avoided in young children because of its blocking effects on mitochondrial metabolism. General anesthesia under electroencephalographic (EEG) control, to obtain a burst suppression pattern, may be effective in refractory status epilepticus.

   f. Outcome: With appropriate use of anticonvulsants and airway management, the mortality of status epilepticus has fallen from greater than 10 per cent to less than 1 per cent over the last four decades. Morbidity from prolonged status epilepticus remains a problem. However the long-term effects of seizures lasting only a few hours remain unclear.

Key Treatment

- Secure airway
- Infuse 50% glucose if cause unknown or likely
- Pyridoxine for infant <18 months
- Lorazepam or diazepam IV
- Phenytoin IV or fosphenytoin

Prevention

1. Patient education to maintain compliance with the use of anticonvulsant drugs, and to prevent the patient from suddenly stopping medication, is the most important preventive tool.

2. Prevention of etiologic factors causing status epilepticus such as head trauma, central nervous system infections, and severe metabolic disorders is also important.

Bibliography

Aicardi J: Epilepsy in Children. New York, Raven Press, 1986.

Engel J: Seizures and Epilepsy. Philadelphia, FA Davis Co, 1989.

Holmes GL: Diagnosis and Management of Seizures in Children. Philadelphia, WB Saunders, 1987.

Kotagal P (ed): Status epilepticus. J Clin Neurophys 1995;12:315–362.

Sperling MR (ed): Status epilepticus. Epilepsia 1993;34(Suppl 1):S1–S81.

290 Coma

David L. Coulter

Critical State

Definition

Coma is a state of unresponsiveness from which the patient cannot be aroused; the eyes are closed and spontaneous movement is absent.

Etiology

1. The most important clinical distinction is between etiologies of coma that reflect focal versus diffuse pathologies. This distinction is reflected in the clinical presentation and laboratory assessment.
2. Common focal pathologies causing coma include tumors, abscesses, empyemas, hemorrhages (traumatic, spontaneous, or arising from a vascular malformation), and large infarcts (strokes). Less common causes include traumatic focal edema and unilateral hydrocephalus.
3. Common diffuse pathologies causing coma include anoxia, trauma with diffuse axonal injury, meningoencephalitis, intoxications, and metabolic disturbances. Increased intracranial pressure due to diffuse cerebral edema or bilateral hydrocephalus may be present and reflect one of these pathologies.

Epidemiology

The incidence and prevalence of coma is a function of the underlying conditions.

Pathophysiology

1. Coma occurs when there is either bilateral cerebral dysfunction or dysfunction of the reticular activating system in the upper brainstem.
2. Focal cerebral lesions cause coma by compression of the opposite hemisphere or by inducing diffuse increased intracranial pressure. Focal lesions in the upper brainstem, such as small traumatic hemorrhages, can cause coma directly, however, even in the absence of more extensive pathology.
3. Diffuse pathologies induce coma by altering neuronal metabolism. Neuronal activity is reduced, which can be measured by positron emission tomography (PET) scanning as decreased cerebral metabolic activity.

Clinical Findings

1. Coma should be distinguished from the locked-in state, in which patients are awake but cannot respond except by simple eye movements or blinking, and from the vegetative state, in which patients have spontaneous eye opening but are not aware of the environment and do not respond to it.
2. The history should be probed for clues to the etiology of coma. Complete general physical examination includes vital signs, inspection of the skin, head, and extremities, and examination of internal organs.
3. Neurologic examination of the patient in coma includes observation of the pattern of respiration (Cheyne-Stokes, central neurogenic hyperventilation, cluster and ataxic breathing), assessment of the size and reactivity of the pupils to light, examination of extraocular movements (for gaze palsies and evidence of cranial nerve III, IV, or VI abnormality), testing of oculocephalic (doll's eyes) and caloric reflexes, determination of motor response patterns (asymmetric postures, decorticate or decerebrate postures or flaccidity), and testing of tendon reflexes and plantar responses for evidence of asymmetry.
4. Transtentorial (uncal) herniation is marked by malfunction of the ipsilateral third (oculomotor) cranial nerve with a fixed, dilated pupil and medial rectus paralysis. Herniation through the foramen magnum is marked by apnea and bradycardia with relatively preserved eye movements.

Key Clinical Findings

- Unarousable unresponsiveness

Laboratory Findings

1. If the history, physical examination, or neurologic examination suggest diffuse pathology, blood and urine should be obtained for glucose, blood urea nitrogen (BUN), creatinine, electrolytes, liver function tests, ammonia level, and toxicologic studies.
2. Electroencephalography is helpful when subclinical or electrical status epilepticus is suspected.
3. Lumbar puncture is indicated if the patient is febrile. A febrile patient with evidence of focal pathology should have an imaging study done before a lumbar puncture is performed. If imaging cannot be performed promptly in a comatose febrile patient with focal signs, antibiotic treatment should be started without waiting for the results of lumbar puncture.

Key Laboratory Findings

- Examine CSF in febrile patient
- Obtain imaging study prior to lumbar puncture if focal signs are present

Radiographic Changes
1. Cranial imaging (computed tomography or magnetic resonance imaging) may be helpful, especially when the etiology of coma is not otherwise apparent.
2. If the history, physical examination, or neurologic examination suggests focal pathology, or if signs of herniation are present, a cranial imaging study should be performed immediately.

Treatment
1. Treatment is directed to the underlying cause of coma whenever possible. Neurosurgical consultation should be obtained when focal pathology is present.
2. General supportive measures include maintenance of vital signs including treatment of hypothermia or hyperthermia, respiratory support if indicated, correction of metabolic abnormalities (glucose, electrolyte, and acid-base), and treatment of increased intracranial pressure if present.
3. Anticonvulsants are appropriate to terminate seizure activity. Intravenous levocarnitine may be helpful when coma is present in a patient with an inborn error of metabolism.

Key Treatment
- Treat underlying cause

Prevention
Preventive strategies must be directed at the specific conditions that may cause coma. (See also Chapter 348.)

Bibliography

Plum F, Posner JB: Diagnosis of Stupor and Coma, 3rd ed. Philadelphia, FA Davis, 1980.
Simon RP: Coma in childhood. *In* Berg BO (ed): Neurologic Aspects of Pediatrics. Boston, Butterworth-Heinemann, 1992, pp 627–638.
Vannucci RC, Wasiewski WW: Diagnosis and management of coma in children. In Pellock JM, Myer EC (eds): Neurologic Emergencies in Infancy and Childhood, 2nd ed. Boston, Butterworth-Heinemann, 1993, pp 103–122.

291 Increased Intracranial Pressure
David L. Coulter

Critical State

Definition
Intracranial pressure greater then 15 mmHg (15 torr) or 200 mmH$_2$0.

Etiology
1. Intracranial volume is relatively fixed, so intracranial pressure will rise with an increase in the volume of any of the normal intracranial components (blood, brain tissue, extracellular fluid, and cerebrospinal fluid [CSF]) or with the addition of a mass lesion (tumor, abscess, or hematoma).
2. Increased blood volume can occur when there is cerebral vasodilatation or cerebral venous obstruction. Blood volume is normally maintained by autoregulation, so vasodilatation implies abnormal autoregulation. Hypoxia, hypercapnia, hyperthermia, seizure activity, and certain drugs (such as halothane) can increase cerebral blood volume. Venous sinus thrombosis, superior vena cava obstruction, and right heart failure can obstruct venous blood flow and cause increased intracranial pressure.
3. Increased volume of brain tissue or extracellular fluid may be due to cerebral edema, which may be either vasogenic or cytotoxic.
   a. Vasogenic edema reflects impairment of the blood-brain barrier with leakage of fluid out of blood vessels into the interstitial space and is commonly seen surrounding mass lesions.
   b. Cytotoxic edema reflects neuronal damage with impairment of membrane ion pumping and entry of fluid into the neuron and is commonly seen following anoxia or ischemia.
4. Increased CSF volume occurs when hydrocephalus is present.
   a. If the increase in CSF volume reflects loss of brain tissue (hydrocephalus ex vacuo), intracranial pressure usually remains normal.
   b. Intracranial pressure is usually raised when the increased CSF volume reflects increased production of CSF (such as from a choroid plexus tumor), obstruction to CSF flow (such as from aqueductal

Critical State *Continued*

stenosis or arachnoiditis), or impaired CSF resorption (such as from sagittal sinus thrombosis).

Epidemiology

Incidence and prevalence are related to the specific underlying disease entities.

Pathophysiology

1. The relation of intracranial pressure to volume is not linear but rather hyperbolic. Pressure remains relatively normal until the increased volume passes a critical point, after which pressure rises steeply. Thus symptoms and signs of a progressive disease process causing increased intracranial pressure may be minimal at first but then may suddenly become dramatic or catastrophic when this critical point is passed.
2. Cerebral perfusion pressure (CPP) is the difference between mean arterial pressure (MAP) and intracranial pressure (ICP): CPP = MAP − ICP. (Note that all units of pressure are in mmHg.)
3. Autoregulation describes the intrinsic compensatory processes by which the brain tries to maintain cerebral blood flow (CBF) when CPP is decreased due to either decreased MAP or increased ICP. CBF can be maintained by intact autoregulation until CPP falls below approximately 40 mmHg in children and adults or 30 to 40 mmHg in infants.
4. When autoregulation is impaired, the level of CPP below which CBF cannot be maintained is substantially greater than 40 mmHg. Since many diseases causing increased ICP such as trauma or anoxia also impair autoregulation, the threshold of clinically acceptable CPP must be raised to not less than 50 to 70 mmHg.
5. When CBF falls below the critical level necessary to maintain tissue integrity (CPP is below the threshold), neuronal damage occurs. When ICP equals or exceeds MAP (CPP is zero or negative), CBF is absent and neuronal damage is irreversible (brain death).
6. Neurologic status reflects CBF most closely and does not depend only on the level of ICP. Thus clinical assessment must also include assessment of the MAP, an understanding of the disease process causing increased ICP, and the likelihood that autoregulation is intact.

Clinical Findings

1. Clinical signs and symptoms typically reflect the underlying disease process causing increased ICP.
   a. In benign ("pure") intracranial hypertension, pseudotumor cerebri, headache predominates and neurologic signs may be limited to papilledema and an enlarged blind spot in the visual fields.
   b. In symptomatic intracranial hypertension, clinical signs and symptoms of the underlying disease process may predominate. Worsening of these signs and symptoms, or exacerbation of seizures, may reflect increased ICP.

2. Headache and vomiting, which need not be projectile, are common but nonspecific. Altered consciousness (lethargy) and behavioral changes are especially significant, however, and should always suggest increased ICP.
3. In infants with an open fontanelle, increased ICP causes the fontanelle to bulge. The cranial sutures will also separate if ICP is raised for a period of time. These mechanisms may relieve ICP to an extent, but they are inadequate when rapid and severe elevation of ICP occurs. For example, severe trauma with brain swelling can cause herniation and death even in an infant with an open fontanelle.

Key Clinical Findings

- Headache
- Vomiting
- Altered consciousness
- Papilledema
- Separate sutures and bulging fontanelle (infant)

Laboratory Findings

1. The best way to detect increased ICP is to measure it directly. This is usually done during lumbar puncture, which should always include measurement of the opening pressure.
2. When increased ICP is present, continuous ICP monitoring is often desirable in order to detect changes and to provide treatment promptly. A variety of techniques are available for continuous ICP monitoring.
   a. Direct methods for ICP monitoring include placement of a catheter, bolt, or pressure transducer into the subdural or subarachnoid space or into the ventricular system.
   b. An indirect method for ICP monitoring in infants involves placement of an external transducer over the fontanelle. This is generally not as reliable as a direct method, however.
3. The principal indication for continuous ICP monitoring is altered consciousness (obtundation, stupor, or coma) in a patient with known increased ICP or with a disease process known to cause increased ICP.

Key Laboratory Test

- Measure pressure when safe to do so

Radiographic Changes

1. Specific radiographic changes are related to the underlying disease process.

2. Computed tomography (CT) scan, magnetic resonance imaging (MRI), and ultrasound in a child with an open anterior fontanelle are useful to demonstrate hydrocephalus. CT and MRI also may show findings consistent with cerebral edema.
3. Skull radiographs in young children may show spreading of sutures or thinning of areas of the bony calvarium.

Treatment

1. Treatment of a patient with increased ICP often must be directed toward the underlying etiology (for example, surgical evacuation of a traumatic hematoma) as well as toward the ICP itself (see below).
2. General measures include elevation of the head of the bed to 30 to 45 degrees to facilitate venous return.
3. Fear, anxiety, and agitation may accompany intubation and further increase ICP, so sedation and muscular paralysis should be utilized as necessary to prevent this. (Sedation should always accompany muscular paralysis.)
4. Hyperventilation to maintain P_{CO_2} between 25 and 30 mmHg effectively reduces ICP. Further reduction below this range provides no additional benefit.
5. If a ventricular catheter is in place, 1 to 2 ml of CSF may be removed to reduce ICP.
6. Several drugs can be used as needed to reduce ICP:
   a. An intravenous injection of a 20% solution of mannitol at a dose of 0.25 to 1.0 mg/kg is effective in many cases and reduces ICP within a few minutes. The effect lasts for 2 to 4 hours and the dose can be repeated for several days. The effect weakens when the serum osmolality is too high, so serum osmolality should be maintained below 310 mOsm by appropriate fluid management.
   b. Steroids are useful in cases of vasogenic edema, particularly to reduce the edema that surrounds a mass lesion such as a tumor, abscess, or hematoma. Dexamethasone 1 mg/kg or its equivalent may be used in these cases. Corticosteroids are not very helpful in cases of cytotoxic edema, however.
7. High-dose barbiturates can reduce cerebral metabolic activity and thereby reduce CBF and consequently ICP as well. A separate neuroprotective effect of barbiturates is often suggested but remains unproven. A short-acting barbiturate such as pentobarbital is often used, but it may cause decreased cardiac function and severe hypotension requiring pressor supports. Phenobarbital, a long-acting barbiturate, is easier to use because it causes fewer systemic effects and blood levels are readily available, but central nervous system (CNS) depression is more prolonged.

Key Treatment

- Manage underlying cause

Prevention

Preventive strategies would have to be directed towards the specific conditions associated with increased ICP.

Bibliography

Fishman RA: Cerebrospinal Fluid in Diseases of the Nervous System. Philadelphia, WB Saunders, 1980.
Miller JD, Ward JD: Increased intracranial pressure: Theoretical considerations. *In* Pellock JM, Myer EC (eds): Neurological Emergencies in Infancy and Childhood, 2nd ed. Boston, Butterworth-Heinemann, 1993, pp 56–69.
Trauner DA: Increased intracranial pressure. *In* Swaiman KF (ed): Pediatric Neurology: Principles and Practice. St Louis, CV Mosby, 1989, pp 169–175.

292 Neurologic Examination

Gerald S. Golden

Procedure

General Aspects

1. A complete physical examination should be part of the neurologic examination. This should include measurement and plotting of height, weight, and head circumference.
2. Most information can be obtained from general observation of the child at rest, playing, and interacting with parents, siblings, or other children. The "hands-on" portion of the examination should be limited and should be done last.

Procedure *Continued*

3. Sensory examination of children is difficult to do and difficult to interpret, and so should usually be limited.
4. All components of the examination are tailored to the child's age and general medical status. An ill child will be unable to cooperate.

Cognitive Screening

- General level of alertness and activity
- Response to the examiner's presence
- Interactions with others
- Orientation should be tested (age appropriate)
  Person (self-identity, identifying others)
  Place (physician's office, hospital)
  Time (day/night, season, year, day of week, date)
- Age-appropriate developmental tasks

General Neurologic Examination

Components of the Neurologic Examination

1. Head, neck, spine, and extremities
2. Cranial nerves
   (a) Visual acuity
   (b) Eye movements
   (c) Symmetry and response of pupils
   (d) Facial symmetry and movement
   (e) Hearing
   (f) Swallowing and gag reflex
   (g) Tongue bulk, movements, fasciculations
3. Motor
   (a) Muscle bulk and symmetry
   (b) Muscle tone
   (c) Strength
4. Coordination
5. Gait and station
6. Involuntary movements
7. Reflexes
   (a) Tendon
   (b) Babinski sign
8. Sensation

Infantile Responses

1. Many of the normal reflex responses of early infancy disappear over time, and a number of new responses appear (Table 292–1).
2. Failure of the timely appearance or disappearance of these responses raises the suspicion of abnormal development of the central nervous system.

TABLE 292–1. DISAPPEARANCE OF NORMAL REFLEX RESPONSES

RESPONSE	DISAPPEARS
Stepping	1.5 months
Grasp	3 months
Suck	4 months
Moro	5 months
Tonic neck	6 months
Traction	Persists
Response	Appears and persists
Lateral propping	7 months
Parachute	9 months

 Bibliography

Ouvrier RA, Goldsmith RF, Ouvrier S, Williams IC: The value of the Mini-Mental State Examination in childhood: a preliminary study. J Child Neurol 1993;8:145–148.

Swaiman KF: Neurologic examination after the newborn period until 2 years of age. *In* Swaiman KF (ed): Pediatric Neurology: Principles and Practice, 2nd ed. St Louis, CV Mosby, 1994, pp 43–52.

Swaiman KF: Neurologic examination of the older child. *In* Swaiman KF (ed): Pediatric Neurology: Principles and Practice, 2nd ed. St Louis, CV Mosby, 1994, pp 19–41.

293 Neurologic Examination of the Neonate

Gerald S. Golden

General Aspects

1. Results of the examination vary with the infant's state (awake and quiet, awake and hungry, asleep, agitated). The most useful examination is with the infant awake and quiet.
2. If the child is systemically ill, the examination has little predictive validity.
3. If the infant suffered neurologic damage during parturition, the examination can define the current status, but predictive validity is low. Follow-up examinations to define changes are more useful than examination at a single point in time.
4. The examination should be structured so that the infant is handled as little as possible and more intrusive procedures are left for last. These include the fundoscopic examination, sensory examination, and evaluation of the child's cry.

Initial Observations

1. A number of useful observations can be made before the infant is manipulated.
   a. The infant's state
   b. Frequency, quality, and symmetry of spontaneous movements made by the awake infant
   c. The presence of abnormal spontaneous movements, especially seizures. These can be quite subtle and consist of nothing but transient changes in the infant's spontaneous activity.
2. Note should be made of the infant's general medical status.
   a. Skin color, particularly jaundice or cyanosis
   b. Respiratory rate and effort
   c. The presence of intravenous lines, ventilators, or other medical devices.

Supine Position

1. The child should be uncovered; it is important that the environment be comfortably warm.
2. Moderate flexor tone of all limbs should be present. Attempts to straighten a limb are resisted, and the limbs should return to the flexed posture after being released.
3. Spontaneous movements should be noted.
4. The head and face should be symmetric and the face should move symmetrically.
5. The awake, alert child will fixate briefly on the examiner's face.
6. The head should be turned gently to one side and then the other. The eyes will lag behind and then follow the head, the so-called "doll's eye" response.

7. The child should blink when a bright light is shined into the eyes. A loud noise will cause either a blink or an alerting response. Observations should be made carefully, as both of these responses attenuate with repeated stimuli.

Prone Position

1. The child is turned prone and observed. The normal infant should be able to turn his head and breathe adequately if placed face down.
2. Predominant flexor tone is also present in this position.
3. Some children will make crawling movements.

Prone Suspension

1. The infant is lifted and supported under the chest and abdomen by the examiner's hand.
2. Limb flexion is still present.
3. The child may attempt to extend the neck and lift the head.
4. Stroking the paraspinous area causes flexion of the spine to that side, and stroking up the midline of the back causes extension of the spine and lifting of the hips.

Vertical Suspension

1. The infant is supported under the arms and held in a vertical position.
2. Muscle strength and tone at the shoulders should be sufficient to prevent the infant from slipping through the examiner's grasp.
3. Some flexion of the legs will still be present.
4. Placing the soles of the feet on a flat surface produces extension of the knees and hips so that the infant appears to stand. Rocking the child slowly side-to-side will produce walking movements.
5. If the dorsum of a foot is touched to a hard object, the child will flex the leg and then step onto the surface.

Infantile Responses

1. A number of stereotyped responses can be elicited in the healthy neonate. These should disappear at varying times during the first year of life. These responses can be elicited during appropriate portions of the examination.
2. Touching the child's lip will cause rooting, opening of the mouth, and movement of the head in that direction. A finger placed in the child's mouth will produce sucking movements although these will be attenuated in a child who has been fed recently.
3. Attempts to pull the child up from a supine position by his hands (the traction response) produces resistance, and the child may flex his neck and pull his head forward. The child will also reflexly grasp the examiner's finger.

Procedure *Continued*

4. The Moro response is best elicited by holding the child supine on the examiner's forearm and allowing the head to suddenly drop backwards a small amount. The arms will extend and abduct, and then resume the normal flexed posture. Legs may flex. The infant will frequently be startled and begin to cry at this point.

Issues Related to Examination of the Premature Infant

1. The infant should be handled as little as possible, and not allowed to become hypothermic. The same general observations are made as with full-term infants.
2. Premature infants will have less flexor tone and less muscle strength than infants born at term.
3. Infantile responses can be expected to begin at specific gestational ages and then become fully developed after a period of several weeks (Table 293–1).
4. The examination of a premature infant at the child's expected date of birth is not identical to that of a normal full-term neonate. Tone and muscle strength are less well developed, and the child may seem to be somewhat less responsive.

TABLE 293–1. APPEARANCE OF INFANTILE RESPONSES

INFANTILE RESPONSE	AGE OF APPEARANCE	AGE OF FULL DEVELOPMENT*
Moro	28 weeks	34 weeks
Suck	28 weeks	36 weeks
Grasp	28 weeks	38 weeks
Traction	32 weeks	40 weeks
Stepping	32 weeks	40 weeks

*See Chapter 292 for time of disappearance.

Bibliography

Swaiman KF: Neurologic examination of the preterm infant. *In* Swaiman KF (ed): Pediatric Neurology: Principles and Practice, 2nd ed. St Louis, CV Mosby, 1994, pp 61–72.

Swaiman KF: Neurologic examination of the term infant. *In* Swaiman KF (ed): Pediatric Neurology: Principles and Practice, 2nd ed. St Louis, CV Mosby, 1994, pp 53–59.

294 Lumbar Puncture

Gerald S. Golden

Procedure

Indications

1. To obtain cerebrospinal fluid for examination if an intracranial infection is suspected
2. To obtain cerebrospinal fluid for examination to determine the presence of blood
3. To obtain cerebrospinal fluid to assist in the diagnosis of a number of metabolic disorders
4. To determine and monitor intracranial pressure intermittently

Contraindications

1. Clinical suspicion of markedly elevated intracranial pressure
2. The presence of a large mass lesion in one cerebral hemisphere
3. The presence of a posterior fossa mass lesion
4. Infection at the site through which the lumbar puncture will be performed
5. The presence of a bleeding disorder is a relative contraindication.

Preparation

1. Make certain that all equipment, including tubes for specimens, is ready and that sterility is maintained.
2. Have adequate personnel to restrain the child during the procedure.
3. Have basic resuscitation equipment available.
4. Scrub hands and put on sterile gloves.

Equipment

1. Lumbar puncture tray including a manometer to measure pressure
2. Several different size and length needles with stylets
3. Solution for sterile skin preparation
4. Sterile specimen tubes

Anesthesia

1. Anesthesia is rarely required. Most children can be adequately restrained by trained personnel.
2. An older child who is extremely uncooperative may require sedation or, rarely, a short-acting anesthetic.

Procedure *Continued*

3. Local anesthesia may be used, although this may be more upsetting to young children than the procedure itself.

Precautions

1. Precipitation of temporal lobe or cerebellar tonsil herniation may occur in the patient with increased intracranial pressure or a significant mass lesion.

2. Avoid airway obstruction with apnea, especially in an infant who is held too tightly in a flexed position.

3. A needle with a stylet should be used to prevent implantation of skin in the spinal canal. In rare instances this can cause an epidermoid tumor.

Technique

1. The procedure can be performed with the patient upright or in the lateral decubitus position. The spine should be moderately flexed anteriorly to open the intervertebral spaces, but should not be flexed laterally or rotated.

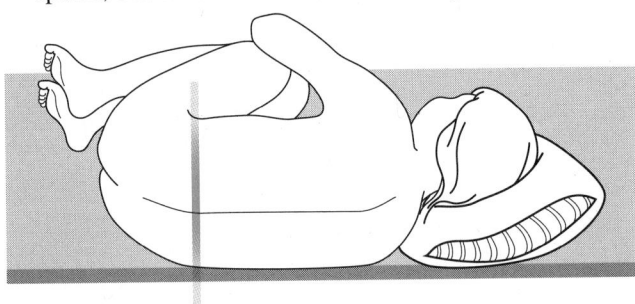

2. After sterile preparation of the skin the needle is inserted in the midline and advanced; a slight "pop" may be felt when the ligamentum flavum is pierced.

3. The stylet is removed. If no fluid is present, the needle should be rotated 90 to 180 degrees. If this does not produce a flow of fluid, the needle is slowly withdrawn. If no fluid is obtained, another attempt should be made.

4. If pressure is to be measured, the flexed position should be carefully relaxed to reduce venous pressure, which could translate into increased spinal fluid pressure. Unless the pressure is significantly above normal, specimens are collected in sterile tubes.

Follow-up

1. Serious complications are rare, but the child should be monitored for several hours for deterioration in the state of consciousness or the onset of focal neurologic signs, especially pupillary inequality.

2. Postlumbar puncture headache is self-limited, although it may last for several days. Lying down and increased fluid intake may be helpful. Mild analgesics such as aspirin or acetaminophen are sometimes required.

 Bibliography

Portnoy MJ, Olson LC: Normal cerebrospinal fluid values in children: another look. Pediatrics 1985;75:484–487.

Swaiman KF: Spinal fluid examination. *In* Swaiman KF (ed): Pediatric Neurology: Principles and Practice, 2nd ed. St Louis, CV Mosby, 1994, pp 123–130.

295 Normal Neonatal Skin

Robert H. Johr and
Lawrence A. Schachner

It is important to be aware of how the skin looks in full-term, premature, and postmature infants. Transient physiologic and self-limited dermatosis should be recognized so that unnecessary invasive interventions, with resultant potentially increased morbidity or mortality, can be prevented. Innocuous dermatoses can be widespread and dramatic, whereas potentially life-threatening infections can have a deceptively banal clinical appearance.

> Life-threatening infections can have few lesions, whereas self-limited dermatosis can be disseminated.

Normal Skin

At Birth
1. The newborn is transiently cyanotic but quickly becomes pink. Acral areas can still appear cyanotic (acrocyanosis).
2. Persistent pallor may represent asphyxia, anemia, shock, or edema.

> Early diagnosis of pallor can be lifesaving (erythroblastosis fetalis, fetomaternal or twin-twin transfusion reactions).

3. Skin appears soft, velvety, and covered with greasy yellowish-white material (vernix caseosa).
4. Desquamation begins within a few days and lasts several weeks.
5. Physiologic dehydration can cause a decrease in tissue turgor and loose wrinkled skin.
6. There may be a good amount of subcutaneous fat, which creates a pudgy appearance.
7. Hyperpigmentation of certain areas, such as the linea alba, areolae of the nipples, ear tips, scrotum, and fingertips.
8. Palpable breast masses and localized areas of edema are common.
9. The baby is usually covered with lanugo, soon replaced by vellus hairs.
10. Skin is easily abraded.

Premature Infant
1. The premature infant has a more transparent or even gelatinous appearance of the skin compared with full-term infants.
2. The premature infant is free of wrinkles.
3. The premature infant is covered with fine lanugo (immature) hairs.
4. Less hyperpigmentation is present in the linea alba, the areolae of nipples, and other areas.
5. Less palpable breast tissue exists.

Postmature (Dysmature) Infant
1. The body usually appears pale and lean, with thin extremities because of the relative lack of subcutaneous fat.
2. Skin is parchment-like, scaly, or desquamating and is often meconium stained.
3. The nails are abnormally long and meconium stained.
4. Abundant hair is present.
5. Vernix caseosa is decreased or absent.

Physiologic Skin Changes
1. *Acrocyanosis*
   a. A purplish discoloration of the hands, feet, and lips is seen during periods of crying, breath holding, or chilling.
   b. Acrocyanosis should not be confused with true cyanosis seen with cardiac or pulmonary pathology.
2. *Cutis marmorata*
   a. This is seen as a response to chilling and disappears when the infant is warmed.
   b. A reticulated bluish mottling of the skin is seen, usually on the trunk and extremities.
   c. If persistent, it can be associated with serious conditions, such as Down syndrome, or it can be a primary skin condition that is called cutis marmorata telangiectatica congenita.
   d. Cutis marmorata alba; this is a white pattern similar to cutis marmorata that is transitory and of no clinical significance.
3. *Harlequin color change*
   a. This change is usually seen in normal children, but it can be associated with intracranial pathology.
   b. A peculiar red color is seen on the dependent half of an infant when the infant is placed flat on one side. The coloring has an obvious demarcation that runs the entire length of the baby's body. The other, or nondependent, half of the body appears pale.
   c. It can be seen at birth or within the first few days of life, lasting from seconds to up to a half hour or more. It usually resolves spontaneously.

296 Neonatal Skin Abnormalities

Robert H. Johr and *Lawrence A. Schachner*

1. *Sclerema neonatorum*
   a. This disorder is seen in premature, debilitated, or otherwise gravely ill neonates. It has a mortality rate of 50 to 70 per cent.
   b. Often, there is a neonatal history of sepsis, respiratory distress, or heart disease.
   c. There is an abrupt onset of a rapidly progressive waxlike hardening of the skin; this hardening can quickly spread to involve the entire body.
   d. The skin appears yellowish, white, cold, and mottled; this infant has immobile limbs and a masklike face.
   e. Antibiotics, fluid and electrolyte corrections, and judicious use of systemic corticosteroids can sometimes decrease morbidity and mortality. Some cases have a complete recovery without permanent sequela.

2. *Subcutaneous fat necrosis*
   a. This condition can be differentiated from sclerema neonatorum by the lack of a systemically ill child.
   b. Asymptomatic to tender, reddish purple plaques and nodules develop suddenly on the face, trunk, and extremities.
   c. Subcutaneous fat necrosis is a self-limited condition that clears spontaneously within a few weeks.
   d. Occasionally, therapy is needed for draining calcium deposits or hypercalcemia.

3. *Bronze baby*
   a. A diffuse, grayish brown discoloration is seen in infants undergoing phototherapy for hyperbilirubinemia.
   b. The condition begins shortly after therapy begins and clears spontaneously a few weeks after phototherapy is completed.

4. *Milia, Bohn nodules, and Epstein pearls*
   a. These are whitish yellow small papules found at birth in up to 85 per cent of infants.
   b. Milia are found on the face.
   c. Bohn nodules and Epstein pearls are found in the mouth.
   d. No treatment is necessary because these usually disappear spontaneously, within a few weeks of their appearance.

5. *Sebaceous gland hyperplasia*
   a. These transient lesions are thought to be caused by the transplacental passage of maternal androgens.
   b. Two- to 3-mm yellowish papules are located on the face.
   c. This disorder resolves spontaneously a few weeks to months after onset.

Bibliography

Fanaroff AA, Martin RJ: Neonatal-Perinatal Medicine: Diseases of the Fetus and Infant, 6th ed. St. Louis, CV Mosby, 1997.

Hurwitz S: Cutaneous disorders of the newborn. *In* Clinical Pediatric Dermatology, 2nd ed. Philadelphia, WB Saunders, 1993, pp 7–17.

Wagner AM, Hansen RC: Neonatal skin and skin disorders. *In* Schachner LA, Hansen RC, (eds): Pediatric Dermatology, 2nd ed. New York, Churchill Livingstone, 1995, pp 263–346.

297 Seborrheic Dermatitis

Robert H. Johr and *Lawrence A. Schachner*

1. Seborrheic dermatitis is an exceedingly common dermatitis seen in the neonatal period. It is characterized by pinkish to erythematous, greasy, scaly dermatitis.
2. The dermatitis is often located on the scalp (cradle cap) or the diaper area. Widespread lesions are common.
3. Lack of pruritus, early onset during the first month of

> Early onset in the neonatal period of a characteristically greasy-appearing dermatitis with lack of pruritus or a family history of atopy separates seborrheic dermatitis from atopic dermatitis.

life, and a negative family history of *atopy* differentiate this condition from *atopic* dermatitis.

4. Psoriasis, Letterer-Siwe disease, Leiner disease, or Wiskott-Aldrich syndrome should be considered in treatment-resistant, severe cases associated with systemic manifestations.

5. Treatment consists of mild- to midpotency topical corticosteroids or preparations that can be used against *Pityrosporum*, such as topical ketoconazole. Stubborn scales in

---

WARNING

Strong corticosteroids should not be used on the face or in intertriginous areas.

---

the scalp can be removed with warm mineral oil or similar liquid rubbed into the scalp, followed by antiseborrheic shampoos.

---

298 Vesiculopustular Rashes

Robert H. Johr and *Lawrence A. Schachner*

---

1. More then 30 diverse conditions need to be considered in the differential diagnosis of vesiculopustular lesions in the neonate.

2. The history should begin at conception, not at parturition. Often, the maternal, obstetric, family, prenatal, and perinatal history are needed to make the diagnosis. Important historical data include

   a. A history of any skin or mucous membrane disease or infections in the mother during the pregnancy or at the time of delivery.

   b. A family history of genetic, mechanobullous or collagen vascular disease that could be transmitted to the neonate.

   c. Positive serologic findings for syphilis or human immunodeficiency virus.

   d. The time frame in terms of hours, days, or weeks that the rash began.

3. Primary lesions include vesicles, bullae, and pustules. A monomorphous presentation is possible; however, most commonly, there are

   a. Combinations of lesions, such as papulovesicles and vesiculopustules.

   b. Secondary changes with erosions, ulcerations, and crusting.

   c. Secondary infection that is obviously present (honey-colored crusting, oozing, flaccid bullae) or subclinical. Failure to identify and treat secondary infection can decrease the effectiveness of therapy.

Secondary bacterial infection needs to be identified and treated.

---

4. Classification of vesiculopustular lesions in the neonatal period.

   a. *Mild noninfectious causes*

      (1) *Neonatal acne:* Seen in up to 20 per cent of newborns, characterized by classic open and closed comedones (black and white heads) and inflammatory lesions seen in the typical acne distribution (face).

      (2) *Acropustulosis of infancy:* severely pruritic vesiculopustular lesions seen more commonly in African American males and recurring in crops every 2 to 4 weeks. Primarily located in an acral distribution. Tzanck preparation demonstrates a predominance of neutrophils.

      (3) *Eosinophilic pustular folliculitis:* recurring crops of pruritic crusted papules, vesicles, and pustules located primarily on the scalp and face, chiefly in males. The process lasts for a few years. Tzanck preparation reveals a predominance of eosinophils.

      (4) *Erythema toxicum neonatorum:* combinations of red macules, papules, wheals, vesicles, and pustules seen in 20 to 60 per cent of full-term infants. Usually not present at birth. The rash is typically evanescent and disappears within a week. Tzanck preparation shows eosinophils.

Serious conditions should be considered in a premature infant with the clinical picture of erythema toxicum neonatorum.

---

      (5) *Miliaria crystallina:* myriads of monomorphous tiny flaccid vesicles filled with clear fluid on otherwise normal appearing skin; seen in the context of high environmental temperature and humidity.

      (6) *Miliaria rubra:* tiny scaly red papulovesicular lesions also seen in the context of high temperature and humidity.

Non–air-conditioned nurseries, incubators, fevers, and occlusive clothing can cause miliaria.

(7) *Transient neonatal pustular melanosis:* a distinctive rash, often present at birth with pustules that transform into scaly hyperpigmented macules of the same size, seen in 2 to 5 per cent of African Americans and a smaller number of neonates of other races. Tzanck preparation demonstrates neutrophils.

(8) *Sucking blisters:*

    (a) These are rarely seen bullae that are present at birth in areas highly accessible to the sucking action of the baby in utero and in the neonatal period.

    (b) They are characteristically located on the hands, wrists, or fingers.

    (c) When normal feeding begins, the desire to suck usually ceases, and lesions spontaneously disappear.

b. *Mild infectious causes*

(1) *Congenital candidiasis* is a rare disorder with widespread vesiculopustular lesions. Usually self-limited but dangerous in low birth weight infants.

(2) *Neonatal candidiasis:*

    (a) This disorder is seen in 4 to 5 per cent of neonates delivered through an infected birth canal.

    (b) It is a characteristic vivid beefy red, glazed, weeping dermatitis with satellite lesions in the genital area beginning after the first week of life.

    (c) Widespread scaly dermatitis, often with oral mucosal involvement (thrush), can develop.

    (d) Potassium hydroxide demonstrates budding yeasts and pseudohyphae.

    (e) Topical therapy with anticandidal cream is usually rapidly curative.

    (f) If disorder is resistant to treatment, suspect immunosuppression.

> Potentially serious local and systemic side effects can be iatrogenically produced with preparations containing strong topical steroids and should be avoided.

(3) *Impetigo neonatorum*

    (a) *Staphylococcus aureus* can be colonized in up to 30 to 40 per cent of newborns.

    (b) It can begin within the first days of life.

    (c) The spectrum of disease depends on the elaboration of varying exfoliative exotoxins from localized disease (bullous impetigo) to the generalized scalded skin syndrome. Organisms that do not form exotoxin produce only vesicles and pustules.

    (d) These vesicles, pustules, and/or bullae on normal to erythematous skin favor moist opposing surfaces (kissing lesions). Lesions rupture easily, forming red, glazed, oozing, peripherally spreading lesions with a collarette of scale.

> A collarette of scale seen with red oozing areas is a good indication of a *Staphylococcus aureus* infection, especially when obvious bullae are not present.

    (e) A Gram stain and bacterial cultures usually confirm the diagnosis.

> A growing number of organisms are resistant to commonly used antibiotics. Therefore, cultures and sensitivity testing are often very helpful.

> Cultures of the anterior nares should be considered so that an occult focus of infection can be ruled out. This can be the source of recurrent problems.

(4) *Scabies*

    (a) Often called the great imitator, scabies can be the easiest or the most difficult diagnosis to make.

    (b) The incubation period is from 3 to 6 weeks; therefore, scabies can be seen in the neonatal period.

    (c) In the neonate, a diffuse rash with vesicles, papules, burrows, eczematization, and secondary infection is found. Burrows, which are considered the classic primary lesion of scabies, are less frequently found in the neonate, whereas nodular lesions are more frequently found in the neonate.

> Burrows, which are the classic primary lesions in scabies, are found less often in the neonatal period.

    (d) Although scabies is classically thought of as a rash from the neck down, in the neonatal period lesions are commonly found on the face, scalp, palms, and soles.

> Classically in neonatal scabies, lesions are generalized and include the face and scalp.

    (e) When others have been in close contact with the neonate and have an itchy rash, scabies should be considered.

    (f) A definitive diagnosis can be made if the scabies mite, eggs, or stool are identified with a scabies scraping. However, most of the rash is a hypersensitivity reaction, and often the mite is hard to find.

The mite, eggs, or stool does not always have to be identified for a clinical diagnosis of scabies to be made.

(g) Lindane has been associated with central nervous system toxicity and treatment resistance; therefore, permethrin cream (Elimite) is now considered the treatment of choice. It has been approved for use in 2-month-olds and appears to be safe when it is used in neonates.

c. *Potentially serious noninfectious causes*

(1) When should a potentially serious cause of vesiculopustular lesions be considered?

(a) When there is a characteristic clinical presentation, such as linear streaks of erythematous papules and vesicles (incontinentia pigmenti).

(b) When other family members have lifelong chronic illnesses, such as bullae, erosions, and ichthyosis (epidermolytic hyperkeratosis).

(c) When the neonate appears systemically ill, with such problems as sharply demarcated scaly plaques with vesicles and bullae in a periorificial and acral distribution, diarrhea, and failure to thrive (acrodermatitis enteropathica).

d. *Potentially serious infectious causes*

(1) These causes are divided into three groups.

(a) Bacterial infections: *Chlamydia trachomatis, Escherichia coli, Haemophilus influenzae, Listeria monocytogenes, Pseudomonas* species, *Staphylococcus aureus* (sepsis, scalded skin syndrome), Group A and B beta-hemolytic streptococci, and congenital syphilis

(b) Fungal infections: congenital candidiasis

(c) Viral infections: herpes simplex, varicella-zoster.

(2) *When should potentially life-threatening infections be considered?*

(a) When there is evidence of systemic involvement, such as hyperthermia, hypothermia, irritability, respiratory distress, meningeal signs, lethargy, history of maternal infections, maternal fever, and premature labor.

(b) When there is extreme prematurity, an immunocompromised state (human immunodeficiency virus), or congenital abnormalities.

(c) When classic clinical presentations are present, such as grouped vesicles, crusts, and erosions on erythematous skin (neonatal herpes simplex infection).

(d) When serologic findings are positive for syphilis or human immunodeficiency virus.

Infections should always be considered first and appropriate therapy should be initiated, pending the results of confirmatory laboratory testing.

Bibliography

Frieden IJ: The dermatologist in the newborn nursery: Approach to the neonate with blisters, pustules erosions, and ulcerations. Curr Probl Dermatol 1992;4:123–166.

Sahn EE: Vesiculopustular diseases of neonates and infants. Curr Opin Pediatr 1994;G:442–446.

Van Praag MCG, Van Rooij RWG, et al: Diagnosis and treatment of pustular disorders in the neonate. Pediatr Dermatol 1997;14:131–143.

299 Alopecias

Neil S. Prose and *Richard Antaya*

Some common causes of patchy hair loss in children are alopecia areata (AA), trichotillomania, and tinea capitis. The first two are outlined in this chapter, and the last is covered under Infections in Chapter 305.

Alopecia Areata

Definition

Alopecia areata is common disorder characterized by the sudden appearance of sharply defined round or oval solitary or multiple patches of hair loss. The disorder may slowly progress to involve a band of hair across the posterior scalp (ophiasis), all scalp hair (alopecia totalis), or all body hair (alopecia universalis).

Etiology

The etiology is unknown; however, an autoimmune process is thought to be likely.

Epidemiology

Alopecia areata is common, with an prevalence of roughly 0.1 to 0.2 per cent of the population. It can occur at all ages;

the first episode appears when the person is younger than 20 years of age in 50 per cent of cases. About 20 per cent of patients have a family history of AA.

Pathophysiology

1. All theories are speculative and include an autoimmune process (the most accepted one), inheritance, exposure to chemicals or infectious agents, and neuronal defects. Most recently, there is evidence that genetically abnormal keratinocytes or melanocytes may play a role in the pathogenesis.
2. Alopecia areata has been associated with atopy, thyroiditis, vitiligo, and diabetes, as well as various other autoimmune diseases.
3. There is an increased incidence of AA in patients with trisomy 21 and an increased association with cataracts.

Clinical Findings

1. Alopecia areata is diagnosed by its characteristic clinical picture of rapid (overnight to a few days) and complete loss of hair in one or more round or oval patches, mostly on the scalp (but may occur on other body sites as well).
2. The bald patches are smooth, soft, and without scale or crust and may be pink or violaceous. They are usually well demarcated but may be atypical in children and occasionally may have long hairs emanating from the patches. Peripheral spread may result in bizarre patterns. Older patches may contain depigmented hairs.
3. "Exclamation mark" hairs are loose hairs that may be easily extracted by gentle traction from the margin of active patches. By use of low-power microscopy, an attenuated (or catagen) bulb is demonstrated at the base of a tapered, hypopigmented shaft, resembling an exclamation mark. These are pathognomonic for AA.
4. The course is extremely variable, and the prognosis is varied. The initial patch may regrow in a few weeks to months, or new patches may continue to appear for months as others resolve. Hair is usually fine and hypopigmented on regrowth, but normal contour and color return gradually. When AA is limited to a few patches, prognosis is generally good, with complete regrowth within 1 year in 95 per cent of cases. Very young age and extensive or total alopecia portend a worse prognosis for complete and permanent recovery, and about 30 per cent of patients have future episodes of AA.
5. Dystrophy of the nails is seen in 10 to 20 per cent of patients with AA. The most common presentations are fine gridlike stippling of the nails and nail pits, which are smaller and more shallow than those associated with psoriasis.

Treatment

1. There is no single best therapy and no overwhelming evidence that pharmacotherapy alters the final outcome of AA.
2. Topical and intralesional steroids have been shown to hasten hair regrowth. The most favored treatments are topical corticosteroids, such as betamethasone diproprionate (Diprosone) lotion applied twice a day or at bedtime without occlusion, and triamcinolone acetonide, in concentrations of 3 to 10 mg/ml, injected intradermally into individual lesions with a 30-gauge needle (maximum of 1 to 2 ml per month) at 4- to 6-week intervals. These treatments usually effect initial regrowth of tufts in 3 to 4 months and 4 to 6 weeks, respectively. Intralesional steroids are impractical in young children.
3. Treatment is difficult to evaluate because of the unpredictable and usually self-limiting nature of AA. Patients and their families should be reassured that spontaneous resolution usually occurs. Psychological implications are well recognized, and wigs may be helpful for patients with extensive alopecia. The National Alopecia Areata Foundation is a valuable source of information and support for patients and their families.

Trichotillomania

Definition and Etiology

Trichotillomania is a self-limiting form of alopecia produced by conscious or subconscious habitual pulling, plucking, twirling, or rubbing hair, resulting in breakage of hair shafts.

Epidemiology

Trichotillomania is seen in both sexes and in children and young adults (most commonly from 4 to 10 years of age and in early adolescence). Although it may be a manifestation of severe underlying psychological disturbances, most cases present in normal children who are reacting to emotional stress (most commonly disturbances in parent-child relationships, fear of being left alone, or recent object loss) or are simply the result of habit.

Clinical Findings

1. Trichotillomania can usually be diagnosed by its characteristic configuration and distribution. Scalp biopsy of the involved area is indicated for more difficult cases.
2. Affected areas are usually single and located on the parietal or occipital areas of the scalp; however, any hair-bearing area, such as eyelashes and eyebrows, may be involved.
3. The disorder is characterized by irregular patches of incomplete hair loss that demonstrate short, broken, or blunt-tipped as well as long strands of hair in the affected area. The underlying scalp is normal. Tinea capitis and AA should always be considered in the differential diagnosis of trichotillomania.
4. Shaving a small patch of hair in the center of the affected area (to prevent manipulation) and observing normal regrowth of hair in approximately 3 to 4 weeks confirm the diagnosis.

Treatment

1. Management is often difficult and mandates a strong physician-patient-parent relationship.
2. Patients rarely admit to touching or manipulating the affected areas, and direct confrontation or accusation is more often detrimental than helpful.
3. Most cases respond to a combination of reassurance, opportunity to express the patient's emotional needs, and reasonable plan of therapy, such as a topical 1 per cent hydrocortisone ointment to relieve "itching" or "irri-

tation." It is also helpful to make the hair more difficult to grab.

4. Trichophagia with resultant trichobezoar should be considered, particularly in young girls with long hair and persistent alopecia.

5. For severe, long-standing cases associated with obsessive-compulsive or emotional disturbances, antidepressants or psychiatric consultation, or both, are reasonable options.

Bibliography

Hordinsky MK: Alopecia areata. *In* Olsen EA (ed): Disorders of Hair Growth: Diagnosis and Treatment. New York, McGraw-Hill, 1994, pp 195–222.

Hurwitz S: Hair disorders. *In* Schachner LA, Hansen RC (eds): Pediatric Dermatology, vol 1, 2nd ed. New York, Churchill Livingstone, 1995, pp 583–614.

Levy ML: Disorders of the hair and scalp in children. Pediatr Clin North Am 1991;38:907–909.

300 Diaper Dermatitis

Bernice R. Krafchik

Irritant Diaper Dermatitis

Definition

The term *irritant diaper dermatitis* includes all eruptions that occur in the area covered by a diaper.

Etiology

1. Conditions caused directly by the wearing of diapers—irritant contact dermatitis, Jacquet erosive diaper dermatitis
2. Conditions that are aggravated by diapers—psoriasis
3. Conditions that occur whether diapers are worn or not—acrodermatitis enteropathica.

Epidemiology

1. In Great Britain in the 1970s, diaper dermatitis accounted for 20 per cent of all skin consultations in the zero- to 5-year age group.

2. In most societies, diapers are not worn, and infants escape a common condition seen in pediatric practice in Western societies.

3. Three methods of diapering are presently in use in the Western world.

   a. Cloth diapers, which are laundered at home, may be used. This method tends to leave chemicals in the diaper, despite numerous rinses, and the number of diaper changes is less than with diaper services and disposable diapers. Irritant diaper dermatitis occurs most often with this method, making it the least desirable manner of diapering.

   b. A second means of diapering is the use of a diaper service. This has become extremely popular since it was recognized that disposable diapers cause 1 to 2 per cent of the nonbiodegradable waste in North America.

   c. Disposable diapers were first used in the 1960s and have become increasingly popular. They have changed from paper to those with an absorbable

cellulose center to the most modern, which have a gel absorbent center that carries the wetness from the inside to the outside of the diaper, leaving the skin dry. These newer diapers probably cause the least problem with diaper dermatitis.

4. Irritant diaper dermatitis usually occurs from 3 to 18 months of life, peaking between 6 and 9 months.

Pathophysiology

1. The crucial factor in preventing irritant diaper dermatitis appears to be the number of diaper changes.

2. Maceration, occlusion, and possibly candidal and bacterial infections may all play a role in the pathogenesis of irritant diaper dermatitis. It has been shown that fecal bacteria may have a synergistic effect with *Candida* in producing the eruption.

3. Damage to the epidermis results in loss of the normal barrier function; this loss fosters increased susceptibility to irritation. The diaper covering the perineal area is an impervious layer because of the plastic covering. This milieu is continuously wet from urine or from hydration caused by occlusion. This makes the skin susceptible to friction from movement under the diaper, which does not occur with a dry diaper.

4. Elevations in the pH of the diaper area activate fecal lipases and proteases; this phenomenon influences the onset of irritant diaper dermatitis. The irritancy of feces has been shown to increase when mixed with urine, producing an increase in ammonia and hence pH.

5. Certain infants are constitutionally more susceptible to irritant contact dermatitis.

Clinical Findings

1. Chafing of the diaper area may occur on the convex surfaces, and a "tide mark" dermatitis occurs at the margin of the diaper. This is caused by friction from the diaper and wet skin and responds well to the use of emollients.

2. In irritant diaper dermatitis, erythema is noticed on the

convex surface of the inner, upper thigh area and buttock. The creases are spared, as is the area over the mons pubis in boys. The eruption subsequently becomes deeply erythematous, with a typical glistening or glazed appearance and a wrinkled surface.

3. An eruption consisting of well-demarcated punched-out ulcers and erosions is seen with home-laundered diapers. This is known as Jacquet erosive diaper dermatitis.

Key Clinical Findings: Irritant Diaper Dermatitis

- Erythematous lesions over diaper area, often with a glistening appearance
- Ulceration and erosion, maybe fever

Treatment

1. Emollients, particularly zinc oxide preparations and petrolatum, eliminate the effect of hydration and provide protection from urine and feces. Initially, a nonfluorinated corticosteroid (hydrocortisone 1 per cent ointment) should be used three times a day until improvement is noticed. This preparation is covered by the emollient. The use of strong corticosteroid preparations and of mixtures of antibiotics and corticosteroids is not recommended in the diaper area, because the occlusion effect from the diaper may cause atrophy and striae, and scrotal absorption is higher than in any other area.

2. Jacquet erosions respond well to change from home-laundered diapers. The fastest cure is to leave the child without any diapers, but this is usually not practical. The ulcers heal quickly with a mild corticosteroid preparation, after compresses with Burow's solution diluted 1/40, three times a day, and the use of thick emollients, which act as a barrier. These ulcerations are not seen with the same frequency since the introduction of newer diapering methods.

Key Treatments: Irritant Diaper Dermatitis

- Zinc oxide preparation
- Steroid ointment

Candidal Diaper Dermatitis

Definition

Candidal diaper dermatitis is caused by infections with *Candida* organisms from the feces, producing a typical clinical picture in the diaper area.

Epidemiology

1. The infant is particularly prone to candidal infection.
2. With the more frequent use of oral antibiotics in infants,

an overgrowth of *Candida* occurs in the feces, leading to the colonization of *Candida* in the diaper area.

3. The significance of recovering *Candida albicans* is at times difficult to interpret because the organism may be recovered from the diaper area in any skin condition after 72 hours and may even be grown in small amounts from normal skin. The organism appears to have the ability to invade through the epidermal barrier, possibly by liberating keratinases. *Candida* is recovered in much larger numbers from the skin and feces when clinical candidiasis occurs.

Clinical Findings

The clinical picture of candidiasis takes two forms.

1. It may present with a diffuse erythematous patch that extends over the genitalia with a peripheral scale and satellite pustules.
2. Small pink papules may be surmounted by a scale. These lesions may coalesce in some areas. The anterior perineal and perianal area are either both or separately involved, as are the creases, which helps differentiate this from an irritant diaper dermatitis. The more classic picture of a beefy red diaper area with satellite pustules is infrequently seen. This is possibly because of earlier treatment with antifungal and anti-inflammatory agents.

Key Clinical Finding: Candidal Diaper Dermatitis

- Diffuse pink erythema perigenitally

Treatment

1. Topical anticandidal therapy, such as nystatin, clotrimazole, and ketoconazole two or three times daily, is successful.
2. Adding hydrocortisone 1 per cent to the aforementioned agents provides an anti-inflammatory effect and promotes more rapid healing.
3. Potent corticosteroids should be avoided.
4. Compresses may be useful with very inflammatory lesions.
5. In a double-blind study, the oral use of nystatin (to eliminate *Candida* from the bowel) in conjunction with topical treatment did not affect the outcome of the dermatitis more favorably than the use of topical nystatin alone.

Key Treatment: Candidal Diaper Dermatitis

- Nystatin
- Clotrimazole
- Ketoconazole

301 Atopic Dermatitis (Eczema)

Bernice R. Krafchik

Definition

Atopic dermatitis (AD) is a chronic inherited skin disease that begins early in life, has a variable prognosis, and is often associated with or followed by other atopic diseases (asthma and hay fever).

Etiology

The precise cause is unknown.

1. Genetic factors
   a. There is often, particularly in severe cases, a history of one or both parents with atopic disease. If one parent has atopy, there is a 60 per cent chance that their offspring will have atopy, and if both parents are affected, there is an 80 per cent chance.
   b. Investigators have attempted to find the atopic gene. It has been localized to chromosome 11q13 (there is still controversy regarding this finding).
2. Environmental factors
   a. Since 1936, food has been implicated in the cause or exacerbation of AD. These studies have grave methodologic flaws, and the argument is still unresolved. Patients with AD have an increased incidence of anaphylactic reactions, particularly to peanuts and eggs. The incidence of hives (urticaria) appears to increase after ingestion of certain foods, and there is also an acute contact reaction to foods such as oranges and tomatoes.
   b. In recent years, the house dust mite antigen has been implicated in worsening AD, causing pruritus in affected individuals.
   c. Dryness in the winter, heat in the summer, wools, and nylon have all been implicated in exacerbating the disease.

Epidemiology

1. The disease begins early in life, with 80 per cent beginning in the first year and 95 per cent by 2 years of age. It often begins before the age of 3 months, at which stage the lesions are not pruritic, and xerosis is the only sign. It is when the itch-scratch cycle evolves that parents seek advice.
2. The incidence of AD has increased from 3 to 5 per cent in the 1970s to 10 per cent in the 1980s and, most recently, to 12 per cent. Most of these figures have been obtained from questionnaires.
3. There is a female:male preponderance of 2:1.
4. No human leukocyte antigen association exists.
5. The incidence of viral (herpes simplex), fungal, and bacterial (*Staphylococcus aureus*) skin infections is increased.

Pathophysiology

1. An increase in gamma E immunoglobulin (IgE) level occurs in more than 80 per cent of patients with AD. The reason for the increase is not known, and IgE has been found at birth in the umbilical cord blood. The increase is correlated with severity and extent.
2. An overall decrease in T cells occurs, with an absolute decrease in suppressor T cells. This finding is also related to the severity and the extent of the disease.
3. Abnormalities of cytokines exist. Two types of T cells, TH1 and TH2 cells, have been cloned. TH2 cells cause an increase in interleukin-2 (IL-2) and IL-4, with a concomitant decrease in interferon gamma. Increased IL-4 is also associated with increased IgE production. Dysregulation of IL-4 appears to occur in AD.
4. An abnormal chemotaxis occurs in AD that is also related to the severity and extent of the disease and affects the polymorphonuclear leukocytes, lymphocytes, and monocytes.
5. Abnormalities in monocytes in AD result in abnormal production of IL-10 and prostaglandin E_2. IL-10 is known to inhibit T cell–mediated reactions and interferon gamma.
6. The production of histamine in AD skin is increased, possibly indicating mast cell degranulation from antigen-antibody reactions. Patients with severe AD have increased basophil releasability of histamine than occurs in patients with mild AD.
7. *Staphylococcus aureus* is almost invariably colonized in patients with AD. The cause of this finding is unknown, but it is thought to be the result of abnormal chemotaxis. The possibility that *S. aureus* acts as a superantigen and drives the eczematous process or produces anti-staphylococcal IgE antibodies and produces a dermatitis has recently been raised as a pathogenetic mechanism.

Clinical Findings

1. History and physical examination
   a. Atopic dermatitis is usually the first manifestation of atopic disease and presents in 85 per cent of cases during the first year of life, usually around 3 months of age, and in 38 per cent of cases even earlier. In 95 per cent of cases, the disease develops by 5 years of age.
   b. The disease usually presents at 2 to 3 months of age on the cheeks, scalp, and lateral extensor areas of the legs, although any part of the body may be involved. The characteristic and only symptom is pruritus, which is a major cause of morbidity and often interferes with normal sleep patterns. Lesions are usually symmetrical and appear as a dermatitis with erythema and scaling or eczema (erythema, scaling, vesicles and crusts). Generalized xerosis, including dry hair and scalp, is an important feature. The diaper area is often spared.
   c. In the childhood phase from the age of 2 years, the flexural areas are involved, particularly the antecu-

bital and the popliteal fossae. The neck, the flexures of the wrists and ankles, and the buttock-thigh crease are also commonly involved. These areas are particularly prone to sweating, which leads to increased itching. Lesions tend to be exudative. Lichenification occurs, consisting of thickening of the skin and increase in skin markings. It is thought to be pathognomonic of AD. The nails may be shiny and buffed from constant rubbing, and the eyebrows may be sparse and broken off (Hertoghe sign). Lymphadenopathy is often a notable feature.

d. At puberty, the clinical features once again involve the face, neck, and body. The lesions tend to be more widespread, with erythema and scaling but with less exudation. Xerosis and lichenification are still prominent features. The face has a typical central pallor. A distinctive rippled, brown, macular discoloration around the neck has been recognized in older patients with AD. This appearance is similar to macular amyloid.

e. In black children, the lesions of AD are often more papular and follicular.

f. Postinflammatory hypopigmentation and hyperpigmentation is often present and particularly visible after treatment. This disappears without scarring.

g. A variant of AD, called the inverse pattern, affects the extensors of the elbows and knees and the dorsa of the hands. This pattern occurs more commonly in boys than in girls. It has a poorer prognosis than other forms of AD.

h. Nummular dermatitis is a chronic exudative discoid form of the disease that occurs in children. Unlike the adult variety, which presents with dry patches, the lesions in children are moist and oozing and respond to antibiotics.

2. Associated findings
   a. Ichthyosis vulgaris that mainly affects the legs occurs in 20 to 37 per cent of patients with AD.

   b. Hyperlinear palms and soles frequently exist, particularly in patients with ichthyosis.

   c. Keratosis pilaris is an extremely common condition that is seen on the extensor aspect of the arms and the anterior thighs in many healthy young children. The lesions tend to be worse in patients with AD. In young children, these findings are also often seen on the lateral aspects of the cheeks. The lesions consist of asymptomatic hyperkeratotic follicular papules, which may have an underlying erythematous telangiectatic background. Keratosis pilaris tends to persist in a mild form for life and presents no more than a cosmetic problem. Treatment is aimed at hydrating the affected area with oil baths and emollients.

   d. Pityriasis alba is found in children with and without AD. It is identified by hypopigmented, ill-defined, scaly patches on the cheeks, particularly toward the end of summer, when the rest of the face is tanned. Pityriasis alba is thought to represent a subclinical dermatitis, resulting in postinflammatory hypopig-

mentation. The patches often recur yearly until puberty. The lesions repigment slowly after treatment with low-potency topical corticosteroid preparations (hydrocortisone 1 per cent ointment two to three times a day) for 2 to 3 weeks. Parents should be reassured that complete repigmentation will eventually occur. This condition is often confused with tinea corporis.

e. The Dennie-Morgan fold is a double fold found under the lower eyelids of patients with AD. It may be present at birth or soon thereafter. Although it is thought to be pathognomonic of AD, it also occurs in other inflammatory conditions around the eye. It tends to disappear with age.

f. Lichen spinulosus is identified by round, occasionally pruritic, follicular plaques on the trunk of patients with AD. It may also occur in children who do not have the disease and is common in black skin. At times, the lesions are hypopigmented, but their diagnostic feature is the presence of grouped hyperkeratotic follicular spines.

g. Eye findings in AD include keratoconjunctivitis, which may occur in a painful form known as vernal conjunctivitis. Cataracts, which may be anterior or posterior subcapsular, have been described in more severe cases. Keratoconus (abnormally shaped cornea) is extremely rare and is associated with very severe cases of AD.

h. Dyshidrotic eczema consists of vesicles on the palms and soles and is often associated with hyperhidrosis. The lesions consist of small, pruritic, multiloculated vesicles along the sides of the fingers, on the toes, and on the palms and soles, resembling "sago grain vesicles." These rupture, leaving crusts and erythema with scaling.

i. Juvenile plantar dermatitis is seen before puberty and presents with scaling, cracking, and painful fissuring on both feet. The big toe and heel are often involved. Hyperhidrosis is associated and responds to barrier creams.

j. Patients with AD are susceptible to infections with herpes simplex and vaccinia (when the latter was used for vaccination). The vesicular or bullous lesions begin on areas of dermatitis, and an associated fever may be present. The eruption is usually seen with a primary herpes infection but has been seen more than once in a patient. After a day or two, the eruption generalizes and involves normal skin (eczema herpeticum or Kaposi varicelliform eruption).

3. Differential diagnosis. The differential diagnosis of AD includes other eczematous disorders, scabies, seborrheic dermatitis, contact dermatitis, psoriasis, and tinea infection.

   a. It is often difficult to distinguish scabies from AD, particularly in infants. Both diseases are extremely pruritic. Recent onset of itching in family members is helpful in the diagnosis of scabies. Xerosis and facial involvement are common findings in infants with AD, although scabies commonly affects the face in infancy. If a child presents for the first time with a pruritic eruption at the age of 5 years, scabies would be more likely to be present than AD.

b. Seborrheic dermatitis occurs in infants at about 6 weeks of age. It is asymptomatic and involves the scalp and intertriginous areas, with a yellow greasy scale on an erythematous base. The diaper area is often affected in seborrheic dermatitis, whereas it is usually spared in AD. The differentiation from AD is not always obvious, because pruritus may at times be prominent in seborrheic dermatitis. Some physicians believe that seborrheic dermatitis is a variant of AD, although the classical clinical picture and excellent prognosis allow them to be distinguished.

c. In infants and young children, an allergic dermatitis is rare. In infants, the most common allergen is nickel snaps on undershirts. A well-demarcated line of dermatitis is present in the central chest area.

d. Psoriasis is uncommon in the early years of life. It is most common on the scalp, elbows, and knees, but it may occur anywhere. In infants and young children, it is common in the diaper area.

e. Atopic dermatitis may be so severe that the whole body becomes erythrodermic. It is important to distinguish this from other causes of erythroderma, like epidermolytic hyperkeratosis, Netherton syndrome, psoriasis, pityriasis rubra pilaris, nutritional deficiencies and drug eruptions.

f. One of the most difficult conditions to differentiate from AD in infancy is immunodeficiency. Children with immunodeficiency present with failure to thrive and dermatitis, which may be present in the same areas as AD, or as an erythroderma. Recurrent infections should help to distinguish the two conditions.

g. Fungal infections in children usually manifest as single plaques, mainly on the extremities. At times, more than one lesion may be present, and a dermatitis may be the presenting primary eruption. Tinea infections are not so widespread as in AD and have a specific peripheral edge with central clearing.

Key Clinical Findings

• Infancy
   Erythematous lesions on face scalp and legs first, followed by any body surface. May show scaling, vesicles, and crusts.

• Childhood
   Flexural areas—may lichenify

Laboratory Findings

1. Mild peripheral eosinophilia may be present in patients with AD. The eosinophil cationic protein level is increased; this is useful as a marker in the serum of AD patients and is indicative of eosinophil activation.

2. Low serum zinc levels have been detected, possibly as a result of chronic inflammation.

3. Complement levels have been found to be low in some patients with AD. The intensity of the complement changes seemed to be correlated to the severity of the disease.

4. Prostaglandin E_2 levels produced by peripheral blood mononuclear cells are increased in AD.

5. Mast cells have enhanced release of histamine that increases in plasma and skin.

Key Laboratory Finding

• Eosinophilia (sometimes)

Treatment

1. General measures. The most important aspect of the treatment is the establishment of an honest, trusting relationship with the parents, explaining the nature of the disease. The health care provider should particularly stress that treatment is aimed at good control of the pruritus, xerosis, and eczematous lesions, but that cure is not possible.

2. Specific measures.

a. Topical treatment.

(1) The inflammation is best treated with corticosteroid ointments. Potent corticosteroids should never be used on the face, where hydrocortisone 1 per cent ointment applied three times a day is very effective. This regimen should be used until improvement occurs, and then it should be withdrawn. The ointment base acts as an emollient for the dry skin but may be substituted for a cream in humid weather or if troublesome folliculitis occurs. For the dermatitis on the body, a more potent corticosteroid ointment, such as betamethasone 17-valerate 0.05 per cent, is applied to the affected areas three times a day until improvement occurs. As soon as the dermatitis resolves, a lubricating ointment should be substituted. When the scalp is involved, application of a corticosteroid cream three times a day and a bland or tar shampoo daily is helpful. Lotions are more aesthetic but tend to burn open excoriated areas. Topical corticosteroids have few side effects.

(2) The xerosis is treated with emollients rather then corticosteroids. Numerous emollients are available, some containing urea. Parents should be warned to apply urea products only when the skin is moist because burning and irritation may otherwise occur. Urea-containing products are usually too strong to use on the face. These compounds are difficult to mix and should be heated before they are incorporated into the vehicle. The dryness is best treated with a bathing regimen consisting of agents such as non-perfumed bath oils with emulsifiers and oilated oatmeal powder to soothe the skin. Bathing should only take 5 to 15 minutes because dehy-

dration of the skin may occur if it is continued longer.

(3) Tar preparations are useful in certain instances. When prescribed as liquor carbonis detergens, 5 to 10 per cent combined with a corticosteroid, they may be of great benefit, particularly in the treatment of nummular patches.

b. Oral agents.

(1) Antihistamines, such as hydroxyzine hydrochloride in an appropriate dosage, may alleviate the incessant itch and allow the patient some peaceful hours of sleep. Doses of hydroxyzine higher than the normal 2 mg/kg/day should be prescribed for the treatment of AD. Babies aged 9 months and older should begin therapy with 10 mg three times a day. Ketotifen (benzocyloheptathiophene) may be useful.

(2) Oral antibiotics are used to treat clinical infection. The infection is almost always caused by *S. aureus* because this organism is known to colonize the skin of patients with AD. Whether prolonged antibiotics should be used to prevent recolonization of the skin is controversial because resistant bacterial strains may emerge. Both erythromycin and cloxacillin may work adequately in *S. aureus* infections. Although antibacterial scrubs may reduce the staphylococcal colony count, they are irritating, and their use is not routinely advised. A study on the use of topical antibiotics has shown a marked decrease in the *S. aureus* colony count and clinical improvement in AD with the use of mupirocin. Topical corticosteroids also reduce the *S. aureus* count.

(3) Systemic corticosteroids have been found to control particularly severe exacerbations, but in view of their multiple side effects and an unwanted rebound flare when they are discontinued, they are rarely indicated. Occasionally, a 2-week tapering dose should be used. Prednisone is given as 1 mg/kg/day for 4 days, 0.75 mg/kg/day for 4 days, and 0.5 mg/kg/day for 4 days after which the medication is stopped. It should be stressed that continued use of systemic corticosteroids is unwarranted and dangerous.

c. Newer agents. As understanding of the pathogenesis of the disease increases, newer agents are being used with variable success.

(1) Ultraviolet (UV) light. It has been known for many years that AD lesions improve in the summer months. Numerous studies have defined the benefits of exposure to both UVA and UVB, either alone or together. In many studies, relapse occurs quite soon after the therapy has been stopped. However, Atherton treated 15 adolescents with severe AD with oral psoralen and UVA and obtained clearing in 14 of the 15 patients. Long-term remission was achieved in nine patients. Other studies have corroborated the beneficial effects of psoralen plus UVA and UVA alone and have stressed the increased effect of UVA over that of UVB. In view of the increased skin malignancies that have been shown after these treatments, they should be prescribed with caution.

(2) Disodium cromoglycate. Oral and topical disodium cromoglycate preparations have been used in Europe, leading to improvement in patients in whom there is a positive correlation between AD and food allergy. A good effect with a topical solution of cromolyn has been reported. The chemical is thought to act by reducing histamine release from mast cells in the gut and skin. Trials in the United States have been less successful.

(3) Cytotoxic agents. In adults with severe intractable AD, oral cyclophosphamide and azathioprine have both been used with marked improvement and remissions that lasted for an average of 24 months. These drugs are not usually necessary for children, given their known side effects.

(4) Oral evening primrose oil. This agent is a source of essential fatty acids, but a recent double-blind study showed no significant benefit of evening primrose oil over placebo.

(5) Thymopoietin. Thymopentin pentapeptide and thymostimulin are immunostimulatory substances that affect the function of mature T cells. Thymopoietin was used by Hanifin in a small group of patients with AD and proved useful in a double-blind prospective study.

(6) Cyclosporine. In both oral and topical form, cyclosporine has been used in the treatment of AD. Topical cyclosporine was used by De Prost in a 10 per cent gel twice per day; 10 of 18 patients showed marked improvement. However, in another study, topical cyclosporine was not efficacious, because absorption of cyclosporine through the skin appears to be poor. Oral cyclosporine has been effective in treating AD in adults, but the lesions recur as soon as the drug is stopped, and the side effects seldom warrant its use in children.

(7) Chinese herbs. These have been used in children with widespread AD, leading to a good response over placebo. Few side effects, except in palatability, occurred. The decoction consists of 10 different herbs, although they are variously formulated, depending on the individual patient. The mechanism by which these herbs produce improvement is not known. They are expensive and difficult to procure in the United States.

Key Treatment

- Corticosteroid ointment

Prevention and Prognosis

1. The effect of food withdrawal during pregnancy in deterring the onset or elimination of AD has not been sufficiently studied. However, in one well-controlled study, a decrease appeared to occur in the incidence of AD at 1 year in the food withdrawal group, but no significant difference occurred at 4 years.
2. There is a marked tendency for the lesions to improve with age. Thirty per cent of patients with AD have persistent disease as adults. A similar number have allergic rhinitis, asthma, or both.

Bibliography

Hanifin JM: Atopic dermatitis in infants and children. Pediatr Clin North Am 1991;38(4):763–789.

Krafchik BR: Eczematous dermatitis. *In* Schachner LA, Hansen RC (eds): Pediatric Dermatology, vol 1, 2nd ed. New York, Churchill Livingstone, 1995, pp 685–721.

Leung DYM: Atopic dermatitis: The skin as a window into the pathogenesis of chronic allergic diseases. J Allergy Clin Immunol 1995;96(3):302–318.

302 Urticaria

Bernice R. Krafchik

Definition

Urticaria represents a reaction in the dermis and subcutaneous tissue to various stimuli. The lesions are pruritic, erythematous wheals that appear in crops anywhere on the body. Acute urticaria continues to erupt for about 10 days, whereas in chronic urticaria, lesions may last for longer than 2 years. Angioedema represents the subcutaneous form of urticaria.

Etiology

1. Many apparent causes exist. A dominant inheritance is associated with the hereditary form of angioedema.
2. Drugs
3. Infections
4. Physical exercise or cold-induced
5. Collagen vascular disease, such as lupus and dermatomyositis
6. Metabolic, such as thyrotoxicosis
7. Idiopathic

Epidemiology

1. At least 15 to 20 per cent of children have at least one episode of urticaria by adolescence.
2. The incidence is equal among the sexes.

Pathophysiology

1. Immunologic
   a. Antigen attachment to a specific antibody of the gamma E immunoglobulin (IgE) class results in activation and subsequent release of mediators from mast cells. Histamine is one of the major chemicals produced by the mast cell on degranulation. It circulates in the blood and attaches to receptors on the blood vessels. This results in dilatation and escape of fluid into the surrounding tissue.
   b. Complement activation through immune complex formation is another mechanism whereby the mast cell is degranulated and mediators are released.

2. Nonimmunologic. Direct pharmacologic degranulation of mast cells through drugs or endogenous prostaglandins.

Clinical Findings

1. History
   a. Evaluation of etiologic agents and organ systems is important.
   b. If the urticaria is acute (first 6 weeks), it is more likely that the etiology can be established.
   c. It is important to establish whether sun, cold, or exercise may be related.

2. Physical examination
   a. Wheals, which are the typical lesions of urticaria, are areas of dermal erythema and swelling that are usually multiple and measure 2 to 5 mm. In young children, the wheals often enlarge over a few hours to form areas with dusky violaceous centers and a peripheral red border, known as giant urticaria. This is often seen as a result of a drug reaction, particularly to cefaclor. These lesions are often confused with erythema multiforme. Urticarial lesions resulting from sun, cold, or exercise are often much smaller and have a white center.
   b. Angioedema is characterized by skin-colored swelling with indistinct borders. The hands, feet, eyelids, and lips are commonly involved. Angioedema may occur concurrently with urticaria and may result in anaphylaxis from laryngeal edema and hypotension.
   c. In acute urticaria, the lesions are extremely pruritic, occur in crops, and usually last for 10 to 14 days. Each individual lesion lasts for 24 to 36 hours.
   d. Chronic urticaria is the persistence of urticaria for 6 weeks or longer. The cause of these lesions is difficult to ascertain, and if the patient is otherwise well, it is not always rewarding to embark on nu-

merous diagnostic tests. The wheals tend to be less numerous than in the acute form.

Key Clinical Finding

- Erythematous, pruritic papules or wheals

Treatment

1. Etiologic agents should be removed if there is a clear-cut history of their involvement.
2. Antihistamines of the H_1 variety are helpful. They act by blocking the action of histamine on the receptors on blood vessels.
3. A combination of an H_1-blocker with an H_2 blocker sometimes works better than an H_1-blocker alone.
4. Doxepin is a tricyclic antidepressant that in low doses

has been shown to be useful in urticaria. A topical form of doxepin is available as an antipruritic.
5. Occasionally, systemic steroid therapy may be warranted in severe acute urticaria but should not be used in chronic urticaria.

Key Treatment

- Antihistamines
- Systemic steroids (rarely needed)

Bibliography

Legrain V, Taieb A, Sage T, Maleville J: Urticaria in infants: A study of forty patients. Pediatr Dermatol 1990;7:101–107.

303 Erythema Multiforme and Stevens-Johnson Syndrome

Bernice R. Krafchik

Definition

1. Erythema multiforme (EM) is a reaction in the skin, usually to a viral infection. The lesions appear as symmetrical, fixed, erythematous papules that evolve into characteristic target lesions.
2. Although Stevens-Johnson syndrome (SJS) was initially thought to be part of the spectrum of EM, it is now recognized to be completely different, with a different etiology and clinical presentation. The disease starts abruptly, with fever and lesions that rapidly become bullous. Toxic epidermal necrolysis is a more severe part of the spectrum of SJS.

Etiology

1. In most cases, a herpes infection precedes EM by up to 10 days.
2. In most cases, SJS is preceded by the ingestion of drugs. The most common are nonsteroidal anti-inflammatory, sulfa drugs, and anticonvulsant drugs, although many others have been implicated.

Epidemiology

1. Erythema multiforme is uncommon in childhood, although 20 per cent of all cases occur in this age group.
2. Stevens-Johnson syndrome, which is more common in children, occurs more frequently in the spring and summer.

Pathophysiology

1. The viral genome has been isolated from the lesions of EM and may be directly involved in the pathogenesis.
2. An enzymatic abnormality has been implicated in the etiology of SJS.

Clinical Findings

1. History
   a. Patients with EM often have a clear-cut history of a cold sore 1 week to 10 days before the development of the lesions, although it is unusual to have a prodrome.
   b. Stevens-Johnson syndrome starts abruptly after the development of a high fever, often while the patient is still receiving the offending drug.
2. Physical examination
   a. The lesions of EM usually appear within 24 to 48 hours and consist of about 100 red papules, which are widespread and predominantly acral. They evolve into typical target lesions that have concentric rings of different colors. The center of the lesion may become bullous and crusted. The mouth is involved in half the patients, with ulceration of the mucous membrane and tongue. Occasionally, EM occurs primarily in the mouth with only a few lesions on the body. No other mucous membranes are involved.

Key Clinical Finding: Erythema Multiforme

- Target or ring erythematous lesion over any part of the body

   b. In SJS, 1 day to 1 week after a prodrome of fever, malaise, and a nonspecific upper respiratory illness, the lesions develop abruptly.
      (1) The eyes are often the first organ to be involved

in SJS, with erythema and pain. Patients with SJS are at risk for synechiae, and blindness has followed severe eye involvement.

(2) Other mucous membranes are also involved.

(3) The individual body lesions are centrally located. They consist of symmetric red macules that rapidly become bullae before sloughing. Areas of raw eroded skin become evident, and in toxic epidermal necrolysis, practically the whole body may be involved.

Key Clinical Findings: Stevens-Johnson Syndrome

• Target lesions and papules may become bullous.

• Ulcerations are present in the oral mucosa (50 per cent).

• Fever is present.

Laboratory Findings

1. Erythema multiforme: none
2. Stevens-Johnson syndrome:
   a. Fluid and electrolyte imbalance
   b. Elevated erythrocyte sedimentation rate
   c. Leukocytosis

Key Laboratory Tests: Stevens-Johnson Syndrome

• Electrolyte levels

• Serum albumin level

Treatment

1. Treatment of EM
   a. Erythema multiforme may be prevented by the prompt treatment of herpes simplex infection with acyclovir.

Key Treatment

• Erythema multiforme
  Administer acyclovir if herpes simplex lesions are present.

• Stevens-Johnson syndrome
  Discontinue drug.
  Restore fluid and electrolyte balance.
  Administer systemic steroids.

   b. Although systemic steroids have been used to treat EM, their use is usually not warranted.
2. Treatment of SJS
   a. Discontinue the probable offending drug.
   b. Correct fluid and electrolyte status.
   c. Promptly treat secondary infection.
   d. Provide good ophthalmologic care.
   e. Use of systemic steroids is controversial, although the symptoms are alleviated by the prompt use of a short course of steroids.
   f. The high mortality associated with SJS decreases with good nursing care.
   g. Some clinicians recommend burn unit care for patients with SJS.

Prognosis and Prevention

1. Erythema multiforme tends to recur. The prognosis is excellent, and the lesions heal with no scarring.
2. In SJS
   a. The offending drug must be avoided because occasional recurrences have been reported.
   b. Long-term eye problems are a source of morbidity.
   c. Although the skin does not scar, unsightly marks may persist for many years.

Bibliography

Assier S, Bastuji-Garin S, Revuz J, Roujeau J-C: Erythema multiforme with mucous membrane involvement and Stevens-Johnson syndrome are clinically different disorders with distinct causes. Arch Dermatol 1995;131:539–543.

Huff JC, Weston WL, Tonnesen MG, et al: Erythema multiforme: A critical review of characteristics, diagnostic criteria, and causes. J Am Acad Dermatol 1983;8:763–775.

304 Hemangioma and Vascular Malformation

Bernice R. Krafchik

Hemangioma

Definition

Hemangiomas are the most common benign tumor of childhood. They are characterized by a proliferative phase and an involutional phase, leading to complete, spontaneous regression in most cases.

Etiology

The etiology of hemangiomas is unknown—abnormal angiogenesis related to estrogen receptors has been implicated.

Epidemiology

1. Hemangiomas occur in approximately 2.5 per cent of neonates.

2. Hemangiomas occur in 10 to 12 per cent of white infants by 1 year of age.
3. The ratio of girls:boys is 3:1.
4. The disorder is more common in twins, premature infants, and families with a history of the disorder.

Clinical Findings

1. History. In 30 per cent of patients, hemangiomas are present at birth. In the remainder of cases, hemangiomas usually appear within the first 3 to 4 weeks of life.
2. Physical examination. The initial lesion may be either a discrete white macule with central telangiectases or a red macule. Within a few days, the lesion rapidly becomes elevated and enlarges. The size, shape, and color vary, so that the appearance may be that of a lobulated, bright red superficial tumor or a deeper, smooth, blue tumor.
3. Course. During the first 6 months of life, hemangiomas proliferate at a rapid rate, slowing in growth between 6 and 10 months and peaking in size at approximately 12 months. Involution begins at 18 months to 2 years; 50 per cent resolve by 5 years, 70 per cent by 7 years, and 90 per cent by 9 years.
4. Complications. Most complications arise during the proliferative stage.
   a. Complications include bleeding, ulceration, infection, and compromise of vital functions.
   b. High-output congestive heart failure may occur.
   c. In large hemangiomas, Kasabach-Merritt syndrome may develop, associated with thrombocytopenia and consumptive coagulopathy.

Key Clinical Finding: Hemangioma

• Growing, raised erythematous papular lesion(s)

Treatment

1. Most patients require no treatment. Parents should have this explained in detail, with photographs illustrating the natural evolution of the disorder.
2. Systemic corticosteroids are used for extensive hemangiomas, diffuse hemangiomatosis, Kasabach-Merritt syndrome, and hemangiomas that compromise vital functions. The dose of prednisone is 2 to 4 mg/kg/day. Response is usually seen within 1 to 2 weeks, at which time the medication is either maintained or slowly tapered.
3. Intralesional corticosteroids may be used for periorbital hemangiomas when vision is threatened.
4. Ulcerations are treated with compresses soaked in Burow's solution or topical and systemic antibiotics. Immediate treatment with the pulsed dye laser alleviates the pain of the ulceration promptly, but healing occurs rapidly, even if the laser is not available.
5. Interferon alfa-2a has been successful in inducing early regression of life-threatening, corticosteroid-resistant hemangiomas.

Key Treatment: Hemangioma

• Usually no treatment required
• Systemic steroids for extensive lesions

Vascular Malformation

Definition

A vascular malformation is the result of a structural abnormality of blood vessels. It is present at birth and grows in proportion to the growth of the child. These lesions do not resolve spontaneously.

Etiology

The etiology is unknown. Recent studies have demonstrated a decrease in the number of nerves surrounding the abnormal blood vessels and impaired neural regulation of blood flow.

Epidemiology

1. Occurs in 0.3 per cent of newborns
2. Equal sex distribution
3. Present at birth

Pathophysiology

Lesions may be composed of ectatic mature capillaries, veins, and lymphatic vessels. Rarely arteriovenous malformations may occur.

Clinical Findings

1. Port-wine stains (nevus flammeus) are usually flat and pink in infancy and darken to a purple hue in adults. Soft tissue and bony hypertrophy can be associated with overlying port-wine stains.
2. On the limbs, the lesion is known as the Klippel-Trenaunay syndrome.
3. The Sturge-Weber syndrome consists of a port-wine stain in the ophthalmic division of the trigeminal nerve, with seizures and an underlying, ipsilateral cerebral vascular lesion.
4. Tumors of various blood vessels are present at birth and may slowly enlarge as new vessels open. The vessels in these lesions are usually obvious.

Key Clinical Finding: Vascular Malformation

• Port-wine stain appearance

Treatment

Treatment is particularly important for patients with facial port-wine stains because of their psychological impact.

Treatment has been revolutionized with the advent of the 585-nm flashlamp-pumped pulsed dye laser. This treatment can result in a marked clearing of the port-wine stain. Early treatment of the lesion is preferable. Treatments are performed every 2 to 3 months. For infants and young children, a general anesthetic is used, and for older children, local anesthesia is obtained with the use of Emla cream (eutectic mixture of local anesthetic).

Key Treatment: Vascular Malformation

- Laser therapy

Bibliography

Esterly NB: Cutaneous hemangiomas, vascular stains and associated syndromes. Current Probl Pediatr 1987;17(1):1–69.

Rabinowitz LG, Esterly NB: Vascular birthmarks and other abnormalities of blood vessels and lymphatics. *In* Schachner LA, Hansen RC (eds): Pediatric Dermatology, vol 2, 2nd ed. New York, Churchill Livingstone, 1995, pp 953–989.

305 Skin Infections

Teresita A. Laude

Bacterial Skin Infections

Impetigo

Etiology

1. Group A β-hemolytic streptococcus (*Streptococcus pyogenes*)
2. *Staphylococcus aureus*, phage 2, type 71 or 52

Clinical Findings

1. Impetigo contagiosa (streptococcal impetigo)
   a. Yellow or honey-colored crusted lesions
   b. Usually on exposed areas of the skin
   c. May have regional lymphadenopathy
   d. May be preceded by minor trauma, e.g., insect bite, cut
   e. More common during summertime
   f. Complication: post-streptococcal glomerulonephritis
2. Bullous impetigo (staphylococcal impetigo)
   a. Flaccid blisters containing pus
   b. More common in young infants
   c. More common in covered areas

Key Clinical Findings: Impetigo

- Honey-colored crusted lesions (group A streptococcus)
- Bullous purulent lesions (*Staphylococcus*)

Laboratory Diagnosis

1. Culture
2. Streptozyme test

Treatment

1. Mupirocin ointment for stable, solitary lesions
2. Oral β-lactamase–resistant antibiotic for 7 to 10 days

Key Treatment: Impetigo

- Antibiotics

Staphylococcal Scalded Skin Syndrome

Etiology

Staphylococcus aureus, phage 2, type 71 colonizes the mucous membranes of the eyes and nasopharynx and selected areas of the skin and produces an epidermolytic toxin called exfoliatin.

Clinical Findings

1. Staphylococcal scalded skin syndrome is most common in children younger than 6 years of age. Called Ritter disease in newborns, it may follow omphalitis or infection of the circumcision site. It may be seen in older children with kidney failure who cannot eliminate the toxin.
2. Crusting around the eyes and mouth occurs.
3. Generalized tenderness and erythema occurs, then exfoliation of the skin in sheets, leaving a scalded-looking surface. The borders are rolled like wet tissue paper.
4. The patient has a positive Nikolsky sign: slight rubbing of the normal-looking adjacent skin results in blistering.
5. Mild-to-moderate constitutional symptoms are present.

Key Clinical Findings: Staphylococcal Scalded Skin Syndrome

- Generalized erythema
- Exfoliation of skin in sheets
- Positive Nikolsky sign

Laboratory Diagnosis

1. Culture from colonized sites.
2. Histologic examination of the exfoliated skin showing partial split of the upper epidermis. (In toxic epidermone-

crolysis due to drugs, the exfoliation involves full thickness of the epidermis.)

Treatment

1. Intravenous (IV) β-lactamase–resistant antibiotic
2. Fluids and electrolytes for support

Key Treatment: Staphylococcal Scalded Skin Syndrome

- Intravenous antistaphylococcus antibiotic
- Fluid and electrolyte support

Folliculitis, Furunculosis, and Carbunculosis

Etiology

Staphylococcus aureus

Clinical Findings

1. Folliculitis (Bockhart impetigo)—scattered small pustules involving hair follicles
2. Furuncle—a tender deep-seated nodule around a hair follicle with signs of "pointing"
3. Carbuncle—several confluent furuncles

Key Clinical Findings: Folliculitis, Furunculosis, Carbunculosis

- Pustules
- Multiple coalesced pustules

Laboratory Diagnosis

1. Culture of the lesion
2. Culture of the nasopharynx or perineum in a *Staphylococcus* carrier

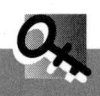

Key Laboratory Test: Folliculitis, Furunculosis, Carbunculosis

- Culture pus

Treatment

1. β-Lactamase–resistant antibiotic
2. Incision and drainage
3. Antibacterial wash
4. Intranasal mupirocin for 5 days for *Staphylococcus* carrier

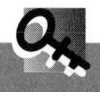

Key Treatment: Follicutitis, Furunculosis, Carbunculosis

- Antistaphylococcus antibiotic

Erysipelas (St. Anthony's Fire)

Etiology

Group A β-hemolytic streptococcus

Clinical Findings

1. Rapidly spreading, well-defined tender and painful erythema and swelling
2. May be preceded by minor skin trauma, like an insect bite or a cut
3. May recur if an underlying local lymphatic dysfunction is present.

Key Clinical Finding: Erysipelas

- Rapidly spreading erythema with defined border

Laboratory Diagnosis

Key Laboratory Test: Erysipelas

- Blood culture

Treatment

Key Treatment: Erysipelas

- IV penicillin

Cellulitis

Etiology

1. Group A β-hemolytic streptococcus
2. *Staphylococcus aureus*
3. *Haemophilus influenzae*, type b
4. *Pneumococcus*

Clinical Findings

1. May have antecedent minor trauma or break in the skin
2. Tender, erythematous, inflamed area
3. Borders are ill defined because of involvement of the deeper subcutaneous tissue.
4. Purplish discoloration in *H. influenzae* cellulitis

Key Clinical Findings: Cellulitis

- Swollen, tender skin and subcutaneous tissue
- Purplish color (*H. influenzae* type b)

Laboratory Diagnosis

Key Laboratory Test: Cellulitis

- Culture lesion and blood

Treatment

Key Treatment: Cellulitis

- IV Antibiotic

Perianal Dermatitis/Cellulitis

Etiology

Group A β-hemolytic streptococcus

Clinical Findings

1. More common in infants and younger children, especially boys
2. Vivid perianal erythema, swelling, and irritation
3. Pain, pruritus
4. Misdiagnosed as candidiasis, child abuse, inflammatory bowel disease, psoriasis
5. May precipitate or worsen guttate psoriasis

Key Clinical Finding: Perianal Dermatitis

- Vivid perianal erythema

Laboratory Diagnosis

Key Laboratory Test: Perianal Dermatitis

- Culture lesion

Treatment

Key Treatment: Perianal Dermatitis

- Course of penicillin or erythromycin

Blistering Distal Dactylitis

Etiology

Group A β-hemolytic streptococcus

Clinical Findings

1. More common in school children, less so in preschoolers
2. Tender blisters over the anterior fat pad of the thumb or fingers

Laboratory Diagnosis

Diagnosis is obtained from culture from the lesion; a third of patients may have a positive throat culture.

Treatment

Oral penicillin or erythromycin

Erythrasma

Etiology

Corynebacterium minutissimum

Clinical Findings

1. Well-defined, brown discoloration, with fine scales
2. Distribution in the intertriginous areas, especially the axillae and interdigits

Laboratory Diagnosis

Wood lamp examination reveals coral pink fluorescence resulting from a porphyrin metabolite.

Treatment

Imidazole cream or oral erythromycin

Fish-Tank and Swimming Pool Granuloma

Etiology

The disorder is caused by infection with *Mycobacterium marinum* via a skin abrasion in contaminated water of fish tanks or swimming pools.

Clinical Findings

1. Purple red nodules exist at the site of injury, usually the finger, hand, or face.
2. Lesions may be distributed along the line of lymphatic drainage from the inoculation site.

Key Clinical Finding: Fish Tank or Swimming Pool Granuloma

- Purplish red nodules at the site of trauma

Laboratory Diagnosis

Key Laboratory Tests: Fish Tank or Swimming Pool Granuloma

- Punch skin biopsy
- Culture

Treatment

Key Treatment: Fish Tank or Swimming Pool Granuloma

- Rifampicin
- Minocycline

Viral Skin Infections

Herpes Simplex

Etiology

Herpes simplex virus (HSV-1 and HSV-2)

Clinical Findings

1. Most infections in children are subclinical.
2. Primary clinical infections.
   a. Herpetic gingivostomatitis—painful shallow ulcers on the buccal mucosa, tongue, gums, palate, and lips; swollen gums; fever; foul breath; regional lymphadenopathy; inability to eat

b. Herpetic dermatitis
  (1) Grouped vesicles on any skin surface
  (2) May invade the eye, producing dendritic corneal ulcers, if the vesicles are periorbital
  (3) May recur in the same site.
c. Eczema herpeticum (Kaposi varicelliform eruption)—disseminated HSV on atopic dermatitis
d. Herpes neonatorum
  (1) HSV-2 acquired from the birth canal of a woman who usually has primary genital herpes
  (2) Grouped vesicles on the presenting part (scalp) and other areas
  (3) May involve the brain and the eye
e. Herpetic vulvovaginitis—painful ulcers in the genitalia; may result from sexual abuse.

Key Clinical Findings: Herpes Simplex

• Vesicles, rash
• Gingivostomatitis

Laboratory Diagnosis

1. Tzanck test—the clinician unroofs a vesicle, scrapes the base onto a slide, airs it dry, fixes it with alcohol, and stains it with Giemsa or Wright stain. Positive findings are multinucleated giant cells, balloon degeneration of the epidermal cells, and intranuclear inclusion bodies.
2. Viral culture
3. Cerebrospinal fluid examination in newborns

Key Laboratory Test: Herpes Simplex

• Tzanck test

Treatment

Acyclovir, 20 mg/kg/dose, 5 times/day for 5 days orally or IV

Key Treatment: Herpes Simplex

• Acyclovir

Herpes Zoster (Shingles)

Etiology

Varicella-zoster virus reactivated after lying dormant in a sensory ganglion following varicella infection

Clinical Findings

1. The patient has a past history of varicella.
2. Grouped vesicles on an erythematous base are distributed along one or two dermatomes supplied by a spinal nerve or cranial nerve, commonly the fifth cranial nerve.
3. Lesions do not cross the midline.
4. In children, pain is minimal.
5. Lesions may disseminate in immunocompromised individuals.

6. A susceptible individual may contract varicella after exposure to herpes zoster.

Key Clinical Finding: Herpes Zoster

• Vesicles following pattern of dermatomes

Laboratory Diagnosis

Key Laboratory Tests: Herpes Zoster

• Tzanck test
• Viral culture

Treatment

Acyclovir if the patient is immunocompromised

Key Treatment: Herpes Zoster

• Acyclovir

Molluscum Contagiosum

Etiology

A pox virus

Clinical Findings

1. The disorder is more common in children and is mildly contagious.
2. Multiple dome-shaped, flesh-colored, 2- to 5-mm waxy papules are present, with central umbilication; the latter phenomenon is sometimes absent in very small lesions.
3. The lesions are usually localized on the face, neck, or upper torso.
4. The lesions involute faster after they are irritated.
5. The disseminated form may be seen in human immunodeficiency virus infection.

Key Clinical Finding: Molluscum Contagiosum

• Small, waxy, dome-shaped umbilicated lesions

Laboratory Diagnosis

Microscopic examination of the material (intracytoplasmic inclusion [molluscum] bodies) squeezed out of the delling or umbilication

Key Laboratory Finding: Molluscum Contagiosum

• Intracytoplasmic inclusions in expelled material of lesion

Treatment

1. Conservative—no treatment
2. Tretinoin (Retin-A) solution applied to individual lesions
3. Cantharone solution applied to individual lesions
4. Manual curettage of large lesions

Key Treatment: Molluscum Contagiosum

- Treatment usually unnecessary
- Curettage of lesions

Warts (Verrucae)

Etiology

Human papillomavirus. Specific strains are trophic to regional areas.

Clinical Findings

1. Common wart (verruca vulgaris)
   a. Discrete, skin-colored single or multiple papules with a rough surface
   b. More common on the hands but may occur anywhere
2. Flat warts (verruca plana)
   a. Grouped flat-topped, skin-colored, or pigmented papules with a smooth surface
   b. Common on the face
3. Anogenital wart (condyloma acuminatum)
   a. Cauliflower-like or pink filiform sessile papules with a rough surface.
   b. May be acquired from the birth canal or may result from sexual abuse.
4. Plantar wart—painful, grows inward on the sole of the foot
5. Periungual wart—around the nail

Key Clinical Finding: Warts

- Rough wrinkled surface papules

Laboratory Diagnosis

Human papillomavirus typing is not practical.

Treatment

1. Conservative—no treatment
2. Preparations containing salicylic acid and lactic acid
3. Cryotherapy (liquid nitrogen)
4. Cimetidine orally for 3 months for recalcitrant warts
5. Twenty per cent podophyllin in tincture of benzoin for anogenital warts

Key Treatment: Warts

- Observation
- Salicylic acid
- Podophyllin (condyloma acuminatum)
- Surgery

Fungal Infections

Candidiasis

Etiology

Candida albicans, a yeast

Clinical Findings

1. Clinical forms
   a. Oral thrush
   b. Candidal diaper dermatitis—beefy red, sharp border, satellite lesions, scrotum always involved in boys
   c. Congenital cutaneous candidiasis
      (1) Results from ascending maternal infection
      (2) Generalized, scaly papulovesicles
      (3) Benign course
   d. Candidal paronychia
   e. Chronic mucocutaneous candidiasis in patients with immunologic defects
2. Oral antibiotic use possibly a predisposing factor for candidosis

Key Clinical Findings: Candidiasis

- White patches on tongue, buccal mucosa (thrush)
- Pink lesions in diaper area

Laboratory Diagnosis

1. Potassium hydroxide preparation
2. Culture

Key Laboratory Test: Candidiasis

- Potassium hydroxide preparation
- Culture

Treatment

1. Nystatin cream, imidazole cream
2. Nystatin suspension
3. Parenteral ketoconazole for chronic mucocutaneous candidiasis

Key Treatment: Candidiasis

- Nystatin cream or ointment

Tinea Capitis

Etiology

Trichophyton tonsurans is the most prevalent organism in the United States. Other causative dermatophytes include *Microsporum canis* and *M. audouinii*.

Clinical Findings

1. Contagious, more common in black children
2. Clinical forms

a. Noninflammatory "black dot" tinea—single or multiple patchy hair loss
b. Inflammatory—kerion; painful, tender abscess
c. Seborrheic—diffuse crusting and scaling with minimal hair loss

3. A diffuse skin hypersensitivity reaction may be seen in children with kerions.

Key Clinical Findings: Tinea Capitis

- Patchy hair loss
- Kerion

Laboratory Diagnosis

1. Potassium hydroxide preparation
   a. *Trichophyton tonsurans*: endothrix (fungal spores inside the hair shaft)
   b. *Microsporum* spp: ectothrix (fungal spores outside the hair shaft)
2. Culture on dermatophyte test medium, Mycosel, or Sabouraud medium
3. Wood lamp examination: *T. tonsurans* tinea capitis does not fluoresce; *Microsporum* tinea capitis does, with an apple green color.

Key Laboratory Tests: Tinea Capitis

- Potassium hydroxide preparation
- Culture

Treatment

1. Griseofulvin
   a. Dose: 15 to 20 mg/kg/day in one or two doses
   b. Given with milk or fatty meal
   c. Duration: 4 to 6 weeks
   d. Laboratory monitoring unnecessary
2. Prednisone, 1 mg/kg/day for 5 days for kerions
3. Selenium sulfide shampoo

Key Treatment: Tinea Capitis

- Griseofulvin

Tinea Corporis

Etiology

Trichophyton, *Microsporum*, and *Epidermophyton* species of dermatophytes

Clinical Findings

1. Single or multiple variably pruritic annular lesions with active, raised, scaly, advancing papulovesicular border, and central clearing.
2. Tinea incognito resulting from treatment with topical ste-

roid, which suppresses the inflammation but not the infection
3. Other conditions mistaken for tinea corporis: herald patch of pityriasis rosea, granuloma annulare, nummular eczema

Key Clinical Findings: Tinea Corporis

- Annular lesions with raised border

Laboratory Diagnosis

Key Laboratory Findings: Tinea Corporis

- Potassium hydroxide preparation
- Fungal culture

Treatment

1. Topical imidazole twice a day for 7 to 10 days
2. Griseofulvin for 1 week for extensive tinea corporis

Key Treatment: Tinea Corporis

- Griseofulvin
- Topical imidazole

Tinea (Pityriasis) Versicolor

Etiology

Pityrosporum orbiculare (*P. ovale, Malassezia furfur*)

Clinical Findings

1. The disorder is common in tropical climates and in summer months.
2. The lesions are distributed on the upper chest, back, shoulder, neck, and upper arms.
3. Active lesions may be either hypopigmented or tan-colored macules with scales. Lesions tend to become confluent.
4. Hypopigmentation resolves slowly.
5. Recurrence is common.

Key Clinical Finding: Tinea Versicolor

- Macular, confluent lesions over trunk

Laboratory Diagnosis

Key Laboratory Tests: Tinea Versicolor

- Wood lamp examination—yellow fluorescence
- Potassium hydroxide preparation

Treatment

1. Selenium sulfide 2.5 per cent solution is mixed with some water, applied over the affected areas, left overnight, then washed off. The process is repeated 1 week later.
2. Imidazole cream is applied twice a day for 2 weeks.
3. Ketoconazole, 200 mg, is taken once daily orally for 1 to 7 days, in adolescents (contraindication: hepatic disease).
4. Selenium sulfide shampoo is used.

Key Treatment: Tinea Versicolor

- Imidazole cream
- Oral ketoconazole
- Selenium sulfide solution

Infestations

Scabies

Etiology

Sarcoptes scabiei, a mite

Clinical Findings

1. The disorder causes an intensely pruritic papular eruption; excoriations are common, and pruritus is worse at night.
2. The lesions are generalized but occur more in the genitalia, interdigital webs; axillae, feet, and hands in young infants; the face and scalp may be spared.
3. Hyperpigmented nodules may be seen in young infants.
4. The lesions may become eczematized from chronic scratching.
5. Common contacts are household members, baby sitters, and playmates.
6. Norwegian or crusted scabies consists of thick psoriasiform crusted lesions seen in patients with Down syndrome, immunocompromised hosts, or institutionalized individuals.

Key Clinical Findings: Scabies

- Intensely pruritic eruption anywhere on body
- Interdigital webs common site

Laboratory Diagnosis

Light microscopic examination of scraping from the burrow or lesion that demonstrates the mite, egg, or excretions

Key Laboratory Test: Scabies

- Scraping of burrow to show mite or eggs

Treatment

1. Permethrin 5 per cent cream is applied from the neck down and left overnight; all the clothes and bed sheets are changed. The regimen is repeated 1 week later for best results. All contacts are treated.
2. An alternate drug for older children is gamma benzene hexachloride cream or lotion used as described earlier.
3. Pruritus may remain for a while after treatment.
4. Norwegian scabies requires several courses of topical permethrin or gamma benzene hexachloride. Ivermectin has also been used successfully.

Key Treatment: Scabies

- Permethrin 5 per cent cream
- All contacts treated

Pediculosis

Etiology

Pediculus humanus, *Phthirus pubis* (crab louse)—blood-sucking wingless insects

Clinical Findings

1. Pediculosis capitis is highly communicable. It causes an intensely itchy scalp; lice and nits attached to hairs may be visible. It is rarely seen in black patients.
2. Nits of *P. pubis* may attach to eyelashes; this may result from sexual abuse.

Key Clinical Findings: Pediculosis

- Itching scalp
- Lice visible, as are nits

Treatment

1. Permethrin cream rinse (1% for head lice, 5% for body lice)
2. Gamma benzene hexachloride (lindane) shampoo
3. Nits on scalp hair may be removed with fine-toothed comb.
4. Nits on the eyelashes may be treated with petroleum jelly (Vaseline) ointment and then removed manually.

Key Treatment: Pediculosis

- Permethrin 5 per cent cream rinse
- Remove nits

Cutaneous Larva Migrans (Creeping Eruption)

Etiology

Larvae of the dog or cat hookworm *Ancylostoma braziliense*, which penetrate the skin from contaminated soil in endemic areas (e.g., southeastern United States, Carribean islands)

Clinical Findings

1. Serpiginous mobile track in the upper epidermis
2. Common distribution: foot, buttock, hand
3. Intensely pruritic

Key Clinical Findings: Cutaneous Larva Migrans

- Serpiginous track in epidermis

Treatment

Key Treatment: Cutaneous Larva Migrans

- Topical application of 10 per cent thiabendazole for 10 days

Insect (Arthropod) Bites

Etiology

Flying or crawling insects

Clinical Findings

1. Bites are more common during summertime.
2. They are commonly on exposed areas of the body.
3. Lesions are scattered pruritic edematous papules surmounted by puncta (flying insects).
4. Lesions may be in a linear array—"breakfast, lunch, dinner" bites (crawling insects).
5. Papular urticaria, hypersensitivity to the bites, may exist.

Key Clinical Findings: Insect bites

- Small urticarial lesions, pruritic

Treatment

1. Preventive—use of insect repellent containing less than 10 per cent diethyltoluamide (DEET), light-colored clothing
2. Colloidal oatmeal baths
3. Pramoxine cream
4. Aqueous epinephrine and oral diphenhydramine for severe local reactions

Key Treatment: Insect Bites

- Colloidal oatmeal baths

- Pramoxine cream

Bibliography

Bergfeld WF, Elewski BE, Hay RJ, et al: Cutaneous mycoses: An update for the 90s (monograph). Califon, NJ, Gardiner-Caldwell SynerMed, 1993.

Busso M, Berman B: Antivirals in dermatology. J Am Acad Dermatol 1995;32:1031–1040.

Darmstadt GL, Lane AT: Impetigo: An overview. Pediatr Dermatol 1994;11:293–303.

Roth RR, James WD: Microbiology of the skin: Resident flora, ecology, infection. J Am Acad Dermatol 1989;20:367–390.

306 Psoriasis

Bernice R. Krafchik

Definition

Psoriasis is a chronic skin disease of unknown etiology, characterized by erythematous, scaly papules and plaques and a tendency to exhibit a Koebner phenomenon (isomorphic response).

Etiology

1. Genetic factors. A family history of psoriasis is evident in 35 per cent of patients. It is more frequently associated with early-onset psoriasis than in older patients. The disease has been found to occur with certain human leukocyte antigen (HLA) types: BW13, B17, and B27 in pustular psoriasis and particularly HLA-Cw6 in early-onset disease.
2. Infections. The occurrence of guttate psoriasis after group A streptococcal infection has long been recognized. It has been proposed that a streptococcal proliferative factor acts as a superantigen, causing keratinocyte proliferation. Guttate flares may result from the streptococcal proliferative factor, causing a Koebner effect.

Epidemiology

1. Psoriasis affects girls more frequently than boys in a 2:1 ratio.
2. The prevalence is 1 to 3 per cent.
3. Two per cent of cases occur before the age of 2 years, 10 per cent before the age of 10 years, 27 per cent before the age of 16 years, and 35 per cent before the age of 20 years.
4. The disorder is common in whites; it is rare in blacks and Asians.
5. No association between age of onset and prognosis.

Pathophysiology

1. The characteristic finding in psoriasis is increased cell turnover, with its attendant increase in DNA synthesis. The epidermal cell transit time is normally 28 days, whereas in psoriasis, the turnover time is 3 to 4 days. In addition, the cell cycle is shortened, from the norm of 457 hours to 37 hours.

2. The cyclic guanosine monophosphate in the involved epidermis is increased. The levels of cyclic adenosine monophosphate are correspondingly low. These findings may denote a role for the cyclic nucleotide pathway in the pathogenesis of the lesions.

3. Immunologic abnormalities occur in psoriasis. Whether these findings are implicated in the pathogenesis is unknown. The ratio of T-helper to T-suppressor cells is increased in the serum, and the T lymphocytes may also be functionally defective. Circulating immune complexes and increased immunoglobulin levels have been demonstrated.

Clinical Findings

1. History

   a. It is important to ask about a family history of psoriasis or arthritis, because of the known familial association.

   b. Although lesions may begin at any time, the fall and winter are particularly common times to present.

   c. Patients often give a history of seborrheic dermatitis or diaper dermatitis in infancy.

   d. Pruritus is very variable in psoriasis but in the majority of patients the lesions tend to be asymptomatic.

   e. A history of trauma followed by a persistent lesion is often an important presenting sign.

   f. A history of a recent sore throat may precede a guttate flare in children by a number of weeks.

2. Physical examination

   a. Areas that are most commonly involved include the elbows, knees, scalp, and lumbosacral area. The lesions are usually chronic and symmetric and consist of well-demarcated papules and plaques surmounted by a silvery scale; the area demonstrates small bleeding points when the scale is removed (Auspitz sign). Patients with psoriasis tend to demonstrate the Koebner phenomenon (the presence of typical lesions in the affected areas in response to trauma).

   b. Scalp involvement is commonly seen with childhood psoriasis. It affects 80 per cent of patients. The lesions present as well-demarcated, erythematous plaques with a thick scale that often involves the hair line and nuchal area. The whole scalp may be involved.

   c. Nails are affected in 25 to 50 per cent of patients. In infants and young children, this may be the first and only manifestation of the disease. Pitting is the diagnostic feature of nail involvement in psoriasis. The pits are superficial and numerous. Another classic appearance of the nails is a distal onycholysis and a smudge of yellowish-brown discoloration; this is known as the "oil drop" sign. Other findings include subungual hyperkeratosis, which is more common in adolescents and adults. The nails may become completely dystrophic.

   d. Thirty-four per cent of children present with guttate lesions, preceded by a sore throat a few weeks before. These lesions appear as small erythematous plaques surmounted by a thin scale, which mainly affects the trunk.

   e. Other presentations include an inverse pattern in which the lesions affect the folds—the groin and the genitalia, the axillae, and the umbilicus. A scale is always present, but this is usually not as silvery or thick as in classic psoriasis.

   f. In infants, the diaper area may show the first manifestation of the disease. The lesions may occur anywhere in the diaper area and are well-demarcated erythematous plaques with a scale.

   g. Pustular psoriasis is a condition that occurs either in well-established psoriasis or de novo. Pustular psoriasis may be either localized or generalized.

      (1) In the generalized form known as the von Zumbusch variety, the onset is often preceded by an infectious episode, and patients are often febrile at presentation. A family history of psoriasis is present in 25 per cent of cases. Twenty-seven per cent of patients present before the age of 1 year. Lesions often occur in crops every few hours to days. The individual lesions are erythematous plaques studded with superficial pustules. These may also occur in a peripheral pattern at the edge of the lesions. Geographic tongue is common in this form.

      (2) Localized pustular psoriasis is uncommon in children. It symmetrically affects the palms and the soles. The lesions are deep, pin-head pustules and should be distinguished from dyshidrotic dermatitis and fungal infections. Occasionally these lesions have been reported in association with chronic recurrent sterile osteomyelitis.

   h. Arthritis occurs in approximately 10 per cent of patients. The arthritis precedes the psoriasis in 50 per cent of patients. It is seronegative, has a strong association with HLA-B27, and is erosive. The joints are tender and swollen. Any joint may be involved, particularly the distal phalangeal joints, but also large joints, such as the elbows and knees, in which case the arthritis is pauciarticular. In the fingers and toes, the extraarticular tissues may be involved, producing a sausage-like deformity. Nail pitting is frequently associated with psoriatic arthritis. When the arthritis becomes chronic, flexion deformities may occur.

3. Differential diagnosis

   a. In infancy, when the scalp and diaper area are involved, it is easy to confuse psoriasis with seborrheic dermatitis. The lesions of seborrheic dermatitis present with asymptomatic, yellow, greasy scales in the scalp, typified by "cradle cap," scaling and erythema of the eyebrows and cheeks, and erythematous, scaling lesions in the intertriginous areas, including the diaper area. The lesions are easy to treat with a mild steroid preparation.

   b. Pityrisis rubra pilaris is a rare condition that presents as either a generalized eruption involving the trunk, palms, and soles or as a localized eruption affecting the elbows and knees with papular, scaling lesions. The etiology is unknown.

c. Lichen planus is important to differentiate from psoriasis. The condition may occur with an acute onset in children, and pruritic, papular scaly lesions that are a distinct purple with a polygonal shape and a lacy pattern known as Wickham striae are seen. Any area may be involved, but typically, the lesions involve the wrists, ankles, penis, and mouth, where the lesions form a white, reticulated pattern on the buccal mucosa.

Key Clinical Findings

- Silvery scale papules on exterior surfaces
- Bleeding when scale is removed
- Pitted nails

Laboratory Findings

1. The histologic findings of psoriasis are typical and consist of elongation of the rete ridges and dermal papillae, absence of the granular layer, parakeratosis, collections of polymorphonuclear leukocytes in the stratum corneum, dilated dermal papillary capillaries, and lymphohistiocytic infiltrate in the upper papillary dermis.
2. No chemical marker exists. In pustular psoriasis, leukocytosis and rarely hypocalcemia may be present.

Key Laboratory Tests

- Biopsy and histologic testing—usually unnecessary

Radiographic Findings

1. An erosive arthritis may be seen on x-ray study.
2. Soft tissue swelling may be evident when extraarticular tissue is involved.

Treatment

1. Topical therapy.
   a. Tar products and their derivatives are used for the treatment of plaque-type psoriasis.
      (1) In cases with limited involvement, the use of a refined tar product known as liquor carbonis detergens is more practical than crude coal tar, which is usually reserved for use in hospitalized patients. A combination of 10 per cent liquor carbonis detergens and a topical midstrength steroid should be applied to body areas three times a day. A lower percentage of liquor carbonis detergens, such as 5 per cent in a mild topical steroid, may be used three times a day on the face.
      (2) When large areas of the body are involved, hospitalization is the most practical approach. Crude coal tar is an extremely messy topical agent. It is effective in combination with ultraviolet B light treatment, known as the Goeckerman regimen.
      (3) Anthralin (a tar by-product) is used according to the Ingram regimen—a daily coal tar bath, ultraviolet B phototherapy, and a 24-hour application of an anthralin paste containing salicylic acid to prevent oxidation of the anthralin. Anthralin is messy and causes staining of both the skin and the clothing. A short-contact regimen has been used in which anthralin is applied for 1 hour and promptly removed. This is as effective as the overnight application and is much more cosmetically acceptable.
   b. Salicylic acid (5 to 10%) preparations are used to lift the scale, which is usually thick and difficult to penetrate, particularly in the scalp. It is applied in an oil base and left on overnight, followed by a tar shampoo to remove the oil and the scale. Salicylic acid can also be combined with liquor carbonis detergens and topical steroids for thick plaques on the body.
   c. Topical corticosteroids are the most widely used modality because of patient acceptance and relative low cost. A midstrength topical corticosteroid ointment under occlusion is beneficial for short-term treatment, although this is not usually used in children.
   d. Calcipotriol, a derivative of vitamin D, has been used topically with success for mild-to-moderate plaque psoriasis. Side effects include irritation.
2. Phototherapy.
   a. Phototherapy (ultraviolet B irradiation) in combination with coal tar preparations is effective in treating patients with moderate-to-severe disease. Application of 2 to 4 per cent crude coal tar in a hydrophilic ointment before daily irradiation with minimal erythrogenic doses of ultraviolet B is effective within 2 to 3 weeks. Caution should be exercised with the use of ultraviolet B irradiation in children because of the cost, inconvenience, and risk of later malignancies.
   b. Photochemotherapy combines the photosensitizing drug methoxsalen with ultraviolet A phototherapy. The drug is given in a dosage of 0.6 mg/kg body weight 2 hours before exposure to ultraviolet A. Treatments are repeated up to 3 times weekly and are valuable in controlling extensive disease, but again, the risk of malignancy in later years should be considered.
3. Systemic therapy. Systemic treatment should be limited to patients with severe psoriasis, which is present in large areas on the body and is unresponsive to topical therapy.
   a. Methotrexate is given orally 0.3 to 0.5 mg/kg/day in three doses at 12-hour intervals once weekly. The patient's hematologic status and renal and liver functions must be monitored to avoid acute side effects. It is particularly useful in pustular psoriasis.
   b. Etretinate (a trans-retinoic acid) is useful in erythrodermic and in generalized pustular psoriasis, and more recently, the short-acting acitretin has become available.

Key Treatment

- Tar products
- Phototherapy
- Methoxsalen/methoxsalen with ultraviolet A phototherapy
- Methotrexate

c. Systemic corticosteroids are contraindicated in psoriasis, except in erythrodermic patients who are acutely ill.

d. Cyclosporine should be reserved for patients with extensive psoriasis that is refractory to other treatment regimens. It is almost never used in children.

Bibliography

Elder JT, Nair RP, Guo S-W, et al: The genetics of psoriasis. Arch Dermatol 1994;130:216–224.

Greaves MW, Weinstein GD: Treatment of psoriasis. N Engl J Med 1995;332(9):581–588.

Henseler T, Christophers E: Psoriasis of early and late onset: Characterization of two types of psoriasis vulgaris. J Am Acad Dermatol 1985;13:450–456.

307 Pityriasis Rosea

Bernice R. Krafchik

Definition

Pityriasis rosea is an acute inflammatory dermatosis of unknown etiology. It is usually characterized by the appearance of a solitary oval lesion (herald patch), followed by a generalized eruption on the upper trunk and extremities.

Etiology

Infections agents, particularly viral, have been implicated although this is unproved.

Epidemiology

1. The female:male ratio is 3:2.
2. Most cases are reported in fall, winter, and spring.
3. The childhood age group (zero to 19 years) makes up approximately 45 per cent of all cases. Fourteen per cent of all cases occur before 10 years of age, and 4 per cent occur in children younger than 4.

Pathophysiology

1. The histologic findings are nondiagnostic, usually showing intraepidermal microvesicles, focal parakeratosis, and superficial perivascular lymphohistiocytic infiltrate, with mild exocytosis.
2. Cytolytic changes in the keratinocytes adjacent to Langerhans cells have been seen in biopsy specimens. Increased gamma M immunoglobulin (IgM)– and IgD-bearing B lymphocytes within lesions in the acute stages and the presence of serum anticytoplasmic IgM suggest that this cytoplasmic antibody may be produced as a result of partial cytolytic degeneration of the keratinocytes.

Clinical Findings

1. History
   a. An initial single lesion usually appears anywhere on the trunk, and within 7 to 14 days, numerous papules and plaques develop on the trunk, extremi-

ties, and neck. These are usually asymptomatic and last for 6 to 8 weeks. Recurrences are seen.
   b. Occasionally, prodromal symptoms precede the onset of the lesion, including headache, malaise, arthralgias, chills, gastrointestinal upset, and pharyngitis.
2. Physical examination
   a. Physical examination usually reveals a resolving 2- to 5-cm scaling plaque on the trunk or proximal extremities (herald patch), associated with numerous smaller, oval, scaling pink papules. The long axis of the lesions follows the lines of skin cleavage, resembling an inverted Christmas tree.
   b. The entire trunk is usually involved, and the hands, feet, and face are spared.
   c. The typical lesion has a peripheral erythematous halo in the center of which is an oval, slightly brownish area. When scratched, this area exhibits "branny desquamation."
   d. Oral lesions are rare but are more common in children. They consist of asymptomatic discrete or confluent white or hemorrhagic erosions, covered with a grayish desquamation, particularly on the buccal mucosa near the back molars.
3. Course of disease. The generalized eruption occurs quickly over a few days, persists for 2 weeks, and then gradually fades over 2 to 4 weeks. Rarely, the lesions last for 6 to 8 weeks.
4. Differential diagnosis
   a. The herald patch may be mistaken for nummular dermatitis or tinea corporis; a potassium hydroxide scraping may be helpful.
   b. Other papulosquamous disorders, including psoriasis, seborrheic dermatitis, secondary syphilis, lichen planus, and pityriasis lichenoides, should be ruled

out. A serologic test for syphilis should be obtained in sexually active teenagers or in infants and in children with signs of sexual abuse.

   c. Pityriasis rosea–like drug eruptions may occur. The drugs most commonly reported to produce this type of eruption include gold, metronidazole, bismuth, and arsenic.

Key Clinical Findings

- Herald patch
- Oval-shaped lesion with erythematous halo
- Lesions follow lines of cleavage; Christmas tree

Laboratory Findings

No specific laboratory abnormalities are seen in pityriasis rosea.

Treatment

1. In most cases, no specific treatment is recommended. Reassurance should be given that the condition is self-limited and that complete remission will occur.
2. The pruritus can be relieved by the use of topical lubricants in mild cases and midpotency topical corticosteroid ointments in more severe cases. Although these measures relieve the pruritus, they do not prevent the development of new lesions or lead to a more rapid resolution of the eruption.
3. Ultraviolet B irradiation is of benefit in accelerating remission.

Bibliography

Caputo RV: Papulosquamous disease. *In* Schachner LA, Hansen RC (eds): Pediatric Dermatology, vol 1, 2nd ed. New York, Churchill Livingstone, 1995, pp 744–745.

Parsons JM: Pityriasis rosea update: 1986. J Am Acad Dermatol 1986;15:159–167.

Telfer NR, Chalmers RJG, Whale K, et al.: The role of streptococcal infection in the initiation of guttate psoriasis. Arch Dermatol 1992;128:39–42.

308 Genodermatoses

Penina Burnstein and *Teresita A. Laude*

Anhidrotic Ectodermal Dysplasia (Christ-Siemens-Touraine syndrome)

1. Inheritance: X-linked recessive
2. Cutaneous features
   a. Hypotrichosis
   b. Anhidrosis, resulting in bouts of fever
   c. Radiating furrows from buccal commissures
3. Associated findings
   a. Facies: high cheekbones, saddle nose, narrow lower face, scant eyebrows
   b. Anodontia or peg-shaped teeth
4. Prognosis
   a. Early mortality due to severe illnesses
   b. Improved prognosis with childhood survival
5. Foundation:
   National Foundation for Ectodermal Dysplasia (NFED)
   219 East Main Street, Box 14
   Mascoutah, IL 62258
   (618) 566-2020

Ataxia-Telangiectasia (Louis-Bar syndrome)

1. Inheritance: autosomal recessive
2. Cutaneous features
   a. Mucocutaneous telangiectasias
   b. Premature graying
3. Associated findings
   a. Cerebellar ataxia
   b. Sinopulmonary infections
   c. Deficient thymus development
   d. Increased alpha-fetoprotein and carcinoembryonic antigen
   e. Total gamma A immunoglobulin (IgA) deficiency
4. Prognosis
   a. May improve with gamma globulin therapy
   b. Death secondary to lymphoreticular malignancies
5. Foundation:
   National Ataxia Foundation
   750 Twelve Oaks Center
   15500 Wayzata, MN 55391
   (612) 473-7666

Bloom Syndrome

1. Inheritance: autosomal recessive
2. Cutaneous features
   a. Photosensitivity
   b. Telangiectatic erythematous plaques on the cheeks, neck, and forearms

c. Café-au-lait macules

3. Associated findings
   a. Dwarfism
   b. Prominent ears
   c. Increased frequency of sister chromatid exchange
   d. Increased incidence of leukemia, lymphoma, and colon cancer

4. Prognosis: decreased life expectancy secondary to severe bacterial infections and malignancies

5. Registry:
   Bloom Syndrome Registry
   c/o Laboratory of Human Genetics
   The New York Blood Center
   310 East 67th Street
   New York, NY 10021
   (212) 570-3075

Darier Disease
(Keratosis follicularis, Darier-White disease)

1. Inheritance: autosomal dominant

2. Cutaneous features
   a. Verrucous, malodorous, papular excrescences on symmetric areas in a seborrheic distribution
   b. Face, trunk, and flexures show vegetating lesions
   c. Oroleukokeratosis
   d. Fissured, swollen lips
   e. Punctate keratoses on palms
   f. Wedge-shaped subungual hyperkeratosis
   g. Photosensitivity
   h. Worse in summertime

3. Associated findings
   a. Immunology: anergic to concanavalin A
   b. Increased risk of Kaposi varicelliform eruption

4. Treatment and prognosis: normal life span; good response to retinoids

5. Foundation:
   National Foundation for Ectodermal Dysplasia (NFED)
   219 East Main Street, Box 14
   Mascoutah, IL 62258
   (618) 566-2020

Dyskeratosis Congenita
(Zinsser-Cole-Engman syndrome)

1. Inheritance: X-linked recessive

2. Cutaneous features
   a. Nail dystrophy (first sign)
   b. Reticular pigmentation over upper trunk, neck, and face
   c. Leukoplakia
   d. Palmar and plantar hyperhidrosis

3. Associated findings
   a. Pancytopenia (aplastic anemia)
   b. Bullous conjunctivitis
   c. Dysphagia

d. Mental retardation
   e. Splenomegaly
   f. Increased risk of neoplasms—squamous cell carcinoma
   g. Increased sister chromatid exchange

4. Prognosis
   a. Complications decrease life span.
   b. Bone marrow transplantation may be helpful.
   c. Mucosal lesions may resolve with retinoids.

Epidermolysis Bullosa

Epidermolysis Bullosa Simplex (EBS)
EBS of Hands and Feet (Weber-Cockayne Variant, Localized EBS)
1. Inheritance: autosomal dominant
2. Cutaneous features
   a. Trauma-induced acral blistering
   b. No scarring
   c. Onset: early infancy or childhood
   d. Improves with age
   e. Worse in summertime

Koebner Variant (Generalized EBS)
1. Inheritance: autosomal dominant
2. Cutaneous features
   a. Trauma-induced generalized tense blisters
   b. No scarring
   c. Onset: birth, infancy, early childhood
   d. Improves with age
   e. Worse in summertime

EBS Herpetiformis (Dowling-Meara Variant)
1. Inheritance: autosomal dominant
2. Cutaneous features
   a. Herpetiform (grouped) blisters diffusely
   b. Palmar and plantar keratoderma
   c. No scarring
   d. Improves with age

EBS with Neuromuscular Involvement (EBS Letalis)
1. Inheritance: autosomal recessive
2. Cutaneous features
   a. Widespread erosions at birth
   b. Cutaneous scarring and atrophy
3. Associated findings
   a. Muscular dystrophy
   b. Myasthenia gravis
4. Prognosis: poor

Junctional Epidermolysis Bullosa (JEB)
JEB Gravis (Herlitz Variant, JEB Letalis)
1. Inheritance: autosomal recessive
2. Cutaneous features
   a. Generalized blisters on trunk, extremities, and mucosa
   b. Hands and feet spared

c. Nonscarring

d. Nail involvement

e. Well-circumscribed exuberant granulation tissue on the face

3. Associated findings

a. Blisters in the gastrointestinal and respiratory tract

b. Pyloric atresia

c. Growth retardation

4. Prognosis: death secondary to sepsis

Dystrophic Epidermolysis Bullosa (DEB)

DEB Albopapuloid (DEB of Pasini)

1. Inheritance: autosomal dominant

2. Cutaneous features

a. Generalized blisters at birth

b. Mucosal involvement

c. Atrophic scarring

d. Papular scars (albopapuloid lesions) at puberty

3. Associated findings

a. Squamous cell carcinoma

b. Growth retardation

DEB Gravis (DEB of Hallopeau-Siemens)

1. Inheritance: autosomal recessive

2. Cutaneous features

a. Generalized trauma-induced hemorrhagic blisters at birth

b. Scarring and atrophy

c. "Mitten hands" caused by digits' fusing on healing

3. Associated findings

a. Mucosal lesions with scarring and stenosis of gastrointestinal and respiratory tracts

b. Squamous cell carcinoma

c. Dental and nail abnormalities

d. Eye abnormalities and scarring

4. Prognosis: shorter life span due to complications

Laboratory Diagnosis of Epidermolysis Bullosa

1. Skin biopsy

2. Immunofluorescent mapping

3. Electron microscopy

Dystrophic Epidermolysis Bullosa Research Association of America, Inc. (DEBRA)
141 Fifth Avenue, Suite 7-S
New York, NY 10010
(212) 995-2220

Focal Dermal Hypoplasia (Goltz syndrome)

1. Inheritance: X-linked dominant; females predominate

2. Cutaneous features

a. Gold-colored nodules

b. Tan, atrophic, linear, cribriform patches on buttocks, axillae, and thighs

c. Papillomas around orifices

3. Associated findings

a. Osteopathia striata (linear streaks on long bone radiographs)

b. Ocular coloboma, yellow fat pads in the sclerae

c. Teeth, hair, and nail abnormalities

4. Prognosis: normal life span

Ichthyosis Varieties

Ichthyosis Vulgaris

1. Inheritance: autosomal dominant

2. Cutaneous features

a. Diffuse fine scales over extensors

b. Sparing of flexures

c. Hyperlinear palms

3. Associated finding: atopic dermatitis

X-Linked Ichthyosis

1. Inheritance: X-linked recessive

2. Cutaneous features

a. May be a collodion baby at birth

b. Dirty-looking scales

c. Sparing of palms, soles, and flexures

3. Associated findings

a. Corneal opacities

b. Cryptorchidism

c. Increased risk of testicular carcinoma

d. Decreased skin steroid sulfatase

Lamellar Icthyosis/Nonbullous Congenital Ichthyosiform Erythroderma (CIE)

1. Inheritance: autosomal recessive

2. Cutaneous features

a. "Collodion baby" at birth

b. Platelike scales (lamellar ichthyosis); fine white scales (nonbullous CIE)

c. Erythroderma (nonbullous CIE)

d. Palmar hyperkeratosis

3. Associated findings:

a. Premature birth

b. Ectropion

Epidermolytic Hyperkeratosis (Bullous CIE)

1. Inheritance: Autosomal dominant

2. Cutaneous features

a. Bullae at birth and early infancy

b. Verruciform or quill-like scales

c. Flexures involved

d. Keratoderma of palms and soles

3. Associated finding: secondary bacterial infection

Syndromes Associated with Ichthyosis

1. Netherton syndrome

a. Inheritance: autosomal recessive

b. Cutaneous features

   (1) Ichthyosis linearis circumflexa (double-edged scale)

   (2) Atopic dermatitis

   (3) Trichorrhexis invaginata (bamboo hair)

2. Sjögren-Larsson syndrome

  a. Inheritance: autosomal recessive

  b. Cutaneous feature: ichthyosis

  c. Associated findings

   (1) Spasticity

   (2) Mental retardation

3. Rud syndrome

  a. Inheritance: autosomal recessive

  b. Cutaneous feature: ichthyosis

  c. Associated findings

   (1) Dwarfism

   (2) Mental retardation

   (3) Hypogonadism

4. CHILD syndrome (congenital hemidysplasia, ichthyosis, limb defect)

  a. Inheritance: X-linked dominant; females predominate

  b. Cutaneous feature: ichthyosis involving half of the body

  c. Associated finding: unilateral limb defect

5. KID syndrome (keratitis, ichthyosis, deafness)

  a. Inheritance: autosomal recessive

  b. Cutaneous feature: ichthyosis

  c. Associated findings

   (1) Keratitis

   (2) Deafness

6. Refsum disease

  a. Inheritance: autosomal recessive

  b. Cutaneous feature: ichthyosis

  c. Associated findings

   (1) Retinitis pigmentosa

   (2) Polyneuritis

7. Conradi-Hünermann syndrome

  a. Inheritance: X-linked dominant, females predominate

  b. Cutaneous feature: whorled ichthyosis

  c. Associated finding: punctate bone densities (chondrodysplasia punctata)

Foundation for Ichthyosis and Related Skin Types (FIRST)
P.O. Box 20921
Raleigh, NC 27619-0921
(919) 782-5728
(800) 545-3286

Incontinentia Pigmenti (Bloch-Sulzberger syndrome)

1. Inheritance: X-linked dominant, females predominate

2. Cutaneous features

a. First stage: linear vesicular lesions at birth

b. Second stage: verrucous lesions

c. Third stage: whorled hyperpigmented macular lesions following Blaschko line

d. Fourth stage: hypopigmented atrophic lesions

3. Associated findings

  a. Patchy alopecia

  b. Eyes: cataract, strabismus, retinal atrophy

  c. Teeth: delayed dentition, pegged teeth

  d. Central nervous system anomalies

4. Prognosis: normal life span

5. Foundation:
National Foundation for Ectodermal Dysplasia (NFED)
219 East Main Street, Box 14
Mascoutah, IL 62258
(618) 566-2020

Neurofibromatosis (von Recklinghausen disease, type I neurofibromatosis) (see Chapter 316)

1. Inheritance: autosomal dominant, gene defect in chromosome 17

2. Cutaneous features

  a. Multiple café-au-lait macules (more than six)

  b. Neurofibromas (more than three)

  c. Axillary freckling (Crowe sign)

3. Associated findings

  a. Lisch nodules (iris hamartomas)

  b. Endocrine disorders

  c. Bone changes—scoliosis

  d. Seizure disorder

  e. Hemihypertrophy

4. Prognosis: shorter life span

5. Foundation:
National Neurofibromatosis Foundation, Inc.
141 5th Avenue, Suite 7-S
New York, NY 10010
(800) 323-7938

Pachyonychia Congenita

1. Inheritance: autosomal dominant

2. Cutaneous features

  a. Thick nails

  b. Palmar and plantar hyperkeratosis and hyperhidrosis

  c. Follicular keratosis on elbows and knees

  d. Leukokeratosis of mucous membranes

  e. Friction blisters on weight-bearing areas

3. Associated findings

  a. Natal teeth

  b. Steatocystoma multiplex

  c. Corneal leukokeratosis

4. Prognosis

a. Nail avulsion may provide temporary relief.

b. Life span is normal.

Rothmund-Thomson Syndrome (Poikiloderma congenitale)

1. Inheritance: autosomal recessive
2. Cutaneous features
   a. Poikiloderma (atrophy, telangiectasia, hypopigmentation) on face and extremities
   b. Photosensitivity
3. Associated findings
   a. Short stature
   b. Hypogonadism
   c. Sparse hair
   d. Juvenile cataracts
   e. Skeletal defects and malignancies
4. Prognosis: normal life span

Tuberous Sclerosis (Bourneville disease, epiloia) (see Chapter 316)

1. Inheritance: autosomal dominant
2. Cutaneous features
   a. Hypopigmented (ash-leaf) macule
   b. Adenoma sebaceum (angiofibromas) on face
   c. Shagreen patch—leather-like skin with knobby surface
   d. Periungual fibromas (Koenen tumor)
3. Associated findings
   a. Central nervous system—seizure disorder, intracranial calcification, mental retardation
   b. Eyes: retinal phakomas
   c. Cardiac rhabdomyomas
   d. Renal hamartomas
4. Prognosis: decreased life span secondary to other system complications
5. Foundation:
   National Tuberous Sclerosis Association (NTSA)
   8000 Corporate Drive, Suite 120
   Landover, MD 20785
   (800) 225-6872

Werner Syndrome (Adult progeria)

1. Inheritance: autosomal recessive
2. Cutaneous features

   a. Premature graying of the hair
   b. Premature skin wrinkles
   c. Scleroderma-like changes
3. Associated findings
   a. Arrested growth at puberty
   b. Senile cataracts
   c. Muscle wasting
   d. Diabetes mellitus
   e. Increased risk of carcinomas
4. Prognosis: fatal by age 30

Xeroderma Pigmentosum

1. Inheritance: autosomal recessive
2. Cutaneous features
   a. Photosensitivity
   b. Senile changes in sun-exposed skin
   c. Increased risk of cutaneous carcinomas
3. Associated findings
   a. Photophobia, lacrimation, corneal opacities
   b. Failure to repair ultraviolet radiation–induced DNA damage
   c. Increased sister chromatid exchange
   d. De Sanctis-Cacchione syndrome: microcephaly, dwarfism, gonadal hypoplasia, xeroderma pigmentosum
4. Prognosis
   a. Better prognosis with sun avoidance
   b. Early death secondary to malignancy

Xeroderma Pigmentosum Registry
UMDMJ, New Jersey Medical School
Department of Dermatology, Room H576
Medical Science Building
185 South Orange Avenue
Newark, NJ 07103
(201) 982-6255

B Bibliography

Alper J: Genetic Disorders of the Skin. Philadelphia, WB Saunders, 1990.

Mallory SB, Leal-Khouri S: An Illustrated Dictionary of Dermatologic Syndromes. New York, Parthenon Publishing Group, 1994.

Novice FM, Collison DW, Burgdorf WHC, Esterly NB: Handbook of Genetic Skin Disorders. Philadelphia, WB Saunders, 1994.

Micali G, Bene-Bain MA, Guitant J, et al: Genodermatoses. In Schachner LA, Hansen RC (eds): Pediatric Dermatology, 2nd ed. New York, Churchill Livingstone, 1995, pp 347–411.

309 Sarcoidosis

Robert H. Johr and *Lawrence A. Schachner*

Definition

1. Multisystem granulomatous disorder of unknown etiology.
2. Uncommonly seen in the pediatric age group with two major presentations:
   a. White children younger than 6 years of age present with polyarthritis (similar to rheumatoid arthritis), severe uveitis, often without lung involvement, and they have a chronic progressive course.
   b. Older children and adolescents can have a clinical picture that is similar to that of adults, with fever, weight loss, cough, abdominal pain, adenopathy, and rash.

Epidemiology

1. Seventy-five per cent of cases seen in the United States are in African American children living primarily in the southeastern section of the country; the so-called sarcoid belt.
2. Twenty per cent of cases are seen in whites and the rest in other groups.
3. Sarcoidosis is rarely seen in Africa.

Pathophysiology

1. Signs and symptoms are due to specific organ infiltration with sarcoidal granulomas.
2. Impaired delayed hypersensitivity or anergy is often present.
3. Immunoregulation abnormal.
4. Specific agents, such as mycobacteria, fungi, viruses, and bacteria, have been implicated in the pathogenesis, but their association has not been proved.

Clinical Findings

1. Cutaneous findings
   a. Most commonly violaceous papules, nodules, or plaques, often with central clearing that forms annular and circinate patterns.
   b. Other cutaneous presentations include subcutaneous tumors, ichthyosis, hypopigmentation, and scaly erythematous patches.
   c. Skin lesions are most commonly found on the face and extremities, especially around the nose, eyes, ears, and mouth. However, lesions can be found anywhere on the cutaneous surface.
   d. Lesions can be asymptomatic or pruritic and are at times disfiguring.
   e. With diascopy (pressing down with a slide on a lesion), a characteristic "apple jelly" yellowish brown color is seen. This is not pathognomonic for sarcoidosis, and it can also be seen with lupus vulgaris (tuberculosis of the skin).

> Diascopy reveals a characteristic "apple jelly" color.

2. Systemic involvement
   a. The lungs, eyes, liver, spleen, lymph nodes, bones, muscles, nervous system, and endocrine glands can be involved.
   b. Pulmonary involvement is seen less often in children than in adults. Bilateral hilar lymph node enlargement with or without detectable lung changes is the most common radiographic finding.
   c. Ocular involvement is common in children. Uveitis and iritis are most commonly seen and often lead to partial or total blindness.
   d. Parotid gland enlargement and adenopathy are also commonly seen in children.

Key Clinical Findings

- Violaceous papules on the face and extremities
- Diascopy reveals a characteristic "apple jelly" color

Laboratory Findings

1. A skin biopsy is needed to confirm the diagnosis of sarcoidosis; however, the histologic findings are not diagnostic. Epithelioid granulomas with a sparse lymphocytic involvement, the so-called naked tubercles, are suggestive of sarcoidosis. The following diseases are included in the histologic differential diagnosis of sarcoidosis: infectious granulomas, tuberculoid leprosy, lupus vulgaris, berylliosis, and other foreign body granulomas.
2. Classic laboratory findings (which are not always seen) include elevated erythrocyte sedimentation rate, hyperglobulinemia, hypercalcemia, leukopenia, and eosinophilia.
3. Up to 80 per cent of children have elevated serum levels of angiotensin-converting enzyme. This finding is nonspecific, and the serum level can be elevated in normal children and is seen with other granulomatous conditions.
4. The Kveim test is rarely used and is felt to be unreliable.

Key Laboratory Findings

- Skin biopsy showing naked tubercles

Treatment

1. Topical and intralesional corticosteroids are used to treat skin lesions.
   a. Stronger topical preparations are the most effective

yet are contraindicated for facial lesions where the skin is very thin.

b. Intralesional corticosteroid injections, such as triamcinolone suspension 5 to 10 mg/ml, are often effective in clearing lesions. Treatments can be repeated every 3 to 4 weeks.

2. Systemic therapy is indicated for uncontrolled, progressive systemic disease.

a. Systemic corticosteroids are given in a tapering dose to control symptoms, starting with a dose of 1 mg/kg/day.

b. Antimalarial agents and immunosuppressive therapy are sometimes used with varying efficacy.

Key Treatment

• Corticosteroid

Prognosis

1. The natural course in childhood can be insidious and smoldering or rapidly progressive. Most cases, even if severe, can be controlled with appropriate therapy.
2. Mortality rates of up to 5 per cent have been reported.

Bibliography

Bondi EE, Jegasothy BV, Lazarus GS: Dermatology Diagnosis and Therapy, 1st ed. Norwalk, CT, Appleton and Lange, 1991, pp 121–122.

Hurwitz S. Sarcoidosis. *In* Hurwitz S (ed): Clinical Pediatric Dermatology, 2nd ed. Philadelphia, WB Saunders, 1993, pp 649–652.

Johnson BL, Honig PJ, Jawarshy C: Pediatric Dermatopathology: Clinical and Pathologic Correlations. London, Butterworth-Heinemann, 1994, pp 177–178.

Mallory SB: Infiltrative diseases. *In* Schachner LA, Hansen RC (eds): Pediatric Dermatology, 2nd ed. New York, Churchill Livingstone, 1995, pp 865–868.

310 Mastocytosis

Robert H. Johr and *Lawrence A. Schachner*

Definition

An idiopathic, usually sporadically occurring group of disorders characterized by the infiltration of the skin and/or internal organs with mast cells.

Epidemiology

Seventy-five per cent of patients are seen in the pediatric age group and often present at birth; lesions can also be seen within the first few years of life.

Pathophysiology

1. Ten to 30 per cent of children diagnosed after the age of 10 years can have systemic involvement. Less than 5 per cent of children diagnosed before the age of 10 years have systemic involvement.

2. Multiple organ system involvement can include bone, liver, spleen, lymph nodes, peripheral blood, gastrointestinal tract, and skeletal and cardiac muscle.

3. Mast cell degranulators (which can precipitate signs and symptoms) include

a. Physical stimuli: Rubbing, temperature extremes, exercise

b. Medications: Aspirin, codeine, opiates, NSAIDs, procaine, alcohol, medications used during surgical procedures, polymyxin B

c. Miscellaneous: Hymenoptera venom, bacterial toxins, shellfish, alcohol (which can be found in cough medications), radiographic dyes

4. There are four major categories of mast cell products that are thought to be involved in the pathogeneses of this skin disease.

a. Vasoaction and smooth muscle contraction agents (prostaglandin-D2, serotonin, histamine, leukotrienes)

b. Chemotactic factors (eosinophil and neutrophil chemotactic factor)

c. Enzymes (tryptase)

d. Proteoglycans (heparin)

WARNING

Too vigorous attempts to elicit a positive Darier sign can precipitate serious systemic reactions.

5. Mastocytosis can be associated with hypomagnesemia and hypocalcemia (secondary to malabsorption) leukemia, reticulum cell sarcoma, Hodgkin disease, and polycythemia vera

Clinical Findings

1. Mastocytomas—Seen in 10 to 15 per cent of patients

a. The lesions are 1 to 5 cm, solitary or multiple, skin-colored to light brown yellow-orange nodules located on the trunk, extremities, neck, and occasionally the face.

b. Bullae formation is possible and is referred to as bullous mastocytomas.

2. Urticaria pigmentosa

a. Two thirds of patients with mastocytosis present with this clinical picture.

b. Multiple yellow-orange hyperpigmented macules, papules, or nodules ranging in size from a few millimeters to a few centimeters are located on the trunk, extremities, and face.

c. Bullous urticaria pigmentosa is the bullous variant of this clinical presentation.

3. Diffuse cutaneous mastocytosis

a. This is the rarest and potentially most serious form of mastocytosis.

b. There is diffuse skin involvement with skin-colored, reddened (erythrodermic) or yellow-orange-brown lesions, causing the skin to feel thickened, boggy, or doughy.

c. The bullous variant is called bullous mastocytosis. With this clinical presentation, systemic involvement is common.

4. Telangiectasia macularis eruptiva perstans

a. Seen in adolescence or adulthood

b. Characterized by diffuse, hyperpigmented, telangiectatic macules

5. A positive Darier sign is highly suggestive but not pathognomonic of mastocytosis, which may be confused with dermatographism.

Key Clinical Findings

- Yellow-orange nodules on trunk and extremities

- Bullae may be present

- Darier sign is seen in 90 per cent of patients with cutaneous mastocytosis and consists of localized erythema and urticarial wheals that develop after a firm single fingernail scratch across a lesion

Laboratory Findings

1. A skin biopsy is often necessary to confirm the diagnosis.

a. Mast cell infiltration of the skin can range from a few cells, which could be easily missed by an inexperienced pathologist, to diffuse infiltration of the skin and subcutaneous tissues.

b. Special stains are often needed to identify mast cell granules.

2. Serum and urine histamine levels are often elevated.

Key Laboratory Test

- Skin Biopsy

Treatment

All of the following have been used to treat mastocytosis.
1. Antihistamines, both H$_1$ and H$_2$ blockers
2. Antiseritonin agents (Periactin)
3. Oral cromolyn sodium
4. Calcium channel blockers
5. Potent topical and intralesional corticosteroids
6. Photochemotherapy (PUVA)
7. Surgical excision of localized tumors.

Key Treatment

- Many methods—all sometimes effective

Prognosis

1. Solitary mastocytomas usually regress spontaneously within a few years.

2. Urticaria pigmentosa—When diagnosed before the age of 10 years, this tends to go into remission spontaneously by adolescence; however, cases do persist into adulthood.

3. Diffuse mastocytosis—The prognosis is related to the age of onset of bullous lesions. The earlier the onset of bullae, the more likely that there will be serious systemic involvement.

4. Telangiectasia macularis eruptiva perstans: This usually persists into adulthood with the potential for systemic involvement.

5. Death has occurred secondary to sepsis, recurrent GI bleeding, histamine-induced shock, bronchospasm, and electrolyte and fluid loss.

Bibliography

Hurwitz S: Mastocytosis. *In* Clinical Pediatrics Dermatology. 2nd ed. Philadelphia, WB Saunders, 1993, pp 663–669.

Johnson BL, Honig PJ, Jawarshy C: Pediatric Dermatopathology: Clinical and Pathologic Correlations. London, Butterworth-Heinemann, 1994, pp 43–44.

Mallory SB: Infiltrative diseases. *In* Schachner LA, Hansen RC (eds): Pediatric Dermatology, 2nd ed. New York, Churchill Livingstone, 1995, pp 852–853.

311 Granuloma Annulare

Robert H. Johr and *Lawrence A. Schachner*

Definition

Granuloma annulare is a commonly seen, nonscarring, self-limited dermatosis.

Etiology

The etiology is unknown; however, granuloma annulare has been associated with trauma, insect bites, and rarely diabetes mellitus, the last association occurring chiefly in adults.

Epidemiology

1. The female:male ratio is 2:1.
2. No racial or ethnic predilection exists.
3. Granuloma annulare occurs most often in children and young adults. Forty per cent of cases are seen in children younger than 15 years of age.

Clinical Findings

1. Discrete, confluent, asymptomatic to slightly pruritic papules can remain solitary or can slowly spread peripherally, with central clearing. Often, different types of lesions will be seen.
2. Most often, the lesions are reddish or pink; skin-colored or purplish lesions can also be found.
3. Circular, oval, or irregular papules and plaques ranging in size from a few millimeters to centimeters are found. Subcutaneous nodules can also be seen.

> One to several lesions are present on areas considered to be subject to minor trauma, such as the dorsal surface of the hands and fingers or around joints such as the elbows or knees.

4. Clinical variants exist, including disseminated small papules. This variant can be associated with diabetes mellitus.
5. Fifty to 70 per cent of lesions clear spontaneously in several months to less than 2 years. Up to 40 per cent can have a waxing and waning course with recurrences.
6. Most often, diagnosis depends on a pattern recognition diagnosis that is based on the typical morphologic features, color, and distribution of lesions.
7. No scaling occurs with granuloma annulare; this characteristic separates granuloma annulare from tinea corporis, for which the former is often mistakenly diagnosed and treated.

Pathology

When the diagnosis is in doubt, a skin biopsy should be performed. "Necrobiotic collagen," surrounded by an infiltrate of lymphocytes, histocytes, and giant cells, is present. A pathologist not familiar with dermatopathology could confuse the histologic picture of granuloma annulare with a foreign body reaction or an infectious granuloma, such as tuberculosis, deep fungus, and leprosy.

> Lack of scaling or ulceration is a major clinical differentiating point seen in granuloma annulare.

Treatment

1. If the patient is asymptomatic and there is no cosmetic concern, reassurance that in most cases the process is self-limited is the only treatment necessary.
2. Midpotency to high-potency topical corticosteroids can be used. The potential for local side effects is great because the response is slow at best.
3. Intralesional corticosteroids, such as triamcinolone suspension, 5 mg/ml, works well. Often, one series of injections clears the lesions.
4. Systemic corticosteroids, antimalarials, dapsone, niacinamide can be given. Alkylating agents and photochemotherapy have been used for disseminated or cosmetically deforming lesions.

B Bibliography

Bondi EE, Jegasothy BV, Lazarus GS: Dermatology Diagnosis and Therapy, 1st ed. Norwalk, CT, Appleton and Lange, 1991, pp 106–107.

Hurwitz S: Sarcoidosis. *In* Clinical Pediatric Dermatology, 2nd ed. Philadelphia, WB Saunders, 1993, pp 598–599.

Johnson BL, Honig PJ, Jawarshy C: Pediatric Dermatopathology: Clinical and Pathologic Correlations. London, Butterworth-Heinemann, 1994, pp 321–322.

Mallory SB: Infilltrative diseases. *In* Schachner LA, Hansen RC (eds): Pediatric Dermatology, 2nd ed. New York, Churchill Livingstone, 1995, pp 834–836.

312 Acne

Neil S. Prose and *Richard Antaya*

Definition

Acne is a chronic inflammatory disease of the pilosebaceous follicles that is characterized by comedones, papules, pustules, cysts, nodules, and scarring that is usually limited to the face, neck, upper back and chest, and arms.

Etiology

Formation of a keratinous plug (or comedo) in the sebaceous follicle is the primary lesion which, when inflamed, results in the formation of erythematous papules, pustules, and cysts.

Epidemiology

1. Heredity plays a role, but the pattern of inheritance is lacking. Familial trends are frequently demonstrated by a history of active disease or residual scarring in first-degree relatives.
2. Prevalence in American teenagers aged 15 to 17 years is approximately 85 per cent. Although acne occurring in the teenage years improves by the late teens or early twenties, about 10 per cent of 25- to 34-year-olds and 3 per cent of 44-year-olds report significant outbreaks.

Pathophysiology

1. Formation of keratinous plugs in the lower infundibulum of the hair follicle caused by the following factors:
   a. Androgenic stimulation of the sebaceous glands
   b. Colonization of the follicles by *Propionibacterium acnes*, which metabolizes sebum to produce free fatty acids (strongly comedogenic substances)
   c. "Stickiness" of the shed epithelial cells of the follicle that fail to be properly discharged from the follicular orifice, creating a plug, or comedo.
2. Increased sebum production has been closely correlated with the risk of developing acne (puberty, stress, menstrual cycle).
3. Diet, poor hygiene, and sexual practices have no role in the development of acne.

Clinical Findings

Patients present with the following skin lesions, usually distributed over the face, neck, and upper chest and back:

1. Closed comedones appear as 1- to 3-mm pale papules with inconspicuous pores.
2. Open comedones appear as large pores with a central brown or black core of sebum and keratin.
3. Erythematous papules and pustules arise secondary to inflammation of comedones.
4. Cysts and nodules are inflammatory reactions that are larger, deep seated, and tender.
5. Scarring may be keloidal, "ice pick"–like, broad, pitted, or widely depressed.

Key Clinical Findings

- Comedones of face, neck, and upper back
- Pustules
- Cysts or nodules (uncommon)

Laboratory Findings

Laboratory findings are completely normal. Serum androgen screening is controversial and should be restricted to females with severe acne when it is associated with other signs of androgen excess or when acne is suspected to be the presenting sign of other conditions associated with androgen excess (e.g., congenital adrenal hyperplasia, Cushing disease).

Treatment

1. The goal in therapy is the avoidance of both the physical and the psychological scarring so frequently associated with acne.
2. Winning the confidence of the patient is essential to effective management. Office visits should provide enough time for hearing the patient's concerns and providing a simple explanation of the causes and course of acne, the side effects of the medication, and the treatment expectations, emphasizing the time course (usually 4 to 6 weeks for significant improvement and 3 to 5 months for maximal benefit).
3. No standard treatment plan exists for acne; however, different strategies exist, depending on the severity of the condition.
4. Medications
   a. Benzoyl peroxide
      (1) Action: decreases *P. acnes* comedones, mild comedolytic
      (2) Preparations: 2.5, 5, and 10 per cent topical gels, creams, and washes (no significant difference in efficacy between concentrations)
      (3) Side effects: localized dryness and peeling
      (4) Indication: mild-to-severe papulopustular acne
      (5) Regimen
         (a) Apply a pea-sized dot to each area
         (b) Initially may use on alternate days, then daily
   b. Tretinoin (Retin-A)
      (1) Action: the only topical preparation available that decreases comedones, increases turnover of follicular epithelial cells, decreases stickiness of cells shed into follicular lumen
      (2) Preparations: 0.025, 0.05, and 0.1 per cent creams; 0.01 and 0.025 per cent gels; 0.05 per cent liquid (begin with lowest concentrations)

(3) Side effects: local drying, peeling, and erythema; increases sensitivity to sunlight (inform patients of apparent worsening of acne in early weeks of treatment.)

(4) Indication: comedonal acne, mild-to-moderate papulopustular and severe inflammatory acne

(5) Regimen

(a) Apply a pea-sized dot to each area (e.g., forehead) nightly (may start with or use on alternating nights to limit irritation).

(b) Avoid eyes, corners of the mouth, and nose.

(c) Apply at least 20 minutes after washing to allow skin to dry.

c. Topical antibiotics: erythromycin and clindamycin

(1) Actions: decreases *P. acnes*, inhibits neutrophil chemotaxis

(2) Preparations: erythromycin, 1.5 and 2 per cent topical solutions; clindamycin, 1 per cent topical solution, lotion, and gel

(3) Side effects: drying, erythema, and peeling; clindamycin may rarely cause pseudomembranous colitis

(4) Indication: mild-to-moderate papulopustular and severe inflammatory acne

(5) Regimen: apply to affected areas in the morning

d. Systemic antibiotics: tetracycline, erythromycin, and minocycline

(1) Actions: same as topical antibiotics

(2) Preparations

(a) Tetracycline: 250-mg and 500-mg tablets, 100-mg, 250-mg, 500-mg capsules

(b) Erythromycin: 250-mg, 333-mg, 500-mg tablets; 125-mg and 250-mg capsules

(c) Minocycline: 50-mg and 100-mg tablets and capsules

(3) Side effects:

(a) Tetracycline and minocycline: gastrointestinal upset, phototoxicity, decreased effectiveness of oral contraceptives, candidal vulvovaginitis in females, hyperpigmentation, staining of permanent teeth (in children < 8 years of age) and gram-negative folliculitis (last two items occurring after long-term use).

(b) Erythromycin: gastrointestinal irritation

(4) Indication: severe inflammatory and nodulocystic acne

(5) Regimen

(a) Use for a least 4 to 6 weeks, then taper over several months while adding topical antibiotics.

(b) May require repeated short courses for flares.

(c) Doses: tetracycline, 500 mg twice a day (bid) on empty stomach; erythromycin, 500 mg bid or 333 mg three times a day; minocycline, 50 or 100 mg bid (may be taken with food *except* dairy products)

e. Isotretinoin (Accutane)

(1) Actions: decreases sebum production and stickiness of cells shed into follicular lumen, inhibits neutrophil migration

(2) Preparations: 10-mg 20-mg, 40-mg capsules

(3) Side effects: *severe teratogen!* Increases serum triglyceride levels; diminishes night vision; causes dry skin, eyes, lips, and mucous membranes; epistaxis; hyperostosis; pseudotumor cerebri

(4) Indication: severe inflammatory, nodulocystic, and recalcitrant acne only

(5) Regimen:

(a) Because of potentially severe side effects, this agent is best administered in consultation with a dermatologist.

(b) Dose: 1 mg/kg/day divided bid (0.5 to 2.0 mg/kg/day)for 15 to 20 weeks

(c) Document absence of pregnancy before starting therapy, and ensure adequate contraception for girls and women.

Key Treatment

- Benzoyl peroxide
- Tretinoin
- Antibiotics

Bibliography

Cohen BA, Prose N, Schachner LA: Acne. *In* Schachner LA, Hansen RC (eds): Pediatric Dermatology, vol 1, 2nd ed. New York, Churchill Livingstone, 1995, pp 661–684.

Rothman KF, Lucky AW: Acne vulgaris. Adv Dermatol 1993;8:347–375.

Winston MH, Shalita AR: Acne vulgaris. Pediatr Clin North Am 1991;38:4:889–903.

313 Damaging Effects of Solar Radiation

Neil S. Prose and *Richard Antaya*

Etiology and Epidemiology

1. The ultraviolet (UV) component of solar radiation is responsible for many untoward effects in the skin of children and adults. A dramatic increase in skin cancers, including malignant melanoma, has been directly associated with exposure to the sun. Sun exposure during childhood has substantial ramifications, ranging from painful sunburn to photoaging and skin cancers (which usually present later in life).
2. The lifetime risk of malignant melanoma is one in 90 for infants born in the 1990s, with 2 per cent of melanomas occurring in patients younger than 20 years.

Pathophysiology

1. Solar radiation can be divided into infrared, visible light, and UV radiation. UV radiation can further be divided into UVA (wavelengths of 320 to 400 nm), UVB (wavelengths of 290 to 320 nm), and UVC (wavelengths of 200 to 290 nm). UVC radiation is absorbed in the ozone layer and never reaches Earth. UVA and UVB radiation penetrate skin at different depths because of their energy differences. UVB radiation is absorbed by window glass, whereas UVA freely passes through it. UVA radiation is responsible for most photosensitivity and photoallergic reactions. UVB radiation, which is largely absorbed in the epidermis, has been shown to be most responsible for the damage of skin that results in sunburn, photoaging, and skin cancers.
2. Excessive sun exposure in the first 20 years of life greatly increases the risk of skin cancer. Animal studies suggest that younger skin is more susceptible to UVB-induced skin cancers.
3. Basal and squamous cell carcinoma appear to be associated with cumulative sun exposure. Because the average child receives three times the UVB radiation exposure of the average adult, most UVB radiation exposure occurs in childhood, making it the opportune time to target prevention.
4. Melanoma has been associated with short, intense sun exposure. Severe and/or blistering sunburns in childhood more than double the risk of developing melanoma later in life, but the tendency to sunburn easily seems to be more strongly associated with melanoma risk than the actual number of sunburns. A positive family history of melanoma, multiple acquired or dysplastic nevi, and large congenital nevi increases the risk of melanoma.

Clinical Findings

1. Sunburn presents as red, tender, edematous skin with occasional blister formation in sun-exposed areas. Effects begin 6 to 12 hours after exposure, peak at about 24 hours, and subside over the ensuing 3 to 5 days, often with superficial desquamation.
2. Characteristics of melanoma are easiest remembered by using the ABCDs of melanoma: *a*symmetry, *b*order irregularity, *c*olor variegation, and *d*iameter greater than 6 mm. Signs of malignant degeneration in pigmented nevi are rapid growth; bleeding; ulceration or crusting; tenderness, itching, or pain; loss of overlying skin lines; inflammation; satellite lesions or changes of any type.

Key Clinical Finding

- Red, tender, edematous skin in exposed areas

Treatment

Sunburn can be treated with cool water compresses, topical corticosteroids, and oral prostaglandin inhibitors, such as aspirin and indomethacin. Proprietary topical anesthetics are generally ineffective and may cause contact dermatitis. Emollients are helpful during the desquamation phase.

Key Treatment

- Cold compresses
- Topical steroids

Prevention

1. Protection from the damaging effects of solar radiation is preferred to treatment. The best measures are listed below.
   a. Limit outdoor activities from 10 AM to 3 PM during summer.
   b. Use sunscreens of sun protection factor 15 or greater in children older than 6 months.
   c. Keep infants younger than 6 months of age out of direct sunlight.
   d. Apply sunscreens at least 30 minutes before exposure.
   e. Wear broad-rimmed hats and tight-weaved clothing.
   f. Reapply sunscreens after swimming, sweating, or toweling.
2. Sunscreens are of two main varieties: those that reflect the sun's visible and UV radiation, such as zinc oxide, titanium oxide, and red petroleum formulations, and those composed of chemicals that primarily absorb UVB wavelengths, the most common and effective being para-aminobenzoic acid (PABA).

3. Para-aminobenzoic acid may cause a contact or photocontact dermatitis, and patients with this condition may benefit from a PABA-free sunscreen that contains cinnamates, benzophenones, or other sunscreen ingredients. These chemicals also may cause contact sensitivity.

4. Broad-spectrum sunscreens protect against both UVB and UVA radiation.

Bibliography

Hebert AA: Photoprotection in children. Adv Dermatol 1993;8:309–325.

Hurwitz S: Photosensitivity and photoreactions. *In* Clinical Pediatric Dermatology, 2nd ed. Philadelphia, WB Saunders, 1993, pp 83–85.

Truhan AP: Sun protection in childhood. Clin Pediatrics 1991;30(12):676–681.

314 Melanoma

Robert H. Johr and *Lawrence A. Schachner*

Epidemiology

1. The incidence of melanoma per 100,000 persons in the United States is increasing at a rate of approximately 4.2 per cent each year. This is faster than any other cancer.

2. There has been a 3 to 9 per cent increase in the incidence worldwide per year.

3. National mortality data for 1973 through 1992 indicate that the overall rate of increase in the rate of deaths from melanomas was 34.1 per cent, which was the third highest of all cancers.

4. Two per cent of all melanomas occur in patients younger than 20 years of age.

5. Melanoma is rare before puberty. It is seven times more frequent in the second decade of life, and most pediatric cases are diagnosed toward the end of the second decade.

Melanoma is rare before puberty; however, it does occur and can be fatal.

Risk Factors for the Development of Melanoma

1. Patients with xeroderma pigmentosa are at risk for developing single or multiple tumors, which can present as early as 6 years of age.

2. Congenital nevi of any size are potential sources of melanoma.

3. Acquired nevi can be histologically contiguous with melanoma in up to 50 per cent of cases. The presence of large numbers of nevi are associated with increased melanoma risk.

4. Dysplastic nevi (atypically pigmented nevi or moles) occurring sporadically or in a familial setting put patients at great risk. Eight to 12 per cent of melanomas occur in a familial setting.

5. Melanoma occurs more often in those with fair skin and freckles, red or blond hair, or blue or green eyes.

6. Propensity to sunburn or lack of ability to tan increases the risk of melanoma. Sun sensitivity has been strongly associated with the development of melanoma.

7. Melanoma is more likely to occur in patients who are immunosuppressed.

8. The incidence of melanoma is increased in people who use indoor tanning parlors.

Melanoma occurs most often in whites; it is seen less frequently in Latin Americans and rarely in African Americans or in darker-skinned children of any race.

9. Genetic factors—familial melanoma locus on chromosome 9p and the short arm of chromosome 1 (7p36).

Clinical Findings

1. Melanoma can be present at birth.
   a. Congenital melanoma. More than 90 per cent of cases develop during pregnancy through the transplacental spread of metastatic melanoma from the mother. This is invariably fatal.
   b. Present at birth in congenital melanocytic nevi.

2. Melanoma can develop during childhood.
   a. One third of all childhood melanomas occur in congenital lesions. The prognosis is poor; the 5-year survival rate is zero to 5 per cent,.
   b. Sixty-five per cent of all melanomas arise in noncongenital nevi sites; patients with these have a 34 per cent overall survival rate.

Besides the commonly recognizable precursor lesions, melanoma can also develop de novo, in normal-appearing skin.

---

   c. Superficial spreading, nodular, amelanotic, and acrolentiginous melanomas are the types found in children.

d. Melanomas in children are most commonly found on the extremities, nail beds, palms, soles, or mucous membranes.

e. The same clinical criteria that are of value for the diagnosis of melanoma in adults are used for that in children. The ABCDs of moles and melanomas are helpful.

(1) Asymmetry (A): refers to the shape of the lesion. This can be determined by dividing the lesion into two axes and noting if the outlines of the sides of the divided lesion are similar. The more asymmetric the lesion, the greater the chance that a high-risk pigmented lesion is present.

(2) Borders (B): jagged, scalloped, or irregular borders.

(3) Color variegation (C): red, white, light and dark brown, slate gray, or black. The more colors present, the greater the chance that the lesion is a melanoma.

(4) Diameter (D): at least 6 mm. A significant number of melanomas have been found to be larger than 6 millimeters.

> The ABCDs of moles and melanoma are guidelines that are not 100 per cent sensitive or 100 per cent specific. Nodular melanomas can be perfectly symmetric with regular borders, a single color, and a diameter less than 6 mm.

f. A change in size or color is the most common sign of malignant change in a nevus. Nevi have a natural life cycle that involves an increase in size or color; this phenomenon is in most cases not indicative of malignant change.

Signs That Favor Melanomas in Children

- Rapid increase in size
- Color change
- Bleeding
- Ulceration
- Pruritus
- Lymph node enlargement
- Subcutaneous mass

---

g. Early diagnosis is crucial to survival. Depth of tumor penetration into the dermis of as little as 1 to 2 mm can result in a fatal outcome. Dermatoscopy is a relatively new technique for diagnosing melanoma. It is a noninvasive in vivo examination of pigmented skin lesions in which a hand-held microscope and some type of oil-fluid immersion are used. With the naked eye, an experienced clinician can diagnose melanoma 60 to 80 per cent of the time. The diagnosis increases with dermatoscopy into the 90 per cent to 95 per cent range.

h. Not all melanomas are pigmented. A number of melanomas in children appear pink or red without the classic ABCDs.

i. Melanomas during childhood have been overdiagnosed and underdiagnosed both clinically and histologically. Spitz nevi, formerly called benign juvenile melanoma, can be misdiagnosed as melanoma. Conversely, melanoma has been mistakenly diagnosed as Spitz nevi, with disastrous outcomes.

Key Clinical Findings

- Macular pigmented lesions, especially in nail beds, palms, and soles
- May also be amelanotic

Treatment

Key Treatment

- Surgery
- Immunotherapy

Bibliography

McLean DI, Gallagher RP: Sunburn freckles, cafe-au-lait macules, and other pigmented lesions of schoolchildren: The Vancouver Mole Study. J Am Acad Dermatol 1995;32:565–570.

Novakovic B, Clark WH, Fears TR, et al: Melanocytic nevi, dysplastic nevi, and malignant melanoma in children from melanoma-prone families. J Am Acad Dermatol 1995;33:631–636.

Roth ME, Grant-Kels JM, Kuhn MK, et al: Melanoma in children. J Am Acad Dermatol 1990;22:265–274.

Spencer JM, Amonette RA: Indoor tanning: Risks, benefits, and future trends. J Am Acad Dermatol 1995;33:288–298.

Weinstock MA: Dysplastic nevi revisited. J Am Acad Dermatol 1994;30:807–810.

315 Nevocellular (Melanocytic) Nevi

Robert H. Johr and *Lawrence A. Schachner*

Definition

Nevus cells can be located at different levels in the skin.

Junctional nevi—Have nevus cells located at the dermal-epidermal junction.

Compound nevi—Have nevus cells located at the dermal-epidermal junction and in the dermis.

Intradermal (dermal) nevi—Have nevus cells located entirely in the dermis.

Clinical Findings

1. These are the most common acquired neoplasms found in humans that appear after the first year of life.
2. The number of melanocytic nevi increases throughout infancy and adulthood, with a peak at puberty and adolescence. By the age of 25 years, most people have their maximum number of lesions. There is a peak of 43 nevi in men and 27 nevi in women.

> The more nevi present, the greater is the risk of developing melanoma.

3. Changes in size and/or color of melanocytic nevi can occur during puberty, pregnancy, following systemic treatment with estrogen or corticosteroids, and with malignant transformation.

> Up to 50 per cent of melanomas have been found to arise in melanocytic nevi.

4. The natural history of nevi is that they tend to disappear with time. By the age of 80 years, most nevi will totally disappear.
5. Melanocytic nevi can occur anywhere on the cutaneous and mucocutaneous surface. The greatest number are found on areas that are maximally exposed to the sun.
6. The scalp, breasts, buttocks, feet, and finger or toe web spaces are areas that normally do not develop nevi. Before puberty, dysplastic nevi often present in these locations.

> ## WARNING
>
> **Beware of pigmented lesions in unusual locations, such as the scalp, breasts, buttocks, feet, or digital interspaces.**

7. Junctional nevi are usually flat, small (<0.5 cm), round to oval, well-circumscribed symmetric lesions with uniform borders and color. The colors range from different shades of brown to black. Junctional nevi can also appear similar in color to the surrounding skin.

> Junctional nevi can appear clinically atypical, displaying many of the clinical characteristics of dysplastic nevi and melanoma.

8. Compound nevi often have the same clinical characteristics as junctional nevi with the exception that they tend to be raised off the skin's surface.
9. Intradermal nevi are raised and usually the color of the patient's skin or slightly browner.

> Size alone is not enough to separate benign from malignant melanocytic pigmented lesions. Many other clinical criteria should be evaluated before that determination is made.

10. The clinical differential diagnosis of acquired melanocytic nevi includes congenital nevi, dysplastic nevi, melanoma, pigmented Spitz nevi, blue nevi, and pigmented basal cell carcinoma.

 Key Clinical Finding

- Pigmented small lesions

Pathology

The histologic diagnosis of melanocytic nevi is usually straightforward; however, there are certain instances in which the dermatopathologist can have difficulty. Junctional nevi with lentiginous changes can be confused with dysplastic nevi, melanoma, or Paget disease. Dermal nevi can have a similar appearance to mast cell tumors.

Treatment

1. It is not recommended to excise nevi simply because they exist. This is not a practical approach and should be discouraged.
2. Indications to remove melanocytic nevi include suspicious changes and location of the lesion in a hidden area, such as the scalp, where early malignant changes could be easily missed and cosmesis warrants removal.
3. The optimal method of excision is controversial; choices include simple ellipse, punch biopsy, or shave excision.

Nevi that recur after excision can be mistaken for melanoma both clinically and histologically (pseudomelanoma).

4. At the present time the removal of nevi with lasers is not recommended because nevus cells are often left behind and their malignant potential is not known.

Key Treatment

- Excise those suspected of being melanomas.

Bibliography

McLean DI, Gallagher RP: Sunburn freckles, café-au-lait macules, and other pigmented lesions of schoolchildren: The Vancouver Mole Study. J Am Acad Dermatol 1995;32:565–570.

Novakovic B, Clark WH, Fears TR, et al: Melanocytic nevi, dysplastic nevi, and malignant melonoma in children from melanoma-prone families. J Am Acad Dermatol 1995;33:631–636.

Roth ME, Grant-Kels JM, Kuhn MK, et al: Melanoma in children. J Am Acad Dermatol 1990;22:265–274.

Ruiz-Maldonado R, Orozo-Covarrúbias L: Malignant melanoma in children. A review. Arch Dermatol 1997;133:363–371.

Spencer JM, Amonette RA: Indoor tanning: Risks, benefits, and future trends. J Am Acad Dermatol 1995;33:288–298.

316 Miscellaneous Pigmented Lesions

Robert H. Johr and *Lawrence A. Schachner*

Nevus Spilus

1. This is a relatively common pigmented skin lesion that can be present at birth or develop in infancy, in childhood, or at any age.
2. It presents as a well-demarcated, brown, nonhairy patch usually located on the face, trunk, or extremities, with characteristic smaller dark speckled macules and papules throughout the lesion.
3. The clinical differential diagnosis includes café-au-lait macules, Becker nevus, congenital melanocytic nevus, plexiform neuroma, and nevi of Ota and Ito.
4. The histologic differential diagnosis includes lentigo and compound nevi. Nevus spilus is essentially a lentigo in which nevus cells are found.

Nevus spilus has the same potential for neoplastic change into melanoma as any other melanocytic nevus.

5. Routine excision is not necessary or practical owing to the typically large size of these lesions. If any area changes and appears to be clinically suggestive of a melanoma, immediate excision is indicated. Patients should follow the same guidelines for periodic self-examination and professional examination as with other melanocytic lesions.

Becker Nevus

1. Becker nevus, usually seen in male patients, develops shortly after puberty. It can, however, be present at birth. It is a relatively common disorder that is also known as pigmented hairy epidermal nevus.
2. Located primarily on the upper trunk (shoulders, chest, or scapula), are areas of macular hyperpigmentation measuring 10 to 15 cm, which can present with coarse dark hair or can develop hair over time.
3. The hypertrichosis persists for life, whereas the hyperpigmented areas can fade with time.
4. Skin biopsy demonstrates changes suggestive of a lentiginous process without the pressure of nevus cells. Since nevus cells are not present, the potential for melanomatous transformation does not exist.
5. Treatment is primarily cosmetic. Laser treatment or complete excision can be used.

Dysplastic Nevi and Dysplastic Nevus Syndrome

Definition

Dysplastic nevi, atypical nevi, B-K moles, Clark nevi, and nevi with architectural and cytologic atypia are all names to describe clinically atypical pigmented melanocytic lesions.

Etiology

1. The syndrome is an autosomal dominant trait in which family members display a phenotype characterized by the presence of distinctive unusual nevi (dysplastic nevi) and are at a markedly increased risk of developing melanoma.
2. Some dysplastic lesions are sporadic.

Epidemiology

1. Approximately 32,000 people in the United States are affected by the dysplastic nevus syndrome.
2. There are many reports of melanoma developing before the age of 20 years, including children as young as 10 or 12 years of age.

The median age at which the diagnosis of melanoma is first made is markedly younger than the average in patients with the dysplastic nevus syndrome.

3. First-degree relatives of those with dysplastic nevi should all be examined even if the patient claims that none has similar moles. Commonly, they are found to also have dysplastic nevi. It is possible to diagnose in these relatives melanomas of which they were not aware.

Up to 68 per cent of apparently sporadic cases of dysplastic nevi are actually familial.

4. People with solitary or many clinically atypical nevi or dysplastic nevi are at an increased risk of developing melanoma, especially in a familial setting.

5. It is estimated that 5 to 7 per cent of the United States population have dysplastic nevi.

6. There are substantial epidemiologic data to suggest that dysplastic nevi not only identify people who are at risk of developing melanoma but can become melanomas themselves.

Dysplastic nevi are regarded as markers and potential precursors for increased melanoma risk.

7. In people having two or more family members with melanomas and who have dysplastic nevi, the risk of their developing melanoma in their lifetime approaches 100 per cent. In this clinical setting, 90 per cent of diagnosed melanomas arise in dysplastic nevi.

8. Dysplastic nevi usually make their appearance during puberty; however, it is not uncommon to find atypically pigmented skin lesions at a much younger age.

9. Sun-exposed areas, such as the trunk and extremities, have the most lesions. Dysplastic nevi are also found in areas normally hidden from the sun, such as the scalp, breasts, buttocks, and feet. Melanomas developing in dysplastic nevi in hidden areas, such as the scalp, have been reported in children.

10. In contrast to ordinary melanocytic nevi, which are symmetric, round to oval, and uniform in color, dysplastic nevi often demonstrate the following clinical characteristics:

   a. Asymmetry in contour or color.

   b. A very dark uniform color that stands out from neighboring nevi or more commonly, different shades of light and dark brown and black. An erythematous hue is also commonly seen.

   c. Irregular, angulated or scalloped borders which are either well demarcated or fade into the surrounding skin.

Dysplastic nevi can demonstrate the same clinical characteristics as melanomas. Often the clinical differentiation is impossible with the naked eye.

   d. The average size of these lesions ranges from 6 to 15 mm. With increased awareness of the existence of dysplastic nevi, lesions <6 mm are often identified.

   e. The number of nevi present can range from solitary or a few lesions to as many as 75 to 100 or more.

Clinical Findings

1. The development of an increased number of morphologically normal-appearing nevi at the age of 5 or 6 years

2. Typically, these patients develop 20 to 40 nevi, which is a markedly higher number than is common in children of this age.

3. An atypical distribution of nevi is common.

4. At puberty there is an accelerated development of nevi, and their atypical characteristics often become identifiable for the first time.

5 The syndrome is usually fully manifest by the late teens and early twenties, with the development of new nevi throughout life.

6. The first step in diagnosing dysplastic nevi is to clinically identify atypically pigmented skin lesions with the naked eye.

7. Dermatoscopy (see under Melanoma) can be performed on all atypically pigmented lesions to help identify high-risk nevi and melanomas that need to be excised.

8. There are normal changes in nevi with time. Compare suspicious lesions with their neighbors. If they differ with respect to size and color, excision should be considered.

The vast majority of dysplastic nevi never become melanomas. It is not necessary to excise all atypically pigmented skin lesions.

Treatment

1. As a general rule, it is not advisable to sample one area of a dysplastic or atypical mole. It should be completely excised so that the dermatopathologist can examine the entire lesion. This may be accomplished by an ellipse, punch biopsy, or shave excision.

2. Dysplastic nevi on the scalp or in other areas that are difficult to monitor are also often excised.

Any lesion suspected to be a melanoma should be totally excised, never shaved off.

Pathology

The histologic criteria to diagnose dysplastic nevi are not universally agreed upon. However, the World Health Organization (WHO) criteria of architectural and cytologic changes are accepted by most pathologists experienced in dealing with pigmented lesions.

Prevention

1. The frequency of follow-up depends on the individual's personal and family history.

2. A person with one dysplastic nevus and a negative family history of melanoma can be seen once a year.

3. Patients with multiple dysplastic nevi with or without a personal or family history of melanoma must follow much stricter guidelines to prevent the development of melanoma or to identify early melanomas in a thin and more curable stage.

   a. Completely avoid sunburns, and use strict sun protection measures.

   b. Professional skin examinations for dysplastic nevi before 10 years of age

   c. Monthly self- or parental total body nevus examinations

   d. Professional comprehensive skin examinations every 3 to 6 months

   e. Shorter follow-up intervals are suggested during puberty and pregnancy, when lesions may change rapidly, or for persons with dysplastic nevi and Hodgkin disease, AIDS, or a transplanted organ, because immunosuppression may increase the risk of melanoma.

   f. Routine ophthalmoscopy to identify and monitor ocular nevi

   g. Early excision of nevi that are changing in a manner suggestive of melanoma.

Patients should be taught to watch for nevi that change in size, color, shape, elevation, pruritus, and ulceration.

Congenital Melanocytic Nevi

Definition

1. Four per cent of the population are born with pigmented skin lesions; of these, 1 per cent are melanocytic in origin. By definition, congenital melanocytic nevi are present at birth or appear within the first year of life.

2. Various criteria have been used to classify congenital melanocytic nevi according to size. The best classification uses actual measurements.

   a. Small congenital melanocytic nevi are <1.5 cm.

   b. Medium-sized nevi range in size from 1.5 to 20 cm.

   c. Large congenital nevi are >20 cm.

   d. Rarely, children are born with melanomas already present in congenital melanocytic nevi.

3. One third of all melanomas arising in childhood develop in congenital melanocytic nevi. It has been estimated that there is a 6 per cent chance of a large congenital melanocytic nevus becoming malignant. Giant lesions represent less of a national health problem, since they are found much less frequently: <1 in 20,000 births, approximately. However, for the patient and family, it is a potentially life-threatening situation.

Clinical Findings

1. Small to medium-sized congenital melanocytic nevi have the following clinical characteristics.

   a. They can present as flat tan lesions that are similar in appearance to café-au-lait macules.

   b. Most commonly, they present as well-demarcated, raised, uniformly pigmented lesions. Their colors range from tan, to light and dark brown, to black.

Darker, irregularly pigmented congenital melanocytic nevi are more worrisome than lighter lesions.

---

   c. Secondary morphologic findings include a verrucous or papillomatous surface with coarse dark hairs.

2. Giant congenital melanocytic nevi are usually easily identifiable and demonstrate the following clinical characteristics.

   a. They often lie in a dermatomal distribution, covering large areas such as an arm, leg, or trunk. Descriptive terminology, such as coat sleeve, stocking, capelike, bathing-trunk, or garment type is often used.

   b. The surface can be verrucous or papillomatous, with irregular borders and satellite nevi present at the periphery. Over 95 per cent have a hairy component.

   c. Lesions present over the scalp, neck, or spine can be associated with leptomeningeal involvement, with potential neurologic manifestations such as epilepsy or focal neurologic abnormalities. If found over the vertebral column, they can be associated with spina bifida or meningomyelocele.

3. Congenital pseudomelanoma is seen in <1 per cent of congenital melanocytic nevi. It presents as rapidly growing nodules, often with ulceration within the nevus. These clinical changes can be present at birth or develop within the first 6 months of life. The nodules simulate melanoma clinically and histologically but act biologically in a benign fashion.

Treatment

1. Small congenital melanocytic nevi (SCMN)—There are many reports in the literature of melanoma arising in small lesions. The risk of malignancy is greatest after puberty; therefore, the excision of such lesions can be postponed until that time. If small lesions are clinically atypical or demonstrate changes suggestive of melanoma, they should be excised immediately.

2. Giant congenital melanocytic nevi (GCMN)—Many clinical features of large lesions make the recognition of melanoma difficult, thereby resulting in late diagnosis and a dismal prognosis. The greatest risk of malignant degeneration exists before the age of 10 years. If possible, prophylactic excision of the entire lesion is recommended during infancy or early childhood. This approach is often impossible owing to the large size of the lesions, and close observation is recommended.

Neurocutaneous Melanosis (NCM)

Definition

Neurocutaneous melanosis is a rare nonhereditary disorder characterized by one or more giant congenital melanocytic nevi and/or multiple small or medium-sized congenital melanocytic nevi accompanied by neurologic signs and symptoms related to benign or malignant tumors of the central nervous system.

Clinical Findings

1. Typical giant congenital melanocytic nevi are present, with smaller satellite congenital melanocytic nevi scattered over the entire body surface.
2. Other skin lesions and assorted anomalies associated with this syndrome include café-au-lait macules, neurofibromas, nevus of Ota, blue nevus, and aberrant mongolian spots, Meckel diverticulum, renal malformations, syringomyelia, and rhabdomyosarcoma.
3. CNS manifestations are essential to making the diagnosis and usually develop within the first 2 years of life. Signs and symptoms secondary to increased intracranial pressure, nerve palsies, generalized seizures, developmental delay, sensory motor defects, spinal cord compression, and psychiatric symptoms are often found.
4. Melanoma is the most feared consequence of NCM. It may arise primarily in the skin or in the meninges.
5. Evaluation of every patient with giant congenital melanocytic nevi should include a thorough neurologic examination and MRI scans to detect CNS involvement, especially when lesions are on the scalp or over the vertebral column.
6. Cytologic study of the cerebrospinal fluid may reveal melanocytes, which suggests the diagnosis.

Treatment

1. Treatment is directed at reducing the risk of development of melanoma in giant congenital melanocytic nevi by their complete excision. This, however, does not eliminate the risk of primary melanoma arising in the leptomeninges.

> The development of melanoma has been reported in >50 per cent of all patients with neurocutaneous melanosis.

2. Neurologic symptoms can sometimes be relieved by the insertion of a ventriculoperitoneal shunt and surgical decompression of a CNS or spinal cord mass lesion.
3. The treatment of melanoma in these patients is usually unsuccessful, and the long-term prognosis is poor. Seventy per cent of affected patients die before the age of 10 years.

Halo Nevi

Definition

Halo nevi are junctional, dermal, or compound lesions that undergo an inflammatory or immunologic event. This response causes destruction of melanocytes and nevus cells, giving lesions their characteristic clinical appearance. Immunophenotyping demonstrates a high number of cytotoxic-suppressor T lymphocytes (CD8 cells).

Clinical Findings

1. Located most commonly on the trunk, a pigmented nevus becomes surrounded by a 1 to 5 mm round halo of depigmentation, often appearing milky white.
2. With time there is complete destruction of the nevus. The halo often persists for months to years, with the skin eventually returning to its normal color.
3. The halo phenomenon can also occur around the following skin lesions: dysplastic, blue, congenital, and Spitz nevi; flat warts; molluscum contagiosum; melanoma; and metastatic melanoma.

> Melanoma at distant sites can cause halo nevi to develop on benign lesions.

Treatment

1. No treatment is needed if the pigmented lesion is not atypical in its clinical appearance.
2. Any lesion suspected of being a dysplastic nevus or melanoma should be excised.

Eczematous Halo Nevus (Meyerson Nevus)

Definition

A melanocytic nevus with an associated eczematous halo reaction surrounding it.

Clinical Findings

1. The typical halo is symmetric, indurated, erythematous, and scaly. In contrast to halo nevi, which are commonly associated with the complete disappearance of the pigmented lesion, eczematous nevi tend to persist.
2. Halo dermatitis has been associated with the following skin lesions: congenital and dysplastic nevi, seborrheic keratosis, lentigines, keloids, insect bites, and with basal and squamous cell carcinoma.

> Eczematous halo nevi can be seen in patients who have dysplastic nevi and melanoma. They can be associated with metastatic disease.

3. The diagnosis is based on the clinical findings and skin biopsy that demonstrates a spongiotic dermatitis.
4. Immunophenotyping demonstrates CD4 (helper-inducer) lymphocytes in the infiltrate.

Treatment

Excision is the treatment of choice.

Spitz Nevus

Definition

1. Spitz nevus, formerly called benign juvenile melanoma, is now referred to as spindle cell nevus or spindle and epithelioid nevus.

2. Spitz nevus is a variant of a common melanocytic nevus that histologically can be confused with melanoma but behaves in a benign fashion.

Clinical Findings

1. These lesions most commonly occur on the head, neck, or extremities in children in the 3- to 13-year age group.
2. Solitary or multiple dome-shaped, smooth-surfaced lesions ranging in size from 0.6 to 1 cm develop, having a characteristic reddish brown color with prominent surface telangiectasia.
3. The clinical differential diagnosis includes hemangiomas, pyogenic granuloma, verruca, melanocytic nevi, or amelanotic melanoma. At times Spitz nevi have irregular borders and mottled pigmentation suggestive of a dysplastic nevus or melanoma.
4. With dermatoscopy, Spitz nevi often demonstrate a characteristic "targetoid" pattern, which helps with the clinical diagnosis.

Treatment

Once the diagnosis has been established, the lesion can be observed; however, conservative excision is frequently recommended.

There have been many cases in which Spitz nevi were mistakenly diagnosed as melanoma and melanoma misdiagnosed as Spitz nevi, often with disastrous results.

Blue Nevi, Mongolian Spots, Nevus of Ota, and Nevus of Ito

Definition

All these pigmentary disorders are thought to represent hamartomas of melanocytes that are bound for the dermal-epidermal junction. Histologically they are characterized by collections of greatly elongated, spindle-shaped melanocytes at different levels of the dermis.

Clinical Findings

1. *Blue nevi*
   a. Blue nevi are usually small, ranging in size from 2 to 10 mm.
   b. They can be flat or raised lesions with distinctive uniform dark blue or slate gray color.
   c. Blue nevi can develop at any age and can occur on all areas of the body without relation to sun exposure.
2. *Mongolian spots*
   a. Mongolian spots are usually present at birth and are seen in >90 per cent of African American and Native Americans and in <10 per cent of Caucasian infants.
   b. Clinically they appear flat, deep brown to slate gray or blue-black, poorly circumscribed lesions ranging in size from a few millimeters to >10 cm.
   c. The lumbosacral area, back, flanks, and shoulders are the areas where these lesions are most often found.

   d. With time, usually 7 to 13 years, they can fade significantly or disappear.
3. *Nevus of Ota*
   a. These present as unilateral irregularly speckled areas of bluish gray discoloration located on the face. More specifically, the discoloration can be seen in the periorbital area, temple, forehead, cheek, nose, and eye.
   b. Eighty per cent of cases of nevus of Ota are found in families of African American or Asian ancestry.
   c. In contrast to mongolian spots, which usually clear with time, nevus of Ota persists throughout the patient's life time.
   d. Areas in the lesions may darken and form raised areas. Melanoma has been reported to arise in these lesions.
4. *Nevus of Ito*
   a. This is similar in appearance to nevus of Ota, differing only in its distribution.
   b. Nevus of Ito may be found on the shoulder, upper extremity, or neck.

Treatment

1. *Mongolian spots and blue nevi*—Therapy is not necessary for blue nevus. When the diagnosis of blue nevus is in doubt, a skin biopsy should be performed.
2. *Nevi of Ota and Ito*
   a. Darker areas suggestive of malignant change should be biopsied.
   b. Excellent cosmetic results have been reported with Laser therapy or cosmetic cover-ups.

Café-au-Lait Spots

Definition

1. Café-au-lait spots are seen in 10 to 20 per cent of the normal population. They present clinically as flat tan macular lesions, ranging in size from a few millimeters to >10 to 20 cm.
2. The borders are often regular and have been described as appearing similar to the coast of California.
3. Café-au-lait spots may be present at birth. They tend to increase in size and number throughout childhood and can be found on any area of the body. Even though they are not induced by sunlight as ephelides (freckles), they do darken with sun exposure.
4. Crowe sign is seen in neurofibromatosis and consists of small grouped freckle-like café-au-lait spots measuring 1 to 4 mm, which are found principally in the axilla or groin.

Café-au-Lait Spots Are Associated with the Following Clinical Syndromes

- Neurofibromatosis
- McCune-Albright syndrome
- Tuberous sclerosis
- Epidermal nevus syndrome

Ephelides and Lentigines

Definitions
1. Ephelides (Freckles)
   a. Well-demarcated, tan to brown flat macules usually <5 mm that appear in childhood on sun-exposed areas such as the face and upper trunk.
   b. Inherited as an autosomal dominant trait linked with fair skin and red hair, freckles are considered a phenotypic sign that identifies people at great risk of developing skin cancer in adulthood.
   c. Sunburn freckles
      (1) They are found mainly in children with light skin, pronounced facial freckling, a propensity to burn in the sun, a history of frequent sunburns, and many melanocytic nevi.
      (2) Sunburn freckles are larger and darker then simple freckles, usually a macule 0.5 to 1 cm, with evenly distributed pigmentation, irregular borders, and location on the face, upper trunk and arms.
      (3) The significance of these lesions is that they indicate intense sun exposure at an early age, which has been shown to be a major risk factor for the development of melanoma and nonmelanoma skin cancers in adulthood.
2. Lentigines (Lentigo)
   a. Tan, dark brown, or black, 1 to 2 mm, oval, circular, or irregular macules that can be located on any mucocutaneous surface.
   b. Lentigines can be present at birth or may develop in childhood or adulthood.

Differentiation of Freckles from Lentigines
1. Freckles usually develop at 3 to 5 years of age; lentigines may be present at birth or occur later in childhood.
2. Freckles darken following sunlight exposure; lentigines are equally dark in winter and summer.
3. Lentigines persist into adulthood, whereas freckles generally fade with age.

Syndromes Associated with Lentigines and Ephelides

- LEOPARD syndrome: Lentigines (*L*), primarily upper truncal and facial; ECG abnormalities (*E*); ocular hypertelorism (*O*); pulmonary stenosis (*P*); abnormalities of genitalia (*A*); retardation of growth (*R*); and deafness (*D*).
- Peutz-Jeghers syndrome: The lentigines can be located on mucocutaneous surfaces with a characteristic periorificial distribution and hamartomas (polyposis) of the entire bowel, with little tendency for malignant change.
- NAME syndrome: Nevi (*N*), atrial myxomas (*A*), myxoid neurofibromas (*M*), and ephelides (*E*).
- LAMB syndrome: Lentigines (*L*), atrial myxomas (*A*), cutaneous papular myxomas (*M*), and blue nevi (*B*).
- Moynahan syndrome: Multiple symmetric lentigines, genital hypoplasia, dwarfism, congenital mitral stenosis, and mental deficiency.

Treatment
1. Other than for cosmetic reasons, treatment is not indicated.
2. When desired, lesions can be excised or destroyed with cryosurgery or laser therapy.
3. Children with sunburn freckles should follow strict precautions with regard to sunlight exposure.

Postinflammatory Hyperpigmentation

Definition
Postinflammatory hyperpigmentation is an extremely common clinical finding in the pediatric age group, occurring most often in children with a darker skin phenotype. It can occur after one case of severe inflammation of the skin; at times it occurs after several episodes of dermatitis.

Clinical Findings
1. Well-demarcated hyperpigmented macules or patches occur over sites of previous inflammation.
2. Often the shape of the hyperpigmented lesions will be the only clue to the patient's past problem. For example, a perfectly round lesion with central lighter areas can be seen after bullous impetigo caused by *Staphylococcus aureus* infection or erythema multiforme. With the presumptive clinical diagnosis in mind, planning for potential future episodes of dermatitis can be made.

Treatment
1. If the diagnosis is not obvious by the clinical presentation, a skin biopsy can be performed to look for other dermatosis that are characterized by hyperpigmented macular lesions.
2. Postinflammatory hyperpigmentation can improve with a formula that contains tretinoin (Retin-A), hydroquinone, and corticosteroid.
3. Lasers often improve appearance.

Bibliography

McLean DI, Gallagher RP: Sunburn freckles, café-au-lait macules, and other pigmented lesions of schoolchildren: The Vancouver Mole Study. J Am Acad Dermatol 1995;32:565–570.

Novakovic B, Clark WH, Fears TR, et al: Melanocytic nevi, dysplastic nevi, and malignant melonoma in children from melanoma-prone families. J Am Acad Dermatol 1995;33:631–636.

Roth ME, Grant-Kels JM, Kuhn MK, et al: Melanoma in children. J Am Acad Dermatol 1990;22:265–274.

Spencer JM, Amonette RA: Indoor tanning: Risks, benefits, and future trends. J Am Acad Dermatol 1995;33:288–298.

Weinstock MA: Dysplastic nevi revisited. J Am Acad Dermatol 1994;30:807–810.

317 Potassium Hydroxide (KOH) Preparation

Robert H. Johr and *Lawrence A. Schachner*

Procedure

Technique

1. A number 15 scalpel blade, the side of a glass slide, or a toothbrush can be used to scrape the lesion. The area to be sampled depends on the etiology of the disorder; care in the choice of area increases the chances of a positive scraping.
   a. Dermatophyte: scrape the active border of the lesion.
   b. *Candida albicans*: if pustular lesions are present, unroof the pustule and scrape the undersurface of the lesion.
   c. Tinea versicolor: scrape any scaly area.
   d. Tinea capitis: pluck hairs.
2. Place the specimen on a clean slide and add several drops of 10 to 30 per cent potassium hydroxide (KOH) with or without dimethyl sulfoxide.
3. Place a coverslip over the specimen and gently heat for 30 seconds. If the solution contains dimethyl sulfoxide, heating is not necessary.
4. View the specimen under the microscope. Decreased light makes spores and hyphae easier to identify.
5. Alternative stains are available for providing color contrast, making fungal/yeast elements quickly and easily identifiable. Chlorazol black E and methylene blue are two such stains; these can be purchased from special dermatologic supply houses.

Results
1. Dermatophytes: septate hyphae
2. Candida/yeast: grapelike clusters of spores
3. Tinea versicolor: monomorphous clusters of spores surrounded by thin hyphae ("spaghetti and meatballs").

A KOH preparation is not 100 per cent sensitive or specific. A negative KOH result does not always rule out infection, and when doubt exists, fungal cultures should be performed.

318 Patch Testing

Robert H. Johr and *Lawrence A. Schachner*

Procedure

Technique

1. Allergens are placed on special disks and are affixed to the skin of the upper back or arms.
2. The test sites must be kept dry and are read at 2 days, 3 days, and 1 week.

Up to 40 per cent of positive reactions can be missed if patch tests are checked only after 2 days.

Test scores range from

- Negative (−)
- Doubtful reaction (?)
- Weak (+) nonvesicular positive reaction
- Strong (+ +) edematous and vesicular reactions
- Extreme (+ + +) bullous positive reactions

319 Scabies Preparation

Robert H. Johr and *Lawrence A. Schachner*

Procedure

Selection of Lesion

1. In most cases of scabies, most of the rash is a hypersensitivity reaction, and very few mites are present.
2. The chances of a positive result are increased if as many primary, untouched lesions are scraped as possible (papules and burrows).
3. Burrows, the classic scabies lesion, are found less frequently in children, whereas nodules are found with increased frequency.

Technique

1. Use mineral oil and not potassium hydroxide.
2. Place a drop of oil on a clean slide.
3. Moisten a number 15 scalpel blade with the oil, then scrape the lesions.
4. Place the material in the oil on the slide and cover it with a coverslip.
5. View the preparation under a microscope.

Results

1. Female mite: the mite is usually seen moving in mineral oil and appears as a translucent pearly gray, oval, eight-legged organism.
2. Eggs: these ovoid translucent structures can be empty or contain larva.
3. Excreta (scybala): these single or groups of small oval solid brown structures appear smaller than the eggs.

> It is not always necessary to find the mite to make the diagnosis of scabies. A diagnosis can be made by the finding of eggs and/or excreta.

320 Tzanck Preparation

Robert H. Johr and *Lawrence A. Schachner*

Procedure

Selection of Lesion

Fresh vesicles and bullae (not more than 24 to 48 hours old) are the ideal lesions to scrape. Excoriated, crusted, or secondarily infected lesions should not be sampled.

Technique

1. Unroof the vesicle or bulla with a large-bore needle, scalpel, or iris scissor.
2. Gently scrape the base of the lesion with a number 15 blade.
3. Spread the material over a clean glass slide and air dry.
4. Molluscum contagiosum consists of solid lesions that can be scraped with a scalpel or curetted off and the contents spread over a glass slide.

5. The classic Tzanck preparation uses the Giemsa or Wright stain; however, other stains are available and include methylene blue, crystal violet, Papanicolaou, and paragon multiple stain.

Results

1. Viral infections: multinucleated giant cells (balloon cells) contain four to 10 nuclei within a single cell. The differentiation between herpes simplex, herpes zoster, or varicella-zoster is not possible with a positive Tzanck result.
2. Molluscum contagiosum: eosinophilic (pink) ground glass ovoid bodies.
3. Pemphigus: acantholytic squamous cells appear as free-floating round cells with large nuclei.

---

321 Wood Lamp Examination

Robert H. Johr and *Lawrence A. Schachner*

Definition

The Wood lamp is a low-intensity ultraviolet light (black light) that can convert the invisible to the visible. It is an extremely easy device to use, and it has many practical clinical applications.

Technique

1. Ensure that the area to be examined is free of any cosmetics or medications that could give false-positive results.
2. For optimal viewing, make the room totally dark. Wait a few minutes to adapt to the darkness, and set the light at full power.

> It is often necessary to bring the patient to a totally darkened area to get the full benefits of the Wood lamp examination.

3. Hold the lamp 6 inches from the patient and totally scan the body from the head to the feet, including all intertriginous areas.
4. Depending on the etiology of the problem, look for areas of fluorescence, pigmentary changes, and potentially unnoticed lesions.

Results

1. Dermatophytes: the most common cause of tinea capitis today is *Trichophyton tonsurans*, which does not fluoresce under the Wood light. However, other potential causes of tinea capitis, such as *Microsporon audouinii*, and tinea corporis fluoresce a blue-green color.
2. Tinea versicolor: a yellowish-white or copper-orange fluorescence can be seen and is due to the elaboration of porphyrins.

> A false-negative result on Wood light examination may occur in a patient with active lesions of tinea versicolor who recently bathed and washed the porphyrins off the skin.

3. Erythrasma: this superficial bacterial infection causes a brilliant coral-orange fluorescence (porphyrins) in the groin, toe web spaces, and axillae.

> Erythrasma can be easily misdiagnosed as a dermatophyte infection if scaly areas in the groin do not undergo a Wood light examination

4. *Pseudomonas aeruginosa*: fluorescein produces a blue color when this bacterium colonizes and/or infects the ear canals, toe web spaces, groin, or wounds.
5. Hypopigmented or depigmented macular (flat) skin lesions: These are commonly seen in children. Caused by partial or total loss of epidermal melanin, they appear lighter under the Wood light.

Procedure *Continued*

a. Vitiligo: complete loss of melanin occurs, and the lesions appear "milky" or "bone" white.

b. Hypopigmented macular lesions: these can be seen in tuberous sclerosis and other conditions; they become light and more easily detected but do not appear "milky white."

> Use the Wood light to scan the patient to help find other inconspicuous hypopigmented areas.

6. Porphyrias: a reddish-orange fluorescence can be seen in the teeth, urine, stool, and blood in the various porphyrias and indicates that large amounts of porphyrins are present.

Bibliography

Elewski BE, Silverman RA: Clinical pearl: Diagnostic procedures for tinea capitis. J Am Acad Dermatol 1996;3:498–499.

Hurwitz S: Disorders of pigmentation. *In* Hurwitz S: Clinical Pediatric Dermatology, 2nd ed. Philadelphia, WB Saunders, 1993, pp 457–479.

Levy ML: Principles of diagnosis. *In* Schachner LA, Hansen RC (eds): Pediatric Dermatology, 2nd ed. New York, Churchill Livingstone, 1995, pp 151–163.

322 Amblyopia

Julia L. Stevens

Definition

Amblyopia is a unilateral or bilateral reduction in vision that cannot be directly attributed to a structural abnormality of the eye or the posterior visual pathways.

Etiology

Amblyopia can be classified into four groups:

1. Strabismic amblyopia—Approximately 30 per cent of patients with strabismus develop amblyopia in the deviated eye (e.g., the eye that is turned inward in a child with esotropia).

2. Anisometropic amblyopia—due to optical blur in one eye caused by an asymmetry of the refractive error between both eyes

   a. It is more common in children with asymmetric hyperopia (farsightedness) than myopia (nearsightedness).

   b. It can also be induced by astigmatism present only in one eye or present to a greater degree in one eye.

   c. This type of amblyopia is difficult to detect when associated strabismus is not present and requires careful monocular vision testing.

   d. Patients can have a combination of strabismic and anisometropic amblyopia.

3. Isoametropic amblyopia—A bilateral reduction in acuity resulting from a large, fairly equal, uncorrected refractive error in both eyes.

4. Deprivation amblyopia—Unilateral or bilateral amblyopia precipitated by any ocular media opacity occuring during the amblyogenic period of childhood.

   a. The relative amount of occlusion of the visual axis and the age of onset of the occlusion dictate the level of amblyopia that develops.

   b. Typical disorders causing this condition are congenital or juvenile-onset cataracts, infantile corneal clouding, and lid lesions obscuring the visual axis, such as ptosis and eyelid hemangiomas.

Epidemiology

1. Amblyopia is the most common cause of unilaterally reduced visual acuity in childhood, with a prevalence of 2 to 4 per cent. Nearly all visual loss due to amblyopia can be prevented with appropriate identification and treatment.

2. Risk factors for amblyopia:

   a. A history of premature birth, especially children with a history of retinopathy of prematurity

   b. Neurologic disorders, most commonly with cerebral palsy and hydrocephalus

   c. Down syndrome

   d. A family history of amblyopia or strabismus.

Pathophysiology

1. Amblyopia is due to a disruption of the maturation of the normal cortical visual pathways during the critical period for visual development.

2. Animal studies have documented that visual blurring or deprivation during the critical period for humans (birth to approximately 10 years of life) will produce changes in the number and function of neurons in the lateral geniculate nucleus and the visual cortex.

3. Complete occlusion of an eye from birth, as in the case of a congenital cataract, can produce irreversible amblyopia if the cause for the visual deprivation is not corrected by 1 to 2 months of age.

4. The window of time for treatment is larger for strabismic, anisometropic, and isoametropic amblyopia (birth to 8 years), though the amblyopic visual cortex changes become progressively irreversible with the advancing age of the child within the critical period. Hence, early identification and intervention in the treatment of amblyopia are imperative.

Clinical Findings

1. A child should be evaluated for suspected amblyopia if he or she has an ocular condition with significant obscuration of the visual axis, including the following disorders.

   a. Cataract

   b. Ptosis

   c. Opaque cornea

   d. Anterior chamber or vitreous chamber hemorrhage.

2. A rule of thumb is that if the examiner cannot "see in" the eye (i.e., a poor red reflex), the patient cannot "see out" and is at risk for the development of amblyopia.

3. Any child who has a two-line or greater difference in visual acuity between the eyes, even within the typical passing range for a child of that age (i.e., 10/12.5 and 10/20 or 20/25 and 20/40) or a visual acuity of <20/40 (10/20) at a distance of 20 feet (10 feet) should be evaluated for amblyopia.

4. For preverbal children, specialized screening techniques or ophthalmologic evaluations are necessary to identify amblyopia in cases of anisometropic or isoametropic amblyopia (see under *Prevention*).

5. Any child with strabismus has an increased risk for the development of amblyopia.

Key Clinical Findings

- Any child with lesion obscuring visual axis

- Any child with two-line chart difference in visual activity

Treatment

1. The likelihood of restoring visual acuity lost to amblyopia varies significantly because of the age at which the amblyopia is diagnosed, the compliance of the patient with the treatment regimen, and the source of the amblyopia.

2. Amblyopia requires ongoing management until approximately age 8 to 9 years. The goal of this long-term treatment protocol is to achieve the maximum vision possible with the least amount of social and psychological burden to the child and the family.

3. Treatment protocols often include combinations of the following choices:

   a. Optical correction—Glasses are used for correction of the optical blur that causes amblyopia in children with uncorrected refractive errors of high magnitude or high degrees of asymmetry. In some patients, especially if treatment is begun at an early age, glasses alone may correct the amblyopia.

   b. Occlusion therapy—Occlusion of the sound eye by an opaque adhesive patch is a well-documented, highly successful method of correcting unilateral loss of vision due to amblyopia.

      (1) Initially, the patient is typically required to wear the patch over the sound eye 80 to 100 per cent of waking hours until visual acuity has returned to the expected best level.

      (2) Frequent reevaluations are indicated to assess the improvement in acuity as well as to ensure that the occluded sound eye does not develop a reduction in visual acuity (occlusion amblyopia).

      (3) Typically, occlusion therapy requires weeks to months of full-time patching therapy, with a reduction to part-time, or maintenance, patching therapy once the endpoint has been reached.

      (4) Maintenance patching therapy may be required until the patient reaches the nonamblyogenic age range (after age 9 to 10 years).

   c. Optical penalization

      (1) Optical blur can be induced in the sound eye by pharmacologically inducing paralysis of accommodation with cycloplegic medications, such as atropine eye drops.

      (2) The optical blur produced in the sound eye has an effect similar to that of occlusion therapy—to promote the preferred use of the amblyopic eye.

      (3) Because absolute occlusion is not achieved, lengthier treatment periods are required.

      (4) This method is successful only if the amblyopia is not severe, since the pharmacologically blurred vision in the "good" eye must be worse than that of the amblyopic eye to cause the child to switch fixation.

      (5) Strict warnings are required regarding the risks of accidental ingestion of atropine eye drops.

4. Correction of the underlying disorder—In patients with disorders producing an opacity in the ocular media, surgery may be indicated for a clear visual axis to allow for optimal visual development and treatment of the associated amblyopia.

Key Treatment

- Optical correction of refractive error
- Occlusion therapy
- Cycloplegic therapy
- Restoration of clear visual axis

Prevention

1. Early diagnosis and treatment of the underlying disorder inducing amblyopia (e.g., congenital cataract, corneal opacity) will often prevent the development of amblyopia.

2. In children with high or unequal refractive errors, early identification of the refractive error and correction with glasses will often prevent or reduce the need for amblyopia therapy.

3. The identification of children with amblyopia or at risk for amblyopia at a young age by appropriate screening techniques that could be implemented in primary care offices or preschool programs would enhance the prospects for optimal treatment of amblyopia.

   a. Photographic refraction techniques, used to identify abnormalities in the red reflex caused by asymmetry in refractive error and strabismus, have been suggested as a screening method.

   b. Even the best photographic screening system fails to recognize some individuals with significant amblyopia.

   c. Currently, the best evaluation consists of a careful evaluation of fixation behavior by a qualified observer.

Bibliography

Kushner BJ: Amblyopia. *In* Nelson LB, Calhoun JH, Harley RB (eds): Pediatric Ophthalmology, 3rd ed. Philadelphia, WB Saunders, 1991, pp 107–121.

Navon SE, McKeown CA: Amblyopia. Int Ophthalmol Clin 1992;32:35–50.

Stager DR, Birch EE, Weakley DR: Amblyopia and the pediatrician. Pediatr Ann 1990;19:301–305.

323 Strabismus

Miles J. Burke

Definition

Strabismus is any misalignment of the eye: in, out, up, down, or twisted (cyclotorsional).

Etiology

Strabismus results from an imbalance between the innervational input to the extraocular muscles, refractively induced accommodative convergence not offset by fusional mechanisms, and/or congenitally or disease-induced structural abnormality of the eye muscle(s) and/or orbital structures.

Epidemiology

1. Manifest strabismus, that type of ocular misalignment that is present most of the time, is found in 3 to 5 per cent of children under the age of 18 years.
2. Most cases are either "congenital" (onset under age 6 months) or "acquired" after 18 months and before age 5 years.
3. Up to 50 per cent of these strabismic problems are esotropia. Approximately 30 per cent of the ocular misalignment problems are exotropia. Ten per cent of the deviations are vertical misalignments described as hypertropia, and the remainder are unusual strabismic problems, some of which will be described later.
4. A family history of strabismus in one or both parents significantly increases the likelihood that their offspring will develop strabismus. Most reports suggest a fourfold increase in the likelihood of developing strabismus. This would suggest that positive family histories raise the incidence of strabismus to between 10 and 20 per cent.

Pathophysiology

1. The causes of strabismus are multifactorial.
   a. Innervational imbalances may upset the relationship between the active convergence and divergence mechanisms.
   b. Abnormalities in the interplay between the fusional mechanisms of the eye may lead to misalignment.
   c. Anatomic and mechanical factors either may be very specific restrictive eye muscle(s) problems or may be thought of as a more general mechanical imbalance involving not only eye muscle(s) but also orbital tissues.
   d. Innervational abnormalities cause varying amounts of extraocular muscle paresis.
2. Infantile or congenital esotropia is much more complex than just crossed eyes in an infant.
   a. Research suggests that congenital esotropia results from a failure of cortical motor fusion to stabilize ocular alignment during the critical developmental period between 2 and 4 months of age.
   b. The varying degree of abnormalities in the balance

of these systems contributes to the additional eye movement and alignment problems that often develop between 1 and 4 years of age.
   c. The associated "baggage" is dissociated vertical deviation (DVD), oblique muscle dysfunction (A or V pattern), latent nystagmus, and optokinetic nystagmus asymmetry.

Clinical Findings

1. Infantile esotropia
   a. By definition, this crossed-eye problem must occur prior to 6 months of age.
   b. These infants usually have a relatively large angle of crossing. The child will either alternately fixate or cross fixate. Cross fixation occurs when both eyes appear esotropic and the left eye is used for right-gaze interests and the right eye is used for left-gaze interests. These patients often appear to have an abduction weakness when none really exists.
2. Accommodative esotropia
   a. Most patients with this disorder present between the ages of 18 months and 5 years.
   b. The crossed eyes are caused by an imbalance between the accommodative convergence and the divergence mechanisms. Most children have a moderate to high amount of farsightedness. The deviation is usually noticed first for near-fixation, although the crossing usually becomes obvious for both distance and near-fixation. When the crossing is intermittently controlled, the deviation is much more likely to be present with fatigue, illness, and stress.
   c. These children often develop an ocular preference leading to amblyopia.
3. Intermittent exotropia
   a. The patient with an intermittently outwardly deviating eye usually presents between the ages of 18 months and 5 years.
   b. The deviation is most noticeable for distance fixation. The deviation is more likely to occur with fatigue, illness, or daydreaming. Bright lights frequently cause the child to squint the deviating eye. Since the accommodative convergence mechanisms are very active for near-fixation, the near position is controlled until very late in the natural history of this disorder.
4. Superior oblique palsy

   The most common vertical misalignment problem in a child is congenital superior oblique palsy. Superior oblique muscle dysfunction gradually causes multiple imbalances to occur. The primary imbalance is ipsilateral inferior oblique overaction. This causes an upward drifting of the involved eye. The vertical misalignment seems to be much worse when looking in the side gaze opposite from the eye involved (the field of action of the inferior oblique muscle). As a way of attempting to keep the eyes straight, the child often assumes a tilted head position toward the shoulder opposite the eye involved.

5. Traumatic strabismus

The most common orbital injury to cause an extraocular muscle restriction is an orbital floor blowout fracture. The inferior orbital contents with or without some of the inferior rectus muscle become entrapped in a fracture on the floor of the orbit. This restricts upgaze and occasionally may injure the muscle and/or nerve, actually causing some downgaze restriction as well.

6. Neuro-ophthalmic causes of partial or complete paralysis of the extraocular muscles

   a. Virus-induced sixth nerve damage

   (1) Is a common cause in a child who presents with an esotropia and/or complaint of double vision, the onset of which is remarkably abrupt. The viral incident usually precedes the extraocular muscle imbalance by 1 to 3 weeks.

   (2) When the crossing is caused purely by a viral encephalic problem, most problems resolve spontaneously over 1 to 2 months.

   b. Gradenigo syndrome

   An inner ear infection, with or without mastoiditis, may cause enough surrounding inflammation or infection to involve the nearby abducens nerve, leading to lateral rectus muscle weakness, esotropia, and/or diplopia.

   c. Central nervous system abnormalities, through trauma and/or tumor, often may affect any of the cranial nerves that supply the extraocular muscles, leading to many types of strabismus.

7. Endocrine

   a. Thyroid orbitopathy

   (1) The orbital tissues often become inflamed by an autoimmune process usually associated with thyroid disease. The most common clinical sign is proptosis of the globes—exophthalmos. Extraocular muscle inflammation leads to thickening and inelasticity. These changes cause restrictive eye movements, strabismus, and diplopia.

   (2) Although this disease usually involves female adults, thyroid orbitopathy should always be in the differential diagnosis of a child of any age with proptosis and/or restrictive incomitant strabismus.

   b. Diabetes mellitus

   Ocular muscle palsy is a very rare manifestation in children with diabetes.

8. Syndromes

   a. Duane retraction syndrome

   (1) Duane retraction syndrome is characterized by an absence of abduction (outward movement of an eye) together with some retraction of the globe on attempted adduction (noticed primarily by narrowing of the palpebral fissures).

   (2) The retraction is caused by paradoxical innervation of the lateral rectus muscle.

   (3) This disorder more often involves the left eye and more often involves females. It is a congenital miswiring but may go unnoticed for months to years.

   (4) About a third of Duane patients have an associated esodeviation most often eliminated by a face turn toward the involved eye.

   b. Brown superior oblique tendon sheath syndrome

   (1) Brown superior oblique tendon sheath syndrome is observed by the parents to be an over-elevation of the normal eye. Actually, the involved eye has a limitation of elevation in adduction. This elevation gradually improves to normal as the eye moves into an abducted position.

   (2) This disorder is caused by a sheath abnormality or adhesion of the superior oblique tendon that catches or restricts the tendon movement through the trochlea, which is necessary to allow the eye to elevate in adduction.

   (3) Most children do not have an associated strabismus. However, some will eventually develop a hypotropia causing a compensatory chin-up position, a tilt of the head, or diplopia awareness.

   c. Möbius syndrome

   (1) This syndrome presents congenitally with facial diplegia causing a masklike facies and a poor suck reflex. There is also an inability to abduct the eyes beyond the midline.

   (2) These problems are generally attributed to aplasia of the VI and VII brainstem nuclei.

   (3) Lingual palsy, brachial malformations, musculoskeletal anomalies, and mental deficiency may also occur.

   d. Double elevator palsy

   (1) This is a monocular elevation deficit in both adduction and abduction. It means that the involved eye does not look upward. It may or may not be associated with an ipsilateral ptosis.

   (2) It is most often associated with a hypotropic position of the involved eye, sometimes causing a vertical deviation of the eye. Alternatively, the misalignment may be offset by the chin-up position to compensate for the elevation anomaly of the involved eye and to thereby obtain fusion.

Key Clinical Findings

- Alternated fixation with cross fixation
- Ocular muscle palsies

Laboratory Findings

Neuroradiologic and/or orbital imaging may be helpful with orbital blowout fractures, endocrine or inflammatory strabismus, presumed viral or infectious paretic strabismus, or a central nervous system or brainstem abnormality or tumor.

Treatment

1. The primary care practitioner's responsibility is to refer to a pediatric ophthalmologist whenever strabismus is identified or suspected.

2. The pediatric ophthalmologist's responsibility

   a. Do a complete eye examination, including best corrected visual acuity, ocular alignment or misalignment, detailed cycloplegic refraction, and careful funduscopic examination.

   b. The first effort is to eliminate any amblyopia and maximize the visual acuity. Once the vision is as good as can be obtained, any significant residual ocular misalignment should be surgically eliminated.

   c. Follow-up of all strabismus and/or amblyopia patients needs to be carried out by the pediatric ophthalmologist through the first 10 years of life. It is only then that one can be sure that the visual developmental system has matured.

3. Eye exercises play no part in the treatment of strabismus.

Key Treatment

- Eliminate amblyopia
- Surgical correction of strabismus

Prevention

1. One must maintain a constant suspicion of strabismus to help make the diagnosis. Listen to parents when they describe problems, such as unusual eye positions or squinting.

2. The primary care practitioner must learn strabismus-detecting skills, mastering the corneal light reflex test and learning to use the cover-uncover and alternate-cover strabismus evaluation techniques.

3. Maintaining a high level of suspicion does not prevent the onset of the strabismus. Keep in mind the significantly increased likelihood of development of strabismus and/or amblyopia associated with a positive family history.

4. The goal is to identify the strabismus as soon as possible in hope of preventing or treating the amblyopia as soon as possible. Proper refractive correction may decrease or eliminate some types of strabismus.

Bibliography

Asbury T, Burke MJ: Strabismus. *In* Vaughn DG, Asbury T, Riordan-Eva P (eds): General Ophthalmology, 14th ed. Norwalk CT, Appleton & Lange, 1995, pp 226–244.

Helveston EM: 19th Annual Frank Costenbader Lecture—The origins of congenital esotropia. J Pediatr Ophthalmol Strabismus 1993;30:215–232.

324 Nystagmus

Karl C. Golnik

Definition

1. Nystagmus, a repetitve, to-and-fro movement of the eyes, is characterized by three factors:

   a. Direction of eye movement
      (1) Vertical
      (2) Horizontal
      (3) Torsional

   b. Involvement of one or both eyes
      (1) Monocular
      (2) Binocular

   c. Pattern of eye movement
      (1) Pendular—to-and-fro oscillations of equal velocity
      (2) Jerk—slow drifts in one direction followed by corrective, fast movements in the other direction. Jerk nystagmus is named for the direction of the fast eye movement.

2. Nystagmus may be constant regardless of eye position, or it may vary depending on direction of gaze. A patient whose eyes both move slowly 5 degrees to the right and then quickly 5 degrees back to the left as he or she is looking straight ahead may have a similar, but larger-amplitude, repetitive movement of 10-degree excursion when he or she looks to the left. This would be described as horizontal, left beating, jerk nystagmus worse on left gaze.

3. Opsoclonus, also known as the dancing eye syndrome, is not true nystagmus. It occurs in the first 5 years of life and consists of episodes of rapid, conjugate, random eye movements. This may be idiopathic, related to infection (varicella, poliovirus, coxsackievirus B), or a paraneoplastic manifestation of neuroblastoma.

Etiology

1. Nystagmus may be normal or abnormal.
2. Pathologic nystagmus has a variety of causes (see Patho-

physiology). In general, nystagmus results from processes that affect ability to hold fixation steady.

3. If nystagmus does not occur until after the first several years of life, an underlying central nervous system (CNS) abnormality should be suspected.

4. Nystagmus present from birth or developing early in life could be idiopathic or related to any ophthalmic abnormality resulting in poor visual acuity.

Epidemiology

Nystagmus may be a result of numerous diverse conditions, most with no definite epidemiology.

Pathophysiology

1. Nystagmus that develops after the first several years of life often indicates the presence of a structural lesion in the CNS. The pattern of nystagmus can predict the lesion's location:

   a. Monocular—third ventricle, optic chiasm

   b. Pendular—brainstem, cerebellum

   c. See-saw (alternating elevation and intorsion of one eye and depression and extorsion of the other eye)—parasellar/chiasmal

   d. Horizontal, jerk—cerebellum, brainstem

   e. Downbeat, jerk—craniocervical junction

   f. Upbeat, jerk—brainstem, cerebellum

   g. Gaze-evoked—brainstem, cerebellum

2. Nystagmus present in infancy may be due to any of the conditions just listed, but most often it will be either idiopathic or a result of ophthalmologic abnormalities causing poor visual acuity.

   a. Idiopathic

      (1) Congenital—jerk or pendular, damps on convergence, null point present

      (2) Latent—binocular jerk, present only when one eye is occluded; beats toward viewing eye

      (3) Spasmus nutans—triad of head nodding, head posturing, disconjugate asymmetric pendular nystagmus; self-limited

   b. Decreased visual acuity

      (1) Media opacity (cataract)

      (2) Retinal abnormality

         (a) Foveal hypoplasia—ocular albinism

         (b) Photoreceptor abnormality—Leber congenital amaurosis, congenital stationary night blindness, cone dystrophy

      (3) Optic nerve hypoplasia

3. Nystagmus does not always represent a pathologic process. Horizontal, jerk nystagmus present only in extreme gaze positions ("endpoint" nystagmus) can often be elicited in normal individuals. Occasionally, an individual can voluntarily produce nystagmus ("voluntary" nystagmus). It is usually conjugate, horizontal, and rapid and is difficult to maintain for more than a few seconds at a time.

4. Certain medications can cause nystagmus. Horizontal, downbeat, and upbeat nystagmus have each been reported as side effects of sedatives and anticonvulsants. Lithium carbonate is a particularly notorious cause of downbeat nystagmus.

Clinical Findings

1. Patients with nystagmus may be completely asymptomatic, or they may complain of to-and-fro movement of their environment (oscillopsia) or decreased vision.

   a. Onset of nystagmus in early childhood usually produces no symptoms. Vision should be checked if possible. Direct ophthalmoscopy is essential to rule out gross retinal or optic nerve abnormalities. Visually significant anterior segment abnormalities (cataract, corneal opacity) will limit the view to the retina. Photoreceptor abnormalities may severely limit vision but produce no visible retinal abnormalities; an electroretinogram is necessary to establish the diagnosis.

   b. Nystagmus acquired in late childhood or adolescence may cause oscillopsia. This symptom should raise suspicion of an underlying CNS abnormality unless the patient is taking one of the aforementioned medications.

   c. Although nystagmus can result from congenitally poor vision, it can also *cause* decreased vision. Significant eye movement destabilizes the image on the retina. Thus, nystagmus can decrease vision in the absence of other ocular pathology.

2. Patients with nystagmus may have clinical signs other than inappropriate eye movements.

   a. An abnormal head position (turn, tilt) is often subconsciously adopted if the nystagmus improves in a certain gaze position. The head position minimizes eye movement, thus maximizing vision.

   b. Ocular misalignment is frequently present in patients with congenital nystagmus. However, a full range of ocular movement should be present. Any ophthalmoplegia should alert the physician to possible CNS abnormality.

   c. Bilateral optic nerve head swelling (papilledema) may be present if the nystagmus results from a space-occupying CNS lesion.

   d. CNS lesions of the brainstem and cerebellum may cause ataxia and imbalance in addition to nystagmus.

 Key Clinical Finding

• Repetitive to-and-fro eye movements

Treatment

1. Asymptomatic nystagmus does not need to be treated. The best treatment for symptomatic nystagmus is to eliminate its cause. Unfortunately, nystagmus may persist despite removal of CNS lesions or cessation of the inciting medication. Most congenital causes of low vision leading to nystagmus cannot be corrected.

2. There is no absolutely reliable way to eliminate persistent

nystagmus. Oral medications including phenytoin, baclofen, clonazepam, and carbamazepine have been tried with very limited success. Contact lenses have been reported to improve vision in patients with nystagmus, but it is unclear why this may occur. Extraocular muscle surgery can be done to realign the eyes if there is a gaze position where the nystagmus is significantly minimized.

3. Retrobulbar injection of botulinum toxin has been used to paralyze the extraocular muscles, thereby eliminating eye movement. Although this eliminates the nystagmus, patients then have unacceptable diplopia. At present, treatment of nystagmus is frustrating for both patient and physician.

Key Treatment

- Eliminate cause if known and possible

Bibliography

Dell'Osso LF: Nystagmus, saccadic intrusions/oscillations and oscillopsia. *In* Lessell S, van Dalen JTW (eds): Current Neuro-Ophthalmology. St. Louis, Mosby–Year Book, 1991, pp 153–192.

Miller NR: Nystagmus and related ocular motility disorders. *In* Miller NR (ed): Walsh and Hoyt's Clinical Neuro-Ophthalmology, vol 2. Baltimore, Williams & Wilkins, 1985, pp 892–931.

325 Retinopathy of Prematurity

Julia L. Stevens

Definition

Retinopathy of prematurity (ROP), previously termed retrolental fibroplasia (RLF), is a condition in which retinal abnormalities occur as a result of prematurity and oxygen therapy in infants.

Historical Background

1. Retinopathy of prematurity was first identified in 1942, with the observation that premature infants requiring oxygen therapy in incubators had a high degree of childhood blindness.
2. The incidence of blindness was later observed to be linked to the duration and degree of oxygen therapy required in premature infants.
3. The increased survival rate of very low birth weight infants in the 1970s and 1980s has significantly increased the number of children with ROP, though appropriate identification of children at risk, intervention, and management have decreased the percentage of premature infants with subsequent severe visual loss.

Etiology

1. Supplemental oxygen therapy and gestational age are the main known causes of ROP.
2. The earlier the gestational age and the lower the birth weight, the more likely the development of ROP.

Epidemiology

1. Infants with ROP are more likely to have concurrent disorders associated with prematurity, including hyaline membrane disease, bronchopulmonary dysplasia, patent ductus arteriosus, apnea, bradycardia, intracranial hemorrhage, and sepsis.
2. Infants at high risk for development of ROP
   a. Low birth weight, with a 40 per cent incidence of ROP between 1000 and 1250 g birth weight and a 75 per cent incidence in infants <1000 g birth weight
   b. Low gestational age at birth
   c. Products of a pregnancy with multiple births
   d. Prolonged hypercarbia in the neonatal period.
3. The incidence of ROP is greater in Caucasians than in African Americans.
4. Ninety per cent of infants with ROP have complete regression of the retinal disease without sequelae. However, 50 per cent of patients who reach threshold ROP (see under *Clinical Findings*) have progression of their disease with retinal scarring and potential visual impairment.

Pathophysiology

1. At 16 weeks of gestation, mesenchymal sheets of retina spread outward toward the retina from the optic nerve, with a precursor of the capillary network following the mesenchymal tissue. In experimental studies, hyperoxia causes capillary vaso-occlusion, with ischemia and prevention of normal vascularization of the peripheral retina. Therefore, the earlier the gestational age at birth, the less retina that is vascularized and the larger the area of the retina that is at risk for abnormal development.
2. The interface between vascularized and avascular retina is the location of the development of neovascular tissue, with sequelae of intraocular hemorrhage, retinal cicatrization (scarring), and retinal detachment.
3. Left untreated, severe ROP often leads to a total retinal detachment with a fibrovascular mass behind the lens of the eye.

Clinical Findings

1. All prematurely born infants weighing <1500 g or with a gestational age of <30 weeks at birth should

have an initial eye examination at 4 to 6 weeks of age or 30 weeks' postconceptional age. Reexamination is performed at least weekly in high-risk infants. Eye examinations are recommended on a biweekly basis in children at lower risk for ROP, with an increase in frequency if signs of progression are noted.

2. Infants remain at risk for the development of ROP until the entire retina is vascularized. This normally occurs at 40 weeks postconception, though it may be delayed in infants born prematurely.

3. Cyclomydril (cyclopentolate 0.25% and phenylephrine 1.0%), given 30 minutes prior to the examination, is the recommended dilating drop for retinal examination in premature infants.

4. The anterior portion of the globe is examined for signs of "plus" disease, including a cloudy cornea, iris neovascularization, and hazy ocular media.

5. The retina is examined carefully by indirect ophthalmoscopy. Infants may demonstrate only an immature retina in the first few examinations, with the potential for development of ROP if the retina has not fully vascularized. See Table 325–1 for the retinopathy classification scheme.

6. Prethreshold ROP must have the following:

   a. Disease in Zone I or II

   b. Stage 2 or 3 disease, any number of clock-hours

   c. Plus disease.

7. Threshold ROP must have the following:

   a. Disease in Zone I or II

   b. Stage 3 ROP involving 5 contiguous clock-hours or 8 cumulative clock-hours

   c. Plus disease.

TABLE 325–1. INTERNATIONAL CLASSIFICATION OF RETINOPATHY OF PREMATURITY

STAGE
1. Demarcation line between vascular and avascular retina
2. Formation of a ridge; can have neovascular tufts posterior to the ridge within the retina
3. Extraretinal fibrovascular proliferation extending from the retina into the vitreous cavity
4. Subtotal retinal detachment
5. Total retinal detachment

LOCATION
Zone I: A circle with a radius of 30 degrees, twice the distance from the disc to the macula, extending radially from the optic nerve
Zone II: From the edge of zone I to the nasal retinal margin (ora serrata) and to the temporal equator of the retina
Zone III: Temporal retina from the retinal equator to the temporal retinal margin (ora serrata)

EXTENT
Measured in clock-hours (30 degree sectors) in a radial pattern centered on the optic nerve

PLUS DISEASE
Corneal haze
Iris rigidity or neovascularization
Vitreous haze
Dilatation and tortuosity of retinal vessels

Key Clinical Findings

- Vascular dilation/tortuosity
- Neovascular proliferation visible on funduscopic examination
- Retinal detachment
- Retinal cicatricial disease

Treatment

1. Infants with immature retinas or prethreshold retinopathy of prematurity require frequent eye examinations, up to twice weekly if they are very near threshold.

2. Once either one eye or both eyes reach threshold ROP, retinal cryotherapy or laser therapy significantly reduces the incidence of the cicatricial sequelae of ROP. Retinal laser or cryotherapy must be performed within 24 hours after an eye reaches threshold, to avoid progression to the cicatricial stage, which often leads to retinal detachment. Threshold usually develops between 32 and 50 weeks' postconceptional age (gestational age at birth plus chronological age) or 6 to 24 weeks chronological age.

3. In patients who develop a retinal detachment, scleral buckling procedures with vitrectomy as well as lensectomy may be indicated. The child's likelihood of useful vision is limited once retinal detachment occurs.

4. Long-term sequelae of ROP—in increasing order of incidence, patients with a history of prematurity, a history of regressed ROP, and a history of cicatricial ROP are at risk for the development of high refractive errors, strabismus, and amblyopia. Long-term ophthalmic follow-up is recommended for infants with a history of prematurity, as these secondary sequelae may not occur until years later.

Key Treatment

- Retinal laser photocoagulation
- Cryotherapy
- Retinal detachment repair
- Observation for late sequelae

Prevention

1. The incidence of ROP is directly related to the incidence of premature births; hence any intervention that reduces prematurity will reduce the incidence of ROP.

2. Maintenance of arterial PO_2 at the minimum level necessary for maintenance of normal lung and CNS development and avoidance of extremely high arterial PO_2 have been shown to reduce the incidence of ROP. However, maintenance of optimal arterial PO_2 at a steady state with sophisticated monitoring techniques has not shown a substantial improvement in the incidence of ROP.

3. Vitamin E therapy—Studies have suggested a reduction in the incidence of ROP with the use of high-dose vitamin E. Since high doses of vitamin E may be harmful to premature infants and may actually increase

the risk of serious sequelae from ROP, current recommendations are for maintaining physiologic serum vitamin E levels in neonates from the first or second day after birth.

4. Others
   a. Reduction in the exposure to high ambient and supplemental light levels to which the premature infant is exposed may inhibit the development of ROP.
   b. Placing infants with acute ROP on supplemental O_2

or higher levels of O_2 has also been suggested as beneficial for the treatment of severe disease.

Bibliography

Cryotherapy for Retinopathy of Prematurity Cooperative Group: Multicenter trial of cryotherapy for retinopathy of prematurity: preliminary results. Arch Ophthalmol 1988;106:471–476.

Phelps DL: Retinopathy of prematurity. Pediatr Rev 1995;16:50–56.

Pierce EA, Mukai S: Controversies in the management of retinopathy of prematurity. Int Ophthalmol Clin 1994;34:121–148.

326 Nasolacrimal Duct Obstruction

Constance E. West

Definition

Most commonly, the lacrimal drainage system is not patent because of an obstruction of the distal nasolacrimal duct.

Etiology

1. Most instances of nasolacrimal duct obstruction are due to failure of the distal duct to establish patency before birth.
2. Others are due to canalicular stenosis or atresia, lacrimal sac abnormalities, or nasolacrimal duct stenosis.

Epidemiology

Nasolacrimal duct obstruction is a common ophthalmic problem in infants, affecting perhaps as many as 15% of newborns. A higher incidence occurs in patients with craniofacial malformations.

Pathophysiology

1. Tears normally drain through the lacrimal puncta (located on the upper and lower lids at the medial canthus) into the canaliculus, then the lacrimal sac, then the nasolacrimal duct, and finally into the nasal cavity under the inferior turbinate.
2. Tears fail to drain from the eye because of an obstruction of the lacrimal drainage system, usually located at the distal nasolacrimal duct where it opens into the nasal cavity under the inferior turbinate.
3. Epiphora (tearing) and discharge usually begin at 2 to 6 weeks of age.
4. The majority of patients with nasolacrimal duct obstruction experience resolution of symptoms before their first birthday.
5. One third of obstructions are bilateral.
6. Dacryocystocele (amniocele, dacryocele, mucocele) results when fluid (amniotic or tears) becomes trapped in the nasolacrimal drainage system and distends it.
7. Dacryocystitis is an infection of the lacrimal sac and can complicate nasolacrimal duct obstruction or dacryocystocele.

Clinical Findings

1. Epiphora (watery discharge) typically develops during the first month of life and is exacerbated by wind, dust, and nasal congestion.
2. Mucoid or mucopurulent discharge can be found if conjunctivitis develops and may be expressed from the lacrimal sac.
3. Dacryocystocele is a bluish, often about 1-cm cystic mass below the medial canthus. Clear, mucoid material can sometimes be expressed through the puncta.
4. If a dacryocystocele becomes infected (dacryocystitis), purulent material can sometimes be expressed from the puncta, and the mass becomes erythematous with surrounding soft tissue swelling.

Key Clinical Findings

- Watery to purulent discharge
- Dacryocystocele

Differential Diagnosis of Epiphora

Congenital glaucoma
Conjunctivitis (allergic or infectious)
Contact lens related
Crocodile tears
Foreign body
Keratitis
Nasolacrimal duct obstruction

Radiographic Findings

1. Computed tomography with bony windows can assist in the evaluation of patients with dacryocystocele who may have extension of the mass into the nose.

2. A dacryocystogram (radiopaque fluid is injected into the puncta and radiographs are taken) can be performed in unusual cases of nasolacrimal duct obstruction when traditional treatment modalities have failed.

Treatment

1. Spontaneous resolution occurs in 50 to 90 per cent of patients by 6 months of age. The probability that an affected 6-month old will experience relief of symptoms by the age of 1 is about 70 per cent.

2. Antibiotics may be necessary if conjunctivitis accompanies the nasolacrimal duct obstruction. Some physicians prefer ointment to aid in removing crusting from the skin and lashes. Others prefer drops because they believe the liquid reaches the lacrimal sac better than ointment. Medicine should be instilled one to four times a day, depending on symptoms.

3. Digital massage of the lacrimal sac to increase hydrostatic pressure, and possibly relieve the obstruction, is sometimes recommended. Most parents find it difficult to accomplish because of poor patient cooperation.

4. When symptoms do not resolve by an age that the parents and physician are comfortable with, probing and irrigation are performed. A lacrimal probe is passed through the lacrimal system into the nose after the superior or inferior punctum or both puncta are dilated. Many surgeons irrigate saline solution through the system at the conclusion of the procedure to verify patency. Eighty to 90 per cent of first probings are successful.

5. The timing of probing and irrigation is controversial.

   a. Proponents of early, in-office probing cite the reduction of duration of symptoms, the reduced cost of office probing, and the avoidance of general anesthesia. The child is restrained during the procedure; some surgeons allow the parents to be present. Respiratory arrest has been reported.

   b. Probing performed after 6 months of age (late probing) is done in the operating room and avoids surgery in the majority of cases. In addition, the risk of complications may be lower because the child is asleep and may avoid the psychological trauma of being restrained for an early probing. However, the procedure is more costly when performed in the hospital.

6. Silicone intubation is reserved for children who have failed at least one simple probing and irrigation. A loop of thin silicone tubing is passed through the upper and lower canaliculi and through the sac and duct. The loop is fastened in the nose and usually left in place for several months. Depending on technique and the cooperation of the child, tubing is removed in the office or may require general anesthesia.

7. Dacryocystorhinostomy may be performed if repeated silicone intubation fails or if there is a significant anatomic abnormality of the nasolacrimal duct that precludes egress of fluids from the lacrimal sac. In this procedure a direct opening from the lacrimal sac into the nasal cavity is made under the middle turbinate. This can be accomplished through the skin or with a nasal endoscope.

8. The management of dacryocystocele is evolving. Immediate probing used to be the treatment of choice, but many clinicians are recommending massage and conservative treatment as long as dacryocystitis does not develop. Physicians must look for signs of respiratory distress, because dacryocystoceles can extend into the nasal cavity and obstruct the airway.

9. Dacryocystitis can complicate nasolacrimal duct obstruction or dacryocystocele and usually requires systemic antibiotics. Probing should not be performed during the acute infection, because false passages can be created and orbital cellulitis can ensue. Incision and drainage can result in a fistula, an undesired outcome.

Key Treatment

- Usually spontaneous resolution
- Digital massage
- Antibiotics for infection
- Probing and irrigation if no resolution

Bibliography

Day S: Lacrimal system. *In* Taylor D (ed): Pediatric Ophthalmology. Cambridge, Blackwell Scientific Publications, 1990, pp 199–206.

Kushner BJ: Congenital nasolacrimal system obstruction. Arch Ophthalmol 1982;100:597–600.

Mansour AM, Cheng KP, Mumma JV, et al: Congenital dacryocele: a collaborative review. Ophthalmology 1991;98:1744–1751.

327 Conjunctivitis

Sean P. Donahue

Definition

Conjunctivitis is inflammation of the conjunctiva of the eye.

Etiology

1. Infection
   a. Viral
      (1) Adenovirus (most common)
      (2) Herpesvirus.
   b. Bacterial
      (1) *Staphylococcus* species (*S. epidermidis or S. aureus*)
      (2) *Streptococcus* species (usually *S. pneumoniae*)
      (3) *Neisseria gonorrhoeae*
      (4) *Chlamydia*
      (5) *Moraxella, Pseudomonas, Proteus,* coliforms.
2. Allergic
3. Secondary
   a. To corneal disease
      (1) Associated with corneal abrasion
      (2) Associated with corneal ulcer (infectious keratitis).
   b. To orbital disease
   c. To iritis
   d. To acute glaucoma.

Epidemiology

1. Viral conjunctivitis is more common during influenza season, is highly contagious, and is often associated with pharyngitis and/or fever.
2. *Neisseria gonorrhoeae* and *Chlamydia* eye disease are sexually transmitted and are seen in sexually active teenagers, in young adults, and following vaginal delivery in neonates of infected mothers.
3. Corneal ulcers are common in debilitated patients whose ocular surface is compromised (tear deficiency, proptosis with exposure, diabetes, collagen vascular disease) and in wearers of soft contact lenses.
4. Neonatal conjunctivitis is a separate topic (see Chapter 28).

Pathophysiology

1. Viral conjunctivitis occurs as part of a syndrome of viral upper respiratory disease, usually associated with pharyngitis or fever.
2. Breakdown in the ocular surface predisposes to corneal infection. Overwear of contact lenses causes hypoxia and loss of corneal epithelial cells.

Supported in part by an unrestricted grant from Research to Prevent Blindness.

3. The tear film contains IgA, lysozyme, lactoferrin, and β lysin. All are important antimicrobial constituents. Interferon is also present in tears.
4. Acute conjunctivitis begins with histamine release from mast cells. This and other chemical mediators induce local vascular changes that result in increased vascular permeability. This manifests in conjunctival injection, chemosis, and either follicles or papillae.

Clinical Findings

1. Adenoviral conjunctivitis
   a. Starts unilateral, becomes bilateral in 50 per cent
   b. History of upper respiratory tract infection, contact with person having red eye
   c. Watery discharge, photophobia, itching, red and edematous lids
   d. Preauricular adenopathy (suggestive of viral or chlamydial disease or *Neisseria* infection)
   e. Conjunctival signs: follicles, chemosis, pinpoint or larger subconjunctival hemorrhages, membranes, watery tear film.
2. Herpes keratoconjunctivitis (HSV 1)
   a. Primary infection is characterized by clear eyelid or skin vesicles on erythematous base; may have associated conjunctivitis; there is usually no corneal involvement.
   b. Recurrent disease
      (1) Always unilateral
      (2) Usually involves cornea
      (3) Epithelial disturbance of varying appearance; not always a classic dendrite (stains with fluorescein)
      (4) Preauricular adenopathy
      (5) Decreased corneal sensation
      (6) Conjunctival follicles and injection.
3. Allergic conjunctivitis
   a. Bilateral itching is the most prominent symptom
   b. Mild watery to mucoid discharge
   c. Moderate diffuse conjunctival injection
   d. Conjunctival papillae
   e. Moderate conjunctival chemosis
   f. Cats and cigarette smoke are often offending allergens; pollens less likely
   g. May be associated with allergic sinusitis and rhinorrhea.
4. Hyperacute conjunctivitis (*Neisseria* species)
   a. Severe purulent discharge, often bilateral
   b. Marked conjunctival injection and chemosis
   c. Preauricular adenopathy

d. Look specifically for corneal disease during slit lamp examination because corneal perforation can occur in up to 10 per cent of cases.

5. Acute conjunctivitis

  a. It is often difficult to determine if the cause is bacterial or viral, especially when the discharge is scant and mucoid and preauricular adenopathy is absent.

  b. One- to 4-week history of mild to moderate discharge, injection, and chemosis

  c. No history of upper respiratory tract infection

  d. Often bilateral

  e. No preauricular adenopathy.

6. Chronic conjunctivitis

  a. History of awakening with crusty lids

  b. Mild conjunctival injection

  c. Scant mucoid discharge; prominent crusting on lashes

  d. Duration of symptoms for more than 4 weeks.

7. Secondary conjunctivitis (slit lamp examination needed)

  a. Corneal abrasion

    (1) Epithelial defect stains with fluorescein

    (2) Diffuse conjunctival injection

    (3) Marked photophobia and tearing

    (4) Nearly always unilateral

    (5) History of trauma or present on awakening

    (6) Foreign body may be under upper lid.

  b. Infectious keratitis

    (1) Epithelial defect with associated corneal stromal infiltrate

    (2) History of contact lens wear or other factors predisposing to altered ocular surface

    (3) Conjunctival injection and mucoid discharge

    (4) Symptoms of photophobia and ocular pain.

  c. Iritis

    (1) Marked photophobia

    (2) Perilimbal injection

    (3) No discharge

    (4) Nearly always unilateral

    (5) Cells and flare in anterior chamber when evaluated with slit lamp.

  d. Acute glaucoma

    (1) Cornea usually hazy

    (2) Patient has marked eye pain

    (3) Intraocular pressure is high.

Key Clinical Findings

- Unilateral or bilateral depending on etiology—some may be either
- Watery or purulent discharge
- Photophobia
- Reddened conjunctiva

Laboratory Findings

1. Hyperacute conjunctivitis and severe acute conjunctivitis should have Gram stain and culture and sensitivity to guide therapy.

2. Infectious keratitis requires adequate corneal scraping (performed by an ophthalmologist) for Gram stain and culture.

3. Mild acute conjunctivitis and chronic conjunctivitis are treated empirically.

Key Laboratory Test

- Gram stain and culture for severe forms

Radiologic Findings

Radiologic study is not indicated unless the disorder is associated with penetrating ocular trauma or optic nerve involvement.

Treatment

1. Adenoviral conjunctivitis

  a. Supportive therapy; antiviral agents are not effective.

  b. Relief of symptoms with cold compresses, artificial tears, and topical vasoconstrictors

  c. Period of virus shedding extends up to 10 days. External contacts should be limited during this period.

  d. Topical corticosteroids (or antibiotic-corticosteroid combinations) are contraindicated. Both fungal and herpetic corneal disease can masquerade as adenoviral conjunctivitis. Corticosteroids exacerbate these conditions and can cause serious ocular complications, including vision loss. In addition, topical corticosteroids prolong the period of virus shedding by up to 50 per cent.

  e. Because the virus is transmitted through contact, tissues, towels, and pillowcases should not be shared.

  f. Consider a topical antibiotic for prophylaxis against bacterial infection. Vasosulf combines sulfacetamide with phenylephrine and thus also alleviates symptoms.

  g. Oral antibiotics are not effective.

2. Hyperacute conjunctivitis

  a. Corneal perforation can occur. This disease threatens vision, and the patient must be referred to an ophthalmologist.

  b. Treat sexual contacts.

  c. Consider other superimposed sexually transmitted diseases.

  d. *Chlamydia* eye disease can be superimposed.

  e. Perform Gram stain and culture as necessary.

  f. Perform frequent saline lavage of conjunctival cul-de-sac.

  g. In absence of corneal involvement, give single dose of ceftriaxone (1 g intramuscularly) and observe for corneal involvement.

h. With corneal involvement:

  (1) Corneal scrapings and cultures by ophthalmologist

  (2) Intramuscular therapy with ceftriaxone daily for 5 days

  (3) Topical fortified cefazolin and topical fortified tobramycin.

3. Herpetic conjunctivitis

  a. Primary infection. Have ophthalmologist evaluate eye for corneal involvement. Consider topical broad-spectrum antibiotic ointment (erythromycin) to prevent bacterial infection.

  b. Secondary (recurrent disease). Refer to ophthalmologist for management. Prescribe topical cycloplegics (scopolamine or homatropine) for pain control and topical antiviral agents (trifluorothymidine).

4. Bacterial conjunctivitis

  a. Severe: very symptomatic with moderate to severe purulent discharge, severe injection, and eye pain

    (1) Perform culture and Gram stain to guide treatment.

    (2) Give broad-spectrum topical agent (polymyxin-trimethoprim) or fluoroquinolone until results of sensitivity study are available.

    (3) Advise hygiene precautions to prevent spread of infection.

  b. Mild: mild to moderate symptoms, moderate injection and discharge

    (1) Cultures not needed

    (2) Prescribe broad-spectrum antimicrobial agents; sulfacetamide 10 per cent is primary choice. Erythromycin or gentamicin are also useful.

5. Secondary conjunctivitis (all cases of conjunctivitis require a slit lamp examination to rule out secondary causes)

  a. Corneal abrasion

    (1) Look for infection.

    (2) Rule out contact lens overwear or trauma.

    (3) Evert upper lid to evaluate for foreign body.

    (4) Consider patching in non–contact lens wearer older than age 10.

    (5) Prescribe topical cycloplegic (homatropine 5 per cent) for pain.

    (6) Prescribe topical microbial (sulfacetamide 10 per cent).

    (7) Follow-up with ophthalmologist.

      (a) Small defects—in 48 hours if not improved

      (b) Defects greater than 50 per cent—next day

      (c) Defects with infiltrate—immediately

      (d) All contact lens wearers—immediately

  b. Corneal ulcer

    (1) Refer immediately to ophthalmologist.

    (2) Culture and Gram stain to guide treatment.

    (3) Treat with fortified cefazolin and tobramycin topically as prescribed by ophthalmologist.

  c. Iritis

    (1) Refer immediately to ophthalmologist.

    (2) Prescribe cycloplegics for pain.

    (3) Prescribe topical corticosteroids for inflammation.

    (4) Perform systemic work-up for etiology of iritis.

  d. Acute glaucoma

    (1) Measure intraocular pressure.

    (2) Refer to ophthalmologist.

Key Treatment

- Varies with etiology
- Antibiotics locally for bacterial causes

Complications

1. Adenoviral: Patient can develop corneal infiltrates with pain and decreased vision.
2. Herpes: Recurrent disease can cause blindness and is one of the leading causes of corneal blindness in the United States.
3. Hyperacute gonococcal conjunctivitis: Corneal perforation and loss of the eye may occur.
4. Corneal abrasion: Infection; nonhealing defect
5. Infectious keratitis: Perforation and sight loss; scarring and permanent vision loss.

Prevention

1. Avoid affected individuals.
2. Remember hygiene, especially hand washing, after examining patients. Consider wiping hands with washcloth soaked in isopropyl alcohol after contact with infected individuals.
3. Wipe equipment with isopropyl alcohol after each use.
4. This disease may be highly contagious and can reach epidemic proportions. The ophthalmologist's office can often be a source of infection.

 ## Bibliography

Baum JL: Antibiotic use in ophthalmology. *In* Tasman W (ed): Clinical Ophthalmology, vol 4, chapter 25. Philadelphia, Lippincott-Raven, 1995.

Donahue SP, Khoury JM: Common ocular infections. Drugs 1996; 52:526–540.

Mannis MJ: Bacterial conjunctivitis. *In* Tasman W (ed): Clinical Ophthalmology, vol 4, chapter 5. Philadelphia, Lippincott-Raven, 1995.

Schein OD, Blynn RJ, Poggio EC, et al: The relative risk of ulcerative keratitis among users of daily-wear and extended-wear soft contact lenses. N Engl J Med 1989;321:773–778.

Ward JB, Siojo LG, Waller SG: A prospective, masked clinical trial of trifluridine, dexamethasone, and artificial tears in the treatment of epidemic keratoconjunctivitis. Cornea 1993; 12:216–221.

328 Orbital and Preseptal Cellulitis

Janet Loch-Donahue and *Sean P. Donahue*

Orbital Cellulitis

Definition

1. *Orbital cellulitis* is active infection of the orbital tissue posterior to the orbital septum.
2. *Orbital septum* is a continuous diaphanous structure contiguous with the periosteum of the superior and inferior orbital rim that runs vertically to attach to the tarsus of the upper and lower lids. It serves as an anatomic landmark to delineate preseptal (periorbital) cellulitis from orbital cellulitis.

Epidemiology

1. Highest incidence in children and young adults
2. Greater frequency in winter—presumed relationship with increased frequency of upper respiratory tract infections.

Etiology

1. Neonates: *Staphylococcus aureus* and gram-negative bacilli
2. Six months old to 9 years old: *Streptococcus pneumoniae* primarily, other gram-positive cocci; non–spore-forming anaerobes are rare in this age group.

    Before the introduction of conjugated *Haemophilus influenzae* b vaccine in 1988, *H. influenzae* type b was the most common agent in this age group.
3. Age 9 to 14 years: *S. aureus,* streptococci, gram-negative organisms, non–spore-forming anaerobes
4. Older than 14 years: Complex polymicrobial infections with anaerobes are typical.
5. Diabetics/immunocompromised: Same etiology as for those older than 14 years plus *Zygomycetes* (mucormycosis) and *Aspergillus.*

Pathophysiology

1. Extension of infection from paranasal sinusitis—primarily ethmoiditis—is the most frequent cause; it is often associated with subperiosteal abscess.
2. Orbital tissue trauma, orbital fractures
3. Foreign body: infection may develop several months after initial injury.
4. Local orbital infection: dacryoadenitis, dacryocystitis, endophthalmitis, panophthalmitis
5. Bacteremia
6. Eye or orbit surgery
7. Extension from dental infection.

Clinical Findings

1. Almost always unilateral
2. Eyelids have edema, warmth, erythema, tenderness
3. Bulbar conjunctival chemosis (edema) and injection
4. Proptosis: vertical and/or lateral displacement of globe
5. Restriction of ocular motility with pain on testing eye movements
6. Optic neuropathy
    a. Indicates damage to optic nerve
    b. Threatened vision
    c. Characteristics
        (1) Decreased vision
        (2) Decreased color perception
        (3) Afferent pupillary defect (Marcus Gunn sign).
7. Systemic signs: fever, headache, varying degrees of lethargy
8. Purulent drainage from nose and/or conjunctival cul-de-sac
9. Late and more ominous signs: meningeal irritation, ophthalmoplegia, decreased sensation of the ophthalmic division of the fifth cranial nerve, retinal venous congestion, optic disc edema, large afferent pupillary defect, markedly restricted motility (Table 328–1).

Key Clinical Findings: Orbital Cellulitis

- Unilateral
- Edema, erythema, tenderness
- Proptosis
- Drainage

Laboratory Findings

1. Leukocytosis is usually present.
2. Blood cultures are very helpful if positive but are positive

TABLE 328–1. DISTINGUISHING FEATURES OF BACTERIAL PRESEPTAL AND ORBITAL CELLULITIS

FEATURE	PRESEPTAL CELLULITIS	ORBITAL CELLULITIS
Vision	Normal	Often decreased
Pupillary reaction	Normal	Often abnormal; afferent pupillary defect present if vision decreased
Proptosis	Absent	Present
Orbital pain	Absent	Present
Pain on motion	Absent	Present
Motility	Normal	Decreased
Chemosis	Rarely present	Common
Corneal sensation	Normal	May be reduced
Ophthalmoscopy	Normal	May be abnormal (venous congestion or disc edema)
Systemic signs (fever, malaise)	Mild	Commonly severe

From Tasman W (ed): Duane's Clinical Ophthalmology, vol 4. Philadelphia, Lippincott-Raven, 1995, p 4.

Supported in part by an unrestricted grant from Research to Prevent Blindness.

less than 50 per cent of the time (possibly because patients are started on oral antibiotics for primary infection several days before developing orbital cellulitis).

3. Obtain cultures and Gram stain of wound and any drainage from conjunctiva and nasopharynx.

4. Consider Gram stain and culture of cerebrospinal fluid from lumbar puncture in infants. For children older than 2 years of age, lumbar puncture should probably be reserved for those patients exhibiting signs of meningitis.

Key Laboratory Tests: Orbital Cellulitis

- Culture and Gram stain of discharge
- Blood culture

Radiographic Findings

1. Plain films of the orbits are of limited help in detecting foreign body.

2. Computed tomography confirms the diagnosis.
   a. True coronal and axial views of the orbit should be ordered.
   b. Detects orbital and subperiosteal abscesses and sinusitis
   c. May need to be repeated if patient is not improving once treatment is started, to rule out new or enlarging abscess, development of sinusitis, and intracranial spread of infection.

Treatment

1. Examination by an ophthalmologist to assess vision, ocular motility, proptosis, intraocular pressure, and ocular status

2. Intravenous antibiotics
   a. Nafcillin and ceftazidime; consider adding clindamycin when anaerobic infection is suspected (patient older than 9 years of age with subperiosteal abscess).
   b. If patient is allergic to penicillin, use vancomycin and gentamicin, possibly adding clindamycin.
   c. Measure drug levels and adjust dosage appropriately in patients with renal insufficiency.

3. Other medications
   a. Topical and/or oral decongestants in case of sinusitis
   b. Lubricating eyedrops or ointment if proptosis causes corneal exposure

4. Switch to oral antibiotics when the orbital cellulitis is consistently improving on intravenous antibiotics and any optic neuropathy has resolved.
   a. Amoxicillin/clavulanic acid or cefaclor
   b. Total time on antibiotics (intravenous and oral) of 14 days

5. The majority of large subperiosteal abscesses are drained by an ophthalmologist or otorhinolaryngologist soon after presentation; small abscesses without an optic neuropathy may be watched carefully, especially if improvement is occurring on intravenous therapy.

6. Consider consulting otorhinolaryngologist to evaluate sinuses in patients with sinusitis.

7. Patients with suspected or known fungal infection should get otorhinolaryngology consultation to debride necrotic tissue; systemic acidosis should be corrected and intravenous amphotericin B administered. These infections can be fatal, especially if caused by *Zygomycetes*.

Key Treatment: Orbital Cellulitis

- Intravenous antibiotics

Complications

1. Corneal exposure, keratitis
2. Subperiosteal or cerebral abscess
3. Cavernous sinus thrombosis
4. Meningitis
5. Death

Preseptal Cellulitis

Definition

Preseptal cellulitis is an inflammatory process—most often infectious—of the tissues anterior to the orbital septum.

Epidemiology

1. Children and young adults have a more rapidly progressive course than do adults.
2. Frequency is higher in winter.

Etiology

1. Inflammatory periorbital edema secondary to paranasal sinusitis (usually sterile)
2. After skin trauma associated with lacerations, puncture wounds, and human and animal bites (*Staphylococcus* and *Streptococcus* species, anaerobes)
3. Associated with bacteremia in young children without other signs of infection (*S. pneumoniae*, *Haemophilus influenzae type b* [see comment on orbital cellulitis]).

Pathophysiology

1. Associated with otitis media and/or upper respiratory tract infection
2. Extension from sinusitis, dacryocystitis, chalazion
3. Periorbital or orbital soft tissue trauma or foreign body
4. Bacteremia.

Clinical Findings

1. Unilateral or (less likely) bilateral
2. Eyelid edema, erythema, warmth, tenderness
   a. In preseptal cellulitis, inflammation extends over the superior orbital rim onto the brow, whereas in orbital cellulitis the attachment of the orbital septum to the superior orbital rim prevents edema from extending over the brow.
   b. Patient may be unable to open lid secondary to edema
   c. Fluctuant lymphedema of the eyelid.
3. Systemic signs: fever, irritability, malaise
4. The eye is quiet (i.e., no conjunctival injection, good ocular motility, normal pupil examination).

5. Localizing signs of infection: otitis media, upper respiratory tract infection, foreign body, laceration, pus, puncture wound

In preseptal cellulitis, there is no proptosis, no decrease in motility, no pain with eye movement, and no signs of optic nerve involvement. These are all characteristics of orbital involvement and must be excluded in all patients suspected of having preseptal cellulitis (see Table 328–1).

Key Clinical Findings: Preseptal Cellulitis

- Eyelid edema extending onto the brow
- Eye is quiet
- No proptosis

Laboratory Findings

1. Leukocytosis is often present.
2. Perform Gram stain and culture drainage from wound or conjunctiva.
3. Blood cultures may be helpful in those with no localized infection.

Key Laboratory Test: Preseptal Cellulitis

- Gram stain and culture of discharge

Radiologic Findings

Computed tomography is usually not indicated unless there is a history of major trauma or the examination is equivocal for orbital cellulitis.

Treatment

1. Refer for ophthalmologic examination if orbital involvement is questionable.
2. Explore and debride any periorbital or eyelid abscess or fluctuant mass.
3. Apply warm compresses to area at least three times a day.
4. Prescribe oral antibiotics (14-day course).

a. Oral therapy is preferred for mild cases in nontoxic patients older than 5 years.

b. Amoxicillin/clavulanic acid or cefaclor is first choice; trimethoprim/sulfamethoxazole or erythromycin is used when there is a contraindication to first choice.

5. Ceftriaxone (1 g/day) can be given intramuscularly for moderate diseases in an outpatient setting with daily follow-up.

6. Inpatient treatment

a. Consider if patient is younger than 5 years old or in infection by *H. influenzae* type b (remember, this is becoming increasingly rare). Intravenous antibiotics are also indicated for patients who are toxic, unable to follow up daily as outpatients, noncompliant, or not improving after 48 hours of oral antibiotics.

b. Use nafcillin or oxacillin plus ceftazidime.

c. Begin on oral antibiotics to achieve 14 days of treatment when consistent improvement is noted.

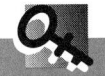

Key Treatment: Preseptal Cellulitis

- Antibiotics

Complications

Orbital cellulitis may occur.

Bibliography

Cullom RD, Chang B (eds): The Wills Eye Manual: Office and Emergency Room Diagnosis and Treatment of Eye Disease, 2nd ed. Philadelphia, JB Lippincott, 1994.

Dagan R, Phillip M, Watemberg NM, Kassis L: Outpatient treatment of serious community-acquired pediatric infections using once daily intramuscular ceftriaxone. Pediatr Infect Dis J 1987;6:1080–1084.

Donahue SP, Khoury JM: Common ocular infections. Drugs 1996;52:526–540.

Hill GT: Subperiosteal abscess of the orbit: Age as a factor in the bacteriology and response to treatment. Ophthalmology 1994;101:585–595.

Jones DB, Steinkuller PG: Microbial preseptal and orbital cellulitis. *In* Tasman W (ed): Duane's Clinical Ophthalmology, vol 4, chapter 25. Philadelphia, Lippincott-Raven, 1995.

329 Retinoblastoma

Constance E. West

Definition

Retinoblastoma is the most common primary intraocular tumor in childhood. It may manifest as a single tumor in one eye or multiple tumors in both eyes.

Etiology

Retinoblastoma results from loss of both copies of an antioncogene on chromosome 13 in both hereditary and nonhereditary forms of the disease.

Epidemiology

The incidence is 1:17,000 live births.

Pathophysiology

1. Retinoblastoma results when there is a loss, point mutation, deletion, or rearrangement of the retinoblastoma gene, which functions as an antioncogene and is located on chromosome 13. In the hereditary form, the mutation is inherited in an autosomal dominant fashion with at least 90 per cent penetrance. A second hit results in loss of heterozygosity at the retinoblastoma locus and leads to tumor formation. Familial and bilateral cases are due to a germinal mutation.
2. Unilateral lesions are usually due to a somatic mutation, but 15 per cent of patients with unilateral retinoblastoma have a germinal mutation, complicating genetic counseling.

Clinical Findings

1. Retinoblastoma most commonly presents as leukocoria but may also present as strabismus, glaucoma, decreased acuity, cellulitis, heterochromia, or hyphema or be detected on routine examination.

Differential Diagnosis of Leukocoria

Cataract
Coats disease
Coloboma
Congenital retinal folds
Hamartoma
Hemangioma
Medulloepithelioma
Myelinated nerve fiber layer
Retinal detachment
Retinal dysplasia
Retinoblastoma
Retinopathy of prematurity
Toxocariasis
Toxoplasmosis
Uveitis
Vitreous hemorrhage

2. An abnormal red reflex is seen with ophthalmoscopy, and larger tumors can be directly visualized through the pupil. The ophthalmologist can detect tumors in the retinal periphery using indirect ophthalmoscopy.
3. Patients with bilateral disease present with leukocoria at an average age of 12 months and those with unilateral disease present at 24 months.
4. Metastatic disease
   a. Children whose diagnosis is delayed may present with symptoms of metastatic disease.
   b. Metastasis occurs by means of the optic nerve to the brain or by means of the optic nerve sheath to the cerebrospinal fluid.
   c. Metastases can also occur during enucleation to the orbit if there is extension of tumor into the optic nerve.
   d. Hematogenous spread leads to involvement of the bone marrow, bone, liver, and lymph nodes.
5. One to 3 per cent of retinoblastomas result from a deletion of the q14 region of chromosome 13; these patients are mentally retarded and have other congenital malformations.
6. Parents and siblings should be examined by an ophthalmologist to find retinoma (nonmalignant manifestation of the retinoblastoma gene), regressed tumor, or retinoblastoma.

Key Clinical Findings

- Leukocoria ("white eye")
- Abnormal red reflex

Laboratory Findings

1. Some centers recommend lumbar puncture and bone marrow aspirate to find metastatic disease during the patient's initial examination under anesthesia.
2. The levels of lactate dehydrogenase in the aqueous are elevated and may be helpful in reaching a diagnosis, and aqueous cytology may be helpful. Vitreous biopsy should be avoided because of the risk of extraocular spread of the tumor.
3. In 95 per cent of families with two or more affected members, genetic testing can accurately identify individuals with the retinoblastoma mutation. Some families can receive useful counseling using linkage studies to the enzyme esterase D.

Radiographic Studies

1. Computed tomography of the head and orbit may show calcification of the intraocular mass or in the pineal gland in the case of a trilateral retinoblastoma.

2. Ocular ultrasonography is used to measure tumor size and assess response to treatment.

Treatment

1. Treatment depends on size and location of the tumor or tumors and involves a multidisciplinary approach (ophthalmologist, oncologist, pediatrician, and geneticist).
2. Enucleation is indicated for eyes with tumors that are too large to treat with other modalities and results in a surgical cure if the tumor is unilateral and confined to the eye.
3. Smaller tumors are treated with radiotherapy (external beam or focal irradiation with a radioactive plaque sewn to the eye), cryotherapy, laser treatment, and chemotherapy.
4. Frequent examination under anesthesia is necessary to find recurrence of disease or to assess treatment success.
5. Long-term ocular sequelae include the need for an ocular prosthesis if the eye is enucleated or cataract formation and orbital contracture if radiation therapy is used.
6. Survivors of hereditary retinoblastoma are at increased risk for the development of second malignancies, even if they do not receive external-beam irradiation.

Key Treatment

- Enucleation (large tumor)
- Radiation therapy
- Cryotherapy

TABLE 329–1. RISK OF DEVELOPING RETINOBLASTOMA

RELATIONSHIP TO PROBAND	RISK OF DEVELOPING RETINOBLASTOMA IN RELATIVE OF PATIENT WITH BILATERAL OR FAMILIAL DISEASE	RISK OF DEVELOPING RETINOBLASTOMA IN RELATIVE OF PATIENT WITH UNILATERAL DISEASE
Offspring	0.45	0.057
Sibling	0.027	0.004
Offspring of an affected sibling	0.0027	0.0004
First cousin	0.00027	0.00004
Monozygotic twin	0.9	0.081
Dizygotic twin	0.027	0.004

Prevention

Genetic counseling is useful after the birth of a child with retinoblastoma or to those with a family history of retinoblastoma (Table 329–1).

Prenatal diagnosis is possible in some familial cases.

See also Chapter 147.

Bibliography

Moore A: Retinoblastoma. *In* Taylor D (ed): Pediatric Ophthalmology. Cambridge, Blackwell Scientific Publications, 1990, pp 348–364.

Musarella MA, Gallie BL: A simplified scheme for genetic counseling in retinoblastoma. J Pediatr Ophthalmol Strabismus 1987;24:124–125.

Shields JA, Shields CL: Current management of retinoblastoma. Mayo Clin Proc 1994;69:50–56.

330 Ocular Trauma

Constance E. West

Definition

Injury to the eyes and or adnexal structures may be secondary to blunt, penetrating, chemical, or thermal trauma.

Etiology

Injuries may be accidental or nonaccidental.

Epidemiology

Ocular trauma is more common in males than females.

Pathophysiology

1. Laceration of the eyelids can result from blunt or sharp trauma and may involve the lacrimal drainage system if the injuries involve the nasal aspects of the lids.
2. Corneal, scleral, and corneoscleral laceration are found after blunt or penetrating trauma. Smaller penetrating injuries may be self-sealing, but larger ones may result in prolapse of the intraocular contents.
3. Eyelid, conjunctiva, cornea, and sclera can be damaged with thermal or chemical burns and lead to scarring, glaucoma, and blindness.
4. Hyphema is a result of trauma to the blood vessels of the anterior segment of the eye and is seen after either blunt or penetrating trauma.
5. Orbital fractures are seen after facial blunt trauma.
6. Optic nerve laceration, avulsion, or hemorrhage can occur with either penetrating orbital trauma or blunt head injuries owing to direct injury or shearing forces.

Clinical Findings

1. Eyelid lacerations are usually obvious, although the extent of damage may not be immediately apparent.
2. Large corneoscleral lacerations are readily apparent but smaller ones may not be. Signs of an occult laceration include hyphema, uveal prolapse, or a peaked or distorted pupil.

3. Orbital fractures are accompanied by contusions, swelling, limited extraocular movement, and enophthalmos.
4. Hyphema results in blood in the anterior chamber, which may obscure visualization of the anterior and posterior segments.
5. Optic nerve damage results in decreased vision and a relative afferent pupillary defect (Marcus Gunn pupil).

Key Clinical Findings

- Lacerations
- Orbital fractures
- Hyphema

Laboratory Findings

There may be evidence of ethanol or drug ingestion on blood or urine testing.

Radiographic Findings

1. Orbital fractures are best evaluated with high-resolution computed tomography of the orbits, preferably with direct coronal views. It may be acceptable or preferable to delay imaging for several days to obtain the most useful studies for evaluation and treatment.
2. Orbital fracture should be assumed if there is air in the orbit.
3. Bony fragments can be seen in proximity to the optic nerve and canal with traumatic optic neuropathy, although their absence does not preclude optic nerve damage.
4. Intraocular foreign bodies can be located with plain films. Magnetic resonance imaging should not be done if the foreign body is metallic.

Treatment

1. Eyelid lacerations can be sutured within 24 hours.
   a. Never trim tissue.
   b. Give tetanus toxoid if necessary.
   c. Consider antibiotic prophylaxis if the wound is dirty. Preseptal and orbital cellulitis may follow eyelid lacerations.
2. Conjunctival lacerations usually do not require suturing. A ruptured globe should be sought.
3. Corneoscleral lacerations require evaluation and treatment by an ophthalmologist and usually require hospitalization.
   a. Patients should not be given anything by mouth in anticipation of going to the operating room.
   b. A protective shield should be placed over the eye, and sedation given, if necessary, to prevent further injury to the eye.
   c. Even if repair is anatomically successful, visual recovery may be limited because of deprivation amblyopia in children younger than 8 years of age.
4. Hyphema is treated with
   a. Bed rest with or without hospital admission
   b. Strong cycloplegic eyedrops (e.g., atropine) to keep the iris from moving and possibly rebleeding
   c. Corticosteroid eyedrops are usually given to de-

crease intraocular inflammation and prevent formation of synechiae.
   d. Oral aminocaproic acid is prescribed by some physicians to delay clot resorption and possibly prevent rebleeding.
   e. A protective shield should be applied to prevent further trauma, particularly eye rubbing.
   f. The head of the bed should be elevated to allow blood to settle in the inferior anterior chamber and not to occlude the pupil.
   g. Aspirin and nonsteroidal antiinflammatory (NSAID) medications should be avoided to decrease the chance of another hemorrhage.
   h. Long-term ophthalmic follow-up is necessary because of the risk of traumatic cataract, retinal detachment, and glaucoma.
5. Orbital fractures are not necessarily repaired surgically if there is no extraocular muscle entrapment or early enophthalmos.

Key Treatment For Hyphema

- Protective shield
- Bed rest
- Cycloplegic eyedrops
- Topical ocular steroid

   a. Assessment of eye movements can be hindered by poor patient cooperation and periorbital swelling.
   b. Patients with suspected orbital fractures should be discouraged from blowing their noses to prevent orbital emphysema and contamination with sinus contents. Orbital emphysema can increase the pressure of the orbital contents and lead to vascular compromise and blindness.
   c. Similarly, orbital hemorrhage can also increase the pressure of the orbital contents and lead to vascular compromise and blindness.
   d. Patients should generally receive antibiotic prophylaxis because of the possibility of contamination of the orbital contents with upper respiratory tract flora.
   e. The timing of surgical repair depends on the patient's general condition, the extent of orbital damage, and the preference of the surgeon.
6. Traumatic optic neuropathy is sometimes successfully treated with high doses of intravenous corticosteroids in adults, but no clinical studies have been done in the pediatric population. Surgical decompression is performed if bony fragments seem to be causing optic nerve dysfunction and is only effective if done soon after the injury.
7. Chemical injuries should be treated with immediate and copious irrigation with isotonic saline solution. A pH strip can be used to assess efficacy of irrigation. An ophthalmologist should be called immediately. A white eye is a particularly ominous sign after a chemical injury and can represent significant ischemia.
8. Thermal injuries to the eyelids and eye can lead to loss

of tissue or damage to tissue. Corneal exposure should be prevented with copious lubrication with ophthalmic ointments.

Prevention

1. Penetrating injuries can be prevented by limiting children's access to, and supervising use of, guns, bullets, and sharp objects.
2. Blunt injuries are often associated with sporting activities, and appropriate protective eyewear and headgear can prevent or limit injuries.
3. Protective eyewear is readily available in pediatric sizes with and without corrective lenses.
4. Parents and physicians should consider limiting participation in at-risk activities for children with certain ocular conditions (pathologic myopia, after retinal detachment surgery, or after corneal transplant) or those with only one sound eye (including dense amblyopia).

 ## Bibliography

Good WV: Accidental and non-accidental trauma. *In* Taylor D (ed): Paediatric Ophthalmology. London, Blackwell Science, 1997, pp 840–870.

331   Symptoms of ENT Disorders

Etiology

1. Earache or otalgia is usually due to an infection in the enteral auditory canal and/or the middle ear. Occasionally there is referred pain coming from the oropharynx probably by means of the glossopharyngeal nerve, which has a middle ear branch called the nerve of Jacobson. Very rarely, in children, will it be associated with dental malocclusion or disorders of the temporomandibular joint.
2. Otalgia is almost always associated with otitis media. It will resolve when the ear drains or the inflammation has subsided.
3. The most frequent source of referred pain from the oropharynx to the external and middle ear is that which is found postoperatively in patients who have undergone a tonsillectomy. Care must be taken to ensure that the postoperative pain is referred and does not represent otitis media or otitis externa.
4. A child who has a draining ear who then develops otalgia should be considered as having an aggressive and dangerous mastoiditis that needs prompt medical and probable surgical treatment.
5. Otalgia that is accentuated by touching the tragus or gently moving the pinna is most often associated with otitis externa.

Clinical Findings

1. History
   a. Otalgia will become manifest within an hour or less of an acute infection of the external or middle ear. This symptom will remain until the infection had subsided or there has been draining of the middle ear either by a spontaneous perforation of the tympanic membrane or by tympanocentesis.
   b. Otalgia that has diminished and then become accentuated in a child with otitis media suggests that the infection has stopped draining or has spread to other portions of the middle ear and mastoid. The sequence of otalgia, ear discharge, diminution/cessation of ear discharge, and the return of the otalgia is a grave sign of severe mastoid involvement.
2. Physical findings
   a. Otitis externa is diagnosed when the external auditory canal is either erythematous, swollen, or filled with debris. Gentle movement or palpation of the tragus will cause discomfort and if moved too much will result in severe pain in many patients with an external otitis. The patients will usually not have fever but may have a leukocytosis.
   b. Acute otitis media will be associated with either an inflamed or bulging tympanic membrane. There may be some mucus discharge in the external auditory canal. Movement of the tragus will usually not result in the patient's discomfort. The patient may have systemic signs of the illness, including temperature, change in disposition, leukocytosis, nausea, and vomiting. The pain will be severe and constant.
   c. Otoscopic examination is the most accurate way to determine whether the patient's otalgia is the result of an otitis externa or media or if it is referred pain.
   d. If there is no edema of the external auditory canal and the tympanic membrane is normal, then the pain is referred and the nasopharynx and/or the oropharynx should be examined to find a source for the referred pain.

Management

1. Otitis externa should be gently cultured. Most of the infections will be caused by *Pseudomonas,* and the culture is used to confirm the bacterial diagnosis so as to ensure optimal local antibiotic therapy.
2. If the canal is extremely edematous, or is closed or almost closed, then Burow solution should be applied for 24 hours. The pain from the otitis externa will stop within a few minutes of the application of the Burow solution.
   a. The action of the Burow solution is to dehydrate the lining of the external auditory canal, reducing the edema and the pressure on the nerve fibers, innervating the external auditory canal and reducing the otalgia, and also providing acetic acid that halts growth of *Pseudomonas.* This is done by taking a small piece of cotton, soaking it in the Burow solution, and then placing it in the affected ear. The cotton serves as a wick.
   b. The cotton is kept wet with the Burow solution for the next 24 hours. The cotton wick is removed and the patient is placed on one of a number of commercial preparations for otitis externa. Also all of these medications contain ototoxic antibiotics and an acid pH. They should only be used when there is an intact tympanic membrane to prevent ototoxic antibiotic from reaching the inner ear by means of the middle ear. These commercial preparations also contain corticosteroids to reduce inflammation. The drops should be used four times a day for 10 days.
   c. The patient is seen in 2 weeks to ensure that the ear has healed and that the diagnosis was correct and that there are no other causal factors such as a foreign body or tumor of the external auditory canal.
3. Acute otitis media may or may not be treated with an appropriate antibiotic after a culture is taken.
   a. The most accepted form of care is to give an antibi-

otic, orally if tolerated, and treat the fever and pain symptomatically.

b. Some clinicians advise doing a tympanocentesis to relieve the pain.

Patient Education

The parents (or caregivers) need to be informed that the pain should go away with effective treatment. If the pain is referred, as found in a postoperative tonsillectomy, then the pain may not subside for 1 or 2 days. The referred pain is not severe, and an understanding of its course and that it does not represent an ear infection is reassuring to the parents.

Follow-up

1. All cases of otalgia need to be observed to determine if the pain has stopped. If the pain is still present, then there has been either an incorrect diagnosis or an inadequate therapy.

2. Often a painless discharge from the ear may be mistaken as an otitis externa when it is coming from a chronic otitis media or as mastoiditis with a cholesteatoma. If the ear drains for more than a few days to a week, and the child is on what is presumed to be adequate therapy, then another diagnosis for the draining must be considered.

3. A rare cause of persistent, or intermittent, discharge from the ear is granulation tissue of the external canal and the tympanic membrane. See Chapter 86.

Bibliography

Rosenfield RM: Comparison of three strategies for the initial empiric therapy of acute otitis media in children. *In* Mogi G, Honjo I, Tetsuo I, Takasaka T (eds): Recent Advances in Otitis Media. Amsterdam/New York, Kugler, 1994, pp 175–178.

| Symptom | **Hearing Loss** | *Robert J. Ruben* |

General Considerations

The symptom of hearing loss may be articulated either by the parent or the child. *All pediatric patients who have this symptom must be assumed to actually have a hearing loss until proven otherwise.* Often the symptom is ignored or dismissed. The child is not recognized as being hearing impaired, and as a consequence of delayed diagnosis, he or she suffers permanent language impairment that decreases the child's opportunity to achieve his or her potential in this communication-based society. Hearing loss and the resultant communication disability is associated, with other factors, in aberrant juvenile behavior.

The symptom of hearing loss may be confused with developmental variability in that all children do not attend to sound in the same manner at the same age. Before this distinction is made it is necessary to make sure that the child's hearing is normal. Only then can the label of possible developmental variability be considered as a cause for a lack of responsiveness to sound. Other causes will be developmental delay and, in older children and adolescents, an occasional patient will be less responsive for some form of secondary psychological gain.

Etiology

The differential diagnosis of hearing loss must consider the location of the loss in the auditory system. Hearing loss can come about from a pathologic process in the external auditory canals, the middle ear, the inner ear, the statoacoustic nerve, the brainstem, the thalamus, the cortex, or any combination of these anatomic sites. The location of the site of the loss is determined so that the correct intervention may be instituted.

The time at which the hearing loss began must be determined for a complete diagnosis. Hearing losses early in life, during the first 24 months, will have a greater effect on the language of a child than those that occur later. The effect of the loss will be dependent on the extent of the loss. Information needs to be obtained as to the amount of the loss and whether it is fluctuating and/or progressive.

Clinical Findings

1. History

a. The most important part of the history is the parent's suspicion that the child may have a hearing loss. Whenever there is a statement by a caretaker that he or she believes the child may have a hearing loss it is mandatory that the child have complete testing. Centers that care for hearing-impaired children consistently report that the parent has been the first to notice the hearing loss and has been ignored or not taken seriously by the physician.

b. Abnormal development of speech or language is another critical portion of the history that occurs with children who have a hearing loss. Although the abnormal speech and language are not always associated with hearing loss, a hearing loss must be ruled out before speech and/or language therapy can be instituted.

c. As the child becomes older, he or she will be able to report the problems of hearing loss. The parents will also note in the older child that the television set is turned louder or the child appears to be ignoring them. At times, the parents will report that the child's hearing appears to be normal. The parents may be reporting that the child has a fluctuating hearing loss. Fluctuating hearing losses may occur in neurosensory hearing losses and in the more common types of hearing loss associated with otitis media with effusion.

d. Unilateral hearing losses have a significant morbidity and are usually diagnosed late. The patient will have a history of using the telephone with one ear and a history of delayed or abnormal language. Most of the children with unilateral hearing loss will have relatively good speech.

e. One of the most important aspects of the hearing loss is when the parent relates that their child appeared to have normal hearing at birth or during the first few months or year of life and then they noted a decrease in hearing. These progressive losses are usually not diagnosed until they have become obvious, and by then the child is profoundly deaf. The late diagnosis is a deterrent to the care of the child because a number of the progressive losses are treatable either by medical or surgical means.

f. A significant part of the history of the child with a hearing loss will be family history of hearing loss. Approximately half of all hearing losses are genetic, and many of these are progressive. The autosomal dominant cases have variable expressivity, with hearing loss beginning early in life or later in life.

g. Infants and toddlers who have even had slight head trauma have been found to have dislocation of the stapes with loss of inner ear fluid of the middle ear, resulting in a rapidly progressive hearing loss. The history of head trauma is also associated with temporal bone fractures, as noted by bleeding from the ear.

h. An uncommon but treatable cause of hearing is that which concerns perilymphatic fistula. Often the major historical event will be nausea and vomiting. Children have been hospitalized for fluid replacement because of the vomiting secondary to the fistula. They will also have a hearing loss. The hearing loss may be in one ear and may not be obvious. A child with repeated episodes of vomiting who also has a history of vertigo and unsteadiness should be considered as having a probable hearing loss.

2. Physical findings

a. The most common forms of hearing loss are those associated with otitis media with effusion. The clinical finding will be a retracted or bulging eardrum with fluid.

b. Hearing loss may be associated with impacted cerumen.

c. Those hearing losses that are associated with congenital malformations of the ear are detected by the observation of lack of development of the external auditory canal.

d. The sensorineural hearing losses, for the most part, usually do not have any associated stigmata.

e. There are a number of easily recognizable syndromes:

(1) Waardenburg's disease with a white forelock or heterochromia

(2) Pendred's disease associated with goiter

(3) All of the patients with craniofacial malformations such as the Treacher Collins sequence, the Pierre Robin sequence, velocardiofacial (Shprintzen) syndrome, and others must be assumed to have a hearing loss until proven otherwise.

3. Tests

a. The most important aspect of testing is to determine whether there is a probability of a hearing loss. The use of a language screen, the Early Language Milestone Scale, has proven satisfactory for screening of all children up to the age of 36 months. If there is a failure in the language examination, then the child will be suspected of having hearing loss. This test is able to detect children with modest to moderate, severe, and profound hearing losses.

b. Children younger than 6 months of age should be tested with physiologic testing.

(1) Most common and widespread is the use of auditory evoked brainstem responses. Unfortunately, this is usually done with a click and not pure tones. Auditory evoked brainstem potential examination is available and should be used to determine the threshold.

(2) Another technique that assesses the integrity of the outer hair cells of the ear is evaluation of spontaneous evoked cochlear emissions. This is also being used as a screening test and has been found to be effective in some environments.

c. All children who are developmentally 6 months of age or older are able to be tested behaviorally with each ear with different pure tones and by air and bone. This test is called visual reinforced audiometry and is readily available. Any child 6 months or older who is suspected of having a hearing loss or who has a speech and/or language abnormality should undergo visual reinforced audiometry testing to determine his or her thresholds at the various frequencies for both bone and air conduction.

d. The use of immittance function for the assessment of the characteristics of the middle ear also contributes to the cause of the hearing loss, but this is not a hearing test. The tympanogram from the immittance function gives information concerning the stiffness and movements of the tympanic membrane. The pressure measures tell about the middle ear pressure. Together this information is empirically correlated with whether there is fluid in the ear that becomes an etiologic factor but does not tell the extent of the hearing loss. Children with middle ear effusion with flat tympanograms can have a hearing loss of several decibels to a rather significant hearing loss of 40 to 45 dB.

e. Other tests can be done that look at the way in which the child processes auditory information both in the midbrain and in the cerebral cortex. These tests are usually used to determine more complex functions of hearing and also to determine the efficacy of interventions such as hearing aids.

Management

1. As soon as the child is determined to have a hearing loss the cause of the hearing loss must be determined. The most common cause of hearing loss in young children is a middle ear effusion. If this hearing loss is believed to have an effect on the child's language, an appropriate intervention should be carried out. The treatment of otitis media with effusion in children without cleft palates or submucosal clefts of the palate is adenoidectomy and insertion of short-acting tympanostomy tubes. If the child has a cleft palate or submu-

cosal cleft of the palate or other abnormalities of the pharynx, then long-acting tympanostomy tubes are put in place. Antibiotics and decongestants have no effect on the hearing of children with otitis media with effusion.

2. Children with sensorineural hearing losses need to have the cause of the loss determined because there are a few treatable forms of sensorineural hearing loss.

   a. If the child has autoimmune disease, then indicated therapy is corticosteroids.

   b. If the child has a perilympathic fistula, then the child is managed with closure of the fistula.

   c. However, even the previous two disorders will usually result in a significant permanent sensorineural hearing loss. The child will need to have hearing amplification and be immediately enrolled in a special educational environment so that he or she can begin to overcome the disability.

3. Children with profound sensorineural hearing losses are now able to be treated with the use of a cochlear implant. The child is seen in a center that has the proper evaluation, interventional follow-up, and educational facilities to care for the child.

4. Children with unilateral hearing losses have a significant defect. They have a decreased ability to detect signals in noise. This disability has been shown to have a significant morbidity, as exemplified by having a 20 times greater chance of being left back in their early school years than matched controls. These children need to be cared for with speech and language intervention and an FM system. The FM system is used in the school to allow for a least restrictive educational environment. The FM system works by having the teacher wear a microphone that broadcasts directly to the child's hearing aid worn in the child's good ear.

Thus, there is no problem with signals in noise because the teacher is "always whispering in the child's ear."

Follow-up

1. All hearing losses need to be treated. Children with otitis media with an effusion, who have had intervention with tympanostomy tubes, must be observed until the tubes have been extruded or removed.

2. Audiometric and language assessments need to be done to see if the hearing has returned to normal and if the language is normal.

3. Children with sensorineural hearing losses need to be checked audiometrically at different schedules depending on the disease. Ten to 20 per cent of sensorineural hearing losses show progressive losses, and these need to be documented so that intervention can be adjusted. These children must be followed periodically to determine if their language has improved and is at an expected level.

The most important aspect of the care of the hearing impaired is early diagnosis. The parents' observation that their child may not be hearing well or their observation of even slight abnormalities in speech and language must always be considered as a hearing loss until proven otherwise.

Bibliography

Aram D, Ruben RJ: Report of the workshop on Communication Disorders and Juvenile Behaviors. Bethesda, MD, NIDCD, 1994.

Bess FH, Klee T, Culbertson JL: Identification, assessment, and management of children with unilateral sensorineural hearing loss. Ear Hear 1986;7:43–51.

Gorlin RJ, Toriello HV, Cohen MM Jr: Hereditary Hearing Loss and Its Syndromes. New York, Oxford University Press, 1995.

Ruben RJ: Early identification of hearing impairment in infants and young children. Int J Pediatr Otolaryngol 1993;27:207–213.

| Symptom | **Vertigo** | | *Robert J. Ruben* |

Definition

1. *Vertigo* is defined as the patient perceiving that he or she is moving in space. It is usually a rotary sensation and is often reported as a violent spinning in one or another direction. Vertigo is commonly accompanied by nausea, vomiting, unsteadiness, loss of balance, and falling. The symptom of vertigo will be manifested differently at different ages. The infant and toddler will fall, stop crawling or walking, and have signs of nausea. The older child will manifest the physical signs and report a feeling of movement, described as spinning, turning, or being on a merry-go-round. The symptom of vertigo can be very frightening to a child and the child's insecurity can be accentuated by the adult not realizing what the child is experiencing.

2. Almost all true vertigo is a result of a pathologic process occurring in the balance (vestibular) portion of the inner ear. This includes the three semicircular canals and the otolith organs of the saccule and utricle. The vertigo may be confined to a signal episode or may be episodic.

Etiology

1. Perilymphatic fistula, a connection between the inner ear and the middle ear, is the most frequently encountered cause of true episodic vertigo in childhood.

   a. The vertigo is frequently but not invariably associated with a sensorineural sudden hearing loss.

   b. The initial manifestation of a perilymphatic fistula can be an isolated episode of true vertigo.

2. Uncommon diseases and disorders that are considered in children with episodic vertigo include

   a. Progressive labyrinthitis from congenital infections such as rubella

   b. Traumatic labyrinthitis from head injury

   c. Fistulization of a semicircular canal in a child with chronic mastoiditis usually with a cholesteatoma

   d. Meniere syndrome

   e. Tumors of the statoacoustic nerve most commonly found in children with neurofibromatosis type 2.

f. All of the these conditions if left untreated will result in substantial morbidity. The recognition of the symptom of vertigo in a child will result in timely intervention that will reduce or prevent morbidity and, in the rare case, mortality. Episodic vertigo is a symptom of a potentially serious disease.

3. A signal episode of vertigo may be associated with a viral or bacterial labyrinthitis. Children who have postmeningitic labyrinthitis will have many of the symptoms of vertigo.

Clinical Findings

1. History
    a. Vertigo will be revealed differently at different ages. The infant and the toddler will have symptoms of nausea and vomiting without any other gastrointestinal signs. Additionally, they will appear clumsy, stop walking, and stop crawling. They will show regression in their locomotion. They may also be upset when a person changes his or her position, because this is aggravating the child's sense of motion.

    b. The older child will have all of the symptoms of the infant and toddler and additionally will complain of the sensation of movement. He or she may compare it to the feeling of twirling or being on a merry-go-round or another ride in an amusement park. The child will not feel that it is a pleasant sensation and will, for the most part, be very frightened. Older children will not be able to ride a bicycle, go skating, or participate in any number of activities while undergoing a vertiginous episode.

    c. The vertigo may last only a few seconds and can persist for 1 to 2 days. The longer the vertigo persists, usually, the more the likelihood that it is related to severe underlying disease of the vestibular labyrinth. However, short, intermittent, episodes of vertigo are associated with tumors of the statoacoustic nerve and fistula of the semicircular canals.

    d. Many children with vertigo will be found not to have any associated diseases or disorder, and the vertigo will be classified as idiopathic.

2. Physical findings
    a. A child who is undergoing an episode of vertigo will have dramatic clinical findings. The child will have difficulty standing with eyes open and when the eyes are closed will fall. The toddler and infant will not be able to move from one position to the other without holding onto a structure such as a crib rail.

    b. The eyes will often show a marked nystagmus, most often horizontal. The nystagmus will persist and sometimes become more intense when the eyes are closed. This may be determined by having the child close his or her eyes and gently palpating the closed upper eyelid. One will easily feel the rapid involuntary eye movements.

    c. Many children with vertigo will have associated sensorineural hearing loss. This is documented by audiographic testing of the hearing in each ear.

d. Between the episodes of vertigo the child will have no clinical signs that are especially associated with the vertigo.

3. Evaluation of the auditory and vestibular systems must be carried out in all children who have the symptom of vertigo. Vestibular testing is done in two ways:
    a. The most common is to access the vestibular system by recording the child's eye movements from known quantities of vestibular stimulation.
        (1) The recording is not invasive and is most commonly done with surface electrodes recording changes in the electroretinogram with eye movements.
        (2) Alternatively, testing is done by using an infrared sensor on the eye and recording the eye movements when the child is in the dark.
        (3) The vestibular stimulation is done by positioning of the head, controlled rotation, and the use of caloric stimulation. The results from the evaluation of the eye movements can determine whether the vestibular abnormalities are peripheral (i.e., in the inner ear) or central. A number of patients with vertigo will have normal vestibular function after the vertiginous episode, and a normal test result will not preclude the child having vertigo.

    b. The second form of testing is to examine the child's posture in a controlled manner. The posture test (postulography) looks at the entire body's ability to orientate in space and gives valuable information as to the child's vestibular function. This form of evaluation uses a posture pressure platform. It has had limited use in the evaluation of children's vertigo.

WARNING

A signal episode of vertigo in a child can be the manifestation of a perilymphatic fistula for which there is effective intervention that may prevent hearing loss and occasionally restore hearing. These children have perilymph leaks (perilymph is a fluid that is in continuity with cerebrospinal fluid) into the middle ear. The leak exposes the central nervous system to the middle ear and outside world. Many of these children will have *recurrent* meningitis. The early diagnosis and repair of the perilymphatic fistula may prevent the child from acquiring meningitis.

Management

The acute episode of vertigo is cared for by bedrest and, in the more severe cases, fluid replacement. Some children may have substantial and prolonged episodes of vomiting that will result in dehydration and significant electrolyte disturbance. The symptoms may be controlled with antinausea medications.

Patient Education

1. The parents need to realize that their child is undergoing a real sensory experience. They must be informed as to

the potential gravity of the symptom of vertigo and the need for further evaluation of their child.

2. The child needs to be reassured that the movement will stop.

Follow-up

The patient is followed until the significant associated disorders of vertigo have been investigated. The follow-up of an initial episode of vertigo must include the need to note any further episodes and a periodic hearing test to ensure that the vertigo is not associated with a progressive sensorineural hearing loss.

Bibliography

Cyr DG, Brookhouser PE, Valente M, Grossman A: Vestibular evaluation of infants and preschool children. Otolaryngol Head Neck Surg 1985;93:463–468.

Ruben RJ, Yankelowitz SM: Spontaneous perilymphatic fistula in children. Am J Otol 1989;10:198–207.

332 Otitis Media

Robert J. Ruben

Etiology

1. Acute otitis media results from bacterial infection of the middle ear. The most common causative bacteria are *Haemophilus influenzae, Streptococcus pneumoniae, Branhamella catarrhalis,*, and other organisms.

2. The susceptibility to the infection and its effect on the individual child are variable. Those who appear to be most susceptible are
   a. Those with immune deficiencies
   b. Those with major or minor abnormalities of the skull base that result in abnormal eustachian tube function
   c. Those who are bottle fed
   d. Those who are in an environment that has tobacco smoke
   e. Those in daycare.

Epidemiology

1. Acute otitis media occurs most frequently during the first 3 to 4 years of life.
2. It affects boys somewhat more than girls.
3. The most recent studies show that in North America there appears to be no racial predominance.
4. American Indians have a higher incidence of acute otitis media, which is, in part, thought to be associated with the high prevalence of submucosal clefts of the palate.
5. There is an increased incidence of otitis media in children in daycare centers. The daycare children are more often infected with antibiotic-resistant organisms than children in the general population.
6. Acute otitis media is seen more commonly in children with immunodeficiencies, especially children infected with the human immunodeficiency virus.

Clinical Findings

1. History. Acute otitis media presents as pain, nausea, vomiting, and fever.
2. Physical findings

a. Occasionally, the pinna will be erythematous.

b. Examination of the external auditory canal with an otoscope may show minimal debris.

c. The tympanic membrane has lost its landmarks and is either erythematous or white. A normal tympanic membrane is a translucent membrane through which the malleus, incus, incudostapedial joint, chorda tympani, eustachian tube orifice, and round window can be seen. Nearly all of these landmarks will not be visible.

d. A light reflex can be seen in children with acute otitis media, and the presence of the light reflex does not connotate normality.

e. The tympanic membrane may be bulging, and/or, on occasion, it will have ruptured and there will be mucopurulent material expelled into the external auditory canal. Of significance is that the canal is not tender and palpation of the tragus is not tender as it is in otitis externa.

Key Clinical Findings

- Fever
- Earache
- Loss of anatomic landmarks on tympanic membrane
- Bulging tympanic membrane

Laboratory Findings

1. The laboratory findings will be a fever and leukocytosis with immature cells. Culture will usually reveal the bacteria.
2. Cultures of the pharynx should be taken to determine whether the offending organism is antibiotic resistant.

Key Laboratory Findings

- Leukocytosis
- Positive pharyngeal culture

Radiographic Findings

1. Unless mastoiditis is suspected, no radiographs are required.
2. Acute otitis media is associated with a clouding of the middle ear cleft and the mastoid. However, of importance is that the bony septa and the mastoid are intact.

Treatment

1. Most children are treated with antibiotics.
2. There are controlled studies that have shown that most cases of acute otitis media will be self-limiting and do not require antibiotic therapy. When antibiotic therapy is not given, the child is given an analgesic.
3. If the child is not given antibiotics, then there must be follow-up of the child. If the child continues to have a fever or shows more symptomatic signs, then antibiotic therapy with or without a tympanocentesis is used.
4. If follow-up cannot be ensured, then appropriate antibiotic therapy is indicated at the initial encounter.
5. There will be an occasional child who will continue to have pain and fever for 12 or more hours after the commencement of antibiotic therapy. These children are candidates for a tympanocentesis.
6. The widespread use of antibiotics for otitis media is considered to be a significant cause for the worldwide increased prevalence of antibiotic-resistant bacteria. Antibiotics should be used with caution and in a controlled fashion.

Key Treatment

- Acute otitis media can be managed with an analgesic if there is excellent follow-up because this appears to be a self-limiting disease. However, if the follow-up is not available or is questionable, then antibiotic therapy is used.

See also Chapter 86.

Bibliography

Breiman RF, Butler JC, Tenover FC, et al: Emergence of drug-resistant pneumococcal infections in the United States. JAMA 1994;271:1831–1835.

CDC Morbidity, Mortality Weekly Report: Drug resistant *Streptococcus pneumoniae*—Kentucky and Tennessee, 1993. JAMA 1994;271:421–422.

Van Buchem FL, Dunk JH, Van't Hof MA; Acute otitis media: myringotomy, antibiotics, or neither? Lancet 1981;2:883–887.

---

333 Serous Otitis Media

Robert J. Ruben

Etiology

Serous otitis media with effusion is caused by abnormal eustachian tube function, or it is a sequela of acute otitis media. Any interference with the eustachian tube results in a change in the environment of the middle ear cleft that causes a redifferentiation of the mucosa and the secretion of serous fluid. If the eustachian tube function is returned to normal or if the middle ear is allowed to aerate, then the mucosa returns to its normal state and will not secrete the abnormal amounts of serous fluid.

Epidemiology

1. Otitis media with effusion most commonly occurs in children younger than 3 years of age.
2. There is a higher incidence in children who have malformations of the skull base, such as cleft palate and submucosal cleft of the palate.
3. Otitis media with effusion is found more frequently in children in daycare centers and in children who have immunodeficiencies.
4. Acute otitis media is seen more commonly in children with immunodeficiencies, especially in children who are infected with the human immunodeficiency virus.

Clinical Findings

1. History. Otitis media with effusion is "a quiet disease." A child will occasionally have symptoms of some fullness or hearing loss and occasionally some unsteadiness. The parents will usually note that the child is not listening to them. There will also be substantive deficiencies in language. This is especially true for expressive language in children younger than 2 years of age.
2. Physical findings
   a. Otoscopic examination will show a variety of different abnormalities of the tympanic membrane. Among the most common is retraction of the tympanic membranes with yellowish fluid. There can be bulging fluid, and there can be very severe retraction of the tympanic membrane where it is touching the medial portion of the middle ear cleft. If the tympanic membrane is adherent to the long process

of the incus, it will result in necrosis of the incus. This will cause a permanent conductive hearing loss of 40 to 50 dB.

b. Severe atelectasis associated with otitis media with effusion will also result in retraction pockets of the cephalad and dorsal portion of tympanic membrane. This may lead to cholesteatoma, destruction of middle ear and mastoid, and mastoiditis.

Key Clinical Findings

- Retracted tympanic membrane with fluid
- Hearing loss

Laboratory Findings

Audiometric findings may or may not show conductive hearing loss. Tympanometric finds show negative middle ear pressure and flattened tympanograms.

Radiographic Changes

Radiographic changes show a cloudy mastoid, but the bony septa are intact.

Prevention and Treatment

Prevention of otitis media with effusion can be done through the establishment of normal aeration of the middle ear.

1. If the child does not have a malformation of the palate or the pharynx, then adenoidectomy with insertion of short-acting tympanostomy tubes is done.

2. If there is malformation, then the use of long-acting tympanostomy tubes will allow the middle ear to aerate and prevent recurrence of the otitis media with effusion.

Children with otitis media with effusion should be suspected of having recurrent and persistent:

1. Immunologic deficiency
2. Skull base malformation
3. The possibility of incus necrosis and/or cholesteatoma
4. Language deficiencies, especially in expressive language associated with the hearing loss.

Key Treatment

- Short-acting tympanostomy tubes

Bibliography

Gates GA, Avery CA, Prihoda TJ, Cooper JC Jr: Effectiveness of adenoidectomy and tympanostomy tubes in the treatment of chronic otitis media with effusion. N Engl J Med 1987; 317:1444–1451.

Mogi G, Honjo I, Ishii T, Takasaka T: Recent Advances in Otitis Media. Amsterdam, Kugler, 1994.

Ruben RJ, Bagger-Sjoback D, Downs MP, et al: Recent advances in otitis media: Complications and sequelae. Ann Otol Rhinol Laryngol Suppl 1989;139:46–55.

Sade J: Middle ear mucosa. Arch Otolaryngol 1966;84:137–143.

Wallace IF, Gravel JS, Ganon EC: Two-year language outcomes as a function of otitis media and parental linguistic styles. In Lim DJ, Bluestone CD, Nelson JD, et al (eds): Recent Advances in Otitis Media. Philadelphia, Decker Periodicals, 1993, pp 527–530.

334 Chronic Otitis Media and Mastoiditis

Robert J. Ruben

Definition and Etiology

1. Chronic otitis media and mastoiditis occur as a consequence of persistent infection of the middle ear cleft and mastoid. They are initially associated with the same bacteria as found in acute otitis media. However, as the disease progresses, there will usually be a predominance of *Staphylococcus aureus* and *Pseudomonas aeruginosa*.

2. Chronic otitis media and mastoiditis are also seen in association with cholesteatoma.

Epidemiology

1. Chronic otitis media and mastoiditis is seen in all age groups.

2. Younger children may have an acute mastoiditis as a result of a single episode of otitis media.

3. Other children will have repeated bouts of acute otitis media and then will have continual drainage from the ear.

4. Mastoiditis is most commonly found in children who have had inadequate or no treatment for acute otitis media and otitis media with effusion.

5. Children with immunodeficiencies and/or skull base malformation also have a higher incidence of chronic otitis media and mastoiditis.

Clinical Findings

1. History and physical findings

   a. The clinical picture of chronic otitis media and mastoiditis includes continual intermittent draining ears. The tympanic membrane has a perforation through which the drainage occurs.

   b. Acute mastoiditis is noted by a swelling behind the pinna with tenderness. This usually indicates that the latter portion of the mastoid bone has been destroyed by the infectious process and there is pus and/or tissue edema under the periosteum of the temporalis fascia.

c. Chronic otitis media and mastoiditis also may be accompanied by more severe signs, such as facial nerve paresis or palsy, deafness, and meningitis.

Key Clinical Findings

- Tender swelling over mastoid region
- Chronic otitis media

Laboratory Findings

1. Patients have very few systemic signs of chronic infection. They seldom have fever or leukocytosis.
2. Radiologic changes show loss of the mastoid septa, destruction of the mastoid bone, bony erosion, and fluid throughout the middle ear and mastoid.

Prevention

1. Treatment of chronic otitis media and mastoiditis is with intravenous administration of an antibiotic. Chronic otitis media and mastoiditis is a form of an osteitis and should be treated appropriately.

2. If antibiotic treatment fails, then surgical removal of the dead, infected bone and granulation tissue is done through a mastoid operation.

Ears that have intermittent or chronic drainage have a potential for a serious spread of infection from the middle ear cleft and the mastoid to the surrounding neural tissues or facial nerve and/or into the inner ear to cause deafness. These cases need adequate prompt treatment. Intermittent drainage is also associated with cholesteatoma, which is a benign tumor that can, if untreated, cause further bony erosion and the same sequelae of central nervous system infection, facial nerve paralysis, and/or deafness.

Key Treatment

- Antibiotics
- Surgery

Bibliography

Kenna MA, Rosane BA, Bluestone CD: Medical management of chronic suppurative otitis media without cholesteatoma in children—an update 1992. Am J Otol 1993;14:469–473.

335 Otitis Externa (Swimmer's Ear)

Robert J. Ruben

Etiology

Otitis externa occurs through trauma to the external auditory canal. The skin lining the external auditory canals differs in that there is no adipose tissue and there is very thin epidermis. The skin is directly applied to either the cartilage or bone. Anything that causes trauma to the skin and results in infection causes acute swelling, pain, edema, and discharge.

1. Trauma may result from foreign bodies that enter the external auditory canal or from attempts to remove cerumen.
2. During the summer, when children are swimming, the ear will become wet and the constant exposure to water of this very thin skin causes maceration, followed by infection.

Epidemiology

1. Otitis externa occurs at all ages but is most common in children from age 6 years through adolescence.
2. It is also found quite often in children who wear hearing aids. Because the hearing aid causes further thinning of the skin, infection results.

Clinical Findings

1. History. The child can present with fever.
2. Physical findings
   a. Most importantly, there is either minimal or modest discharge from the ear with exquisite tenderness to touch of any portion of the external auditory canal, especially the tragus.
   b. The ear is swollen and quite painful to touch.

Key Clinical Finding

- Exquisite tenderness of auditory canal

Laboratory Findings

Laboratory findings usually show bacterial infection, most often *Pseudomonas aeruginosa* (usually causing the foul odor), *Staphylococcus aureus, Proteus, Staphylococcus epidermidis, Enterobacter, Escherichia coli,* and *Klebsiella.*

Key Laboratory Finding

- Culture—usually *Pseudomonas* infection

Treatment

1. The initial treatment with the pain and swelling would be the use of Burow solution, which decreases the swelling of the external auditory canal. This is applied on a small cotton wick and kept soaked for 24 hours. Within a few minutes, this relieves the pain. Burow solution has an acid pH that will act against the *P. aeruginosa.*
2. A cortisone-based antibiotic is directed at the *Pseudomonas.* A number of commercial preparations are available, and most of these have antibiotics that are ototoxic. They should be used with caution and only when a nonototoxic agent is not available.

Key Treatment

- Burow solution with a cotton wick

Bibliography

Coser PL, Stamm AEC, Pinto JA: Malignant external otitis in infants. Laryngoscope 1980;90:312–316.
Hirsch BE: Diseases of the external ear. *In* Bluestone CD, Stool SE, Kenna MA (eds): Pediatric Otolaryngology, 3rd ed, vol I. Philadelphia, WB Saunders, 1996, pp 378–387.

336 Hearing Tests

Robert J. Ruben

Procedure

A hearing test is indicated for every child in whom there is the suggestion of a hearing loss and/or any difficulty with voice, speech, or language.

Preparation

1. Children who are tested with auditory evoked potentials when younger than 6 months of age usually need sedation, or this may be done during natural sleep.
2. Most children older than 6 months of age are able to be tested behaviorally with a visual auditory reinforcement technique.
3. All tests of hearing, whether physiologic or behavioral, must be carried out in a sound-controlled environment with calibrated equipment and by a trained, certified audiologist.

Anesthesia

Chloral hydrate has been found to be a safe and effective anesthetic agent when obtaining auditory evoked potentials in younger or uncooperative children.

Techniques

Techniques vary according to the age of the child. Most important is an accurate assessment of the child's hearing acuity to all tones with air and bone conduction.

Follow-up

Children who have a hearing loss need to have follow-up examination to ensure whether the hearing has returned to normal or if there has been no further progression of the hearing loss.

The proper and adequate treatment of every child with a possible communication disorder requires an accurate assessment of hearing with an appropriate hearing test.

Bibliography

Davis H, Hirsh SK, Turpin LL, Peacock ME: Threshold sensitivity and frequency specificity in auditory brainstem response audiometry. Audiology 1985;24:54–70.
Gravel JS (ed): Accessing auditory system integrity in high-risk infants and young children. *In* Seminars in Hearing, vol 10. New York, Thieme Medical Publishers, 1989, pp 213–292.
Gravel JS, Traquina DN: Experience with the audiologic assessment of infants and toddlers. Int J Pediatr Otorhinolaryngol 1992;23:59–71.

337 Tympanocentesis

Robert J. Ruben

Procedure

Indications

Tympanocentesis may be indicated in children when an accurate culture is needed or when severe pain and/or facial nerve paralysis has occurred in conjunction with acute otitis media.

Contraindications

Tympanocentesis should not be attempted in a child who is not still and whose eardrum is not anesthetized because it is possible to destroy the ossicles and/or enter the inner ear through the oval window, which may result in sensorineural deafness.

Preparation

1. General anesthesia with a mask is preferred.
2. Tympanocentesis can be done with phenol as a local anesthetic, but this should only be offered to older children.
3. An infant may be restrained and the procedure done without anesthesia. This should be performed by a physician or surgeon who has obtained experience in performing the procedure on anesthetized children.

Equipment

1. Tympanocentesis should be done with an operating microscope or with an operating otoscope in a sterile field with the use of the appropriate myringotomy knife.
2. Cultures need to be taken.
3. The middle ear fluid needs to be collected with suction.

Technique

A wide ventral, cephalad incision is made just ventral to the long process of the malleus, and the fluid is suctioned and removed for culture. The incision is wide to allow for removal of the fluid and aeration of the middle ear cleft.

Precautions

Tympanocentesis should not be done in an ear in which there is the suggestion of vascular anomalies such as a jugular bulb that is filling the caudal portion of the middle ear cleft.

Follow-up

Children with tympanocentesis should be observed in 1 to 2 weeks to ensure that the incision has healed and there are no sequelae.

Tympanocentesis is rarely indicated in children. It may be necessary when there is a need for an accurate culture of the contents of the middle ear, when pain is present, or when a child has a facial paralysis as a result of acute otitis media.

Bibliography

Edmond CV Jr, Antoine G, Yim D, et al: A case of facial diplegia associated with acute otitis media. Int J Pediatr Otolaryngol 1990;18:257–262.

338 Removing Cerumen

Robert J. Ruben

Removal of cerumen to diagnose acute otitis media is questionable because the acute otitis media causes drainage and seldom does cerumen completely block the ear. The removal of cerumen in a child with acute otitis media may often cause the child to become very uncooperative; and once this happens, especially if the child is crying, the tympanic membrane will become erythematous and the physician will not know whether the erythema was from the acute infection or the child crying during the removal of the cerumen.

Contraindications

Cerumen should not be removed from a child who is struggling. Injury to the external auditory canal may result and/or rupture of the tympanic membrane with destruction of ossicles may occur while the child is moving.

Preparation

The child should be cooperative. If the child is not willing to be cooperative, then mechanical means for removing the cerumen should be discontinued.

Technique

1. Cerumen can be removed gently with a curette.
2. If there is any chance of abrasion to the canal while the child is moving, then the cerumen can be washed out with water at body temperature (so as not to calorically stimulate the vestibular apparatus) or with 5 per cent hydrogen peroxide solution. Both should be delivered under modest pressure.

3. If there is no immediate reason for removing the cerumen, then the child can be placed on medication that contains glycerin hydrogen peroxide or carbamide peroxide. Several drops of the preparation can be used twice a day for a week. After that, the cerumen should be easily wiped out of the external auditory canal or removed gently with irrigation.

Follow-up

If there has been any trauma to the ear canal, the child should be seen to ensure there is no infection and no permanent hearing loss.

> Removal of cerumen may result in lacerations of the external auditory canal and perforations of the tympanic membrane with ossicular destruction. It should not be removed while the child is uncooperative.
>
> Removal of cerumen is rarely necessary to diagnose acute otitis media.

REMOVAL OF A CERUMEN IMPACTION

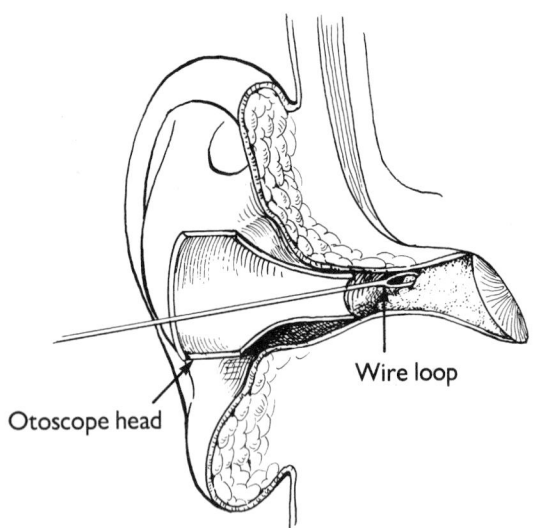

Wire loop

Otoscope head

(From Dunmire SM, Paris PM: Atlas of Emergency Procedures. Philadelphia, WB Saunders, 1994.)

339 Symptoms of Orthopedic Disorders

Symptom **Limp**   *Jack T. Andrish*

Definition

Not all limps are the same. Observation of the child's gait often provides the first clue for the underlying diagnosis.

1. A limp that is the result of *pain* with weight bearing is called an *antalgic gait.* It is characterized by a shortened stance phase of the affected extremity during walking compared with the normal leg. The child attempts to minimize the time spent bearing weight on the painful leg.

2. Some may limp because of *deformity.*

   a. *A leg-length discrepancy* gives a *short leg gait* and is characterized by a pelvic tilt to the side of the affected extremity. There may also be increased knee flexion of the normal extremity. Both of these maneuvers attempt to compensate for the short leg and minimize the vertical translations of the body's center of gravity.

   b. *Bowing* of the tibia or the femur may produce *genu varum* and may be severe enough to cause excessive lateral sway and/or a broad-based gait.

   c. *Genu valgum,* if severe, can result in a stiff gait created by adduction and abrasion of the thighs.

   d. *Coxa vara* is a deformity of the proximal femur that may be congenital or acquired and can produce a *waddling gait.*

   e. *Rotational malalignment,* which includes medial femoral and/or external tibial torsion, may produce a valgus thrust to the knee with the early stance phase portion of gait.

   f. *Rigid foot deformity,* such as that seen with clubfoot (talipes equinovarus) or with a rocker-bottom foot (congenital vertical talus), may alter gait and produce a limp by altering the normal transfer of forces during foot progression.

3. A limp may also be the result of a *joint contracture.*

   a. *Adduction of the hip* produces a short leg gait with the affected leg appearing short (but usually measuring equal to the contralateral extremity).

   b. *Flexion of the hip* produces a shortened stride length.

   c. *Flexion of the knee* produces a short leg gait.

   d. *Equinus* of the foot, if mild, may produce a "back knee" or recurvatum (of the knee) gait but, if severe, may require excessive stance-phase knee flexion of the ipsilateral extremity to compensate for unilateral toe walking.

4. *Weakness* of muscle groups, whether due to myopathic or neurogenic cause, leads to *characteristic* gait patterns and "limp."

   a. Weakness of the *gluteus medius* allows the contralateral ilium to drop during single-leg stance phase of the affected extremity. The body attempts to compensate by leaning over the affected leg. This type of limp is referred to as a *Trendelenburg gait.* The abnormal drooping of the contralateral ilium during single-leg stance on the affected extremity is called the *Trendelenburg sign.*

   b. The *gluteus maximus* affects the strength of the hip extensors. Weakness is compensated for by having the body lean backward over the affected extremity during stance phase. The resulting limp is referred to as a *gluteus maximus lurch.*

   c. The *quadriceps* generate extension of the knee. Significant weakness makes it difficult to walk up, and especially down, hills or stairs. The body compensates by "setting" the knee in full extension during heel strike and maintaining the progression of the center of gravity of the body forward to the center of rotation of the knee. This mechanism works best on level ground. With severe weakness, over time, *genu recurvatum* or *back-knee* can result.

   d. The *hamstring muscles* provide active knee flexion as well as assist with hip extension. Mild weakness can be well compensated, but severe or total loss of function can result in unopposed quadriceps muscle activity and a severe *genu recurvatum gait.*

   e. The *gastrocnemius/soleus muscles* of the calf provide the power of plantarflexion of the ankle. Loss of this power results in a *lack of push off* during walking and a loss of smoothness of gait.

   f. The *muscles of the anterior compartment* provide active dorsiflexion of the foot and ankle. Loss of this power results in a *dropfoot gait.* Excessive hip and knee flexion during the swing-through phase of gait is required to allow clearance of the foot.

Etiology

1. *Trauma* is the most common cause. If severe, it is usually obvious; if the trauma is not severe and the duration of symptoms is short, the condition is usually self-limiting. Examples include

   a. The common *bruise,* which can be obvious or, especially in the very young child or infant, may not be so obvious. Further investigations may be required to rule out associated injury such as fracture.

   b. *A foreign body,* especially the commonly encountered splinter/needle/thorn in the foot, will produce a limp while often remaining surprisingly occult.

   c. *A fracture* that produces a limp is almost invariably a stable fracture or a stress fracture because unstable

983

or displaced fractures are not compatible with weight bearing.

 d. *Internal derangement of the knee,* such as a torn meniscus or loose body, can often lead to an antalgic gait or a stiff-legged gait.

 e. The *slipped capital femoral epiphysis* can present purely as a limp with minimal or no pain and therein lies the treachery of this condition. Fortunately, pain is usually present, although it may be perceived to be knee pain and not hip pain.

2. Although the incidence is low, the presence of *tumor* should always be considered.

 a. *Benign* tumors may be isolated, or they may be multicentric. Examples of the more common childhood benign musculoskeletal tumors include the osteochondroma, the osteoid osteoma, and the neurofibroma. Bone cysts may also be considered and may be lined with a thin fibrous layer and filled with serous fluid or nothing at all; or they may be filled with blood (aneurysmal bone cyst), fibrous tissue (fibrous cortical defect, nonossifying fibroma, fibrous dysplasia), or cartilage (enchondroma).

 b. *Malignant* tumors may be primary or secondary.

 (1) Primary tumors of the lower extremity can include those of hematogenous origin (leukemia), bone (osteosarcoma, Ewing sarcoma), cartilage (chondrosarcoma), or muscle (rhabdomyosarcoma).

 (2) Secondary tumors in children typically include Wilms tumor, neuroblastoma, and melanoma.

3. *Infections* are not uncommon in children and may be superficial or deep, localized or diffuse, and acute or chronic. They may involve the skin and subdermal tissues (cellulitis, lymphangitis) or the deeper soft tissues (myositis, abscess) or the skeletal system (osteomyelitis, septic arthritis). Musculoskeletal infections often include some *combination* of the above description and may frequently be *multicentric.*

 a. The pathogens may be common, such as *Streptococcus, Staphylococcus pneumoniae, Escherichia coli,* and *Salmonella.*

 b. Or, the pathogens may be less commonly encountered, such as from Lyme disease.

 c. Or, the organisms may be fastidious to culture, such as with fungi and *Mycobacterium.*

4. *Inflammatory disease* is most often manifested in children as a synovitis. It may be monarticular, pauciarticular, or polyarticular, and it may be associated with the following:

 a. A systemic disease such as juvenile rheumatoid arthritis or colitis

 b. A nonsystemic disease such as pigmented villonodular synovitis

5. *Metabolic disease* may produce a limp by pain and/or deformity.

 a. Disorders of lipid storage (e.g., Gaucher disease) may affect the hip and lead to avascular necrosis and bony collapse. Disorders of lysosomal storage

(the mucopolysaccharidoses) may lead to deformities such as coxa vara.

 b. Disorders of calcium and phosphorus metabolism can lead to osteomalacia and bone deformity. Often a primary or secondary hyperparathyroidism may coexist. In addition to coxa vara and tibia vara, chronic slipped capital femoral epiphysis may present in children and adolescents with chronic disease of calcium and phosphorus management.

 (1) These disorders may be primary, as in nutritional rickets, and often inheritable, as in hypophosphatemic vitamin D refractory rickets and hypophosphatasia.

 (2) Or, they may be secondary to renal or gastrointestinal disease.

 c. Disorders of blood coagulation (the hemophilias) give pain and limp due to acute bleeding in (the knee) joints and over time can lead to degenerative joint disease with pain and stiffness. Bone infarct from a sickle cell crisis also produces severe bone and/or joint pain.

6. *Neuromuscular diseases* may create a limp by the weakness they produce. They may be congenital or acquired, and they may be neuropathic or myopathic, or they may be mixed. Examples include

 a. Cerebral palsy

 b. Hereditary motor and sensory neuropathies

 c. Trauma

 d. Spinal and intraspinal abnormalities

 e. Muscular dystrophies and the myopathies.

7. The *bone dysplasias* may produce a limp by the deformity of bone and joints they create. They may be classified as being epiphyseal dysplasias, metaphyseal dysplasias, or spondyloepiphyseal dysplasias. Most often associated with short stature, these disorders are frequently characterized by disorganization of the growth plate (physis) and/or inadequate bone remodeling.

8. There may be *congenital deformities* of limbs that result from failures of formation or differentiation. Total or partial absence of parts (absent tibia, absent fibula, proximal femoral focal deficiency) give limb-length discrepancies. Congenital coxa vara, with or without short femur, can produce a "hip limp."

9. Some children are normal at birth and encounter a *developmental dysplasia.*

 a. Legg-Calvé-Perthes disease is a disorder of the proximal femoral epiphysis that can lead to collapse and deformity. Typically first detected in children between the ages of 4 and 8 years, it may occur earlier or later. Intermittent pain usually brought on by weight-bearing activity attracts the attention of the parents, although limp alone may exist.

 b. Tibia vara, or Blount disease, is a disorder of the proximal tibial growth plate that can lead to severe bowing. Indistinguishable below the age of 2 from "physiologic" bowing, the infantile form is usually detectable between the ages of 2 and 4. The adolescent form develops during the adolescent growth spurt and is not associated with the severe epiphyseal destruction and collapse that can occur with the infantile form.

Evaluation

1. Record the history of the limp and include
   a. The time of onset
   b. The presence or absence of pain and the character of the pain
   c. The presence or absence of trauma
   d. Family history of similar problem
   e. Associated systemic disease
   f. Associated systemic symptoms such as fever and malaise
   g. Treatment to date
2. Perform and record a careful physical examination.
   a. Observe and characterize the gait.
   b. Observe the stature of the child.
   c. Observe the limb for gross deformity.
   d. Observe for puncture wounds, scars, bruises, and swelling.
   e. Locate tenderness.
   f. Execute a gentle determination of the range of motion of all joints and assess in relation to the contralateral limb *and* to anticipated normal values.
   g. Record the child's temperature.
3. Order appropriate plain radiographs. This is still probably the most generic and useful test to obtain after the history and physical examination because all entities listed as potential causes may appear as abnormalities seen on plain radiographs. However, the presence or absence of radiographic findings is often determined by the time in the course of the disease that the film is taken. False-negative results are not uncommon.
4. If infection, metabolic disease, or inflammatory disease is suspected, obtain appropriate laboratory studies.
   a. CBC with differential
   b. C-reactive protein (CRP) and/or a sedimentation rate (the CRP will elevate first in the presence of infection)
   c. Cultures of blood and, if possible, aspirations of joint effusions or fluid collections
   d. Immunologic titers (rheumatoid factor, Lyme titer, antinuclear antibody)
   e. Metabolic work-up as appropriate (calcium/phosphorus, kidney panel, lipids, carbohydrates).
5. *Imaging studies* are frequently used to localize and define the lesion.
   a. The bone scan is sensitive but usually nonspecific. It is best used to locate the site of bone or joint infection or the location of an occult fracture.
   b. Computed tomography is best for defining the bone detail of a fracture or a tumor.
   c. Magnetic resonance imaging has become the most powerful tool available for diagnosing and defining the extent of musculoskeletal pathology, such as tumor, occult fracture or stress fracture, avascular necrosis, infection, and internal derangement of the knee.

Bibliography

Dabney K, Lipton G: Evaluation of limp in children. Curr Opin Pediatr 1995;7:88–94.

 Symptom | **Painful Knee**

Jack T. Andrish

Basic to the evaluation of the child with knee pain is the determination as to whether the perception of pain is due to a *primary* condition of the knee or *secondary* to a condition away from the knee.

Secondary Conditions

Knee pain in the child may be a reflection of a problem more proximal in the body. Most commonly, hip pathology may present as knee pain. Usually the pain is medial or anteromedial and is a result of "referred pain" in the distribution of the obturator nerve. Some conditions to be considered include

1. Slipped capital femoral epiphysis
   a. This is probably the most commonly missed diagnosis in the adolescent or preadolescent with hip pathology masquerading as knee pain.
   b. The diagnosis should be suspected if the child prefers to hold the affected leg in external rotation and/or on physical examination attempted hip flexion only occurs if the leg is allowed to fall into progressive external rotation as well.
   c. A plain radiograph will reveal the problem, but a true lateral view of the proximal femur is necessary as well as an anteroposterior view of the hip.
2. Lesions of the femur
   a. Occult fracture or stress fracture can give pain referred away from the site of involvement.
   b. Tumors of the thigh or femur can be deceptive as well. This can include malignant lesions such as osteogenic sarcoma as well as benign lesions such as osteoid osteoma. Plain radiographs will often be diagnostic, but the bone scan helps to localize the problem if the plain films are unremarkable.
3. Lesions of the spine
   a. The herniated lumbar disk in the adolescent can be very deceptive. It may present as lateral or posterolateral knee pain. This can give one the impression of dealing with a torn lateral meniscus, when in reality the problem is radicular.
   b. A high "index of suspicion" is required for this diagnosis, and magnetic resonance imaging will confirm the cause.

Primary Conditions

The classification of primary disorders of the knee may be further labeled as *acute* versus *chronic* and as *traumatic* versus *nontraumatic*.

1. Acute-onset knee pain: traumatic

   a. Contusions are the most common injury to the knee, but not necessarily the most common reason to bring the child to the attention of the doctor. Although simple measures of supportive care suffice for most contusions, the force producing the contusion may have also created a more serious underlying injury, such as a fracture or sprain.

   b. *A sprain* is an injury to a ligament and may be classified as being of first, second, or third degree. The distinction is made by the physical examination.

      (1) With a first-degree sprain, the injury is microscopic and the integrity of the ligament is grossly intact. There is no increased joint laxity.

      (2) With a second-degree sprain, a partial tear is implied, and thus there is some perceptible loss of strength and stability.

      (3) A third-degree sprain is a complete tear of the ligament and thus detectable abnormal laxity will result from this injury.

   c. *Fractures* may be obvious, or they may be not so obvious. Fractures about the knee tend to involve the growth plates in children and even adolescents. In fact, they may be more susceptible to injury than the ligaments.

      (1) Typical fractures to the distal femur and proximal tibia may involve the main growth plate that contributes to longitudinal growth. The distal femur is more commonly involved.

      (2) Avulsion fractures also occur and typically either involve the tibial tubercle or the tibial spine. The former is a traction injury of the insertion of the patellar tendon and the latter involves the anterior cruciate ligament.

   d. *Dislocations* and *subluxations* of the knee may involve the patella (common) or may involve the main knee joint (uncommon). Either case may look dramatic, but the dislocated patella is easily reduced by passive extension of the knee; the true knee dislocation is a medical emergency requiring reduction, observation, and documentation of neurovascular function.

2. Acute-onset knee pain: nontraumatic

   a. High on the list of potential causes for this scenario is *infection*. This may be due to acute osteomyelitis of the distal femur, or it may be a primary septic arthritis. The work-up proceeds as described in the section on the child with a limp and includes aspiration of joint fluid or subperiosteal abscess for Gram stain and culture.

   b. *Synovitis* associated with a systemic inflammatory disease (e.g., juvenile rheumatoid arthritis)

   c. Congenital abnormalities of the meniscus (*discoid meniscus*) may be silent for years and yet eventual degeneration and tearing, even in the absence of recognized trauma, can produce acute-onset knee pain.

   d. *Osteochondritis dissecans* of the knee typically involves the lateral aspect of the medial femoral condyle but may indeed be found on any surface of the knee. Dislodgement of the dissecans lesion may become a *loose body* and can give acute-onset pain.

3. Chronic knee pain: traumatic

   a. Probably the most frequently encountered assorted conditions producing anterior knee pain are those related to the patella. Formerly described as "chondromalacia of the patella," a more appropriate term for the pediatric age group is *patellofemoral stress syndrome.*

      (1) The symptom complex includes anterior knee pain aggravated by activity and relieved by rest. Pain on kneeling, squatting, running, stair climbing, and walking or running hills—especially going down long inclines—characterizes this condition. Even sitting a long time with the knee bent can produce the "aching" pain of this condition.

      (2) *Patellar malalignment*, with or without instability of the patella, is a common feature. Torsional malalignment of the entire lower extremity (medial femoral torsion and/or external tibial torsion) can be the cause of the patellar malalignment, but more often the problem is intrinsic to the patellofemoral articulation itself such as a tight lateral retinaculum.

      (3) *Chondromalacia of the patella* is a pathologic degenerative process of articular cartilage (of the patella). It is characterized by softening, fibrillation, and even at times fragmentation and erosion. Although common in the adult, it is an uncommon cause of anterior knee pain in the child and adolescent. When present, it is usually the result of specific trauma such as a hard fall on the flexed knee or as the result of a patellar dislocation.

   b. Anterior knee pain can also be secondary to a chronic *tendinitis,* and nowhere is this more common than in the active adolescent and preadolescent. The presence of unfused apophyses about the knee serving as attachment sites for tendons also accounts for injury patterns unique to the growing individual. Tight muscle-tendon units, along with tenderness and swelling about the bony insertion sites, are the predominant findings.

      (1) The most commonly recognized apophysitis/tendinitis is Osgood-Schlatter disease. This presents as pain, swelling, and tenderness about the tibial tubercle.

      (2) At the inferior pole of the patella the lesion (tendinitis) of Sinding-Larsen is found. In the young child this may accompany a small fleck of bone from the patella. In the adolescent and adult, this tendinitis is referred to as "jumper's knee."

      (3) The iliotibial band friction syndrome gives pain

with running and is located over the lateral femoral epicondyle.

c. *Osteochondritis dissecans* is a chronic disorder of articular cartilage and subchondral bone with histologic features of avascular necrosis. Although trauma is believed to be the cause, other anatomic and constitutional factors may contribute as well. Pain occurs when there is instability of the "lesion" (subchondral fracture) and mechanical symptoms of catching and even locking occur when the lesion detaches (partial or complete). Loose bodies within the knee can originate from an unstable osteochondritis dissecans lesion.

4. Chronic knee pain: nontraumatic
   a. Here the list of possible etiologies may be extremely obvious or frustratingly obscure.
   b. Especially if there is joint effusion, *synovitis* should be high on the list of possibilities. The general work-up should consider
      (1) Juvenile rheumatoid arthritis
      (2) Infection: mycobacterial, fungal
      (3) Pigmented villonodular synovitis
   c. The "snapping knee syndrome" due to a *congenital discoid meniscus*
   d. *Arthrosis* may be secondary to congenital joint deformity, or it may be due to the ravages of a remote inflammatory or infectious arthritis (synovitis).

Evaluation

1. History
   a. *When* did the pain begin? Is it recent or remote?
   b. *How* did the pain develop? Was it insidious or was it the result of a specific injury or illness? If it was the result of trauma, what was the specific mechanism of injury?
   c. *What is the character* of the pain?
      (1) Constant or intermittent?
      (2) Activity related? Night or rest pain?
      (3) Dull, aching, sharp, well-localized, or diffuse?
   d. *Where* is the pain located?

   e. Do *mechanical symptoms* accompany the pain? Locking, popping, giving way?
   f. Is there *swelling?* A lot? A little? Localized or diffuse?
   g. Is there associated *systemic disease?* Juvenile rheumatoid arthritis, renal disease, gastrointestinal disease?
   h. Is *a recognized knee condition already established*? Discoid meniscus, osteochondritis dissecans?
   i. Are systemic symptoms present? Fever, malaise?
2. Physical findings
   a. The examination of the child's knee should always include an examination of the hip!
   b. Observe for deformity, swelling, bruising, lower-extremity alignment, and, if possible, the gait.
   c. Palpate for tenderness, local swelling, joint swelling (effusion), synovial thickening, cysts, and crepitation (patellofemoral).
   d. Document the range of motion: active versus passive.
   e. Complete with testing of ligamentous stability and provocative testing for meniscus derangement (McMurray test).
3. Plain radiographs are almost always necessary and include
   a. Anteroposterior and lateral views
   b. A tunnel view
   c. A "sunrise view" of the patella (Merchant view).
4. Laboratory findings (see Symptom: Limp).
5. Imaging (see Symptom: Limp).

Bibliography

Englaro E, Gelfand M: Bone scintigraphy in preschool children with lower extremity pain of unknown origin. J Nucl Med 1992;33:351–354.

Ruffin M, Kiningham R: Anterior knee pain: The challenge of patellofemoral syndrome. Am Fam Phys 1993;47:185–194.

Stanitski C, Harvell J: Observations on acute knee hemarthrosis in children and adolescents. J Pediatr Orthop 1993;13:506–510.

Sutherland D, Davids J: Common gait abnormalities of the knee in cerebral palsy. Clin Orthop Rel Res 1993;288:139–147.

340 Flatfeet and Tibial Torsion

Theresa L. Dise

Flatfeet (Flexible Pes Planovalgus)

Definition
The longitudinal arch of the weight-bearing foot fails to develop.

Etiology
Flatfeet is most commonly congenital and familial, although it can be acquired, secondary to muscle imbalance or weakness, accompanied by a shortened heel cord, or caused by bony abnormalities such as tarsal coalition.

Associations
Flatfeet may occur in patients with Ehlers-Danlos, Marfan, and trisomy 21 syndromes, cerebral palsy, osteogenesis imperfecta, muscular dystrophy, myelodysplasia, and obesity.

Pathophysiology
There is an abnormal relationship of the talar, navicular, and the medial cuneiform bones of the foot in the weight-bearing position. Flexible flatfoot has three categories:

1. Mild—on weight bearing the arch is lower than usual but still seen.
2. Moderate—on weight bearing the arch is no longer seen.
3. Severe—on weight bearing the talar head comes out below and anterior to the medial malleolus, making the medial edge of the foot appear convex.

Clinical Findings
1. The flexible flatfoot is painless and asymptomatic. It is brought to the clinician's attention by concerned parents who notice the abnormal position of the bare foot against the floor. The parents may be more aware of this issue if there is a positive family history of flatfeet.
2. Up to the age of 3 years, it is normal for the child's foot to have the appearance of being "flat." Parents may bring the child in because of concerns of in-toeing as well. In-toeing is a posture that the child assumes to counteract the imbalance that flatfeet causes. This should be explained to the parents so that they may be reassured.
3. Shoe examination is very important. Normally, shoe soles are worn slightly to the outer side of the midline of the shoe. If a sole is worn down medially or on the inner side, this is abnormal.
4. Pathologic flatfoot with the following characteristics should be considered for referral if the patient is older than 3 years of age:
   a. Pain is present
   b. "Severe" category
   c. Abnormal shoe wear
   d. The arch of the foot is not restored when the patient stands on tiptoe
   e. The foot is not supple
   f. The longitudinal arch is not present when the foot is dangling (non–weight-bearing).

Key Clinical Findings

- Pain
- Abnormal shoe wear
- Rigidity
- Arch not restored on tiptoe

Radiographic Changes
Lateral views of the weight-bearing foot are obtained. These demonstrate the loss of the typical straight-line relationship seen with the talus, navicular, and medial cuneiform bones. Instead, the talus is flexed. Because mild and moderate categories of flatfeet do not require treatment, routine radiographic studies are not indicated.

Treatment and Referral
1. For the painless, flexible flatfoot of the mild and moderate categories, no treatment is required. Various exercises, pads, supports, and arches have not been shown to change the natural history of this entity.
2. For the painful, flexible flatfoot, a removable, longitudinal arch support may be recommended, after orthopedic evaluation has excluded underlying pathologic causes.
3. Rigid flatfoot should be referred for orthopedic evaluation.

Key Treatment

- Painless variety—no treatment
- Painless flatfoot
- Longitudinal arch support

Tibial Torsion

Definition
Torsion is the twisting of a long bone about its long axis. Medial tibial torsion is an abnormal exaggeration of medial twisting that results in in-toeing of the feet, and lateral tibial torsion is a twisting in the lateral direction that results in out-toeing of the feet.

Epidemiology
Tibial torsion may be congenital, developmental, or acquired.

Associations

1. Medial tibial torsion may be associated with congenital metatarsus varus, developmental genu varum (bowleg), tibia vara (Blount disease), and congenital or acquired bony abnormalities of many causes.
2. Lateral tibial torsion is usually an acquired deformity because of contracture of the iliotibial band; it may be associated with femoral antetorsion, triceps surae muscle contracture, foot deformities such as calcaneovalgus or flexible pes planovalgus, or congenital disorders.

Pathophysiology

1. The amount of tibial torsion varies among individuals and changes with age. At birth, most newborns have a mean lateral torsion of 2.2 degrees. The normal adult has a mean lateral tibial torsion of 23.7 degrees. Therefore, with time, most persons gradually attain about 20 degrees of lateral torsion; and the medial malleolus lies anterior to the lateral malleolus.
2. Abnormal lateral torsion has as its predominant finding patellae that point forward and feet that point outward. It is usually bilateral.

Clinical Findings

1. Medial tibial torsion
   a. The parents are concerned that in-toeing is present or that the child is bowlegged. This is noticed at 6 to 12 months of age. Most commonly there is no varus deformity of the metatarsals. The medial malleolus is posterior instead of anterior to the lateral malleolus.
   b. Gait is first assessed to determine the amount of in-toeing present during ambulation. Then, in the prone position, the relationship of the foot to the thigh is examined. The knee and ankle are flexed to 90 degrees. The examiner stands over the lifted foot and looks down on it. This relationship of the thigh to the foot is called the thigh-foot axis, and the normal range at about 13 years old is -5 to $+30$ degrees. Tibial torsion is present if the foot is medially rotated more than -10 to -20 degrees, keeping in mind the patient's age. It is important to note the absence of metatarsus varus and talipes equinovarus.
   c. It is also important to note the presence of medial tibial torsion in the parents or in siblings. If there is no family history of persistent torsion, then spontaneous correction by age 7 years will most likely occur.
2. Lateral tibial torsion
   a. The parental concern is that out-toeing is present. The child may also exhibit knock-knees.
   b. Gait is assessed to determine the amount of out-

toeing that is occurring. The thigh-foot angle is measured, and measurements greater than $+30$ degrees indicate that abnormal lateral tibial torsion is present.

Radiographic Changes

In general, radiographs are not helpful. The orthopedist may use computed tomography or ultrasonography to determine the degree of torsion.

Treatment and Referral

In general, most medial torsional deformities correct on their own; therefore, observation and reassurance is the best approach.

1. Medial tibial torsion
   a. May be exacerbated by certain postures, but this is controversial. The physician may counsel the family to prevent prone sleeping in the knee-chest position with the feet internally rotated and sitting in the reverse tailor position with the feet tucked underneath the buttocks.
   b. If medial tibial torsion is greater than -20 degrees at age 3 years, referral to an orthopedist is suggested.
   c. The orthopedist may suggest passive stretching exercises, or the use of external rotation splints. Severe cases that persist into late childhood and early adolescence may require surgery.
2. Lateral tibial torsion
   a. There are no postures associated with lateral tibial torsion.
   b. This usually does not spontaneously correct, and if the foot-thigh angle is greater than 30 degrees, early referral to an orthopedist is warranted.

Bibliography

FLATFEET

Craig CL, Goldberg MJ: Foot and leg problems. Pediatr Rev 1993;14:395–400.
Sharrard WJW: Paediatric Orthopaedics and Fractures, 3rd ed. London, Blackwell Scientific Publications, 1993.
Tachdjian M: Pediatric Orthopedics, 2nd ed. Philadelphia, WB Saunders, 1990.

TIBIAL TORSION

Sharrard WJW: Paediatric Orthopaedics and Fractures, 3rd edition. London, Blackwell Scientific Publications, 1993.
Staheli LT: Torsional deformity. Pediatr Clin North Am 1986; 33:1371–1383.
Tachdjian M: Pediatric Orthopedics, 2nd ed. Philadelphia, WB Saunders, 1990.

341 Dysplasia of the Hip

James T. Bennett

Definition

Developmental dysplasia of the hip, previously called congenital hip dislocation, represents a spectrum of disorders characterized by abnormal development of the hip joint. This spectrum includes frank dislocation (Ortolani positive), subluxation (Barlow positive), and simple failure of the hip to develop normally (dysplasia).

1. Dislocation—the hip is frankly dislocated
2. Subluxation—the hip is partially reduced but not necessarily concentrically
3. Dysplasia—the hip/acetabulum is immature, failure for the socket to deepen.

Etiology

Genetic, hormonal, mechanical, and environmental influences predispose the hip joint to dislocation

1. Incidence: 10 per 1000 live births
2. Associated mechanical factors
   a. Breech
   b. Congenital genu recurvation or knee dislocation
   c. Torticollis
   d. Metatarsus adductus
3. Physiologic factors
   a. Sex, girls to boys 6:1
   b. Maternal estrogens

Pathophysiology

In all newborns there is normal laxity of all joints. Later in the older child with persistent dislocation of a hip both soft tissues and bony parts are distorted. Anatomic abnormalities that have been demonstrated include

1. Acetabular labrum—may be infolded
2. Pulvinar—fat and fibrous tissue within the acetabulum
3. Capsule—construction forms an "hourglass" deformity
4. Iliopsoas tendon—indents inferior capsule
5. Transverse acetabular ligament
6. Femoral head deformity—head becomes flattened

If left untreated, developmental dysplasia of the hip may be the cause of 20 to 50 per cent of hip arthritis, although early disability is quite minor.

Clinical Findings

A hip examination should be performed *and recorded* in every newborn and at every subsequent physician office visit to detect development dysplasia of the hip until age 2. The clinical examination is thought to vary with the age at which the patient is examined and the severity of the disorder.

1. Early ("loose phase" or first 6 months)
   a. Ortolani positive: with hip in flexion, abduction reduces the hip with a clunk
   b. Barlow positive: with the hip in flexion and adduction, a posteriorly directed force on the knees causes the hip to dislocate
2. Later ("hip stuck out," irreducible, generally after age 6 months)
   a. Limited abduction—if dislocation is unilateral the dislocated hip will abduct less than the normal side. In bilateral dislocation this may not be apparent
   b. Galeazzi—dislocated side appears shorter: asymmetry of thigh ceases
   c. Trendelenburg limp—painless limp in which the femoral head has migrated proximally, the abductors are redundant and therefore weakened, and the patient leans to the dislocated side (waddles) during stance phase of gait

Key Clinical Findings

- Ortolani sign—positive
- Barlow sign—positive

Radiographic Changes

The choice of imaging is a function of the patient's age. If younger than 6 months the ossification center may not be present, making conventional radiographs unreliable.

1. Ultrasonography
   a. Dynamic—a multipositional evaluation that mirrors the physical examination: normal → dysplastic → subluxated → dislocated
   b. Morphologic—classifies the hip morphology
2. Plain radiography—a "normal" study at birth does not exclude the possibility of dysplasia or even frank dislocation. *Acetabular dysplasia* refers to the immaturity or failure of the acetabulum to thoroughly develop.
   a. Hilgenreiner line—femoral metaphysis should be distal to the line drawn through the triradiate cartilage (central growth plate of the acetabulum)
   b. Perkin line—femoral metaphysis should be medial to the line perpendicular to Hilgenreiner line, drawn from the edge of the acetabulum
   c. Shenton line—an imaginary line drawn along the femoral neck that should be continuous with the obturator foramen
3. Computed tomography—used to confirm reduction after an open reduction
4. Arthrography—used dynamically to assess the cartilaginous components of the hip joint
5. Magnetic resonance imaging—may be used in lieu of computed tomography and may have a role in detection

of avascular necrosis and defining the cartilaginous components

Treatment

Treatment varies according to age at diagnosis and severity of the disorder.

1. Early (before walking age)
   a. Subluxation → Pavlik harness
   b. Dislocation
      (1) Reducible → Pavlik harness
      (2) Irreducible → Pavlik harness trial and if unsuccessful a closed reduction followed by Pavlik or spica cast. Rarely will open reduction be required in this age group
2. Late (after walking age)
   a. Subluxation → pelvic/femoral osteotomy
   b. Dislocation
      (1) Traction with closed reduction is first tried, with open reduction more common here—later open reduction with femoral shortening and or pelvic osteotomy may be required
      (2) Traction with open reduction, which is more common
      (3) Open reduction femoral shortening and/or pelvic osteotomy
3. Reconstructive procedure
   a. Salter—to address residual dysplasia
   b. Pemberton—when the triradiate cartilage is still open with a copious acetabulum

c. Steele ("triple")—when the dysplasia is more severe and the patient is older
d. Other: Sutherland/Tonnis/Chiari

Key Treatment

- Pavlik harness
- Closed surgical reduction

Prevention

There is no known means to prevent this disorder, and all efforts are directed at the earliest possible diagnosis.

Bibliography

Bennett JT, MacEwen GD: Congenital dislocation of the hip: Recent advances and current problems. Clin Orthop 1989; 247:15.

Graf R: Fundamental of sonographic diagnosis of infant hip dysplasia. J Pediatr Orthop 1984;4:735.

Lindstrom JR, Ponseti IV, Wenger DR: Acetabular development after reduction of congenital dislocation of the hip. J Bone Joint Surg Am 1979;61:112.

Ramsey PL, Lasser S, MacEwen GD: Congenital dislocation of the hip: Use of the Pavlik harness in the child during the first six months of life. J Bone Joint Surg Am 1976;58:1000.

Severin E: Contribution to the knowledge of congenital dislocation of the hip joint: Late results of closed reduction and arthrographic studies of recent cases. Acta Chir Scand 1988; 84(Suppl 63):1.

342 Slipped Capital Femoral Epiphysis

Fredric H. Warren

Etiology

The etiology of slipped capital femoral epiphysis (SCFE) is believed to be multifactorial. The following are possible factors in this disorder:

1. Mechanical: Because the growth plate widens with rapid growth and because the upper femoral plate slopes inferiorly it is mechanically susceptible to slipping.
2. Hormonal: Factors are especially common in the child younger than 9 years old. During phases of rapid growth, human growth causes the physis to widen, thus increasing the risk of slip. SCFE is also seen in endocrinopathies, such as
   a. Hypothyroidism
   b. Hypopituitary states
   c. Hypogonadism—decreased testosterone (estrogen strengthens the physis, which is perhaps why SCFE is decreased in females)

d. Chronic renal failure
   e. SCFE is also seen in patients receiving chemotherapy or radiation therapy.
3. Trauma may play a role in cases of repetitive shear stress, and indeed approximately 50 per cent have positive history of an injury.
4. Inflammatory changes in the form of synovitis are common. There are documented abnormalities in the immune complexes in children with SCFE with the presence of IgG and C3 in the synovial fluid.
5. There is a 5 per cent familial association, and it is thought that SCFE is an autosomal dominant condition but with variable penetrance.

Epidemiology

1. Incidence ranges from 0.71 per 100,000 in New Mexico to 3.41 per 100,000 in Connecticut and Sweden.
2. The average age of occurrence is 13 to 14 years (majority:

10–12 years) in boys and 11–12 years in girls, usually before menarche. These averages are chronological. Early slips are usually indicative of an underlying endocrinopathy. Most occur during the adolescent growth spurts.

3. Males are affected at a ratio of 2 to 3:1.
4. Blacks are affected more than whites. Black boys are affected at a rate of 7.8 per 100,000, whereas black girls are affected at a rate of 6.7 per 100,000. White boys are affected at a rate of 4.7 per 100,000, and white girls are affected at 1.6 per 100,000. Socioeconomic factors are noncontributory.
5. A seasonal distribution occurring more often in spring and summer than fall and winter is not related to the increase in trauma seen during these seasons.
6. A positive family history occurs approximately 5 per cent of the time.
7. Boys are affected on the left hip at a rate of 2:1, whereas girls are equally affected right to left. There is an incidence of bilaterality in 20 to 25 per cent of the cases.
8. The body habitus is a factor in that a majority of affected patients are more than the 90th percentile for weight. There is no statistically valid correlation with height.
9. Trauma is not a causative factor in the majority of slips.

Pathology

1. The articular cartilage of the femoral head is normal; however, the epiphysial plate is abnormal, consisting of disorganized intracellular structure (in the proliferative zone) with clustering of cartilage cells. There are septa and clefts in the physis with extension into the metaphysis. The actual slip occurs through the zone of hypertrophy as is seen in acute fractures; however, the organization of the cells is more atypical.
2. Mechanically, the slip occurs first posteriorly then inferiorly. As a result of the slip the periosteum is intact both posteriorly and inferiorly with disruption anteriorly/superiorly. Because the main blood supply to the capital femoral epiphysis is primarily posterior and medial, the intact periosteum of the slip tends to protect the fragile blood supply, thus preventing avascular necrosis as a result of the actual slip.

Clinical Findings

Affected children present with complaints of thigh or knee pain. The gait is antalgic and usually has a short leg component (50 per cent up to 1 inch shorter on the affected side). Most children have some thigh atrophy. Physical examination reveals decreased internal rotation, with most patients being unable to bring the leg to even neutral internal rotation. Abduction is also limited, as is extension. The presentation can be acute (within 3 weeks—14 per cent incidence) or chronic with symptoms longer than 3 weeks (86 per cent incidence), or an acute episode can follow the chronic. Patients in severe pain with markedly restricted motion are likely candidates for chondrolysis or infection.

Key Clinical Findings

- Pain in thigh or knee
- Thigh atrophy
- Decreased internal rotation

Radiography

1. The diagnosis of SCFE is made by conventional radiographs taken as anteroposterior pelvis, frog-leg lateral (best for minimal slips), and true lateral views. The earliest sign is widening of the physis. The anteroposterior view reveals a double-density effect of the femoral neck overlying the femoral head that has slipped posteriorly, thus giving an appearance of increased radiodensity that is referred to as the Blanche sign of Steele. Because of the slip the epiphysis will appear to be smaller owing to decreased height from the slippage posteriorly. Chronic slips, as one might surmise, will reveal new bone formation in the region of the intact periosteal sleeve. This is seen in combination with metaphyseal callus.
2. Absolute measurements of the slip are made by two methods:
   a. Maximal epiphysial displacement as measured on the anteroposterior and frog-leg views. This is a measurement of the distance from the superior margin of the femoral neck to the superior margin of the epiphysis.
   b. The distance from the axis of the center of the femoral neck to the center of the femoral head
3. Computed tomographic scanning is extremely useful for preoperative planning and is the most reproducible method of evaluation of the slip by allowing measurements of
   a. Head–shaft angle
   b. Percentage of epiphysial slip
   c. Head–neck angle

Classifications

There are two classifications in use:
1. One is by grade.
   a. Grade I: slip less than one-third width of the femoral neck.
   b. Grade II: slip between one-third and one-half width.
   c. Grade III: slip greater than one-half neck width.
2. Another is by severity.
   a. Mild: difference between head–shaft angles—normal to affected side—is less than 30 degrees.
   b. Moderate: difference between head–shaft angle is 30 to 50 degrees.
   c. Severe: Difference between head–shaft angle is more than 50 degrees.

Treatment

1. The goal of treatment is
   a. To prevent further slippage
   b. To stabilize until the physis closes
   c. To do no further harm by the treatment (i.e., avascular necrosis or chondrolysis)
2. Methods of treatment for acute slips
   a. Spica cast immobilization
      (1) Advantages
         (a) Low risk of avascular necrosis (AVN)
         (b) Low morbidity

(c) No surgery

(2) Disadvantages

(a) Excessive duration to allow closure of physis

(b) Chondrolysis can occur as a result of immobilization (theoretical).

(c) Does not necessarily prevent further progression of the slip

b. In-situ pin fixation—most accepted form of treatment

(1) Advantages

(a) Surgeon familiar with technique and instruments

(b) Stabilizes the slip

(2) Disadvantage: It is easy to penetrate the head of the femur with the fixation device.

c. Open epiphysiodesis. This technique was popular regionally but fell out of favor with the success of in-situ pinning. There is now some reinterest secondary to potential problems with in-situ pins and its risk of penetration and chondrolysis.

(1) Advantages

(a) Stops growth by bone grafting the physis

(b) Done under "direct" open vision

(2) Disadvantages

(a) Open arthrotomy, thus potential for stiffness

(b) Requires immobilization postoperatively

(c) Bone graft not as mechanically stable as screw

(d) Technically demanding for inexperienced surgeons

d. Manipulation—not advised because there is a higher risk of AVN that is believed to be iatrogenic. It has the theoretical advantage of restoration of the normal anatomy; however, the risk of AVN as well as the ability of the hips to remodel makes this form of treatment ill advised.

3. Secondary treatment is used as a method to improve the anatomy of the slip.

a. Manipulation can be used "gently" to reduce an acute on chronic slip. This can be done by

(1) Traction—skin traction with possible derotation strap is generally considered "safe."

(2) Manual reduction—hard to judge what is "gentle." Most of the time it will have a forceful component, and it carries the risk of AVN.

(3) Internal rotation maneuvers can affect the reduction.

b. Osteotomy—The rationale for osteotomy is to try to place the hip in a better position in an attempt to reduce the long-term sequelae of osteoarthritis.

4. Tertiary treatment should be used in cases with severe degree of slip or in cases of complications, such as AVN or chondrolysis.

a. Given time most hips will adapt and actually may be better after this adaptive period than the result that an operation can provide. Tertiary treatment procedures should be regarded as "salvage."

b. Osteotomies are still helpful in selected cases but now most patients will opt for either total hip arthroplasty or arthrodesis.

c. Total hip arthroplasty is not indicated in these young patients unless there is severe bilateral involvement. It is unreasonable to expect an arthroplasty to last a lifetime; thus, revisions are to be expected.

d. Because arthroplasty is not the best form of long-term treatment for the young adult, arthrodesis is more advisable but difficult to convince the young adult. It should be emphasized that arthrodesis does have a good long-term result and can be converted to total hip arthroplasty at the appropriate age.

Complications

No discussion of SCFE is complete without considerations of the dreaded complications of this disorder:

1. Chondrolysis is, as the name implies, a progressive atrophy of the articular cartilage. The end result is joint stiffness with joint destruction. Its relationship to SCFE varies in incidence from 1 to 55 per cent.

2. AVN is believed to be iatrogenic because it does not occur with untreated cases.

 Key Treatment

- Spica cast
- Pin fixation

 Bibliography

Chung SMK, Betterman SC, Brighton CT: Shear strength of the human femoral capital epiphyseal plate. J Bone Joint Surg Am 1976;58:94.

Gage JR, Sundberg AB, Nolan DR, et al: Complications after cuneiform osteotomy for moderately or severely slipped capital femoral epiphysis. J Bone Joint Surg Am 1978;60:157.

Harris WR: The endocrine basis for slipping of the upper femoral epiphysis. J Bone Joint Surg Br 1950;32B:5.

Herndon CH, Heyman CH, Bell DM: Treatment of slipped capital femoral epiphysis by epiphysiodesis and osteoplasty of the femoral neck: A report of further experience. J Bone Joint Surg Am 1963;45A:999.

Kelsey JL: Epidemiology of slipped capital femoral epiphysis: A review of the literature. Pediatrics 1973;51:1042.

343 Genu Varum and Genu Valgum
Fredric H. Warren

Definition

1. Genu varum (bowlegs) and genu valgum (knock-knees) are both physiologic and pathologic conditions occurring in childhood. It is imperative that the practitioner be able to recognize the differences between the spectrum of physiologic to pathologic. These entities are generally considered as angular deformities; however, there are usually coexisting rotational components to the deformity.
2. In 1975, Salenius and Vankka reported on the normal physiologic development of the tibiofemoral angle. Infants have varus (bowing) of the knees from birth to age 2 years. From age 2 to 4 years the knees are in a valgus (knock-knee) posture with "hypervalgus" between age 3 and 3 1/2 years, thereafter leveling off by age 7 years at 4 to 7 degrees valgus in males and 5 to 9 degrees valgus in females.

Genu Valgum

The physiologic peak is at age 24 to 36 months.

Pathology

A possible pathologic condition should be suspected in the following situations:

1. Tibiofemoral angle more than 15 degrees valgus
2. Asymmetry
3. Short stature
4. Persistence of deformity past age 6 or 7 years
5. Obesity

Treatment

1. Education and observation are the rule. If the deformities persist, then bracing, usually a night brace, should be considered for deformity greater than 15 to 20 degrees, especially if there is a positive family history.
2. Surgical correction may be indicated in the child with persistence of the deformity past age 10 years or if there is ligamentous instability or patellofemoral instability. Cases selected early (growth remaining) can often be corrected by epiphyseal stapling on the medial femoral side. Later cases usually require formal osteotomy of both the tibia and the fibula to effect satisfactory correction.

Posttraumatic Valgus Deformity

Valgus deformity can develop after isolated proximal tibial fracture. The mechanism of this deformity remains unclear. It is postulated that it is the result of either an occult growth disturbance in the proximal tibial physis or from a tethering effect by the intact fibula. Fortunately, most of these cases resolve with observation. A few may require bracing or even osteotomy.

Varus Deformity of the Lower Extremity

Physiologic Varus

1. This type of varus should be considered as normal until age 3 years.
2. Family history or asymmetry should raise concern for pathologic varus.
3. Varus more than 10 degrees beyond 18 months is physiologic if radiographically there is lateral bowing of the femur and tibia and flaring (or spurring) of the medial metaphysis, both femoral and tibial. Usually there is associated thickening of the medial cortices of the femur and tibia.
4. This physiologic condition may progress to "persistent" or pathologic varus.

"Persistent" Varus

1. Varus continuing after age 2 to 2½ years is considered "persistent."
2. Older children, especially girls, have a poorer prognosis.

Clinical Findings

1. The anatomic changes consist of relative lengthening of the fibula and greater proximal tibial angulation than distal femoral angulation. This condition is considered congenital.
2. At early stages it is very difficult to differentiate from infantile Blount disease (pathologic varus).

Radiographic Changes

Radiographs are usually deferred until it is determined that no improvement in the varus has occurred. Radiographs are needed to differentiate between Blount disease and rickets.

Treatment

1. Bracing may be indicated, especially if Blount disease is suspected.
2. If the condition persists, then physeal stapling is to be considered even without radiographic changes of Blount disease.

Pathologic Tibia Vara (Blount Disease)

There are three distinct periods of onset:

1. Infantile—18 months to 3 years
2. Juvenile—4 to 10 years
3. Adolescent—over 11 years

Epidemiology

An increased incidence of Blount disease occurs in Hispanic, black, and Scandinavian populations. It is correlated with obesity, and it is not unusual for affected children to be early walkers.

Pathology

Blount disease is a pathologic condition affecting the proximal tibia. The origin of the defect is not known, but the disease results in pathologic changes in the proximal tibial involving the medial epiphysis, physis, and metaphysis. These pathologic changes vary in magnitude and are evolutionary with variations in pathologic anatomy. It does appear that the medial tibial metaphysis is the likely origin of the deformity, with the physeal and epiphyseal changes occurring as the disease progresses.

Differential Diagnosis

1. Differential diagnosis include varus tibial deformities secondary to trauma, congenital varus (persistent varus), osteochondromas, and rickets.
2. The main difficulty in the early diagnosis is the differentiation between physiologic varus and Blount disease.
3. The tibial femoral angle cannot predict Blount disease, whereas the tibial metaphyseal angle of Drennan is useful. If a radiographic measurement of more than 11 degrees varus is present, then this finding is suggestive of Blount disease.

Radiographic Findings

Irregularity is evident in the proximal medial tibia metaphysis with medial sloping of the physis and metaphysis. Cystic changes are noted in the metaphysis with a "lateralization" of the tibia. It may be necessary to obtain linear tomography, three-dimensional reconstruction computed tomographic scans, or magnetic resonance imaging to assess the possible coexistence of a partial physeal arrest. These studies are extremely helpful in preoperative planning.

Clinical Presentation

Younger children are usually without symptoms and are brought in specifically for the bowleg deformity. Parents may believe that the deformity interferes with activities, but usually the children have few functional limitations. The older children may have symptoms of stiffness or aching after activities. With this there may be clinical symptoms of joint laxity as the lateral collateral ligaments stretch under the constant varus positioning. There is almost always a persistence of internal tibial torsion with this deformity.

Key Clinical Finding: Blount Disease

- Bowlegs

Classification

Infantile Blount disease progresses in severity with age. Reversible changes can occur through stages I through IV provided an early diagnosis and treatment is started (Table 343–1).

Treatment

1. Infantile Blount disease
   a. Stages I and II usually resolve with bracing if the child is younger than 4 years old and has less than 30 degrees of tibiofemoral angulation.
   b. Stages III and IV usually require proximal tibial osteotomy (with fibular osteotomy) with correction to 5- to 8-degree valgus, preferably done before age 8 years.
   c. Stages V and VI usually result in late sequelae, such as premature osteoarthritis as a result of the long-standing incongruence of the knee joint. Because of the magnitude of deformity at these stages,

TABLE 343–1. STAGES OF BLOUNT DISEASE

STAGE	AGE (YEARS)	RADIOGRAPHS
I	2–3	Irregular medial tibial metaphysis
II	2½–4	Medial fluid metaphysis is depressed with wedging of the epiphysis
III	4–6	Deepening depression of medial beak, skip-off, and medial calcification
IV	5–10	Epiphysis irregular and depressed into the metaphyseal depression
V	9–11	Double epiphyseal plate
VI	10–13	Medial bridge

often the medial plateau must be elevated in addition to correcting the tibial angulation and rotation. Because of relative medial femoral overgrowth, it may also be necessary to perform corrective osteotomies on the femur at the same time. If the knee ligaments are lax, advancement may be needed.

2. Adolescent Blount disease differs in that it only has narrowing of the medial physis with preservation of the epiphysis. Because of this finding it is suspected that it is the result of trauma, either acute or repetitive, leading to a partial growth arrest or delay. The treatment consists of tibial osteotomy as well as completion of the growth arrest by epiphysiodesis. There are rare cases in which the physeal arrest is small enough to allow takedown of the physeal bridge with interposition of fat, Silastic, or methyl methacrylate. Unfortunately, most cases have too large an arrest to allow this form of treatment to be successful. At times the leg-length discrepancy is sufficient to warrant contralateral epiphysiodesis.

Key Treatment: Blount Disease

- Often none

- Bracing

- For severe forms—osteotomy

Tibial Bowing

There are cases of isolated tibial bowing that are noted early in life.

1. Posteromedial bowing is a benign condition that usually resolves spontaneously around age 3 to 4 years. Usually no specific treatment is needed, but the child should be followed for possible leg-length discrepancy.
2. Anterior bowing is often caused by neurofibromatosis and may present as a pre-pseudarthosis of the tibia. This condition is extremely difficult to treat. If no fracture has occurred, it can be managed by protective bracing. Osteotomy can be performed but is fraught with difficulties in healing. If the bone is already fractured, treatment

consists of correction of deformity, intramedullary fixation, and possible vascularized bone graft vs. conventional grafting.

3. Bowing can also be caused by hemimelia of the tibia or fibula, which results in anterior bowing with either lateral bowing (fibular hemimelia) or medial bowing (tibial hemimelia). Treatment is usually directed toward the anatomic location and may require excision of the fibrocartilaginous anlage as well as either centralization of the foot or even amputation of the foot if severe deformity of the foot is present.

Bibliography

Kling TF, Hensinger RN: Angular and torsional deformities of the lower limbs in children. Clin Orthop Rel Res 1983;176:136.

Langenskiold A: Tibia vara: Osteochondrosis deformans tibiae; Blount disease. Clin Orthop Rel Res 1981;158:77.

Levine AM, Drennan JC: Physiological bowing and tibia vara. J Bone Joint Surg Am 1982;64:1158.

Salenius P, Vankka E: The development of the tibiofemoral angle in children. J Bone Joint Surg Am 1975;57:259.

Staheli LT: The lower limb. In Morrissy RT, Weinstein SL (eds): Lovell and Winter's Pediatric Orthopaedics, 4th ed. Philadelphia, Lippincott-Raven, 1996.

344 Legg-Calvé-Perthes Disease

Fredric H. Warren

Etiology

Legg-Calvé-Perthes disease affects the hip or hips of growing children. Many theories have been proposed regarding its cause, but no single cause has been identified. It is thought that this disease is the result of an intermittent transient interference of the blood supply to the developing femoral head, resulting in avascular necrosis of the hip.

Epidemiology

The incidence varies from 1:1,200 to 1:12,500, depending on the geographic area. A higher incidence is evident in urban areas than rural ones. Boys are affected more than girls at a ratio of 4 to 5:1. There is a low frequency among relatives, and there is no obvious pattern of inheritance. Correlations exist between older parents, usually in larger families of lower income. Bilateral presentation occurs in 10 to 12 per cent of patients and must be differentiated between multiple epiphyseal or spondyloepiphyseal dysplasias. The children often have nonfamilial short stature, with skeletal maturity lagging behind chronological age. Approximately 10 per cent have breech or abnormal birth presentation and low birth weight, and 17 per cent present with a history of trauma. Associated congenital anomalies include congenital heart disease, pyloric stenosis, inguinal hernia, undescended testes, and epilepsy.

Pathophysiology

The initiating event is an interference of the blood flow to the hip in the growing child. This results in varying degrees of avascular necrosis, ranging from a small segment to the entire femoral head. This leads to temporary cessation of growth to the ossific nucleus but a continued growth and hypertrophy of the articular cartilage, which is nourished by the synovial fluid. With time, revascularization occurs from the periphery to the center. During this time the necrotic bone is replaced by new bone formation. During this phase the bone is susceptible to subchondral fracture, which is the herald of symptoms. Further resorption occurs and is replaced by fibrous bone, which has biologic plasticity and which in turn can result in permanent alteration of the normal architecture of the femoral head. This change results in deformity in the form of flattening (coxa plana) and enlargement (coxa breva) of the femoral head and growth disturbances leading to cessation of longitudinal growth (coxa breva), which is manifested by varus angulation (coxa vara).

Clinical Findings

1. The average age at onset is 6 years (4–9 years). Girls with the disease usually present earlier and tend to have more serious problems. Even though it is more common in boys the prognosis is better. Bilateral cases usually present at a younger age and have a higher incidence of anomalies. The presentation may be either acute or chronic. The acute presentation may be thought to be irritable hip or transient synovitis, but the symptoms persist or recur. There is a sudden onset of pain in the groin or knee often at night and associated with running, stiffness, or pain with weight bearing. There may be little restriction in motion of the other hip than guarding to flexion, internal rotation, and abduction. Actual restrictions in motion occur later.

2. The chronic presentation is one of insidious limping, which is often more noticeable in the morning and after activities. The pain may be remarkably mild and often described as aching in the anterior thigh or knee and, to less extent, the groin area. As is the limping, stiffness is worse in the morning or after rest.

3. The gait pattern is one of pain, but a component of shortening is also present. This shortening may be real as a result of deformity of the proximal femur or apparent as the result of flexion and adduction contractures. Range of motion of the hip is characterized by decreased abduction, internal rotation, and extension.

Key Clinical Findings

- Pain in groin or knee
- Limp
- Leg shortening, apparent or real

Differential Diagnosis

Acute and chronic infection, acetabular dysplasia, slipped capital epiphysis, Gaucher disease, multiple and spondyloepiphyseal dysplasias, lymphoma, sickle cell disease, eosinophilic granulomas, and hemophilia should all be considered in the differential diagnosis.

Laboratory Findings

Laboratory findings are not useful in the diagnosis of Legg-Calvé-Perthes disease; however, a complete blood cell count, sedimentation rate, and Sickledex studies can be useful in the differential diagnosis.

Radiographic Changes

Radiographic imaging is the hallmark of the confirmation of this disease condition. Routine anteroposterior pelvis and frog-leg lateral radiographic images confirm the diagnosis and help in establishing the stage of disease as well as assisting in classification and prognostication of the disease.

1. In the early phases the x-ray changes consist of smaller epiphysis, increased epiphyseal density, subchondral fracture line, widened medial joint space, or lateralization of the femoral head. As the disease progresses, the femoral head begins to "fragment" as it undergoes resorption and reossification, with partial to complete collapse of the head. The reossification of the femoral head, intact or deformed, heralds the healing phase. Finally, the head progresses to a remodeling definitive phase.

2. Radiographic signs suggestive of poorer results or "head at risk" signs include
   a. Calcification lateral to epiphysis—present when the head has enlarged
   b. Gage sign—decreased ossification in the lateral epiphysis and metaphysis
   c. Diffuse metaphyseal changes such as thickening and irregular ossification
   d. Lateral subluxation
   e. Horizontal growth plate showing fixed subluxation, adduction, and external rotation deformities.

   Two or more of these findings indicate poorer results.

Treatment

The principles of treatment are control of growth disturbances; prevention of propagation of ischemic changes; reduction in synovitis; maintenance and improvement in motion; "containing" the hip to allow molding of, one hopes, a spherical head; and prevention of further injury. The early diagnosis usually allows treatment before irreversible permanent deformity develops.

The preservation of motion usually implies a better result. Clinical "at risk" signs are obesity, loss of motion, age older than 6 years, and presence of adduction contractures.

1. Benign neglect in young children is usually reserved for milder cases.
2. The mainstay of nonoperative treatment has been bracing. Newer braces allow both protection and "containment" while allowing ambulation.
3. The other alternative treatment is "definitive" (surgical). Early definitive treatment is used to prevent deformity. The methods include femoral osteotomy usually incorporating varus and derotation.
4. Nonoperative treatment is best used in the younger child with milder disease, whereas surgical treatment is more useful in the older child with more serious disease.

Key Treatment

- For some, none necessary
- Bracing
- Surgery

Bibliography

Catterall A: Legg-Calvé-Perthes Disease. New York, Churchill Livingstone, 1982.

Gallagher JM, Weiner DS: When is arthrography indicated in Legg-Calvé-Perthes disease? J Bone Joint Surg Am 1983; 65:900.

Lloyd-Roberts GC, Catterall A: Controlled study of the indications for and the results of femoral osteotomy in Perthes disease. J Bone Joint Surg Br 1976;58:31.

Molloy MK: Birth weight and Legg-Perthes disease. J Bone Joint Surg Am 1967;49:498.

Salter RB: The present status of surgical treatment for Legg-Perthes disease—current concepts review. J Bone Joint Surg Am 1984;66:961.

345 Osgood-Schlatter Disease and Other Apophysitides

Paul G. Dyment

Definition

Apophyses are secondary ossification centers with a cellular structure similar to growth plates ("physes") that frequently are the insertion sites of large tendons. When overuse results in microtrauma and then inflammation at one of those sites the condition is called *apophysitis*. The other two growth sites of the developing skeleton, the joint surface and the physeal plate, do not seem to be often involved in overuse injuries of the pediatric or adolescent patient. The two most common apophysitides are *Osgood-Schlatter disease*, affecting the anterior tibial tubercle, and *Sever disease*, affecting the posterior calcaneus. Other apophysitides include *Sinding-Larsen-Johansson syndrome, or "jumper's knee,"* affecting the inferior edge of the patella, *apophysitis of the hip* (the iliac crest or ischial tuberosity), and *medial epicondylitis of the humerus*. The treatment principle of rest is the same for all of these conditions.

Pathophysiology

Before their etiology as being repeated microtrauma was recognized, this group of conditions was considered to be on the list of *osteochondroses*, a group of syndromes including Legg-Calvé-Perthes disease in which some degree of bone necrosis occurred and whose postulated causes included hormonal, genetic, traumatic, and inflammatory findings. However, apophysitis syndromes are caused by repeated traction stress on the apophyseal cartilage at the site of the insertion of the tendon. This causes cartilaginous microfractures, leading to inflammation with pain, tenderness, and swelling.

Osgood-Schlatter Disease

Frequency

1. This is the most common of the apophyseal injuries, and it is also the most common cause of chronic knee pain in the young adolescent.
2. It results from repeated extension of the knee, usually in sports, and occurs in boys more often than girls, although this is now thought to be due to gender differences in physical activity rather than any innate gender-related difference in susceptibility.
3. Its peak age at occurrence is 13 years in boys and 11 years in girls (i.e., early puberty). The disease affects about 15 per cent of boys and 10 per cent of girls, or over 20 per cent of all of those early pubertal children who participate in sports.

Clinical Findings

1. History
   a. A young adolescent complains of pain just below the knee.
   b. It usually commences after sports or running activities and is relieved by rest.
   c. In almost half of the cases it is bilateral.

2. Physical findings
   a. The anterior tibial tubercle is quite tender and usually more prominent than normal.
   b. Pain at that site can be elicited by knee extension against resistance or by full passive knee flexion.

Key Clinical Finding: Osgood-Schlatter Disease

• Pain over tibial tubercle

Radiographic Findings

Radiographs are only necessary to exclude other causes of a tender bone swelling and are therefore probably not necessary if there is bilateral disease. Patients with unilateral presentations should have anteroposterior and lateral radiographs obtained to exclude other bone lesions, the most serious of which would be osteogenic sarcoma, for which the upper tibia is the second most frequent site. The radiograph may show nothing unusual, or there can be fragmentation of the ossified portions of the tibial tubercle. In the unusual case of a skeletally mature patient with persistent disease a small discrete calcification in the tendon may be present.

Treatment

1. Its self-limited nature should be explained to the patient.
2. If pain is intermittent, then the patient need only avoid activities that produce pain. More symptomatic lesions may benefit from applying an ice compress over the site for 15 minutes after playing and from performing hamstring and quadriceps stretching exercises before participation in sports. If the sport results in blows to the inflamed area, as in ice hockey, then a "doughnut" pad can be cut out of felt and taped over the site at the beginning of play.
3. If the pain is more severe and persistent, or is interfering with school or sleep, then complete rest of that joint (not of the other three extremities) is advised; the usual active adolescent will probably require a knee mobilizer to accomplish this. This degree of rest should last for several weeks, after which gradual return to physical activity along with quadriceps and hamstring stretching exercises could be advised. In general, nonsteroidal antiinflammatory drugs are not recommended because the condition lasts several months at least and chronic use of those drugs carries with it the risk of gastrointestinal hemorrhage.

Prognosis

Within a few months the symptom will usually be much better, and the patient can be returned to full activity. A persistent prominent tibial tubercle may remain. Only rarely do the symptoms persist past puberty, and in those cases a radiograph generally shows a separate ossicle in the tendon close to the bone that will need to be surgically excised.

Key Treatment: Osgood-Schlatter Disease

- Usually unnecessary—except for rest

Sever Disease (Calcaneal Apophysitis)

The Achilles tendon inserts into a secondary ossification center on the posterior portion of the calcaneus. Repeated contraction of the gastrocnemius muscle causes microfractures at the apophysis resulting in local inflammation.

Clinical Findings

The usual patient is an athletic child in early puberty. Boys are more frequently affected than girls. Posterior heel pain occurs during or after exercise. Physical findings are tenderness anywhere along the posterior surface of the calcaneus and pain that is reproduced by passive ankle dorsiflexion.

Key Clinical Findings: Sever Disease

- Heel pain
- Tenderness over calcaneus

Radiographic Findings

Radiographs are generally not indicated because there are no specific radiographic abnormalities, and the diagnosis is made clinically.

Treatment

1. A 1/4-inch heel lift pad is used for shock absorption and to reduce the pull on the calcaneal apophysis.
2. Stretching the gastrocnemius muscle before athletic activities and/or applying ice for 15 minutes to the heel area afterward can prevent some of the discomfort.
3. After 1 or 2 weeks of resting the limb as much as possible and receiving a nonsteroidal antiinflammatory drug, the patient can gradually return to full activity, although continuing to use a heel pad for several months is usually advisable to facilitate complete healing.

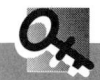

Key Treatment: Sever Disease

- Heel pad

Bibliography

Renstrom P, Johnson RJ: Overuse injuries in sports: A review. Sports Med 1985;2:316–333.

---

346 Scoliosis and Kyphosis

James T. Bennett

Scoliosis

Definition

Scoliosis is a *structural lateral* spinal curvature of more than 10 degrees with *rotation*.

Classification

1. Idiopathic. The cause is unknown but postulated to be equilibrium dysfunction, familial, or asymmetric growth. There are three types classified by age: infantile (age birth–3 years), juvenile (3–10 years), and adolescent (10 years–maturity).
2. Paralytic. Muscle imbalance in growing spine results in scoliosis. Examples include cerebral palsy, muscular dystrophy, and other neuromuscular disorders (e.g., Charcot-Marie-Tooth, Friedrich ataxia, spinal muscular atrophy, polio).
3. Congenital. This occurs when there is a structural anomaly present at birth and includes failure of formation (wedge vertebrae or hemivertebrae), failure of segmentation (bars or block vertebrae), and mixed types.
4. Mesenchymal. Marfan syndrome, Ehlers-Danlos syndrome, osteogenesis imperfecta, and neurofibromatosis are examples.
5. Posttraumatic. Scoliosis can occur as a result of fracture or after irradiation (as after Wilms tumor).
6. Tumors. Osteoid osteoma is the classic example.
7. Causes of scoliosis include dystrophies (diastrophic dwarf, spondyloepiphyseal dysplasia), metabolic disturbances (mucopolysaccharidosis), and many others.

Epidemiology

1. Idiopathic scoliosis
   a. Adolescent
      (1) Most common
      (2) Prevalence—2 to 4 per cent of population have curves of less than 10 degrees, but only 0.1 to 0.3 per cent have curves greater than 20 degrees.
      (3) Female:male ratio 1:1, but for curves more than 21 degrees the ratio is 5:1. Earlier growth spurts

and less muscle development in girls probably account for greater severity of this condition in girls.

    (4) Right thoracic curve most common (90 per cent): any curve other than a right thoracic one should be viewed with great caution.

b. Juvenile

    (1) Uncommon; only 12 to 16 per cent of all idiopathic patients

    (2) More difficult to manage

c. Infantile

    (1) Common in Great Britain, rare in United States

    (2) More common in males, 3:2

    (3) Resolves spontaneously in 90 per cent

    (4) Progressive: Rib vertebral angle difference (Mehta) greater than 20 degree or ribs in phase II suggests progression.

2. Neuromuscular. Prevalence and severity are related to the age at onset, severity, and progression of the neuromuscular disorder. For example, scoliosis would be expected in nearly all patients diagnosed shortly after birth with spinal muscular atrophy (Werdnig-Hoffmann disease) because the neurologic disorder is progressive with early age at onset. Scoliosis occurring after spinal cord injury approaches 90 per cent if the onset of paralysis is early (<10 years) and high (quadriplegia vs. paraplegia).

3. Congenital. A spontaneous abnormality occurs in the embryonic period (3–8 weeks). There is a 1 per cent incidence of a first-degree relative with congenital spinal deformity. Associated anomalies include genitourinary, more than 20 per cent; heart, 7 per cent; and also Klippel-Feil syndrome, radial clubhand, and VATER syndrome.

4. Mesenchymal. The severity and prevalence of scoliosis occurring in various mesenchymal disorder varies. For example, Marfan syndrome, with a prevalence of 0.01 per cent in the general population, has a prevalence of scoliosis of 55 per cent. Similarly, the prevalence of scoliosis in osteogenesis imperfecta varies with severity of the underlying disease.

Pathophysiology

1. Idiopathic. Treatment is based on risk of progression, which is a function of the curve magnitude and immaturity of the patient. For Risser 0 or 1 and curve less then 20 degrees, the risk of progression is approximately 20 per cent. Similarly, for Risser 2, 3, or 4 (mature) and curve in excess of 20 degrees (and less than 29 degrees) the risk of progression is approximately 20 degrees. Rarely do Risser curves 2, 3, or 4 that are less then 20 degrees progress (2 per cent). Risser classification refers to the excursion of the iliac crest: 0, absent (prepubescent); 1, capped by one fourth; 2, half capped; 3, three fourths capped; 4, full capped; and 5, fused. The greatest risk of progression, approximately 70 per cent, is in curves in excess of 20 degrees in immature patients (Risser 0 or 1)

2. Paralytic. Risk of progression is related to maturity and

curve magnitude. In general, paralytic curves tend to be large C-shaped curves that extend to the sacrum

3. Congenital. Risk of progression is largely dependent on the type of deformity, which includes the presence/absence of symmetric growth centers.

    a. Hemivertebrae and contralateral bar. The side on which the hemivertebra occurs has an additional growth area, and this growth area is opposite the bar where there is no growth potential. This pattern, if recognized, should be treated surgically as soon as possible.

    b. Multiple hemivertebrae. Deformity can be severe depending on the extent and asymmetry of the vertebrae.

    c. Unilateral bar (congenital unilateral fusion of vertebral body)

    d. Block vertebrae. This rarely causes significant deformity (complete fusion of two adjacent vertebrae).

4. Mesenchymal

    a. Neurofibromatosis. Typically, a short, sharp, and rapidly progressive curve occurs once progression is recognized. Surgery is generally recommended.

    b. Marfan syndrome. This may be characterized by severe kyphoscoliosis.

    c. Osteogenesis imperfecta. The brittle bones do not tolerate bracing well.

5. Tumor. The prototypical example, osteoid osteoma, causes a "painful scoliosis." Removal of the painful focus before the curve becomes structural results in spontaneous correction of the deformity.

Clinical Findings

1. Idiopathic. The effectiveness of school screening continues to be debated. The Adams forward bend test is based on detecting rib asymmetry, which occurs as a result of spinal rotation. Inclinometry measurements greater than 5 degrees are associated with scoliosis greater than 20 degrees. A careful neurologic examination should include normal reflexes (including abdomen), motor, sensory, and position testing.

2. Paralytic. Long C-shaped curves that typically include the pelvis are common.

3. Congenital. Look for cutaneous abnormalities posteriorly such as sacral dimple or hairy patches.

Key Clinical Findings: Scoliosis

• Spinal curvature greater than 10 degrees with rotation

Radiographic Changes

1. Routine views. Anteroposterior and lateral views on trifold full-length films are performed with patient sitting if unable to stand. Posteroanterior projection reduces breast exposure in females.

2. Special views. Bending views are used to detect curve flexibility and fusion levels but are unnecessary initially. Magnetic resonance imaging is the standard for excluding intraspinal anomalies (astrocytoma/syrinx).

Bone scan may confirm the suspicion of osteoid osteoma.

3. Curve assessment
   a. Appearance. Look for congenital anomalies and short angular curves (neurofibromatosis) or long C-shape patterns. Widening of the interpedicular distance suggests intraspinal pathology. The most typical pattern is right thoracic; a left thoracic pattern suggests a neuropathic process.
   b. Measurement
      (1) Error: ± 5 degrees intraobserver, ± 9 degrees interobserver
      (2) Cobb
         (a) Superior end vertebrae. Last vertebrae to have superior border points toward the concavity of the curve.
         (b) Lower end vertebrae. Inferior border points toward concavity.
         (c) Vertebral rotation. Pedicles and spinous processes are rotated.
   c. Maturity. Bone age: wrist or iliac apophysis–ossification proceeds from anterior iliac spine (Risser 1) to the posterior iliac apophysis (Risser IV). Fusion of the apophysis is Risser V.

Treatment

In general, treatment is directed at prevention of further deformity. This can be accomplished through bracing or surgery; however, most patients with idiopathic scoliosis require only observation. Bracing is only effective in the immature spine. The effectiveness of bracing in paralytic curves is controversial. Exercise, physical therapy, or chiropractic manipulation has not been shown in any study to alter the natural history of scoliosis, nor has electrical stimulation shown any value. However, because the great majority of curves *do not* progress, the lack of curve progression when these modalities were used has been used as justification of their effectiveness. Bracing arrests curves at the point magnitude at which it is applied. Although there is curve correction within the brace, the curve returns to the same arc as when the brace was applied. Only surgery can reduce a curve's magnitude.

Key Treatment: Scoliosis

- Most patients may require only observation.
- Bracing
- Surgical correction of large curves only

1. Idiopathic
   a. No treatment: curve less than 25 degrees
   b. Brace: curve greater than 25 degrees but less than 45 degrees (immature spine)
   c. Surgery: curve greater than 45 degrees
2. Paralytic
   a. Brace: controversial

   b. Surgery: curve greater than 40 degrees: instrumentation: Lugue/Galveston with sublaminar wires with fusion to the pelvis. No bracing is usually required.
3. Congenital
   a. Brace: no role (except for the compensatory curves)
   b. Surgery: generally done quite early (age < 5 years)
   c. Miscellaneous: autogenous blood donation, spinal cord monitoring, allograft and bone substitutes (bone morphogenetic proteins)
4. Instrumentation
   a. Harrington rods. This is the standard and may still be used if primarily thoracic fusion only is needed; postoperative bracing is required.
   b. Cotrel-Dubosset/Texas Scottish Rite/Miami Moss. Newer instrumentation systems provide better correction, are more stable, and do not require bracing.
   c. Anterior fusion. Short segment fusion prevents crank shaft phenomenon (curve progression resulting from continued anterior growth).

Prevention

There is no known mechanism to prevent scoliosis, but early detection makes it possible to prevent further progression.

Kyphosis

Normally the thoracic spine is kyphotic (40 ± 10 degrees). An increase in kyphosis can occur and may be confused with scoliosis.

1. Congenital. In a manner similar to congenital scoliosis, failure of formation of the vertebral body occurs, and when the posterior elements (spinous process, lamina, and pedicles) do form, a very sharp kyphosis results. This is an extremely dangerous condition because paralysis due to cord compression will occur. Treatment is anterior and posterior fusion.
2. Scheuermann kyphosis. This is often seen in adolescent males. A thoracic kyphosis is caused by wedging of multiple (>3) vertebrae. If left untreated, there is a cosmetic, and later a functional, problem (low back pain from increased compensatory lumbar lordosis). Treatment is with bracing and, unlike scoliosis, if the brace is properly applied, a permanent correction can be achieved.
3. Postural round back. A long nonstructural kyphosis is important to differentiate from Scheuermann kyphosis because it is nonstructural and typically nonprogressive.

Bibliography

Bradford DS, Lonstein JE, Moe JH, et al: Moe's Textbook of Scoliosis and Other Spinal Deformities, 2nd ed. Philadelphia, WB Saunders, 1987.
Bishoff R, Bennett JT, Stuecker R, et al: The use of Texas Scottish Rite instrumentation in idiopathic scoliosis: A preliminary report. Spine 1993;18:2452–2456.
Terminology Committee Scoliosis Research Society: A glossary of scoliosis terms. Spine 1976;1:57–58.
Waugh TR, Levine DB, Keim HA, Edmonson AS: Scoliosis. Instr Course Lect 1975;24:56–80.

347 Skeletal Dysplasias

Michael Marble

The skeletal dysplasias constitute a large heterogeneous group of genetic conditions. Dramatic progress has been made in delineating the genetic etiology of many of these conditions. There has also been substantial progress in defining their natural history, complications, and management. Some of the more common skeletal dysplasias are reviewed here.

Achondroplasia

This condition is characterized by rhizomelic dwarfism, relatively normal trunk, midface hypoplasia, frontal bossing, trident hands, and exaggerated lumbar lordosis.

Etiology
A mutation occurs in the gene for fibroblast growth factor receptor type 3 (*FGFR3*).

Inheritance
Inheritance is autosomal dominant, with about 80 per cent of cases due to new mutation.

Pathophysiology
FGFR3 is a cell surface receptor for fibroblast growth factors, which play a mediating role in growth and development of skeletal tissues. It is not well understood how the altered *FGFR3* leads to the achondroplasia phenotype.

Clinical Findings
1. Patients have a large head, prominent forehead, and hypoplastic midface.
2. The limbs are rhizomelic, and the hands are short and trident shaped. Elbow extension is limited.
3. Exaggerated lumbar lordosis is common, and a lumbar gibbus is possible.
4. Some patients have complications, including cervical medullary compression caused by the narrow foramen magnum, that can cause permanent neurologic sequelae and death.
5. Some patients require neurosurgical intervention.
6. Other potential problems include hydrocephalus, central and/or obstructive sleep apnea, frequent otitis media, conductive hearing loss, obesity, bowing of extremities, spinal deformities, and claudication of the spinal cord.

Key Clinical Findings: Achondroplasia
- Large head
- Rhizomelic limbs

Radiographic Findings
1. The foramen magnum is small, the thorax is narrow, and the ribs are short.
2. The posterior vertebral bodies show mild platyspondyly and scalloping, and the interpediculate distance of the lumbar spine shows narrowing.
3. The iliac wings are squared, the acetabular roof is horizontal, and the sacrosciatic notches are narrow.
4. The tubular bones are short, and the fibulas are relatively long.

Hypochondroplasia

A condition marked by disproportionate short limb dwarfism, hypochondroplasia is similar to achondroplasia but has milder features. The face is essentially normal. Some patients have macrocephaly.

Etiology
The cause is probably heterogeneous. A mutation has been found in *FGFR3* in many patients.

Inheritance
Inheritance is autosomal dominant, with the majority of cases due to new mutation.

Pathophysiology
The abnormal *FGFR3* is different from that in patients with achondroplasia because of a different mutation in the gene. As in achondroplasia, it is not understood precisely how this leads to the specific phenotype.

Clinical and Radiographic Findings
1. The short stature may not be recognized until the patient reaches 2 to 3 years of age.
2. The limbs are short with relatively normal trunk. Lower extremities may be bowed, and there is exaggerated lumbar lordosis.
3. Radiographs show an essentially normal skull with slight frontal bossing and a mildly hypoplastic midface.
4. Other findings include mild platyspondyly; short, squared ilia; relatively long fibulas; short tubular bones with slight metaphyseal flare; and lack of caudal widening of the interpediculate distance.

Key Clinical Findings: Hypochondroplasia
- Short limb dwarfism
- Lumbar lordosis

Thanatophoric Dysplasia

The term *thanatophoric* is from the Greek and means "death bringing." Thanatophoric dysplasia (TD) is thought to be the most common skeletal dysplasia that is lethal in the neonatal period. TD type I is characterized by short, curved femurs with or without a cloverleaf skull. TD type II is characterized by relatively long and straight femurs and a severe cloverleaf skull.

Etiology

Both types are caused by mutations in *FGFR3*.

Inheritance

Inheritance is sporadic and due to new dominant mutations.

Pathophysiology

The distinct phenotypes of TD types I and II are due to different abnormalities in *FGFR3* caused by different mutations. It is not well understood how these alterations cause these severe phenotypes.

Clinical and Radiographic Findings

1. These newborns have extremely small limbs and chest.
2. The head is relatively large with a depressed nasal bridge. There may be brain anomalies.
3. Radiographs show short ribs, a relatively long trunk, "handlebar clavicles," cloverleaf skull in some, marked platyspondyly (flat vertebrae) with U- or H-shaped appearance, abnormal pelvis and scapulas, and extremely short tubular bones.
4. Femurs in TD type I are shaped like telephone receivers, but they are relatively straight in TD type II.
5. Neonatal death due to respiratory failure occurs in most patients. Foramen magnum stenosis may be involved in the respiratory failure.

Key Clinical Findings: Thanatophoric Dysplasia

- Large head
- Small limbs and chest
- Usually death in neonatal period

Metaphyseal Dysplasias

The metaphyseal dysplasias constitute a group of conditions in which the predominant skeletal abnormality involves the metaphyses. The vertebrae are relatively normal. There are several types.

Schmid Type

Etiology
Mutation occurs in the gene for type X collagen.
Inheritance
Inheritance is autosomal dominant.
Clinical and Radiographic Findings
1. Short stature, exaggerated lumbar lordosis, and waddling gait are noted.
2. Significant bowing may occur.
3. The face is generally normal.
4. Radiographs show wide irregular metaphyses, short tubu-

lar bones, and tibial and femoral bowing. The vertebrae and hands are normal (see Chapter 66).

Key Clinical Findings: Schmid Type

- Short stature
- Waddling gait

Jansen Type

Etiology
The cause is unknown.
Inheritance
Inheritance is autosomal dominant.
Clinical and Radiographic Findings
1. The patient has severe short stature and enlarged joints with flexion contractures.
2. There is often a waddling gait.
3. Cranial sclerosis occurs, which can cause hearing loss.
4. Frontonasal dysplasia and micrognathia are common.
5. Radiographs show abnormal metaphyses, including those of the hands and feet (unlike Schmid type).
6. Other findings include small air sinuses, undermineralized mandibles, short tubular bones, and bowing of lower limbs.

Key Clinical Findings: Jansen Type

- Severe short stature
- Flexion contracture
- Waddling gait
- Hearing loss

McKusick Type (Cartilage-Hair Hypoplasia)

Etiology
The cause is unknown.
Inheritance
Inheritance is autosomal recessive.
Clinical and Radiographic Findings
1. These patients have short stature with fine, light hair and short fingernails.
2. There is joint hypermobility in the fingers, and the legs are often bowed.
3. Patients have an increased risk of leukopenia and a high susceptibility to fatal varicella infection. Therefore, it is recommended to administer varicella zoster immune globulin in these patients after varicella exposure.
4. Other reported clinical problems include aganglionic megacolon, intestinal malabsorption, and an increased risk of malignancy.
5. Radiographs show abnormal metaphyses, especially at the knees; small, irregular carpal and tarsal bones; very short phalanges, metacarpals, and metatarsals; and lumbar lordosis.

Key Clinical Findings: McKusick Type

- Short stature
- Fine, light hair
- Short fingernails

Camptomelic Dysplasia

Camptomelic dysplasia (CD) is characterized by bowing of the long bones, especially the tibia. Many patients with CD with normal male 46XY karyotype have female genitalia.

Etiology
Mutation occurs in the gene that encodes for the SOX9 protein.

Inheritance
Inheritance is autosomal dominant.

Pathophysiology
The normal SOX9 protein is thought to be involved in testicular and skeletal development. Deficiency of this protein presumably leads to abnormal development of the skeleton and the genitalia in males.

Clinical Picture and Radiographic Findings
1. Prenatal onset growth deficiency, large head, bowing of the tibias, flat face, cleft palate, micrognathia, tracheobronchial hypoplasia, heart defects, absent olfactory bulbs, and renal anomalies are seen.
2. The majority of patients die in the neonatal period of respiratory failure.
3. Radiographs show long, bent femurs, short bent tibias, hypoplastic fibulas, high iliac wings, hypoplastic scapulas, nonmineralized thoracic pedicles, and a bell-shaped chest.
4. In the 46XY individual with camptomelic dysplasia, the genitalia may be normal male, ambiguous, or normal female.

Key Clinical Findings: Camptomelic Dysplasia

- Bowed legs
- Failure of male genitalia development in 46 XY patients
- Tracheobronchial hypoplasia

Diastrophic Dysplasia

Patients with diastrophic dysplasia have short stature, clubfoot, "hitchhiker" position of thumb, and hypertrophy of auricular cartilage.

Etiology
Mutation occurs in a gene that encodes for DTDST, a protein involved in cellular sulfate transport.

Inheritance
Inheritance is autosomal recessive.

Clinical and Radiographic Findings
1. The "hitchhiker" position of the thumb is caused by a short first metacarpal bone. Some of the proximal interphalangeal joints are fused.
2. Severe clubfoot is seen.
3. Most patients develop an inflammatory process in the auricles during infancy that is followed by hypertrophy and ossification in some.
4. Spinal deformities, which may lead to spinal cord compression and neurologic problems, are common.

Key Clinical Findings: Diastrophic Dysplasia

- Severe club foot
- "Hitchhiker" thumb
- Hypertrophied ear cartilage

Hyperphosphatasia

A rare disorder, hyperphosphatasia causes bowing of the long bones, short stature, and a large head.

Etiology
The cause is unknown.

Inheritance
Inheritance is autosomal recessive.

Clinical and Radiographic Findings
1. Skeletal deformity is progressive, and tubular bones and skull are thickened.
2. Elevations occur in levels of serum acid and alkaline phosphatase, leucine aminopeptidase, and urine hydroxyproline.

Hypophosphatasia

Hypophosphatasia is a disorder involving undermineralization of the bones and premature loss of deciduous teeth. It has been divided into six types.

Etiology
Mutation occurs in the gene for tissue-nonspecific alkaline phosphatase, which is involved in bone metabolism.

Inheritance
Inheritance is autosomal recessive.

Pathophysiology
It is not known how decreased tissue-nonspecific alkaline phosphatase causes the hypophosphatasia phenotype.

Clinical and Radiographic Findings
1. There are six different types, which range from the perinatal lethal type with virtual absence of mineralization of the skeleton and stillbirth to milder forms with only premature loss of teeth.

2. Increased intracranial pressure due to functional cranio-synostosis occurs in some cases despite apparently wide-spaced sutures owing to undermineralization.

McCune-Albright Syndrome (Polyostotic Fibrous Dysplasia)

The McCune-Albright syndrome is a sporadic disorder characterized by the triad of polyostotic fibrous dysplasia, café-au-lait spots, and endocrine hyperfunction.

Etiology
Activating mutations occur in the Gs alpha gene in a mosaic pattern.

Inheritance
Inheritance is sporadic.

Pathophysiology
Gs alpha is a subunit of the stimulatory G protein, which increases intracellular cyclic adenosine monophosphate (AMP) (an intracellular second messenger). Activating mutations lead to excess cyclic AMP, causing excess endocrine gland function. The mutations have also been identified in the bone lesions and the café-au-lait spots. The mutation is harbored in some cells but not others (mosaicism), accounting for the characteristic distribution of lesions.

Clinical and Radiographic Findings
1. Limb deformity and bone pain are often unilateral. Other features include chest and spine deformities, facial asymmetry, and temporal bone dysplasia with hearing loss.
2. Café-au-lait spots with "coast of Maine" configuration (irregular edges) that are often unilateral occur on the side of the bony lesions.
3. Precocious puberty in females, hyperthyroidism, excess growth hormone, hypercortisolism, hypophosphatemia, and gynecomastia have been noted.
   See also Chapter 263.

Key Clinical Findings: McCune-Albright Syndrome
• Limb deformity
• Café-au-lait spots
• Endocrine hyperfunction

Caffey Disease (Infantile Cortical Hyperostosis)

Caffey disease is usually a self-limiting condition characterized by cortical hyperostosis with swelling over the affected bone, irritability, and fever.

Etiology
The cause is unknown.

Inheritance
Inheritance is autosomal dominant. The sporadic type (acquired phenotype?) seen with some frequency in the 1940s and 1950s is now exceedingly rare or gone. The mandible invariably is involved.

Pathophysiology
The pathophysiology is unknown.

Clinical and Radiographic Findings
The onset is consistently before 5 months of age (some prenatally), with relatively abrupt soft tissue swelling and tenderness over the affected bone. There is fever and elevated serum alkaline phosphatase and sedimentation rate. Any bone can be affected, most commonly the mandible. Tibial bowing is common. Occasionally, there is residual skeletal deformity or recurrence. Radiographs show subperiosteal cortical hyperostosis that resolves over months to years in most patients.

Key Clinical Findings: Caffey Disease
• Fever
• Irritability
• Swelling of many bones
• Mandibular involvement
• Leukocytosis
• Self-limited course

Type II Collagenopathies

These conditions primarily involve the spine and epiphyses.

The trunk is short, and there may be cleft palate and myopia. The pathophysiology is not well understood. Type II collagen is predominantly located in hyaline cartilage and vitreous humor.

Achondrogenesis Type II
Etiology
Mutation occurs in the *COL 2A1* gene, causing defective type II collagen.
Inheritance
Sporadic inheritance is due to a new mutation in affected patients.
Clinical and Radiographic Findings
1. These newborns have a large cranium, severe micromelia, and a short trunk.
2. Cleft palate is seen in some patients.
3. Death occurs in the neonatal period.
4. Radiographs show extremely short and broad long bones and relatively poor ossification of the axial skeleton.

Kniest Dysplasia
Etiology
Mutation occurs in the *COL 2A1* gene.
Inheritance
Inheritance is autosomal dominant.
Clinical and Radiographic Findings
1. There is marked short stature with short trunk, variable joint contractures, and enlarged joints.
2. Patients have myopia and an increased risk of retinal detachment. Therefore, close ophthalmologic follow-up is imperative.

3. Other features may include cleft palate and frequent otitis media.
4. Radiographs show platyspondyly, kyphosis of thoracolumbar spine, broad hypoplastic ilia, broad metaphyses, and irregular epiphyses.

Spondyloepiphyseal Dysplasia Congenita

Etiology
Mutations have been found in the *COL 2A1* gene.

Inheritance
Inheritance is autosomal dominant.

Clinical and Radiographic Findings
1. The disorder is characterized by short trunk and short stature, pectus carinatum, flat face, and myopia.
2. Retinal detachment may occur; therefore, ophthalmologic monitoring is essential.
3. Some patients have cleft palate.
4. Other features include degenerative arthritis and C1–C2 vertebral subluxation that may lead to cervical cord compression.
5. Radiographs show platyspondyly, ovoid-shaped vertebrae, unossified pubic bone, shortening of the long bones, irregular epiphyses, and odontoid hypoplasia.

Stickler Syndrome

Etiology
Mutation occurs in the *COL 2A1* gene in some patients.

Inheritance
Inheritance is autosomal dominant.

Clinical and Radiographic Findings
1. The patient has a marfanoid habitus, flat face, myopia that may lead to retinal detachment, and sensorineural and conductive hearing loss.
2. Cleft palate is seen in some.
3. Radiographs may show changes in spine and epiphyses.

Management of the Skeletal Dysplasias

There is considerable variability with regard to the natural history and potential complications of the individual skeletal dysplasias. Medical management must be tailored to each patient, accordingly. It is therefore essential that the diagnosis be specific and correct. Medical genetics consultation is important for diagnostic evaluation and genetic counseling. Depending on the specific diagnosis, it will be important for the primary care physician to institute coordinated follow-up with a multidisciplinary approach. Involvement may be required from orthopedics, neurology, neurosugery, ophthalmology, otolarygololology, and other specialties depending on the specific disorder and its complications. It may be important to refer some patients to a center experienced in the multidisciplinary evaluation and management of the skeletal dysplasias. In addition, patients and their families should be made aware of available resources and organizations, such as Little People of America, which can provide valuable information and support.

Bibliography

Francomano CA: Clinical implications of basic research: The genetic basis of dwarfism. N Engl J Med 1995;332:58.

Jones KL: Smith's Recognizable Patterns of Human Malformation, 4th ed. Philadelphia, WB Saunders, 1988.

McIntosh I, Abbott MH, Francomano CA: Concentration of mutations causing Schmid metaphyseal chondrodysplasia in the C-terminal noncollagenous domain of type X collagen. Hum Mutat 1995;5:121–125.

Rimoin D, Lachman RS: Genetic disorders of the osseous skeleton In Beighton P (ed): McKusick's Heritable Disorders of Connective Tissue, 5th ed. St. Louis, CV Mosby, 1993, pp 557–689.

Wynne-Davies R, Hall CM, Apley AG (eds): Atlas of Skeletal Dysplasias. Edinburgh, Churchill Livingstone, 1985.

348 Comatose Child

Binita R. Shah

Consciousness is the state of awareness of self and environment. The spectrum of altered level of consciousness is described by

1. Lethargy—reduced wakefulness and lack of interest in the environment but easily arousable and can communicate
2. Confusion—inattentiveness, mental slowness, dulled perception of the environment, incoherence in thinking
3. Obtundation—severe blunting of alertness with a decreased response to stimuli and increased sleep
4. Delirium—confusion with hallucinations and motor abnormality (tremors/myoclonus). Agitation may alternate with drowsiness.
5. Stupor—unresponsiveness from which the patient can be aroused only by vigorous and repeated stimuli. Patient lapses back into unresponsive state when the stimulus is withdrawn.
6. Coma—unresponsiveness from which the patient cannot be aroused by verbal, sensory, or even vigorous physical stimuli.

Pathogenesis

1. Consciousness requires intact function of both cerebral hemispheres and the brainstem ascending reticular activating system (ARAS) that traverses through diencephalon, midbrain, and upper pons.
2. Stupor/coma results from injury to or dysfunction of either the brainstem ARAS or both cerebral cortices or global dysfunction involving both the brainstem and the cerebral cortices.
3. Unilateral injury or dysfunction of cerebral hemispheres will not cause coma unless the contralateral hemisphere is affected by secondary effects of the primary injury (raised intracranial pressure [ICP] by tumor, trauma, abscess).

Etiology

Stupor or coma is a life-threatening emergency. A therapeutic classification that establishes priorities for both diagnosis and management is helpful at the bedside (Table 348–1).

1. *Immediately treatable toxic-metabolic encephalopathies* that diffusely affect the brain—most common causes in children (70–80 per cent of the cases) (e.g., hypoglycemia, poisonings, meningitis)

    a. Initially—progressive mental changes, symmetric motor signs, brainstem reflex pathways spared, acid–base disturbance

    b. "Dissociation of findings": abnormal respiratory rate (e.g., apnea) with preserved pupillary reflexes

    c. Comatose state—seizures, stuporous state, tremors, myoclonus.

2. *Structural abnormalities of the brain* (20–30 per cent of the cases)

    a. *Rapidly progressive supratentorial lesion* compressing or displacing diencephalon and brainstem (e.g., trauma, tumor)

       (1) Initially—focal/asymmetric motor signs (hemiparesis, hemisensory loss, aphasia), pupillary reflexes abnormal

       (2) Rostrocaudal progression—neurologic signs point to dysfunction at successively lower anatomic areas (diencephalon, midbrain-pons, medulla)

    b. *Rapidly progressive subtentorial destructive or expanding lesions* that damage or compress the ARAS (e.g., posterior fossa tumor, cerebrovascular disease)

       (1) Initially—sudden-onset coma, brainstem abnormalities

       (2) Abnormal respiratory patterns, cranial nerve palsies

3. Nonprogressive "stable" coma. All causes of coma

TABLE 348–1. COMMON CAUSES OF COMA: MNEMONIC "COMATOSE PATIENT"

C: Carbon monoxide poisoning
O: Overdose (anticholinergics, phencyclidine, amphetamines, sedative-hypnotics, narcotics, organophosphates, salicylates, iron)
M: Metabolic: Electrolytes/ions (hypernatremia or hyponatremia, hypercalcemia or hypocalcemia, hypermagnesemia or hypomagnesemia, hypophosphatemia)
A: Abuse
T: Trauma (head: hematomas [intracerebral, subdural, epidural], cerebral edema, severe concussion, contusion, laceration)
O: Organic acidurias, inherited hyperammoninemias and other inborn errors of metabolism
S: Seizures (postictal), nonconvulsive status epilepticus
Stroke (thromboembolism [dehydration, infection, blood dyscrasia, hemoglobinopathy]), arteriovenous malformations
Shunt failure (ventriculoperitoneal shunt infection/obstruction)
Shock (hypovolemic/septic/cardiogenic/neurogenic)
E: Encephalopathy (Reye syndrome, hepatic, uremic, hypertensive, lead, hypoxic-ischemic [drowning, strangulation])
P: Psychogenic/Pseudocoma (conditions mimicking coma—conversion reaction, malingering, catatonia)
A: Alcohols
Acidosis—metabolic (e.g., methanol, ethylene glycol, or salicylate intoxication); respiratory (e.g., sedative-hypnotics intoxication)
Alkalosis—respiratory (e.g., hepatic encephalopathy, salicylate intoxication)
T: Tumor (increased intracranial pressure, secondary hydrocephalus)
I: Insulin (too little/too much—diabetic ketoacidosis/hypoglycemia)
Infection (meningitis, encephalitis, brain abscess, empyema [epidural/subdural])
Intussusception
E: Endocrine: hyperfunction or hypofunction
Thyroid (myxedema or thyrotoxicosis)
Adrenal (Addison or Cushing disease), pheochromocytoma
Parathyroid (hypoparathyroidism or hyperparathyroidism)
N: Narcosis (hypercapnia, e.g., pickwickian syndrome)
T: Temperature (hypothermia, hyperthermia/heat stroke)

(except all emergently treatable causes) are included under this category.

Clinical Findings

1. History
   a. Onset/progression of symptoms
   b. Possible history of trauma, ingestion (medications/illicit drugs/toxins), recent infection or exposure to infection, seizures, chronic diseases (e.g., hepatic, renal, diabetes), and similar episodes in past.
2. Vital signs: Fever (infection, overdose), hypothermia (overdose, hypoglycemia), bradycardia (overdose, increased ICP), tachycardia (shock, overdose), hypotension (hypovolemia, overdose, Addison disease) hypertension (hypertensive encephalopathy, overdose)
3. Respiratory rate/pattern
   a. Tachypnea (hypoxia, toxins)/bradypnea (toxins, increased ICP)
   b. Kussmaul (fast/deep breathing): compensation for metabolic acidosis—diabetic ketoacidosis, toxins (e.g., salicylates)
   c. Cheyne-Stokes (alternating hyperpnea/apnea): hemispheric or diencephalon dysfunction, incipient transtentorial herniation
   d. Ataxic (unpredictable irregularity in rate/depth)—pons/medulla
4. General physical examination
   a. Signs of trauma (see Chapter 349), meningeal irritation (meningitis/subarachnoid hemorrhage), purpura (meningococcemia).
   b. Fundoscopic: papilledema, hemorrhages (cerebral trauma/traumatic subarachnoid hemorrhage, child abuse)
5. Neurologic evaluation to assess the hemispheric dysfunction and the ARAS (ARAS is in the anatomic "neighborhood" of several brainstem reflexes—pupil light reaction [cranial nerves II/III] and reflex eye movements [cranial nerves III/VI/VIII])
   a. Level of consciousness: Glasgow Coma Scale score (Table 348–2).
   b. Pupillary equality, size, reactivity to light. Pupillary pathways are relatively resistant to metabolic insult. Presence/absence of light reflex is the single most important physical sign differentiating metabolic and structural coma.
      (1) Light reflex present: metabolic coma (despite caloric unresponsiveness, respiratory depression, decerebrate rigidity, motor flaccidity). Light reflex is preserved until near-terminal stages of most diseases.
      (2) Light reflex absent: structural coma (in absence of asphyxia, anticholinergic or glutethimide ingestion)
   c. Doll's eyes/oculocephalic reflex indicates comatose patient with
      (1) Intact brainstem—conjugate eyes deviation *opposite* to direction in which head is turned (positive response)
      (2) Pons–midbrain lesion—random eye movements

TABLE 348–2. GLASGOW COMA SCALE

RESPONSE	INFANTS	CHILDREN AND ADULTS	POINTS
Eye opening	No response	No response	1
	To pain	To pain	2
	To voice	To voice	3
	Spontaneous	Spontaneous	4
Verbal	No response	No response	1
	Moans to pain	Incomprehensible sounds	2
	Cries to pain	Inappropriate words	3
	Irritable, cries	Disoriented conversation	4
	Coos, babbles	Oriented and appropriate	5
Motor	No response	No response	1
	Decerebrate posturing	Decerebrate posturing	2
	Decorticate posturing	Decorticate posturing	3
	Withdraws to pain	Withdraws to pain	4
	Withdraws to touch	Localizes pain	5
	Normal spontaneous movement	Obeys commands	6
Total score			3–15

GCS <8: significant neurologic injury.
GCS 9–12: moderate neurologic injury.
GCS >12: mild neurologic injury.
Jennett B, Teasdale G: Glasgow "coma" or unresponsiveness scale. Lancet 1977;1:878. © The Lancet Ltd. 1977.

   d. Cold calorics/oculovestibular reflex indicates comatose patient with
      (1) Intact brainstem—fast nystagmus absent, eyes tonically deviate *toward* irrigated ear, slowly returning to midline
      (2) Brainstem lesions—no response
      (3) Cold calorics may be blocked in comatose patient by cyclic antidepressant, phenytoin, barbiturate, succinylcholine.
   e. Motor response to pain (supraorbital or subungual pressure)
      (1) Speech and/or purposeful withdrawal—cortical preservation
      (2) Decorticate posture—cortical or diencephalon dysfunction
      (3) Decerebrate posture—midbrain or upper pons dysfunction
      (4) Flaccid paralysis—lower pons–medullary dysfunction
6. Signs of herniation: uncal or transtentorial (midbrain-pons)
   a. Regular sustained hyperventilation/Cheyne-Stokes respirations
   b. Asymmetric posture or decorticate/decerebrate posture
   c. Pupils: uncal—ipsilaterally wide/fixed; transtentorial—midsize/fixed
   d. Cushing triad: irregular respiration, hypertension, bradycardia
   e. Doll's eyes and cold calorics: impaired or disconjugate

Key Clinical Findings: Coma with Small Reactive Pupils

- Horner syndrome (unilaterally constricted, anhidrosis, ptosis)—impending transtentorial herniation, hypothermic damage

- Narcotics—bradypnea, bradycardia, hypotension, hypothermia

- Clonidine—bradypnea, bradycardia, hypotension, or hypertension

- Sedative-hypnotics—bradypnea, hypotension, hypothermia

- Phencyclidine—tachycardia, hypertension, hyperthermia, myoclonus, nystagmus, seizures

- Organophosphates—bradypnea or tachypnea, bradycardia or tachycardia, hypotension, "DUMBELS," fasciculations (see Chapter 350)

- Phenothiazines—miosis or mydriasis, tachycardia, hypotension, hypothermia or hyperthermia, extrapyramidal movements

- Pinpoint—narcotics, pontine hemorrhage

Key Clinical Findings: Coma with Small Fixed Pupils

- Pinpoint—narcotics, pontine lesion

Key Clinical Findings: Coma with Dilated Reactive Pupils

- Postictal state

- Amphetamines—tachypnea, tachycardia, hypertension, hyperthermia, tremors, seizures, diaphoresis

- Cocaine—tachycardia, hypertension, hyperthermia, diaphoresis, seizures, hyperactive bowel sounds

- Anticholinergics—tachycardia, hypotension or hypertension, hyperthermia, hot/dry/flushed skin, urinary retention, diminished bowel sounds

- Carbamazepine—bradypnea, tachycardia, hypotension, hypothermia, seizures, extrapyramidal signs, nystagmus

Laboratory Assessment

1. Order Dextrostix; complete blood cell count; determination of serum glucose, electrolytes, urea nitrogen, calcium, phosphorus, magnesium, liver enzymes, and ammonia levels; coagulation studies; arterial blood gas analysis; carboxyhemoglobin concentration; electrocardiogram; and urinalysis.
2. Order toxicology screen (urine/blood/gastric aspirate) if clinically indicated (see Chapter 350)
3. Precontrast computed tomography (CT) of head is indicated for suspected trauma or intracranial mass, bleeding disorders, increased ICP, hydrocephalus, focal seizures, or neurologic signs. Use CT with contrast medium enhancement to evaluate for tumors, herpes encephalitis, or brain abscess.
4. Obtain blood, urine, and cerebrospinal fluid cultures to exclude infection (lumbar puncture should not be performed until structural brain lesion has been excluded by CT scan, except in patients with strongly suspected meningitis or encephalitis).
5. Obtain radiographs of lateral cervical spine, AP of chest and pelvis (for trauma).

Key Clinical Findings: Coma with Dilated Fixed Pupils

- Ipsilaterally dilated—uncal herniation

- Bilaterally dilated—cerebral anoxia, bilaterally compressed third cranial nerves, atropine or scopolamine (large amounts)

- Midposition or moderately wide *unequal* pupils—glutethimide

- Midposition—midbrain damage (transtentorial herniation, hemorrhage), massive barbiturates overdose, severe hypothermia

Treatment

1. Stabilize airway, breathing, and circulation and perform continuous cardiac and pulse oximetry monitoring *before* any diagnostic work-up (for "ABCDE" of primary survey, see Chapter 349).
2. Administer dextrose 25 per cent in water (dextrose 50 per cent diluted 1:1 with water) given intravenously (0.5–1 g/kg [2–4 ml/kg]) to comatose patients without clear evidence of hyperglycemia on bedside Dextrostix testing or without focal signs (awaiting confirmation of hypoglycemia is dangerous). Continuous infusion of 10 per cent dextrose is begun if patient shows dramatic response.
3. Give thiamine, 100 mg, intravenously to patents with ethanol intoxication, especially adolescents, who may be chronic alcohol abusers or thiamine deficient due to chronic disease or eating disorder.

Key Treatment: Naloxone

- For patients with apnea or hypoventilation
  Initial dose: 2 mg (children >5 years and adults); 0.1 mg/kg (birth–5 years [weight, 20 kg])
  Additional dose: 2 mg every 2 to 5 minutes until a therapeutic response or a total of 10 to 20 mg

- Patients with central nervous system depression without respiratory depression
  Initial dose: 0.1 to 0.8 mg. Additional dose (up to 2 mg) as required to a total of 10 to 20 mg

- Failure to respond to 10 mg of naloxone excludes opiate as a major cause of central nervous system depression.

- Opiate-dependent patients who are not apneic
  Use a small dose (0.001 mg/kg) and titrate to avoid opiate withdrawals.

4. Naloxone (intramuscular, intravenous, subcutaneous, or endotracheal). If patient was exposed to opioid, improvement in respiration, central nervous system depression, and pupillary dilatation occurs after therapy. Repeat doses or a continuous infusion may be necessary for several opioids (methadone, propoxyphene, codeine) (shorter half-life of naloxone [20–60 minutes] vs. longer half-life of many opiates [hours]).

5. Treat increased ICP. Immediate therapeutic intervention includes
   a. Prevention of hypoxemia/hypercarbia. Hyperventilate with 100 per cent oxygen to induce cerebral vasoconstriction—$PaCO_2$ 25–30 mmHg. $PaCO_2$ less than 20 mmHg may lead to severe vasoconstriction and cerebral ischemia.
   b. Hyperventilation is the most important acute method and can be titrated to signs of impending herniation (e.g., a fixed and dilated pupil becomes smaller and responds to light).
   c. Osmotherapy with intravenous 25 per cent mannitol: 0.5 g/kg (with normotension)

d. Restriction of fluids
e. Invasive ICP monitoring/neurosurgical consultation

6. Specific therapy for meningitis, antidote for ingestion (see Chapter 350), seizures, electrolytes, and acid–base disturbances.

7. Admit all patients after stabilization to an intensive care unit for continued monitoring and definitive therapy as indicated or to continue work-up for patients whose diagnosis is unclear.

B Bibliography

Silverman BK (ed): Emergencies with altered level of consciousness. *In:* APLS: The Pediatric Emergency Medicine Course. 2nd ed. Elk Grove Village, IL, American Academy of Pediatrics, American College of Emergency Physicians, 1993, pp 177–185.

Plum F, Posner JB: The Diagnosis of Stupor and Coma, 3rd ed. Philadelphia, FA Davis, 1982.

Tait VF, Dean JM, Hanley DF: Evaluation of the comatose child. *In* Rogers MC (ed): Textbook of Pediatric Intensive Care, 2nd ed. Baltimore, Williams & Wilkins, 1992, pp 733–750.

349 Child with Multisystem Trauma
Binita R. Shah

Incidence
1. Trauma remains the leading cause of death in the first four decades of life. In children (ages 1–14 years), accidents account for close to one half of all deaths (exceeding all other causes of childhood mortality). Motor vehicle–related injuries account for most fatalities, followed by falls from heights, drownings, burns, and societal violence (homicide and child abuse).
2. Blunt injuries (86 per cent) are the most frequent type of traumatic injuries sustained by children, followed by penetrating injuries (10 per cent), crush injuries (3 per cent), and drowning (1 per cent).
3. Management of a critically injured child requires a well-rehearsed team approach (surgeons, emergency department physicians). The outcome depends on the care given in the first critical minutes/hour after the injury. Multisystem injury is the rule, and all organ systems are assumed to be injured until proven otherwise.
4. Assessment/management occurs simultaneously through an approach that is divided into two phases: primary and secondary survey.

Primary Survey: Assessment of "ABCDE" and Resuscitation
1. The goals of a *physiological survey* of the vital systems are
   a. Identify and *simultaneously* treat life-threatening injuries.
   b. Identify injuries necessitating operative intervention.
2. Airway and cervical spine (C-spine) protection:
   a. The most common preventable cause of death in an injured child is failure to secure the airway.
   b. C-spine *must* be protected (semi-rigid collar, sand bags, immobilization of entire patient on a long spinal board) until it can be ascertained that no spinal injury exists.
   c. Stabilize C-spine with in-line manual immobilization (a neutral position: neither hyperextended, hyperflexed, nor rotated) to either establish or maintain the airway.
   d. Methods to establish a patent airway
      (1) Suction oropharynx (secretions/food/foreign matter).
      (2) Relieve obstruction (chin lift/jaw thrust maneuver, nasopharyngeal airway [conscious child]/oropharyngeal airway [unconscious child]).
      (3) Orotracheal intubation (*not* nasotracheal in children)
      (4) Needle cricothyroidotomy (<12 years): Complete upper airway obstruction; inability to intubate (e.g., fractured larynx).
   e. Provide 100 per cent oxygen with face mask/reservoir for alert patients and, if not intubated, bag-

valve-mask ventilation to patients with altered sensorium or difficulty in breathing.

3. *Breathing and ventilation:*

a. LOOK: air hunger, cyanosis, rate (rapid/slow/irregular), labored breathing, retractions, bilateral chest expansion

b. LISTEN/PERCUSS: air entry, heart sounds, hyperresonance

c. FEEL: crepitus, tracheal position, neck vein distention

d. Tension pneumothorax—needle decompression (second intercostal space at midclavicular line). For an open pneumothorax, occlusive dressing is taped securely on three sides of the wound's edges to allow egress of entrapped air during exhalation.

e. Massive hemothorax: tube thoracostomy.

Key Indications: Endotracheal Intubation

- Apnea or respiratory failure (flail chest, lung contusion)

- Inability to maintain a patent airway by other means

- Failure to maintain adequate oxygenation by other means

- Need for prolonged ventilatory support (e.g., Glasgow Coma Scale score <8)

- Prevention of aspiration of blood or gastric contents

- Closed-head injury requiring hyperventilation

- Shock unresponsive to fluid therapy

4. *Circulation and control of bleeding*

a. Level of consciousness (brain perfusion)

b. Pulses and blood pressure (BP). Tachycardia and increased systemic vascular resistance are compensatory mechanisms for inadequate cardiac output and may preclude a drop in BP until patient has lost up to 30 per cent of the blood volume. Thus, compromised circulation may exist despite a normal BP.

c. Systolic BP (mmHg) (diastolic BP = two thirds of systolic BP)

(1) 1 to 10 years:
5th percentile: 70 + (2 × age in years);
50th percentile: 90 + (2 × age in years)

(2) 1 month to 1 year: 5th percentile to at least 70th

d. Urine output (renal perfusion). Urinary catheter placement is contraindicated with genitourinary trauma (blood at the urethral meatus, scrotal hematoma, a high-riding prostate).

e. Continuous monitoring: Pulse, pulse oximetry, respiratory rate, BP, electrocardiography, arterial blood gas analysis

Key Points: Circulatory Impairment

- Peripheral pulses: rapid, thready, weak, or absent

- Discrepancy in volume between peripheral and central pulses

- Skin perfusion: color (pale, blue, or mottled), temperature (cool extremities), prolonged capillary refill (more than 2 seconds)

- An injured patient with tachycardia and cool extremities is in hypovolemic shock until proven otherwise

- Isolated head injuries do not cause shock. Sites of internal bleeding: chest, abdomen, retroperitoneum, pelvis/femur

- Volume resuscitation to stabilize BP takes precedence over head injury and possible increased intracranial pressure

5. *Disability* (neurologic examination): A rapid mini-neurologic examination is done to detect the presence of gross neurologic deficits suggesting a mass lesion that may require an urgent surgical evacuation.

a. Pupils: size, symmetry (unequal pupils), and response to light

b. Level of consciousness by AVPU system:

(1) A—Alert

(2) V—responds to Verbal stimuli

(3) P—responds to only Painful stimuli

(4) U—Unresponsive

c. Localizing sign (weakness or paralysis of an extremity)

6. *Exposure/Environmental control:* Completely undress patient to visualize any occult injury (prevent hypothermia: warm blankets, warm ambient temperature, warm fluids [high-flow fluid warmer]).

Key Points: Shock Management

- Direct pressure control of external hemorrhage

- Peripheral or central venous access (hematocrit, type and crossmatch)

- Crystalloid bolus: 20 ml/kg—*reassess*—may repeat bolus 20 ml/kg, one time—*reassess*—surgical consultation—*reassess*. Packed red blood cells: 10 ml/kg (type-specific or O-negative)—*reassess*—further studies and/or operation

Secondary Survey and Definitive Care

1. An *anatomic survey* (head-to-toe evaluation)

a. Identify presence, type (blunt or penetrating), and severity of non–life-threatening injuries and initiate therapy.

b. Prepare for transport or definitive care.

c. Be alert for any unexpected physiologic deterioration during this survey. Immediately repeat primary survey in same order of priority.

2. History: Mnemonic "AMPLE" for: *A*llergies, *M*edications, *P*ast medical history, *L*ast meal, *E*vents leading to the injury.

3. Physical examination

   a. Head and maxillofacial region: Pupils; eyes for conjunctival or fundal hemorrhages and visual acuity; head and face for lacerations, fractures, and dislocations.

   b. C-spine and neck: Trachea deviation, subcutaneous emphysema, vertebral injuries (pain, muscle spasm, head tilt, edema, ecchymosis, visible or palpable deformity, tenderness)

   c. Chest: Flail chest, open pneumothorax, contusions/hematomas

   d. Abdomen: Abdominal wall/lateral flank bruises, contusions, distention, bowel sounds, rebound tenderness, seat-belt marks

   e. Pelvis: Palpate bony prominences for instability, tenderness.

   f. Rectum: Sphincter muscle tone, rectal wall integrity, blood, prostate position (distortion/displacement), bony fragments

   g. Genitalia: Lacerations, hematoma in the vaginal vault, scrotal hematoma, blood at the urethral meatus

   h. Musculoskeletal: Palpation of long bones circumferentially for crepitation, tenderness, deformity, abnormal movement, perfusion, and pulses. Angulation deformity is straightened and immobilized.

Key Findings: Basilar Skull Fracture

- Battle sign (retroauricular or mastoid ecchymosis)
- "Raccoon eyes" (periorbital ecchymoses)
- Hemotympanum (bluish discoloration and bulging)
- Cerebrospinal fluid or bloody otorrhea or rhinorrhea

---

   i. Neurologic status: Glasgow Coma Scale score, see Chapter 348), sensorimotor and cranial nerve examination. Suspect spinal cord trauma: hypotension and bradycardia (without hypovolemia), flaccid areflexia, priapism, lack of bladder or rectal control.

   j. Back (patient log-rolled): Penetrating injuries, hematomas

   k. Skin: Petechiae (traumatic asphyxia), bruises, burns

   l. Gastric tube: Orogastric or nasogastric tube to decompress stomach and reduce the risk of aspiration. Contraindications for nasogastric tube: Cribriform plate fracture (suspect this with facial fractures or with evidence of basilar skull fracture).

4. Laboratory assessment: Complete blood cell count; urinalysis; determination of glucose in serum, electrolytes, and urea nitrogen, coagulation studies, liver and cardiac enzymes, and amylase (as indicated).

5. Radiographic studies (during or after resuscitation phase)

   a. Initial screening: Three radiographs (by portable unit)

      (1) A crosstable lateral C-spine (*most important*), anteroposterior (AP) chest, and AP pelvis

      (2) Indications: Multisystem trauma, injury above the clavicle (facial, head), unconsciousness, hypotension, torso trauma (blunt/penetrating), pelvic instability, gross hematuria, gross blood on vaginal or rectal examination.

      (3) Base of the skull, all seven cervical and first thoracic vertebrae *must* be visualized for an acceptable lateral C-spine radiograph.

      (4) A normal radiograph does not exclude all C-spine injuries. If spinal cord injury is suspected based on history or neurologic examination, *assume* that injury exists.

   b. Open-mouth odontoid, AP, and oblique cervical views for any patients with suspected cervical injury and a normal lateral C-spine radiograph; AP thoracolumbar spine views for any patient with multiple trauma or torso trauma

   c. Abdominal AP, cross-table lateral decubitus views for intraabdominal injury (free air, foreign body, bony abnormality)

   d. Extremities: AP, lateral views of fracture sites (including joint above and below the injury and comparison view of other extremity).

6. Computed tomography (CT) scan of head. Indications: All patients with head injury (except minor injury), Glasgow Coma Scale score less than 13, depressed or basilar skull fracture, focal neurologic signs, posttraumatic seizures, an infant with bulging fontanelle

7. Abdominal CT scan (with intravenous and oral contrast medium enhancement)

   a. Indications: Signs of intraabdominal injury, gross hematuria, hypovolemic shock that responded to fluids, major trauma (head/pelvis), altered sensorium precluding abdominal examination

   b. Detects presence and extent of injuries to specific organs including retroperitoneal and pelvic organs. Limited in diagnosis of hollow viscus injury (e.g., bowel perforation)

   c. Contraindications: Hemodynamically unstable patient or a patient with already determined need for celiotomy.

8. Diagnostic peritoneal lavage may be considered for

   a. Evaluation of a hemodynamically unstable patient (in deciding whether immediate celiotomy is indicated)

   b. Patient with multiple injuries requiring general anesthesia for nonabdominal surgery (e.g., penetrating upper chest injuries, evacuation of an epidural hematoma).

c. It is neither organ nor injury specific and cannot reliably assess retroperitoneal injuries.

9. Definitive care/disposition: After stabilization, admit patient to local hospital (availability of consultative services) or transfer to a regional pediatric trauma center. Communication among physicians and nurses is vital. All pertinent medical records and radiographs are sent with the patient. Communication and moral support to the family is important.

B **Bibliography**

American College of Surgeons Committee on Trauma. *In* Advanced Trauma Life Support Course Student Manual, 5th ed. Chicago, American College of Surgeons, 1993.
APLS: The Pediatric Emergency Medicine Course, 2nd ed. Elk Grove Village, IL, Joint Task Force On Advanced Pediatric Life Support. American Academy of Pediatrics and American College of Emergency Physicians, 1993.

350 Child Poisoned by Unknown Substance

Binita R. Shah

Epidemiology

1. There is a biphasic curve in the incidence of pediatric poisonings. The first peak occurs between 1 and 6 years of age and accounts for 85 to 90 per cent of cases. The second peak occurs during adolescence and accounts for 10 to 15 per cent of cases.

2. Single agents (frequently nontoxic household products) are ingested accidentally in a small amount by young children. Multiple pharmaceutical drugs in larger amounts are intentionally ingested (a suicidal intent) by adolescents (Table 350–1).

Clinical Findings

1. Poisoning can occur as a result of ingestion, inhalation, absorption (dermal/rectal/ocular), or exposure (parenteral, transplacental) to foreign products. Often when a patient presents with an intoxication, the nature of the poison or even the existence of a poisoning may be uncertain.

TABLE 350–1. EXAMPLES OF POISONS AND THEIR ANTIDOTES

POISON	ANTIDOTE
Acetaminophen	*N*-Acetylcysteine
Anticholinergics	Physostigmine
Benzodiazepines	Flumazenil
Beta blockers	Glucagon
Carbon monoxide	Oxygen/hyperbaric oxygen
Cyanide	Cyanide antidote kit
Digoxin	Digibind
Ethylene glycol	Ethanol
Iron	Desferoxamine
Isoniazid	Pyridoxine
Methanol	Ethanol
Methemoglobinemia	Methylene blue
Narcotics	Naloxone
Organophosphate insecticide	Atropine and pralidoxime
Carbamate insecticide	Atropine
Phenothiazines	Diphenhydramine
Tricyclic antidepressants	Sodium bicarbonate

2. The clinician must consider poisoning when a patient presents with any of the following: cyanosis, shock, vomiting, diarrhea, hypothermia or hyperthermia, abnormal behavior, or unusual odor. Life-threatening presentations include coma, seizures, bradyarrhythmias or tachyarrhythmias, hypotension or hypertension, and respiratory failure.

3. History
   a. What, when, how much (number of pills or the amount of liquid missing)
   b. Symptoms since ingestion
   c. Any treatment before arrival
   d. Know all medications at home and potentially toxic household products. Assume that all that cannot be readily accounted for has been ingested.
   e. Contact poison control center or the manufacturer if the ingredients of a product are unknown.
   f. In adolescents, utilize the data but remain skeptical (silent ingestion, e.g., acetaminophen).
   g. Suspect child abuse: Ingestion in child younger than 1 year; repeated episodes of ingestion; or child's developmental level and the skills required to perform the events described are inconsistent.

4. Physical examination: *Toxidromes* are characteristic constellation of signs and symptoms seen with certain classes of poisons. Toxidromes help in the diagnosis and management of acutely ill patients, in whom a history of poisoning is lacking (Table 350–2).
   a. Anticholinergic: Atropine, tricyclic antidepressants, antihistamines, phenothiazines, antispasmodics, mushrooms
   b. Sympathomimetic: Amphetamines, phenylpropanolamine, cocaine, crack cocaine, phencyclidine, ephedrine, aminophylline
   c. Narcotic: Heroin, methadone, morphine, codeine, meperidine
   d. Sedative-hypnotic: Barbiturates, benzodiazepines
   e. Cholinergic: Insecticides (organophosphate, carba-

TABLE 350–2. THE MNEMONICS OF POISONINGS

Increased Anion Gap Metabolic Acidosis: "ACIDOSIS"

Alcohols (methanol, ethylene glycol), Carbon monoxide or Cyanide, Iron, Other (uremia, paraldehyde), Seizures or Shock (lactic acidosis), Isoniazid, Salicylates

Anticholinergics:

HOT as a hare (febrile), RED as a beet (flushed skin), BLIND as a bat (mydriasis), MAD as a hatter (delirium), DRY as a bone (decreased secretion)

Cholinergics: "DUMBELS"

Diarrhea, Urination, Miosis, Bronchorrhea/Bronchospasm, Emesis, Lacrimation, Salivation

Miosis: "COPS"

Clonidine, Opiates (except meperidine and diphenoxylate/atropine sulfate), Organophosphates, Phenothiazine-Phencyclidine, Sedative-hypnotic coma (barbiturates, benzodiazepines, ethanol)

Mydriasis: "SHAW"

Sympathomimetic, Hallucinogen, Anticholinergic, Withdrawal (sedative-hypnotic, opioid, ethanol)

Radiopaque Medications: "COCAINE"

Cocaine packets, Opiates packets, Chloral hydrate, Arsenic (heavy metals—lead, mercury), Iron, Neuroleptics (phenothiazines, cyclic antidepressants), Enteric-coated preparations (e.g., aspirin)

Drugs or Chemicals Producing Seizures: "CAMPHOR BALLS"

Camphor, Cocaine, Carbon monoxide, Cyanide, Caffeine, Clonidine, Carbamazepine
Amphetamines, Anticholinergics (cyclic antidepressants, antihistamines), Aspirin
Methylxanthines (theophylline)
Phenothiazines or Phencyclidine
Hypoglycemic agents (oral insulin), Heavy metals (e.g., lead)
Opioids (propoxyphene, meperidine), Organophosphates
Rodenticides (strychnine, thallium, arsenic)
Barbiturates, Benzodiazepines (withdrawal seizures)
Alcohols (methanol, ethylene glycol), ethanol (withdrawal seizure)
Lidocaine
Lithium
Salicylates

Key Points: Toxicologic Clues/Tests at the Bedside

- Therapeutic response to glucose or naloxone

- Dextrostix:
  Hyperglycemia—salicylates, iron, isoniazid
  Hypoglycemia—hypoglycemic agents, alcohols, salicylates

- Arterial blood gases:
  Decreased hemoglobin saturation with normal/increased PO_2—carbon monoxide, methemoglobinemia; carboxyhemoglobin and methemoglobin levels

- Skin:
  Cherry red = carbon monoxide, anticholinergics
  Blue = cyanosis, methemoglobinemia

- Blood:
  Chocolate brown or cyanosis unresponsive to O_2—methemoglobin

- Odor:
  Acetone = isopropyl alcohol, methanol
  Oil of wintergreen = methyl salicylate
  Alcohol = ethanol, methanol
  Garlic = organophosphates
  Coal gas = carbon monoxide
  Bitter almond = cyanide
  Rotten eggs = hydrogen sulfide
  Fruity = isopropanol

- EKG:
  Terminal 40 msec frontal plane QRS vector—tricyclic antidepressants

- Urine ferric chloride:
  Purple—salicylates, phenothiazines

- Urine:
  Calcium oxalate crystals = ethylene glycol
  Ketones = acetone, isopropyl alcohol, salicylates

- Urine fluorescence under Wood's lamp:
  Ethylene glycol from antifreeze (fluorescent substance in antifreeze)

- Gastric contents deferoxamine test: (deferoxamine + hydrogen peroxide added to gastric contents)
  Vin rosé color = iron

mate): coma, seizures. Nicotinic effects: fasciculation, weakness, paralysis, weakness. Muscarinic effects: "DUMBELS" (see Table 350–2).

   f. Hypermetabolic: Salicylates: hyperpnea, tachycardia, convulsions, coma, hyperthermia, vomiting, tinnitus

   g. Extrapyramidal: Phenothiazines: rigidity, dysphonia, torticollis, oculogyric crisis, anticholinergic signs

   h. Withdrawal: Opioids, benzodiazepines, alcohols: tachycardia, diarrhea, restlessness, hallucinations, sweating, abdominal cramps, lacrimation

Laboratory Assessment

If clinically indicated:

1. Serum: Electrolytes, osmolality (anion/osmolal gap). Increased osmolal gap: ethanol, methanol, isopropanol, ethylene glycol.
2. Quantitative serum level (for management decisions/predicting severity of exposure) of salicylate, iron, acetaminophen, theophylline, alcohol, methanol, lithium, and ethylene glycol. "Drug screens" are not helpful in the acute management.
3. All patients with intentional overdose: Serum acetaminophen and salicylate levels and pregnancy test for teenage girls
4. Urine for qualitative detection: Benzodiazepines, opioids, barbiturates, cocaine, amphetamines, marijuana
5. Chest radiograph (aspiration pneumonitis or pulmonary edema)
6. Abdominal radiograph for radiopaque substances. The absence of visible tablets does not rule out ingestion. With a high index of suspicion (e.g., iron), it may confirm the diagnosis and help to evaluate the efficacy of gastric decontamination.
7. Gastric aspirate/vomitus: Save for possible qualitative detection. Note appearance, pills, odor (e.g., camphor).

Treatment

1. Resuscitation and stabilization. The cornerstone of the care of a poisoned patient is stabilization of airway,

Key Points: Comparison of Sympathomimetics and Anticholinergics

	Sympathomimetics	**Anticholinergics**
Vital signs	Tachyarrhythmias	Tachyarrhythmias
	Hypertension/tachypnea	Hypertension/hypotension
	Hyperthermia	Hyperthermia
Pupils	Mydriasis	Mydriasis
Central nervous system	Hyperalert/agitation	Coma/agitation
	Hallucinations	Hallucinations
	Delirium/psychosis	Extrapyramidal movements
Skin	Severe sweating	Dry, hot, flushed
Urine	Normal	Retention
Gastrointestinal	Increased bowel sounds	Decreased bowel sounds

breathing, and circulation (ABCs) based on abnormal vital signs *before* any diagnostic test. Seizures are controlled by diazepam or, when indicated, with a specific therapy (e.g., pyridoxine therapy for acute isoniazid toxicity).

2. Any patient with an altered sensorium: Therapeutic trial of glucose or naloxone, as clinically indicated (see Chapter 348).

3. Surface decontamination of external toxin: Irrigation of eyes (caustics), removal of the clothes, and washing of skin (insecticides)

4. Gastrointestinal tract decontamination methods include

   a. Emesis: Syrup of ipecac: Rarely used in emergency department but still an important first-aid management of poisoning at home. Contraindications: Caustics, coma, petroleum distillates, seizures

   b. Orogastric lavage: Usually indicated for a patient presenting within 1 to 2 hours of a potentially toxic ingestion seizing or in coma (intubate before lavage).

      (1) A large-bore orogastric tube (large enough to evacuate particulate matter) is used, and position of the tube in the stomach is confirmed.

      (2) With the patient in the left lateral decubitus position, a saline lavage (aliquot: child, 50–100 ml; adolescents, 200 ml) is performed until effluent solution is clear.

      (3) Contraindications: Ingestion of corrosives/caustics, hydrocarbons/petroleum distillates

   c. Activated charcoal adsorbs almost all toxins. It is

given orally as a slurry in water or fruit juice or by nasogastric or orogastric tube, if refused.

   (1) Usual dose (children/adults): 1 g/kg or 10:1 ratio of activated charcoal:drug. Multiple-dose activated charcoal (0.5–1 g/kg every 4–6 hours) for theophylline, phenobarbital, salicylate, tricyclic antidepressants, carbamazepine

   (2) Complications: aspiration, intestinal obstruction.

Key Points: Activated Charcoal

- A single dose to patients with potentially toxic ingestion

- Ineffective for iron, lithium, alcohols, and caustics

- Contraindications: Intestinal obstruction or perforation, altered sensorium (absent gag reflex/unprotected airway), caustics (endoscopy difficult—accumulates in burned area)

   d. Cathartics (sorbitol, magnesium sulfate, or magnesium citrate) are not warranted in routine management of pediatric ingestion. A single dose may be given to an adolescent with a large amount of ingested drugs when desorption from activated charcoal is a possibility. Do not use repeated doses with multiple-dose activated charcoal (could cause fluid and electrolyte disturbances). Contraindications for cathartic use include absent bowel sounds and ingestion of caustics or gastrointestinal irritants.

5. Antidotes are usually not used prophylactically. Life-threatening toxidromes (opioid, cholinergic, methemoglobinemia, tricyclic antidepressants), carbon monox-

Key Points: Comparison of Narcotics and Sedative-Hypnotics

	Narcotics	**Sedative-Hypnotics**
Vital signs	Bradypnea/bradycardia	Bradypnea/bradycardia
	Hypotension/hypothermia	Hypotension/hypothermia
Pupils	Miosis (except meperidine)	Mydriasis, miosis (early)
Central nervous system	Lethargy to coma	Coma, nystagmus
Other	Pulmonary edema	Bullae
Antidote	Naloxone	Flumazenil (benzodiazepine)

ide, and cyanide poisonings require *simultaneous* use of an antidote with the initial stabilization of vital functions. Other antidotes are not usually required immediately and, if indicated, can be administered once the diagnosis is confirmed (see Table 350–1).

6. Hospitalize:

 a. Patients with a suicidal intent (psychiatric/social services intervention)

 b. Patients in whom identification of poison is unclear or acutely ill patients requiring emergency stabilization

 c. Patients requiring further management such as urinary alkalinization (salicylate), hemodialysis (methanol, ethylene glycol, salicylate), whole-bowel irrigation (iron).

7. Discharge home: Patients with accidental nontoxic ingestion after counseling and social service intervention if:

 a. The product or drug has been identified.

 b. The time and the exact amount of ingestion is known.

 c. The amount ingested is less than the smallest amount known to produce toxicity.

 d. Patient has no signs of toxicity since the time of ingestion.

 e. The time elapsed since the ingestion is greater than the longest interval known between ingestion and peak toxicity.

 f. Child abuse/neglect has been excluded.

 Bibliography

Committee on Injury and Poison Prevention: Handbook of Common Poisonings in Children, 3rd ed. American Academy of Pediatrics, Elk Grove Village, IL, 1994.

Goldfrank LR, Flomenbaum NE, Lewin NA, et al (eds): Goldfrank's Toxicologic Emergencies, 5th ed. Norwalk, CT, Appleton & Lange, 1994.

351 Poisonings and Environmental Hazards

Laurence Finberg

Poisonings

In the narrow sense, a poison is a toxic substance that when contacted by ingestion, inhalation, or absorption through the skin in small quantity harms the person. In a more general sense, any substance, even those essential for life, in sufficiently large quantity (e.g., water, oxygen, salt) is toxic. Here the focus is on the narrower definition and on the more common examples for pediatrics, or when a principle of therapy is illustrated. Accidental ingestion is most common in the toddler age group in whom physical skills have advanced more rapidly than cognitive restraints. For all but a few agents (see later), emesis followed by 15 to 30 g of activated charcoal slurry ingestion is useful in the first hours after ingestion.

Drugs

The following discussion includes examples of poisonings that may occur after accidental contact or mistaken overdose with certain drugs.

1. Acetaminophen
   a. Source: analgesic remedies alone or in combination
   b. Toxic single dose and serum levels
      (1) Dose more than 50 mg/kg or 4 g
      (2) Serum level more than 1300 μM/L (200 μg/ml). Toxicity is possible at lower levels (e.g., 350 μM/L [50 μg/ml]) and is enhanced by alcohol ingestion.
   c. Symptoms: Nausea and vomiting, followed by abdominal pain

Key Clinical Findings: Acetaminophen

- Nausea
- Vomiting

   d. Pathophysiology: The drug is metabolized by the cytochrome P_{450} system to sulfate (primarily in children younger than age 6) and to a glucuronide (older children and adults). The glucuronide path depletes liver glutathione, and then intermediate metabolites damage hepatic cells. Chronic usage may lead to renal damage.
   e. Useful laboratory information
      (1) Liver tests: aspartate transaminase (AST), alanine transaminase (ALT), bilirubin, and prothrombin time. AST levels more than 100 μm/L indicate toxicity.
      (2) Serum level greater than 1300 μM/L (200 μg/ml) at 4 hours or 325 μM/L (50 μg/ml) at 12 hours is in toxic range.

   f. Treatment
      (1) Emesis or lavage followed by activated charcoal if less than 6 hours after ingestion.
      (2) N-acetylcysteine—140 mg/kg initially of 5 per cent solution orally, followed by 70 mg/kg every 4 hours for 17 additional doses. Therapy is most effective before 16 hours after ingestion and possibly is of benefit up to 36 hours after ingestion.
      (3) In the most severe poisonings, liver transplant may be necessary.

Key Treatment: Acetaminophen

- N-Acetylcysteine

2. Boric acid
   a. Source: Eyewash, ant poison, household cleaners
   b. Toxic dose: Less than 5 g in infants has been lethal, as has 5 to 20 g in older children and adults.
   c. Symptoms: Anorexia, vomiting, lobster-red color of skin, oliguria leading to anuria

Key Clinical Findings: Boric Acid

- Lobster-red skin
- Vomiting
- Oliguria/anuria

   d. Pathophysiology: Diffuse systemic poisoning with renal tubular necrosis is most prominent. Skin, cardiac, pancreatic, and liver injury may occur.
   e. Laboratory findings: Turmeric paper test of urine turns reddish brown. Follow urea nitrogen and creatine levels in serum.
   f. Treatment
      (1) Emesis or lavage if within 3 hours of ingestion
      (2) Supportive; may require dialysis because of anuria—not useful to remove bound toxin.
3. Captopril
   a. Source: Medication for adult members of family for hypertension. It is one of the most common medication ingestions by toddlers.
   b. Toxic dosage: Fortunately, margin of safety is great. As much as 500 mg ingested by a toddler has been asymptomatic.
   c. Symptoms: Uncommon; hypotension occurs with massive ingestion.

d. Pathophysiology: The drug is an angiotensin-converting enzyme (ACE) inhibitor.

e. Laboratory findings: Occasional hyponatremia and hyperkalemia

f. Treatment: Usually none required other than observation. If hypotension occurs, use volume expanding fluid administration.

4. Cyclic antidepressants

a. Source: Medication for patient or family member

b. Toxic dosage: The therapeutic dose for an adult may be toxic for a toddler.

c. Symptoms

(1) Anticholinergic signs, tachycardia, pupillary dilatation, dry mucous membranes, retention of urine

(2) Cardiovascular: Initial hypertension followed by hypotension, arrhythmias, electrocardiographic changes

(3) Central nervous system (CNS): Hallucinations, myoclonus, coma.

Key Clinical Findings: Cyclic Antidepressant

- Tachycardia
- Dilated pupils
- Urinary retention

d. Pathophysiology: Drug is tightly bound to plasma proteins and acts as an anticholinergic, adrenergic, and α-adrenergic blocking agent.

e. Laboratory findings: Usually nonspecific or normal; blood levels are usually not helpful.

f. Treatment

(1) Avoid emesis if CNS symptoms are present.

(2) Use activated charcoal, 30 g, for toddlers, 100 g for adolescent, and repeat in 2 hours.

(3) Add laxative (e.g., magnesium sulfate).

(4) Supportive for cardiac and CNS manifestations.

5. Ibuprofen and other nonsteroidal antiinflammatory drugs (NSAIDs)

a. Source: Analgesic over-the-counter preparations.

b. Toxic dose: Variable, but definitely anything more than 100 mg/kg/day or producing a level greater than 80 μg/ml at 3 hours past ingestion

c. Symptoms

(1) Initially nausea, abdominal pain, and gastrointestinal bleeding

(2) Oliguria, anuria

(3) Lethargy, seizures, apnea (≥300 mg/kg dosage)

(4) Acidosis

d. Pathophysiology: The drug is bound to plasma protein with a half-life of 2 hours. Metabolism is in the liver. About 10 per cent of a therapeutic dose is excreted unchanged.

e. Treatment

(1) Emesis must be early after ingestion to be of any help.

(2) Activated charcoal should be given.

(3) Cardiovascular and respiratory support if needed

(4) Hemoperfusion (charcoal) should be useful.

6. Iron

a. Source: Prescribed pills for patient or family member

b. Toxic dose: More than 60 mg/kg of elemental iron

c. Symptoms

(1) Initially, vomiting, abdominal pain, hematemesis

(2) Hypotension occasionally in first 2 hours

(3) Latent period 2 to 8 hours after ingestion with no symptoms

(4) Hypoglycemia and acidosis/acidemia more than 6 hours after ingestion

(5) Hepatic necrosis more than 2 to 3 days after ingestion

(6) Late (weeks after ingestion) pyloric scarring and obstruction.

Key Clinical Findings: Iron

- Vomiting
- Hypotension
- Gastrointestinal hemorrhage

d. Pathophysiology

(1) Initially iron is corrosive to the gastric mucosa and may cause hemorrhage with significant blood loss.

(2) Circulating hypotensive factor may add to shock from blood loss.

(3) Iron enters mitochondria, producing disturbance of many organs, chiefly kidney, lung, and cardiovascular systems. Multiple enzyme systems are poisoned with metabolic derangements.

e. Laboratory findings

(1) Toxicity if free iron greater than 90 μM/L (500 μg/dl).

(2) A test dose of deferoxamine (15 mg/kg in 50 ml of 5 per cent glucose intravenously) will turn urine a reddish color. Failure to obtain the color 2 to 3 hours after ingestion means the absence of a toxic dose. A positive test does not foretell severity.

Key Laboratory Findings: Iron

- Deferoxamine test
- Serum iron

f. Treatment
   (1) Emesis and lavage generally not useful and contraindicated if hematemesis has occurred.
   (2) Charcoal does not bind iron.
   (3) Undissolved tablets may be removed by colonic lavage.
   (4) Deferoxamine, 10 to 15 mg/hr intravenously for 24 hours or 90 mg/kg every 8 hours intramuscularly, not to exceed 6 g.

Key Treatment: Iron

• Deferoxamine

7. Salicylate (aspirin)
   a. Source: Analgesic over-the-counter preparations solely or in combination
   b. Toxic dose: Single ingestion—100 to 200 mg/kg results in possible toxicity; more than 200 mg is always toxic if absorbed.
   c. Symptoms
      (1) Nausea and vomiting early
      (2) Hyperventilation
      (3) Tinnitus in subacute or chronic poisoning
      (4) Lethargy and rarely convulsions.

Key Clinical Findings: Salicylate

• Nausea

• Vomiting

• Hyperventilation

• Tinnitus

d. Pathophysiology
   (1) Direct stimulation of the respiratory center reduces P_{CO_2}. In children older than 6 years this will cause an early respiratory alkalosis.
   (2) Poisoning of Krebs cycle enzymes α-ketoglutarate and succinic dehydrogenases leads to ketosis and acidemia.
   (3) Uncoupling of oxidative phosphorylation causes fever and increased O_2 consumption.
   (4) In chronic poisoning (several days) there is reduction of prothrombin production.
   (5) In toddlers, the ketoacidosis overwhelms the respiratory alkalosis so that the primary metabolic disturbance in them is an acidemia, unlike the adolescent in whom the respiratory alkalosis may predominate for a number of hours.
   (6) Aspirin also may injure hepatic and renal cells, although these are unusual manifestations after a single toxic dose.
   (7) Salicylate is detoxified in the liver by glycination and glucuronidation, both relatively slow processes.
   (8) Free salicylic acid is relatively insoluble, but the ionized form (sodium or potassium salicylate) is highly soluble. Therefore, if the renal tubular fluid is alkaline, excretion can be enhanced almost 100-fold by raising the pH from 6 to 8.

e. Laboratory findings
   (1) Salicylate levels in serum are biphasic after a toxic ingestion. About 90 minutes after ingestion on an empty stomach the level peaks. Up to 70 mg/dl may be nontoxic at the peak, but more than 50 mg/dl at 6 hours will be toxic because the body distribution space is increasing from the plasma, where it is bound to albumin, to the extracellular fluid as a whole.
   (2) Urine: Salicylate will give a strong purple color with ferric chloride within 15 minutes after ingestion. Aspirin (acetylsalicylic acid) does not give that result; therefore, the test is not useful on stomach contents if aspirin has been ingested. The acetyl group is removed in the liver within minutes.
   (3) Prothrombin time is not prolonged after a single toxic ingestion but will be increased in chronic poisoning.
   (4) Ketoacidosis (primarily in children younger than age 3 to 4) and also alkalosis in older children.

Key Laboratory Findings: Salicylate

• Electrolytes

• Salicylate level

• Urine ferric chloride test

f. Treatment
   (1) Emesis and activated charcoal are helpful in first hours only.
   (2) Forced diuresis is usually by the intravenous route with sodium bicarbonate to alkalinize the urine, enhancing excretion.
   (3) Glucose is important because hypoglycemia may occur from Krebs cycle inhibition.
   (4) Potassium losses may be profound, so that this ion should be replaced from the onset.
   (5) Vitamin K administration in chronic poisoning; not needed for single ingestion.
   (6) Use of the carbonic anhydrase inhibitor acetazolamide, 5 mg/kg intramuscularly, every 5 hours for three doses as a facilitator for sodium bicarbonate intravenously. This therapy has been controversial and is not recommended by standard texts because given by itself acetazolamide will, while producing an alkaline urine, return hydrogen ions to the extracellular fluid, producing a metabolic acidosis. I disagree with this judgment both for theoretical considerations and based on empirical data. The metabolic acidosis

will not be enhanced by the acetazolamide *if M/6 (167 mEq/L) sodium bicarbonate in 5 per cent glucose solution is begun first.* (In adolescents during the alkalosis phase, the acetazolamide may be given at once, but the sodium bicarbonate should begin soon after). After the urine is alkaline, the bicarbonate concentration may be reduced to 40 to 50 mEq/L and potassium chloride should be added to the intravenous solution, 20–30 mEq/L. The advantage in this therapy is that the excess salicylate is excreted promptly (usually in 24 hours or less) without the risk of producing hypernatremia. Hypernatremia commonly occurs if sodium bicarbonate is alone pushed to produce an alkaline urine in the toddler and in the past produced serious damage. Experience with this procedure in over 1000 patients in the past 35 years without adverse consequences has convinced me of both its efficacy and safety.

Key Treatment: Salicylate

- Forced diuresis
- Glucose and potassium administration
- Acetazolamide—controversial but preferred by author

Pesticides

1. Organophosphate (OP) and carbamate; cholinesterase inhibitors. Examples: parathion, malathion.
   a. Source: Insecticides; may be absorbed through the skin or ingested
   b. Toxic dose: Very small amount varying with the specific product
   c. Symptoms: Salivation, lacrimation, miosis, fasciculations

Key Clinical Findings: Pesticides

- Salivation
- Lacrimation
- Miosis

   d. Pathophysiology: Inhibition of cholinesterase, permanent with OPs, reversible with carbamate, leads to excess acetylcholine and parasympathetic actions.
   e. Laboratory findings: Reduction of red cell cholinesterase activity for OP; this finding is not useful for carbamate because reversal occurs in the blood sample for analysis.
   f. Treatment
      (1) Atropine, 0.5 mg/kg intravenously every 10 to 20 minutes until respiratory symptoms and secretions have abated; may be needed periodically for several days.
      (2) Wash skin with detergent if route of poisoning is by cutaneous absorption.

      (3) Pralidoxime, 25 to 50 mg/kg intravenously every 8 hours, not exceeding rate of 500 mg/min.
      (4) Supportive

Key Treatment: Pesticides

- Atropine
- Pralidoxime

2. Paraquat
   a. Source: Herbicide
   b. Toxic dose: Very small amount usually by ingestion
   c. Symptoms
      (1) Corrosive to mouth, pharynx, esophagus
      (2) Causes proliferate bronchiolitis and alveolitis, leading to fibrosis
   d. Pathophysiology: Impairs gas exchange in the lung, leading to progressive pulmonary failure
   e. Laboratory findings: Fall in P_{O_2}; rise in P_{CO_2}
   f. Treatment: Symptomatic and supportive; spontaneous improvement may occur after months. Lung transplant is a last resort.

Environmental Hazards

Pollutants

1. Polychlorinated biphenyls (PCBs) and polybrominated biphenyls (PBBs). Compounds are used as fire retardants in electrical insulation and clothing.
   a. Source: Polluted streams from industrial waste carried in fat of fish who have swallowed them; contaminated cooking oils.
   b. Symptoms: Discoloration of skin in newborn after in utero exposure plus contaminated breast milk ingestion; defects in skin, teeth, hair, and nails
   c. Treatment: None
2. Asbestos
   a. Source: Insulation for fire proofing; brake linings.
   b. Toxic dose
      (1) Although rare, a single long fiber may act as a physical toxin if it reaches the bloodstream and then pierces a cell, causing a mesothelioma as much as 20 to 30 years later.
      (2) In cigarette smokers, asbestos exposure predisposes to bronchogenic carcinoma in adult life.

Household Products and Hazards

1. Carbon monoxide (CO)
   a. Source: Defective (leaking) heating units, automobile exhaust, house fires
   b. Toxic dose: More than 5 per cent saturation of hemoglobin
   c. Symptoms: Drowsiness, cherry-red lips, headaches, nausea, dyspnea, confusion, coma

Key Clinical Findings: Carbon Monoxide

- Lethargy, drowsiness
- Confusion, coma
- Cherry-red lips

   d. Pathophysiology: CO binds to hemoglobin preferentially to oxygen, displacing the oxygen and leading to asphyxiation.

   e. Laboratory findings: Measurement of carboxyhemoglobin saturation. More than 40 per cent is serious poisoning; more than 60 per cent is quickly fatal.

Key Laboratory Findings: Carbon Monoxide

- Carboxyhemoglobin

   f. Treatment
     (1) 100 per cent oxygen administration
     (2) Possible use of a hyperbaric chamber if not at excessive distance
     (3) Supportive

Key Treatment: Carbon Monoxide

- Oxygen

2. Caustics (e.g., strong alkalis and acids)
   a. Source: Drain cleaners, dishwasher detergents, disc batteries
   b. Toxic dose: Any amount may burn the lips, mouth, pharynx, and esophagus. Acids may concentrate at the pylorus and cause scarring.
   c. Symptoms: Pain, dysphagia
   d. Pathophysiology: These agents cause liquefaction necrosis and lesser burns. Scarring causes strictures.
   e. Laboratory findings: Not useful
   f. Treatment
     (1) If patient can swallow, a few sips up to 2 cups of water may be helpful.
     (2) Neutralizing acids or bases by mouth is contraindicated.
     (3) After 12 hours, if there are mouth and pharyngeal burns, flexible esophagoscopy should be performed.
     (4) Unless there is an esophageal perforation, antibiotics have not been helpful.
     (5) Use of corticosteroids is controversial and probably not helpful.

3. Hydrocarbons: Kerosene, gasoline, lighter fluid
   a. Source: Heaters, lighter for charcoal, automobile fuel
   b. Toxic dose: 15 ml up to 100 ml or more.
   c. Symptoms: Cough, vomiting, CNS symptoms with lighter fluid or gasoline

   d. Pathophysiology
     (1) Because of very low surface tension, some of the liquid is invariably aspirated, causing a chemical pneumonia.
     (2) Lighter fluid and gasoline are absorbed from the intestine and cause anesthetic-like CNS suppression.
   e. Laboratory findings: Not useful
   f. Treatment
     (1) Kerosene
       (a) Do not produce emesis and do not lavage, both of which will increase aspiration.
       (b) Use antibiotic for bacterial complications of chemical pneumonia.
     (2) For gasoline or lighter fluid, lavage to remove CNS toxin is often justified even though it worsens the pulmonary problem.

4. Naphthalene
   a. Source: Usually from moth balls or moth flakes.
   b. Toxic dose: For persons deficient in glucose-6-phosphate dehydrogenase (G6PD), even a whiff of air in a closet where the product is in use; for a susceptible newborn, wearing a diaper treated by moth proofing with naphthalene causes hemolysis.
   c. Susceptibility: G6PD deficiency is inherited as an X-linked trait. American and African blacks have a 13 per cent prevalence in boys and men and a 1 per cent prevalence in girls and women. Asiatic and people of Mediterranean origin (Italian, Greek) also have a high prevalence.
   d. Symptoms: Sudden hemolytic anemia, pallor, hemoglobinuria.

Key Clinical Findings: Naphthalene

- In patients with G6PD deficiency
- Pallor

   e. Pathophysiology: The genetic defect of deficient G6PD lowers the concentration of reduced glutathione in older red cells, which lessens the protection of the red blood cell membrane SH groups from oxidizing chemicals such as naphthalene. When oxidization occurs, hemoglobin is denatured, forming precipitates (Heinz bodies) and initiating a hemolytic process followed by splenic removal of damaged cells.

   f. Laboratory findings: Anemia, sometimes profound, Heinz bodies on smear, hemoglobinuria; reticulocytosis. During the anemic stage the remaining (young) red blood cells may have normal levels of G6PD. Patient's mother will have reduced (heterozygote) levels of G6PD.

Key Laboratory Findings: Naphthalene

- Anemia
- Hemoglobinuria
- Heinz bodies on blood smear

g. Treatment
   (1) Transfusion with packed red blood cells to restore hematocrit to 30 per cent
   (2) Removal of naphthalene products from environment

Key Treatment: Naphthalene

- Packed red blood cell transfusion

h. Prevention
   (1) No naphthalene products in home
   (2) Persuade regulators and legislators to ban naphthalene to be sold as a moth repellent because a much less toxic product, paradichlorobenzene, is available, equally effective, and as low in cost

Miscellaneous Environmental Chemicals

1. Cyanide (CN)
   a. Source: Acetonitrile compounds for removing glue that secures acrylic fingernails; industrial uses; laboratory supplies
   b. Toxic dose
      (1) A few milligrams of cyanide or 5 ml of acetonitrile glue remover
      (2) If acetonitrile is ingested, sufficient toxic cyanide release occurs 3 to 12 hours later.
   c. Symptoms: Nausea, headaches, dyspnea, convulsions, coma

Key Clinical Findings: Cyanide

- Nausea, dyspnea
- Convulsions, coma

   d. Pathophysiology
      (1) If acetonitrile, the compound is metabolized in the liver by cytochrome P_{450} enzymes to hydrocyanic acid.
      (2) Cyanide inactivates many enzymes, including, most importantly, the cytochrome oxidases blocking electron transport, making oxygen unavailable to tissue. Cyanide also binds to the ferrous ion of hemoglobin, which then does not carry oxygen.
   e. Laboratory findings
      (1) Venous blood has excessively high P_{O_2}.
      (2) Calculated oxygen saturation from arterial blood gas measurement is higher than measured oxygen by oximeter. If the difference is greater than 5 per cent, suspect cyanhemoglobin.
      (3) Acidemia

Key Laboratory Findings: Cyanide

- Venous blood oxygen excessively high
- Acidemia

   f. Treatment
      (1) Sodium thiosulfate, 1.65 ml/kg of 25 per cent solution intravenously to produce thiocyanate.
      (2) Amyl nitrate inhalant
      (3) 100 per cent oxygen.
      (4) Correct acidemia.

Key Treatment: Cyanide

- Sodium thiosulfate intravenously
- Amyl nitrate inhalant

2. Lead (Pb)
   a. Source
      (1) Crumbling painted (prior to 1978) plaster and peeling paint from wood surfaces
      (2) Soil in cities and along roads from leaded gasoline, now diminishing
      (3) Lead smelters—affecting air and surrounding soil
      (4) Glazed pottery, primarily from outside United States
      (5) Medications for diarrhea from Mexico and China
   b. Toxic dose
      (1) Variable but more than 30 μg/dl level in blood
      (2) Threshold for possible harm, 10 to 20 μg/dl
      (3) Encephalopathic level usually more than 90 μg/dl, but more than 70 μg/dl represents danger.
   c. Symptoms
      (1) History of deteriorating plaster or paint availability and possible ingestion
      (2) Anorexia, constipation; ataxia; encephalopathy; mild anemia
      (3) Cognitive deficits and behavior disorders (late)

Key Clinical Findings: Lead

- Pica history
- Anorexia, constipation
- Ataxia
- Convulsions

d. Pathophysiology
(1) Lead chelates sulfhydryl groups, reducing enzyme efficacy in many systems.
(2) Reduced hemoglobin synthesis
(3) Toxic intermediary metabolite of hemoglobin synthesis (and other systems) causes cerebral cell swelling.
(4) Metaphyseal bone formation is interrupted.
(5) Renal tubular damage may lead to Fanconi syndrome.

e. Laboratory findings
(1) Pb levels in whole blood are elevated.
(2) Erythrocyte protoporphyrin (EP) levels indicate toxicity—not useful for screening because not sensitive at levels now thought dangerous.
(3) Radiographs of long bones (anteroposterior view of knee) show increased density, lead line, a failure of osteoblastic expansion with denser calcium apatite deposition, not lead atoms
(4) Abdominal film (optional) showing plaster (calcium sulfate) particles and rarely lead particles from unusual ingestion

Key Laboratory Findings: Lead

- Anemia
- Lead levels in blood
- Increased erythroprotoporphyrin

f. Treatment
(1) Removal from source. For mild exposure, this is the only treatment necessary.
(2) Calcium sodium ethylenediaminetetraacetic acid (EDTA)
(a) 20 mg/kg/day intravenously over several hours for 5 days to mild elevation with no symptoms
(b) 50 mg/kg IV for higher (>70 g/dl) Pb levels
(3) Dimercaprol (BAL), 4 mg/kg every 4 hours × six doses for Pb levels more than 70 μg/dl; first dose before EDTA.
(4) Succimer, 30 mg/kg/day, orally × 5 days, used after removal from source for outpatient usage.

Key Treatment: Lead

- Dimercaprol (BAL)
- EDTA
- Succimer

g. Prevention
(1) Keep toddlers from living in *deteriorating* housing built before 1978.
(2) Screen housing built before 1978 for lead content in plaster and wood surfaces and ensure either excellent maintenance or implement removal of lead in safe (for workers and residents) manner.
(3) Screen children from area of high risk until removal program has been completed.

3. Mercury (Hg)
a. Source
(1) Laboratory; elemental Hg, especially vapor. Liquid Hg is not very toxic.
(2) Mercury salts—medicinal and in fungicides
(3) Organic (e.g., methyl mercury formed by microorganisms when elemental mercury is released into the environment); may be ingested by and stored in tissue of fish after pollution of various bodies of water.
b. Toxic dose: For adults, 1 g of Hg can be lethal; precise dosage data for children are not known, but clearly more than 100 mg would be dangerous.
c. Symptoms: Mouth ulcers, acrodynia, renal tubular necrosis, nephrotic syndrome, ataxia, convulsions, coma

TABLE 351–1. TOXIC FOODS

TOXIN	COMMENT
Mushrooms	
Amanita family	Most deadly, may require liver transplant
Gyromitra family	Methylene blue infusion may help
Muscarine group	Atropine useful, 0.1 mg/kg
Solanine (sprouted potatoes)	May produce shock, though usually mild
Fish	
Ciguatera poisoning From reef-feeding fish caught for sport or illegally (e.g., grouper, snapper, amberjack, kingfish, dorardo, barracuda): larger fish = more toxin	Toxin from a dinoflagellate eaten by fish near coral reef; severe CNS toxin—may cause coma and ascending paralysis
Scombroid poisoning Albacore, tuna, mackerel	Histamine release during aging of fish flesh when not eaten fresh
Shellfish	
Mollusk Contaminated by a "red tide"	Caused by a dinoflagellate (paralytic neurotoxin)
Amnesic Mussels, clams, crabs, and anchovies	Vomiting, diarrhea, headache, seizures, and coma; short-term memory loss
Neurotoxic Mussels and most plankton feeders	Diarrhea, vomiting, ataxia, and paresthesias
Paralytic Mussels and clams	Vomiting, diarrhea, facial paresthesias, and respiratory paralysis

TABLE 351–2. VENOMOUS ANIMALS

VENOMOUS ANIMAL	COMMENT AND TREATMENT
Snakes (United States only)	
Pit viper	For management, block circulation proximal to the bite with a tourniquet.
Rattlesnake	
Copperhead	Apply suction to bite. Use antivenin for serious viper and coral snake bites.
Water moccasin	
Coral snake	
Spiders	
Latrodectus (black widow)	Neurotoxin causes muscle spasm; rarely severe enough to cause hypertension, shock, coma, and death. Antivenin is available.
Loxosceles (brown recluse)	Cytotoxin causes a necrotic ulcer after vesiculation; rarely, hemolysis, disseminated intravascular coagulation, and renal failure have occurred. Treatment is supportive.
Scorpions	Local pain; uncommonly, agitation, tachycardia, nystagmus, and convulsions
	Treatment is supportive. Antivenin gives high serum sickness rate.
Hymenoptera (bees, wasps, etc.)	Local reaction and anaphylaxis.
	Treatment is supportive with antihistamine, epinephrine, and corticosteroids
Marine Envenomations	Intense local pain—analgesia
Stingrays	Local pain-antihistamines and corticosteroids may be helpful.
Jellyfish	
Cnidaria (larvae sea anemone)	Antihistamines and corticosteroids
Swimmer's itch	
Seabather's eruption	

Key Clinical Findings: Mercury

- Mouth ulcers
- Acrodynia
- Edema
- Ataxia

   d. Pathophysiology: Chelates SH—enzymes in kidney, CNS, and gastrointestinal tract

   e. Laboratory: Blood and urine levels

Key Laboratory Findings: Mercury

- Mercury levels
- Serum albumin
- Electrolytes

  f. Treatment

    (1) Succimer: oral 10 mg/kg/dose, every 8 hours × 5 days, plus every 12 hours × 14 days

    (2) Dimercaprol (BAL) (not for methyl mercury): 4 mg/kg every 4 hours for 4 days plus 2.5 mg/kg every 4 hours for 7 days

Key Treatment: Mercury

- Succimer
- Dimercaprol

Toxins in Food and Plants
See Table 351–1.

Envenomations
See Table 351–2.

Bibliography

Committee on Drugs, American Academy of Pediatrics: Treatment guidelines for lead exposure in children. Pediatrics 1995; 96:155–159.

Finberg L, Kravath RE, Hellerstein S (eds): Water and Electrolytes in Pediatrics, 2nd ed. Philadelphia, WB Saunders, 1995, pp 230–233.

Gosselin RE, Hodge HC, Smith RP, Gleason MN: Clinical Toxicology of Commercial Products, 4th ed. Baltimore, William & Wilkins, 1976.

Rumack BH, Hess AJ (ed): Poisindex. Denver, 1995.

Index